WILLIAM A. SODEMAN, Jr., M.D., F.A.C.P.

Associate Professor of Medicine;
Chief, Division of Gastroenterology,
Medical College of Ohio at Toledo

WILLIAM A. SODEMAN, M.D., F.A.C.P.

Professor of Medicine, Emeritus; Dean Emeritus and
Vice President for Medical Affairs, Emeritus,
Jefferson Medical College,
Thomas Jefferson University, Philadelphia

fifth edition

PATHOLOGIC PHYSIOLOGY
MECHANISMS OF DISEASE

W. B. SAUNDERS COMPANY • PHILADELPHIA • LONDON • TORONTO

W. B. Saunders Company: West Washington Square
Philadelphia, Pa. 19105

12 Dyott Street
London, WC1A 1DB

833 Oxford Street
Toronto, Ontario M8Z 5T9, Canada

Pathologic Physiology: Mechanisms of Disease   ISBN 0-7216-8472-6

© 1974 by W. B. Saunders Company. Copyright 1950, 1956, 1961, 1967 by W. B. Saunders Company. Copyright under the International Copyright Union. All rights reserved. This book is protected by copyright. No part of it may be reproduced, stored in a retrieval system, or transmitted in any form or by any means, electronic, mechanical, photocopying, recording, or otherwise, without written permission from the publisher. Made in the United States of America. Press of W. B. Saunders Company. Library of Congress catalog card number 72-90728.

Print No.:   9   8   7   6   5   4   3

CONTRIBUTORS

Peter Abramoff, Ph.D. Professor and Chairman, Department of Biology, Marquette University, Milwaukee, Wisconsin.

J. A. Abildskov, M.D. Professor of Internal Medicine, University of Utah College of Medicine, Salt Lake City, Utah.

Ezra A. Amsterdam, M.D. Assistant Professor of Medicine, Assistant Professor of Pharmacology, Director of Coronary Care Unit, Section of Cardiovascular Medicine, Departments of Medicine and Pharmacology, University of California School of Medicine, Davis, California.

Charles E. Billings, M.D., M.Sc. Professor and Director, Division of Environmental Health, Department of Preventive Medicine, The Ohio State University; Attending Physician, Ohio State University Hospitals, Columbus, Ohio.

George A. Bray, M.D. Professor of Medicine, UCLA School of Medicine; Director, Clinical Study Center, Harbor General Hospital, Torrance, California.

Thomas W. Burns, M.D. Professor of Medicine and Director, Division of Endocrinology, University of Missouri School of Medicine; Attending Endocrinologist, University of Missouri Medical Center; Consultant in Endocrinology, V.A. Hospital, Columbia, Missouri.

Bertram D. Dinman, M.D., Sc.D. Medical Director, Aluminum Company of America, Pittsburgh, Pennsylvania.

Harold T. Dodge, M.D. Professor of Medicine, University of Washington; Co-Director, Division of Cardiology; Director, Cardiovascular Research and Training Center, Seattle, Washington.

Leonard S. Dreifus, M.D. Clinical Professor of Medicine and Senior Attending Physician, Hahnemann Medical College, Philadelphia, Pennsylvania.

René J. Duquesnoy, Ph.D. Assistant Professor of Microbiology, The Medical College of Wisconsin, Milwaukee, Wisconsin.

Louis J. Elsas, II, M.D. Associate Professor of Pediatrics, Assistant Professor of Internal Medicine, Assistant Professor of Biochemistry, Chief, Section of Medical Genetics (Department of Pediatrics), Emory University School of Medicine. Attending Physician, Emory University Hospital, Grady Memorial Hospital, and the Henrietta Egleston Hospital for Children, Atlanta, Georgia.

Allan J. Erslev, M.D. Cardeza Research Professor of Medicine, Jefferson Medical College of Thomas Jefferson University; Attending Physician (Medicine), Thomas Jefferson University Hospital, Philadelphia, Pennsylvania.

Robert E. Forster, II, M.D. Isaac Ott Professor and Chairman of the Department of Physiology, University of Pennsylvania School of Medicine; Physiologist, Hospital of the University of Pennsylvania and Children's Hospital; Consultant, Philadelphia Naval Hospital and Philadelphia General Hospital.

Thomas G. Gabuzda, M.D. Professor of Medicine, Jefferson Medical College of Thomas Jefferson University; Chief, Department of Hematology, Lankenau Hospital; Consulting Staff, Roxborough Memorial Hospital, Philadelphia, Pennsylvania.

Benjamin Robert Gendel, M.D. Professor and Associate Chairman, Department of Medicine, University of Tennessee College of Memphis; Chief, Medical Service, V.A. Hospital, Memphis, Tennessee.

CONTRIBUTORS

Ray W. Gifford, Jr., M.D. Head, Department of Hypertension and Nephrology, Cleveland Clinic Foundation, Cleveland, Ohio.

Franz Goldstein, M.D. Professor of Medicine, Jefferson Medical College of Thomas Jefferson University; Chief, Department of Gastroenterology, Lankenau Hospital, Philadelphia, Pennsylvania.

Arthur C. Guyton, M.D. Professor of Physiology and Biophysics, University of Mississippi School of Medicine, Jackson, Mississippi.

W. Proctor Harvey, M.D. Professor of Medicine; Director, Division of Cardiology, Georgetown University Medical School; Georgetown University Hospital; Consultant, Washington V.A. Hospital; Bethesda Navy Hospital; Walter Reed Army Medical Center; National Heart and Lung Institute, Washington, D.C.

Frank L. Iber, M.D. Professor of Medicine, University of Maryland; Chief of Gastroenterology, University Hospital, Baltimore; Chief of Gastroenterology, Loch Raven Veterans Administration Hospital, Baltimore, Maryland.

J. Ward Kennedy, M.D. Associate Professor of Medicine, University of Washington; Chief, Department of Cardiology, Veterans Administration Hospital, Seattle, Washington.

John H. Killough, Ph.D., M.D. Associate Professor of Medicine and Associate Dean, Jefferson Medical College; Attending Physician, Thomas Jefferson University Hospital, Philadelphia, Pennsylvania.

Joseph B. Kirsner, M.D., Ph.D. Louis Block Professor of Medicine, Deputy Dean for Medical Affairs, University of Chicago; Attending Physician, A. M. Billings Hospital, University of Chicago, Chicago, Illinois.

Herbert C. Mansmann, Jr., M.D. Professor of Pediatrics, and Associate Professor of Medicine, Jefferson Medical College; Medical Director, Children's Heart Hospital of Philadelphia; Pediatrician, Thomas Jefferson University Hospital, Philadelphia, Pennsylvania.

Dean T. Mason, M.D. Professor of Medicine, Professor of Physiology, Chief, Section of Cardiovascular Medicine, Departments of Medicine and Physiology, University of California, School of Medicine, Davis, California.

Rashid A. Massumi, M.D. Professor of Medicine, Director, Electrophysiology, Section of Cardiovascular Medicine, Department of Medicine, University of California, School of Medicine, Davis, California.

Paul H. Maurer, B.S., Ph.D. Professor of Biochemistry and Chairman of the Department, Jefferson Medical College of Thomas Jefferson University, Philadelphia, Pennsylvania.

William W. Parmley, M.D. Associate Professor of Medicine, UCLA School of Medicine; Associate Director, Department of Cardiology, Cedars-Sinai Medical Center, Los Angeles, California.

Spencer O. Raab, M.D. Associate Professor of Medicine, University of Arkansas School of Medicine; Attending Physician, University Hospital; Consultant (Hematology), Veterans Administration Hospital, Little Rock, Arkansas.

William D. Robinson, M.D. Professor and Chairman, Department of Internal Medicine, University of Michigan Medical Center, Ann Arbor, Michigan.

David B. Skinner, M.D. Dallas B. Phemister Professor and Chairman, Department of Surgery, University of Chicago; Chief of Surgery, University of Chicago Hospitals and Clinics (Billings Hospital), Chicago, Illinois.

William A. Sodeman, Jr., M.D., F.A.C.P. Associate Professor of Medicine; Chief of the Division of Gastroenterology, Medical College of Ohio at Toledo, Toledo, Ohio.

John F. Stapleton, M.D. Professor of Medicine, Georgetown University Medical School; Medical Director, Georgetown University Hospital, Washington, D.C.

H. J. C. Swan, M.D., Ph.D. Professor of Medicine, UCLA School of Medicine; Director, Department of Cardiology, Cedars-Sinai Medical Center, Los Angeles, California.

Morton N. Swartz, M.D. Professor of Medicine, Harvard Medical School; Chief, Infectious Disease Unit, Massachusetts General Hospital, Boston, Massachusetts.

Robert C. Tarazi, M.D. Staff Member, Research Division, Cleveland Clinic Foundation, Cleveland, Ohio.

Milton Toporek, B.A., M.A., Ph.D. Professor of Biochemistry, Jefferson Medical College of Thomas Jefferson University, Philadelphia, Pennsylvania.

Yoshio Watanabe, M.D. Professor of Medicine, Fujita Garken University School of Medicine, Toyo-Ake-Shi, Japan.

CONTRIBUTORS

DAVID W. WATSON, M.D. Associate Professor of Medicine, University of California, Davis; Attending Physician, Sacramento Medical Center; Consultant in Gastroenterology, San Joachin General Hospital, California.

LOUIS WEINSTEIN, Ph.D., M.D. Professor of Medicine, Tufts University School of Medicine; Lecturer in Medicine, Harvard Medical School; Chief, Infectious Disease Service, Tufts-New England Medical Center; Associate Physician, Medical Service, Massachusetts General Hospital, Boston, Massachusetts.

JOHN M. WELLER, M.D. Professor of Internal Medicine, University of Michigan; Director, Nephrology Division, University Hospital, Ann Arbor, Michigan.

K. LEMONE YIELDING, M.D. Professor, Biochemistry, University of Alabama School of Medicine, Birmingham, Alabama.

ROBERT ZELIS, M.D. Associate Professor of Medicine, Associate Professor of Physiology, Director, Clinical Physiology and Cardiac Catheterization Laboratories, Section of Cardiovascular Medicine, Departments of Medicine and Physiology, University of California, School of Medicine, Davis, California.

PREFACE TO THE FIFTH EDITION

This edition of *Pathologic Physiology*, the fifth, represents a complete rewriting of the text. This restructuring coincides with an extensive turnover in the list of contributors. It is in the spirit of the dramatic changes and staggering advances in medical science that the editors accepted the fact that many of the contributors who had remained with the book since the First Edition in 1950 should now give way to a younger group. Thus, the text has undergone a complete rewriting and reorientation of approach, especially in fields such as immunology, genetics, and molecular biology. Importantly, these new contributors have joined with us in capturing the concept presented in the First Edition, the goal of the text being to present and interpret the clinical picture of disease and the genesis of symptoms and signs as physiologic dysfunctions.

The W. B. Saunders Company and its staff have been more than patient and cooperative as the work has progressed. We are grateful and thank them. The Editors also wish to thank their wives, Marjorie Christian Sodeman and Mary Agnes Sodeman, for their support and tolerance as the work on the text and the reading of manuscripts progressed.

WILLIAM A. SODEMAN, JR., M.D.
WILLIAM A. SODEMAN, SR., M.D.

PREFACE TO THE FIRST EDITION

This volume, a collaborative effort by 25 authors, approaches problems of disease in the field of internal medicine from the standpoint of disturbed physiology. Unlike the usual text, which is devoted to discussions of etiology, pathology, symptoms and treatment, this work analyzes symptoms and signs and the mechanisms of their development. The monograph is not intended to take the place of standard texts on physiology or textbooks of medicine. It does not aim at the completeness of either, but does try to bridge the gap between them by presenting a clinical picture of disease seen as physiologic dysfunction. An attempt is made to promote understanding of how and why symptoms appear, so that the student or physician may have a reasonable explanation for the findings he elicits. Neurologic problems are considered only as they are related to the various disease groups. The same is true of metabolic disturbances and disorders of acid-base balance.

The Editor thanks the contributors for their ready cooperation in covering certain aspects of disease in which presentation of material is at times most difficult. He thanks the Saunders Company for their help and guidance, and also Miss Brent S. Robertson for her long hours of hard work and patience in reading and checking manuscripts.

WILLIAM A. SODEMAN, M.D.

CONTENTS

SECTION I. SCIENTIFIC FOUNDATIONS

Chapter 1
METABOLIC BIOCHEMISTRY 3
Milton Toporek and Paul H. Maurer

Chapter 2
MOLECULAR BIOLOGY 27
K. Lemone Yielding

Chapter 3
MEDICAL GENETICS 40
Benjamin R. Gendel and Louis J. Elsas, II

Chapter 4
IMMUNOBIOLOGY 97
Peter Abramoff and René J. Duquesnoy

Chapter 5
IMMUNODEFICIENCY DISEASES AND TUMOR IMMUNOBIOLOGY 124
René J. Duquesnoy and Peter Abramoff

SECTION II. CARDIORENAL AND RESPIRATORY SYSTEMS

Chapter 6
INTEGRATIVE HEMODYNAMICS 149
Arthur C. Guyton

Chapter 7
SYSTEMIC ARTERIAL PRESSURE 177
Robert C. Tarazi and Ray W. Gifford, Jr.

xiii

Chapter 8
MECHANISMS OF CARDIAC CONTRACTION: STRUCTURAL, BIOCHEMICAL, AND FUNCTIONAL RELATIONS IN THE NORMAL AND DISEASED HEART 206
Dean T. Mason, Robert Zelis, Ezra A. Amsterdam, and Rashid A. Massumi

Chapter 9
CARDIAC OUTPUT, CARDIAC PERFORMANCE, HYPERTROPHY, DILATATION, VALVULAR DISEASE, ISCHEMIC HEART DISEASE, AND PERICARDIAL DISEASE 235
Harold T. Dodge and J. Ward Kennedy

Chapter 10
CONGESTIVE HEART FAILURE 273
H. J. C. Swan and William W. Parmley

Chapter 11
HEART SOUNDS, MURMURS, AND PRECORDIAL MOVEMENTS 295
John F. Stapleton and W. Proctor Harvey

Chapter 12
THE ELECTROCARDIOGRAM 312
J. A. Abildskov

Chapter 13
ARRHYTHMIAS—MECHANISMS AND PATHOGENESIS 329
Yoshio Watanabe and Leonard S. Dreifus

Chapter 14
RENAL DISEASE: WATER AND ELECTROLYTE BALANCE 345
John M. Weller

Chapter 15
PULMONARY VENTILATION AND BLOOD GAS EXCHANGE 371
Robert E. Forster

Chapter 16
PROTECTIVE MECHANISMS OF THE LUNGS; PULMONARY DISEASE; PLEURAL DISEASE 393
John H. Killough

SECTION III. RHEUMATOLOGY, ALLERGY, INFECTIOUS DISEASE, AND HEMATOLOGY

Chapter 17
RHEUMATIC DISEASES 417
William D. Robinson

Chapter 18
ALLERGY: ITS NATURE AND RELATIONSHIP TO OTHER IMMUNOLOGICALLY INDUCED DISEASE STATES 445
Herbert C. Mansmann

Chapter 19
PATHOGENIC PROPERTIES OF INVADING MICROORGANISMS 457
Louis Weinstein and Morton N. Swartz

Chapter 20
HOST RESPONSES TO INFECTION 473
Louis Weinstein and Morton N. Swartz

Chapter 21
PATHOPHYSIOLOGIC CHANGES DUE TO LOCALIZATION OF INFECTIONS IN SPECIFIC ORGANS 489
Louis Weinstein and Morton N. Swartz

Chapter 22
PATHOPHYSIOLOGY OF HEMATOLOGIC DISORDERS 511
Allan J. Erslev and Thomas G. Gabuzda

Chapter 23
THE SPLEEN AND RETICULOENDOTHELIAL SYSTEM 665
Spencer O. Raab

SECTION IV. GASTROENTEROLOGY, ENDOCRINOLOGY, AND METABOLISM

Chapter 24
THE ESOPHAGUS 697
David B. Skinner

Chapter 25
THE STOMACH 709
Joseph B. Kirsner

Chapter 26
THE SMALL INTESTINE 734
David W. Watson and William A. Sodeman, Jr.

Chapter 27
THE LARGE INTESTINE 767
William A. Sodeman, Jr., and David W. Watson

Chapter 28
NORMAL AND PATHOLOGIC PHYSIOLOGY OF THE LIVER 790
F. L. Iber

Chapter 29
PATHOPHYSIOLOGY OF GALLBLADDER DISEASE.. 818
Franz Goldstein

Chapter 30
PATHOPHYSIOLOGY OF THE PANCREAS... 827
Franz Goldstein

Chapter 31
NUTRITIONAL FACTORS IN DISEASE.. 839
George A. Bray

Chapter 32
ENDOCRINOLOGY.. 865
Thomas W. Burns

SECTION V. TOXIC PHYSICAL AND CHEMICAL AGENTS

Chapter 33
EFFECTS OF PHYSICAL AGENTS.. 917
Charles E. Billings

Chapter 34
CHEMICAL AGENTS AND DISEASE 949
Bertram D. Dinman

INDEX 973

SECTION I

SCIENTIFIC FOUNDATIONS

CHAPTER 1

METABOLIC BIOCHEMISTRY

MILTON TOPOREK
PAUL H. MAURER

The ultimate goal of metabolic biochemistry or intermediary metabolism is to determine all the reactions undergone by the various molecules which enter the body, by normal or other means, from the time they enter until they or their derivatives leave the body. Although much has been accomplished in this field in the last 25 years since radioactive isotopes became available, much more remains to be learned. However, much of the information available has already provided the medical profession with many useful procedures for diagnosis and therapy based on objective criteria of clinical laboratory determinations which, when compared to normal metabolic patterns, can indicate the health status of the patient. It is therefore the purpose of this chapter to review, in limited form, the major metabolic pathways, with some examples of abnormal changes correlated with clinical conditions.

CARBOHYDRATE METABOLISM

A general summary of carbohydrate metabolism is presented in Figure 1-1. This diagram shows the possible uses of glucose in the liver and muscle to be as follows:

Liver	*Muscle*
Storage as glycogen	Storage as glycogen
Oxidation for energy purposes	Oxidation for energy purposes
Conversion to other metabolites:	
Fat	
Amino Acids	
Other carbohydrates	

USES OF GLUCOSE

Storage as Glycogen (Glycogenesis)

Glucose not used for other purposes as listed below may be converted to glycogen and deposited in the liver or muscle tissues in relatively small and limited amounts. Remaining available glucose is disposed of in pathways discussed below.

Oxidation for Energy Purposes

Complete oxidation of glucose to CO_2 and H_2O can furnish energy for the body as required. This is accomplished in two stages: (1) glycolysis (Embden-Meyerhof pathway), taking glucose to the 3-carbon pyruvate or lactate point; and (2) the tricarboxylic acid cycle (Krebs, or citric acid cycle), which converts the 3-carbon pyruvate to CO_2 and H_2O. Under anaerobic conditions, as in muscle after prolonged or strenuous exercise, glycolysis produces lactic acid, a reduction product of pyruvic acid. By way of the blood, the lactic acid reaches the liver for reprocessing or further oxidation. Under aerobic conditions, lactate is converted back to pyruvate, and the oxidation of pyruvate is completed in liver and muscle by way of the tricarboxylic acid cycle.

Liver and adipose tissue can also degrade glucose by the pentose phosphate pathway (pentose shunt), a pathway which is relatively unimportant in skeletal muscle.

Conversion to Other Metabolites

Fat. Excess glucose may be converted to fatty acids and glycerol and deposited as triglycerides

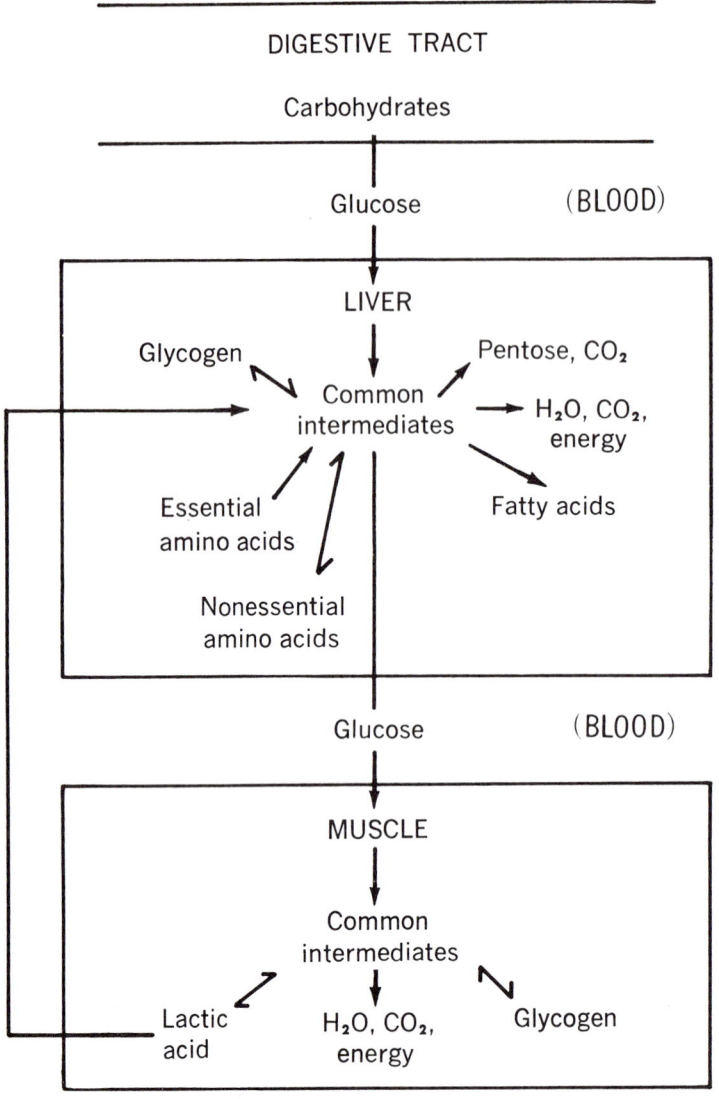

Figure 1–1 General summary of carbohydrate metabolism. (From Toporek: Basic Chemistry of Life, 1968. Courtesy of Appleton-Century-Crofts, Inc.)

in adipose tissue, a process which, to the sorrow of many, is unlimited except by restrictions on intake of carbohydrates. As will be noted later, there are certain features common to the metabolic pathways of glucose and the fatty acids, but the conversion of glucose to fatty acids is irreversible on the basis of energy accounting, i.e., it would require a net expenditure of energy to convert fatty acids to glucose.

Amino Acids. The carbon skeletons of the nonessential amino acids may be derived from glucose in a reversible process. The essential amino acids can also contribute to the carbon skeleton of glucose, but the reverse is not possible in this case.

Other Carbohydrates. Some glucose is used for the synthesis of other important sugars such as ribose and deoxyribose, components of the nucleic acids, and galactose, a component of cerebrosides, gangliosides, and glycolipids.

OXIDATION OF GLUCOSE

The complete oxidation of glucose is divided into two major phases: (1) glycolysis (Embden-Meyerhof pathway), an anaerobic pathway (does not require oxygen but can occur in its presence) which includes glycogenesis and glycogenolysis, interconversions of galactose, fructose, and glucose, and ends with the production of pyruvate (under aerobic conditions) or lactate (under anaerobic conditions) and a small amount of energy; and (2) the tricarboxylic acid cycle (Krebs cycle, citric acid cycle), an aerobic pathway which completes the oxidation of glucose to H_2O and CO_2, with the production of a much larger amount of energy.

Glycolysis

The metabolic reactions of glycolysis are outlined in Figure 1-2. The solid line arrows indicate the reactions in the direction of glycogenesis and the anaerobic metabolism of glucose to the pyruvate or lactate stage (glycolysis). A single-headed arrow (⟶) indicates a reaction which is irreversible as written. A double-headed arrow (⟷) indicates a reversible reaction. A broken arrow (---→) indicates a reaction which has the effect of reversing an irreversible reaction by a reaction which is different from the forward reaction. Thus, there is complete *biologic reversibility*, but it occurs at the price of a loss of energy, i.e., since the reactions in the direction of glucose to pyruvate generate energy, the reactions in reverse must require an input of energy. The individual reactions are listed below by numbers corresponding to those in Figure 1-2.

Reactions to Glycolysis

Reaction 1 – Glucose is converted to glucose-6-phosphate (G-6-P) under the influence of hexokinase and adenosine triphosphate (ATP). This is an irreversible reaction because a high-energy phosphate group in ATP is used to form a low-energy ester phosphate bond in G-6-P.

Reaction 2 – G-6-P is converted back to glucose in the liver by glucose-6-phosphatase, not by reversal of reaction 1. Muscle does not have this phosphatase.

Reaction 3 – G-6-P is converted to glucose-1-phosphate (G-1-P) by phosphoglucomutase.

Reaction 4 – This summarizes a series of reactions resulting in the formation of glycogen, as follows:

G-1-P + UTP $\xrightarrow{\text{Pyrophosphorylase}}$ UDPG + pyrophosphate

UDPG $\xrightarrow[\text{Branching enzyme}]{\text{Glycogen synthetase}}$ Glycogen + UDP

UDP + ATP $\xrightarrow{\text{Phosphokinase}}$ UTP + ADP

UTP = uridine triphosphate
UDP = uridine diphosphate
UDPG = uridine diphosphate-glucose
Glycogen synthetase: forms 1,4-linkages between glucose moieties, making straight chains
Branching enzyme: forms 1,6-linkages between glucose moieties, making branches between straight chains

Reaction 5 – Glycogen is broken down to G-1-P in the presence of a debranching enzyme (breaks 1,6-linkages) and phosphorylase (breaks 1,4-linkages). Reaction 3 converts G-1-P to G-6-P. If required for blood sugar, G-6-P can be converted back to glucose by reaction 2.

Reaction 6 – G-6-P is converted to fructose-6-phosphate (F-6-P) in a reversible reaction catalyzed by phosphohexose isomerase.

Reaction 7 – F-6-P is phosphorylated to fructose-1,6-diphosphate (F-1,6-P_2) in an irreversible kinase reaction in the presence of phosphofructokinase.

Reaction 8 – Reaction 7 can be biologically reversed by way of a phosphatase reaction.

Reaction 9 – F-1,6-P_2 is split into two triose phosphate molecules, glyceraldehyde-3-phosphate (glycerald-3-P) and dihydroxyacetone phosphate [$(OH)_2$-acetone-P], in a reversible reaction catalyzed by fructose diphosphate aldolase.

Reaction 10 – The triose phosphates, glycerald-3-P and $(OH)_2$-acetone-P, are in equilibrium with each other in the presence of an isomerase. Thus, both halves of the original glucose molecule are available for subsequent reactions.

Reaction 11 – The conversion of glycerald-3-P to 1,3-diphosphoglycerate (1,3-P_2-glycerate) is catalyzed by glycerald-3-P-dehydrogenase in a reversible reaction. The carboxyl phosphate bond is a high-energy bond, the energy coming from the oxidation of the aldehyde to a carboxyl group.

Reaction 12 – In the conversion of 1,3-P_2-glycerate to 3-phosphoglycerate (3-P-glycerate) under the influence of phosphoglycerate kinase, the energy of the carboxyl phosphate bond is captured in the concomitant conversion of ADP to ATP.

Reaction 13 – 3-P-glycerate forms 2-P-glycerate in the presence of phosphoglyceromutase in a reversible reaction.

Reaction 14 – The dehydration of 2-P-glycerate to phosphoenolpyruvate (P-E-pyr) with the production of a high-energy phosphate bond is catalyzed by enolase.

Reaction 15 – The high energy in P-E-pyr is captured in the formation of ATP from ADP in an irreversible reaction in the presence of pyruvate kinase, resulting in the formation of pyruvate.

Reaction 16 – Under anaerobic conditions, pyruvate is converted to lactate in the presence of lactate dehydrogenase in a reaction which reverses itself under aerobic conditions. This concludes the glycolysis reactions.

Reaction 17 – In the liver, reaction 15 can be

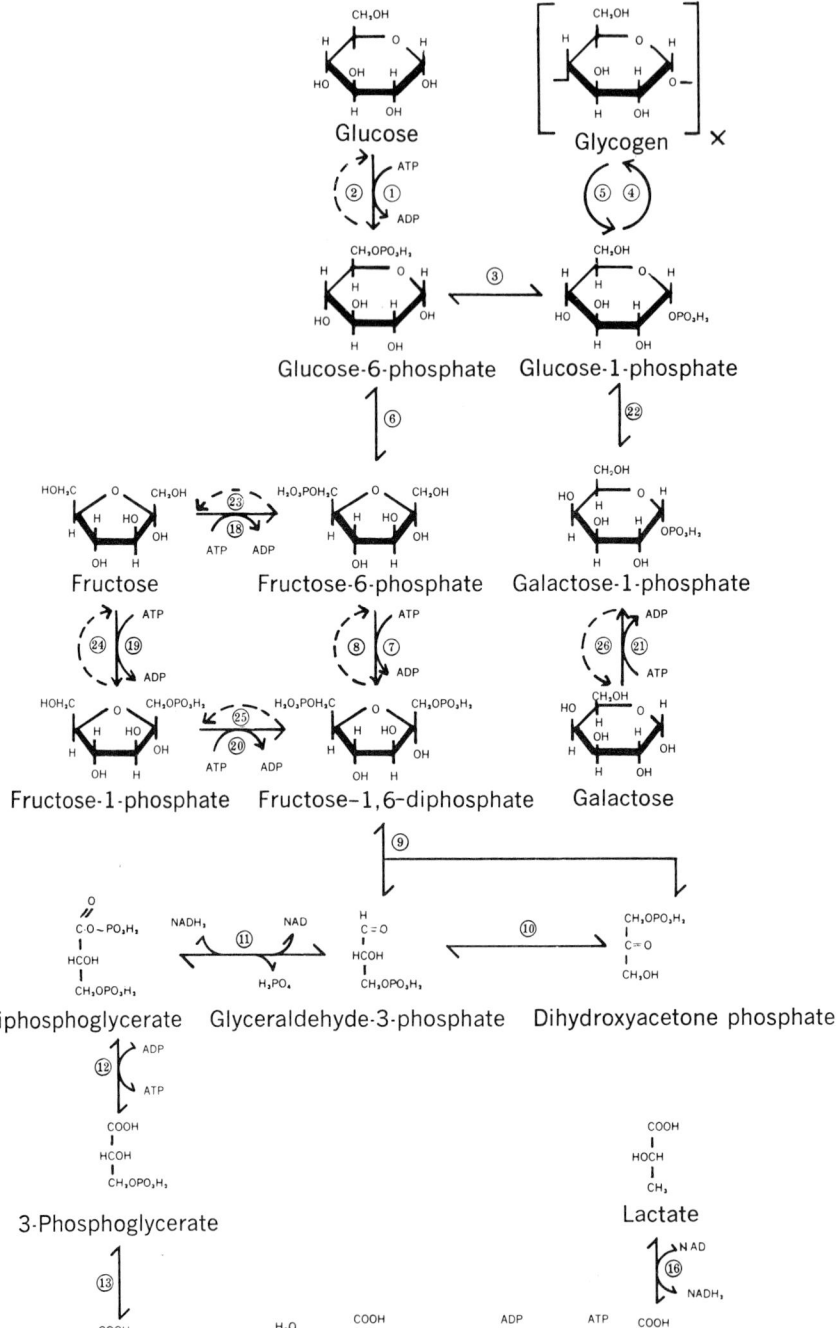

Figure 1-2 Anaerobic metabolism of glucose (glycolysis) and related hexoses. ($\sim$ = high energy bond.) (Adapted from Toporek: Basic Chemistry of Life, 1968. Courtesy of Appleton-Century-Crofts, Inc.)

Condition	Deficient Enzyme	Reaction Involved
Glycogen storage diseases		See Figure 1-2
I von Gierke's disease	Glucose-6-phosphatase	1-2
II Pompe's disease	Alpha-1,4-glucosidase (acid maltase)	
III Limit dextrinosis	Amylo-1,6-glucosidase (debranching enzyme)	1-5
IV Andersen's disease (Amylopectinosis)	Amylo-(1,4 to 1,6)-transglucosidase (branching enzyme)	1-4
V McArdle's disease	Muscle phosphorylase	1-5
VI	Liver phosphorylase	1-5
VII	Muscle phosphofructokinase	1-7
VIII	Liver phosphorylase kinase	(1-5)

reversed (bypassed) with a set of two reactions with the expenditure of energy:

$$\text{Pyruvate} \xrightarrow{\text{Pyruvate carboxylase}} \text{Oxaloacetate}$$

$$\text{Oxaloacetate} \xrightarrow{\text{Phosphoenolpyruvate carboxykinase}} \text{P-E-pyr}$$

Reaction 18 – In the presence of a kinase, fructose (F) can be converted to F-6-P, which is directly on the glycolytic pathway.

Reaction 19 – In another kinase reaction, F can be converted to F-1-P.

Reaction 20 – F-1-P, in the presence of a phosphofructokinase, is converted to F-1,6-P_2, also directly on the glycolytic pathway.

Reaction 21 – Galactose (Gal) is converted to Gal-1-P in a kinase reaction.

Reaction 22 – Gal-1-P can be converted to G-1-P in a reaction involving uridine diphosphate glucose and a transferase. G-1-P can then be converted to G-6-P by reaction 3.

Reactions 23 to 26 – All the phosphorylations in reactions 18 to 21 can be biologically reversed with appropriate phosphatase reactions.

Energy Accounting in Glycolysis. Of approximately 50,000 calories of free energy liberated per mole of glucose catabolized in glycolysis, 15,000 calories are recovered with a net gain of two high-energy phosphate bonds, or an efficiency of about 30 per cent.

Clinical Conditions Related to Glycolytic Reactions. With so many reactions and so many enzymes working in proper sequence required for the proper functioning of the glycolytic pathway, there are many possibilities for the introduction of clinical difficulties. It is not intended to discuss the many disease states associated with derangements in carbohydrate metabolism but rather to cite a few typical examples. The first glycogen storage disease recognized to be genetically caused, known as von Gierke's disease, results from the lack of the enzyme glucose-6-phosphatase. This leads to hypoglycemia (glucose can enter the glycolytic pathway by reaction 1, but it cannot be regenerated because of lack of enzyme for reaction 2), enlargement of the liver to accommodate increased stores of glycogen (glycogen cannot be converted back to glucose because of lack of enzyme for reaction 2), and elevation of blood lactate concentration (more glucose than normal reaches the lactate stage).

It is important to realize that although clinically we can observe a single condition of excess glycogen storage, the disturbance can have various sources. Eight different glycogen storage disease conditions and the enzymes involved are listed in a table of disorders in which deficient activities of specific enzymes have been demonstrated in man. (See table above.)

Tricarboxylic Acid Cycle

The completion of the oxidation of pyruvate to H_2O and CO_2, with the production of much more energy than in the glycolytic segment, is accomplished under aerobic conditions by way of the tricarboxylic acid cycle. Before entering the tricarboxylic acid cycle, pyruvate is converted to acetyl-CoA by a complicated set of reactions involving the pyruvate dehydrogenase system of enzymes, vitamin B_1, coenzyme A, and nicotinamide adenine dinucleotide (NAD). The net reaction is as follows:

$$\underset{\text{Pyruvate}}{CH_3COCOOH} + \underset{\text{Coenzyme A}}{CoASH} \xrightarrow[CO_2]{NAD \quad NADH_2} \underset{\text{Acetyl-CoA}}{CH_3CO{\sim}SCoA} + H_2O$$

At this point it is important to note that fatty acid metabolism, to be discussed later, is another source of acetyl-CoA molecules, indicating the close link between the metabolism of carbohydrates and that of fatty acids.

Reactions of the Tricarboxylic Acid Cycle. The reactions of the tricarboxylic acid cycle are outlined in Figure 1-3.

Reaction 1 — Acetyl-CoA is taken into the tricarboxylic acid cycle in an irreversible reaction by way of a condensation with oxaloacetate to form citrate as CoA is regenerated. Oxaloacetate is a member of the cycle which is regenerated with each turn of the cycle.

Reactions 2-1 and *2-2* — These reactions involve an equilibrium between citrate, cis-aconitate, and isocitrate. The net result, under the influence of aconitase, is the production of isocitrate, an isomer of citrate, by moving the —OH group from the central carbon atom to an end carbon atom.

Reactions 3-1 and *3-2* — In this two-stage reaction, apparently catalyzed by a single enzyme, isocitrate dehydrogenase, the net reaction is an oxidative decarboxylation of isocitrate to α-ketoglutarate, the oxalosuccinate apparently not being free during the reactions. The decarboxylation makes the net reaction irreversible.

Reaction 4 — α-Ketoglutarate is oxidatively decarboxylated to succinate in an irreversible reaction involving NAD, vitamin B_1, and CoA.

Reaction 5 — In a reversible reaction catalyzed by succinic dehydrogenase and iron-flavin prosthetic groups acting as hydrogen acceptors (instead of NAD), succinate is oxidized to fumarate.

Reaction 6 — The reversible hydration of fumarate to malate is catalyzed by fumarase.

Reaction 7 — Malate is dehydrogenated in a reversible reaction involving malate dehydrogenase and NAD, and oxaloacetate is regenerated as a result, in preparation for the next turn of the cycle.

The dotted lines in Figure 1-3 indicate the production and capture of energy as high-energy phosphate bonds as the hydrogen atoms are fully oxidized to H_2O by way of the oxidative chain. The net reaction for the oxidation of pyruvic acid may be written as follows:

$$CH_3COCOOH + 5(O) \rightarrow 2H_2O + 3CO_2 + Energy$$

Energy Accounting in Aerobic Oxidation. In the aerobic oxidation of glucose, of the maximum available free energy of 688,500 calories per mole of glucose, 285,000 calories, or 41 per cent, are conserved. This makes it quite clear that in efficiency and absolute amount, aerobic oxidation of glucose is much more beneficial than anaerobic oxidation.

Pentose Phosphate Pathway

In liver and adipose tissue, glucose can also be oxidized by a series of reactions known as the pentose phosphate pathway (pentose shunt). Energy production does not seem to be the primary purpose of this pathway. The more important products seem to be ribose and ultimately deoxyribose, for RNA and DNA synthesis, and $NADPH_2$, which is used for reducing purposes as required in other reactions, such as the synthesis of fatty acids.

In net terms, one molecule of CO_2 is produced per turn of this cycle (the aldehyde carbon, C-1, of glucose is lost in a decarboxylation reaction) and glucose is regenerated. Therefore, six turns of the cycle are required to completely degrade one molecule of glucose. This means that if six molecules of glucose go through six turns of the cycle, six molecules of CO_2 are produced and five molecules of glucose are regenerated.

Glucose-6-phosphate and fructose-6-phosphate are involved in the pentose shunt as well as in the glycolytic scheme. Therefore, these two metabolic pathways must be in some kind of equilibrium in tissues in which both pathways are operating.

BLOOD SUGAR CONCENTRATION

The processes and substances involved in the maintenance of the blood sugar concentration within normal levels are briefly reviewed in this section.

Factors Contributing to Blood Sugar

Intestinal Absorption. Because of the rapid absorption of sugars from the small intestine after meals, and depending on the type of meal, there may be temporary increases in blood sugar.

Glycogenolysis. In periods of hypoglycemia, the rate of glycogenolysis in the liver increases in order to put more glucose into the blood.

Gluconeogenesis. When the intake of carbohydrates is restricted or absent, gluconeogenesis increases in an attempt to maintain the required concentration of blood sugar.

Factors Removing Sugar from Blood

Liver, Muscle, and Other Tissues. After absorption, glucose goes first to the liver, where, as noted before, it may be used for storage as glycogen, oxidized for energy purposes, or converted to other metabolites. Some is released for use by other tissues of the body. Muscle also uses glu-

METABOLIC BIOCHEMISTRY

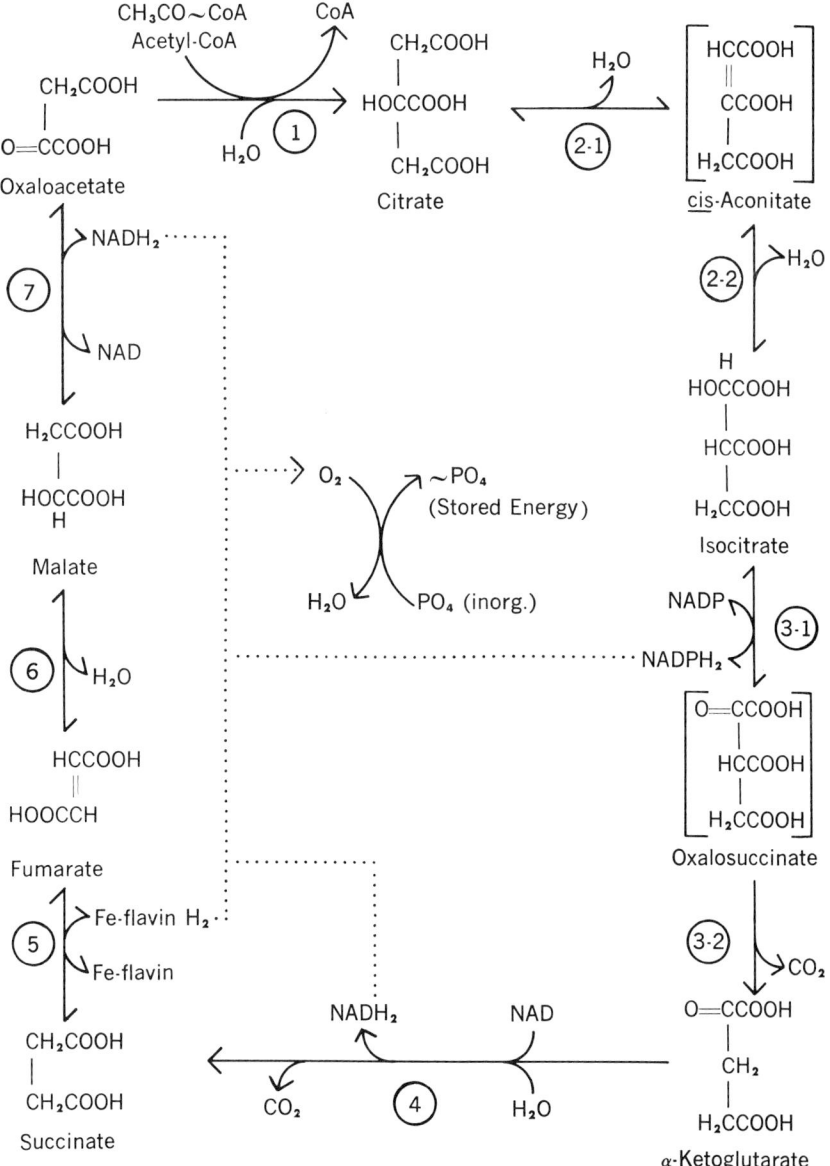

Figure 1-3 The tricarboxylic acid cycle (also known as the citric acid cycle or the Krebs cycle). ($\sim$ = high energy bond.) (From Toporek: Basic Chemistry of Life, 1968. Courtesy of Appleton-Century-Crofts, Inc.)

cose for storage as glycogen, and, with all other tissues, uses glucose for energy production.

Amino Acid Synthesis. At times, glucose may serve to supply the carbon skeleton of nonessential amino acids.

Fatty Acid and Glycerol Synthesis. As noted before, during periods of excessive intake of carbohydrates, glucose may be diverted to the synthesis of fatty acids and glycerol, and the resulting lipids may be stored in adipose tissue.

Kidney. Since the kidney has a limited ability to reabsorb sugar during the formation of urine, the renal threshold being exceeded when the blood sugar concentration rises above approximately 160 mg. per 100 ml., glucose in excess of this concentration begins to spill out into the urine. This occurs in uncontrolled diabetes mellitus and some other conditions.

Hormonal Effects on Carbohydrate Metabolism

Insulin. Insulin acts to decrease blood sugar by stimulating glycogenesis in the liver and increased metabolism of glucose by other tissues. (Other insulin actions are discussed in Chapter 33.)

Epinephrine. Epinephrine favors glycogenolysis in liver and muscles by stimulating phosphorylase activity and appears to decrease the uptake of glucose by tissue cells.

Glucagon. Glucagon stimulates glycogenolysis in the liver, thereby increasing blood sugar concentration.

Glucocorticoids. The 11-oxygenated adrenocortical hormones tend to increase gluconeogenesis and act generally in a manner opposite to that of insulin, thereby exerting a hyperglycemic effect.

Thyroid Hormone. Thyroxine stimulates glycogenolysis in the liver, resulting in an increase in blood sugar.

Adenohypophyseal Hormones. By their actions in stimulating the production of the glucocorticoids and thyroxine, adrenocorticotropic and thyrotropic hormones also have hyperglycemic effects.

Diabetes Mellitus

The classic clinical condition resulting from deranged carbohydrate metabolism is diabetes mellitus. Only the important metabolic considerations will be reviewed at this point (see Ch. 32). In the face of a partial or total lack of insulin, or a defective response of target cells to insulin, diabetic patients become hyperglycemic because of decreased glycogenesis (see glycolytic scheme, Figure 1-2). Another major metabolic problem is the possible excess production of ketone bodies that results from an imbalance in the supply and utilization of acetyl-CoA (see oxidative decarboxylation of pyruvate). Because of the limited ability of the extrahepatic tissues to oxidize the acidic ketone bodies, excessive production of these substances may lead to acidosis, ketonuria, fruity breath odor, and ultimately diabetic coma. As noted earlier, acetyl-CoA is also supplied or utilized in fatty acid metabolism. The relationships between carbohydrate and lipid metabolism will be discussed in the next section.

SUMMARY OF CARBOHYDRATE METABOLISM

A scheme summarizing carbohydrate metabolism in simplified form is presented in Figure 1-4. This diagram will be amplified in subsequent sections to illustrate the relationships between carbohydrate, lipid, and protein metabolism.

LIPID METABOLISM

The lipids include a number of diverse types of chemical substances. The major types to be discussed here are generally classified as follows:

  I. Simple Lipids
    A. Fats (glycerides)
 II. Compound Lipids
    A. Phospholipids
       1. Lecithins
       2. Cephalins
       3. Sphingomyelins
    B. Glycolipids
       1. Cerebrosides
III. Steroids
    A. Sterols

Fat Metabolism

Fats are structurally composed of glycerol esterified with three fatty acids. The synthesis and catabolism of fatty acids both involve acetyl-CoA, an important intermediate in carbohydrate metabolism. Glycerol may also be derived from carbohydrate metabolism. It should be obvious, therefore, that there must be some close relationships between lipid and carbohydrate metabolism.

Synthesis of Fatty Acids. Synthesis of the fatty acids may be accomplished either in or outside of the mitochondria. The extramitochondrial pathway in simplified form is shown in Figure 1-5. In the first step, acetyl-CoA is converted to malonyl-CoA in a carbon dioxide assimilation reaction. Then, after condensation of acetyl-CoA with malonyl-CoA, involving a decarboxylation reaction, and subsequent reactions, including two reductions with a dehydration in between, the result is the production of butyryl-CoA. If butyryl-CoA now condenses with malonyl-CoA and

METABOLIC BIOCHEMISTRY 11

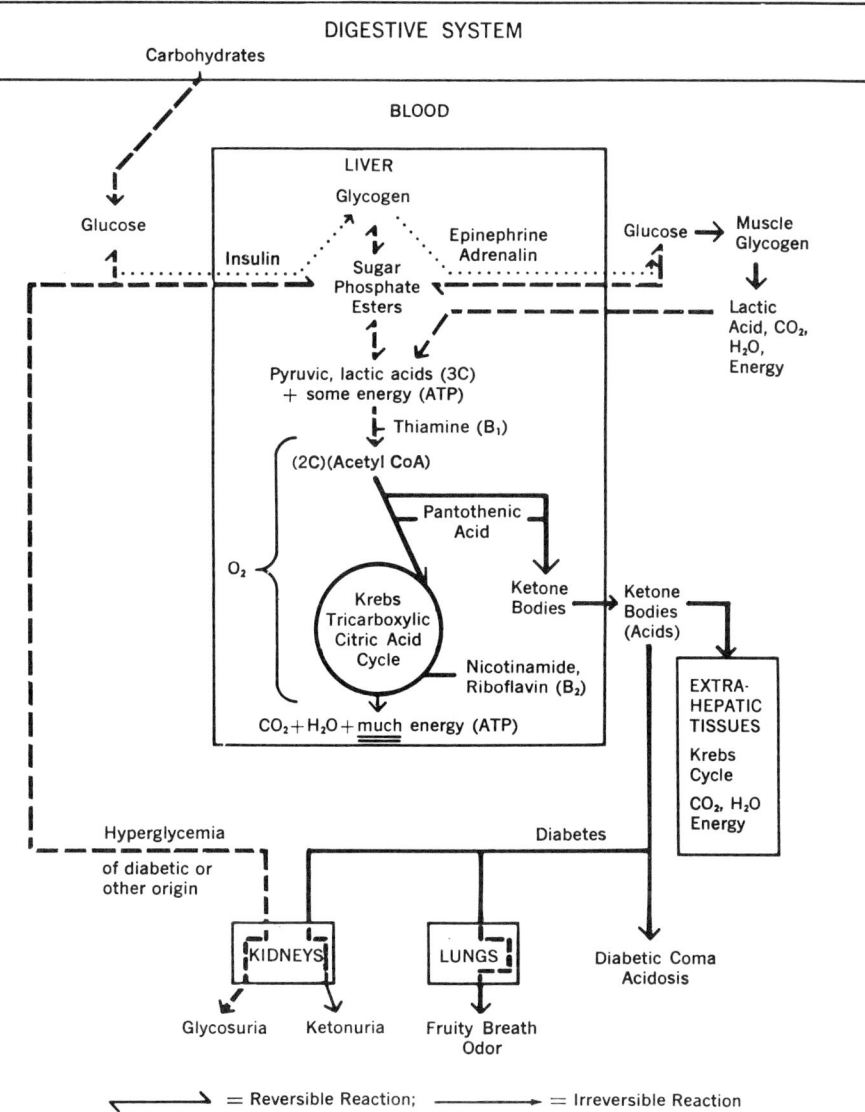

Figure 1-4 Flow chart of carbohydrate metabolism. (Pathways: – – – – = carbohydrate; ──── = common.) (From Toporek: Basic Chemistry of Life, 1968. Courtesy of Appleton-Century-Crofts, Inc.)

the same series of reactions is repeated for a total of seven times, palmityl-CoA, or palmitic acid (16-carbon acid – 14 from acetyl-CoA and 2 from malonyl-CoA), is the end product. This metabolic pathway has a high requirement for NADPH$_2$, which is produced in the pentose shunt (p. 8), a process which is quantitatively significant in liver and adipose tissue.

The mitochondrial pathway is presented in Figure 1-6. In this series of reactions, *malonyl-CoA is not involved*, and NADH$_2$ is used instead of NADPH$_2$ in one of the reduction steps. This mitochondrial pathway appears to serve mainly for lengthening of existing fatty acid chains rather than for complete synthesis.

The energy required for the synthesis of fatty acids is provided by the breakdown of carbohydrates (p. 3). The rate of turnover or replacement of fatty acids, as studied in radioactive tracer experiments, is high in liver, adipose tissue, and intestinal mucosa, and low in muscle, skin, and nervous tissue.

Interconversions. Interconversions between fatty acids can be accomplished by the addition or removal of 2-carbon units in reactions such as those discussed earlier. Some unsaturated fatty acids may also be synthesized, but the essential fatty acids, linoleic, linolenic, and arachidonic, must be obtained from the diet.

Breakdown of Fatty Acids. The reactions resulting in the breakdown of fatty acids are presented in simplified form in Figure 1–7. This metabolic pathway uses reactions which are similar to those used in the synthesis of the fatty acids but in reverse, the products being acetyl-CoA, the ever-present 2-carbon unit of fatty acid metabolism, and the parent fatty acid minus 2 carbon atoms.

As shown in Figure 1–7, the acetyl-CoA can then enter the tricarboxylic acid cycle for further oxidation and production of energy. CoA is produced in the first reaction of the tricarboxylic acid cycle along with citrate (p. 8). Since CoA is produced in fatty acid synthesis, and required for fatty acid breakdown, the functioning of the tricarboxylic acid cycle can influence the supply of CoA and, thereby, fatty acid metabolism, again illustrating the close interrelationship between carbohydrate and fatty acid metabolism.

Ketone Body Formation. There is a small, normal accumulation of acetyl-CoA from the metabolic pathways discussed above. As a result, the following reaction may occur:

$$2CH_3CO{\sim}CoA \longrightarrow CH_3COCH_2CO{\sim}CoA + CoA$$
Acetyl-CoA   Acetoacetyl-CoA

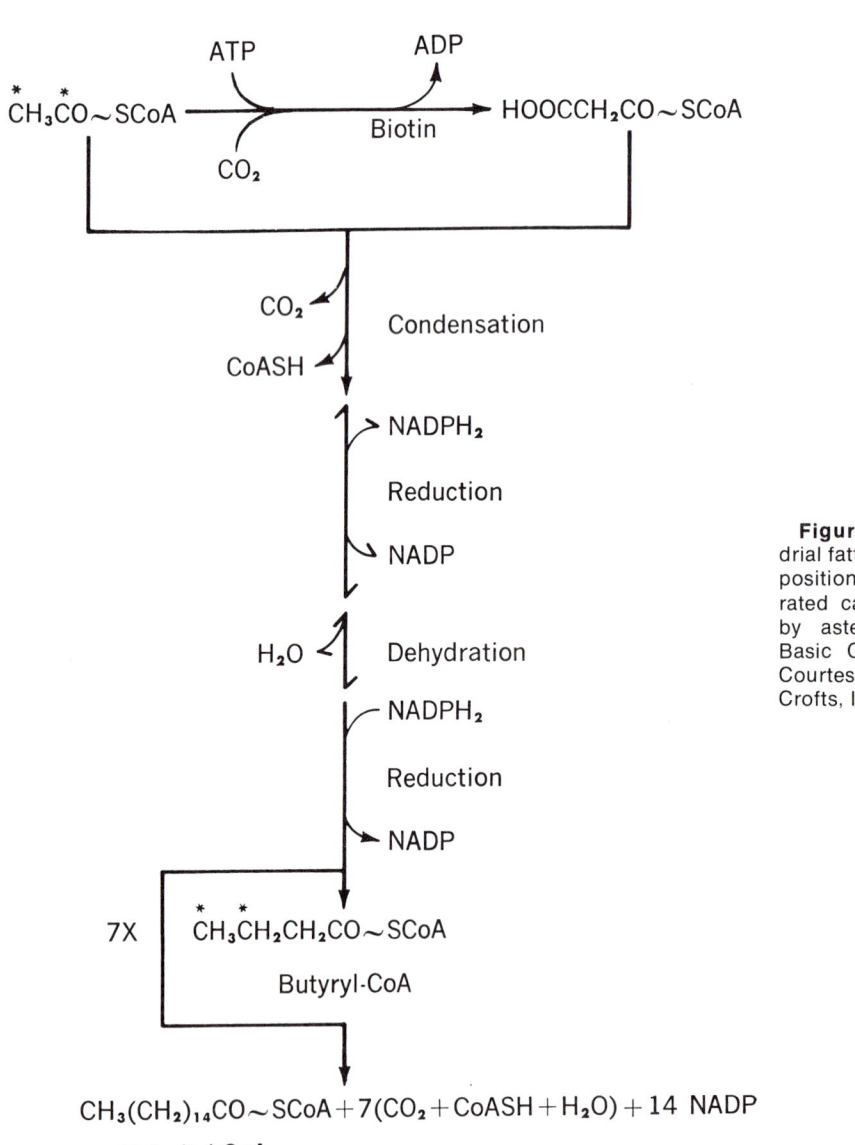

Figure 1–5 Extramitochondrial fatty acid synthesis. Note the positions of the newly incorporated carbon atoms (designated by asterisks). (From Toporek: Basic Chemistry of Life, 1968. Courtesy of Appleton-Century-Crofts, Inc.)

METABOLIC BIOCHEMISTRY 13

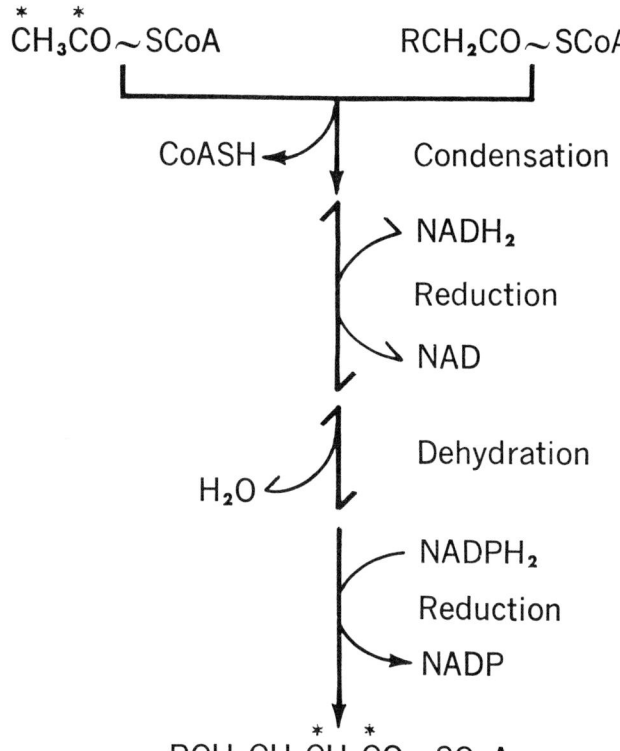

Figure 1-6 Mitochondrial fatty acid synthesis. Note the positions of the newly incorporated carbon atoms (designated by asterisks). (From Toporek: Basic Chemistry of Life, 1968. Courtesy of Appleton-Century-Crofts, Inc.)

In the liver there is a thiolesterase which catalyzes the hydrolysis of acetoacetyl-CoA to acetoacetate, a reaction which is irreversible in the liver but not in extrahepatic tissues:

$$CH_3COCH_2CO\sim CoA \rightarrow CH_3COCH_2COOH + CoA$$
    Acetoacetyl-CoA   Acetoacetate

Subsequent reactions in the liver result in the production mainly of β-hydroxybutyrate and some acetone, as follows below.

The three compounds shown below are the ketone bodies which the liver releases to the blood to be carried to extrahepatic tissues, where they are put back on the tricarboxylic acid pathway to complete their oxidation. The concentration of ketone bodies in the blood normally remains quite low. However, under circumstances in which fat metabolism may increase as carbohydrate metabolism decreases, as in diabetes mellitus (Ch. 32), ketonemia, ketonuria, and ketosis of varying degrees may result.

Energy Accounting in Fatty Acid Oxidation. Taking palmitate (16 carbon atoms) as an example, its complete oxidation produces approximately 2,340,000 calories per mole, of which 975,000 are conserved in the form of high-energy phosphate. This represents an efficiency of about 42 per cent, approximately the same as that for glucose (p. 8).

Synthesis of Triglycerides. The fatty acid portion of the triglycerides (fats) can be synthesized as described above. The glycerol portion is de-

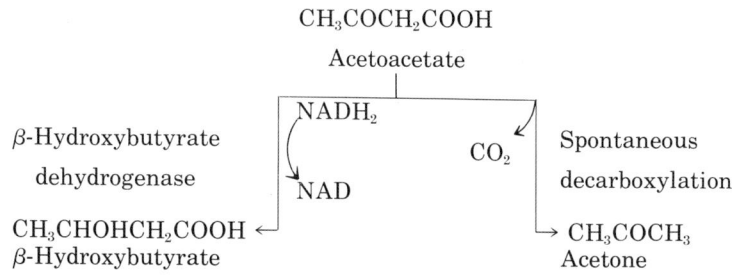

rived from an intermediate in glycolysis (p. 5), according to the following reaction:

$$\begin{array}{c} CH_2OH \\ | \\ C=O \\ | \\ CH_2O\,\text{\textcircled{P}} \end{array} \xrightarrow{NADH_2 \quad NAD} \begin{array}{c} CH_2OH \\ | \\ HOCH \\ | \\ CH_2O\,\text{\textcircled{P}} \end{array}$$

Dihydroxyacetone-phosphate   L-Glycerol-phosphate

\textcircled{P} = Phosphate

Synthesis of triglycerides is completed when the two components are combined in the series of reactions shown in Figure 1–8.

Breakdown of Triglycerides. Triglycerides are hydrolyzed by intracellular lipases before they can be oxidized further. The glycerol enters the glycolytic scheme (p. 5) by reversal of the reaction forming L-glycerol-phosphate, and the fatty acids are oxidized in 2-carbon segments by way of the tricarboxylic acid cycle (p. 8) as described above (p. 12).

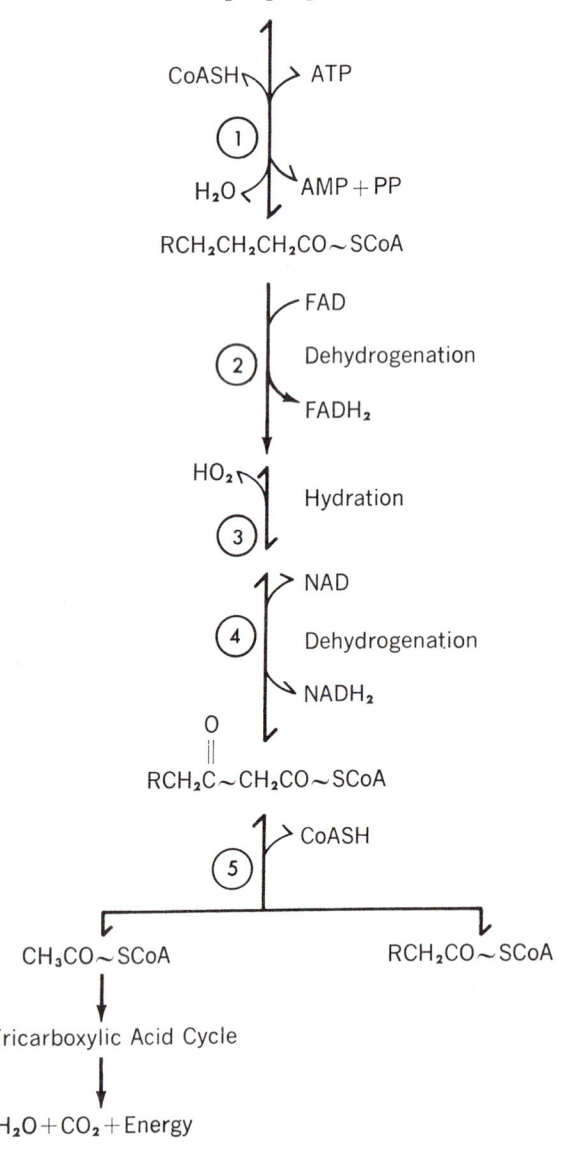

Figure 1–7 Breakdown of fatty acids to acetate and further oxidation via the tricarboxylic acid cycle. (Enzymes for reaction ① = acyl-CoA synthetase, ② = acyl-Coa dehydrogenase, ③ = enoyl-CoA hydratase, ④ = β-hydroxyacyl-CoA dehydrogenase, ⑤ = β-ketoacyl-CoA thiolase.) (From Toporek: Basic Chemistry of Life, 1968. Courtesy of Appleton-Century-Crofts, Inc.)

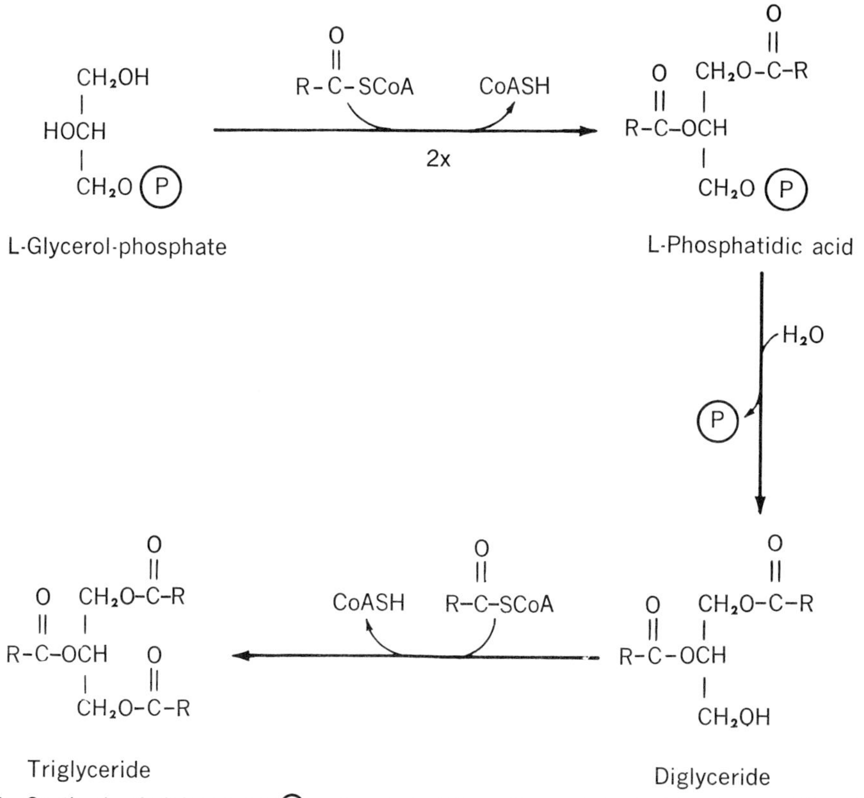

METABOLIC BIOCHEMISTRY

Figure 1-8 Synthesis of triglycerides. (Ⓟ = phosphate.) (From Toporek: Basic Chemistry of Life, 1968. Courtesy of Appleton-Century-Crofts, Inc.)

Phospholipid Metabolism

Synthesis of Lecithins and Cephalins. The lecithins (containing the nitrogenous base choline) and the cephalins (containing the nitrogenous base ethanolamine) may be synthesized from a diglyceride intermediate (see triglyceride synthesis, p. 13) in a reaction with the appropriate base in activated form as a cytidine-diphosphate base (CDP-base):

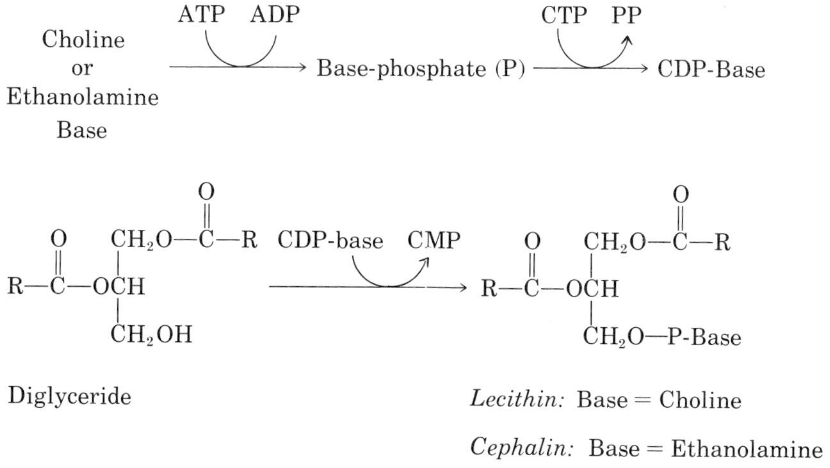

$$\text{Choline or Ethanolamine Base} \xrightarrow{\text{ATP} \quad \text{ADP}} \text{Base-phosphate (P)} \xrightarrow{\text{CTP} \quad \text{PP}} \text{CDP-Base}$$

Diglyceride

Lecithin: Base = Choline

Cephalin: Base = Ethanolamine

Although all tissues can synthesize phospholipids for their own use, the liver exports large amounts as plasma phospholipids.

Synthesis of Sphingomyelins. Sphingomyelins are synthesized, as we know, from sphingosine (an amino alcohol derived from a fatty acid and serine), including a reaction with CDP-choline (as shown below for the lecithins and cephalins). The sphingomyelins are concentrated in brain and nervous tissue.

Breakdown of Phospholipids. The phospholipids can be hydrolyzed completely by appropriate hydrolases, the components being degraded by pathways already described above, except for the bases. A number of clinical conditions have been recognized resulting from defects in the hydrolytic reactions, e.g., *Niemann-Pick disease*. In this disease, the sphingomyelinase enzyme (in spleen, liver, and kidney) responsible for the hydrolysis of sphingomyelin to ceramide and phosphorylcholine (P-choline) is markedly reduced or virtually absent. As a result, sphingomyelin accumulates in excessive amounts in the tissues of patients suffering from *Niemann-Pick disease*. In the normal breakdown process, ceramidase hydrolyzes ceramide to sphingosine and a fatty acid.

Glycolipid Metabolism

Glycolipids include in their structure both lipid and carbohydrate moieties.

Synthesis and Breakdown of Cerebrosides. Cerebrosides, incorporating glucose or galactose as the carbohydrate moiety, can be synthesized as shown at the top of the following page.

Appropriate hydrolases are available for the complete hydrolysis of the cerebrosides. Here also, as with the breakdown of the phospholipids, deficiencies in hydrolytic enzymes lead to clinical conditions, e.g., *Gaucher's disease*. A deficiency in the splenic glucocerebrosidase, which normally breaks down glucocerebroside to glucose and ceramide, leads to the abnormal accumulation of glucocerebroside in the reticuloendothelial tissue of such patients.

Sterol Metabolism—Cholesterol

Cholesterol is the most important sterol in animal metabolism. It is synthesized from small molecules in a long series of steps which include condensations, transformations, and ring closures. The first important reaction involves the condensation of acetyl-CoA with acetoacetyl-CoA, thereby establishing a close relationship with carbohydrate and fatty acid metabolism. A general outline of cholesterol metabolism is presented in Figure 1–9. Cholesterol is probably synthesized in all tissues, the liver and intestines being major sites for production of circulating cholesterol.

Intensive investigations of the relationship between cholesterol metabolism and atherosclerosis have been under way for some years and are still continuing. One very interesting observa-

$$CH_3-(CH_2)_{12}-CH=CH-\underset{OH}{\underset{|}{CH}}-\underset{NH_2}{\underset{|}{CH}}-CH_2OH + R-\overset{O}{\underset{\|}{C}} \sim CoA \longrightarrow$$

Sphingosine

$$CH_3-(CH_2)_{12}-CH=CH-\underset{OH}{\underset{|}{CH}}-\underset{\underset{R}{\underset{|}{C=O}}}{\underset{|}{\underset{|}{NH}}}-CH_2OH + CoA$$

Ceramide (N-acylsphingosine)

$$\begin{array}{c}\text{Ceramide}\\+\\\text{CDP-Choline}\end{array} \longrightarrow CH_3-(CH_2)_{12}-CH=CH-\underset{OH}{\underset{|}{CH}}-\underset{\underset{R}{\underset{|}{C=O}}}{\underset{|}{\underset{|}{NH}}}-CH_2-O-\text{P-choline} \quad + \text{ CMP}$$

Sphingomyelin

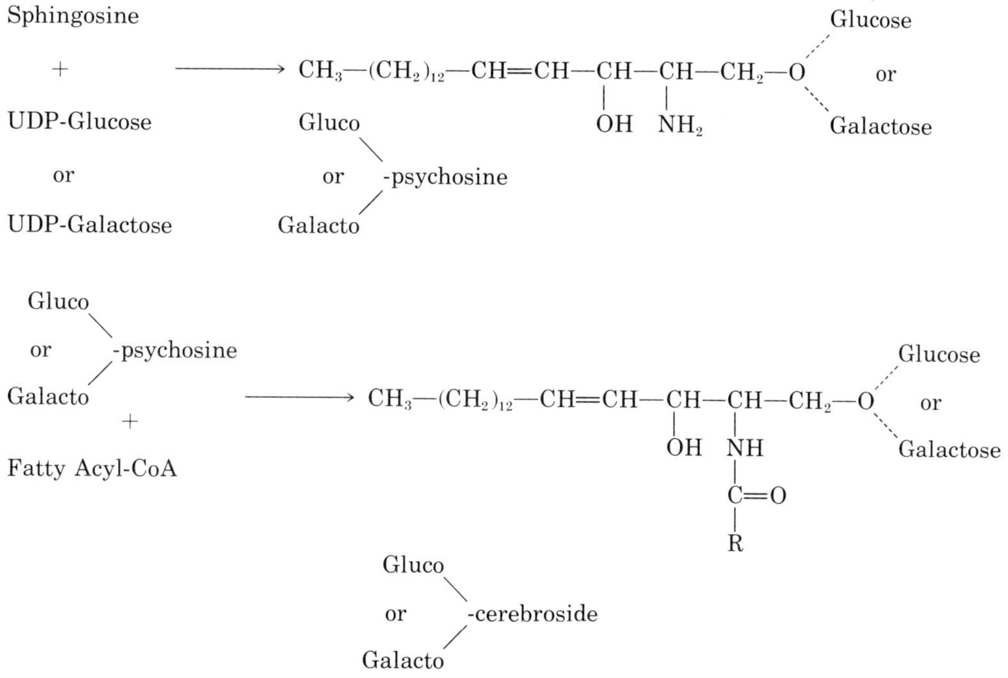

METABOLIC BIOCHEMISTRY

Sphingosine + UDP-Glucose or UDP-Galactose ⟶ CH₃—(CH₂)₁₂—CH=CH—CH(OH)—CH(NH₂)—CH₂—O—Glucose or Galactose (Gluco- or Galacto-psychosine)

Gluco- or Galacto-psychosine + Fatty Acyl-CoA ⟶ CH₃—(CH₂)₁₂—CH=CH—CH(OH)—CH(NH—C(=O)—R)—CH₂—O—Glucose or Galactose (Gluco- or Galacto-cerebroside)

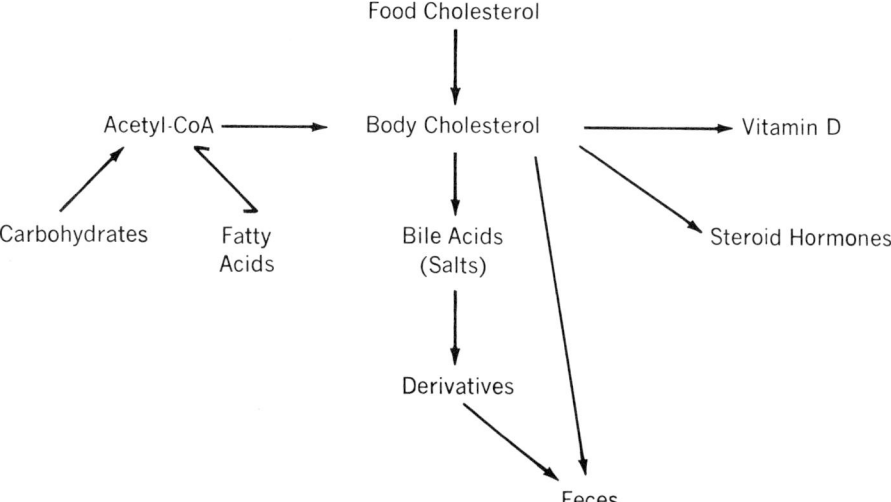

Figure 1–9 Cholesterol metabolism. (From Toporek: Basic Chemistry of Life, 1968. Courtesy of Appleton-Century-Crofts, Inc.)

tion that has led to much work in this field is that synthesis of cholesterol by the liver is inversely related to the intake of dietary cholesterol. However, attempts to control the cholesterol concentration in blood by dietary manipulations or drug administrations have thus far not led to much in the way of spectacular results. This is largely reflected by the fact that there is as yet little definitive information available with regard to the regulation of cholesterol metabolism.

Hormonal Effects on Lipid Metabolism

Insulin. Insulin stimulates the increased utilization of glucose, including the increased production of $NADPH_2$, via the pentose shunt (p. 8), thereby leading to an increase in fatty acid synthesis, a process which requires adequate supplies of $NADPH_2$. Triglyceride synthesis in liver and adipose tissue is increased on insulin administration and the rate of release of fatty acids from adipose tissue is decreased. These factors lead to a decrease in ketone body formation (p. 12).

The reverse situations occur in insulin deficiency, including an increased synthesis of cholesterol resulting from the increased availability of 2-carbon fragments (p. 10).

Adrenocortical Hormones. The glucocorticoids tend to increase the rate of release of fatty acids from adipose tissue. If at the same time there is a deficiency of insulin or impaired carbohydrate metabolism, an increase in ketone body formation and synthesis of cholesterol and fatty acid-containing lipids may result because of the increased availability of 2-carbon fragments (see above).

Anterior Pituitary Hormones. ACTH increases the release of fatty acids from adipose tissue, also leading to increased ketone body formation (see above).

Epinephrine. Epinephrine, in the presence of adrenocortical and thyroid hormones, also increases mobilization of fatty acids from adipose tissue, thereby leading to increased ketogenesis (see above).

Thyroid Hormone. Thyroid hormone tends to cause a decrease in plasma cholesterol and other lipids. However, in conjunction with impaired carbohydrate metabolism or an inadequate insulin supply, fatty acid mobilization from adipose tissue is increased, again leading to increased ketogenesis (see above).

SUMMARY OF LIPID METABOLISM AND ITS RELATIONSHIP TO CARBOHYDRATE METABOLISM

A simplified summary of lipid metabolism is outlined in Figure 1-10, and Figure 1-11 shows the general relationships between lipid and carbohydrate metabolism.

A few important points should be noted here. Although the metabolic flow is usually from carbohydrate to lipid in both glycerol and fatty acid moieties, lipids can contribute to carbohydrate metabolism in a net sense only by way of glycerol. Glycerol can shuttle up and back between the carbohydrate and lipid metabolic pathways in a reversible manner but fatty acids are synthesized from acetyl-CoA units arising from the oxidative decarboxylation of pyruvate (p. 8), an irreversible reaction.

A key branching point in the metabolic pathways occurs at the acetyl-CoA stage. As noted several times before, there is a delicate balance between the rate of carbohydrate metabolism and the synthesis or mobilization of fatty acids for oxidation, all these processes depending on or contributing to the rate of production and utilization of acetyl-CoA. An imbalance in these processes often results in an increase in ketone body formation and accompanying problems (see hormonal effects on this page and diabetes mellitus, p. 10).

Protein metabolism, which will be discussed later, provides the intermediates for the formation of the nitrogen bases—ethanolamine, choline, and serine—which are used in the synthesis of phospholipids.

PROTEIN METABOLISM

The concept of the dynamic nature of intermediary metabolism was first proposed after investigations on protein metabolism. Both stable and radioactive isotopes were used in these experiments which traced the actual chemical reactions undergone by protein metabolites. It quickly became obvious that an equilibrium existed between dietary intake and synthetic and catabolic processes, by way of metabolic pools, with body constituents being replaced constantly and relatively rapidly. Such a general scheme for protein metabolism is shown. These concepts of intermediary metabolism were rapidly extended to studies concerned with all other types of metabolites.

$$\text{Dietary Protein} \xrightarrow[\text{Absorption}]{\text{Digestion}} \text{Amino Acid Pool} \xrightarrow[\text{Catabolism}]{\text{Anabolism}} \text{Body Protein}$$

$$\text{Amino Acid Pool} \xrightarrow{\text{Catabolism}} NH_3 \rightarrow \text{Urea}$$

$$\text{Body Protein} \xrightarrow{\text{Catabolism}} \text{Carbon Skeleton} \rightarrow CO_2, H_2O$$

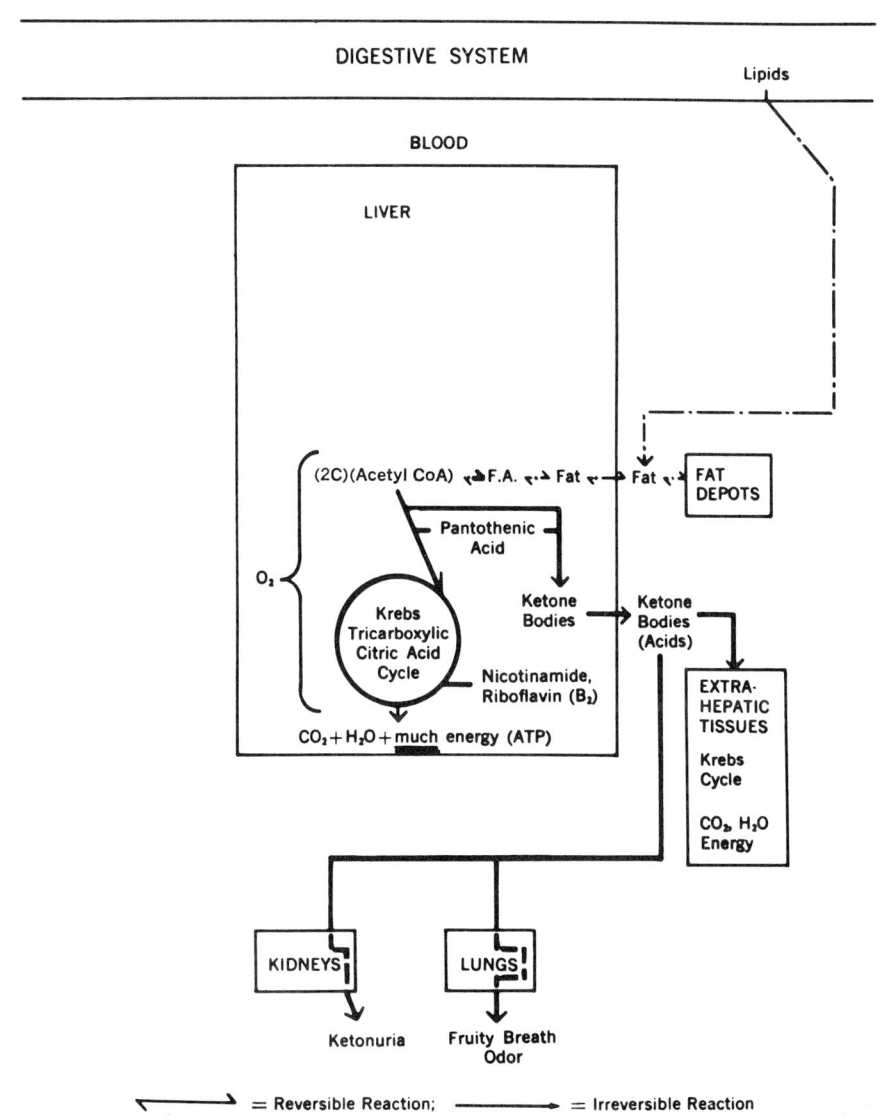

Figure 1-10 Flow chart of lipid metabolism. (Pathways: —·—·— = lipid; ——— = common.) (From Toporek: Basic Chemistry of Life, 1968. Courtesy of Appleton-Century-Crofts, Inc.)

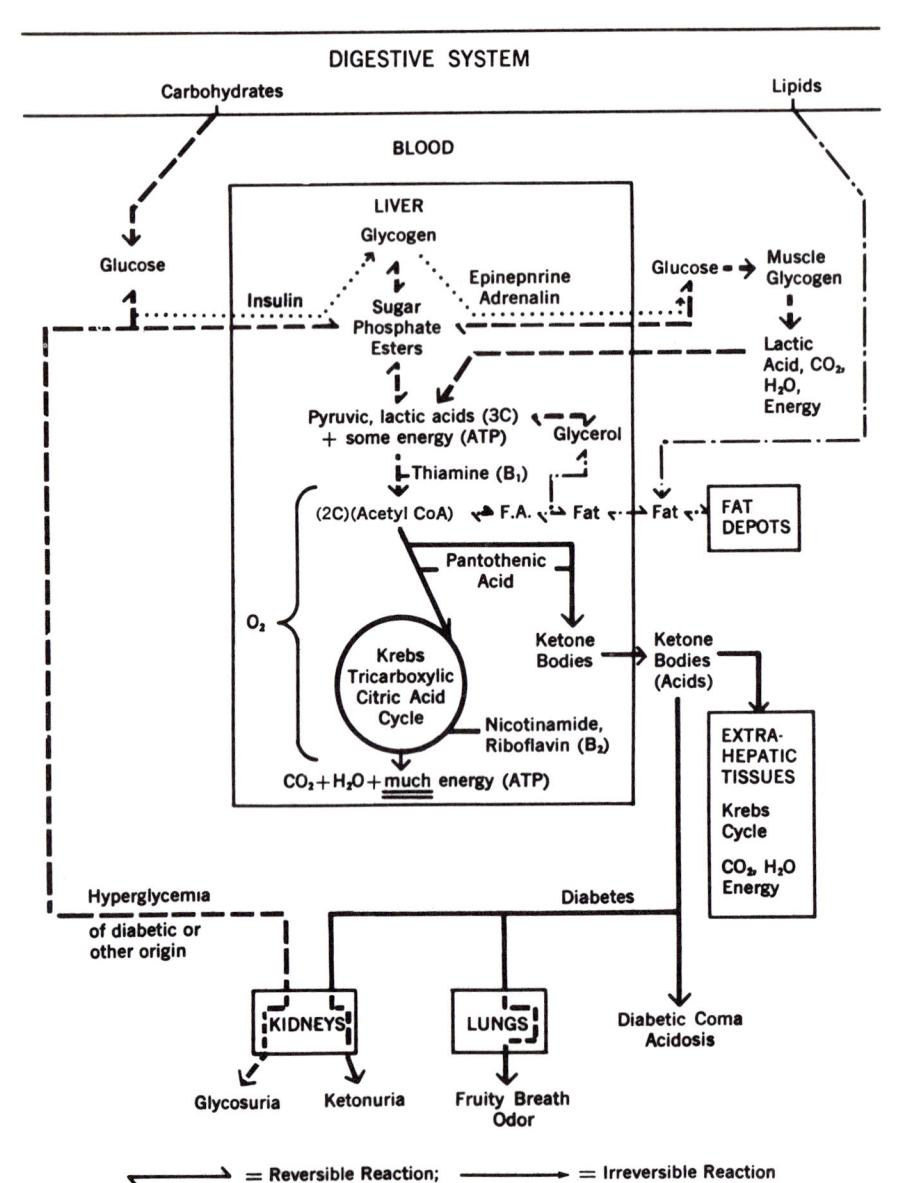

Figure 1-11 Flow chart showing interrelationships of carbohydrate and lipid metabolism. (Pathways: ---- = carbohydrate; —·—·— = lipid; ——— = common.) (From Toporek: Basic Chemistry of Life, 1968. Courtesy of Appleton-Century-Crofts, Inc.)

Protein Synthesis

The key chemical reaction in protein synthesis is the formation of the peptide bond, for which the net reaction may be written as follows:

In addition to amino acids, protein synthesis requires the concerted action of ribosomes, messenger RNA (mRNA), transfer RNA (tRNA), and supporting factors such as amino acid activating

$$R_1-\underset{\underset{NH_2}{|}}{CH}-COOH + R_2-\underset{\underset{NH_2}{|}}{CH}-COOH \longrightarrow R_1-\underset{\underset{NH_2}{|}}{CH}-\underset{\underset{\text{Peptide bond}}{\underbrace{\overset{O}{\overset{\|}{C}}-NH}}}-\underset{\underset{R_2}{|}}{CH}-COOH + H_2O$$

enzymes (aminoacyl-tRNA synthetases) and initiating, transfer, and terminating factors.

Figure 1-12 presents in simplified form the generally accepted mechanism for cytoplasmic protein synthesis. The information required to produce proteins of specified composition is derived from DNA. In the upper part of Figure 1-12, representing the nucleus, an mRNA molecule is being synthesized on a DNA template by a process known as transcription. The important feature of this process is the complementary base-pairing which occurs, e.g., wherever a guanine (G) appears on the DNA template, a cytosine (C) must take its place on the growing mRNA molecule in a position facing the G on the DNA template. The possible base pairs are listed below:

DNA Template	*mRNA Molecule*
Guanine (G)	Cytosine (C)
Cytosine (C)	Guanine (G)
Adenine (A)	Uracil (U)
Thymine (T)	Adenine (A)

In this way, the information related to the specific order of bases in the DNA template is preserved in the transcribed mRNA molecule. The mRNA molecule then moves to the cytoplasm, where, in association with the ribosome, it becomes the site of protein synthesis.

An input of energy is required for the formation of the peptide bond. This occurs in a synthetase reaction in which an amino acid is said to be activated. Using glycine as an example, the reaction occurs as shown in the middle of Figure 1-12.

The aminoacyl portion of the complex formed in this reaction is then transferred to the —C—C—A end of an appropriate tRNA molecule, as shown in Figure 1-12, the glycine synthetase being regenerated and ready for further use. The tRNA molecules are presumably synthesized in a manner analogous to the process described for the synthesis of mRNA molecules, i.e., on the basis of information derived from DNA.

In the next stage (the lower portion of Figure 1-12), the tRNA carrying the glycine residue must position itself in the proper place on the mRNA. This is accomplished on the basis of a trinucleotide codon (codeword) system, i.e., a specific sequence of three nucleotides specifies the amino acid required in a certain position. Therefore, a portion of the tRNA molecule must have in its structure an anticodon (complementary) sequence which will recognize the codon sequence on the mRNA molecule. Then under the guidance of initiating, transferring, and terminating factors, the peptide chain is synthesized from the free amino end toward the carboxyl end as the ribosome travels along the mRNA molecule. This process is known as translation. Evidence now indicates that interactions among amino acids grouped in a specific sequence is sufficient to allow the completed peptide molecule to assume its final, characteristic, three-dimensional shape.

As noted with several examples on Figure 1-12, there are antibiotics and analogues available which interfere with the process of protein synthesis at specific points. These substances may be used in two ways: (1) to investigate ever more critically the processes involved in protein synthesis, and (2) to interfere with protein synthesis, hopefully on a differential basis, in certain clinical conditions such as tumor growth or leukemia.

Breakdown of Proteins

Enzymes known as cathepsins are believed to be responsible for the intracellular breakdown of proteins. There is a constant breakdown and renewal of tissue proteins, the two processes being approximately at equilibrium in the adult under normal conditions. The final disposition of the amino acids resulting from protein breakdown will be discussed below.

Protein Turnover

High rates of protein turnover are usually associated with high metabolic rates in such tissues as liver, kidney, and intestinal mucosa. Lower rates of turnover are found in tissues such as muscle, brain, and skin. Listed below are some representative turnover rates in man:

Protein	*Half-Life (Days)*
Whole body	80
Liver	10
Serum albumin	15–25
Muscle	180

Hormonal Effects on Protein Metabolism

Growth Hormone and Testosterone. Growth hormone and testosterone exert a protein anabolic effect, i.e., a net increase in deposition of proteins in the tissues.

$$\text{Glycine synthetase} + \text{Glycine} + \text{ATP} \rightleftharpoons \text{Gly-AMP-Synthetase}_{\text{Gly}}$$
$$\text{PP}$$

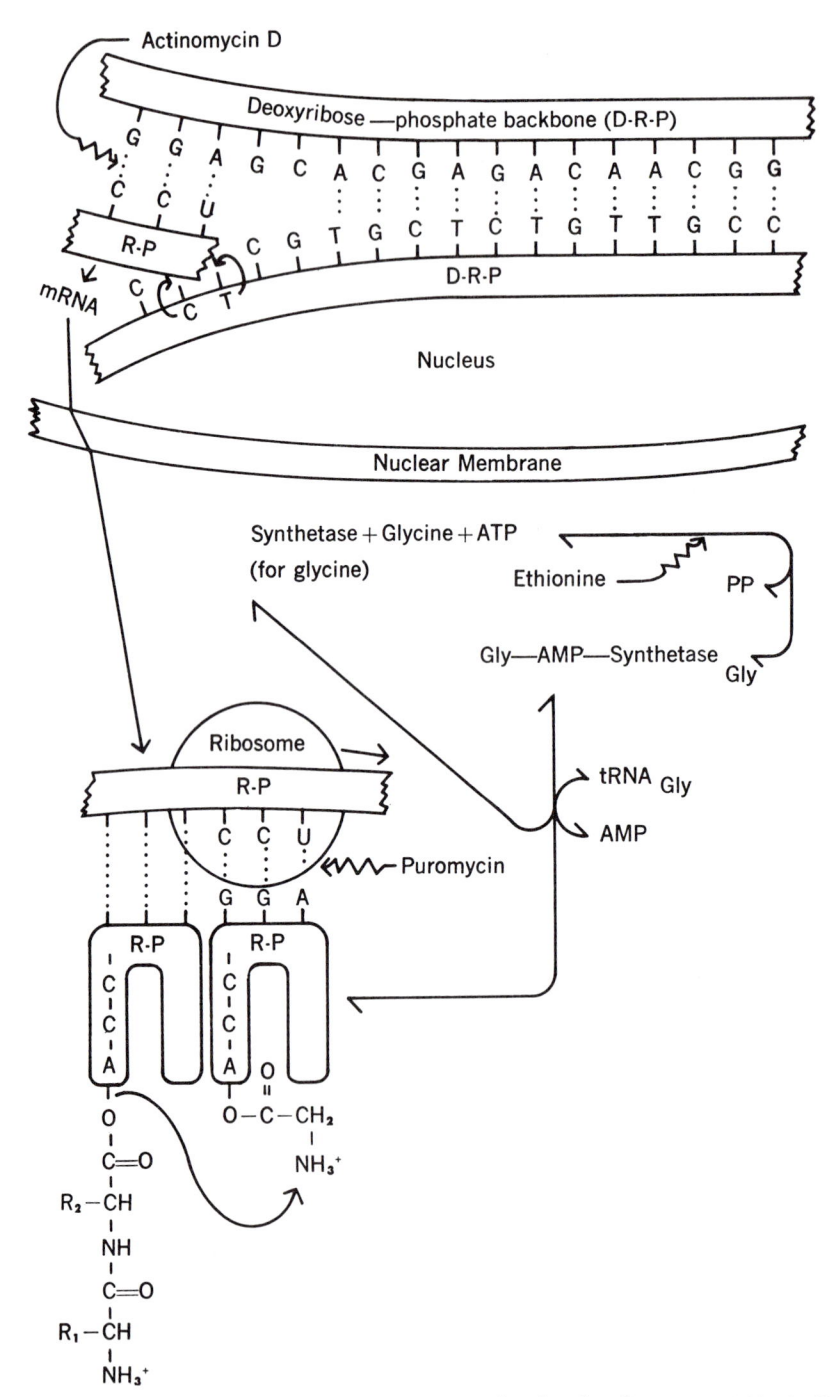

Figure 1-12 Proposed mechanism of protein synthesis (⌐⌙⌙⌙→ = inhibition). (From Toporek: Basic Chemistry of Life, 1968. Courtesy of Appleton-Century-Crofts, Inc.)

$$\underset{R_1-CH-COOH}{\overset{NH_2}{|}} + \underset{R_2-C-COOH}{\overset{O}{\|}} \underset{\text{Pyridoxal phosphate}}{\overset{\text{Transaminase}}{\rightleftharpoons}} \underset{R_1-C-COOH}{\overset{O}{\|}} + \underset{R_2-CH-COOH}{\overset{NH_2}{|}}$$

Insulin. Insulin appears to increase the rate of entry of amino acids into cells and subsequently incorporation into proteins by stimulating the synthesis of mRNA. The protein anabolic effect of growth hormone requires the presence of insulin.

Glucocorticoids. Because of their effect in increasing gluconeogenesis, i.e., conversion of amino acids to carbohydrates, the glucocorticoids tend to cause a negative nitrogen balance.

Thyroid Hormone. Administration of thyroid hormone doses in the physiologic range has a protein anabolic effect, but large doses have been found to exert a protein catabolic effect.

Metabolism of Amino Acids

A complete presentation of the metabolism of each amino acid is beyond the scope of this section. Instead, the general metabolic reactions undergone by most of the amino acids will be reviewed briefly, including some selected examples of clinical conditions directly related to derangements in amino acid metabolism.

Disposition of the Nitrogen

OXIDATIVE DEAMINATION. The oxidative deamination of most L-amino acids is catalyzed by L-amino acid oxidase:

$$\underset{R-CH-COOH}{\overset{NH_2}{|}} \xrightarrow{\text{Oxidase}} \underset{R-C-COOH}{\overset{O}{\|}} + NH_3$$

Further disposition of the α-keto acid and the ammonia will be discussed below.

TRANSAMINATION. Transamination is a reaction in which an amino group is transferred from one amino acid to an α-keto acid, forming a new amino acid and a new α-keto acid. Pyridoxal phosphate is required as a coenzyme, the ammonia does not appear free at any time, and the reaction is readily reversible (see formula above). These are very active metabolic reactions, specific transaminase reactions being quantitatively more prevalent in certain tissues. Should tissue injury occur, the transaminases may find their way into the blood, where their concentration may be measured. Thus, in cases of damage to heart tissue, the amount of serum glutamic-oxaloacetic transaminase (SGOT) may rise to high levels, whereas damage to liver tissue may result in high serum levels of glutamic-pyruvic transaminase. Determination of these enzyme levels may therefore be of help in diagnosing certain clinical conditions.

SYNTHESIS OF PURINES, PYRIMIDINES, AND AMINO ACIDS. The ammonia arising from deamination of amino acids (see above) may be used for the synthesis of purines and pyrimidines, important constituents of the nucleic acids, DNA and RNA. Ammonia may also be used in the formation of amino acids by the reductive amination of α-keto acids, which arise from carbohydrate metabolism:

$$\underset{R-C-COOH}{\overset{O}{\|}} \xrightarrow{NH_3} \underset{R-CH-COOH}{\overset{NH_2}{|}}$$

DETOXIFICATION OF AMMONIA: GLUTAMINE FORMATION. Since free ammonia is toxic to cells, it must be removed or somehow detoxified. Glutamine formation from glutamic acid is one detoxification process (see formula below). The glutamine, formed largely in the liver, is carried in the blood to the kidney, where it is hydrolyzed and the regenerated ammonia is excreted. Hepatic coma may result if the load of ammonia presented to the liver is excessive or if the metabolic functions of the liver fail or are interfered with.

EXCRETION AS AMMONIA. Ammonia may be excreted directly into the urine if amino acids are deaminated in the kidneys.

UREA FORMATION: ORNITHINE CYCLE. Ammonia and carbon dioxide are converted to urea, the major nitrogenous waste product of protein catabolism, by way of a series of reactions known as the ornithine cycle. These reactions are shown in Figure 1–13. Since all the reactions in the cycle take place on the carbon atom farthest from

$$\underset{\text{Glutamic acid}}{\overset{O}{\|}\atop{HO-C-CH_2CH_2-\overset{NH_2}{\underset{|}{C}H}-COOH}} \xrightarrow[NH_3 \quad H_3PO_4]{ATP \quad ADP} \underset{\text{Glutamine}}{\overset{O}{\|}\atop{H_2N-C-CH_2CH_2-\overset{NH_2}{\underset{|}{C}H}-COOH}} + H_2O$$

the carboxyl group of ornithine, the 5-carbon chain structure of ornithine, which remains untouched, is referred to as the R group in the diagram. The liver appears to be the sole site of formation of urea. Clinical conditions directly related to deficiencies of each of the enzymes involved in the conversion of NH_3 and CO_2 to urea have been recognized and are listed below:

Condition	Deficient Enzyme
Hyperammonemia II	Carbamoyl phosphate synthetase
Hyperammonemia I	Ornithine transcarbamylase
Citrullinemia	Argininosuccinic acid synthetase
Argininosuccinic-aciduria	Argininosuccinase
Argininemia	Arginase

EXCRETION AS CREATININE. Creatinine is one of the end products of muscle metabolism and is excreted in a rather constant daily amount by a given individual, apparently because of its direct relationship to the muscle mass.

Disposition of the Carbon Skeleton

SYNTHESIS OF AMINO ACIDS. As noted above, α-keto acids may be reductively aminated to form amino acids.

GLUCONEOGENESIS: FORMATION OF CARBOHYDRATE INTERMEDIATES. Some of the α-keto acids formed by transaminations involving amino acids may enter carbohydrate pathways. These amino acids are said to be glucogenic, e.g., alanine ⟶ pyruvate ⟶ glucose. Gluconeogenesis requires pyridoxal phosphate as a coenzyme and is reversible for the nonessential amino acids but not for the essential amino acids.

FORMATION OF KETONE BODIES. Amino acids which give rise to ketone bodies are known as ketogenic amino acids. Included in this group are leucine, isoleucine, phenylalanine, and tyrosine. Only leucine is exclusively ketogenic, the others being glucogenic as well.

ENERGY ACCOUNTING FOR AMINO ACID OXIDATION. Taking glutamic acid as an example, and assuming that the nitrogen is excreted as urea while the carbon skeleton is oxidized to CO_2 and H_2O via the tricarboxylic acid cycle, one mole of glutamic acid would give a maximum of 490,000 calories. Since 191,000 calories are conserved in the form of ATP, this represents an efficiency of 39 per cent, which is similar to that achieved in carbohydrate and fatty acid oxidations.

Disposition of Sulfur

FORMATION OF SULFATE. The sulfur that occurs in the amino acids cystine and methionine is eventually oxidized to sulfate, which is excreted in the urine mainly as inorganic sulfate. Cystinuria occurs when the ability of the kidney to reabsorb cystine is impaired as the result of an inborn error of metabolism.

Clinical Problems Related to Amino Acid Metabolism. In this section only, several examples of metabolic problems encountered in individual amino acid pathways will be reviewed briefly.

PHENYLKETONURIA. One of the normal metabolic pathways open to phenylalanine is its conversion to tyrosine. This reaction involves a specific hydroxylase, a less specific second enzyme, oxygen, Fe^{++}, $NADPH_2$, and a pteridine-like cofactor. In individuals with phenylketonuria, the specific hydroxylase is missing, thus leading to the excretion in the urine of excessive amounts of phenylalanine and its conversion products, mainly phenylpyruvate. One or more of these substances are toxic, especially in infants, when present in high concentrations in the blood, and brain damage occurs unless the condition is detected very early and adequate steps are taken, usually dietary, to lower the blood concentration of phenylalanine and its derivatives.

ALKAPTONURIA. Homogentisic acid is an intermediate along the catabolic pathway for tyrosine. In some individuals the enzyme homogentisic acid oxidase is missing, thus interrupting the further catabolism of tyrosine and allowing the buildup of higher concentrations of homogentisic acid, which is excreted in the urine. The urine darkens if left standing for some time. Phenylalanine is also involved by way of its normal conversion to tyrosine.

MAPLE SYRUP DISEASE. This condition involves the branched-chain amino acids, valine, leucine, and isoleucine, all of which are catabolized in similar pathways. The deficient enzyme in this case is the one required to oxidatively decarboxylate the α-keto acids resulting from transamination of the branched-chain amino acids. As usual, this leads to accumulation of the parent compounds and the α-keto acids in the blood and subsequently in the urine, where these compounds and possibly their decomposition products give rise to the maple syrup odor which gives this condition its name.

SUMMARY OF PROTEIN METABOLISM AND RELATIONSHIP OF PROTEIN TO CARBOHYDRATE AND LIPID METABOLISM

A simplified summary of protein and amino acid metabolism is presented in Figure 1–14.

Figure 1–15 is a flow diagram incorporating the more important aspects of metabolic biochemistry, involving relationships between protein, carbohydrate, and lipid pathways.

The major branching or transfer point is at the pyruvate stage. All the pathways are probably operating to some extent at the same time, the net metabolic flow being determined by the state

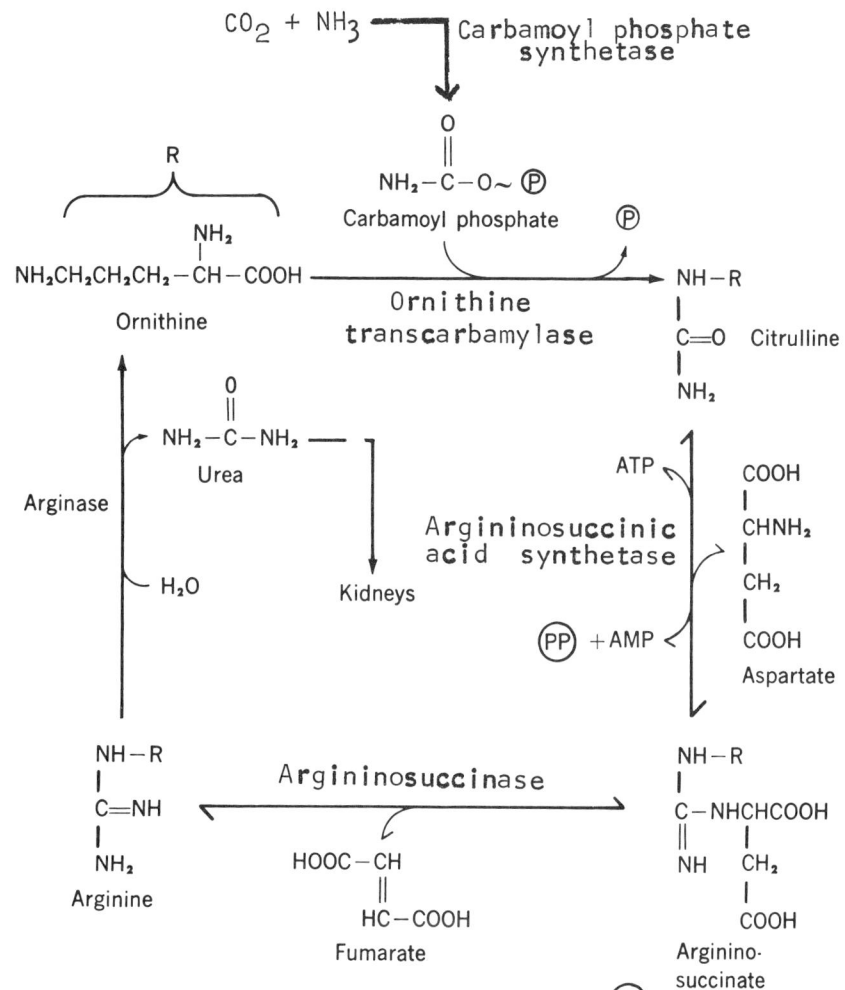

Figure 1-13 Production of urea via the ornithine cycle. (Ⓟ = phosphate; ⓅⓅ = pyrophosphate.) (Adapted from Toporek: Basic Chemistry of Life, 1968. Courtesy of Appleton-Century-Crofts, Inc.)

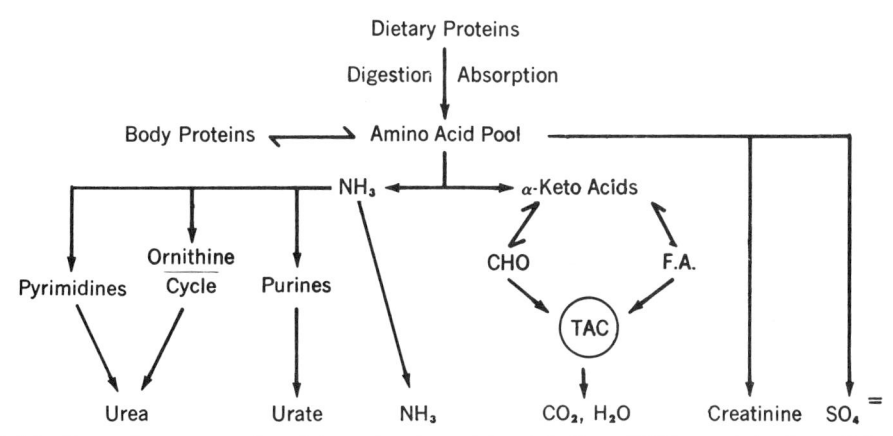

Figure 1-14 General summary of protein and amino acid metabolism. (CHO = carbohydrate; F.A. = fatty acid; TAC = tricarboxylic acid cycle.) (From Toporek: Basic Chemistry of Life, 1968. Courtesy of Appleton-Century-Crofts, Inc.)

Figure 1-15 Flow chart summarizing interrelationships of carbohydrate, lipid, and protein metabolism. (Pathways: — — — — = carbohydrate; — · — · — = lipid; ▬▬▬ = protein; ——— = common.) (From Toporek: Basic Chemistry of Life, 1968. Courtesy of Appleton-Century-Crofts, Inc.)

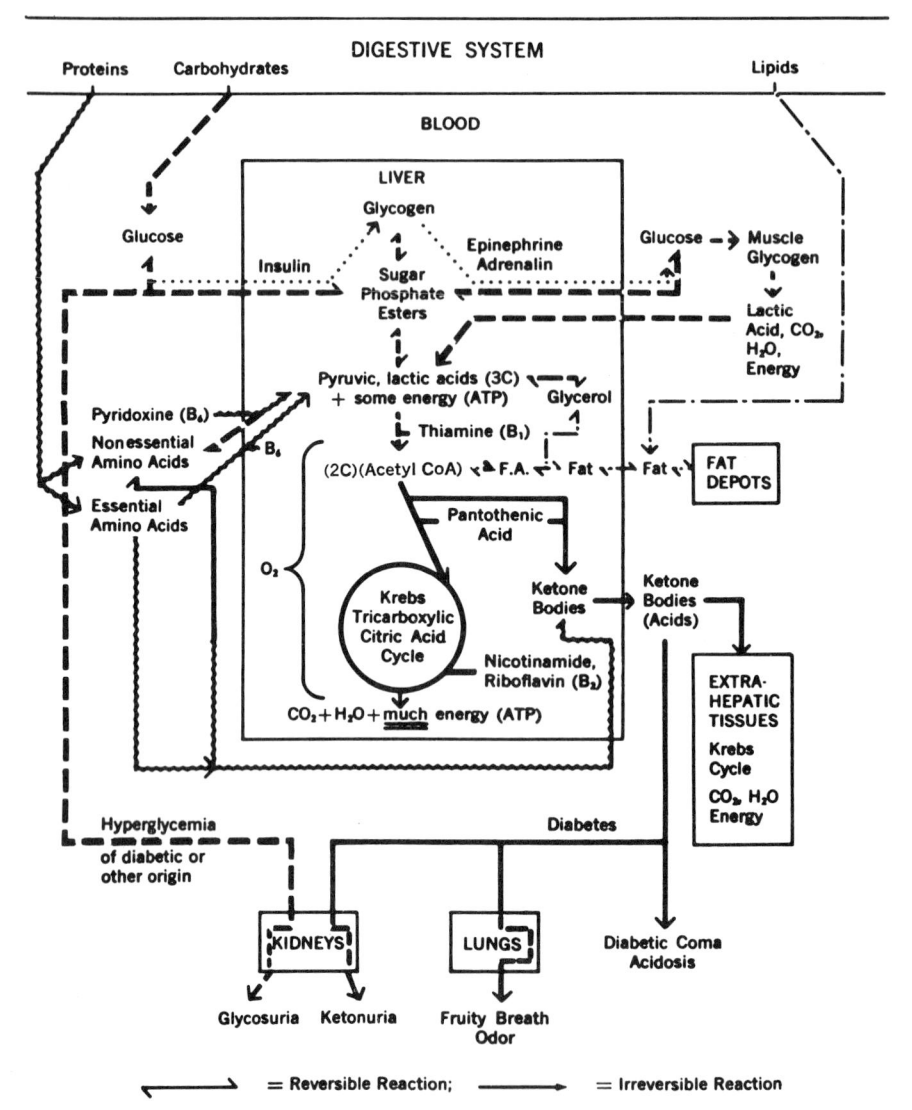

and requirements of the body at a particular time and under the guidance of a sensitive, finely tuned system of coordination and controls. It is at times of stress, when deviations from the normal occur, that the efficiency of this complicated metabolic machinery is truly appreciated, for it is not always a simple task, nor is it always possible, to get things back on the right track.

REFERENCES

Bittar, E. E., and Bittar, N.: The Biological Basis of Medicine. Vols. 1 to 6. New York, Academic Press, 1968–1969.

Cantarow, A., and Schepartz, B.: Biochemistry. 4th ed. Philadelphia, W. B. Saunders Co., 1967.

Goodman, R. M.: Genetic Disorders of Man. Boston, Little, Brown and Co., 1970.

Kaldor, G.: Physiological Chemistry of Proteins and Nucleic Acids in Mammals. Philadelphia, W. B. Saunders Co., 1969.

Lehninger, A. L.: Biochemistry. New York, Worth Publishers, Inc., 1970.

Levine, R., and Luft, R.: Advances in Metabolic Disorders. New York, Academic Press, series starting in 1964.

Masoro, E. J.: Physiological Chemistry of Lipids in Mammals. Philadelphia, W. B. Saunders Co., 1968.

McGilvery, R. W.: Biochemistry. Philadelphia, W. B. Saunders Co., 1970.

CHAPTER 2 MOLECULAR BIOLOGY

K. LEMONE YIELDING

INTRODUCTION

The contemporary understanding of the chemistry of biological processes now makes it possible to consider human diseases and their management in terms of molecular derangements. For some years interests in molecular disease were concerned with the description of examples of genetically determined molecular defects such as hemoglobinopathies, enzyme deficiencies, storage diseases, and the like; but now the whole array of biological processes involved in human diseases and their treatment should come into focus. These include, of course, all aspects of the function of the human organism as well as those for the variety of parasites which impose their effects.

A major insight into biological processes derives from the realization that they are straightforward chemical processes governed by conventional thermodynamic and kinetic rules. Any process can occur spontaneously only if it is accompanied by a decrease in "free energy" of the system and may be driven either through an increase in entropy (paraphrased as "disorder") or a decrease in enthalpy ("heat" or "work" energy). Such considerations involve the *total* system—for example, solvent effects are extremely important in biosystems because of the large entropy effects which are possible from the ordering and disordering of the structure of liquid water at temperatures of living systems. While thermodynamic considerations govern whether a reaction *can* occur, kinetics are concerned with route, rate, and, therefore, probability of occurrence. Thus, a cell accomplishes its chemistry through a decrease in free energy of the system as in any process which occurs spontaneously, and its total economy requires that it capture energy from the environment for survival. Individual "uphill" (thermodynamically unfavorable) reactions are promoted only by tight "coupling" with reactions which are highly favored—a form of energy transduction which permits the cell to perform a large variety of rather unexpected chemical transformations. Kinetically, two general points are important. First, biological processes consist of many complicated and interrelated steady state systems or pathways, with slow and fast steps to provide rate limiting control points. Predictably a simple perturbation in one system (e.g., an enzyme deficiency or a simple toxic effect) may be amplified into a variety of biological results. The second point is that reactions are catalyzed by enzymes which provide reaction acceleration as great as 10^{12} times and extraordinarily sensitive and effective regulation mechanisms. Biological processes are also compartmentalized and organized by the variety of discriminating boundaries which exist internally between cell organelles and externally between cells and the environment. Thus, a cell is a highly organized structure which conducts a variety of chemical reactions in a manner appropriate to maintain its own structure and internal steady state in relation to a changeable environment. Moreover, the cell must carry the complete mechanisms for self-assembly and self-replication.

The remarkable features of living cells depend largely on the complex structures and interactions of macromolecules which not only account for the precise structural and boundary characteristics of cells and the various effector roles served (catalysis, transport, energy transduction, and so on) but also provide the essential information content, communication, and regulation. It is the structure-function relationships of these "informational" macromolecules on which molecular biology is focused. While the study of model systems and simple organisms has provided the major progress in this understanding, the study of molecular diseases by pointing up specific molecular defects also serves in a reciprocal way to enhance our fundamental knowledge. The basic questions to be asked, then, are

1. What molecules and molecular arrangements account for the unique structural and functional features of biological systems?
2. How are these complex structures and functions regulated?
3. How may disease result from changes in molecular structure and regulation?
4. How may understanding of molecular processes result in rational approaches to therapy?

STRUCTURE OF INFORMATIONAL MACROMOLECULES

Nucleic Acids

The roles of nucleic acids in providing the stable storage form for information in cells as well as the templating mechanisms for information readout (transcription, translation, replication, reverse transcription, repair) are well known and need not be discussed in great detail here. These macromolecules illustrate one of the basic premises of molecular biology, i.e., that knowledge of molecular structure can lead to an understanding of function. The double-helical structure of DNA deduced by Watson-Crick led to confirmation of the two-dimensional readout nature of cellular information storage and retrieval, to an understanding of the stable nature of and replicative mechanism for the information system, and to a precise understanding of the chemical nature of genetic variability and mutations. The structures of DNA and RNA, paraphrased in Figure 2–1, result in several predictable properties for these molecules. The chemical natures and specific interactions of the purine and pyrimidine bases of nucleic acids and their sequential arrangement provide the information coding mechanism. These specific reactive properties of the bases also account for the modifications known to impair or change function. For example, the bases are susceptible to modification by alkylating drugs, formation of various adducts, simple chemical cleavage of the glycosidic bond, or modification by absorption of radiant energy. Their specific functions and interactions may also be disrupted by binding of various aromatic heterocyclic drugs which show avidity for ordered sequences of purines and pyrimidines. This is particularly true for binding to the "core" of purine and pyrimidine base pairs in double-stranded DNA. The polyanionic backbone of the nucleic acid is also important in binding and, because of its repetitive character, encourages cooperativeness in binding. Thus, polycations such as basic proteins and certain drugs and antibiotics may bind tightly either to the charged backbone alone or to both the backbone and the purine and pyrimidine bases. Table 2–1 summarizes various agents known to bind and modify nucleic acids.

In addition to their common features, DNA and RNA also show several important differences. First, there is a single copy of DNA made for each chromosome at each cell replication, whereas RNA may be synthesized in multiple copies. Second, DNA is much larger in size and represents a larger "target" for various insults. Both these factors combine with the critical role of DNA to make the cell particularly vulnerable to DNA damage. Third, the deoxysugar and thymine are unique to DNA and represent specific loci where DNA synthesis can be regulated, a point of considerable importance to chemotherapy. At the same time, the deoxysugar makes the DNA backbone more stable chemically by protecting it against alkaline hydrolysis. Its double-helical structure also lends stability, as well as providing a complementary strand for use in replication and repair. The large target size of DNA also accounts for the major lethal effects of ionizing radiation, whereas UV irradiation kills cells largely owing to the efficient and specific capture of radiant energy by the thymine in DNA, with formation of dimers and consequent disruption of its information role.

Based on the realization that the information responsible for a cell's characteristics is encoded in the sequence of DNA, it follows simply that a qualitative change in a DNA locus by removal, addition, or change in a nucleotide base information bit can result in a mutation or change in cell properties. Since the sum total of an organism's properties depends also on the dynamic interplay of all its systems, it is not surprising that normal information expression requires a correct quantitative balance between the different elements of expression, particularly in highly complex organisms which go through a precisely timed sequence of differentiation. When the genetic load is disrupted by a change in chromosomal number, gross errors in differentiation occur (for example, the various human abnormalities associated with the occurrence of extra chromosomes) (see Ch. 3). It is also noteworthy that changes in the information content of the cell can result from the imposition of external genetic material, such as that resulting from virus infections, which may simply disrupt cell functions or may cause heritable changes in cell properties such as neoplastic transformation.

The variety of steps involved in information storage and processing in nucleic acids is summarized in Figure 2–2. These processes are especially pertinent to biological regulation and can be exploited to explain disease processes or used for therapeutic applications. Sites for regulation are also indicated in Figure 2–2.

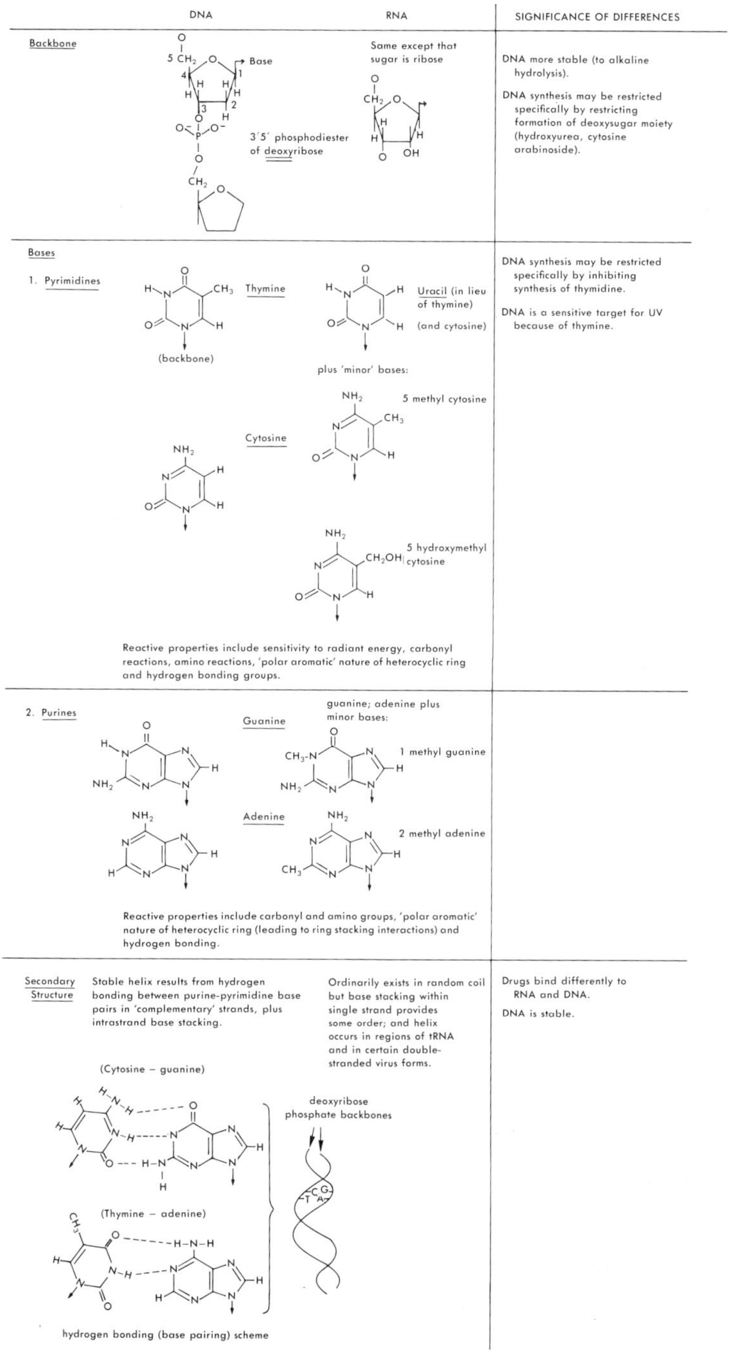

Figure 2-1 Diagram of primary and secondary aspects of DNA and RNA structure (with abbreviated structural formulas—Emphasis on 3D arrangement).

TABLE 2-1 INTERACTION OF CHEMICAL AGENTS WITH NUCLEIC ACIDS

Type of Interaction	Drug	Nucleic Acid Structural Site(s) Involved	Effects on DNA Properties and Function	Clinical Use
Covalent	Alkylating agents: nitrogen mustard, such antibiotics as mitomycin, etc.	Adds to N-7 position of guanine	Inhibits cell replication; also mutagenic	Cytotoxic agent
	Certain reactive aromatic hydrocarbons (fluorenylacetamide, for example)	Adds to N-8 position of guanine	Mutagenic, carcinogenic	
	Hydrazine and hydroxylamine	Reacts with C=O groups	Mutagenic	
	Nitrous acid	Reacts with NH_2 groups	Mutagenic	
Noncovalent	Polyamines (spermine, spermidine)	Backbone (PO_4)	Stabilizes	
	Basic proteins (histones)	Backbone (PO_4)	Stabilizes	
	Ions	Backbone, and polar groups of bases	Backbone binding stabilizes, base binding disrupts DNA helix	
	Hydrocarbons	Stacks with purine bases	Mutagenic, carcinogenic	
	Heterocyclic drugs and antibiotics			
	1. Actinomycin	Ring stacking and charge interaction with backbone (minor groove)	Inhibits RNA synthesis, and to a lesser extent DNA synthesis	Cytotoxic agent
	2. Streptomycin	Ribosomal RNA	Inhibits protein synthesis	Antibiotic
	3. Aminoquinoline antimalarial drugs	Ring stacking and charge interaction with backbone	Stabilizes DNA helix, inhibits DNA synthesis and repair; inhibits RNA synthesis poorly	Antiparasitic
	4. Acridines (including quinacrine)	Ring stacking and charge interaction with backbone	Same spectrum of action as aminoquinolines	Antiparasitic
	5. Furocoumarins	?	Photosensitivity	Vitiligo therapy

DNA replication is a tightly controlled and precisely ordered process in which each strand of double-helical DNA serves as a template for the synthesis of a new DNA strand for distribution to daughter cells. Each parent strand and its complementary newly synthesized strand are segregated into the daughter cells by a precise process of mitosis which distributes identical loads of genetic material to each cell. Uncontrolled and inappropriate replication and cell proliferation are obviously detrimental and provide the basis for disease. For example, the growth of neoplastic tissues, the proliferation of pannus in the joints in rheumatoid arthritis, keloid formation, and psoriasis may all represent excessive or inappropriate cell proliferation. Conversely, depression of the bone marrow and ulceration of the intestinal mucosa consequent to the administration of a variety of toxic drugs or in the course of radiation represent examples of inadequate replication and proliferation of cells.

An understanding of the specific structures and processes involved in replication also provides the rational basis for regulation. Thus, limitation of the synthesis of thymidine by folic acid antagonists and certain fraudulent nucleotides or inhibition of reductive formation of deoxyribose nucleotides by hydroxyurea or cytosine arabinoside restricts replication at the precursor level. The process of DNA copying by the DNA polymerase can be interfered with by a variety of drugs and antibiotics which interact with the DNA template, such as daunomycin, ethidium bromide, various antimalarials, mitomycin, nitrogen mustard, and to some extent actinomycin D. Subsequent to DNA synthesis the segregation process for the newly synthesized DNA in mitosis can be blocked by the administration of specific mitotic inhibitors such as vincristine or colchicine. At the present time it is not clear what the signal is in a cell for the start of DNA synthesis and cell division and no exploitation of this mech-

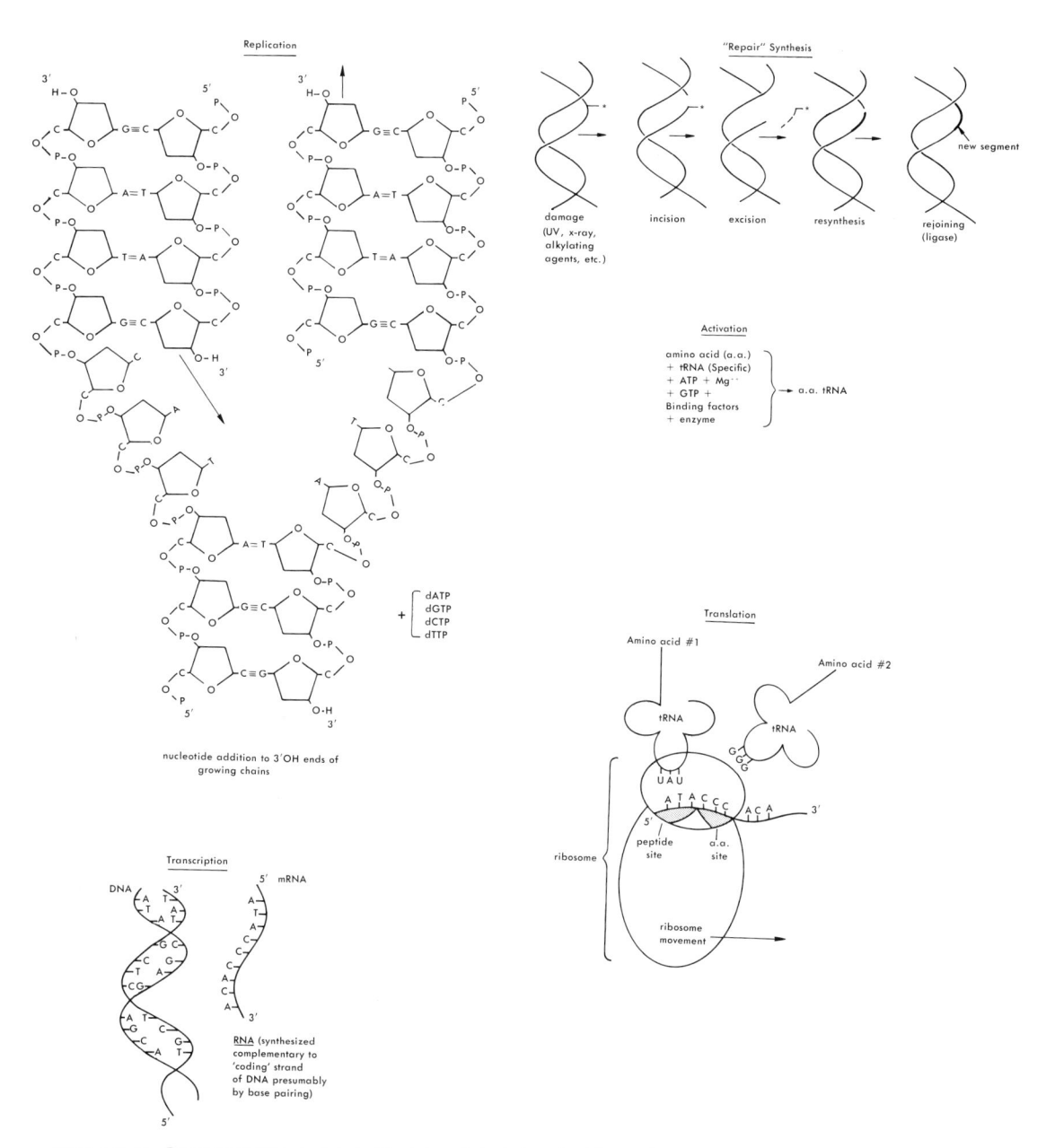

Figure 2-2 Diagrammatic sketch (with abbreviated chemical formula) to follow fate of DNA and RNA structure through replication, repair, transcription, and translation.

anism has been possible for therapeutic purposes. However, cells can be stimulated to divide in vitro by the administration of certain agents such as phytohemagglutinin and pokeweed mitogen, illustrating the potential for regulation at this locus.

Another type of DNA synthesis has been described during the past few years in which localized segments of DNA are excised and replaced to reverse the lethal and mutational effects of a variety of agents. This so-called *repair synthesis* reverses such insults as UV and x-ray irradiation, alkylating agents, and perhaps thermal damage. It appears to represent, therefore, an important homeostatic mechanism by which the cell preserves the integrity of its basic information system. The possibility also exists that this is the means by which the cell can undergo biological variations by modification of limited regions of DNA without the necessity for undergoing cell division. Predictably, disease can result from a defect in this repair system. Cleaver has shown that patients with *xeroderma pigmentosum* who show an extraordinary sensitivity to sunlight with frequent and extensive skin cancer are defective in their ability to repair UV damage to their skin cell DNA. The possible role in other precancerous lesions must also be questioned. This system may also be exploitable therapeutically for modifying the sensitivity of cancer cells to radiation and alkylating agents, since such therapy works by introducing lesions into cellular DNA which are repairable.

The orderly readout of stored information in the cell occurs through the processes of transcription (synthesis of a messenger RNA) followed by translation of this messenger into protein structure. Transcription represents the appropriate and timely templating of the information strand of the helical DNA into a single strand of messenger RNA which is the vector for cytoplasmic expression. Studies with model systems in simple organisms have revealed that transcription is a tightly controlled process in which messenger RNA is made appropriate to the needs of the cell. For each gene, transcription must start at a precise initiation point and continue in a sequential fashion to the end of the gene. The details of the control of this process in cells, particularly mammalian cells, are not yet worked out, but it is clear that the initiation process involves both negative and positive control factors and that more than one gene may be controlled coordinately, possibly because a single large messenger is transcribed for several genes (polycistronic messengers). Transcription may be repressed by the binding of some recognition molecule to the initiation region on DNA, so that it cannot occur unless an appropriate signal in the form of a small molecule interacts with this repressor to impede its binding. This permits small molecules to turn on transcription. In a similar fashion, small molecules may serve to turn off transcription in the event that the DNA binding repressor binds more tightly when it is bound to the small molecular signal. These processes of induction and repression are illustrated in Figure 2–3 and are essential to the understanding of enzyme induction and enzyme repression, both of which offer potential for exploitation in therapy.

Transcription offers three specific sites for regulation. First, induction and repression may be accomplished either by the use of the appropriate small molecular signal, usually a product for the gene action in question or a related system, or by the use of fraudulent small molecules which serve to mimic their action. Second, the templating function of DNA may be interfered with by the binding of specific agents such as actinomycin D that bind to the DNA template and prevent copying. Third, the action of the RNA polymerase itself may be blocked (in bacteria) by such agents as the antibiotic rifamycin.

The process of translation of the genetic message into protein structure is a complex sequence of events offering multiple points for potential regulation. The structures and stability of ribosomes, tRNA, or messenger may be modified; the availability of amino acids may be impaired; the growing protein chain may be displaced; or any one of the enzymic steps may be blocked (amino acid activation, peptide bond synthesis, and so on). A variety of antibiotics, such as streptomycin, chloramphenicol, puromycin, and cycloheximide, inhibit translation.

The action of interferon is particularly intriguing. These specific proteins are synthesized by mammalian cells in response to the presence of virus nucleic acids, and they appear to interfere specifically with the process of translation of virus messengers without interfering with host messenger. Since interferon production is host specific but not virus specific, it can be stimulated in host cells by the administration of synthetic polynucleotides as well as virus nucleic acids and represents a potential means of controlling virus infections. The role of hormones and various other biological regulators in modifying the process of translation is also under intensive investigation.

Information storage and processing are important keys, therefore, for the understanding and control of human diseases. It is especially significant that most of our present knowledge was acquired in a brief period of less than 20 years.

Proteins

Proteins constitute the work molecules for biological systems. They provide structural integrity and specificity, appropriate solution properties and barrier functions (buffers, and the like) as well as effector roles such as transport, energy

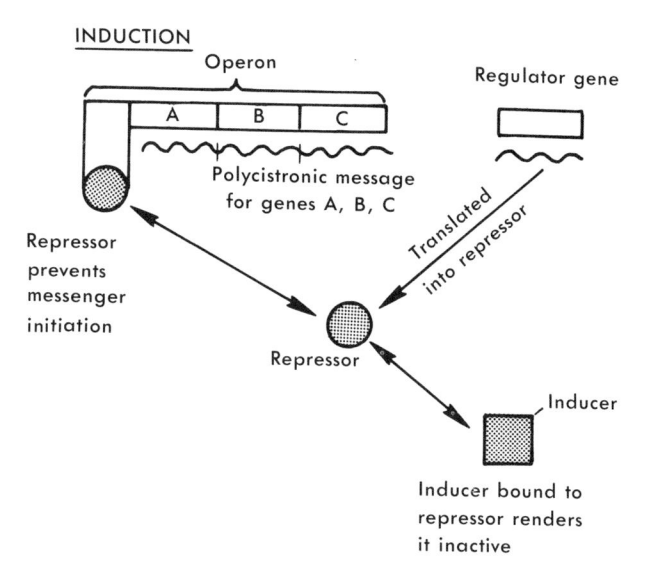

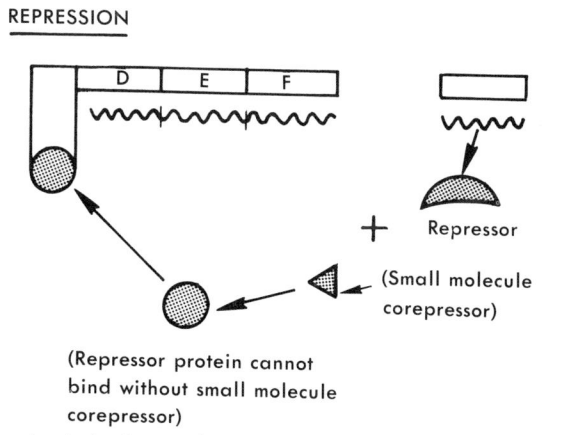

Figure 2-3 Model scheme for induction and repression of protein synthesis operating at the level of RNA transcription.

transduction, and catalysis. They are in the strictest sense informational molecules in that their unique three-dimensional structures provide the basis for all their discriminating interactions and functions. Proteins are especially well suited for biological diversity because of the endless number of structures which can be generated from sequences of the 20 amino acids available. The most important insight into protein structure and function is the recognition that the primary covalent sequence of amino acids dictates the most favorable secondary structure (hydrogen bonding between peptide bonds in the chain), and tertiary structure (interactions between amino acid side chains) based on the lowest (and most favorable) free energy state of the protein and its surrounding medium. Because of this important governing thermodynamic principle, the readout of two-dimensional information encoded in nucleic acids into a two-dimensional protein sequence is transformed into a unique three-dimensional structure. Furthermore, the association of this protein into aggregates (quaternary structure) or other more complicated macrostructures such as virus coats, ribosomes, membranes, and so on can also occur spontaneously according to the same simple principle. The role of water structure is a most important consideration. The so-called hydrophobic interactions of the amino acid side chains are the most important quantitatively in protein tertiary structure. Such interactions derive their stability from the fact that removal of hydrophobic groups from solution results in a considerable increase in entropy of the water. Protein denaturation and renaturation are governed by both thermodynamic and kinetic considerations. The protein, once formed, may be extremely stable even when the surrounding medium is changed, because the energy of activation for a structure transition is high owing to the combined effects of its many weak interactions or because of the imposition of covalent restraints in the form of the covalent disulfide bonds. Conversely, a protein may become quite labile or refuse to renature because of transport into an environment different from the site of synthesis or if a portion of the peptide backbone is removed. An example of the latter mechanism is insulin, for which proteolytic removal of a portion of the backbone of the precursor, proinsulin, prior to secretion removes its ability to renature following denaturation. Such proteolysis, in addition to providing biologically active structures at the time and site of need, also provides a limitation on their stability and turnover. Other pertinent examples are clotting factors, the complement system, digestive enzymes, and various kinins. In contrast, some of the effector and regulatory roles of proteins would require that structure transitions be rather freely reversible in the course of their function.

Individual amino acids in a protein chain may be viewed as serving two types of roles. First, they determine the unique structural features required for the discriminating functions of proteins, and, second, they provide the structural basis for interacting with the environment and determining protein structure and stability. Therefore, modifying a protein (for example, by genetic "error") may either interfere with its functional and regulatory capacity or change its structural stability or both. Defects in red blood cells provide excellent examples of these different defects. Sickle hemoglobin, because of a single amino acid change (glutamate → valine), shows a tertiary structure lability, so that although it can still bind O_2, its tertiary structure in the deoxygenated state is so distorted that it forces gross deformity of the red blood cells. A variety of other hemoglobin defects in contrast have a decreased capacity to bind O_2. Certain mutants for glucose-6-PO_4 dehydrogenase in the red cell show substantial changes in catalytic properties. This also illustrates an excellent example of the seemingly remote biological effects which may result from an enzyme deficiency due to perturbation of interrelated steady-state systems. The ultimate result of this enzyme deficiency is red blood cell fragility, apparently because the decreased reduction of NADP by glucose-6-PO_4 restricts availability of reduced glutathione for reduction of methemoglobin. Pyruvate kinase deficiency associated with hemolytic anemias appears to result from a defect in enzyme stability which is expressed as the cell ages. It may well be that some instances of apparent complete enzyme absence may instead represent highly labile though potentially active enzyme, a point of considerable therapeutic interest.

Certain toxic effects may also be explained on the basis of modifications of protein structure, in terms of either functional capacity or structural integrity. Thus, amino acid-specific reagents such as heavy metals and thiols which react with —SH groups in proteins, or reactive organophosphates which react with "active" serines in enzyme catalytic sites, would be expected to have extensive biological consequences. Modification of the protein environment can also be important in biological systems. Cryoglobulins, for example, precipitate as the temperature is lowered because of the change in water structure, which in turn promotes protein aggregation. Another physical effect on proteins results from their natural tendency to unfold at interfaces owing to their content of both hydrophobic and hydrophilic groups. This is an important concept to consider, for example, in the construction of heart-lung machines and prosthetic heart valves or arteries, or during the infusion into the blood of chemical agents in order to prevent denaturation of blood elements and resulting toxic effects.

Nonprotein moieties in proteins also deserve special consideration, since they impart important properties and functions for structural and effector proteins. The covalent attachment of carbohydrate (via serine, threonine, and arginine covalent bonds) provides special binding properties such as immunologic specificity, cell recognition, and perhaps aspects of cell communication related to regulation. The process of attachment of carbohydrate to proteins in the Golgi apparatus may also serve an important secretory role. Transport lipoproteins have attracted clinical attention since the recognition of specific diseases such as Tangier disease, in which abnormal lipid deposits in tissues result from deficient transport (for review, see Ch. 30). Lung surfactant is a lipoprotein which normally maintains the unique properties of the gas exchange surfaces of the lung and may provide major insight into understanding and treating lung disease. Lung surfactant appears to be lacking in hyaline membrane disease of the newborn and is a critical target for study in a variety of pulmonary diffusion difficulties (see Ch. 16). Lipoproteins also serve a variety of other functions such as the construction of membranes and cell organelles, and the lipid as well as the protein moieties provide extensive means of varying structure. The recent discovery of the many effects of prostaglandins has emphasized how potent lipid-protein interactions may also be in regulating biological systems. A variety of specific small prosthetic molecules, such as heme, pyridoxal, nucleotides, metals, and even PO_4, also provide regulatory and functional properties for catalytic and carrier proteins and illustrate one of the ways minor dietary substances can influence biological function.

The description and management of diseases in terms of deficiencies or abnormalities of proteins provide an interesting challenge to medical science, the approach to which will require thorough understanding of protein structure and function.

ASSEMBLY OF COMPLEX BIOLOGICAL STRUCTURES

The state of knowledge about macromolecules combined with the current sophistication of electron microscopy provides promising background information on such complex structures as cell membranes, cell organelles, and parasites. The principle of "self assembly" demonstrated for tertiary and quaternary structure of proteins, based on the structures of the component molecules, also operates for more complex systems, as shown by the reassembly in vitro of previously disrupted virus capsules, ribosomes, bacterial flagellae, and membrane components of animal cells.

Membranes

The discriminating barrier, transport, and regulatory functions of biological membranes are essential for the properties of living cells, and the structural basis for their functions is under intensive investigation. Membranes do not appear to be simple barriers but complex aggregates of macromolecules which show structural variability depending on functional requirements. Thus, a myelin sheath, while similar to the plasma membrane of a liver cell, will also display distinct chemical differences. The concept that a membrane in any site is a dynamic complex of individually synthesized macromolecules is important to the question of assembly, stability, turnover, and function, and the structures of the individual component molecules are of critical interest. The lipid bilayer has served as a useful experimental model for the structural features of a membrane, particularly because molecules may be intruded into its structure and serve there as the "catalytic" or "carrier" units. For example, simple models for ion transport by both carrier and channel mechanisms can be demonstrated using peptide antibiotics which bind specific ions. A wide variety of genetic defects in amino acid, sugar phosphate, and ion transport result from specific defects in membrane function. Similarly, membranes are clearly important end organs for the action of specific drugs and hormones, as well as for acute toxic diseases and more chronic processes such as demyelination or chronic renal disease. Unfortunately, our knowledge of membrane structure still does not allow mechanistic discussions, but this will be an area of active discovery in the next few years. Genetic diseases may again serve as important study systems to identify the biochemical basis for function in much the same way as in intermediary metabolism.

Cell Organelles

A detailed discussion of organelles is beyond the scope of this chapter, but a few cogent points should be made for ribosomes and mitochondria as examples of the potential of the molecular approach.

Ribosomes, complex aggregates of RNA and specific proteins, are the site of protein synthesis as outlined above and therefore are rate limiting for many biological processes. They display self-assembly from experimentally disrupted molecular components and are the site of action of several antibiotics and other drugs. Abnormal or "mutant" ribosomes occur in microorganisms but probably preclude survival in higher forms, although the possibility that they may provide disease mechanisms cannot be excluded. In animal cells, the endoplasmic reticulum to which the ribosomes are attached is also a major concentration of a variety of enzymes which serve such varied functions as drug metabolism and detoxification.

Mitochondria are complex organelles with extensive responsibility for metabolic and energy support of the cell. They consist of membranous structures into which are incorporated a variety of catalytic and structural macromolecules. In addition, mitochondria contain DNA and can account for the phenomenon of cytoplasmic inheritance, since they carry the information for synthesizing some of their own components. Mitochondria apparently are self-replicating structures but there is a complex interplay between them and the nucleus, since some of their components are also dictated by nuclear DNA and are synthesized in the cytoplasm. Their structure and self-assembly are further complicated by the fact that their stability varies considerably from tissue to tissue (half-life of 3 days in liver and 30 days in brain); moreover, their various components show different turnover rates. At least one disease appears to represent a defect in mitochondrial morphogenesis (central core myopathy), and experimentally the resistance of malaria to certain chemotherapeutic agents seems to bear an inverse relationship to frequency of mitochondrial bodies in the parasites.

Lysosomes are of special interest as examples of the important role of compartmentalization of biological function. These organelles contain a rather extensive variety of degradative enzymes and represent potential "suicide packages." On release, these enzymes are involved in digestion of phagocytosed or pinocytosed material, self-resorption in the event of cell death, and maintaining the normal steady-state concentrations of a variety of tissue components. It has been suggested that "storage diseases" can result from deficiencies of lysosomal function, and tissue disruption can occur from excessive lysosomal activation as might occur as a consequence of chemical toxicity.

MOLECULAR BASIS FOR BIOLOGICAL REGULATION

One of the most remarkable features of a living system is the precision with which its numerous chemical processes are integrated and regulated appropriately in response to signals from the environment. To this end, both simple and direct mechanisms exist as well as rather extensive and complex systems such as the endocrine glands. Based on an understanding of the structure and function of macromolecules and cell organelles these control phenomena may now be discussed in terms of molecular interactions. The result of perturbing a particular biochemical process depends on the nature of the process, what its role is in each system involved, whether it plays the rate-limiting role, and whether there are other compensating or amplifying mechanisms involved. It is also clearly important whether the perturbation is temporary or chronic.

Regulation of Protein Function

The effector roles of proteins plus the precise discrimination provided by protein binding sites make this class of macromolecules ideal for monitoring small molecular "signals" from the environment. The strength of such molecular signals (extent of binding) depends simply on their concentration in the milieu. The simplest type of regulation is through competition at the functional site (for example, at the catalytic site of an enzyme or transport site of a membrane) by fraudulent "substrates." Methotrexate, an analog of folic acid and a powerful inhibitor of dihydrofolate reductase, a rate-limiting enzyme for thymine (and therefore DNA) synthesis, is an example of such a competitive inhibitor which binds even tighter than the normal substrate. The search for useful competitive inhibitors is a straightforward process based simply on knowledge of substrate structure. For example, allopurinol was developed as a xanthine oxidase competitive inhibitor so that uric acid production could be reduced in gout. By blocking terminal formation of the highly insoluble uric acid, the much more soluble and excretable hypoxanthine becomes the terminal product. Fraudulent substrates also may be metabolized. For example, ingested glycols are oxidized to highly insoluble oxalic acid by alcohol dehydrogenase with catastrophic results, because the normal substrate is not available to saturate the enzyme. Similarly, drugs may compete at receptor sites for a natural "regulator" and either produce blockade of normal function or may themselves provoke a response. Table 2-2 lists several examples of well-known competitive inhibitors which have relevance to clinical medicine.

Many proteins also have specific sites, other than the effector or functional sites, which serve as sensors for monitoring the environment through binding a variety of specific regulatory substances. The consequence of such binding is a change in tertiary structure, with resulting change in functional properties. A regulator can thus serve to stimulate or inhibit a reaction and it need not bear any structural similarity to the substrate for the protein. This provides the molecular mechanism for appropriate regulation of a system by end product (feedback inhibition), cross-linked control between collateral systems, as well as hormonal and drug control. It also represents another type of macromolecular defect which could lead to disease, i.e., defective regula-

TABLE 2-2 EXAMPLES OF COMPETITIVE INHIBITORS

Drug	Enzyme or Receptor	Reaction or Natural Substrate Inhibited	Examples of Clinical Use
Neostigmine	Acetylcholinesterase	Acetylcholine	Myasthenia gravis; Glaucoma
Atropine	Parasympathetic nerve endings (cholinergic endings)	Acetylcholine	Parasympathetic blockade
Guanethidine	Adrenergic endings	Catecholamines	Hypertension
Methyldopa	Dopa decarboxylase	Dopa, 5—OH tryptophan	Hypertension
Ganglionic blocking drugs	Ganglionic receptor	Acetylcholine	Hypertension
Neuromuscular blocking agents (curare, etc., succinylcholine)	Neuromuscular junction	Acetylcholine	Anesthesia (muscle relaxation), spastic disorder
Antihistamine	"Histamine receptors"	Histamine	Allergy
Isocarboxazid (Marplan) Nialamide (Niamid) Phenelzine sulfate (Nardil) Tranylcypromine (Parnate)	Monoamine oxidase	Epinephrine, norepinephrine, dopa	Depressive disorders
Tetraethylthiuram disulfide (Antabuse)	Aldehyde dehydrogenase	NAD, acetaldehyde	Alcoholism
Ethanol	Alcohol dehydrogenase	Methanol→formaldehyde and glycol→oxalic acid by alcohol dehydrogenase	Methanol and glycol poisoning
Clomiphene	Estrogen receptor site	Estradiol	Infertility
Allopurinol	Xanthine oxidase	Xanthine, hypoxanthine	Gout

tor binding sites with resulting inadequate or inappropriate control. This regulation by binding at nonsubstrate sites has been discussed extensively as "allosteric" regulation. The additional fact that the enzymes thus regulated are usually composed of subunits also tends to promote cooperative binding of the regulator and substrate molecules with the result that the system may be very sensitive to small concentration changes over a critical range. This type of regulation, then, results from the detection of small changes in the environment through discriminating binding by proteins and consequent changes in the three-dimensional structure on which their functional properties depend.

Therapeutically, allosteric regulation offers extensive potential for exploitation. For example, fraudulent feedback inhibitors can be employed to turn off metabolic pathways (as with certain nucleic acid precursors in cancer therapy) or abortive inhibitors can be used which bind but do not inhibit and therefore release a system from normal inhibition.

The simplest type of protein regulation involves detection by the enzyme or other effector molecule of changes in concentration of a small molecular signal. There are also secondary or remote mechanisms involved in regulation. For example, some proteins are modified covalently by specific enzymes to produce more stable changes in structure and function, with the primary regulatory signal operating on the modifying enzyme. The concept of a so-called "secondary messenger" in regulatory processes has also become quite important, although the choice of terms leads to some confusion with the "messenger" role of RNA. This concept, so beautifully established with cyclic AMP, interposes an additional, strictly regulatory enzyme between the environmental signal and the target enzyme(s), with the resulting regulatory enzyme product serving as the final enzyme stimulator or inhibitor. Thus, adenyl cyclase is stimulated or inhibited by a variety of drugs or metabolic products in its catalysis of cyclic AMP production. The levels of the cyclic AMP, in turn, are responsible for the regulation of an extensive array of biological processes, with consequent amplification and orchestration of the environmental stimulus into function. It is particularly interesting that this mechanism has already been used to rationalize the defect in regulation of the kidney tubule in pseudohypoparathyroidism. A thorough understanding of such secondary regulation mechanisms is of great importance both for understanding diseases and for therapy.

Protein structure may also be modified in less specific ways by changes in the solvent environment. For example, the sickling of red blood cells due to hemoglobin S can be antagonized by urea, which is thought to modify protein structure by increasing solubility of hydrophobic groups through changes in water structure.

While function is the major consideration in the types of regulation discussed above, the influence of such changes on the structural stability of proteins is also very important.

Regulation of the Concentration of Proteins

The steady-state concentration of a protein or other macromolecule is the sum of all the processes involved in formation and breakdown. Regulation, then, depends on which step is rate limiting.

Enzyme induction, or environment-stimulated increase in enzyme level, and enzyme repression, a converse decrease in level, were first elucidated in bacteria and are outstanding examples of mechanistic biology. The models for these processes, as illustrated in Figure 2-3, show transcription to be the rate-limiting process and assume protein stability to be relatively unimportant in these short-lived organisms. Classically, enzymes are induced by substrate and repressed by end products, so that function is linked to metabolic need. In higher organisms, control signals such as hormones must also be included, and, most importantly, all aspects of synthesis and breakdown must be considered. Thus, in addition to transcriptional control, translation, and assembly of final tertiary and quaternary structure (including any covalent modifications, or additions of nonprotein moieties), protein stability and consequent turnover are important. Each potential control point provides a locus for malfunction, and each offers a possible site for therapeutic manipulation. It is also clear that regulation may be imposed through secondary effects much in the same way as allosteric regulation (secondary messenger, and so on).

There has been considerable speculation about whether inherited deficiency diseases might become treatable based on such mechanisms as gene transfer by viruses (transduction), since such transfers have been accomplished in vitro. In fact, much less drastic methods may be applicable if the defect is not a complete deletion of the gene but one of depressed level and may be achieved through alterations in the regulation machinery or structure for the macromolecule.

Several diseases are already explicable based on faulty control of protein levels. For example, delta-aminolevulinic acid synthetase is excessive in porphyria, and chemical induction by drugs such as barbiturates results in disease exacerbation. Thalassemia appears to result from depressed (and unbalanced) levels of one of the two types of hemoglobin chains which normally must be available in equal amounts for normal assembly of the protein. Polycythemia results from overactivity of erythropoiesis.

The ability of drugs to perturb steady-state levels of enzymes by interacting at any of the control points is important therapeutically in explaining drug toxicity, and for developing insight into such regulatory effects. The ability of barbiturates to induce glucuronyl transferase and mixed-function oxidases has found application in treatment of both congenital jaundice of *Crigler-Najjar syndrome* and physiologic jaundice of the newborn. It is also well known that tolerance to drugs may be induced through the mechanism of increasing levels of metabolizing enzymes and that "cross tolerance" may be observed (for example, the tolerance to alcohol evoked by barbiturates and vice versa).

Therapeutic approaches based on regulation of macromolecular levels are limited chiefly by our lack of information about specific disease defects and about mechanisms for producing the appropriate perturbations. Our knowledge about both these points is increasing rapidly, however, and it is clear that this type of thinking will dominate therapeutics. Cancer chemotherapy illustrates how regulatory principles can be applied when the chemical objective is clear and many of the mechanisms known. Since the problem is one of uncontrolled cell growth, therapy is aimed at preventing cell proliferation and viability, both of which are ultimately dependent on DNA directed processes. A summary of current chemotherapy reveals that DNA synthesis is inhibited by limiting precursors; by fraudulent feedback inhibition; competitive inhibition; and by interference with the DNA template through simple or covalent drug binding and the destructive effects of radiation. The ultimate aim of chemotherapy to spare normal cells, of course, can be realized only through sufficient knowledge of regulation in both populations of cells.

COMMENTS ON THE MOLECULAR BASIS FOR DISEASE

In order to understand the consequence of molecular derangements in terms of disease, it is clearly essential to define the full role(s) for the molecule involved. For example, an enzyme deficit (or toxic damage) could result in a deficiency state in the case of a synthetic enzyme; an excess of some cell component if it is a degradative enzyme; seemingly remote or widespread effects if it is a regulatory enzyme; or no expression of disease if compensating regulatory mechanisms are called into play or if there is no current demand for the particular biological role played. Thus, a pseudocholine esterase deficiency is not expressed unless the individual is given the appropriate toxic drug; Hurler's and Hunter's syndromes result from defects in normal mucopolysaccharide degradation and turnover, and patients with McArdle's syndrome cannot synthesize glycogen normally. Certain other defects prevent normal cross-linking of metabolic pathways; for example, in galactosemia, galactose cannot be converted to glucose. The disturbance, however, results from accumulation of the substrate rather than from a metabolic deficiency. Diseases also result from excesses, as pointed out in the example of acute intermittent porphyria. In all instances, there may also be far-reaching consequences of a defect resulting from the secondary regulatory roles served by enzyme products. An excellent example of this is the *adrenogenital syndrome*, in which the molecular defect is hydroxylation of the 11-position of the steroid nucleus to form active adrenal corticoids. These individuals not only show severe adrenal insufficiency but also are severely masculinized, because the normal hydroxysteroid product is not present to regulate (inhibit) early steps in steroid biogenesis, with resultant overproduction of androgens.

It is also interesting to consider the kinetics of disease development and recovery in terms of perturbation of steady-state concentrations of molecules. Whereas some alterations are manifested immediately owing to rapid achievement of new steady states, others develop slowly even over the course of many years, either through cumulative defects (arteriosncleroses, for example) or through slow achievement of a new steady state owing to low rates of synthesis and turnover.

REFERENCES

Ashwell, M., and Work, T. S.: The biogenesis of mitochondria. Ann. Rev. Biochem., *39*:251, 1970.

Burgess, R. R.: RNA polymerase. Ann. Rev. Biochem., *40*:711, 1971.

Cleaver, J. E.: Defective repair replication of DNA in xeroderma pigmentosum. Nature, *218*:652, 1968.

Gerduschek, E. P., and Haselkorn, R.: Messenger RNA. Ann. Rev. Biochem., *38*:647, 1969.

Goldberg, I. H., and Friedman, P. A.: Antibiotics and Nucleic acids. Ann. Rev. Biochem., *40*:775, 1971.

Goulian, M.: Biosynthesis of DNA. Ann. Rev. Biochem., *40*:855, 1971.

Holzer, H., and Duntzl, W.: Metabolic regulation by chemical modification of enzymes. Ann. Rev. Biochem., *40*:345, 1971.

Korn, E. D.: Cell membranes: Structure and synthesis. Ann. Rev. Biochem., *38*:263, 1969.

Lark, K. G.: Initiation and control of DNA synthesis. Ann. Rev. Biochem., *38*:569, 1969.

Lengyel, P., and Söll, D.: Mechanism of protein biosynthesis. Bacteriol. Rev., *33*:264, 1969.

The Molecular Basis of Life — an Introduction to Molecular Biology. Readings from Scientific American, introduced by R. H. Hayne and P. C. Hanawalt, San Francisco, W. H. Freeman and Co., 1968.

Pestka, S.: Inhibitors of ribosome functions. Ann. Rev. Biochem., *40*:697, 1971.

Schimke, R. T., and Doyle, D.: Control of enzyme levels in animal tissues. Ann. Rev. Biochem., *39*:929, 1970.

Watson, J. D.: Molecular biology of the gene. 2nd ed. Menlo Park, California, W. A. Benjamin, Inc., 1970.

CHAPTER 3 MEDICAL GENETICS

BENJAMIN R. GENDEL
LOUIS J. ELSAS, II

INTRODUCTION

The application of genetics to medicine has profoundly increased man's understanding of the pathologic physiology of inherited human disease and his desire to predict these disease processes and to prevent them from becoming manifest. Genetic engineering, environmental engineering, genetic counseling, and prenatal diagnosis are some clinical realities and expectations resulting over the last decade from this applied body of information. The incidence and recurrence figures for pathologic processes caused by the interaction of multiple genes and the environment provide empiric recurrence risk figures to families seeking counseling for diseases such as cleft palate, pyloric stenosis, and spina bifida. Other diseases are presumably caused by single mutant genes of large effect, since they conform to a mendelian pattern of inheritance. Pedigree analysis provides information regarding recurrence risks for subsequent offspring even when the molecular mechanisms producing the disease are unknown.

The chromosome is now recognized as the nuclear structure responsible for the physical transmission of genetic information. Abnormalities of chromosome structure are associated with a number of clinical syndromes. New techniques using Giemsa banding and fluorescent staining now enable identification of individual chromosomes and their subparts. Translocations, deletions, and inversions can now be confirmed and related to abnormal phenotypes.

The description of etiology, prediction of recurrences, and prevention of disease have become possible in the group of mendelian disorders known as the "inborn errors of metabolism."

The assumption of A. E. Garrod that an abnormal gene product resulted in impaired cellular metabolism and produced an "inborn error of metabolism" has been verified in many disorders. Over the last two decades, his "block-in-reaction sequence" definition has been expanded to include other mutant polypeptides affecting metabolic function. The molecular concepts derived from microbial systems by Watson and Crick for the biochemical transmission of genetic information through deoxyribonucleic acid (DNA); by Jacob and Monod for the regulation of gene expression; and by Nirenberg for the translation of triplet codons in nucleic acids to specific amino acids in a peptide chain are finding application in human disease. Single amino acid changes occur in sickle hemoglobin and can be explained by a single base pair substitution (point mutation) in the DNA triplet codon. These and other observations in mutant α and β hemoglobin chain synthesis and structure provide direct evidence that the genetic concepts derived from microbial systems apply to man. The genetic axiom "one gene – one enzyme" now extends to "one gene – one polypeptide."

The concept of "inborn errors of metabolism" includes defects of structural proteins, subunits of functioning proteins, transport proteins, proteins regulating gene expression, proteins involved with coenzyme function, and proteins involved in the repair of DNA itself. Replacement of abnormal enzymes, deficient enzyme products, or coenzymes; addition of inducers or feedback inhibitors; restriction of toxic precursors, or by-products; and replacement of the deficient genes themselves are therapeutic maneuvers being studied or used to treat this group of disorders. The use of quinacrine fluorescence and man-mouse cell hybridization techniques enabled the delineation of at least one gene locus on the human chromosome. By use of these techniques, thymidine kinase was localized to chromosome number 17. It is predicted that many more gene loci will be located and associated with linkage groups. Thus, the disciplines of population genetics, biochemical genetics, and cytogenetics align in studying, defining, counseling, and treating inherited pathologic processes.

This chapter will review basic mendelian genetics as a necessary prerequisite to the principles of human genetics. Three general categories of genetic disorders will then be discussed: (1) diseases caused by multiple genes and the environment, (2) diseases associated with chromosomal abnormalities, and (3) diseases caused by single genes of large effect. All genetic diseases cannot be discussed in this chapter and examples are arbitrarily used to illustrate a category of a presumed pathophysiologic mechanism.

MENDELIAN INHERITANCE

Mendel's Experiments

Although Rabbi Simon ben Gamaliel (Talmud of Maimonides, A.D. 100) excused brothers of "bleeders" from circumcision, it was not until 1900 that Mendel's laws were discovered and a formal study of patterns of inheritance in man began. Today, 1876 traits are catalogued in patterns conforming to mendelian inheritance and are presumably caused by single genes of large effect. It is important to begin our discussion of pathologic physiology with Mendel's principles of inheritance. Mendel's observations were made while experimenting with *Piscum sativum* or garden pea plant between 1856 and 1865. Mendel selected 34 varieties of true-breeding plants and studied discontinuous characters such as the length of the stem, the position of the flowers relative to the stem, the seed color, and the coat texture. Since the flower could fertilize itself and be protected from outside artifact, Mendel could cross hybrids derived from true breeders and make quantitative calculations of those disparate characteristics which appeared in subsequent generations. In one such experiment, the texture of the seed coat was either wrinkled or smooth. When he crossed true-breeding wrinkled plants with true-breeding smooth plants, he found that in the F_1 generation, only smooth-coated seeds were found. When he self-fertilized these smooth-seeded (F_1) plants, he found 25 per cent (1/4) true-breeding smooth plants, 25 per cent (1/4) true-breeding wrinkled plants, and 50 per cent (2/4) smooth, impure breeders, which, when self-fertilized, reproduced the same 1:2:1 ratio.

Phenotype

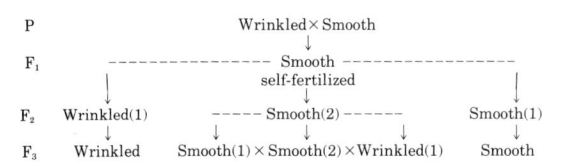

P   Wrinkled × Smooth
F_1 Smooth self-fertilized
F_2 Wrinkled(1)   Smooth(2)   Smooth(1)
F_3 Wrinkled   Smooth(1) × Smooth(2) × Wrinkled(1)   Smooth

He recognized that the wrinkled coat was transmitted from the F_1 to the F_2 generation in an unchanged state, although it was not phenotypically evident in the F_1 hybrid plant. To explain the disappearance of this hereditary trait in the F_1 hybrid and its predictable recurrence, he recognized that the physical expression (phenotype) differed from the genetic constitution (genotype), which must be composed of two genes. Mendel's *first law* stated that the alternate forms of this gene (later called alleles) must segregate during gamete formation and recombine independently in the offspring to provide this 1:2:1 ratio. From the phenotypic expression of these discontinuous traits, the concepts of dominance and recessivity were derived. In the F_1 hybrid derived from two pure-breeding strains, that allele which is expressed is dominant (smooth, S). The unexpressed allele is recessive (wrinkled, w). The genotypes in this experiment can now be written:

Genotype

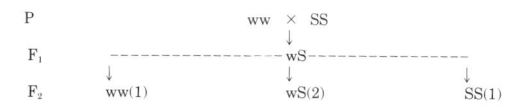

P   ww × SS
F_1 wS
F_2 ww(1)   wS(2)   SS(1)

In another set of experiments Mendel compared the textures of the seeds with their internal color. If he crossed true-breeding plants having smooth seeds and yellow interiors with plants having wrinkled seeds and green interiors, all the F_1 hybrids were smooth and yellow. When this hybrid was self-fertilized, he found a ratio of 9 smooth-yellow seeds, 3 smooth-green, 3 wrinkled-yellow, and 1 wrinkled-green out of a total of 16. These ratios (9/16; 3/16; 3/16; 1/16) were the product of the probability that either trait would appear independent of the other. Thus, for the two dominant traits (smooth seeds with yellow interiors), there was a 3/4 × 3/4 probability, or 9/16. For the recessive traits (wrinkled seeds with green interior), the probability was 1/4 × 1/4, or 1/16. Mendel recognized that the texture of the seed and the color of its interior were independent traits which were not allelic. Thus, his *second law* stated that nonallelic traits do not segregate but assort randomly and recombine with the product of their independent probabilities.

Because the botanists of Mendel's time were observing continuous rather than discontinuous traits, his concepts of a unit of inheritance lay dormant until 1900, when they were rediscovered independently by several different geneticists. By 1902, his observations had been applied in a pedigree analysis of man to explain the patterns of recurrence of brachydactyly. It should be remembered that the concepts of dominance and recessivity were derived from phenotypes and not from biochemical or molecular mechanisms of inheritance. However, the analyses of pedigrees using mendelian concepts are used to predict and test genetic control and may offer insights into the abnormal genetic mechanisms producing disease even when the biochemical mechanisms are unknown.

Autosomal Dominant Inheritance

This pattern of inheritance is the most common mode of transmission in man, although recessive traits are gaining in prevalence as new metabolic disorders are discovered through modern screening techniques. Most autosomal dominant traits exhibit distinct phenotypic abnormalities, making them relatively easy to detect. From mendelian concepts, one can predict the pedigree pattern for expression of a single dominant gene.

Consider the mating A in Figure 3-1. The heterozygote is affected and, by definition, expresses the dominant trait. If such a parent mates with a homozygous normal, on the average, one half the progeny will be affected heterozygotes and one half will be normal. In mating B, two affected heterozygotes mate. Their alleles segregate during gamete formation and recombine randomly. It could be predicted that one fourth of their offspring would be affected homozygotes, one half affected heterozygotes, and one fourth normal homozygotes. Seventy-five per cent (3/4) of this mating would be affected by the dominant trait. A schematic pedigree representing an autosomal dominant pattern of inheritance is indicated in Figure 3-2. Since the heterozygote expresses this trait, there is direct parent-to-offspring transmission, and a vertical pattern of abnormal individuals is produced. Since the mutant gene is located on an autosome, there is an approximately equal distribution of males and females. On the average, 50 per cent of a patient's offspring are affected.

Important in genetic counseling is the fact that if an individual does not express a dominant trait, he cannot transmit it to subsequent generations. This reassuring fact must be tempered against the difficulty in differentiating the disease from other similar diseases, the age at which the genetic determinant is expressed, and the spectrum of expression. For example, the fact that an offspring of a patient with familial colonic polyposis (an autosomal dominant trait) does not demonstrate polyps by sigmoidoscopy at age 5 years does not mean that polyps will not occur later in life or that they are not present in regions above the sigmoidoscope.

Currently, there are 943 dominant traits catalogued, including acute intermittent porphyria, Huntington's chorea, hemorrhagic telangiectasia, Marfan's syndrome, hypertrophic subaortic stenosis, polycystic kidney disease, neurofibromatosis, hereditary nephritis with deafness, familial polyposis, brachydactyly, tuberous sclero-

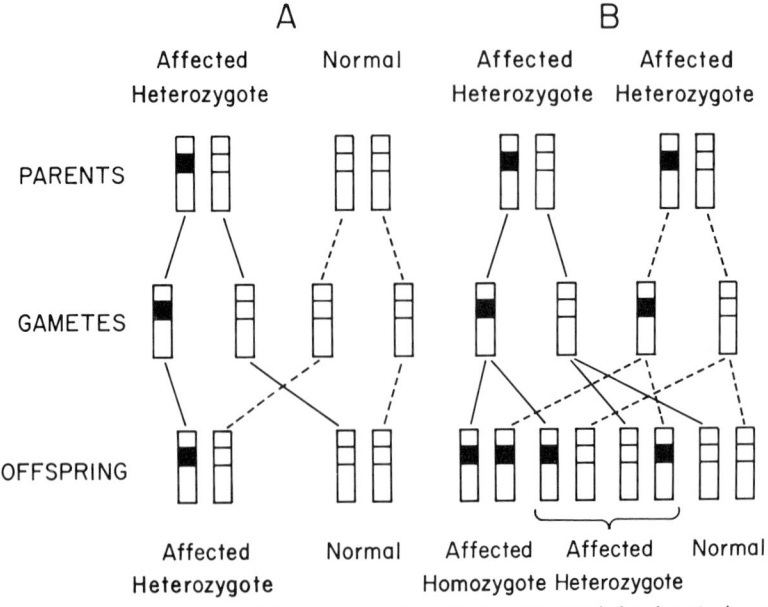

Figure 3-1 Schematic representation of the transmission of an autosomal dominant phenotype. A and B represent separate matings.

LEGEND:

☐, ○ Normal male, female
⊕ Deceased
■, ● Heterozygote, Phenotypically affected
I Generation
¹○₂ Superscript = position in pedigree
   Subscript = age in years

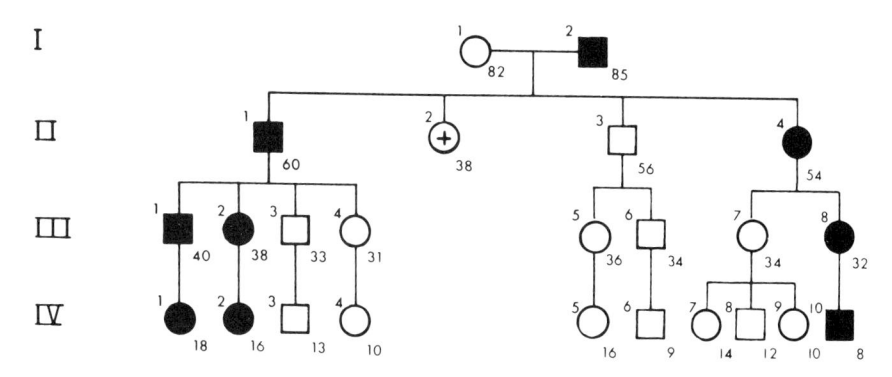

Figure 3-2 Pedigree conforming to an autosomal dominant pattern of inheritance.

sis, and so on. Despite our current lack of knowledge regarding the basic defect in many of these disorders, the dominant pattern of inheritance suggests several mechanisms for their expression and molecular control. In a dominant trait the heterozygote expresses the mutant allele. Thus, the mutant gene product could interfere with the function of the normal gene product by producing an abnormal subunit in a protein complex rendering the intact complex less effective. An example of this concept would be dysfibrinogenemia. Dominant mutant alleles might produce proteins which interfere with the regulation of gene expression (repression or feedback control). These concepts will be considered in more detail later when *inborn errors of metabolism* are discussed.

Autosomal Recessive Inheritance

From the scheme represented in Figure 3-3, one can predict the pattern of inheritance for an autosomal recessive trait. In mating A, a normal homozygote marries a phenotypically normal carrier of an autosomal recessive trait. In accordance with mendelian principles, the heterozygote does not express the trait. The offspring of such a mating are all phenotypically normal, although, on the average, 50 per cent (1/2) are heterozygotes. The mating in Figure 3-3, labeled B, is the more common situation requiring genetic counseling for an autosomal recessive trait. Here, two phenotypically normal parents carry an autosomal recessive mutation and produce an affected child. A recurrence of this phenomenon can be predicted from Mendel's hybridization experiments. On the average, a 1:2:1 ratio of homozygous normal:heterozygous:homozygous abnormal is expected and produces the classic ratio of 3 phenotypic normals to 1 affected. A schematic pedigree conforming to these predictions is outlined in Figure 3-4.

Several differences from the autosomal dominant pedigree outlined in Figure 3-2 are obvious. There is no direct parent-to-offspring transmission of the phenotypic trait but siblings are affected, and a horizontal pattern as compared to the vertical pattern of dominant inheritance is produced. Twenty-five per cent rather than 50 per cent recurrence in siblings is seen. Since recessive traits are rare in the population, consanguineous matings are more likely to produce the affected homozygote. Subjects III-3 and III-4 are first cousins and their consanguineous mating is indicated by the horizontal double bar. Recessive traits may have identifiable biochemical abnormalities.

In several of the recessive traits, heterozygotes can be detected by appropriate studies, although they are phenotypically normal under normal environmental conditions. The partially closed symbols represent phenotypically normal heterozygotes detectable by biochemical tests. Unlike the situation for the dominant traits, a

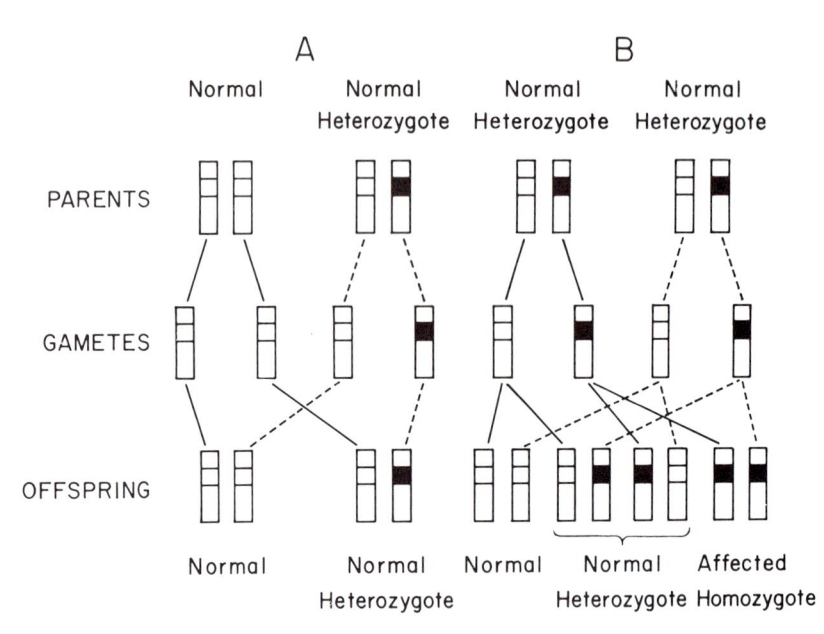

Figure 3-3 Schematic representation of the transmission of an autosomal recessive trait. A and B represent separate matings.

LEGEND:

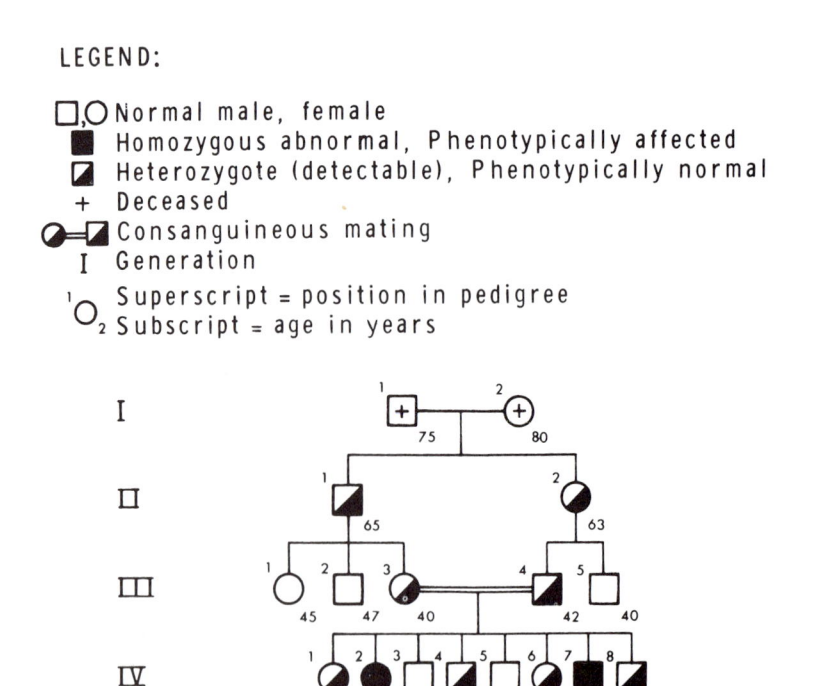

☐,○ Normal male, female
■ Homozygous abnormal, Phenotypically affected
◨ Heterozygote (detectable), Phenotypically normal
+ Deceased
○─◨ Consanguineous mating
I Generation
¹○₂ Superscript = position in pedigree
Subscript = age in years

Figure 3-4 Pedigree conforming to an autosomal recessive pattern of inheritance.

phenotypically unaffected member in this pedigree cannot be assured that he has no greater risk than the general population for transmitting the disorder. The risk of having an affected offspring is based on the product of the probability that the unaffected member carries the mutant gene, that he will marry a carrier, and that both mutant genes will be transmitted to the offspring. If heterozygotes can be detected by biochemical means, more precise information can be given. Suppose patient IV-1 (Fig. 3-4) seeks counseling regarding recurrence risks and is found to carry the mutant gene by biochemical testing. Her mate is then tested. If he carries the mutation, the risk of producing a phenotypically affected child is 25 per cent ($1/2 \times 1/2 = 1/4$). If her mate is normal, all their children will be unaffected, though each has a 50 per cent risk of being a carrier. Since both recessive and dominant traits occur on autosomes, males and females are equally affected.

There are 783 diseases of man classified as autosomal recessive traits. Most of the inborn errors of metabolism are included in this category as compared to autosomal dominant traits, which are more easily identifiable by their morphologic appearance.

X-Linked Inheritance

In both of the previous patterns of inheritance, the mutant gene was located on one of the 22 autosomes of man. Let us now consider a mutation residing on the X chromosome. In Figure 3-5A, a female carrying an X-linked mutation marries a normal male. The expectations of such a mating are that 50 per cent of the female offspring and 50 per cent of the male offspring will inherit the maternal X chromosome containing the mutant gene. If the mutant allele is recessive to the normal allele, the carrier female will not express the trait, but the male, who has only one X chromosome, is hemizygous for the trait and has no normal allele. He, therefore, would express the disorder. The prediction is that one half the sons will be affected and the other half will be unaffected and unable to transmit the mutation. One half the daughters will be heterozygotes and carry the mutation and one half will be homozygous normal, but all will be phenotypically normal.

Let us turn now to the critical mating (Fig. 3-5B). The mutation is located on the X chromosome of an affected male; all his daughters will inherit this X chromosome containing the mutation, but none of his sons can inherit this disorder because they must all receive his Y chromosome. The pattern of inheritance for an X-linked trait is illustrated by the pedigree in Figure 3-6. Heterozygotes for X-linked traits are indicated by a symbol with a darkened inner circle. If the trait is recessive, only hemizygous males are affected phenotypically. Since maternal uncles of affected males are commonly affected, an oblique pattern of inheritance, like the move of the knight in the game of chess, can be imagined. Subject II-1 is an affected male and does not transmit the trait to any of his sons. Both his daughters are carriers and the trait reappears in his grandson, subject IV-2. On the average, half the sons of a carrier female are affected and half the daughters are carriers. A homozygous affected female may appear in a pedigree for an X-linked recessive trait if a hemizygous affected father marries a heterozygous carrier female, or rarely if the X-chromosome containing the normal allele is inactivated during lyonization, leaving only cells with the mutant X-chromosome (see later, the Lyon Hypothesis). There are 150 diseases of man catalogued as X-linked recessive traits.

If the X-linked trait depicted in Figure 3-6 were familial hypophosphatemic rickets, heterozygous females would have abnormally low tubular reabsorption of phosphate and perhaps rickets. This is a dominant X-linked trait and twice as many females are affected as males, presumably because there is twice the risk for a female to inherit the mutant X chromosome. Direct parent-to-offspring transmission is seen. The progeny of subject II-1 provide a critical test of this hypothesis. In this situation, neither of his sons (III-1, III-3) but all his daughters (III-2, III-4) are affected. If such a critical mating were not present, an X-linked dominant trait might be mistaken for an autosomal dominant. Prediction and prevention in this disease is critical. Treatment with oral phosphates and vitamin D should be instituted before weight-bearing age to preserve normal bone growth. An accurate pedigree analysis is therefore imperative to aid in prediction, early diagnosis, and prevention.

There are many problems in analyzing pedigrees for "mendelizing phenotypes." Mendelian inheritance may be simulated by environmental mechanisms. Women with phenylketonuria may produce retarded children with microcephaly and other congenital anomalies even though the children are genotypically heterozygotes. The retardation presumably is caused by the effect of high concentrations of phenylalanine on the developing fetus. Phenocopies may be produced by intrauterine infections. Rubella virus may produce a syndrome of deafness and chorioretinal degeneration simulating Usher's syndrome, an autosomal recessive trait. Environmentally caused diseases may masquerade as mendelian traits. At least one instance is known of a mother affected by the rubella syndrome who produced a child with a similar syndrome. Recessive traits which usually are not clinically manifest may produce disease under unusual stressful circumstances. When heterozygotes for sickle cell hemoglobin

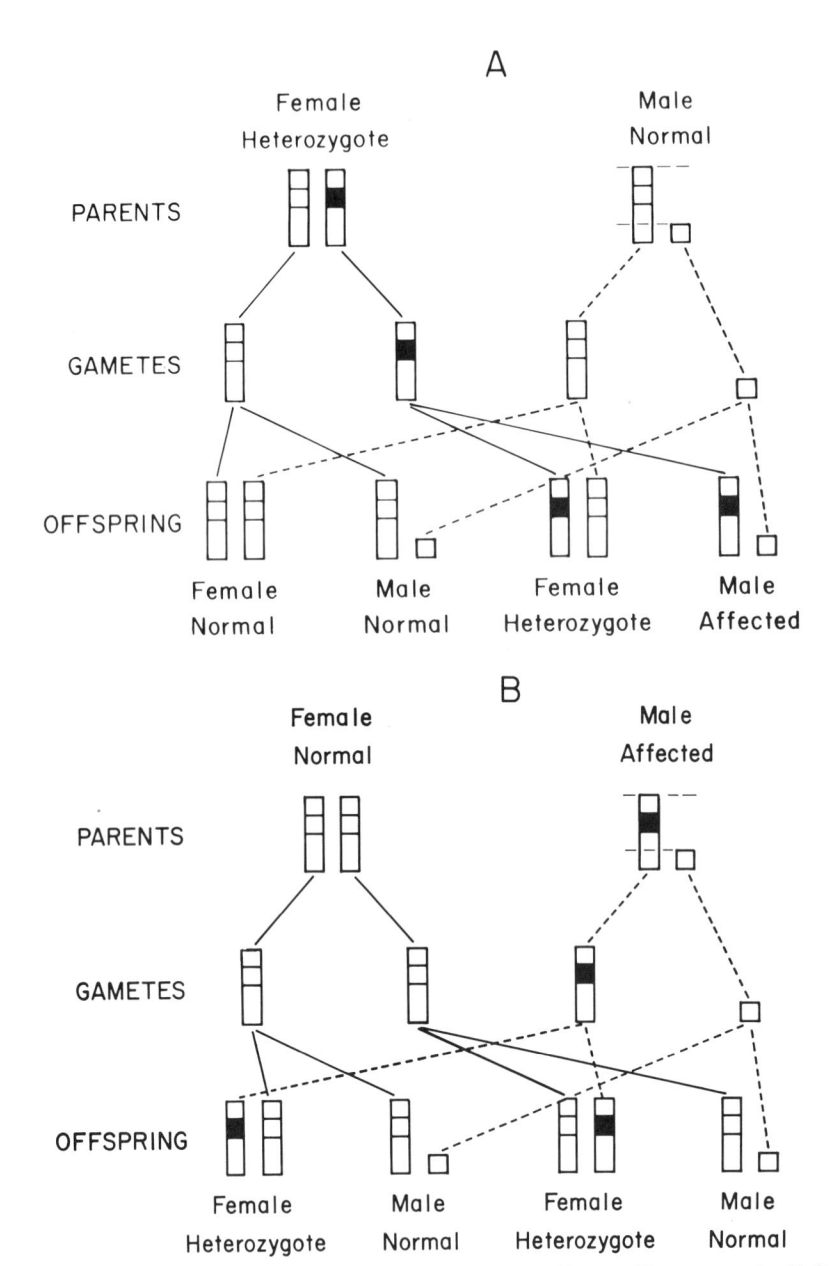

Figure 3-5 *A,* Schematic representation of X-linked transmission: Maternal heterozygote. *B,* Schematic representation of the critical mating in X-linked transmission: Paternal hemizygote.

LEGEND:

☐ Normal male
○ Normal female
⊙ Heterozygous female, Phenotypically normal or abnormal
■ Hemizygous male, Phenotypically abnormal
+ Deceased
I Generation
¹○ Superscript = position in pedigree
○₂ Subscript = age in years

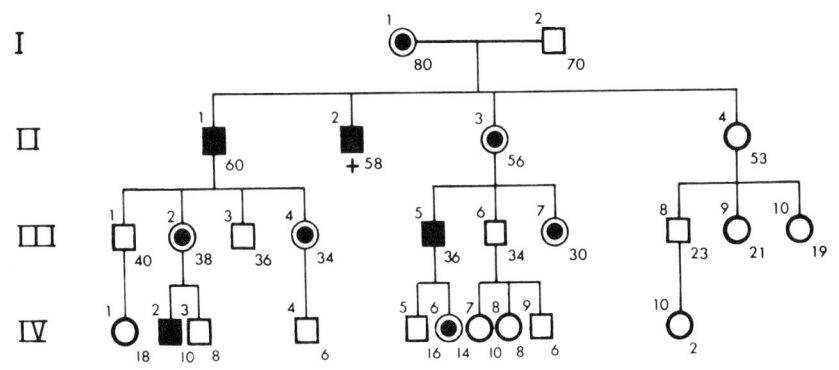

Figure 3-6 Pedigree conforming to an X-linked pattern of inheritance. If heterozygous females are phenotypically normal, the trait is recessive, as in hemophilia. A. If she is phenotypically affected, the trait is dominant, as in familial hypophosphatemic rickets.

(AS) are subjected to lowered atmospheric pressure, such as in nonpressurized aircraft flights, a "sickle crisis" may occur. Similarly, if the genetic determinant used in a pedigree analysis of sickle cell disease is erythrocyte sickling upon in vitro exposure to sodium metabisulfite, a dominant rather than recessive pattern of inheritance would emerge. Despite these problems, pedigree analysis and mendelian classification aid in establishing a probable genetic cause in predicting high-risk individuals and in suggesting basic genetic mechanisms. The problems raised by phenotypic expression will be solved by more precise information concerning the mutant gene product.

MULTIFACTORIAL GENETIC DISORDERS

Although Mendel's hybridization studies were quantitated using discontinuous traits, he also made some observations on traits which blended into a continuum between the parental phenotypes. He recognized that when purple-petaled and white-petaled plants were crossed, an intermediate mauve color was found in the hybrid. When this F_1 hybrid was self-fertilized, a range of color from purple to white was produced in the progeny. These observations seemed to contradict the concept of single gene effects, but Mendel suggested that flower petal color was determined by more than a single gene and that the expressed color resulted from a blending of these genes. Such common conditions as diabetes, schizophrenia, cleft palate, intelligence quotient, height, club foot, spina bifida, and pyloric stenosis recur in populations and families, with frequencies suggesting some genetic influences. Falconer interpreted these observations in the following manner: (1) there are both heritable and environmental influences acting upon the final phenotypic expression; (2) the hereditary component is polygenic and represents a continuum of genetic expression within the population; and (3) the small affected fraction of the population exceeded a threshold liability produced by both a larger number of "risk genes" and the environmental influences to produce the disease (Fig. 3-7). These hypotheses meet certain predicted conditions:

1. If these traits are not monogenic in causation, they will not conform to a mendelian pattern of recessive or dominant inheritance. Therefore, if one looked at the recurrence in first-degree relatives, one would *not* expect to find either a 25 per cent recurrence (autosomal reces-

sive) or a 50 per cent recurrence (autosomal dominant) but rather some other calculable increased risk over the general population. There should be a marked reduction in its recurrence from the first-degree relatives to the second-degree relatives but some definable increased risk over the general population. This contrasts sharply with either recessive or dominant inheritance. In mendelian recessive traits, one would expect no increased risk to second-degree relatives, barring consanguinity.

2. A second condition tests the recurrence of traits in monozygous and dizygous twins. In either recessive or dominant mendelian traits, the phenotype must be present in both monozygotic twins (100 per cent concordance). In these forms of inheritance, the recurrence rates in dizygous twins are the same as in first-degree relatives. In a multifactorial trait, one would expect an increased incidence in monozygous twins, but not 100 per cent concordance because of different nongenetic influences. The increased incidence found in dizygous twins should reflect this environmental effect. The recurrence rate found in first-degree relatives should be the same in dizygous twins.

3. One might expect that the more severe the disease expression, the greater the recurrence, since more "risk genes" must be present.

4. One might also expect that if the disease is more frequent in one sex, then the sex with the lower incidence figure would have a higher threshold and would require more "risk genes" to manifest disease.

5. Finally, one might anticipate that in families in which more than a single sibling is affected, the recurrence risks for a third affected offspring would be greater, since, again, more of the "risk genes" must be present in the parents and the probability of transmission is increased.

Carter's data for cleft lip with or without cleft palate satisfy these criteria. Other known familial causes of cleft lip and palate were excluded, i.e., cleft lip and palate with lower lip mucous pits (Van der Woude's syndrome, an autosomal dominant trait; trisomy 13, oral-facial-digital syndrome; and so on). Table 3–1 gives the combined data from four different studies in populations with cleft lip. The general incidence of cleft lip is 0.1 per cent. Monozygous twins were both affected in 40 per cent of cases, whereas in dizygous twins both were affected in only 4 per cent. Neither of these values would be consistent with a monogenic disorder. The first-degree relatives had a fortyfold increase over the general population. The second-degree relatives had a ninefold increase, and the third-degree relatives had a fourfold increase. When a more severe form of the disease was present, such as bilateral cleft lip with cleft palate, a higher recurrence risk figure for first-degree relatives was found (6 per cent). When the milder form of the disease, unilateral cleft lip without cleft palate, was present, a lower recurrence risk of 2.5 per cent was found. When two siblings were affected, the recurrence risk for a third affected individual within that family rose to 12 per cent. These data can be explained on the basis of a continuously distributed liability produced by multiple genes and the environment, with a threshold beyond which the disease is manifest (Fig. 3–7).

Several other relatively common disorders of man conform to a multifactorial mode of inheritance (Table 3–2). In some instances, the environmental influences are greater than the heritable component. For example, Carter reminds us that Laplanders and the American Indians swaddle their infants with legs extended and adducted. In

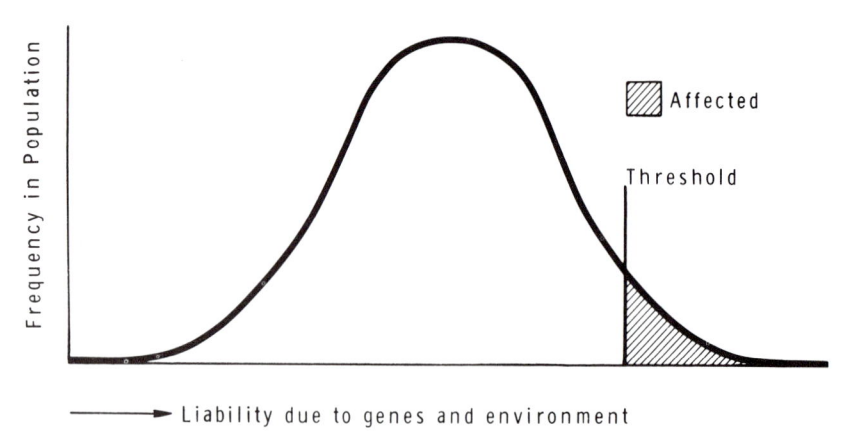

Figure 3–7 Multifactorial inheritance. The continuous distribution of liability to develop a multifactorial disease is determined by many genes and the environment. A threshold of liability indicates the limit beyond which disease is expressed.

TABLE 3-1 MULTIFACTORIAL INHERITANCE OF CLEFT LIP WITH OR WITHOUT CLEFT PALATE

Condition	Incidence in General Population (Per cent)	Monozygous Twin	First Degree (Siblings)	First Degree (Children)	Second Degree (Aunts and Uncles)	Second Degree (Nephews and Nieces)	Third Degree (First Cousins)
Overall recurrence risk for cleft lip ± cleft palate	0.1	40 (400X)	4.4 ± 0.7 (40X)	3.3 ± 1.2	0.7 ± 0.1 (9X)	1.1 ± 0.5	0.4 ± 0.1 (4X)
Bilateral cleft lip + palate	--	--	6.0		--		--
Unilateral cleft lip − palate	--	--	2.5		--		--
Two affected siblings	--	--	12.0		--		--

Data taken from Carter, C. O.: Hosp. Pract., 5:45, May, 1970.
Blanks (--) indicate insufficient data.
Numbers in parentheses followed by X (400X) indicate the increased risk relative to the general population.

both these groups, the incidence of dislocation of the hip is higher than the negligible incidence in certain Asiatic groups such as the Chinese, in which the infant is held on a back sling with hips flexed and abducted. The incidence in a population in which neither of these environmental extremes is present is approximately 0.2 per cent. At least two genetic factors (acetabular dysgenesis and familial joint laxity) and at least two environmental factors (breech positioning at birth and swaddling) have been described which adversely affect the incidence and recurrence risk figures for dislocation of the hip. A twenty-fivefold increase over the incidence in the general population is found in first-degree relatives of patients with congenital dislocation of the hip. There is only a threefold and twofold increased risk to second- and third-degree relatives, respectively. In pyloric stenosis, a sex predilection has been demonstrated. Although pyloric stenosis occurs more commonly in males than in females (0.5 vs. 0.1 per cent), the recurrence risk to the

TABLE 3-2 MULTIFACTORIAL INHERITANCE—EMPIRICAL DATA FROM FAMILIES WITH CONGENITAL MALFORMATIONS

Condition	Incidence in General Population (Per cent)	Monozygous Twin	First Degree	Second Degree	Third Degree
Dislocation of hip (Females)	0.2	200X	25X	3X	2X
Pyloric stenosis (Males)	0.5	80X	10X (Males)	5X	1.8X
Pyloric stenosis (Females)	0.1	--	200X (Males)	20X	1.8X
Spina bifida cystica	0.2	--	10X	--	--
Talipes equinovarus	0.1	300X	25X	5X	2X
Ankylosing spondylitis (Males)	0.02	--	35X	10X	3X
Early-onset ischemic heart disease (Males)	0.15	--	6X	--	--

Blanks (--) indicate insufficient data.
Numbers in parentheses followed by X (200X) indicate the increased risk relative to the general population.
Data compiled from Carter, C. O.: Hosp. Pract., 5:45, May, 1970, and Falconer, D. S.: Ann. Human Genet., 29:51, August, 1965.

sons of affected fathers is ten times the general population risk. In keeping with the postulates for a multifactorial mode of inheritance, the female may require more "risk genes" before manifesting the trait if perhaps hormonal influences protect her. If an increased number of "risk genes" is required for her to express the disease, a recurrence risk should be higher in her hormonally unprotected male offspring. Sons of females with pyloric stenosis have a two-hundredfold increased incidence relative to the general population. Cater has determined that in the London area, the incidence of spina bifida cystica is approximately 0.2 per cent. The recurrence is 2 per cent in families in which one member has been affected. After two children in a family are affected, the risk rises to 12.5 per cent.

These kinds of data are useful in relating recurrence risk figures to families, but the concept of a continuous distribution and "multifactorial" disease should not inhibit attempts to find specific causes within these heterogeneous groups. The "continuous" expression of an enzyme function in population studies may be related to multiple genotypes in that population. Harris clearly demonstrated the continuous distribution of serum cholinesterase (pseudocholinesterase) activity if serum hydrolytic activity alone were the genetic determinant (Fig. 3-8A). Only a small portion of the population (closed squares) was functionally defective and no mendelian pattern was delineated. When other characteristics of the gene products were examined, such as resistance to dibucaine, three phenotypes become evident: "usual," "intermediate," and "atypical" (Fig. 3-8B). This trimodal distribution then suggested mendelian rather than multifactorial inheritance in which "usual" was homozygous normal, "intermediate" was heterozygous, and "atypical" was homozygous abnormal. The discriminant, "dibucaine resistance," resolved the genetic control mechanisms for this enzyme function into a mendelian pattern. Since this earlier description, other parameters of resistance, inheritance, and separation of isozymes have demonstrated at least two loci for pseudocholinesterase activity and 10 genotypes to account for the continuous polygenic distribution in the population. Environmental factors such as liver disease, general nutrition, and renal glomerular integrity contribute further to the "multifactorial" pattern of enzyme activity originally found.

CYTOGENETICS

Another mechanism for disease in man is that which results from chromosomal abnormalities, which may be of two types. There may be a numerical variation from the normal number or

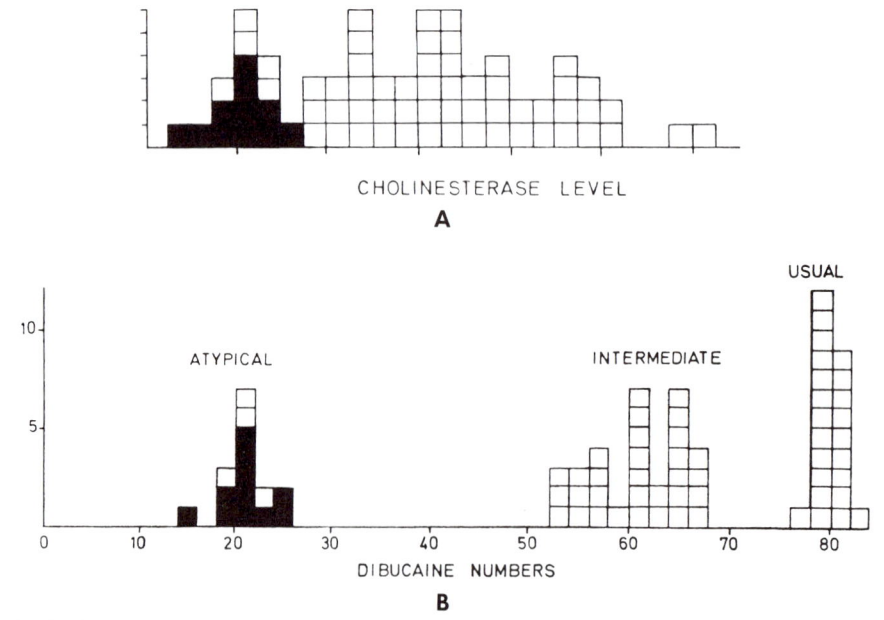

Figure 3–8 *A*, Continuous distribution of serum cholinesterase (pseudocholinesterase) activity. Each square represents one individual. Suxamethonium-sensitive individuals are marked in black. *B*, Distribution of dibucaine numbers (per cent inhibition) on identical serum specimens. Discrimination of three phenotypes is evident. (From Harris, H., et al.: Acta Genet. (Basel), *10*:1, 1960.)

the normal number may be present but gross structural abnormalities of individual chromosomes may exist. Chromosomal aberrations have been known to occur in plants and animals for a long time, but only in recent years have human cytogenetic techniques been advanced sufficiently to demonstrate that they occur in humans as well.

The Chromosomes

The chromosomes are the paired structures which carry the hereditary information in the form of DNA in each cell of the body. The number of chromosomes varies in plants and animals; in man, the normal number, 46, was definitively established only as recently as 1956. There are 22 pairs of autosomes, which are identical in both sexes, and one pair of sex chromosomes. The latter two chromosomes have a similar appearance in the female, XX, but are dissimilar in the male, one being like the X chromosome of the female and the other, Y, being smaller and seen only in the male. The chromosomes appear in metaphase as double rod-shaped structures, the *chromatids*, which lie adjacent to each other and are connected at a constriction called the *centromere*. An analysis of the chromosomes has permitted their classification based on their size and shape, the latter being determined by the position of the centromere. The chromosome is called metacentric when the centromere is approximately in the middle of the chromosome, in which case the chromatid arms are about equal in length. The centromere may be toward one end, in which case the arms on opposite sides of the centromere are unequal, one arm being longer than the other. *Acrocentric* chromosomes are those in which the position of the centromere may be very close to one end, making them almost V-shaped (Fig. 3-9).

The autosomes are divided into seven groups, A to G, depending upon their size and the position of the centromere (Table 3-3). They are numbered in descending order from 1 to 22, based on their size within the groups. The X chromosome is of the size of the larger chromosomes of group C, but cannot be differentiated from them with the older techniques; the Y chromosome is small and acrocentric and cannot be easily differentiated from those in group G (Fig. 3-10).

The earlier techniques made it possible to group the chromosomes in a satisfactory way, but only within group A and to some extent within group E was it possible to separate the individual members of a group. The X chromosome could not be differentiated from the larger members of group C, and the Y could not be easily distinguished from group G chromosomes. At times the Y could be separated by virtue of the fact that it tended to be slightly larger, the long arms were longer and more closely approximated, and it did not have satellites.

Other techniques have helped to better delineate the individual chromosomes. The use of tritiated thymidine, which labels newly synthesized DNA, demonstrated differences in the labeling time of the various chromosomes and aided in their differentiation. The two members of group B could be separated, as well as one of the two X chromosomes of the female which was late-labeling. Chromosomes in other groups could be differentiated as well. Interpretation, however, was difficult with respect to the separation in some groups and was not universally accepted. Recently, several new techniques have increased the cytogeneticist's ability to distinguish the chromosomes. It was discovered that quinacrine mustard would cause the chromosomes to fluoresce, a finding of great value in delineating the Y chromosome, which fluoresces intensely (Fig. 3-11A). It also provides differing fluorescent banding patterns in other chromosomes and permits delineation of the X from other members of the C group. Figure 3-11B demonstrates the usefulness of the fluorescent karyotype in a patient with translocation type of Down's syndrome. Other recent innovations involve modifications of technique using Giemsa staining, which also provides different banding patterns for individual chromosomes and is of great help in more accurate karyotyping.

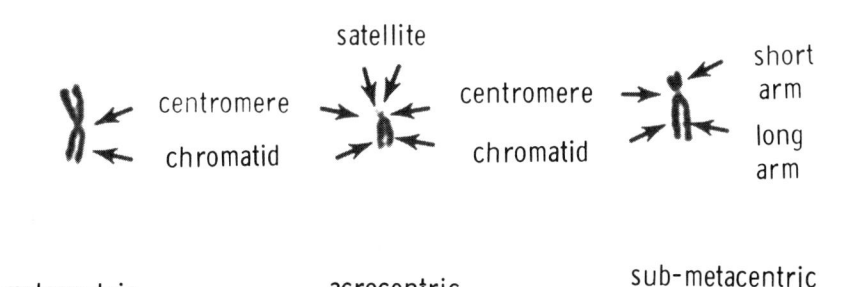

Figure 3-9 Types of human metaphase chromosomes.

TABLE 3-3 MORPHOLOGIC CHARACTERISTICS OF THE HUMAN METAPHASE CHROMOSOMES

Groups	Chromosome Number	Characteristics
A	1, 2, 3	Largest chromosomes, metacentric; #3 smaller than #1; #2 is more submetacentric.
B	4, 5	Large chromosomes, submetacentric.
C	6 to 12, and X	Medium-sized metacentric and submetacentric; X is one of the longer chromosomes of this group.
D	13 to 15	Larger, acrocentric chromosomes; may have satellites.
E	16 to 18	Smaller than above groups; #16 is metacentric; #17 and #18 submetacentric with 18 having smaller short arms.
F	19, 20	Four small chromosomes which appear like the letter x.
G	21, 22, Y	Short acrocentrics; may be satellited; Y is similar but usually slightly larger; longer arms, closer together and with occasional constriction; no satellites.

Data compiled from references cited in bibliography under Cytogenetics.

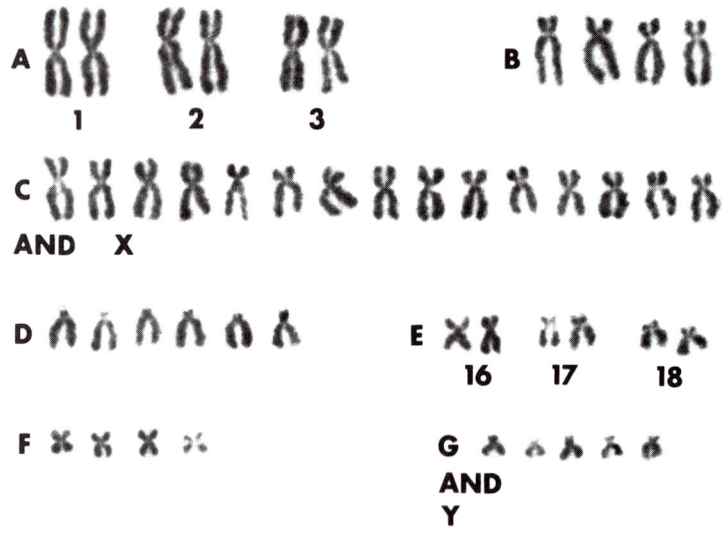

Figure 3-10 Normal male karyotype using standard staining techniques. Forty-six chromosomes are arranged in 7 groups (A to G). Note that the X chromosome cannot be differentiated from the C group; the Y is very similar to the others of the G group. (Courtesy of Dr. Jean H. Priest.)

MEDICAL GENETICS

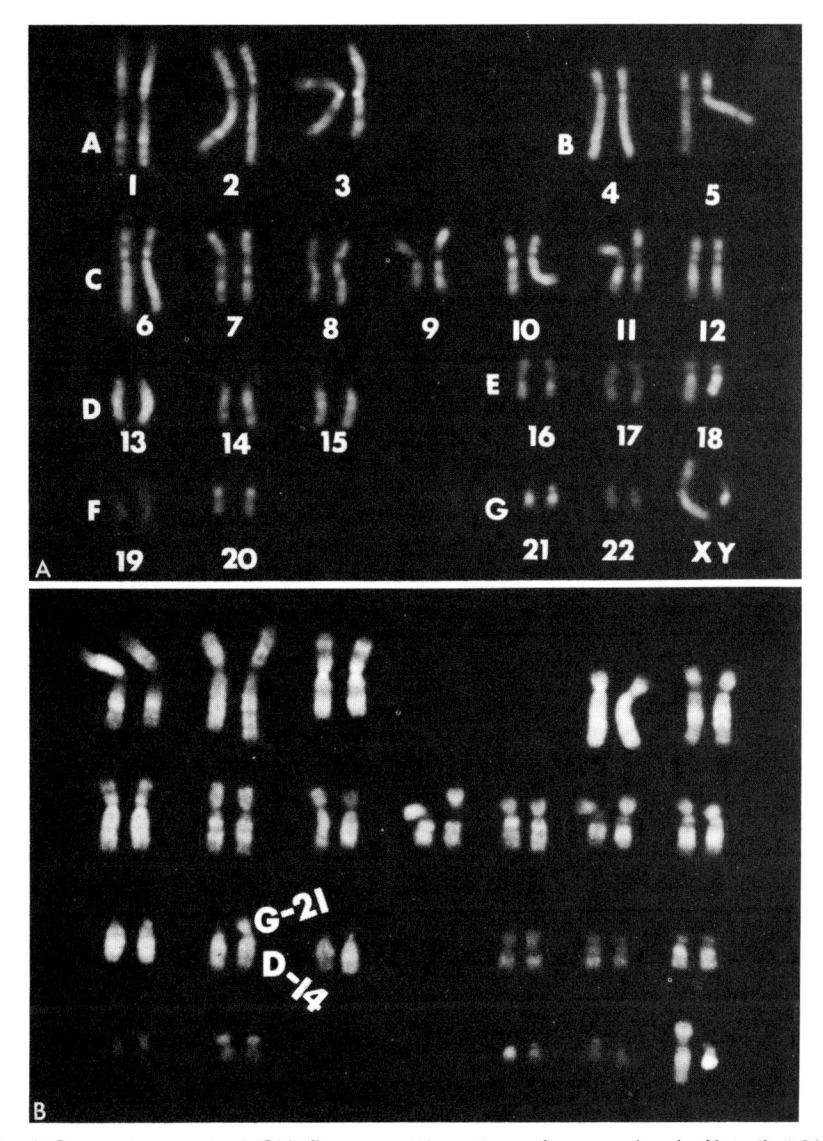

Figure 3-11 *A*, Quinacrine mustard (QM) fluorescent karyotype of a normal male. Note that 21 and 22 can be separated by different fluorescence. The long arm of the Y chromosome shows intense fluorescence, distinguishing it from others in the G group. Chromosome pairs in other groups can also be identified. (Courtesy of Dr. W. Roy Breg.) *B*, Quinacrine mustard (QM) fluorescent karyotype from a patient with the translocation type of Down's syndrome. Note the D/G translocation chromosome which could be identified as 21/14 based on fluorescent banding patterns. (Courtesy of Dr. W. Roy Breg.)

Mitosis and Meiosis

The many cells of the body are derived from the division of preceding cells; hence, it is essential that we review briefly mitosis and meiosis. In mitosis, the resting cell is referred to as being in the *interphase*. The term "resting cell" is a misnomer carried over from early morphologic observations, when it appeared that little or no activity was occurring in the nucleus at that time. Subsequent physiologic studies showed that the chromosomes were indeed metabolically active and that doubling of the DNA occurred at this time. The remainder of the actual cell division comprised only a small portion of the time of the cell cycle. During the interphase, the chromosomes are elongated, thin filaments; however, as the cell prepares to divide and enter the *prophase*, the chromosomes condense and become thicker and more discrete. In the *metaphase*, the next stage, the chromosomes, which have doubled their DNA, now consist of two parts, the chromatids, held together at the centromere. After this, the chromosomes independently migrate to the equatorial plate, and some of the mitotic spindle fibers, which extend from the centrioles, attach to the centromere. During the next phase, the *anaphase,* the chromatids move apart, apparently pulled by the spindle fibers to each pole of the dividing cell. Each chromatid becomes the chromosome of the daughter cell. The *telophase* is the stage during which the nuclear membrane forms about each group of daughter chromosomes, and the cell divides into two daughter cells. Thus, each newly formed cell nucleus has the same number and kind of chromosomes as the original cell from which it was derived. This paired number of chromosomes in each cell is called the *diploid* number.

During the formation of the reproductive cells, a modification of the above process occurs called *meiosis.* Here, during the course of two successive cell divisions, the duplication of the chromosomes occurs only once, so that the germinal cells have only one of each pair of chromosomes. This number or set of individual chromosomes is called the *haploid* number. The chromosomes, instead of remaining independent as in mitosis, line up in pairs during the division of either the primary spermatocyte or primary oocyte. When the cell divides in the first meiotic division, the chromosomes are not duplicated. Instead, during this reduction division, one of each pair goes to each newly formed cell, giving rise to the haploid number. In the second meiotic division, the haploid number of chromosomes is duplicated in each daughter cell, just as in a mitotic division. The meiotic division and its reduction of the diploid number of chromosomes to a haploid number is essential in sexual reproduction because fertilization joins two haploid sets from the father and mother and thus re-establishes the diploid number of chromosomes. If this were not the case, fertilization would result in a doubling of the diploid number with each event and the chromosomes would double with each generation. Meiosis serves to keep the chromosome number constant for the species.

CHROMOSOMAL ABNORMALITIES

The normal diploid number of chromosomes in man is 46 and they are present in all the somatic cells. In the gametes, however, the haploid number is 23 and includes one of each pair. Since the genes are located on the chromosomes, one could suspect that a variation in number, or variation in gross structure, would add or subtract many genes from the individual cell and lead to an abnormality. One must bear in mind, however, that minor structural changes may occur as normal variations in man without any significant phenotypic expression. Gross chromosomal abnormalities are associated with a number of clinical disorders. The relationship of the chromosomal abnormality to the disease state in terms of the precise pathophysiologic mechanism for the production of the effect is not known.

Before considering the specific syndromes associated with chromosomal abnormalities, it is necessary to review a cytogenetic shorthand which was suggested in 1966 and which is now in common usage. A brief synopsis of this is presented, using only the common terms or terms used in this chapter. The karyotype is written by noting the total number of chromosomes followed by the sex chromosomes. For example, 46,XY is the normal male and 46,XX is the normal female karyotype.

In considering the numerical aberrations, 45,X indicates a total number of 45 chromosomes with only one X chromosome; 47,XXY indicates a total of 47, the extra chromosome being one of the sex chromosomes which consist of two X chromosomes and a Y; 47,XY,D+ indicates a male with trisomy of one of the D group chromosomes; 47,XX,18+ indicates a female with 47 chromosomes due to trisomy of chromosome 18; 45,XY,C− indicates a male with 45 chromosomes, the missing one being of the C group.

Chromosomal mosaics are shown by separating the several cell lines by a diagonal slash. For example, 45,X/46,XY indicates a chromosome mosaic with two cell lines: one has 45 chromosomes and a single X; the other is normal with 46 chromosomes and XY. The mosaic karyotype, 46,XY/47,XY,21+ indicates a mosaic with one normal male cell line and the other with one additional chromosome 21.

In defining structural abnormalities, the short arm of the chromosome is designated with a small "p"; the long arm with a "q." Therefore, 46,XY,5p− indicates a male with 46 chromosomes, but chromosome 5 has a deletion of the short arm. The karyotype 46,XX,22q− shows a female with a normal chromosome number, but a deletion of the long arm of chromosome 22. A plus sign (+) is used to designate an increase in material in either the short or long arm. An isochromosome of the X chromosome is shown in the karyotype 46,XXqi which designates a female with one normal X chromosome and an abnormal X, consisting of an isochromosome (i) of the long arms (q) of the X. A ring chromosome is designated by a small "r" after the chromosome involved, e.g., Gr is a ring chromosome of one of the G group.

Translocations are indicated by the letter "t" followed by parentheses which include the chromosomes involved. One type of translocation can be designated 45,XX,D−,21−,t(Dq21q)+ and indicates that the individual is a female with 45 chromosomes; one of the 21 chromosomes is missing as is one of the D group. The long arms of these two chromosomes are united in a translocation (t). There are other types of translocation, but these will not be discussed.

Chromosome abnormalities may lead to a number of consequences: (1) They have been found in association with *fetal loss.* Spontaneously aborted fetuses have a variety of chromosomal abnormalities. The incidence has been found to be 46 per cent in the first trimester, falls to 15 per cent in the second trimester, and is only 1 to 2 per cent in the last trimester of pregnancy. (2) Several types of *congenital malformations* result from chromosomal abnormality. (3) *Mental retardation* is associated with several trisomic states, especially that of chromosome 21. (4) *Neoplasia* is associated with aneuploidy, and a specific chromosomal abnormality occurs in chronic granulocytic leukemia. The chromosomal abnormalities will be discussed in relation to the two major groups, numerical abnormalities and structural abnormalities (Table 3-4).

NUMERICAL ABNORMALITIES OF THE CHROMOSOMES

Polyploidy

This refers to an abnormal number of chromosomes in multiples of the haploid number, 23. As mentioned previously, the diploid state, 46 is normal for the somatic cells. Triploidy is a form of polyploidy in which 69 chromosomes are present, three of each chromosome instead of the normal pair (Fig. 3-12); in tetraploidy, 92 chromosomes, four of each individual chromosome are present. Polyploidy is found normally in some liver cells and in the megakaryocytes of the bone marrow. It, along with other aneuploid states, is found also in spontaneously aborted fetuses. Polyploidy accounts for about 17 per cent of all the aborted fetuses with demonstrated chromosomal abnormalities. The frequency of aneuploidy in association with spontaneous abortion early in pregnancy suggests that there is a cause and effect relationship, but the mechanism is not clear. One can think of this as a safeguarding mechanism to eliminate grossly abnormal fetuses.

Aneuploid States

Aneuploidy is the term applied to an increase or decrease in the normal (euploid) number of chromosomes, but not involving a full haploid set. The aneuploid state may involve the autosomes, the sex chromosomes or sometimes both. *Trisomy,* a form of aneuploidy with 47 chromosomes in which one chromosome of a pair is present three times instead of in the normal paired state, is clearly established as an important cause of clinical disease. Sometimes it is difficult to specify the chromosome which is the trisomic one. Under these circumstances, the condition is referred to as trisomy for a particular group (e.g., trisomy D). If the trisomic chromosome is definitely known, this is designated (e.g., trisomy 13). There are three trisomic conditions which have been clearly established. These are (1) trisomy for chromosome 21, which results in Down's syndrome or mongolism; (2) trisomy for chromosome 13, which produces a rare form of congenital malformation (designated previously as D_1 trisomy because it was the first trisomy of the D group to be described); and (3) trisomy 18 which also produces a syndrome of congenital malformation.

Monosomy is the state in which only one of a particular chromosome pair is present instead of two. Autosomal monosomic conditions have not been clearly established. Monosomy for the X chromosome is well known, however, and is the basis for Turner's syndrome. Other aneuploid states may occur which are more complex; some involve trisomy of two chromosomal pairs, which produces a karyotype with 48 chromosomes. An example is the combination of both Down's syndrome and Klinefelter's syndrome in the same individual (48,XXY,21+).

Nondisjunction

Trisomy and monosomy may be explained in part by biologic experiments on the fruit fly in which chromosomal accidents called nondisjunction were found. During the reduction division in meiosis, the chromosomes initially form in pairs and then separate or disjoin from each other. This phenomenon is known as a disjunction. Ordinarily, this separates the two chromosomes of any pair and we would expect each gamete formed after the reduction division to contain only a single chromosome of each pair. Nondisjunction occurring in the gonads of normal individuals is

TABLE 3-4 CLASSIFICATION OF CHROMOSOMAL ABNORMALITIES

1. Numerical
   A. Polyploidy
   B. Aneuploidy
      (1) Autosomal
      (2) Sex chromosomal
2. Structural
   A. Translocations
   B. Deletions
   C. Isochromosomes
   D. Ring chromosomes
   E. Inversions

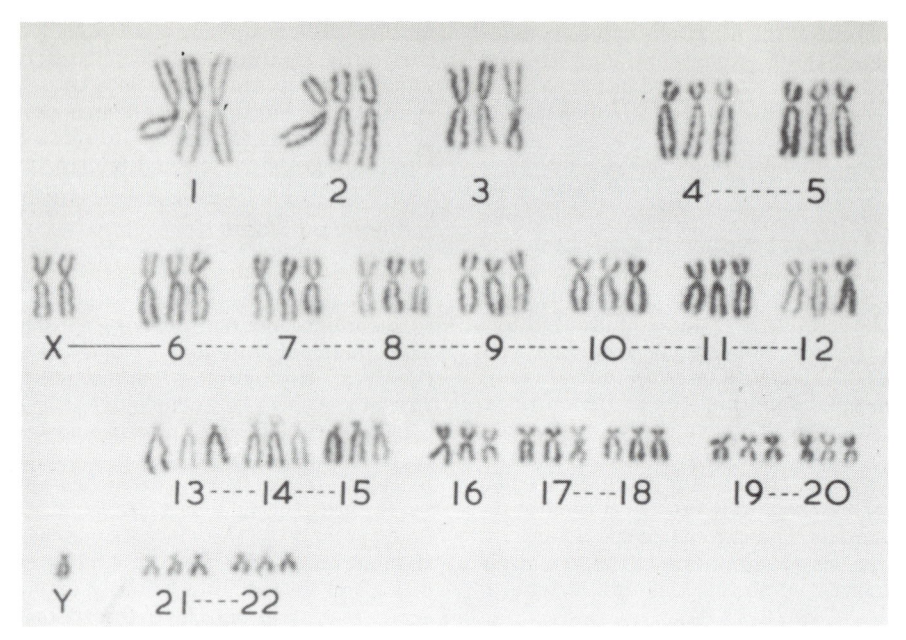

Figure 3–12 A karyotype of a spontaneously aborted fetus, 69,XXY. All autosomes are present in triplicate; the sex chromosomes consist of two X chromosomes and a Y. (Courtesy of Professor Paul E. Polani.)

called *primary nondisjunction.* If we take as an example only the sex chromosomes, X and Y, the X would go to one daughter cell and the Y to the other. This would mean the resulting sperm would be either X chromosome-containing or Y chromosome-containing. If nondisjunction were to occur, the sex chromosomes would not separate and it would be possible for sperm to contain both the X and Y chromosomes or neither. Similarly in oogenesis, nondisjunction of the two X chromosomes results in ova containing no sex chromosomes or ova which have both. The same process may involve the autosomes as well.

There are several other forms of nondisjunction. *Secondary nondisjunction* is that which occurs during meiosis in those individuals who are already trisomic because of a previous nondisjunctional event. This will be discussed later in connection with offspring of mothers with Down's syndrome due to trisomy 21.

The factors which lead to the production of primary nondisjunction are not understood. In Down's syndrome, the incidence of the condition increases with advancing age of the mother. Similar but less marked maternal age effect is noted also in other forms of trisomy. A possible explanation for this is that at birth the female already has all the oocytes needed for the rest of her life. The primordial germ cells have become the primary oocytes and have entered the prophase of the first meiotic division. They then remain suspended in this state for many years. The remainder of meiosis is not completed until after ovulation many years later. Thus the ova have remained dormant for many more years in the older mother than in the younger mother and there would be more opportunity for damage to the chromosomes by infection, drugs, or other environmental factors.

Mitotic nondisjunction, a third form, is that which occurs in mitosis. When it has its origin early in the embryo, a particular division results in some daughter cells having 47 chromosomes instead of 46; other daughter cells lack one chromosome and have only 45. This would produce individuals who are mosaics with two distinct cell lines, 45/47.

Anaphase Lag

Anaphase lag is another phenomenon which may account for mosaics or other chromosomal abnormalities of the types discussed. This occurs when a chromosome lags behind in cell division and is lost. The two daughter cells, therefore, have nuclei which differ in their chromosomal number, some with 45 and the others with 46 chromosomes. Each daughter cell with a different chromosomal number then perpetuates that number by continued mitosis. The individual in these circumstances will have some somatic cells with a normal number of chromosomes and other somatic cells with the deficient number of chromosomes. This would account for mosaics with cell lines of 45/46.

AUTOSOMAL ANEUPLOIDY

Trisomy 21

In 1959, Lejeune was the first to find that patients with Down's syndrome had one extra chromosome. The additional one was an acrocentric chromosome belonging to the smallest group (G) and is now accepted as chromosome 21. Subsequently, many other workers have confirmed that the basic defect in this condition is trisomy 21. Down's syndrome is more frequent with advancing age of the mother, and meiotic nondisjunction is believed to be the mechanism responsible for the trisomic state.

While most children with Down's syndrome are born of older mothers, some exceptions to this were soon discovered. These had the following characteristics which permitted their separation from the more common classic cases produced by trisomy 21: (1) there was a familial occurrence; (2) the mothers were younger; (3) the affected children had 46 instead of 47 chromosomes, but one was a peculiar large one (Fig. 3–11B); (4) the mother had 45 chromosomes but one of these was the same peculiar large chromosome which the child also had. It became apparent from a study of the normal mother that she had only 5 chromosomes in the D group instead of 6 and only one chromosome 21. It was deduced that the abnormal chromosome consisted of a translocation of chromosome 21 to chromosome 14 (or 15). In effect, therefore, the mother really had a diploid complement of chromosomes including two 14's and two 21's, one of each chromosome separately and the other two making up the translocation chromosome. Since the mother was normal, she was said to have a "balanced translocation." If the mother's oocyte were to split to form two possible ova (Fig. 3–13), it is possible for some of her children to receive a separate 21 and also the 14 with the translocated 21. Therefore, in effect, the ovum would have two 21's and one 14. If such an ovum were fertilized by a sperm containing a 21 and a 14, the zygote would be trisomic for 21 and

Figure 3–13 The mechanism for the production of a 14/21 translocation Down's syndrome (see text for detailed explanation). It should be noted that only the split of the primary oocyte which could produce Down's syndrome of the translocation type is shown. Other splits of the oocyte are possible, but for the sake of simplicity are not depicted.

In earlier work, the identity of the D group chromosome could not be established definitely and this had been designated as chromosome 13, 14, or 15, for the most part arbitrarily. The D group chromosome may vary in different families, but it is now possible to determine specific chromosomes using fluorescence or special Giemsa staining. (See Fig. 3–11B.)

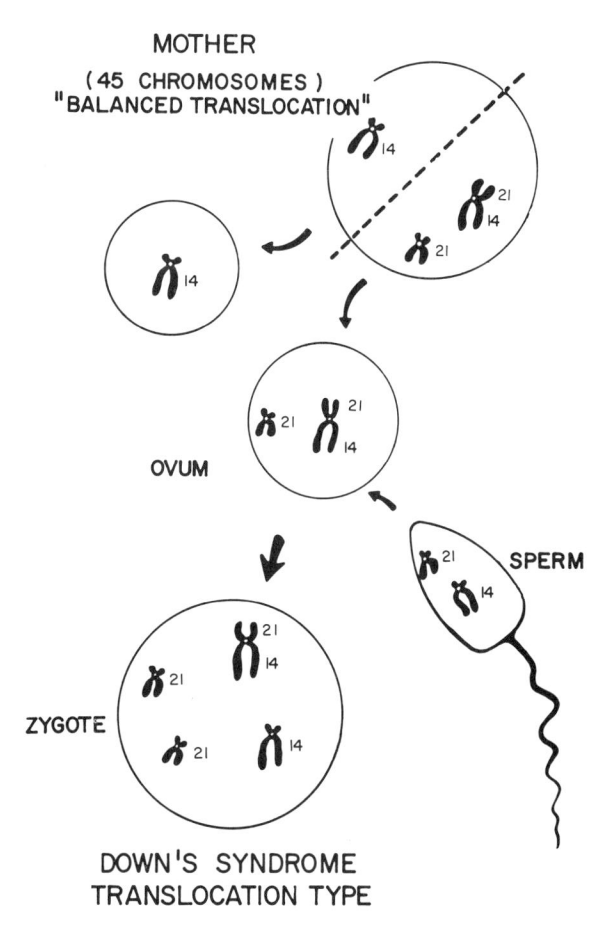

have a pair of chromosome 14. This would result in Down's syndrome owing to the translocation (translocation mongolism or interchange trisomy).

Another type of translocation mongolism is due to the translocation of one chromosome 21 to another chromosome 21. This has been called a G/G translocation because of the difficulty in determining whether it represents a 21/21 or 21/22 translocation. The difference, however, is considerable in that all the children receiving the translocation, if it were a 21/21, would have Down's syndrome. This is important in genetic counseling, and the new fluorescent or Giemsa techniques should prove to be helpful in making this distinction. Three and one-half per cent of patients with Down's syndrome are associated with translocations.

In addition to the classic and translocation types of mongolism, there are other patients who have milder forms of the disease and who have two or more cell lines, only some of which are trisomic. The normal cell lines in these mosaics appear to ameliorate the severity of the disease. Another unusual variety of Down's syndrome is double trisomy with 48 chromosomes. This occurs in the patient with trisomy 21 combined with Klinefelter's syndrome (XXY sex chromosomal constitution). This form of double trisomy has a higher frequency in the newborn period as compared to later in life. This is because of the high mortality rate early in life. Other forms of double trisomy combining Down's syndrome with the other trisomic states have also been reported.

A rare basis for Down's syndrome is the situation of the female with trisomy 21 who survives long enough to bear children. In Penrose's review of this subject, five children were born with Down's syndrome and four were normal. It appears that when separation of the three maternal 21 chromosomes occurs, the ova of the mother have two 21 chromosomes half the time. This obligatory unequal separation of the three chromosomes has been called secondary nondisjunction.

Trisomy 13 (D₁) Syndrome

Patau and his coworkers described a patient with retarded development, failure to thrive, and a very striking constellation of congenital malformations including harelip, cleft palate, microphthalmia, polydactyly, congenital heart defects, and mental retardation. The child had an extra chromosome which had the appearance of one of the D group. These chromosomes are the long acrocentrics, 13 to 15, and the chromosome involved is thought to be number 13. The syndrome is rare, occurring about 1 per 7600 births. In addition to the manifestations noted above, congenital heart disease, deafness, iris colobomas, seizures, hypotonicity, horizontal palmar creases, and capillary hemangiomas also may occur.

A new hemoglobin of embryonic origin which persisted into the neonatal period has been found in some of these cases. This hemoglobin is called Gower II and consists of two α-chains and two chains of an embryonic hemoglobin designated as ϵ-chains ($\alpha_2\epsilon_2$). This hemoglobin which is normally produced in the early embryo had not been discovered previously because it usually disappeared about the third month of intrauterine life. Peculiar nuclear projections of the polymorphonuclear leukocytes may also be found, but these are not specific.

Meiotic nondisjunction is probably the basis for this trisomic condition, but the pathophysiologic mechanism for the production of the various defects is not understood. While trisomy 13 is responsible for most cases of this syndrome, some have D/D interchange trisomy or are mosaics.

Trisomy 18 (E₁) Syndrome

A slightly more common type of congenital malformation was described by Edwards. In this, there is trisomy of chromosome 18, the smallest of the E group. These patients have developmental and mental retardation; hypertonicity; low-set ears; a peculiar flexion deformity of the fingers, with the index finger overlapping the third finger; and various congenital cardiac abnormalities. Of 143 cases of this syndrome collected by Taylor, 113 were female and only 30 were male. The reason for this abnormal sex distribution is not understood. These patients usually live for only a few months, although some survive longer. The karyotype of a patient with trisomy 18 is shown in Figure 3–14.

Other Trisomies

Theoretically, trisomies of all the other chromosomes are possible. Some have been seen in spontaneously aborted fetuses, possibly because these abnormalities are not compatible with life.

SEX CHROMOSOMAL ANEUPLOIDY

Determination of Sex

The primitive gonad is bipotential and can develop into either an ovary or a testis depending upon sex determining genes present on the sex chromosomes. Human cytogenetic studies have shown that the Y chromosome carries the male determining genes which promote testicular development from the medullary portion of the primitive gonad. In the female, normally the absence of a Y chromosome and in the presence of

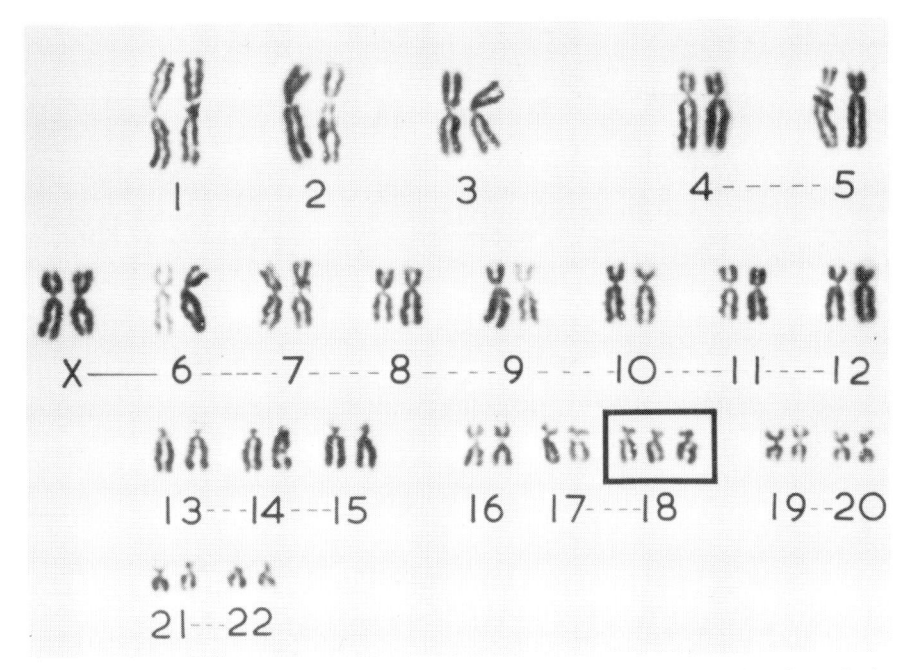

Figure 3–14 Karyotype showing 47,XX,18+ (Edwards' syndrome). The patient is a female, as is the case in the majority of reported instances. (Karyotype supplied through the courtesy of Professor Paul E. Polani.)

two X chromosomes, the cortex of the primitive gonad develops into an ovary. The importance of the Y chromosome is underlined by the fact that the XXY individual is a male despite the presence of two X chromosomes. In fact, the XXXY and the XXXXY individuals are also phenotypic males despite the additional X chromosomes which are present. On the other hand, the 45,X individual is phenotypically a female, but one with failure of ovarian differentiation, and has Turner's syndrome. This suggests that the second X chromosome is necessary for the primitive gonad to develop into an ovary.

The Sex Chromatin

Some years before the modern techniques of human chromosome analysis were developed, Barr and Bertram in 1949 discovered the presence of a condensed chromatin mass in the nuclei of females. A similar body was not present in males. The sex chromatin body (Barr body) usually appears as a plano-convex condensation of chromatin about 1μ in diameter under the nuclear membrane. Examination for the sex chromatin is a very useful and simple technique to estimate the number of X chromosomes present in the individual. In clinical practice, smears of the buccal mucosa are readily available, and these are usually studied. The sex chromatin body is seen in about 30 per cent of intact nuclei of the female. Its presence indicates that there are two X chromosomes in the cell, one of which is "inactivated" to form the Barr body. The sex chromatin body is not seen in the normal male (XY) or in the patient with classic (chromatin-negative) Turner's syndrome (XO). Subsequently, it was found that the XXX female had some cells with two chromatin bodies and the XXXX individual had some cells with three chromatin bodies (Fig. 3–15). Examination for the chromatin body provides a simple method of determining the number of X chromosomes. The number of X chromosomes would be $1+n$, where n is the number of Barr bodies.

Lyon Hypothesis

Observations on the sex chromatin body along with other biologic studies on the genetics of mice led to the Mary Lyon hypothesis that only one X chromosome is active in each cell during the interphase. The second X chromosome, if we can use an analogy from sports, "takes to the sidelines" as an inactive condensed chromatin body. Furthermore, any additional X chromosome also becomes inactive and appears as a Barr body. This helps to explain the reason that additional X chromosomes do not have the same devastating effects which the presence of extra autosomes have in Down's syndrome and the other autosomal trisomies.

The basic features of the Lyon hypothesis are that (1) in the female, all or part of one X chromosome is genetically inactive and forms the Barr body; (2) the decision about whether the maternally derived (X^M) or the paternally derived X chromosome (X^P) is the inactive one is made early in embryonic life and is random in each cell; and (3) all cells subsequently derived from each cell at the time of lyonization of the X chromosome continue to have the same inactive X chromosome, either maternal (X^M) or paternal (X^P). Therefore these cells and all their descendants have the same active X chromosome.

The Lyon hypothesis clarifies some confusing clinical and biologic problems pertaining to quantitative gene expression. Why does the male with only one X chromosome have the same amount of gene product for genes carried on the X chromosome as a female who has two X chromosomes? The level of G6PD, an enzyme in the erythrocytes and many other tissues of the body, is controlled by an X-linked gene and is approximately the same in normal males and females. Levels of coagulation Factor VIII (antihemophilic globulin) are also about the same in normal men and women despite the presence of two X chromosomes in the female. The mechanism for this "dosage compensation" can be understood in light of the Lyon hypothesis if one of the two X chromosomes of the female were inactive.

Occasionally a heterozygous female for the hemophilia trait has a bleeding disorder manifested by reduced circulating Factor VIII. Why is this X-linked recessive trait expressed? The Lyon hypothesis provides one explanation. Since inactivation of one X chromosome is a random event, occasionally almost all X chromosomes containing the normal allele for Factor VIII are inactivated, leaving only the X chromosomes containing the mutant allele.

Turner's Syndrome (Ovarian Dysgenesis)

This syndrome is a form of primary hypogonadism in phenotypic females who have gonadal aplasia with infantile genitalia, amenorrhea, short stature, and a lack of secondary sex characteristics. A variety of congenital defects, includ-

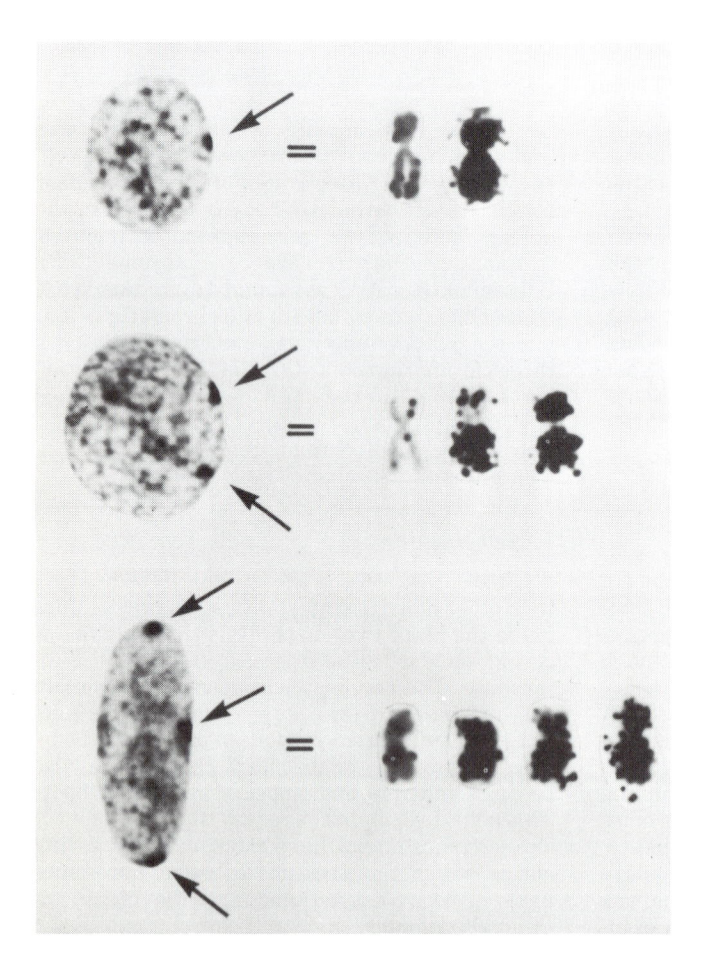

Figure 3-15 Three cell nuclei from XX, XXX, and XXXX individuals are shown. These demonstrate the number of Barr bodies designated by the arrows. Alongside each nucleus are the X chromosomes from metaphase plates after labeling with tritiated thymidine. Note that all X chromosomes in excess of one are late-labeling. (Photograph supplied through the courtesy of Professor Paul E. Polani.)

ing webbing of the neck and coarctation of the aorta may accompany the syndrome. The nipples are widely spaced on the chest and pigmented nevi are frequently present on the skin. Lymphedema has been described when the syndrome occurs in the early weeks of life. The syndrome is accompanied by high gonadotropin excretion in the urine and low urinary estrogens, as would be expected in primary gonadal failure. About 60 to 80 per cent of these individuals are chromatin-negative and cytogenetic studies have shown that their karyotype is 45,X.

The number of patients with Turner's syndrome is believed to be only a small fraction of the total number of conceptions with the 45,X karyotype. Many studies show that this karyotype occurs frequently in spontaneously aborted fetuses. The frequency with which it is found suggests that over 90 per cent of such conceptuses are aborted and only less than 10 per cent survive to be born and show Turner's syndrome.

Interesting associations with Turner's syndrome are the clinical accompaniment of Hashimoto's thyroiditis and the even more frequent finding of circulating antibodies to thyroglobulin. These associations may be more common in patients with the syndrome produced by the isochromosome X. Studies of thyroid function in patients with Turner's syndrome showed that even in the absence of clinical hypothyroidism, patients with Turner's syndrome who had thyroid antibodies had a low thyroid reserve. The association of thyroid antibodies in these patients brings up the question of whether the development of antibodies is the consequence of the chromosomal abnormality or whether the reverse might be true. Engel and Forbes found a high incidence of thyroid antibodies in the families of these patients and speculated that the tendency to autoantibody formation in the parents might affect the germ cell development or in some other way be related to the chromosomal abnormalities of the children.

In contrast to the majority of patients with Turner's syndrome, some patients are chromatin positive and have a normal number of chromosomes. In some of the patients, the 44 autosomes were all normal, as would be expected, and a single normal-appearing X chromosome was present. The other (46th) chromosome was a large metacentric chromosome that looked more like chromosome 3 than like any other (Fig. 3-16). This structurally abnormal chromosome was called an isochromosome X. This abnormal chromosome is believed to arise as a result of misdivision through the centromere rather than the normal longitudinal division (Fig. 3-17). This concept of the origin of the isochromosome X is now capable of being studied by newer techniques and verification of this hypothesis should be possible. If this proves to be correct, each chromatid would be composed of long arms of the X which are mirror images of each other. Thus, in individuals who have a normal X and an isochromosome X, the short arms of the X are represented only once on the normal X chromosome, whereas the long arms are represented three times, once on the normal X and twice on the arms of the isochromosome. Isotopic studies show that the isochromosome X is the late-labeling one (i.e., the normal X chromosome synthesizes its DNA first). In the decision as to which X chromosome becomes the Barr body at the time of lyonization, the isochromosome X becomes the inactive one.

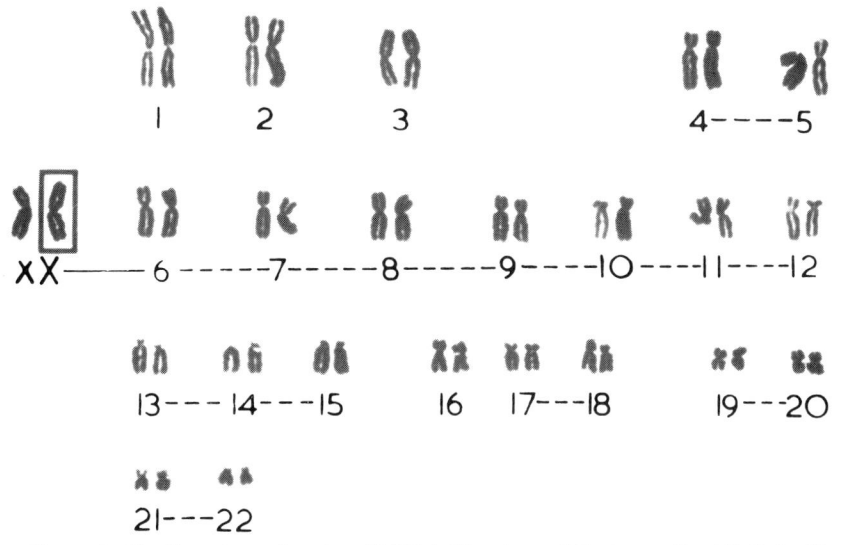

Figure 3-16 Karyotype showing 46,XXqi. (Courtesy of Professor Paul E. Polani.)

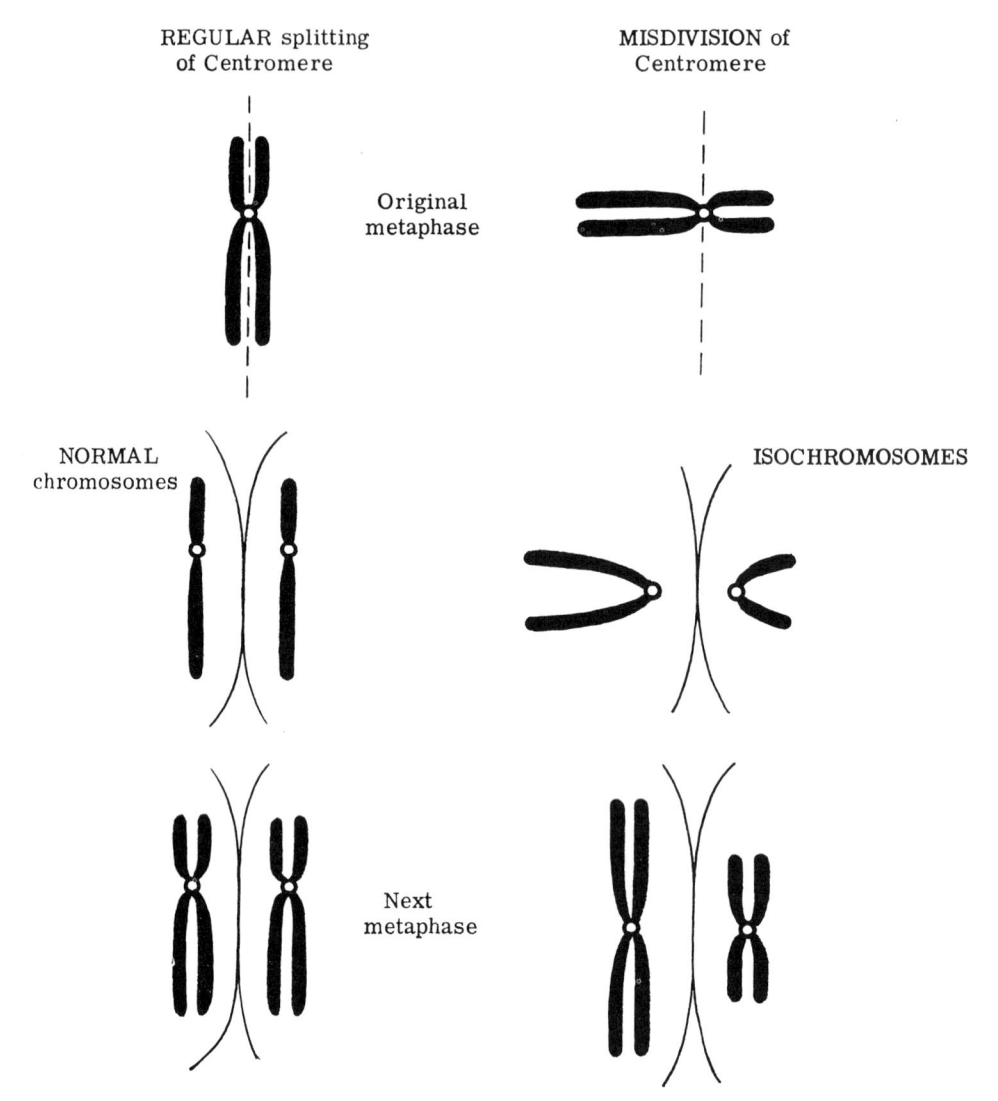

Figure 3–17 The mechanism for production of an isochromosome. (From Hamerton, J. L. (Ed.): Chromosomes in Medicine. London, William Heinemann Medical Books, Ltd., 1962.)

MEDICAL GENETICS

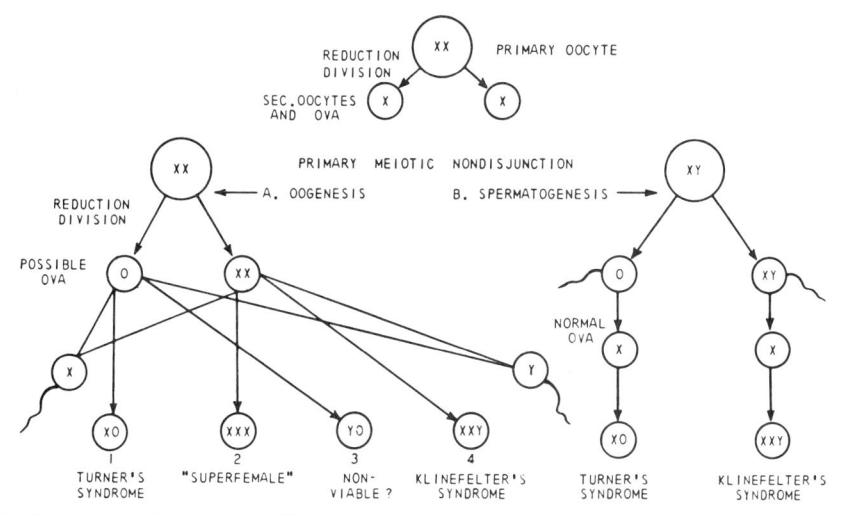

Figure 3-18 Meiotic division and nondisjunction. In normal meiotic division of a primary oocyte, each of the secondary oocytes and ova contains one X chromosome. For simplification, the polar bodies are ignored. The same process in spermatogenesis leads to X or Y chromosome-containing sperm. *A*, In primary meiotic nondisjunction involving oogenesis, an ovum with no X chromosomes and another with both X chromosomes are shown. In each instance, the result of fertilization by an X-containing sperm and the result of fertilization by a Y-containing sperm are depicted. The possible combinations could lead to Turner's syndrome, an XXX "superfemale," or Klinefelter's syndrome. The YO offspring has not yet been shown for humans and is nonviable in the Drosophila. *B*, Primary meiotic nondisjunction is shown occurring in spermatogenesis. Each possible sperm is shown fertilizing a normal ovum.

The chromatin body produced may sometimes be seen as larger than usual because of the greater amount of material involved.

Turner's syndrome with one normal X and another chromosome which appears to be a smaller X has been described (Xx). Since some of the classic features are lacking, this condition has been called "partial Turner's syndrome." Other patients with an abnormal X chromosome in the shape of a ring have also been described (XXr).

In addition to these two rarer varieties of the syndrome, a form due to mosaicism has been described frequently. Among these have been mosaics with 45/46 chromosomes, XO/XX or XO/XY; 45/47 chromosomes, XO/XXX, or XO/XYY, and even more complex mosaics with three different cell types of 45/46/47 chromosomes, XO/XX/XXX. The mosaics may be chromatin positive or negative, depending upon the number of X chromosomes present in the cells studied. Originally, it was felt that the syndrome had its origin in meiotic nondisjunction (Fig. 3-18), but another explanation for the occurrence of the chromosomal abnormalities found in Turner's syndrome has its basis in the relative frequency of these mosaic types. This hypothesis suggests that it occurs after the formation of the zygote rather than before. During a mitotic division, the diploid zygote, which is either XX or XY, loses either the second X or the Y and becomes monosomic, 45,X. Support for this mechanism is suggested by the fact that advanced maternal age is less obvious in Turner's syndrome than in either Down's syndrome or Klinefelter's syndrome.

Klinefelter's Syndrome

This syndrome is one of the common forms of primary hypogonadism and infertility in the male. It occurs about once in every 400 live male births and does not appear to be a cause of spontaneous abortion. It is estimated that 8.5 per cent of all males attending infertility clinics have Klinefelter's syndrome. The condition was described in 1942 in phenotypic males who had small, firm testes, azoospermia, and elevated levels of gonadotropin in the urine. Gynecomastia occurs in 40 to 50 per cent of the cases, and mental abnormalities occur in about 25 per cent. Its association with some degree of mental retardation is evident, in that about 1:100 inmates in institutions for the mentally retarded have Klinefelter's. In the mid 1950's it was discovered that these individuals were chromatin positive, as were normal females. Soon after the application of cytogenetic techniques, it was found that these patients had a karyotype of 47,XXY. Several mosaic varieties of Klinefelter's syndrome such as 46,XY/47,XXY and 46,XX/47,XXY have been described. The syndrome in these patients tends to be milder.

The origin of the abnormal karyotype is not clear but probably occurs as a result of primary meiotic nondisjunction (Fig. 3–18). There is some degree of association with advanced maternal age in this syndrome, but it is less pronounced than in Down's syndrome. Pedigree studies using color vision and other X-linked genes as markers show that more XXY individuals have both XX from the mother. This favors the mechanism of meiotic nondisjunction as the mechanism for its occurrence.

Another theoretical mechanism is its occurrence in mitotic nondisjunction in division of the zygote. In this situation, the X and Y replicate to form two X's and two Y's before cell division takes place. At this point, if the nondisjunctional division results in the separation of the chromosomes so that one daughter cell gets XXY and the other only the Y, the cell line with the single Y (and no X chromosomes) would be nonviable and therefore only the XXY line would survive.

Additional varieties of Klinefelter's syndrome other than the chromatin-positive type with one Barr body have been described. One type has 48 chromosomes, two Barr bodies, and the sex chromosomes are XXXY; another has three Barr bodies, XXXXY, and a total of 49 chromosomes. The clinical picture of hypogonadism is present, but there seems to be a greater degree of mental retardation with each additional X chromosome. In addition, the XXXXY variety may have several additional features, including skeletal anomalies. Radioulnar synostoses have occurred, and the condition is characterized by a more severe hypogonadism, with hypoplasia of the penis and scrotum. Neither the explanation for the more marked mental retardation with increasing numbers of X chromosomes nor the explanation for the associated skeletal anomalies is known.

Another variety of Klinefelter's syndrome is that resulting from the karyotype 48,XXYY. It is similar to the usual Klinefelter's but the patients may be somewhat taller. This brings up the YY syndrome, which will now be discussed.

YY Syndrome

In 1965, a syndrome was described in males with two Y chromosomes. These men were found in maximum security institutions and (1) were unusually tall, usually over 6 feet, (2) were mentally subnormal, and (3) showed antisocial aggressive behavior. Many were incarcerated because of crimes of a violent nature. Recent studies have shown that the incidence of this karyotype is not as infrequent as was originally thought. Also, many of these individuals did not manifest the aggressive behavior problems which were noted at first. Some of the crimes perpetrated by these YY individuals have been minor and have not involved violence. The explanation for the tall stature is unknown. Since growth hormone is one of the factors influencing body growth, it was studied in four cases and in each case the levels were within normal limits. It is estimated to occur in about 1:1000 male births. One recent prospective study of newborn infants reported an even greater incidence, 1:250. The medicolegal aspects of the YY syndrome are quite complex and beyond the scope of this chapter. They are in urgent need of clarification.

The technique of fluorescent staining of mitotic chromosomes with quinacrine has been of great help in studies of the Y chromosome. The distal portion of the long arm of the Y chromosome fluoresces brightly and it can be detected easily (Fig. 3–19). The technique has been adapted to human interphase nuclei so that it is now possible to detect the presence of the Y chromosome in the interphase nuclei of peripheral blood lymphocytes. This enables the clinician to screen for Y chromosomes as simply as he can estimate the number of X chromosomes by studying Barr bodies. The fluorescent spot of the Y chromosome has been called the Y-body (Fig. 3–20). Buccal mucosa can be studied, as in the case of the Barr bodies, but caution must be exercised in interpretation, because fluorescence of bacteria in the mouth flora may be confusing.

Multi-X Females

The normal female has two X chromosomes, but females with more than two X chromosomes have been described. The triple-X female (47,XXX) has two Barr bodies. Although the first patient with this disorder had secondary amenorrhea, no characteristic clinical picture has been defined.

Although about one third of the triple-X females have shown a variety of congenital defects, the majority are normal except for some tendency to show mental subnormality. Most have a normal reproductive system and are fertile. Children born to such mothers are usually normal but in a few instances have had chromosomal abnormalities. In these cases, the mothers have been mosaics. The fact that the majority of the children have normal chromosome complements is in contrast to the situation in children of mothers with Down's syndrome.

Tetra-X females with XXXX, three Barr bodies, and 48 chromosomes, and the penta-X state with XXXXX, four Barr bodies, and 49 chromosomes, have also been described. There is a greater degree of mental subnormality with the progressive increase in number of X chromosomes for reasons unclear at present.

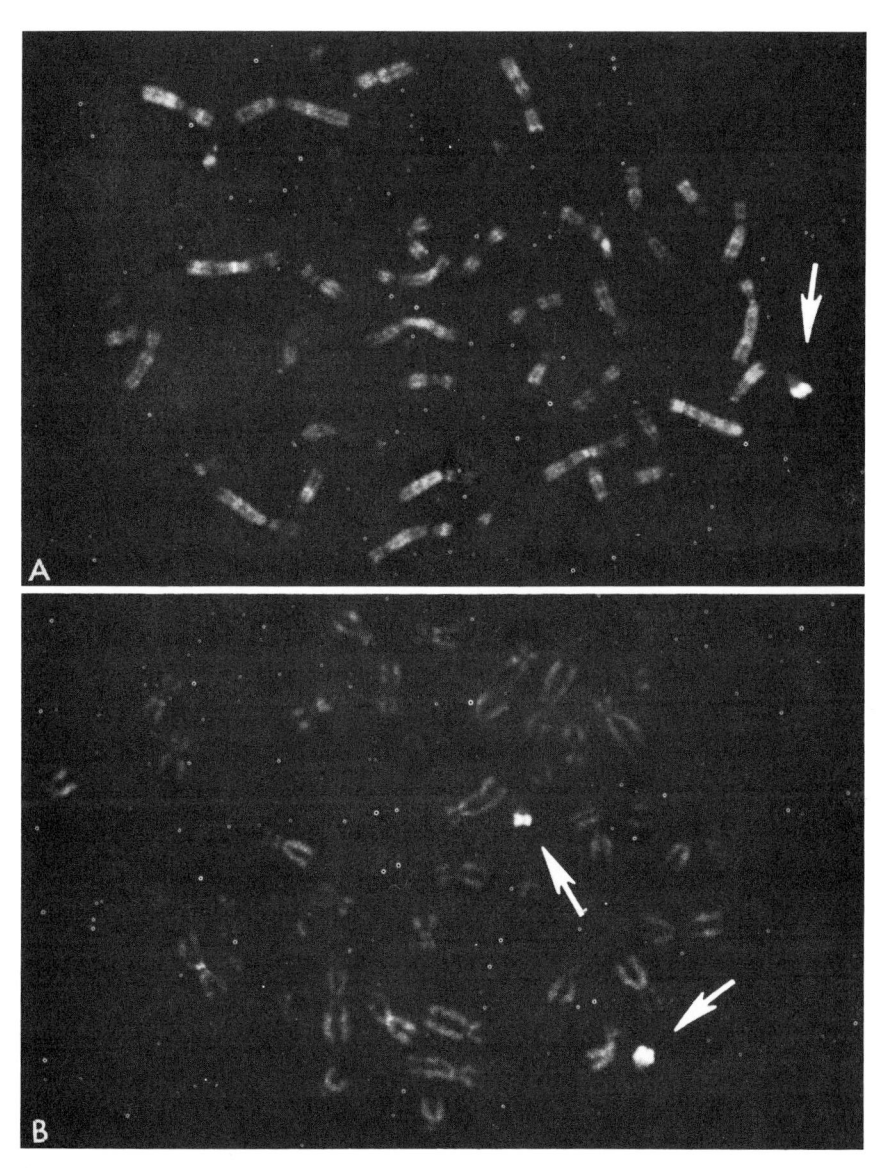

Figure 3-19 *A,* Metaphase plates stained with quinacrine mustard (QM). This plate shows the Y chromosome in a normal male, 46,XY. *B,* This plate shows two fluorescent Y chromosomes in a male with 47,XYY.

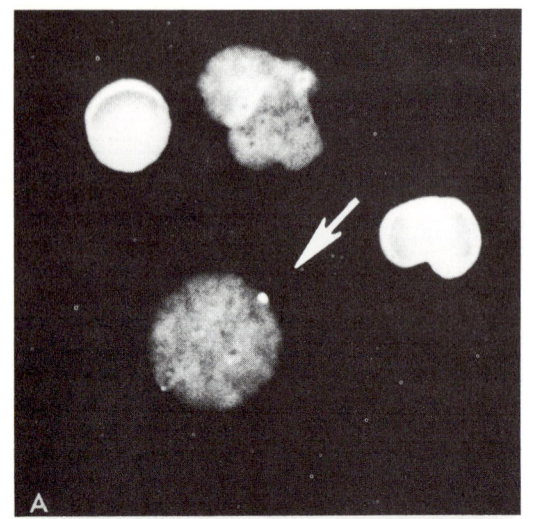

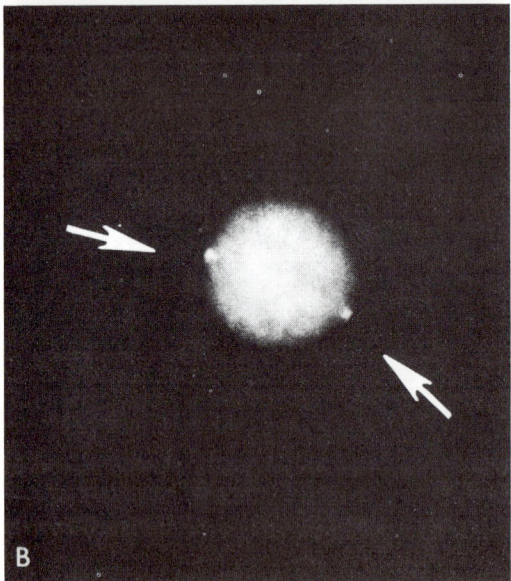

Figure 3-20 *A,* Peripheral blood lymphocytes stained with quinacrine mustard (QM). This plate shows a single Y-body. These are seen in from 25 to 50 per cent of cells. Sometimes the body may be divided into two parts and these may be separated, simulating the situation when two Y chromosomes are present. *B,* Peripheral blood lymphocytes stained with quinacrine mustard (QM). This plate shows two Y-bodies in a patient with the YY chromosome, 47,XYY.

STRUCTURAL ABNORMALITIES OF THE CHROMOSOMES

Although the total number may be normal, the chromosomes may be abnormal in structure. This may result from chromosome breakage. Probably in most instances the broken pieces are repaired and rejoin normally, so that there is no basic change. If this does not happen, the separated fragment of a chromosome becomes attached to another chromosome or it is not viable and is lost. This produces deletions. If the broken piece attaches to another chromosome, a translocation is produced.

Translocations

If the separated chromosomal fragment becomes attached to another chromosome, it is said to be translocated. Sometimes parts of two different chromosomes exchange places with each other, producing a reciprocal translocation. If the translocated piece is large enough, the chromosome to which it is attached will be morphologically altered and can be recognized as abnormal. If, however, the translocated piece is very small, it may not be possible to recognize this under the microscope using conventional techniques, and it may be overlooked. It is possible that many small translocations are undetected for this reason. Translocations which have clinical significance in human cytogenetics involve either a whole chromosome or the major portion of one. These have been discussed previously in connection with Down's syndrome and the 21/14 and 21/21 translocations.

Deletions

A number of syndromes associated with the deletion of a piece of chromosome have now been reported. The most common and best characterized is the 5p− syndrome or the *cri du chat syndrome* described by Lejeune in 1963. This is produced by a deletion of the short arm of chromosome number 5 and is characterized by failure to thrive and microcephaly, associated with a round face, severe mental retardation, wide-set eyes, epicanthic folds, and a simian crease. The major feature of this disorder is the characteristic weak mewing cry like that of a suffering kitten. The peculiar cry results from delayed maturation of the larynx and this feature is lost as the infant grows older.

The factors involved in the break of the chromosome are not known. Maternal and paternal ages are not apparently increased, as is the case in Down's syndrome. About 10 to 15 per cent of cases are due to a translocation analogous to translocation Down's syndrome. Under these circumstances, one of the parents is a carrier of the translocation and transmits the 5p− chromosome to the child.

A brief summary of the data on the other deletion syndromes is presented in Table 3–5.

TABLE 3-5 THE DELETION SYNDROMES

Chomosome Deletion	Brief Clinical Description	Appearance of Chromosome
4p—	Low birth weight No cat cry Cleft palate Carp mouth Beaked nose Preauricular dimples Hypospadias	Abnormally long acrocentric; late replicator with H^3 thymidine.
5p—	More common Mental retardation Cat cry Hypertelorism	Abnormally long acrocentric; only 3 normal B group chromosomes present; early replicator.
Dq—	Very rare Some features like trisomy 13	Like an extra 18 but only 5 D's present.
18p—	More common Microcephaly Mental and growth retardation	Like an 18 without short arms.
18q—	As common as 18p— Microcephaly, hypotonia Carp mouth—central facial dysplasia Ear abnormalities Congenital heart disease in one third	Only one 18 present; an extra chromosome like a G group but patient does not have Down's syndrome.
Gq—	Called "antimongolism" Eyes slant downward Hypertonia	A minute chromosome, but with variable G structure; Gq— or Gr; often mosaics.

Other Structural Changes

Inversions result from two breaks along the course of a chromosome and re-alignment after a 180-degree reversal of the order of the chromosome. This subject has been reviewed by Polani. If the breaks are on the same side of the centromere, a *paracentric* inversion occurs and the re-alignment does not change the shape of the chromosome. If the breaks occur on opposite sides of the centromere, a *pericentric* inversion occurs and if the segments are unequal in size, the position of the centromere may be altered.

Chromosomes and Leukemia

In 1960, Nowell and Hungerford in Philadelphia reported the association of a G-group chromosomal abnormality with chronic granulocytic leukemia. They found that what they considered to be chromosome 21 had lost about one half the material of its long arm. This was believed to be a deletion, although a translocation of the deleted piece to another larger chromosome could not be ruled out. The abnormality was designated as the Ph^1 chromosome, or the Philadelphia chromosome (Fig. 3-21). This finding represented a milestone in that, although chromosomal abnormalities in malignant disease were known for many years, this was the first time that a *specific* chromosomal abnormality was associated with a specific malignant condition. The Ph^1 chromosome is believed to be a somatic mutation which takes place in a relatively undifferentiated hemopoietic cell. The abnormal chromosome appears only in cells of the granulocytic, erythrocytic, and megakaryocytic series. Cultures of other tissues such as skin or even lymphocytes have not shown the Ph^1 chromosome. It is present in 80 to 90 per cent of cases of chronic granulocytic leukemia. The Ph^1 negative cases show atypical features and tend to be either older patients or young children, do not respond as well to treatment, and have a shorter survival. The Ph^1 negative cases show a predominance of males over females.

It is also noteworthy that the abnormality can be found in cells in the marrow even when treatment induces a complete remission of the disease, characterized by normalization of blood counts, regression of splenomegaly, and the return to normal of leukocytic alkaline phosphatase level. The Ph^1 chromosome has been found also in the terminal phase of chronic granulocytic leukemia when an acute blast crisis has supervened. Aneuploidy may then become manifest and two Ph^1 chromosomes may be present.

Since the Ph^1 chromosome is a long arm deletion of a G-group chromosome, it can be written as Gq—, which indicates the deletion of the long arm of one of the G-group (21 to 22) chromosomes. Originally, it was thought that chromosome 21 was the one involved, the same chromosome which was implicated in Down's syndrome. This led to a number of speculations because of the known frequency of leukemia in patients with Down's syndrome. The locus for the gene for leukocytic alkaline phosphatase (LAP) was thought to be located on the 21 chromosome, since the LAP is very low in chronic granulocytic leukemia and it was found to be elevated in trisomic Down's syndrome. These speculations may now be laid to rest. It seems fairly well established that the G-group chromosome involved in chronic granulocytic leukemia is different from the one involved in Down's syndrome. Most authorities and worldwide usage have designated the chromosome involved in Down's syndrome as 21; the Ph[1] chromosome, therefore, should now be designated as 22. This conclusion is based on two sets of evidence. First, in a patient with chronic granulocytic leukemia whose Ph[1] chromosome had long satellites, Prieto et al. showed with tritiated thymidine labeling that the chromosome had labeling times different from those of the chromosome in Down's syndrome. Second, Caspersson, using the quinacrine mustard fluorescent technique, also showed that the Ph[1] chromosome belonged to the pair which had the lighter fluorescent staining, whereas the 21 chromosome had the brighter fluorescence. Whether the abnormality is a pure deletion or whether the deleted piece is translocated to one of the other larger chromosomes could not be clarified by these studies.

Chromosomal studies in other types of leukemia have not been as fruitful as those in chronic granulocytic leukemia. In chronic lymphocytic leukemia, the karyotype has been found to be normal, or abnormalities found have not been consistent. A possible exception to this was described by Gunz and Fitzgerald, who found an abnormal G-group chromosome resulting from a deletion of the short arm in two siblings with chronic lymphocytic leukemia and in several normal members of their family. This chromosome was designated Ch[1] (Christchurch, New Zealand) and was thought possibly to be related to familial cases of chronic lymphocytic leukemia. This finding has not been confirmed by other studies and a similar chromosomal abnormality has been found in normal individuals. At the moment, the status of the Ch[1] chromosome and its relationship to chronic lymphocytic leukemia is not clear, but most authorities consider it to be a coincidental association.

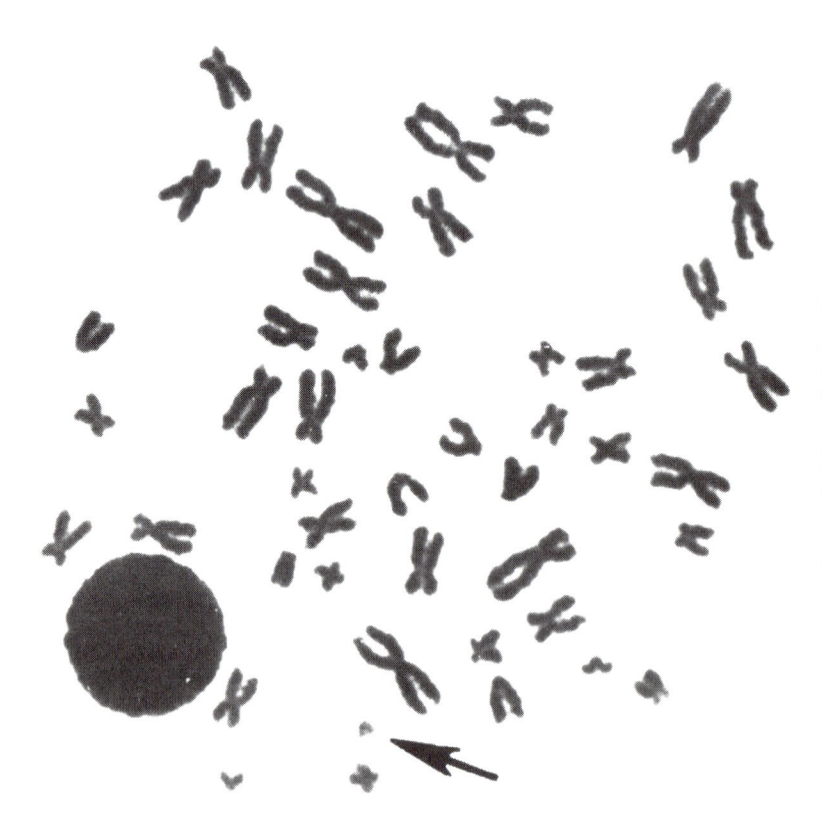

Figure 3–21 A metaphase plate from a patient with chronic granulocytic leukemia, 46,XY,-Gq—. The Philadelphia chromosome is shown by the arrow and results from a deletion of about one half the long arm of a G group chromosome. Originally it was thought to be chromosome 21, the same one as is involved in Down's syndrome. Recent studies indicate that it is chromosome 22 (see text).

In acute leukemia, many cytogenetic abnormalities have been found, but these have not been consistent. Numerical and structural abnormalities of the chromosomes have been noted. The abnormalities have been found to disappear when complete remission of the disease has been induced by treatment. Subsequent relapse of the disease has resulted in the reappearance of the same chromosomal abnormalities which existed originally. The abnormalities included various types of aneuploidy, but these were not the same in different patients.

CHROMOSOME BREAKAGE

Chromosome breakage is induced by or associated with a number of factors. These are (1) radiation, (2) viruses, (3) chemicals and drugs, and (4) some rare diseases associated with spontaneous chromosome breakage. In examining routine normal cultures, a small number of metaphase cells may show a few simple breaks. The frequency of these varies from one laboratory to another and even at different times in the same laboratory. The significance of these is unknown and they may be in-vitro phenomena related to the manipulations in culturing the chromosomes.

When a chromosome breaks in vivo, it is believed that under most circumstances the broken ends of the chromosomes reunite without incident, and there is no residual evidence of the previous defect. Alternatively, the break may persist as an obvious displacement in the continuity of the chromosome. Aside from actual breaks, one may also see lighter areas with no apparent displacement along the course of the chromatid. These areas are called *gaps* and their relationship to breakage is not clear except for the fact that they are more frequent when obvious breakage is present. Sometimes the broken ends join in a positional rearrangement to produce a striking structural abnormality in the form of translocations, ring chromosomes, or dicentric chromosomes.

The effect of radiation on chromosomes has been known for a long time, and the abnormalities produced may persist for many years after the exposure. Small amounts of radiation such as are incurred during routine chest x-ray examination or other brief procedures do not appear to cause any significant damage to the chromosomes. Greater degrees of exposure such as those associated with gastrointestinal series are accompanied by changes in the chromosomes. Some of these are transient and disappear in a period of weeks.

Viruses may damage the chromosomes, and this is seen when some viruses are added to cultures. Chemotherapeutic agents such as nitrogen mustard, methotrexate, and others used in treating hematologic malignant conditions produce chromosome damage. A more controversial subject is whether LSD damages the chromosomes.

Several inherited diseases associated with chromosomal breaks have stimulated a great deal of interest in recent years. This is particularly the case because of the apparent association of some of these diseases to either leukemia or lymphoma. *Bloom's syndrome* is a rare disease of children characterized by a sun-sensitive telangiectatic erythema, low birth weight, stunted growth, and presumed recessive inheritance pattern. These children have cytogenetic abnormalities resulting from increased chromosome breakage. There is also a high risk for the development of leukemia. *Fanconi's anemia* is another disease with presumed recessive inheritance and is characterized by bone marrow failure with pancytopenia; pigmentation of the skin; congenital malformations of the skeleton, eye, or kidney; hypogonadism; and an increased risk of leukemia. This syndrome also is associated with an increase in chromosome breakage. Information on several other diseases is less well documented and more study is needed. One of these is the *ataxia-telangiectasia* syndrome, which is characterized by progressive cerebellar ataxia, multiple telangiectasia of the skin and eye, and recurrent sinopulmonary infections. It appears also to be inherited in a recessive manner. About 70 per cent of the patients have an absence of IgA and there is an increased risk for the development of lymphoma. The greater risk for the development of either leukemia or lymphoma gives these rare conditions a greater importance than their relative frequency would otherwise warrant.

CHROMOSOMES AND CANCER

Neoplasia has been associated with a number of factors including the oncogenic viruses, ionizing radiation, and various carcinogenic chemicals. As has been noted already, these agents also produce chromosome breakage which can be the basis for chromosomal rearrangements. Abnormal mitotic figures resulting from chromosomal rearrangements have been noted as a hallmark of malignancy for many years. In fact, the idea of specific chromosomal changes as a cause of cancer was suggested by Boveri as early as 1914. The discovery of the Ph[1] chromosome and its association with chronic granulocytic leukemia has led to renewed interest in this subject. The association of leukemia and Down's syndrome (trisomy 21) is well known. The risk of leukemia in patients with Down's syndrome is increased twentyfold, and this has led to speculations concerning the relationship of aneuploidy to the development of leukemia. Rare instances of leukemia developing in aneuploid individuals with trisomy 13, Klinefelter's syndrome, and Turner's syndrome have been reported. Interest in the possible relationship of chromosome breakage to leukemia was stimulated by the finding of the Ph[1] chromosome. Several instances of leukemia occurring in individuals who reportedly used LSD have been noted and these findings have supported the speculations concerning the possible leukemogenic effects of chromosomal abnormalities.

Studies of other tumors show that in these cases there are marked chromosomal changes, but the question of whether there is a cause and effect relationship is not settled. In view of developments in leukemia, it is an attractive hypothesis to consider the chromosomal changes as primary and the malignant condition to result from the chromosomal change. It has been hypothesized not only that the chromosomal aberrations may be produced by viruses, radiation, and chemicals but that immunologic influences and autoimmune disease may be an added factor in the sequence of chromosomal aberrations to leukemia. The entire subject is in need of further study and clarification.

CHROMOSOMES AND AGING

Several studies have shown that a small proportion of human somatic cells become aneuploid with advancing age. This occurs particularly over 60 years of age but is more common in women, in whom about 10 to 13 per cent of the cells appear to lose a C-group (?X) chromosome. In the male, the number of aneuploid cells is less and the lost chromosome appears to be a Y chromosome. Not all investigators are in full agreement on the occurrence of hypodiploidy in the aged, but the subject is important because of its possible significance to the aging process.

The relationship of the chromosomal abnormalities to the various disease states and the other conditions discussed above is not clear. Large deletions may result in the loss of genes located on the deleted part of the chromosome. Additional genes made available by trisomy or duplications also would have some effect. Even inversions, by altering the linear order of genes, could have an effect on the individual. These changes could result in biochemical disturbances which are obscure at the present time. These disturbances may be elucidated in due course and a clearer understanding of the pathophysiology will be available at that time.

BIOCHEMICAL BASIS FOR INHERITANCE

The basic unit of inheritance first postulated by Mendel must have at least three properties. It must control a specific function in the organism. It must replicate and transmit this function from one generation to the next. It must mutate and produce variations in this function. This basic unit of inheritance should be present in all cells of the organism. The physical basis for these properties is satisfied by the chromosome. Reduction division seen during meiosis and gamete formation, recombination during zygote formation, chromosome replication preceding mitosis, and phenotypic aberrations associated with abnormal chromosomes satisfy these requirements.

Watson and Crick, in 1953, first pointed out that deoxyribonucleic acid (DNA) was a biochemical contained in bacteria and in the cell nucleus of mammals and satisfied the requirements at a molecular level. Since the concepts of the inborn errors of metabolism relate to primary defects in gene structure and the function of their protein products, a brief review of the structure of DNA and of the regulation of gene expression is useful. The Watson-Crick model for DNA proposed that it consisted of two antiparallel polynucleotide chains coiled around a common axis to form a double helix (Fig. 3–22). A continuous

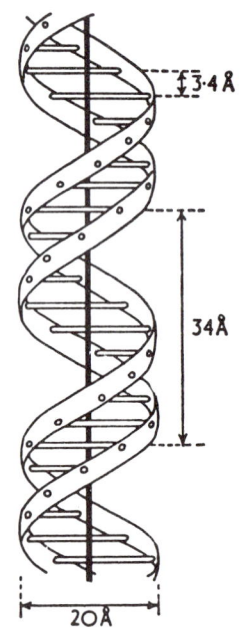

Figure 3–22 The double helical model of DNA as proposed by Watson and Crick. Each helical strip is composed of deoxyribose linked by phosphate bonds at 3 and 5 position. Paired bases joined by hydrogen bonding provide a loose association between the two chains. Each full turn of the double helix (34 Å) contains 10 base pairs. (From Watson, J. D., and Crick, F. H. C.: Nature, *171*:737, 1958.)

chain is formed, consisting of alternating molecules of deoxyribose joined at their 3 and 5 position by phosphate. The two single strands appear like the banisters of a spiral staircase. The steps or horizontal bars represent a paired purine and pyrimidine, loosely bound by hydrogen bonds. Guanine (G) is paired with cytosine (C), and adenine (A) with thymine (T). This complementary base pairing must be purine with pyrimidine, and only adenine pairs with thymine and only guanine with cytosine. The double-helical model, with its base pairs oriented internally and joined by noncovalent bonds, provides a molecular method of replication. Each strand can unwind, separate, and serve as a template for replication of a new thread derived from substrates in the cell. A single strand of DNA permits only the insertion of that base complementary to it on the new strand of DNA as it grows alongside the original strand. This semiconservative model for replication of the DNA molecule was confirmed by Meselson and Stahl (Fig. 3-23). The original parent molecule of DNA dissociates and each strand directs the synthesis of a new strand complementary to itself. Thus, the first generation daughter molecules contain one original and one newly synthesized helical strand. In the second generation, one half the molecules are composed of two new strands and one half contain an original and a newly formed strand. In microbial systems, purified DNA polymerase can use a primer single strand of DNA and replicate by matching one of the four deoxyribose triphosphates (GTP, ATP, CTP, or TTP) with the complementary base on the primer strand. The chain grows by adding appropriate bases at the 3' hydroxy group and releasing pyrophosphate. DNA replication in chromosomes of higher organisms is more complex and less well understood. Autoradiographic studies indicate that several points along the chromosome may replicate.

The double helix model provides several possibilities for error or mutation. For instance, the base might exist in its tautomeric form and, during replication, pair with a new base not complementary to the original strand. This erroneous base would then direct the insertion of a new base complementary to itself in the second and subsequent generations. Mutations are produced also by chemicals which are structurally similar to the bases. Bromodeoxyuridine is structurally similar to thymine but pairs with guanine rather than adenine. If this pyrimidine analog were incorporated into the DNA strand, guanine would replace adenine in subsequently formed strands. Many other mutagenic agents are known such as

Figure 3-23 Model for semiconservative DNA replication. Solid, black helical strands represent original DNA molecules; open, white strands represent DNA freshly synthesized from the media. In the first generation, there is a 1:1 ratio of old to freshly synthesized strands. In the second generation, only 2 of 8 or one fourth are original strands. (From Meselson, M., and Stahl, F. W.: Proc. Nat. Acad. Sci., 44:671, 1958.)

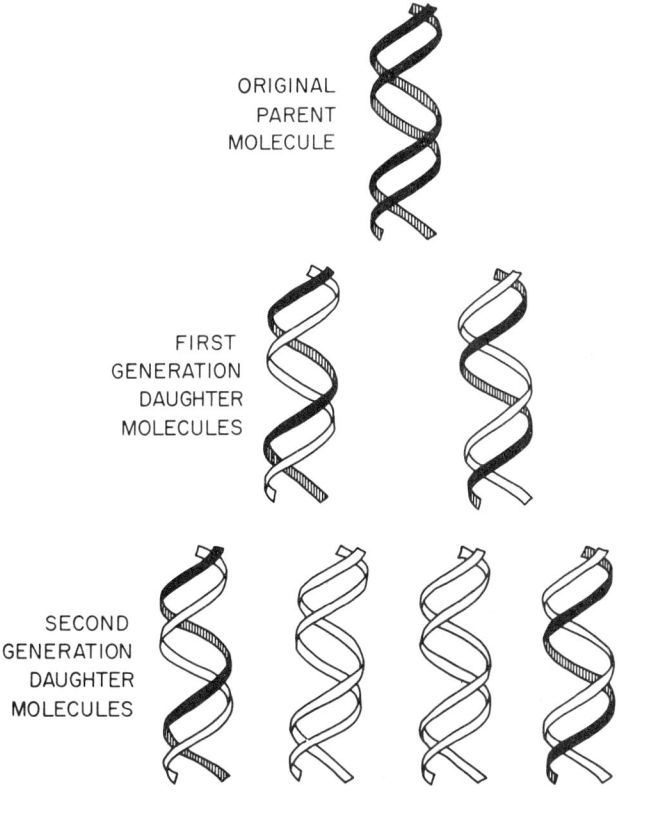

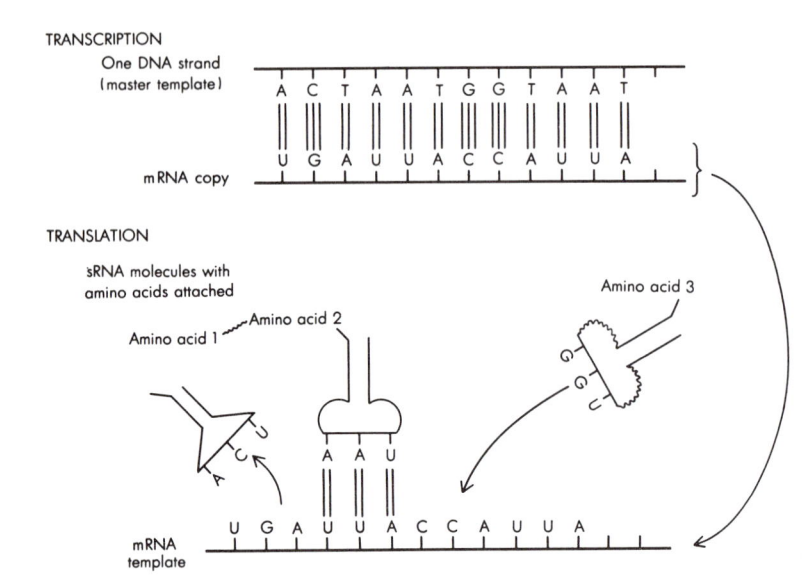

Figure 3-24 A model for the transcription and translation of DNA into proteins. (From Hartman, P. E., and Suskind, S. R.: Gene Action. Foundations of Modern Genetics Series, Englewood Cliffs, Prentice-Hall, Inc., 1965.)

acridine dyes, nitrogen mustards, nitrous acid, and ultraviolet light. Ultraviolet light increases the incidence of interaction between bases on the same strand. These dimers (thymine-thymine) are excised in one process (dark repair). Using the other DNA strand as a template, new bases are then inserted. Abnormalities in this repair mechanism are reflected in man by the disease *xeroderma pigmentosum*. In this autosomal recessive trait, an endonuclease necessary to initiate repair is defective, and thymine-thymine dimers are not excised at a normal rate.

The DNA molecule can replicate and undergo variation. How does it relate to the organ or cell function? It is probable from bacteria and from a few examples in mammalian systems that the amino acid sequence of a polypeptide chain is determined by the sequence of bases on a single strand of DNA. The operational scheme by which genetic information coded on a single DNA strand is transcribed to messenger RNA and translated into a sequence of amino acids on a growing peptide chain is outlined in Figure 3-24. The mechanisms involved are detailed in another chapter, but the events will be summarized briefly here.

There are three classes of ribonucleic acid (RNA) which enable DNA to direct the synthesis of polypeptides. Messenger RNA (mRNA) is formed upon a template of single-stranded DNA. Messenger RNA is a single-stranded nucleic acid similar to DNA but contains ribose rather than deoxyribose, and uracil (U) instead of thymine (T). Messenger RNA associates with a second class of stable RNA, ribosomal RNA in the cytoplasm. Amino acids in the cytoplasm are activated by "activating enzymes" and "recognized" by a third class of RNA, soluble or transfer RNA (sRNA). Soluble RNA has an additional recognition site which binds to complementary bases on the mRNA strand. Each amino acid has a specific sRNA which attaches to its carboxy end and to the mRNA-ribosomal complex at the complementary site on the mRNA template. The sequence of amino acids is determined by the mRNA strand and the amino acids are covalently bound at their carboxy terminal. The length of this peptide is determined by punctuation marks in the genetic code. Thus, a sequence of DNA results in the production of a peptide chain which may have many functions.

Various control mechanisms between DNA and its expression as a polypeptide chain have been postulated from microbial systems. The operon model of Jacob and Monod is indicated in Figure 3-25. In their negative control hypothesis, a repressor protein prevents the structural genes from producing mRNA by binding to a site on the DNA molecule called an operator. In the presence of an inducer, the repressor protein is inactivated and does not bind to the operator, and the structural genes in the operon are transcribed. Ptashne has isolated a protein from bacteria with characteristics predicted for a repressor substance including the ability to bind to genetically competent DNA. Other models of positive control systems have been postulated.

There is indirect evidence for the existence of these working models of protein biosynthesis and DNA regulation in mammalian cells. This evidence is derived from cultured liver cells, some of whose enzymes are induced by cortisol. When cells are stimulated with cortisol, there are more enzymes produced and new nuclear RNA species (mRNA) are found. The process of induction is prevented by inhibiting DNA transcription with

Figure 3-25 The operon model for the regulation of mRNA synthesis. Normally a regulator gene produces a repressor protein which binds to an operator portion of DNA, preventing other genes in the operon from transcribing mRNA. An inducer inactivates the repressor protein, allowing expression of structural genes. (From Davidson, J. N.: The Biochemistry of the Nucleic Acids. 5th ed. New York, Methuen and Co., 1965.)

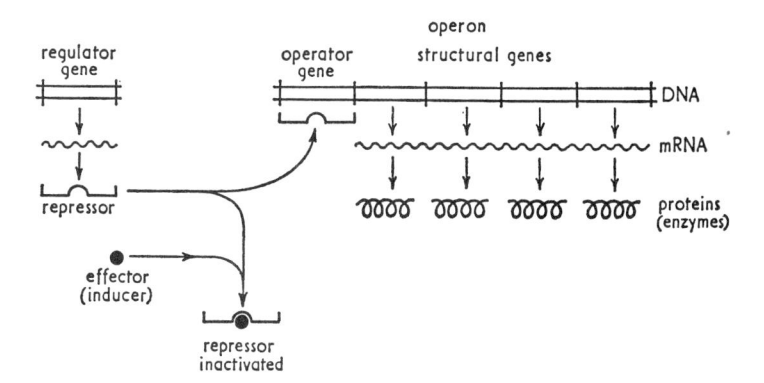

actinomycin D before adding cortisol. These data are interpreted to indicate that cortisol induces the transcription of normally repressed genes. There are many controls not only at transcription but also at the translational and post-translational events. Mammalian protein biosynthesis differs from microbial systems, since mammalian cells have a nuclear membrane which is not present in microbial systems. Newly formed messenger RNA must cross this nuclear membrane to associate with ribosomes located in the cytoplasm. It is probable that many nuclear RNA species are prevented from reaching the sites of protein synthesis in the cytoplasm by selectivity across this potential barrier. It is known that RNA species complementary to DNA are present in a wider variety in the nucleus than in the cytoplasm of mammalian cells even though nuclear RNA is degraded more rapidly. Regulatory mechanisms may exist not only at the transcription of messenger RNA from DNA but also at levels of nuclear membrane transport, at translation of mRNA into peptides, and with the interaction of the peptides with others to form functioning proteins.

A precise definition of the mRNA code for specific amino acids was possible following the discovery by Nirenberg that polyphenylalanine is formed when an artificial mRNA, polyuridylic acid, is added to bacterial ribosomes. The genetic code described in microbial systems probably functions in higher organisms including man (Fig. 3-26). The essential features of the genetic code are that each amino acid is dictated by a sequence of three bases (triplet codons). These triplet codons are arranged in a linear fashion and do not overlap, so that one group of three specifies one amino acid, the next group of three specifies a second amino acid, and so on. The four bases of an mRNA strand (UCAG) can occur in 64 different triplet sequences. Sixty-one triplet combinations are known to specify one of the 20 amino acids. There are three triplet codons which do not specify amino acids but act as punctuation and result in termination (term) of the growing polypeptide chain. These so-called nonsense codons are UAA, UAG, and UGA. Most of the amino acids have more than one code word and therefore the genetic code is said to be degenerate. Thus, the process of gene expression in mammalian cells proposes a sequence of events by which single strands of nuclear DNA transcribe their triplet codons to messenger RNA. Messenger RNA proceeds through the nuclear membrane and associates with cytoplasmic ribosomal complexes. Specific "activated" amino acids bound to sRNA are then added in a linear fashion to form polypeptide chains. These polypeptide chains must interact with each other, with different peptide chains and with the environment to form functioning proteins which may be expressed in a variety of cellular, metabolic processes.

Hemoglobin Variants: A Human Model of Molecular Disease

The first direct evidence that gene mutations result in altered human proteins came from observations in sickle cell anemia. This disease occurs in a small percentage (1 to 2 per cent) of black populations. It is expressed by severe anemia, infarctions of various organs such as the kidney and lungs, susceptibility to bone infections, and death, frequently in the second decade of life. Erythrocytes subjected to low oxygen tensions became elongated, filamentous, and sickle shaped. Sickling of the erythrocytes can be demonstrated in 8 per cent of the Negro population of the United States and this may occur in the absence of disease. These individuals are said to have sickle trait. Neel suggested that individuals with the sickle trait were heterozygous and those expressing disease were homozygous for an abnormal gene. Family studies further supported this hypothesis. In 1949, Pauling demonstrated that normal hemoglobin and hemoglobin S differed in their electrophoretic properties. Red cells from normal individuals contained only hemoglobin A, but cells from patients with sickle cell trait contained both hemoglobin A and the abnormal sickle hemoglobin (hemoglobin S). A third abnormal hemoglobin, hemoglobin C, was discovered by Itano and Neel. In family studies, this hemoglobin was also determined by a single gene and heterozygotes for this gene had both hemoglobin A and hemoglobin C in their red blood cells. Homozygotes for the mutant C gene formed only hemoglobin C but clinically had only a mild anemia. That the two mutations were allelic became evident when patients with both mutant hemoglobins were found (double heterozygotes). Since the two hemoglobins were readily differentiated by electrophoresis, pedigree analysis of the two mutations (hemoglobin C and hemoglobin S) could be made. When one parent was a double heterozygote (SC) while the other was normal (AA), offspring were produced with either hemoglobin C trait (AC) or sickle cell trait (AS). No offspring were doubly heterozygous (SC) or homozygous normal (AA). Thus, hemoglobin S, C, and A segregated during meiosis and were presumably alleles.

A molecular basis for these pedigrees became evident when the structure of the variant hemoglobins was determined. Normal hemoglobin A was found to contain four polypeptide chains, two alpha (α_2) and two beta (β_2) chains, each with a characteristic amino acid sequence. The α-chain contains 141 amino acids, the β-chain 146 amino acids, and their precise sequences have been established. The nature of the difference between hemoglobin A and hemoglobin S was determined by Ingram in 1957 when he found that one amino acid in the β polypeptide chain at position 6 was occupied by glutamic acid in hemoglobin A and by valine in hemoglobin S. This position was subsequently found to be occupied by a lysine residue in hemoglobin C (Table 3–6). In all three of these β polypeptide chains, the sequence of the other 145 amino acids was identical. Thus, not only were the mutations occurring at the same locus, but at the same amino acid position of the chain. In molecular terms, the gene can be defined as that sequence of DNA which produces a functional polypeptide. The mutations for S and C hemoglobin occur within the gene at identical codon sites (point mutations) and are homoallelic. The messenger RNA triplet codon, GAA, and its complementary DNA codon, CTT, are the code for glutamic acid (Table 3–6). A single base change from A to U produces GUA, the codon for

	Second base				
First base	U	C	A	G	Third base
U	UUU, UUC } Phe UUA, UUG } Leu	UCU, UCC, UCA, UCG } Ser	UAU, UAC } Tyr UAA term. UAG term	UGU, UGC } Cys UGA term UGG Try	U C A G
C	CUU, CUC, CUA, CUG } Leu	CCU, CCC, CCA, CCG } Pro	CAU, CAC } His CAA, CAG } Gln	CGU, CGC, CGA, CGG } Arg	U C A G
A	AUU, AUC, AUA } Ile AUG Met	ACU, ACC, ACA, ACG } Thr	AAU, AAC } Asn AAA, AAG } Lys	AGU, AGC } Ser AGA, AGG } Arg	U C A G
G	GUU, GUC, GUA, GUG } Val	GCU, GCC, GCA, GCG } Ala	GAU, GAC } Asp GAA, GAG } Glu	GGU, GGC, GGA, GGG } Gly	U C A G

Figure 3–26 Codon assignments. (Modified from Woese, C. R.: The Genetic Code. New York, Harper and Row, 1967.)

TABLE 3-6 MUTANT CODONS THAT COULD PRODUCE OBSERVED VARIANTS IN HUMAN HEMOGLOBIN

Variant Hemoglobin	Amino Acid (Position 6)	mRNA Triplet	DNA Triplet
A	Glutamic	GAA	CTT
S	Valine	GUA	CAT
C	Lysine	AAA	TTT

valine and hemoglobin S. The substitution of A in the first position for G results in AAA, the genetic codon for lysine and hemoglobin C. These observations provide strong support for the concept that genetic mutations in mammals represent changes of bases in the DNA sequence of a particular gene.

Structure-function relationships between normal hemoglobin A, hemoglobin S, and hemoglobin C provide some insight into how a single base substitution can result in the expression of a systemic disease. Perutz and Mitchison observed that deoxygenated sickle cell hemoglobin is less soluble in aqueous solutions than deoxygenated normal hemoglobin. These observations suggested a molecular mechanism for the sickling phenomenon. Murayama demonstrated that substitution of valine for glutamic acid at the 6th position in the two β chains of tetrameric hemoglobins allowed intermolecular hydrophobic bonding and molecular stacking between hemoglobin molecules. Perutz and Lehmann suggested that the 6th position of the β polypeptide chain of hemoglobin occupies the surface of the tertiary structure and that normally the polar group (glutamic acid) adheres to a complementary site on its neighboring hemoglobin molecule. In the absence of this polar group, linear aggregates of hemoglobin S occur. In homozygotes for sickle cell disease, the intracellular concentration of hemoglobin S is high and leads to intermolecular stacking. Deoxygenated red blood cells sickle in the venous circulation, increase blood viscosity, impede the circulation of the venous capillaries, block smaller blood vessels, and form thrombi leading to tissue infarction. The sickled red cells are less well able to withstand the stresses of the circulation and have a shorter survival time leading to hemolytic anemia. A pathologic structural-functional relationship is also seen in patients homozygous for hemoglobin C. These patients have only mild hemolysis as compared to the severe fatal disease produced by hemoglobin S. Substitution of another polar amino acid, lysine, in the 6th position of the β-chain (hemoglobin C) does not produce intermolecular stacking and high viscosity, although a tendency to gel is observed under reduced oxygen tension. It is still not clear how a lysine substitution produces this functional defect in hemoglobin C.

Over 100 different variants of the α or β chains of hemoglobin have been identified. The functional expression of these mutant gene products depends on the charge and location of the amino acid substitution, the resultant conformational change in the tetrameric hemoglobin molecule, and the interaction of these polypeptides with their four prosthetic heme groups. Genetic control of the rate of protein synthesis is reflected by observations on variations in the rate of hemoglobin synthesis. Impaired enzyme function may be caused by a reduction in the rate of protein synthesis, either absolute or relative, rather than by structural changes. The *thalassemias* represent a group of chronic hemolytic anemias caused by a reduction in the rate of α- or β-chain synthesis. Although, strictly speaking, the β- or α-chain of hemoglobin is not an enzyme, the concepts of control in inherited metabolic diseases of man are derived from studies in these disorders. Homozygotes for β-chain thalassemia manifest severe hemolytic anemia from birth and have a deficiency of normal β-chain production and consequently of normal tetrameric hemoglobin A $(\alpha_2\beta_2)$. Other normal polypeptide chains δ or γ are produced in excess. The resultant red cells contain both increased amounts of hemoglobin F $(\alpha_2\gamma_2)$ and A_2 $(\alpha_2\delta_2)$, are deformed, and are subject to increased hemolysis. There are several reviews on this subject.

INBORN ERRORS OF METABOLISM

Enzymes as Mutant Gene Products

Few mutant proteins other than the hemoglobin peptide chains have had adequate analysis of amino acid sequence to demonstrate single amino acid substitutions. Most inherited metabolic diseases of man are characterized by the functional derangement imposed on the organism by its mutant gene products. A. E. Garrod first introduced the term "inborn error of metabolism" and described four diseases: alkaptonuria, albinism, cystinuria, and pentosuria, which conformed to mendelian patterns of inheritance and presumably resulted from a block in a major metabolic pathway. He noted that when protein or other precursors of homogentisic acid were administered orally to patients with alkaptonuria, the urinary excretion of homogentisic acid increased. He theorized that this "block-in-reaction sequence" was under genetic control, since pedigree analyses were consistent with an autosomal recessive mode of inheritance. The enzyme defect in alkaptonuria was not discovered until 50 years later when homogentisic acid oxidase activity was found missing in the liver and kidneys of patients affected with alkaptonuria. Garrod's concepts have been extended from the "one gene–one enzyme" to "one gene–one polypeptide" or "one cistron–one functional polypeptide."

A mutant gene product does not necessarily result in an inborn error of metabolism. A number of normally functioning protein variants including hemoglobins, phosphoglucomutase, lactate dehydrogenase, red cell acid phosphatase, and haptoglobin have been discovered during routine electrophoretic surveys in various normal populations. The vast array of "structural" gene loci in normal individuals has been described in detail by Harris. Using electrophoretic surveys, he has described the considerable protein polymorphism present in normal populations. He has classified the genetic control of these multiple molecular forms into three categories: (1) there may be several gene loci coding for structurally distinct polypeptide chains of a protein; (2) there may be only one gene locus, but many different alleles at this locus; and, finally, (3) there may be secondary "post-translational" modifications of the basic protein. When the mutant gene product results in functional derangement, an inborn error of metabolism exists. The functional defect may be expressed by many different pathogenic mechanisms. The mutant protein may transport substrates across the plasma membrane, catalyze a reaction in a metabolic pathway, interact with other proteins to affect hemostasis, provide active coenzymes from precursor vitamins, excise thymine dimers from normal DNA, and so on. The severity of the clinical pathologic condition produced will depend on the degree of alteration and the metabolic role of the mutant gene product.

The discussion of inherited pathologic physiology will be subdivided into eight categories according to the metabolic role played by the mutant gene product in the intact organism. These categories include diseases caused by defective proteins which (1) catalyze plasma membrane transport; (2) catalyze major metabolic pathways with disease caused by accumulation of toxic precursors; (3) catalyze a major pathway with disease caused by overproduction of toxic by-products from a minor pathway; (4) catalyze a needed end product in the pathway with disease caused by a deficiency of this product; (5) catalyze products in the major pathway which act as feedback inhibitors and cause disease by overproduction of precursors; (6) circulate in the blood and have many different functions (clotting, metal binding, maintenance of erythrocyte structure, and so on); (7) catalyze the production of specific coenzymes involved in a major pathway; and (8) catalyze the removal of potentially toxic pharmacologic agents (Table 3–7).

TABLE 3–7 CLASSIFICATION OF INBORN ERRORS OF METABOLISM BY DEFECTIVE GENE PRODUCTS

Defective Gene Products Act As Follows:
1. Catalyze plasma membrane transport
2. Catalyze major cellular metabolic pathways
   a. Disease is caused by accumulation of toxic precursors
   b. Disease is caused by toxic by-products from a normally minor pathway
   c. Disease is caused by deficiency of end product
   d. Disease is caused by overproduced intermediates through loss of feedback control
3. Circulate in blood and provide and maintain various functions (clotting; metal transport; red cell structure; and so on)
4. Produce or bind coenzymes involved in specific enzymatic reactions
5. Catalyze the removal of potentially toxic pharmacologic agents

Inherited Disorders Caused by Defective Membrane Transport

The jejunal epithelium and the proximal renal tubular epithelium have cells which have differentiated for the transport of essential substrates from outside the cell to its interior. This transport step shares several characteristics with enzymes such as saturation, steric specificity, energy dependence, competitive and noncompetitive inhibition, and concentrative ability. Direct evidence for the existence of substrate-specific permeases has been obtained from microbial systems. In man, evidence for their existence is obtained from pedigree analysis of inherited diseases in which this transport function is defective and can be studied. Most of these inherited transport defects have been defined in the intestine or kidney. Table 3–8 lists some inborn errors of membrane transport, the tissues affected, substrates malabsorbed, and the proposed mode of inheritance.

Garrod first recognized the familial occurrence of cystine stone formation, which he ascribed to a block in metabolic reaction sequence. In 1951, Dent and Rose suggested that *cystinuria* was caused by an error in the renal tubular transport

TABLE 3-8 SOME DISEASES CAUSED BY PLASMA MEMBRANE TRANSPORT MUTATIONS

Disease	Tissues Affected	Malabsorbed Substrate	Mode of Inheritance	Clinical Expression
Cystinuria	Kidney ± gut	Cystine ± lysine, arginine, ornithine	Autosomal Recessive	Renal lithiasis (cystine)
Hartnup disease	Gut + kidney	Neutral amino acids	Autosomal Recessive	Nicotinic acid deficiency (pellagra)
Blue diaper syndrome	Gut	Tryptophan	Autosomal Recessive	Hypercalcemia
Methionine malabsorption	Gut	Methionine	Autosomal Recessive(?)	Mental retardation, white hair, failure to thrive
Glucose-galactose malabsorption	Gut + kidney	Glucose and galactose	Autosomal Recessive	Refractory diarrhea
Renal glycosuria	Kidney	Glucose	Autosomal Recessive	Benign glycosuria
Hypophosphatemic rickets	Kidney	Phosphate	X-linked Dominant	Rickets
Congenital chloridorrhea	Gut	Chloride	Autosomal Recessive	Diarrhea, alkalosis
Hereditary spherocytosis	Erythrocyte	Sodium	Autosomal Dominant	Hemolytic anemia
B_{12} malabsorption	Ileum	B_{12}	Autosomal Recessive	Juvenile pernicious anemia

mechanism for cystine, arginine, ornithine, and lysine. These four dibasic amino acids were found in excess in affected patients' urine. An autosomal recessive mode of inheritance was confirmed by Harris. Rosenberg defined three different forms of cystinuria. Types I, II, and III were distinguished by comparing, in a pedigree analysis, differences in dibasic amino acid transport across the gut in homozygous affected individuals, and in heterozygotes by variation found in urinary excretion of the dibasic amino acids. These three genetically distinct types of cystinuria were subsequently demonstrated to be allelic. Type II–III double heterozygotes expressed the clinical phenotype and produced offspring who were either Type II or Type III heterozygotes, but none were normal nor clinically affected. Disease is caused by malabsorption of cystine in the proximal renal tubule. When the urine contains greater than 30 mg. of cystine per 100 ml., cystine crystallizes and forms stones. Cystinuric homozygotes and double heterozygotes excrete over 600 mg. of cystinine in 24 hours. Cystinuria is the most common cause of bladder calculi at birth and may account for 5 per cent of all nephrolithiasis. It is most commonly expressed during the third and fourth decades of life. The urine from members of an affected family should be screened for asymptomatic stone formation. Cystine is more soluble in dilute urine and in an alkaline pH. Stone formation may be decreased by maintaining water diuresis and a urinary pH above 7.5. Renal stones once formed may be dissolved by the administration of D-penicillamine (β,β-dimethylcysteine), which forms soluble penicillamine-cystine disulfides.

Renal stone formation is but one of many clinical manifestations produced by heritable defects in membrane transport permeases. In *Hartnup disease*, malabsorption of the neutral amino acids by the intestinal mucosa may have no ill effects. However, if the defect is severe and enough tryptophan is malabsorbed, intracellular nicotinamide deficiency may result. The disease is then expressed as a pellagra-like syndrome with ataxia, sun-sensitive rashes, and dementia. Treatment consists of administration of the deficient vitamin, niacin. In *familial glucose-galactose malabsorption*, severe osmotic diarrhea occurs in infants from the inability of their jejunal mucosa to transport glucose and other sterically similar monosaccharides. Direct evidence for the genetic control of intestinal glucose transport was obtained by in-vitro studies of jejunal biopsy material. As seen in Figure 3–27, epithelial cells from an affected homozygote were unable to accumulate glucose over a 60-minute incubation period, whereas cells from her clinically normal brother and normal controls concentrated glucose to levels 15 times that in the ex-

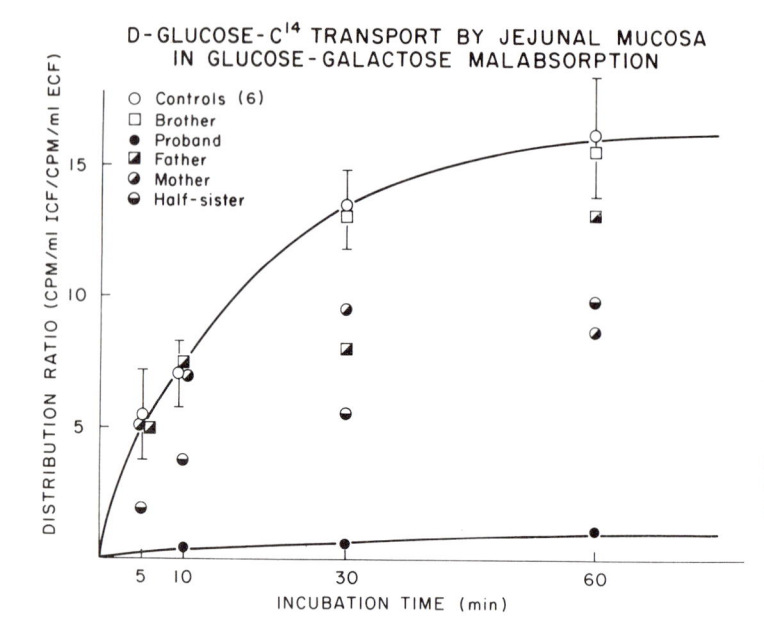

Figure 3-27 Jejunal mucosa from the affected proband (●) is unable to accumulate glucose, whereas normals (○) and her brother (□) concentrate to levels 15 times more. Both parents and a half sister (◐◨◒) accumulate intermediate amounts of glucose, indicating a partial transport defect and identifying them as heterozygotes for the mutant gene. Distribution ratio is calculated from the ratio of counts per minute per milliliter of intracellular space to counts per minute per milliliter of extracellular space (CPM/ml ICF:CPM/ml ECF).

tracellular space. Biopsies from both parents demonstrated partial impairment of this transport function. These data indicate that the proband is homozygous for the glucose transport mutation; that her brother is homozygous for the normal allele, and that both parents and her half-sister are heterozygotes, each carrying one mutant and one normal allele. The osmotic diarrhea induced by ingested glucose is prevented by substituting fructose as the dietary carbohydrate source. This monosaccharide has a different steric configuration and membrane transport requirements. In familial glucose-galactose malabsorption, absent intestinal glucose transport is shared by a partial defect in the kidney. In *renal glycosuria*, the kidney tubule is unable to reabsorb glucose, but this genetic defect is not expressed by the intestine. In one family, renal glucose transport was quantitated using in-vivo titration techniques, and an autosomal recessive mode of inheritance was defined (Fig. 3-28). Heterogeneity for renal glucose transport is evidenced by the different types of abnormal curves found in other families with familial glycosuria. In contrast to glucose-galactose malabsorption, renal glucose malabsorption produces no ill effects unless iatrogenic disease arises from a misdiagnosis of diabetes mellitus.

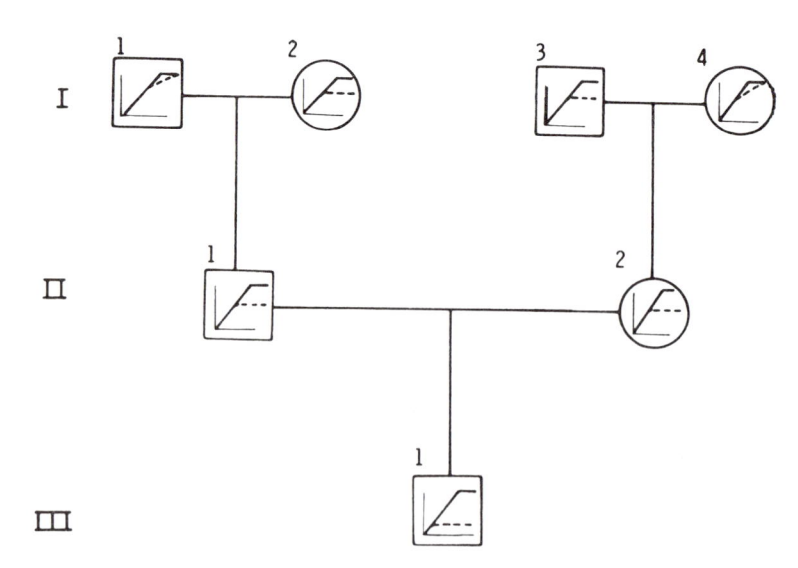

Figure 3-28 Autosomal recessive inheritance of renal glycosuria. The results of renal glucose titration are inscribed within the pedigree symbols. Broken lines (– – –) represent observed deviation from the theoretical curve (——). The proband (III-1) expresses severe Type A glycosuria and his parents (II-1, II-2) and grandparents (I-2, I-3) have milder forms. Grandparents (I-1) and (I-4) have normal curves.

Defective accumulation of phosphate, vitamins, sodium, and chloride may result from other heritable membrane transport mutations. The changes resulting from these defects vary. In *familial hypophosphatemic rickets,* the best genetic determinant of this X-linked dominant trait is defective phosphate reabsorption by the proximal renal tubule. If this is the initiating event, it is postulated that hypophosphatemia results, followed by bone resorption to maintain normal serum phosphate levels. In addition, shortened lower body segments, rickets in children, and osteomalacia in adults may be present. In *congenital chloridorrhea,* adults may manifest malabsorption of chloride by the colon, resulting in watery diarrhea, hypochloremia, and decreased renal chloride filtration. Bicarbonate ion is reabsorbed in the absence of tubular chloride to maintain a normal electropotential gradient. Increased bicarbonate reabsorption by the kidney tubule results in continued metabolic alkalosis. In *hereditary spherocytosis,* impaired erythrocyte membrane permeability to sodium results in a shortened survival of the erythrocyte and hemolytic anemia. This condition is inherited as an autosomal dominant trait with parent-to-offspring transmission. In *vitamin B_{12} malabsorption,* juvenile pernicious anemia results. This autosomal recessive trait is seen in children with normal gastric acid secretion in whom intrinsic factor can be demonstrated.

Inherited Disorders Resulting from Precursor Accumulation

The most commonly described inborn error of metabolism results from a metabolic block in a major pathway and the accumulation of toxic precursors. One such disease is *alkaptonuria,* a defect in homogentisic acid oxidase activity. This enzyme normally catalyzes the conversion of homogentisic acid to maleylacetoacetic acid in the oxidative catabolic pathway of tyrosine (Fig. 3-29). Virtual absence of this enzyme in kidney and liver results in the accumulation of homogentisic acid in tissues and excretion into the urine. Ho-

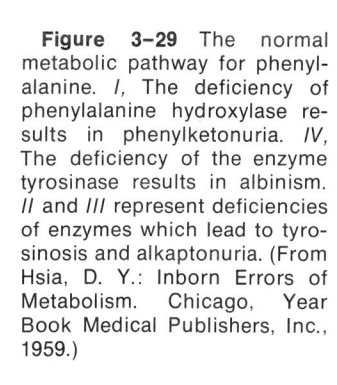

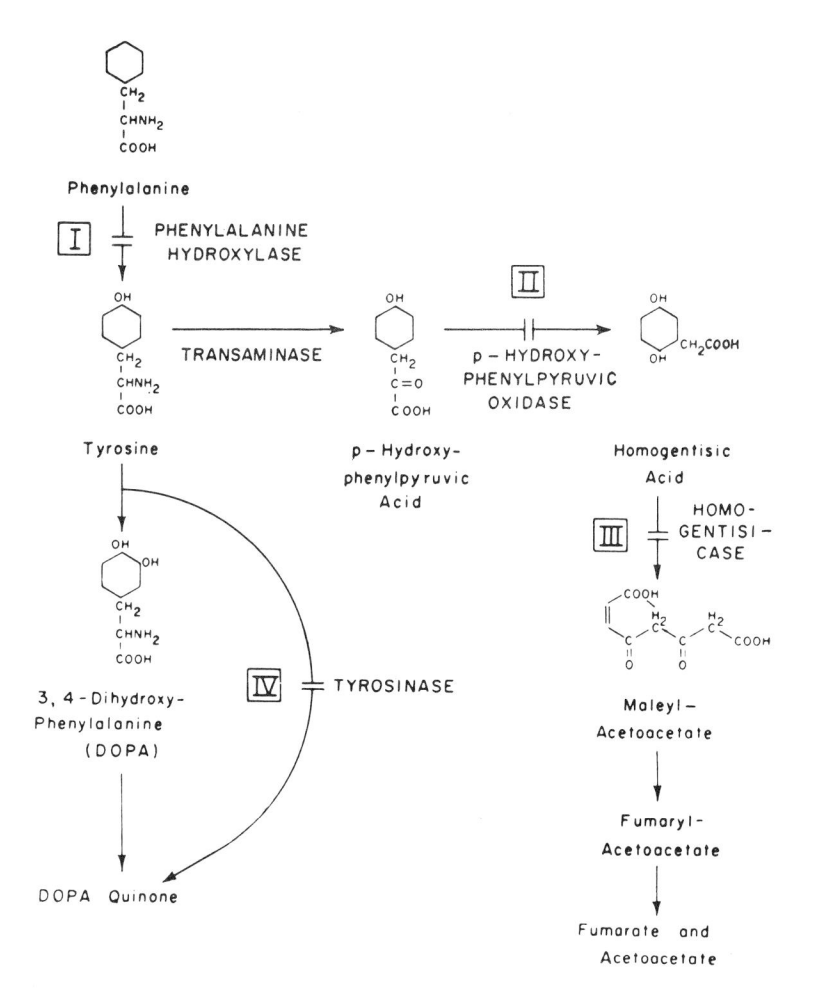

Figure 3–29 The normal metabolic pathway for phenylalanine. *I,* The deficiency of phenylalanine hydroxylase results in phenylketonuria. *IV,* The deficiency of the enzyme tyrosinase results in albinism. *II* and *III* represent deficiencies of enzymes which lead to tyrosinosis and alkaptonuria. (From Hsia, D. Y.: Inborn Errors of Metabolism. Chicago, Year Book Medical Publishers, Inc., 1959.)

mogentisic acid accumulation in cartilaginous tissue is associated with premature arthritis and provides this tissue with the characteristic dark tinge caused by its oxidation. The disease is not usually manifest until after 30 years of age, and whether tissue deposition could be delayed or prevented with restricted phenylalanine and tyrosine intake is unknown.

An array of storage diseases have been delineated, in which glycogen, sphingolipids or mucopolysaccharides are found in excess in tissues. The deposition of these compounds presumably results from a block in their normal catabolic pathway and in varied types of precursor accumulation and organ disease. The precise mechanisms by which intracellular storage of these compounds produces clinical disorders are not as yet clear.

In classic *galactosemia,* a defect in galactose-1-phosphate uridyl transferase results in accumulation of the hexose monophosphate, galactose-1-phosphate and its precursor galactose. Because different errors exist in this catabolic pathway, the pathogenesis of disease in this disorder is somewhat better understood. Galactose-1-phosphate accumulates in liver, kidney, and brain and produces cirrhosis, renal tubular malabsorption, and mental retardation. The molecular mechanism by which galactose-1-phosphate accumulation interferes with normal cellular function is not clear. In another defect in galactose utilization, *galactokinase deficiency,* galactose is accumulated in the blood and tissues but galactose-1-phosphate is normal or reduced. In this disorder, cataracts are manifest without impairment of kidney, liver, or brain. Cataract formation in both classic galactose-1-phosphate uridyl transferase deficiency and galactokinase deficiency presumably results from excessive accumulation of galactose and conversion in the lens by aldose reductase in the presence of triphosphopyridine nucleotide to galactitol. This poorly effluxed alcohol is trapped in the lens, creates an osmotic gradient, and produces degeneration of lens fibers. The pathologic condition created by both enzyme defects can be ameliorated if detected early and if dietary restriction of nonessential galactose-containing sugars is instituted.

Maple syrup urine disease or branched-chain α-keto acidemia results from defective decarboxylation of the branched-chain α-keto acids. The reaction sequence is indicated in Figure 3–30. Isoleucine, leucine, and valine, the branched-chain amino acids, are reversibly transaminated to their branched-chain α-keto acid derivatives, α-keto-β-methyl valeric, α-keto isocaproic, and α-keto isovaleric acids. Subsequent decarboxylation of all three of these organic acids to their coenzyme A derivatives is blocked in maple syrup urine disease. The α-keto acids and their branched-chain amino acid precursors accumulate in tissue and blood and are excreted in the urine. Racemers of these branched-chain α-keto acids impart a fragrant odor of maple syrup to the patient's urine. The enzyme defect is expressed in leukocytes isolated from the peripheral blood and in fibroblasts cultured from patient's skin. By analogy to pyruvic acid decarboxylation, three different enzyme proteins may be involved in branched-chain α-keto acid decarboxylation. These include a thiamine-dependent α-keto acid decarboxylase; lipoic acid reductase transacylase; and lipoamide oxidoreductase. Five coenzymes may also be required in this reaction: thiamine pyrophosphate (Thp~p); reduced coenzyme A (CoASH); oxidized lipoic acid $\left(\text{La}\begin{smallmatrix}S\\|\\S\end{smallmatrix}\right)$; flavoprotein (FAD); and oxidized nicotinamide adenine dinucleotide (NAD+). The complex of these three enzymes and their cofactors which decarboxylate α-keto isocaproic acid and α-keto-β-methyl valeric acid (6-carbon compounds) resides in the mitochondria of bovine liver, whereas the complex which oxidizes the α-keto isovaleric acid (a 5-carbon compound) is found in microsomal cell fractions. It is not surprising that at least four different forms of the disease have been described, since there are many possible mutant proteins which could produce a block in this reaction. In the "classic" form, keto acid decarboxylase activity is absent in the white cells and fibroblasts obtained from homozygous affected patients. Severe central nervous system depression may occur during the first few days of protein ingestion and apnea and coma result. If infants survive this initial insult, permanent neurologic damage may persist. Quantitatively different reductions in parental (obligatory heterozygotes) decarboxylase activity by cultured fibroblasts were seen in one family. Thus, different non-complementing mutant gene products may commonly result in absent function producing affected double heterozygotes. The "intermittent" form is differentiated from the classic phenotype by its later onset in childhood, by its episodic remitting and nonprogressive course, and by leukocyte and fibroblast enzyme activity in homozygotes which retain up to 20 per cent of activity. Environmental insults such as protein ingestion and infections induce intermittent episodes characterized by branched-chain α-keto acidemia and death, if the stress persists. In reported cases, only one parent, usually the father, has reduced α-keto acid oxidase activity in peripheral leukocytes. An "intermediate" variant is characterized by persistent branched-chain α-keto aciduria, mild nonprogressive psychomotor retardation, hyperuricemia, and reduced enzyme activity in leukocytes and fibroblasts. Leukocyte activity

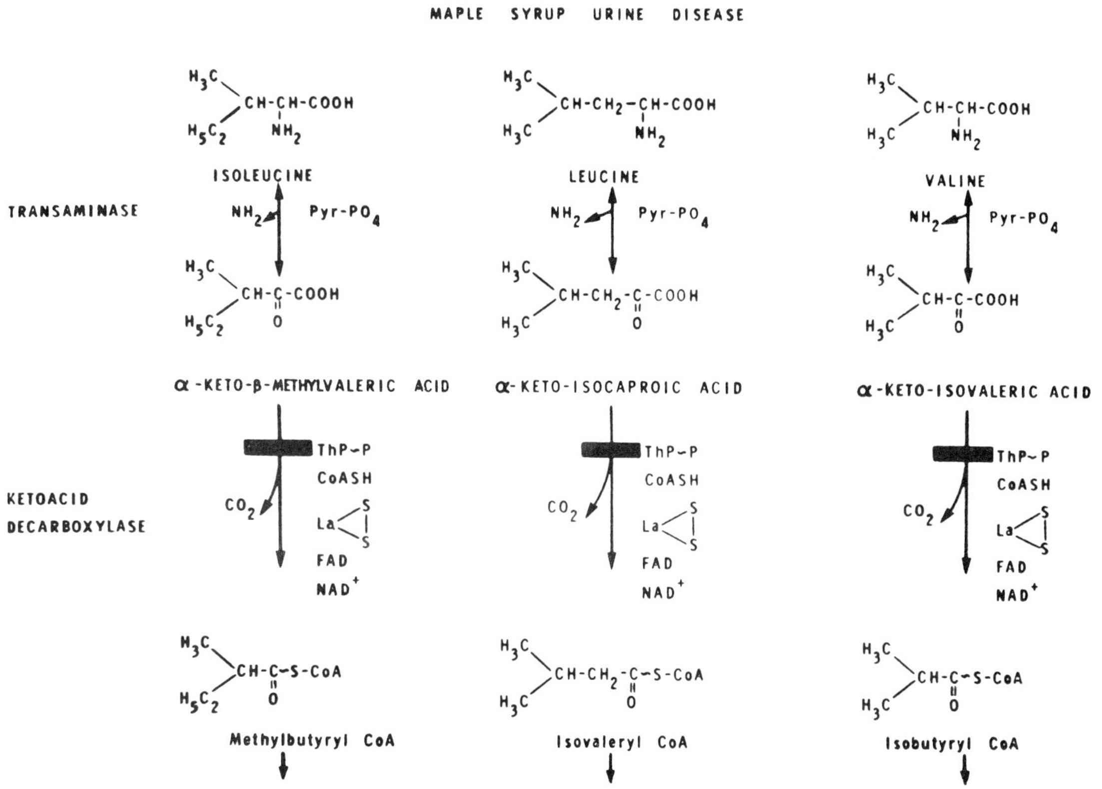

MAPLE SYRUP URINE DISEASE

Figure 3-30 Catabolic pathway for branched-chain amino acids. Bar ▬ represents block in maple syrup urine disease. ThP~P, CoASH, La$<^S_S|$, FAD, and NAD+ are coenzymes implicated in the oxidative decarboxylation of α-keto acids. At least three proteins are also involved.

was 15 to 20 per cent of normal, and fibroblast activity 42 to 47 per cent of normal. Both parents had greater than normal activity in cultured fibroblasts, and homozygotes did not respond to thiamine administration. A fourth phenotype characterized by branched-chain amino aciduria and delayed development responded dramatically to oral thiamine. Thus, at least one variant of maple syrup urine disease has been defined, in which the administration of large amounts of cofactor involved in the keto acid decarboxylase step augmented defective enzyme function.

The pathologic physiology in all four variants is presumably caused by the effects of α-keto isocaproic acid on myelin formation and central nervous system mitochondrial oxidation. Examination of the myelin suggests that changes in myelin formation do not occur before birth. The acute reversible aspects of the disease support this concept, since normal development will occur in affected children who are treated during the neonatal period with diets restricted in branched-chain amino acids. High concentrations of α-keto isocaproic acid inhibit decarboxylation of pyruvic acid, protein synthesis, and amino acid transport by neural tissue in various animal systems. The severity of these insults is related to the tissue concentrations of α-keto isocaproic acid which determine reversibility or continued interference in function. The disease process is caused by the toxic effects of these immediate precursors, accumulated as a result of defects in the major decarboxylation pathway of branched-chain α-keto acids.

Inherited Diseases Caused by Products of Minor Pathways

The precursor in the metabolic block of a major pathway may not be the immediate cause of the disease. Instead by-products of an alternate minor pathway may cause the disease. The activity of such a pathway is normally minimal, but is enhanced by abnormal precursor accumulation. For example, cataracts in *galactosemia* are caused not by galactose or galactose-1-phosphate. Rather the increased concentration of galactose in lens fibers results in excessive amounts of non-diffusible galactitol produced as a result of an alternate pathway through aldose reductase. A second example is *phenylketonuria*. A deficiency in phenylalanine hydroxylase results in the accumulation of phenylalanine. It is, however, the deaminated by-product of phenylalanine, phenylpyruvic, which produces the characteristic ferric chloride reaction in the urine and metabolic acidosis. Since a moderate elevation of phenylalanine alone is not toxic, these by-products in high concentrations may interfere with central nervous system processes. Although mental retardation and demyelination are consequences of the untreated disease, the basis for their pathogenesis remains an enigma.

A third example is *hyperoxaluria*, which is characterized by the excretion of large amounts of oxalic acid, nephrolithiasis, nephrocalcinosis, and early renal failure. The stones are formed from calcium oxalate, a nonessential end product of glycine degradation. This disorder is caused by excessive biosynthesis of oxalic acid which is formed from glycine through the irreversible oxidation of glyoxilic acid. Two causes for excessive accumulation of glyoxilic acid and its insoluble by-product, oxalic acid, have been postulated. In Type I, a defect in the soluble enzyme glycolic acid α-ketoglutarate carboligase blocks conversion of glyoxilic acid to α-OH-β-ketoadipic (one of six alternate routes for glyoxilic acid) and results in accumulation of glyoxilic acid and conversion to oxalic acid. In Type II, Williams described excessive D-glyceric aciduria as well as hyperoxaluria and found deficient D-glyceric acid oxidase in the leukocytes of affected patients and of the mother but not of the father. These authors postulate that a deficiency in this enzyme reduces conversion of glyoxilic acid to glycolic acid. Both types lead primarily to excesses of glyoxilic acid by blocking normal dissimilation and secondarily to increased biosynthesis of oxalic acid normally present but in smaller amounts. These examples then represent inborn errors of metabolism, the manifestations of which are caused not by the precursor in the metabolic block but by the overproduction of by-products from the accumulating precursor.

Inherited Diseases Caused by Deficiencies of End Product

A pathologic condition may result from a mutant gene product which reduces the intracellular concentration of essential end products in its pathway. *Albinism* represents a group of disorders caused by impaired production of melanoprotein from tyrosine. A specialized cell, the melanocyte, is the source of pigment in hair, skin, and eyes. Hydroxylation of L-tyrosine to 3,4-dihydroxyphenylalanine (DOPA) and its subsequent oxidation to dopa-quinone utilize the same enzyme, tyrosinase (Fig. 3–29). Nonenzymatic reactions then occur in the melanocyte, resulting in polymerization of dopa-quinone derivatives and reaction with a specialized protein to form melanoprotein. Melanocytes are present in albinism but do not contain melanin. Many different clinical forms of albinism exist with different genetic patterns of inheritance. Classic oculocutaneous albinism (Type I) is expressed as diffuse hypopigmentation of the hair, skin, fundus oculi, and iris. It is inherited as an autosomal recessive trait. Melanocytes are present but are presumably deficient in tyrosinase. The disease expression therefore is due to a deficiency of the end product melanin, which normally acts as a sunscreen and protects cells from light energy. In albinism, instead of tanning, affected individuals burn on exposure to light. Exposed skin has an increased tendency to develop malignant melanomas. Photophobia, nystagmus, and visual impairment result from melanin deficiency in the eye.

Defective formation of thyroid hormone represents another group of inborn errors of metabolism in which deficiency of the product of the enzyme pathway results in expression of disease. Several different enzymatic defects have been described which produce a deficiency of functioning thyroid hormone. These include (1) an iodide transport defect; (2) iodide organification defects; (3) a defect in the coupling of iodotyrosyl to form thyroxine; (4) failure to synthesize normal thyroglobulin; and (5) failure to dehalogenate organic iodide. Mental retardation or cretinism is caused by a deficiency in the end product, thyroid hormone.

Congenital adrenal hyperplasia results from an inherited, relative or absolute, loss in one of the enzymes which produces normal hormonal steroids from cholesterol. When this block in the normal biosynthetic pathway results in insufficient production of salt-retaining mineralocorticoids and anti-inflammatory glucocorticoids, persistent loss of sodium in the urine, vomiting, dehydration, hypotension, shock, or sudden death may occur. At least five different enzyme deficiencies in this pathway have been described including 21-hydroxylase, 11-hydroxylase, 3 β-hydroxysteroid dehydrogenase, 17-hydroxylase, and 18-hydroxylase. Salt wasting may occur in all except the 11-hydroxylase deficiency, in which salt retaining hormones 11-deoxycortisol and 11-deoxycorticosterone are formed in excess and protect the organism against deficient aldosterone production. An autosomal recessive pattern of inheritance is presumed for these disorders.

Inherited Diseases Caused by Loss of Feedback Inhibition

In the preceding section, it was shown that deficiency of essential end products in the major metabolic pathway produces abnormalities directly. The failure to synthesize thyroxine results in mental retardation. The total phenotype is due not only to deficient hormone but also to loss of feedback inhibition of hypothalamic thyrotropin releasing factor, excess secretion of TSH, and the formation of excessive thyroid parenchyma. The goiter expressed in familial hypothyroidism results from the loss of end product inhibition of TSH regulatory control mechanisms.

In the adrenogenital syndrome, particularly in 11-hydroxylase deficiency, the end product deficiency may not in itself produce the entire syndrome. A precursor, 11-deoxycorticosterone, is accumulated in one group (the 11-hydroxylase deficiencies), conserves renal sodium, and may even produce hypertension. However, the major pathologic process in this disorder is masculinization. Normally, cortisol and corticosterone regulate hypothalamic-pituitary ACTH secretion by acting as depressants on corticotropin-releasing factor. Corticotropin-releasing factor acts to stimulate synthesis and release of ACTH. When cortisol production is reduced, as in 11-hydroxylase deficiency, this negative feedback control is lost, more ACTH is produced, and excessive androgenic steroids in the pathway are formed. Levels of ACTH, 17-ketosteroids, and potent androgens such as testosterone are elevated in plasma and tissues. This pathologic process occurs during intrauterine development and may cause clitoromegaly or ambiguous genitalia in the female infant, macrogenitosomia in the male, and virilization with epiphyseal closure in both. The whole process is reversed by providing exogenous cortisol in physiologic amounts, returning feedback inhibition to the hypothalamic-pituitary-ACTH axis.

In most inborn errors of metabolism, a diminution in enzyme function is present. An exception to this rule is the defect in *acute intermittent porphyria*. This inborn error is characterized by hepatic overproduction of porphyrin precursors δ-aminolevulinic acid and porphobilinogen. Increased activity of hepatic δ-aminolevulinic acid synthetase has been described in patients affected with this disorder. Family studies in 600 patients from Sweden describe direct parent-to-offspring transmission, with both sexes equally affected. This indicates an autosomal dominant pattern of inheritance. A dominant mutation with increased enzyme activity led to the hypothesis that the gene mutation involves regulation of an operator gene repressed by normal biosynthesis of heme. Granick found that hepatic δ-aminolevulinic acid synthetase is an inducible enzyme. Studies in intact animals and cultured liver cells indicate that both carbohydrate and heme act to repress δ-aminolevulinic acid synthetase production. Acute intermittent porphyria is characterized by intermittent episodes of severe abdominal pain, psychoses, and paralysis. A number of factors are known to provoke acute attacks in patients with this disorder including certain drugs, infections, female sex hormones, and starvation. During attacks, the urine contains excessive amounts of porphobilinogen, which on standing in an acid pH will polymerize to form porphyrins and other dark reddish pigments. There is no quantitative correlation between acute clinical episodes, increased enzyme activity, and excessive production of porphobilinogen. This inborn error is unique in resulting from increased activity of an enzyme. Although this activity could result from decreased catabolism or increased production of the enzyme, the latter concept is currently favored. If heme acts as a corepressor with an aporepressor to provide negative control, a block in heme synthesis could result in loss of feedback regulation of δ-aminolevulinic acid synthetase and in overproduction. Evidence for such a mechanism has recently been advanced by Marver and associates. A mutation in the aporepressor or at the operator level of DNA could also result in loss of normal repression at the transcriptional level and cause overproduction of gene products.

In an inborn error of pyrimidine biosynthesis, *orotic aciduria*, a single rare mutant gene produces a deficiency of two enzyme functions: orotic acid phosphoribosyl transferase (O-PRT) and orotidine-5′-phosphate decarboxylase (ODC). This block results in the accumulation and excretion of a relatively insoluble pyrimidine nucleotide precursor, orotic acid, and reduced synthesis of its mononucleotide product, uridylic acid. Orotic acid is found in the urine of affected children and produces needle-shaped crystals and obstructive urinary tract symptoms when affected individuals become dehydrated. Children also manifest megaloblastic anemia and psychomotor retardation, presumably caused by "pyrimidine deficiency." A deficiency of this end product, uridylic acid (uridine-5′-monophosphate) results in overproduction of orotic acid, since it acts as a feedback inhibitor of carbamyl phosphate synthetase and aspartate transcarbamylase, initial enzymes in the biosynthetic pathway of uridylic acid production. If the feedback inhibitor uridine is provided, reduction in the rate of orotic acid overproduction is seen in patients and in cells cultured from their skin. Uridine replacement also improves the anemia and growth retardation.

Another inborn error of nucleotide feedback control is exemplified by defects in purine biosynthesis. The enzyme hypoxanthine-guanine-phosphoribosyltransferase (HGPRTase) acts to catalyze the formation of the mononucleotides inosinic and guanylic acid from hypoxanthine and guanine using phosphoribosyl pyrophosphate (PRPP). Defects in this enzyme result in reduced feedback inhibition of the de-novo synthesis of uric acid, increased cellular concentrations of PRPP, and marked overproduction of uric acid. Patients affected with complete HGPRTase deficiency have severe mental retardation, chorea, spasticity, and a bizarre compulsion to self-mutilation. They also exhibit hyperuricemia, urinary uric acid stones, and clinical gout. The gene is located on the X chromosome. Female heterozygotes demonstrate mosaicism for HGPRTase activity in fibroblasts cultured from their skin. Approximately half their cells are unable to incorporate tritiated hypoxanthine into nucleic acids (HGPRTase deficient), while the other half have normal enzyme activity. These observations support the Lyon hypothesis for early random and continued X-inactivation. The mechanism by which HGPRTase deficiency interrupts normal brain biochemistry and function is unknown. Two possibilities exist: that an important purine nucleotide is deficient or that an abnormal purine intermediate is overproduced. Neither of these possibilities is confirmed, but uric acid is clearly overproduced and the disease can be classified as an inherited defect resulting in loss of feedback control of de-novo purine biosynthesis.

Inherited Disease Associated With Deficient or Abnormal Circulating Proteins

A wide variety of genetically controlled proteins circulate in the blood. In some, changes in concentration, structure, or function may have no effect on the organism as a whole; in others, such changes may have distinctly deleterious results. Reduction in the concentration of *thyroxine-binding globulin*, a protein controlled by a locus on the X chromosome, reduces the serum protein-bound iodide but does not alter metabolic function. Dominantly inherited variants of the iron-binding protein, *transferrin*, have been described but none of these structural mutations have a known effect on iron metabolism. On the other hand, a recessively inherited *atransferrinemia* has been described in which there is a transferrin deficiency with a refractory hypochromic anemia. In *Wilson's disease*, reduction in circulating ceruloplasmin, a polyamine oxidase which is induced by and binds 95 per cent of serum copper, is associated with copper deposition in almost all tissues of the body. The deposition of copper in liver, brain, eyes, and kidney results in cirrhosis, extrapyramidal tract degeneration, pathognomonic corneal Kayser-Fleischer rings, and renal tubular dysfunction. Removal of copper from these organs with chelating agents such as penicillamine will prevent impairment and in some instances improve organ malfunction. Although reduction in circulating ceruloplasmin remains the best genetic determinant of affected homozygotes, approximately 2 to 3 per cent of patients with phenotypic Wilson's disease have chemically and functionally normal ceruloplasmin. The basic mutant gene product and the relationship between tissue copper and reduced levels of ceruloplasmin still remain unsolved.

The hemostatic mechanism in man is provided by several different factors under genetic control. In *classic hemophilia A,* an X-linked recessive trait, hemizygous males have diminished functional antihemophilic globulin (Factor VIII, AHG). *Vascular hemophilia* or Von Willebrand's disease is an autosomal dominant trait in which there is also a deficiency of Factor VIII. It is interesting that the more serious coagulation defect (classic hemophilia A) more commonly has detectable immunologic AHG which is hemostatically defective, whereas "vascular" hemophilia A (Von Willebrand's disease) has no immunoreactive material but the disease is characterized by a less severe defect in hemostasis. Hemophilia B or *Christmas disease* is a defect in Factor IX (plasma thromboplastin component) and, like Factor VIII, deficiency is also transmitted in an X-linked recessive pattern. Studies in families in which classic hemophilia A and hemophilia B were segregating showed that the two disorders were clearly nonallelic.

Several families have been reported with hemostatic defects expressed as mild prolongation of blood and plasma coagulation times and by the presence of abnormal fibrinogens. These *dysfibrinogenemias* are inherited in an autosomal dominant pattern when prolonged prothrombin time is used as the genetic determinant. Three different abnormal fibrinogens have been described: Fibrinogen-Detroit, -Baltimore, and -Cleveland. All three abnormal fibrinogens are immunologically distinct. Affected individuals have two populations of fibrinogen, normal and mutant. Mammen suggested that a substitution of a stongly basic amino acid (arginine) for serine in Fibrinogen-Detroit changed the conformational site for active polymerization and resulted in interference with the clotting properties of the normal fibrinogen which was also present. Another disorder, *congenital afibrinogenemia,* has been described. In this disorder, there is absent coagulation of blood in the affected individuals, and parents have mild coagulation defects. This disorder is inherited as an autosomal recessive trait. The dominant pattern of inheritance in dysfibrinogenemia and the expressed coagulation defects in "afibrinogenemic" heterozygotes indicate that in both disorders the mutant gene product (fibrinogen) is altered, so that it interferes with the product of its normal allele and results in phenotypic expression.

Congenital β-lipoprotein deficiency is characterized by reduced levels of circulating β-lipoprotein. This disease is inherited as an autosomal recessive trait and is expressed by abnormal red blood cell structure (acanthocytes); steatorrhea; diffuse central nervous system abnormalities (cerebellar, posterior column, peripheral nerve); and low serum cholesterol, phospholipid, and triglyceride levels. β-lipoprotein functions to transport triglycerides in the blood and it is absent in congenital a-beta-lipoproteinemia. Accumulation of triglycerides is seen in those tissues which normally synthesize the β-lipoproteins. Fatty acids are readily absorbed from the intestine and esterified to triglycerides by the intestinal mucosa, but because chylomicrons do not form, the triglycerides remain in the intestinal mucosa. Although diets low in fat decrease steatorrhea, the hematologic and neurologic defects in this disorder are not affected. The mechanism by which β-lipoprotein deficiency produces these pathologic findings is unknown.

Inborn Errors Caused by Reduced Coenzyme Binding or Production

Renewed interest in cofactor interaction with enzymes has resulted from the immediate therapeutic effects of administering supraphysiologic doses of vitamins whose coenzyme products augment defective enzyme pathways. Rosenberg defined the "vitamin dependent inborn errors" as genetic disturbances leading to specific biochemical abnormalities, affecting one reaction catalyzed by a vitamin and responding only to pharmacologic amounts of that vitamin. This definition thus clearly differentiates vitamin dependency from vitamin deficiency, which affects many pathways, responds to physiologic amounts of the vitamin, and is acquired. Frimpter first demonstrated decreased cystathionase activity in the liver from patients with *cystathioninuria.* When liver homogenates were incubated with its coenzyme, pyridoxal phosphate, activity was markedly increased. He also showed that cystathionine excretion in patients was lowered significantly by the administration of large amounts of vitamin B_6. Vitamin B_6 is phosphorylated to pyridoxal-5'phosphate or pyridoxamine-5'-phosphate by specific kinases requiring adenosine triphosphate. These phosphorylated compounds act as coenzymes for a large number of apoenzymes which regulate the catabolic pathways for fatty acids, amino acids, and glycogen. Since cystathionase activity alone was impaired in cystathioninuria, a vitamin deficiency was unlikely. Frimpter's work suggested that the mutation in cystathioninuria altered that portion of the specific apoenzyme which bound its active coenzyme, pyridoxal phosphate. Other inborn errors of metabolism demonstrating vitamin B_6 dependency include *infantile convulsions, pyridoxine-responsive anemia, xanthurenic aciduria,* and *homocystinuria.* In homocystinuria, B_6 may either augment cystathionine synthetase or provide alternate metabolic pathways for the degradation of homocystine and methionine to inorganic sulfate.

Only two reactions in mammalian systems have demonstrated a requirement for B_{12} coenzymes. The best example from man comes from studies of vitamin B_{12} responsive *methylmalonic aciduria.* This disorder arises from impairment in the conversion of methylmalonyl CoA to succinyl CoA. The reaction is catalyzed by the enzyme methylmalonyl CoA-mutase and its coenzyme 5'-deoxyadenosylcobalamin, a vitamin B_{12} derivative. Metabolic ketoacidosis accompanied by coma and shock was a common finding during the early weeks of life in six patients described. Other findings included hypotonia, hepatomegaly, osteoporosis, neutropenia, and thrombocytopenia. The appearance of long-chained ketones, including butanone and hexanone in the urine; intermittent hyperglycinemia and glycinuria; and the excretion of large amounts of the unusual organic acid methylmalonic acid characterized the biochemical phenotype. Biochemical studies in vitro revealed that peripheral blood leukocytes and cultured skin fibroblasts from affected patients were unable to convert methylmalonic acid to succinic acid. Normal levels of tissue and plasma vitamin B_{12} were found. When 1-mg. doses of hydroxycobalamin were given to one child with this disease, methylmalonic acid excretion fell and white blood cell utilization of methylmalonate rose. Continued administration of these large doses of vitamin B_{12} lowered this child's sensitivity to valine, a precursor of methylmalonic acid and prevented the appearance of ketosis. If fibroblasts were grown in tissue culture media containing physiologic concentrations of vitamin B_{12}, very low intracellular concentrations of the active coenzyme 5'-deoxyadenosylcobalamin were produced. However, when the cells were grown in medium with 10,000-fold increases of vitamin B_{12}, 5'-deoxyadenosylcobalamin rose to normal levels. Methylmalonate CoA mutase activity and its ability to bind coenzyme was normal in fibroblast homogenates from two patients, indicating that the apoenzyme was normal and had a normal affinity for its coenzyme. A primary genetic defect was thus postulated in the production of the coenzyme 5'-deoxyadenosylcobalamin from its precursor, vitamin B_{12} (Step 2, Fig. 3–31).

In these metabolic disorders, defects occur not in the primary apoenzyme structure but in the binding or the production of coenzymes involved in the major catalytic reaction. Only a few of the vitamin dependency syndromes have been adequately evaluated at the molecular level, but many possible abnormalities exist (Fig. 3–31); the vitamin may not be (1) transported into a specialized cell; (2) converted to its active coenzyme; or (3) bound to its apoenzyme to form a holoen-

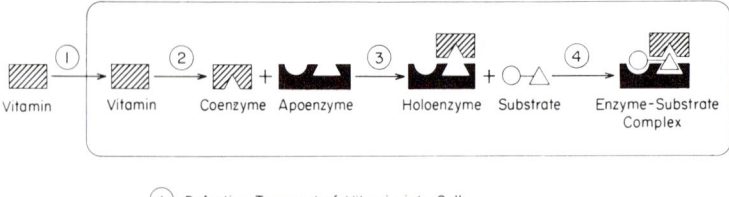

Figure 3-31 Inborn errors of metabolism expressing vitamin dependency could arise from any of the four biochemical blocks represented. (From Rosenberg, L. E.: New Eng. J. Med., *281*:145, 1969, with permission of author.)

① Defective Transport of Vitamin into Cell
② Defective Conversion of Vitamin to Coenzyme
③ Defective Formation of Holoenzyme
④ Inhibition of Formation of Enzyme-Substrate Complex

zyme; and, finally, (4) an inhibitor produced from an unrelated process may interfere with the formation of the enzyme-substrate complex. Therapeutic importance of this type of pathologic physiology is evident. In certain instances, administration of high concentrations of the precursor vitamin may augment the defective coenzyme or enzyme pathway and provide the individual with some protection against the toxic precursor or deficient product resulting from the altered pathway.

Diseases Caused by Enzymes Regulating Drug Metabolism

Some inherited disorders are not expressed until the organism is stressed by the administration of certain drugs. Such a disorder might arise if a mutant gene product did not remove a potentially toxic drug. A well-known example of this disorder is *serum cholinesterase* deficiency. As described previously, this enzyme hydrolyzes choline esters, notably the muscle relaxant succinyldicholine. Different types of mutant gene products can be analyzed in pedigrees by their resistance to inhibitors. A silent allele has also been described which results in the complete loss of enzyme activity in the homozygous condition. Immunochemical studies suggest that this "silent allele" produces a true absence of the total enzyme protein, whereas other mutant alleles produce products which differ only in their kinetic properties for the binding of cholinesterase and various inhibitors. The abnormal enzymes, however, have similar immunochemical properties, electrophoretic mobilities, and molecular size. Pedigree analyses suggest ten different phenotypes from three alleles at one locus (E_1). A second locus (E_2) has been described for this protein when examined by starch gel electrophoresis. The (E_2) locus is characterized by an isozyme with a fifth subunit (C_5) which is seen in approximately 10 per cent of European people. The functional attributes of this electrophoretic variation are as yet unknown. Individuals who are homozygous for an atypical allele or doubly heterozygous for the atypical silent allele are unable to hydrolyze succinyldicholine, a drug used to induce transient muscular paralysis during surgery. Normally, it is removed in minutes, but in affected individuals the drug persists in its pharmacologically active form for a prolonged period of time.

The use of a pedigree and biochemical analysis in the diagnosis and prevention of this disorder in a family is illustrated in Figure 3–32. The 19-year-old proband (III–1) is a healthy football player who had a molar tooth extracted. During surgery, succinyldicholine was administered and he remained paralyzed for six hours. A family history indicated that his mother had a similar respiratory arrest four years earlier following hysterectomy. Serum from the mother (II–2), proband, and siblings (III–2, III–3) had reduced hydrolytic activity as well as resistance to dibucaine and fluoride consistent with the homozygous atypical genotype (AA). This initial family history evaluation suggested direct parent-to-child transmission of an autosomal dominant trait which was contrary to the usual recessive mode of inheritance for serum cholinesterase deficiency. Serum from the clinically normal father (II–1) had normal enzyme activity but increased resistance to dibucaine and fluoride, suggesting that he was heterozygous (AU). This finding provided evidence for an autosomal recessive mode of inheritance. The mother and siblings were advised to avoid drugs of this type in the future. The normals and heterozygotes were reassured that they were not sensitive.

Another group of inborn errors caused by drug administration resulted from the observations of Hockwald that American Negroes develop an acute hemolytic anemia after receiving synthetic antimalarial drugs such as primaquine. This abnormal hemolytic response to the drug was caused by a deficiency of the enzyme *glucose-6-phosphate dehydrogenase* (G6PD), which normally catalyzes the oxidation of glucose-6-phosphate to 6-phospho-gluconate with reduction

PSEUDOCHOLINESTERASE DEFICIENCY
(Pedigree Mi)

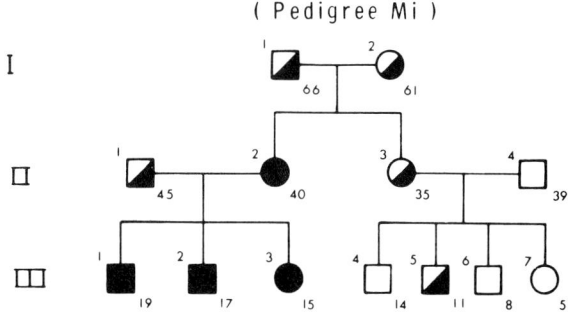

Figure 3-32 An example of combined pedigree and biochemical analysis in a family with pseudocholinesterase deficiency. Members represented by closed symbols are sensitive to succinyldicholine. "A" is atypical and "U" is the usual allele. Dibucaine and fluoride numbers indicate per cent inhibition of hydrolytic activity. (Assays were performed through the courtesy of B. N. LaDu, M.D., Ph.D.)

Patient	Activity*	Dibucaine Number	Fluoride Number	Probable Genotype
I-1	0.573	61.3	48.9	UA
I-2	0.700	64.0	51.5	UA
II-1	0.849	60.7	47.7	UA
II-2	0.421	20.8	23.0	AA
II-3	0.550	57.7	45.0	UA
II-4	1.140	83.0	60.5	UU
III-1	0.394	18.8	26.6	AA
III-2	0.391	12.4	23.2	AA
III-3	0.418	9.8	17.3	AA
III-4	1.054	81.2	64.6	UU
III-5	0.922	59.0	52.0	UA
III-6	1.070	80.3	63.8	UU
III-7	1.140	78.8	62.8	UU
(Normal)	(0.6-1.2)	(77-83)	(57-68)	(UU)

*μmoles benzoylcholine hydrolyzed / min / ml

of the coenzyme NADP to NADPH. This is the first step in the oxidation of glucose via the pentose shunt pathway, which serves to maintain the intracellular concentration of reduced coenzyme NADPH and glutathione. It is postulated that the interaction of primaquine with mutant G6PD results in failure to maintain reduced NADPH, diminution of reduced glutathione, fragility of red cell membrane, and hemolysis. Other drugs can produce these hemolytic crises; these include the sulfonamides, antimalarials, and fava beans (favism). Different mutant G6PD proteins occur in Negroes, Mediterranean, and Middle Eastern populations. They are all X-linked recessive traits. Of 21 variants which have been described, six are associated with hemolytic disease and presumably have specific properties which render red blood cells unstable. Female heterozygotes may be sensitive to these drugs, depending on lyonization effects and the quantitative impairment in G6PD.

Another inherited disease produced by drugs was found after isoniazid (INH) was introduced for tuberculosis therapy. Initial studies revealed two distinct groups of individuals with different rates of removal of INH from the plasma. Evans demonstrated that six hours after a 40 mg. per kg. dose, a group of subjects known as "slow inactivators" had plasma INH concentrations above 4 mcg. per ml., whereas the "rapid inactivators" had levels below 3 mcg. per ml. Rapid inactivators had a higher proportion of the drug in the urine in an acetylated form as compared to slow inactivators who excreted the drug unchanged. Acetylation of INH occurs in the liver as a consequence of the enzyme *acetyl-coenzyme A transferase*. The activity of this enzyme is much greater in the livers of rapid inactivators as compared to slow inactivators. This enzyme is also concerned with the acetylation of drugs such as sulfamethazine and sulfadiazine. This pathologic physiology has some significance in the use of the drug for the treatment of tuberculosis. Slow inactivators of INH are more likely to develop peripheral neuropathy after prolonged administration, but this rare complication of INH treatment can be prevented by the simultaneous administration of pyridoxine. Rapid inactivators may require higher doses to provide adequate circulating levels of the unacetylated active form. It is presumed from pedigree analyses that slow inactivators are homozygous for a "slow allele" and that rapid inactivators are either heterozygous or homozygous for the "rapid allele."

All three of the above examples of genetically determined enzyme defects are related to the metabolism of drugs and emphasize again the interrelationships of genetic and environmental factors in the pathogenesis of disease. Since the underlying genetic differences are brought out by drugs, these and several conditions of a similar nature have been called pharmacogenetic disorders.

APPLICATIONS TO MANAGEMENT OF INHERITED DISEASE

Although knowledge in the field of human genetics has grown rapidly, our concern as physicians has been to find applications for this knowledge even in its present sketchy state. Table 3-9 represents a composite of both factual and speculative approaches to the management of inherited diseases. These therapeutic approaches have been categorized according to the level of recognition of the pathogenic mechanisms. Thus, if all we recognize at present is an abnormal phenotype as in Down's syndrome, muscular dystrophy, or spina bifida, therapeutic approaches are limited to genetic counseling regarding the recurrence risks and to rehabilitation of the patient. In some instances the clinical phenotype may be expressed in cultured fetal cells, and more precise counseling such as antenatal diagnosis can be offered. The diagnosis of a male fetus in the case of X-linked recessive disorders or a chromosome abnormality in the cytogenetic disorders may be made and termination of pregnancy considered. In Hurler's and Hunter's syndromes, the rate of accumulation of S^{35}-labeled chondroitin sulfate by cultured amniotic cells provides a diagnostic handle in tissue culture even though the specific enzymatic defect is not recognized. Genetic counseling will become more precise as techniques of antenatal diagnosis improve. At this level of recognition, treatment of the affected individual must also be considered. Let us assume that a patient with phenylketonuria was not detected early enough in life to prevent mental retardation. Dietary restriction, controlled educational programs, and specific training may potentiate the patient's remaining capabilities such that he can take part in our complex society.

Many of the inborn errors of metabolism are detected by the presence of abnormal concentrations of potentially toxic precursors in an impaired reaction sequence and can be treated before the disease is clinically manifest. The best example of this is the statewide screening of newborns for elevated blood phenylalanine levels to diagnose phenylketonuria. Treatment of this group of disorders involves a form of environmental engineering in which the potentially toxic precursor, phenylalanine is restricted in the diet to prevent manifestations of the clinical phenotype. In other diseases such as Hartnup disease, the pellagra-like symptoms are preventable by the administration of the deficient end product nicotinic acid. In vitamin dependency syndromes such as vitamin responsive methylmalonic aci-

TABLE 3-9 THERAPY OF INHERITED DISEASE

Level of Recognition	Treatment

1. Clinical Phenotype	1. Genetic Counseling
	    a. Antenatal diagnosis
	    b. Rehabilitation

2. Impaired Reaction Sequence
    a. Toxic precursor
    b. Deficient product
    c. Deficient coenzyme
    d. Sensitivity to environment
	2. Environmental Engineering
	    a. Restriction
	    b. Replacement
	    c. Vitamin administration
	    d. Exposure prevention

3. Defective Gene Product
    a. Enzyme
    b. Structural protein
    c. Regulation
	3. Genetic Engineering
	    a. Replacement
	    b. Prevention of structural changes
	    c. Provision of inducer, repressor, or feedback inhibitor

4. Mutant DNA	4. Genetic Engineering
	    a. Transformation
	    b. Transduction

duria, the administration of massive amounts of the vitamin precursor will increase the deficient coenzyme and ameliorate the blocked reaction sequence and clinical problems attendant to the untreated condition. Environmental engineering may also be provided in circumstances in which an individual has a mutant gene product reflected only under stressful environmental conditions. The group of pharmacogenetic disorders is a good example of this situation in which patients are sensitive to the administration of primaquine (G6PD deficiency) or succinyldicholine (pseudo-cholinesterase deficiency). Prediction and prevention can be affected through pedigree analysis and chemical evaluation of "high-risk" members. Speculation in this area grows as we analyze the complex alleles of circulating blood proteins such as the α_1-antitrypsin. Fagerhol has pointed out that functional defects in antitrypsin activity and protein phenotypes may be associated with increased susceptibility to pulmonary disease, cirrhosis, and clotting disorders. As more knowledge is collected relating the structural and functional defects of this group of proteins and as populations are screened for their protein genotype, physicians may offer specific suggestions concerning the best type of environment in which an individual should live. For instance, a presymptomatic patient with α_1-antitrypsin deficiency and a protein genotype of ZZ (deficient) or MZ (40 per cent activity) may be advised to live in a rural rather than urban area to retard the development of lung disease resulting from the polluted environment.

In some of the inborn errors alluded to previously, the defective gene product has been defined as a functional or regulatory impairment of cell metabolism. At this level of recognition, therapy can be considered in terms of genetic engineering in which the objective is the replacement of a defective enzyme. This concept is not novel, since we all recognize the value of insulin or antihemophilic globulin in inherited disorders such as diabetes mellitus or hemophilia A. However, the administration of specific enzymes involved in intracellular function remains at present in the area of research. Purified enzymes can be enclosed in semipermeable inert nylon microspherules to protect the enzyme from immune host response. Catalase has been injected intravenously to revert the abnormal biochemical phenotype in acatalasemic mice, and urease has raised the blood ammonia in dogs. If the enzyme is lysosomal or cytoplasmic, its eventual deposition in liver may provide function to the organism in which this enzyme is deficient. Purified α-1,4-glucosidase from *Aspergillus niger* has reduced liver glycogen in patients dying from glycogen storage disease, Type II. In other instances, the defective gene product may be a structural protein whose molecular structure is recognized. The administration of urea to patients with sickle cell disease is a form of genetic engineering aimed at correcting the molecular aggregation of sickle hemoglobin. The use of the cyanate ion and carbamyl phosphate to inhibit the sickling phenomenon is also under study. In some disorders, the defective enzyme function may be inducible. Thus, in hepatic glucuronyl transferase deficiency, sodium phenobarbital has enhanced this enzymatic pathway and the perinatal utilization of bilirubin. Steroid hormones may also be effective inducers of some enzymes. In one patient with Type III glycogen storage disease, a double enzyme deficiency involving amylo-1,6-glucosidase and glucose-6-phosphatase was described. A fourfold increase in glucose-6-phosphatase activity occurred upon administration of triamcinolone. Repression of an overactive pathway may also become a form of genetic engineering. In orotic aciduria the administration of uridine represses the initial step of this pathway and reduces the formation of insoluble orotic acid.

Finally, the most intriguing aspect of therapy in inherited disease of man involves the recent approaches to gene insertion into mammalian cells. Although many of the fundamental genetic and regulatory processes of mammalian cells remain unknown, transduction using bacterial viruses and transformation using cell fusion techniques have demonstrated science's ability to introduce new functional genes into mammalian cells. Although transformation per se has not been used in mammalian cells derived from humans, Harris' group has demonstrated that by fusing a chick red blood cell whose nucleus carries the gene for inosinic acid pyrophosphorylase with a mouse fibroblast A_9 cell which is deficient in this enzyme function, transformation of the mutant mouse cell line is accomplished. Transduction has been utilized in one human disease, galactosemia. Merril's group has produced a λ-phage (λpgal) lysogenic for *E. coli* which carries part of the bacterial galactose operon coding for α-D-galactose-1-phosphate uridyl transferase (UDPGal-1-P). This λ-phage will infect cultured fibroblasts derived from the skin of patients lacking this enzyme function (galactosemia) and return UDPGal-1-P activity. The infected fibroblasts retain this activity for at least 8 population doublings (40 days in culture) and manufacture new λ-specific RNA. Whether other side-effects from λ-pgal infection will be seen in intact mammals is currently under investigation. Although these new developments do not provide practical genetic engineering, it is now clear that science has provided means by which genes can be transferred and inserted into mammalian cells. These basic tools will provide answers to many questions concerning gene function and perhaps in the future, a method for treating the inborn errors of metabolism.

GLOSSARY OF GENETIC TERMS

Acrocentric — Chromosomes with the centromere close to one end.

Alleles — Alternate forms of a gene occurring at the same locus.

Aneuploid — Deviation from the basic diploid number or from exact multiples of the basic (haploid) number in a chromosome series (aneuploidy).

Arm (chromosome) — The portion of a chromatid located on either side of the centromere of a metaphase chromosome.

Autosome — Any chromosome other than the sex chromosomes (22 pairs in humans).

"Balanced translocation" — Rearrangement of chromosomal material, without genetic effect because the loss of part of one chromosome is compensated for by its attachment to another chromosome of the individual.

Break (chromosome) — Interruption in staining of the chromosome arm, with displacement in the alignment of the portions on either side of the interruption.

Cell cycle (cell life cycle) — The cycle in the life of a cell which includes mitosis (M) and the interphase.

Centromere (also kinetochore or primary constriction) — A nonstaining area on a chromosome, separating the chromosome arms; the point of attachment of the chromosome to the mitotic spindle.

Chromatid — One of two structurally distinguishable (by light microscopy) longitudinal subunits of a metaphase chromosome.

Chromatin — Areas of a cell nucleus that stain with a DNA stain. (See also *Sex chromatin*.)

Cis — Two genes on the same chromosome are cis to each other or coupled.

Cistron — The gene considered on a functional basis as defined by the cis-trans complementation test. Two mutants in the same cistron do not complement; two mutants in different cistrons do.

Codon — A triplet of three bases in a strand of DNA which codes for a specific amino acid.

Complementation — Interaction of two cytoplasmic products to produce a normal phenotype.

Crossing-over — The exchange of genetic material between members of a pair of homologous chromosomes that leads to the formation of recombinants.

Daughter cell — One of the two products of mitosis.

Deletion (chromosome) — Absence of part of a chromosome.

Diploid — Possessing two genomes. In man, the somatic cells contain the diploid number of chromosomes: 46 (2n).

Discontinuous traits — Two clearly different phenotypes which do not blend with one another.

DNA — Deoxyribonucleic acid; a constituent of chromosomes.

Dominant — The phenotype expressed in the F_1 heterozygote resulting from a cross between two true-breeding strains. The dominant allele determines the phenotype expressed by a heterozygote.

F_1 — The first filial generation (the progeny) of a cross between two individuals.

Fragment (chromosome) — A portion of a chromosome.

Gap (chromosome) — Interruption in staining of a chromosome arm, without disturbance of alignment of the portions on either side of the interruption.

Gene — (a) Classic mendelian definition: The fundamental biologic unit of heredity transmitted from generation to generation unchanged;
    (b) Molecular definition: Unit of function of a cistron. One gene codes for one polypeptide chain.

Genome — One copy of each allele.

Genotype — The genetic constitution of an individual.

Haploid — A haploid cell contains one copy of a genome. The normal gamete contains only one member of each chromosome pair and is therefore haploid. In man, the haploid chromosome number (n) is 23.

Hemizygous — A special term used in designating the genotype of the male. Since human males have only one X chromosome, they are said to be hemizygous with respect to the X-linked genes.

Heterochromatin (heterochromatization; heterochromatic) — Nuclear areas that stain "differently" with DNA stains.

Heterogeneity — A trait whose phenotypic expression can be produced by a number of different genetic mechanisms is heterogeneous.
Heterokaryon — Cell with two or more genomes of different types.
Heterozygote — An individual who has two different alleles for a given gene.
Homozygote — An individual possessing a pair of identical alleles for a given gene.
Hyperdiploidy (hypodiploidy) — More (or less) than the diploid number of chromosomes — a form of aneuploidy.
Isochromosome — A chromosome consisting of identical arms on either side of the centromere.
Karyotype — The chromosome set of an individual.
Linkage — Association of genes on one chromosome.
Locus — A cluster of genes located in a linkage group.
Meiosis — That form of cell division occurring in the formation of gametes producing the haploid chromosome number (n) from a diploid cell (2n).
Metacentric — Chromosomes with the centromere located in the center, making the two arms on either side of it equal in length.
Mitogenic — Capable of inducing mitosis.
Mitosis — Somatic cell division resulting in the formation of two cells, each with the same chromosome complement as the parent cell.
Monosomic — The double basic number in a chromosome series minus one; one pair contains 1 instead of 2 chromosomes (monosomy).
Monozygotic — Twins derived from a single fertilized ovum (identical twins).
Mosaic — An individual or tissue with at least two cell lines, differing in genotype or karyotype, derived from a single zygote.
Mutant — An altered gene, or an individual bearing such an altered gene.
Mutation — An alteration in genetic material that is transmitted from one generation to the next.
Nonsense mutation — A change in a gene resulting in the formation of one of the "stop" codons in place of a codon for a particular amino acid and leading to formation of a partial protein that is terminated at the site of the mutation.
Operon — A genetic unit consisting of an operator and the cistrons whose actions it controls.
Phenocopy — An individual whose appearance is produced by an environmental effect, but whose phenotype is similar to one produced by a genetic effect.
Phenotype — The physical constitution of an individual. This includes physical, biochemical, and physiologic makeup of an individual as determined by his genotype and the environment in which he develops.
Pleiotropy — The situation in which a single gene or gene pair produces multiple effects.
Point mutation — A change in a single base pair.
Polypeptide — A chain of amino acids held together by peptide bonds.
Polyploidy — The designation for the occurrence of chromosome numbers in multiples of the basic haploid number (n), other than the diploid number (2n), e.g., triploidy (3n), tetraploidy (4n), and so on.
Proband — Same as *propositus*.
Propositus — Also called index case, or proband; the family member who first draws attention to a pedigree of a particular trait.
Protein polymorphism — The occurrence of two or more different forms of the same protein.
Recessive — That phenotype which is *not* expressed in the F_1 heterozygote resulting from a cross between two true breeding strains.
Recombination — The formation of new combinations of linked genes by crossing-over between them.
Replication, DNA — The process by which new DNA is made from a DNA template.
Ring (chromosome) — Attachment of opposite ends of a chromosome to form a ring resulting from two breaks with joining of both ends (a deletion is implied in this situation).
RNA — Ribonucleic acid.
Satellite — DNA staining structure on the distal end of a chromosome arm and separated from it by a secondary constriction.
Secondary constriction — A nonstaining area on a chromosome arm.
Segregation — The separation of alleles and chromosomes during meiosis.

Sex chromatin, female (Barr body) — A characteristic area in the interphase nucleus, composed of X-chromosome material that stains heavily with a DNA stain.

Sex chromatin, male (Y body) — A characteristic area in the interphase nucleus composed of Y-chromosome material that fluoresces brightly.

Sex chromosomes — XX in human female; XY in human male: 1 pair is normally present in each individual.

Silent allele — An allele which has no detectable product, presumably produced by a nonsense mutant.

Somatic — Pertaining to cells other than germ cells.

Tetraploid — The quadruple basic number in a chromosome series (4n).

Trans — Two genes on different chromosomes are trans to each other, or in repulsion.

Transcription, RNA — The process by which new RNA is made from a DNA template.

Transduction — A change in the genetic constitution of a cell in which a bacteriophage carries DNA from one cell to another.

Translation — The process by which genetic information contained in DNA is carried by mRNA from the nucleus to the cytoplasm and affects amino acid sequences in the synthesis of proteins.

Translocation — The transfer of a piece of one chromosome to a nonhomologous chromosome.

Triploid — The triple basic number in a chromosome series (3n).

Trisomy — The state of having one extra chromosome per cell. Instead of the usual pair of chromosomes, there are now three of a particular pair.

X-linked — Genes on the X chromosome or traits determined by such genes are X-linked.

Zygote — The first product of the union of sperm and egg.

REFERENCES

INTRODUCTION

Garrod, A. E.: Inborn errors of metabolism (Croonian Lectures). Lancet, 2:1, 73, 142, and 214, 1908.

Ingram, V. M.: Gene mutations in human haemoglobin: the chemical difference between normal and sickle cell haemoglobin. Nature, 180:326, August 10, 1957.

Jacob, F., and Monod, J.: On the regulation of gene activity. Cold Spring Harbor Symposia on Quant. Biol., 26:193, 1961.

Miller, O. J., Allderdice, P. W., Miller, D. A., Breg, W. R., and Migeon, B. R.: Human thymidine kinase gene locus: assignment to chromosome 17 in a hybrid of man and mouse cells. Science, 173:244, 1971.

Nirenberg, M. W., and Matthaei, J. H.: The dependence of cell-free protein synthesis in *E. coli* upon naturally occurring or synthetic polyribonucleotides. Proc. Nat. Acad. Sci. (U.S.A.), 47:1588, October 15, 1961.

Watson, J. D., and Crick, F. H. C.: Genetical implications of the structure of deoxyribonucleic acid. Nature, 171:964, May 30, 1953.

Weiss, M. C., and Green, H.: Human-mouse hybrid cell lines containing partial complements of human chromosomes and functioning human genes. Proc. Nat. Acad. Sci. (U.S.A.), 58:1104, September, 1967.

MENDELIAN INHERITANCE

Edwards, J. H.: The simulation of mendelism. Acta Genet. (Basel), 10:63, 1960.

Haws, D. V., and McKusick, V. A.: Farabee's brachydactylous kindred revisited. Bull. Johns Hopkins Hosp., 113:20, July, 1963.

Huntley, C. C., and Stevenson, R. E.: Maternal phenylketonuria. Course of two pregnancies. Obstet. Gynec., 34:694, November, 1969.

Kerr, G. R., Chamove, A. S., Harlow, H. F., and Waisman, H. A.: "Fetal PKU": the effect of maternal hyperphenylalaninemia during pregnancy in the rhesus monkey *(Macaca mulatta)*. Pediatrics, 42:27, July, 1968.

Kirkman, H. N.: Dominant mutations — biochemical basis for phenotype. *In* Fraser, F. C., and McKusick, V. A. (Eds.): International Conference on Congenital Malformations III, Netherlands, The Hague, 1969. Excerpta Medica (New York), No. 204, p. 209.

Mendel, G.: Versuche über Pflanzenhybriden. Leipzig, Engelmann, 1901. Translated in J. Heredity, 42:1, 1951.

McKusick, V. A.: Mendelian Inheritance in Man: Catalogs of Autosomal Dominant, Autosomal Recessive, and X-linked Phenotypes. 3rd ed. Baltimore, Johns Hopkins Press, 1971.

Menser, M. A., Slinn, R. F., Dods, L., Herzberg, R., and Harley, J. D.: Congenital rubella in a mother and son. Aust. Paediat. J., 4:200, September, 1968.

Schoen, E. J., and Reynolds, J. B.: Severe familial hypophosphatemic rickets. Normal growth following early treatment. Amer. J. Dis. Child., 120:58, July, 1970.

Winters, R. W., Graham, J. B., Williams, T. F., McFalls, V. W., and Burnett, C. H.: A genetic study of familial hypophosphatemia and vitamin D resistant rickets with a review of the literature. Medicine, 37:97, May, 1958.

MULTIFACTORIAL GENETIC DISORDERS

Carter, C. O., David, P. A., and Laurence, K. M.: A family study of major central nervous system malformations in South Wales. J. Med. Genet., 5:81, June, 1968.

Carter, C. O., and Evans, K. A.: Inheritance of congenital pyloric stenosis. J. Med. Genet., 6:233, September, 1969.

Harris, H., Whittaker, M., Lehmann, H., and Silk, E.: The pseudocholinesterase variants. Esterase levels and dibucaine numbers in families selected through suxamethonium sensitive individuals. Acta Genet. (Basel), 10:1, 1960.

Carter, C. O.: Multifactorial genetic disease. Hosp. Pract., 5:45, May, 1970.

Falconer, D. S.: The inheritance of liability to certain diseases, estimated from the incidence among relatives. Ann. Human Genet., 29:51, August, 1965.

Carter, C. O.: Genetics of common disorders. Brit. Med. Bull., 25:52, January, 1969.

CYTOGENETICS

Chicago Conference: Standardization in Human Cytogenetics. Birth Defects: Original Article Series, II:2, 1966. New York, The National Foundation.

Dhadial, R. K., Machin, A. M., and Tait, S. M.: Chromosomal anomalies in spontaneously aborted human fetuses. Lancet, 2:20, July 4, 1970.

Priest, J. H.: Human cell culture: An important tool for the diagnosis and understanding of disease. J. Pediat., 72:415, March, 1968.

NUMERICAL ABNORMALITIES OF THE CHROMOSOMES

Barr, M. L., Sergovich, F. R., Carr, D. H., and Shaver, E. L.: The triple-X female: An appraisal based on a study of 12 cases and a review of the literature. Canad. Med. Assoc. J., 101:247, September 6, 1969.

Carr, D. H.: Chromosome anomalies as a cause of spontaneous abortion. Amer. J. Obstet. Gynec., 97:283, February 1, 1967.

Caspersson, T., Farber, S., Foley, G. E., Kudynowski, J., Modest, E. J., Simonsson, E., Wagh, U., and Zech, L.: Chemical differentiation along metaphase chromosomes. Exp. Cell. Res., 49:219, January, 1968.

Court Brown, W. M.: Males with an XYY sex chromosome complement. J. Med. Genet., 5:341, December, 1968.

Edwards, J. H., Harnden, D. G., Cameron, A. H., Crosse, V. M., and Wolff, O. H.: A new trisomic syndrome. Lancet, 1:787, April 9, 1960.

Engel, E., and Forbes, A. P.: Cytogenetic and clinical findings in 48 patients with congenitally defective or absent ovaries. Medicine, 44:135, March, 1965.

Fine, R. N., Wang, M. F., and Heath, C. W., Jr.: Nuclear projections of neutrophils in the 13-15 trisomy syndrome. Pediatrics, 35:712, April, 1965.

Hamerton, J. L., Giannelli, F., and Polani, P. E.: Cytogenetics of Down's syndrome (mongolism). I. Data on a consecutive series of patients referred for genetic counseling and diagnosis. Cytogenetics, 4:171, 1965.

Jacobs, P. A., Brunton, M., Melville, M. M., Brittain, R. P., and McClemont, W. F.: Aggressive behavior, mental subnormality and the XYY male. Nature, 208:1351, December 25, 1965.

Lundberg, P. O., and Wahlström, J.: Hormone levels in men with extra Y chromosomes. Lancet, 2:1133, November 28, 1970.

McHardy-Young, S., Doniach, D., and Polani, P. E.: Thyroid function in Turner's syndrome and allied conditions. Lancet, 2:1161, December 5, 1970.

Patau, K., Smith, D. W., Therman, E., Inhorn, S. L., and Wagner, H. P.: Multiple congenital anomaly caused by an extra autosome. Lancet, 1:790, April 9, 1960.

Pearson, P. L., Bobrow, M., and Vosa, C. G.: Technique for identifying Y chromosomes in human interphase nuclei. Nature, 226:78, April 4, 1970.

Penrose, L. S., and Smith, G. F.: Down's Anomaly. London, J. & A. Churchill, Ltd., 1966.

Polani, P. E.: Sex Chromosome Anomalies in Man. *In* Hamerton, J. L. (Ed.): Chromosomes in Medicine. London, William Heinemann Medical Books, Ltd., 1965.

Polani, P. E.: Autosomal imbalance and its syndromes, excluding Down's. Brit. Med. Bull., 25:81, January, 1969.

Sergovich, F., Valentine, G. H., Chen, A. T., Kinch, R. A. H., and Smout, M. S.: Chromosome aberrations in 2159 consecutive newborn babies. New Eng. J. Med., 280:851, April 17, 1969.

Taylor, A. I.: Autosomal trisomy syndromes: A detailed study of 27 cases of Edwards' syndrome and 27 cases of Patau's syndrome. J. Med. Genet., 5:227, September, 1968.

Zaleski, W. A., Houston, C. S., Pozsonyi, J., and Ying, K. L.: The XXXXY chromosome anomaly: report of 3 new cases and review of 30 cases from the literature. Canad. Med. Assoc. J., 94:1143, May 28, 1966.

STRUCTURAL ABNORMALITIES OF THE CHROMOSOMES

Bloom, A. D., and Tjio, J. H.: In vivo effects of diagnostic x-irradiation on human chromosomes. New Eng. J. Med., 270:1341, June 18, 1964.

Breg, W. R., Steele, M. W., Miller, O. J., Warburton, D., deCapoa, A., and Allderdice, P. W.: The cri du chat syndrome in adolescents and adults: Clinical findings in 13 older patients with partial deletion of the short arm of chromosome No. 5 (5p−). J. Ped., 77:782, November, 1970.

Buckton, K. E., Jacobs, P. A., Court Brown, W. M., and Doll, R.: A study of the chromosome damage persisting after x-ray therapy for ankylosing spondylitis. Lancet, 2:676, October 6, 1962.

Caspersson, T., Gahrton, G., Lindsten, J., and Zech, L.: Identification of the Philadelphia chromosome as a number 22 by quinacrine mustard fluorescence analysis. Exp. Cell Res., 63:238, November, 1970.

Dosik, H., Hsu, L. Y., Todaro, G. J., Lee, S. L., Hirschhorn, K., Selirio, E. S., and Alter, A. A.: Leukemia in Fanconi's anemia: Cytogenetic and tumor virus susceptibility studies. Blood, 36:341, September, 1970.

Ezdinli, E. Z., Sokal, J. E., Crosswhite, L., and Sandberg, A. A.: Philadelphia-chromosome-positive and -negative chronic myelocytic leukemia. Ann. Intern. Med., 72:175, February, 1970.

German, J.: Human chromosomal breakage. J. Pediat., 72:440, March, 1968.

Hirschhorn, K.: Cytogenetic alterations in leukemia. *In* Dameshek, W., and Dutcher, R. M.: Perspectives in Leukemia. New York, Grune and Stratton, 1968.

Miller, O. J., Breg, W. R., Warburton, D., Miller, D. A., deCapoa, A., Allderdice, P. W., Davis, J., Klinger, H. P., McGilvray, E., and Allen, F. H., Jr.: Partial deletion of the short arm of chromosome No. 4 (4p−): Clinical studies in five unrelated patients. J. Pediat., 77:792, November, 1970.

Prieto, F., Egozcue, J., Forteza, G., and Marco, F.: Identification of the Philadelphia (Ph¹) chromosome. Blood, 35:23, January, 1970.

Sawitsky, A., Bloom, D., and German, J.: Chromosomal breakage and acute leukemia in congenital telangiectatic erythema and stunted growth. Ann. Intern. Med., 65:487, September, 1966.

Schroeder, T. M., and Kurth, R.: Spontaneous chromosomal breakage and high incidence of leukemia in inherited disease. Blood, 37:96, January, 1971.

Tjio, J. H., Carbone, P. P., Whang, J., and Frei, E., III: The Philadelphia chromosome and chronic myelogenous leukemia. J. Nat. Cancer Inst., 36:567, April, 1966.

Tjio, J. H., Pahnke, W. N., and Kurland, A. A.: LSD and chromosomes: A controlled experiment. J.A.M.A., 210:849, November 3, 1969.

CANCER AND AGING

Fialkow, P. J.: "Immunologic" oncogenesis. Blood, 30:388, September, 1967.

Court Brown, W. M.: Frontiers of Biology: Human population cytogenetics. Vol. 5. Amsterdam, North-Holland Publishing Co., 1967.

Hamerton, J. L., Taylor, A. I., Angell, R., and McGuire, V. M.: Chromosome investigations of a small isolated human population: Chromosome abnormalities and distribution of chromosome counts according to age and sex among the population of Tristan da Cunha. Nature, 206:1232, June 19, 1965.

Pierre, R. V., and Hoagland, H. C.: 45,X cell lines in adult men: Loss of Y chromosome, a normal aging phenomenon? Mayo Clin. Proc., 46:52, January, 1971.

Sandberg, A. A., Cohen, M. M., Rimm, A. A., and Levin, M. L.: Aneuploidy and age in a population survey. Amer. J. Human Genet., 19:633, September, 1967.

Spriggs, A. I., Boddington, M. M., and Clarke, C. M.: Chromosomes of human cancer cells. Brit. Med. J., 2:1431, December, 1962.

BIOCHEMICAL BASIS FOR INHERITANCE

Braunitzer, G., Hilse, K., Rudloff, V., and Hilschmann, N.: The hemoglobins. Advanced Protein Chem., 19:1, 1964.

Cleaver, J. E.: Defective repair replication of DNA in xeroderma pigmentosum. Nature, 218:652, May 18, 1968.

Granner, D. K., Hayashi, S. L., Thompson, E. B., and Tomkins, G. M.: Stimulation of tyrosine aminotransferase synthesis by dexamethasone phosphate in cell culture. J. Molec. Biol., 35:291, 1968.

Ingram, V. M., and Stretton, A. O.: Genetic basis of the thalassaemia diseases. Nature, *184*:1903, December 19, 1959.

Itano, H. A., and Neel, J. V.: A new inherited abnormality of human hemoglobin. Proc. Nat. Acad. Sci. (U.S.A.), *36*:613, November 15, 1950.

Kornberg, A.: Enzymatic synthesis of DNA. New York, John Wiley and Sons, Inc., 1962.

Krieg, D. R.: Specificity of chemical mutagenesis. Progr. Nucleic Acid Res., *2*:125, 1963.

Lehmann, H., and Carrell, R. W.: Variations in the structure of human haemoglobin with particular reference to the unstable haemoglobins. Brit. Med. Bull., *25*:14, January, 1969.

Meselson, M., and Stahl, F. W.: The replication of DNA in *Escherichia coli*. Proc. Nat. Acad. Sci. (U.S.A.), *44*:671, July 15, 1958.

Murayama, M.: Structure of sickle cell hemoglobin and molecular mechanism of the sickling phenomenon. Clin. Chem., *14*:578, 1967.

Neel, J. V.: The inheritance of sickle cell anemia. Science, *110*:64, July 15, 1949.

Neel, J. V.: The inheritance of sickling phenomenon with particular reference to sickle cell disease. Blood, *6*:389, May, 1951.

Nirenberg, M. W., and Matthaci, J. H.: The dependence of cell-free protein synthesis in *E. coli* upon naturally occurring or synthetic polyribonucleotides. Proc. Nat. Acad. Sci. (Wash.), *47*:1588, 1961.

Pauling, L., Itano, H. A., Singer, S. J., and Wells, I. C.: Sickle cell anemia, molecular disease. Science, *110*:543, November 25, 1949.

Perutz, M. F., and Lehmann, H.: Molecular pathology of human haemoglobin. Nature, *219*:902, August 31, 1968.

Perutz, M. F., and Mitchison, J. M.: State of haemoglobin in sickle-cell anaemia. Nature, *166*:677, October 21, 1950.

Prescott, D. M.: The structure and replication of eukaryotic chromosomes. *In* Prescott, D. M., Goldstein, L., and McConkey, E. (Eds.): Advances in Cell Biology. Vol. 1. New York, Appleton-Century-Crofts, 1969, pp. 57–117.

Ptashne, M.: Specific binding of the λ-phage repressor to λ-DNA. Nature, *214*:232, April 15, 1967.

Speyer, J. F.: The genetic code. *In* Taylor, J. H. (Ed.): Molecular Genetics. Part II. New York, Academic Press, Inc., 1967, pp. 137–191.

Sullivan, D. T.: Molecular hybridization used to characterize the RNA synthesized by isolated bovine thymus nuclei. Proc. Nat. Acad. Sci. (U.S.A.), *59*:846, March, 1968.

Weatherall, D. J.: Genetics of the thalassaemias. Brit. Med. Bull., *25*:24, January, 1969.

Woese, C. R.: The present status of the genetic code. Progr. Nucleic Acid Res. and Molec. Biol., *7*:107, 1967.

Inborn Errors of Metabolism

Enzymes

Harris, H.: Genes and isozymes. Proc. Roy. Soc. Lond., *174*:1, October 7, 1969.

LaDu, B. N., Zannoni, V. G., Laster, L., and Seegmiller, J. E.: The nature of the defect in tyrosine metabolism in alcaptonuria. J. Biol. Chem., *230*:251, January, 1958.

Membrane Transport

Bowden, J. A., and Connelly, J. L.: Branched-chain α-keto acid metabolism. II. Evidence for the common identity of α-ketoisocaproic acid and α-keto-β-methyl-valeric acid dehydrogenases. J. Biol. Chem., *243*:3526, June 25, 1968.

Crane, R. K.: Intestinal absorption of sugars. Physiol. Rev., *40*:789, October, 1960.

Crawhall, J. C., Scowen, E. F., and Watts, R. W.: Further observations on use of D-penicillamine in cystinuria. Brit. Med. J., *1*:1411, May 30, 1964.

Dancis, J., Hutzler, J., and Rokkones, T.: Intermittent branched-chain ketonuria, variant of maple-sugar-urine disease. New Eng. J. Med., *276*:84, January 12, 1967.

Dancis, J., Hutzler, J., and Cox, R. P.: Enzyme defect in skin fibroblasts in intermittent branched-chain ketonuria and in maple syrup urine disease. Biochem. Med., *2*:407, 1969.

Dent, C. E., and Rose, G. A.: Amino acid metabolism in cystinuria. Quart. J. Med., *20*:205, July, 1951.

Elsas, L. J., and Rosenberg, L. E.: Familial renal glycosuria: a genetic reappraisal of hexose transport by kidney and intestine. J. Clin. Invest., *48*:1845, October, 1969.

Elsas, L. J., Hillman, R. E., Patterson, J. H., and Rosenberg, L. E.: Renal and intestinal hexose transport in familial glucose-galactose malabsorption. J. Clin. Invest., *49*:576, March, 1970.

Elsas, L. J., Busse, D., and Rosenberg, L. E.: Autosomal recessive inheritance of renal glycosuria. Metabolism, *20*:968, October, 1971.

Elsas, L. J., Pask, B. A., Wheeler, F. B., Perl, D. P., and Trusler, S.: Cofactor resistant maple syrup urine disease. Metabolism, *21*:929, 1972.

Evanson, J. M., and Stanbury, S. W.: Congenital chloridorrhea or so-called congenital alkalosis with diarrhoea. Gut, *6*:29, February, 1965.

Goedde, H. W., and Keller, W.: Metabolic pathways in maple syrup urine disease. *In* Nyhan, W. L. (Ed.): Amino-acid Metabolism and Genetic Variations. New York, McGraw-Hill, 1967, pp. 191–214.

Goldberg, L. S., and Fudenberg, H. H.: Familial selective malabsorption of vitamin B_{12}. Re-evaluation of an *in vivo* intrinsic-factor inhibitor. New Eng. J. Med., *279*:405, August 22, 1968.

Harris, H., Mittwoch, U., Robson, E. B., and Warren, F. L.: Phenotypes and genotypes in cystinuria. Ann. Human Genet., *20*:57, August, 1955.

Hsia, D. Y.: Galactosemia. Springfield, Ill., Charles C Thomas, 1969.

Jacob, H. S., and Jandl, J. H.: Increased cell membrane permeability in the pathogenesis of hereditary spherocytosis. J. Clin. Invest., *43*:1704, August, 1964.

Kalckar, H. M., Braganca, B., and Munch-Petersen, A.: Uridyl transferases and the formation of uridine diphosphogalactose. Nature, *172*:1038, December 5, 1953.

Kinoshita, J. H., Futterman, S., Satoh, K., and Merola, L. O.: Factors affecting the formation of sugar alcohols in ocular lens. Biochem. Biophys. Acta, *74*:340, 1963.

Menkes, J. H., Hurst, P. L., and Craig, J. M.: New syndrome: progressive infantile cerebral dysfunction associated with an unusual urinary substance. Pediatrics, *14*:462, November, 1954.

Menkes, J. H.: Maple syrup disease: investigations into the metabolic defect. Neurology, *9*:826, December, 1959.

Milne, M. D., Crawford, M. A., Girao, C. B., and Loughridge, L. W.: The metabolic disorder in Hartnup disease. Quart. J. Med., *29*:407, July, 1960.

O'Brien, W. M., LaDu, B. N., and Bunim, J. J.: Biochemical, pathologic and clinical aspects of alcaptonuria, ochronosis and ochronotic arthropathy. Review of World Literature (1584–1962). Amer. J. Med., *34*:813, June, 1963.

Pardee, A. B.: Crystallization of a sulfate-binding protein (permease) from *Salmonella typhimurium*. Science, *156*:1627, June 23, 1967.

Rosenberg, L. E., Downing, S., Durant, J. L., and Segal, S.: Cystinuria: biochemical evidence for three genetically distinct diseases. J. Clin. Invest., *45*:365, March, 1966.

Rosenberg, L. E.: Genetic heterogeneity in cystinuria. *In* Nyhan, W. L. (Ed.): Amino-acid Metabolism and Genetic Variations. New York, McGraw-Hill Book Co., Inc., 1968, pp. 341–349.

Schulman, J. D., Lustberg, T. J., Kennedy, J. L., Museles, M., and Seegmiller, J. E.: A new variant of maple syrup urine disease (branched-chain ketoaciduria): Clinical and biochemical evaluation. Amer. J. Med., *49*:118, July, 1970.

Scriver, C R., and Hechtman, P.: Human genetics of membrane transport with emphasis on amino acids. *In* Harris, H., and Hirschhorn, K. (Eds.): Advances in Human Genetics. New York, Plenum Press. Vol. 1, 1970, pp. 211–274.

Scriver, C. R., Clow, C. L., MacKenzie, S., and Delvin, E.: Thiamine-responsive maple syrup urine disease. Lancet, *1*:310, 1971.

Silberberg, D. H.: Maple syrup urine disease metabolites studies in cerebellum cultures. J. Neurochem., *16*:1141, July, 1969.

Snyderman, S. E.: The therapy of maple syrup urine disease. Amer. J. Dis. Child., *113*:68, January, 1967.

Products of Minor Pathways

Koch, J., Stokstad, E. L., Williams, H. E., and Smith, L. H.: Deficiency of 2-oxo-glutarate: glyoxylate carboligase activity in primary hyperoxaluria. Proc. Nat. Acad. Sci. (U.S.A.), *57*:1123, April, 1967.

Waisman, H. A.: Induced phenylketonuria in experimental animals – opportunities and limitations. *In* Anderson, J. A., and Swaiman, K. F. (Eds.): Phenylketonuria and Allied Metabolic Diseases. Washington, U.S. Department of Health, Education and Welfare, Children's Bureau, 1967, pp. 21–31.

Williams, H. E., and Smith, L. H., Jr.: L-glyceric aciduria. A new genetic variant of primary hyperoxaluria. New Eng. J. Med., *278*:233, February 1, 1968.

End Product Deficiency

Biglieri, E. G., Herron, M. A., and Brust, N.: 17-hydroxylation deficiency in man. J. Clin. Invest., *45*:1946, December, 1966.

Bongiovanni, A. M.: The adrenogenital syndrome with deficiency of 3 β-hydroxysteroid dehydrogenase. J. Clin. Invest., *41*:2086, November, 1962.

Childs, B., Grumbach, M. M., and Van Wyk, J. J.: Virilizing adrenal hyperplasia: a genetic and hormonal study. J. Clin. Invest., *35*:213, February, 1956.

Fitzpatrick, T. B., Seiji, M., and McGugan, A. D.: Melanin pigmentation. New Eng. J. Med., *265*:328, 374, and 430, 1961.

Gabrilove, J. L., Sharma, D. L., and Dorfman, R. I.: Adrenocortical 11 β-hydroxylase deficiency and virilism first manifest in the adult woman. New Eng. J. Med., *272*:1189, June 10, 1965.

Seiji, M., Fitzpatrick, T. B., Simpson, R. T., and Birbeck, M. S.: Chemical composition and terminology of specialized organelles (melanosomes and melanin granules) in mammalian melanocytes. Nature, *197*:1082, March 16, 1963.

Stanbury, J. B., and DeGroot, L. J.: The clinical chemistry and pathologic physiology of thyroid tissue. Clin. Chem., *13*:542, 1967.

Visser, H. K., and Cost, W. S.: A new hereditary defect in the biosynthesis of aldosterone: Urinary C_{21}-corticosteroid pattern in three related patients with a salt-losing syndrome, suggesting an 18-oxidation defect. Acta Endocr., *47*:589, December, 1964.

Loss of Feedback Inhibition

Fujimoto, W. Y., and Seegmiller, J. E.: Hypoxanthine-guanine phosphoribosyltransferase deficiency: Activity in normal, mutant, and heterozygote – cultured human skin fibroblasts. Proc. Nat. Acad. Sci. (U.S.A.), *65*:577, March, 1970.

Granick, S., and Urata, G.: Increase in activity of δ-aminolevulinic acid synthetase in liver mitochondria induced by feeding of 3,5-dicarbethoxy-1,4-dihydrocollidine. J. Biol. Chem., *238*:821, February, 1963.

Haggard, M. E., and Lockhardt, L. H.: Megaloblastic anemia and orotic aciduria. A hereditary disorder of pyrimidine metabolism responsive to uridine. Amer. J. Dis. Child., *113*:733, June, 1967.

Huguley, C. M., Jr., Bain, J. A., Rivers, S. L., and Scoggins, R. B.: Refractory megaloblastic anemia associated with excretion of orotic acid. Blood, *14*:615, June, 1959.

Meyer, U. A., and Marver, H. S.: Intermittent acute porphyria: Clinical demonstration of a genetic defect in porphobilinogen metabolism. Clin. Res., *19*:398, 1971.

Rosenbloom, F. M., Henderson, J. F., Caldwell, I. C., Kelley, W. N., and Seegmiller, J. E.: Biochemical bases of accelerated purine biosynthesis *de novo* in human fibroblasts lacking hypoxanthine-guanine phosphoribosyltransferase. J. Biol. Chem., *243*:1166, March 25, 1968.

Seegmiller, J. E.: Diseases of purine and pyrimidine metabolism. *In* Bondy, P. K., and Rosenberg, L. E. (Eds.): Duncan's Diseases of Metabolism. Vol. 1. Philadelphia, W. B. Saunders Co., 1969, pp. 516–599.

Tschudy, D. P., Perlroth, M. G., Marver, H. S., Collins, A., Hunter, G., Jr., and Rechcigl, M., Jr.: Acute intermittent porphyria: the first "overproduction disease" localized to a specific enzyme. Proc. Nat. Acad. Sci. (U.S.A.), *53*:841, 1965.

Waldenström, J., and Haeger-Aronsen, B.: The porphyrias: a genetic problem. Progr. Med. Gen., *5*:58, 1967.

Welland, F. H., Hellman, E. S., Gaddis, E. M., Collins, A., Hunter, G. W., Jr., and Tschudy, D. P.: Factors affecting the excretion of porphyrin precursors by patients with acute intermittent porphyria. I. The effect of diet. Metabolism, *13*:232, March, 1964.

Deficient or Abnormal Circulating Proteins

Beck, E. A., Charache, P., and Jackson, D. P.: A new inherited coagulation disorder caused by an abnormal fibrinogen (fibrinogen Baltimore). Nature, *208*:143, October 9, 1965.

Elsas, L. J., Hayslett, J. P., Spargo, B. H., Durant, J. L., and Rosenberg, L. E.: Wilson's disease with reversible renal tubular dysfunction. Ann. Intern. Med., *75*:427, September, 1971.

Forman, W. B., Ratnoff, O. D., and Boyer, M. H.: An inherited qualitative abnormality in plasma fibrinogen: fibrinogen Cleveland. J. Lab. Clin. Med., *72*:455, September, 1968.

Heilmeyer, L., Keller, W., Vivell, O., Keiderling, W., Betke, K., Wohler, F., and Schultze, H. E.: Congenital transferrin deficiency in a seven-year-old girl. German Med. Monthly, *6*:385, 1961.

Holtzman, N. A., Naughton, M. A., Iber, F. L., and Gaumnitz, B. M.: Ceruloplasmin in Wilson's disease. J. Clin. Invest., *46*:993, June, 1967.

Levy, R. I., Fredrickson, D. S., and Laster, L.: The lipoproteins and lipid transport in a-beta-lipoproteinemia. J. Clin. Invest., *45*:531, April, 1966.

Mammen, E. F., Prasad, A. S., Barnhart, M. I., and Au, C. C.: Congenital dysfibrinogenemia: fibrinogen Detroit. J. Clin. Invest., *48*:235, February, 1969.

Prichard, R. W., and Vann, R. L.: Congenital afibrinogenemia: report on a child without fibrinogen and review of the literature. Amer. J. Dis. Child., *88*:703, December, 1954.

Rapaport, S. I., Patch, M. J., and Moore, F. J.: Antihemophilic globulin levels in carriers of hemophilia A. J. Clin. Invest., *39*:1619, November, 1960.

Robertson, J. H., and Trueman, R. G.: Combined hemophilia and Christmas disease. Blood, *24*:281, September, 1964.

Scheinberg, I. H., and Sternlieb, I.: Metabolism of trace metals. *In* Bondy, P. K., and Rosenberg, L. E. (Eds.): Duncan's Diseases of Metabolism. Vol. 2. Philadelphia, W. B. Saunders Co., 1969, pp. 1321–1326.

Stites, D. P., Hershgold, E. J., Perlman, J. D., and Fudenberg, H. H.: Factor VIII detection by hemagglutination inhibition: Hemophilia A and Von Willebrand's Disease. Science, *171*:196, January 15, 1971.

Reduced Coenzyme Binding or Production

Frimpter, G. W.: Cystathioninuria: Nature of the defect. Science, *149*:1095, September 3, 1965.

Frimpter, G. W.: Cystathioninuria. *In* Nyhan, W. L. (Ed.): Amino Acid Metabolism and Genetic Variation. New York, McGraw-Hill Book Co., 1967, pp. 315–323.

Mahoney, M. J., and Rosenberg, L. E.: Inherited defects of B_{12} metabolism. Amer. J. Med., *48*:584, May, 1970.

Rosenberg, L. E.: Inherited amino-acidopathies demonstrating vitamin dependency. New Eng. J. Med., *281*:145, July 17, 1969.

Drug Metabolism

Bell, J. C., and Riemensnider, D. K.: Use of serum microbiologic assay technique for estimating patterns of isoniazid metabolism. Amer. Rev. Tuberc., *75*:995, June, 1957.

Evans, D. A., Manley, K. A., and McKusick, V. A.: Genetic control of isoniazid metabolism in man. Brit. Med. J., *2*:485, August 13, 1960.

Harris, H., Robson, E. B., Glenn-Bott, A. M., and Thornton, J. A.: Evidence for non-allelism between genes affecting human serum cholinesterase. Nature, *200*:1185, December 21, 1963.

Harris, H.: Principles of Human Biochemical Genetics. New York, Elsevier Publishing Co., Inc., 1970, pp. 107–121.

Hockwald, R. S., Arnold, J., Clayman, C. B., and Alving, A. S.: Status of primaquine: toxicity of primaquine in Negroes; report to council on Pharmacy and Chemistry. J.A.M.A., *149*:1568, August 23, 1952.

Jenne, J. W.: Partial purification and properties of the isoniazid transacetylase in human liver. Its relationship to the acetylation of P-aminosalicylic acid. J. Clin. Invest., 44:1992, December, 1965.

Kirkman, H. N.: Glucose-6-phosphate dehydrogenase variants and drug-induced hemolysis. Ann. N.Y. Acad. Sci., 151:753, July, 1968.

APPLICATION TO MANAGEMENT OF INHERITED DISEASE

Cerami, A., and Manning, J. M.: Potassium cyanate as an inhibitor of the sickling of erythrocytes *in vitro*. Proc. Nat. Acad. Sci., 68:1180, June, 1971.

Fagerhol, M. K.: Quantitative studies on the inherited variants of serum α_1-antitrypsin. Scand. J. Clin. Lab. Invest., 23:97, 1969.

Fagerhol, M. K.: The serum α_1-antitrypsin polymorphism. Abstract in symposium delivered at the 4th International Congress of Human Genetics, Paris, Excerpta Medica: International Congress Series, No. 233, p. 3, 1971.

Fratantoni, J. C., Neufeld, E. F., Uhlendorf, B. W., and Jacobson, C. B.: Intrauterine diagnosis of the Hurler and Hunter syndromes. New Eng. J. Med., 280:686, March 27, 1969.

Hug, G., and Schubert, W. K.: Lysosomes in Type II glycogenosis. Changes during administration of extract from *Aspergillus niger* J. Cell Biol., 35:C1, October, 1967.

Kraus, L. M., and Kraus, A. P.: Carbamyl phosphate mediated inhibition of the sickling of erythrocytes *in vitro*. Biochem. Biophys. Res. Comm., 44:1381, 1971.

Lauer, R. M., Mascarinas, T., Racela, A. S., and Diehl, A. M.: Administration of a mixture of fungal glucosidases to a patient with Type II glycogenosis (Pompe's disease). Pediatrics, 42:672, October, 1968.

Merril, C. R., Geier, M. R., and Petricciani, J. C.: Bacterial virus gene expression in human cells. Nature, 233:398, October 8, 1971.

Milunsky, A., Littlefield, J. W., Kanfer, J. N., Kolodny, E. H., Shih, V. E., and Atkins, L.: Prenatal genetic diagnosis (three parts). New Eng. J. Med., 283:1370, 1441, and 1498, 1970.

Moses, S. W., Levin, S., Chayoth, R., and Steinitz, K.: Enzyme induction in a case of glycogen storage disease. Pediatrics, 38:111, July, 1966.

Nadler, H. L., and Gerbie, A. B.: The role of amniocentesis in the intrauterine detection of genetic disorders. New Eng. J. Med., 282:596, March 12, 1970.

Nalbandian, R. M. (Ed.): Molecular Aspects of Sickle Cell Hemoglobin. Springfield, Ill., Charles C Thomas, 1971.

Rabovsky, D.: Molecular biology: gene insertion into mammalian cells. Science, 174:933, November 26, 1971.

Schwartz, A. G., Cook, P. R., and Harris, H.: Correction of a genetic defect in a mammalian cell. Nature New Biol., 230:5, March 3, 1971.

Scriver, C. R.: Treatment of inherited disease: realized and potential. Med. Clin. N. Amer., 53:941, July, 1969.

Yaffe, S. J., Levy, G., Matsuzawa, T., and Baliah, T.: Enhancement of glucuronide-conjugating capacity in a hyperbilirubinemic infant due to apparent enzyme induction by phenobarbital. New Eng. J. Med., 275:1461, December 29, 1966.

CHAPTER 4 IMMUNOBIOLOGY

PETER ABRAMOFF
RENÉ J. DUQUESNOY

INTRODUCTION

Few scientific disciplines have equaled the rapid growth of immunobiology in the last twenty years. Historically, immunology had its origins in microbiology, pathology, and biochemistry. It now has important implications for all of the basic biological sciences as well as for many clinical specialties. While the application of immunologic phenomena has enhanced the field of biology, immunology has become a specialty within this field with its own language and dogmas.

In classic usage, immunology was concerned with the general field of resistance to infectious diseases, both naturally existing and artificially induced. It is now evident that immune responses are not always beneficial nor are they solely associated with resistance to infection. On the contrary, they can cause very harmful effects on the host, as experienced in hypersensitivity or allergy. Furthermore, the immune system is designed not only to defend against infectious agents, but also to remove worn-out "self" components (homeostasis) and to monitor the recognition of abnormal cell mutants which constantly arise in the body (surveillance).

The first function, that of defense against invasion by microorganisms, is effective if the cellular elements of the immune system are deployed successfully. However, when these elements are hyperactive, certain undesirable features may be expressed, such as allergy or hypersensitivity. When these elements are hypoactive, there may be increased susceptibility of the host to repeated infections, as observed in the immunodeficiency disorders.

The second function, homeostasis, is concerned with the normal degradation and removal of used or damaged cellular elements. Aberrations of this homeostatic function may lead to autoimmune diseases in which there is a self-destructive process directed by the host's immune system.

The third and most recently recognized function of the immune system is surveillance, which recognizes the origin of abnormal or mutant cell types within the body. These mutants may occur spontaneously or they may be induced by certain viruses or chemicals. Failure of this immune surveillance mechanism to recognize and dispose of these abnormal cells may be the cause of malignancy. Some investigators now believe that, were it not for the evolution of immune surveillance, no vertebrate could long escape death from neoplastic disease.

Types of Immunity

It is clear that the acquired immunity, which is brought about by the introduction of foreign materials into the organism, is not the only way in which the organism protects itself against foreign substances. A natural immune state can be demonstrated to exist in individuals who have had contact with an antigen.

Innate Immunity. Nonspecific or innate immunity ranges from complete nonsusceptibility to certain diseases to a resistance so low that every individual exposed to the disease will contact it. Such constitutional or "genetic" immunity is brought about by anatomic and physiologic features associated with the species. It is inherited in the same way as any other characteristic of the species. The concept of nonsusceptibility is illustrated by the occurrence of infections in some species but not in others. Man, for example, will not be infected by a large number of animal pathogens (such as distemper, hog cholera, or cattle plague). On the other hand, many human diseases such as cholera, dysentery, measles, syphilis, and mumps do not affect lower animals. Nonsusceptibility appears to depend upon a barrier to the penetration of organisms at the level of the skin or integuments, inhibition of growth and reproduction of organisms after penetration into the tissues, inactivation of toxins liberated by such microorganisms, and the processes of phagocytosis and inflammation.

Natural Immunity. Natural immunity may be present in animals that have not been immunized and have not been infected with the disease to which they are immune. This form of immunity is probably brought about by substances which cross-react with the infectious agent involved or with some of its by-products. These substances, which are very much like specific antibodies in their behavior, are called normal or natural antibodies. For instance, normal human serum contains naturally occurring antibodies to erythrocytes of other individuals in the human species as well as to the red blood cells of other species (e.g., rabbit, sheep, ox, horse, guinea pig, and pigeon).

Some of these antibodies are probably induced by subclinical infections or in response to organisms that have entered the body by abnormal routes (e.g., gastrointestinal absorption). Others may be induced by exposure to closely related materials, as appears to be the case for the isohemagglutinins (antibodies to blood group substances), which may be developed as a result of exposure to enteric bacteria which contain substances resembling blood group antigens in their structure.

Acquired Immunity. The immunity acquired by the introduction of substances (immunogens) depends upon the ability of the animal to recognize these substances and to produce antibodies to some of its components. Thus, infection is not the only way in which immunity can be acquired or the antibody-producing mechanism stimulated. Immunity can be conferred by purified substances which are only a part of the original immunogen. Active immunity usually develops following a natural or artificial stimulation of the antibody-producing mechanism. "Natural stimulation" means the type of stimulus which is imparted by contracting a disease and recovering from it. This will usually result in a long-lasting immunity to another attack of the same organism. Artificial stimulation is accomplished by introducing microorganisms or some of their component products into the body.

Passive Immunity. This type of immunity is achieved by the transfer of antibodies that have been produced in another individual. Its duration is brief, since these antibodies are catabolized like normal globulins and therefore will soon be eliminated. Such antibodies may be naturally acquired by transplacental passage from mother to fetus or via the colostrum (first milk of the mother) shortly after birth. Passive immunity may also be acquired by the injection of sera obtained from artificially immunized animals or from humans that have been exposed to the antigenic determinants of the organism.

Adoptive Immunity. Adoptive immunity is a passive immunity acquired by the transfer of antibody-producing cells from one individual to another.

ANTIGENS AND IMMUNOGENICITY

The generally accepted definition of an antigen is functional in that it is considered to be a substance which, when introduced into an organism, will elicit an immune response. Secondly, this substance must react in some demonstrable way with the antibody that is produced. More recently the term "antigenicity" has been restricted to those characteristics of a molecule which deal with its capacity to interact with antibodies. The term "immunogenicity" is used to refer to those characteristics of molecules (immunogens) which stimulate a specific immune response. However, there are a number of substances (haptens) which, although they combine with antibodies, are unable to induce antibody production by themselves. These incomplete immunogens need to be covalently bound to carrier molecules (e.g., proteins) to become immunogenic.

Considerable experimental evidence has accumulated in recent years regarding the specific chemical characteristics of immunogenic molecules and the properties which determine the extent of their immunogenicity. Some of the generalizations which can be stated regarding the factors that determine immunogenicity are:

1. The most important requirement for immunogenicity is the recognition of a substance or cell as foreign or "nonself" to the host. Ordinarily a host does not produce an immune response to its own constituents. However, under certain circumstances an organism will develop immunity to "self" constituents (autoimmunity).

2. There is a certain minimum molecular weight (about 5000) below which substances are not in themselves immunogenic. Furthermore, the larger the molecular weight, the more immunogenic the molecule.

3. Size alone is not enough to insure immunogenicity. A rigid structure of the determinant groups appears to be a prerequisite for immunogenicity. For example, gelatin, which is poorly immunogenic because it has no fixed molecular configuration, can be made highly immunogenic by the addition of aromatic groups such as tyrosine and tryptophan which stabilize the molecule and give it rigidity.

4. The solubility of a molecule also influences its immunogenicity. Soluble proteins may actually induce a refractory state or tolerance

when present in monomeric form although they are highly immunogenic in their polymeric states. Several molecules, which when isolated in pure form are nonimmunogenic, become immunogenic when they are combined with artificial particles to form a larger complex. Such substances which enhance immunogenicity are called adjuvants.

5. The metabolism of immunogens may regulate antibody formation by controlling the amount of immunogen left intact and capable of stimulating antibody formation. For example, pneumococcal polysaccharides at low doses induce antibody formation, whereas at high doses they render the animal incapable of responding to the type-specific pneumococcus (immune paralysis). Good immunogens are rapidly degraded, so that over a wide range of doses, optimal amounts of immunogen are available to stimulate antibody formation. Thus, there appears to be a balance between stimulation and paralysis for every immunogen, such that a poor antigen induces paralysis easily and good antigens stimulate antibody formation under a wide variety of conditions.

The overwhelming majority of immunogens are proteinaceous substances ranging in size from glucagon (M.W. 3800) to tobacco mosaic virus (M.W. about 40,000,000). These may exist as pure proteins or combined with others such as lipids (lipoproteins), nucleic acids (nucleoproteins), or carbohydrates (glycoproteins such as the blood group substances). The most important immunogenic polysaccharides are those that are present in the capsules of bacteria, since antibodies directed against them may provide protective immunity (e.g., antipneumococcal antibody). Although there have been many reports of the functional immunogenicity of lipids, there is no undisputed proof of any purified lipid being immunogenic. However, the ability of lipids to induce specific antibody formation when mixed with a foreign serum is fairly well established. Under certain conditions, nucleic acids may serve as immunogens, particularly when single-stranded. In systemic lupus erythematosus, antibodies to DNA are detected, and the various forms of tissue damage in this disease are thought to result from DNA–anti-DNA complexes.

IMMUNOGLOBULINS

Antibodies in man and other animals are associated with a family of proteins called immunoglobulins. These proteins share many antigenic, structural and biologic similarities, but differ in primary amino acid sequence, thus permitting their antibody function to be highly specific.

In man there are five different classes of immunoglobulins, each with a distinct chemical structure and, in most cases, a specific biologic function. These are designated by the letters G, A, M, D, and E, either after the symbol γ (indicating their electrophoretic mobility as γ globulins) or after the abbreviation Ig (indicating their immunoglobulin function). Table 4-1 summarizes some of the major properties of each of these immunoglobulin classes.

Structure of Immunoglobulins

All known classes of immunoglobulins have the same unit structure consisting of two identical heavy chains (M.W. 50,000–70,000) and two identical light chains (M.W. 22,000) held together by disulfide bonds (Fig. 4-1). A chemically different kind of heavy chain exists for each class of immunoglobulin and is responsible for the antigenic and biologic differences which have been observed between classes. As indicated in Table 4-1, the five kinds of heavy chains are designated by the Greek letter equivalent to their class name, i.e., γ, α, μ, δ, and ϵ. The two different types of light chains which exist in common with all classes of immunoglobulins are called kappa (κ) and lambda (λ). Thus, there are ten possible combinations of heavy and light chains, and all ten are normally found in each individual.

By antigenic reactivity and subsequent immunochemical analysis, minor differences (subclasses) within immunoglobulin classes have been identified. Thus, four different subclasses of IgG have been designated γG1, γG2, γG3 and γG4. Similarly, two subclasses of IgA and IgM have recently been detected and are called γA1 and γA2, and γM1 and γM2, respectively. Important biologic differences have been demonstrated between the activities of these subclasses.

IgG molecules are composed of two identical halves, each consisting of a light and a heavy chain, joined together by two disulfide bonds. This basic four chain structure exists in common with all of the immunoglobulin classes. However, the IgM molecules consist of a pentamer of four basic four chain units, with each of the subunits held together by weak disulfide bonds (Fig. 4-2). IgA and, occasionally, IgG may also exist in a polymeric form in serum, but they are usually joined by electrostatic forces rather than disulfide bonds. On the other hand, the IgA which appears in the secretory fluids consists of two IgA molecules linked together by a secretory component to form secretory IgA (M.W. 400,000). The IgA monomers are synthesized by plasma cells localized in the submucosa of the respiratory and gastrointestinal tracts. Two of these molecules are joined with the secretory piece as they pass through these epithelial cells.

Studies of the amino acid sequences of both

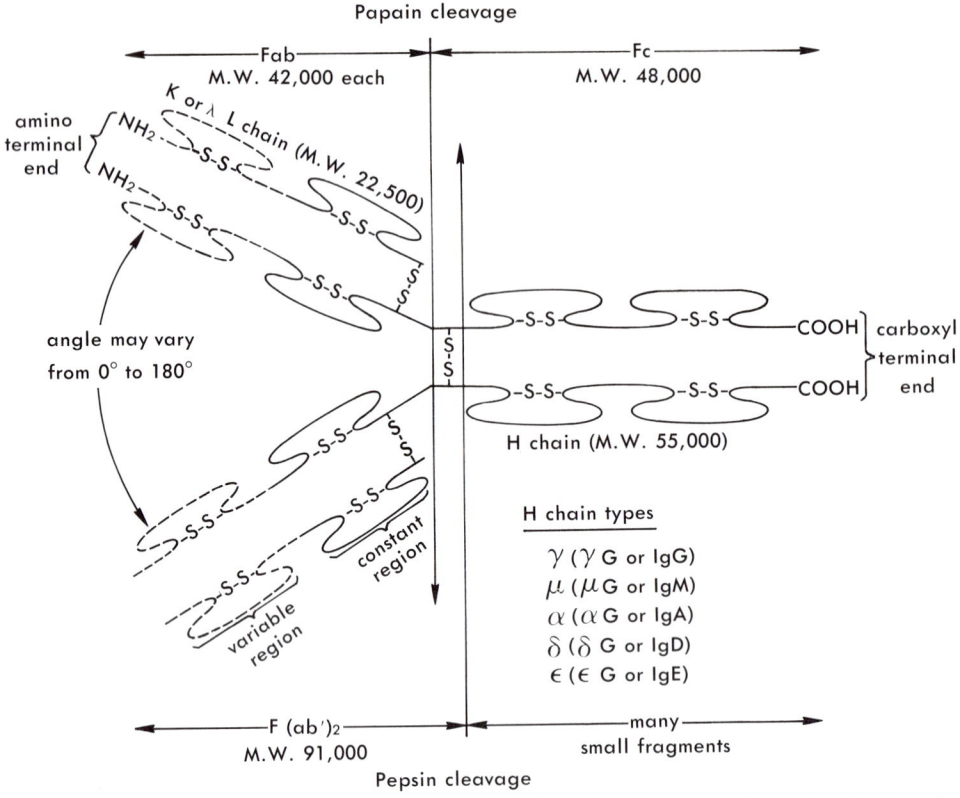

Figure 4-1 Basic four-chain structure of the immunoglobulin molecule showing the probable sites of cleavage by papain and pepsin.

light and heavy chains have revealed that their amino terminal ends comprising the first 110 or so amino acids are variable and specific for each type of antibody. The remaining carboxyl terminal regions of both types of chains are constant in the amino acid sequence. However, the constant region of the heavy chain (C_H) is about three times (approximately 300 amino acids) larger than the heavy variable region (V_H). The region of the antibody that combines with an antigenic determinant (antigen-binding or antibody active site) includes the variable parts of both light and heavy chains. In IgG molecules two antigen-binding sites exist, while in IgM molecules there are ten sites.

The constant carboxyl terminal region of the heavy chains appears to be responsible for the different biological properties of the various classes of immunoglobulins. These properties include the ability to activate the complement and anaphylactic systems of immunobiological amplification, to react with surfaces of various cell types, and to cross placental and other membrane barriers.

The genetic markers which differentiate those antigenic specificities (allotypes) which differ in various groups of individuals within the same species are localized on the constant region of light and heavy chains. These allotypic specificities are revealed by immunizing a large number of individuals with immunoglobulins from other individuals of the same species. In humans the allotypic specificities designated InV are associated with the constant regions of κ light chains of all the immunoglobulin classes. The human Gm allotypes are confined exclusively to the constant regions of the γ chains. Recently, allotypic variants have also been identified for λ, α, and μ chains.

Biological Properties of the Immunoglobulins

The biological properties of the immunoglobulins can be grouped into two categories: antigen binding and biological function. Combination with the antigen is specific, and each molecule of antibody can bind only to the specific antigen, or to antigens very closely related to it. The biological properties of the immunoglobulins are independent of the specificity and are common to all the molecules belonging to a given class. Some of these biological properties are activated after com-

IMMUNOBIOLOGY

TABLE 4-1 PROPERTIES OF THE HUMAN IMMUNOGLOBULINS

Immunoglobulin Class	Serum Concentration (mg./100 ml.)	Approximate Molecular Weight	Heavy-Chain Type	S_{20} Value	Heavy-Chain Allotype Markers	Biological Function
γG or IgG	1275 ± 280	150,000	γ	7S	Gm	Fix complement Cross placenta Heterocytotropic antibody Cytophilic antibody
γA or IgA	225 ± 55	180,000	α	7–11S	Am	Secretory antibody
γM or IgM	125 ± 45	900,000	μ	19S	present	Fix complement Efficient agglutination and hemolysis Virus neutralization
γD or IgD	3	150,000	δ	7S	—	?
γE or IgE	0.03	200,000	ε	8S	—	Reaginic antibody Homocytotropic antibody

bination with antigen (complement fixation, cytolysis, opsonization, phagocytosis, immune adherence, chemotaxis, hypersensitivity); others do not depend on that combination (distribution in the body, transmission across membranes, cytophilia). The heterogeneity of the immunoglobulins is the consequence of diverse functional requirements. One of the major problems is to define the particular biological properties and the physiologic roles of the various families of immunoglobulins.

IgG. The IgG antibodies are the most abun-

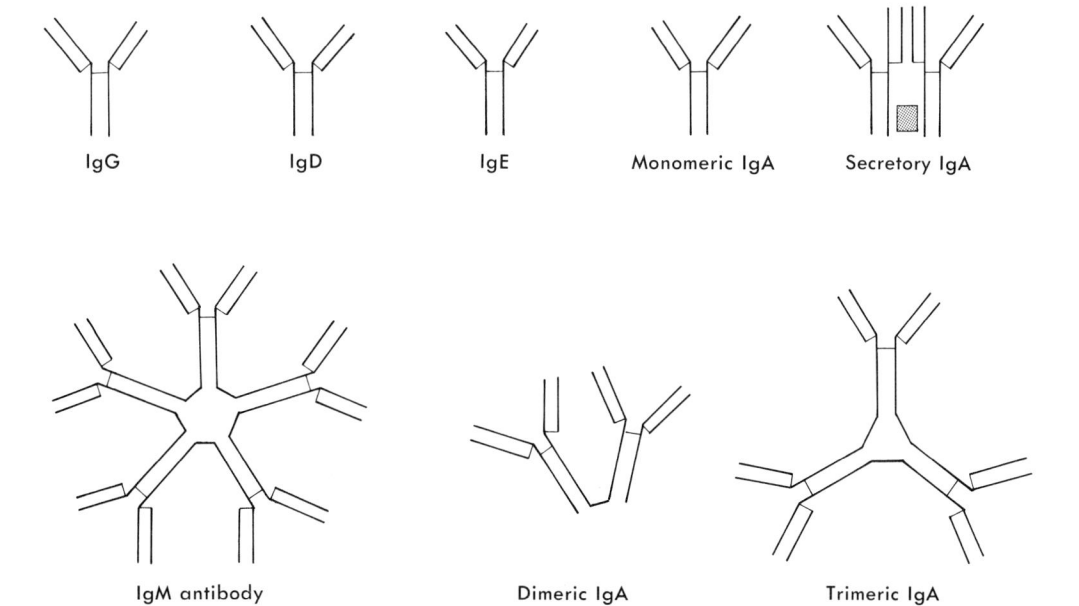

Figure 4-2 Schematic structure of the various classes of immunoglobulin molecules.

dant of the immunoglobulins, being found in high concentrations in both the vascular and extravascular spaces. This class of immunoglobulins provides the bulk of immunity to most infecting agents which have a blood-borne dissemination. Furthermore, IgG or some of its subclasses possess cytophilic activity (i.e., cell fixation) for homologous macrophages. The biological usefulness of cytophilic antibody appears to be its capacity to bind soluble or particulate antigens so as to promote their phagocytosis by macrophages (a process called opsonization). IgG antibodies can also activate complement and thus enhance phagocytic activity.

IgA. This class is the second most abundant serum immunoglobulin. It is produced in high concentrations by lymphoid tissues lining the gastrointestinal, respiratory, and genitourinary tracts. In these secretions, IgA is combined with a protein called the secretory or transport piece, which appears to endow the molecule with some protection against effects of proteolytic enzymes normally found in these regions. It has been suggested that one of the functions of IgA antibodies may be to keep harmful antigens out of the body by forming nonabsorbable complexes in the human external secretory system (saliva, tears, nasal and bronchial fluid, bile, intestinal secretions, and mammary secretions). This may explain why patients deficient in IgA have unusually high titers of circulating antibodies against food antigens. Bound IgA antibody after interaction with antigen can cause release of histamine and other pharmacologic agents at the local site of interaction. It is possible that these biologic attributes of IgA may play a role in defending exposed body cavities to penetration by infective agents.

IgM. This class of antibodies includes the largest of the immunoglobulin molecules with an average molecular weight of about 900,000. They constitute about 5 to 10 per cent of the total serum γ-globulins and, because of their large size, are restricted almost exclusively to the intravascular spaces. The formation of IgM antibodies is generally transient, and within 2 to 3 weeks, IgG is the principal class of specific antibody produced. Furthermore, IgM antibody to red blood cells, bacteria, and bacteriophage is extremely efficient (avid) in binding these particulate antigens, causing hemolysis and neutralization, respectively. On the basis of these observations, it has been suggested that the IgM system might be regarded as a first line of defense, capable of prompt production of large numbers of antibody molecules which can readily eliminate particulate antigens. In contrast, the IgG system may be initially incapable of an immediate vigorous response, but is eventually able to synthesize more efficient (higher affinity) antibody molecules for long periods of time and to participate in the development of a persisting immunologic memory.

IgD. This minor component of the immunoglobulins has not yet been assigned a specific biological role, but antibody activity has been associated with it, including cases of penicillin hypersensitivity in humans.

IgE. This immunoglobulin is present in only trace amounts in serum. Produced chiefly in the linings of the respiratory and intestinal tracts, it is localized in the external secretory system. It has the ability to attach to human skin (homocytotropic antibody) and to initiate aspects of the allergic reaction (reaginic antibody). IgE antibody is responsible for activation of the anaphylactic system of immunobiological amplification.

INDUCTION OF THE IMMUNE RESPONSE

The production of antibody in response to an immunogenic stimulus is a complex response that can be divided into three major phases: (1) afferent, with "processing" of antigen and induction of the immune response; (2) central, with multiplication and differentiation of antibody-producing cells and synthesis of antibody or the development of cell-mediated reactivity; (3) efferent, with interaction of antibody or effector cells with antigen, the ultimate purpose of which is to eliminate the antigen.

Antibody does not appear immediately in the circulation following exposure of the animal to immunogen. Instead, a latent or induction period occurs in which most of the immunogen is rapidly catabolized before the ensuing antibody response. For intravenously injected immunogens three phases of removal are easily detected (Fig. 4–3). The first phase requires only 10 to 20 minutes if particulate antigens are used and represents the time required for equilibration of antigen with tissues and fluids. Because of extensive phagocytosis in the liver, lung, and spleen nearly 90 per cent of the antigen is removed from the circulation in its first passage from these organs. Soluble antigens are not removed from the blood as quickly because of their slow pinocytotic uptake by cells. The second phase of antigen elimination is the gradual catabolic degradation and removal of the antigen (nonimmune catabolism). This phase continues for 4 to 7 days and depends upon the enzymatic capability of the host for the particular antigen being metabolized. In animals that fail to produce antibody against the antigen, this second phase is extended for several weeks. With the onset of antibody production, the remaining circulating antigens are rapidly catabolized and disappear from the circulation,

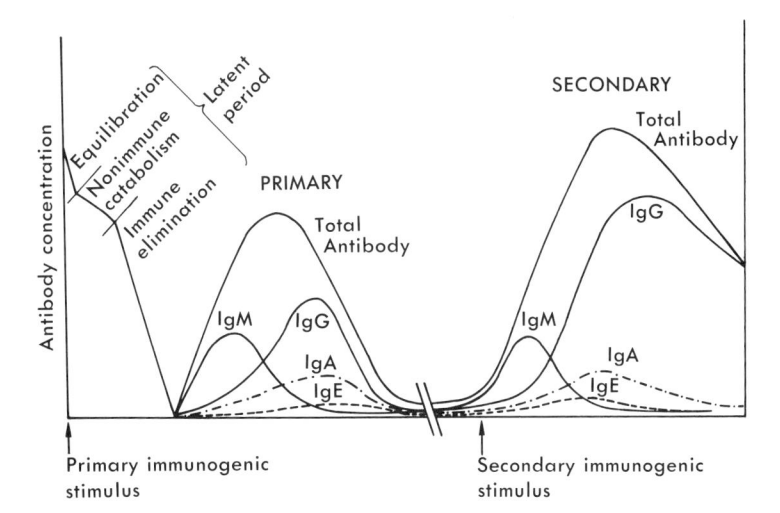

Figure 4-3 Primary and secondary antibody response curves.

after which antibody appears in the circulation. This third phase (immune catabolism) is the result of the newly formed antibody molecules combining with the antigen to form immune complexes which enhance phagocytic engulfment, digestion, and removal of the antigen. The absolute removal of all antigen from an immunized individual may take many months or years.

It has been suggested that during this induction period macrophages "process" immunogenic materials by reducing them to immunogenic fragments which are combined with macrophage RNA. Such complexes may serve to enhance the cellular uptake of the immunogenic fragments by antibody-forming cells. It is not known whether a macrophage-processing step, that is, the linkage of an immunogenic fragment to the immunogen-carrier RNA, is a necessary step for the production of antibody to all antigens. However, in the case of the high molecular weight antigens studied to date, it seems clear that antigen processing takes place.

The induction period of an immune response is followed by a three-part production phase (Fig. 4-3). First to occur is a logarithmic increase in the amount of antibody in the serum. This is followed by a plateau phase which can be transitory or even nonexistent. Last to occur is a decline phase. During the log phase, production of antibody exceeds catabolism; during the plateau phase, they are equal; and during the decline, catabolism exceeds synthesis.

The course of antibody synthesis during a secondary response differs significantly from that seen during the primary response. At first, the secondary response evokes a sharp drop in circulating antibody because it is complexing with the newly injected antigen. Immediately thereafter there is a marked increase in circulating antibody which may continue for several days, so that the ultimate titer far surpasses that of the primary response. This phase is followed by a gradual decline in antibody titer which is probably the result of two factors; one is that more cells appear to be involved in the secondary response, and the second is that the immunoglobulins involved in the secondary response appear to be qualitatively different from those produced in a primary immune response. It has been demonstrated that the classes of immunoglobulins are formed in a characteristic sequence during the primary immune response. Depending upon the type of immunogen, its mode of introduction, the dosage employed, and various other factors, the earliest detectable serum antibodies are of the IgM class, while the other classes of immunoglobulins appear later. The formation of IgM antibodies is generally transient, and within about 1 to 2 weeks of immunogenic challenge, IgG is the principal class of immunoglobulin produced (Fig. 4-3). In some instances, when the immunogen is a polysaccharide, IgM is the predominant class of immunoglobulins during the entire immune response.

The significance of the heterogeneity of the immune response appears to be the fact that during immunization a progressive change occurs in the quality of IgG immunoglobulins produced, resulting in an increased efficiency in their capacity to bind to specific antigen. Furthermore, IgM antibody to erythrocytes, bacteria, and bacteriophage can be extremely efficient in binding these particulate antigens and causing hemolysis and neutralization, respectively. Thus, it has been suggested that the IgM system is the first line of defense, capable of prompt elimination of particulate antigens. The IgG system may be initially represented by a small population of cells not capable of an immediate vigorous response but eventually able to synthesize more efficient antibody molecules for long periods of time and to participate in the development of a persisting immunologic memory.

CELLULAR ASPECTS OF ANTIBODY SYNTHESIS

The vertebrates have evolved a ubiquitous cell system, the lymphoreticular system, in order to carry out the functions of immunity. This collection of cellular elements, distributed strategically throughout the body, also lines lymphatic and vascular channels. Its cells are located in primary (thymus and avian bursa of Fabricius) and secondary or peripheral lymphoid organs (spleen; lymph nodes; Peyer's patches; tonsils; appendix; and diffuse lymphoid tissues in gut, skin, uterus and ovaries; and so on). A number of effector systems involving soluble serum factors as well as several cell types and products may be called into play by the host following immunogenic stimulation. The cellular constituents include macrophages, plasma cells, and lymphocytes. Immunologic reactions may also involve other humoral factors which can augment or amplify the immune response without direct participation of cells. These biological amplification systems are composed of primary and secondary components. The primary components consist of products of the specific immune response (antibody and cell-mediated factors), while the secondary components include complement, prostaglandins, and the coagulation kallikrein, and fibrinolytic systems.

Cells of the Immune System

Macrophages are mononuclear cells found in most organs of the body (e.g., Kupffer cells of the liver, sinusoidal and dendritic cells of the spleen, glial cells of the central nervous system, and alveolar macrophages of the lungs) and in the blood, where they are called monocytes. These cells are characterized by having a large amount of cytoplasm and a medium-sized nucleus containing tightly packed heterochromatin (Fig. 4-4). The macrophages are highly specialized for the ingestion and destruction of all particulate

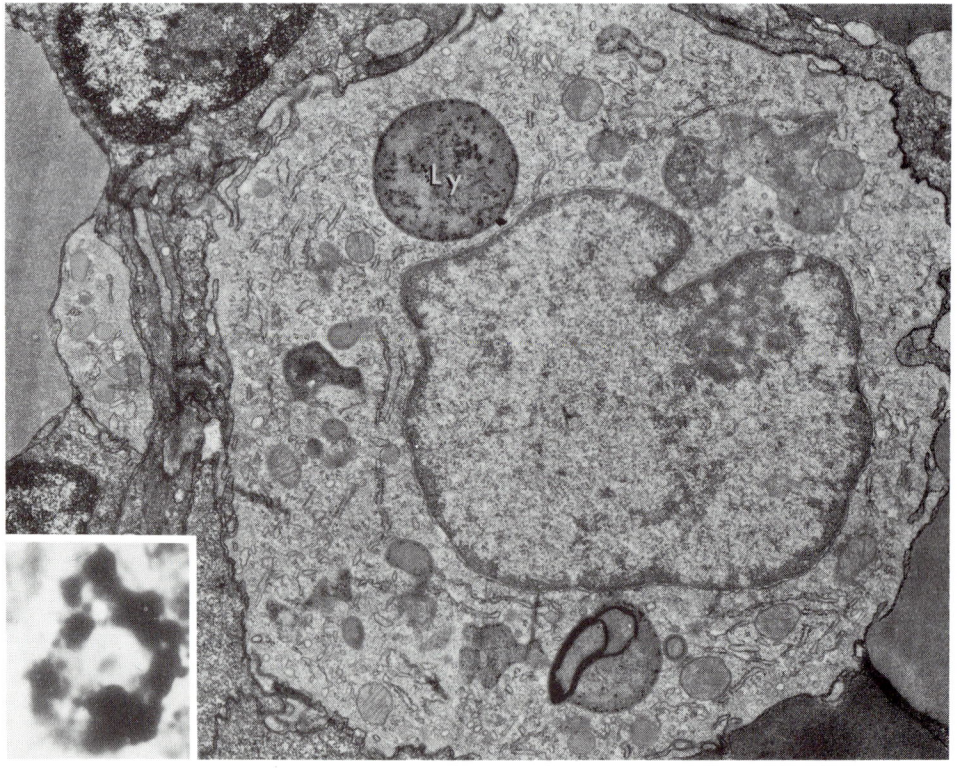

Figure 4-4 Typical macrophage from the rat spleen. The cytoplasm contains a granular endoplasmic reticulum, several mitochondria, and lysosomes (Ly) in various stages of development. Insert at lower left shows a macrophage as observed by light microscopy. (Courtesy of Dr. M. F. La Via, Emory University.)

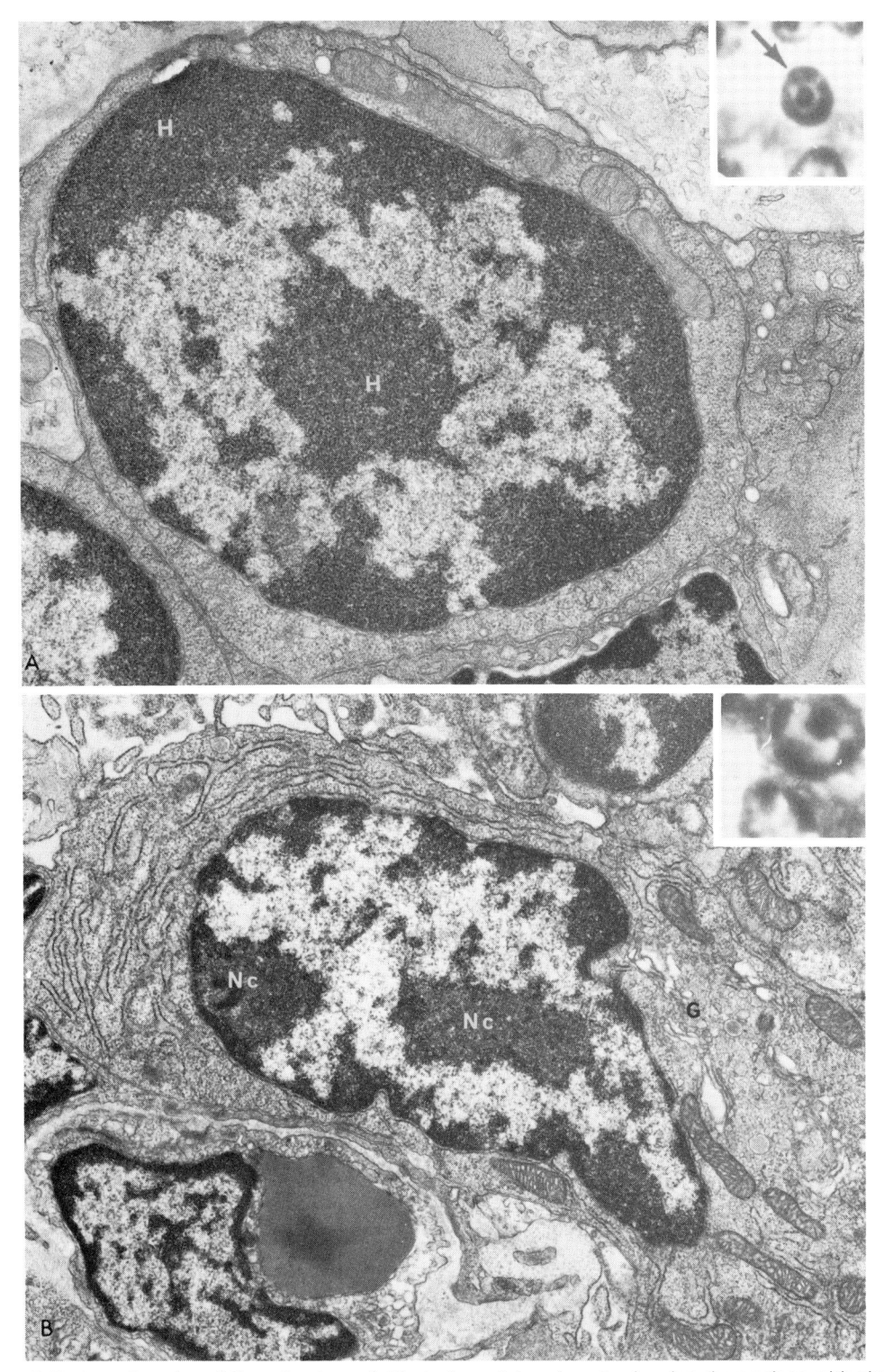

Figure 4–5 Lymphocytes of the rat spleen. *A,* Typical small lymphocyte showing the nucleus with clump of heterochromatin fibers (H) packed close to the nuclear envelope and in the center. A thin cytoplasmic rim with a few ribosomes and mitochondria surrounds the nucleus. Insert at upper right shows the same cell viewed with the light microscope. *B,* A medium lymphocyte with prominent nucleoli (Nc) and well-developed Golgi region (G). The cytoplasm is greatly expanded and cisternae of granular endoplasmic reticulum are apparent. Insert at upper right shows the same cell as seen by light microscopy.

(Figure 4–5 continued on opposite page.)

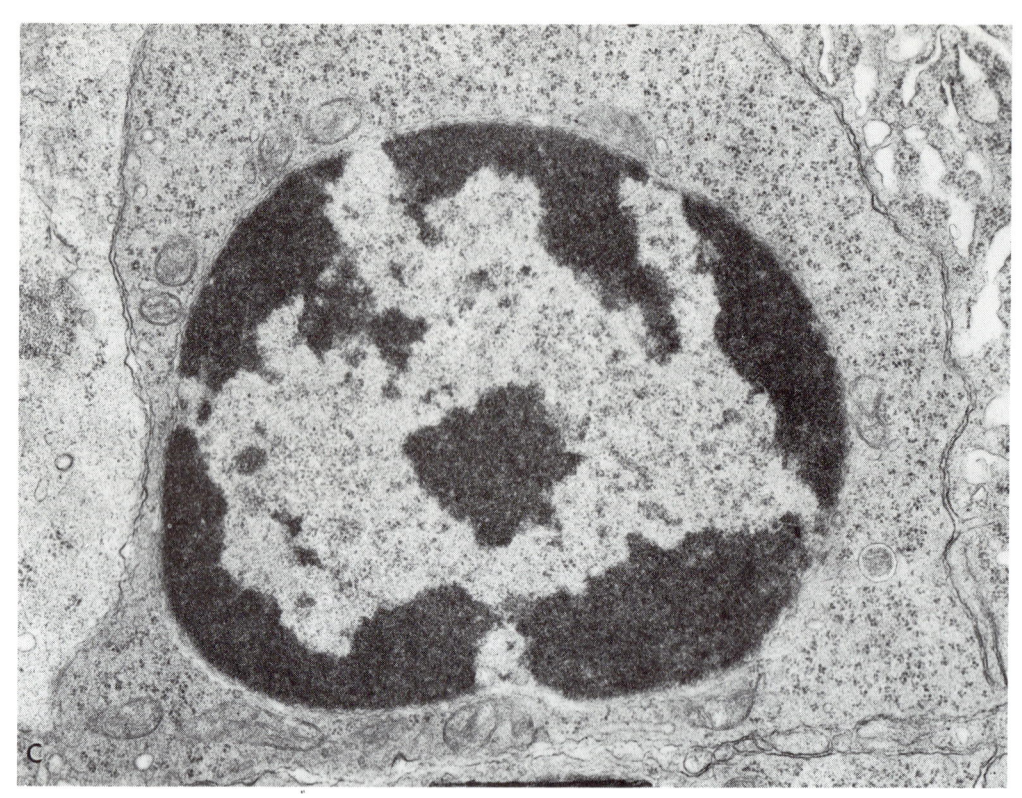

Figure 4-5 Continued *C,* A large lymphocyte showing extensive cytoplasm and numerous clusters of ribosomes. (Electron micrographs courtesy of Dr. M. F. La Via, Emory University.)

matter by the process of phagocytosis. These cells remove and destroy certain bacteria, damaged or effete cells, neoplastic cells, colloidal material, and macromolecules. The phagocytic activity of macrophages can be amplified by antibodies (opsonins) which coat particles and complement. The circulating monocytes are involved in delayed hypersensitivity reactions and are attracted to an area of injury by chemotactic factors. The macrophage system also appears to be important in the initial recognition and processing of antigen.

The lymphoid cells of the immune system include lymphocytes and plasma cells which differ from the preceding group of cells by their ability to react specifically with antigen and to elaborate specific cell products. These may be specific antibody or a cell-mediated event such as delayed hypersensitivity.

The *plasma cell* is characterized by an extensive endoplasmic reticulum, an eccentrically placed nucleus, and highly developed Golgi apparatus (Fig. 4-5). These cells store and release antibody and are believed to be of primary importance in antibody synthesis.

The *lymphocytes* consist of a family of small, medium, and large cells. The small lymphocyte is the most characteristic cell of this series and the most numerous (Fig. 4-6). Usually measuring up to 7 μ in diameter, it consists of a nucleus surrounded by a thin rim of cytoplasm. The medium and large lymphocytes are larger than the small lymphocytes; their cytoplasm contains many polysomes, varying amounts of rough endoplasmic reticulum, a Golgi apparatus, and many mitochondria.

In addition to the production of antibodies, lymphocytes produce a variety of factors which trigger inflammatory or cell-damaging reactions, leading to a series of cell-mediated events that result in the destruction of foreign target cells or the damage and destruction of host tissues. Lymphocytes thus possess the most diversified functions of all the cells of the immune system.

Primary Lymphoid Organs

Only two organs can be designated as primary lymphoid organs—the thymus in all vertebrates and the bursa of Fabricius in birds. Certain fundamental features distinguish primary from secondary lymphoid organs:

1. The primary lymphoid tissues are the first to become lymphoidal during development. In these organs lymphocytes differentiate from stem

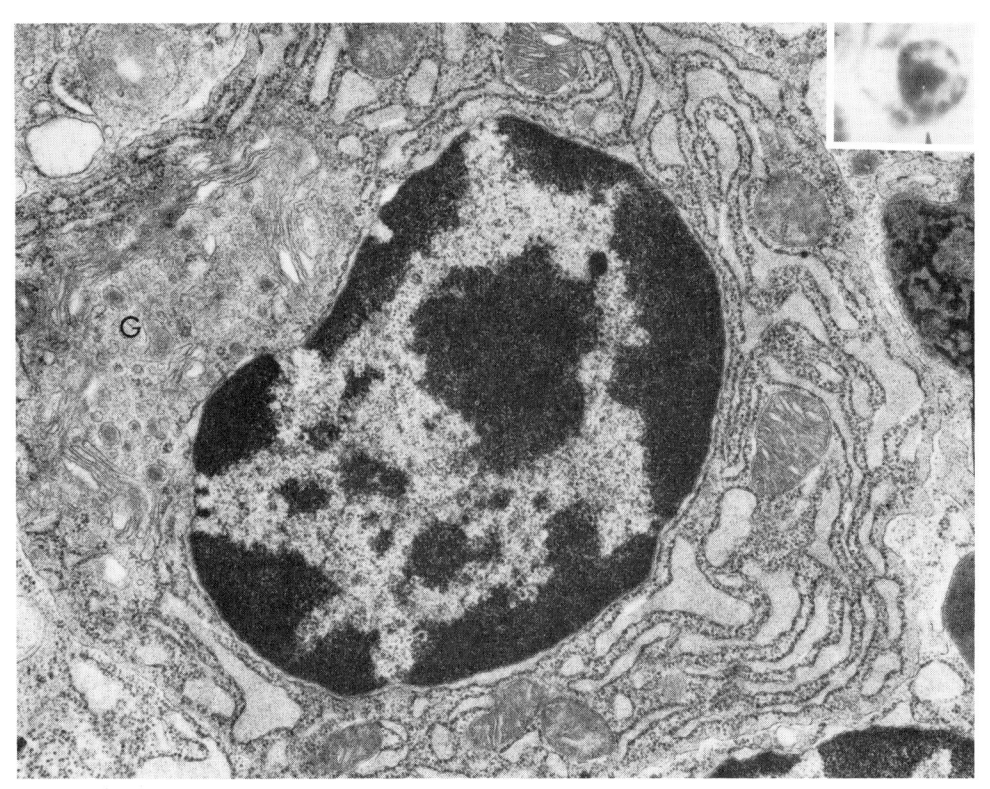

Figure 4-6 Plasma cell with a highly developed Golgi region (G) and abundant cytoplasm packed with granular endoplasmic reticulum cisternae. Mitochondria are tightly bound by the endoplasmic reticulum. Insert at upper right shows a plasma cell seen by light microscopy. (Electron micrograph courtesy of Dr. M. F. La Via, Emory University.)

cells that have migrated into the epithelial rudiment of thymus and bursa from a stem cell pool which changes from primitive blood islets of the yolk sac to fetal liver to bone marrow during ontogenetic development. Lymphoid development in secondary tissues occurs later with the lymphocytes originating from cells that have already been wholly or partially differentiated in the primary organs.

2. Lymphopoiesis in primary lymphoid organs is independent of immunogenic stimulation. Lymphoid cell proliferation in the secondary lymphoid organs such as lymph nodes, splenic white pulp, and Peyer's patches, on the other hand, is normally immunogen dependent.

3. Repopulation of primary lymphoid organs following irradiation is dependent upon a supply of stem cells and cannot be accomplished by differentiated lymphocytes from the thymus, bursa, thoracic duct, or lymph nodes. However, repopulation of secondary lymphoid tissues can be achieved by populations of lymphocytes lacking stem cells.

4. Extirpation of primary lymphoid tissues under defined conditions leads to defects in immune capacity. Removal of these tissues prior to maturation of immune capability of the host leads to permanent impairment of immunologic competence. Removal of the same organs in the adult does not influence immunologic capacity unless the pool of immunocompetent lymphocytes is depleted as a result of aging or following destruction by irradiation, drugs, or antilymphocytic measures. Under these conditions the maintenance or recovery of immune capacity is dependent upon the existence of primary lymphoid organs.

In the chicken, there is a definitive separation between thymus-dependent cellular immunity and bursa-dependent production of humoral antibodies. Neonatal chickens hormonally or surgically bursectomized are characterized by a deficiency of both IgG and IgM immunoglobulins and by the absence of both primary and secondary antibody production. However, they do exhibit cell-mediated immune responses such as graft rejection and delayed hypersensitivity reactions. On the other hand, thymectomy at hatching does not depress immunoglobulin synthesis but does impair cell-mediated immunity. In mammals, thymectomy impairs cell-mediated immunity but does not appear to directly influence immunoglobulin production. Thus, there must be a nonthymus-dependent homolog of the avian bursa that controls the differentiation of immunoglobulin-synthesizing cells. To date, no single or multifocal organ has been identified, although certain gut-associated lymphoid tissues (appendix, sacculus rotundus, and Peyer's patches) have been implicated as exerting bursa-like functions in the control of the humoral immune response.

Man has several immunodeficiency syndromes (congenital and acquired hypogammaglobulinemias) which are associated with the humoral immune system. They are characterized by hypogammaglobulinemia and deficient antibody synthesis, although cellular immunity is normal or only slightly impaired. Patients with congenital absence of the thymus (DiGeorge's syndrome) have deficient cell-mediated immunities but normal immunoglobulin levels and little impairment of humoral antibody production. In combined immunodeficiency disease (Swiss agammaglobulinemia) both humoral and cellular immune systems are defective as a consequence of lymphoid stem cell abnormality. These clinical observations indicate that the immune system in man is also composed of (1) a thymus-dependent system responsible for the development of small lymphocytes capable of initiating cell-mediated immune responses; (2) a system equivalent to the bursa-dependent system and responsible for the production of plasma cells and lymphoid follicles and the synthesis of immunoglobulins and antibodies; and (3) a population of lymphoid stem cells responsible for populating the primary lymphoid organs.

Secondary Lymphoid Organs

The cells that populate the secondary or peripheral lymphoid tissues (lymph nodes, spleen, Peyer's patches) are derived originally from stem cells that have been influenced by the thymus or avian bursa (or its mammalian homolog). The secondary lymphoid organs are compound structures made up of distinctive anatomic compartments, each of which is populated by populations of "thymus-dependent" or "bursa-dependent (thymus-independent)" lymphocytes. These terms are used to indicate that these cells are dependent upon the existence of the thymus and bursa for their origin; they do not imply a dependence on the primary lymphoid organs for the functioning of these cells once they are produced.

The thymus-dependent ("T") cells are localized in the paracortical areas of lymph nodes, periarteriolar lymphocyte sheaths of the spleen, and diffuse lymphoid tissues of Peyer's patches. The T cells are responsible for the initiation of cellular immune responses such as graft-versus-host reactions (GVHR) and host-versus-graft (homograft) reactions. These immune responses are diminished by thymectomy and by any measures that deplete the recirculating pool of long-lived small lymphocytes such as thoracic duct drainage and irradiation of the spleen or of the blood in an extracorporeal circuit. Thus, cells released from the thymus and circulating in the thoracic duct accumulate to constitute a larger pool of effective thymus cells that can be recruited directly from the thymus. These thymus-derived or T cells do, in fact, originate from the bone marrow as stem cells and migrate to the thymus. There, under the influence of the thymic environment, they proliferate and differentiate into immunocompetent lymphocytes.

Chickens that have been neonatally bursectomized and irradiated lack follicles and plasma cells but not small lymphocytes in the periarteriolar sheaths of the spleen. Thus, the bursa-dependent lymphoid tissues include lymphoid follicles and plasma cells. In mammals there is also a "thymus-independent" pathway for lymphocyte production, since thymectomy does not affect the population of cells in lymphoid follicles and white pulp of the spleen and cortex of the lymph nodes. Bone marrow cells can repopulate these areas in thymectomized irradiated mice. These marrow-derived, thymus-independent cells are called "B" cells. It is believed that in mammals some gut-associated epithelial tissue analogous to the chicken bursa may influence the differentiation of these bone marrow-derived cells to become immunocompetent cells in the secondary lymphoid organs.

Cellular Kinetics and Interactions

Following a primary immunogenic stimulus, large pyroninophilic cells appear in the periarteriolar lymphatic sheaths of the spleen. These cells, evidently immunoblasts, increase in number and move to the periphery of the sheath. After 48 hours clusters of immunoblasts appear in the splenic cords and by 4 days the splenic cords and sinuses of the red pulp contain many plasma cells. At 3 days, germinal center formation begins in the white pulp and by 7 to 9 days these centers are rather large and contain many mitotic cells. During the next 10 to 20 days these centers gradually diminish in size but remain larger than normal for about 4 weeks. A secondary antibody response is accompanied in the spleen by intensive antigen localization in the germinal centers and by an enlargement of these structures.

The cellular events that take place in a lymph node after primary immunogenic stimulation are of two kinds, depending upon whether the stimulus predominantly causes a humoral immunoglobulin response or cell-mediated immunity. In the first case, the first antibody-producing cells appear in the cortex, which includes a germinal center response. Later antibody-producing cells are found in large numbers in the medulla. Thus, the lymph node reactions typically parallel those of the spleen, where the red pulp, comparable in many ways to the lymph node medulla, shows a sustained cellular response following the response in white pulp. The cells in the white pulp and cortex, moreover, represent relatively early stages in plasma cell formation. The cells in the red pulp and medulla include many mature plasma cells. During a secondary response the involvement of lymph node germinal centers is much more pronounced, with a rapid and intensive uptake of antigen and enlargement of the centers. It appears that this involvement of the secondary response is connected with the establishment of immunologic memory through the production of "memory" cells. Memory cells, primed and capable of an immediate vigorous proliferation and antibody production, are the basis of the secondary or anamnestic responses.

A different kind of cellular reaction develops in lymph nodes following immunogenic stimuli which lead to the cell-mediated immunities characteristic of homograft reactions and delayed hypersensitivity. In these cases, there is an impressive immunoblast transformation in the thymus-dependent paracortical zone of lymph nodes. This is followed by a decline in the number of immunoblasts as a result of their transformation into small and medium lymphocytes. In the immune response of the delayed type there is no participation of germinal centers or of cells of the plasma cell series unless the response is accompanied by the production of humoral immunoglobulins.

Recent studies have demonstrated that the antibody response depends upon at least two and possibly three cell types, depending upon the immunogen. Tissue culture studies have indicated that one of these cells adheres to the surface of plastic culture dishes (probably macrophages), while the others remain unattached and free-floating in the culture medium. When adherent and nonadherent cells are separated and cultured apart, little antibody production above background is observed. When they are combined in the same culture, considerable antibody production is seen. Furthermore, it has been observed that cell clusters appear to be necessary for antibody formation. Preliminary electron microscopic study of these clusters has revealed them to be complex formations of macrophages, lymphocytes, and plasma cells, all with surface microvilli (Fig. 4-7).

A cooperation between cells released from bone marrow and thymus has been observed in the production of antibody by mice against sheep erythrocytes and albumin. In these experiments cell suspensions were injected singly and in different combinations into animals rendered incapable of antibody production by irradiation. Spleen or lymph node cells, which contain a mixture of cells derived from marrow and thymus, are capable of conferring antibody production in the irradiated recipient. However, a suspension of thymus cells alone is incapable of restoring immune capacity as is a suspension of bone marrow cells. On the other hand, a mixture of thymus and marrow cells produces a considerable restoration of antibody production. Thus, it appears that cells released from the marrow (B cells) and those released from the thymus (T cells) interact synergistically in the humoral immune response. The observation that T cells react with antigen through specific cellular receptors and yet do not release antibody leads to the idea that they may be required to capture and present the immunogen in some way before it can stimulate B cells to produce antibody. In those systems involving macrophages it is believed that these cells "process" particulate antigens for presentation to these T cells. These T cells, called "antigen-reactive" or "antigen-sensitive" cells, also play an essential role in cell-mediated immune responses. This antigen-handling function may be mediated by a cell-bound immunoglobulin which is not normally found in serum. The bone marrow cells (B cells) are both antigen-reactive and antibody-producing. The nature of the interaction or exchange between T and B cells is unknown. Cytoplasmic bridges and emperipolesis between macrophages and immunocompetent cells have been observed. Furthermore, cells in antibody-producing clusters often have cytoplasmic processes which interdigitate with or indent contiguous cells (Fig. 4-7). Thus, the physical relationships of these cell types is such as to permit passage of information from one cell to another.

IMMUNOLOGIC MEMORY

Immunologic memory may be described as the altered immune reaction of an organism to an immunogenic stimulus as a result of having experienced this stimulus before. This memory exists in two forms. With positive memory, the organism produces a greater immune response to the second immunogenic stimulus than it did to the first. With negative memory, the organism generally fails to react to the first or subsequent immunogenic stimuli.

Positive Immunologic Memory

Secondary immune responses are generally characterized by shorter latent periods, steeper

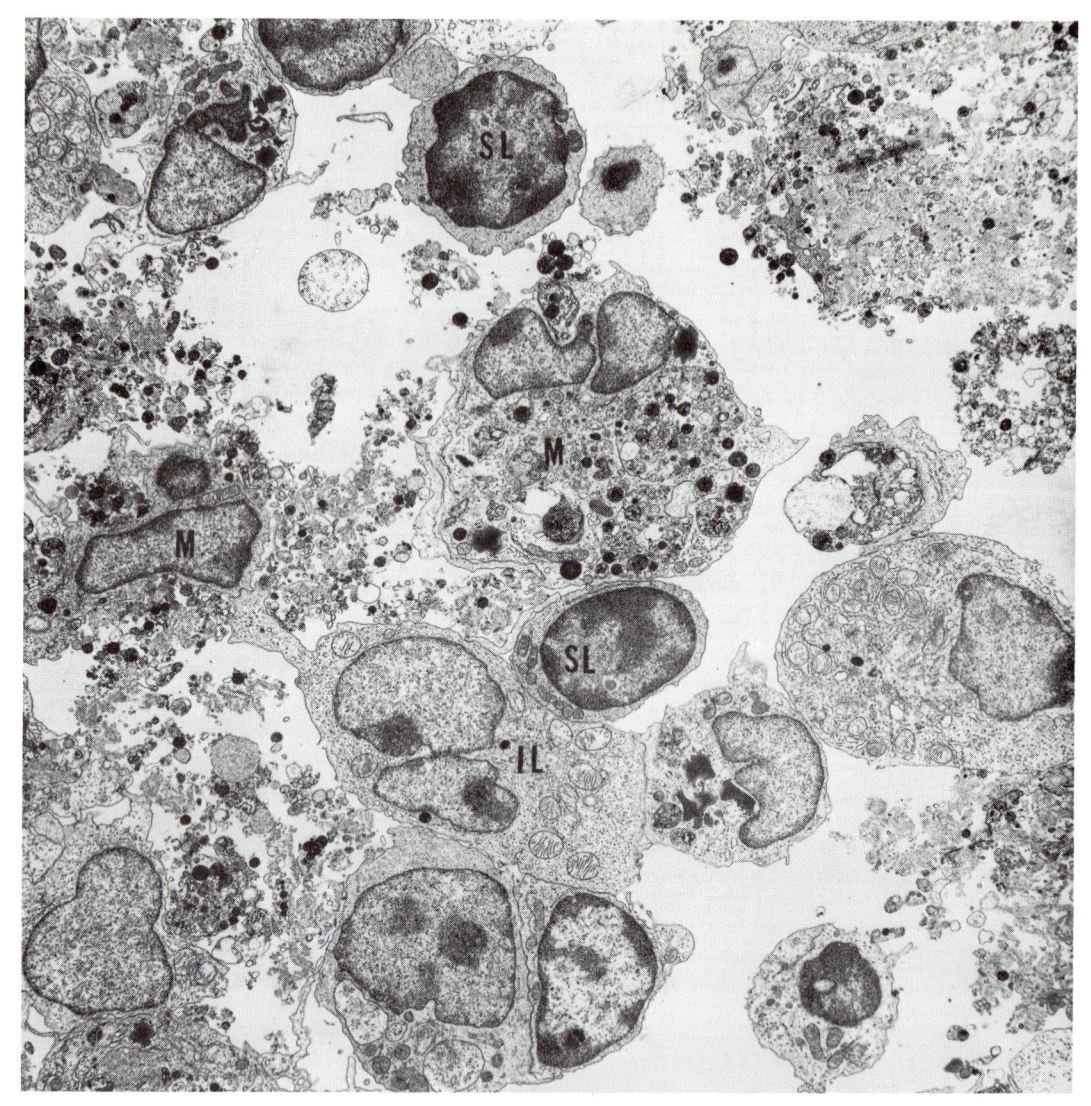

Figure 4–7 Cluster of cells from a 24 hour culture of mouse spleen cells immunized with sheep erythrocytes. It shows three distinct cell types: macrophages (M) and two types of immunologically different lymphocytes (small lymphocytes [SL] and immature lymphocytes [IL]). (Courtesy of Dr. M. F. La Via, Emory University.)

rises in antibody production, and higher peaks of antibody than homologous primary responses. Furthermore, the threshold dose of immunogen required to elicit a secondary response is far smaller than that required to stimulate a primary response to the same immunogen. The secondary response is extremely durable and can be evoked many months, and even years, after the primary injection. As the interval between primary and secondary stimulation increases, the magnitude of the secondary response increases; it is usually maximal 3 to 12 months after primary stimulation, though it may persist without diminution for many years and sometimes for the life of the individual. Antibodies produced during the secondary response are predominantly IgG antibodies with increasingly high affinity. The specificity of the secondary response is pronounced but not absolute and is usually elicited most strongly with the same immunogen as that used for primary stimulation. In some systems, however, it can be evoked by a structurally related immunogen; the antibodies then usually have as high an affinity for the first immunogen as for the second. This phenomenon, called "original antigenic sin," indicates that a population of antigen-sensitive cells can be cross-stimulated by structurally similar immunogens.

A variety of conditions will influence the establishment of immunologic memory. There is a striking variation among antigens in their capacity to induce memory; polysaccharides are relatively deficient in this capacity, whereas most proteins are highly effective. When relatively high doses of immunogen are used to elicit a pronounced primary response, they may diminish the capacity to give a good secondary response, at least within a reasonably short time. Secondary responses can be modified by agents that interfere with cell multiplication. Adjuvants, endotoxin, and oligonucleotides enhance secondary responses, whereas x-irradiation or 6-mercaptopurine can selectively inhibit the establishment of IgG memory without abolishing a primary IgM response. Furthermore, immunologic memory is not readily established in old animals because their proliferative capacities are diminished.

The observations described above are believed to reflect the following cellular events associated with secondary responses:

1. The specific reaction of immunogen with receptors on antigen-sensitive cells leads to cell proliferation. Those progeny cells that react again with immunogen go on to differentiate into antibody-producing cells, whereas others, not further reacting with immunogen, continue to proliferate, forming a colony of memory cells.

2. This colony of memory cells is larger than the one that responds to primary stimulation and it is relatively enriched with cells whose progeny can form highly avid immunoglobulins. The data to date indicate that memory to heterologous erythrocytes can be carried by both T and B cells and that B cells require T cells, but not necessarily primed T cells, for expression of IgG memory. Similar evidence is lacking for the role of T and B cells in secondary immune responses to soluble antigens.

Negative Immunologic Memory (Tolerance)

Negative immunologic memory or tolerance is a type of immune unresponsiveness which is mediated by the introduction of immunogen into an immunologically immature or incompetent host, or by the introduction of immunogen which is qualitatively or quantitatively nonoptimal. It may occur as a natural or acquired phenomenon. Unresponsiveness of this type has been defined as a central failure of immune responsiveness brought about by exposure to immunogen, so that immunologically competent cells become unable to initiate antibody synthesis. There is no apparent failure of immunogen to react with such cells (afferent block) or of synthesis of immunoglobulins that are subsequently blocked (efferent block). Another essential feature of tolerance is specificity, that is, a central failure of immune competence only to the specific immunogen used to induce tolerance.

Tolerance is most readily induced if immunogens are introduced in fetal or neonatal animals, because the ability to make antibody occurs slowly during embryonic development and such animals are generally immunologically incompetent. It is believed that clones of immunologically competent lymphoid cells which contact "self" immunogens in embryonic life are destroyed. Any "sequestered" self immunogens which do not have an opportunity to meet lymphoid cells will have corresponding intact lymphoid clones able to synthesize antibodies against these immunogens. Under ordinary circumstances, these immunogens remain sequestered and the lymphoid clones unstimulated. Conditions such as trauma or infection might make these immunogens available to the lymphoid cells and thus lead to autoantibodies against these immunogens. Such sequestered immunogens are believed to include the cornea of the eye, thyroglobulin, and spermatic tissue.

Tolerance induction is also conditioned by the dose and physical characteristics of the immunogen. It has been found that for a wide variety of immunogens very low (low-zone tolerance) and very high doses (high-zone tolerance) will induce a specific immune unresponsiveness to these immunogens. High-zone tolerance tends to be more complete and longer lasting than low-zone tolerance, which is usually partial and more transient. Highly soluble immunogens, free of aggregates, prepared by high-speed centrifugation of protein solutions or in-vivo screening of proteins leave immunogenic products that tend to induce tolerance. These procedures remove aggregates that would ordinarily be taken up and processed by macrophages. One interpretation of these observations is that aggregate-free immunogens reach lymphocytes and directly induce tolerance, while particulate or aggregated immunogens processed through macrophages induce antibody formation. This information becomes clinically important in cases in which specific immune suppression is desirable. Thus, attempts are being made to inject solubilized histocompatibility antigens of donor tissue into prospective recipients in order to prevent graft rejection through this mechanism of tolerance induction.

In tolerance induced by living cells, the tolerant state may last indefinitely if it is induced in neonatal animals and a stable chimeric state is established. This relatively stable form of tolerance may be terminated by the injection (adoptive transfer) of cells specifically sensitized to the tolerant immunogen. When tolerance to nonliving immunogens is produced, it may be abrogated by the injection of normal lymphoid cells from compatible animals. This is strong evidence that the tolerant state is indeed a central failure of the immune system and not some general alteration of the cellular environment of the tolerant animal.

Tolerance to nonliving immunogens such as serum albumins and globulins can be terminated by the injection of cross-reacting immunogens. This, too, has important clinical significance to man, who is subjected to structurally similar antigens from a variety of disease-bearing pathogens. Thus, the introduction of a cross-reacting immunogen could terminate a state of natural tolerance to self immunogens, with the resultant induction of an autoimmune disease. This may be the case in the well-established sequence of rheumatic heart disease following a hemolytic streptococcal infection, since cross-reacting immunogens have been demonstrated between this organism and heart tissue.

IMMUNOSUPPRESSION

Immunosuppressive agents may be divided into two groups: those which are nonspecific and lead to a broad suppression, and those which are restricted in their suppression.

Nonspecific Immunosuppressants

1. CYTOTOXIC DRUGS AND RADIATION. Since a characteristic feature of the immune response is cell proliferation, antiproliferative agents have been exploited as nonspecific immunosuppressants.

X-irradiation, when used in sublethal doses (300 to 500 r), will suppress immune responses depending upon when the x-rays are given in relation to immunogenic stimuli and whether the response is primary or secondary. If immunogenic stimulation has begun, x-irradiation may depress, but not suppress, a primary immune response. However, irradiation preceding immunogenic stimulation will suppress or abolish primary immune responses. Secondary immune responses are relatively resistant to x-irradiation. This effect on antibody synthesis is apparently due to the destruction of lymphocytes, since sensitized lymphocytes are apparently radioresistant. Since the dangers of using whole body irradiation in clinical medicine far outweigh any benefits, this method has been largely abandoned. However, the work being done by some transplant groups with extracorporeal irradiation of the blood carries considerably reduced risks to the patient, but has proved cumbersome and difficult to manage in human beings.

Cytotoxic drugs can exert an effect on many components of an immune response, including phagocytosis, mitosis, and DNA and RNA replication. One of the most recently developed and clinically useful cytotoxic drugs is cyclophosphamide, which appears to be an extremely active and powerful immunosuppressant. Several of the cytotoxic drugs are purine antimetabolites (6-mercaptopurine, azathioprine, 6-thioguanine), and pyrimidine analogs (5-fluorouracil, 5-bromodeoxyuridine). Folic acid antagonists (amethopterin and its methylated derivative, methotrexate) have the same effect of blocking DNA and RNA synthesis by blocking a number of essential precursors. In general, azathioprine (Imuran) and methotrexate appear to be of greatest value for prolonging the survival of allografts because they are less toxic than many of the immunosuppressant drugs. Some of the antibiotics (puromycin, mitomycin, actinomycin D, chloramphenicol) and proved less useful clinically than experimentally because of their extreme toxicity.

2. CORTICOSTEROIDS. In addition to their potent immunosuppressive properties, corticosteroids are anti-inflammatory and can thus suppress some of the secondary consequences of the immune response, including delayed and immediate-type hypersensitivities. In large doses they can also interfere with the initiation of both cellular immunity and immunoglobulin formation. They cause lymphopenia and deplete lymphoid tissue, especially the thymus, of lymphocytes. For these reasons corticosteroids are widely used for the treatment of autoimmune disease and for the suppression of rejection phenomena in organ transplantation.

3. ANTILYMPHOCYTE SERUM (ALS) is a powerful immunosuppressive agent which inhibits cell-mediated immunity primarily, although it does impair some humoral antibody responses. It is prepared by immunizing an animal of one species, such as the horse, with lymphocytes from animals of another species, such as man. ALS selectively depletes lymphoid organs of migrant lymphocytes, the depletion occurring mainly in the paracortical area of the lymph node and periarteriolar lymphocyte sheaths of the spleen, sites of extensive lymphocyte recirculation. There are several serious problems associated with the use of ALS. ALS suppresses the entire delayed hypersensitivity capability of an individual, not just the response to the particular reaction one wishes to suppress. Cell-mediated immunity is particularly important in the defense against viruses, and ALS has been found to inhibit host-responses to vaccinia, herpes simplex, and oncogenic viruses. Furthermore, ALS-treated patients often respond to ALS as a foreign protein, because their humoral antibody mechanisms are left intact while their delayed hypersensitivity responses are effectively suppressed. Therefore, there are risks of serum sickness and

anaphylaxis following continuous ALS treatment. It is for these reasons that the continued use of ALS in clinical medicine must be approached with extreme caution.

Specific Agents

SPECIFIC ANTIBODY. The ability of specific antibody to inhibit the induction of an immune response has recently been illustrated in the suppression of erythroblastosis fetalis by an anti-Rh antiserum. It is an example of a nontoxic, highly specific, biological form of immunosuppression. The mechanism of action of such specific antibodies is not fully understood but is believed to act by combining with antigenic sites on the immunogen, either prior to or following the processing by macrophages. Another possible mode of action, particularly true in transplantation immunity, is that antibody may coat the target graft and thereby prevent the cell-mediated rejection by lymphocytes.

DRUG-INDUCED TOLERANCE. Drug-induced tolerance is the most recent form of specific immunosuppression. This method involves the injection of the specific immunogen against which antibody suppression is to be directed in combination with cytotoxic drugs. The immunogen selectively stimulates the proliferation of cells producing specific antibody to the immunogen. The cytotoxic drugs then destroy these cells with a resultant tolerance to the immunogen in question. This approach has been used effectively in the suppression of autoimmune thyroiditis in guinea pigs following treatment with thyroglobulin and cyclophosphamide. Furthermore, these animals appear to be specifically tolerant to further injections of thyroglobulin. This approach therefore has definitive implications for clinical medicine, since it is the least toxic and most immunogen-specific form of suppression known to date.

EFFECTOR MECHANISMS OF THE IMMUNE RESPONSE

The efferent limb of the immune response refers to the ability of antibodies and sensitized lymphocytes to interact with antigen in vivo and to initiate a series of events which ultimately leads to the elimination of that antigen. In essence, all antibodies and sensitized lymphocytes contain two functional units: the antigen-reactive or antigen-combining site and a biologically active component.

The antigen-combining site serves to recognize and to form a complex with the antigen. This site is responsible for the in-vitro antigen-antibody reactions which result in precipitation or agglutination of the antigen and in some instances, when the antigen is a bacterial toxin or a virus, neutralization of some biological activity. These manifestations are generally of limited importance in the in vivo situation, although they may contribute in the phagocytosis of antigen by the cells of the reticuloendothelial system. The interaction between the antigen-combining site and the antigen mainly serves to activate the biologically active portion of the antibody molecule or lymphocyte. Subsequently, a very effective biological amplification system is initiated which is capable of inducing an inflammatory reaction and eventually causes the elimination of antigen. At least three biological amplification systems of immunity are known, each of which follows a specific pattern of biochemical and physiological events and induces a characteristic inflammatory lesion. The complement system and the anaphylactic system are related to humoral immunity; the third is the biologic amplification system of cellular immunity.

Anaphylactic System

The anaphylactic system is mediated by cytotropic antibodies which bind to the surface of two types of cells: the tissue mast cell and the circulating basophilic granulocyte. Interaction of these cell-bound antibodies with antigen induces the cells to release a number of bioactive substances which have pronounced effects on inflammatory processes. This amplification system is responsible for the manifestations of immediate hypersensitivity, such as local and systemic anaphylaxis, and allergy (see Chapter 18).

Local cutaneous anaphylactic reactions are induced with intradermal injections of antigens in the skin of sensitive individuals and occur within minutes as the wheal and flare reaction. Anaphylactic reactivity can be transferred to nonsensitive recipients by serum from sensitive persons. In passive cutaneous anaphylaxis, a latent period is required between injection of antiserum and antigen challenge, allowing the fixation of cytotropic antibodies to the tissue of the recipient.

Cytotropic antibodies belong to two immunoglobulin classes, IgE being far more important than IgG. There are marked differences between the cytotropic activities of these types of antibody. In passive anaphylactic sensitization much smaller amounts of antibody are required for IgE than for IgG. The latent period is 2 to 4 hours for IgG and 24 to 72 hours for IgE. In contrast to the relatively loose binding of IgG, antibodies of the IgE class are firmly fixed to mast cells and persist in tissue for several weeks. IgE has also been referred to as homocytotropic or reaginic antibody. By definition, homocytotropic antibody from a given species is only capable of passive anaphylactic sensitization of a member of the same species. Human IgE cannot be considered a true homocytotropic antibody, because it fixes not only to human but also to monkey and rat mast cells. Antibodies of IgG classes capable of tissue binding in different species have been called heterocytotropic antibodies.

Cytotropic antibodies should not be confused with cytophilic antibodies. Certain subclasses of IgG display cytophilic activity for macrophages. The interaction of macrophage-bound cytophilic antibody with antigen serves to enhance phagocytosis of antigen by macrophages. No soluble bioactive mediators are released.

The structures responsible for the fixation of cytotropic antibodies to mast cells and basophils reside in the F_c portion of the IgE molecule. They are sensitive to heat and reductive agents like 2-mercaptoethanol; however, it is not clear whether they involve disulfide bonds. The nature of the IgE receptor site on the mast cell surface is still obscure. The release of bioactive factors from mast cells or basophils involves the initial interaction of at least two proximate membrane-bound IgE antibody molecules with antigen. This interaction induces structural changes in the F_c region of the antibody molecules whereby biologically active sites are exposed which activate an unknown biochemical system in the cell membrane in which adenyl cyclase and cyclic AMP appear to be involved. Subsequently, a variety of bioactive factors are released by the cell (Fig. 4-8). The release of these mediators is concurrent with a loss of the metachromatic cytoplasmic granules, a process known as degranulation. The quantity released as well as the biological activity of each mediator varies from one species to another.

The most important mediator of the anaphylactic system is histamine (β-imidazolylethylamine). Its biological effects include increase of vascular permeability of small venules; contraction of bronchiolar and other smooth muscle; and increased gastric, nasal, and lacrimal secretions. The effects are transient because histamine is rapidly broken down by plasma enzymes. The second vasoactive amine released by mast cells is

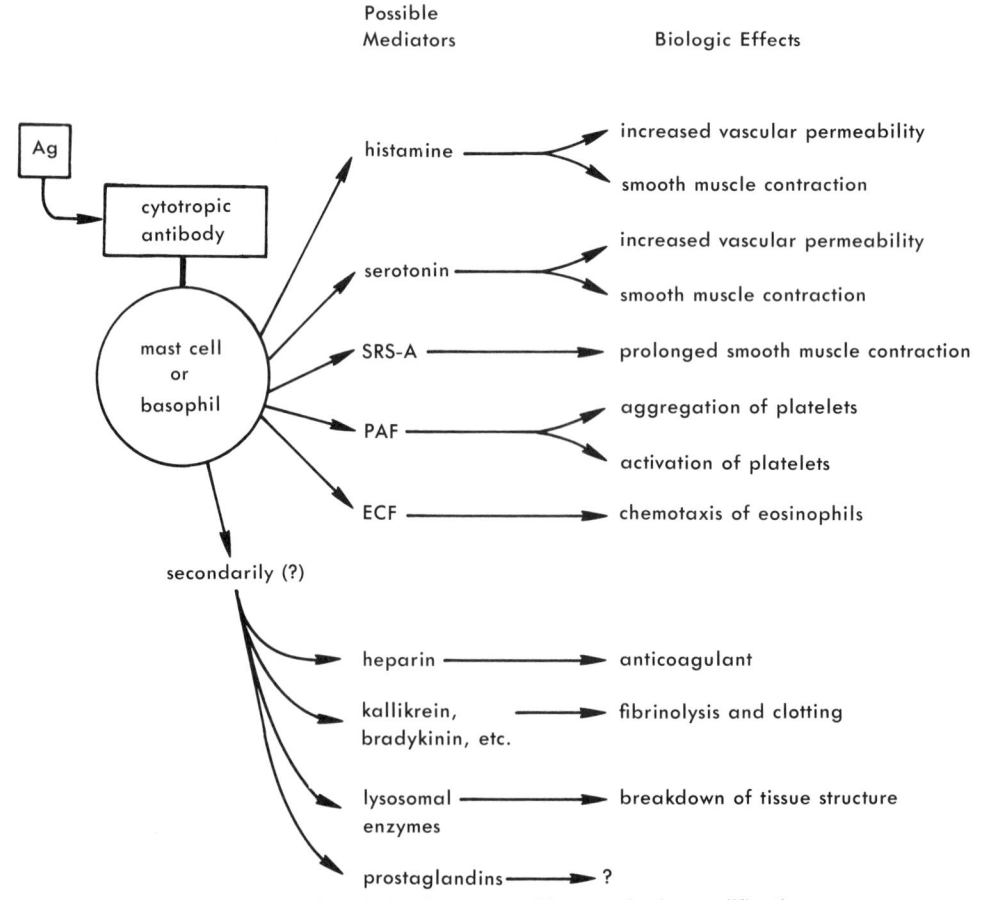

Figure 4-8 Anaphylactic system of immunologic amplification.

serotonin (5-hydroxytryptamine), which also causes increased vascular permeability and smooth muscle contraction. Slow reacting substance of anaphylaxis (SRS-A), an acid lipid with a molecular weight of about 1000, also induces smooth muscle contraction and may partly be responsible for the prolonged bronchospasm seen in asthma. (The biological effects of these mediators are discussed in greater detail in Chapter 18.)

Two factors active in the anaphylactic system have recently been identified. Rabbit basophils have been shown to release a soluble factor called platelet activating factor (PAF), which induces aggregation of platelets and release of vasoactive substances. An eosinophilic leukocyte chemotactic factor (ECF) has been described in diffusates of lung tissue fragments sensitized with IgE antibody and challenged with antigen. The biological significance of PAF and ECF has not yet been fully evaluated.

Several other mediators of the anaphylactic system have been detected. These include kallikrein, bradykinin, and other substances of the kinin system as well as heparin, lysosomal enzymes, and prostaglandins. Direct IgE-mediated release of these mediators by mast cells or basophils has not yet been demonstrated. It is possible that they arise as secondary factors in the anaphylactic system.

The pathophysiologic effects of the anaphylactic system include increased vascular permeability affecting venules and small veins, smooth muscle contraction, glandular secretion, and frequently eosinophil granulocytic infiltration of affected tissue. Other effects are incoagulability of blood, increased heart rate, bronchoconstriction, diarrhea, hypothermia, and shock.

The physiologic significance of the IgE-mediated anaphylactic system is unclear. Its detrimental effects to the individual, exemplified by allergic reactions and other forms of anaphylaxis when exposed to an apparently innocuous antigen, seem to contradict the usefulness of the anaphylactic system in immunologic homeostasis. Recent evidence has also indicated the possible role of IgE in the pathogenesis of immune vasculitis and other forms of immune complex disease. However, from an evolutionary standpoint, IgE-mediated immunity should have a useful purpose, since IgE has persisted in higher vertebrates. It is possible that the anaphylactic system offers a first line of defense against extraneous agents, including microorganisms. This is indicated in patients with certain parasitic infections who often have markedly elevated levels of IgE. Also, selective IgE deficiency with normal levels of all other immunoglobulins is associated with frequent sinopulmonary infections leading to chronic pulmonary disease.

Complement System

Complement refers to an important biological amplification system of humoral immunity. It consists of nine enzyme precursors (C1 to C9) which can be activated to interact in a sequence of restricted proteolytic reactions that affect immune lysis and the generation of bioactive factors critical to mechanisms of inflammation and phagocytosis (Table 4-2). The ability of many types of antibody to activate the complement system has been utilized in various serologic tests for antibody such as hemolysis, bacteriolysis, and the complement-fixation reaction.

The first step in the complement sequence involves the binding and activation of the recognition unit C1, which is a complex of three subunits C1q, C1r, and C1s (in a ratio of 1:2:4) held together by a calcium ion (Table 4-2). The interaction of antibody with its corresponding antigen is required to reveal a specialized molecular structure (the complement-fixation site) on the F_c portion of the antibody molecule which then combines with the C1q subunit of the C1 complex.

Complement component C1 is fixed by immunoglobulins of the IgG and IgM classes, but not all subclasses display this property equally well. In man, IgG1 and IgG3 antibodies generally bind C1 very efficiently in contrast to the low binding ability of IgG2 antibodies. IgG4 does not fix complement. Similar differences have been found in IgM and IgG subclasses in animals. Single antibody molecules of IgM in combination with antigen are capable of fixing C1. The fixation of C1q by IgG requires the close proximity or aggregation of at least two IgG molecules in the antigen-antibody complex. The nature of the antigen plays an important role in determining whether the immune complex will fix C1. Antibodies to haptenic groups will not bind C1 when only reacted with simple haptens or with bivalent haptens.

The concentration and distribution of the antigenic groups at the cell surface to which antibodies are directed also have a great influence on the complement-fixing ability. A low density of antigenic groups on a cell surface is generally associated with decreased efficiency of binding of C1 by IgG antibodies, since the chance is small that antigen-bound IgG molecules are sufficiently proximate to another. In this situation IgM antibodies in combination with cell-bound antigens may fix complement quite well, although IgG antibodies may be more efficient than IgM antibodies when antigen is presented in a soluble form.

Upon binding of C1q to antibody, a spatial rearrangement of the subunits of the C1 complex occurs which induces C1r to activate the proenzyme subunit C1s to become C1 esterase.

TABLE 4-2 THE COMPLEMENT SYSTEM

Step	Complement Component	Reaction in Complement Sequence	Properties of Membrane-bound Fragment*	Properties of Fragment in Fluid Phase
1	C1	AgAb ⇅ C1q ↔ 2C1r ↔ 4C1s ↔ Ca^{++} → C1s	C1q: Recognition of CF site of antibody C1s: Becomes C1 esterase	
2	C4 C2	AgAbC1qr—C1s C4 → C4a, C4b Mg^{++} C2 → C2a, C2b	C4b: Virus neutralization Immunoconglutination C2a: Becomes C3 convertase	C4a: Kinin-like activity C2b: Kinin-like activity
3	C3	AgAbC14b—C2a C3 → C3a, C3b	C3b: Many molecules on membrane Conglutination Immune adherence Enhanced phagocytosis Binding of B lymphocytes Immune conglutination	C3a: Anaphylatoxin I Increased vascular permeability Contraction of smooth muscle Release of histamine Degranulation of mast cells Chemotaxis of leukocytes
4	C5	AgAbC14b2aC3b C5 → C5a, C5b		C5a: Anaphylatoxin II Increased vascular permeability Contraction of smooth muscle Release of histamine Requires cocytotaxin for chemotactic activity for leukocytes
5	C6 C7	AgAbC14b2a3b5b C6 → ? C7 → ?		$\overline{C567}$: Chemotactic activity
6	C8 C9	AgAbC14b2a3b5b67 C8 → ? C9 → ?	C8: "Partial" membranolysis C9: Complete membranolysis	

*Other than activation of the next component in the complement sequence.

The second step in the complement sequence involves the interaction of C1 esterase ($\overline{C1s}$) with C4 and C2 (magnesium-dependent) whereby each component is enzymatically split into two fragments. The fragments C4b and C2a form a bimolecular complex which attaches to membrane or immunoglobulin receptors while two low molecular weight fragments C4a and C2b appear in the fluid phase. The $\overline{C4b2a}$ complex becomes an enzyme which acts on C3 and is called C3-convertase. This complex has also been shown to play a role in the neutralization of herpes simplex virus sensitized by IgM antibody. Little is known about the biological properties of the C4a and C2b fragments except that they may have a kinin-like activity.

The enzyme $\overline{C4b2a}$ cleaves the third component C3 into fragments C3a and C3b. The larger fragment C3b attaches itself to the antigen-antibody-C14b2a complex and a new enzyme is formed, of which C5 is a substrate. Many C3b molecules (up to a few hundred) also become attached to the membrane surface at varying distances of the complex. The great number of C3b on the membrane surface allows histochemical detection of complement with fluorescent antibodies to C3 or serum β1C-globulins which contain C3.

The presence of C3b on the surface of cells will promote conglutination (or clumping) of these cells and immune adherence, in which process the cells will adhere or attach themselves to other cells. Fragment C3b also renders the cell more susceptible to phagocytosis by neutrophils. Both immune adherence and enhanced phagocytosis may be important in the clearance of C3b-coated particles such as erythrocytes, leukocytes, bacteria, rickettsiae, and viruses by the reticuloendothelial system.

Recent evidence has indicated that B lymphocytes are capable of binding to antigen-antibody-complement complexes. It appears that B lymphocytes have C3b specific receptor sites on their membranes.

Many pathobiological activities relevant to inflammatory processes have been ascribed to the low molecular weight fragment C3a present in the fluid phase. This fragment, also called anaphylatoxin, causes increased vascular permeability, contraction of smooth muscle, and degranulation of mast cells with release of vasoactive amines. A low molecular weight protein called chemotaxin has been identified as a cleavage product of C3 and has been shown to promote chemotaxis of neutrophils and other leukocytes.

The activation of C5 by $\overline{C4b2a3b}$ results in the formation of C5a and a larger fragment C5b, which becomes loosely attached to the membrane surface. Low molecular weight C5a is also an anaphylatoxin similar but not equal to C3a and causes increased vascular permeability, smooth muscle contraction, and release of histamine. C5a is not chemotactic by itself but needs the presence of another fragmentation product of C5 called cocytotaxin to display chemotactic activity for neutrophils.

Attachment of C5b leads to activation of the enzyme $\overline{C4b2a3b5b}$ which interacts with C6 and C7 in a not clearly understood manner. A trimolecular complex $\overline{C567}$ is formed which has chemotactic activity for neutrophils. The binding of the trimolecular complex $\overline{C567}$ to the membrane induces a conformational change in $\overline{C567}$, thereby exposing the binding site for one molecule of C8. Upon interaction with C8 the resulting tetramolecular complex reveals multiple binding sites for up to six molecules of C9. Interaction with C9 leads to damage of the membrane of the cell, exemplified by hemolysis in the case of red blood cells.

Although discrete alterations of the membrane are observed early in the complement sequence, functional lesions are largely produced by C8 and C9 which allow influx of extracellular fluid and egress of intracellular ions and macromolecules. It is not known whether the mechanism of membrane lesion production is mediated directly through complement enzymes or by activation of intrinsic enzymes by the complement system. It appears that upon completion of the complement sequence the entire antigen-antibody-complement complex, together with a part of the membrane, is transported toward the inside of the cell, thereby producing a "hole" in the membrane and causing a disturbance of the osmotic balance. Under certain conditions it has been shown that regenerative processes can repair the membrane damage.

Alternate Pathways of Complement Activation. The activation of the complement sequence is induced not only by suitable antigen-antibody combinations but also by a variety of other substances. For instance, aggregation of immunoglobulins may activate complement.

Of pathobiological importance is the recognition and activation mechanism that acts on C3 in the complement sequence, thus bypassing the requirement of C1, C4, and C2. The C3-activator system (also called the complement activation bypass system or the properdin system) can be triggered through the activation of a noncomplement serum proenzyme called C3-proactivator (C3PA) (Fig. 4-9). This protein was first demonstrated through its ability to form a complex enzyme with a protein from cobra venom, a substance known to cause C3 depletion in animals. The C3PA-cobra factor complex can cleave C3 into C3a and C3b and in the presence of C5 through C9 initiate the lysis of unsensitized erythrocytes. The discovery of this artificial pathway of C3 activation stimulated research of the physiologic role of C3PA. It was shown that

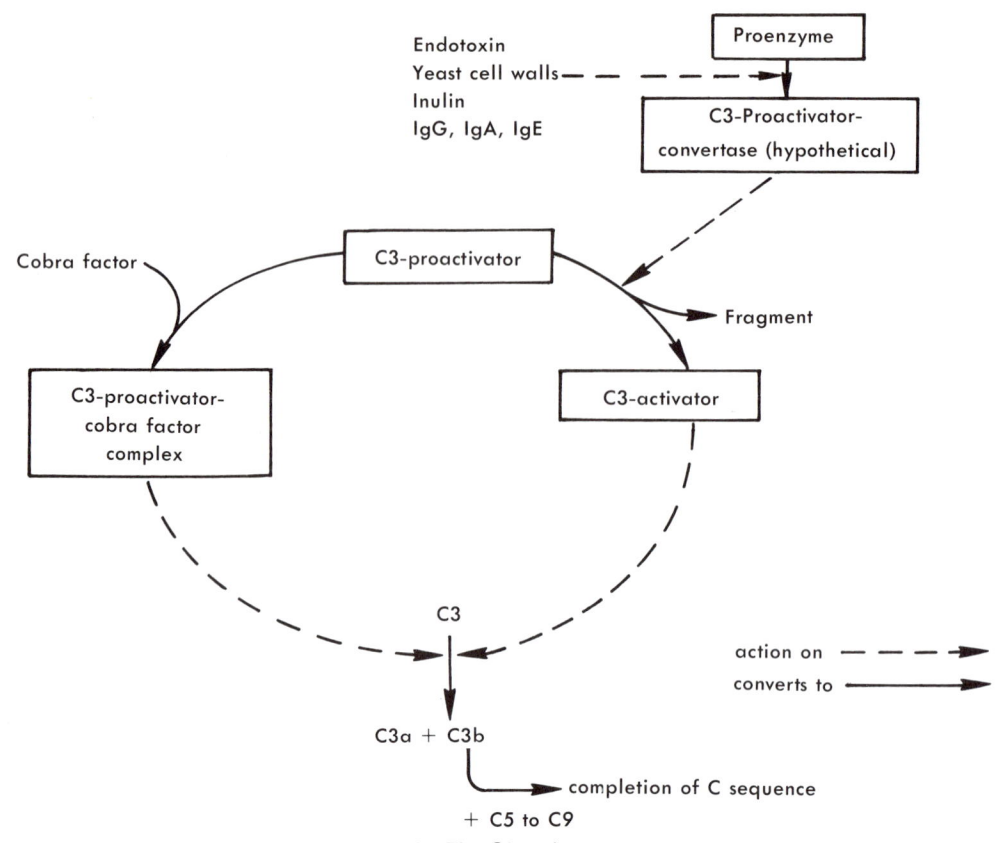

Figure 4-9 The C3 activator system.

C3PA can be enzymatically converted into an enzyme called C3 activator, which splits C3 into pathobiologically active fragments C3a (anaphylatoxin, chemotaxin) and C3b.

A varied group of substances can initiate this pathway of C3 activation. Endotoxins from gram-negative bacteria, yeast cell wall extracts (zymosan), and polysaccharides like inulin are potent stimulators of this complement activation system. Also, proteolytic enzymes like trypsin and papain and aggregates of IgG and IgA myeloma proteins have been shown to activate the bypass activation mechanism. Recent evidence has indicated the involvement of IgA and IgE antibodies in the utilization of late components of the complement system through the C3 activation pathway.

The alternate pathway of C3 activation shows a resemblance with the properdin system. Properdin was originally described as a heat labile beta globulin which, in the presence of magnesium ions, could interact with zymosan, endotoxins, and other polysaccharides to form a complex capable of preferential inactivation of late complement components. In addition, the properdin system participated in the antibacterial and antiviral properties as well as in the lysis by normal serum of erythrocytes from patients with paroxysmal nocturnal hemoglobulinuria. Several investigators questioned the bioactive nature of properdin, suggesting that it was an IgM type of antibody against polysaccharides of gram-negative bacteria of the intestinal flora. However, recent studies have demonstrated a close resemblance between the properdin system and the C3PA activation system.

Another mechanism of activation of C3 is the direct effect of trypsin and other lysosomal enzymes on C3, thereby causing cleavage and the formation of low molecular weight fragments with chemotactic activity for neutrophils. Lysosomal enzymes have also been shown to activate C1 and C5 directly. In infectious inflammatory lesions bacterial enzymes may also act directly on complement components, especially C3. These direct pathways are primarily simple enzyme-substrate reactions which do not initiate the completion of the remaining complement sequence.

The alternate pathways of complement activation, in particular of C3, may be important pathobiological mechanisms of immunity during the preantibody phase of host defense against infections.

The relationship between the clotting system and complement has been demonstrated by the ability of the Hageman factor, via activation of plasmin, to initiate the complement sequence. Plasmin acts to convert C1s into C1 esterase without participation of C1q and C1r. Thus $\overline{C1s}$ can interact with C3 and C2 to activate the other components of the complement system.

Homeostatic Control of the Complement System. There are many mechanisms of activation of the complement sequence or the various segments of the complement system. To ensure a normal functioning of the complement system a variety of inhibitory mechanisms for each component must be readily available. Our understanding of the homeostatic control mechanisms of the complement system is rather limited. It is generally believed that the products resulting from cleavage of complement components have a relatively short half-life in the fluid phase and are somehow readily converted into an inactive form. The attachment of complement fragments to cell membranes is reversible and such fragments are rapidly inactivated in the fluid phase.

Only a few homeostatic control mechanisms have been defined for the complement system. Best known is the C1 esterase inhibitor which blocks the activity of C1s and is therefore capable of suppressing the progression of the complement sequence beyond C1. This enzyme also blocks the activity of several enzymes active in the clotting system including Hageman factor, plasmin, and prekallikrein. Patients with hereditary angioneurotic edema who lack C1 esterase inhibitor suffer from episodic triggerings of the complement system and experience severe angioedematous reactions in various tissues, particularly of the upper respiratory tract.

Another homeostatic control mechanism in the complement system is mediated by anaphylatoxin-inactivator, which is an enzyme that cleaves the C-terminal lysine or arginine groups of C3a and C5a. Lysosomal enzymes have also been shown to inactivate complement components.

Biological Amplification of Cellular Immunity

Cellular or cell-mediated immunity refers to those manifestations of the immune response which are mediated through specifically sensitized lymphocytes. An example is the delayed hypersensitivity reaction which is characterized by the relatively slow development of an inflammatory lesion following local injection of antigen into an appropriately sensitized host. This inflammatory reaction occurs in the absence of antibodies and can be transferred to nonsensitive recipients by mononuclear cells but not by serum from sensitive donors. Cellular immunity plays an important role in maintaining resistance to intracellular infections, in contact sensitivity to low molecular weight chemicals, in allograft rejections, in restricting tumor growth, and in autoallergic disease.

Delayed hypersensitivity reactions are demonstrable in varying degrees in different species and are especially pronounced in man and guinea pig. When an antigen is introduced in a tissue of an appropriately sensitized host, there ensues a slowly evolving inflammatory reaction which is mainly characterized by induration and erythema, and reaches its peak within 24 to 48 hours. The extent of the inflammatory lesion resulting from a delayed hypersensitivity reaction is determined not only by the hypersensitive state of the host but also by the amount and distribution of the antigen in the tissue. In the skin test for delayed hypersensitivity, like the tuberculin test, intradermally injected antigen diffuses throughout the dermis to the blood vessels and lymphatics and may become attached to tissue constituents like collagen fibers. The tissue distribution of antigen is different in skin tests for contact sensitivity in which the chemical is applied percutaneously. Here the chemical penetrates only in the uppermost layers of the dermis and reacts there with host protein constituents to form a complete antigen.

The inflammatory reaction of delayed hypersensitivity is characterized by progressive perivascular infiltrations by mononuclear cells. The perivascular lesions affect only small and medium-sized veins and occur only in areas where antigen is present. A small proportion of the infiltrating mononuclear cells are lymphocytes while the great majority are formed by monocytes derived from the bone marrow. These monocytes are highly motile phagocytic cells which may assume the appearance of histiocytes and macrophages. In other instances they may form masses of epithelioid cells, giant cells, or granulomas. Parenchymal damage is seen particularly in areas of cellular infiltration blood vessels. Disseminated lesions tend to occur around venous plexuses. Intense delayed hypersensitivity reactions may result in additional tissue necrosis, infiltration of polymorphonuclear leukocytes, and hemorrhage.

Because of the complex pathobiological manifestation of the in-vivo reaction of delayed hypersensitivity, numerous experimental procedures have been designed to study biological effects of cellular immunity in vitro. In these procedures, lymphocytes from a sensitized host were incubated with specific antigen in suitable culture media. After a period of incubation which varied from one hour to several days, both lymphocytes and supernatant fluids were tested for certain biological activities using different bioassays. It was found that following reaction with its specific antigen the lymphocyte undergoes a series of morphologic and physiochemical changes, releasing a number of soluble bioactive substances.

The morphologic changes of antigen-stimulated lymphocytes include blast cell transformation and mitosis. Mitogenic agents like phytohemagglutinin, pokeweed mitogen, and concanavallin A can also nonspecifically stimulate lymphocytes to undergo blastogenesis and produce bioactive factors. Blastogenesis is associated with increased synthesis of nuclear DNA and RNA and can be quantitated by the uptake of radioactive precursors of DNA and RNA as a means of determining the reactivity of lymphocytes.

When the antigen is present on the membrane of a cell, the antigen-stimulated lymphocyte becomes involved in a series of reactions which ultimately lead to the elimination of that cell. Destruction of this target cell may occur either as a result of direct contact with cytotoxic antigen-activated lymphocytes, through soluble cytotoxic mediators produced by these lymphocytes, or by phagocytic cells which have been activated by soluble factors.

A direct cytotoxic effect of activated lymphocytes on target cells bearing the specific antigen has been observed in transplantation, tumor immunity, and autoallergies. One sensitized lymphocyte is able to destroy several target cells at one time and move along to new cells. The cytotoxicity of these activated lymphocytes is specific and requires close contact with the antigen-bearing target cells; specific antibody will inhibit the cytotoxic effect. The mechanism of destruction of specific target cells by immune lymphocytes is unknown. It appears that lysosomal enzyme-like proteins in the membrane play an important role in the cytotoxic properties of lymphocytes. These membrane proteins are susceptible to carboxypeptidase and trypsin but are resistant to neuraminidase.

Following the interaction with antigen the sensitized lymphocyte is capable of producing a variety of soluble factors which are of great importance in the biological amplification system of cellular immunity. These effector substances of cellular immunity have been demonstrated by many investigators using different in-vitro systems of lymphocytes incubated with specific antigen or nonspecific mitogenic stimulators like phytohemagglutinin. These mediators can be classified into three major groups according to their biological properties: the mitogenic factors which act on other lymphocytes, the cytotoxic and metabolism inhibitory factors, and the group of factors which activate the macrophage system (Fig. 4–10).

At least two types of blastogenic and mitogenic lymphocyte factors have been identified which act on nonsensitive lymphocytes. Delayed hypersensitivity in man, and perhaps in lower animals, can be transferred with extracts from peripheral blood leukocytes. A transfer factor (TF) identified in extracts from peripheral human leukocytes has been shown able to confer delayed hypersensitivity to a specific antigen either in vivo or in vitro. Transfer factor is a relatively stable, dialysable substance of protein and polynucleotide composition with a molecular weight of less than 10,000. It can be prepared from leukocytes of antigen-sensitive individuals by lysis of these cells or by short-term in-vitro incubation with antigen. Although unrelated to immunoglobulins, transfer factor is immunologically specific for the antigen. For instance, when tuberculin-negative persons are injected with transfer factor prepared from tuberculin-sensitive leukocytes, they will convert to a tuberculin-positive state which may persist for years. Lymphocytes from individuals injected with transfer factor, when incubated with antigen, will undergo blast transformation and produce a clone of sensitized lymphocytes. In-vitro incubation of nonsensitized lymphocytes with transfer factor makes these lymphocytes susceptible to antigen-induced blast transformation and proliferation of sensitized cells. Transfer factor is immunologically specific for antigen in its release as well as in its activity. For example, lymphocytes from persons sensitive to tuberculin and diphtheria toxoid will only release transfer factor specific for tuberculin when incubated with tuberculin, and only release transfer factor specific for diphtheria toxoid when incubated with diphtheria toxoid. Lysis of these cells by freeze-thawing procedures or in hypotonic solution will liberate transfer factors with both specificities.

Incubation of sensitive lymphocytes with antigen has led to the identification of two soluble mediators, a lymphocyte transforming factor (LTF) and a blastogenic factor (BF), which are both capable of inducing blastogenesis of nonsensitive lymphocytes.

Besides the specific cytotoxicity through direct contact with target cells, lymphocytes are also capable of releasing soluble cytotoxic factors and other inhibitors of cellular metabolism. For example, lymphotoxin (LT) has been demonstrated to be in the supernatant fluid of cultures of PHA and antigen-stimulated lymphocytes. Human lymphotoxin, a heat-labile protein of a molecular weight between 80,000 and 90,000, is capable of destroying different human and animal cell cultures while others appear unaffected. The selective cytotoxic effect of lymphotoxin remains unexplained. Other lymphocyte factors have been shown to inhibit growth and other aspects of cellular metabolism without actually killing the target cell. These factors have been called

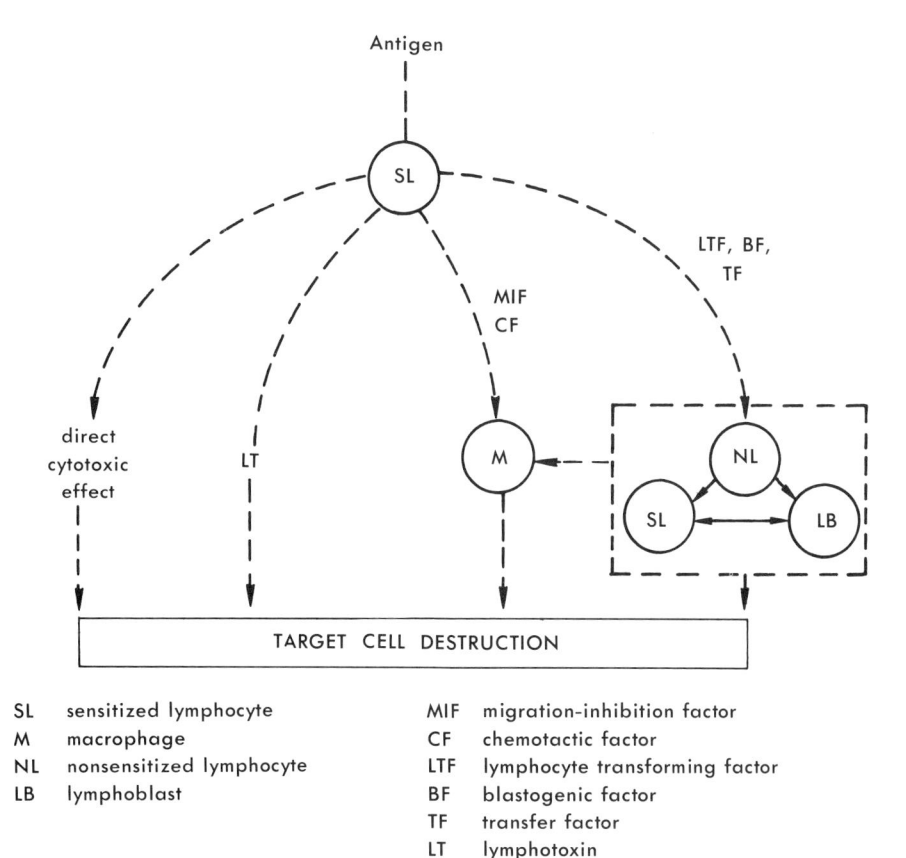

Figure 4–10 Biologic amplification of cellular immunity.

SL	sensitized lymphocyte	MIF	migration-inhibition factor
M	macrophage	CF	chemotactic factor
NL	nonsensitized lymphocyte	LTF	lymphocyte transforming factor
LB	lymphoblast	BF	blastogenic factor
		TF	transfer factor
		LT	lymphotoxin

cloning-inhibitory factor, proliferation-inhibitory factor, and inhibitor of DNA synthesis. It is not known whether all these activities are produced by one single substance.

The third group of lymphocyte mediators deals with factors which have profound effects on the macrophage system. The best example is the migration-inhibition factor (MIF), which can be demonstrated through its ability to inhibit the migration of macrophages from a capillary tube containing a peritoneal exudate to an incubation medium in which the capillary was placed. This phenomenon has been observed in several species, including man, and the activity of MIF does not depend on the immune status of the host from which the macrophages were obtained. For example, the MIF produced by tuberculin-sensitive human lymphocytes inhibits the migration of leukocytes from tuberculin-positive as well as tuberculin-negative individuals and, to a different extent, of guinea pig macrophages. Through the release of MIF, the immune lymphocyte exerts a very efficient influence on the macrophage system. It has been estimated that one lymphocyte is capable of producing enough MIF to immobilize 1000 macrophages. MIF not only inhibits the mobility but also increases the phagocytic capacity, the intracellular metabolism (through the hexose-monophosphate shunt), and the membrane activity of macrophages. In addition to MIF, other factors active in the macrophage system have been shown in supernatants of antigen-stimulated lymphocytes, macrophage activating factor, macrophage aggregating factor, and macrophage spread inhibiting factor. These factors may not represent separate entities but could merely be different expressions of the biological activity of MIF.

Chemotactic factors for macrophages and neutrophils have been shown to be released from antigen-stimulated guinea pig lymphocyte cultures. The macrophage chemotactic factor (CF), like MIF, is heat-stable, with a molecular weight between 35,000 and 55,000. It differs from MIF in its faster electrophoretic mobility and resistance to neuraminidase treatment. Whereas guinea pig MIF acts well in guinea pig macrophages but poorly in rabbit macrophages, guinea pig chemotactic factor is equally effective in attracting macrophages from guinea pigs and rabbits.

Other lymphocyte mediators of the amplification system of cellular immunity include a lymph node permeability factor, a skin reactive factor which produces erythema, and an interferon-like factor which interferes with virus pathogenicity in cell culture.

REFERENCES

GENERAL IMMUNOBIOLOGY

Abramoff, P., and La Via, M. F.: Biology of the Immune Response. New York, McGraw-Hill, 1970.
Amos, B. (Ed.): Progress in Immunology (Proceedings of the First International Congress of Immunology, Washington, D.C., 1971). New York, Academic Press, 1971.
Bellanti, J. A.: Immunology. Philadelphia, W. B. Saunders, 1971.
Burnet, Sir Macfarlane: Cellular Immunology. London, Cambridge University Press, 1969.
Factors Regulating the Immune Response, Technical Report No. 448, World Health Organization, Geneva, 1970.
Good, R. A., and Fisher, D. W. (Eds.): Immunobiology. Stamford, Conn., Sinauer, 1971.
Nossal, G. J. V., and Ada, G. L.: Antigens, Lymphoid Cells, and the Immune Response. New York, Academic Press, 1971.
Smith, R. T., and Landy, M.: Immune Surveillance. New York, Academic Press, 1971.
Waksman, B.: Atlas of Experimental Immunobiology and Immunopathology. New Haven, Conn., Yale University Press, 1970.

ANTIGENS AND IMMUNOGENICITY

Bretscher, P., and Cohn, M.: A theory of self-nonself discrimination. Science, 169:1040, 1970.
Goodman, J. W.: Immunochemical specificity: Recent conceptual advances. Immunochemistry, 6:139, 1969.
Kabat, E. A.: Structural Concepts in Immunology and Immunochemistry. New York, Holt, Rinehart and Winston, 1968.
Maurer, P.: Use of synthetic polymers of amino acids to study the basis of antigenicity. Progr. Allergy., 8:1, 1964.
Sela, M.: Antigenicity: Some molecular aspects. Science, 166:1365, 1965.
Sela, M.: Studies with synthetic polypeptides. Advances Immun., 5:29, 1966.

IMMUNOGLOBULINS

Bennichi, H., and Johansson, S. G. O.: Structure and function of human immunoglobulin E. Advances Immun., 13:1, 1971.
Bernier, G. M.: Structure of human immunoglobulins. Progr. Allerg., 14:1, 1970.
Binaghi, R. A.: Biologic activities of IgG in mammals. In Amos, B. (Ed.): Progress in Immunology. New York, Academic Press, 1971.
Cunningham, B. A., Gottlieb, P. D., Pfumm, M. N., and Edelman, G. M.: Immunoglobulin structure: Diversity, gene duplication, and domains. In Amos, B. (Ed.): Progress in Immunology. New York, Academic Press, 1971.
Dayton, D. H., Jr., Small, P. A., Jr., Chanock, R. M., Kaufman, H. E., and Tomasi, T. B., Jr. (Eds.): The Secretory Immunologic System. Washington, D.C., U.S. Government Printing Office, 1970.
Green, M.: Electron microscopy of the immunoglobulins. Advances Immun., 11:1, 1969.
Haurowitz, F.: Immunochemistry and the Biosynthesis of Antibodies. New York, Interscience, 1968.
Hood, L., and Talmage, D. W.: On the mechanism of antibody diversity: Germline basis for variability. Science, 168:325, 1970.
Hood, L., and Prahl, J.: The immune system: A model for differentiation in higher organisms. Advances Immun., 14:291, 1971.
Killander, J.: Gamma Globulins: Structure and Control of Biosynthesis. New York, Interscience, 1967.
Merler, E. (Ed.): Immunoglobulins. Washington, D.C., National Academy of Sciences, 1970.
Metzger, H.: Structure and function of γM macroglobulins. Advances Immun., 12:57, 1970.
Putnam, F. W.: Immunoglobulin structure: Variability and homology. Science, 163:633, 1969.

INDUCTION OF THE IMMUNE RESPONSE

Fishman, M.: Induction of antibodies. Ann. Rev. Microbiol., 23:199, 1970.
Uhr, J. W., and Finkelstein, M. S.: The kinetics of antibody formation. Progr. Allerg., 10:37, 1967.
Waldmann, T. A., and Strober, W.: Metabolism of immunoglobulins. Progr. Allerg., 13:1, 1969.

CELLULAR ASPECTS OF ANTIBODY SYNTHESIS

Abdou, N. I., and Richter, M.: The role of bone marrow in the immune response. Advances Immun., 12:202, 1970.
Makinodan, T., and Albright, J. F.: Proliferative and differentiative manifestations of cellular immune potential. Progr. Allerg., 10:1, 1967.
Metzger, H.: The antigen-receptor problem. Ann. Rev. Biochem., 39:889, 1970.
Möller, G. (Ed.): Antigen Sensitive Cells. Their Source and Differentiation. Vol. 1, Transplantation Reviews. Baltimore, Williams and Wilkins, 1969.
Möller, G. (Ed.): Antigen-Binding Lymphocyte Receptors. Vol. 5, Transplantation Reviews. Baltimore, Williams and Wilkins, 1970.
Osoba, D.: The regulatory role of the thymus in immunogenesis. In Cinader, B. (Ed.): Regulation of the Antibody Response. Springfield, Ill., Charles C Thomas, 1968.
Siskind, G. W., and Benacerraf, B.: Cell selection by antigen in the immune response. Advances Immun., 10:1, 1969.
Talmage, D. W., Radovich, J., and Hemmingsen, H.: Cell interaction in antibody synthesis. Advances Immun., 12:271, 1970.
Taylor, R. B., and Iverson, G. M.: Hapten competition and the nature of cell-cooperation in the antibody response. Proc. Roy. Soc. London (Biol.), 176:393, 1971.
Weiss, L.: The Cells and Tissues of the Immune System. Englewood Cliffs, N.J., Prentice-Hall, Inc., 1972.
Wennberg, E., and Weiss, L.: The structure of the spleen and hemolysis. Ann. Rev. Med., 20:29, 1969.

IMMUNOLOGIC MEMORY

Bosman, C., and Feldman, J. D.: Cellular events during the expression of immunologic memory. Clin. Exp. Immun., 7:565, 1970.
Cunningham, A. J.: Studies on the cellular basis of IgM immunological memory. Immunology, 16:621, 1969.
L'Age-Stehr, J., and Herzenberg, L. A.: Immunological memory in mice. J. Exp. Med., 131:1093, 1970.
Landy, M., and Braun, W. (Eds.): Immunological Tolerance. New York, Academic Press, 1968.
Nossal, G. J. V.: Recent advances in immunological tolerance. In Amos, B. (Ed.): Progress in Immunology. New York, Academic Press, 1971.
Weigle, W. O., Chiller, J. M., and Habicht, G. S.: Immunological unresponsiveness: Cellular kinetics and interactions. In Amos, B. (Ed.): Progress in Immunology. New York, Academic Press, 1971.

IMMUNOSUPPRESSION

Batchelor, J. R.: Hormonal control of antibody formation. *In* Cinader, B. (Ed.): Regulation of the Antibody Response. Springfield, Ill., Charles C Thomas, 1968.

Dresser, D. W., and Mitchison, N. A.: The mechanism of immunologic paralysis. Advances Immun., 8:129, 1968.

Gabrielson, A. E., and Good, R. A.: Chemical suppression of adaptive immunity. Advances Immun., 6:91, 1967.

Greaves, M. F.: Biological effects of anti-immunoglobulins: Evidence for immunoglobulin receptors on 'T' and 'B' lymphocytes. Transplant. Rev., 5:45, 1970.

James, K.: Anti-lymphocytic antibody—A review. Clin. Exp. Immun., 2:615, 1967.

Sorkin, E. (Ed.): The Immune Response and Its Suppression. Antibiot. Chemother. (Basel), 15:1970.

EFFECTOR MECHANISMS OF THE IMMUNE RESPONSE

Alper, C. A., and Rosen, F. S.: Genetic aspects of the complement system. Advances Immun., 14:252, 1971.

Benacerraf, B., and Green, I.: Cellular hypersensitivity. Ann. Rev. Med., 20:141, 1969.

Bloom, B. R., and Glade, P. R.: In Vitro Methods in Cell-Mediated Hypersensitivity. New York, Academic Press, 1971.

Dumonde, D. C., and Maini, R. N.: The clinical significance of mediators of cellular immunity. Clin. Allerg., 1:120, 1971.

Effectors of cellular immunity. President's Symposium, Amer. Soc. Exp. Path. Amer. J. Path., 60:407, 1970.

Humphrey, J. H., and Dourmashkin, R. R.: The lesions in cell membranes caused by complement. Advances Immun., 11:75, 1969.

Ishizaka, K.: Experimental anaphylaxis. *In* Immunological Diseases. Boston, Little, Brown and Co., 1968.

Lawrence, H. S., and Landy, M. (Eds.): Perspectives in Immunology: Mediators of Cellular Immunity. New York, Academic Press, 1969.

Movat, H. Z. (Ed.): Inflammation, Immunity and Hypersensitivity. Hagerstown, Md., Harper and Row, 1961.

Movat, H. Z. (Ed.): Cellular and Humoral Mechanisms in Anaphylaxis and Allergy. Basel and New York, S. Karger, 1969.

Müller-Eberhard, H. J.: Chemistry and reaction mechanisms of complement. Adv. Immunol., 8:1, 1968.

Orange, R. P., and Austen, K. F.: Slow reacting substance of anaphylaxis. Adv. Immunol., 10:106, 1969.

Pick, E., and Turk, J. L.: The biological activities of soluble lymphocyte products: A review. Clin. Exp. Immun., 10:1, 1972.

Rapp, H. J., and Borsos, T.: Molecular Basis of Complement Action. New York, Appleton-Century-Crofts, Inc., 1970.

CHAPTER 5

IMMUNODEFICIENCY DISEASES AND TUMOR IMMUNOBIOLOGY

RENE J. DUQUESNOY
PETER ABRAMOFF

INTRODUCTION

Basic progress toward an improved understanding of the relation of structure to function of cells, tissues, and organs of the lymphoid system has taught us about the significance of the immune apparatus in the pathogenesis of many disease processes. The classic definition of immunity as being an exemption from disease has traditionally been related to resistance to infection. Until the turn of the century, the immune system was considered to have evolved as a homeostatic mechanism specifically directed against infectious agents. It is now recognized that the immune system participates in many processes of tissue injury elicited by hypersensitivity reactions against a great variety of innocuous substances. These immunologically mediated hypersensitivity reactions of tissue injury are divided into four major categories: (1) The immediate-type of hypersensitivity reactions mediated by the humoral immune system. (2) The delayed-type of hypersensitivity reactions which are manifestations of cellular immunity. (3) The immune complex diseases which result from the deposition of circulating soluble antigen-antibody complexes in the walls of blood vessels and the glomeruli. (4) Autoallergic disorders which may occur as a consequence of immunologic reactivity against the host's own tissue components. These hypersensitivity reactions will be discussed in greater length in Chapters 17 and 18.

This chapter deals with the immunopathologic mechanisms which underlie certain abnormalities of the lymphoid system. We will discuss those primary immunodeficiency disorders due to a developmental defect of the lymphoid system as well as the immunodeficiency states secondary to various diseases.

In the section on tumor immunology, malfunction of immunologic processes in patients with malignant disease will be analyzed in terms of the surveillance function of the lymphoid system of malignant growth.

IMMUNODEFICIENCY DISEASES

Development of the Lymphoid System

The hematopoietic system develops from hematopoietic stem cells residing at different locations during ontogenesis; these locations are in the primitive blood islets of the yolk sac, the fetal liver, and finally in the bone marrow. These stem cells can proliferate and differentiate along the hematopoietic pathways of the erythroid, monocytic, granulocytic, megakaryocytic, or lymphoid systems.

In the lymphoid system, the lymphoid stem cells may differentiate to form two lymphocyte populations: the T lymphocytes, which are dependent upon the thymus, and the B lymphocytes, which are dependent upon an undefined bursa equivalent (Fig. 5–1). Under the influence of the inductive microenvironments of the

THYMUS SYSTEM DEVELOPMENT

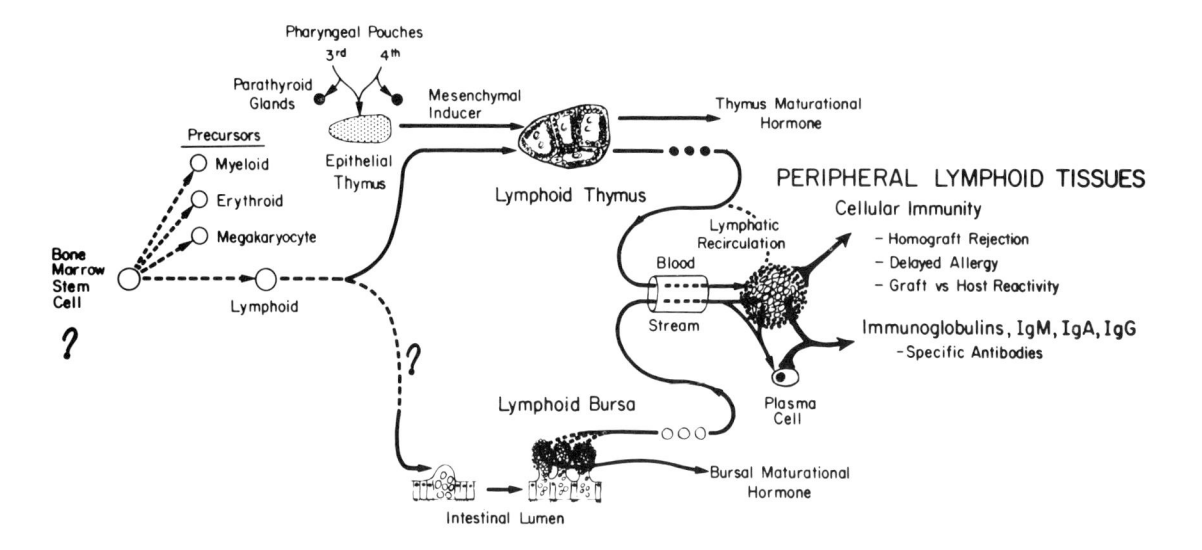

BURSAL SYSTEM DEVELOPMENT

Figure 5-1 Two-component concept of the lymphoid system. Lymphoid stem cells may proliferate and differentiate under influences of the thymus or a bursa equivalent to give rise to populations of T and B lymphocytes, respectively. (Courtesy of Dr. Robert A. Good, Director of Sloan-Kettering Institute, New York.)

thymus cortex and medulla, the prethymic lymphoid stem cells proliferate and differentiate into T lymphocytes (T cells). The lymphocytes which reside in the thymus and which have different stages of lymphoid development are called thymocytes. It is not certain whether differentiation of a thymocyte into a T cell takes place within the thymus before emigration or in the peripheral tissues. Recent experiments with mice indicate that certain medullary thymocytes have properties similar to peripheral T lymphocytes. Further, it appears that subpopulations of T lymphocytes exist, each with a different stage of immunologic development, life span, and immunologic function.

Upon immunogenic stimulation, certain T cells can proliferate and differentiate to become sensitized T cells. These sensitized T cells can be activated by antigen to become "killer" lymphocytes, which produce soluble factors called lymphokines and give rise to the so-called amplification system of cellular immunity. T cells have also been shown to interact synergistically with B cells in the immune response of mice and a limited number of other species, but not in man. These T lymphocytes may express immunologic memory.

T lymphocytes are found in the deep cortical regions of lymph nodes, the periarteriolar sheaths of splenic follicles, the diffused lymphoid tissue of the gastrointestinal tract, the thoracic duct lymph, and the circulating blood.

In the chicken, the organ responsible for the differentiation of lymphoid stem cells into B lymphocytes (B cells) is the bursa of Fabricius. It has yet to be identified in the mammalian species. The appendix, Peyer's patches, and gut-associated lymphoid tissue as well as tonsils, bone marrow, and even skin have been implicated as the mammalian bursa equivalent; however, these postulates lack sufficient experimental evidence.

There are two categories of B cells: the nonsecreting and the secreting B cells. B cells of the first group are capable of synthesizing antibody but are not specialized for antibody secretion in large amounts. These cells carry immunoglobulin receptors for both light and heavy chains and, in mice, also have receptors for C3. They can be found in the far cortical areas of lymph nodes, the perifollicular zones of the malpighian corpuscles of the spleen, and the circulating blood.

Upon interaction with antigen, nonsecreting B cells can transform into secreting B lymphocytes or plasma cells. These cells are specialized for production and secretion of antibody. They can be found in the medullary cords of lymph nodes, in the red pulp of the spleen, in the lamina propria of the gastrointestinal tract and secretory glands, in the interstitial tissue of the bone marrow, and, occasionally, in the peripheral blood and lymph.

The two-component concept of the lymphoid system implies that there are two basic syndromes of immunodeficiency: one, a deficiency of humoral immunity as a consequence of an abnormality of the B cell system, and the other, a defect of the T cell system of cellular immunity. Patients with immunodeficiency diseases manifest parts of each syndrome, depending upon the type and extent of their deficiency. Careful diagnostic evaluation of both B and T cell systems is mandatory in the proper management and treatment of the disease in these patients.

Evaluation of the T Cell System

Generally, a T cell deficiency is indicated with increased susceptibility to infection by fungi, viruses, atypical acid-fast organisms, and some of the so-called lower-grade pathogens. Causative organisms include *Candida albicans,* vaccinia and mumps viruses, Mycoplasma, Staphylococcus, and *Pneumocystis carinii.* On the other hand, fewer problems are encountered with high-grade encapsulated pathogens, such as Pneumococcus, Haemophilus, Streptococcus, and Meningococcus.

Pneumocystis carinii deserves special attention, since it frequently causes severe pulmonary disease in patients with immunodeficiency. In these patients, pneumocystis pneumonia shows characteristic accumulations of foamy, pink-staining exudates containing many pneumocystis organisms (Fig. 5-2A and B). This protozoan produces disease in patients with B and T cell deficiencies and has also caused plasma cell pneumonia epidemics in neonates and premature and debilitated infants in central Europe. The diagnosis of pneumocystis infections in patients with immunodeficiency disease is hampered by the absence of any demonstrable specific immune response. Demonstration of specific antibodies in close relatives of the patient may provide an indication of pneumocystis infection; otherwise, a lung biopsy is a better diagnostic measurement. Early pneumocystis infection can be effectively treated with pentamidine isethionate.

The laboratory evaluation of the T cell system in patients with suspected immunodeficiency is given in Table 5-1. An effective test for the analysis of the T cell population is a quantitation of the responsiveness of peripheral blood lymphocytes or lymph node cells to blastogenic stimulation with phytohemagglutinin (PHA). The capability to develop delayed allergic reactions may be analyzed by the ability to develop contact allergy after stimulation with dinitrochlorobenzene (DNCB). Skin tests for delayed hypersensitivity to ubiquitous antigens such as mumps, Candida, Trichophyton, tuberculin, histoplasmin, and streptokinase-streptodornase may be of little value in young children who have had little opportunity to develop cell-mediated immune responses to these antigens. However, negative skin tests to Candida antigens in children suffering from infection with this fungus may have diagnostic usefulness. Tests for the ability to reject allogeneic skin grafts are no longer commonly used.

Morphologic analysis of the number of small lymphocytes in peripheral blood and in the deep cortical areas of biopsied lymph nodes may provide some quantitation of the T cell system. Since T lymphocytes do not have immunoglobulin receptors on their cell surface, membrane immunofluorescence methods with fluorescent labeled antiglobulin antibodies should give a higher ratio of positively staining lymphocytes in T cell deficient patients than in normal persons. Although T cells in mice have specific membrane markers (e.g., theta and TL antigens), such markers have not been demonstrated on human T cells.

Several tests for lymphokine production have been developed which are of potential usefulness in the evaluation of the amplification system of cellular immunity. In particular, the capillary test for migration inhibitory factor has become a routine procedure in many laboratories.

Evaluation of the B Cell System

A deficiency of the B cell system is generally indicated with frequent occurrences of infection causing pneumonia, otitis media, conjunctivitis, meningitis, and sepsis. Causative microorganisms include Pneumococcus, Streptococcus, Haemophilus, Meningococcus, *Pseudomonas aeruginosa,* hepatitis virus, and *Pneumocystis carinii.* These patients experience fewer problems with handling of Staphylococcus, most enterobacteria, mycobacteria, fungi, and viruses.

Most laboratory tests for evaluation of the B cell system are carried out on the products of B lymphocytes, i.e., the antibodies and immunoglobulins (Table 5-2). Electrophoretic and immunoelectrophoretic analyses of serum and secretions provide qualitative information about the presence or absence of the various immunoglobulins, as well as the presence of homogeneous immunoglobulin populations seen in monoclonal gammopathies.

A variety of immunologic methods are currently available for determining immunoglobulin levels. Most commonly used is the radial immunodiffusion technique by which the test serum is allowed to diffuse in a layer of agar gel containing antiserum specific to one of the immunoglobulins. The concentration of each immunoglobulin is determined by comparing the diameter of the precipitin ring with that given by an immunoglobulin standard solution of defined concentration. When special precautions are

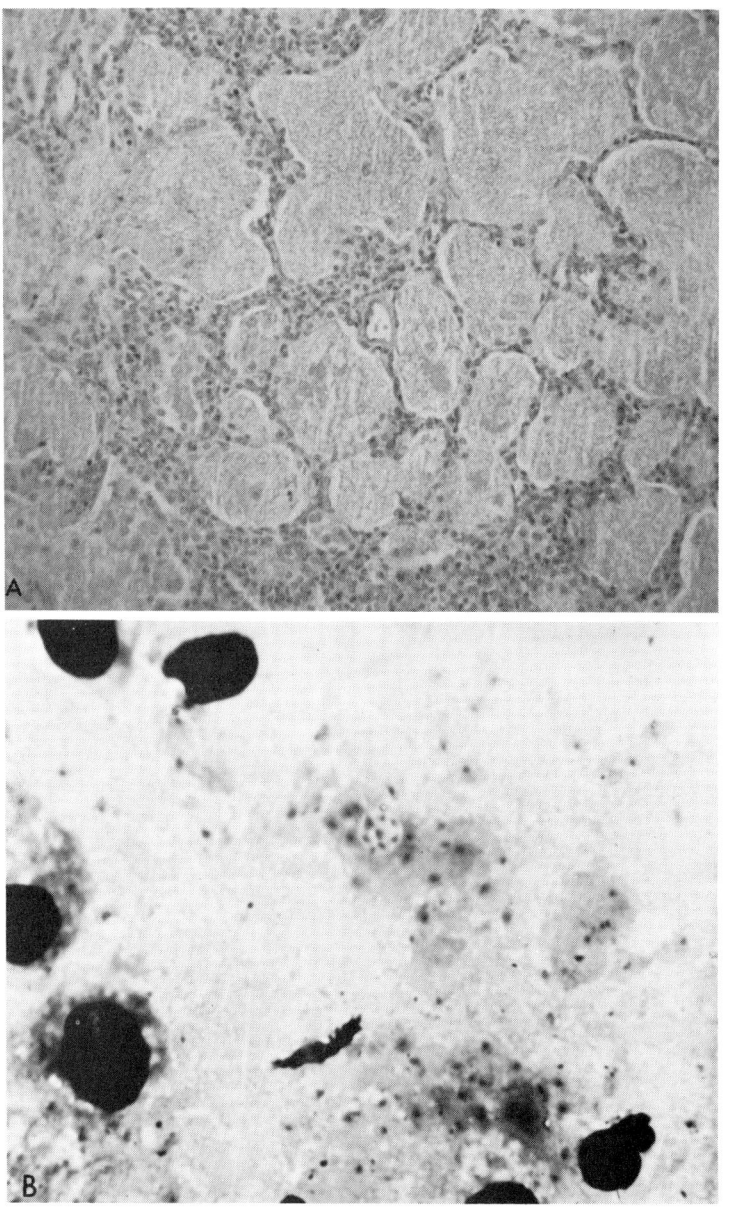

Figure 5–2 Pneumocystis pneumonia in an agammaglobulinemic patient. *A,* Eosinophilic accumulations in pulmonary lesion. *B, Pneumocystis carinii* organisms in pulmonary exudate. (Courtesy of Dr. Robert A. Good, Director of Sloan-Kettering Institute, New York.)

TABLE 5-1 LABORATORY EVALUATION OF T CELL FUNCTION

1. Microbiological studies, history of infections.
2. Quantitation of PHA-induced lymphocyte blastogenesis.
3. Skin tests for delayed hypersensitivity to ubiquitous antigens.
4. Development of contact allergy to DNCB.
5. Blood lymphocyte count.
6. Allogeneic skin graft rejection.
7. Histologic analysis of lymphocyte populations in thymus-dependent areas of lymph nodes.
8. Immunoglobulin receptors on lymphocytes.
9. Amplification of cellular immunity, MIF test.

taken to ensure that the immunoglobulins in the standards and the sera are not split or aggregated, the radial immunodiffusion method can be used to measure, with some accuracy, the levels of IgG, IgM, IgA, and IgD. Serum IgE levels are measured with the radioimmunoassay method. The normal values for each of these immunoglobulins are given on p. 101. Caution should be given in the evaluation of immunoglobulin levels in adult serum, since they may vary greatly from individual to individual and are related to age, sex, environment, and racial background. No threshold for values can be set for the diagnosis of immunoglobulin deficiencies unless associated with clinical symptoms. Reliable measurements cannot be made with such proteins as low molecular weight IgM and secretory IgA unless a standard immunoglobulin is available in the same form.

Special attention should be given to analysis of the subclasses of immunoglobulins. Using appropriate antisera, the levels of immunoglobulin subclasses are measured by radial immunodiffusion or direct hemagglutination-inhibition tests. The approximate percentages in American Caucasians of normal serum IgG are IgG_1, 66 per cent; IgG_2, 23 per cent; IgG_3, 7 per cent; and IgG_4, 4 per cent. The importance of determining immunoglobulin subclasses has been demonstrated in certain patients with normal total IgG serum levels, but lacking one of the IgG subclasses, and showing great susceptibility to pneumococcal and other high-grade, extracellular, pyogenic pathogens, similar to patients with generalized B cell immunodeficiency diseases.

Humoral immune function of the B cell system can be evaluated by tests for existing antibody to antigen to which man is commonly exposed or by humoral antibody assays following active immunization. Antibodies to ubiquitous antigens include type A and B isohemagglutinins and antibodies to infectious agents, e.g., antistreptolysin O, antiviral antibodies and agglutinins of typhoid, paratyphoid, brucella, diphtheria, tetanus, Candida, and Staphylococcus. The antigens used for active immunization should be proteins as well as polysaccharides. Quantitation of antibody responses may be carried out following injection of poliovirus vaccines, diphtheria, tetanus, and pertussis toxoid, and pneumococcal or meningococcal polysaccharide antigens. The use of live vaccines (e.g., Bacillus of Calmette-Guerin (BCG) or attenuated viruses) should always be avoided. However, more than just the total amount of antibody produced should be considered. The induction, logarithmic, plateau, and decline phases of antibody production should be measured whenever possible. The normal maturation of the immune response (from predominantly IgM to predominantly IgG) ought to be followed.

Absence of low serum levels of one or more immunoglobulins may have three possible causes: (1) absence or decreased numbers of B cells in the circulation and lymphoid tissue, (2) a defect in immunoglobulin secretion by B cells, and (3) an increased rate of immunoglobulin catabolism. The following tests need to be carried out to distinguish between these possibilities. Determination of lymphocyte membrane immunofluorescence with fluorescent antibodies against the various immunoglobulins can be used to analyze the B cell population in the circulation as well as in the lymph nodes. In addition, one can look for the presence of germinal centers and plasma cells in lymph nodes. The evaluation of immunoglobulin catabolism can be determined by measurement of the rate of disappearance of radioactivity from the circulation following injection of radio-labeled immunoglobulins.

A complete evaluation of the B cell system should include analysis of the amplification systems belonging to the various types of antibodies. For instance, analysis of complement-fixing antibodies can be carried out to detect those types of

TABLE 5-2 LABORATORY EVALUATION OF B CELL FUNCTION

1. Microbiological studies, history of infections.
2. Electrophoresis and immunoelectrophoresis of serum.
3. Concentration of immunoglobulin classes and subclasses in serum and secretions by radial immunodiffusion.
4. Tests for antibodies to ubiquitous antigens.
5. Quantitation of humoral immune response.
6. Immunoglobulin receptors on lymphocytes by membrane immunofluorescence.
7. Histology of lymph node biopsies, germinal center formation.
8. Analysis of immunoglobulin catabolism.
9. Amplification of humoral immunity. Complement system.

IgG antibody which are unable to activate the complement system. Evaluation of the complement system may also be necessary to determine the levels of complement components and some of the homeostatic control mechanisms of the complement system, such as C1 esterase inhibitor.

Primary Immunodeficiencies

Primary immunodeficiency results from a failure to produce the effectors of the immune response, i.e., antibodies and sensitized lymphocytes. Excluded from this definition are the hypercatabolic states and disorders in the amplification systems, such as the complement deficiencies. Secondary immunodeficiencies may occur in patients with a variety of diseases.

The variability of immunologic findings presents a major difficulty in classification of the primary immunodeficiencies. Often neither etiologic nor functional or structural considerations, taken alone or together are satisfactory for adequate classification of immunodeficiency diseases in man. Well-characterized diseases associated with primary immunodeficiency are listed in Table 5–3. However, the majority of patients with immunodeficiency cannot be unequivocally classified and are therefore grouped under the heading of variable immunodeficiency. The probable levels at which various primary immunodeficiency diseases interfere with normal lymphoid development are shown in Figure 5–3. Only a few will be selected for discussion.

Patients with infantile, sex-linked agammaglobulinemia (Bruton's agammaglobulinemia) have an immunodeficiency exclusively involving the B cell system while the functions attributable to the T cell system appear to be intact. Concentration of each of the immunoglobulins in serum or secretions is very low or absent, and humoral antibody responses are absent even to repeated injections of potent antigens. Histologic studies show that lymph nodes and spleen of these patients lack germinal centers, and that plasma cells are absent from lymph nodes, spleen, bone marrow, and connective tissue including the lamina propria (Figs. 5–4A and B, 5–5A and B). The tonsils have poorly developed lymphoid elements which lack follicular components (Fig. 5–6A and B). By contrast, these patients have normal or nearly normal levels of circulating lymphocytes, normal numbers of lymphocytes in the thymus-dependent regions of lymph nodes and spleen, and a normal thymus. Membrane immunofluorescence methods show absence of immunoglobulin receptors on these lymphocytes.

These patients usually have recurrent bacterial infections which begin during the second six months of life. They show extraordinary susceptibility to infection with certain extracellular pyogenic pathogens like Pneumococcus, Streptococcus, and Haemophilus, but infections with other organisms like Staphylococcus and Pseudomonas occur only occasionally. Many patients develop pneumocystis infections. They suffer repeatedly from acute episodes of otitis, sinusitis, skin infection, conjunctivitis, and pulmonary disease. Such patients are also prone to septicemia and meningitis. In striking contrast, these patients can resist infections by many other microorganisms including viruses, fungi, and most enterobacteria, even when they appear to produce little or no antibody to these microorganisms. They seem unable to resist infection with hepatitis virus, and such infections usually cause either massive liver destruction or chronic active hepatitis with steady progression to complete destruction of the liver. Patients with sex-linked agammaglobulinemia are prone to develop connective tissue diseases such as arthritis, dermatomyositis, and diffuse vasculitis. Furthermore, they often develop malignant conditions, especially in the lymphoreticular and gastrointestinal tissues.

Certain selective immunoglobulin deficiencies have been described which seem to be associated with defective development of a single immunoglobulin class. One of the most common primary immunodeficiency diseases is the isolated (or selective) deficiency of IgA which affects 1 out of 700 persons. Most patients are clinically asymptomatic but some may have recurrent gastrointestinal infections and a spruelike syndrome. The incidence of rheumatoid arthritis, lupus erythematosus, tenosynovitis, and other

TABLE 5–3 SELECTED PRIMARY IMMUNODEFICIENCY DISEASES*

Disorder	B Cells	T Cells	Stem Cells
Infantile sex-linked agammaglobulinemia (Bruton's)	+		
Selective immunoglobulin deficiency (IgA)	+		
Thymic hypoplasia (DiGeorge syndrome)		+	
Combined immunodeficiency	+	+	+
Ataxia-telangiectasia	+	+	
Wiskott-Aldrich syndrome	+	+	
Immunodeficiency with thymoma	+	+	
Variable immunodeficiency (unclassified)	+	(+)	

*A complete classification is given in Fudenberg, H., et al.: Pediatrics, 47:927, 1971.

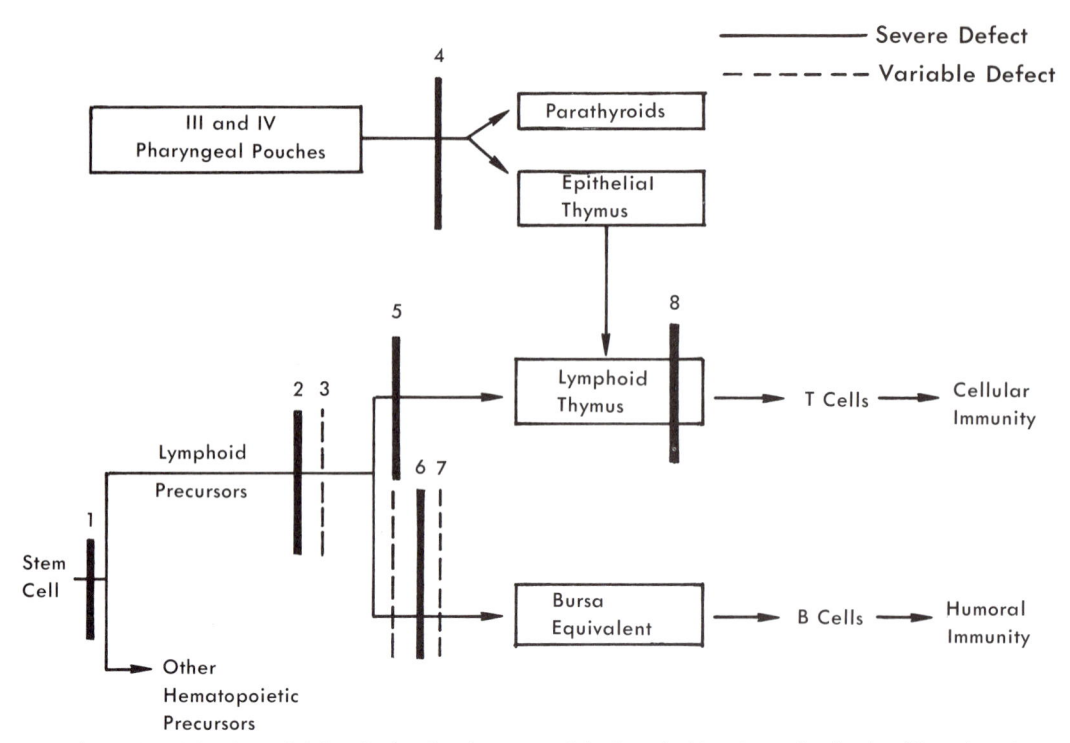

Figure 5–3 Possible sites of defect in the development of the lymphoid system of patients with various types of primary immunodeficiency. (1) Immunodeficiency with generalized hematopoietic hypoplasia, reticular dysgenesis. (2) Autosomal recessive combined immunodeficiency. (3) Sex-linked and sporadic types of immunodeficiency. (4) Thymic hypoplasia (DiGeorge). (5) Ataxia-telangiectasia. (6) Infantile sex-linked agammaglobulinemia. (7) Selective immunoglobulin deficiency (IgA), transient hypogammaglobulinemia of infancy. (8) Thymus dysplasia with normal immunoglobulins (Nezelof).

mesenchymal diseases is higher in patients with selective IgA deficiency. A number of patients with low levels of IgA produce anti-IgA antibodies which lead to decreased survival rate of serum IgA. Blood products containing IgA given to these individuals may result in anaphylactic reactions. Selective IgA deficiency causes low levels of IgA in serum as well as in secretions. The two subclasses, A_1 and A_2, are usually reduced in equal proportions. However, in certain patients, low serum IgA levels are accompanied by normal concentrations of secretory IgA. The reverse situation may be present in other patients with IgA deficiency.

Selective IgE immunoglobulin deficiencies have been described in children and are associated with frequent episodes of respiratory infections developing into a progressive sinopulmonary disease.

Severe immunodeficiency disease of the thymus-dependent system is present in patients with thymic hypoplasia (DiGeorge syndrome). In these patients there is a congenital arrest in the development of the thymus and parathyroids from the epithelial anlage derived from the III and IV pharyngeal pouches. Such infants with hypocalcemic tetany at birth are unable to survive because they lack the capacity to develop the T cell system and to express cell-mediated immunity. Circulating lymphocyte counts are usually near normal at birth but soon decline to a significantly low level. These patients fail to express any of the functions of cellular immunity and have a high susceptibility to fungal and viral infections. By contrast, their levels of immunoglobulin are normal, plasma cells are present in normal numbers in the lymphoid tissues in bone marrow, and the thymus-independent regions of lymph nodes and spleen are well preserved. The thymus-dependent, deep cortical areas of lymph nodes and periarteriolar sheaths of splenic follicles are depleted of lymphocytes (Fig. 5–4C). Infections usually begin early in life and may be caused by fungi, viruses, atypical acid-fast organisms, low-grade and high-grade encapsulated bacteria, and *Pneumocystis carinii.*

Severe combined immunodeficiency disease affects both B and T cell systems. The autosomal recessive variant of this alymphocytic agammaglobulinemia has been called Swiss type agammaglobulinemia. These patients have severe cellular defects in the development of hu-

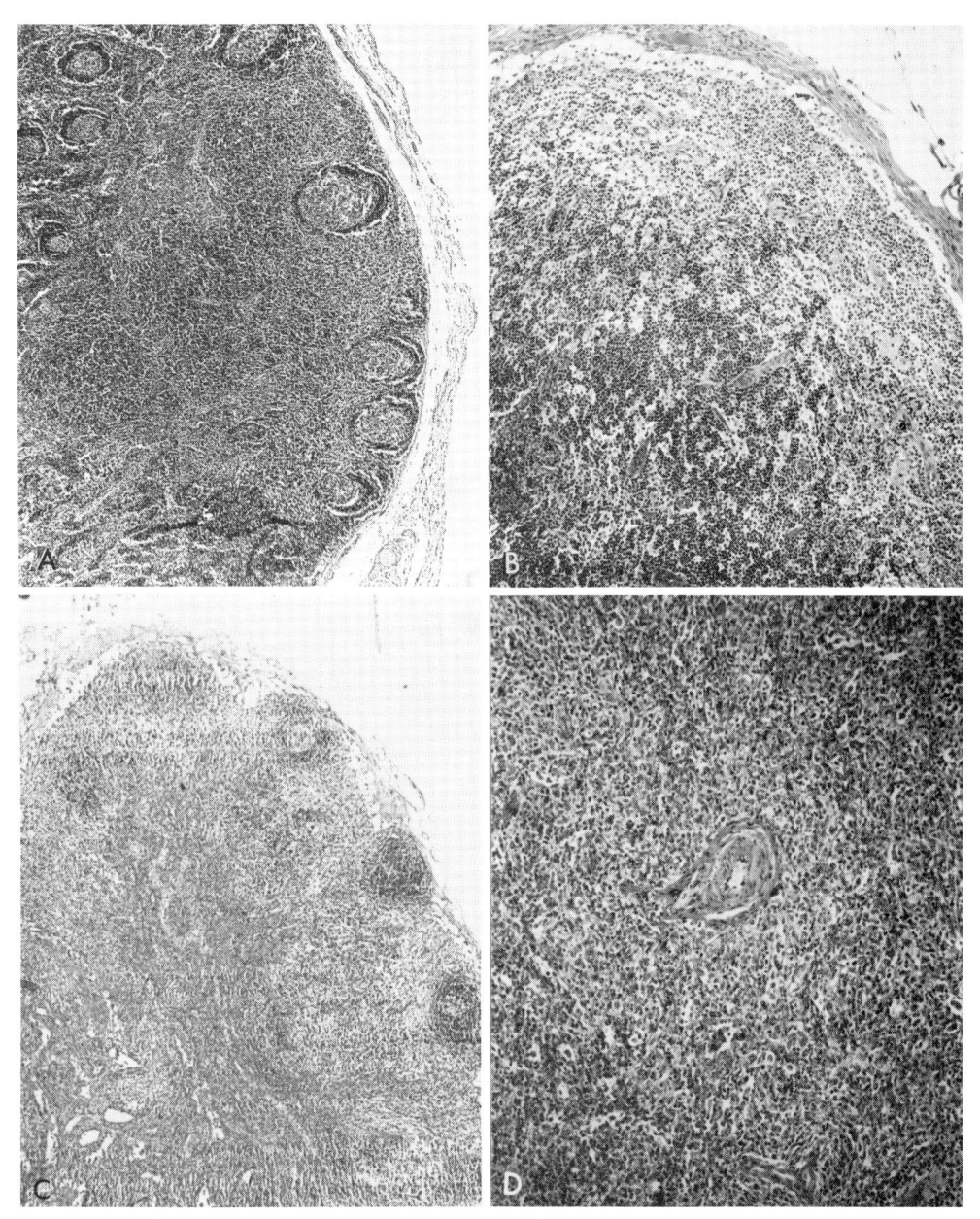

Figure 5–4 Lymph node histology in primary immunodeficiency. A, Stimulated lymph node of a normal 11-month-old child. Well-developed germinal centers and abundance of plasma cells. The cortical and deep cortical regions are densely populated by lymphocytes. B, Lymph node from a boy with infantile sex-linked recessive agammaglobulinemia 5 days after secondary antigenic stimulation. Absence of cortical germinal centers and plasma cells, dense populations of small lymphocytes in the deep cortical regions, and lymphocyte depletion in cortex. C, Lymph node from a patient with thymic hypoplasia. The thymus-dependent deep cortical regions are depleted of small lymphocytes. Lymphoid follicles, germinal centers, and plasma cells are present. D, Lymph node from a child with autosomal recessive combined immunodeficiency disease. Severe depletion of lymphocytes and plasma cells accompanied by histiocytosis and stromal hyperplasia. (Courtesy of Dr. Robert A. Good, Director of Sloan-Kettering Institute, New York.)

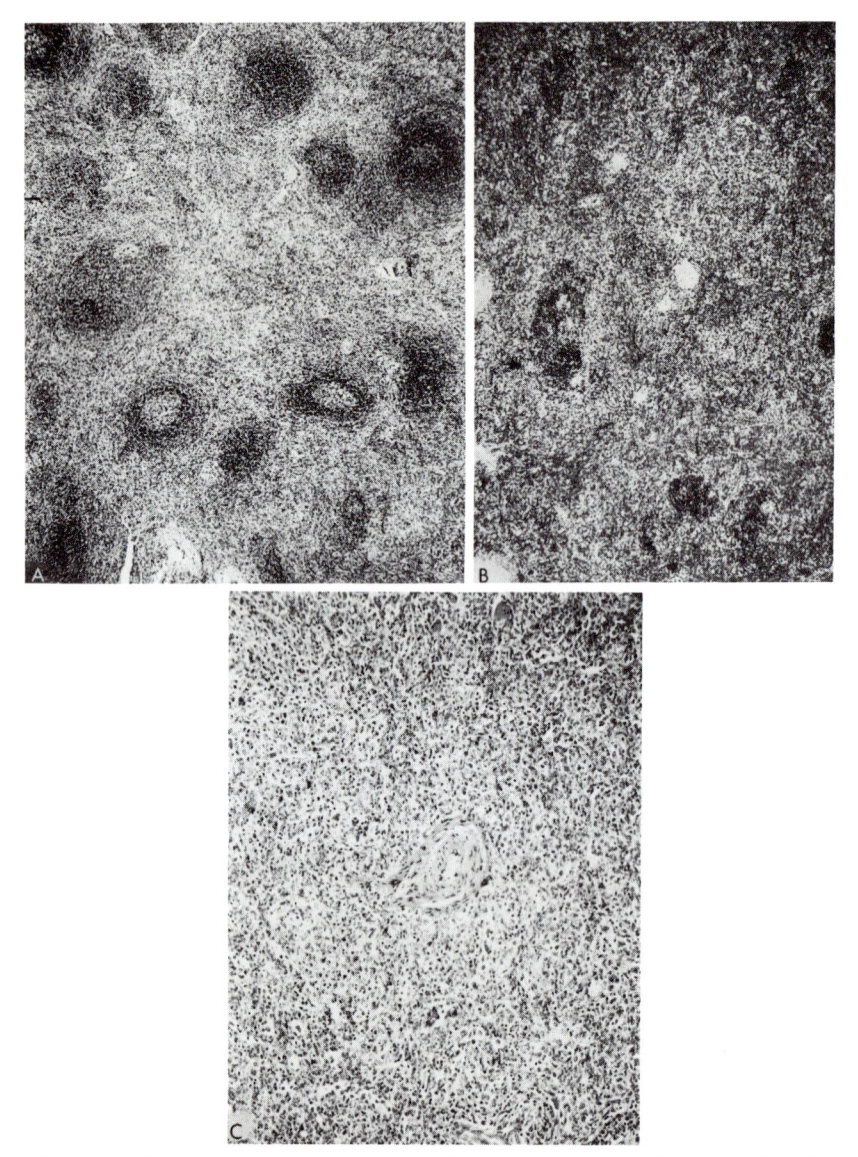

Figure 5-5 Histology of spleen in primary immunodeficiency. *A,* Spleen of a child who died of congenital heart disease at 3 months of age. Note the normal dense lymphoid cellularity of the malpighian follicles and several germinal centers. *B,* Spleen from child with sex-linked agammaglobulinemia. Note the primitive development of lymphoid follicles and absence of germinal centers and plasma cells. *C,* Severe depletion of lymphocytes and plasma cells in spleen from patient with autosomal recessive combined immunodeficiency disease. (Courtesy of Dr. Robert A. Good, Director of Sloan-Kettering Institute, New York.)

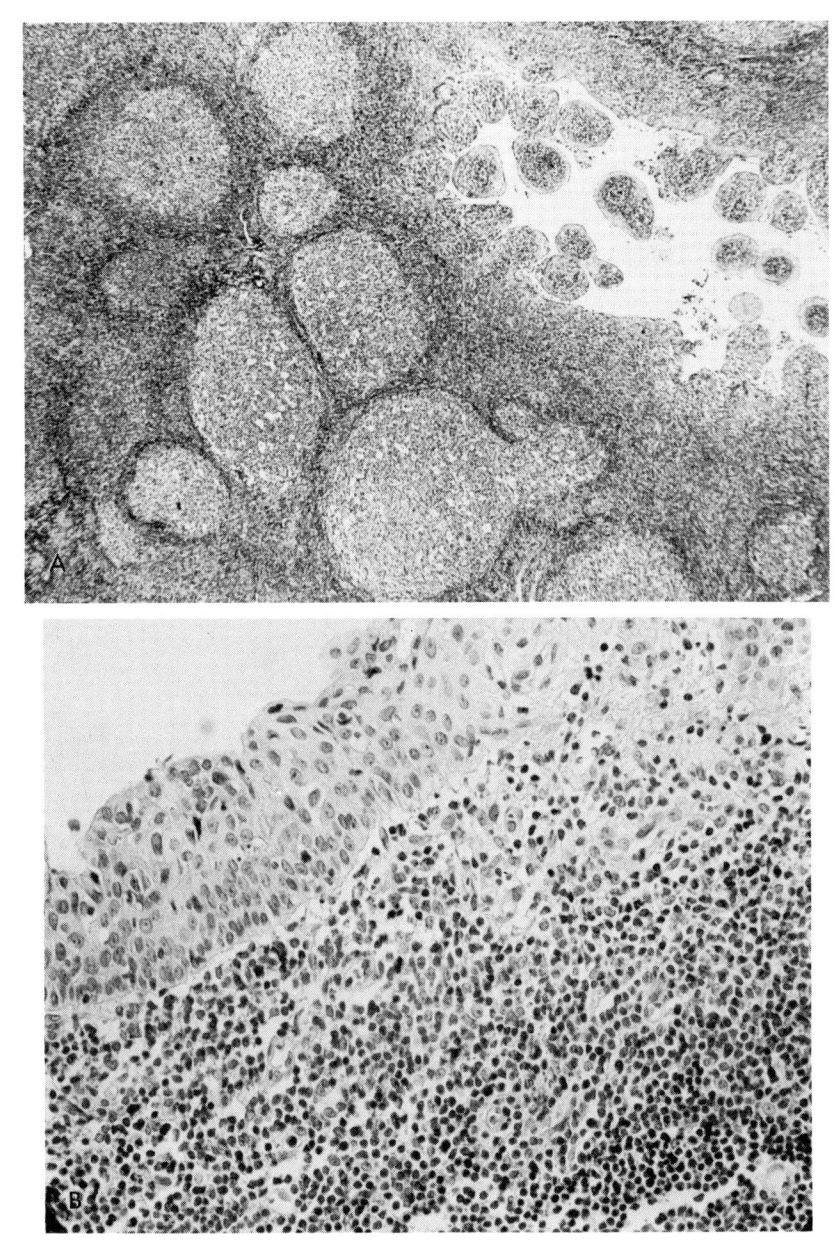

Figure 5-6 *A,* Normal tonsillar tissue with abundance of lymphoid elements. *B,* Tonsil from a patient with infantile sex-linked agammaglobulinemia. (Courtesy of Dr. Robert A. Good, Director of Sloan-Kettering Institute, New York.)

moral as well as cell-mediated immunity as a consequence of a lymphoid stem cell defect. Very young infants are affected by this disease and suffer recurrent infections with a great variety of microorganisms. They generally succumb during the first year of life to low-grade, opportunistic pathogens such as Pseudomonas, Staphylococcus, the common enterobacteria, *Pneumocystis carinii,* and *Candida albicans.* If exposed to measles virus, they may die of a characteristic giant cell pneumonia (Hecht's pneumonia); they do not show the characteristic measles rash. Also, progressive, generalized vaccinia will occur after dermal smallpox vaccination.

Serum levels of all immunoglobulin classes are either absent or extremely low. The thymus is hypoplastic and lacks lymphoid cells and Hassall's corpuscles (Fig. 5–7). These patients have severe lymphopenia and an absence or marked deficiency of lymphocytes in the thymus-dependent as well as the thymus-independent regions of peripheral lymphoid tissues (Fig. 5–4C and D).

In addition to the Swiss type of agammaglobulinemia, a large number of patients have lymphopenic immunodeficiency syndrome which varies greatly in the clinical and laboratory manifestations. Some of these patients are clearly of sex-linked recessive inheritance, others seem to be inherited as autosomal recessive traits, and still others have thus far not revealed any hereditary patterns. Laboratory evaluation of both T and B cell systems show variability of immunodeficiency. Some patients with these forms of combined immunodeficiency possess nearly normal amounts of IgM, little IgG, and no IgA. Different degrees of defective development of peripheral lymphoid organs and thymus have also been observed.

Immunodeficiency of the B cell system, and especially of the T cell system, is encountered in ataxia-telangiectasia (Louis-Bar syndrome). These patients develop a progressive cerebellar ataxia which usually begins during the first few years of life. They often have recurrent pulmonary infections and develop prominent telangiectases in the sclerae, the skin of the eyelids, the ear lobes, the neck, and the popliteal and antecubital spaces. These patients have variable degrees of deficiency of the cell-mediated immune responses. In some instances they show deficient antibody production to certain relatively weak immunogens. A large percentage have low levels of IgA and IgE as a consequence of decreased rate of synthesis of the immunoglobulins. Several patients have an increased rate of IgA catabolism because of the presence of anti-IgA antibodies. Histologically, the thymus-dependent regions of the peripheral lymphoid tissue show a depletion of small lymphocytes. The thymus is small, lacks Hassall's corpuscles and is poorly organized into a cortex and medulla (Fig. 5–8). Female children with ataxia-telangiectasia frequently show ovarian dysgenesis. The etiology of this autosomal recessive disease is not well understood, but may be due to a neuroendocrine abnormality. These patients have a relatively high susceptibility to malignant disease, in particular, lymphosarcoma, reticulum cell sarcoma, or reticuloendotheliosis.

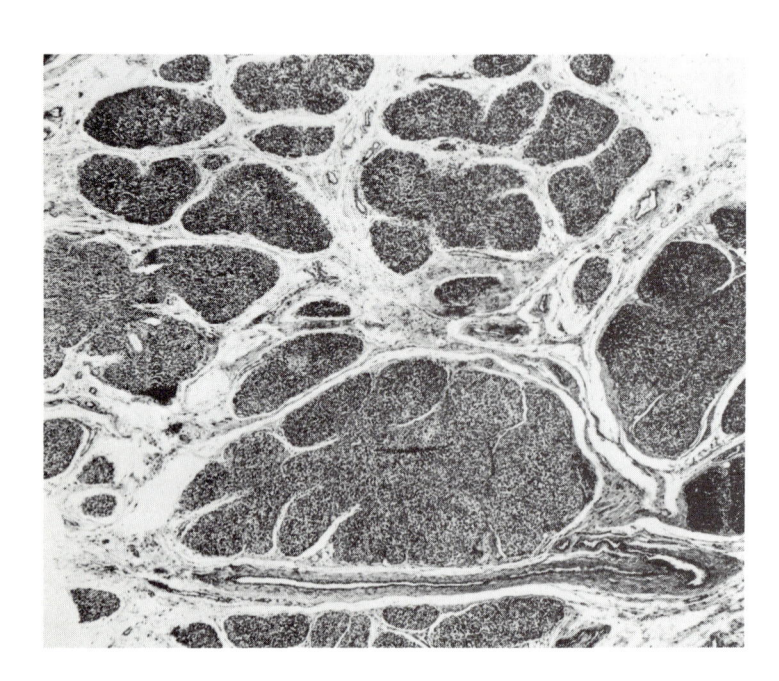

Figure 5–7 The hypoplastic thymus lacking lymphoid elements and Hassall's corpuscle is a salient feature of autosomal recessive combined immunodeficiency disease. (Courtesy of Dr. Robert A. Good, Director of Sloan-Kettering Institute, New York.)

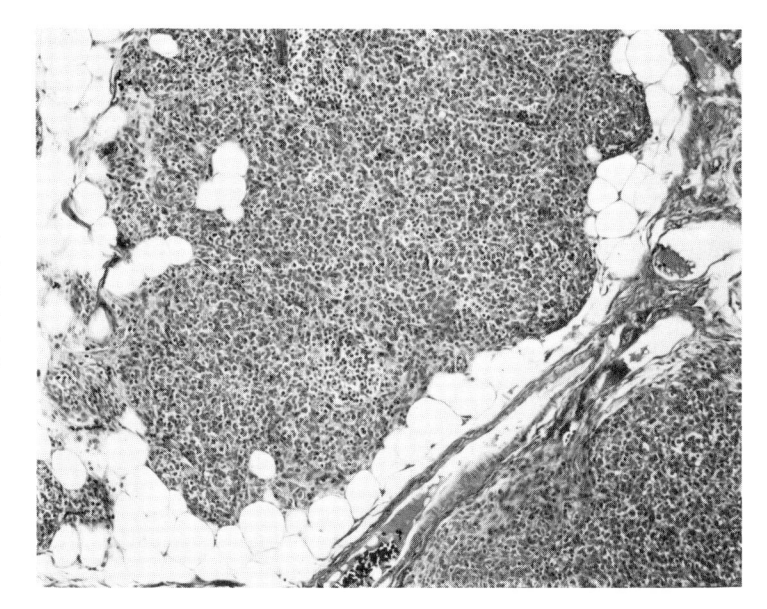

Figure 5-8 Thymus in ataxia-telangiectasia. Severe lymphoid depletion in both cortex and medulla. Hassall's corpuscles are absent. (Courtesy of Dr. Robert A. Good, Director of Sloan-Kettering Institute, New York.)

The Wiskott-Aldrich syndrome is a sex-linked disease characterized by a central thrombopenia, eczema, and marked susceptibility to many infections. Patients with this syndrome lack the normal isohemagglutinins and hemolysins and fail to produce antibodies to polysaccharide antigens. By contrast, the humoral antibody response to antigens such as tetanus toxoid is normal. In these patients a progressive deficiency of cell-mediated immunity develops. Like the patients with ataxia-telangiectasia, a high incidence of lymphoreticular malignant conditions is found. These malignant conditions may rapidly become widespread and seem to have great propensity to invade the central nervous system. It appears that the basic immunologic defect in these patients involves the afferent limb of the immune response and perhaps resides primarily in the macrophage processing of antigen.

Patients with a benign spindle cell tumor of the thymus have been described as having hypogammaglobulinemia, antibody deficiency syndrome, defects of cellular immunity, and often an absence of eosinophils. As with other hypogammaglobulinemic patients, they are prone to develop arthritis and other autoallergic and mesenchymal diseases.

The group of variable immunodeficiency disorders includes many syndromes which are not well understood. Included in this group are cases previously classified as "congenital" nonsex-linked or sporadic hypogammaglobulinemia, primary "dysgammaglobulinemia" of both childhood and adult life, and "acquired" primary hypogammaglobulinemia.

Treatment of Immunodeficiency

Considerable improvement is achieved in patients with B cell deficiency by replacement therapy with gamma globulins. Special precautions should be taken to avoid infection by hepatitis virus which frequently causes lethal liver disease in these patients. Some patients with thymic hypoplasia have been successfully treated with fetal thymus transplants. Although these transplants came from histoincompatible donors, they were able to reconstitute T cell function for a considerable time. Combined immunodeficiency disease can be corrected by transplanting a source of lymphoid stem cells, usually the bone marrow. The development of graft-versus-host disease is a serious complication, because the bone marrow gives rise to a population of immunocompetent lymphoid cells which make an immune response against the histoincompatible and immunologically incompetent host. Identity across the HL-A histocompatibility locus is generally required for the successful acceptance of these bone marrow transplants.

Disorders of Immunoglobulin Metabolism

These may occur secondarily to a variety of pathophysiologic mechanisms. As has been discussed above, hypogammaglobulinemia may be due to a primary immunodeficiency of the B lymphocyte system affecting one or more classes of immunoglobulins. Alternatively, hypogammaglobulinemia may be secondary to excessive loss of immunoglobulins into the urinary or gastrointestinal tracts. Finally, abnormal immunoglobulin levels may be secondary to disorders of endogenous immunoglobulin catabolic pathways. Accelerated catabolism may affect one or more immunoglobulin classes.

Accelerated catabolism of IgG has been observed in patients with myotonic dystrophy. This autosomal dominant disorder is characterized by myotonia, muscle wasting, premature baldness and testicular atrophy, cataracts, and electrocardiographic abnormalities. The serum levels and metabolism of albumin, IgM, IgA, IgD, and IgE are normal. In contrast, serum levels of IgG are markedly reduced as the result of an accelerated catabolism.

An increased rate of catabolism of IgA has been observed in patients with isolated IgA deficiency or ataxia-telangiectasia, when they produce anti-IgA antibodies.

Alternatively, generalized hypercatabolism of many serum proteins, including immunoglobulins, is often present in patients with Wiskott-Aldrich syndrome or with familial hypercatabolic hypoproteinemia. Elevated urinary or serum levels of immunoglobulin light chains are observed in patients with tubular proteinuria or uremia when the normal site of catabolism of these molecules, the proximal convoluted tubules, is damaged.

Disorders of the Complement System

A variety of genetically determined abnormalities of the complement system have been described. These can be classified as (1) defects in inhibitors which result in the spontaneous consumption of complement components, (2) synthesis of defective complement molecules, and (3) absence of a complement component.

Hereditary angioedema is caused by a defective synthesis of C1 esterase inhibitor. In normal persons, C1 esterase inhibitor blocks the activity of C1s and is therefore capable of suppressing the progression of the complement sequence beyond C1. This enzyme also inhibits the activity of certain enzymes active in the clotting system, including the Hageman factor, plasmin, and prekallikrein. Patients with hereditary angioedema suffer from episodic triggerings of the complement system and develop severe angioedematous reactions in various tissues, particularly those of the upper respiratory tract. It is unclear why these patients have episodic disease, but trauma, menstruation, and infections may precipitate clinical crises. This disease may be observed at any age but usually first manifests itself during late adolescence or early adult life. The recurrent attacks of edema are mostly confined to skin, gastrointestinal tract, and respiratory mucosa. The edema is nonpitting and nonpruritic. The episodes last for about 48 to 72 hours. The involvement of the larynx is most serious and many patients may die from suffocation. Hereditary angioedema exists in two genetic variants. In one type no C1 esterase is produced and in the other the protein is made but is not functional.

Patients with a defect in C3 catabolism as the result of an abnormal activity of C3-proactivator suffer from frequent recurrent pyogenic infections. Familial C5 dysfunction has been described in patients with Leiner's syndrome who suffer from generalized seborrheic dermatitis, intractable severe diarrhea, recurrent local and systemic bacterial infections usually of gram-negative etiology, and a marked wasting and dystrophy. Deficient opsonic activity of the patient's serum with yeast cells is the diagnostic laboratory finding in this disease.

Autosomal recessive C2 deficiency is usually not associated with any clinical disease. Although the sera of these patients are extremely defective in hemolytic activity, many biological functions of the complement system, like immunoadherence and facilitation of phagocytosis, seem unimpaired. It appears that C2 deficient individuals have an unusually high incidence of hypersensitivity disease.

Patients with the autosomal recessive form of combined immunodeficiency disease have extremely low serum levels of C1q. Since C1q has an electrophoretic mobility of a gamma globulin, it is particularly interesting that this protein should be defective in patients lacking both B and T lymphoid cells. In contrast, patients with sex-linked, recessive combined immunodeficiency as well as the various forms of hypogammaglobulinemia show only slight to moderate reduction of C1q levels.

Experimental strains of mice and rabbits have been described which lack C5 and C6, respectively. Low serum levels of complement can also be observed secondary to a variety of diseases, particularly in immune complex diseases such as acute glomerulonephritis, systemic lupus erythematosus, and poststreptococcal glomerulonephritis.

Secondary Immunodeficiency Diseases

Although primary immunodeficiencies have received considerable attention, these diseases are rather uncommon. In contrast, depressed immune function occurs quite frequently as a consequence of various disease states, especially those that cause disturbances in general metabolism and which induce stress. These secondary immunodeficiencies are frequently observed in certain infections, malignant conditions (especially of the lymphoid system), excessive loss of proteins or cells from the body, drug therapy, debilitating diseases, and aging. Clinically, immunodeficiency is first indicated by more frequent and persisting infections with one specific microorganism or a variety of microorganisms. Secondary immunodeficiencies may affect both humoral and cellular immune systems, and may operate at the induction (afferent limb) or expression (efferent limb) of immunity. The methods of evaluation of humoral and cellular immune function in patients with suspected secondary immunodeficiency are listed in Tables 5-1 and 5-2.

Certain infections may lead to decreased immune function. For example, secondary immunodeficiency is usually present in infants with congenital rubella syndrome. Infection with rubella virus is contracted during the second and third month of gestation. These patients have a continuing active viral infection from birth up to 18 months of age and produce antiviral antibodies, primarily of the IgM type. Increased serum IgM levels are frequently accompanied by markedly reduced IgG concentrations; occasionally there is a generalized hypogammaglobulinemia. During active rubella infection, peripheral blood lymphocytes may fail to undergo phytohemagglutinin-induced blastogenesis. Infections with measles (rubeola) virus frequently induce a temporary loss of delayed hypersensitivity. Tuberculin-positive patients may temporarily lose their ability to express a delayed allergic reaction to tuberculin protein during a measles infection. Lymphocytes from these patients are unable to respond with blastogenesis to antigen, although their responsiveness to phytohemagglutinin or other mitogens is unaltered. Lymphocytes infected by Mycoplasma also have diminished ability to respond to antigenic and mitogenic stimulation.

Most immunoproliferative diseases are accompanied by a secondary immunodeficiency state. Abnormal proliferation may affect the B and T cell immune systems. Best known are the secreting B cell tumors, which include multiple myeloma, Waldenström's macroglobulinemia, and heavy chain disease. These disorders have often been called the monoclonal gammopathies because these plasma cell tumors produce excessive amounts of an immunoglobulin of sharply restricted molecular heterogeneity. These paraproteins may be of any one of the immunoglobulin classes and may have the same basic molecular structure as their normal counterparts. An exception is a paraprotein of heavy chain disease which lacks a portion of the Fd fragment of the heavy chain (see p. 100). Since numerous myeloma proteins have been found to have antibody specificity for certain antigens, it is currently believed that all myeloma proteins are antibodies of restricted molecular specificity. Light chains of either kappa or lambda types may be produced in excess of heavy chains and may circulate as free dimers of homogeneous light chains. Because of their small size they are rapidly excreted in the urine (Bence Jones proteins).

Patients with multiple myeloma often suffer from recurrent infections with Pneumococcus and other highly pathogenic bacteria. They have no unusual susceptibility to infections with staphylococci, enterobacteria, or fungi. Severe deficiency of the B cell immune system can be demonstrated by the low levels of serum immunoglobulin and seems to be a result of decreased synthesis of normal immunoglobulin molecules. Antibody synthesis against exogenously administered antigen is markedly deficient. In contrast, cellular immune function is grossly normal.

Patients with Waldenström's macroglobulinemia have excessively high serum levels of a high molecular weight protein which has the chemical and immunochemical characteristics of IgM. Because of the high intrinsic viscosity of IgM protein, these patients have increased viscosity of the serum, which leads to sluggish blood flow, thrombosis, central nervous system disturbances, and bleeding. Most commonly affected are the skin, nasal mucosa, and gastrointestinal tract. Sluggish blood flow of the retinal vessels may eventually cause thrombosis of retinal veins and blindness. Frequently, the patient's red cells, granulocytes, and particularly platelets may be coated with macroglobulins, which results in impaired survival and function of these elements. Lymphadenopathy and hepatosplenomegaly are salient features. Hyperproduction of IgM macroglobulin is often accompanied by decreased synthesis of other immunoglobulins. Many patients produce detectable amounts of monomeric, low molecular weight macroglobulins (7S IgM). Approximately 10 per cent have demonstrable Bence Jones proteinurea.

The recent elucidation of the structure of the immunoglobulins (see p. 101) and the detailed characterization of the proteins in serum and urine of patients with proliferative disorders of plasma cells and lymphocytes have led to a better understanding of the biosynthetic alterations accompanying these disorders. These diseases are now frequently classified on the basis of the products of the neoplastic cells. Multiple myeloma is defined by the type of immunoglobulins produced (G, A, D, and E myeloma), and the biosynthetic processes in myeloma and macroglobulinemia can be either the balanced synthesis of heavy and light chains, resulting in homogeneous serum immunoglobulin, or the unbalanced synthesis manifested by the presence of light and occasionally heavy chains as an additional, or at times, the sole detectable product. In addition, the recognition of several new disorders of immunoglobulin synthesis has resulted in the identification of a number of new syndromes. Best described among these are the group of heavy chain diseases which represent examples of abnormal immunoglobulin synthesis and assembly. Three types of heavy chain diseases corresponding to the heavy chains of IgG (gamma), IgA (alpha), and IgM (mu) are now recognized. Gamma chain disease is most frequently seen in the middle aged and elderly. A rather characteristic clinical picture which resembles a malignant lymphoma rather than multiple myeloma includes lymphadenopathy and hepatosplenomegaly. Involvement of the nodes of Waldeyer's ring resulting in palatal edema is particularly striking. Almost all patients suffer from frequent episodes of infection. Anemia, leukopenia, eosinophilia, and hyperuricemia are common but are relatively nonspecific laboratory findings. Definitive diagnosis of gamma chain disease can only be made by immunochemical analysis of serum and urine proteins. Characteristically, there is a broad peak with a mobility of a beta globulin present in both serum and urine. Amino acid sequence analysis of gamma chain disease proteins has demonstrated deletion of most of the Fd fragment as a consequence of loss of interchain disulfide bridges. Alpha chain disease has been found in patients with malignant lymphoma involving the small intestine and is usually associated with severe malabsorption. A few cases of mu chain disease have been described in patients with chronic lymphocytic leukemia.

Patients with Hodgkin's disease develop a progressive immunodeficiency of the cellular immune system while humoral immune function appears essentially normal. Both the afferent and efferent limbs of T cell-mediated cellular immunity are deficient. Although patients with Hodgkin's disease have a normal resistance to infections with Pneumococcus, Haemophilus, and Streptococcus, they are susceptible to tuberculosis and fungal infections.

Patients with chronic lymphocytic leukemia develop deficiencies of both the T and B cell immune systems. Both immune systems are essentially normal in acute lymphocytic leukemia. In later phases of these lymphoreticular malignant conditions, apparently as a consequence of continuous anticancer chemotherapy, defective host defense mechanisms allow recurrent infections to become an immense problem.

The lymphoreticular malignant conditions, like the lymphocytic leukemias, the lymphomas, reticulum cell sarcomas, and Hodgkin's disease, have thus far been classified on the basis of morphologic and clinical observations. However, with respect to our rapidly expanding knowledge of the immune lymphoid system, it is advisable to classify these proliferative disorders according to functional characteristics of B and T lymphocytes. Experimental evidence indicates that chronic lymphocytic leukemia is probably a non-secreting B cell leukemia and certain forms of malignant lymphoma are T cell tumors.

Patients with nephrotic syndrome have low serum levels of albumin and gamma globulin because the excessive amounts of these proteins are lost in the urine. Consequently, these patients are very susceptible to infections by encapsulated microorganisms as well as gram-negative bacteria. Nephrotic patients respond well to immunogenic stimuli but specific antibody is rapidly lost in the urine. The most affected immunoglobulin is IgG, while IgM and the beta and alpha globulins of the complement system are normal. This is also the case in classic lipoid nephrosis of children. In contrast, patients with acute glomerulonephritis and certain forms of chronic glomerulonephritis not only lose protein in the urine but also deposit immune complexes and complement in their kidneys. These patients may have complement deficiencies because of an excessive rate of utilization. Some patients with hypocomplementemic forms of chronic renal disease may have a decreased rate of synthesis of complement components, especially C3. These patients have a diminished ability to develop inflammatory responses.

Protein losses from the intestinal tract during certain acute and chronic diseases of the bowel may lead to hypogammaglobulinemia. In intestinal lymphangiectasia, both serum proteins and lymphocytes are lost in the stool. Such patients have low immunoglobulin levels, lymphopenia, and deficient immune function of both B and T cell systems.

Patients who have sustained major burn injuries develop immunodeficiencies. A transient hypogammaglobulinemia may occur during the first week because of losses through the burn lesions. Increased synthesis of immunoglobulins overcompensates for these losses one week later. Lymphocyte depletion occurs as a result of destruction of lymphocytes under the influence of a stress-induced increase of adrenocorticosteroid production. The markedly decreased resistance of burn patients to infections is mainly due to the relative inability of their neutrophils to kill phagocytosed bacteria.

TUMOR IMMUNOLOGY

Tumor-Associated Antigens (Tumor-Specific Antigens)

The majority of tumors, including those induced by chemical carcinogens and viruses, as well as spontaneously arising tumors, carry antigens which elicit immune responses in the host. Tumors induced by chemical or physical agents express individually distinct antigens so that cross-immunization is rarely possible even in tumors of similar morphology induced by the same carcinogen. In contrast, virus-induced tumors contain cross-reacting antigens showing virus-related specificities. Immunization against one tumor may lead to protection against other tumors induced by the same virus. This difference in the specificities of antigens associated with tumors induced by chemical carcinogens and oncogenic viruses has provided a method for determining the etiology of spontaneous tumors. Since several virus-induced tumors have recently been shown to have individually specific antigens besides the common antigens coded for by the virus, this distinction is less clear and definition of the antigenic tumor specificities does not provide conclusive evidence of its etiology. In addition, several chemical carcinogen-induced tumors stimulate the production of antibodies which cross-react with antigens associated with certain viruses.

There are two major categories of tumor-associated antigens in virus-induced neoplasms: (1) the virus-specific antigens and (2) the newly formed antigens, i.e., the antigens that were not present in the normal cells before neoplastic transformation, or on the virions. Antigens belonging to the latter category may arise as (a) products of a specific interaction of the viral genome with the host genome, (b) a specific uncovering of normal or preexisting (embryonic?) cell products, or (c) as a consequence of derepression of intracellular type-C RNA viruses.

The virus-specific antigens may be structural components of the virion or virus-coated products synthesized by the neoplastic cells. Although viral antigens are frequently demonstrable in RNA virus-induced neoplasms, they are rarely seen in tumors induced by DNA viruses. In leukemias induced by RNA viruses, cell surface antigens may be shared with those of the virion. The viruses mature at the cell membrane by budding and the virus particles which are continuously shed by the leukemic cells receive an outer coat from the cell membrane.

Tumor-specific antigens in DNA virus-induced neoplasias are not identical with the antigens of the mature virion and are present even when infectious virus production by the transformed cells cannot be demonstrated. Since these antigens relate specifically to the inducing virus, their presence and permanence suggest that viruses leave at least part of their genetic information in a cell after neoplastic transformation. In view of the cross-reactivity of cells of different types and between tumors in different species, it is likely that the new antigens on the surface of DNA virus-induced tumor cells are determined by the viral genome. On the other hand, tumors induced by different viruses do not cross-react, even when these tumors are morphologically similar and are present in the same species. Exceptions to these rules for cross-reactivity of chemical- or virus-induced neoplasms may occur when the transformed cells express new antigens related to derepression of certain host genomes or of intracellular virogenes.

Derepression of cell genome-coated products occurs in certain types of tumors giving rise to tumor-associated antigens which cross-react with antigens found in embryonal tissue but not in adult host tissue. Most frequently described are the carcinoembryonic antigen of carcinoma of the colon and the alpha fetoprotein associated with hepatic malignant disease in man. The relation between the appearance of these embryonal antigens and neoplastic transformation is not clear, since carcinoembryonic antigen has recently been found in colonic and other gastrointestinal tissue in patients with various non-neoplastic disorders. Several experimentally induced tumors also express embryonal tissue antigens.

Recent studies support the concept that vertebrates contain the genetic information for producing type-C RNA tumor virus in an unexpressed form in their somatic cells as well as in their germ cells. The viral oncogene theory proposes that the endogenous virogenes (the genes for production of type-C viruses) and the oncogenes (that portion of the virogene responsible for transforming a normal cell into a neoplastic cell) are maintained in an unexpressed form by repressors in normal cells. Various agents, including radiation, chemical carcinogens, and exogenously added viruses, may transform cells by "switching on" the endogenous oncogene information. It is under these conditions that the major internal antigen of type-C virus, the group specific or gs antigen can be detected in tumorous tissue.

One approach to studying the etiology of human malignant disease has been the detection of immunologic cross-reactivity in a variety of human tumors. Since all tumors induced by the same virus contain common tumor-associated antigens, while neoplasms induced by different viruses or by nonviral carcinogens usually lack a common antigenicity, one would anticipate a common viral etiology from neoplasms possessing common tumor-associated antigens. However, immunologic cross-reactivity between tumors can be due to the presence of embryonic and gs antigens or antigens induced by virus infection of tumor cells. Patterns of cross-reactivity have been demonstrated between antigens associated with a variety of tumors. Various human cancers originating in the same organs appear to share antigens recognized as foreign by the immune system of the patient while being undetectable in normal cells of the same organ. Certain human tumors share common antigens not found on other tumors. They include neuroblastoma, mammary carcinoma, endometrial cancer, colonic carcinoma, bladder tumors, and malignant melanomas. These observations suggest a viral etiology for the majority of human neoplasms, provided that one postulates that there is a large array of viruses, each of which is associated with neoplasms of a certain origin. This could be the case for RNA viruses, which are usually specific for the type of tumor and organ affected. Unfortunately, there are no data to support the hypothesis that these human tumors are induced by tumor viruses. On the other hand, there is evidence that common antigens detected in Burkitt's lymphoma and nasopharyngeal tumor are associated with the presence of Epstein-Barr (EB) herpes type virus in these neoplasms. The question to be resolved for these neoplasms is whether they carry EB virus as an etiologic agent or as a passenger virus.

Demonstration of Tumor Immunity

It is generally accepted that both cell-mediated and humoral immune response play a major role in host-tumor relationships. Histologic evidence of tumor immunity is indicated by the infiltration of several types of tumor by mononuclear lymphoid cells, which is frequently accompanied by increased cellularity of the regional lymph nodes. For instance, in malignant melanoma, this appearance is most frequently found around primary tumors and early tumors. The lymphocellular response usually decreases as time elapses and the tumor grows. Increased proliferation of mononuclear cells in the regional lymph nodes and infiltration of lymphocytes and plasma cells around the periphery of the tumor have often been associated with a favorable prognosis of patients with various types of malignant disease (e.g., mammary carcinoma, gastric carcinoma, malignant melanoma, testicular seminoma, and urinary bladder tumor).

Several in-vitro tests have been developed to analyze humoral and cellular immunity to tumor cells. Humoral antibodies can be demonstrated by tests for cytotoxicity, membrane immunofluorescence, and mixed hemadsorption and immune adherence. Cytotoxicity tests determine tumor-specific antibodies which, in the presence of complement, exert a cytolytic effect on tumor cells. Although these cytotoxicity tests may be useful in determining humoral immunity to lymphoma and leukemia cells, they rarely work for sarcomas and carcinomas. Cell surface antigens are demonstrable by membrane immunofluorescence in Burkitt's lymphoma and nasopharyngeal carcinoma in which cross-reacting antigens associated with the EB virus can be detected.

Cell-mediated immunity to malignant disease has been demonstrated by use of in-vitro assays with tumors from experimental animals as well as in man. These tests are based on the fact that tumor-specific immune lymphocytes, upon interaction with tumor cells, can be activated to produce soluble factors, lymphokines, which participate in the amplification system of cell-mediated immunity and which may lead to destruction of the tumor cell. The major evidence for cell-mediated immune reactions against human tumors has come from studies performed with the colony-inhibition technique. Tumor cells are first grown in vitro and are then exposed to tumor-specific immune lymphocytes. The inhibitory effect of these lymphocytes is assessed by a reduction in the number of tumor colonies as compared to the effect with nonimmune lymphocytes.

The first human tumor to be studied by the colony-inhibition technique was neuroblastoma. It was found that peripheral blood lymphocytes from patients with such tumors inhibited colony formation of neuroblastoma cells, whether they were of autochthonous or allogeneic origin. Normal skin fibroblasts from tumor donors were not inhibited. Lymphocytes from patients with tumors other than neuroblastomas and from donors not having cancer did not inhibit these neuroblastoma cells. Thus, the lymphocyte effect was specific and could not be attributed to immunity to normal alloantigens. These observations also implied that neuroblastomas have a common tumor-associated antigen.

Similar results have been obtained with the colony-inhibition test in a large variety of human malignant conditions (Table 5-4). In many in-

TABLE 5-4 ANTIGENIC CROSS-REACTIVITY BETWEEN TUMORS OF THE SAME TYPE

Tumor Type	Number of Patient-Tumor Cell Combinations Positive Per Number of Combinations Tested*
Melanoma	41/41
Colon cancer	25/31
Breast cancer	12/14
Lung cancer	5/6
Sarcoma	2/3
Endometrial cancer	2/3
Ovarian cancer	3/5
Testicular tumor	8/10
Squamous cell cancer	2/2
Kidney cancer	1/1
Wilms' tumor	1/2
Parotid tumor	1/1
Total	103/119 (87%)

*Tumor patient lymphocytes were tested on target tumor cells derived from different donors all having the same type of neoplasm. Information courtesy of Dr. K. E. Hellström.

stances, the specific inhibition of colony formation by lymphocytes from patients with a certain type of tumor has provided evidence of antigenic cross-reactivity within (but not between) groups of tumors of the same morphology.

Several neoplasms in experimental animals (e.g., Shope papilloma in rabbits and Moloney virus-induced sarcomas in mice) and man (e.g., neuroblastoma) undergo spontaneous regression. This was not due to alteration of cellular immunity to the tumor cells, since lymphocytes from both persistors (in whom tumors were growing) and regressors (in whom the tumors had regressed) had the same inhibitory effect on colony formation. On the other hand, incubation of the tumor cell cultures with serum from persistors abolished the tumor-inhibiting effect of both persistor and regressor lymphocytes (Fig. 5-9). Serum from regressors did not interfere with the antitumor activity of these lymphocytes.

The serum of tumor-bearing individuals has often been shown to block the activity of tumor-specific immune lymphocytes in the colony-inhibition technique. This serum blocking activity has been associated with tumor-specific antibodies or with antigen-antibody complexes. Provided that these antibodies or complexes have a similar effect in vivo as in vitro, the presence of serum blocking activity would be a powerful mechanism of escape from an efficient lymphocyte-mediated immune surveillance of tumor growth. If the development of blocking antibodies plays an important role in enabling tumors to grow in an immunologically sensitized host, it should be possible to inhibit tumor growth by measures that counteract the blocking activity, either by the prevention of blocking antibody formation or by intervention with its action. In this respect, it was found that in Moloney sarcomas of mice and other tumor systems admixture of regressor serum to persistor serum abolishes the blocking activity of regressor serum, and the blocking activity of persistor serum is not well understood.

Host-Tumor Relationships and Immunosurveillance

From a teleologic standpoint, it is generally accepted that the lymphoid system may have evolved in vertebrates for the purpose of seeking out, recognizing, and destroying malignantly al-

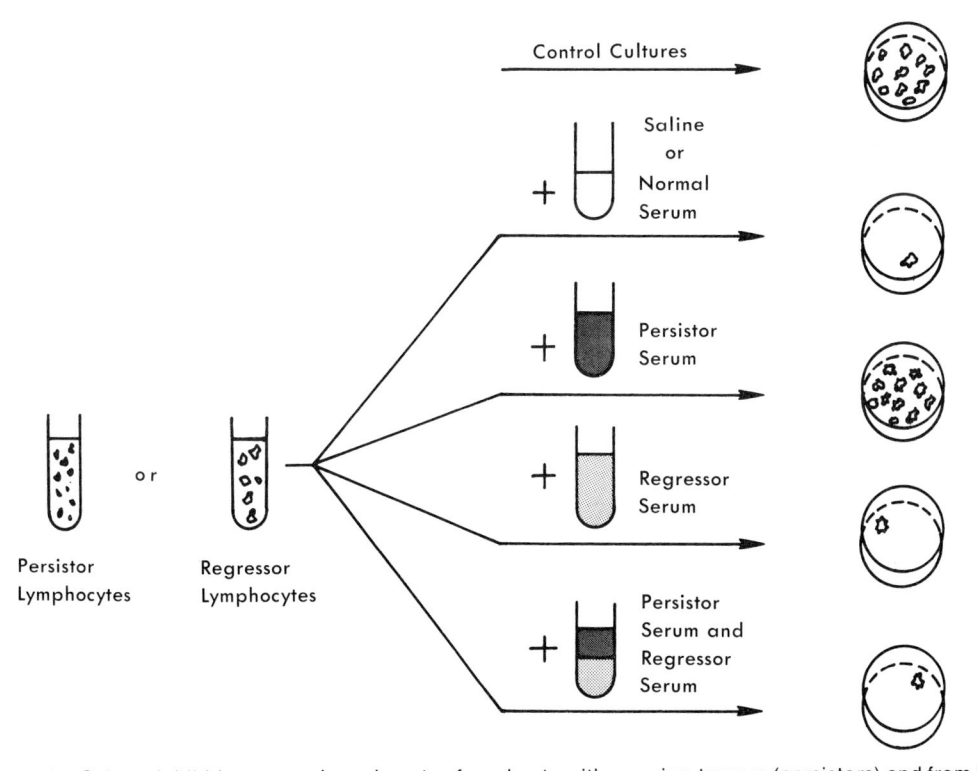

Figure 5-9 Colony-inhibition assay. Lymphocytes from hosts with growing tumors (persistors) and from hosts with regressed tumors (regressors) inhibit the in-vitro formation of tumor colonies. Serum from persistors block the tumor-inhibiting effect of both persistor and regressor lymphocytes. In contrast, serum from regressors does not exhibit this blocking effect and may even have the capability to "unblock" the blocking activity of persistor serum.

TABLE 5-5 MALIGNANT CONDITIONS IN PATIENTS WITH IMMUNODEFICIENCY*

Primary Disease	Number of Patients Who Developed Malignant Condition	Types of Malignant Conditions	Percentage of Patients With Cancer
Infantile sex-linked agammaglobulinemia	5	Leukemia	5 to 10 per cent
Ataxia-telangiectasia	42	Many	10 to 15 per cent
Wiskott-Aldrich syndrome	13	Mostly lymphoreticular	> 10 per cent
Common variable immunodeficiency	30+	Many	5 to 10 per cent
Severe combined immunodeficiency	3	— —	1 to 10 per cent

*Observations by Dr. R. A. Good.

tered tissue. This surveillance system may be just another homeostatic control mechanism through which the host maintains its integrity. Faulty immunosurveillance is generally associated with increased incidence of malignant disease. Decreased immune function normally present in immature or aging animals or experimentally induced by irradiation, neonatal thymectomy, and administration of immunosuppressive drugs or antilymphocyte serum is often associated with an increased susceptibility to malignancy. In addition, much clinical evidence links the lymphoid system inextricably with malignant change in man. Regardless of the nature of the disorder, all forms of primary immunodeficiency of man have shown evidence of increased susceptibility to malignant disease. For example, patients with a sex-linked recessive Bruton type agammaglobulinemia are inordinately susceptible to the development of leukemia. A high incidence of malignant disease is also found in ataxia-telangiectasia. These diseases are frequently reticulum cell sarcomas, lymphosarcomas, and leukemias, but epithelial malignant diseases, especially of the gastrointestinal tract and of other supporting and mesenchymal tissues, have also been reported. Patients with the Wiskott-Aldrich syndrome have a high frequency of malignant disease, the most common form of which is a reticulum cell tumor which often affects the brain as well as the lymphoid and hematopoietic organs. A high incidence of malignant disease is encountered in most other immunodeficiency syndromes (Table 5-5).

Conversely, malignant disease of the lymphoid system such as Hodgkin's disease, multiple myeloma, and chronic lymphatic leukemia all manifest severe malfunction of humoral or cellular immunity, or both. Such deficiencies have also been described in patients with malignant diseases of nonlymphoid organs. These patients respond subnormally to immunogenic stimulation with tetanus toxoid, dinitrochlorobenzene (DNCB), and tuberculin. For instance, the inability of breast cancer patients to become sensitized to DNCB has been associated with a poor prognosis. It is quite likely that the immune defect in these cancer patients is a consequence of advanced disease and not its cause.

The concept of immunosurveillance should by no means be construed as the only mechanism serving to control neoplastic change. For instance, the role of hormones in the surveillance of endocrine tissue and their tumors is well documented. Contact inhibition of isolated aberrant cells provides another mechanism of surveillance. Closely resembling contact inhibition is the phenomenon of allogeneic inhibition, by which cells with different structures on their cell surfaces mutually inhibit their growth when in contact with each other. A newly formed neoplastic cell may be eliminated by the normal cells around it long before it becomes recognized by the immune system. The significance of these nonimmunologic mechanisms of surveillance against malignancy is difficult to assess.

The combined surveillance mechanisms appear to be most effective in the control of malignant change. In spite of the continuous and extensive exposure to carcinogenic agents, cancer is very uncommon in most age groups. In addition, we probably carry oncogenic viruses (e.g., type-C RNA viruses) which may induce neoplasms under certain conditions.

Although the association between immunodeficiency and the increased incidence of malignant disease is well documented, most cancer patients have no history of apparent immunodeficiency disorders. It is in these instances that the relation between immunologic aberration and neoplastic growth is poorly understood. Several mechanisms have been proposed by which tumors can overcome immunosurveillance by the lymphoid system. The escape of neoplastic growth from immunosurveillance may occur at the level of induction of the immune response (afferent limb) or at the level of expression of immunity (efferent limb).

In the afferent limb of the immune response, the tumor antigens should be regarded as tumor immunogens. The structure and physiochemical nature of these immunogens, as well as the amounts present in the tumor and available for immunogenic stimulation, obviously have great influence on the outcome of the tumor-specific immune response. When a cell undergoes a neoplastic change, it seems quite likely that sufficient amounts of tumor-specific antigen must be present on that cell to stimulate the immune system. Therefore, this neoplastic cell will probably have to undergo a number of divisions before sufficient quantities of tumor-specific antigens are present to elicit an immune response. Immunogenic stimulation of the lymphoid system is probably induced by the antigenic structures present on tumor cell break-down products, such as cell membranes, which enter the regional lymph nodes by way of the draining lymphatics. When the immunogenicity of the tumor is low, or when the tumor has a high cellular proliferation rate, the tumor may outgrow its susceptibility to the effects of the immune system and thus escape immune surveillance.

In experimental studies, it has been shown that exposure of the animals to an oncogenic virus or a carcinogen will temporarily suppress the immune response. With reference to the unknown etiology of most human cancers, it is not known whether this potential suppression of the immune response is relevant to the development of human malignant disease.

Immunologic factors may suppress those cells with the most surface immunogenicity and "select" those cells with the least immunogenicity. This immunoselection may represent a mechanism by which a neoplastic cell with low immunogenicity "sneaks through" the immunosurveillance of the host.

The genetic background of the host may also influence his immune system. It has been demonstrated that the quantity as well as the quality of the immune response is controlled by "immune response genes," some of which appear to be associated with transplantation genes. Several investigators have observed that these operate at the level of the antigen-reactive thymus-derived lymphocyte, but others have indicated that antibody-producing B cells may also be involved. Evidence suggests that these genes may be one of several genetic factors affecting a variety of neoplastic and autoallergic diseases. For instance, the resistance of mice to Gross virus leukemogenesis is under the influence of two genes, one of which is the immune response gene, the other a histocompatibility gene. In this respect it is interesting to note that certain types of malignant disease occur in higher frequency in patients having specific combinations of transplantation antigens. For instance, the presence of HLA-5 antigen is associated with an increased incidence of Hodgkin's disease.

It is possible that the host has developed immunologic tolerance to his tumor, similar to the chimeric state seen after transplantation of hematopoietic and other tissues, so that rejection does not occur. Pregnancy represents a comparable balanced immunologic relationship whereby the graft, the fetus, survives in an immunologically incompatible host, the mother. In chimerism, as in the host-tumor relationship, we appear to be dealing with a complex set of biological problems involving the potentiality for adaptation by the graft or tumor and the host. Our attention in tumor immunology has been focused on immunologic adaptation by the host. Attention must be given to the possible contribution of the tumors in this process.

Even when a host develops a vigorous immune response against the tumor, i.e., an effective cellular immunity which may be accompanied by humoral cytotoxic antibody formation, the possibility still exists that the tumor survives in the host. This situation is prevalent in many tumor systems as demonstrated by the presence of blocking factors which interfere with the antitumor activity of tumor-specific immune lymphocytes in the colony-inhibition technique. These blocking factors resemble the antibody molecules responsible for the phenomenon of immunoenhancement. Experimental studies have shown that passive transfer of tumor-specific antibodies into a syngeneic host exerts an enhancing effect on the growth of a transplant of that tumor. Also, mixing of humoral antibody with tumor cells in vitro made possible their development into tumors under conditions which otherwise precluded such events. Several explanations have been proposed about the mechanism of immunoenhancement by humoral antibodies. An essential component is that such protective action by humoral antibodies is likely to take place in situations in which the host defense is primarily mediated by immune lymphocytes. One explanation is that immunoenhancement is active at the efferent limb of the immune response. The antigenic determinants on the tumor cell surface are blocked by antibody so that immune lymphocytes do not recognize these antigens and therefore do not attack tumor cells. These humoral antibodies may also prevent tumor antigens from sensitizing lymphocytes or they may interfere with proliferation of new reactive populations of immune lymphocytes. These postulates for the mechanism of action of enhancing antibodies may also apply to those factors which block the activity of tumor-immune lymphocytes in the colony-inhibition assay. However, recent evidence seems to indicate that the blocking factors are circulating complexes between antibody and tumor-associated antigens.

An important consideration should be given to the role of tumor-associated antigens in the efferent limb of the host immune response to the tumor. They can be classified into two groups: (1) those antigens present on the cell surface that have been called tumor-rejection antigens, and (2) the soluble antigens localized in the cell cytoplasm and nucleus to which specific immunity has little effect on tumor growth. The availability of tumor-rejection antigens to the effector mechanisms of humoral and cellular immunity greatly influences their efficiency. For instance, tumor antigens deeply embedded in the cell surface are inaccessible to antibodies as well as to immune lymphocytes. Also, the density of tumor-rejection antigens on the cell surface is relevant to the effectiveness of certain types of immune responses. For example, IgG complement-fixing antibody requires a relatively high density of tumor antigen to induce a cytotoxic effect on the tumor cell because of the requirement of the close proximity of at least two IgG molecules on the surface to activate the complement sequence (see Chapter 4). The same cytotoxic complement-fixing antibody does not exhibit this effect when the density of the tumor-rejection antigen is low. In this situation, by combining with the antigens on the tumor cell, this antibody may interfere with the effector mechanisms of tumor-specific cellular immunity.

Clinical Applications of Tumor Immunobiology

Our rapidly expanding knowledge of tumor immunology has provided a basis for the immunologic approach in the diagnosis and treatment of malignant disease. Since the demonstration of tumor-specific antigens in a great variety of human malignant diseases, many attempts are underway to isolate and purify these substances. The development of practical tests for tumor antigen detection should enhance diagnosis and permit detection of residual tumor after therapy.

Tumor-specific immunity, both cell-mediated and humoral, can now be assessed in vitro on an experimental basis. However, most of the methods involved are technically difficult and not practical for routine use.

Evaluation of the general status of the immune system of the tumor patient can be of prognostic value. For example, total lymphocyte counts are low, delayed hypersensitivity reactions to common antigens are less frequent, phytohemagglutinin-induced transformation of lymphocytes is reduced, and susceptibility to sensitization to DNCB is impaired in cancer patients who have extensive and disseminated disease. Unfortunately, these observations are applicable to some tumors but not to others.

Another important application of tumor immunology is the use of immunologic principles in the treatment of cancer. In most cases the central problem of tumor immunotherapy is not that of inducing the patient to become immune to his tumor, but rather to make existing immunity more effective in controlling tumor growth. Immunotherapy must attempt to direct the interaction between tumor growth and tumor immunity in favor of the host, either by quantitative augmentation of immunity or by qualitative alteration of the immune response so as to expose new tumor vulnerabilities. The approach of augmenting tumor-specific cell-mediated immune mechanisms or depression of the humoral immune response should be considered with some skepticism, since many of the immunologic aspects of the interaction between host and tumor are still poorly understood.

Attempts to increase cell-mediated immunity by adoptive transfer of allogeneic leukocytes from other individuals who had spontaneous regression or who had been tumor-immunized has had limited success. This may be attributed to the relatively short life span of the histoincompatible lymphocytes or to a graft-versus-host reaction occurring in patients receiving immunosuppression by their tumor or by chemotherapy. On the other hand, adaptive transfer through the use of transfer factor obtained from tumor-specific immune lymphocytes may be a potentially useful approach.

Another approach to augmentation of active tumor immunity is to increase or alter the immunogenicity of tumor cells. For example, tumor cells have been altered chemically or enzymatically so that they become more immunogenic. Painting of skin sensitizers such as DNCB on superficial squamous skin cancers of DNCB-sensitized patients, has induced selective tumor rejection. This method represents a new approach to the control of dermal cancers.

In addition to the specific augmentation methods mentioned above, nonspecific augmentation of tumor immunity appears to have been achieved through immunization with BCG. Clinical trials using this approach to immunotherapy of leukemia have been relatively successful.

Finally, cautious manipulation of the humoral immune response of the cancer patient (e.g., from blocking antibody to unblocking antibody) or administration of unblocking antibody with tumor specificity may offer a promising approach to immunotherapy.

REFERENCES

GENERAL REFERENCES

Alexander, J. W., and Good, R. A.: Immunobiology for Surgeons. Philadelphia, W. B. Saunders Co., 1970.

Amos, B. (Ed.): Progress in Immunology. New York, Academic Press, 1971.

Bellanti, J. A.: Immunology. Philadelphia, W. B. Saunders Co., 1971.

Forscher, B. K., and Houck, J. C.: Immunopathology of Inflammation. Amsterdam, Excerpta Medica, 1971.

Freedman, S.: Clinical Immunology. New York, Harper and Row, 1971.

Miescher, P. A., and Mueller-Eberhard, H. J. (Eds.): Textbook of Immunopathology. New York, Grune and Stratton, 1969.

Movat, H. Z.: Inflammation, Immunity and Hypersensitivity. New York, Harper and Row, 1971.

Samter, M. (Ed.): Immunological Diseases. Boston, Little Brown and Co., 1971.

Waksman, B. H.: Atlas of Experimental Immunobiology and Immunopathology. New Haven, Connecticut, Yale University Press, 1970.

IMMUNODEFICIENCY DISEASES

Alper, C. A., and Rosen, F. S.: Genetic aspects of the complement system. Adv. Immunol., 14:252, 1971.

Bergsma, D., and Good, R. A. (Eds.): Immunologic Deficiency Disease in Man. The National Foundation of Birth Defects, Original Article Series, Vol. IV, No. 1, 1968.

Bortin, M. M.: A compendium of reported human bone marrow transplants. Transplantation, 9:571, 1970.

Buckley, R. H.: Reconstitution: grafting of bone marrow and thymus. In Amos, B.(Ed.): Progress in Immunology. New York, Academic Press, 1971.

Franklin, E. C.: Some protein disorders associated with neoplasms of plasma cells and lymphocytes: heavy chain diseases. In Amos, B. (Ed.): Progress in Immunology. New York, Academic Press, 1971.

Fudenberg, H., Good, R. A., Goodman, H. C., Hitzig, W., Kunkel, H. G., Roitt, I. M., Rosen, F. S., Rowe, D. S., Seligmann, M., and Soothill, J. R.: Primary immunodeficiencies. Report of a World Health Organization Committee. Pediatrics, 47:927, 1971.

Good, R. A., Biggar, W. D., and Park, B. H.: Immunodeficiency diseases in man. In Amos, B. (Ed.): Progress in Immunology. New York, Academic Press, 1971.

Hoyer, J. R., Cooper, M. D., Gabrielsen, A. E., and Good, R. A.: Lymphopenic forms of congenital immunologic deficiency diseases. Medicine, 47:201, 1968.

Kagan, B. M., and Stiehm, E. R.: Immunologic Incompetence. Chicago, Year Book Medical Publishers, Inc., 1971.

Merler, E. (Ed.): Immunoglobulins. Biologic Aspects and Clinical Uses. Washington, D.C., National Academy of Sciences, 1970.

Waldman, T. A., Strober, W., and Blaese, R. M.: Metabolism of immunoglobulins. In Amos, B. (Ed.): Progress in Immunology. New York, Academic Press, 1971.

TUMOR IMMUNOLOGY

Association Française pour l'Étude du Cancer: Cancer et Immunité. Ann. Inst. Pasteur, 122:589, 1972.

Gold, P.: Antigenic reversion in human cancer. Ann. Rev. Med., 22:85, 1971.

Good, R. A.: Relations between immunity and malignancy. Proc. Nat. Acad. Sci. (U.S.A.), 69:1026, 1972.

Hellström, I., Hellström, K. E., Sjögren, H. O., and Warner, G. A.: Demonstration of cell-mediated immunity to human neoplasms of various immunological types. Int. J. Cancer, 7:1, 1971.

Hellström, K. E., Hellström, I., Sjögren, H. O., and Warner, G. A.: Cell-mediated immunity to human tumor antigens. In Amos, B. (Ed.): Progress in Immunology. New York, Academic Press, 1971.

Klein, E., and Cochran, A. J.: Immunology and malignant disease. Haematologia, 5:179, 1971.

Law, L. W.: Studies of tumor antigens and tumor-specific immune mechanisms in experimental systems. Transpl. Proc., 2:117, 1970.

McDevitt, H. O., and Bodmer, W. F.: Histocompatibility antigens, immune responsiveness and susceptibility to disease. Amer. J. Med., 52:1, 1972.

Sjögren, H. O., and Bansal, S. C.: Antigens in virally induced tumors. In Amos, B. (Ed.): Progress in Immunology. New York, Academic Press, 1971.

Smith, R. T.: Potentials for immunologic intervention in cancer. In Amos, B. (Ed.): Progress in Immunology. New York, Academic Press, 1971.

Todaro, G. J., and Huebner, R. J.: The viral oncogene hypothesis: New evidence. Proc. Nat. Acad. Sci. (U.S.A.), 69:1009, 1972.

SECTION II

CARDIORENAL AND RESPIRATORY SYSTEMS

CHAPTER 6   INTEGRATIVE HEMODYNAMICS

ARTHUR C. GUYTON

It would be pointless to review in this chapter all the details of hemodynamics, such as the interrelationships between pressure, resistance, and flow, or the problems of blood viscosity, or the differences between streamline and non-streamline blood flow, because these are found in every textbook of medical physiology. On the other hand, the integrative aspects of hemodynamics are extremely important to the clinician and, yet, are rarely found in physiology texts. It is these aspects that will be covered in this chapter.

Basic Philosophy of the Circulatory System

The purpose of the circulatory system is to provide transport for nutrients, excreta, and other substances to and from the cells. To do this there are two major groups of hemodynamic systems. One of these is geared to provide a continuous pressure head in the arterial tree and the other to control blood flow in each individual section of the circulation in accord with local needs. It will be the aim of this chapter to show how these different mechanisms operate together to provide continuous automatic function of the circulation and how dysfunction can lead to circulatory inadequacy.

INTEGRATION OF HEMODYNAMIC FACTORS IN OVERALL CIRCULATORY REGULATION

Figure 6-1 depicts the principal hemodynamic factors in overall function of the circulation and also shows their interrelationships. First, let us describe the six factors located on the periphery of the diagram in Blocks 1 through 6, beginning with arterial pressure. (1) When the arterial pressure increases, this causes the renal output of water and electrolytes also to increase. (2) Increased loss of water and electrolytes from the kidneys reduces the extracellular fluid volume, which (3) causes a similar effect on blood volume. (4) The decrease in blood volume decreases the circulatory filling pressure (the tightness with which the circulation is filled with blood). (5) Decreasing this factor decreases venous return and cardiac output, and (6) the decrease in cardiac output obviously decreases arterial pressure.

Thus, one sees that an initial increase in arterial pressure causes a series of events which in turn tend to reduce the arterial pressure back toward normal. Conversely, a decrease in arterial pressure will cause exactly the opposite events, this time raising the diminished pressure back toward normal.

As one studies this circuit of Figure 6-1 still further (Blocks 1 through 6) one sees that it is a negative feedback hemodynamic mechanism that tends always to return the functional variables of the circulation back toward their normal levels. It is negative feedback loops such as these that provide most control functions in the body, and this specific hemodynamic negative feedback loop of Figure 6-1 is the most basic control loop of the circulatory system. Furthermore, complete understanding of this mechanism can help to explain many clinical circulatory abnormalities, as we shall see in subsequent pages.

Effects of Water and Electrolyte Intake. The two inside blocks of Figure 6-1 also deserve special mention. Block 7 shows that one's intake of water and electrolytes also plays a major role in overall control of the circulation, obviously counterbalancing renal output of water and electrolytes.

Effects of Total Peripheral Resistance and Autoregulation. Block 8, total peripheral resis-

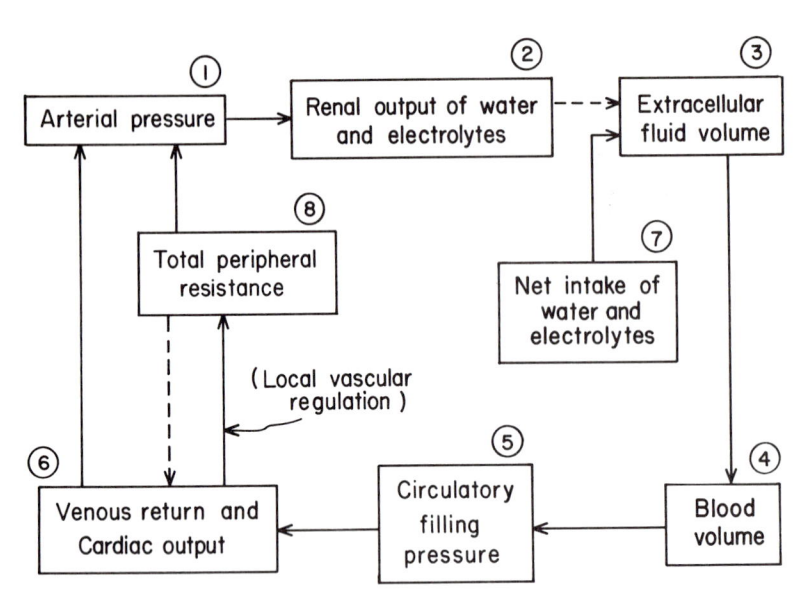

Figure 6-1 The major hemodynamic factors of circulatory function and their interrelationships.

tance, has two very significant effects on circulatory regulation: (1) An increase in total peripheral resistance tends to increase arterial pressure, but (2) an increase in total peripheral resistance also tends to decrease venous return and cardiac output. The second one of these two effects is often forgotten; sometimes it is even more potent than the effect of the resistance on arterial pressure. For instance, when the total peripheral resistance increases because of venous constriction, the tendency to decrease cardiac output is much greater than the tendency to increase arterial pressure. Therefore, in this instance, the arterial pressure actually decreases instead of increasing because of the greatly decreased cardiac output. This interplay between the positive and negative effects of total peripheral resistance on pressure is mentioned here merely to illustrate one of the falsities that has crept into much understanding of the circulatory hemodynamics, namely, a widespread impression that total peripheral resistance and arterial pressure are almost always directly related to each other.

It is also noted in Block 8 that an increase in cardiac output can increase total peripheral resistance. This effect is frequently overlooked in schemes of circulatory function. It results from the ability of tissues to control their own local blood flows, which will be discussed later in this chapter. When the cardiac output becomes too great, blood flows through the tissues in excessive amounts and the tissues attempt to return their flows back to normal. As a result, the local blood vessels constrict, thereby increasing total peripheral resistance. Conversely, whenever the cardiac output falls too low and blood flow in the tissues diminishes, the local vasculature dilates. This effect of cardiac output on vascular resistance is called *autoregulation*. As a result of it, there is a tendency for the total peripheral resistance to change in the same direction as the change in cardiac output. The effect, however, is not an instantaneous one. Part of it occurs within the first minute or so, still more within the next hour, and much more over a period of days and weeks, as will be discussed later in this chapter in relation to local blood flow regulation.

With this rapid introduction to the major hemodynamic factors in circulatory control, now let us turn to one of the more specific circulatory functions.

LOCAL BLOOD FLOW AND ITS REGULATION

Every clinician is familiar with the ability of local tissues to protect their own blood flows. For instance, if a femoral artery suddenly becomes occluded, within 60 to 90 seconds collateral blood vessels open to supply blood to the leg. Then, during the next several weeks to several months, the collaterals become progressively larger, until finally blood flow is almost as adequate as before, particularly in very young persons.

On the other hand, exactly the opposite effects occur when blood flow to the tissues becomes too great, for acute constriction of the blood vessels occurs within the first minute or so, and this is followed gradually over days, weeks, and months by actual decrease in vascular dimensions.

Mechanisms of Local Blood Flow Regulation: Role of Oxygen

Different tissues have different mechanisms for control of local blood flow, depending on their specific local needs. However, the majority of the tissues control local blood flow in relation to their need for oxygen. This is particularly true in all types of muscle—skeletal, cardiac, and smooth—which make up approximately one half the body. Diminished oxygen delivery causes up to fourfold increase in blood flow within seconds to minutes; then, additional vasodilatation occurs during the ensuing half hour to hour.

In some tissues this effect of oxygen lack is subservient to other more potent local factors controlling blood flow. For instance, in the brain the factor that normally plays the most potent role is carbon dioxide, an increase in carbon dioxide causing increased blood flow and thereby providing increased removal of the excess carbon dioxide from the brain tissue. However, when the brain becomes extremely hypoxic, vasodilatation occurs as a result of the hypoxia itself in exactly the same way as it occurs in muscle.

Possible Vasodilator Substances. The basic mechanism by which decreased oxygen delivery to the tissues causes vasodilatation is still unknown. Some research workers believe that diminished oxygen causes release of some humoral vasodilator material that in turn actively dilates the local vessels. The substance that has received widest attention in recent years has been *adenosine*, one of the breakdown products of adenosine triphosphate that is released in small quantities into the tissue fluid in hypoxic states. Other possible vasodilator substances that have been suggested include potassium, osmotic substances of any nature, adenosine triphosphate, carbon dioxide, lactic acid, histamine, and others. All these can indeed cause vasodilatation in large enough quantities, but to date none of them has been proved to be formed in the quantities required to cause the dilatation that occurs in hypoxia.

Vasodilatation Caused By Oxygen Deficiency Per Se. More recently, experiments have shown that the vasodilating effect of tissue hypoxia could result from simple decrease of oxygen itself in the tissues rather than from the presence of vasodilator substances. Absence of oxygen prevents formation of significant quantities of ATP and other high-energy compounds in the smooth muscle cells of the vascular walls, so that the strength of contraction of these cells is diminished in exactly the same way that the strength of contraction of skeletal muscle is also diminished in hypoxia. Obviously, this could easily cause local vasodilatation when too little oxygen is available to the tissues.

Long-term Changes in Blood Vessels During Ischemia or Hypoxia. In animals kept for months at high altitudes, the actual sizes and numbers of vessels in the tissues increase, causing a phenomenon called increased vascularity. Furthermore, return of these animals to normal altitudes causes the vascularity to return toward normal. Essentially the same effects also occur when the tissues are made ischemic. Unfortunately, the causes of these changes in vascularity are not yet known, but the vascularity changes themselves help to maintain proper delivery of oxygen and other nutrients to the tissues.

Other Normal and Pathologic Factors in Local Blood Flow Regulation. In the skin, local blood flow is controlled almost entirely by the body temperature control mechanism, acting mainly by means of nervous constriction or dilatation of the skin vessels.

In the kidneys, blood flow is controlled primarily by the renal excretory loads, especially by the presence of excess sodium and possibly other electrolytes in the plasma; it is also possible that some of the end products of metabolism help to control renal blood flow. Only when the kidneys become extremely hypoxic does the hypoxia mechanism play any significant role in renal blood flow regulation.

Finally, any pathologic state that causes direct communication between the arteries and the veins increases the local blood flow and contributes to the overall control of the circulation. Thus, either minute pathologic arteriovenous fistulae or major A-V fistulae are factors that increase local blood flow.

Local Blood Flow Regulation During Increased Tissue Activity. The local blood flow regulating mechanisms also respond to increased cellular activity. To give an example, Figure 6–2 shows the effect of progressive increase in work output during exercise on both oxygen consumption and cardiac output, illustrating that as tissue metabolism increases (indicated by increasing oxygen consumption), blood flow through the entire body also increases (indicated by the increasing cardiac output). Other examples in which increased tissue activity causes vascular dilatation include (1) increased metabolism of the tissues caused by thyrotoxicosis, (2) increased tissue activity caused by excessive catecholamines, and (3) increased metabolism caused by fever. Therefore, the increased local blood flows and increased cardiac outputs observed in these conditions can all be ascribed to the increased activities in the local tissue cells themselves.

CARDIAC OUTPUT: HEMODYNAMIC FACTORS IN ITS REGULATION

When one thinks of cardiac output regulation, he almost immediately thinks of the heart, but

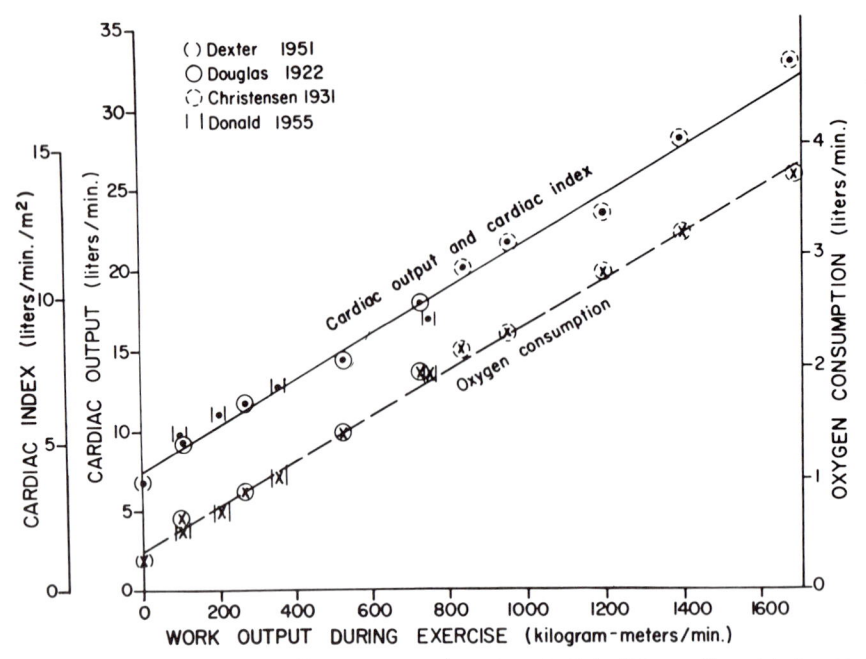

Figure 6-2 Relationship between cardiac output and work output (solid curve) and between oxygen consumption and work output (dashed curve) during exercise. Reprinted from Guyton, A. C., et al.: Circulatory Physiology: Cardiac Output and its Regulation. 2nd ed. Philadelphia, W. B. Saunders Co., 1973.)

normally 90 to 95 per cent of cardiac output regulation is effected by peripheral circulatory factors, and not more than 5 to 10 per cent by the heart itself. On the other hand, when the heart becomes diseased and is then unable to provide adequate pumping capacity, the limiting factor in cardiac output regulation becomes the heart.

Role of the Heart in Cardiac Output Regulation

Even under resting conditions the normal human heart is capable of pumping between 10 and 15 liters of blood per minute, though it actually pumps only 5 to 6 liters. The simple reason for this difference is the following: only this smaller amount of blood flows into the heart from the veins, and, however much pumping capacity the heart may have, it can never pump more blood than flows into it. The normal heart merely keeps the input veins pumped almost dry, which can be illustrated by injecting a contrast medium into any of the peripheral veins and noting the slitlike character of the veins where they empty into the thorax.

Effect of the Nervous System on the Heart's Pumping Capacity. In dog studies, maximal sympathetic stimulation of the heart can increase the pumping capacity of the heart about 70 to 100 per cent. On the other hand, maximal vagal stimulation can stop the heart for a few seconds until the ventricles begin to beat at a very slow rate, driven by a ventricular pacemaker. After the ventricles have thus "escaped" from the vagal stimulation, the maximum pumping capacity of the heart is reduced to about 50 per cent of normal. Therefore, the total range of nervous control of heart pumping is probably between −50 per cent and +100 per cent.

Effect of Cardiac Hypertrophy on Heart Pumping Capacity. In athletes who train for endurance, the maximum cardiac output can be increased 50 to 100 per cent by the training procedure. At least part of this effect is caused by cardiac hypertrophy. Likewise, from study of certain disease conditions, such as left-to-right shunts, in which the heart must pump greatly increased amounts of blood indefinitely, one can also come to the conclusion that heart hypertrophy can increase the heart's pumping capacity as much as 100 per cent.

Cardiac Reserve. The difference between the heart's pumping capacity and the actual amount of blood pumped by the heart under resting conditions is called the "cardiac reserve." Thus, if the heart of an exceedingly well-trained athlete is capable of pumping 30 liters per minute but under resting conditions pumps only 5 liters, the cardiac reserve is 25 liters. Expressing this in percentage, which is the usual method, this person has a cardiac reserve of 500 per cent above normal.

Role of Peripheral Circulation in Cardiac Output Control

If the peripheral blood vessels were rigid tubes, the peripheral circulation would play essentially no role in cardiac output regulation, because whenever the heart should pump increased quantities of blood into a peripheral vessel an equal amount of blood would be returned instantaneously to the input side of the heart. However, the fact that the peripheral vessels are highly distensible prevents this instantaneous increase in venous return. Instead, the extra blood pumped by the heart at first simply distends the arterial tree. Then it is allowed to flow through the small tissue vessels into the veins and, finally, back again to the heart only at the will of the tissues. Consequently, it is frequently said that cardiac output is controlled by venous return and that venous return is controlled by the tissues. This means simply that whatever amount of blood is allowed to flow through the small vessels of the tissues into the veins and thence into the heart is also the amount of blood that the heart pumps.

Cardiac Output Regulation as the Sum of Local Blood Flow Regulations. The factors that control local blood flow in the peripheral circulation change from minute to minute in accord with the needs of the tissues, as already discussed, and these effects simultaneously alter venous return and cardiac output. Therefore, another way of looking at normal cardiac output regulation is simply to state that it is the sum of all the local blood flow regulations. If return of blood to the heart from any single tissue increases, cardiac output increases by approximately a similar increment.

This principle is illustrated very forcefully when one studies the effects of an arteriovenous fistula on circulatory function, as illustrated in Figure 6-3. This figure shows an instantaneous increase in cardiac output resulting from opening the fistula. The primary effect is to allow direct flow of blood from the arteries into the veins, and the surge of blood returning to the heart instantaneously increases the cardiac output. Within another few seconds, the nervous reflexes further compensate for the fistula by causing blood reservoirs to constrict throughout the body, thereby making still more blood available to be pumped by the heart. Then, during the next several days, renal retention of water and salt (for reasons discussed earlier in this chapter in relation to Figure 6-1) causes the blood volume to increase slightly, making even more blood available to the heart. Thus, within two to three days, there is full compensation to opening the A-V fistula, and *the cardiac output is increased by an amount exactly equal to the fistula flow*, if the heart does not go into failure.

Role of Blood Volume and "Circulatory Filling Pressure" in Cardiac Output Regulation. Another peripheral factor that even normally plays a supporting role in cardiac output regulation (and under certain abnormal conditions plays the major role) is the blood volume and its ability to fill the circulatory system, as measured by the "circulatory filling pressure." When the blood vol-

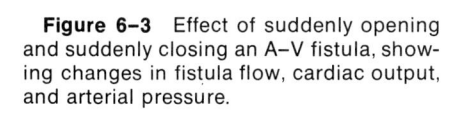

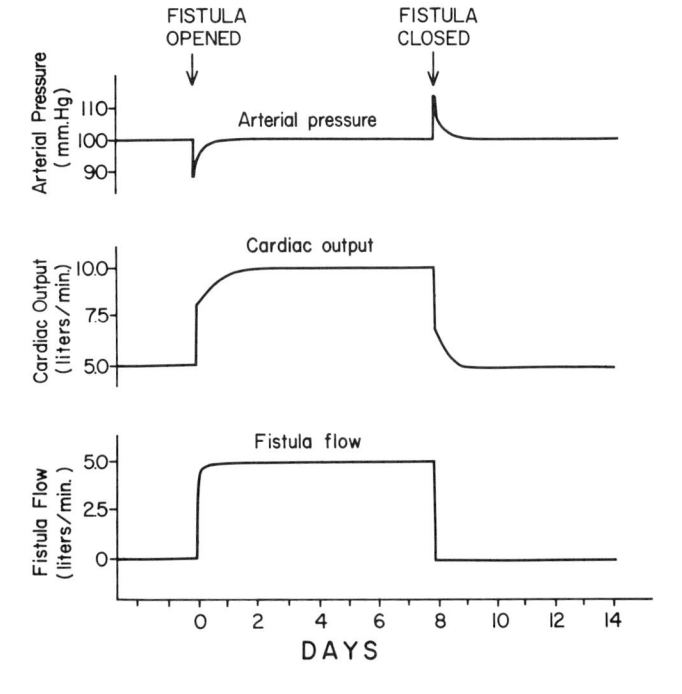

Figure 6-3 Effect of suddenly opening and suddenly closing an A-V fistula, showing changes in fistula flow, cardiac output, and arterial pressure.

ume is increased, the quantity of blood in each vessel in the body tends also to increase. Therefore, the pressure in each vessel becomes slightly greater than normal. The algebraic sum of these pressures, weighted in proportion to the capacitances of the respective vascular segments, is the circulatory filling pressure, and its normal value is 7 mm. Hg, as estimated from measurements in dogs. This is also the average pressure in the peripheral circulation that tends to push blood toward the venous input side of the heart. Both mathematically and experimentally, it has been demonstrated that venous return increases directly in proportion to an increase in circulatory filling pressure. On the other hand, the right atrial pressure exerts a back pressure to reduce flow of blood into the heart. Putting both these factors together, one finds that *return of blood to the heart is directly proportional to the circulatory filling pressure minus the right atrial pressure.*

EFFECT OF VASCULAR CAPACITY ON FILLING PRESSURE. The capacity of the circulatory system itself is another factor that helps to determine the circulatory filling pressure. Obviously, the greater the capacity, the greater must be the blood volume to create the same degree of filling pressure. Furthermore, the capacity of the circulatory system can be changed by nervous stimulation, hormonal effects, fever, and so forth. Some of these factors will be discussed later in the chapter in relation to blood volume regulation, but it is very clear that the tightness with which the circulatory system is filled with blood is determined by the ratio of the blood volume to the capacity of the system itself. Therefore, from the point of view of control of the circulation, one needs to think in terms of circulatory filling pressure and not in terms of blood volume itself.

Role of Circulatory Filling Pressure in Circulatory Shock and in Heart Failure. There are two very important applications of the concept of circulatory filling pressure to clinical medicine—one to help explain circulatory shock and the other to explain one of the compensations in congestive heart failure. In circulatory shock, the blood volume is usually greatly decreased, but shock can also result from excessive dilatation of the vasculature, which simply increases the capacity of the system. That is, either decreased blood volume or increased vascular capacity decreases the circulatory filling pressure below its normal value and can correspondingly reduce venous return and cardiac output. In the early stages of some types of shock, such as hemorrhagic shock, the pumping capacity of the heart actually increases far above normal because of reflex nervous stimulation of the heart. Yet, despite this, the venous return is still too low, and the cardiac output cannot rise above the venous return; hence, the patient is in circulatory shock despite massive pumping effort by the heart. Thus, the concept of circulatory filling pressure is an exceedingly important one in understanding abnormal control of the circulation in circulatory shock.

In congestive heart failure, the primary abnormality occurs in the heart itself, but even a very weak heart can often pump normal cardiac output if it is constantly primed with excessive amounts of blood attempting to enter the right atrium. In severe congestive heart failure, the kidneys function very poorly, causing diminished urinary output and consequent increase in extracellular fluid volume and blood volume. As a result, the circulatory filling pressure sometimes rises to as high as 20 to 30 mm. Hg. This excessive pressure plays a significant role in pushing extra quantities of blood toward the heart, often compensating completely for the weak heart, so that cardiac output is normal (even though the excess fluid might be harmful in other ways because of the edema that it causes). This is an example in which one hemodynamic factor, an increase in blood volume and circulatory filling pressure, opposes another factor, decreased pumping ability of the heart, to afford almost normal delivery of blood to the tissues despite a severe abnormality in the circulation.

Quantitative Method for Assessing Respective Roles of the Heart and Peripheral Circulation in Cardiac Output Regulation

Figure 6–4 presents a graphic procedure that can be used to determine the relative hemodynamic roles of the heart and of the peripheral circulation in cardiac output regulation. Note first the curve labeled "cardiac output curve." This illustrates the effect of increasing right atrial pressure on cardiac output, showing that as the pressure rises from about −4 mm. Hg up to 6 mm. Hg the cardiac output rises from zero to a plateau level of about 13 liters per minute.

The curve labeled "venous return curve" shows the effect on venous return of increasing right atrial pressure. As the right atrial pressure rises to approach approximately 7 mm. Hg (the circulatory filling pressure), the venous return falls to approach zero.

Now, let us see what happens when the two curves interact with each other. First, let us assume that the right atrial pressure is 7 mm. Hg. At this pressure, the cardiac output is 13 liters per minute and venous return is zero. Therefore, blood will be pumped rapidly out of the right atrium, and the right atrial pressure will decrease. Venous return will increase upward along the venous return curve while cardiac output will decrease downward along the cardiac output curve. As long as there is greater cardiac output than venous return, the blood volume in the heart will be decreasing and the right atrial pres-

Figure 6-4 Interrelationship between cardiac output and venous return, showing (1) that the ability of the heart to pump blood can be expressed by *cardiac output curves*, (2) that the ability of blood to flow into the heart can be expressed by *venous return curves*, and (3) that the actual operating conditions of the circulation are expressed by the equilibrium point at which the two curves cross. The point labeled CFP represents the circulatory filling pressure of the system. (Modified from Guyton, A. C., et al.: Circulatory Physiology: Cardiac Output and Its Regulation. 2nd ed. Philadelphia, W. B. Saunders Co., 1973.)

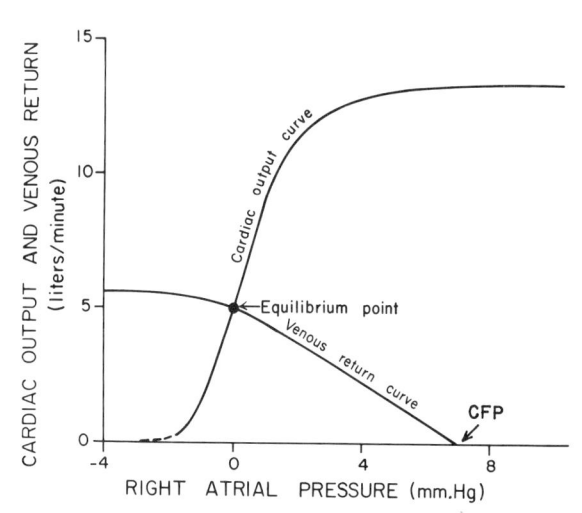

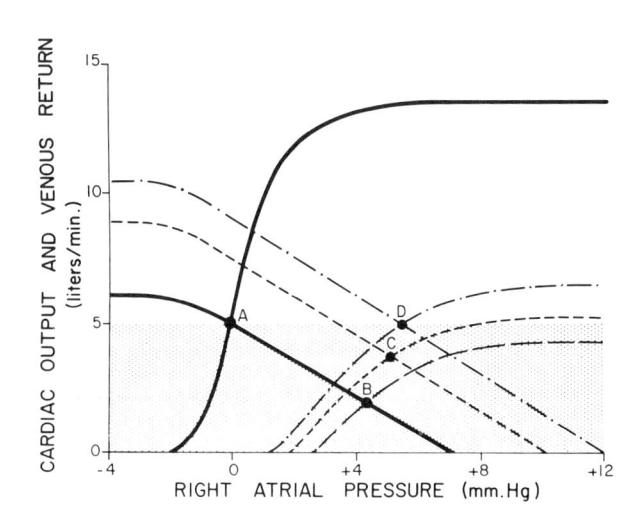

sure will be falling. But when the right atrial pressure reaches that point at which the two curves cross each other, venous return and cardiac output become equal, and the right atrial pressure also becomes stable. Therefore, this point is called an "equilibrium point," depicting the steady-state operational state of the circulation. In Figure 6-4, which represents the normal state of the circulation, the equilibrium point shows a cardiac output of approximately 5 liters per minute and a right atrial pressure of approximately 0 mm. Hg (with reference to atmospheric pressure).

Analysis of Sequential Events Following Acute Heart Failure. We can now use the principle of equating venous return and cardiac output curves to analyze the sequence of events following an acute heart attack. In Figure 6-5 the two dark curves represent the same normal curves as those in Figure 6-4. Immediately after the heart attack, the peripheral circulation has not yet been changed at all. However, the strength of the heart has been reduced to the long-dashed curve of the figure. This equates with the normal venous return curve at point B, showing that instantaneously the cardiac output falls to 2 liters per minute while the right atrial pressure rises to 4 mm. Hg. At this low cardiac output, the person is likely to faint and is certain to become very weak.

EFFECT OF CIRCULATORY REFLEXES. Within seconds the cardiovascular reflexes become active, and they change both the venous return curve and the cardiac output curve to the small-dashed curves. The venous return curve is changed because sympathetic stimulation tightens the blood vessels around the blood, thereby increasing the circulatory filling pressure, and in turn promoting greater tendency for blood to flow from the peripheral vessels to the

Figure 6-5 Use of cardiac output and venous return curves to analyze changes in cardiac output and right atrial pressure following acute onset of cardiac failure, showing complete cardiac output compensation at equilibrium point D after a week or more of recovery. (Reprinted from Guyton, A. C., et al.: Circulatory Physiology: Cardiac Output and Its Regulation. 2nd ed. Philadelphia, W. B. Saunders Co., 1973.)

heart. The cardiac function curve is increased because sympathetic stimulation increases the strength of contraction of the undamaged portions of the heart. These sympathetic reflexes begin to act within two to three seconds and reach full development in 30 seconds to one minute. Therefore, the cardiac output rises by this time from point B to the new equilibrium point, C, which represents a cardiac output of 3.5 liters per minute and an atrial pressure of 5.5 mm. Hg.

EFFECT OF HEART RECOVERY AND FLUID RETENTION. During the next week, the strength of the heart improves because of (a) increase in collateral circulation to the ischemic areas of the heart, (b) some degree of hypertrophy of the undamaged heart muscle, and (c) stiffening of the infarcted portion of the myocardium to reduce aneurysmal bulging of this area. Simultaneously, the low cardiac output causes the kidneys to retain water and salt for a variety of different reasons, thereby increasing the circulatory filling pressure still further, and further elevating the venous return curve. Therefore, the respective venous return and cardiac output curves become those represented by the dot-dashes, and the new equilibrium point becomes point D in Figure 6-5. By this time, the cardiac output has returned to normal, and renal output of water and salt is again in balance with the intake of water and salt. However, in the meantime, the body has accumulated fluid, the blood volume has increased a small amount, and the right atrial pressure has now risen to 6 mm. Hg. Yet, despite the fact that the pumping capacity of the heart is only one half normal, the cardiac output has returned essentially to normal. This demonstrates again the importance of the peripheral circulatory system in long-range control of cardiac output.

Cardiac Output Regulation in Abnormal States

Figure 6-6 illustrates the effects of different abnormal states on cardiac output. One can readily understand most of the different factors that decrease the cardiac output in such states as myocardial infarction, hemorrhagic shock, traumatic shock, valvular heart disease, and cardiac shock. On the other hand, the factors that increase the cardiac output above normal are not so readily understood.

High Output States. Each one of the high output states illustrated in Figure 6-6 is associated with reduced total peripheral resistance. For instance, in beriberi, the total peripheral resistance is often reduced to as low as 50 per cent of normal, and in patients with A-V shunts the total peripheral resistance is rarely reduced to as low as 30 to 40 per cent of normal. In anemia, blood viscosity

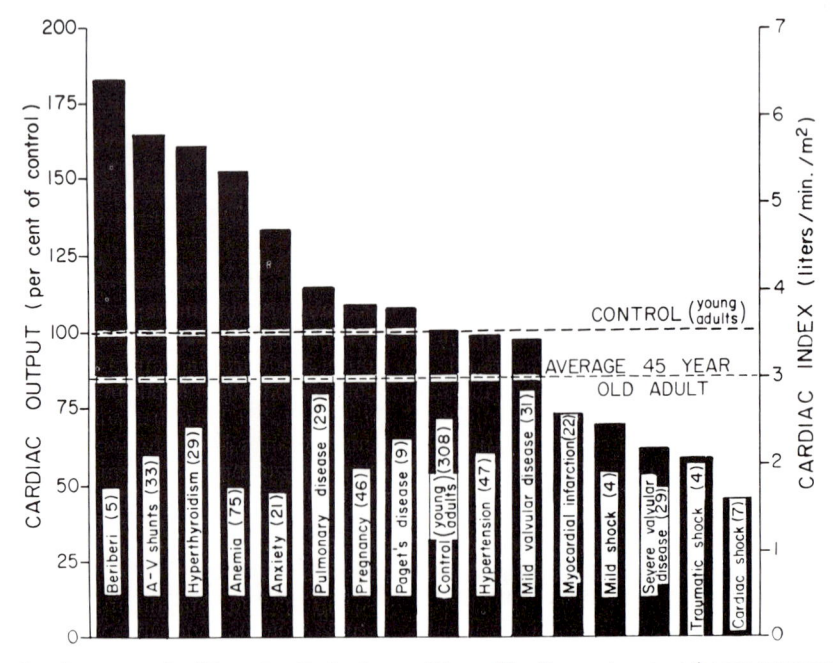

Figure 6-6 Cardiac output in different pathologic conditions. The figures in parentheses represent numbers of patients from which the average values were obtained. (Constructed from data in National Academy of Sciences: Handbook of Circulation, Philadelphia, W. B. Saunders Co., 1959.)

is greatly reduced and, also, diminished delivery of oxygen to the tissues causes vasodilatation; thus, two different effects decrease the total peripheral resistance. In pulmonary disease, diminished delivery of oxygen to the tissues can dilate the peripheral vessels and, also, increased metabolism because of extra respiratory effort dilates the blood vessels in the respiratory muscles; both these effects reduce the total peripheral resistance. And, finally, in pregnancy and in Paget's disease, increased vascular shunting in both these conditions decreases total peripheral resistance.

Thus, in none of these high cardiac output conditions can one ascribe the high output to excess pumping capacity of the heart. Instead, one finds the total peripheral resistance to be decreased and the cause of the increased cardiac output to be increased venous return. Indeed, in many of these conditions, the pumping capacity of the heart is actually reduced rather than increased.

One might suspect hyperthyroidism and anxiety to be exceptions to this rule that high output is caused by peripheral factors, because the heart becomes hyperactive in both these states. However, increasing heart activity caused by pacing it at a high rate in a normal resting person or in an animal does not significantly alter cardiac output, even though this procedure does indeed increase the pumping capacity of the heart itself. Therefore, at present, there is no proved condition in which higher than normal cardiac output is caused by increased pumping capacity of the heart itself. The increased pumping capacity merely increases the cardiac reserve, not the cardiac output.

Low Output Caused by Cardiac Insufficiency. The above principles illustrate once again that so long as the heart has unused cardiac reserve, the cardiac output is controlled almost entirely by factors in the peripheral circulation. However, when the cardiac reserve approaches zero, and particularly when the cardiac pumping capacity actually falls below the needs of the body's tissues, the heart becomes the limiting factor in the control of cardiac output. This is illustrated in Figure 6-6 by the cardiac outputs in patients with myocardial infarction, severe valvular heart disease, and cardiac shock. All these conditions impose limits on the amount of blood that the heart can pump. Note also that in these conditions the peripheral tissues lose their ability to control their own local blood flows because the heart does not supply enough blood flow to allow this luxury. Therefore, the flows in the respective tissues will no longer be distributed according to the needs of the tissues. As a consequence, one would expect some tissues to deteriorate more than others. The one most notably affected is usually the kidneys, which can cause death of the person even if all the other tissues do survive.

VENOUS PRESSURE, ITS REGULATION, AND ITS ABNORMALITIES

Venous pressure regulation is inextricably tied to the regulation of cardiac output, which one can see by referring to both Figures 6-5 and 6-6. At the same time that venous return interacts with the cardiac pumping capacity to determine cardiac output it also determines right atrial pressure, which is the central venous pressure. Therefore, any factor that affects either the heart's pumping capacity or venous return from the systemic circulation will also affect central venous pressure. In general, increased pumping capacity of the heart is associated with reduced central venous pressure, while diminished pumping capacity is associated with elevated central venous pressure. Also, any peripheral circulatory factor that increases venous return is associated with increased central venous pressure, while any factor that reduces venous return is associated with diminished central venous pressure. However, when factors affect both the heart and the peripheral circulation simultaneously, the central venous pressure is then determined by a balance between the two respective factors; the only way to determine this balance accurately is by use of some quantitative method such as the graphic method illustrated in Figures 6-5 and 6-6.

Circulatory Filling Pressure as the Upper Limit to Central Venous Pressure. Referring again to Figure 6-5, one will note that as the right atrial pressure rises to approach the circulatory filling pressure, venous return approaches zero. Therefore, the upper limit to which the central venous pressure can rise is the circulatory filling pressure. The normal value for this filling pressure in the dog (it has never been measured in human beings) is 7 mm. Hg. However, when the venous return and cardiac output fall below normal, nervous reflexes can increase the filling pressure up to levels as high as 18 to 20 mm. Hg. Therefore, if the normal heart is weakened slowly enough for the reflexes to develop completely, cardiac output will decrease to zero only when the right atrial pressure rises to a maximum value of 18 to 20 mm. Hg.

In pathologic conditions that cause retention of body fluids and consequent increase in blood volume, the circulatory filling pressure, even without reflex stimulation, can be as high as 20 to 30 mm. Hg — in congestive failure, for instance. Therefore, progressive deterioration of the heart under these conditions can cause the central venous pressure to rise to maximum values of 20 to 30 mm. Hg, or perhaps even higher than this for short periods of time because of superimposed action of sympathetic reflexes.

Peripheral Venous Pressure versus Central Venous Pressure. Unfortunately, the peripheral venous pressure does not always correlate well with central venous pressure. The reason for this is that veins are frequently compressed in their courses to the heart, and the pressure beyond each compression point must rise enough to overcome the compression before the blood vessel will open enough to allow blood flow. The peripheral venous pressure, therefore, is more often a measure of the degree of venous compression than a measure of the central venous pressure. For this reason, to obtain meaningful venous pressure measurements, it is usually necessary to pass a catheter into a central vein. The tip of this catheter need not pass all the way into the right atrium, however, because the negative intrathoracic pressure keeps the central veins widely open so that central venous pressure measured anywhere inside the thoracic cavity will be within 1 mm. Hg of the right atrial pressure itself.

When the central venous pressure rises above 6 to 10 mm. Hg, the pressure in many or most of the peripheral veins then becomes great enough to overcome external compression on the veins. When this happens, the peripheral veins remain filled essentially all the time, and the resistance between the peripheral veins and the central veins becomes very slight. Therefore, now, the pressure measured in the peripheral veins becomes nearly equal to the pressure in the central veins (except for hydrostatic pressure difference). Furthermore, pressure waves generated in the right atrium as a result of cardiac pumping are now transmitted with ease along the veins. This accounts for the obvious pulsation of the veins in the neck in congestive heart failure.

Hydrostatic Reference Level for Measuring Venous Pressure. Extremely minute changes in central venous pressure can have marked effects on the output of the heart, which can be understood by referring to the cardiac output curve in Figure 6-5. In this figure, an increase in right atrial pressure from 0 to 1 mm. Hg is shown to increase the cardiac output approximately 30 per cent. Therefore, all central venous pressures must be measured at a very exact hydrostatic pressure level to be meaningful. Different reference levels have been suggested, such as one third the thickness of the chest behind the sternum, 10 cm. anterior to the back, and so forth. However, physiological studies have shown that there is one point in the heart at which the central venous pressure changes less than 1 mm. Hg, regardless of the position of an animal. This is the very midpoint of the tricuspid valve. A basic physiological reason for the constancy of pressure at this point is the following: Whenever the pressure at the tricuspid valve rises above its normal control value, the right ventricle fills more than normally and automatically pumps the increased quantity of blood out of the right ventricle; this obviously decreases the tricuspid pressure back toward normal. Conversely, decreased pressure at the tricuspid valve decreases the filling of the ventricle so that less blood is pumped; therefore, the pressure rises once again back to its normal control value at the tricuspid valve level.

Thus, a physiologic hydrostatic reference point for measurement of venous pressure is the midpoint of the tricuspid valve. However, if the venous pressure is always measured with the patient in precisely the same position from one time to another and from one patient to another, any of the hydrostatic reference points—such as 10 cm. in front of the patient's back—will usually serve adequately. One of the most unforgivable mistakes, however, is to refer the measured pressure to the level of the catheter tip, because it makes no significant difference where the tip of the catheter lies in the central veins; the hydrostatic column of blood inside the veins beyond the tip of the catheter compensates for changes in position of the catheter tip, still making it essential that the pressure be measured in relation to the tricuspid valve.

ARTERIAL PRESSURE AND HEMODYNAMIC FACTORS IN ITS REGULATION*

Fortunately, our bodies possess a large number of arterial pressure control mechanisms, no one of which can regulate arterial pressure under all conditions, though the total consortium of these mechanisms performs admirably. Eight of the best known arterial pressure control systems are described in the following sections. Three of these are strictly hemodynamic controls: the stress relaxation, the capillary-fluid shift, and the renal-body fluid mechanisms. The last of these is a crucial one in the long-term control of arterial pressure.

1. The Baroreceptor Reflex. An increase in arterial pressure stretches the *baroreceptors* (also called pressoreceptors) located in the carotid sinuses, in the arch of the aorta, and in other large central arteries. Signals from these are transmitted to the brain stem and thence back to the peripheral blood vessels to dilate them and also to the heart to decrease its pumping activity; both these effects reduce the arterial pressure back toward normal.

2. The Chemoreceptor Reflex. A decrease in arterial pressure decreases blood flow to the *chemoreceptors* in the carotid and aortic bodies. The decreased flow decreases the available oxygen to the chemoreceptors and also enhances the

---

*Further discussions in this area are presented in Chapter 7.

buildup of carbon dioxide in these receptors. Both these effects stimulate the chemoreceptors, causing them also to transmit signals by way of the brain stem to the blood vessels and the heart, this time raising the arterial pressure back toward normal.

3. The Central Nervous System Ischemic Response. When the arterial pressure is reduced below approximately 50 mm. Hg, the brain stem becomes ischemic and elicits the so-called central nervous system ischemic response. This sends powerful signals through the sympathetic nerves to the blood vessels to cause vasoconstriction and to the heart to enhance its pumping activity, thus bringing the arterial pressure back up to a level that will prevent brain ischemia.

4. Stress Relaxation. When the arterial pressure rises above normal, the pressure frequently is increased in all or most of the vessels of the circulation as well as in the arteries. The smooth muscle cells of these vessels gradually become stretched, a phenomena called "stress relaxation." This increases the capacity of the vascular tree, thereby decreasing the circulatory filling pressure, decreasing cardiac output, and decreasing arterial pressure back toward normal. Conversely, when the pressures in all the respective vessels fall below normal, the blood vessels slowly contract around the blood and return the pressure back upward toward normal.

5. The Renin-Angiotensin-Vasoconstrictor Mechanism. Decrease in arterial pressure below normal causes the kidneys to release renin. The renin in turn enzymatically splits angiotensin from renin substrate in the plasma proteins. The angiotensin then causes peripheral vasoconstriction, and it also causes secretion of aldosterone. The vasoconstriction causes a direct effect to increase total peripheral resistance and thereby returns the arterial pressure back upward toward normal.

6. The Aldosterone Pressure Regulating Mechanism. Decrease in arterial pressure increases aldosterone secretion both because angiotensin stimulates the adrenal cortex and also because of other not yet understood effects of decreased arterial pressure acting either directly or indirectly on the adrenal glands. The increased aldosterone in turn causes the kidneys to retain salt, which then has several indirect effects to cause the kidneys also to retain water. The increased water and salt increases the extracellular fluid volume, which increases blood volume, which increases cardiac output, which in turn increases arterial pressure back toward normal.

7. The Capillary-Fluid Shift Mechanism. Increase in arterial pressure is frequently accompanied by an increase in capillary pressure. When this occurs, excess fluid begins to filter from the capillaries into the tissue spaces thereby reducing the blood volume, reducing cardiac output, and reducing arterial pressure back toward normal. This effect also operates in the opposite direction when the capillary pressure falls below normal.

8. The Renal-Body Fluid Pressure Regulating Mechanism. A decrease in arterial pressure has a direct effect on the kidneys to reduce renal output of water and salt. This results primarily from (a) decreased glomerular filtration rate caused by decreased glomerular pressure, and (b) increased tubular reabsorption caused by reduced peritubular capillary pressure. The result is retention of water and salt in the body and consequent progressive increase in extracellular fluid volume and blood volume as the person ingests additional quantities of water and salt. The increase in blood volume increases cardiac output and thereby returns the arterial pressure back toward normal. This mechanism is essentially the important hydrodynamic feedback control system illustrated at the outset of this chapter in Figure 6-1.

Interaction of Different Pressure Control Systems—The Concept of Feedback Gain

The greatest problem in understanding arterial pressure regulation has been to understand how all the different pressure regulating mechanisms interact with each other and under what conditions the different ones are important. To understand this, it is first necessary to explain the concept of feedback gain in control systems.

Let us assume that the normal arterial pressure is 100 mm. Hg and that some abnormal factor suddenly increases this pressure to 180 mm. Hg. The baroreceptors become stretched, and within seconds the baroreceptor reflex returns the arterial pressure to about 110 mm. Hg. Thus, 70 mm. Hg compensation occurs, and there is still 10 mm. Hg abnormality. The ratio of these two values is a mathematical measure of the ability of the control system to control arterial pressure; this ratio is also the feedback gain of the system. In this case the feedback gain is 70 divided by 10, or a gain factor of 7.

To give another example, if the arterial pressure is increased above its control value by sudden closure of a large arteriovenous fistula, the kidneys begin to excrete more water and salt than the net intake of these. Consequently, the body fluid volumes decrease, cardiac output decreases, and arterial pressure returns to normal. Furthermore, the arterial pressure will not stop falling until urinary output of water and salt returns exactly to equal the intake, which means that the arterial pressure must return all the way back to its control value and not merely a certain proportionate way. Therefore, the correction is some finite value, and the final abnormality is zero. A finite value divided by zero is infinity. Therefore, the renal-body fluid feedback mechanism for control of arterial pressure has a feedback gain of infinity when allowed long enough time to respond fully.

In a similar manner, we can derive gains for the eight well-known arterial pressure control mechanisms. The values for these are approximately the following when each is operating under optimum conditions:

CNS ischemic response	11.0
Baroreceptor reflex	7.0
Chemoreceptor reflex	4.0
Stress relaxation mechanism	2.8
Capillary-fluid shift mechanism	2.5
Renin-angiotensin-vasoconstrictor mechanism	1.6
Aldosterone, body fluid pressure control mechanism	4.0
Renal-body fluid pressure control mechanism	∞

Response Times of Respective Arterial Pressure Control Mechanisms. Figure 6-7 illustrates the response times of the different pressure control mechanisms. Note that the time scale is a logarithmic one, beginning with seconds and then extending to minutes, hours, and days. The three nervous feedback mechanisms—the baroreceptor, the chemoreceptor, and the CNS ischemic effects—all begin to act within seconds and reach full gains within 30 seconds to a minute. Therefore, these are the mechanisms that are most important for control of arterial pressure from second to second or from minute to minute. They are the mechanisms that prevent sudden death following rapid bleeding and that prevent fainting when a person stands up. Each of the three nervous pressure control mechanisms operates in a different pressure range. The baroreceptors function most effectively at pressures between 80 and 180 mm. Hg, the chemoreceptors between 40 and 100 mm. Hg, and the CNS ischemic response mainly below 40 to 50 mm. Hg. The extreme gain of the CNS ischemic response at very low pressures causes it to resist strongly any final decrease of pressure below about 30 mm. Hg. It causes the sympathetic nervous system to become stimulated to its maximum, causing the heart to beat very forcefully and causing the highest possible degree of sympathetic constriction of the peripheral vessels. Therefore, this mechanism is frequently called the "last-ditch stand" against final circulatory collapse.

At least three non-nervous pressure control mechanisms begin to operate within minutes and continue to operate perhaps for hours or days. These are the stress relaxation mechanism, the renin-angiotensin-vasoconstrictor mechanism, and the capillary-fluid shift mechanism. None of them has a major amount of gain, but when multiplied by the gains of the other mechanisms they play very significant roles in maintaining normal arterial pressure temporarily in such conditions as slow bleeding, dehydration, and loss of the nervous controls of the circulation.

Finally come the long-term controls of arterial pressure, which are based primarily on retention of water and salt by the kidneys. The aldosterone mechanism has a finite gain while the direct renal-body fluid pressure control mechanism has

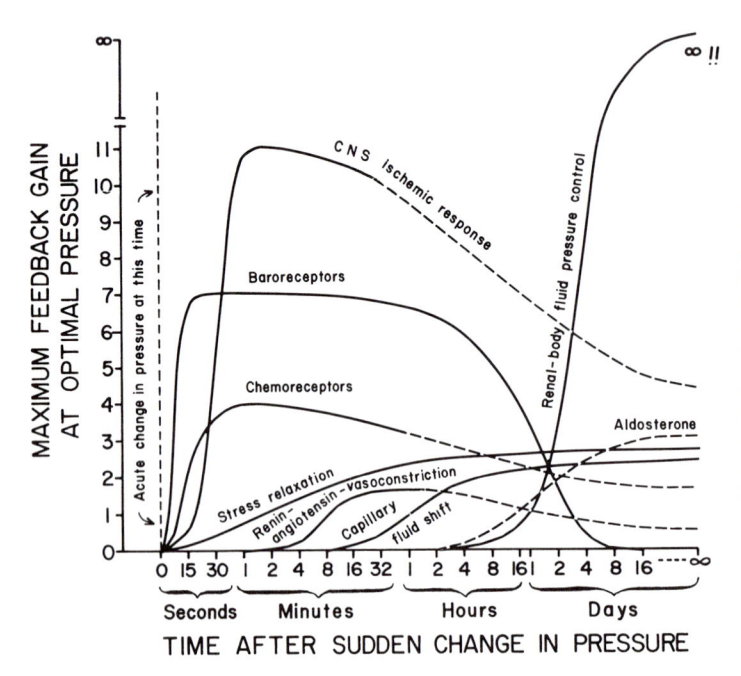

Figure 6-7 Response times of the major arterial blood pressure regulating mechanisms. This figure also shows approximate feedback gains of these mechanisms at different times after their responses have been initiated. Note especially the infinite gain that occurs in the renal-body fluid pressure control mechanism at infinite time. (Preprinted from projected publication by Guyton, A. C., Coleman, T. G., and Cowley, A. W., Jr.: Arterial Pressure Regulation and Hypertension. Philadelphia, W. B. Saunders Co.)

infinite gain if given adequate time to come to full equilibrium, which in practice is several weeks. Because of this infinite gain, the renal-body fluid pressure control mechanism is the one that under long-term conditions dominates arterial pressure control for reasons that will be discussed in more detail in the following section.

Importance of Infinite Gain in Renal-Body Fluid Pressure Control Mechanism and Its Significance in Long-term Arterial Pressure Regulation

When two or more control systems attempt to control the same factor at the same time, the contribution of each of the systems toward the final level of control is determined by the ratio of their gains. Note in Figure 6–7 that, at infinity time, the renal-body fluid pressure control system has infinite gain while all the others have finite gains. Therefore, the ratio of the renal-body fluid pressure control system to all the others is infinity divided by some finite value, which is still infinity. Consequently, the long-term arterial pressure level calculates to be entirely in the hands of the renal-body fluid pressure control system. Let us explain this mechanism more fully.

Renal output of water and electrolytes is highly dependent on arterial pressure. A decrease in arterial pressure from its normal mean value of 100 mm. Hg to 60 mm. Hg decreases renal output essentially to zero, while, on the other hand, an increase in pressure to twice normal (to 200 mm. Hg) increases renal output of water and salt to 6 to 8 times normal. Using this information one can easily understand the renal-body fluid pressure control mechanism if he will refer back to Figure 6–1 showing the interrelationships of the major circulatory hemodynamic factors. Note that two separate factors determine whether or not extracellular fluid volume will at any given instant be increasing or decreasing. These are the renal output of water and electrolytes and the net intake of water and electrolytes (intake by mouth minus that lost by nonrenal routes). If these two are exactly in balance, the extracellular fluid volume will be stable. Likewise, the blood volume, circulatory filling pressure, venous return, arterial pressure, and renal output of water and electrolytes will all be stable. However, if the arterial pressure becomes artificially altered, the renal output of water and electrolytes also becomes out of balance with the net intake of these, and the extracellular fluid volume will be changing. Furthermore, all the other factors in the control loop shown in Figure 6–1 will also change until the intake and output become equal again, which is the only stable state for the system. This occurs when the arterial pressure returns exactly to its original level.

Determinants of the Long-term Level of Arterial Pressure.

It is axiomatic that the renal output of water and electrolytes must in the long run exactly balance the net intake of water and electrolytes. Figure 6–8 illustrates all the factors that affect this balance. These include (a) changes in intake of water and salt; (b) changes in nonrenal loss of water and salt, such as through dehydration, diarrhea, or dialysis; and (c) that collection of different factors that control renal output of water and salt. One notes from the figure that arterial pressure is only one of the factors that determine fluid balance. Furthermore, if any other factor changes, the arterial pressure must change to a new value to re-establish the steady-state balance between fluid intake and output, and this is accomplished automatically by the renal-body fluid feedback system. Therefore, all the other factors shown in Figure 6–8 besides arterial pressure itself are long-term determinants of the arterial pressure.

Lack of Correlation Between Arterial Pressure and Cardiac Output, Total Peripheral Resistance, and Blood Volume. For years investigators have argued the importance of total peripheral resistance, cardiac output, blood volume, and extracellular fluid volume in the regulation of the long-term level of arterial pressure. However, one will note in Figure 6–8 that none of these four factors is listed as a primary determinant of the long-term steady-state level of arterial pressure. To give an example, a change in cardiac output can obviously cause a temporary change in arterial pressure. But if this causes the renal output to become unequal to the intake of water and salt, the extracellular fluid volume, blood volume, and cardiac output will all be altered up or down until that level of arterial pressure is achieved as required by the determinants shown in Figure 6–8. Therefore, extracellular fluid volume, blood volume, and cardiac output are nothing more than *dependent variables* in the system.

It is exceedingly important to understand the difference between the determinants of the long-term arterial pressure level and the dependent variables because a change in a determinant will always of necessity alter the long-term pressure. On the other hand, a change in one of the dependent variables will simply throw the system out of balance temporarily, but the system will automatically readjust the variables until the arterial pressure comes back exactly to where it was. Therefore, it is mainly fruitless to argue whether or not one of the dependent variables correlates with arterial pressure. For instance, in the type of hypertension that occurs immediately after a massive transfusion, the total peripheral resistance is greatly reduced while cardiac output is greatly elevated. On the other hand, in hypertension caused by a pheochromocytoma, the total peripheral resistance is greatly increased while the cardiac output is often reduced. Thus, these fac-

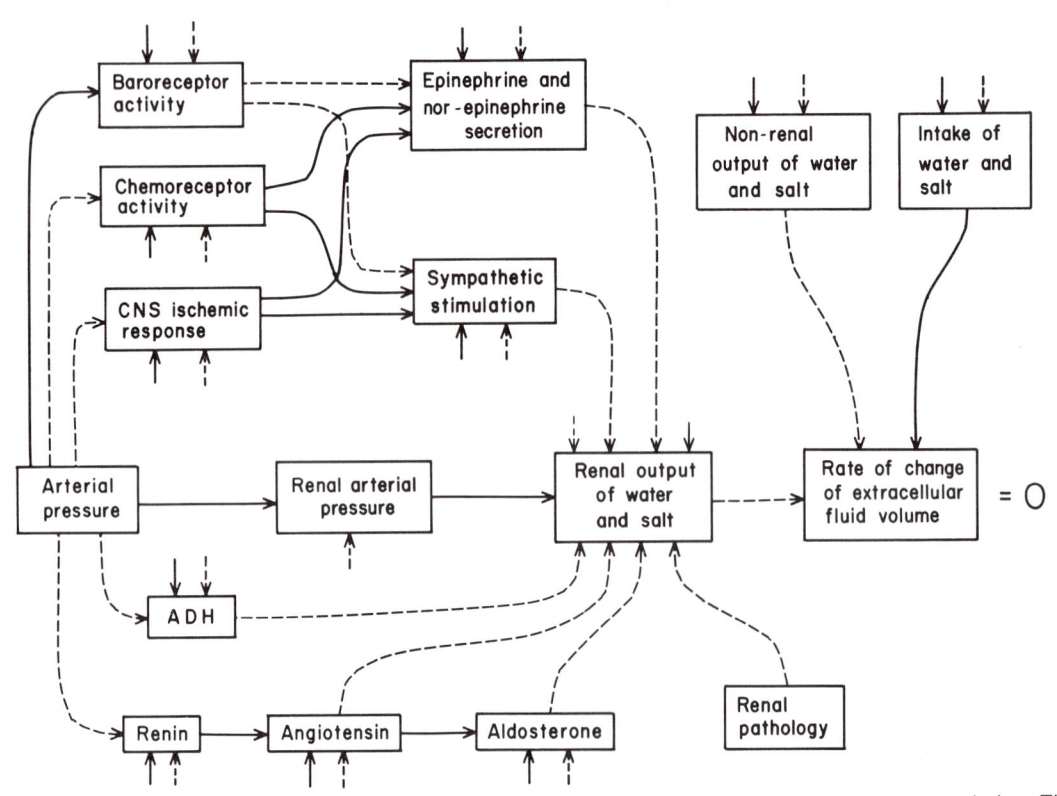

Figure 6-8 Diagrammatic representation of the determinants of long-term arterial pressure regulation. This figure shows that only those factors which determine the relationship of arterial pressure to the balance between renal output of water and electrolytes, on the one hand, and net intake of these (intake minus nonrenal output), on the other hand, can be determinants of long-term arterial pressure regulation. (Preprinted from projected publication by Guyton, A. C., Coleman, T. G., and Cowley, A. W., Jr.: Arterial Pressure Regulation and Hypertension. Philadelphia, W. B. Saunders Co.)

tors are nothing more than manipulated pawns in the regulation of arterial pressure.

CAPILLARIES AND CAPILLARY EXCHANGE

The body has roughly 50 billion capillaries, and their total cross-sectional area is a thousand or more times the total cross-sectional area of the aorta. It is rare that any cell of the body lies more than 30 to 50 microns from the nearest capillary. These facts bespeak the functions of the capillaries, namely, to deliver nutrients or humoral agents to the cells and to remove excreta from the cells.

The principal means for capillary exchange of both water and nutrients between the blood and the interstitial fluid is by the process of *diffusion*. In fact, diffusion is so great through the capillary walls that water molecules diffuse in each direction several thousand times as rapidly as the blood itself flows in the capillaries. Therefore, there is constant mixing of most of the constituents of the interstitial fluids with those of the blood.

Dynamic Equilibrium at the Capillary Membranes

Figure 6-9 illustrates a capillary in juxtaposition to its surrounding tissues. It also shows colloid osmotic pressures and hydrostatic pressures on each side of the capillary membrane. It is the dynamic equilibrium at this capillary membrane that prevents excessive quantities of fluid from filtering through the capillary membranes into the interstitial spaces. This can be explained as follows.

Since plasma proteins leak through the capillary membrane only to a slight extent, their concentration in the blood remains relatively high, causing a normal plasma colloid osmotic pressure of about 28 mm. Hg in the human being. The plasma protein that does leak into the interstitial spaces creates an average interstitial fluid colloid osmotic pressure of about 5 mm. Hg, varying from as little as 1 to 2 mm. Hg in some tissues with only slightly porous capillary membranes, such as in the brain, to as high as 20 mm. Hg in tissues with extremely porous membranes, as in the liver. The colloid osmotic pressure of the plasma is so much greater than that of the interstitial fluid that it creates a continual force for movement of fluid from the interstitial spaces into the capillaries. In Figure 6–9 this difference between the two colloid osmotic pressures is shown to be 23 mm. Hg, that is, a *net* colloid osmotic absorptive force of this amount.

On the other hand, the average "functional" capillary pressure in the capillaries, as measured in several different ways, averages about 17 mm. Hg. This value is considerably lower than the 25 mm. Hg so often taught in the past. This hydrostatic pressure tends to force fluid outward through the capillary membrane. Yet, when it competes with the 23 mm. Hg colloid osmotic absorptive force attempting to move fluid inward, one finds 6 mm. Hg more absorptive force than hydrostatic force tending to force fluid outward. Therefore, under normal circumstances, there seems to be a net absorptive capability of the capillaries, which theoretically can create a *negative* pressure (less than atmospheric pressure) in the interstitial spaces averaging about −6 mm. Hg. On studying Figure 6–9 once again, a hydrostatic pressure of −6.5 mm. Hg is shown in the tissue spaces rather than the theoretical value of −6. The extra 0.5 mm. Hg is caused by the pumping action of the lymphatics, which causes a minute trickle of fluid to flow from the tissue spaces into the lymph vessels and thereby creates slightly more negative pressure in the interstitial spaces than can theoretically be accounted for by the colloid osmotic and hydrostatic forces at the capillary membrane.

If we now add separately the colloid osmotic and the hydrostatic forces on the two sides of the membrane, we find a colloid osmotic pressure difference of 23.0 mm. Hg (28 minus 5) attempting to cause absorption and a hydrostatic difference of 23.5 mm. Hg (17 minus −6.5) attempting to force fluid outward from the capillaries. Summing these values there is a net *filtration pressure* averaging about 0.5 mm. Hg at the capillary membrane. This 0.5 mm. Hg represents a continual state of nonequilibrium at the membrane, and it causes net filtration of fluid out of the capillaries into the tissue spaces, thereby providing the small trickle of fluid that flows into the lymph vessels. The lymph vessels in turn transport the fluid back into the circulation, so that a steady state develops, with neither loss of fluid out of the circulation nor gain of fluid.

LYMPHATIC DRAINAGE FROM THE TISSUES

In a sense, the lymphatic system is older than the venous system because in lower phylogenetic levels whole blood is discharged directly from small blood vessels into the tissue spaces; the blood cells, along with other tissue fluid constituents, are then drained into lymphatic type vessels that pump the mixture back toward the heart. In higher animals some of these early vessels have

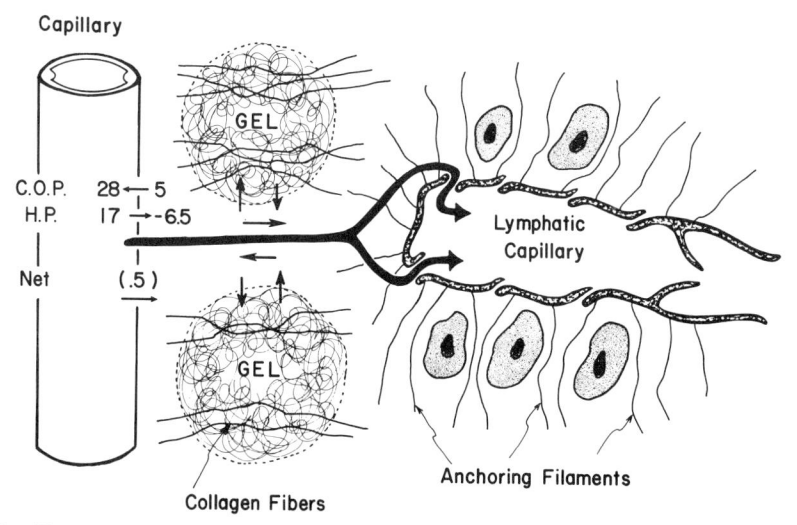

Figure 6–9 Capillary, tissue fluid, and lymph vessel relationships, illustrating dynamics at the capillary membrane, net outflow of fluid from the capillaries into the lymph vessels, and diffusional exchange of fluid and dissolved substances within the free fluid of the interstitial spaces and between the free fluid and the gel fluid.

become the lymph vessels while others have become a less porous tubular system that is composed of the capillaries and veins. The lymph vessels still perform the same function that they did in the lower animals, namely, they drain any excess fluid, cells, and debris that collect in the interstitial spaces.

Determinants of Lymph Flow

The rate of lymph flow is determined by three major factors: (1) pumping action of the lymph vessels themselves, (2) pumping effect of tissue motion, and (3) the pressure of fluid in the tissue spaces.

Lymphatic Valves and Pumping Action of the Lymph Vessels. The lymph vessels undergo continual rhythmic contraction, this occurring in all lymph vessels from the lymph capillaries up to the thoracic duct itself. Also all lymph vessels larger than the lymph capillaries have valves which are all oriented toward the point of discharge from the lymphatic system into the circulation at the junctures of the jugular and subclavian veins. Because of this orientation of the valves, contraction of a section of a lymph vessel will propel fluid toward the circulation but never backward toward the tissues. Combining this valve function with the natural rhythmic contraction of the lymph vessels, the larger lymph vessels can pump against a pressure head of at least 15 to 20 mm. Hg.

Lymphatic Pumping Caused by Tissue Motion. Obviously, any tissue motion that compresses the lymph vessels from the outside can also compress fluid from one lymph vessel segment to another, but only in the direction that the valves are oriented. Therefore, tissue motion provides another propelling force to cause flow in the lymph vessels.

The Terminal Lymphatic Capillary Pump. Lymphatic motion also causes lymphatic pumping at the very tips of the lymphatic capillaries, which can be understood by referring again to Figure 6–9. The endothelial cells lining the lymphatic capillary are shown in this figure to overlap each other. At the point of overlap, the cells are not attached, but instead, their inner edges can flap to the interior. Therefore, if the pressure outside the capillary is greater than that inside, fluid can push the flaps open and move to the interior. On the other hand, if the capillary is compressed so that the pressure inside becomes greater than that on the outside, any attempt of the fluid to escape from the capillary will close the flaps. Thus, the junctures between the endothelial cells are actually valves, allowing fluid to move into the lymphatic capillary but not in the outward direction.

Other structures important to terminal lymphatic pumping are the *anchoring filaments.* These are shown attached to the outside surfaces of the endothelial cells. They extend into the surrounding tissues where they are held tightly between the cells by the hyaluronic acid gel that fills the intercellular space. When the tissues are compressed, the cells compress the lymphatic capillary and cause fluid to move away from the capillary toward the larger lymphatics. Then, when the tissues recoil because of the tissue turgor, the anchoring filaments pull the lymphatic capillary to an open position. Experiments indicate that this creates a negative pressure inside the capillary and causes fluid to flow from the surrounding tissue areas into the lymphatic capillary. Once filled, another cycle of compression of the capillary will again force fluid into the larger lymph vessels. Thus, tissue motion of any type creates actual sucking at the very tips of the terminal lymphatic capillaries, and it is this sucking action that keeps the trickle of fluid flowing from the tissue spaces into the lymphatic system and from there back into the blood circulation.

Recent motion pictures have shown that even the terminal lymphatic capillaries undergo rhythmic contraction several times a minute, presumably caused by myofibrillae in the cytoplasm of the endothelial cells themselves. Obviously, this contraction also aids in the suction pump action of the terminal lymphatic capillaries. It is still a question whether this rhythmic motion is strong enough to be of significant value in comparison with the tissue motion itself.

Effect of Interstitial Fluid Pressure on Lymph Flow. Though the large lymph vessels can pump against a pressure head of 15 to 20 mm. Hg, the suction pump at the tips of the vessels seems to be a relatively weak one, having in most tissues a suction limit of about −7 mm. Hg. In other words, if the interstitial fluid pressure falls below −7 mm. Hg, flow becomes essentially zero despite full pumping by the terminal suction pump.

When the interstitial fluid pressure rises above −7 mm. Hg, the lymphatic suction pump begins to function, and the rate of lymph flow increases almost linearly until the interstitial fluid pressure rises to equal atmospheric pressure. The normal rate of lymph flow from a typical peripheral tissue at a normal interstitial fluid pressure of approximately −6.5 mm. Hg is about 0.1 ml. of lymph per 100 grams of tissue per hour, illustrating the extremely slow trickle of fluid that normally flows in the lymphatics. However, when the interstitial fluid pressure rises to approach 0 mm. Hg (atmospheric pressure level), lymph flow increases 10- to 50-fold, now delivering as much as 1 to 5 ml. per 100 grams of tissue per hour.

INTERSTITIAL FLUID DYNAMICS AND EDEMA

There is a very common misbelief that the interstitial spaces are large baggy chambers filled with freely mobile fluid. Even though the interstitial fluid spaces do represent about one sixth of the total tissue by volume, this concept is still far from the truth. Instead, the interstitial compartment is highly structured, filled primarily with two types of structural elements: (1) collagen fibers and (2) a gel matrix composed mainly of hyaluronic acid. The amount of freely mobile fluid in normal tissue spaces is probably a fraction of 1 per cent.

Figure 6–9 illustrates two gel masses lying between a blood capillary and a lymphatic capillary and also surrounded by tissue cells. Actually, this diagram is very disproportionate because it shows a large free fluid space between the two gel bodies, while in normal tissues this space is nothing more than minute sluices along the cell surfaces. This figure also shows two types of fluid mobility that occur within the interstitial spaces. The large arrows show a net trickle of fluid from the capillary through the tissue free fluid sluice and thence into the lymphatic capillary. The small arrows illustrate diffusion of substances into and out of the blood capillary and also back and forth between the free fluid space and the gel. Thus, continual dynamic equilibria exist between the different fluid compartments of the tissues.

Interstitial Pressures—Interstitial Fluid Pressure, Solid Tissue Pressure, and Total Tissue Pressure. In an earlier section of this chapter we have already pointed out that the normal *interstitial fluid pressure* in the free fluid of the interstitial spaces is about –6.5 mm. Hg, which is caused by the terminal lymphatic suction mechanism and by a tendency for the colloid osmotic pressure of the plasma to cause absorption of fluid from the tissue spaces.

However, another type of pressure also occurs in the interstitial spaces. This is pressure exerted by the solid elements of the tissues and is called *solid tissue pressure*. When fluid is removed from the free fluid spaces by capillary osmosis or by lymphatic pumping, the decreased pressure in the free fluid immediately sucks fluid from the gel into the free fluid, and this fluid also is removed. Therefore, suction occurs in the entire interstitial space. In consequence, the walls of the interstitial spaces crowd toward each other only to be held apart by the positive solid tissue pressure exerted by the solid structures in the spaces.

The solid structures in the interstitial spaces that exert solid tissue pressure are mainly the collagen fibers plus the reticulum of the hyaluronic acid gel. At present we do not know how much of the solid tissue pressure is caused by the gel and how much by the collagen and other fibers. However, the sum of these pressures must be great enough to oppose the negative suction effect of the interstitial fluid pressure, and it must also be great enough to overcome any other compressional forces that exist on the tissues such as pressure exerted by a blood pressure cuff, pressure caused by turgor of the skin, pressure caused by compression points on the surface of the body, and so forth. When the skin and other tissues exert zero turgor and there is no compression from outside the body, the algebraically averaged solid tissue pressure must exactly equal the negative of the interstitial fluid pressure. If the fluid pressure is –6.5, then the solid tissue pressure must be 6.5. If we assume a skin turgor of another 2 mm. Hg, then the solid tissue pressure would be 8.5 mm. Hg.

Finally, one can sum the interstitial fluid pressure and the solid tissue pressure to determine still another quantity, the *total tissue pressure*, which is the pressure acting on any surface in a tissue by the summated effects of both the fluid and the solid elements. Assuming an average interstitial fluid pressure of –6.5 mm. Hg and a solid tissue pressure of 8.5 mm. Hg, then the total tissue pressure would be 2.0 mm. Hg.

Significance of the Different Types of Tissue Pressure. Because the above three different types of tissue pressure all exist in the tissue spaces, and because different methods for measuring tissue pressure measure different ones of these pressures, major confusion has developed regarding the true tissue pressure and its significance. However, if one will follow the logic of the above discussion, one can readily see that each of the different types of tissue pressure has its own peculiar significance, as follows:

Interstitial fluid pressure is the pressure that promotes fluid movement (a) from one part of a tissue to another part, (b) through the pores of a capillary membrane, or (c) from the tissue spaces into the lymphatics. In other words, interstitial fluid pressure relates to the fluids themselves and the forces that cause their mobility in the tissues.

Solid tissue pressure is pressure caused by contact points between solid elements of the tissues. Therefore, the greater the solid tissue pressure, the greater will be the forces exerted by these contact pressure points and, therefore, also the greater will be the distortional forces caused in the tissues. It is solid tissue pressure that causes the shapes of cells to be irregular, causes at least part of the folding of the fibers in the tissue spaces, and distorts such structures as capillaries, and so forth.

Interstitial fluid pressure and solid tissue pressure can be summated with each other by any structure that is capable of summating forces over a spatial domain. For instance, if fluid is compressing a capillary at one point and a fiber at a slightly different point, the elastic coefficient of the capillary membrane allows it to summate these two compressional forces even though they are not acting at precisely the same point. This is also true of cell membranes and of any other solid surface in a tissue. Therefore, total tissue pressure can act on any solid surface in a tissue. One of the most important of these solid surfaces is the blood vessels. Thus, the compressional force of the tissues against the blood vessels is equal to the total tissue pressure and is not equal to either the interstitial fluid pressure or the solid tissue pressure alone except when one of these is zero.

If we recognize, in accord with the discussion in the above section, that interstitial fluid pressure, solid tissue pressure, and total tissue pressure are usually very different from each other, one can understand the importance of distinguishing them. In clinical medicine the two that are especially important are the interstitial fluid pressure, which is related primarily to the problem of interstitial fluid edema, and total tissue pressure, which is related primarily to the problem of blood vessel collapse.

Measurement of the Different Types of Tissue Pressure. MEASUREMENT OF TOTAL TISSUE PRESSURE. Methods are now available for measuring both interstitial fluid pressure and total tissue pressure. From these two values one can calculate the algebraically averaged solid tissue pressure.

The time-honored method for measuring tissue pressure has been to insert a minute needle into the tissue, then to inject about 1 cu. mm. of fluid at the tip of the needle, and, finally, to measure the pressure in this minute bolus of injected fluid using an extremely low compliance pressure measuring device. When pressure is measured in this manner, it gives a value of 1 to 3 mm. Hg, which is equal to the total tissue pressure. One might ask why this method measures total tissue pressure rather than interstitial fluid pressure, particularly in view of the fact that fluid is at the tip of the needle. The answer to this is that the fluid injected into the tissue temporarily displaces the solid tissue elements, so that the solid tissue pressure at this point is temporarily zero. Therefore, so long as the small bolus of fluid remains at the tip of the needle, its surface with the tissue is pressed against by the total tissue pressure, so that the pressure measured is total tissue pressure and not interstitial fluid pressure. If, however, one waits 30 seconds to several minutes after injecting the bolus of fluid and then records the pressure, it will likely be extremely erratic, depending upon whether the tip of the needle has become occluded with tissue and upon many other factors. Sometimes it still measures the positive value and sometimes it measures values as low as -20 to -30 mm. Hg (particularly when there is motion in the tissues and a ball-valve action develops at the tip of the needle).

Therefore, this method can be used for measuring total tissue pressure only so long as the bolus of fluid is still present at the tip of the needle. Unfortunately, it cannot measure the true interstitial fluid pressure, which develops in the spaces surrounding the tip of the needle only after a few minutes is allowed for absorption of the bolus of fluid. Further proof that this method measures total tissue pressure is afforded by pressures measured in minute flaccid balloons implanted in the tissues. These balloons, because of their continuous surface structure, certainly measure total tissue pressure, and they too measure a pressure of 1 to 3 mm. Hg in most tissues.

MEASUREMENT OF INTERSTITIAL FLUID PRESSURE. To measure interstitial fluid pressure, some device must be inserted into the tissue that can remain there long enough for the fluid in the interstitial spaces to come to equilibrium with fluid in the device. The method that has been used most successfully thus far has been to implant a small hollow but porous capsule, 0.5 to 2.0 cm. in diameter, in the tissue. Over a period of days, the fluid inside the capsule comes to equilibrium with the fluid in the surrounding spaces. When pressure is measured inside this capsule, it is found to average about -6.5 mm. Hg in most tissues of the body (though not this low in tissues with tight capsules such as the kidneys, which give higher pressure).

Unfortunately, the implanted capsule method is often not applicable to clinical patients, though it has been applied in a few instances in human beings. A newer method has recently been developed which gives an indication of the interstitial fluid pressure but probably does not measure its true value in all instances. This is a wick method in which a small wick of cotton protruding from the tip of a 1 mm. Teflon tube is inserted into the tissue and allowed to come to equilibrium for about one half hour. A low displacement manometer connected to the Teflon tube then records a pressure of about -2 to -5 mm. Hg, a less negative pressure than that usually measured with the perforated capsule. However, the fact that this method does measure a negative pressure demonstrates that other methods besides the porous capsule method can also be used for measuring negative interstitial fluid pressure. Furthermore, the wick method can be applied to the human being, though the problem of bleeding around the inserted wick is likely to nullify the validity of the pressure measurements. Those who have employed this method thus far in human beings have used it primarily for determining *changes* in interstitial fluid pressure rather than for measuring true value of the pressure.

Regulation of Interstitial Fluid Protein

Since interstitial fluid protein is one of the major factors in controlling the dynamic equilibrium of capillary exchange, it is important to understand how interstitial fluid protein concentration itself is regulated. The above discussions can now be used to explain this. When the interstitial fluid protein concentration rises to a high value, a high colloid osmotic pressure is created in the interstitial fluid. This in turn causes the dynamic equilibrium at the capillary membrane to be unbalanced toward the tissue space, increasing the quantity of fluid transuding through the capillary membrane into the tissue space. As a result, interstitial fluid volume increases, and interstitial fluid pressure also increases, causing increased lymph flow, as discussed earlier. The increased lymph flow carries fluid away from the tissue spaces, and this fluid is replaced by fluid transuding through the capillary membrane having a protein concentration only about 0.1 gram per 100 ml. in comparison with 2.0 grams per 100 ml. average concentration in the fluid removed by the lymphatic vessels. Therefore, replacement of the high-protein interstitial fluid by low-protein interstitial fluid returns the interstitial fluid protein concentration back to its normal level.

Conversely, if the tissue fluid protein concentration falls too low, lymph flow decreases and most of the fluid transuding into the interstitial spaces from the capillaries is reabsorbed as a result of the colloid osmotic forces at the venous ends of the capillaries. The protein is not reabsorbed along with the water. In this process, the protein concentration rises progressively until it once again returns to its normal value.

In clinical conditions in which the capillaries become highly permeable, such as in burns, occasionally in severe chronic hypoxia, in allergies, and so forth, the greatly enhanced tendency for proteins to transude into the tissue spaces biases the protein control mechanism in favor of increased tissue fluid protein. However, a factor that will increase tissue protein concentration to its greatest extent is lymphatic blockage. When this occurs, the lymphatic protein removal mechanism discussed above becomes incapable of diluting the proteins in the interstitial fluids; yet, the venous capillary reabsorptive mechanism for removing fluid (but not protein) will cause continual buildup of protein in the tissue spaces until its concentration approaches that of the plasma.

Regulation of Interstitial Fluid Pressure

Almost identically the same mechanism regulates interstitial fluid pressure as that which regulates interstitial fluid protein. That is, if the pressure becomes too great, lymph flow increases. The lymph flow in turn drains some of the excess fluid from the interstitial spaces and reduces the pressure. However, the pressure is reduced even more in still another way, as follows: The increased lymph drainage carries increased quantities of protein away from the interstitial spaces, thereby reducing the interstitial fluid colloid osmotic pressure. When this happens, the still high colloid osmotic pressure of the plasma causes osmotic reabsorption of fluid from the interstitial spaces into the blood. This second effect normally accounts for nine tenths or more of the reabsorption of excess fluid from the usual tissue space, while the lymphatic drainage mechanism accounts for less than one tenth. In severe edematous states, on the other hand, the lymphatic drainage mechanism becomes progressively more important, sometimes outdoing the osmosis mechanism because of the extreme rates of lymph flow that occur at high interstitial fluid pressures.

Regulation of Interstitial Fluid Volume

Obviously, the regulation of interstitial fluid volume is also closely related to the regulation of both interstitial fluid pressure and interstitial fluid protein, because whenever the interstitial fluid volume increases, the tissue spaces expand and correspondingly the interstitial fluid pressure increases. The same sequence as that described earlier for both interstitial fluid pressure and interstitial fluid protein regulation ensues once more: namely, increased pressure increases lymph flow, decreases tissue colloid osmotic pressure, increases capillary osmotic absorption of fluid from the tissue spaces, and thereby returns interstitial fluid volume back toward normal. Therefore, all these factors operate together in a simple but extremely important basic control system to keep the interstitial fluid pressure, protein concentration, and fluid volume all regulated to very exact levels.

Physiologic Basis of Edema

Positive Interstitial Fluid Pressure as Cause of Edema. In several thousand measurements of interstitial fluid pressure using the perforated capsule technique and encompassing both nonedematous and edematous tissues, it has been found that loose areolar subcutaneous tissues will invariably be edematous if the interstitial fluid pressure is positive—that is, above atmospheric pressure; on the other hand, the tissues will be nonedematous if the pressure is negative (less than atmospheric pressure). Therefore, whether or not edema exists in these tissues seems to be determined by a simple factor: whether or not the interstitial fluid pressure is above atmospheric pressure or less than atmospheric pressure.

The Normally "Dry" State of the Interstitial "Free" Fluid Compartment. The free fluid volume and the volume of nonmobile fluid in the gel state of both normal and edematous tissues has been estimated by studying the mobility of fluids in the tissue spaces. Figure 6–10 illustrates these findings. At a normal interstitial fluid pressure of −6.5 mm. Hg there is essentially zero free fluid, as shown in the figure, while, on the other hand, there are approximately 12 liters of nonmobile gel fluid in the adult human being.

Thus, in the normal interstitial fluid spaces, the interstitial fluid volume is regulated to essentially zero free fluid. Furthermore, whenever any significant amount of free fluid begins to develop in the tissues, the lymphatic and capillary osmotic mechanisms normally return this free fluid to the circulatory system almost immediately. Thus, in effect, the mechanisms for regulating interstitial fluid volume normally maintain an almost completely "dry" state in the *free* fluid compartment of the interstitial spaces. The fluid that does exist in the interstitial spaces is almost entirely that fluid which is bound in the form of a gel.

Character of the Interstitial Fluids in Edema—Pitting Edema. Note also in Figure 6–10 the changes in both free fluid and nonmobile fluid volumes when the interstitial fluid pressure rises. The nonmobile fluid volume increases about 30 per cent as the interstitial fluid pressure rises from −6.5 mm. Hg up to zero—that is, before frank edema occurs. This is caused by the natural tendency of the gel reticulum to expand and thereby to pull fluid into the gel. However, when the free interstitial fluid pressure rises above zero, the gel has by then expanded to its limit, so that thereafter the nonmobile gel fluid volume does not increase further. Instead, above this very critical level of zero pressure the free interstitial fluid volume increases drastically.

The sudden increase in *free* fluid volume as the interstitial fluid pressure rises above atmospheric pressure accounts for the pitting phenomenon observed in most forms of extracellular fluid edema. Free fluid is highly mobile in the tissue spaces, while the gel fluid is almost completely nonmobile. Therefore, in the normal state of the interstitial spaces, pitting does not occur. On the other hand, when vast amounts of free fluid de-

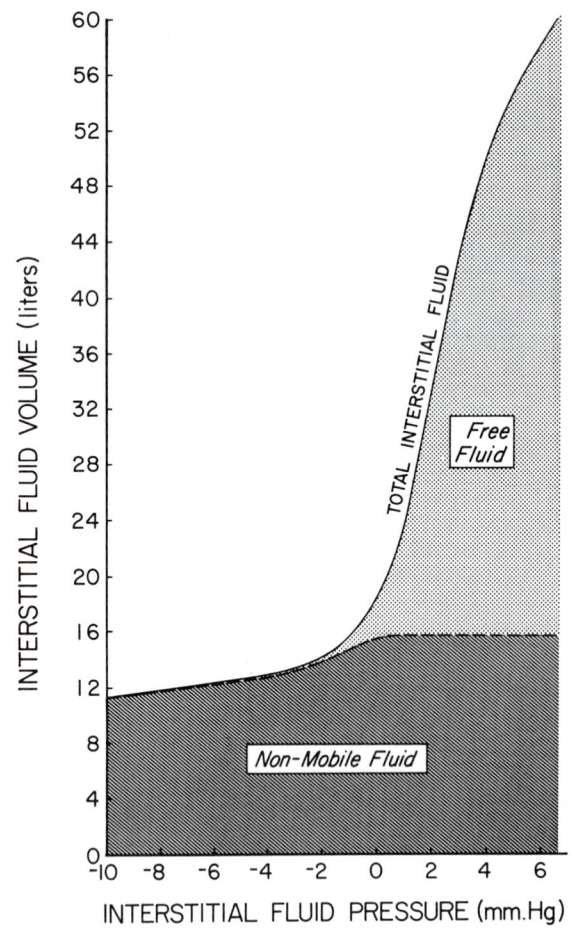

Figure 6–10 Changes in total interstitial fluid volume, free fluid volume, and nonmobile fluid volume (gel fluid) and the tissue spaces as the interstitial fluid pressure rises from a negative value of −10 up to a positive value of 7 mm. Hg. Note the rapid appearance of free fluid in the interstitial spaces as the interstitial fluid pressure crosses from the subatmospheric pressure range into the supra-atmospheric pressure range. (Reprinted from Guyton, A. C., Granger, H. J., and Taylor, A. E.: Physiol. Rev., *51*:527, 1971.)

velop, the fluid can be made to flow freely from one sector of the tissues to another. Thus, pressure with a finger on an edematous area will translocate fluid from the point of compression, and a pit will remain for a few seconds to a minute or more after the finger is removed—that is, until the fluid has time to flow back into the pitted area.

The high mobility of free fluid in edema also explains several other clinical phenomena such as the continual weeping of wounds in edematous tissues and the failure of wounds to heal in edematous tissues. It explains, too, at least part of the dependent nature of edema. For instance, if a person has generalized edema, fluid can actually flow through the tissues from the top side of the body to the low side, such as from one breast to the other in a patient lying on her side. Obviously, another cause of dependent edema is high pressure in the dependent capillaries in the edematous state.

Role of Gel in the Interstitial Spaces. Though still too little research has been performed on the functional importance of gel in interstitial spaces, it probably has at least three very valuable functions. One of these is to prevent dependent edema even in the normal person. Measurements of fluid flow in free fluid versus fluid flow through hyaluronic gel have shown a difference of several millionfold. In other words, the fact that the tissue spaces are normally filled with gel and not with free fluid prevents the fluid from flowing from the upper parts of the body to the lower parts. With one sixth of our body composed of interstitial fluid, one can readily understand that if the fluid were not in a gel state, both legs would almost certainly be perpetually edematous.

Second, the nonmobile nature of the gel prevents spread of infection in the tissues. Indeed, some bacteria are extremely pathogenic simply because they secrete hyaluronidase to dissolve the gel and allow movement of the local fluids with consequent spread of the bacteria.

Third, the gel probably is important to keep the formed elements of the tissues separated appropriate distances from each other. Since most nutrients are transported from the capillaries to the cells and most excreta from the cells to the capillaries by the process of diffusion, it is essential that appropriate avenues be maintained for adequate diffusion through the spaces. If the cells should be crowded completely upon each other, enough space would not be available for the diffusion process and one would expect outlying cells to be deficient in certain nutrients. For instance, glucose will not diffuse through cells because it becomes trapped inside cells. Therefore, it is essential that glucose diffuse *between* cells if it is to reach those cells far removed from the capillaries. Fortunately, such substances diffuse in tissue gel almost equally as rapidly as in the free fluid. On the other hand, the diffusion process operates most efficiently for short distances of diffusion. Therefore, it is important that the mechanism for controlling interstitial fluid volume maintain the volume only at a certain level—not too little, not too much. This is accomplished by the mechanism that maintains the tissue fluid compartment normally dry of free fluid and limits the volume to the gel fluid.

Tissue Nutrition in Edema. One of the major problems in edema is nutrition of the tissue cells, because expansion of the tissue spaces increases the distances required for diffusion. Every physician becomes cognizant of this when treating varicose ulcers of the leg, because it is almost impossible for these to heal in a continuously edematous leg. Also, nutrition of essentially any tissue of the body can be compromised at least to some extent by edema. Indeed, functional measurements in the heart have even shown that an edematous myocardium has considerably decreased pumping capability.

Aside from the decreased nutrition caused by increased diffusion distances, edema fluid can reduce nutrition in still another way: by compressing the blood vessels. This phenomenon is especially striking when the tissues are in a tight binder, such as in a cast, or when fibrin clots block the lymph vessels, causing interstitial fluid pressure to rise to very high levels.

Role of Capillary and Lymphatic Dynamics in Causation of Edema. The roles of the capillaries and of the lymphatics in causing edema are so well known that they require only transient mention at this point. There are basically four dynamic abnormalities that can theoretically cause edema: (1) high capillary pressure, (2) low plasma colloid osmotic pressure, (3) increased permeability of the capillaries, and (4) blockage of the lymphatics. All these tend to increase the interstitial fluid pressure, and when this pressure rises above the atmospheric pressure level, edema occurs. Increased permeability of the capillaries increases the tendency for edema in three ways: (a) by allowing more rapid leakage of fluid into the tissue spaces; (b) by decreasing the effectiveness of the proteins to cause colloid osmotic pressure at the capillary pores (that is, the proteins leak through the pores rather than create colloid osmotic pressure); and (c) by buildup of protein in the interstitial spaces and loss of protein from the blood to cause greatly enhanced tissue colloid osmotic pressure as well as reduced plasma colloid osmotic pressure. Though the literature frequently refers to all three of these as being important, one can show mathematically that only the last of the three is of real significance, namely, increased tissue colloid osmotic pressure and decreased plasma colloid osmotic pressure because of protein leakage. Long before the other two can possibly become important, this last effect will have killed the patient because of massive edema and volume depletion.

Safety Factor Against Edema

Fortunately, the human being has tremendous capability for resisting the development of edema. For instance, the capillary pressure in a usual tissue must rise to approximately two times normal before edema will appear, or the colloid osmotic pressure of the plasma must fall from the normal level of 28 mm. Hg to below 10 mm. Hg before edema will occur. From the previous discussion of interstitial fluid dynamics and of edema, one can readily understand how these tremendous safety factors come about.

Basically, edema cannot occur until the interstitial fluid pressure rises above atmospheric pressure, and there are three different mechanisms that come into play to prevent this from occurring. These are the following:

1. The normal negative interstitial fluid pressure of approximately −6.5 mm. Hg must be lost before edema can occur. Therefore, the mechanisms discussed above for maintenance of the normal negative interstitial fluid pressure constitute the first safety factor.

2. When the interstitial fluid pressure begins to rise, lymph flow increases rapidly, increasing an average of 20- to 25-fold by the time the interstitial pressure reaches atmospheric pressure. This greatly enhanced lymph flow constitutes a second safety factor against edema. Approximately 7 mm. Hg excess filtration pressure is required across the capillary membrane to form the amount of lymph that can be carried away by the normal lymph vessels.

3. When the lymph flow increases, the rapid flushing of fluid through the interstitial spaces toward the lymph vessels washes protein out of the interstitial spaces. This decreases the colloid osmotic pressure in normal interstitial fluid from about 5 mm. Hg down to approximately 1 mm. Hg. Therefore, the plasma colloid osmotic pressure becomes 4 mm. Hg more effective for absorbing fluid from the tissue spaces. This adds another 4 mm. Hg of safety factor.

Adding the above safety factors, 6.5 + 7.0 + 4.0, one finds a total safety factor of approximately 17.5 mm. Hg. This explains the necessary decrease in colloid osmotic pressure from a normal value of 28 down to 10 mm. Hg before edema will occur. It also explains the doubling of capillary pressure required before edema occurs, an increase from 17 to 34 mm. Hg, or a safety factor of 17 mm. Hg. Finally, recent experiments have also shown that edema can be caused in an arm exposed to an external vacuum greater than 18 mm. Hg but cannot be caused by a vacuum less than 18 mm. Hg.

There, obviously, is a clinical state which one might call "pre-edema," which means a state in which much of the safety factor has been dissipated even though the edema state itself has not yet been reached.

BLOOD VOLUME AND ITS REGULATION

Hemodynamic Factors. The basic hemodynamic mechanisms for blood volume regulation can be understood by combining the discussions from previous sections of this chapter. First, referring again to Figure 6–2, one notes that an increase in blood volume increases cardiac output, which increases arterial pressure, which increases urinary output, which decreases extracellular fluid volume, which finally returns the blood volume back toward normal. All steps of this mechanism have been proved in individual physiological experiments. Also, in animals with the nervous system completely destroyed, infusion of several hundred milliliters of saline causes approximately a 10-fold increase in urinary output within less than one minute. This increase continues, but with progressive decrement, for several hours until the urinary output gradually dwindles back to its control value. In the meantime, essentially all the excess saline infused is recovered in the urine.

Nervous Factors. Dilatation of the atria of the heart initiates potent nervous vasodilating reflexes to the kidneys and also transmits signals to the neurohypophysis to diminish the secretion of antidiuretic hormone. Both these effects increase the output of urine. Therefore, it is frequently said that the atrial receptors are "volume receptors" that detect increases in blood volume and in turn help to rectify the abnormality. However, this mechanism seems to be important in volume regulation only transiently, because the high atrial pressures occurring in heart failure do not cause continued excessive urinary output, as the mechanism would suggest.

Relationship Between Blood Volume Regulation and Interstitial Fluid Volume Regulation

Retention of fluid by the kidneys does not mean that the fluid will necessarily remain in the blood, because extracellular fluid is partitioned between the plasma compartment of the blood and the two interstitial fluid compartments, the free fluid compartment and the gel compartment. Under normal circumstances, in the absence of edema, the free fluid compartment volume of the interstitial spaces is essentially zero, and it is only the gel compartment with which we are concerned. When extra amounts of fluid are available, the recoil effect of the gel reticulum causes the gel to absorb moderate amounts of the extra fluid. On the other hand, in dehydration states—that is, when the interstitial fluid pressure falls to a very low level—fluid is pulled out of the gel and returned to the circulation either by capillary osmosis or through the lymphatics. Therefore, there is a dynamic equilibrium between the plasma volume and the interstitial gel volume.

Measurements have shown that infusion of a balanced electrolyte solution into the circulatory system of a nonedematous person will cause approximately two thirds of the fluid to enter the gel compartment of the tissue spaces and one third to remain in the blood. Therefore, in the pre-edema state, retention of water and salt by the kidneys increases both blood volume and interstitial fluid volume. Conversely, dehydration decreases both of these; indeed, severe dehydration can cause shock.

Tissue Compliance Change in Edema. An entirely different effect occurs once the edema stage is reached, that is, once the interstitial fluid pressure rises above atmospheric pressure level. Referring again to Figure 6-10, one notes that the total interstitial fluid volume now increases extremely rapidly but with almost no additional rise in the interstitial fluid pressure. This is in contrast to a marked rise in pressure occurring along with the volume increase in nonedematous tissues. The reason for this difference is that the walls of normal tissue spaces are tightly collapsed around the gel, and the volume cannot change without simultaneous marked changes in the negative pressure that is dehydrating the gel. On the other hand, once the interstitial fluid pressure rises into the positive pressure range, there is not a significant restraining force to prevent outward stretching of the tissue spaces. The only major restraining force is the skin, and measurements show that the skin exerts less than one twenty-fifth as much restraining force on changes in the interstitial fluid volume as do the elastic forces of the gel. To express this another way, in the negative interstitial fluid pressure range, the compliance of the tissue space is slight, while in the positive interstitial fluid pressure range the looseness of the skin and other tissue elements allows the compliance to increase 25-fold.

Therefore, once the interstitial pressure rises to a positive value, tremendous quantities of free fluid begin to collect in the tissue spaces, and this fluid collects despite extremely little additional rise in interstitial fluid pressure.

Safety Valve Function of the Interstitial Fluid Spaces for Blood Volume. The significance of edema to the circulatory system probably has escaped most physiologists and clinicians alike, because the ability for tremendous quantities of fluid to collect rapidly in tissue spaces when the blood volume rises above a certain critical level is actually an important safety valve for the circulatory system. Were it not for this, it would be impossible to infuse more than 1 to 3 liters of electrolyte solution into a normal patient without killing him, which one can demonstrate anytime he wishes by simply infusing several liters of fluid into a person at a rate too rapid for the fluid to transude out of the capillaries into the interstitial spaces. Pressures throughout the system rise to extreme values and can cause rupture of vessels, arrhythmias of the heart, and typical signs of acute cardiac failure.

Therefore, the edema mechanism is an important safety valve for blood volume control in the human being. Furthermore, this "safety valve" functions at a very exact capillary pressure level—at exactly that capillary pressure at which the total safety factor against edema has been dissipated.

Significance of Blood Volume Measurements and of Circulatory Filling Pressure

Because it is very easy to measure blood volume by injecting any type of indicator material that will stay in the circulatory system and then measuring the degree of dilution of the indicator, blood volume measurements are frequently made, yet they are rarely of great significance. The reason for this is elementary: blood volume is automatically adjusted to fit the capacity of the circulatory system itself, and even such oddities as varicose veins can change both the capacity of the circulatory system and the blood volume markedly. Likewise, a state of vasoconstriction, as occurs in patients with pheochromocytomas, can greatly reduce the capacity of the circulation. Or vasodilatation, as caused by block of the sympathetic nervous system, can increase the capacity of the system.

The tightness with which the blood volume fills the circulatory system is measured by the circulatory filling pressure, and this can change as a result of a change in either blood volume or circulatory capacity. From our earlier discussion of cardiac output regulation, it is clear that it is not blood volume per se that affects venous return and cardiac output but, instead, the circulatory filling pressure. Therefore, alteration of the circulatory filling pressure, whether it be caused by changing blood volume or by a change in capacity of the system, has essentially the same effect on the circulation.

Consequently, the factor that needs to be measured, so far as the dynamics of the circulation are concerned, is not blood volume but, instead, circulatory filling pressure. In animals, in which it is possible to stop the heart and to bring pressures to equilibrium throughout the system, it is possible to measure this pressure, the normal value for which is 7 mm. Hg. In human beings, this measurement has never been achieved. In the meantime, one can understand why blood volume measurements are much less useful in explaining hemodynamic function of the circulation than are such functional measurements as arterial pressure and cardiac output.

Effect of Right Atrial Pressure on Blood Volume

Every clinician is very familiar with the fact that an increase in right atrial pressure, as occurs in heart failure, is usually associated with increased blood volume. This can also be understood on the basis of hemodynamics already discussed in this chapter. When the heart fails and the right atrial pressure increases, venous return immediately decreases, thereby reducing cardiac output, arterial pressure, and urinary output. Consequently, the body fluid volumes begin to increase and continue to increase until the circulatory filling pressure has risen enough to oppose the negative effect of right atrial pressure on venous return. When this has been achieved, a new steady state will have been reached. But, in the meantime, since the circulatory filling pressure has been greatly increased—for instance, an increase in right atrial pressure of 6 mm. Hg will cause almost a 6 mm. Hg rise in circulatory filling pressure, from the normal value of 7 up to 13 mm. Hg—one can readily understand how this increases blood volume.

In acute conditions, an increase in circulatory filling pressure of 1 mm. Hg increases blood volume a little over 2 per cent. However, in chronic conditions, in which the phenomenon of stress relaxation allows slow stretching of the circulatory system, a rise in circulatory filling pressure of 1 mm. Hg is associated with as much as 5 per cent increase in blood volume. Therefore, in patients with long-standing congestive heart failure, in which the circulatory filling pressure can rarely be as high as 25 mm. Hg, the blood volume can sometimes increase to as much as 50 to 100 per cent above normal.

PULMONARY CIRCULATION

Many of the same hemodynamic principles that apply to the systemic circulation also apply to the pulmonary circulation, but because of special functions of the lungs, this is not entirely true. For instance, the pulmonary system is a low pressure system, for which reason it has correspondingly thinner arterial and arteriolar vasculature, as well as less smooth muscle in the vessel walls. This is very fortunate, because the pulmonary vasculature receives the same stroke volume output from the right heart that the entire systemic arterial tree receives from the left heart. The high degree of distensibility of the pulmonary arteries, despite their short length, is of major advantage in allowing the pulmonary vascular tree to absorb the large thrust of blood with each heart beat. Also, because of very low pulmonary vascular resistance from the arteries to the veins, only about one tenth that of the systemic circulation, there is marked runoff of blood from the pulmonary arteries to the left atrium even before systole is complete, which decreases the quantity of blood that must be accommodated in the pulmonary arterial tree. These two factors acting together cause the pulmonary arterial pulse pressure to be only about 14 mm. Hg, in contrast to 40 mm. Hg in the aorta.

One might also ask himself why the pulmonary circulatory system can operate with a very low pressure while the systemic system must have a much higher pressure. This can be answered by simply considering the function of the pulmonary circulation. In general, each alveolus subserves the same function as all the other alveoli. Therefore, it is not nearly so important in the lungs as in the systemic circulation to control blood flow differentially in different parts of the lungs.

Effect of Alveolar Hypoxia on Local Vascular Resistance. There are three important exceptions to the usual rule that blood flow is distributed indiscriminately to all alveoli. The first of these exceptions occurs when some alveoli are ventilated to less extent than others. If the poorly ventilated alveoli were perfused with blood to the same extent as the other alveoli, the oxygen in the poorly ventilated alveoli would become depressed, thereby creating hypoxia in the blood of adjacent blood vessels. However, the effect of hypoxia on these vessels is exactly opposite to its effect on systemic vasculature, causing in this instance vasoconstriction instead of vasodilatation. The vasoconstriction reduces the perfusion of the affected alveolar walls and thereby shunts blood flow to other alveoli that are better ventilated. Unfortunately, though, this mechanism is a very weak one—that is, it does not have a very high feedback gain, having a maximum gain of perhaps one. Therefore, it is not as important a mechanism as one might wish it to be to control distribution of blood flow to the respective alveoli.

Pulmonary physiologists have also pointed out that hypoxia of all the alveoli can sometimes cause enough vasoconstriction of the total pulmonary vasculature to elevate pulmonary arterial pressure significantly. In some instances, the rise in pulmonary arterial pressure seems to be enough to cause right heart failure with corresponding reduction in right ventricular output and, therefore, also reduction in cardiac output. Oxygen therapy often aids this condition, presumably by decreasing the pulmonary vascular resistance.

Effect of Atelectasis on Local Blood Flow. The second condition in which unequal distribution of alveolar blood flow occurs to a significant extent is atelectasis. When a bronchus is blocked, the alveoli beyond the block begin to collapse within minutes, and whole segments of the lung can become collapsed over a period of hours. The mechanical collapse of the alveoli causes the solid tissues between the alveoli to close tightly around the local blood vessels, in some cases actually kinking the vessels. As a result, in total atelectasis over 80 per cent of the blood flow is usually shunted to the normal lung tissue. This is a very fortunate mechanism because it ensures that essentially all the blood flow passing through the lungs will flow in juxtaposition to ventilated alveoli and will bypass nonventilated alveoli.

Effect of Hydrostatic Pressure on Local Blood Flow in the Lung. Still a third hemodynamic factor that causes nonuniform blood flow in the pulmonary circulation is the different hydrostatic levels of the different parts of the lung. When a person is in a standing position, the apex of his lung lies as much as 10 to 15 cm. above the midlevel of the heart, which means that the pulmonary arterial pressures are only barely high enough to pump blood through the apical vessels. Indeed, only the systolic pressure is high enough, so that blood flows through the apical vessels in spurts synchronized with cardiac systole. At the base of the lung, on the other hand, located some 10 cm. below the level of the heart, the pulmonary vessels are subjected not only to normal pulmonary vascular pressure but also to an additional 7 mm. Hg hydrostatic pressure. Therefore, both the diastolic and systolic pressures are considerably elevated in the base of the lung, and blood flows through this region continuously throughout systole and diastole. This difference creates another problem, namely, that in the standing, quiet state the base of the lung is overperfused while the apex is underperfused. This effect is partially compensated by the fact that the base of the lung is, for mechanical reasons, ventilated to a greater extent than is the apex. Fortunately, during exercise, when the fullest functional capacity of the lungs is needed, the pulmonary pressures rise throughout the lungs, and all portions now reach almost optimal ventilation-perfusion ratios.

Pulmonary Edema

Principles almost identically the same as those discussed earlier for the systemic circulation apply to capillary dynamics in the lungs, but a few differences are important.

Normal Mechanism for Keeping the Alveoli "Dry." To keep the alveoli in their normal "dry" state—that is, filled with air rather than with fluid—the pulmonary interstitial fluid pressure is almost certainly negative in the same way that it is in peripheral tissues. Though this interstitial fluid pressure has not been measured with accuracy, measurements from implanted perforated capsules in the lungs have given a negative pressure value averaging about −5 mm. Hg. Negative pressure in the interstitial spaces of the lungs would obviously keep the alveolar membrane pulled tightly against the capillaries and their supporting structures. It would also provide an absorptive force for causing absorption of any stray fluid that might occur in the alveoli, thus returning the alveoli to their normal dry state.

On the other hand, if the interstitial fluid pressure of the lungs should ever rise into the positive range, one would expect pulmonary edema to result in the same way as edema results in peripheral tissues.

Safety Factor Against Pulmonary Edema. The safety factor against edema in the lungs is greater than in systemic tissues. The pulmonary capillary pressure must be increased acutely to approximately 30 mm. Hg, or to about 2 mm. Hg greater than the colloid osmotic pressure of the blood, before pulmonary edema will ensue. Since the normal pulmonary capillary pressure in the human being is about 7 mm. Hg, the safety factor against pulmonary edema can be calculated to be approximately 23 mm. Hg, which compares with 18 mm. Hg in the systemic circulation. An acute increase in pulmonary capillary pressure above 30 mm. Hg will cause a proportionately increased rate of fluid transudation into the lungs (based on studies in dogs), and when the pressure is raised acutely to 50 mm. Hg it can cause lethal pulmonary edema in as little as one half hour.

Role of Lymphatics in Chronic Pulmonary Edema. In chronic pulmonary edema, still another safety factor occurs. Even a few weeks of elevated left atrial pressure causes great overgrowth of the pulmonary lymphatics, increasing their lymph carrying capacity sometimes as much as 6- to 10-fold. Therefore, one would expect that pulmonary capillary pressure would have to rise much higher than the 30 mm. Hg required in acute conditions before pulmonary edema would occur. This corresponds to the finding in many catheter laboratories that patients with chronic mitral stenosis frequently have chronic elevations of pulmonary capillary pressure in the 35 to 45 mm. Hg pressure range without evident pulmonary edema.

Alveolar Membrane Leakage and Alveolar Fluid in Pulmonary Edema. Another primary difference between pulmonary edema and systemic edema is that the limiting boundary of the pulmonary interstitial spaces, the alveolar membrane, is a very thin and weak one-cell layer membrane. Therefore, in contrast to the skin on the surface of the body, the alveolar membrane cannot withstand significant amounts of positive pressure in the interstitial spaces of the lungs. Evidence at present indicates that these alveolar membranes begin to break when the interstitial fluid pressure rises above approximately 1 to 2 mm. Hg positive pressure. When this happens, fluid in the interstitial spaces of the lungs simply flows immediately into the alveoli. Therefore, only very early pulmonary edema can be confined to the interstitial spaces; if this edema develops to any significant extent, a major share of the edema fluid immediately flows through the broken alveolar membranes into the alveoli themselves.

ARTERIAL PULSATION

Arterial pulsation is so well understood by most clinicians that it hardly deserves comment at this point. However, it is important to review a few simple principles.

Arterial Elasticity and Net Stroke Volume as Determinants of Arterial Pulse Pressure. The basic determinants of arterial pulse pressure are twofold: (1) the elasticity of the arteries; and (2) the net stroke volume output of the heart, which is defined as the stroke volume of the heart minus the volume runoff through the small vessels during the period of systole. In other words, the greater the net gain of blood volume in the arterial tree between the beginning of systole and the end of systole, the greater also will be the arterial pulse pressure. Also, the higher the volume elasticity coefficient of the arterial vessels—that is, the less distensibility—the greater will be the pulse pressure.

Obviously, a large number of other factors can affect one or both of these two basic determinants of the pulse pressure. These include the presence or absence of arteriosclerosis, the degree of active vasoconstriction or vasodilatation of the arterial tree, and the sizes of the arteries themselves, all of which affect the volume elasticity coefficient of the arterial system. Factors that can affect the net stroke volume output include cardiac output, heart rate, and degree of peripheral vasodilatation. That is, stroke volume output is equal to cardiac output divided by heart rate, and net stroke volume output is stroke volume diminished by the amount of blood runoff during systole.

Diminished Peripheral Pulsation. The clinical habit of feeling the peripheral pulse can be a highly valuable art, even to the extent that a few clinicians can estimate arterial pressure quite accurately by feeling the radial artery, though, in general, this art is no longer developed significantly by most clinicians. Only two features of the peripheral arterial pulse are noted by the usual clinician—the pulse frequency pattern and the intensity of pulsation.

The significance of diminished intensity of the peripheral pulse is illustrated in Figure 6-11, which shows a recorded arterial pulse curve from the dorsalis pedis artery before and after stimulation of the sympathetic nerves. Note that the pulse pressure diminished markedly following the vasoconstriction and that the mean pressure level also diminished. This figure demonstrates that there is a high degree of correlation between the intensity of peripheral arterial pulsation and tissue perfusion. Consequently, the clinical dictum that diminished pulsation means diminished tissue perfusion is indeed a well-founded one, though, of course, this also has its exceptions, especially when collateral vessels have taken over the function of a normally pulsatile artery.

Some physiologists have claimed that arterial pulsation per se plays a significant role in maintenance of peripheral perfusion. However, this is still a very doubtful concept and has been both supported and denied by different investigators. The only value of peripheral arterial pulsation that has thus far been proved beyond doubt is its capability, in at least some instances, to promote lymph flow. In a completely pulseless tissue, lymph flow is greatly diminished, particularly when an animal is under the influence of anesthesia such as sodium pentobarbital that blocks lymph vessel vasomotion.

The Hemodynamic Anomaly of Pulsus Alternans. Pulsus alternans is a condition in which the arterial pulse alternates usually every other heart beat, first strong, then weak, then strong, and continuing in this alternating pattern. Thus far, it has never been appropriately explained. It is mentioned here because several basic studies of circulatory hemodynamics have recently offered an explanation. One of these was a computer

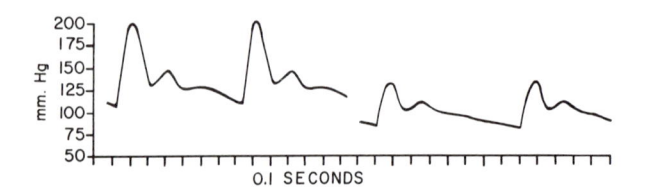

Figure 6-11 Pressure contour in the dorsalis pedis artery recorded, first, under normal conditions and, second, during stimulation of the sympathetic nerves supplying the femoral artery. (Modified from Alexander, R. S., and Kantrowitz, A.: Surgery, *33*:42, 1953.)

study in which the systemic circulation and the pulmonary circulation were simulated mathematically to operate in a complete circuit. In performing different experiments with the simulation, several conditions were found in which typical pulsus alternans occurred. One of these was abnormality of ventricular response to changes in atrial pressure. When the computer was programed so that a minute change in atrial pressure would cause marked change in ventricular output, the left ventricle would first pump an excessively large quantity of blood into the systemic circulation during one heart beat, but during the next heart beat the right ventricle would pump an excessively large quantity into the lungs, the blood volume oscillating back and forth between the pulmonary circulation and the systemic circulation. It was also possible to cause oscillation of the blood volume between the central circulation of the chest region and the more peripheral circulation. Furthermore, the system frequently would be working completely normally and would then be thrown into pulsus alternans by some transient event that occurred in the simulated circulation. This is completely in accord with typical findings in the clinical catheter laboratory that a sudden event related to the catheterization procedure itself can often throw a person into pulsus alternans.

This phenomenon and its possible explanation have been discussed here because, if the explanation is correct, the phenomenon is strictly a hemodynamic problem resulting from resonance within the mechanical system itself, not too unlike the resonance that occurs in the pipe of a pipe organ, with pressure waves reflecting back and forth from one end of the pipe to the other.

HEMODYNAMIC CORRELATES OF PERIPHERAL VASCULAR DISEASE

A clinical understanding of peripheral vascular disease is usually based on knowledge of vascular disease, and only rarely is it difficult to understand the physiology involved once the disease is understood. For instance, in arteriosclerosis and in Buerger's disease, in which actual blockage of peripheral vessels occurs, the physiological problems are almost entirely associated with diminished perfusion. However, in one peripheral vascular disease, Raynaud's disease, knowledge of the basic physiology is essential to an understanding of the disease itself.

Raynaud's Disease. For reasons not yet understood, the blood vessels in the hands (and less frequently the feet) of certain patients, particularly young adult women, exhibit extreme sensitivity to cold and to sympathetic stimulation. Ischemic episodes of the hands or feet are initiated by exposure to cold, either cold applied to the entire body or cold applied to the extremities themselves. Also, such episodes can be caused by emotional disturbances or other psychic stresses that cause either mass discharge of the sympathetic nerves throughout the body or release of epinephrine and norepinephrine into the circulating blood from the adrenal medullae.

In most normal persons even the strongest degree of sympathetic stimulation cannot cause severe ischemia of the tissues. One of the reasons for this is that the local, intrinsic tissue blood flow regulating mechanisms discussed earlier in this chapter oppose extreme vasoconstriction. That is, as the tissues approach ischemia, local effects in the tissues themselves cause opposing vasodilatation. A balance is achieved between sympathetic constriction of the vessels and the opposing vasodilatation, and, usually, this balance is such that the tissues do not undergo damaging ischemia.

In persons with Raynaud's disease, on the other hand, the appropriate balance between local vasodilatation and sympathetic constriction unfortunately does not occur. Instead, the sympathetic component greatly overbalances the local component to the extent that almost total cutoff of blood flow occurs. Upon exposure to cold, the initial stage of the reaction is extreme blanching of the fingers, followed a few minutes later by dilatation of the capillaries which then fill with intensely cyanotic, almost nonflowing blood. In this stage, the fingers are very painful.

Unfortunately, the cause of the pain in Raynaud's disease is not known. However, studies of pain mechanisms per se have demonstrated that pain is almost always associated with tissue damage, presumably because of release of deterioration products from damaged cells. Though in most persons with Raynaud's disease the tissue damage is mild, in severe degrees of the disease the tissue damage can lead to sclerosis of the terminal digits and occasionally even to gangrene.

An obvious physiological therapy for severe and debilitating Raynaud's disease is local sympathectomy. However, this too presents physiological problems for several reasons. First, there is extreme tendency for regrowth of the sympathetic nerve fibers; yet, with appropriate operative procedures this can be minimized. Second, circulating epinephrine and norepinephrine can still elicit Raynaud episodes. In fact, the local blood vessels, deprived of their sympathetic nerves, frequently become hypersensitive to circulating catecholamines, so that the condition may not have been remedied as much as desired by the operative procedure. Therefore, another obvious element of therapy is to prevent the causes of the episodes, particularly emotional crises and exposure to cold. It is theoretically possible to achieve some benefit by use of blocking drugs, but appropriate regimens for this type of therapy are yet to be optimized.

REFERENCES

Berne, R. M.: Regulation of coronary blood flow. Physiol. Rev., *44*:1, 1964.

Bevegard, B. S., and Shepherd, J. T.: Regulation of the circulation during exercise in man. Physiol. Rev., *47*:178, 1967.

Bishop, V. S., and Stone, H. L.: Quantitative description of ventricular output curves in conscious dogs. Circ. Res., *20*:581, 1967.

Braunwald, E., Ross, J., and Sonnenblick, E.: Mechanism of Contractility of the Normal and Failing Heart. Boston, Little, Brown and Co., 1968.

Dahl, L. K., Knudsen, K. D., Heine, M. A., and Leitl, G. J.: Effects of chronic excess salt ingestion: modification of experimental hypertension in the rat by variations in the diet. Circ. Res., *22*:11, 1968.

Duling, B. R., and Berne, R. M.: Propagated vasodilation in the microcirculation of the hamster cheek pouch. Circ. Res., *26*:163, 1970.

Fishman, A. P., and Hecht, H. H. (Eds.): The Pulmonary Circulation and Interstitial Space. Chicago, University of Chicago Press, 1969.

Gauer, O. H., Henry, J. P., and Behn, C.: The regulation of extracellular fluid volume. Ann. Rev. Physiol., *32*:547, 1970.

Gregg, D. E.: Coronary Circulation in Health and Disease. Philadelphia, Lea and Febiger, 1950.

Guyton, A. C.: Circulatory Physiology: Cardiac Output and Its Regulation. Philadelphia, W. B. Saunders Co., 1963.

Guyton, A. C., and Coleman, T. G.: Quantitative analysis of the pathophysiology of hypertension. Circ. Res. *24*(Suppl. 1):1, 1969.

Guyton, A. C., Granger, H. J., and Taylor, A. E.: Interstitial fluid pressure. Physiol. Rev., *51*:527, 1971.

Herd, J. A.: Overall regulation of the circulation. Ann. Rev. Physiol., *32*:289, 1970.

Jones, C. E., Crowell, J. W., and Smith, E. E.: A cause-effect relationship between oxygen deficit and irreversible hemorrhagic shock. Surgery, *127*:93, 1968.

Kezdi, P.: Baroreceptors and Hypertension. New York, Pergamon Press, Inc., 1968.

Korner, P. I.: Circulatory adaptations in hypoxia. Physiol. Rev., *39*:687, 1959.

Reeve, E. B., and Guyton, A. C.: Physical Bases of Circulatory Transport: Regulation and Exchange. Philadelphia, W. B. Saunders Co., 1967.

Starling, E. H.: The Linacre Lecture on the Law of the Heart. London, Longmans Green and Co., 1918.

Wayland, H.: Rheology and the microcirculation. Gastroenterology, *52*:342, 1967.

Weil, M. H., and Shubin, H.: Shock. Baltimore, Williams and Wilkins Co., 1967.

Wood, E.: The Veins. Boston, Little, Brown and Co., 1965.

Yoffey, J. M., and Courtice, F. C.: Lymphatics, Lymph, and Lymphoid Tissue. Baltimore, Williams and Wilkins Co., 1967.

CHAPTER 7

SYSTEMIC ARTERIAL PRESSURE*

ROBERT C. TARAZI
RAY W. GIFFORD, JR.

The pressure in arteries and veins was first measured in 1733 by Stephen Hales, who inserted a cannula into an artery and into a vein of a mare and noted the rise of the blood column in a tube. The arterial column rose approximately 8 feet, whereas the venous column rose only 12 inches. Since that time, tubes have been successfully inserted into various segments of the circulation of conscious unrestrained subjects and the pressure determined by sensitive manometers with high frequency of response. Thus, a map could be drawn of pressure variations along the circulatory circuit and of its fluctuations with different phases of the cardiac cycle (Fig. 7-1). The marked drop of pressure observed at the systemic arteriolar level led to a subdivision of the circulation into a "high-pressure" (resistance) segment and a "low-pressure" (capacitance) segment. The first is thought to be mainly concerned with flow distribution and regulation, and the second with priming of the cardiac pump and control of its output and possibly with regulation of intravascular volume. Important as these subdivisions are, the essential unity of the circulation must not be forgotten. A greater transmission of pressure from arteries to capillaries (as by arteriolar vasodilation) may increase capillary ultrafiltration and reduce intravascular volume while concomitantly increasing venous return. Conversely, venoconstriction may, under certain conditions, relocate blood to the cardiopulmonary area, enhance cardiac output, and thus influence arterial pressure. Blood pressure in capillaries, veins, and the lesser circulation is discussed elsewhere in this text and will be referred to here only insofar as it influences systemic arterial pressure.

Left ventricular contraction provides a phasic output of energy for the circulation; during systole, the intraventricular pressure rises from an average of 8 mm. Hg to about 120 mm. Hg under normal conditions. Blood is ejected into the aorta when the intraventricular pressure forces open the semilunar valves; during that portion of the cycle, systolic pressure is practically equal in the ventricle and aorta. At the end of systole, the heart muscle relaxes, and as intraventricular pressure falls steeply, the semilunar valve is closed. While blood is running from the arterioles into capillaries and veins, the large arteries, which had absorbed part of the energy of systole, now recoil on the diminishing volume of blood left by ventricular ejection, so that arterial pressure falls gradually during diastole. Thus, the arterial pressure pulse results from the ejection of a small volume of blood into a partly filled container of limited distensibility. This ejection distends at first only the proximal portion of the aorta, but the pressure wave generated is then rapidly transmitted to the rest of the arterial tree, with a velocity inversely proportional to the distensibility of the

---

*Many concepts and mechanisms described in this chapter are related to general concepts discussed in Chapter 6.

vessels involved. Since compliance of the arterial tree is less far out from the central aorta, the pulse wave velocity increases the farther it travels. When the wave reaches the main branching sites, but especially the precapillary resistance barrier, it is reflected back. Summation of the advancing waves with reflected waves may alter pulse tracings to a greater or lesser extent, depending on the particular artery considered, the speed of wave transmission, and the degree of peripheral vasoconstriction at that time. Particularly obvious is the peaking of pulse waves in the femoral arteries when the size of the wave often becomes greater than in more central vessels, and phasic backflow may occur. Conditions stiffening arterial walls such as hypertension or sclerosis will also increase pulse wave velocity.

Pulse wave velocity must not be confused with the velocity of blood flow. The actual volume of blood yielded by the heart will have moved only a few centimeters by the time the pressure wave has reached the distal ends of the arterial system. Blood movement can be likened to the result of pushing a series of billiard balls: applying force on a ball at one end displaces another at the other end. As total surface area of the vasculature increases with repeated branching of the vessels, blood flow velocity decreases; simultaneously, the pulse wave velocity increases. This explains why the velocity of the pressure pulse is approximately 15 times that of blood flow in the aorta but may be as great as 100 times the velocity of blood flow in the distal arteries.

DETERMINATION OF ARTERIAL PRESSURE AND DEFINITION OF TERMS

Arterial pressure can be determined either directly (intra-arterial insertion of a needle or tube connected to a manometer) or indirectly, usually by auscultation over an artery to which pressure is applied proximally (sphygmomanometer). The choice of method will depend on purpose; the accuracy of determinations does not depend on the method used as much as on the attention given to seemingly minor but really quite important details.

Direct Method

The pressure determined in this way depends on the type of manometer to which the intra-arterial cannula is connected. The older U-tube mercury manometer has so much inertia that it cannot rise and fall rapidly and therefore simply oscillates around a mean level of pressure. To record faithfully rapidly changing pressures, manometers with higher frequency responses are currently used with optimal damping to ensure a uniform output throughout the range of frequencies expected. The records obtained are illustrated in Figure 7–2. The difference between the highest (systolic) and lowest (diastolic) pressure of a cycle is called the pulse pressure (PP). An integrated mean for the pressure developed throughout a whole cardiac cycle can either be recorded by electronically damping the response of the recording system or be determined by planimetry. The *mean arterial pressure* (MAP) thus obtained reflects the average pressure pushing blood through the systemic circulation and is therefore used to calculate peripheral resistance (see later discussion); it is not equal to the arithmetic mean of the systolic and diastolic pressures but depends in part on the heart rate and relative duration of systole and diastole; a close approximation is obtained as follows: MAP = DBP + ⅓ PP. The *mean systolic pressure* (MSP) is determined by integrating the area under the systolic part of the cycle; its main use is in calculations of cardiac work and tension-time indices; it is closely related to myocardial oxygen consumption, since pressure work is more costly to the heart than volume work.

Indirect Method

The instrument universally used is the sphygmomanometer; the arterial pressure is usually measured in man at the brachial artery with the subject seated or lying down, with the arm slightly flexed and at heart level. Time should be allowed for recovery from recent exercise or excitement; clothing should not constrict the arm and the patient should be put as much at ease as possible. A cloth-covered rubber bag is placed firmly and snugly around the upper arm with its lower edge about an inch above the antecubital space. The bag should be 20 per cent wider than the diameter of the limb on which it is to be used (12 to 14 cm. for the average adult but wider for obese patients) and should be long enough (25 to 30 cm.) to encircle the limb almost completely. There should be no bulging or displacement of the bag when inflated. The air pressure inside the bag is determined by a mercury manometer or by an aneroid manometer calibrated against a mercury manometer. While the brachial or radial pulse is palpated, the bag is inflated to a pressure 30 mm. Hg higher than that required to obliterate the pulse. The pressure is then gradually reduced at a rate approximately 2 to 3 mm. Hg per second while a stethoscope, which is applied firmly but with as little pressure as possible over the previously palpated brachial artery, is em-

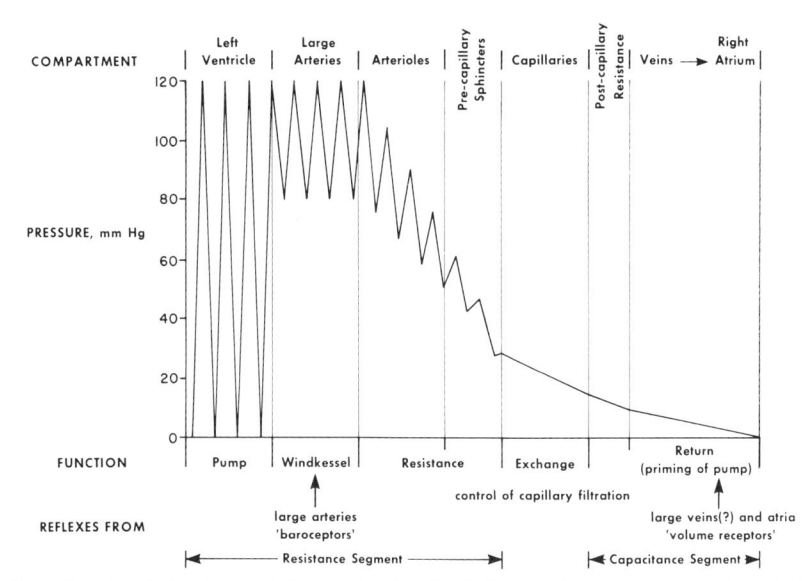

Figure 7-1 Functional subdivisions of the systemic circulation and pressure variations in its different segments. (After Folkow and Neil.)

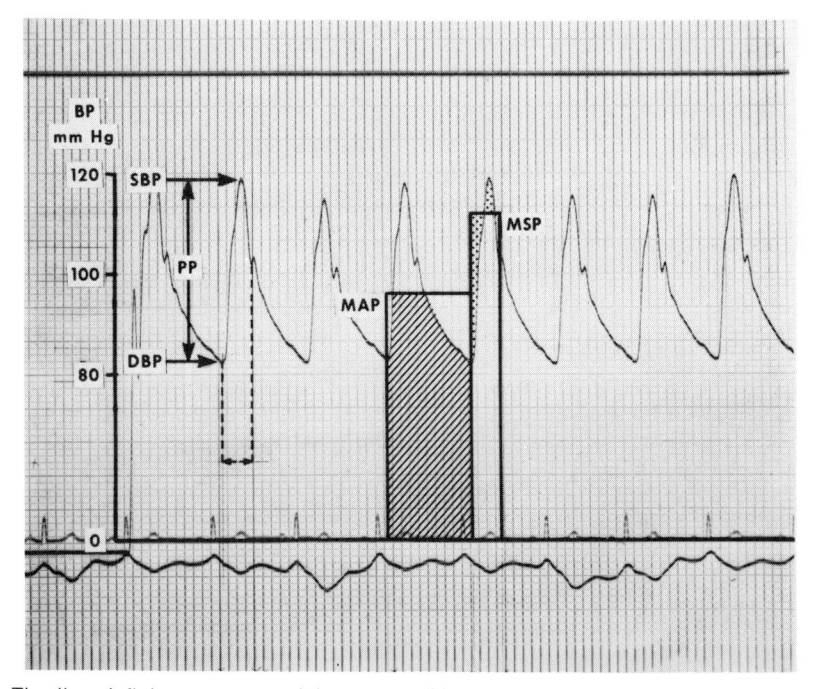

Figure 7-2 The line defining mean arterial pressure (MAP) can be drawn so that the area added (blank) is equivalent to the area subtracted (blank) from the whole cardiac cycle. Similarly, mean systolic pressure (MSP) can be estimated by adding an area (stippled) equivalent to that subtracted (stippled) from the ventricular ejection period only (from onset of pulse to incisure).

ployed. As the pressure in the bag falls, a series of sounds—the Korotkoff sounds—are heard as follows:

Phase I: Sudden appearance of a clear, sharp, snapping sound that grows louder
Phase II: Sound is softened and becomes prolonged into a murmur
Phase III: Sound again becomes crisper and increases in intensity
Phase IV: Distinct abrupt muffling of the sound
Phase V: The point at which sounds disappear

The first appearance of the sound (phase I) indicates the breakthrough of the pulse wave and gives the systolic pressure. Phase IV is currently recommended by the American Heart Association as the best index of diastolic pressure, mainly on the basis that there is no logical connection between phase V and diastolic pressure, whereas the abrupt muffling of the arterial sound signals that blood flow is no longer impeded during diastole by the cuff pressure. Usually there is little difference between the two phases, but they may become widely separated when arterial flow is increased. In such cases it is best to record both phases, so that blood pressure is recorded as, for example, 128/88/76. The first figure represents the systolic (phase I); the second, the diastolic (phase IV); and the third, phase V pressure.

Sometimes, particularly in some hypertensive patients, the usual sounds heard over the brachial artery when the cuff pressure is high disappear as the pressure is reduced and then reappear at a lower level. This early, temporary disappearance of sound is called the *auscultatory gap* and occurs during the latter part of phase I and phase II. Because this gap may cover a range of 40 mm. Hg, one can seriously underestimate the systolic pressure or overestimate the diastolic pressure, unless its presence is excluded by first palpating for disappearance of the radial pulse as the cuff pressure is raised.

When all sounds have disappeared, the cuff should be deflated rapidly and completely. One to two minutes should elapse for the release of blood trapped in the veins before further determinations are made.

An important sign to be looked for actively, especially in patients with some indication of cardiac dysfunction, is *pulsus alternans.* This is detected by noting that after the first sounds are heard and as pressure is reduced, their rate suddenly doubles, strong sounds alternating with weak sounds. It is an important sign of left ventricular failure and should be carefully distinguished from arrhythmia (irregular intervals between sounds) or respiratory variations of arterial pressure; the degree of alternans (interval between phase I and level of doubling of the sounds) and the heart rate at the moment should be carefully noted. The wider the alternans and the slower the heart rate at the time, the more seriously must it be viewed; minor degrees of alternation are not uncommon with marked tachycardia.

Blood pressure can also be determined during sphygmomanometry in two other ways. The first, the *palpatory,* involves palpating the radial pulse and noting the pressure at which it returns, after it has been obliterated by elevation of the pressure in the cuff above the pressure in the brachial artery. This method is not used extensively for several reasons. In the first place, only the systolic pressure can be determined, and, in general, it is inaccurate, being too low by approximately 5 to 10 mm. of mercury. However, the method is useful, in part at least, in assuring from the absence of the radial pulse that the brachial pulse is exceeded, a point that cannot always be settled by the auscultatory method. The second is the *oscillometric.* In the Pachon type oscillometer two rubber bags are contained in the cuff, and the pressure in these bags is transmitted to a recording manometer. The mechanism is so arranged that when the column of blood reaches the lower cuff, the pulsation is reversed on the record. The entrance of the column of blood into the artery under the second cuff and the reversal of the record signal the systolic pressure. As the pressure is further reduced, the oscillations become greater and greater until they suddenly diminish markedly in size. This point is commonly taken as the diastolic pressure, but the precise point on the record at which the change occurs is not always evident.

The blood pressure may be taken in other parts of the body, particularly in the leg. When this is done, the patient rests in the horizontal position and the cuff is placed around the thigh, the sound being elicited over the artery in the popliteal space by application of the diaphragm of the stethoscope there. A special wide "thigh-cuff" should be used, wrapped firmly, but not tightly, with the compression bag over the posterior aspect of the midthigh. The systolic pressure thus recorded in the thigh is higher by 10 to 40 mm. Hg than that in the arm, but the diastolic is essentially the same. This difference is mainly spurious (uncomfortable position, difficulty of proper compression), though a minor part may be related to the effect of reflected pulse waves. It is accentuated in aortic insufficiency (Hill's sign), but more importantly it disappears or becomes reversed (arm pressure > thigh pressure) in coarctation of the aorta or obstruction at the aortic bifurcation, and sometimes in abdominal aortic aneurysms.

Correlation Between Direct and Indirect Methods

Cuff readings are closely related to direct measurements, though levels are on the average 5 mm. Hg too low for the systolic and 8 mm. Hg too high for the diastolic (taken as phase IV). Actually, the disappearance of sounds (phase V) often coincides with diastolic pressure measured directly but it is less easy to define in some cases than phase IV and admits of wider variations. One of the most important factors affecting the accuracy of indirect recordings is the size of cuff used and its proper application to ensure adequate and even compression of the artery. The smaller the cuff in relation to the arm circumference, the higher the recorded pressure and the greater the error.

In both methods, the relation of the arm and manometer to the "heart level" is crucial; lowering or raising the arm from that level will increase or reduce recorded pressure because of hydrostatic factors involved, hence the importance of keeping the arm level with the fourth intercostal space whenever blood pressure is determined while the subject is sitting or standing.

BASIC FACTORS DETERMINING ARTERIAL PRESSURE

Pressure, Flow, and Resistance

Blood flow through vessels depends on two factors—the pressure head driving it and the resistance it meets. The relationship between these factors is defined by some basic hydrodynamic laws developed by Newton, Hagen, Poiseuille, and others. Translated into clinical terms, these laws have become essential for the understanding of arterial pressure variations in health and disease.

As just stated, the flow of any liquid along a tube is associated with a pressure gradient along that tube dependent on the rate of flow and on the resistance it meets. Because resistance (R) cannot be measured directly, it is calculated as the ratio of the pressure gradient (ΔP) to the rate of flow (F):

$$R = \Delta P/F \qquad (1)$$

The rate of flow of liquids within cylindrical vessels can be mathematically deduced from Newton's principles on laminar movement of fluids. If the liquid is of uniform viscosity and its flow streamlined and nonpulsatile, then

$$F = \frac{\Delta P \times r^4}{l \times v} \times \frac{\pi}{8} \qquad (2)$$

(r = radius of vessel, l = its length, and v = the fluid viscosity; $\frac{\pi}{8}$ is a constant, arising from calculus derivations).

Strictly speaking, these conditions are not met in the circulation, but despite the obvious differences, this fundamental law (Poiseuille) is largely valid for hemodynamic studies. The calculations derived from it are very useful in assessing the relative parts played by blood flow and peripheral resistance in changes of arterial pressure. It is important, however, to realize the approximations and reservations involved in its application to the intact organism. MAP (mean arterial pressure) is considered the equivalent of ΔP; the marked difference between systemic arterial and central venous pressure as well as the relatively small fluctuations of the latter allows its disregard in calculations of resistance in the systemic circulation. This simplification is naturally not possible for the pulmonary circulation; CO (cardiac output) is the equivalent of F, and TPR, the "total peripheral resistance."

Hence, the basic equation expressing the relationship of arterial pressure, cardiac output, and peripheral resistance is

$$MAP = CO \times TPR \qquad (3)$$

Cardiac output and arterial pressure are determined directly and TPR is calculated as their ratio. However, since cardiac output is related to body size whereas MAP is not, it seems preferable to use the "cardiac index" (CI = cardiac output/body surface area) rather than output for calculations.*

The simplicity of this formula must not lure one into simplistic interpretations of calculated changes in peripheral resistance. Total peripheral resistance is the composite of the vascular resistance of each organ. Resistances to flow obey the same laws as electric resistances for combinations of series and of parallel arrangements. Therefore, a change in TPR does not necessarily indicate that similar quantitative or even similar directional changes are occurring in all individual vascular territories. Within the usual physiological limits of blood viscosity and assuming a constant vascular length in the same individual, variations in resistance will usually result from active, passive, or structural changes of vessel diameter. Since the radius is magnified

---

*Resistance can be expressed either in arbitrary units, PRU (peripheral resistance units) = $(\frac{mm.\ Hg}{L./min./M.^2})$, or in fundamental units of force. For the latter, pressure in mm. Hg is converted to dynes/cm.^{2} (1 mm. Hg = 1333 dynes/cm.^{2}) and flow to cm.^{3}/sec. (1 L. = 1000/60 cm.^{3}/sec.); the calculated resistance is then expressed in dynes. sec./cm.^{5} This can be achieved practically by multiplying PRU by 80.

to the fourth power in equation 2, flow and pressure are markedly affected by relatively small changes in vessel size. However, a word of caution is needed against unqualified translation of TPR into an index of peripheral arteriolar vasoconstriction, with failure to recognize the important role that large and small arteriovenous shunts, precapillary sphincters, passive arterial variations, structural changes, and collateral vessels may sometimes play in that respect.

Factors Determining Pulse Pressure

Aside from forces regulating the average level of arterial pressure, a number of factors determine the width of pulsations around the mean. This discussion concerns those factors affecting central pulse pressure rather than the local variations already mentioned, resulting from reflected waves and altered distensibility of various peripheral portions of the arterial tree.

The aorta and its main branches take up a relatively large volume of blood under pressure during systolic ejection; during diastole, the pressure energy thus stored is gradually used to press blood onward. This "Windkessel function" helps transform an intermittent input to a more even outflow (Wiggers). The factors determining pulse pressure will therefore relate mainly to (1) quantity of blood ejected per beat (stroke volume); (2) compliance of the aorta and large vessels; and to a lesser degree (3) speed of ejection of blood. The aortic wall is not a perfectly elastic material and its viscous components imply that the more rapidly blood is ejected, the larger the rise in pulse pressure. Obviously, the larger the stroke volume, the wider the pulse pressure; the causes of increased stroke volume are usually evident (aortic insufficiency, complete heart block, various high output states). In contrast, conditions associated with diminished aortic compliance are not often clinically evident but are suspected from the resultant systolic hypertension and wide pulse pressure.

The effects of altered compliance can be readily appreciated from the physical definition of the term:

Vascular compliance (or volume distensibility) = $\frac{\text{Increase in volume }(\Delta V)}{\text{Increase in pressure }(\Delta P)}$

Translated into clinical terms,

Aortic compliance = $\frac{\text{Stroke volume}}{\text{Pulse pressure}}$

from which follow:
 (a) Stroke volume = Pulse pressure × Aortic compliance
 (b) Pulse pressure = $\frac{\text{Stroke volume}}{\text{Aortic compliance}}$

If compliance were constant, stroke volume could be deduced from pulse pressure and cardiac output could then be calculated by multiplying pulse pressure by heart rate. Unfortunately, variables are too great for useful interpretations of the formula.

It is readily seen that decrease in compliance will result in wider pulse pressure per ml. of blood ejected. Compliance decreases slightly as arterial pressure increases or with sympathetic stimulation; it is markedly reduced by loss or fragmentation of aortic elastic and muscular tissue, as occurs with age or extensive atheromatous involvement with secondary medial fibrosis or intimal calcification. Reduction of aortic distensibility per se leads to a slight decline in diastolic and a marked rise in systolic pressures. Diastolic hypertension even with a very wide pulse pressure cannot therefore be ascribed to reduce aortic compliance alone. Conversely, with aortic distensibility held constant, increasing peripheral resistance will be associated with declining pulse pressure. The wide pulse pressures found in many hypertensive subjects may therefore reflect a secondary loss of large vessel distensibility.

Effect of Age and Environmental Factors on Arterial Blood Pressure

Definition of a "normal" arterial blood pressure is so closely linked to the discussion of the nature of hypertension that it is better reviewed later, in the section on hypertension. Suffice it here to point out the often wide variations in both systolic and diastolic pressures encountered from moment to moment in the same subject. Most are related to such obvious causes as bodily movement, position, pain, emotional stress, and the like. Under ordinary conditions, blood pressure measured even after a few minutes' rest in the doctor's office (casual pressure) is markedly higher than that recorded under basal conditions. Smirk defined "basal pressure" as the one recorded in the morning 10 to 12 hours postprandially; after an additional half hour rest in a warm room, repeated recordings are obtained over 30 to 45 minutes in a monotonous, silent atmosphere to the lowest attainable levels. Home blood pressures recorded by the patient himself or by a lay relative often approximate basal levels. The difference (casual minus basal) is called supplemental pressure. Though the basal pressure might be statistically more closely related to the clinical consequences of hypertension, it has found little clinical acceptance. Most epidemiologic and clinical experience has been derived from studies of casual pressure.

Age, Sex, and Body Build. Until adult life is reached, the factor of age may make a remarkable difference (Fig. 7–3); subsequent changes with age vary in different communities and from subject to subject. In some, pressure does not rise with age, in others the rate of rise is quite

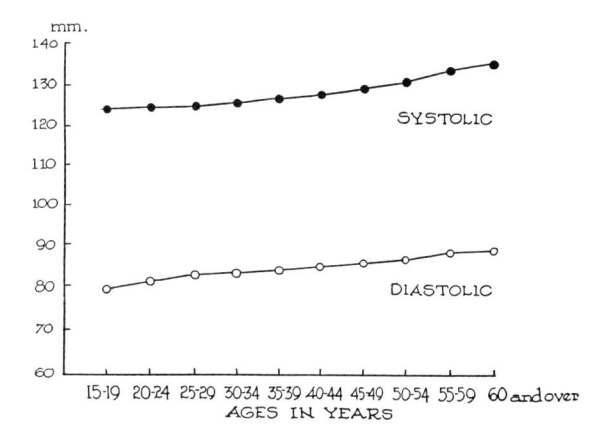

Figure 7-3 Blood pressure and age. (From data by Symonds: J.A.M.A., *80*:232, 1923.)

marked. Studies in Wales suggest that the rate of rise in Western populations, at least, correlates with the initial level of blood pressure. Young men tend to have higher pressures than young women, but between ages 35 and 45, the curves for systolic pressure cross and women's pressures subsequently rise more steeply with age than men's. There is no evidence that menopause is associated with a particular type of hypertension. Obese subjects tend to have higher blood pressure that cannot be accounted for by systematic errors due to increased arm circumference.

Posture and Exercise. With standing, pulse pressure narrows as the systolic drops slightly and the diastolic rises by about 5 mm. Hg, so that mean arterial pressure does not vary by more than ± 5 to 10 mm. Hg. Changes in arterial pressure with dynamic exercise (cycling, walking) are proportional to the severity of exercise; it may reach 200/100 when exercise becomes strenuous. Static exercise, e.g., sustained contraction of forearm muscles, is associated with an abrupt reflex rise in pressure proportional to the muscular tension developed.

Variations With Daily Activities. The size of these variations as recorded by automatic recorders is quite impressive, averaging in one study 24 mm. Hg (range 15 to 40) for systolic and 14 mm. Hg (5 to 20) for diastolic in normotensive subjects. Arterial pressure falls profoundly during sleep but is most unstable in REM (rapid eye movement) sleep. Relation of pressure variations to nocturnal cardiovascular accidents is still conjectural.

SOME ASPECTS OF ARTERIAL PRESSURE REGULATION

Arterial blood pressure is only one aspect in a highly integrated cardiovascular control system. Accordingly, to understand its disturbances one should consider the cardiovascular system as a whole, including cardiac performance and peripheral resistance, but also the indirect effect of capacitance vessels on blood flow and the ways in which hemodynamic functions can be modified by sympathetic neural activity and hormonal factors. Control of circulatory pressure must be closely associated with control of the volume distending the circulation, and arterial pressure reflects, in part, this relationship between container (blood vessels) and content (blood volume). Hence, the mechanisms regulating the size and distribution of extracellular fluids must be considered along with factors controlling hemodynamic functions.

Hemodynamic Aspects

Physical bases of mean arterial and pulse pressure have already been discussed. Arterial pressure can be regulated by variations of either cardiac output or peripheral resistance or both.

Interrelationship Between Output and Resistance. In acute studies, cardiac response to changes in peripheral resistance is to increase output for a decrease in peripheral resistance and to decrease output for an increase in resistance. Thus, any effect on pressure is at least attenuated. This relationship underlines the importance of peripheral factors in determining cardiac output (given normal myocardial contractility) by controlling the flow of blood from arteries to veins. Conversely, primary changes in output lead to reciprocal changes in peripheral resistance, tending to maintain pressure constant. This relationship is probably mediated principally through baroceptor reflexes (see later discussion).

Chronic changes in blood flow unrelated to local needs of tissues will lead to a different type of long-term readjustment. In such cases, a persistent inappropriate increase of cardiac output would induce a progressive constriction of local vessels over a period of days or months until finally blood flow through the tissues would return to near normal. Return of output to normal is associated with increased peripheral resistance (Fig. 7-4). The ability of tissues, even when denervated, to restore experimentally altered blood flow to normal is called "autoregulation." There is no consensus regarding the exact definition of the term. Local regulation of blood flow to the needs of the tissues depends on (a) concentration of local metabolites and (b) myogenic response of vessel wall to stretch (Bayliss mechanism). Development of collateral vessels has also been viewed as a phenomenon of long-term flow regulation (Ch. 6). Whatever its exact mechanism, the concept behind it supposes that regulation of flow has been disassociated from, and in a way has superseded, pressure regulation.

Blood Vessels and Arterial Blood Pressure. All systemic vessels—arteries, veins, and capillaries—participate each in its way in arterial blood pressure regulation. The following classification of blood vessels is based on the functional characteristics of each segment (Folkow):

1. "Windkessel" vessels (aorta and its large branches) damp the pulsatile output from the left ventricle and help steady the blood flow to the periphery; their main effect is on pulse pressure.

2. Resistance vessels (small arteries and arterioles) furnish most of total resistance to flow and regulate the distribution of cardiac output. Their high intrinsic (myogenic) tone is continuously modified by physical, chemical, and neural influences. As flow is proportional to the fourth power of the radius, seemingly minor changes in diameter may exert a powerful influence on blood pressure (Poiseuille).

3. Exchange vessels (capillaries) are guarded by precapillary sphincters and postcapillary resistance vessels (venules and small veins). Diffusion, filtration, and reabsorption occur through the capillary walls but the capillaries themselves have no active influence on this exchange. The net fluid transfer between plasma and interstitial fluid, given normal plasma oncotic pressure, depends on the ratio of precapillary to postcapillary resistance which is controlled by sphincters and resistance vessels at either end of the capillaries. Changes in this ratio affect primarily blood volume and indirectly arterial pressure. A fall in pressure at the arteriolar end will favor intravascular shift of fluid and thus help to some degree in restoring arterial pressure.

4. Capacitance vessels (veins) add little to peripheral resistance but accommodate the larger portion of blood volume and thus play an important role in circulatory regulation. They are well supplied by sympathetic nerves and may react differently from resistance vessels to nervous and humoral stimuli. To ascribe a role to veins in regulation of arterial pressure may look paradoxical but cardiac output depends on venous return. Venoconstriction resulting from sympathetic stimulation will not significantly alter peripheral resistance but it will lead to decreased venous capacity. This will enhance a translocation of blood out of systemic veins into the cardiopulmonary area, raise cardiac output, and thus help prevent or correct falls in arterial pressure due to blood loss or excessive peripheral pooling.

Intravascular Volume and Arterial Pressure

The vascular circuit just described is obviously not a homogeneous system; each of its subdivisions has its own pressure/volume characteristics. The arterial segment has limited distensibility and is maintained at high pressure and low volume; it is thought to contain about 20 per cent of the total blood volume. Although the capillary bed is of considerable length, it contains only 5 per cent of the total blood volume. Capillary pressure is determined by the balance of constriction between precapillary arterioles and postcapillary venules. The venous side of the circulation is a low pressure, highly distensible compartment which contains about 75 per cent of the intravascular volume.

Both the arterial and venous compartments

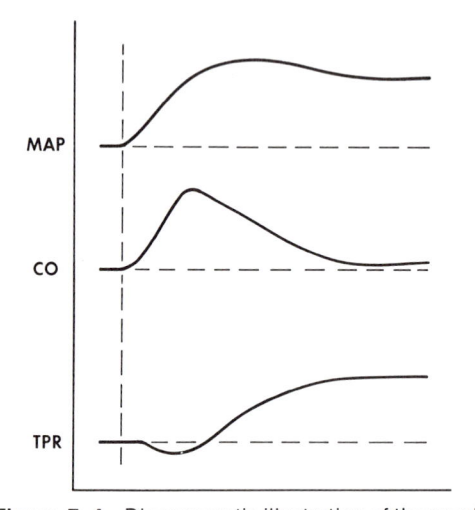

Figure 7-4 Diagrammatic illustration of the results of a sustained increase in cardiac output (CO) unrelated to peripheral demands; as output rises, mean arterial pressure (MAP) increases while total peripheral resistance (TPR) remains unchanged or even decreases slightly. Within a few weeks, however, TPR increases and cardiac output returns toward normal; MAP remains elevated because of the persistent increase in resistance.

are importantly affected by sympathetic vasomotor outflow but, characteristically, these effects are different. Neural influences alter arterial capacity and volume but little, but small changes in that segment may affect arterial pressure directly. In contrast, sympathetic vasomotor activity plays a large role in determining venous capacity but the contribution of veins to total peripheral resistance is small. More important is their control of venous return and influence on cardiac output. In that respect and within certain limits, the distribution of intravascular volume may be more important than its magnitude; thus it is possible to have, on the one hand, a large blood volume, venous pooling, low central blood volume, and low cardiac output or, on the other, a small blood volume, diminished venous capacity, a disproportionately high central blood volume, and a normal or slightly increased cardiac output.

The potential of vascular adaptability is such that changes in blood volume are not normally reflected to any important degree in arterial pressure variations, unless the change is acute or excessive (hemorrhage). Conditions marked by hypervolemia (polycythemia vera) are not necessarily associated with hypertension. This efficacy of adaptation implies that important disturbances in regulation may lead to only subtle changes in pressure/volume relationships. On the other hand, arterial pressure becomes quite sensitive to blood volume changes when neural reflexes are interfered with. A small blood loss that would normally be well tolerated may lead to profound hypotension if suffered by a patient treated with neural blocking agents. Conversely, fluid retention and plasma volume expansion will nullify an initial good response to such hypotensive agents as ganglion blockers, guanethidine, reserpine, and similar drugs.

Factors regulating blood volume are beyond the scope of this discussion; they include renal excretory mechanisms, balance between interstitial and intravascular component of extracellular fluid volume, and neurohumoral control mechanisms (see appropriate sections).

Principles of Vascular Control

The inherent myogenic activity of vessel walls is responsible for a *basal vascular tone* which is locally regulated by the vasodilator action of tissue metabolites. Superimposed on this, neurogenic mechanisms exert a "remote" control to adjust the circulation to the requirements of the body as a whole. Various circulating hormones add their excitatory or inhibitory influences.

Vascular innervation is not restricted to arteries; all vessels except capillaries are innervated. Arterioles are supplied by two sets of nerves—sympathetic vasoconstrictors (alpha-adrenergic) and different vasodilator fibers.

Sympathetic nerve fibers reach the vessels either from plexuses along their walls or through somatic nerve trunks. This distribution is important, for stripping the greater vessels of their nerve supply will not affect the smaller vessels. The more important neural influence on the arterial side is vasoconstriction; similarly, the overriding effect of sympathetic stimulation on veins is alpha-adrenergic venoconstriction. Thus, the main effects of sympathetic stimulation are increases in resistance and enhancement of venous return.

Vasodilator fibers are less widespread and not tonically active. Beta-adrenergic receptors are found in arteries and probably in veins; their functional importance is debated. Cholinergic sympathetic vasodilator nerves supply only the larger resistance vessels of skeletal muscle and are activated mainly when the animal is alerted (defense reaction); as most other regions are vasoconstricted, the muscles may thus be provided with near maximum blood supply. Parasympathetic vasodilator nerves supply some specialized tissues such as salivary glands and external genitalia.

Hormonal influences include circulating epinephrine (from adrenal medulla), which stimulates both alpha- and beta-receptors, so that it usually causes a redistribution of blood flow; myocardium, muscle, and liver receive more blood at the expense of other circuits (kidney, skin, gastrointestinal tract) which are vasoconstricted. Angiotensin is discussed later. Many other "vasoactive agents" are known (prostaglandins, histamine, serotonin, vasopressin); specialized reviews should be consulted for details of their effects.

Finally, especially in the context of blood pressure regulation, it is important to remember that salt-water equilibrium profoundly affects the activity and responsiveness of smooth muscles. Changes in sodium gradient across cell membrane may enhance constriction (if extracellular sodium is increased) or relaxation (if sodium is depleted).

Neural Reflexes and "Central" Reactions

Neural circulatory reflexes act mainly to stabilize arterial pressure at the levels set for a particular subject. They help buffer the impact of stimuli by raising arterial pressure when it is lowered or decreasing it when it rises. When neural activity is impaired by drugs or disease, arterial pressure may fluctuate widely between hypertension in the supine position and hypotension and fainting on standing.

Like all neural reflexes, they comprise an afferent and an efferent limb joined through a center (the vasomotor center). They are activated from sensory receptors in different parts of the circulation; the most important are located in the carotid sinus and aortic arch. These stretch receptors are sensitive to expansion or deformation of the arterial wall and respond more to a pulsatile than to an equivalent steady pressure (the term *baroreceptor* is inaccurate because they do not respond to pressure per se). Fibers from the carotid sinus travel cephalad in the glossopharyngeal nerve and those from the aortic arch, in the vagus. The carotid sinus reflex is normally the more powerful, possibly because it guards the blood supply to the central nervous system. But other sensitive vascular areas, e.g., the mesenteric, can also induce compensatory blood pressure responses in anesthetized animals with cut sinus nerves and vagi (Heymans). Apart from reflexes originating from the "high-pressure" circuit, it seems clear that there are also sensory endings in the thorax from the "low-pressure" segment, the fibers from which are vagal in location. They respond to shifts in blood volume, or rather to distention in vessel walls related to these shifts. These endings are almost certainly part of the mechanisms concerned in counteracting the high G force developed in centrifugation experiments or with sudden acceleration or changes in direction.

The stretch receptors are activated when arterial pressure rises and the consequent impulses inhibit the tonic activity of the vasomotor center. This latter term is applied to a group of neurons located in the upper medulla and lower pons which maintain normally a slow rate of firing to essentially all sympathetic vasoconstrictor fibers. Baroreceptor impulses normally exert an inhibitory influence on the center; when blood pressure tends to fall, their activity is reduced, thus liberating the vasomotor center, and the consequent increase in sympathetic discharge helps restore pressure to normal. The vasomotor center influences the heart as well as the peripheral vessels, so that increase or reduction of cardiac activity (chronotropic and inotropic) parallels the increase or decrease in vasoconstrictor impulses. Efferent impulses travel along the two components of the autonomic system—sympathetic and parasympathetic. Of these the sympathetic is of greater importance because of its wider distribution to the peripheral vasculature and in the heart, going to both atria and ventricles. Vagal fibers supply mainly the sino-auricular and atrioventricular nodes and the atria; there is evidence, however, of a significant parasympathetic influence on ventricular function as well.

These reflexes play a major role in circulatory adjustments to postural changes (see discussion of hypotension). Both sides of the reflex are demonstrated in responses to the Valsalva maneuver (a sustained increase in intrathoracic pressure obtained by blowing against some resistance for 20 to 30 seconds). During the period of straining, venous return is sharply curtailed and cardiac output decreased, so that systolic pressure falls. Resultant reflex sympathetic stimulation increases heart rate and limits fall in diastolic pressure. When straining is suddenly stopped, blood rushes into the thorax and the resurgent cardiac output is thrust into an arterial system whose outflow resistance has been increased. This results in a brief overshoot of arterial pressure; the opposite reflex readjustment then leads to bradycardia and a decline of pressure to prestrain levels.

These sequential variations with the Valsalva maneuvers are usually classified into four phases (Fig. 7–5): phase 1 is a brief rise in pressure with onset of straining; phase 2 is the reduction in pulse pressure and increase in heart rate; phase

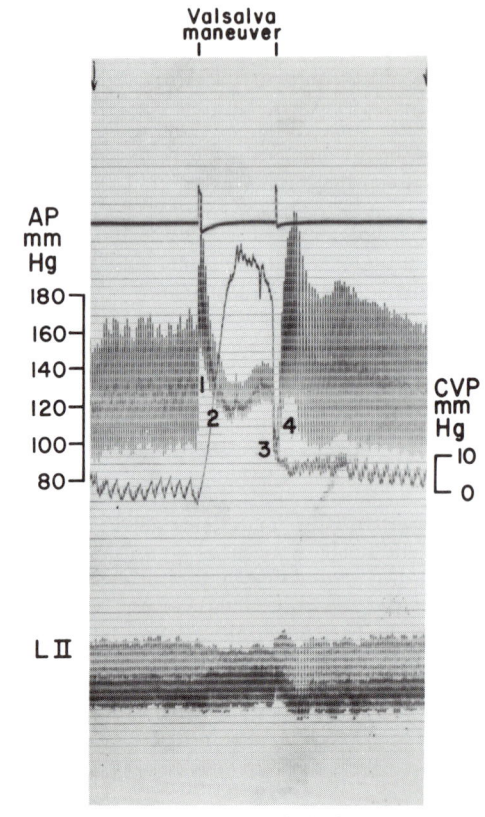

Figure 7–5 Response to a Valsalva maneuver performed for 20 seconds. From above downward are shown (a) signal indicating beginning and end of straining; (b) arterial pressure (AP) showing four phases: *1*, initial rise with onset of straining; *2*, the fall in pulse pressure as venous return is temporarily diminished; *3*, a further fall in pressure with the first deep breaths on cessation of strain; and *4*, the pressure overshoot as an increased left ventricular output is now thrown in a constricted vascular bed; (c) central venous pressure (CVP) tracing showing the marked increase during straining; (d) electrocardiogram (lead II), which shows the slowing in heart rate with phase 4 after its increase during phase 2.

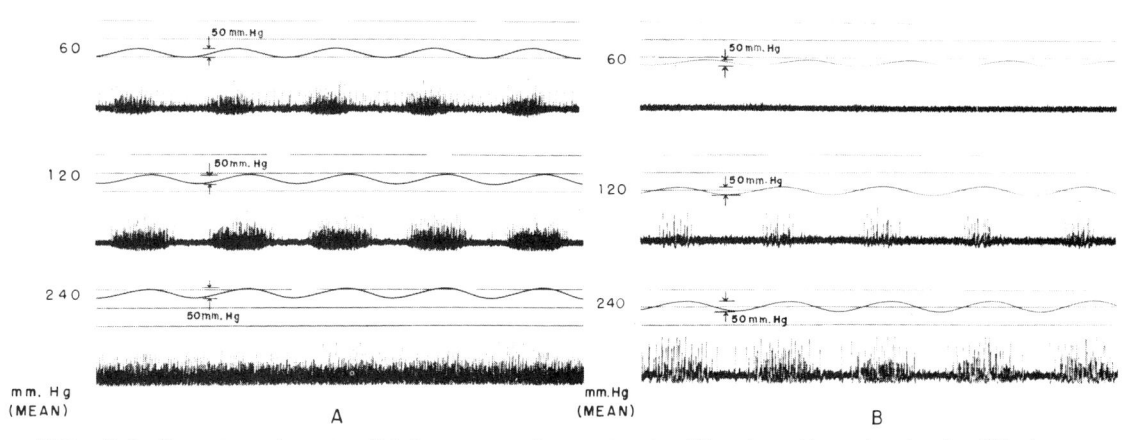

Figure 7-6 Neurogram from carotid sinus nerve of normotensive (A) and renal hypertensive dog (B): at a mean arterial pressure of 60 mm. Hg, nerve activity was clearly present in dog A but absent in the hypertensive animal. At 240 mm. Hg MAP, firing was continuous in A but still intermittent in B, suggesting that the normal range of baroceptor response had been shifted upward in the hypertensive animal. (After McCubbin, J., et al.: Baroceptor function in chronic renal hypertension. Circ. Res., 4:205, 1965, by permission of The American Heart Association, Inc.)

3 is a further drop in pressure as straining is suddenly stopped and the resultant increased pulmonary vascular capacity momentarily reduces return to the left ventricle further; phase 4 refers to the overshoot in arterial pressure and reflex bradycardia. These responses, however, depend not only on the integrity of neural reflexes but also on the degree of volemia and on cardiac compensation; in heart failure, blood pressure actually rises during straining, and phase 4 is abolished.

The effectiveness of this system in controlling excessive pressure fluctuations immediately raises the question of its inability to prevent hypertension. This failure is related to the fact that the receptors eventually adapt to whatever pressure level they are exposed to if this pressure is maintained long enough (Fig. 7-6). This resetting of baroreceptors not only prevents the reflex from functioning as a long-term control system but may also act in reverse, increasing the difficulties of initiating antihypertensive therapy.

Of less importance for arterial pressure control are chemoreceptor reflexes; they are not very effective in the normal pressure range, but in hypertensive states diminished arterial oxygen concentration excites the carotid and aortic bodies, thus reflexively elevating arterial pressure.

"**Central Reactions.**" In contrast to the feedback system of baroreceptor reflex, these reactions do not serve to control arterial pressure. The circulatory response to hypothalamic stimulation is a marked blood pressure rise with profound inotropic and chronotropic excitation of the heart. It represents a full mobilization of the organism for fight or flight. It is mentioned here because its frequent repetition or its possible evolution into a conditioned reflex has been proposed as a possible cause for hypertension. Conversely, the "playing dead" reaction (profound bradycardia, hypotension, and fainting occurring in some animals when cornered) may be analogous to some cases of emotional fainting. In these conditions, the muscle cholinergic vasodilator system is markedly activated.

The Kidney and Blood Pressure Regulation

There are two aspects of the close relationship existing between systemic arterial pressure levels and renal function. The first relates to the excretory function of the kidney; diminished excretion of salt and water in the face of maintained intake leads to hypervolemia and hypertension to achieve greater filtration and a new equilibrium between intake and output.

The second mechanism is related to a more "active" process, a renal pressor system capable of raising pressure directly when activated. Though these two mechanisms are often associated, they can also be disassociated in both clinical and experimental situations. This is discussed at greater length under Mechanisms in Hypertension; at this point only the *renal pressor system* will be described.

The importance of this system in regard to hypertension is that its end product, angiotensin II, is the most potent pressor substance known and also a stimulator of aldosterone. The system itself is really two enzyme systems in series (Fig. 7-7). In the first reaction, a proteolytic enzyme of renal origin called *renin* reacts with a circulating alpha-2-globulin (renin substrate or angiotensinogen) to release the decapeptide

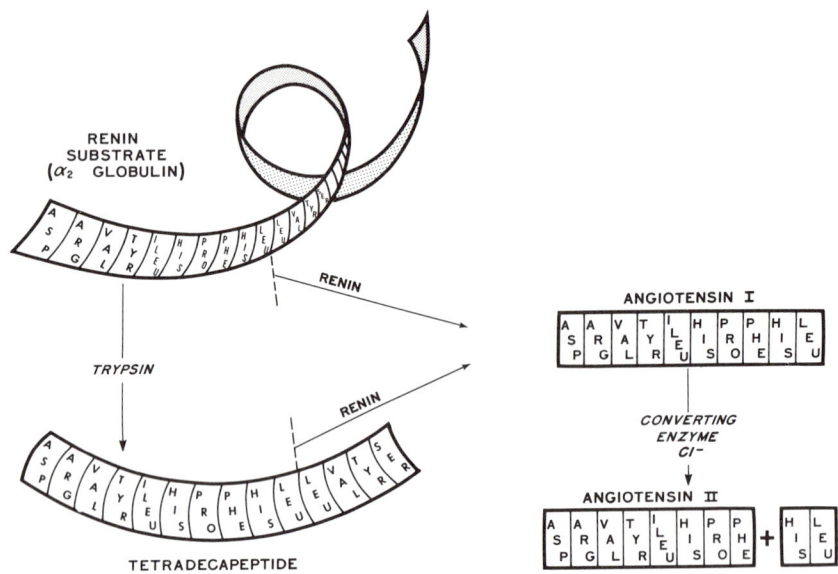

Figure 7-7 Renin-angiotensin system. (After F. M. Bumpus. *In* Page, I. H., and McCubbin, J.: Renal Hypertension. Chicago, Year Book Medical Publishers, 1969.) The normal amino acid sequence of angiotensin II is essential for its biological action; recently, analogs obtained by substitution of some amino acids have been shown to block, through competitive inhibition, various effects of the octapeptide. They are therefore very useful tools for investigation (? treatment) of some types of hypertension.

angiotensin I. This serves as substrate for converting enzyme which, by releasing two amino acids, produces the octapeptide, angiotensin II; the converting enzyme is present in plasma and tissues and there is evidence to suggest that in some species the major conversion of angiotensin I to II occurs in the lung. Angiotensin II is inactivated by plasma and tissue angiotensinases. Renin not only is active in circulating blood but is also stored in arterial walls; the importance of this local storage and possible later activation is yet to be determined. Still under investigation too is a phospholipid renin inhibitor system dependent on a renal phospholipase and a circulating phospholipid inhibitor.

Angiotensin I has no direct effect on arterial pressure, whereas only nanogram amounts of angiotensin II can produce substantial elevations. Information currently available suggests that the plasma concentration of angiotensin II is usually less than 100 picograms per ml. Because of difficulties in measuring circulating angiotensin, current information concerning the renal pressor system comes from studies of plasma renin activity (PRA); it should be emphasized that the methods widely used provide an estimate of the activity of renin but do not measure it directly.

Source of Renin—The Juxtaglomerular Apparatus. Renin comes from the kidney, hence the term renal pressor system. It is formed and stored in the juxtaglomerular (JG) apparatus, or complex, at the vascular pole of the glomerulus. At this point the macula densa portion of the distal tubule is in close proximity to the afferent and efferent arterioles. The JG complex is composed of granular cells in the afferent arterioles, the macula densa and the polkissen, a group of cells in the triangle formed by the afferent and efferent arteriole and the distal tubule. The complex is richly innervated by sympathetic nerve fibers.

Renin seems to be primarily located in the granular cells of the afferent arteriole; experimentally there is a close relationship between the granularity of these cells and renal renin content. The role of the macula densa in renin production has not yet been exactly defined. However, its cells are in close contact with JG cells and their cytologic characteristics are distinct from those of other cells in the distal tubule, suggesting a difference in function at this site. The strategic location of the JG apparatus between an arteriole and a tubule seems particularly suited for a system apparently related to both arterial pressure and sodium excretion.

It was first assumed that the factor stimulating *renin release* was renal ischemia but this was later disproved, since release could be stimulated by alterations in sodium balance that do not produce ischemia and by reductions in perfusion pressure too small to decrease renal blood flow significantly. Two concepts regarding the mechanism of renin release were then developed, the intrarenal baroreceptor hypothesis and the macula densa theory. According to the first, the renal afferent arterioles and JG cells respond to changes in stretch which could be secondary to changes in intravascular volume or in arterial pressure. For others, the macula densa is a primary sensing element responding to changes in the sodium load reaching it. Neither theory can explain all experimental observations and it seems possible that both types of receptor exist and that they influence each other. In addition to these intrarenal mechanisms, sympathetic nerves and circulating humoral agents may play important modifying roles.

A common denominator for the many stimuli that affect renin release is "effective blood volume"; its apparent correlates in clinical situations include serum sodium as well as actual blood volume. Rapid reduction of intravascular volume by controlled bleeding increases PRA, as does the reduction produced by a low-sodium diet or diuretic drug treatment. Conversely, plasma volume expansion turns off the stimulus for renin release and reduces PRA. So predictable are these responses that dietary sodium restriction and intravenous sodium chloride infusion are used as standard tests of the renal pressor system. These maneuvers alter both blood volume (and extracellular fluid volume) and sodium balance; under normal conditions both stimuli act in the same direction on renin release. Under experimental conditions the two stimuli can be dissociated and it would seem that changes in intravascular volume predominate over changes in serum sodium in determining PRA. That is not to say that serum sodium plays no role in influencing renin release. On the contrary, this has been clearly shown in animal experiments utilizing renal perfusion techniques with which it is possible to vary sodium concentration of the perfusate without varying that of the whole body. Hyponatremia increased renin release and hypernatremia diminished it. It has been suggested that the reason why diuretic drugs increase PRA is not only because they decrease plasma volume but also because they diminish sodium transport by macula densa cells. In this connection, changes in serum potassium must be taken into account in the interpretation of renin data. Hypokalemia may stimulate and hyperkalemia may inhibit PRA, independent of associated alterations in either aldosterone secretion or sodium balance.

Though it is not essential for renin release, the sympathetic nervous system may alter it directly or indirectly. Conditions associated with rise in PRA are usually those associated with increased sympathetic activity (upright posture, hypovolemia). Both alpha- and beta-adrenergic blocking drugs have been shown to diminish PRA. As well as manipulations of sodium intake, upright posture is frequently used as a clinical test of renin release. Patients with idiopathic orthostatic hypotension sometimes fail to show the expected increase of PRA with standing.

Pressor Effects of the Renin-Angiotensin System. Though angiotensin II is the most powerful vasoconstrictor agent, its direct effect on resistance vessels might not be its most important contribution to arterial pressure regulation except in special cases. Possibly of greater significance for circulatory control are its effects on aldosterone secretion and sympathetic functions.

Infusions of even small subpressor doses of angiotensin lead to marked increase in aldosterone secretion. The resultant fluid retention and increase in sodium stores set the stage for blood pressure elevation, water retention by increasing extracellular fluid volume, and sodium retention by increasing vascular responsiveness to vasoconstrictor agents.

On the other hand, angiotensin has major effects on sympathetic nervous activity. It enhances activity through a direct stimulatory action on the vasomotor center; the area postramus is one place where blood-brain barrier against angiotensin breaks down. Peripherally, it enhances sympathetic nerve effects by diminishing neuronal norepinephrine uptake, thus allowing a greater concentration of the neurohormone to reach vascular receptor sites. Angiotensin is also a potent stimulus for catecholamine release from the adrenal medulla. Thus, it is obvious that no matter how potent a vasoconstrictor angiotensin may be in its own right, it has the potential for affecting arterial pressure in many other ways. Its effects on nerve function are suggesting that angiotensin may eventually prove to be an important modulator of neural activity.

Renal Pressor System and Hypertension. It is obvious by now that "renin" has emerged as a very complex system as regards both its control mechanisms and the extent of its effects. Estimates of peripheral plasma renin activity (PRA) cannot therefore be expected to define all disturbances of this system. A normal PRA does not rule out the possibility of important minor variations in circulating angiotensin II. Conversely, an elevated PRA can be found in normotensive states such as hepatic cirrhosis or the nephrotic syndrome, showing that there is more to any hypertension than the renal pressor system. The number of factors affecting renin release make it clear that reported levels of renin activity cannot, therefore, be interpreted out of context and should be evaluated only in relation to clinical setting, posture of patient at time of sampling, level of arterial pressure, sodium balance (24 hour urinary sodium), serum electrolytes, and some estimate of intravascular volume.

The renal pressor system has been implicated in malignant hypertension, renovascular hypertension, and the hypertension induced by oral contraceptives. In most other hypertensions, there is no clear evidence of its participation. In primary aldosteronism, aldosterone alone is increased while PRA is suppressed. Animal studies have suggested that excess renin may cause vascular injury but it is not yet evident if this applies to man.

Each type of hypertension is discussed separately, so that we will refer here only to that related to the use of oral contraceptive agents. The estrogen component of these medications increases renin substrate, and although renin itself is not necessarily increased, more angiotensin is formed, and circulating angiotensin is usually increased. Since there is no way (in man) to block the enzymes of the renal pressor system, there is no way of knowing the exact nature of the hypertension that occurs in only a few of the women so treated. However, when treatment is discontinued, the components of the renal pressor system return to normal levels and the hypertension disappears.

HYPERTENSION*

Hypertension means elevated arterial pressure, either systolic or diastolic or both, as is often the case. Diastolic elevation had been considered the hallmark of hypertension while systolic blood pressure was thought to be more variable and its elevation inconsequential. Recent evidence has shown both assumptions to be false; diastolic pressure levels vary as much as the systolic, and systolic hypertension is associated with increased morbidity and mortality. The close relation between mean systolic pressure and myocardial oxygen requirements shows that systolic hypertension is not hemodynamically insignificant; it imposes a costly load on the heart and seems as closely related to cardiac hypertrophy as diastolic hypertension, if not more so. The basic mechanisms of systolic hypertension have been reviewed and this discussion will deal with what is called diastolic hypertension, although systolic pressure is elevated as well.

Hypertension by itself is not a diagnosis. It is the result of a number of diseases and disturbances—some serious and progressive, others transient—and it can be classified in many ways. The following is modified from Pickering:
1. By kind
    a. Systolic hypertension
    b. Diastolic hypertension
2. By degree
    a. Nonmalignant
    b. Malignant
3. By cause
    a. Primary or unexplained—essential hypertension
    b. Secondary hypertension

A list of causes is given in Table 7-1.

*See also Chapter 6.

Definition of Hypertension

To speak of elevated arterial pressure begs the question of what constitutes "normal" pressure levels. Mathematical limits can be defined by population surveys (means, standard deviations) but the absence of a demonstrable cause for deviation from the norm in the vast majority of cases has led to a re-examination of basic concepts regarding the nature of hypertension. Put simply, the question is, is there a natural dividing line between normal and raised arterial pressure, or is hypertension a purely quantitative alteration of a biophysical measurement (pressure)? In the first case, hypertension would be a specific disease leading to pressure elevation; in the second, it would be a simple quantitative deviation from normal with no specific point at which the disease can be said to begin.

The controversy is not yet completely settled. One school of thought (Platt and coworkers) is that hypertension is a specific disease entity. Two groups exist—those whose pressures do and those whose pressures do not increase with age—and the difference between them is determined by monogenic inheritance. Pickering and coworkers have argued very strongly that arterial pressure is a biophysical characteristic, like height, whose frequency distribution curves show no natural subdivision into separate groups and which is governed by a graded multifactorial or polygenic inheritance. Arguments are based on complicated statistical analysis of population surveys but also fundamentally, we think, on the persistent failure to uncover "the fault" that would explain essential hypertension.

A very important benefit from these discussions has been the attention drawn to the quantitative aspects of hypertension. Whatever its basic nature, there is no doubt about the importance of the actual level of pressure. Perhaps in no other disease does the quantitative deviation of a single variable so influence the course and complications of the disorder. Studies by life insurance companies have shown an impressive relationship between mortality and blood pressure levels extending over the whole range of arterial pressures, with no sudden break at any point. Aside from specific characteristics of diseases associated with hypertension, high blood pressure has consequences of its own. Many are closely related to the level of pressure itself and are prevented or reversed by adequate pressure control. These would include left ventricular failure, hypertensive encephalopathy, and the malignant phase. Fibrinoid necrosis can occur in any form of hypertension, with the possible exception of aortic coarctation, if the pressure is high enough. The relationship with pressure is less clear-cut for other complications; atherosclerotic complications are more frequent in

TABLE 7–1 AN ETIOLOGIC CLASSIFICATION OF HYPERTENSION

I. *Arterial Hypertension (elevation of systolic and diastolic blood pressures)*
  A. Essential hypertension
    1. Labile (intermittent)
    2. Established ("fixed")
  B. Renal hypertension
    1. Kidney disease
      a. Glomerulonephritis
      b. Chronic pyelonephritis
      c. Congenital polycystic kidneys
      d. Obstructive uropathy
      e. Diabetic glomerulosclerosis
      f. Interstitial nephritis due to analgesics, gout, hypercalcemia
      g. Connective tissue diseases, periarteritis nodosa, scleroderma, lupus erythematosus
      h. Renal tumor
      i. Renal amyloidosis
      j. Radiation nephritis
      k. Hereditary nephritis
    2. Renal arterial disease
      a. Fibrous dysplasias
      b. Atherosclerotic disease
      c. Embolic obstruction
      d. Traumatic arterial dissection or occlusion
    3. Compression of kidney
      a. Perinephritis
      b. Perirenal hematoma, usually post-traumatic
  C. Endocrine hypertension
    1. Catecholamine excess: pheochromocytoma
    2. "Steroid" hypertension
      a. Mineralocorticoid excess
        (1) Primary aldosteronism
        (2) Functional enzymatic block leading to adrenal hyperplasia (e.g., 11-hydroxylase deficiency in adrenogenital syndrome, 17-hydroxylase deficiency, androgen-induced hydroxylase deficiency in masculinizing tumors)
        (3) Iatrogenic: Excess DOC or fluorinated steroid administration
      b. Glucocorticoid excess—various causes of Cushing syndrome (adrenal, pituitary, ectopic ACTH syndromes, ovarian tumors)
    3. Oral contraceptives
    4. Condition associated with hypertension
      a. Acromegaly
      b. Thyroid disorders
        (1) Myxedema
        (2) Thyrotoxicosis, usually a cause of systolic, not diastolic, hypertension
  D. Neurogenic hypertension
    1. Anxiety states (?)
    2. Intracranial disease
      a. Increased intracranial pressure
      b. Encephalitis
      c. Diencephalic syndrome
      d. Lead encephalopathy
    3. Disturbances in vasomotor center
      a. Bulbar poliomyelitis
      b. Disturbances in vascular supply
    4. Spinal cord and peripheral nerves
      a. Transection of the cord, transverse myelitis
      b. Polyneuritis
      c. Porphyria
  E. Hypertension of coarctation of the aorta
  F. Hypertension of toxemia of pregnancy
    1. Preeclampsia
    2. Eclampsia
II. *Systolic Hypertension*
  A. Caused mainly by an increased stroke output of the left ventricle
    1. Complete heart block
    2. Aortic regurgitation
    3. Patent ductus arteriosus
    4. Thyrotoxicosis
    5. Arteriovenous fistula
    6. Paget's disease of bone
  B. Caused mainly by a decreased distensibility of the aorta
    1. Arteriosclerosis of aorta
    2. Coarctation of aorta

hypertensive patients but may develop in normotensive subjects. In this case the duration of hypertension may be more important than its level. Though strokes are prevented to a certain extent by control of arterial pressure, myocardial infarction does not seem to be.

General Pathophysiologic Aspects in Hypertension

The number of unrelated diseases associated with hypertension indicates that there must be a variety of ways to produce a chronic rise of blood pressure. These are called pressor mechanisms. In a sense, this term is a misnomer because, with the exception of pheochromocytoma, the physiologic abnormalities associated with hypertension have not been shown to be causal. Although these abnormalities represent distinct aberrations of a number of cardiovascular control systems, the degrees to which they participate in arterial pressure elevation are not known. There is a real difference between recognizing the "cause" of a particular hypertension and describing its mechanism.

Hypertension is a disease of regulation; the mosaic theory proposed by Page in 1949 stressed the multifactorial response of the body to environmental influences. A disturbance of one factor will lead to automatic involvement of others, so that a whole new set of relationships may be established, often making it very difficult to decide which came first.

Some of these secondary alterations may be responsible for what might be termed post-causal hypertension, meaning persistence of hypertension even after removal of its primary cause. This can be shown experimentally in hypertension produced by renal arterial constriction; removal of the ischemic kidney will reduce blood pressure only if performed within a certain time after the provoking maneuver; if nephrectomy is delayed, hypertension will not be relieved. A clinical counterpart of this situation might be surmised when removal of apparently primary causes (e.g., adrenocortical tumor, pheochromocytoma, renal arterial stenosis) fails to relieve the patient of his hypertension. It is, however, very difficult in man to ascertain whether one is not dealing with the coexistence of two separate causes for the hypertensive disease, e.g., renal arterial stenosis in a patient with essential hypertension.

Of the possible factors helping to perpetuate hypertension, three are of particular interest.

1. The vulnerability of the renal vessels to increased pressure loads, leading to development of arteriolar nephrosclerosis.

2. The structural adaptation of vessel walls to hypertension; the thickened wall amplifies the luminal reduction produced by even normal stimuli (Folkow).

3. Resetting of baroreceptors: the fact that carotid sinus reflexes are active in hypertensive patients led to questioning why they did not prevent hypertension. McCubbin et al. showed in dogs with chronic renal hypertension that there is a shifting upward in response of baroreceptors, i.e., an adaptation resetting the reflex to operate normally at higher pressure levels (Fig. 7-6). Once developed, this resetting may well militate for a time against attempts at reducing arterial pressure.

SECONDARY HYPERTENSION

The mechanisms responsible for a secondary hypertension are not completely known in all cases. The following is a summary of some of the main types. A certain degree of overlapping is unavoidable and this section should be read along with that on essential hypertension.

Renal Hypertension*

One of the important results of recent studies has been the differentiation of hypertensive states associated with renal disease into two types—one related, at least initially, to activation of some pressor mechanism, and the other related to loss of renal substance and possibly of an antipressor effect. The first is exemplified by renal arterial stenosis and the second by the anephric state. In a schematic form that admits of many exceptions, the first type is characterized in man by elevated plasma renin activity (especially in recent hypertension), low plasma volume, and indices of increased neurogenic activity. The second type is marked by a positive correlation between blood volume and arterial pressure and very low or absent circulating renin; neurogenic activity fluctuates inversely with the degree of volemia. Patients with parenchymal kidney disease show varying mixtures of these two extremes, with either the "renal" or "renoprival" element predominating according to the type or stage of the lesion (Fig. 7-8).

Renovascular Hypertension. A large body of knowledge has been accumulated concerning this type of hypertension since the classic experiments of Goldblatt in dogs. Essential to proper evaluation of experimental studies is the realization of the extent of differences that may result from variation in techniques, timing of observations, and animal species used. Studies in many have shown that cardiac output was elevated in many patients with renovascular hypertension, but also that this increase was not alone responsible for the maintenance of their hypertension. Total peripheral resistance was raised in patients with both normal and elevated outputs; successful surgical repair or nephrectomy was associated with reduction in resistance more often than with reduction in output. This common participation of varying degrees of increased output and resistance in the maintenance of renovascular hypertension in man corresponds to recent experimental studies in rats and dogs. Though the early rise of arterial pressure following clipping of renal arteries or cellophane wrapping of the kidney is primarily due to increased cardiac output, later stages are characterized by a delayed rise in peripheral resistance with a return of output toward normal. The change in hemodynamic pattern with time has been related to autoregulatory mechanisms (see earlier discussion).

The increase of output and initiation of hypertension following renal arterial clipping have been related to fluid retention consequent on the reduction in renal perfusion pressure. However, no change in blood volume was noted in the initial stages of perinephritic hypertension in dogs when cardiac output was rising; indeed, in both man and dogs with chronic renovascular hypertension plasma volume is slightly reduced. The combination of lower intravascular volume and increased cardiac output suggested an increased tone of the capacitance vessels shifting

---

*See also Chapter 14.

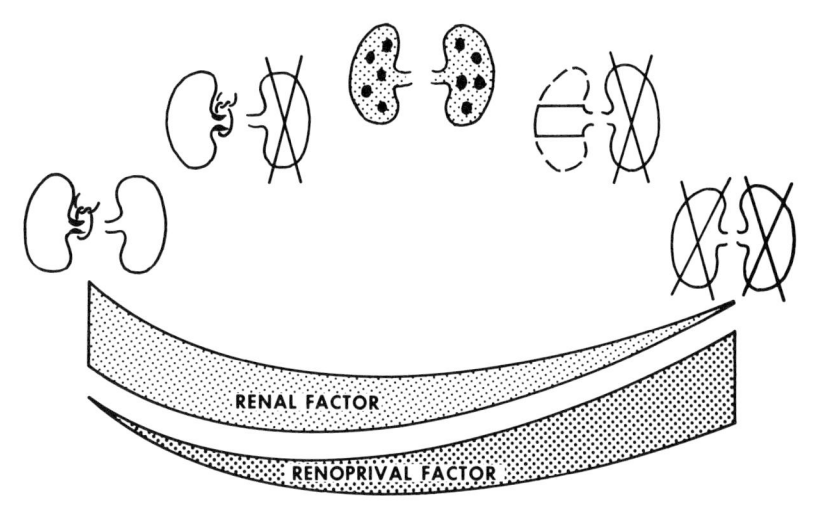

Figure 7–8 Renal and renoprival mechanisms in various types of "renal" hypertension; at one extreme is the renal mechanism activated by critical narrowing of one renal artery, the other remaining intact. At the other, removal of both kidneys leads to a renoprival volume-dependent state. In between these two extremes, both renal and renoprival factors participate in different combinations in the development of hypertension, depending on amount of renal tissue lost and on impairment of circulation through the remainder. (Modified from Tarazi, R. C., et al.: Pathol. et Biol. *16*:547, 1968.)

blood toward the heart. This is presumably related to enhanced sympathetic activity by angiotensin, since the latter has little, if any, direct effect on veins. Simultaneous stimulation of arterioles directly or indirectly (Fig. 7–9) helps set the stage for increased peripheral resistance. Once established, hypertension may be perpetuated by the development of secondary factors obscuring the initial disturbance (see later discussion).

It is generally agreed that the renal pressor system plays an important role in the early stages of renovascular hypertension; its participation in the chronic stage is much more debatable. This is probably because of the number of factors involved in any hypertension of sufficient duration and because of the wide spectrum of effects of angiotensin II, even in minute doses. However, peripheral plasma renin activity is not infrequently elevated in patients with renal arterial stenosis and seems to be directly related to the height of diastolic arterial pressure. This is important to remember, since these patients in a hospital setting often have mild labile hypertension and a finding of normal PRA does not mean that the hypertension is nonrenal. Because peripheral PRA is inconsistently elevated in renovascular hypertensive subjects, measurements in renal venous blood have been advocated. This is based on the likelihood that in unilateral renal arterial stenosis the affected kidney will produce, either spontaneously or in response to adequate stimulation, more renin than the unaffected kidney.

Hypertension and Renal Parenchymal Disease. This type of hypertension is so often complicated by the features attendant on diminished kidney function that acceptable studies of its mechanism in man have been very difficult to obtain. Furthermore, the time course of renal decompensation can be compressed into a few days or extended over several years, so that hypertensive mechanisms may be quite different from one case to the other. Whether the diseased kidneys are still present or have been removed is another important factor; in some instances the characteristics of hypertension are radically altered by bilateral nephrectomy, even though the removed organs had practically no excretory function left.

The dependence of arterial pressure on volume expansion characterizes the hypertension associated with loss of renal tissue. In contrast with the slight plasma volume contraction seen in essential and renovascular hypertension is the direct correlation between arterial pressure and intravascular volume found in many patients with renal parenchymal disease (Fig. 7–10). In each one, however, the hypertensive features will depend on the individual proportion of the renal and renoprival elements outlined earlier.

The hypertension of acute glomerulonephritis has been related to hypervolemia with consequent circulatory congestion, high ventricular filling pressure, and increased cardiac output, the total peripheral resistance remaining inappropriately normal in the face of increased blood flow.

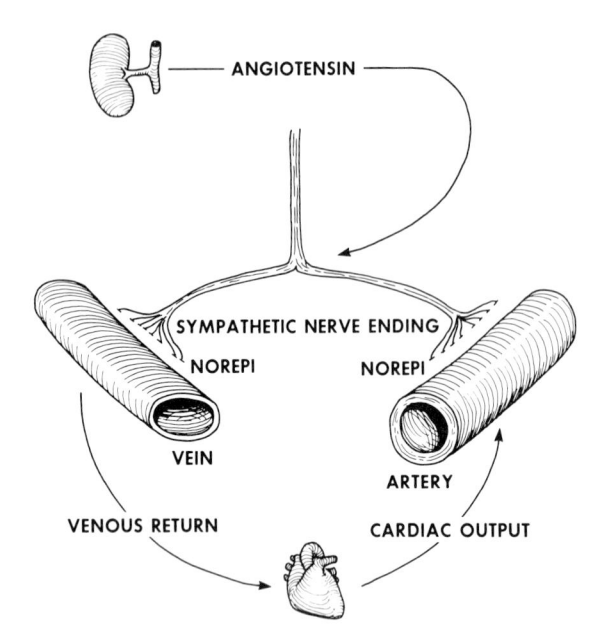

Figure 7-9 Diagram of possible ways by which angiotensin may raise arterial pressure, apart from a direct vasoconstrictor effect. It may act centrally (stimulation of vasomotor center) or peripherally (inhibiting re-uptake of norepinephrine (norepi) by sympathetic nerve endings, thus potentiating its action); arterial pressure is raised by a combination in different proportions of increased peripheral resistance (arteriolar constriction) and increased cardiac output (venoconstriction enhancing venous return).

In patients with end-stage kidney disease, two varieties of hypertension may be seen. The first and more common is volume-dependent; the height of the arterial pressure is related to the degree of volemia and can be controlled by diuretics (if still effective) or by dialysis; PRA is not elevated. The second group of patients do not respond well to dehydration or vasopressor agents; their hypertension seems to depend on continued activation of the renal pressor system and is markedly reduced (or made easier to manage) by nephrectomy.

Hemodynamic findings in the hypertension of renal parenchymal disease are quite variable because of the number of complicating factors present, such as degree of anemia, fluid balance, myocardial status, and so on. However, when conditions are strictly controlled, the increase in pressure is found to depend on an absolute or relative increase in total peripheral resistance. It differs from essential hypertension in the absence of a preferential redistribution of blood flow to the muscles. Brod et al., who reported these findings, interpret them as a definite qualitative difference from the "patterns of persistent stress or preparedness to exercise characteristic of essential hypertension."

Coarctation of the Aorta

The hypertension associated with coarctation of the aorta is an experiment of nature of considerable hemodynamic interest. It has demonstrated that the body can adjust peripheral resistance differently in organs above and below the coarctation so as to provide all of them with a normal blood flow. Unfortunately, the mechanism of this precise adjustment has not yet been determined, though it offers the best possible example for autoregulation of blood flow.

Though the renal arteries are usually below the aortic constriction, there is no unequivocal evidence for activation of a renal pressor mechanism. The hypertension is probably related to the mechanical obstruction. Cardiac output in coarctation is usually increased; the ejection of a large stroke volume into an aorta with decreased capacity and relatively limited runoff accounts for the large pressure found in vessels above the area of constriction. As output and rate of ejection are increased with exercise, so is the systolic blood pressure, often to alarming levels, even in patients who have near normal blood pressure at rest. By diminishing this increase of cardiac output with intravenous propranolol, blood pressure rise with exercise is attenuated despite the significant increase in total peripheral resistance induced by the drug.

The importance of adaptive changes to hypertension can be seen in the occasional complications that follow surgical repair. When the obstruction is removed, vessels below the coarctation are suddenly exposed to higher pressures than they are used to; concomitantly baroreceptor reflexes are activated by the drop of pressure in their area. The result may be a hypertensive crisis with arteriolar necrosis in the lower body parts.

Pheochromocytoma

Most interesting and unusual is the hypertensive state associated with pheochromocytoma, a tumor of the medullary portion of the adrenal gland. It is one of the rare types in which the actual pressor mechanism is known. The tumors contain large amounts of epinephrine and norepinephrine in varying proportions. Hypertension may be persistent but is often paroxysmal. Symptoms result from release of the hormones from the tumor, causing sudden rapid rises in blood pressure, tachycardia, anxiety, headache, perspiration, nausea, and epigastric and precordial pain. All symptoms do not always appear but it would be a most unusual patient who would not have at least one or two. Norepinephrine produces no tachycardia and does not affect the cardiac output. Epinephrine does both and produces hypermetabolism and hyperglycemia as well. Variations in the clinical picture depend in large part on these variables, but there are exceptions. The only definitive means of making the diagnosis are biochemical tests showing increased catecholamine excretion; these include determination of urinary vanillylmandelic acid (VMA), metanephrines, and catecholamines either during a hypertensive period or following a provocative test. Intravenous histamine (0.025 mg.) may bring on an attack and is probably still the more reliable provocative agent as regards both blood pressure response and urinary excretion of catecholamine metabolites. Adrenergic blocking agents such as phentolamine or dibenzyline will reduce the elevated pressure. Phentolamine is especially useful for hypertensive episodes; dibenzyline is preferred for medical treatment if tumors are inoperable.

Beta-adrenergic blockers may be needed to control tachycardia or ventricular irritability induced by excess catecholamines.

Primary Aldosteronism (Conn's Disease)

The frequency of this condition as a cause of hypertension is not known for certain. It is certainly a more frequent cause than is pheochromocytoma; however, it is less common than autopsy findings of small adrenocortical nodules might suggest. It results from autonomous hypersecretion of aldosterone by small single or multiple tumors of the adrenal cortex zona glomerulosa; sometimes only bilateral hyperplasia is found, with no strictly definitive tumor (see Chapter 32). Its importance stems from the possibility of specific therapy or surgical cure for this type of hypertension.

The diagnosis is suggested by finding hypokalemia and inappropriate kaliuresis (> 30.0 mEq. daily urinary potassium excretion with a serum potassium < 3.5 mEq./L.) in a hypertensive patient with no history of recent diuretic therapy; the clinical picture is otherwise very similar to essential hypertension. The specific endocrine derangement is indicated by (1) low plasma renin activity that cannot be stimulated by low sodium intake (thus excluding secondary aldosteronism), and (2) more specifically, increased aldosterone excretion that cannot be suppressed by high sodium intake (thus reflecting the abnormality in regulation). Adrenal venography has been recommended for localization of the lesion.

The metabolic abnormalities in primary aldo-

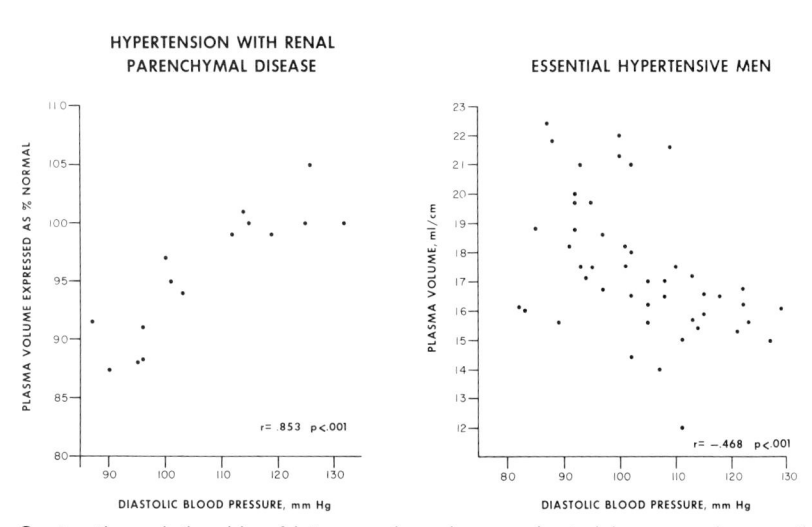

Figure 7–10 Contrasting relationship of intravascular volume and arterial pressure in essential hypertensive men and patients with renal parenchymal disease. (After Tarazi, R. C., et al.: Arch. Int. Med., 125:835, 1970. Copyright 1970, American Medical Association.)

steronism are better understood than the mechanism of its hypertension. Increased aldosterone excretion leads to sodium and water retention; stimulation of potassium-for-sodium exchange in the distal tubule leads to hypokalemia from excessive potassium loss in the urine. Increase in extracellular sodium and relative expansion of plasma volume probably account for the suppression of plasma renin activity, since administration of spironolactone can stimulate it. Initial investigations have shown a normal or somewhat increased cardiac output and an elevated total peripheral resistance.

There are other causes of hypertension due to *mineralocorticoid excess,* all sharing the same pattern of suppressed plasma renin activity and easily induced hypokalemia (see diagram). Some result from excess administration of sodium-retaining steroids or steroid-like substances (e.g., licorice) and simply require discontinuing the drug or readjusting its dose. Others are due to enzymatic blocks (congenital or acquired) in hydroxylation of adrenal steroids at the 11 or 17 position. These blocks interfere with the production of cortisol and hence with its negative feedback control over ACTH production. The resultant excessive ACTH drive leads to adrenal hypersecretion of mineralocorticoids and consequent hypertension. Treatment consists of ACTH suppression by dexamethasone. Still other cases result from disordered hormonal production by adrenal and extra-adrenal tumors.

ESSENTIAL HYPERTENSION

By far the commonest type, essential hypertension still remains a diagnosis by exclusion, reached only by ruling out the various causes of elevated arterial pressure. It is characterized by a strong hereditary element and a long natural course, so that in early phases the subject appears normal except for the high blood pressure.

All the mechanisms discussed earlier have been at one time or another linked with essential hypertension. It is obviously very difficult in slowly developing asymptomatic processes to differentiate primary factors from secondary reactions. Until now no animal model exists for essential hypertension; the relation of genetic strains of spontaneously hypertensive rats to the human disease is still conjectural. Another difficulty is the lack of homogeneity resulting from lack of precision in diagnosis; there are probably different subgroups still included, for want of a better definition, under the overall term of "essential or idiopathic hypertension."

Hemodynamic Characteristics

The main development in this area concerns the relationship between fixed and labile essential hypertension. Well-established essential hypertension is associated with a normal cardiac output and elevated peripheral resistance. The elevated resistance seems to be uniformly distributed in practically all vascular territories except in the kidney, where it may be more intense, and in the skeletal muscular system, where it is slightly less marked. This pattern was likened by Brod to a constant preparedness for exercise or response to unspecified stress. Within this general framework a certain gradation has been described wherein a progressive reduction of resting cardiac output occurred with development of progressive cardiac involvement in the course of the disease. Even before cardiac decompensation occurred, cardiac output was reduced (and total peripheral resistance further increased) in hypertensive patients with definite left ventricular hypertrophy.

Contrasting with the above findings, an increasing number of studies from laboratories in the United States and Europe have established that a large proportion of patients with essential hypertension, especially those with mildly or intermittently elevated arterial pressure, have increased cardiac output and normal, near normal, or subnormal values of total peripheral resistance. The suggestion is that this pattern of "increased output–normal resistance" is the beginning phase leading to increased resistance and fixed hypertension. It is not yet evident from information available whether increase in cardiac output represents an early stage in the development of hypertension or a qualitatively different hemodynamic type of the disease. The answer must await longitudinal clinical studies of labile hypertensive subjects.

The reason for the increased output in borderline hypertension is not clear; oxygen consumption is normal for that level of output in contrast with other idiopathic high output states. Resting heart rate, though slightly faster than normal, is not faster than that in other forms of hypertension. The finding reawakened interest in the old suggestion that an "augmented force" of the heart beat could play a role in the genesis of hypertension; but an increase in output might as well represent a normal cardiac response to constriction of the capacitance vessels and central redistribution of blood. Similarities with hemodynamic findings in renovascular hypertension are obvious; however, the mechanisms involved in essential hypertension are still purely conjectural.

In these considerations of increased output, it must be remembered that in the final analysis, hypertension is the result of failure of the peripheral circulation to adapt to systemic flow. Indeed, some abnormality in peripheral circulatory adjustment is demonstrable even in patients with "normal total peripheral resistance." Though

SIMPLIFIED SCHEME OF MINERALOCORTICOID HYPERTENSIONS

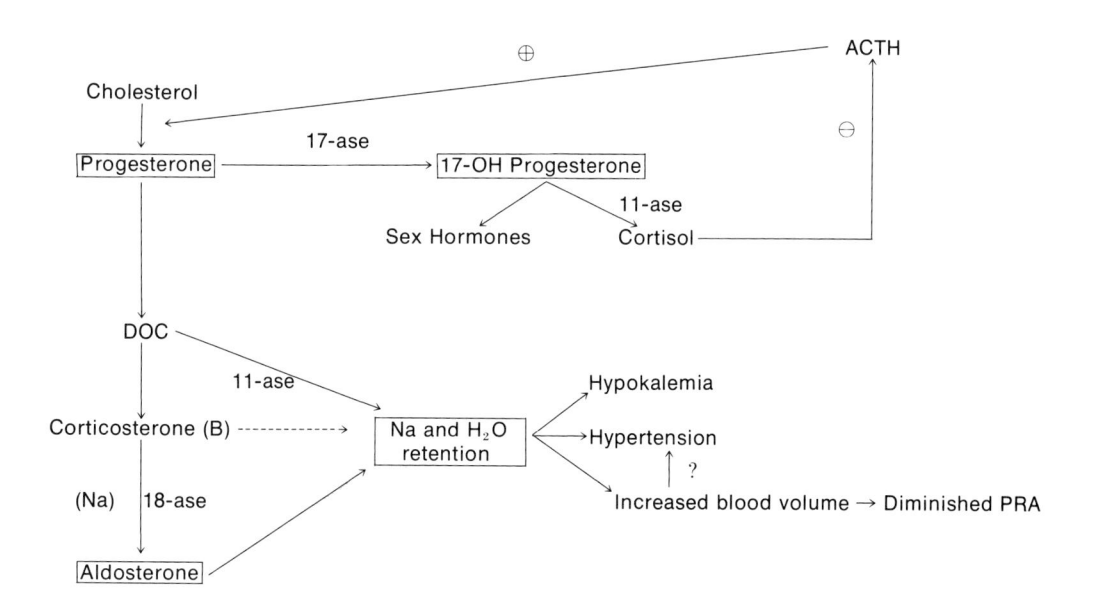

```
                                    ⊕ ────────────────────→ ACTH
    Cholesterol
         │                                              ⊖
         ↓          17-ase
    [Progesterone] ─────────→ [17-OH Progesterone]
         │                           │  11-ase
         │                    Sex Hormones  Cortisol ──────┘
         ↓
        DOC ─────┐
         │        \  11-ase
    Corticosterone (B) ─ ─ ─ ─→ ┌──────────────┐ → Hypokalemia
         │                      │ Na and H₂O   │
    (Na) │18-ase                │  retention   │ → Hypertension
         ↓                      └──────────────┘        ↑ ?
    [Aldosterone] ──────────────────↑            Increased blood volume → Diminished PRA
```

Key:
⊕ Positive stimulus
⊖ Negative feedback
11-ase, 17-ase = 11 beta or 17 alpha-hydroxylase
PRA = plasma renin activity

(a) 11 beta-hydroxylase deficiency leads to decreased cortisol; the increased ACTH drive leads to hypertension secondary to DOC excess and to accumulation of 17 OH-products increasing androgenic hormones.
(b) 17 alpha-hydroxylase deficiency leads to decreased cortisol and therefore to increased ACTH drive, but sex hormones are usually absent owing to lack of 17 hydroxylation; hypertension is related to increased DOC and corticosterone as sodium retention decreases their conversion to aldosterone.
(c) Combined DOC, corticosterone, and aldosterone excess occurs in adrenocortical tumors, especially if malignant, and in disordered ACTH drive (ectopic); cortisol is usually also increased in these cases.
(d) In primary aldosteronism, only aldosterone is increased.
(e) Iatrogenic hypertension usually results from excess DOC or fluorinated cortisol derivatives with unrestricted salt intake.

correctly said to be "within normal range," their resistance is abnormally high for their cardiac output, as is shown by comparison with normotensive subjects with equivalent levels of output. The abnormality is clearly revealed during muscular exercise.

In the absence of cardiac failure, response to dynamic exercise in hypertensive patients is much the same as in normal subjects. Cardiac output increases proportionately to oxygen uptake, and peripheral resistance falls. This fall is never to normal levels, so that blood pressure remains high; although the heart responded normally, the extent of reduction in peripheral resistance was not commensurate with the rise in output, especially in young subjects. The anomaly of peripheral reactions in hypertension is also shown in the pattern of response to stressful interviews. The resultant increase of blood pressure was due to increased cardiac output in 80 per cent of normal subjects, whereas most hypertensive patients responded by an increase in total peripheral resistance.

Neurogenic Factors

The obvious effects of emotional factors on arterial pressure have led to many assumptions regarding the role of *psychogenic factors* in essential hypertension. It has been suggested that frequent psychogenic rises in blood pressure may culminate finally in fixed hypertension. The corticohypothalamic "defense reaction" not only may be activated by manifest threats but is also said to occur whenever "alertness" is raised. Repeated increases in arterial pressure would lead to structural adaptation (hypertrophy) of the arterioles, which in turn would amplify the vasoconstrictive effects of even normal nerve traffic or circulating substances. Various alterations found in essential hypertension—namely, altered regional blood flow, modest increase in basal heart rate, and decrease in plasma volume—have been likened to the pattern of "preparedness to exercise."

Despite its attractiveness, this hypothesis still remains to be proved, since there is no firm evidence that psychogenic stimuli result in chronic sustained hypertension. These stimuli are difficult to quantitate and nerve traffic cannot yet be measured directly in man. Studies showing excessive pressure rise in hypertensive patients in response to stressful experiences do not differentiate between increased sympathetic outflow from vasomotor centers and increased vascular responsiveness to normal outflow. The problem is complicated by the possible influence of such ill-defined factors as personality traits. Pavlov noted that it is easier to produce a neurotic state in "sanguine" than in "melancholic" dogs. Promising studies are being conducted in the area of conditioned blood pressure control and the effects of reticular formation on baroreceptor activity.

The hypertension produced in laboratory animals by sino-aortic denervation does not bear any real resemblance to essential hypertension. It is accompanied by wide swings of blood pressure and marked tachycardia; the pressure falls to normal levels when the animal is quiet or asleep and is unusually sensitive to neural blocking agents. Apart from rare cases of polyneuritis involving the ninth cranial nerve, disturbances of baroreceptor mechanism probably do not have a causative role in essential hypertension. Secondary resetting of their threshold and/or diminished sensitivity of the reflex due to functional or structural changes in the carotid arteries might theoretically play a minor role in its maintenance.

The striking antihypertensive effectiveness of drugs that suppress adrenergic functions is still one of the main evidences that neural factors operate in some way to maintain hypertension. A clinically applicable way to estimate their importance is to determine the immediate pressure response to an intravenous injection of a ganglion blocker. The pressure reduction obtained in essential hypertensive subjects correlated significantly with pre-injection diastolic pressure and total peripheral resistance. Again, the higher the pressure and the resistance, the smaller the plasma volume, so that intravascular volume was inversely related to sympathetic activity. At the present time there is no way of knowing whether intravascular volume is reduced because increased sympathetic tone has reduced vascular capacity or whether increased sympathetic outflow is a compensatory response to a reduced plasma volume.

An important aspect developed over the past decade is the close and reciprocal interaction between the renal pressor and sympathetic nervous systems. The potentiating action of angiotensin on the cardiovascular effects of the sympathetic nervous system has already been discussed. On the other hand, sympathetic hyperactivity may help trigger the renin-angiotensin system by restricting blood flow to the kidney (a part of the "defense reaction"). Thus, whether a neurogenic or a hormonal factor is the initial event, both may inter-react to maintain a more sustained neurohumoral drive on the cardiovascular system (Folkow and Neil). The clinical relevance of these relationships is underlined by the experience that renovascular hypertension can be effectively treated by drugs which suppress adrenergic activity.

Extracellular Fluid and Blood Volume

There now seems little question that plasma volume is quite regularly altered in various forms of hypertension. It is reduced in essential hypertension in relation to the level of diastolic pressure and peripheral resistance, so that the higher the resistance, the lower the volume. Since extracellular fluid volume is usually normal in this condition, the reduction in plasma volume probably reflects a subtle abnormality in the distribution of fluid between its intravascular and interstitial compartments. Hypertension accompanying renal arterial disease or pheochromocytoma is also characterized by reduced plasma volume.

In contrast, plasma volume is modestly expanded in primary aldosteronism, although not as consistently as is usually suggested. The more striking abnormality is the positive correlation between total blood volume and arterial pressure found in patients with renal parenchymal disease (see Renal Hypertension). Finally, a subgroup of essential hypertension has been described with plasma volume either expanded or inappropriately normal for height of diastolic pressure. This group possibly represents the same type of hypertension as is being tentatively characterized by various investigators as having increased extracellular fluid volume, increased exchangeable sodium, and hyporeninemia with no evidence of primary aldosteronism.

The clinical relevance of volume studies is not limited to diagnostic considerations. As indicated above, pressure responsiveness to ganglion blockers is inversely related to degree of volemia, hence the greater sensitivity of patients with low plasma volume (spontaneous or diuretic-induced) to neural blocking drugs. Conversely, pressure response to these drugs is attenuated or lost when hypervolemia develops, as it often does during their administration. The increase in plasma volume during treatment results from diminished tone of capacitance vessels with resultant transfer of fluid from the interstitial to the intravascular compartment and is accentuated by actual fluid retention. This "false tolerance" to the neural blocking drugs is reversed and pressure control is restored by adequate volume depletion with diuretics.

Renal Pressor System

At the present time there is no indication of any gross abnormality of this system in nonmalignant essential hypertension. Plasma renin levels are usually within normal range but occasionally can be quite low and unresponsive to the usual stimuli used to increase circulating renin. In the majority of subjects with essential hypertension aldosterone secretion correlates normally with urinary sodium excretion. In some, however, discrepancies between levels of plasma renin activity and aldosterone excretion have been described, especially under the stimulus of sodium deprivation. The role of this hormonal imbalance is still not clear.

Malignant hypertension—of whatever origin— is associated with marked secondary aldosteronism: high plasma renin activity, hyponatremia, hypokalemia, and great rises of aldosterone excretion. Activation of the renin-angiotensin system in this condition has been viewed as partly responsible for the intensification of the vascular disease and of hyponatremia.

In summary, this review of pathophysiologic mechanisms in essential hypertension has revealed multifactorial disturbances. Any of the numerous changes that occur in hypertension cannot be considered alone; the complexity of relationships and practical impossibility to differentiate primary from secondary factors explain the failure of finding a "single" cause of essential hypertension (Page).

HYPOTENSION

General Considerations and Definition of Terms

Low systemic arterial pressure impairs tissue perfusion; however, the pressure level at which blood flow is critically diminished will vary, depending on the extent and rate of reduction in blood pressure, local condition of the vessels, and adequacy of compensating mechanisms. Hence, a numerical definition of hypotension raises the same problems of "normalcy" as a numerical definition of hypertension. Some normal subjects have arterial pressures below 90/60 mm. Hg with no apparent cause and no sign of ill-effect. The brain can apparently be adequately perfused, even in the upright position, by systolic pressures as low as 60 mm. Hg or less. The symptoms of diminished vitality, easy fatigue, or dizziness that have been sometimes loosely ascribed to hypotension (systolic below 100 mm. Hg) are just as frequently found in normotensive or in hypertensive patients.

A low arterial pressure level by itself is not necessarily a pathologic finding; in fact, chronic "hypotension" in the absence of associated disease may be a favorable condition because of the diminished cardiovascular load. Pathologic hypotension is the level at which blood flow to vital organs (brain, heart, kidneys) is impaired. Obviously perfusion will be more easily impaired by acute hypotension than by a chronic reduction in arterial pressure that may allow time for more effective compensatory adjustments of blood flow. The effects of hypotension may be subdivided into (a) those resulting directly from impaired organ perfusion, e.g., fainting due to cerebral ischemia; and (b) those due to activation of compensatory mechanisms, e.g., sweating and tachycardia from sympathetic stimulation secondary to decreased baroreceptor activity. The resulting clinical picture will therefore vary markedly with the cause of hypotension, its time course, the pattern of blood flow alteration, the activation of compensatory mechanisms or their failure, and any pre- or coexisting disease.

Postural Hypotension. This is characterized by a marked fall in arterial pressure with dizziness and possibly syncope on standing but a quite adequate circulation and pressure when lying down (Fig. 7-11). A more detailed discussion follows.

Though acute hypotension (postural, cardiac, or reflex) is one of the commonest causes of syncope, the two terms are not synonymous. *Syncope* refers to a sudden transient loss of consciousness; it is indeed very frequently due to hypotension and impaired cerebral perfusion but might in other instances result from biochemical derangements like hypoglycemia or reflect cerebral dysfunction as in the cerebral type of carotid sinus syndrome. Most fainting spells (vasovagal attacks or vagodepressor syncope) occur when the subject is standing and are associated with a fall in arterial pressure. They differ from "postural hypotension" in that they may occur when the subject is in the supine position, an extra-provocative factor is usually present (emotional disturbance, sight of blood, pain, hot weather), and signs of vagal activity (slowing pulse, nausea) are evident. Whereas all symptoms associated with postural hypotension quickly disappear as soon as the patient lies or falls down, the vasovagal disturbance clears much more slowly. Vasodepressor syncope is characterized by a sudden reduction in peripheral vascular resistance (Fig. 7-12), venoconstriction rather than dilatation, and little change in cardiac output. There is no evidence for excessive plasma volume contraction.

Shock. Despite its lack of precision, this term does evoke an impressive and readily recognizable picture and will certainly continue to be used clinically. It describes a condition of marked weakness, a variable degree of mental torpor with weak rapid thready pulse, cold clammy skin, and unobtainable or very low arterial pressure by usual method of examination. Many of these signs may not necessarily be found; arterial pressure may occasionally be relatively normal, especially if the patient was previously hypertensive. In some cases central pressure obtained by arterial cannulation may be high while brachial pressure is clinically unobtainable owing to marked peripheral vasoconstriction. Mentation may be unexpectedly clear if peripheral and renal vasoconstriction are intense enough to secure adequate cerebral blood flow. Instead of being cold and clammy, the skin may be dry and hot in cases of bacteremic shock. However, despite these variations, the picture is usually readily recognizable; the basic fault is a gross impairment of tissue perfusion due to marked reduction in cardiac output. The subject is much too extensive to be covered in this chapter; it is important, however, to underline its differences from other types of hypotension and to realize that in any hypotension, the body suffers not from the fall in arterial pressure per se but from the reduced blood flow that hypotension produces or signifies.

Chronic Hypotension. Chronic hypotension with vague or nonspecific symptoms may be associated with a variety of diseases such as aortic stenosis, adrenocortical insufficiency, malabsorption syndrome, severe cardiac failure, and

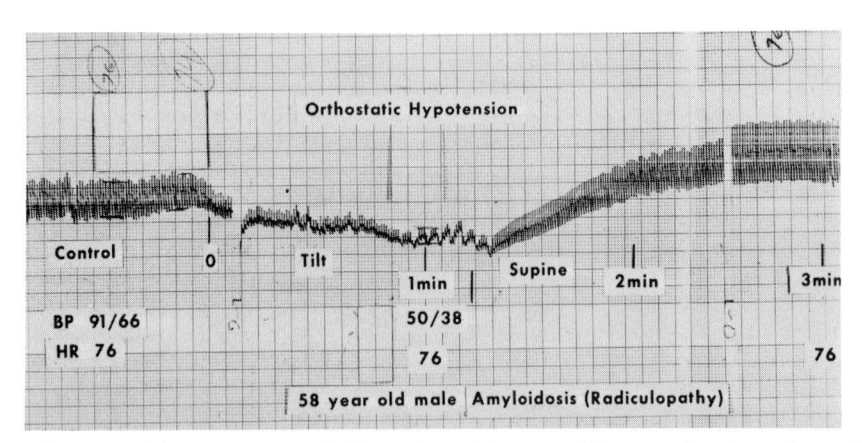

Figure 7-11 Intra-arterial pressure record of a patient with postural hypotension due to loss of sympathetic nerve function; note the rapid (as opposed to sudden) reduction in pressure from the beginning of head-up tilt and the unchanged heart rate despite the fall in pressure. As soon as the patient is returned to the horizontal position, arterial pressure begins to rise to even hypertensive levels; this tilt-back overshoot occurs following head-up tilt in patients with organic or drug-induced sympathetic dysfunction and has been related to liberation of catecholamines.

Figure 7–12 Semidiagrammatic illustration of hemodynamic events in vasodepressor syncope and in orthostatic hypotension due to loss of sympathetic activity. In the former, the drop in blood pressure occurs suddenly after a normal response to tilt (simulated in this case by lower body negative pressure, LBNP); heart rate and total peripheral resistance increase before they suddenly drop. In contrast, arterial pressure is gradually reduced to hypotensive levels in patients with sympathetic paralysis (see Fig. 7–11), with no change in either TPR or heart rate; note also the posttilt overshoot of the arterial pressure.

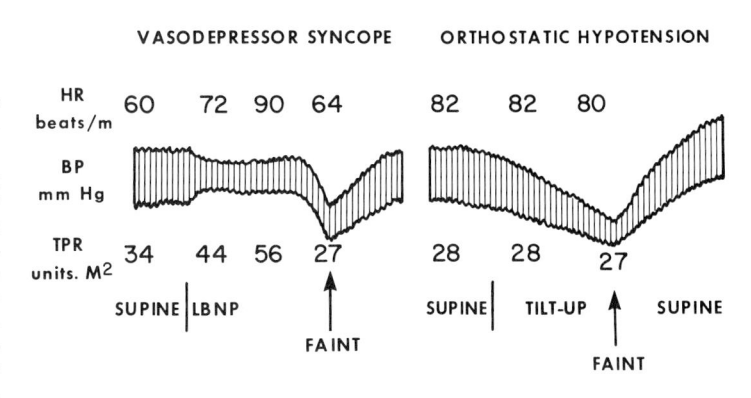

constrictive pericarditis. The clinical picture is dominated by the primary disease of which hypotension is only a sign. Some of these conditions may be associated with postural hypotension also. In contrast with such secondary forms of hypotension, an idiopathic, chronically low arterial pressure is not really a pathologic condition. Indeed, statistical studies would suggest enhanced longevity for apparently healthy people with idiopathic hypotension.

Pathophysiology of Postural Hypotension

Adjustment to Postural Changes. The pressure in a column of fluid depends on its specific gravity and the vertical distance from the point of measurement to the reference level; hence, the pressure at the bottom of a U tube will obviously be higher than that at the top. However, the pressure head required to drive fluid through a system of horizontal tubes will not be altered by the addition to that system of an unyielding U tube dipping below the line of flow. Similarly, if blood vessels were rigid tubes, standing up would not affect arterial or venous blood pressure at the heart's level and cardiac output would not change. The intravascular pressures in the feet would be markedly increased by an amount equal to their distance below the phlebostatic or zero point, but the arteriovenous gradient would not be altered, since arterial and venous pressures would be affected to the same extent.

Vessels, however, are not rigid impermeable tubes. As we stand, the pull of gravity pools blood in distensible veins below the heart and plasma is lost to interstitial fluid as capillary pressure and ultrafiltration increase. Diminished venous return reduces cardiac output and unless compensatory mechanisms perform adequately the subsequent fall in arterial pressure will result in impaired cerebral perfusion and loss of consciousness. Fortunately, adjustment mechanisms are normally quite effective and arterial pressure is maintained (see page 185). Even with passive head-up tilt, which exaggerates the effect of gravity by minimizing the support derived from contraction of the lower limb muscles, mean arterial pressure varies by ±10 mm. Hg.

This stability is due to an almost instantaneous reflex increase in sympathetic vasomotor outflow (see Neural Reflexes). Obviously vasoconstriction must occur in the resistance vessels to offset the effect of reduction in output and in the capacitance vessels to diminish pooling and help hasten venous return. As part of this sympathetic stimulation, heart rate increases slightly. The same reflexes are involved in bleeding or when mechanical factors hinder venous return (e.g., recumbency in late pregnancy).

Associated with this increased sympathetic activity, catecholamine concentration is increased in plasma and urine. The increase in epinephrine is due to reflex sympathetic stimulation of the adrenal medulla, and the increase in norepinephrine is mostly due to increased activity of the sympathetic vasomotor nerves. Other hormones are also involved in the response to upright posture; renin and aldosterone secretion are increased and there is even some evidence that antidiuretic hormone may be released, probably in response to reduced tension or intrathoracic volume receptors. Plasma renin activity was found to be elevated within a few minutes of upright tilt, but its rise lagged behind the reflex increase in pulse rate and diastolic blood pressure. Renin release is markedly affected by sympathetic nerve activity and circulating catecholamines and may be impaired in some patients with autonomic nerve disease or during treatment with adrenergic blocking drugs; however, increased catecholamine production is not an indispensable prerequisite for adequate stimulation of renin and aldosterone in the upright posture.

Whatever the reflex effects on resistance vessels, the capillary vessels in the feet during standing must still contend with a pressure exceeding 100 mm. Hg, far above the maximum colloid osmotic pressure of plasma proteins.

Plasma loss by diffusion may thus be enormous; this is prevented by contraction of precapillary sphincters, thus effectively shutting off filtration from a large number of dependent capillary beds. In addition, counter pressures develop in dependent areas to prevent overdistention of veins and help balance some of the rise in capillary pressure. Intramuscular tissue pressure increases with muscular contraction. Lower limb veins are compressed when leg and thigh muscles contract, and blood is pushed upward; as the muscles relax, backward flow of blood is prevented by intravenous valves. By interrupting the column of blood in the veins at different points, valves also prevent transmission of the full weight of that column to small dependent venules. Thus, "muscular pumping" helps lower both venous pressure and effective capillary filtering pressure; when interfered with, the incidence of fainting is increased. This may happen in normal subjects standing motionless at attention, or tilted passively and then supported in the upright position, or in patients with incompetent venous valves and dilated varicose veins.

Cerebral Circulation. The oxygen requirements of the central nervous system are fairly constant, and cerebral blood flow must therefore be kept constant if consciousness and life are to be preserved. The cerebral vessels are remarkably unresponsive to the usual neural and hormonal stimuli; the constancy of flow is secured by local autoregulatory mechanisms dependent on local production of carbon dioxide and local oxygen needs. Arterial Pco_2 is the most powerful regulator of cerebral flow; doubling Pco_2 approximately doubles cerebral flow, whereas a decrease in oxygen saturation to about 75 per cent increases flow approximately 40 per cent. However, the vasodilator effect of oxygen deficiency increases at very low saturations. This close adaptation of cerebral flow to neuronal metabolic needs ensures an impressively constant flow over wide ranges of arterial pressure down to quite low levels (50 to 60 mm. Hg mean pressure). Thus, whenever widespread sympathetic vasoconstriction develops (shock, hemorrhage, or upright posture), the cerebral vasculature is not materially affected by it but blood is redistributed toward the brain (and heart) from other constricted vascular beds. Moreover, since cerebral vessels and cerebrospinal fluid are enclosed within a rigid cavity, variations in cerebrospinal fluid or extravascular pressure with standing parallel very closely the variations in intravascular pressure, thus increasing the stability of the cerebral circulation. The stability of cerebral flow despite marked fluctuations in arterial pressure may explain why antihypertensive therapy is very rarely associated with cerebral damage even when transient hypotension develops. As soon as blood pressure is increased beyond a minimal level (as by lying down), cerebral blood flow is rapidly restored to near normal.

Pathophysiologic Classification. Orthostatic hypotension is characterized by a fall of at least 20 mm. Hg in both systolic and diastolic pressure on assumption of the standing position; in severe cases the patient cannot even stand up, since simple sitting leads to severe reduction in blood pressure. Severe hypotension may also develop in positions other than standing; women in late pregnancy may faint when lying on their backs, and patients with atrial myxoma or pedunculated intra-atrial thrombus may faint on sitting up. These types of postural hypotension are due to impaired ventricular filling and diminished cardiac output.

Orthostatic hypotension is the commonest form of postural hypotension; the blood pressure in the supine position may be reduced, normal, or even elevated. The patient may feel and look quite normal when lying down or some circulatory disorder may be apparent, e.g., rapid pulse and low arterial pressure as in hemorrhage or adrenocortical insufficiency. However, whatever the cause of the orthostatic fall in pressure, the clinical picture on standing is common to all (Table 7–3). The patient feels dizzy, weak, and faint; ataxia, blurring of vision, or occasionally some dysarthria develops, and unless he lies down rapidly, he ends up falling down unconscious. All symptoms, including syncope, clear up rapidly in the supine position.

Postural hypotension may have different causes (Table 7–2) that can be essentially linked to either of two basic mechanisms. In the first group, cardiac output is so reduced that despite reflex sympathetic stimulation, arterial pressure falls (sympathicotonic type). The second group is characterized by failure of the barostatic mechanism at some point along the reflex arc; hence, there are no or inappropriately few signs of sympathetic activity. Reflexes may be interfered with by disease or simply slowed by such factors as aging, prolonged recumbency, physical exhaustion, or starvation. The commonest cause of orthostatic hypotension, however, is inhibition of sympathetic reflexes by drugs that interfere with ganglionic transmission or with norepinephrine liberation at the nerve endings or block alpha-adrenergic receptors (see Table 7–2). The effects of bed rest on sympathetic activity are particularly important to note, since even short periods of inactivity may aggravate orthostatic hypotension due to other causes. By the same token, repeated head-up tilting may reduce the postural fall in pressure produced by some neurologic lesions.

Clinical differentiation of various types is not always easy. When present, signs of associated disease give helpful clues, but determination of

TABLE 7-2 POSTURAL HYPOTENSION

I. *Diminished Cardiac Output*
  A. Interference with venous return and cardiac filling at the muscular, venous, or cardiac level:
    1. Poor muscular pumping mechanism:
      a. Muscular atrophy
      b. Poor postural adjustment in young asthenic persons standing at strict attention
      c. Passive tilting
    2. Venous disease:
      a. Incompetent valves
      b. Varicose veins
      c. Obstruction (e.g., late pregnancy)
    3. Cardiac: Tamponade, constrictive pericarditis, atrial myxoma, ball valve thrombus
  B. Absolute or relative depletion of intravascular volume:
    1. Relative: Due to dilatation of capacitance vessels by drugs (e.g., nitrites) or disease (e.g., venous angiomatosis)
    2. Absolute:
      a. Hemorrhage, internal or external
      b. Excessive loss of fluid by diuresis, vomiting, diarrhea
      c. Increased capillary permeability with loss of fluid in interstitial spaces
      d. Urinary salt wasting due to selective hypoaldosteronism
  C. Diminished myocardial performance:*
    1. Myocarditis, severe coronary arterial disease
    2. Postural arrhythmias with excessively slow or extremely rapid heart rate
    3. Outlet obstruction as in aortic or pulmonary stenosis (usually leads to exercise rather than orthostatic hypotension)
II. *Impaired Peripheral Resistance*
  A. Arteriolar:
    1. Disease: Relatively rare (e.g., amyloidosis), and then usually associated with neural involvement as well
    2. Arteriolar vasodilators as nitrites or nitroprusside
  B. Neurologic dysfunction:
    1. Lesion in afferent limb: Tabes dorsalis, rarely in polyneuritis
    2. Lesion in central nervous system
      a. Some forms of chronic idiopathic hypotension; possible relationship to Shy-Drager syndrome
      b. Parkinsonism either isolated or part of a more extensive degenerative disease
      c. Cerebral arteriosclerosis
      d. Syringomyelia, various myelopathies, Wernicke's syndrome, tumors
      e. Drugs (e.g., meprobamate)
    3. Lesion in efferent sympathetic limb (parasympathetic may be affected but is not responsible for hypotension)
      a. Some forms of chronic idiopathic hypotension
      b. Polyneuritis (e.g., diabetes, porphyria)
      c. Myelopathies
      d. Iatrogenic:
        (1) Postsympathectomy
        (2) Neural blocking drugs
          (a) Ganglion blocking agents, adrenergic blockers
          (b) Monoamine oxidase inhibitors
          (c) L-dopa
III. *Undetermined or Mixed Mechanisms*
  A. Adrenocortical insufficiency: Possibly related to cardiac dysfunction and aggravated by fluid loss; reactions of resistance and capacitance vessels said to be normal
  B. Diabetic acidosis
  C. Pheochromocytoma (distinctly uncommon)

*Note: Cardiac failure as such is *not* a cause of orthostatic hypotension; in fact, patients in congestive failure tolerate head-up tilt very well, possibly because of their hypervolemia.

---

the mechanism involved and localization of the lesion require a stepwise reasoned approach. Causes listed as Group I are usually readily differentiated from those in Group II-B by the intensity of sympathetic activity in the first group and its relative absence in the second (Table 7-2). Clinical signs of increased sympathetic drive include pallor, sweating, and tachycardia; hemodynamic studies may document the simultaneous increase in peripheral resistance, diminution in forearm blood flow, and venoconstriction. The absence of these signs despite the fall in arterial pressure characterizes neurogenic hypotension (Table 7-3). However, though the absence of tachycardia during hypotension indicates an inadequate neural response, its presence does not necessarily exclude a neurogenic lesion. Thus, heart rate may increase in early idiopathic hypotension before cardiac nerves are involved or in hypotension due to lumbar sympathectomy. The same remarks apply to pallor and sweating. Failure of peripheral resistance to increase is particularly significant. The picture in vasodepressor syncope is quite different; here the pulse actually slows and peripheral resistance suddenly falls as the patient faints (Fig. 7-12).

Lesions in the efferent limb will be characterized by loss of pressure responses to all reflex pressor maneuvers; the Valsalva maneuver, cold stimulus, or stressful mental arithmetic will not raise blood pressure as they normally should, since the final common neural pathway is not functioning. However, arteriolar responsiveness to norepinephrine infusion will be intact or in-

TABLE 7-3 HEMODYNAMIC RESPONSES TO STANDING UP

	Normal	Oligemia or Diminished Venous Return	Idiopathic Orthostatic Hypotension Early	Idiopathic Orthostatic Hypotension Advanced
Blood pressure	Little change; mean arterial pressure varies by < 10 mm. Hg	Reduction in both systolic and diastolic pressures, sometimes quite marked.		
Heart rate	Increases by about 15%	Marked increase	Slight increase	No change
Cardiac output	Reduced, usually 10 to 20%	Reduced to varying degree	Reduced, usually > 25%	Reduced
Total peripheral resistance	Increased by 15 to 20%	Marked increase	Slight increase may occur	No increase
Phenylephrine				
Blood pressure	Increased, depending on dose	Normal response	Response > normal because of denervation hypersensitivity	
Heart rate	Slowed with blood pressure rise	Normal response	Response may be normal	No change despite rise in blood pressure
Valsalva overshoot (phase IV)	Rise in diastolic pressure averages 25 to 35% of control	Normal or increased	Absent	Absent and return from phase III may be quite slow

deed exaggerated (denervation hypersensitivity) in contrast with the impaired responsiveness found in purely arteriolar lesions. Similarly, loss of reflex sweating (warming contralateral limb) despite the presence of responsive sweat glands suggests an efferent or central sympathetic defect. In many but not all cases of efferent limb dysfunction, the cardiac nerves (sympathetic and parasympathetic) are involved; if the heart is functionally denervated, its rate will be slow and fixed, unresponsive to atropine injections, carotid sinus pressure, or increase in arterial pressure by phenylephrine. If neural involvement is not far advanced (early idiopathic postural hypotension) or is localized (as following lumbar sympathectomy), demonstration of reflex cardiac slowing will indicate that afferent nerves, medullary centers, and parasympathetic efferent nerves are intact.

Pathophysiologic localization of central lesions is more difficult; reflex pressor responses are also interfered with. Some help may be derived from the presence of other neural signs (rigidity, parkinsonism, nystagmus, alterations of deep reflexes, and so on) but especially from demonstration of intact peripheral sympathetic innervation. This is most readily achieved by showing increased toe or finger blood flow with local anesthesia of the corresponding nerves. Lesions of afferent baroreceptor nerves may be suspected when orthostatic reflexes are absent (hypotension and unchanged heart rate during head-up tilt), in contrast with normal pressor responses to cold stimulus and mental arithmetic, normal peripheral blood flow response to nerve blockade, and intact vagal supply to the heart (increased rate following atropine injection). The loss of baroreceptor sensitivity may be demonstrated by absence of reflex bradycardia when blood pressure is raised and lack of pressor response to maneuvers lowering arterial pressure.

Idiopathic Orthostatic Hypotension

This syndrome affects men more frequently than women; it is a slowly progressive condition marked by obvious neural autonomic involvement (postural hypotension, loss of sweating, fixed heart rate), subtle neurologic signs (pupillary abnormalities, generalized hyperreflexia, disturbed bladder regulation), and usually intact sensation and mental faculties. Association with parkinsonism is particularly frequent and may be very disabling. In many instances, the disease may represent variants of the syndrome described by Shy and Drager but not all forms are necessarily related to the same pathologic alterations. Some may be due to involvement of sympathetic nerves or spinal centers. The initial description of the syndrome by Bradbury and Eggleston stressed the triad of postural hypotension gradually increasing in severity, anhydrosis slowly spreading to involve most of the body surface, and impotence. Plasma and urinary catecholamines are usually decreased; renin-angiotensin-aldosterone system was impaired in some patients and reported as normal in others.

Cerebrovascular Disease and Hypotension

A sudden fall in systemic blood pressure can cause focal neurologic impairment, especially in patients with atherosclerotic narrowing or occlusion of intracranial vessels or of the carotid or vertebral arteries. On the other hand, cerebrovascular disease may itself cause hypotension and fainting, so that determination of which event came first may be very difficult. The question is particularly relevant in antihypertensive therapy; it is our opinion that hypotension has been grossly overrated as a cause of strokes. Though hypotensive episodes were very frequent in the heroic days of ganglion blocking therapy, the incidence of permanent neurologic damage was not particularly increased. This impression is supported by the rarity of cerebral infarction in patients with idiopathic orthostatic hypotension, many of whom are elderly and subject to frequent hypotensive spells.

Postural hypotension is more common in patients with cerebrovascular disease than in normal controls. Central interference with the baroreceptor reflex may be one cause; pressor response to the Valsalva maneuver is often blunted and may be completely absent in elderly patients with cerebral atherosclerosis. Patients may easily faint while coughing or when straining at stool or during micturition, possibly because of reflex failure of vasoconstriction in the face of diminished venous return rather than because of laryngeal or vesical reflexes. However, anatomic interference with baroreceptor arc may not be the only mechanism; a study of such patients showed that systemic blood pressure could be adequately maintained unless an additional factor such as a sedative drug or prolonged rest was added. Recumbency even for relatively short periods such as a night's rest reduces sympathetic activity; hypotension is therefore aggravated in the early morning hours. Prolonged recumbency adds the additional stress of blood volume contraction.

REFERENCES

Folkow, B., and Neil, E.: Circulation. New York, Oxford University Press, 1971.

Page, I. H., and McCubbin, J. W.: The physiology of arterial hypertension. *In* Hamilton, W. F., and Dow, P. (Eds.): Handbook of Physiology. Vol. III. Circulation. Washington, D.C., American Physiological Society, 1965, pp. 2163–2208.

Pickering, G.: High Blood Pressure. New York, Grune and Stratton, 1968.

CHAPTER 8

MECHANISMS OF CARDIAC CONTRACTION: STRUCTURAL, BIOCHEMICAL, AND FUNCTIONAL RELATIONS IN THE NORMAL AND DISEASED HEART

DEAN T. MASON
ROBERT ZELIS
EZRA A. AMSTERDAM
RASHID A. MASSUMI

The clinician has appreciated for many years that major improvements in the understanding and management of heart disease attend advances in knowledge of the fundamental mechanisms making up and governing contraction of cardiac muscle in normal and pathologic states. Although a complete detailed elucidation of the contractile process is not yet available and controversy remains concerning certain of its aspects, intensive investigation in the past decade has provided a considerable body of new information which has permitted formulation of the events involved in myocardial contraction in health and disease. These advances have been stimulated by contributions from members of several disciplines, including the clinical investigator, physiologist, pharmacologist, biochemist, and anatomist, through the development of a multiplicity of improved techniques and their application to experimental biological systems and to patients.

The purpose here is to present the status of this field and the progress that has recently taken place, particularly at the level of the myocardial cell, in enhancing the clinical understanding of the mechanisms and regulation of contraction of the normal and diseased heart. The discussion that follows is intended to provide an overall integrated conceptual view of the various principal characteristics of the myocardium relating to the complex phenomenon of cardiac contraction. Attention is focused on the subcellular organizational structure of heart muscle and the biochemical processes which control the energy system within the myocardium. Proceeding from this anatomic and metabolic background, the mechanism linking electrical excitation of heart muscle with activation of its contractile machinery is considered, and the molecular biochemical basis of the contractile process itself is analyzed. Finally, the function of the normal and failing heart is assessed in terms of its muscle mechanical properties. Emphasis will be placed on the clinical meaning of the events constituting cardiac contraction in order to translate important, newly perceived basic concepts into improved principles and practical information applicable to evaluation and care of the patient with cardiovascular disease.

MYOCARDIAL ULTRASTRUCTURE

Sophisticated delineation of the microanatomical features of heart muscle has now become possible with the recent development and utilization of modern methods in the examination of cardiac morphology. These studies have shown clearly that there is a definite relationship between the fine architecture of heart muscle and the contractile mechanism of the functioning ventricle. Thus, a subcellular structural basis has been established for myocardial mechanical activity and cardiac pump performance in which the fundamental individual contractile component is recognized to be the sarcomere.

Myocardial Cell and Myofibrils

The gross musculature of the ventricles is traditionally described as being encircled by superficial, middle and deep muscle bundles which arise and insert at the fibrous skeleton of the valve annuli. In the past, the separate nature of these three layers was emphasized, whereas the view currently proposed by Grant holds that the spiral bundles may represent more of a transitional continuum with outer and inner fibers at right angles to those in the midwall. Under the light miscroscope, the muscle bundles are composed of individual branching striated muscle cells or fibers, approximately 50μ in length and 15μ in width, oriented in the same direction within a given bundle (Fig. 8-1A). In turn, the muscle fiber contains multiple parallel rows of longitudinal myofibrils which traverse the entire length of the cell. Each myofibril consists of several of the basic contractile units, sarcomeres, which are joined serially, end-to-end, in a single line (Fig. 8-1B).

Sarcomere and Myofilaments

Further delineation of myocardial morphology or ultrastructure requires the resolution and magnification powers of the electron microscope. The sarcomeres themselves are composed of specific arrangements of two sets of overlapping myofilaments of contractile proteins: *thick filaments* of myosin molecules and *thin filaments* of actin molecules (Fig. 8-1C). It is the biochemical and biophysical interactions that occur at precise sites between these strands of actin and myosin aggregates that ultimately produce contraction with generation of force and shortening of heart muscle. Within an individual myocardial cell, the sarcomere bodies of neighboring myofibrils lie next to each other with their ends adjacent, so that the banded organization of contractile proteins inside the sarcomere imparts a cross-striated appearance to the muscle fiber.

The relative densities of the cross bands identify the location of the contractile proteins within the sarcomere (Figs. 8-1C and 8-2). The myosin filaments are indicated by the broad dark A band of constant length (1.5 μ in the center portion of the sarcomere); the stationary myosin units are held to each other by linkages at the midpoint of their filaments, shown by the dark M line. Surrounding the myosin units are the sliding actin filaments of constant length (1.0 μ) attached at either end of the sarcomere at the dark Z line, which also connects adjacent sarcomeres at this point. Interestingly, the Z band is now thought to have an important generative function in the production of new sarcomeres (Legato, 1969). From the light I band of variable dimension, the actin filaments run centrally to be largely covered by the fixed myosin framework. Under physiologic conditions, overall sarcomere length (Z to Z distance) varies during the cardiac cycle between 1.5 and 2.2 μ, depending on the degree of end-diastolic fiber stretch and the extent of shortening during contraction. Immediately lateral on both sides of the M line is a thin light L line; this central area is the ML complex or pseudo-H zone. In acutely overstretched skeletal muscle and to a lesser degree in myocardium, a pathologic wide H zone appears, indicating partial disengagement of the thick and thin filaments. In contrast, slippage and malalignment of myofibrils appear to be the principal morphologic alterations in chronic excessive dilation of the ventricle (Ross et al., 1971). Alterations in molecular composition and physical structure of the contractile proteins and myofilaments themselves are not found in heart failure.

Contractile Proteins

Concerning the two primary contractile proteins of the sarcomere, the *actin* and *myosin* chains possess distinct structural and functional properties (Katz, 1970) (Fig. 8-3). The thick filament is composed of staggered parallel clusters of a few hundred myosin molecules, each characterized by an elongated rodlike core of interwoven paired helical coils (*light meromyosin*) with globular lateral endings or heads (*heavy meromyo-*

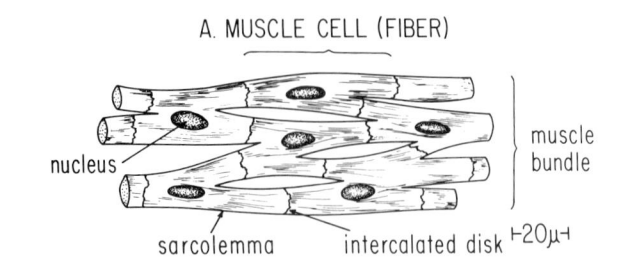

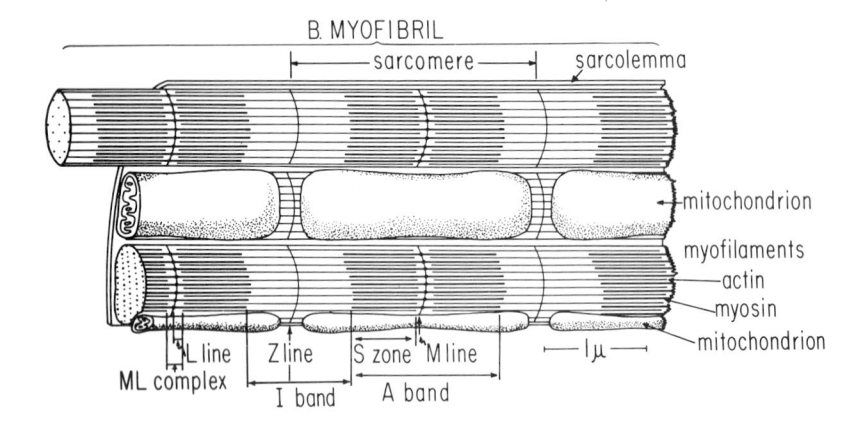

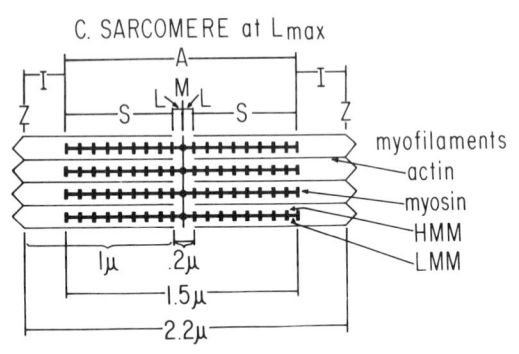

Figure 8-1 *A,* Myocardial structure viewed under light microscope showing syncytium of cells or fibers. *B,* Ultrastructure of longitudinal section of an individual fiber schematized from electron microscope demonstrating parallel myofibrils composed of serially connected sarcomeres in register with sarcomeres of adjacent fibrils. Horizontal rows of mitochondria are situated throughout the cell. *C,* Diagrammatic representation of a sarcomere at L_{max} (resting length at which active tension becomes maximal) showing overlapping arrangement of thick (myosin) and thin (actin) myofilaments. S = S zone (area of actin-myosin overlap); *HMM* = heavy meromyosin; *LMM* = light meromyosin.

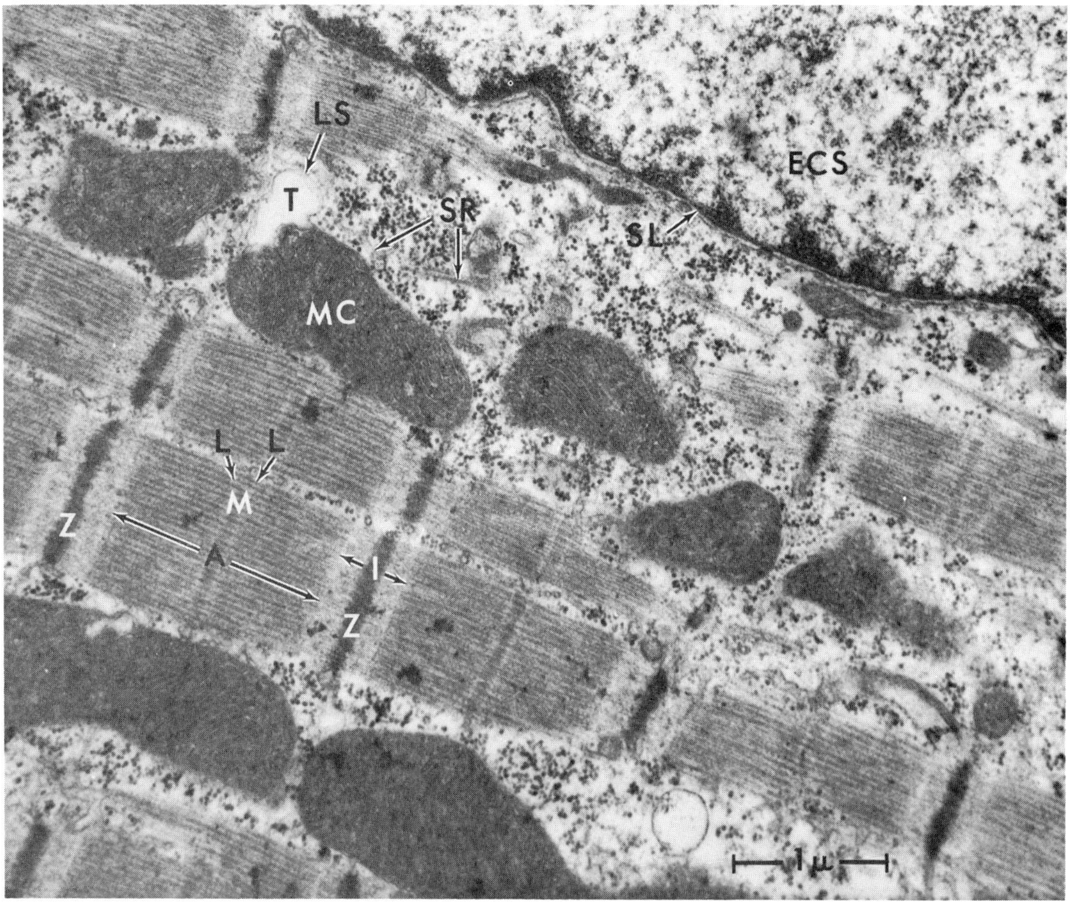

Figure 8-2 Electron micrograph of longitudinal section of canine right ventricle showing characteristic bands (A and I) and lines (Z, M, and L) of sarcomere substructure. Individual sarcomeres are delineated by dark Z lines. MC = mitochondrion; SL = sarcolemma; T = sarcotubule; LS = lateral sac of sarcoplasmic reticulum (SR); ECS = extracellular space.

sin). The globular projection contains the principal functional component of myosin: the cross bridge of the thick filament which interacts with actin of the thin filament to produce contraction. Further, each globular cross bridge is considered to be paired with light myosin subunits at their termination. These light subunits (light chains) of heavy meromyosin are thought to regulate the level of enzyme activity of myosin adenosine triphosphatase (ATPase) in the remaining portion of the heavy meromyosin (heavy chains). Myosin ATPase splits the terminal phosphate bond off ATP and thereby liberates the energy for the contractile process.

The thin filament is principally constituted by two helical chains of globular actin molecules (Fig. 8-3). As observed in cross section of the sarcomere, each thin filament is surrounded by three thick filaments and each thick filament is encompassed by six thin filaments (Fig. 8-3B). Although actin enhances the enzymatic action of myosin ATPase to more active actomyosin ATPase, there is no enzymatic participation of actin itself in the contractile mechanism. Instead, the physiologic role of actin is its ability to combine reversibly at specific binding sites on the thin filament with the myosin cross bridges, one myosin spine attaching to each active actin site. Thus, according to the sliding filament theory of contraction offered by Huxley, formation of cross bridges between active sites of actin and myosin causes inward movement of the thin filament centrally along the fixed thick filament framework. In this contractile process, the lengths of the two filaments remain unchanged while the sarcomere shortens.

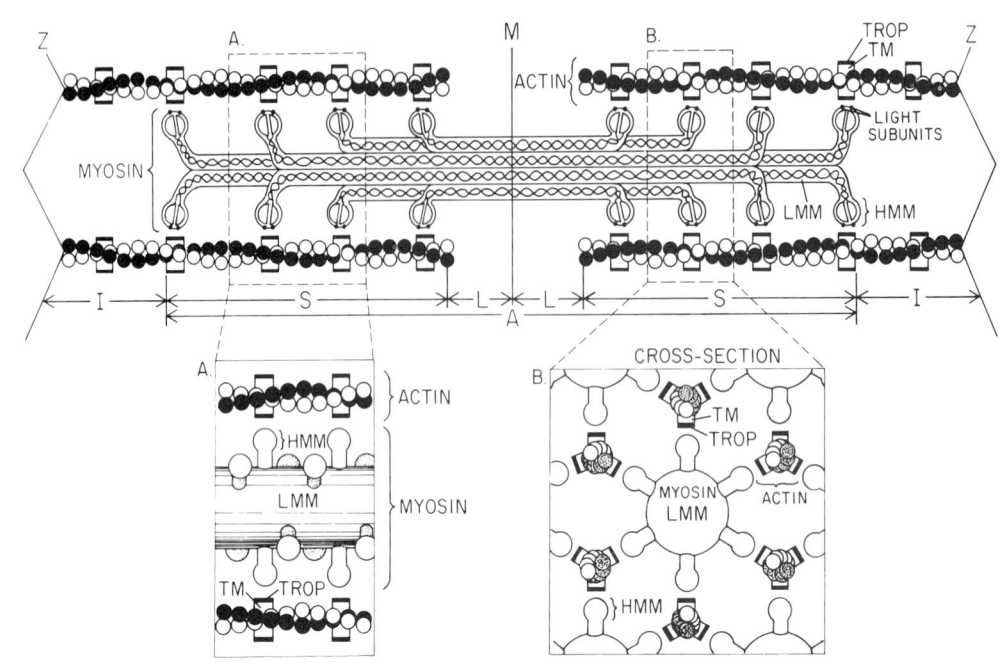

Figure 8-3 Diagrammatic representation of the contractile proteins of heart muscle during relaxation, indicating the relative longitudinal configurations and positions of actin and myosin filaments and modulatory proteins, tropomyosin (*TM*) and troponin (*TROP*), as viewed by electron microscopy. Each thick filament is composed of horizontal aggregations of myosin molecules with long shafts (light meromyosin: *LMM*) and cross-bridge heads (heavy meromyosin: *HMM*) containing light subunits regulating myosin ATPase activity which interact with myosin-binding sites on actin of the thin filament during contraction. Inserts *A* (horizontal view) and *B* (cross-section) indicate three-dimensional orientation of actin-myosin relationships within the S zone, demonstrating hexagonal lattice of six thin filaments arranged around each thick filament, and each thin filament surrounded by three thick filaments.

In addition to the two primary contractile proteins, actin and myosin, two regulatory proteins, *tropomyosin* and *troponin,* are located along the thin actin filament (Fig. 8-3). Tropomyosin and troponin are not contractile proteins as such but rather they serve a modulatory role in the contractile mechanism of inhibiting the actin-myosin interaction. Tropomyosin molecules lie in elongated chains longitudinally along the paired actin strands of the thin filament. Troponin is attached at regular intervals to tropomyosin, coinciding with the grooves of the actin double-helix. During relaxation of cardiac muscle, troponin in consort with tropomyosin prevents cross bridge reaction between actin and myosin. As demonstrated by Ebashi, troponin contains the receptor protein for the specific binding of calcium in the contractile system. Although calcium is considered in the broad sense as the activator of mechanical contraction, this action actually functions as the specific inactivator of the troponin-tropomyosin complex's inhibition of actin-myosin linkage formation. Two further protein subcomponents complete the troponin structure: a tropomyosin-binding protein and an actin-myosin interaction inhibitor.

Superficial Membrane System

In addition to the sarcomere contractile apparatus which occupies approximately one half the myocardial fiber, there are other important specialized subcellular constituents. The individual myocardial fibers are covered by the *sarcolemma* membrane, of which the *intercalated disc* and *transverse tubular system* are derivatives of major significance (Figs. 8-1*B*, 8-2, and 8-4). The intercalated disc is situated at intercellular junctions between the terminal sarcomeres of the cell, thereby locking fibers together at their ends. In the ventricular myocardium, deep invaginations of the sarcolemma at frequent intervals from the fiber surface vertically into the interior of each cell constitute the complex transtubular network or T system. The intercalated disc and transverse tubular membranes provide pathways for rapid transmission of the depolarizing impulses which electrically excite adjacent fibers and the intra-

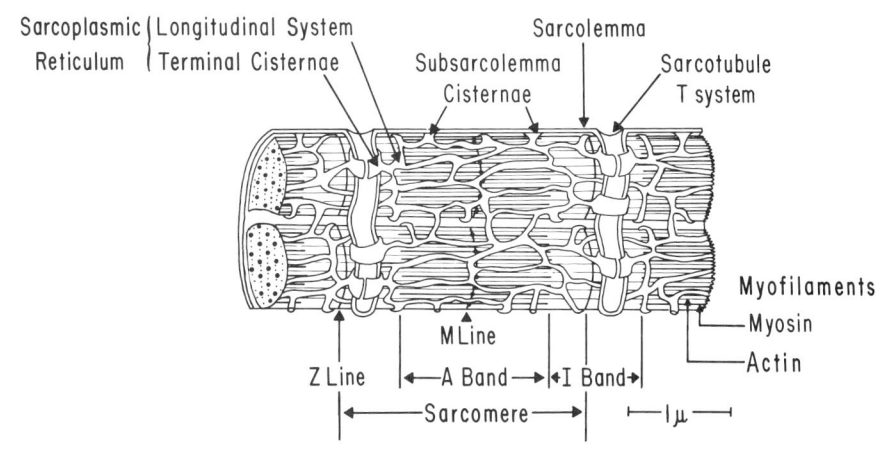

Figure 8-4 Longitudinal diagram of myocardial ultrastructure reconstructed from electron micrographs showing relationships between the superficial (sarcolemma and wide T system) and intracellular (sarcoplasmic reticulum) membranes of the cardiac fiber.

cellular membrane–sarcomere contractile system. In addition to contributing a vehicle for excitation, the transtubular system provides a comprehensive extension of the extracellular space throughout the cell so that transmembrane cation transport of sodium, potassium, and calcium accompanying depolarization, repolarization, excitation-contraction coupling, and relaxation occurs quickly and synchronously within myocardial fibers. Furthermore, the T system furnishes a conduit for ready entry and egress of metabolites and other substances between the interstitial medium and the sarcoplasm, and access is afforded to cardiovascular drugs, such as digitalis and antiarrhythmic agents, for their action on intracellular membranes and related enzyme systems in the vicinity of the contractile apparatus within the entire fiber, even if the drugs do not actually cross the membrane in clinically meaningful doses.

Sarcoplasmic Reticulum

An extensive intracellular tubular membrane system, the sarcoplasmic reticulum, complements the transtubular T system structurally and functionally in support of the process of excitation-contraction coupling and mechanical relaxation (Figs. 8-2 and 8-4). The T-tubular system is in contact with the extracellular environment and runs a vertical pathway through the width of the sarcomere I bands. The sarcoplasmic reticulum is entirely within the cell and its general orientation is at right angles to the T system, so that the sarcotubular structure courses longitudinally along the rows of sarcomeres with multiple branching interconnections. *Lateral sac* cuff modifications or terminal cisternae of the narrow sarcoplasmic reticulum or longitudinal L system occur at its point of contact with the wider T system in the lateral I band on one side of the Z line. The sarcotubular lateral sacs store calcium; the intracellular transport of calcium from this area is important in linking membrane excitation with troponin of the contractile apparatus. Also, lateral sacs abut the intercalated discs and sarcolemma to provide each of the specialized membranes with a complete system for excitation-contraction coupling. An interesting exception is the Purkinje cell, which has no transverse tubular system (Legato, 1969). Perhaps dissimilarities in the electrical and contractile responses of different types of cardiac cells to pharmacologic agents are, in part, the result of variations in the extent and nature of development of the transtubular network and inherent modifications in the characteristics of the superficial membranes.

Mitochondria

The final myocardial substructure to be considered is the mitochondrion, which contains the aerobic biochemical systems of the fiber (Figs. 8-2 and 8-4). The mitochondria, located between the myofibrils, are abundant in accordance with the heart's high requirements for oxygen, and they constitute nearly 30 per cent of the myocardial cell. The mitochondria are the metabolic power plants in which oxygen and appropriate substrates are utilized to produce ATP, the final direct energy source for myocardial contraction and other biochemical reactions. In the cytoplasm or sarcoplasm, glycogen granules are stored and the process of anaerobic glycolysis is operative. Morphologically, the mitochondrion is surrounded by a membrane from which there are numerous cristae infoldings on which the process of oxidative phosphorylation takes place. In addition, the mitochondrial membranes are capable of accumulating calcium, which might serve as an internal buffer against abnormal rises of sarcoplasmic calcium during diastole and perhaps might represent a mechanism influencing myocardial compliance or a source of activator calcium.

MYOCARDIAL METABOLISM

The principal biochemical processes which relate to the ultimate contractile function of the ventricle include those involved in regulation of energy metabolism, contractile machinery of the sarcomere, the muscle relaxing system, electrical and transport activity of the membranes, and protein synthesis within the fiber. It is emphasized that these chemical mechanisms are interrelated, and alterations in any one of them may influence activity in the other pathways. For conceptual purposes, the sequence of reactions important in myocardial energy metabolism is substrate availability and energy production, storage, and utilization.

Energetics

Normal heart muscle is uniquely dependent on *aerobic* metabolism for its energy supply. To satisfy this obligatory need, the myocardium requires the delivery of a continuous supply of large quantities of oxygen via the coronary circulation. The oxygen demand of the heart is considerably greater than for other organs and, since myocardial oxygen extraction is nearly maximal at body rest, increases in oxygen need are primarily accomplished by elevations of coronary blood flow. *Myocardial oxygen consumption* of the ventricle is principally determined by three hemodynamic-related variables: (1) intramyocardial systolic tension (primarily governed by systolic pressure and ventricular volume); (2) contractility; and (3) heart rate (Fig. 8–5). In addition to these three major determinants, external work or ventricular shortening (*Fenn effect*), energy of activation-relaxation, and basal diastolic energy requirements contribute to a relatively minor degree to overall myocardial oxygen requirements (Fig. 8–5). In considering the effects of an intervention on myocardial oxygen consumption, such as with the administration of digitalis or nitroglycerin, it is important to appreciate that the final result quantitatively is dependent on the entire hemodynamic functional status of the heart, an interplay among the more important factors regulating oxygen utilization, and the summation of their individual actions.

Oxidative Phosphorylation. Since ATP is the immediate energy source for the contractile apparatus and biochemical reactions elsewhere in the cell, myocardial energy metabolism is normally directed toward aerobic production of ATP in the mitochondria by substrate oxidation (dehydrogenation of citric acid intermediates requiring nicotinamide adenine dinucleotide), with discharge of carbon dioxide in the *Krebs cycle,* consequent transport of hydrogen and its electrons through the respiratory chain of flavoproteins and cytochromes (resulting in oxygen consumption and making of water), and oxidative phosphorylation in which inorganic phosphate acquires a high-energy bond and combines with adenosine diphosphate (ADP) to form ATP (Fig. 8–6). Schwartz has shown depressed mitochon-

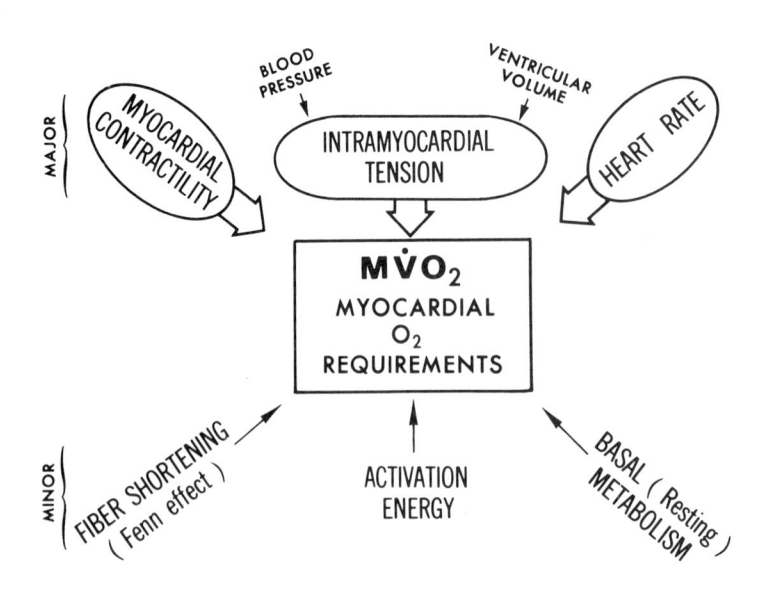

Figure 8–5 Major and minor determinants of myocardial oxygen consumption (MV̇O₂).

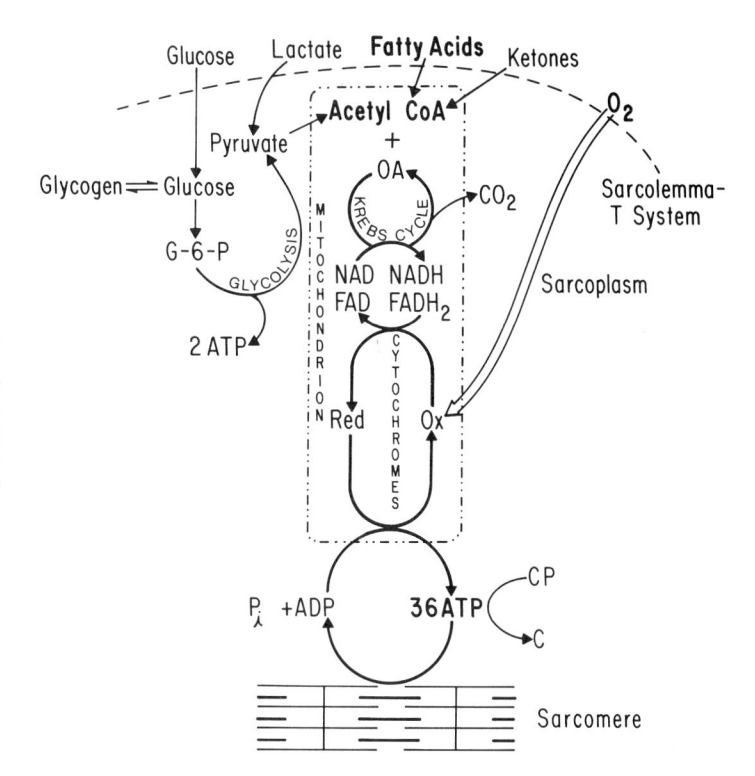

Figure 8-6 Metabolic pathways for energy (ATP) production shown diagrammatically within the cardiac cell. NAD = nicotinamide adenine dinucleotide; FAD = flavin adenine dinucleotide; $NADH$ = reduced NAD; $FADH_2$ = reduced FAD; Ox = oxidation; Red = reduction; CP = creatine phosphate; C = creatine; $G\text{-}6\text{-}P$ = glucose-6-phosphate; P_i = inorganic phosphate. See text for further explanation.

drial energy production in the severely failing myocardium, whereas respiratory function in the mitochondria is increased in the hypertrophied heart prior to failure. While abnormalities in mitochondrial energy metabolism may contribute to myocardial dysfunction in heart failure, these biochemical aberrations are generally not considered causative of failure due to chronic hemodynamic overload.

The predominant substrate fuel for myocardial ATP synthesis consists of the circulating *free fatty acids,* consumption of which accounts for the majority of oxygen extracted by the heart. Concerning other primary substrates, normally *blood glucose* is used preferentially in the postprandial state. Circulating lactate is also an important fuel, particularly when its blood concentration is elevated by prolonged skeletal muscle exercise. Blood pyruvate, like glucose, lactate, and free fatty acids, is readily taken up by the myocardium in proportion to its arterial blood concentration. Blood-borne ketone bodies and even amino acids may serve as substrates in certain abnormal conditions. Conversion of the substrate fuels into acetyl-coenzyme A is necessary for their entry into the citric acid cycle for aerobic ATP production. Concerning blood glucose as substrate in myocardial energy systems, after the substance is transported across the sarcolemma-transtubular membranes and metabolized to glucose-6-phosphate under the influence of insulin, it may be stored as glycogen or undergo anaerobic glycolysis to pyruvate in the sarcoplasm. In normal conditions, pyruvate is oxidized to acetyl-coenzyme A and undergoes aerobic metabolism in the citric acid cycle within the mitochondria. In the absence of hypoxia, the heart does not produce lactate.

Anaerobic Glycolysis. The importance of anaerobic glycolysis as a source of energy varies with the state of oxygenation of the myocardium. Normally, glycolysis is of considerably less significance, since this entire process results in only two ATP molecules for each molecule of glucose, whereas each glucose molecule provides 36 molecules of ATP in the aerobic pathways. When myocardial oxygen delivery falls, there is increased glycolysis, although this is an ineffective process alone for maintaining energy supply, and ATP levels decline. Also, less pyruvate enters the citric acid cycle during enhanced glycolytic metabolism in myocardial hypoxia. Consequently, in the heart relatively deprived of oxygen, pyruvate is reduced to *lactate,* and lactate is not extracted; thereby, the hypoxic myocardium may produce more lactate than it consumes, with the result that coronary sinus blood will contain more lactate than systemic arterial blood. In contrast, lactate concentration is greater in arterial blood than in the coronary venous effluent in the normally metabolizing heart owing to myocardial lactate extraction for aerobic synthesis of ATP. By selective catheterization of the coronary sinus, Gorlin has shown that detection of abnormal myocardial lactate metabolism or balance provides a useful biochemical means for the objective identification of myocardial ischemia in patients with coronary artery disease. Furthermore, when the abnormality is not present at rest in patients with angina pectoris, it can often be revealed by increasing the mechanical and metabolic activity of the heart by the performance of exercise, by increasing heart rate with a pacemaker catheter, or by administration of isoproterenol.

Creatine Phosphate. In regard to myocardial energy storage, creatine phosphate functions as a limited reservoir of high-energy phosphate to maintain ATP. Thus, following the cleavage of ATP by myofibrillar ATPase to ADP and inorganic phosphate in the contraction reaction and by the additional myocardial ATPases in other biochemical processes requiring energy utilization, ADP is replenished with a high-energy phosphate from creatine phosphate or by oxidative phosphorylation to re-form ATP. Creatine phosphate is resynthesized by oxidative phosphorylation. Although creatine phosphate serves as a ready source of auxiliary chemical energy for ADP, it is relatively small in quantity, even in the normal heart. In chronic heart failure, ATP levels are not depleted, although creatine phosphate is often diminished, but this reduction follows rather than precedes abnormal contractile performance.

Protein Synthesis

Protein synthesis in the myocardium provides a continuously operative system for renewal of fiber structure and enzymatic machinery and a rapidly responsive compensatory mechanism for ventricular hypertrophy induced by cardiac mechanical stress. High-energy nucleotides are consumed in the process of protein synthesis, which comprises the stages of (1) replication in the nucleus (deoxyribonucleic acid (DNA)-controlled DNA synthesis by DNA polymerase); (2) transcription in the nucleus in which nucleoli are centers of RNA activity (ribonucleic acid (RNA) nucleotide synthesis by RNA polymerase on the chromosomal DNA template); and (3) translation involving three RNA types in the sarcoplasm (formation of specific proteins on ribosomes, directed by messenger RNA containing the genetic code, from amino acids carried by transfer RNA). Excessive intramyocardial tension appears to be the transducer coupling mechanical systolic overload with increased activity of protein synthesis pathways. Increased muscle mass resulting from elevated hemodynamic burden is due to hypertrophy rather than hyperplasia of myocardial fibers, although there is some proliferation of connective tissue cells. As shown by Meerson, Rabinowitz and Nair, and others, activation of all stages of protein synthesis occurs rapidly following acute stress with increased DNA in connective tissue cells and elevations of RNA and incorporation of amino acids into proteins in myocardial cells. With chronic hemodynamic overload, however, there is some diminution of these processes. It is currently considered that alterations in protein synthesis, as in energy metabolism, do not exert a causative role in heart failure but may contribute to it.

Cyclic AMP

Another important biochemical system in heart muscle is that involved with the intracellular regulatory substance cyclic AMP (adenosine monophosphate), discovered by Sutherland. Cyclic AMP is synthesized in the sarcoplasm from ATP by stimulation of the enzyme adenylate cyclase of the plasma sarcolemma and transtubular membranes. The activity of adenylate cyclase is enhanced by beta-adrenergic receptor stimulation located also in the plasma membranes. It has been suggested that the positive inotropic action of several cardiovascular agents is mediated by activation of this process leading to increased cyclic AMP formation: catecholamines by stimulation of the beta receptor, and glucagon, thyroid hormone, and tolbutamide by direct action on adenylate cyclase. Furthermore, the increased contractility produced by aminophylline has been attributed to the drug's ability to inhibit phosphodiesterase, an intracellular enzyme which inactivates cyclic AMP. Although the mechanism through which cyclic AMP increases skeletal muscle and myocardial glycogenolysis has been established (cyclic nucleotide stimulation of protein kinase causes phosphorylation of phosphorylase kinase from ATP which, in turn, activates the phosphorylase enzyme degrading glycogen), knowledge is incomplete concerning the significance of cyclic AMP in the modulation of cardiac contraction. The possibilities under investigation in heart muscle are that myocardial cyclic AMP-dependent protein kinase might phosphorylate protein components in sarcoplasmic reticulum governing calcium transport or in troponin itself, thereby influencing the effects of calcium in the contractile reaction. Concerning the heart failure state, adenylate cyclase activity is not altered, but its stimulation by certain cardiovascular agents may be impaired.

Norepinephrine

Examination of the biosynthesis of myocardial norepinephrine is important in the consideration of mechanisms governing mechanical performance of heart muscle, since this hormone is the neurotransmitter directly linking cardiac sympathetic activity with beta receptor stimulation, resulting in elevated contractility and heart rate. The sympathetic nervous system normally exerts a major regulatory role in the augmentation of cardiovascular function in response to increased metabolic demands of the peripheral tissues, such as during physical exercise. The rich sympathetic innervation of heart muscle permits the heart to produce the majority of its own norepinephrine requirements. In the terminals of sympathetic nerves, norepinephrine is synthesized through a series of steps from tyrosine, in which tyrosine hydroxylase is the rate-limiting enzyme. The neurotransmitter is stored in the nerve ending in granules which protect it from enzymatic destruction by monoamine oxidase in the neuronal cytoplasm. In response to sympathetic impulses, norepinephrine is released to activate myocardial beta receptors. Importantly, in the failing heart the activity of tyrosine hydroxylase is markedly reduced, thus resulting in severe decrease of myocardial norepinephrine. The depression of norepinephrine appears to be the result of disturbed metabolic function in the neuron rather than actual loss of neural tissue. While this defect deprives the dysfunctioning ventricle of an adaptive mechanism for increasing its contractility, the depletion of myocardial norepinephrine is not responsible for the intrinsic weakness of the failing muscle. In heart failure, there is supersensitivity of myocardial beta receptors to circulating norepinephrine, and blood levels of this hormone are elevated because of its increased synthesis in the peripheral vasculature and the adrenal medulla; thereby, this supporting mechanism is restored, in part, to the failing heart.

It is apparent that a number of highly important biochemical processes are operative in the intact ventricle. Their complete integrity of function and proper integration are essential for normal mechanical and hemodynamic performance of the heart. Although aberrations have been identified in certain of these systems in the failing myocardium, the current view is that abnormalities in myocardial energy metabolism, protein synthesis, cyclic AMP reactions, and norepinephrine production may contribute by encroaching on compensatory mechanisms but do not play the primary causative role in the onset of congestive heart failure induced by chronic hemodynamic overload. A more promising possibility is that the biochemical defect or constellation of abnormalities resides in the mechanism of excitation-contraction coupling and the function of the contractile proteins.

EXCITATION-CONTRACTION COUPLING AND THE CONTRACTILE PROCESS

Sarcoplasmic Reticulum

When the stimulating impulse from the cardiac pacemaker arrives at the surface of the myocardial cell (Fig. 8-7A), an orderly sequence of events is initiated in which *calcium* movement is the chief component linking electrical excitation of the fiber with mechanical activation of the contractile machinery in the sarcomere. Excitation of the individual cell proceeds as the depolarization wave spreads throughout the entire fiber along the sarcolemma and its interior transtubular membrane system (Fig. 8-7B). When the depolarizing current in the transtubular system reaches the intimately apposed cisternae calcium depots of the sarcoplasmic reticulum, ionic calcium release is triggered from the lateral sacs into the sarcoplasm (Fig. 8-7C). Together with an apparently smaller but crucial quantity of ionic calcium influx across the sarcolemma-transtubular membrane occurring during phase 2 of the transmembrane action potential, this discharged calcium immediately diffuses to the sarcomeres, where it binds to the specific troponin calcium-receptor protein on the thin myofilaments in the overlap region between the thick and thin filaments. Mechanical *activation* is achieved by the binding of activator-calcium to troponin which overcomes the troponin-tropomyosin complex inhibition of actin and myosin interaction, with the result that actin-myosin electrostatic cross bridges are formed. The temporal course of the entire excitation-contraction coupling process takes place relatively quickly as indicated clinically by the average 0.06-second delay between the beginning of the scaler electrocardiographic QRS complex and the onset of isovolumic ventricular contraction.

Contractile Proteins

The onset of contraction takes place with development of force and contractile element shortening by the cyclic *interaction* of actin-myosin linkages pulling the thin filaments along the immobile thick filaments (Fig. 8-7D). It is believed that the electrostatic links are next broken as *myosin ATPase* of the heavy meromyosin heavy chains, in the presence of magnesium, hydrolyzes ATP, which is diffused to the sarcomeres from closely neighboring mitochondria, to ADP and

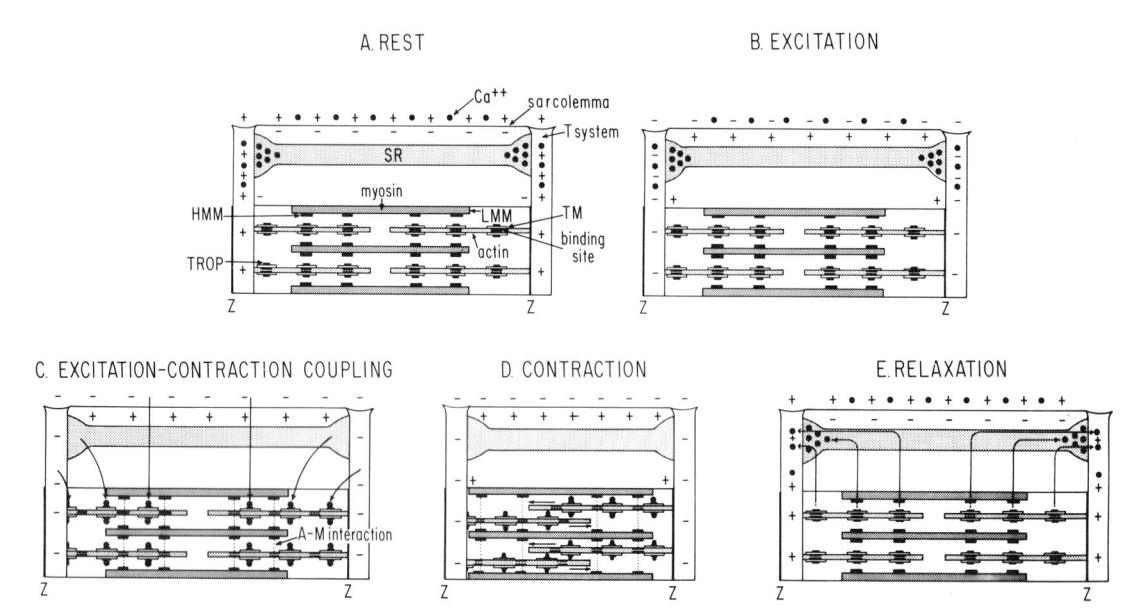

Figure 8-7 Diagrammatic sequence of subcellular events underlying the phases of the cardiac cycle. *A*, At rest, extracellular calcium (solid dots) is concentrated in the interstitial medium around the sarcolemma and in the T system, and intracellular calcium (solid dots) is sequestered in the lateral sacs of the sarcoplasmic reticulum (*SR*). *B*, With electrical excitation, complete depolarization of the fiber occurs by rapid influx of sodium during Phase O of the spike action potential, resulting in positive intracellular voltage. *C*, Excitation-contraction coupling is triggered by excitation, resulting in release of intracellular calcium from the SR and entry of extracellular calcium during Phase 2 of the action potential, with delivery of calcium (arrows) to troponin of the contractile apparatus within the sarcomeres. Calcium binding to troponin derepresses troponin (*TROP*)–tropomyosin (*TM*) inhibition of myosin linkage with specific binding site on actin. Thereby, actin-myosin (*A-M*) interaction initiates contraction. *D*, The process of contraction takes place by sequential making and breaking of A-M interconnections, with consequent sliding of actin centrally (arrows) along the fixed myosin filaments, producing force development and sarcomeric shortening. *E*, Relaxation occurs with removal of calcium by SR (arrows), with calcium returned extracellularly and sequestered in SR lateral sacs. Repolarization takes place by potassium efflux with re-establishment of negative intracellular voltage which, in diastole, is maintained with sodium extrusion and potassium return by sarcolemma-T membrane pump ATPase activity.

inorganic phosphate. Thus, a repetitive sequence of making and breaking cross linkages is established as the actin filament slides past the myosin filament during the entire course of ventricular contraction.

Excitation

The electrical event constituting excitation of the myocardial fiber involves depolarization of the cell by rapid ingress of a small quantity of sodium into the sarcoplasm (phase 0 spike of the action potential), followed by egress extracellularly of an equal amount of potassium (phase 3 repolarization of the action potential). Depolarization and repolarization do not require ATP energy. The large quantity of potassium within the cell is required for general maintenance of fiber electrical and mechanical function; in addition to its other roles, potassium is believed to be taken up by the sarcoplasmic reticulum after calcium release during excitation-contraction coupling. The removal of sodium during diastole (phase 4 resting potential) is accomplished by activity of the sarcolemma-transtubular membrane sodium-potassium pump ATPase, which utilizes energy. Schwartz, Langer, and Repke have proposed this enzyme as the pharmacologic receptor for digitalis, and the increased calcium influx responsible for the positive inotropic effect of the glycoside may result directly from or be associated with the drug's interference with this enzyme pump. There appears to be reduction of membrane sodium-potassium ATPase activity in heart failure.

Calcium Dynamics

The phase of the excitation-contraction coupling process in which calcium is delivered to the contractile apparatus does not require ATP energy. The contractile reaction involving myosin ATPase utilizes the great majority of total myocardial energy which varies according to the muscle loading conditions and contractile state. Following development of the full active contractile state, the active process of relaxation ensues, with calcium departing from the sarcomere and rapidly binding to the sarcoplasmic reticulum (Fig. 8–7E). The cation is then pumped back into the lateral sacs by *sarcotubular calcium pump ATPase* (relaxing factor), the total energy needed for relaxation being relatively small.

Concerning calcium dynamics, essentially no sarcoplasmic calcium is present during diastole, and the quantity of available calcium stored intracellularly is insufficient in itself to activate subsequent systole. Myocardial cells are not able to contract in a calcium-free external medium and, unlike skeletal muscle, some extracellular calcium is indispensable for contraction. The total amount of calcium provided to the sarcoplasm from internal and external sources is normally sufficient to activate all myosin molecules of the thick filament, with contraction taking place when a critical threshold of sarcoplasmic calcium concentration is reached. The greater the rate and quantity of calcium delivered to troponin, the faster the rate and number of activated interactions between actin and myosin, with consequent more rapid rate of tension development, greater maximum tension, and increased contractility.

Heart Failure

Enhancement of the rate and quantity of calcium influx from external sources appears to be an important mechanism for increasing myocardial contractility such as with digitalis. Negative inotropic drugs might diminish this calcium influx, and Briggs has shown their reduction of sarcotubular calcium pump ATPase. Concerning heart failure, there is abnormal transport of calcium by the sarcoplasmic reticulum as evidenced by its impairment of calcium uptake, binding, release, and pump ATPase activity as demonstrated by Schwartz, Gertz, Chidsey, and others. Furthermore, Chidsey has suggested a maldistribution of myocardial intracellular calcium in chronic hemodynamic overload in which depressed sarcoplasmic function leads to increased mitochondrial sequestration of calcium, with total intracellular calcium being unaltered. Katz and Briggs, in independent studies, have shown that the early decline of contractility in myocardial ischemia, with attendant intracellular acidosis due to lactate production, results directly from hydrogen ion inhibition of calcium binding to troponin.

In regard to the function of the contractile proteins in heart failure, attention has been focused on a potentially significant abnormality in energy utilization. Thus, the activity of myofibrillar ATPase is reduced in the failing myocardium as demonstrated by Alpert, Chandler, Luchi, and others. Although myofibrillar ATPase may not be rate limiting in the contractile process, it is conceivable that diminished activity of this enzyme in heart failure might limit the intensity of interaction between actin-myosin linkages and thereby lower contractile state. The failing heart does not appear to be inefficient in its conversion of chemical energy to mechanical work. Katz has pointed out that, although diminished myosin ATPase activity may impair contractile state, the lowered enzyme function may be viewed as a compensatory mechanism keeping energy utilization and production in balance when there is increased energy demand in chronic hemodynamic overloading or reduced energy synthesis in coronary artery disease. In the final phase of ischemic heart disease, exhaustion of ATP supply leads to the development of irreversible ventricular contracture, whereas decreased contractility in the earlier stage of ischemia due to disturbed excitation-contraction coupling may be reversible with reperfusion of the myocardium with oxygenated blood.

Finally, an additional consideration is that dysfunction of hypertrophied muscle may be related to changes in myofibril arrangement and quantitative differences in the generation of subcellular constituents. It is likely that in circumstances in which there is divergence of results and views concerning the causative, contributory, or coincidental nature of certain biochemical abnormalities in the pathogenesis of depressed mechanical function and contractility in the failing myocardium, these dissimilarities reflect basic differences in the types of heart failure studied—acute or chronic, mild or severe, experimental or human, idiopathic, drug-induced, ischemic, or volume or pressure overload.

MYOCARDIAL FUNCTION

Preload

The force of contraction of the myocardium is controlled by two fundamental mechanisms inherent in the contractile machinery of the sarcomere: (1) extent of diastolic stretch (preload) of the myofilaments, and (2) contractility (contractile or inotropic state) related to the intensity of biophysical and biochemical interactions between the myofilaments. Concerning the first mechanism, the length of the sarcomere at end diastole governs the degree of overlap of the movable actin and fixed myosin contractile filaments and thereby determines the number of interaction sites between the heavy meromyosin heads and actin active sites. Since the myosin filament is 1.5 μ long, with all but 0.2 μ of its center containing reactive spines, and the actin filament is 1.0 μ long, the optimal sarcomere length at which each of the possible actin-myosin cross bridges can be established is 2.2 μ (Fig. 8–8) as shown by Sonnenblick in heart muscle and by Huxley in skeletal muscle.

In heart muscle, Sonnenblick has shown that the extent of diastolic overlap of actin and myosin filaments between sarcomere lengths of 1.5 to 2.2 μ is directly related to the force of contraction, the strongest contraction occurring at the maximum overlap of 2.2 μ initial sarcomere length and the weakest at 1.5 μ with the minimum overlap. This relationship between sarcomere resting length and developed force is the ultrastructural basis for the length-active tension curve of isolated cardiac muscle (Fig. 8–8) and the *Frank-Starling principle* of the ventricular function curve of the intact heart (Fig. 8–9), relating end-diastolic volume to performance characteristics of the heart (stroke volume, cardiac output, or stroke work). In the normal left ventricle the upper limit of normal end-diastolic pressure of 12 mm. Hg corresponds to the optimal 2.2 μ individual sarcomere length, while the resting muscle length at which the maximum developed tension occurs (L_{max}) on the length-active tension curve represents the optimal sarcomere length. Thus, a wide spectrum of initial sarcomere lengths ranging from 1.5 to 2.2 μ is operative on the ascending limb of the ventricle function and length-tension curves. Normally the heart works at an intermediate point, usually on the upper portion, of the steep ascending limb of its function curve; thereby, the ventricle can improve its systolic performance by augmenting end-diastolic volume.

Active tension declines in skeletal muscle at sarcomere lengths greater than 2.2 μ, since thick and thin filament overlap diminishes, resulting in fewer actin-myosin linkages when the muscle is acutely overstretched. The relative disengage-

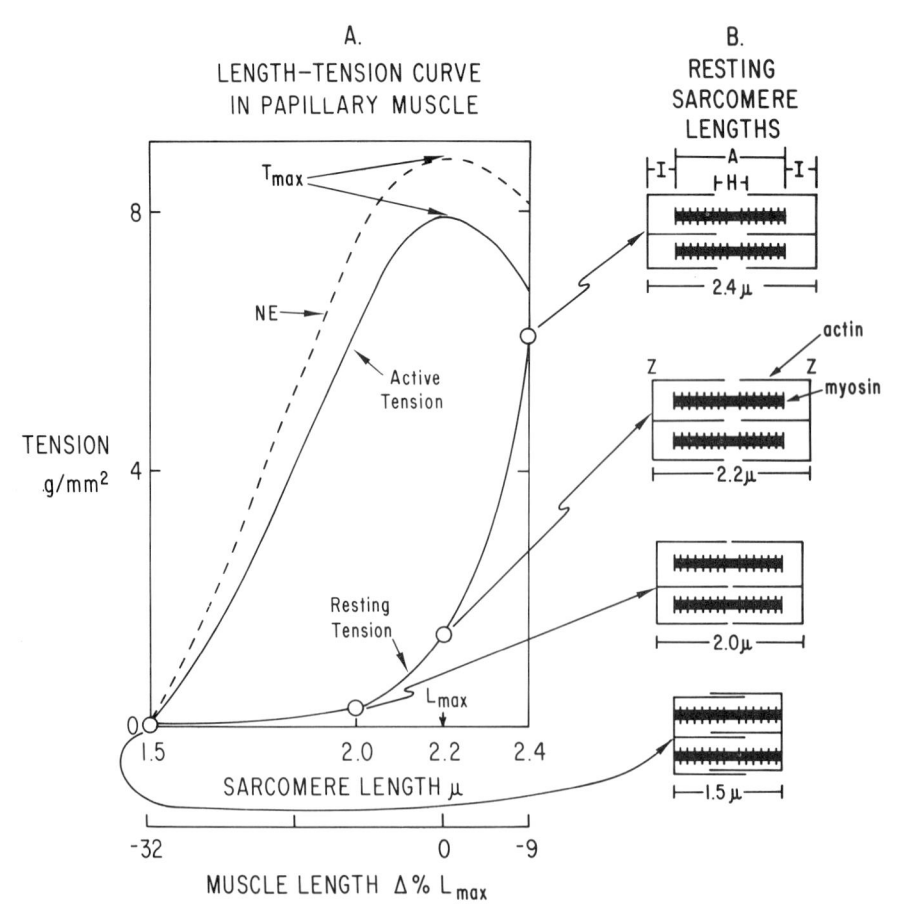

Figure 8–8 *A*, Relationships between active and resting (passive) tension development and sarcomere and papillary muscle length of the feline right ventricle. The active tension curve is elevated by increased contractile state induced by norepinephrine (*NE*). T_{max} = maximal active tension at L_{max}. *B*, Diagrammatic resting sarcomere lengths showing relations between actin and myosin filaments at different preloads.

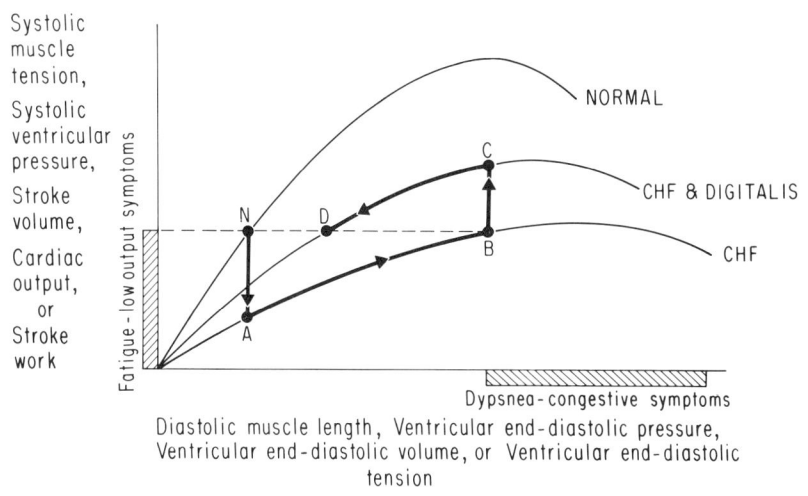

Figure 8-9 Ventricular function curves relating cardiac performance characteristics to extent of preload in the normal state, congestive heart failure (CHF), and CHF treated with digitalis. Points N through D represent in sequence: normal contractile state (N), depression of contractility (A), Frank-Starling compensation (B), increase in contractility toward normal with digitalis (C), and less utilization of preload compensation which digitalis allows (D). Although points N, D and B represent equal stroke volume on the vertical axis, each requires a progressively greater end-diastolic pressure indicated by the horizontal axis. The excessive end-diastolic pressures causing pulmonary congestion and the reduced levels of cardiac performance resulting in low cardiac output symptoms are represented by the cross-hatched areas. (Reproduced with permission from Mason, D. T., et al.: *In* Yu, P. N., and Goodwin, J. F. (Eds.): Progress in Cardiology. Philadelphia, Lea and Febiger, 1972.)

ment of the actin filament from the myosin band is indicated by the abnormal central H zone and expanded I band representing the areas of non-overlap of filaments (Fig. 8-8B). Thus, in acutely overstretched skeletal muscle and to a lesser extent cardiac muscle, sarcomere lengths greater than 2.2 μ are observed on the descending limb of the length-active tension curve. However, the predominant finding on the descending limb of the ventricular function curve of the chronically overdistended heart is slippage of myofibrils, with attendant distortion of orderly vertical register alignment of sarcomeres, rather than excessive elongation of individual sarcomere units with removal of paracentral filament binding sites.

Heart muscle also exhibits a *length-passive tension curve* which determines its diastolic *compliance* or distensibility characteristics (Fig. 8-8B). Thus, passive tension is generated upon stretch of the myocardium in its resting state. In the intact ventricle, this length-passive tension curve is represented by the relation between end-diastolic pressure and end-diastolic volume. Cardiac muscle exhibits considerable resting tension as it is stretched to lengths approaching the physiologic limit of sarcomere length of 2.2 μ or 12 mm. Hg in the intact ventricle. This increase in passive tension contributes to total tension of the myocardium during systole, as does the greater effect of consequent rise in active developed tension at greater muscle lengths, thereby strengthening the force of contraction. The heart becomes extremely stiff when it is overstretched beyond the length corresponding to the apex of its ventricular function curve, resulting in marked elevations of end-diastolic pressure without improvement in ventricular performance. Clinically, alterations in compliance of the whole ventricle occur in certain chronic cardiac disorders. Compliance is reduced in idiopathic hypertrophic cardiomyopathy, myocardial fibrosis, and excessive pressure loading in aortic stenosis. In chronic volume overloading the entire diastolic pressure-volume curve is displaced to the right, usually with reduced functional distensibility at the ventricle's elevated operating end-diastolic pressure.

Contractility

Concerning contractility, this second important basic functional variable of the myocardium which allows intrinsic control of its strength of contraction can be defined mechanically as the unique quality of heart muscle to alter its contractile force and velocity independent of fiber length. As is the case for the Frank-Starling principle, changes in myocardial contractility have a specific subcellular foundation. Although skeletal muscle exhibits a length-active tension relationship similar to heart muscle, skeletal muscle does not possess the physiologic regulatory mechanism of variable contractility characteristic of heart muscle. Whereas length-induced changes in contractile force are determined quantitatively by the number of operative active sites between actin and myosin, the cellular basis of variable myocardial contractility is dependent on alterations in the qualitative nature (intensity and rapidity) of these cyclic force-generating sites between the contractile proteins.

Recently it has been considered by Katz and Brady that the process of actin-myosin interaction at constant myofilament overlap governing contractility appears to comprise two biophysical-chemical components: (1) *activation rate* of actin-myosin binding sites (rate at which activator calcium is delivered to modulator troponin, thereby preventing troponin-tropomyosin inhibition of actin-myosin reactive sites), and (2) *interaction rate* between actin-myosin molecules at the activated binding sites (rate of energy release and conversion of chemical to mechanical energy in the contractile process). These subprocesses are conceived as having two specific mechanical correlates quantifying contractility: (1) peak rate of tension rise or peak dT/dt (binding activation rate controlled by excitation-contraction coupling) and (2) peak rate of contractile element shortening or V_{max} (binding interaction rate regulated by the level of myosin ATPase activity). Furthermore, maximum systolic tension of heart muscle is determined by the number of actin-myosin interactions as governed by myofilament overlap and quantity of calcium bound to troponin.

Afterload

In addition to the fundamental intrinsic preload and contractility mechanisms of the myocardium regulating contractile force, there are two further independent properties of heart muscle determining cardiac performance which are largely under extrinsic control. The first of these is the afterload imposed on the muscle in order to shorten in an isotonic contraction of isolated muscle and to deliver stroke volume during ejection in the intact heart. Ventricular afterload is the myocardial wall tension during ejection defined by the *Laplace relation,* in which tension is directly equated with the product of ventricular systolic pressure and radius and inversely related to wall thickness. Thus, afterload is largely related to aortic pressure, which, in turn, is principally modulated by systemic vascular resistance. In addition, tension is a function of ventricular size and its geometry; a large ventricle must meet a higher afterload than a smaller ventricle at the same level of aortic and ventricular systolic pressures. Thus, when end-diastolic volume is increased, the ventricle generates more systolic tension to develop the same pressure for opening the aortic valve and to eject the same stroke volume. For the dilated ventricle to deliver an increased stroke volume in relation to the elevation of end-diastolic volume, it also moves up the ascending limb of its ventricular function curve, resulting in further rise in systolic tension.

Heart Rate

The final independent property of cardiac muscle normally governing ventricular performance is the heart rate. The frequency of contraction is primarily controlled by the autonomic nervous system through unequal reciprocal changes in activity of its parasympathetic and sympathetic components. Thus, like afterload which is largely determined by changes in peripheral vascular resistance and in turn is regulated by adrenergic activity and regional metabolic factors, the heart rate is principally controlled by means extrinsic to the ventricle. Concerning the role of heart rate in the regulation of cardiac output which is the product of heart rate and stroke volume, normally the frequency of contraction is very important in rapid adjustments of cardiac output, while chronic alterations in cardiac output are more the result of changes in stroke volume governed by the ventricular loading conditions and contractile state.

Dyssynergy

When considering cardiac function in certain clinical heart disorders, it is important to add a fifth principal factor which adversely affects ventricular performance: abnormal temporal sequence or dyssynergy of ventricular contraction as demonstrated by Gorlin. The normal pattern of left ventricular contraction takes place in a coordinated manner, with integrated inward movement of the ventricular wall during ejection (Fig. 8–10A). However, intraventricular conduction defects may cause a disorderly contraction sequence which in itself decreases cardiac function. More importantly, dyssynergy of contraction is also produced by localized disturbances in muscle function. Thus, segmental abnormalities of ventricular contraction occur commonly in coronary artery disease, and dyssynergy per se may contribute greatly to impaired cardiac function, in addition to the regional abnormalities of contractility and compliance accompanying the deranged wall movement (Fig. 8–10B,C, and D). Increased systolic compliance as occurs in ventricular aneurysm and dyssynergy each disturbs ventricular function in terms of the Frank-Starling relation by producing an adverse effect analogous to decline in preload, as has been shown in specialized papillary muscle prepara-

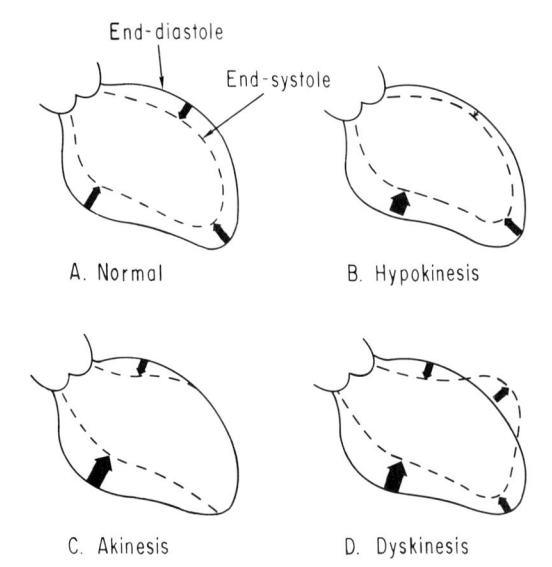

Figure 8–10 Localized patterns of left ventricular (*LV*) dyssynergy. The direction and extent of internal wall movement from end-diastole to end-systole are shown by the arrows. RAO = right anterior oblique view. (Reproduced with permission from Mason, D. T., et al.: *In* Yu, P. N., and Goodwin, J. F. (Eds.): Progress in Cardiology. Philadelphia, Lea and Febiger, 1972.)

tions with increased series elasticity and muscles contracting asynchronously in tandem.

Evaluation of Contractility

From the foregoing discussion concerning the regulation of myocardial contraction it is apparent that the function of the heart is normally determined by the interplay among its preload, contractility, afterload, and heart rate. The terms *cardiac function* and *ventricular performance* are used in the general sense to refer to the integrated action of all these determinants and not necessarily only to the single determinant, contractility itself. The contractile state and function of the heart can be evaluated by two general approaches: (1) its *pump* (hemodynamics), and (2) its *muscle* (mechanics) performance characteristics. In the traditional approach of pump analysis the standard hemodynamic variables of cardiac output, stroke volume, systolic ejection rate, and ventricular end-diastolic pressure and the more complex measurements of ventricular end-diastolic volume, ejection fraction, stroke work, stroke power, and ventricular mass are studied in the basal state and also evaluated within the background of the Frank-Starling principle of initial length changes relative to systolic performance. In addition, cardiac contractility and function have recently been evaluated by the second approach in terms of muscle mechanics which describe the force, velocity, and length characteristics of the myocardium.

Length-Active Tension Curve. An understanding of the property of contractility and its assessment by mechanical and hemodynamic techniques can be achieved by consideration of the mechanics of contraction in isolated muscle. During *isometric contraction,* contractile state can be evaluated by the relative position and shifts of the length-active tension curve (isometric force-length relation) utilizing papillary muscle preparations (Fig. 8–8*A*). The length-active tension curve is obtained by stretching the muscle, electrically stimulating it at a fixed length, and determining the active tension it produces while contracting isometrically; this procedure is carried out throughout a series of muscle lengths to establish the entire curve for a given contractile state. In the study of the inotropic effect of a pharmacologic agent, the entire technique is repeated after bathing the muscle with the drug to assess the new level of contractility. An upward displacement of the ascending limb of the curve indicates qualitatively that an increase in contractility has occurred (Fig. 8–8*A*), and a downward shift identifies a directional decrease in contractility. Thus, alterations of the entire length-isometric tension curve signify changes in inotropism, while movements along a given stationary curve denote variations in fiber length. Depressed length-tension curves are observed in muscles taken from failing hearts. Concepts gained from studies of the myocardial length-tension mechanical relationship can be extended to the clinical evaluation of cardiac function by hemodynamic means. Thus, the systolic force-resting length framework of analysis of the inotropic and preload properties of isolated cardiac muscle also applies to the assessment of these properties in the intact ejecting heart employing Frank-Starling ventricular function curves (Fig. 8–9).

Force-Velocity Curve. A more precise conceptual analysis of myocardial mechanical properties and contractility is provided by consideration of muscle models containing functionally different components: the *contractile element* (CE), *series elastic* component (SE), and *parallel elastic* component (PE) (Fig. 8–11). As originally proposed by Hill in skeletal muscle and extended to cardiac muscle by Abbott and Mommaerts, Sonnenblick, Brady, Hefner, and Parmley, the CE develops force and shortens when activated (CE active state) and represents the intensity of interaction between the cyclic binding sites of the myofilaments; the CE is freely extensible at rest. The SE and PE are conceived as passive inert springs with different stress-strain characteristics. The SE is thought to reside in the myofilaments and cell membranes, while the PE is considered to be in the supporting connective tissue

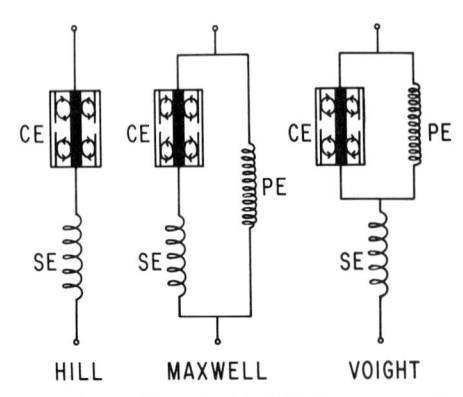

Figure 8-11 The A. V. Hill 2-component and Maxwell and Voight 3-component modifications of mechanical models of heart muscle. CE = contractile element; SE = series elastic element; PE = parallel elastic element.

structures. According to the 3-component model shown (Maxwell adaptation of Hill model), the SE is in series with the CE, and the PE is connected alongside the CE and SE. Diastolic tension (preload) results from stretching the stiff PE. During isometric contraction after electrical stimulation, the rate of CE shortening (V_{CE}) occurs at the same rate the nonlinear, more distensible SE spring elongates (V_{SE}), leading to the generation of active tension without change in muscle length.

In heart muscle preparations allowing *isotonic contraction*, the muscle shortens when the force developed equals the load (afterload) against which it is contracting. During isotonic contraction, tension is constant while the muscle shortens. Since the SE is stationary at the onset of muscle shortening, the initial peak fiber shortening rate (*FSR*) is equal to V_{CE} for the total load encountered (tension or force exerted). By repeating a series of isotonic contractions over a wide range of different loads and graphing the relationship between systolic load and V_{CE} (peak FSR), an inverse *force-velocity curve* is obtained in which V_{CE} declines as force increases (Fig. 8-12). Maximum V_{CE} (V_{max}) is obtained by extrapolation of the curve to zero load. Maximum force (P_0), which is directly related to preload, is achieved at the load at which no fiber shortening takes place (at zero V_{CE}). Since alterations in contractile state change V_{max}, while variations in preload directly affect P_0 but are generally held not to influence V_{max}, V_{max} is considered an independent numerical index of contractility, with the value directly related to inotropic state (Fig. 8-12). Thus, the maximum rapidity of unloaded CE cyclic interactive sites (activity of myosin ATPase) is envisaged as being uninfluenced by sarcomere length or number of linkage sites. Some workers prefer that V_{max} estimated by force-velocity curve extrapolations be considered an empirical index of contractile state because of possible influence on this value by instantaneous changes in CE length, active state, internal viscosities, and muscle model uncertainties, although these concerns have been refuted by others. It is important that from consideration of the force-velocity-initial and shortening length relationship, both peak external work (product of force and extent of muscle shortening) and power (product of force and FSR) are dependent on preload and contractility.

Contractile element velocity can also be determined from isometric contractions of isolated ventricular papillary muscles. Since V_{SE} equals V_{CE} during isometric systole, V_{CE} can be determined from the rate of SE elongation which is defined as the rate of tension development (dT/dt) related to the SE modulus or stiffness factor (dT/dl). The *SE modulus* is described as the product of a constant (K) and muscle tension (T), plus the constant C; C is disregarded because of its relatively small value. From these considerations, V_{CE} is calculated from the equation (dT/dt)/(KT), in which K is 32/muscle length at body temperature. A force-velocity curve is obtained by plotting the relationship of instantaneous V_{CE} to simultaneous tension throughout the course of a single contraction.

The concepts developed from study of isolated cardiac muscle mechanics have recently been extended to the assessment of contractility and performance of the intact heart experimentally and in patients. In the investigation of left ventricular mechanics, the development of chamber force and tension are related to the velocity and extent of contractile element and fiber shortening. The approach utilizing muscle mechanics provides a means for the quantitative analysis of the principal determinants of cardiac performance including the numerical evaluation of contractile state. Although the pump characteristics of stroke volume and mean systolic ejection rate indirectly reflect the extent and velocity of fiber shortening respectively, hemodynamic variables are influenced by alterations in loading in addition to changes in contractility. In the application of the principles of muscle mechanics to the ventricle as a whole, its integrated function is described in terms of representative or average values of force, velocity, and length of the entire ventricle. The methods for evaluation of the mechanics of ventricular contraction have been developed along two different lines: the properties of (1) isovolumic and (2) ejection phases of systole.

Isovolumic Indices. Concerning the techniques for assessment of the mechanics of isovolumic ventricular contraction, an important method is determination of the rate at which intraventricular pressure rises or the first derivative of ventricular pressure (*dp/dt*) (Fig. 8-13). *Peak dp/dt* itself is a valid and sensitive measure for the study of ventricular inotropic state in intrapa-

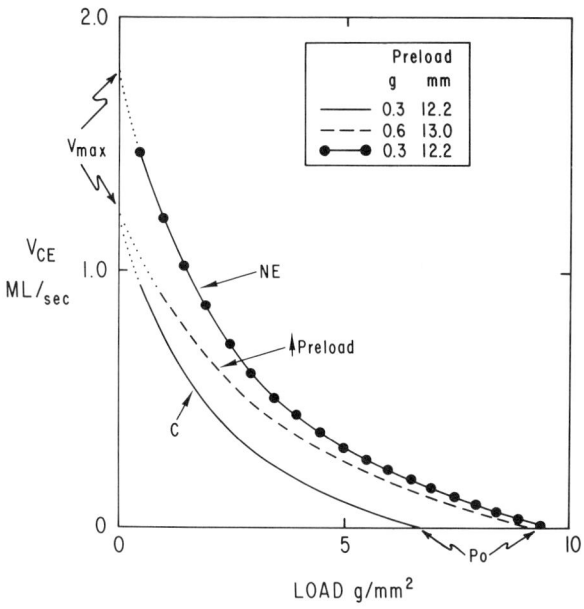

Figure 8–12 Force-velocity relationship in feline right ventricular papillary muscle in control state (C), after increasing initial muscle length (preload), and with augmentation of contractility by norepinephrine (NE) at control initial muscle length. V_{CE} = contractile element velocity expressed in muscle lengths (ML) per second. V_{max} = maximal V_{CE} at zero load obtained by extrapolation of force-velocity curve. P_O = maximal isometric force.

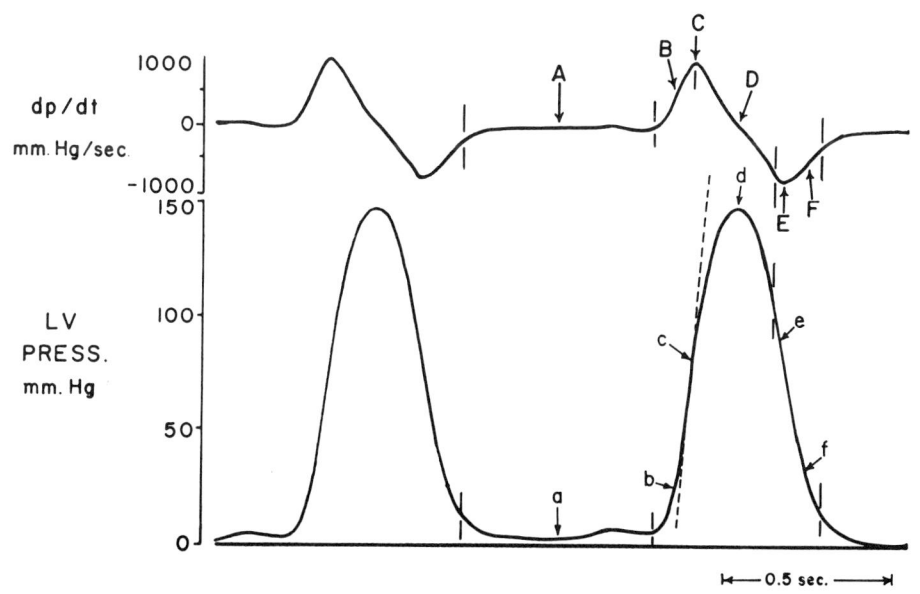

Figure 8–13 Simultaneous recordings of high-fidelity left ventricular pressure (LV) and its first derivative (dp/dt) in a patient with an aortic valve prosthesis. The various portions of the first derivative and corresponding segments of the pressure recording from which they were continuously computed are labeled. During ventricular filling when rate of change of ventricular pressure is minimal, dp/dt is flat at a level near zero (segment A). With the onset of isovolumic contraction, dp/dt rises slowly and then rapidly (segment B) to reach the peak dp/dt (point C), the maximal rate of pressure rise, indicated by slope of the diagonal broken line. Peak dp/dt usually occurs at the instant of opening of the semilunar valves, thus at peak isovolumic ventricular pressure. During early and middle phases of ventricular ejection, dp/dt descends to the baseline, and during late ejection, as intraventricular pressure decreases, dp/dt becomes negative (segment D). The rate of decrease of ventricular pressure is maximal at point E during isovolumic relaxation (segment F). Left ventricular pressure was recorded by direct needle puncture. (Reproduced with permission from Mason, D. T.: Amer. J. Cardiol., 23:516, 1969.)

tient studies when loading conditions are constant. Thus, with ventricular loading stable, peak dp/dt itself correlates directly with the contractile state of the ventricle in the study of interventions in single patients. However, peak dp/dt is a complex function also directly dependent on the preload or left ventricular end-diastolic pressure (LVEDP) and afterload (arterial diastolic pressure in the case of peak dp/dt). An increase in LVEDP causes an elevation of instantaneous dp/dt throughout the course of isovolumic contraction including peak dp/dt, whereas a rise in arterial diastolic pressure elevates only peak dp/dt. Since changes in loading conditions of the ventricle ordinarily occur in response to most physiologic and pharmacologic interventions in individual patients and in the basal state among different patients, usually it is not possible precisely to evaluate changes in ventricular contractile state by the determination of peak dp/dt alone.

The recognition that dp/dt is influenced by preload and afterload variations has led to the development of contractility indices in which dp/dt is modified by certain hemodynamic and mechanical variables which minimize or cancel the changes in dp/dt caused by inconstant loading. Thus, by relating these loading-related correction factors to dp/dt, it is possible to employ dp/dt in the assessment of contractility despite concurrent alterations in loading. One approach which is useful in intrapatient studies is the examination of the time interval from the onset of ventricular contraction to maximum dp/dt (*time-to-peak dp/dt*) in relation to peak dp/dt itself (Fig. 8–14). Alterations in contractility produce opposite changes between time-to-peak dp/dt and peak dp/dt, while variations in loading result in directionally similar changes in these two variables. Although directionally opposite changes between time-to-peak dp/dt and peak dp/dt indicate a qualitative alteration of contractility, large concomitant changes in LVEDP or arterial diastolic pressure might obscure alterations in inotropic state analyzed in this manner. In the presence of changes in LVEDP without associated variations of arterial diastolic pressure, alterations in contractility can be studied using the ratios: peak dp/dt to integrated systolic isovolumic tension (IIT), peak dp/dt to peak isovolumic pressure (PIP), peak dp/dt to maximum isovolumic ventricular tension (MIT), peak dp/dt to LVEDP, and

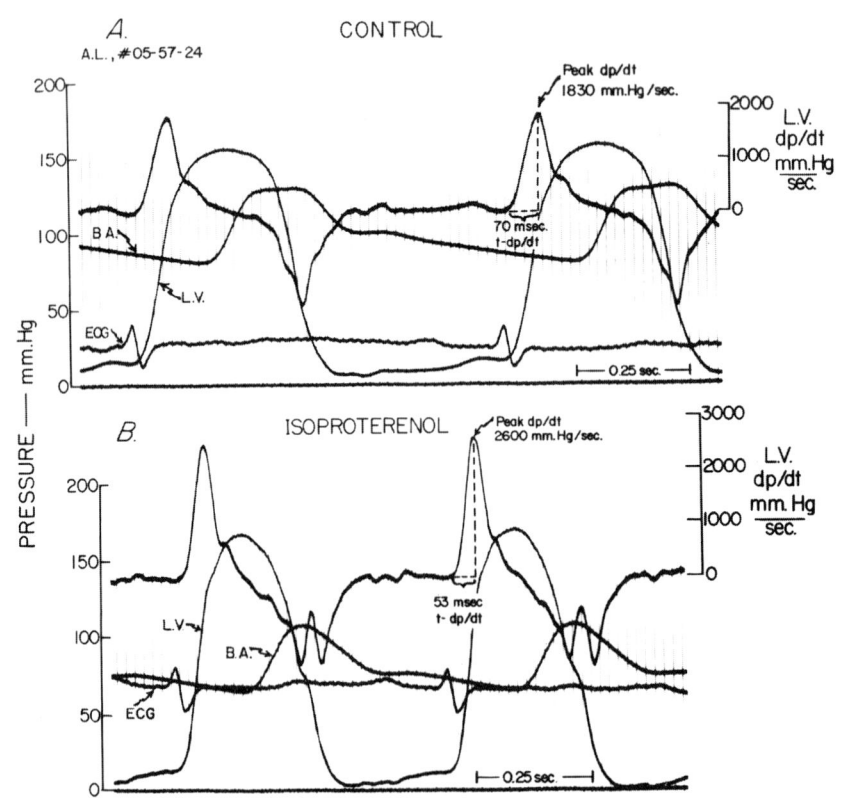

Figure 8–14 Simultaneous recordings of the high-fidelity left ventricular pressure, its first derivative, and brachial arterial pressure (*B.A.*) during the control period (*A*) and after increasing contractility with isoproterenol (*B*) in a patient with an aortic valve prosthesis. The interval from the onset to peak dp/dt (t-dp/dt) is indicated. Left ventricular pressure was recorded by direct needle puncture. (Reproduced with permission from Mason, D. T.: Amer. J. Cardiol., 23:516, 1969.)

(peak dp/dt)/PIP related to left ventricular end-diastolic circumferential fiber length. As with peak dp/dt, these ratios are dependent on arterial diastolic pressure.

When LVEDP is nearly constant and arterial diastolic pressure varies, the relation of dp/dt to peak common developed isovolumic pressure (CPIP) or *(dp/dt)/CPIP* correlates directly with contractile state independent of afterload variations (Fig. 8–15). The relation between dp/dt and simultaneously developed pressure during the course of isovolumic contraction can also be applied in the assessment of basal contractile state among different patients. Thus, dp/dt determined

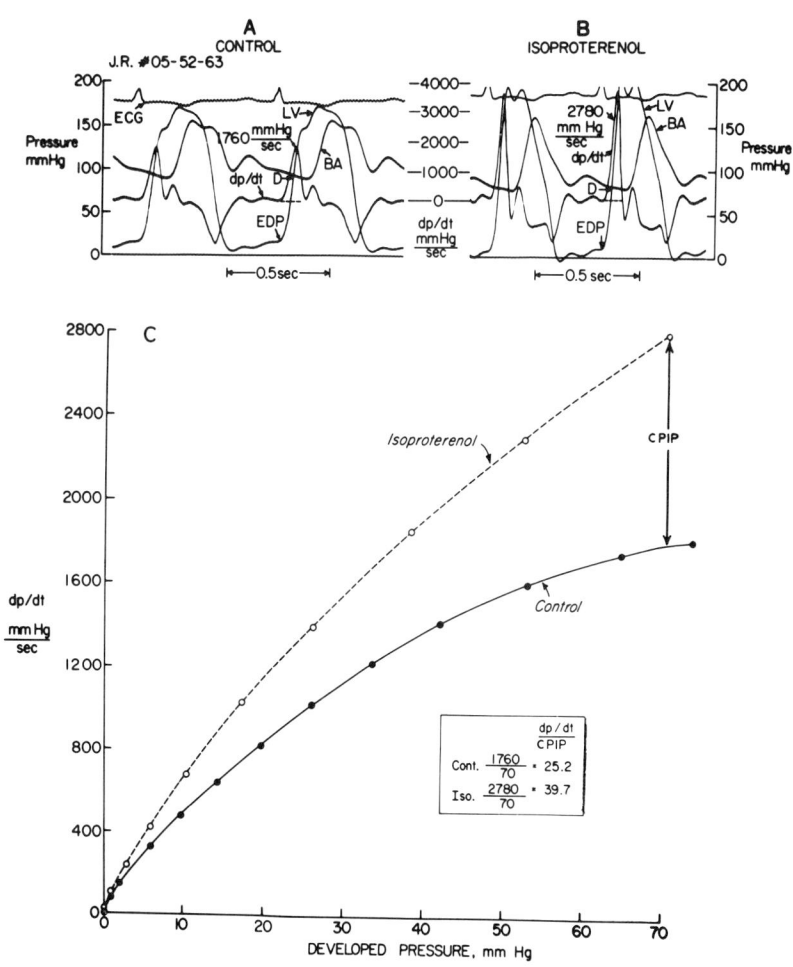

Figure 8–15 *A* and *B,* Simultaneous recording of high-fidelity left ventricular (*LV*) pressure, its first derivative (*dp/dt*), the brachial arterial pressure (*BA*), and electrocardiogram during the control period (*A*) and during isoproterenol (*B*). *EDP* = LV end-diastolic pressure; *D* = peak isovolumic LV pressure. The numerical values of dp/dt indicated are at the highest common developed isovolumic pressure (*CPIP*). *C,* Relation between LV dp/dt and developed isovolumic pressure at 5-msec. intervals throughout isovolumic systole of the contractions shown in *A*, during the control period (*Cont.*), and *B*, during isoproterenol (*Iso.*). The arrows indicating CPIP of both curves are the points at which the ratios of (dp/dt)/CPIP shown in the insert were calculated. (Reproduced by permission of the American Heart Association, Inc., from Mason, D. T., et al.: Circulation, *44*:47, 1971.)

at the developed isovolumic ventricular pressure of 50 mm. Hg common to each of the different ventricles corrects for differences in arterial diastolic pressure. Since the preload of the different ventricles varies widely, dp/dt at common developed isovolumic pressure of 50 mm. Hg is modified by relating it to left ventricular end-diastolic volume index (LVEDVI). This ratio (dp/dt$_{CPIP}$)/LVEDVI is analogous to V_{CE} corrected for its preload-dependence at an isopressure point on the pressure-velocity curve to be described.

It has recently been shown that the contractile state can be quantified clinically by determination of *ventricular pressure-velocity curves* from high-fidelity recordings of isovolumic ventricular systolic dp/dt and pressure (Fig. 8–16). This new method is based on force-velocity concepts derived from study of isometric myocardial mechanics discussed earlier in isolated muscle and, from a single beat, provides segments of isovolumic pressure-V_{CE} curves related to the entire force-velocity relationship. In the intact heart during isovolumic contraction, alterations in ventricular geometry are small and thus V_{CE} can be assumed essentially equivalent to V_{SE}. In the calculation of isovolumic ventricular V_{SE}, and thereby V_{CE}, knowledge of tension is not necessary; only the value of isovolumic pressure is required, since pressure is essentially the only independent variable, and chamber radius and wall thickness cancel in the equation for isovolumic V_{SE}. Therefore, isovolumic V_{CE} in ejecting beats can be determined entirely from isovolumic ventricular pressure (IP) and corresponding dp/dt by use of the equation for isovolumic V_{SE}: $(dp/dt)/(32 \times IP)$ expressed in muscle lengths (ML) per second.

The isovolumic pressure-velocity curve can be constructed from an individual contraction by relating instantaneous V_{CE} to simultaneous total isovolumic pressure from the closure of the atrioventricular valve to the opening of the semilunar valve (Fig. 8–16). Extrapolation of the pressure-velocity descending limb to zero pressure allows estimation of maximum V_{CE} or V_{max}. In practice, the segment of the pressure-velocity curve is averaged from several beats. Like V_{max} obtained from isometric and isotonic contractions in isolated papillary muscle, ventricular V_{max} is related directly to contractile state and is independent of physiologic variations in left ventricular end-diastolic volume and pressure; some dependence is reported with very large preload increases. This practical method of determining pressure-velocity relations in the assessment of contractility obviates the complex angiographic techniques for the calculation of tension. Importantly, ventricular pressure-velocity and tension-velocity curves of a given beat extrapolate to identical values of V_{max}.

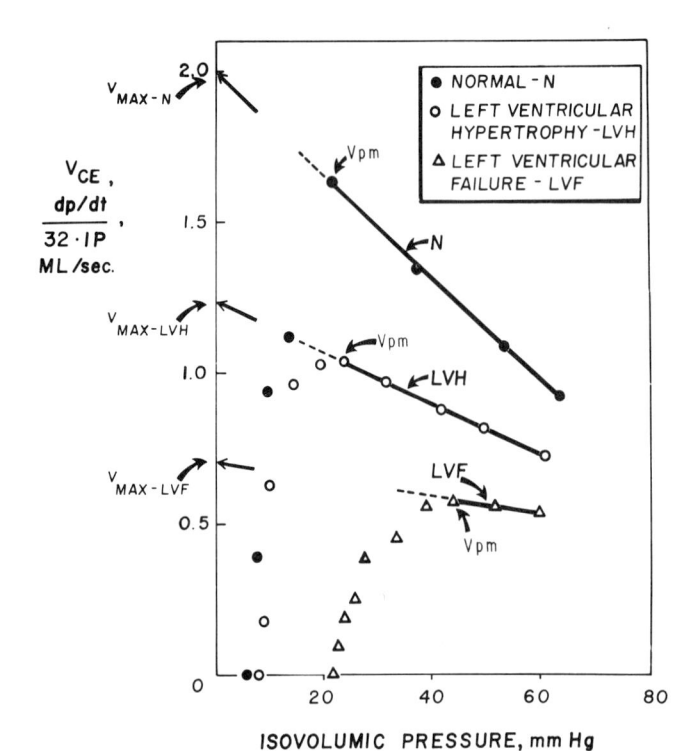

Figure 8–16 Representative comparison of the pressure-velocity relation during isovolumic systole of the left ventricle in a normal patient, in a patient with aortic stenosis with left ventricular hypertrophy in the absence of failure, and in a patient with aortic stenosis with left ventricular hypertrophy and failure. The diagonal broken lines indicate extrapolation of the isovolumic segments to V_{max} at zero load. Vpm = peak measured V_{CE}. IP in the V_{CE} equation and pressure on the horizontal axis are total isovolumic pressure. (Reproduced with permission from Mason, D. T., et al.: *In* Alpert, N. R. (Ed.): Ventricular Hypertrophy. New York, Academic Press, 1971.)

The pressure-velocity method of assessing left ventricular contractile state can be applied both in studies of interventions in individual patients and in the evaluation of basal contractility in different patients, since V_{max} is expressed in terms of muscle units and is independent of loading and wall thickness. Utilizing this method in patients with primary and secondary ventricular hypertrophy, a spectrum of decreasing inotropic state has been demonstrated between those without failure and those with failure (Fig. 8–16). Although determination of V_{max} from isovolumic pressure and its dp/dt has been thought to require a truly isovolumic portion of systole, recent evidence indicates that mitral insufficiency itself has little to no effect on V_{max} obtained from pressure-velocity curves. Abnormal ventricular compliance and dyssynergy such as occur in coronary artery disease have been considered conditions in which the pressure-velocity method is not applicable in the study of contractility. Recent work, however, has demonstrated that when SE stiffness is altered or dyssynergy produced, the determination of V_{max} extrapolated from the isovolumic pressure-velocity relation remains valid. V_{max} does not appear to be influenced by regional myocardial necrosis itself, since maximum velocity is sensitive only to the intensity of operative binding sites between myofilaments. Although compliance variations, altered temporal contraction sequence, non-isovolumic systole, and segmental necrosis may considerably affect loaded V_{CE} prior to aortic valve opening, the accompanying slope change of the pressure-V_{CE} curve is such that the extrapolation to V_{max} is essentially undisturbed. Therefore, in these particular conditions there may be marked disparity between ventricular hemodynamic performance and contractility assessed as V_{max}. In addition to V_{max}, certain other properties of the isovolumic total pressure velocity relation are useful in evaluating contractility such as peak measured V_{CE} (V_{pm}), which is a finite value not requiring extrapolation (Fig. 8–16).

The isovolumic *total pressure*-velocity method for the evaluation of contractile state is based on the 2-component Hill model in which CE and SE are connected in series. It has been suggested that the PE component should also be considered during isovolumic contraction by subtracting LVEDP from total isovolumic pressure to obtain developed isovolumic pressure for use in the V_{CE} equation and on the abscissa of the pressure-velocity curve (Fig. 8–17). With the isovolumic *developed pressure*-velocity curve obtained by utilization of the 3-component model, V_{CE} is infinitely high at very small developed isovolumic pressures and, therefore, the first point on the descending pressure-velocity limb is usually arbitrarily taken at 10 mm. Hg. It is also possible to estimate right ventricular contractility by application of this developed pressure-V_{CE} approach, since this method allows description of a descending limb at relatively low isovolumic pressures. In contrast, the onset of the total pressure-V_{CE} descending curve is delayed until development of full active state of the ventricle (Fig. 8–17); thus the total IP-V_{CE} method may not be applicable in beats with relatively small amplitudes of isovolumic pressure. Comparing the degree of sensitivity to contractility and preload of the principal contractility indices employing isovolumic dp/dt, the order of decreasing inotropic and loading sensitivities is peak dp/dt, (dp/dt)/CPIP, total and then developed pressure V_{CE} methods, with peak dp/dt at the top of the spectrum being very sensitive to inotropism but still somewhat responsive to loading, while developed pressure V_{CE} on the bottom is not altered by large changes in end-diastolic volume but is relatively insensitive to contractility. Contractility indices designed to obviate loading influences become inherently less sensitive to contractility.

Ejection Indices. The systolic ejection techniques applied to analysis of ventricular force-velocity properties and contractile state examine fiber shortening rate or circumferential fiber shortening velocity (V_{CF}) to determine V_{CE} according to the principles of isotonic mechanics elucidated in isolated muscle (see earlier discussion). One approach to the analysis of V_{CF} in intrapatient studies is the cinegraphic method of determining rate of change of epicardial dimensions by measurement of the velocity of movement, frame by frame, of roentgenopaque markers which were previously sutured to the ventricle's surface at therapeutic operation. Other techniques for the study of external border motion are the measurement of epicardial segmental velocity as determined by the movement of branch points of coronary arteries during angiography and noninvasively by radarkymography.

A more promising approach to the evaluation of V_{CE} and contractility during ejection is the study of endocardial wall motion. Angiographic study of instantaneous tension-velocity-length relations provides determination of V_{CF} at peak midwall tension (T) at which V_{SE} is zero; thereby, V_{CF} *at peak T* equals V_{CE} at peak tension. Thus, a single V_{CE}-tension relation is established which identifies a point on the force-velocity curve of the ventricle, similar to the manner in which a point is determined on the isotonic force-velocity curve of papillary muscle by determination of peak FSR at peak T from a single isotonic contraction. The electromagnetic

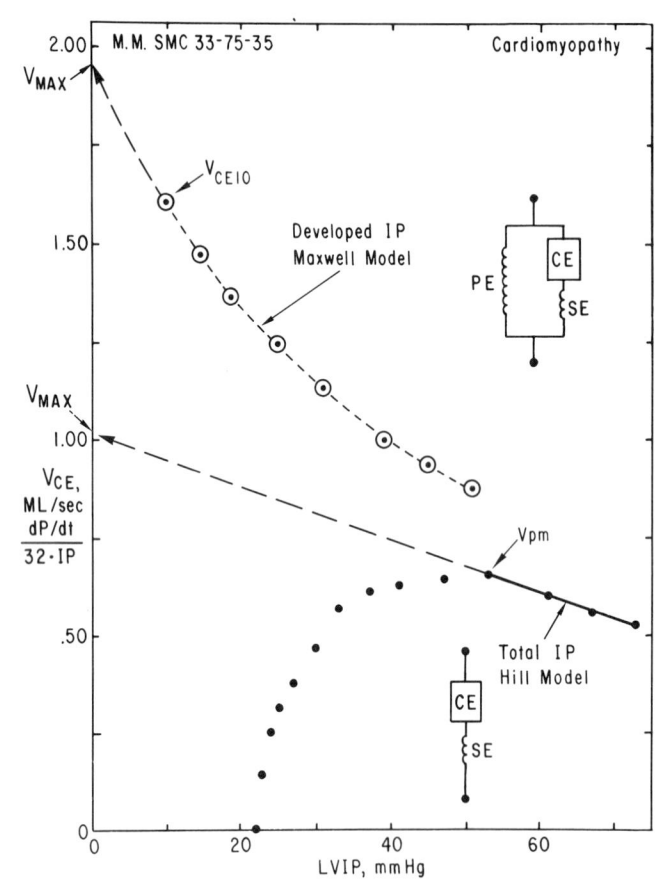

Figure 8–17 Left ventricular (*LV*) pressure-velocity relation during isovolumic contraction obtained by the use of total instantaneous isovolumic pressure, as IP, in the calculation of instantaneous V_{CE} (2-component Hill model) and on the abscissa for LVIP (closed dots and solid lines) compared to the isovolumic pressure-velocity relation determined by employment of developed instantaneous isovolumic pressure in the V_{CE} equation (3-component Maxwell model) and on the abscissa for LVIP (open circles and broken lines). The extrapolations to V_{max} are shown by the long broken lines and arrows. The appropriate muscle models are shown. The two pressure-velocity curves were obtained from the same LV beat in a patient with a cardiomyopathy. *Vpm* = peak measured V_{CE} using total IP; $V_{CE}10 = V_{CE}$ at 10 mm. Hg developed IP. (Reproduced with permission from Mason, D. T., et al.: *In* Yu, P. N., and Goodwin, J. F. (Eds.): Progress in Cardiology. Philadelphia, Lea and Febiger, 1972.)

velocity catheter in the ascending aorta has also recently been used in determining instantaneous V_{CF} related to corresponding tension in the ejecting ventricle. Ventricular V_{CE} at peak T correlates well with cardiac function, and V_{CE} values less than 1.30 circumferences per sec. indicate depressed contractility. Although loading dependent and not V_{max}, V_{CE} at peak T is applicable in nonisovolumic contractions and does obviate the need for the SE constant. It has been shown that *mean V_{CF}*, determined angiographically as the relation of extent of internal wall shortening (end-diastolic volume minus end-systolic volume, corrected for end-diastolic volume) to duration of ejection, provides a good correlation with the more difficult calculation of V_{CE} at peak T. Furthermore, V_{CF} determined by echocardiographic measurements of left ventricular endocardial dimensions relates closely to mean V_{CF} calculated by angiographic means.

SUMMARY

The hemodynamic function of the heart as a pump is dependent on the mechanical properties of its myocardium in which the sarcomere is the basic subcellular contractile unit. The contractile apparatus of the sarcomere consists of four protein aggregates: the primary interacting actin and myosin molecular chains and the modulator proteins troponin and tropomyosin, which inhibit actomyosin reaction. Resting sarcomere length controls the extent of myofilament overlap which determines the number of actin-myosin binding sites, the subcellular basis for the Frank-Starling principle. The intensity of interaction between thick and thin filaments regulates contractility.

Excitation throughout the myocardial fiber takes place by the rapid spread of the depolarization wave along the network of sarcolemma cell membrane invaginations constituting the transverse tubular system. Excitation-contraction coupling is achieved by delivery of calcium from the sarcoplasmic reticulum and from outside the cell to troponin. The combination of calcium with troponin activates the contractile process by releasing troponin-tropomyosin inhibition of actin-myosin binding. Contraction occurs by myosin ATPase-regulated cyclic interactions between the actin-myosin linkages with the development of force (dp/dt) and shortening (V_{CE}). ATP energy for operation of the contractile machinery is produced in surrounding mitochondria by oxidative phosphorylation of circulating free fatty acids and glucose.

Concerning translation of the physicochemical mechanisms mediating contraction to mechanical variables, it is envisaged that peak systolic tension measures the number of active actin-myosin binding sites (muscle length) and that peak dp/dt (maximum rate of ventricular pressure rise) and V_{max} (maximum velocity of contractile element shortening) are properties expressing contractility which are related to two different processes: activation rate of actin-myosin binding or activity of sarcotubular calcium transport (peak dp/dt) and interaction rate of actin-myosin binding turnover or activity of myosin ATPase (V_{max}). Abnormalities in sarcotubular and myosin enzymatic activity are currently considered the most likely biochemical defects to account for depressed contractility in the failing myocardium.

Myocardial mechanical properties and contractile state can be assessed in isolated papillary muscle during isometric (length-active tension curve) and isotonic (force-velocity curves) contractions. Concepts developed from study of heart muscle can be extended to the evaluation of the intact ventricle. Cardiac function is normally governed by four determinants: preload (end-diastolic volume), afterload (systolic tension), contractility (inotropic state), and heart rate, to which dyssynergy is included as a fifth factor in certain types of heart disease. Ventricular function and contractility can be assessed in terms of pump (hemodynamics) and muscle (mechanics) performance of the heart. Concerning analysis of myocardial mechanics in the intact heart, contractility can be quantified by isovolumic indices utilizing dp/dt and ejection indices employing V_{CF} (circumferential fiber shortening rate).

When systolic pressure or volume overloading or a primary defect in contractility is imposed upon the heart, there are three principal *compensatory mechanisms* available for the direct support of cardiac function and its fundamental goal of maintaining normal cardiac output at rest: (1) the Frank-Starling principle, (2) ventricular hypertrophy, and (3) the sympathetic nervous system. Deleterious symptoms necessarily accompany the operation of these compensatory mechanisms in their primary role of sustaining basal stroke volume, and these symptoms (dyspnea due to ventricular dilation, angina pectoris resulting from hypertrophy and tachycardia subsequent to adrenergic activity) limit the extent to which the adaptive systems can be employed. In *compensated* heart failure (Classes I, II, and III Cardiac Functional Classification of the New York Heart Association), these reserve mechanisms achieve normal basal cardiac output from the dysfunctioning ventricle at the expense of increased ventricular end-diastolic, pulmonary, and systemic venous pressures. With bodily exertion, further elevations of these pressures occur, with attendant dyspnea and reduced response of cardiac output with fatigue (Class II). In patients with more advanced depression of ventricular performance, there are symptoms of congestion and fatigue even with ordinary physical activity (Class III), although the resting cardiac output may be normal. Finally, *decompensated* congestive heart failure (Class IV) evolves with chronic low cardiac output causing resting fatigue and oliguria, despite maximum use of compensatory mechanisms with resultant persistent congestive symptoms at rest. Thus, in the decompensated failing heart, marked impairment of contractility exceeds the capacity of preload, hypertrophy, and adrenergic protection for supporting basal cardiac output at normal levels. It is pointed out that the standard clinical functional classification of congestive heart failure is more coupled to symptoms consequent to secondary factors (compensatory mechanisms) in this condition rather than to the crucial hemodynamic variable (cardiac output) and the fundamental cause (depressed contractility) of decompensation.*

---

*The authors gratefully acknowledge the secretarial assistance of Barbara Giles and Karen Sime and medical artistry of Kathryn Marr, Celeste Morrison, and Hal Pullum.

REFERENCES

MYOCARDIAL ULTRASTRUCTURE

Braunwald, E.: Control of myocardial oxygen consumption: physiologic and clinical considerations. Amer. J. Cardiol., 27:416, 1971.
Braunwald, E., Chidsey, C. A., Pool, P. E., Sonnenblick, E. H., Ross, J., Jr., Mason, D. T., Spann, J. F., and Covell, J. W.: Congestive heart failure: Biochemical and physiological considerations. Ann. Intern. Med., 64:4, 1966.
Braunwald, E., Ross, J., Jr., and Sonnenblick, E. H.: In Braunwald, E., et al. (Eds.): Mechanisms of Contraction of the Normal and Failing Heart. Boston, Little, Brown and Co., 1967.
Carney, J. A., and Brown, A. L., Jr.: Human cardiac myosin: electron microscopic observations. Circ. Res., 17:336, 1965.
Davies, R. E.: Molecular theory of muscle contraction: calcium-dependent contractions with hydrogen bond formation plus ATP-dependent extensions of part of myosin-actin crossbridges. Nature (London), 199:1068, 1963.
Ebashi, S., and Endo, M.: Calcium ion and muscle contraction. In Butler, J. A. V., and Noble, N. (Eds.): Progress in Biophysics and Molecular Biology. New York, Pergamon Press, 1968, p. 123.
Grant, R. P.: Notes on the muscular architecture of the left ventricle. Circulation, 32:301, 1965.
Hanson, J., and Lowy, J.: Molecular basis of contractility in muscle. Brit. M. Bull., 21:264, 1965.
Haugaard, N., Haugaard, E. S., Lee, N. H., and Horn, R. S.: Possible role of mitochondria in regulation of cardiac contractility. Fed. Proc., 28:1657, 1969.
Huxley, A. F., and Niedergerke, R.: Structural changes in muscle during contraction: interference microscopy of living muscle fibres. Nature (London), 173:971, 1954.
Huxley, H. E.: Structural arrangements and contraction mechanism in striated muscle. Proc. Roy. Soc. London (Biol.), 160:442, 1964.
Katz, A. M.: Contractile proteins of the heart. Physiol. Rev., 50:63, 1970.
Legato, M. J.: The correlation of ultrastructure and function in the mammalian myocardial cell. Prog. Cardiovasc. Dis., 11:391, 1969.
Ross, J., Jr., Sonnenblick, E. H., Taylor, R. R., Spotnitz, H. M., and Covell, J. W.: Diastolic geometry and sarcomere lengths in the chronically dilated canine left ventricle. Circ. Res., 28:49, 1971.
Sarnoff, S. J., Braunwald, E., Welch, G. H., Jr., et al.: Hemodynamic determinants of oxygen consumption of the heart with special reference to the tension-time index. Amer. J. Physiol., 192:148, 1958.
Spiro, D., and Sonnenblick, E. H.: Comparison of the ultrastructural basis of the contractile process in heart and skeletal muscle. Circ. Res., 14(Suppl. 2):14, 1964.
Wilkinson, J. M., Perry, S. V., Cole, H. A., and Trayer, I. P.: The regulatory proteins of the myofibril. Separation and biological activity of the components of inhibitory-factor preparations. Biochem. J., 127:215, 1972.

MYOCARDIAL METABOLISM

Bing, R. J.: Cardiac metabolism. Physiol. Rev., 45:171, 1965.
Brostrom, M. A., Reimann, E. M., Walsh, D. A., and Krebs, E. G.: A cyclic 3',5'-AMP-stimulated protein kinase from cardiac muscle. Advances Enzym. Regulat., 8:191, 1970.
Chidsey, C. A., Braunwald, E., Morrow, A. G., and Mason, D. T.: Myocardial norepinephrine concentration in man: Effects of reserpine and of congestive heart failure. New Eng. J. Med., 269:653, 1963.
Chidsey, C. A., Weinbach, E. C., Pool, P. E., and Morrow, A. G.: Biochemical studies of energy production in the failing human heart. J. Clin. Invest., 45:40, 1966.
Cohen, L. S., Elliott, W. C., Rolett, E. L., and Gorlin, R.: Hemodynamic studies during angina pectoris. Circulation, 31:409, 1965.
Coleman, H. N., Sonnenblick, E. H., and Braunwald, E.: Myocardial oxygen consumption associated with external work: the Fenn effect. Amer. J. Physiol., 217:291, 1969.
Covell, J. W., Braunwald, E., Ross, J., Jr., and Sonnenblick, E. H.: Studies on digitalis. XVI. Effects on myocardial oxygen consumption. J. Clin. Invest., 45:1535, 1966.
Covell, J. W., Chidsey, C. A., and Braunwald, E.: Reduction of the cardiac response to postganglionic sympathetic nerve stimulation in experimental heart failure. Circ. Res., 19:51, 1966.
Epstein, S. E., Skelton, C. L., Levey, G. S., and Entman, M.: Adenyl cyclase and myocardial contractility. Ann. Intern. Med., 72:561, 1970.
Gold, H. J., Prindle, K. H., Jr., Levey, G. S., and Epstein, S.: Effects of experimental heart failure on the capacity of glucagon to augment myocardial contractility and activate adenyl cyclase. J. Clin. Invest., 49:999, 1970.
Helfant, R. H., Forrester, J. S., Hampton, J. R., Haft, J. I., Kemp, H. G., et al.: Differential hemodynamic, metabolic, and electrocardiographic effects in subjects with and without angina pectoris during atrial pacing. Circulation, 42:601, 1970.
Kramer, R. S., Mason, D. T., and Braunwald, E.: Augmented sympathetic neurotransmitter activity in the peripheral vascular bed of patients with congestive heart failure and cardiac norepinephrine depletion. Circulation, 38:629, 1968.
Levey, G. S., and Epstein, S. E.: Activation of adenyl cyclase by glucagon in cat and human heart. Circ. Res., 24:151, 1969.
Levey, G. S., and Epstein, S. E.: Myocardial adenyl cyclase: Activation by thyroid hormones and evidence for two adenyl cyclase systems. J. Clin. Invest., 48:1663, 1969.
Levey, G. S., Palmer, R. F., Lasseter, K. C., and McCarthy, J.: Effect of tolbutamide on adenyl cyclase in rabbit and human heart and contractility of isolated atria. J. Clin. Endocr., 33:371, 1971.
Levitt, M., Spector, S., Sjoerdsma, A., and Udenfriend, S.: Elucidation of the rate-limiting step in norepinephrine biosynthesis in the perfused guinea pig heart. J. Pharmacol. Exp. Ther., 148:1, 1965.

Lindenmayer, G. E., Sordahl, L. A., Harigaya, S., Allen, J. C., Besch, H. R., and Schwartz, A.: Some biochemical studies on subcellular systems isolated from fresh recipient human cardiac tissue obtained during transplantation. Amer. J. Cardiol., 27:277, 1971.

Lindenmayer, G. E., Sordahl, L. A., and Schwartz, A.: Re-evaluation of oxidative phosphorylation in cardiac muscle from normal animals and animals in heart failure. Circ. Res., 23:439, 1968.

Marcus, M. L., Skelton, C. L., Prindle, K. H., Jr., and Epstein, S. E.: Potentiation of the inotropic effects of glucagon by theophylline. J. Pharmacol. Exp. Ther., 179:331, 1971.

Mason, D. T.: Autonomic nervous system and regulation of cardiovascular performance. Anesthesiology, 29:670, 1968.

Mason, D. T., Spann, J. F., Jr., Zelis, R., and Amsterdam, E. A.: Physiologic approach to the treatment of angina pectoris. New Eng. J. Med., 281:1225, 1969.

Meerson, F. Z., Alekhina, G. M., Aleksandrov, P. N., and Bazardjan, A. G.: Dynamics of nucleic acid and protein synthesis of the myocardium in compensatory hyperfunction and hypertrophy of the heart. Amer. J. Cardiol., 22:337, 1968.

Morkin, E., and Ashford, R. P.: Myocardial DNA synthesis in experimental cardiac hypertrophy. Amer. J. Physiol., 215:1409, 1968.

Namm, D. H., and Mayer, S. E.: Effects of epinephrine on cardiac cyclic 3′,5′-AMP, phosphorylase kinase and phosphorylase. Molec. Pharmacol., 4:61, 1968.

Olson, R. E.: Physiology of cardiac muscle. In Hamilton, W. F., and Dow, P. (Eds.): Handbook of Physiology. Vol. I, Section 2. Washington, D.C., American Physiological Society, 1962, p. 199.

Opie, L. M.: Metabolism of the heart in health and disease, Parts 1 to 3. Amer. Heart J., 76:865, 1968; 77:100 and 383, 1969.

Pool, P. E., Covell, J. W., Levitt, M. Gibb, J., and Braunwald, E.: Reduction of cardiac tyrosine hydroxylase activity in experimental congestive heart failure. Circ. Res., 20:349, 1967.

Pool, P. E., Spann, J. F., Jr., and Buccino, R. A.: Myocardial high energy phosphate stores in cardiac hypertrophy and heart failure. Circ. Res., 21:365, 1967.

Rabinowitz, M., Nair, K. G., and Zak, R.: Cellular and subcellular basis of cardiac hypertrophy. Med. Clin. N. Amer., 54:211, 1970.

Rall, T. W., Sutherland, E. W., and Berthet, J.: The relationship of epinephrine and glucagon to liver phosphorylase. IV. Effect of epinephrine and glucagon on the reactivation of phosphorylase in liver homogenates. J. Biol. Chem., 224:463, 1957.

Scheuer, J.: Myocardial metabolism in cardiac hypoxia. Amer. J. Cardiol., 19:385, 1967.

Scheuer, J.: Metabolism of the heart in cardiac failure. Progr. Cardiovasc. Dis., 13:24, 1970.

Scheuer, J., and Brachfeld, N.: Coronary insufficiency: Relations between hemodynamic, electrical and biochemical parameters. Circ. Res., 18:178, 1966.

Sobel, B. E., Henry, P. D., Robison, A., et al.: Depressed adenyl cyclase activity in the failing guinea pig heart. Circ. Res., 24:507, 1969.

Sobel, B. E., Spann, J. F., Jr., Pool, P. E., Sonnenblick, E. H., and Braunwald, E.: Normal oxidative phosphorylation in mitochondria from failing heart. Circ. Res., 21:355, 1967.

Sordahl, L. A., Wood, W. G., Lazarus, M., and Schwartz, A.: Alterations in heart mitochondria during hypertrophy and progressive failure: Increases and decreases in function and structure. Circ. Res., 42:(Suppl. II):51, 1970.

Spann, J. F., Jr., Buccino, R. A., Sonnenblick, E. H., and Braunwald, E.: Contractile state of cardiac muscle obtained from cats with experimentally produced ventricular hypertrophy and heart failure. Circ. Res., 21:341, 1967.

Spann, J. F., Jr., Chidsey, C. A., Pool, P. E., and Braunwald, E.: Mechanism of norepinephrine depletion in experimental heart failure produced by aortic constriction in the guinea pig. Circ. Res., 17:312, 1965.

Spann, J. F., Jr., Sonnenblick, E. H., Cooper, T., Chidsey, C. A., Willman, V. L., and Braunwald, E.: Cardiac norepinephrine stores and the contractile state of heart muscle. Circ. Res., 19:317, 1966.

Vogel, J. H. K., and Chidsey, C. A.: Cardiac adrenergic activity in experimental heart failure assessed with beta receptor blockade. Amer. J. Cardiol., 24:198, 1969.

Vogel, J. H. K., Jacobowitz, D., and Chidsey, C. A.: Distribution of norepinephrine in the failing bovine heart. Circ. Res., 24:71, 1969.

Wikman-Coffelt, J., Zelis, R., Fenner, C., and Mason, D. T.: Myosin chains of myocardial tissue. I. Purification and immunological properties of myosin heavy chains. Biochem. Biophys. Res. Comm., 51:1097, 1973.

EXCITATION-CONTRACTION COUPLING AND THE CONTRACTILE PROCESS

Beeler, G. W., Jr., and Reuter, H.: Membrane calcium current in ventricular myocardial fibers. J. Physiol. (London), 207:191, 1970.

Besch, H. R., Allen, J. C., Glick, G., and Schwartz, A.: Correlation between the inotropic action of ouabain and its effects on subcellular enzyme systems from canine myocardium. J. Pharmacol. Exp. Ther., 171:1, 1970.

Chandler, B. M., Sonnenblick, E. H., Spann, J. F., and Pool, P. E.: Association of depressed myofibrillar adenosine triphosphates and reduced contractility in experimental heart failure. Circ. Res., 21:717, 1967.

Draper, M., Taylor, N., and Alpert, N. R.: Alteration in contractile protein in hypertrophied guinea pig hearts. In Alpert, N. R. (Ed.): Cardiac Hypertrophy. New York, Academic Press, 1971, p. 315.

Fuchs, F., Gertz, E. W., and Briggs, F. N.: The effect of quinidine on calcium accumulation by isolated sarcoplasmic reticulum of skeletal and cardiac muscle. J. Gen. Physiol., 52:955, 1968.

Fuchs, F., Reddy, Y., and Briggs, F. N.: The interaction of cations with the calcium-binding site of troponin. Biochem. Biophys. Acta, 221:407, 1970.

Gertz, E. W., Hess, M. L., Lain, R. F., and Briggs, F. N.: Activity of the vesicular calcium pump in the spontaneously failing heart lung preparation. Circ. Res., 20:477, 1967.

Gordon, M., and Brown, A. L.: Myofibrillar adenosine triphosphate activity of human heart tissue and congestive failure: Effects of ouabain and calcium. Circ. Res., 18:534, 1966.

Harigaya, S., and Schwartz, A.: Rate of calcium binding and uptake in normal animal and failing human cardiac muscle. Circ. Res., 25:781, 1969.

Hoffman, B. F., and Cranefield, P. F.: Physiological basis of cardiac arrhythmias. Amer. J. Med., 37:670, 1964.

Huxley, H. E.: Mechanism of muscular contraction: Recent structural studies suggest a revealing model for cross-bridge action at variable filament spacing. Science, 164:1356, 1969.

Ito, Y., and Chidsey, C. A.: Intracellular calcium and myocardial contractility. IV. Distribution of calcium in the failing heart. J. Molec. Cell. Cardiol., 4:507, 1972.

Katz, A. M., and Brady, A. J.: Mechanical and biochemical correlates of cardiac contraction. Mod. Conc. Cardiovasc. Dis., 40:39, 45; 1971.

Katz, A. M., and Hecht, H. H.: The early "pump" failure of the ischemic heart. Amer. J. Med., 47:497, 1969.

Katz, A., and Tada, M.: The "stone heart": A challenge to the biochemist. Amer. J. Cardiol., 29:578, 1972.

Langer, G. A.: Ion fluxes in cardiac excitation and contraction and their relation to myocardial contractility. Physiol. Rev., 48:708, 1968.

Langer, G. A., and Serena, S. D.: Effects of strophanthidin upon conduction and ionic exchange in rabbit ventricular myocardium: relation to control of active state. J. Molec. Cell. Cardiol., 1:65, 1970.

Luchi, R. J., Kritcher, E. M., and Thyrum, P. T.: Reduced cardiac myosin adenosine triphosphate activity in dogs with spontaneously occurring heart failure. Circ. Res., 24:513, 1969.

Muir, J. R., Dhalla, N. S., Ortega, J. F., and Olson, R. E.: Energy linked calcium transport in subcellular fractions of the failing rat heart. Circ. Res., 26:429, 1970.

Nayler, W. G.: The significance of calcium ions in cardiac excitation and contraction. Amer. Heart J., 65:404, 1963.
Nayler, W. G., and Merrillees, N. C. R.: Cellular exchange of calcium. *In* Harris, P., and Opie, L. H. (Eds.): Calcium and the Heart. New York, Academic Press, 1971, pp. 24–65.
Pool, P. E., Chandler, B. M., Spann, J. F., Jr., Sonnenblick, E. H., and Braunwald, E.: Mechanochemistry of cardiac muscle. IV. Utilization of high-energy phosphates in experimental heart failure in cats. Circ. Res., 24:313, 1969.
Repke, K.: Effect of digitalis on membrane ATPase of cardiac muscle. *In* Drugs and Enzymes. Proceedings of 2nd International Pharmacology Meeting. New York, Pergamon Press, 1965, pp. 65–87.
Sandow, A.: Excitation-contraction coupling in skeletal muscle. Pharmacol. Rev., 17:265, 1965.
Schwartz, A.: Calcium and the sarcoplasmic reticulum. *In* Harris, P., and Opie, L. H. (Eds.): Calcium and the Heart. New York, Academic Press, 1971, pp. 66–92.
Skou, J. C.: Enzymatic basis for active transport of Na^+ across cell membrane. Physiol. Rev., 45:596, 1965.
Sordahl, L. A., Wood, W. G., and Schwartz, A.: Production of cardiac hypertrophy and failure in rabbits with Ameroid clips. J. Molec. Cell. Cardiol., 1:341, 1970.
Suko, J., Vogel, J. H. K., and Chidsey, C. A.: Intracellular calcium and myocardial contractility. III. Reduced calcium uptake and ATPase in the sarcoplasmic reticular fraction prepared from chemically failing calf hearts. Circ. Res., 27:235, 1970.
Sulakhe, P. V., and Dhalla, N. S.: Excitation-contraction coupling in the heart. VII. Calcium accumulation in subcellular particles in congestive heart failure. J. Clin. Invest., 50:1019, 1971.

MYOCARDIAL FUNCTION

Abbott, B. C., and Mommaerts, W. F. H. M.: A study of inotropic mechanisms in the papillary muscle preparation. J. Gen. Physiol., 42:533, 1959.
Agress, C. M., Wegner, S., Forrester, J. S., Chatterjee, K., Parmley, W. W., and Swan, H. J. C.: An Indirect Method for Evaluation of Left Ventricular Function in Acute Myocardial Infarction. Circulation, 46:291, 1972.
Brady, A. J.: The three element model of muscle mechanics: its applicability to cardiac muscle. Physiologist, 10:75, 1967.
Brady, A. J.: Active state in cardiac muscle. Physiol. Rev., 48:570, 1968.
Braunwald, E., and Ross, J., Jr.: The ventricular end-diastolic pressure: appraisal of its value in the recognition of ventricular failure in man. Amer. J. Med., 34:147, 1963.
Braunwald, E., Ross, J., Jr., Gault, J. H., Mason, D. T., Mills, C., Gabe, I. T., and Epstein, S. E.: Assessment of cardiac function. Ann. Intern. Med., 70:369, 1969.
Brutsaert, D. L., Claes, V. A., and Sonnenblick, E. H.: Velocity of shortening of unloaded heart muscle and the length-tension relation. Circ. Res., 29:63, 1971.
Bunnell, I. L., Grant, C., and Greene D. G.: Left ventricular function derived from the pressure-volume diagram. Amer. J. Med., 39:881, 1965.
Burton, A. C.: Importance of shape and size of heart. Amer. Heart J., 54:801, 1957.
Capone, R. J., Mason, D. T., Amsterdam, E. A., and Zelis, R.: The effect of mitral regurgitation and ventricular aneurysm on Vmax calculated from pressure-velocity data during "isovolumic" systole. Circulation, 44(Suppl. II):96, 1971.
Cohen, L. S., Simon, A. L., Whitehouse, W. C., Schuette, W. H., and Braunwald, E.: Heart motion video-tracking (radarkymography) in diagnosis of congenital and acquired heart disease. Amer. J. Cardiol., 22:678, 1968.
Cooley, D. A.: Ischemic contracture of the heart: "Stone heart." Amer. J. Cardiol., 29:575, 1972.
Cooper, R. H., O'Rourke, R. A., Karliner, J. S., Peterson, K. L., and Leopold, G. R.: Comparison of ultrasound and cineangiographic measurements of the mean rate of circumferential fiber shortening in man. Circulation, 46:914, 1972.
Covell, J. W., Ross, J., Jr., Sonnenblick, E. H., and Braunwald, E.: Comparison of the force-velocity relation and the ventricular function curve as measures of the contractile state of the intact heart. Circ. Res., 19:364, 1966.
DeMaria, A., Bonanno, J. A., Amsterdam, E. A., Massumi, R. A., Zelis, R., and Mason, D. T.: Radarkymography. *In* Weissler, A. M. (Ed.): Noninvasive Techniques in Cardiac Evaluation. New York, Grune and Stratton. 1973.
DeMaria, A., Kamiyama, T., Peng, C. L., Mason, D. T., Amsterdam, E. A., Massumi, R. A., and Zelis, R.: Alterations of ventricular function and myocardial contractility indices induced by ventricular asynchrony. Clin. Res., 21:414, 1973.
Diamond, G., Forrester, J. S., Chatterjee, K., Wegner, S., and Swan, H. J. C.: Mean electromechanical dp/dt. An indirect index of the peak rate of rise of left ventricular pressure. Amer. J. Cardiol., 30:338, 1972.
Dodge, H. T., and Baxley, W. A.: Left ventricular volume and mass and their significance in heart disease. Amer. J. Cardiol., 23:528, 1969.
Dodge, H. T., Sandler, H., Baxley, W. A., and Hawley, R. R.: Usefulness and limitations of radiographic methods for determining left ventricular volume. Amer. J. Cardiol., 18:10, 1966.
Falsetti, H. L., Mates, R. E., Greene, D. G., et al.: Vmax as an index of contractile state in man. Circulation, 43:467, 1971.
Forrester, J. S., Diamond, G., Parmley, W. W., and Swan, H. J. C.: Early increase in left ventricular compliance after myocardial infarction. J. Clin. Invest., 51:598, 1972.
Frank, M. J., and Levinson, G. E.: An index of the contractile state of the myocardium in man. J. Clin. Invest., 47:1615, 1968.
Fry, D. L., Griggs, D. M., Jr., and Greenfield, J. C., Jr.: Myocardial mechanics: Tension-velocity-length relations of heart muscle. Circ. Res., 14:73, 1964.
Gaasch, W. H., Battle, W. E., Oboler, A. A., Banas, J. S., Jr., and Levine, H. J.: Left ventricular stress and compliance in man with special reference to normalized ventricular function curves. Circulation, 45:756, 1972.
Gabe, I. T., Gault, J., Ross, J., Jr., Mason, D. T., Mills, C. J., Shillingford, J. P., and Braunwald, E.: Measurement of instantaneous blood flow velocity and pressure in conscious man with a catheter-tip velocity probe. Circulation, 40:603, 1969.
Gault, J. H., Ross, J., Jr., and Braunwald, E.: Contractile state of the left ventricle in man: Instantaneous tension-velocity-length relations in patients with and without disease of the left ventricular myocardium. Circ. Res., 22:451, 1968.
Gleason, W. L., and Braunwald, E.: Studies on the first derivative of the ventricular pressure pulse in man. J. Clin. Invest., 41:80, 1962.
Glick, G., Sonnenblick, E. H., and Braunwald, E: Myocardial force-velocity relations studied in intact unanesthetized man. J. Clin. Invest., 44:978, 1965.
Gordon, A. M., Huxley, A. F., and Julian, F. G.: Variation in isometric tension with sarcomere length in vertebrate muscle fibres. J. Physiol., 184:170, 1966.
Grossman, W., Brooks, H., Meister, S., et al.: New technique for determining instantaneous myocardial force-velocity relation in the intact heart. Circ. Res., 28:290, 1971.
Grossman, W., Hayes, F., Paraskos, J. A., Saltz, S., Dalen, J. E., and Dexter, L.: Alterations in preload and myocardial mechanics in the dog and in man. Circ. Res., 31:83, 1972.
Herman, M. V., and Gorlin, R.: Implications of left ventricular asynergy. Amer. J. Cardiol., 23:538, 1969.
Hill, A. V.: The heat of shortening and the dynamic constants of muscle. Proc. Roy. Soc. London, Series B, 126:136, 1938.
Karliner, J. S., Gault, J. H., Eckberg, D. E., Mullins, C. B., and Ross, J., Jr.: Mean velocity of fiber shortening. A simplified measure of left ventricular myocardial contractility. Circulation, 44:323, 1971.
Kong, Y., Morris, J. J., Jr., and McIntosh, H. D.: Assessment of regional myocardial performance from biplane coronary cineangiograms. Amer. J. Cardiol., 27:529, 1971.
Levine, H. J., and Britman, M. A.: Force-velocity relations in intact dog heart. J. Clin. Invest., 43:1383, 1964.
Levine, H. J., McIntyre, K. M., Lipana, J. G., and Bing, O. H. L.: Force-velocity relations in failing and nonfailing hearts of

subjects with aortic stenosis. Amer. J. Med. Sci., *259*:79, 1970.

Levine, H. J., Neill, W. A., Wagman, R. J., Krasnow, N., and Gorlin, R.: The effect of exercise on mean left ventricular ejection rate in man. J. Clin. Invest. *41*:1050, 1962.

Mason, D. T.: Usefulness and limitations of the rate of rise of intraventricular pressure (dp/dt) in the evaluation of myocardial contractility in man. Amer. J. Cardiol., *23*:516, 1969.

Mason, D. T., and Braunwald, E.: Studies on digitalis. IX. Effects of ouabain on the nonfailing human heart. J. Clin. Invest., *42*:7, 1963.

Mason, D. T., and Braunwald, E.: Hemodynamic techniques in the investigation of cardiovascular function in man. *In* Gordon, B. (Ed.): Clinical Cardiopulmonary Physiology. 3rd ed. New York, Grune and Stratton, 1969, p. 153.

Mason, D. T., Braunwald, E., Covell, J. W., Sonnenblick, E. H., and Ross, L. L.: Assessment of cardiac contractility: The relation between the rate of pressure rise and ventricular pressure during isovolumic systole. Circulation, *44*:47, 1971.

Mason, D. T., Ross, J., Jr., Gault, J. H., Braunwald, E., and Morrow, A. G.: Combined prosthetic replacement of the mitral and aortic valves: Pre- and post-operative hemodynamic studies including left ventricular responses to muscular exercise. Circulation, *35(Suppl. 1)*:15, 1967.

Mason, D. T., Sonnenblick, E. G., Ross, J., Jr., Covell, J. W., and Braunwald, E.: Time to peak dp/dt: A useful measurement for evaluating the contractile state of the human heart. Circulation, *32(Suppl. 2)*:145, 1965.

Mason, D. T., Spann, J. F., Jr., and Zelis, R.: Quantification of the contractile state of the intact human heart. Maximal velocity of contractile element shortening determined by the instantaneous relation between the rate of pressure rise and pressure in the left ventricle during isovolumic systole. Amer. J. Cardiol., *26*:248, 1970.

Mason, D. T., Spann, J. F., Jr., Zelis, R., and Amsterdam, E. A.: Alterations of hemodynamics and myocardial mechanics in patients with congestive heart failure: Pathophysiologic mechanisms and assessment of cardiac function and ventricular contractility. Prog. Cardiovasc. Dis., *12*:507, 1970.

Mason, D. T., Zelis, R., Amsterdam, E. A., and Massumi, R. A.: Clinical determination of left ventricular contractility by hemodynamics and myocardial mechanics. *In* Yu, P. N., and Goodwin, J. F. (Eds.): Progress in Cardiology. Philadelphia, Lea and Febiger, 1972, pp. 121–154.

Mason, D. T., et al.: Comparison of the contractile state of the normal, hypertrophied, and failing heart in man. *In* Alpert, N. R. (Ed.): Ventricular Hypertrophy. New York, Academic Press, 1971, pp. 433–444.

McCullagh, W. H., Covell, J. W., and Ross, J., Jr.: Left ventricular dilatation and diastolic compliance changes during chronic volume overloading. Circulation, *45*:943, 1972.

McDonald, I. G.: Contraction of the hypertrophied left ventricle in man studied by cineradiography of epicardial markers. Amer. J. Cardiol., *30*:587, 1972.

Mehmel, H. C., Krayenbuehl, H. P., and Wirz, P.: Isovolumic contraction dynamics in man according to two different muscle models. J. Appl. Physiol., *33*:409, 1972.

Mirsky, I., Pasternac, A., and Ellison, R. C.: General index for the assessment of cardiac function. Amer. J. Cardiol., *30*:483, 1972.

Mitchell, J. H., Hefner, L. L., and Monroe, R. G.: Performance of the left ventricle. Amer. J. Med., *53*:481, 1972.

Nobel, M. I. M., Bowen, T. E., and Hefner, L. L.: Force-velocity relationship of cat cardiac muscle, studied by isotonic and quick-release techniques. Circ. Res., *24*:821, 1969.

Parmley, W. W., Chuck, L., and Sonnenblick, E. H.: Relation of Vmax to different models of cardiac muscle. Circ. Res., *30*:34, 1972.

Peterson, K. L., Uther, J. B., Shabetai, R., and Braunwald, E.: Instantaneous left ventricular tension-velocity relations obtained with an electromagnetic velocity catheter in the ascending aorta. Clin. Res., *20*:173, 1972.

Pollack, G. H.: Maximum velocity as an index of contractility in cardiac muscle. Circ. Res., *26*:111, 1970.

Rackley, C. E., Behar, V. S., Whalen, R. E., and McIntosh, H. D.: Biplane cineangiographic determinations of left ventricular function: Pressure-volume relationships. Amer. Heart J., *74*:766, 1967.

Rackley, C. E., Dodge, H. T., Coble, Y. D., and Hay, R. E.: A method for determining left ventricular mass in man. Circulation, *29*:666, 1964.

Ross, J., Jr., and Braunwald, E.: The study of left ventricular function in man by increasing resistance to ventricular ejection with angiotensin. Circulation, *29*:739, 1964.

Ross, J., Jr., Covell, J. W., Sonnenblick, E. H., and Braunwald, E.: Contractile state of the heart characterized by force-velocity relations in variably afterloaded and isovolumic beats. Circ. Res., *18*:149, 1966.

Ross, J., Jr., Gault, J. H., Mason, D. T., Linhart, J. W., and Braunwald, E.: Left ventricular performance during muscular exercise in patients with and without cardiac dysfunction. Circulation, *34*:597, 1966.

Ross, J., Jr., and Sobel, B. E.: Regulation of cardiac contraction. *In* Comroe, J. H., Jr. (Ed.): Annual Review of Physiology. *34*:47, 1972.

Russell, R. O., Jr., Frimer, M., Porter, C. M., and Dodge, H. T.: Left ventricular power in heart disease. Amer. J. Cardiol., *23*:136, 1969.

Salel, A. F., Kamiyama, T., Peng, C. L., Mason, D. T., Amsterdam, E. A., Massumi, R. A., and Zelis, R.: Pressure-velocity curves in the evaluation of right ventricular contractility. Circulation, *46(Suppl. 2)*:216, 1972.

Sarnoff, S. J., and Mitchell, J. H.: Control of function of heart. *In* Hamilton, W. F., and Dow, P. (Eds.): Handbook of Physiology. Vol I, Section 2. American Physiological Society, Washington, D.C., 1962, pp. 489–532.

Siegel, J. H., and Sonnenblick, E. H.: Isometric time-tension relationships as an index of myocardial contractility. Circ. Res., *12*:597, 1963.

Skloven, D., Peterson, K., Uther, J., and Ross, J., Jr.: Comparison of isovolumic and ejection phase indices of contractility in man. Circulation, *46(Suppl. 2)*:45, 1972.

Sonnenblick, E. H.: Implications of muscle mechanics in the heart. Fed. Proc., *21*:975, 1962.

Sonnenblick, E. H.: Instantaneous force-velocity-length determinants in the contraction of heart muscle. Circ. Res., *16*:441, 1965.

Sonnenblick, E. H.: Contractility of cardiac muscle. Circ. Res., *27*:479, 1970.

Sonnenblick, E. H., and Downing, S. E.: Afterload as a primary determinant of ventricular performance. Amer. J. Physiol., *204*:604, 1963.

Sonnenblick, E. H., Ross, J., Jr., Spotnitz, H. M., Covell, J. W., and Spiro, D.: The ultrastructure of the heart in systole and diastole: Changes in sarcomere length. Circ. Res., *21*:423, 1967.

Sonnenblick, E. H., Spiro, D., and Cottrell, T. S.: Fine structural changes in heart muscle in relation to length-tension curve. Proc. Nat. Acad. Sci., *49*:193, 1963.

Sonnenblick, E. H., Spiro, D., and Spotnitz, H. M.: Ultrastructural basis of Starling's law of heart: role of sarcomere in determining ventricular size and stroke volume. Amer. Heart J., *68*:336, 1964.

Sonnenblick, E. H., et al.: Ventricular function: evaluation of myocardial contractility in health and disease. Progr. Cardiovasc. Dis., *12*:449, 1970.

Spann, J. F., Mason, D. T., and Zelis, R.: Recent advances in the understanding of congestive heart failure. Mod. Conc. Cardiovasc. Dis., *39*:73, 79; 1970.

Taylor, R. R., Ross, J., Jr., Covell, J. W., and Sonnenblick, E. H.: A quantitative analysis of left ventricular myocardial function in the intact, sedated dog. Circ. Res., *21*:99, 1967.

Urschel, C. W., Covell, J. W., Sonnenblick, E. H., Ross, J., Jr., and Braunwald, E.: Myocardial mechanics in aortic and mitral valvular regurgitation: the concept of instantaneous impedance as a determinant of the performance of the intact heart. J. Clin. Invest., *47*:867, 1968.

Urschel, C. W., Henderson, A. H., and Sonnenblick, E. H.: Model dependency of ventricular force-velocity relations: importance of developed pressure. Fed. Proc., *29*:719, 1970.

Veragut, U. P., and Krayenbuhl, H. P.: Estimation and quantification of myocardial contractility in the closed-chest dog. Cardiologia, *47*:96, 1965.

Wallace, A. G., Skinner, N. S., Jr., and Mitchell, J. H.: Hemodynamic determinants of the maximal rate of rise of left ventricular pressure. Amer. J. Physiol., *205*:30, 1963.

Wolk, M. H., Keefe, J. F., Bing, O. H. L., Finkelstein, L. J., and Levine, H. J.: Estimation of Vmax in auxotonic systoles from the rate of relative increase of isovolumic pressure: (dP/dt)KP. J. Clin. Invest., *50*:1276, 1971.

Yeatman, L. A., Jr., Parmley, W. W., and Sonnenblick, E. H.: Effects of temperature on series elasticity and contractile element motion in heart muscle. Amer. J. Physiol., *217*:1030, 1969.

Yeatman, L. A., Jr., Parmley, W. W., Urschel, C. W., and Sonnenblick, E. H.: Dynamics of contractile elements in isometric contractions of cardiac muscle. Amer. J. Physiol., *220*:534, 1971.

Zelis, R., Amsterdam, E. A., and Mason, D. T.: "Isometric" Vmax as an index of contractility independent of series elastic and fiber shortening: Implications concerning pressure-velocity data in myocardial fibrosis, valvular regurgitation, ventricular aneurysm and ventricular septal defect. Circulation, *44(Suppl. II)*:89, 1971.

Zelis, R., Salel, A. F., Capone, R. J., DeMaria, A., Choquet, Y., Amsterdam, E. A., and Mason, D. T.: Evaluation of muscle function in the human myocardium by contractility measurements: Coronary artery disease. *In* Proceedings of International Symposium on Chronic Diseases of the Heart. Freiburg, Germany, October, 1972 (in press).

CHAPTER 9

CARDIAC OUTPUT, CARDIAC PERFORMANCE, HYPERTROPHY, DILATATION, VALVULAR DISEASE, ISCHEMIC HEART DISEASE, AND PERICARDIAL DISEASE

HAROLD T. DODGE
J. WARD KENNEDY

CARDIAC OUTPUT

The measurement of cardiac output by what is now known as the Fick principle was first applied in animals at the end of the last century. Since this method requires sampling of mixed venous blood from the pulmonary artery or right ventricle, its application to man followed the development of right heart catheterization in the 1940s. The indicator dilution method for determining cardiac output was developed by Stewart in 1897 and by Hamilton in 1929 and became widely applied in the 1950s. Both the direct Fick and indicator dilution methods have become standard techniques in cardiac catheterization laboratories and have recently been brought into limited use in intensive and coronary care units for the serial measurement of cardiac output during the course of severe illness. More recently, the development of sensitive thermistor probes has allowed modification of the indicator dilution method to the thermo-dilution method, in which warm or cool saline instead of a dye is used as an indicator. The development and wide application of angiocardiography have provided another method for measurement of the output of the heart by analysis of the change in volume (stroke volume) of the left ventricle during the cardiac cycle. Quantitative angiocardiographic methods for measuring left ventricular stroke volume and minute output are particularly useful in evaluating heart ventricular performance in patients with heart disease, as will be discussed later.

In addition to the above methods for directly measuring cardiac output in man there have also been many methods devised to estimate cardiac output indirectly. These include analysis of arterial pulse waves; the ballistocardiogram; systolic time intervals using electrocardiographic, phonocardiographic, and carotid pulse wave data; ultrasonic echocardiography; and, most recently, the development and application of instruments for measuring blood flow velocity with ultrasound by the Doppler shift principle. Although some of these methods are useful in predicting directional changes in cardiac output during the course of illness, they all appear to be less accurate than the direct Fick and indicator dilution methods.

Fick Method

This method depends upon a knowledge of the quantity of oxygen entering the system measured as the oxygen consumption as determined from samples of expired air and the difference in oxygen content between venous and arterial blood. Since venous blood from different parts of the body has a variable oxygen content, it must be mixed to obtain a sample that represents total body venous oxygen content. Such a mixing does not occur in the right atrium; however, when blood passes through the right ventricle, adequate mixing occurs. Blood for Fick cardiac output determination is therefore sampled from the pulmonary artery through a right heart catheter. Occasionally, a right ventricular sampling site is utilized when the pulmonary artery cannot be entered. The arterial sample may be obtained from any convenient peripheral artery in the absence of a right-to-left cardiac shunt. When a shunt is present, the sample must be obtained upstream from the shunt.

The formula for determining cardiac output (CO) is as follows:

$$\text{Cardiac output} = \frac{\text{Oxygen Consumption}}{\text{Arteriovenous oxygen difference}}$$

A typical value for oxygen consumption in an average-sized adult male at rest is 240 ml. per min. The normal resting arteriovenous oxygen difference is in the range of 40 ml. of O_2 per liter of blood. Substituting into the formula,

$$CO = \frac{240}{40} = 6.0 \text{ L./minute}$$

Errors in the measurement of oxygen consumption and oxygen content of arterial and venous blood result in a total error of the method of 8 to 10 per cent. In applying the method, the chief limitations are the necessity of pulmonary artery catheterization and the cooperation of the patient to obtain a representative sample of expired air that can be used for measuring oxygen consumption.

Indicator Dilution Method

The indicator dilution technique is more often used than the direct Fick method because right heart catheterization is not required. A known quantity of indicator (I) is injected into the venous circulation and the resultant time-concentration curve (Ct) is determined by continuous withdrawal of arterial blood through a densitometer, or through frequent sampling at known time intervals.

$$\text{Cardiac output} = \frac{I}{\overline{C} \cdot t}$$

$\overline{C}$ represents the mean concentration of the indicator during the time (t) from the appearance to disappearance of the indicator and is determined from the time-concentration curve. The validity of the method depends on two assumptions: (1) that there is complete mixing of indicator prior to sampling and (2) that the indicator concentration curve with respect to time represents only the first passage of the indicator past the sampling site. Since early recirculation of indicator distorts the terminal portion of the primary curve to a greater or lesser extent, depending upon the injection and sampling sites and the status of circulatory dynamics, various methods have been developed to separate the primary curve from the recirculation curve. These methods are based on the assumption that the fall of concentration in the primary curve follows an exponential time course that can be determined by relating the logarithm of the concentration to time. The time-concentration curve is plotted on a semilogarithmic graph, and the initial position of the primary curve is identified and then extrapolated as a straight line to avoid recirculation and to define the entire primary indicator dilution curve. An adequate portion of the primary curve must be obtained to permit the extrapolation. From the primary curve, values for (C) and (t) are determined. Small special-purpose computers are now available to separate the primary and recirculation curves and give immediate cardiac output results.

The thermo-dilution technique is similar to the indicator dilution technique described above but has the advantage of no significant recirculation, since the temperature difference of the injectate is lost into the tissue prior to recirculation. In general, there is good agreement between the results of the Fick, indicator dilution, and thermo-dilution methods for determining cardiac output in man.

Normal Cardiac Output

Since the cardiac output is a fundamental measurement of cardiac function, it has been the subject of extensive study in normal animals and man, at rest and during various stresses and in patients with all types of heart diseases. This subject is well reviewed in the monograph by Wade and Bishop (1962). Cardiac output is best expressed in terms of body size, and, in general, body surface area is used instead of body weight. The term cardiac index is used to refer to the cardiac output per square meter of body surface area. It is frequently convenient to express the output of the heart per beat as stroke volume or the cardiac index per beat as stroke index. The resting cardiac index in normal man is approximately 3.3 L. per min. per $M.^2$, with a low value of about 2.8 L. per min. per $M.^2$ The upper limit of normal is more difficult to define because anxiety increases the cardiac output. Cardiac output decreases with age at the rate of approximately 25 ml. per min. per $M.^2$ per year after early adulthood. Assuming a resting heart rate of 70 beats per minute, the normal stroke index is 46 ml. per beat for an adult of average size.

Regulation of Cardiac Output

The cardiac output normally increases under the stimulus of muscular exercise up to five times the resting value, depending somewhat upon the age and physical training of the individual. There are many factors which make possible such large changes of flow, some of which will be described below.

The return of venous blood to the right heart is regulated in such a manner that the venous return essentially equals the systemic output of the left ventricle. Venous return to a great extent is regulated by alterations in the tone of the venous capacitance vessels which contain most of the blood volume. Increases or decreases in venous tone therefore have a marked effect on the filling of the right atrium and ventricle and thereby on the output of the left ventricle. Increases or decreases of circulating blood volume also cause respective changes of venous return and cardiac output if not compensated for by changes of venous tone. Cardiac output may increase for a short time with increases in blood volume as occurs with overtransfusion, but compensatory increased volume of venous capacitance vessels soon reduces the right ventricular filling volume, pressure, and output. In patients with chronic heart failure, circulating blood volume is chronically increased owing to retention of sodium and water by the kidneys, and venous tone is increased. As a result, an increased volume of blood is present in the central circulation which elevates the filling volume and pressure of the two ventricles to maintain cardiac output through the Frank-Starling mechanism. Accordingly, venous return is a major factor in the control of cardiac output in both health and disease and is determined by the blood volume and the capacity and tone of the venous bed.

Autonomic Control of Cardiac Output

The autonomic nervous system has a major controlling influence on cardiac output by its effect upon heart rate, myocardial contractility, and vasomotor tone. In general, parasympathetic tone is greater than sympathetic tone when an individual is at rest. Maximal stimuli to sympathetic tone occur during heavy exercise, and tachycardia results. Increased parasympathetic tone as occurs with vigorous carotid sinus massage results in marked cardiac slowing or even cardiac arrest and a marked decrease in the vigor of atrial contraction. Sympathetic nerve stimulation has a considerable positive effect on myocardial contractility, causing increased force, extent, and velocity of myocardial fiber shortening, and results in an increased stroke volume, provided that venous return is adequate to maintain an elevated stroke volume and cardiac output. In contrast to this, increased parasympathetic tone probably has little or no effect on contractility of the ventricles. Peripheral vasculature tone increases with sympathetic stimulation and this results in increased venous return to the right heart, increased ventricular filling pressure, and increased stroke volume. The effects of increased sympathetic tone—i.e., increased heart rate, increased myocardial contractility, and increased venous return—all combine to increase cardiac output.

Peripheral Oxygen Requirement

In general, cardiac output varies according to the requirement of the peripheral tissues for oxygen. Control of regional circulation is maintained so that cardiac output is shunted to the particular organ in need of oxygen. For example, during physical exertion blood flow is preferentially increased to the working muscles and reduced to the splanchnic bed and kidneys. When there is a marked reduction in cardiac output, as in some patients with heart failure, there is reduced blood flow to the skin, muscle, and splanchnic vascular beds. As the cardiac output

Therapeutic Control of Cardiac Output

In situations of high or low cardiac output due to disease, the physician often attempts to control the cardiac output with drugs or by other maneuvers. In several different circumstances, cardiac output is abnormally high as in febrile patients, conditions of increased metabolism such as thyrotoxicosis, arteriovenous shunts, severe anemia, or ineffective oxygen carrying capacity of hemoglobin as in carbon monoxide poisoning. In all these conditions, cardiac output returns toward normal with correction of the abnormality that accounts for the elevated output.

In conditions of abnormally low cardiac output, the physician often is faced with a more difficult problem. Low cardiac output due to inadequate venous return as a result of inadequate blood volume is easily treated with transfusion or fluid replacement. Low cardiac output due to bradycardia may be successfully treated with drugs or an artificial pacemaker. When cardiac output is inadequate due to poor myocardial contraction, sympathomimetic drugs or digitalis glycosides may be used to increase myocardial contractile force. At times, venous filling pressure may be artificially elevated above normal levels by the administration of saline or plasma in an attempt to increase cardiac output. Unfortunately, the depressed cardiac output such as occurs in advanced myocardial failure often remains low in spite of current therapeutic methods.

Vascular Resistance

The peripheral vasculature of the systemic circulation, and to a lesser extent of the pulmonary circulation, is under autonomic nervous system and hormonal control. The vascular resistance, therefore, will vary depending upon the hemodynamic state of the patient. Systemic vascular resistance becomes chronically elevated in idiopathic or renal vascular hypertension. In chronic mitral stenosis, pulmonary vascular resistance is chronically elevated. It is frequently important to determine the systemic and pulmonary vascular resistance.

The resistance of a vascular bed can be calculated if the flow and pressure drop across the bed are known. For these calculations, mean pressures are utilized and the values are reported in dynes-second centimeters^{-5} (dsc.$^{-5}$). In order to calculate resistance in dsc.$^{-5}$, pressure measured in mm. Hg must be converted into dynes per cm.^{2} by multiplying by 1332. Liters per minute are converted to ml. per sec. by multiplying further by 0.06, yielding a conversion factor of 80.

Therefore:

$$\text{Resistance in dsc}^{-5} = \frac{\text{Mean pressure (mm. Hg)} \times 80}{\text{Flow (L./min.)}}$$

Systemic vascular resistance (SVR) is calculated as follows:

$$\text{SVR} = \frac{\text{Mean arterial pressure} \times 80}{\text{Cardiac output (L./min.)}}$$

Total pulmonary artery resistance is calculated in a similar manner. In some instances it is useful also to measure the pulmonary vascular resistance (PVR) in order to separate out the components of total pulmonary resistance which results from the pulmonary vasculature from that component resulting from left atrial pressure. This is, of course, most useful in evaluating patients with left atrial hypertension such as occurs with mitral stenosis or left ventricular failure. Pulmonary vascular resistance is determined by using the pulmonary flow and the difference between the mean pulmonary artery (Pa mean) and mean left atrial pressure (LA mean).

$$\text{PVR} = \frac{(\text{Pa mean} - \text{LA mean}) \times 80}{\text{Pulmonary flow (L./min.)}}$$

Normal values for systemic, total pulmonary, and pulmonary vascular resistance are listed in Table 9-1 as reported by Barratt-Boyes (1958). As is apparent from these values, total pulmonary resistance is mostly the result of left atrial pressure, not resistance in the pulmonary vasculature. In other words, about two thirds of right heart pressure work goes into filling the left heart under normal resting conditions.

TABLE 9-1 NORMAL VALUES — INTRACARDIAC PRESSURES

	Systolic	Diastolic	Mean
Right Atrium	3–7	0–2	0–6
Right Ventricle	15–30	0–5	—
Pulmonary Artery	15–30	6–12	9–17
Left Atrium	—	—	5–12
Left Ventricle	100–140	2–12	—
Vascular Resistance			
Systemic	1130±178 dsc.^{5}		
Total Pulmonary	205± 51 dsc.^{5}		
Pulmonary Vascular	67± 23 dsc.^{5}		

Adapted from data in Barratt-Boyes, B. G., and Wood, E. H.: J. Lab. Clin. Med., *51*:72, 1958.

CARDIAC CATHETERIZATION

The technique of cardiac catheterization merits brief mention in a text of pathologic physiology because much of what is known of altered cardiac function in various disease states has been gained through the use of this technique. Cardiac catheterization was first carried out by Forssmann in 1929 when he passed a catheter into his own right atrium. Although occasional cardiac catheterization procedures were attempted in the 1930s, it was André Cournand and colleagues who introduced the important technique for the study of normal and pathologic physiology. Today, all chambers of the heart and much of the venous and arterial vasculature are regularly catheterized for purposes of blood sampling, pressure recording, and the injection of radiographic contrast material for angiographic visualization. The usual sites of catheter insertion include the veins of the antecubital fossa, the femoral vein, and the brachial and femoral arteries. Large vessels may be entered safely with the percutaneous Seldinger technique. This method involves needle puncture of the vessel with insertion of a flexible guide wire over which the catheter is inserted. When smaller vessels are entered, a small incision with isolation of the vessel for cannulation is required. Cardiac catheterization of the right heart, left heart, and coronary arteries has been shown to be of minimal risk in very ill patients.

Intracardiac Pressure Recordings

Recording pressure in the various chambers of the heart and the great vessels is often a major goal of cardiac catheterization. This is usually accomplished by attaching a fluid-filled catheter to a pressure transducer. The electrical output of the transducer is amplified and displayed on an oscilloscope and recorded on paper or magnetic tape. The system is carefully calibrated and the zero level of the transducers is set at the level of the midthorax. Normal pressures for the various cardiac chambers are given in Table 9–1. At times, it is more convenient to limit catheterization to the right side of the heart. When this is the case, an estimate of pulmonary venous pressure and left atrial pressure can be obtained by passing an end-hole catheter out into a terminal pulmonary artery. When "wedged" in this position, the catheter records the pressure transmitted back across the pulmonary capillary bed from the pulmonary veins. This pressure is termed the pulmonary wedge or pulmonary capillary pressure. The mean pulmonary wedge pressure will generally be within 2 mm. Hg of the mean left atrial pressure, unless pulmonary venous obstruction is present.

In the last several years, various types of catheters have been developed which contain a pressure transducer at the distal end of the catheter. These catheter tip manometers are capable of recording pressures more accurately in the heart because they are free from the hydraulic damping effects, time delays, and catheter motion artifacts which distort pressures recorded through standard fluid-filled catheters. These improved pressure recording systems have allowed the detailed analysis of the rapid pressure changes which occur in the right and left ventricle during early systole and early diastole. The maximum rate of rise of the left ventricular pressure generally referred to as LV dp/dt has been used as an index of left ventricular myocardial performance. Catheter tip manometers make it possible to record LV dp/dt with sufficient accuracy to permit their use for evaluating myocardial contractility in man. Multiple variables influence the LV dp/dt, including heart rate, filling pressure (preload), aortic diastolic pressure (afterload), myocardial inotropic state, and left ventricular diastolic volume. Because of these many influences, LV dp/dt is more useful in evaluating changes of myocardial performance in a single patient than in comparing the myocardial performance in one patient with that of another.

Various types of valvular abnormalities due to congenital and rheumatic heart disease can now be treated surgically, so that it has become important to evaluate precisely the severity of valve stenosis or incompetence or both. Congenital aortic, pulmonary, and postrheumatic mitral and aortic valve stenosis are the most common types of valvular stenosis, although the other cardiac valves may become stenotic on either a congenital or rheumatic basis. Cardiac catheterization is required to measure the pressure on each side of a stenotic valve, so that the pressure gradient across the valve can be determined. Figure 9–1 is taken from the simultaneous recording of left ventricular and aortic pressure in a patient with aortic stenosis. The high-fidelity left ventricular pressure was obtained with a catheter tip manometer. The shaded area represents the gradient across the stenotic aortic valve. The mean gradient can be obtained by dividing the shaded area by the duration of the valve gradient. Figure 9–2 is taken from simultaneous pressure recordings in the left atrium and left ventricle in a patient with mitral stenosis. The left ventricular pressure was recorded through a fluid-filled catheter and there is some oscillation in the pressure during diastole, indicating an underdamped pressure manometer system. The diastolic gradient across the mitral valve is represented by the shaded area. In these two examples, large pressure gra-

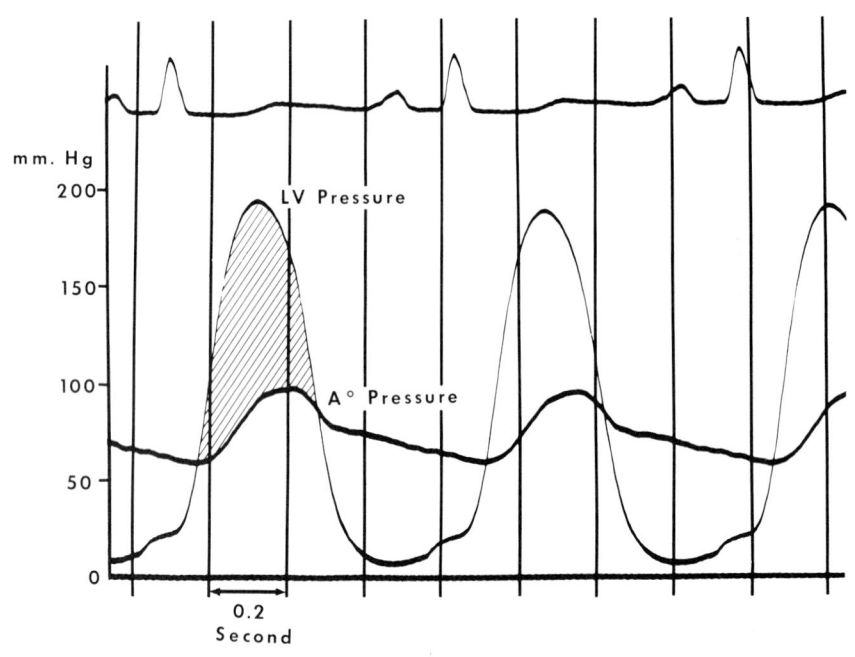

Figure 9-1 Left ventricular and central aortic pressure in a patient with tight valvular aortic stenosis. The shaded area indicates the pressure gradient across the valve during systole.

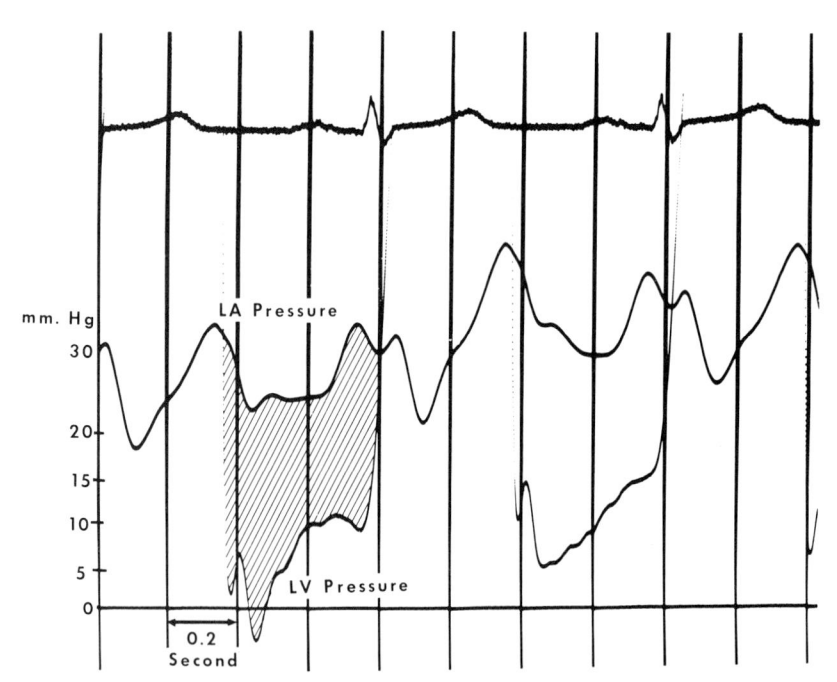

Figure 9-2 Left ventricular and left atrial pressure in a patient with mitral stenosis. Only the lower portion of the left ventricular pressure is seen. The shaded area indicates the pressure gradient across the mitral valve during diastole.

dients are present across these stenotic valves, but since the pressure gradient is a function of both valve orifice size and flow across the valve, the severity of valvular stenosis is best determined by calculation of the cross-sectional area of the valve. This can be done by utilizing the formulas developed by Gorlin and Gorlin. These formulas relate the gradient in pressure across the valve during the period of valve flow and rate of flow across the valve to the area of the valve orifice. Empirical correction factors have been introduced based upon surgical and postmortem observations.

The basic formula is as follows:

$$\text{Valve orifice} = \frac{\text{Valve flow}}{(K) \sqrt{\text{Pressure gradient}}}$$

In the case of the mitral valve the valve flow is measured per diastolic second, whereas when calculating the area of the aortic valve orifice the flow is determined per systolic second. The pressure gradient is the mean difference in pressure across the valve during diastolic filling for mitral stenosis and systolic ejection for aortic stenosis. The K values are 31.0 and 44.5 for the mitral and aortic valves respectively. When there is no valvular incompetence or intracardiac shunt, the flow across the valve is equal to the cardiac output. When valvular incompetence is also present, the flow across the valve is increased and must be taken into account if an accurate valve area is to be obtained. Usually the mitral valve orifice is constricted to less than 1.2 cm.^{2} or the aortic valve to less than 1.0 cm.^{2} before symptoms develop that are significant enough to indicate surgical correction.

Intracardiac Shunts

Cardiac catheterization techniques are used to locate and quantify intracardiac shunts. This is generally done by determining the oxygen content of blood samples from the appropriate cardiac chambers and great vessels. Frequently, the cardiac catheter will pass through the intracardiac defect or abnormal venous or arterial channel directly demonstrating its presence. The introduction of a dye, radiopaque contrast media, or hydrogen gas may also be used to detect or demonstrate abnormal blood flow. The Fick principle or an indicator dilution technique is applied to determine the magnitude of abnormal blood flow.

Left-to-Right Shunts

Abnormal shunting of blood occurs most commonly from the systemic to the venous circulation and is identified by demonstrating oxygenated blood entering the venous circulation. Conditions in which this occurs include patent ductus arteriosus; aorticopulmonary window; atrial septal defect; ventricular septal defect; and anomalous pulmonary venous drainage to the vena cava, coronary sinus, or right atrium. Occasionally, left-to-right shunts may develop following birth, as with the rupture of a sinus of Valsalva aneurysm into the right heart, or the development of a ventricular septal defect following infarction of the interventricular septum. Arteriovenous fistulae may be congenital or acquired and result in a functional arteriovenous shunting of blood.

In general, these defects are easy to recognize at cardiac catheterization by sampling blood from the appropriate sites on the right side of the heart. An increase in oxygen saturation or content occurs at the level of the shunt, thus localizing it anatomically. By comparing the oxygen content of mixed venous blood before and beyond the level of the shunt, the volume of the shunt can be calculated utilizing the Fick principle. As shown below, these formulas yield a value for systemic blood flow and pulmonary blood flow. The difference between the two is the shunt flow. The ratio of pulmonary to systemic flow is often used to express the severity of the shunt. For example, if the pulmonary flow is 10 L. per min. and the systemic flow is 5 L. per min., the magnitude of the shunt would be 2:1.

In the case of a ventricular septal defect and in the absence of right-to-left shunting, for example,

$$\text{Pulmonary blood flow} = \frac{O_2 \text{ consumption (ml./min.)}}{\text{Systemic arterial } O_2 \text{ content} - \text{Pulmonary arterial } O_2 \text{ content}}$$

$$\text{Systemic blood flow} = \frac{O_2 \text{ consumption (ml./min.)}}{\text{Systemic arterial } O_2 \text{ content} - \text{Right atrial } O_2 \text{ content}}$$

Left-to-right shunt flow = Pulmonary blood flow − Systemic blood flow

In the case of an atrial septal defect, the mixed venous O_2 content needs to be obtained from samples taken in the inferior and superior venae cavae. In this situation,

$$\text{Mixed venous } O_2 \text{ content} = \frac{\text{SVC } O_2 + 2 \text{ IVC } O_2}{3}$$

The 2:1 ratio is employed because of the large blood flow in the IVC relative to that in the SVC. In resting subjects the oxygen content of IVC blood is higher than that of SVC samples because of the contribution of renal venous blood which has a relatively high oxygen content.

Cyanotic Heart Disease

The term cyanotic heart disease is used to refer to patients with systemic arterial oxygen desaturation due to a cardiovascular abnormality. Cyanosis is generally the result of the shunting of systemic venous blood into the systemic arterial circulation and occurs in such conditions as tetralogy of Fallot, single ventricle, truncus arteriosus, tricuspid atresia, and transposition of the great vessels.

For right-to-left shunting to occur across a patent ductus, ventricular septal defect, or atrial septal defect, the pressure on the right side of the defect must be higher than on the left side at least at some time during the cardiac cycle and may occur only during physical activity. Cyanosis, for example, may be noted only after exertion. Right-to-left shunting occurs across a patent ductus either because it is located distal to a coarctation of the aorta or because of the presence of pulmonary hypertension of such severity that the total pulmonary resistance is greater than the systemic resistance. In this situation, there may be differential cyanosis, with cyanosis greater in the lower extremities. When right-to-left shunting occurs in patients with ventricular septal defect it is associated with either pulmonary hypertension due to increased pulmonary vascular resistance or pulmonary stenosis of the valvular or infundibular type. Pulmonary stenosis and ventricular septal defect are most often seen as features of the tetralogy of Fallot, the other two features being right ventricular hypertrophy and dextro location of the aorta with overriding of the interventricular septum, so that the aorta communicates more or less directly with the right ventricular outflow tract. Atrial septal defect is less often associated with a right-to-left shunt. When this occurs, pulmonary hypertension has resulted in right ventricular failure and elevation of right atrial pressure to a level higher than the pressure in the left atrium. In the combination of atrial septal defect and tricuspid stenosis, right-to-left shunting at the atrial level will occur without pulmonary stenosis or right ventricular failure.

The calculation of right-to-left shunt is similar to the calculation of left-to-right shunts except that pulmonary venous blood must be either sampled or assumed to be 98 per cent saturated. If the patient is breathing oxygen, it can be assumed that the sample is fully saturated. Pulmonary blood flow (PBF) is then determined by the following formula:

$$\text{PBF} = \frac{O_2 \text{ consumption}}{\text{Pulmonary venous } O_2 - \text{Pulmonary artery } O_2}$$

The systemic flow is calculated as follows:

$$\text{SF} = \frac{O_2 \text{ consumption}}{\text{Systemic arterial } O_2 - \text{Mixed venous } O_2}$$

The mixed venous O_2 should be obtained proximal to the shunt, since a bidirectional shunt may be present. The magnitude of right-to-left shunt is determined by subtracting the pulmonary blood flow from the systemic blood flow. When a bidirectional shunt is present, the effective pulmonary blood flow (Eff Pul BF) must be determined. This is the quantity of blood which picks up oxygen while circulating through the lungs and is determined by the following formula:

$$\text{Eff Pul BF} = \frac{O_2 \text{ consumption}}{\text{Pulmonary venous } O_2 - \text{Mixed venous } O_2}$$

A bidirectional shunt may then be calculated as follows:

Right-to-left shunt =
  Systemic flow − Effective pulmonary flow

Left-to-right shunt =
  Pulmonary flow − Effective pulmonary flow

The validity of flow values determined by these methods depends upon rapid and accurate sampling of blood in the various cardiac chambers and vessels concerned. Blood entering the right atrium from the superior vena cava, inferior vena cava, and coronary sinus varies considerably in its O_2 content. The inferior vena cava blood has a high O_2 content owing to a large component of renal venous blood, whereas the blood draining the coronary circulation has a very low O_2 content. The atrium does not mix the blood well, so that blood flows in a laminar fashion through the atrium and into the right ventricle. Better mixing occurs here, so that the blood entering the pulmonary artery is usually relatively homogeneous. The nonmixing of blood in the right atrium and vena cava results in the possibility of sampling errors and in resultant inaccurate shunt flow calculations. Rapid sampling and duplicate measurements can, however, give good estimates of flow which are of value in the clinical evaluation of patients.

Frequently, a left-to-right shunt is associated with pulmonary hypertension. When the pulmonary vascular resistance reaches systemic levels, right-to-left shunting develops and surgical correction of the defect becomes hazardous, if not impossible. In the presence of pulmonary hypertension due to cardiac shunts, great care must be taken in calculating blood flow and pulmonary artery pressure so that accurate pulmonary resistance values can be obtained. In borderline cases it may be useful to measure pulmonary flow and pressure before and during oxygen administration. If pulmonary vascular resistance falls with oxygen administration, surgical correction may be possible, whereas failure of a drop in pulmonary artery pressure suggests that pulmonary vascular resistance is fixed and not due in part to anoxia.

LEFT VENTRICULAR VOLUME AND MASS

There are two generally used methods of determining left ventricular chamber volumes in man: (1) indicator dilution and (2) angiocardiography. With the indicator dilution methods, an indicator is injected into the left ventricle and sampled immediately above the aortic valves with a sensor which responds rapidly to changes in the concentration of the indicator. The indicator dilution curves show a steplike decrease in indicator concentration, with the change of concentration per beat being a function of the volume of the left ventricle at end systole and the dilution with each stroke (stroke volume). End-diastolic volume (EDV) is computed as follows:

$$\text{EDV} = \frac{\text{Stroke volume}}{\left(1 - \dfrac{Cn}{Cn-1}\right)}$$

where stroke volume is determined by the standard indicator dilution method for measuring cardiac output and $\dfrac{Cn}{Cn-1}$ is the ratio of beat-to-beat changes of concentration of indicator in the aorta. The accuracy of the volume determination is dependent on complete mixing of indicator in the left ventricle, a concentration of dye in the aorta which is equivalent to that in the ventricle, and a sufficiently high-frequency response of the system for indicator detection to determine accurately indicator concentration and ventricular washout as a step function. Various indicators have been used and include dyes, saline, and cold saline with appropriate indicator detection systems. These methods have the advantage of requiring but a small volume of indicator which does not in itself cause physiologic changes, and measurements can be repeated frequently. In general, the indicator dilution methods have given larger end-diastolic and residual volumes than the angiocardiographic methods which may be related to uneven mixing of the indicator.

Left ventricular chamber volumes can also be determined from angiocardiograms and cineangiocardiograms taken in biplane as well as single plane projections (Fig. 9–3). The methods most generally used assume that the left ven-

Figure 9–3 Angiocardiogram with the left ventricle and a segment of left ventricular wall outlined. Wall thickness is indicated by *h* and semidiameter by *b*. (From Dodge, H. T.: Determination of left ventricular mass. Radiol. Clin. N. Amer., 9:459, 1971.)

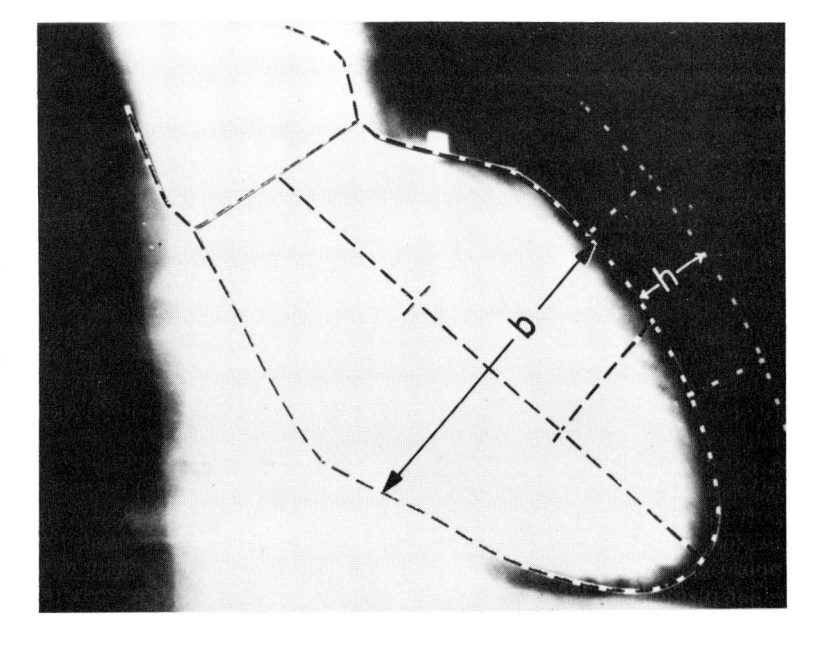

tricle can be represented by an ellipsoid reference figure, with volume computed as

$$V = 4/3 \pi abc$$

where a equals the major semidiameter and b and c equal the two minor semidiameters. The differences in methods used for computing volume by various laboratories are due to differences in the methods applied for determining the chamber dimensions. It has been demonstrated that in most subjects the two minor semidiameters (b and c) are similar. Accordingly, chamber volume can be computed from films taken in a single projection by assuming that b and c are equal, and the formula for computing volume becomes

$$V = 4/3 \pi ab^2$$

When the time of filming is recorded together with the electrocardiogram and left ventricular pressure, as shown in Figure 9–4, the computed volumes can be related to time within the cardiac cycle to construct a left ventricular volume curve as shown in Figure 9–5. From this volume curve, end-diastolic, end-systolic, and stroke volumes can be determined. The portion of the end-diastolic volume ejected with systole $\left(\frac{SV}{EDV}\right)$ has been termed systolic ejection fraction. From the slopes of the ejection and filling limbs, the rates of ventricular ejection and filling respectively can be computed. In addition, the angiocardiographic methods provide information on ventricular shape and dimensions, permit visualization of focal contraction abnormalities as seen in ischemic heart disease, and also provide information on wall thickness. When added to chamber dimensions, the latter has made it possible to compute left ventricular mass as follows:

Vol. LV chamber + Wall =
$$4/3\pi (a + h)(b + h)(c + h)$$

LV mass (g.) = [(Vol. chamber + wall) − Vol. chamber] 1.050

where a, b, and c equal chamber semidiameters as previously defined, h equals wall thickness, and 1.050 is the specific gravity of heart muscle. Normal values for left ventricular chamber volumes, ejection fraction, wall thickness, and mass are given in Table 9–2.

LEFT VENTRICULAR PUMP FUNCTION

The left ventricular end-diastolic volume in the normal adult of average size is in the range of 120 to 130 ml. Approximately two thirds of this end-diastolic volume is ejected with systole. Values for this ejection fraction which are greater than 0.5 are usually accepted as normal (see Table 9–2).

In the presence of lesions that place a chronic volume overload on the left ventricle, the ventricle dilates with the relationship between stroke volume and end-diastolic volume much as

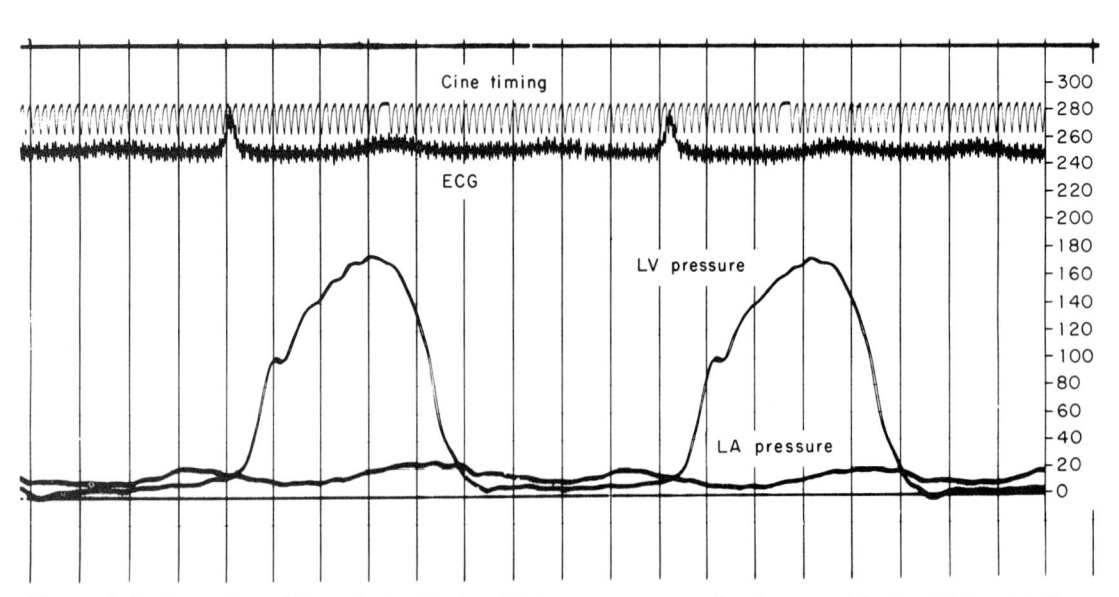

Figure 9–4 Recording of time of cine filming (65 frames per second) with respect to the ECG and left ventricular and atrial pressure in a patient with mitral stenosis.

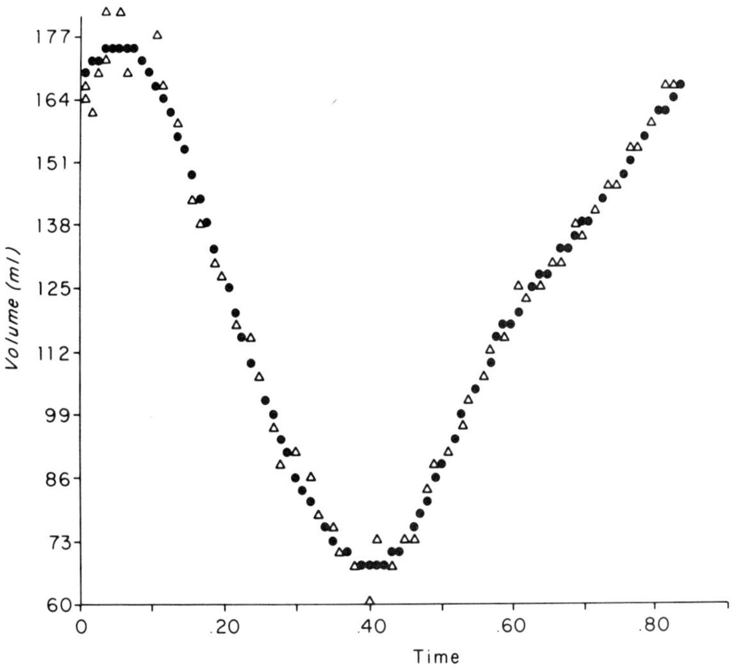

Figure 9-5 Left ventricular volumes computed from cine films taken at 65 frames per second are plotted as triangles with respect to time within the cardiac cycle. From these computed volumes a volume curve has been generated, as shown by the solid circles, through the use of a curve-fitting computer program.

in the normal; namely, greater than one half the end-diastolic volume is ejected with systole. The left ventricular stroke volume with very severe aortic and/or mitral value insufficiency may approach, but rarely exceeds, 300 ml. With lesions that place a chronic pressure overload on the left ventricle, as is observed with aortic valvular stenosis, the left ventricle hypertrophies with a thickened wall but end-diastolic volume and ejection fraction are similar to those observed in normal subjects. This is in contrast to the ventricular dilatation and reduced ejection fraction that are observed with acute pressure loads. Ventricular hypertrophy very likely provides the mechanism whereby the ventricle with a chronic pressure overload functions at a normal volume and with a normal ejection fraction.

With myocardial disease the left ventricle dilates inappropriately for the stroke volume, so that the residual volume is increased and the ejection fraction reduced. In patients with severe myocardial disease, ejection fractions of less than 0.10 are occasionally observed. Even in the presence of mechanical overloads such as those imposed by valvular heart disease, the relationship of stroke volume and end-diastolic volume as expressed by the ejection fraction has proved to be of value in assessing myocardial function.

The difference between left ventricular stroke volume, as determined by the angiocardiographic method and forward flow, or effective cardiac output per stroke, as measured by the Fick or indicator dilution methods, provides a method for quantifying the volume of regurgitant flow in patients with aortic and/or mitral valve insufficiency and shunt flow in patients with ventricular septal defect. An example of findings in a patient with mitral insufficiency is shown in Figure 9-6. Patients with severe valvular insufficiency may have regurgitant volumes per stroke

TABLE 9-2 NORMAL VALUES IN ADULTS AND CHILDREN

	End-Diastolic Volume (ml./M^2)	Stroke Volume (ml./M^2)	End-Systolic Volume (ml./M^2)	Ejection Fraction (SV/EDV)	Wall Thickness (mm.)	Left Ventricle Mass (g./M^2)
ADULTS	70±20	45±13	24	0.67±0.08	10.9±2.0	92±16
CHILDREN AND INFANTS						
Less than 2 Years of Age	42±10	28.6	13.4	0.68±0.05		96±11
More than 2 Years of Age (3 to 16 Years)	73±11	44±5	27±7	0.63±0.05		86±11

From Dodge, H. T.: Determination of left ventricular volume and mass. Radiol. Clin. N. Amer., 9:459, 1971.

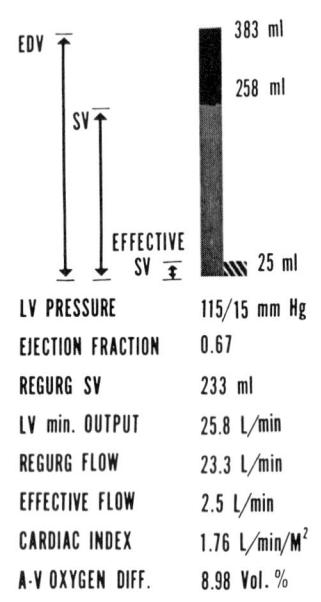

EDV	383 ml
SV	258 ml
EFFECTIVE SV	25 ml
LV PRESSURE	115/15 mm Hg
EJECTION FRACTION	0.67
REGURG SV	233 ml
LV min. OUTPUT	25.8 L/min
REGURG FLOW	23.3 L/min
EFFECTIVE FLOW	2.5 L/min
CARDIAC INDEX	1.76 L/min/M²
A-V OXYGEN DIFF.	8.98 Vol. %

Figure 9–6 Left ventricular pressure, volume, and cardiac output data from a patient with severe mitral valve insufficiency. The end-diastolic volume, stroke volume, and effective stroke volume, or forward flow, are as indicated. (Adapted from Dodge, H. T., and Baxley, W. A. *In* Gordon, B. L. (Ed.): Clinical Cardiopulmonary Physiology. 3rd ed. Grune and Stratton, Inc., 1969. By permission of Grune and Stratton, Inc.)

in the range of 250 ml. which may be in excess of 80 per cent of the left ventricular stroke volume. Left ventricular minute outputs in such patients may be as large as 25 to 30 liters per minute.

From the slopes of the ejection and filling limbs of ventricular volume curves the rates of ventricular ejection and filling respectively can be determined. Figure 9–7 shows a curve of ventricular filling and ejection rates calculated from a ventricular volume curve in a patient with ischemic heart disease. The maximum rates of filling and ejection are usually similar and in the normal resting subject are in the range of 500 ml. per second. With severe aortic and/or mitral valve insufficiency, peak-ejection and filling rates approach 1500 ml. per second. Peak values as low as 200 ml. per second are observed in patients with mitral stenosis, aortic stenosis, or severe myocardial disease.

Chronic disease is often associated with altered left ventricular distensibility. Figure 9–8 shows the left ventricular end-diastolic pressure-volume relationships of patients with chronic heart disease. End-diastolic volumes of as much as four times normal are observed with filling pressures that are within the normal range. With the increased distensibility, the ventricle functions at a large volume with little or no increase in filling pressure or pulmonary venous pressure. This is important because pulmonary venous hypertension secondary to an elevated ventricular filling pressure is associated with dyspnea. In general, patients with the more distensible left ventricles are those with chronic volume overloads or longstanding chronic myocardial disease.

Reduced ventricular distensibility is often observed with thick-walled hypertrophied left ventricles as occurs with aortic valve stenosis or hypertrophic subvalvular aortic stenosis. Here the filling pressure may be elevated in the presence of a normal ventricular end-diastolic volume. Some patients with ischemic heart disease also have elevated filling pressures with normal end-diastolic volumes.

The functional characteristics of the left ventricle as a pump in performing pressure-volume work can be determined from the ventricular pressure-volume relationships as shown in Figure 9–9. By relating pressure and volume with respect to time a pressure volume curve is constructed, with pressure on the vertical axis and volume on the horizontal axis. The height of the curve is determined by the systolic pressure, location on the horizontal axis by the end-diastolic volume, and the excursion along the horizontal axis by the stroke volume. The superior and inferior portions of the curves represent pressure-volume relationships during systole and diastole respectively. The shape of the curve is altered by mechanical defects such as aortic or mitral insufficiency which shorten or abolish the isovolumic contraction and/or relaxation period. Differences in locations and shapes of pressure-volume curves as determined from patients with various heart diseases are illustrated in Figure 9–10.

Left ventricular systolic work is determined from the pressure-volume relations during systole and is illustrated by the area beneath the systolic portion of the curve in Figure 9–9, or

$$\text{Systolic work} = \int_{V_d}^{V_s} P\, dV$$

where V_s and V_d are the end-systolic and end-diastolic volumes respectively and P is the ventricular systolic pressure. Systolic stroke work values as much as three to four times normal are observed with severe mitral and aortic valve insufficiency. Values as much as four to five times normal occur when severe valvular insufficiency is associated with ventricular hypertension from aortic stenosis.

The level of work expended in distending the diastolic left ventricle can be determined from the pressure-volume relationships of the left ventricle during diastole. This is illustrated by the area beneath the pressure-volume curve of Figure 9–9, or

$$\text{Diastolic work} = \int_{V_s}^{V_d} P\, dV$$

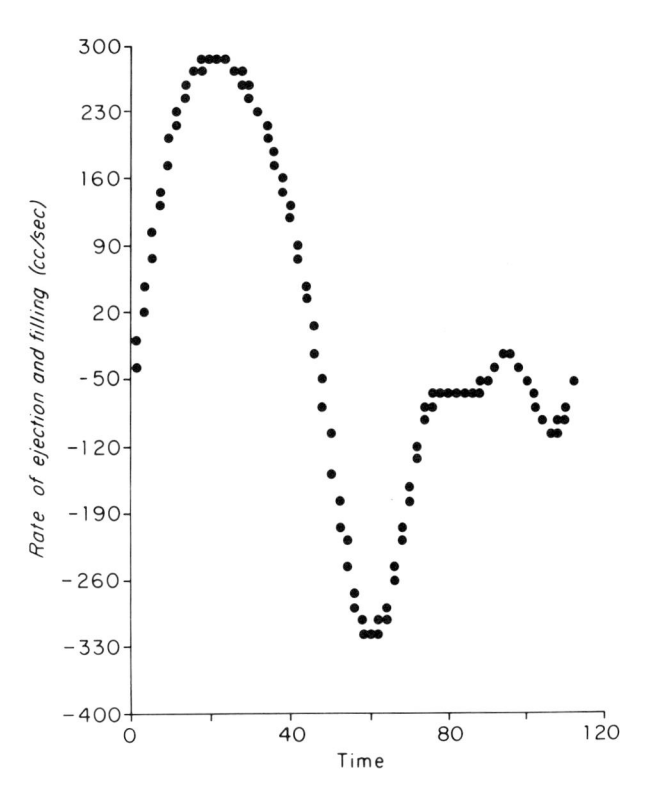

Figure 9-7 Rate of left ventricular ejection and filling with respect to time within the cardiac cycle as determined from the first derivative of a left ventricular volume curve. The positive values are during ejection and negative values during ventricular filling. Zero time is the onset of QRS of the ECG.

where P and V are the pressure and volume respectively during diastole. With left ventricular failure and an elevated left ventricular filling pressure, increased work is performed in distending the diastolic left ventricle. This work is performed by the left atrium and right ventricle and is the physiologic basis for the left atrial dilatation and right ventricular dilatation and hypertrophy that are observed with chronic left ventricular failure.

The difference between the systolic work and diastolic work values has been termed net work and is represented by the area enclosed by the pressure-volume loop shown in Figure 9-9. In considering the left ventricle as a pump, the net work is then the energy delivered as pressure-volume work in systole less the energy expended in distending the left ventricle as pressure-volume work during diastole. With increasing left ventricular failure, net work is decreased relative to systolic and diastolic work. This is illustrated in Figure 9-11, which shows a pressure-volume curve from a patient with a left ventricular end-diastolic volume of 525 ml. and pressure of 20 mm. Hg. Systolic work is 37.5 grammeters per stroke. Diastolic work is nearly 30 per cent of this, and net work is only 26.5 grammeters per stroke.

The most accurate method for computing left ventricular systolic and net work values is from ventricular pressure and volume curves as described above. However, left ventricular stroke work (LVSW) may also be estimated from stroke volume (SV) and left ventricular systolic pressure (LVSP) as follows:

$$LVSW = SV \ (\overline{LVSP} - LVEDP)$$

where $\overline{LVSP}$ equals the mean left ventricular systolic pressure during ejection and LVEDP is left ventricular end-diastolic pressure.

Ventricular power is the rate at which work is performed and can be calculated from the systolic pressure-volume relationships of the left ventricle as $P \times dV/dt$, where P is instantaneous pressure and dV/dt the instantaneous rate of ejection. Peak power values in the range of 500 grammeters per second are observed in normal resting human subjects and values in excess of four times this in patients with severe aortic and/or mitral valve disease.

In chronic heart disease left ventricular hypertrophy is observed as a response to chronic pressure and/or volume overloads and also in association with chronic left ventricular dilatation. In patients with valvular heart disease and as shown in Figure 9-12 where left ventricular weight is related to left ventricular stroke work, the extent of hypertrophy is directly related to

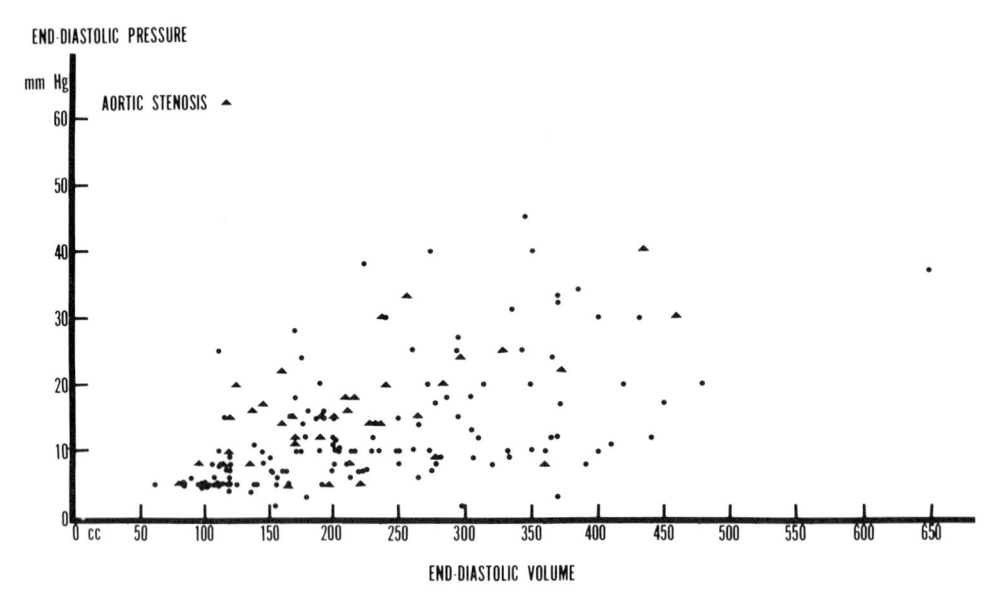

Figure 9–8 Left ventricular end-diastolic pressure and volume are related in 144 patients with various types and durations of heart diseases. Patients with aortic valvular or subaortic stenosis are designated by the triangles. From Dodge, H. T., and Baxley, W. A., Hemodynamic Aspects of Heart Failure. Amer. J. Cardiol., 22:24, 1968.

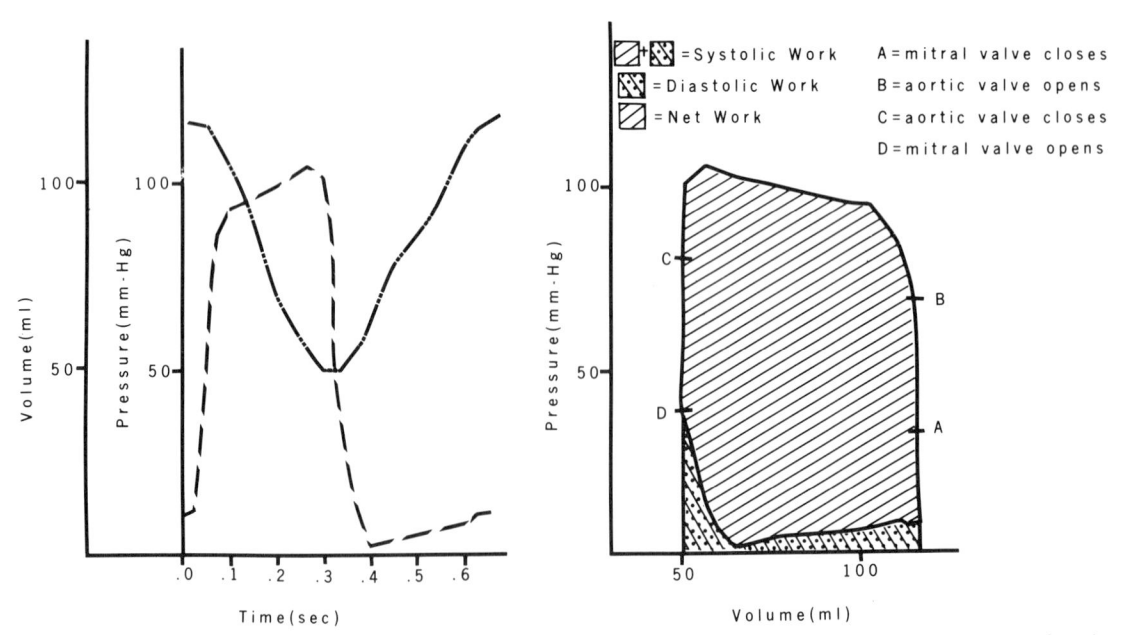

Figure 9–9 On the left are left ventricular pressure and volume curves plotted with respect to time after the QRS of the electrocardiogram. On the right, a pressure-volume curve has been constructed, with work values as indicated by the shaded areas. Mitral valve closure is delayed within the isovolumic contraction period because of an elevated left atrial pressure due to mitral stenosis. The mitral valve opens early in the isovolumic relaxation period also because of an elevated left atrial pressure from mitral stenosis.

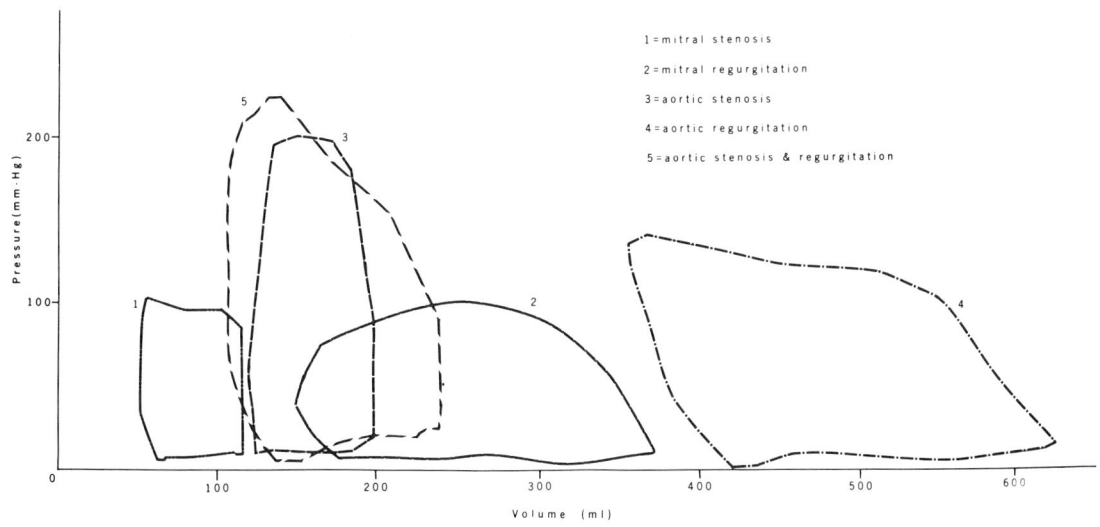

Figure 9-10. Examples of left ventricular pressure-volume curves from patients with different types of heart diseases (mitral stenosis, mitral regurgitation, aortic stenosis, aortic regurgitation, and aortic stenosis and regurgitation). The curve from the patient with mitral stenosis shows well-defined isovolumic contraction and relaxation periods, a normal stroke volume, and relatively normal stroke work. The relatively larger stroke work values in the other patients can be roughly estimated by comparing the areas beneath the systolic limbs of the pressure-volume curves. The patients with aortic regurgitation, mitral regurgitation, and aortic stenosis and regurgitation have greatly elevated stroke work values with large stroke volumes as is evident by the excursion of the curves along the horizontal or volume axis. The abnormality in shape and location of these curves is evident. Patients with valvular insufficiency have a shortening or absence of isovolumic contraction and relaxation periods. Patients with aortic valve stenosis have elevated systolic pressures. Patients with large stroke volumes have elevated end-diastolic volumes.

the workload. The manner in which the heart hypertrophies differs, however, depending upon whether the increased work is a result of a pressure or volume overload. With compensated volume overloads the wall shows only a small amount of thickening as end-diastolic volume is increased, and the ratio of left ventricular mass to end-diastolic volume is close to 1.0. With pressure overloads the wall thickness is considerably increased, with end-diastolic volume being relatively normal so that the ratio of left ventricular mass to end-diastolic volume is greater than 1.0. It has been shown that in compensated valvular heart disease and with either pressure or volume overloads, the wall thickness is increased in proportion to chamber dimensions and systolic pressure, so that systolic wall stress or force per unit of cross-sectional area of ventricular wall remains relatively normal.

Left ventricular hypertrophy is also observed in the presence of chronic left ventricular dilatation, even when left ventricular stroke work is diminished as occurs in patients with myocardial disease. In Figure 9-13 left ventricular end-diastolic volume is related to left ventricular mass and as can be seen, increase in left ventricular weight is roughly proportionate to that of volume. Significant ventricular dilatation is regularly associated with ventricular hypertrophy in man with chronic heart disease. The stimulus to hypertrophy is very likely the increased wall force that occurs with the increased chamber dimensions and reduced wall thickness that accompany ventricular dilatation.

The above observations on increased left ventricular mass in the presence of chronic work overloads and ventricular dilatation are consistent with a growth of myocardium in patients with chronic heart disease. In experimental animals with left ventricular dilatation and hypertrophy from an induced chronic volume overload, maximal sarcomere lengths have been shown to be unchanged from the 2.2μ observed in the normal left ventricle. This together with the observations of increased myocardial mass in man with chronic heart disease suggests that growth of new myocardium and sarcomeres is an important adaptive mechanism in chronic heart disease and that the Frank-Starling mechanism may not be important in these chronic adjustments. There is currently a controversy concerning the contractile state of myocardium which is hypertrophied in response to pressure and volume overloads. Some groups have reported normal and others depressed contractility when expressed per unit of myocardium.

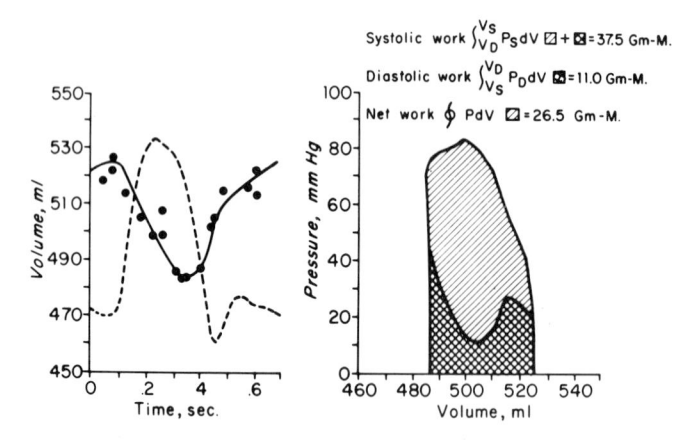

Figure 9-11 Left ventricular pressure, volume, and pressure-volume curves from a patient with ischemic heart disease and left ventricular failure. The various pressure-volume work components are designated and described in the text. (Adapted from Dodge, H. T., and Baxley, W. A.: Hemodynamic aspects of heart failure. Amer. J. Cardiol., 22:24, 1968.)

Figure 9-12 Relationship of left ventricular stroke work and mass in 165 patients with valvular heart disease. (From Dodge, H. T., and Baxley, W. A.: Left ventricular volume and mass and their significance in heart disease. Amer. J. Cardiol., 23:528, 1969.)

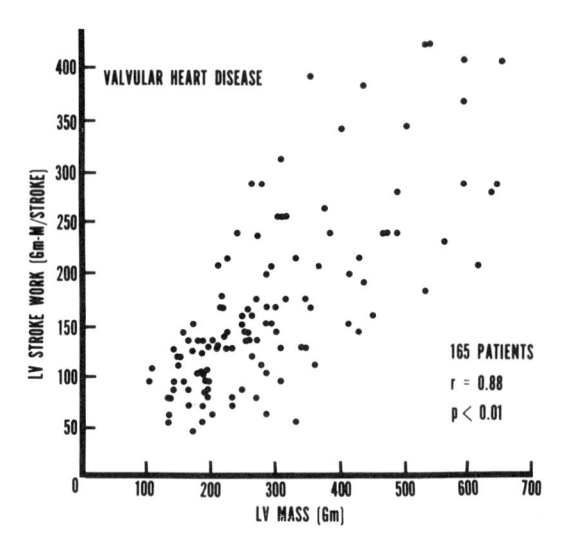

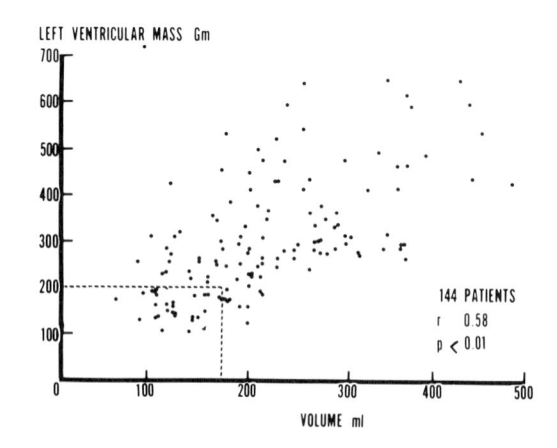

Figure 9-13 Relationship of left ventricular end-diastolic volume and mass in 144 patients with various types of heart diseases. (From Dodge, H. T., and Baxley, W. A.: Hemodynamic aspects of heart failure. Amer. J. Cardiol., 22:24, 1968.)

MYOCARDIAL PERFORMANCE

Myocardial performance can be more directly evaluated in the intact heart through an analysis of wall forces and motion. The forces present within the myocardium of the chamber walls are a function of the chamber pressure, dimensions, and wall thickness. A method for computing these forces for the left ventricle is to assume that the ventricle can be represented as a thin-walled ellipsoid of revolution and to apply the Laplace expression:

$$\frac{T_1}{R_1} + \frac{T_2}{R_2} = P$$

where T_1 and T_2 are mean wall tensions in the meridional and circumferential directions respectively and R_1 and R_2 are the associated principal radii of curvature. P is chamber pressure. Tension is expressed in force per linear cm., if dimensions are expressed in terms of cm., and can be considered as the force acting per cm. of slits in the wall placed perpendicular to the principal radii of curvature. The wall forces also can be expressed in terms of stress (σ) or force per unit area (cm.^{2}) by dividing tension by wall thickness (h). The Laplace expression then becomes

$$\frac{\sigma_1}{R_1} + \frac{\sigma_2}{R_2} = \frac{p}{h}$$

where σ_1 and σ_2 equal wall stress in the directions of the principal radii of curvature. Wall stress or force per unit area is expressed in the same units as those used for chamber pressure. The largest wall force values are in the circumferential direction.

Because of the above relationships between chamber pressure, wall thickness, and wall stress, wall stress increases more rapidly than chamber pressure as chamber dimensions increase and wall thickness decreases as occurs when the diastolic left ventricle is acutely distended. During systole, chamber dimensions decrease and wall thickness increases so that wall stress decreases relative to chamber pressure. As described previously, in compensated heart disease associated with chronic pressure or volume overloads, wall thickness is increased so that wall stress values are similar to those found in normal subjects. In subjects with left ventricular failure, large wall stress values are frequently present, indicating that myocardial hypertrophy has not been adequate to compensate for the increase in dimensions and decrease of wall thickness as the chamber has dilated.

The relationship of wall stresses in the directions of the principal chamber axes to wall motion expressed in terms of change of these axes during systole has provided a method for expressing myocardial performance of the intact ventricle in terms of force, extent, and velocity of shortening. This has been used to apply knowledge concerning the relationships of force to the extent and velocity of myocardial contraction as determined in in-vitro studies to the intact ventricle of experimental animals and man.

In-vitro studies of contractile characteristics of myocardium indicate that the myocardial contractile state can be evaluated independently of preload or the Frank-Starling effect from an analysis of myocardial force and velocity of contraction relationships. With this approach to evaluate myocardial contractility, a model to represent the contractile apparatus of the myocardium is assumed. This model consists of a contractile element (CE), a series elastic element (SE), and, for a 3-component model, a parallel elastic element. Myocardial contractility is expressed in terms of velocity of contraction of the contractile element (VCE) with respect to force to determine force-VCE relationships. These force-velocity relationships, when extrapolated to zero force, provide a measure of VCE under zero load which has been termed V_{max}. Some studies indicated that V_{max} is independent of fiber length, or the Frank-Starling effect. However, there is controversy concerning the validity of this concept when applied to isolated heart muscle preparations and even more controversy when applied to evaluate the myocardial contractile state of the intact ventricle of experimental animals and man. For a further discussion of these concepts refer to the section on heart muscle and its dynamics (Chapter 8).

The preceding studies and concepts are the basis for evaluation of myocardial contractile state of the intact ventricle in experimental animals and man from high-fidelity ventricular pressure data recorded during the isovolumic contraction period and from studies of ejection phase dynamics. During the isovolumic period, if one assumes no change of cardiac dimensions and wall thickness,

$$VCE = \frac{(dp/dt)}{(K \times P)}$$

where K is equal to the elastic modulus of the series elastic element and P the corresponding isovolumic pressure. VCE extrapolated to zero pressure provides a measure of V_{max}, an index of myocardial contractility which is said to be independent of preload and afterload. If a 3-component model with a parallel elastic component is assumed, developed pressure (DP) is substituted for P in the above equation. DP is computed as P less the initial or end-diastolic pressure. The expression (dP/dt) / K × DP is said to be less sensitive to changes of preload and to provide a more precise index of myocardial contractile state.

Indices of myocardial contractile state as determined from the ventricular ejection phase include the velocity of ventricular circumference change (VCF), VCF at peak wall stress which is equivalent to VCE, peak VCE and VCE extrapolated to zero load, or V_{max}. These computations require knowledge of chamber dimensions, pressure and wall thickness, and instantaneous changes of these parameters during systole. The reader is referred to the section on heart muscle and its dynamics for a further discussion of the theoretical basis for these concepts and their application to evaluate the myocardial contractile state (see Chapter 8).

HEMODYNAMICS OF HEART FAILURE

Cardiac enlargement, increased ventricular filling pressure, and a low cardiac output at rest, or relative to the demands of some stress such as exercise, are features of heart failure. Basically, the clinical picture of heart failure is the result of a decreased ability of the heart to contract, an increased pressure-volume load, a combination of increased load and depressed contractility, or occasionally interference with venous return to the heart as occurs with constrictive pericarditis. Figure 9-6 illustrates an example of failure resulting from a large volume overload due to mitral regurgitation. In man with chronic heart disease and ventricular failure there is compensation for the decreased myocardial contractility and increased mechanical pressure and volume loads by cardiac dilatation (Frank-Starling mechanism) and by cardiac hypertrophy as previously described. It is often difficult to determine precisely when in the course of chronic heart disease these mechanisms for compensation become inadequate to maintain cardiac output and heart failure develops. In fact, these mechanisms of chamber dilatation and hypertrophy can be viewed as early manifestations of cardiac decompensation as they represent the initial adjustments of the diseased heart. Because there are limits to the extent of cardiac dilatation and hypertrophy that occur in disease, once these compensatory mechanisms develop there is a diminished capacity of the heart to adjust to further increases in mechanical loads or further decreases of myocardial contractility.

A fundamental mechanism by which the ventricles maintain stroke volume in response to acute increases of systolic pressure (afterload), volume overload, or depression of contractility is through chamber dilatation, which has been termed the Frank-Starling mechanism. The increased fiber length which occurs with chamber

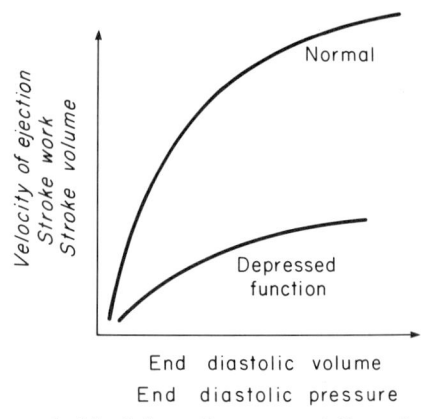

Figure 9-14 Schematic representation of a normal and a depressed ventricular function curve as defined by the relationship of parameters as given on the horizontal and vertical axes.

dilatation is associated with an increased force and extent of contraction. Figure 9-14 shows what have been termed ventricular function curves. With normal myocardial function, chamber volume enlargement is associated with increases of stroke work and stroke volume along a theoretically normal curve. With depressed myocardial function, lower stroke volume and stroke work are generated from a given end-diastolic volume, and stroke volume is maintained through ventricular dilatation. A depressed systolic ejection fraction as is observed in man with myocardial disease is a numerical expression of a depressed ventricular function curve, since it indicates inappropriate chamber enlargement with a low stroke volume and large residual volume relative to end-diastolic volume. Drugs which have a positive inotropic effect elevate a depressed ventricular function curve.

With acute increases of ventricular end-diastolic volume there is an eventual leveling off of the ventricular function curves, so that further increases in volume result in no further increase in stroke work or stroke volume. Indeed, under some conditions a descending limb of the function curves has been demonstrated. With ventricular dilatation, ventricular diastolic pressure is increased and filling pressure is often used as an index of diastolic volume or preload in determining ventricular response to a changing preload. In man with heart failure due to acute myocardial infarction it has been shown that little increase or even a fall of stroke volume occurs with elevation of left ventricular end-diastolic pressure beyond 22 to 25 mm. Hg.

As described previously, chronic increases of ventricular chamber volume or work load are associated with ventricular hypertrophy. There is a question concerning the role of the Frank-Starling mechanism in the adjustments to chronic increases of ventricular volume and pressure, and hypertrophy may be the dominant response to chronic loads.

Measures of ventricular pump performance other than stroke volume relative to end-diastolic volume (ejection fraction) can be used to assess myocardial performance in chronic heart disease. These are stroke work, ventricular ejection rate, or peak power. As with stroke volume, none of these parameters have significance for evaluating myocardial performance unless they are related to ventricular end-diastolic volume. In the presence of myocardial disease, depressed values relative to volume are observed. This is illustrated in Figure 9-15, in which stroke power normalized for end-diastolic volume is related to the ejection fraction.

There is a problem with using stroke work relative to volume to assess myocardial performance in chronic heart disease. As described previously, the adjustment to chronic systolic pressure overload is ventricular hypertrophy rather than dilatation. Accordingly, stroke work relative to chamber volume is high in compensated pressure overload states and decreases with myocardial failure, but it still may be high relative to the stroke work/end-diastolic volume relationships observed in other types of heart disease. As a result stroke work/end-diastolic volume does not appear to provide a very useful index for evaluating myocardial performance in chronic heart disease.

With ventricular failure, abnormally low values for ventricular performance are also obtained by analysis of ventricular pressure changes during isovolumic contraction (dp/dt) and of wall force and motion relationships. The velocity of circumference change relative to end-diastolic circumference (VCF) is depressed. Derived values for peak VCE, VCE at peak stress, and V_{max} are also depressed.

ISCHEMIC HEART DISEASE

Ischemic heart disease results from an inadequate supply of oxygenated blood to the myocardium. For practical purposes this disease is due to atherosclerotic occlusive disease of the large extramural coronary arteries, although disease of these vessels occasionally results from other pathologic processes such as embolization, fibromuscular disease of the arteries, and arteritis of variable etiology. Atherosclerosis, although usually diffusely distributed in the proximal portions of the coronary arteries, tends to cause localized areas of stenosis or occlusion. The localized distribution of highly stenotic or occlusive lesions results in regional areas of ischemic or infarcted myocardium. Myocardial functional abnormalities are therefore usually of a segmental or regional distribution in patients with ischemic heart disease. When myocardial damage becomes very extensive due to multiple sites of high-grade stenosis or occlusions of coronary arteries, the entire left ventricle may exhibit reduced contraction. In order to evaluate left ventricular performance in ischemic heart disease it is necessary to study the extent and severity of regional contraction abnormalities.

Evaluation of regional contraction abnormalities is difficult because it requires that all aspects of the left ventricle including its apex, free wall, anterior and posterior surfaces, and septum be visualized and studied. At this time angiocardiography is the best method available for the detailed evaluation of segmental abnormalities of left ventricular contraction. The evaluation of left ventricular function in patients with ischemic heart disease is best carried out in conjunction with selective coronary arteriography. Indications for study include angina pectoris, symptoms of heart failure, or persistent chest pain following recovery from a myocardial infarc-

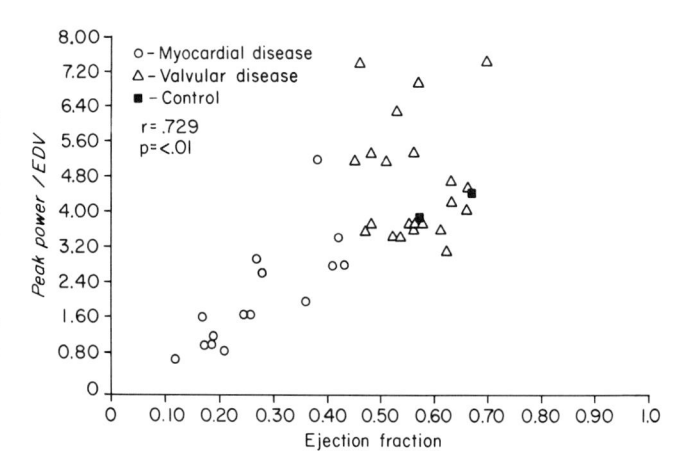

Figure 9-15 A significant correlation is demonstrated for the relationship of left ventricular peak power normalized for end-diastolic volume and ejection fraction in 39 subjects with various types of heart diseases as coded. The subjects indicated as "control" had no demonstrable disease affecting the left ventricle. (From Gensini, G. G. (Ed.): The Study of the Systemic, Coronary and Myocardial Effects of Nitrates. Courtesy of Charles C Thomas, Publisher, Springfield, Illinois. In press.)

tion. Occasionally, patients with heart failure of uncertain etiology are also studied in this manner. Left ventricular angiocardiography may be carried out in single or biplane views with direct or cine filming techniques. In most situations single plane cine angiocardiography is adequate for clinical purposes, although biplane methods are preferable. The pattern of ventricular contraction is evaluated by analysis of end-diastolic and systolic films. This is best carried out by tracing the outline of the opacified chamber and constructing a line from the apex of the left ventricle to the center of the aortic valve. By superimposing systolic and diastolic outlines, the symmetry and extent of contraction can be assessed.

Regional contraction abnormalities can be conveniently divided into five types:

I. *Normal:* The entire ventricular wall moves inward appropriately toward the geometric center of the ventricle. Occasional patients with small volumes and normal ejection fractions have ventricles that appear asymmetrical at end systole due to distortion of the cavity shape by the papillary muscles.

II. *Borderline Abnormal:* The ventricle demonstrates a minor degree of contraction asymmetry involving less than 25 per cent of the wall.

III. *Localized Akinesis or Hypokinesis:* More than 25 per cent but less than 75 per cent of the ventricular wall has diminished or absent contraction.

IV. *Localized Dyskinesis:* More than 25 per cent of the ventricular wall demonstrates paradoxical outward motion during systole.

V. *Diffuse Akinesis or Hypokinesis:* More than 75 per cent of the ventricular surface has diminished or absent contraction.

Selective coronary arteriograms usually demonstrate that the coronary vessels which supply an akinetic or dyskinetic region have severe stenosis or total occlusion. Often, however, severely stenotic or occluded coronary vessels supply areas of myocardium which appear to contract normally. Severe coronary artery disease is not, therefore, necessarily associated with areas of abnormal myocardial contraction, at least in the resting subject. Generally, there has been a good correlation between definite electrocardiographic evidence of myocardial infarction and regional contraction abnormalities as assessed by left ventricular angiocardiography. The opposite, however, is not true. Frequently, a severe myocardial contraction abnormality may be present and the electrocardiogram does not definitely localize an infarct to that region of the heart. Electrocardiography, selective coronary arteriography, and left ventricular angiography are all necessary to evaluate fully the patient with ischemic heart disease. Each method yields information not available from the others and together they give a rather complete picture of the left ventricle, its blood supply, electrical integrity, and contractile function.

Ventricular Performance in Ischemic Heart Disease

The incidence of significant segmental contraction abnormalities in patients with ischemic heart disease varies with the patient group submitted to angiocardiographic studies. The majority of patients with angina pectoris without a history or electrocardiographic evidence of prior myocardial infarction have a normal contraction pattern. Not infrequently, however, these patients have a modest reduction in ejection fraction and an elevation of diastolic pressure. Under the stress of tachycardia induced with right atrial pacing, the end-diastolic pressure often becomes abnormally elevated and abnormal contraction patterns may appear, or become more marked. Diastolic pressure rise is especially likely to occur in those in whom pacing induces anginal pain. Exercise in this group of patients is also associated with increased left ventricular end-diastolic pressure and subnormal increase in cardiac output.

The majority of patients who have suffered a myocardial infarction and have associated electrocardiographic evidence of myocardial scar will have a segmental area of abnormal left ventricular contraction. It has been postulated that akinesis of more than 25 per cent of the ventricular myocardium must result in either ventricular dilatation or reduction in stroke volume. This theory rests upon estimates of the limits of contractile element shortening which can occur under physiologic conditions. Quantitative assessment of the extent of segmental contraction abnormality in large groups of patients suggests that this theory is essentially correct. When more than 25 to 30 per cent of the left ventricular wall is akinetic or dyskinetic, ventricular dilatation and reduced ejection fraction are usually present. The left ventricular end-diastolic pressure is also elevated in most of these patients. Major contraction abnormalities (Type IV or V) are nearly always associated with a history of heart failure and a resting ejection fraction below 40 per cent.

Left ventricular myocardial hypertrophy is frequently present in patients with ischemic heart disease. This appears to be closely related to a history of congestive heart failure and the presence of left ventricular dilatation. There is a close correlation between the increase in left ventricular diastolic volume and the increase in myocardial mass. However, the degree of myocardial hypertrophy relative to diastolic volume is less in ischemic heart disease than in patients with valvular heart disease. This is probably due to the fact that these patients usually do not have an increased volume or pressure load on the left ventricle. In addition, the lesser degree of left ventricular hypertrophy in ischemic heart disease may be related to shorter duration of disease or an expression of inadequate coronary arterial blood supply.

It is of interest that the electrocardiogram is relatively insensitive in detecting the presence of left ventricular hypertrophy in patients with ischemic heart disease. It should be remembered that ventricular hypertrophy as estimated from angiocardiograms or as determined from left ventricular weight at autopsy does not separate normal myocardial tissue from fibrous tissue and scar and is therefore subject to variable error in estimating actual muscle mass, depending upon the extent of ischemic damage present. The presence of considerable fibrosis and scarring may account for the disparity between electrocardiographic and angiocardiographic evidence of ventricular hypertrophy.

Mitral Regurgitation in Ischemic Heart Disease

Mild mitral regurgitation is frequently present in patients with ischemic heart disease. It is often intermittent and associated with the presence of congestive heart failure, or it may be present only during episodes of myocardial ischemia. Mitral regurgitation in ischemic heart disease may be the result of papillary muscle dysfunction, dilatation of the mitral annulus secondary to left ventricular dilatation, or papillary muscle rupture.

The two papillary muscles of the left ventricle receive their blood supply from terminal branches of the anterior descending and posterior descending coronary arteries. Since the terminal portions of these muscles are free in the ventricular cavity they are directly subjected to intercavity pressure. The combination of these two factors may explain why these small muscles are especially vulnerable to ischemia and infarction. The papillary muscles must contract in concert with the ventricle so that the mitral valve is held in a competent position across the mitral orifice. Failure of these muscles to contract will result in prolapse of the mitral valve into the left atrium during the later portion of systole, as indicated in Figure 9-16. Clinically, this will result in a mid and late systolic ejection murmur which is characteristic of papillary muscle dysfunction. When left ventricular dilatation is extensive, the papillary muscles are pulled down and laterally away from the mitral valve. If the muscles contract with systole in a normal manner, the mitral valve will be held down in the ventricle in an incompetent position throughout systole, as illustrated in Figure 9-16B. This situation will usually result in a blowing pansystolic murmur. This type of regurgitation frequently disappears when treatment for congestive heart failure results in reduction in left ventricular volume. It is of interest that patients with long-standing left ventricular dilatation of any cause often develop mitral regurgitation. At surgical or postmortem examination some of these patients have a dilated mitral annulus and normal valve leaflets,

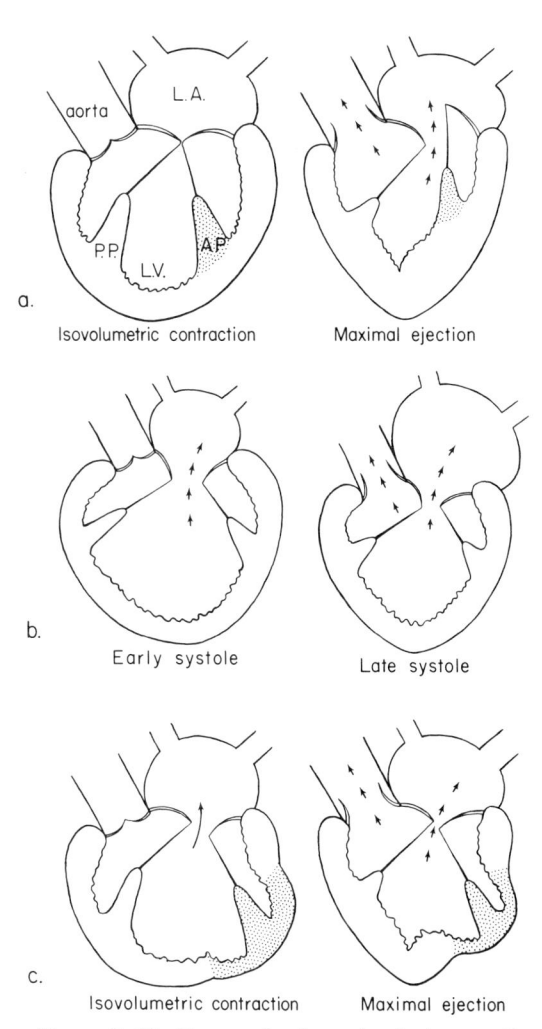

Figure 9-16 The mechanism of mitral regurgitation secondary to ischemia or infarction of the anterior lateral papillary is shown in diagrammatic form (a). During isovolumic contraction and early systole the mitral valve is competent but during the maximal ejection period the anterior valve leaflet prolapses into the left atrium and mitral regurgitation results.

The mechanism of mitral regurgitation secondary to left ventricular chamber dilatation (b).

The mechanism of mitral regurgitation which results from infarction of the papillary muscle and the underlying left ventricular wall (c). In this example the infarcted left ventricular wall is aneurysmal and bulges out during systole. (Adapted from Burch, G. E., DePasquale, N. P., and Phillips, J. H.: Amer. Heart J., 75:399, 1968. Copyright 1968, American Medical Association.)

indicating that mitral incompetence resulted from enlargement of the mitral annulus secondary to ventricular dilatation. It is not certain how often mitral regurgitation is due to displacement of the papillary muscle by a dilated ventricular cavity and how often annular dilatation plays an important role in the production of valve incompetence.

Quantitative angiocardiographic assessment of patients with ischemic heart disease indicates that in those patients with mitral regurgitation there is evidence of extensive ventricular dilatation, with the left ventricular end-diastolic volume greater than 150 ml. per $M.^2$ in the majority of cases. In addition, these patients nearly always give a history of prior myocardial infarction and congestive heart failure. Left ventricular contraction patterns are also nearly always distinctly abnormal. These findings are not consistent with isolated ischemia or infarction of one or the other papillary muscle but are indicative of more widespread damage of the left ventricular myocardium. A number of recent studies have been carried out in an attempt to create papillary muscle dysfunction in dogs. One or both papillary muscles have been injected with sclerosing material and in another study the base of a papillary muscle was ligated. In those animals in which damage was confined to the papillary muscle, mitral regurgitation did not result. When the underlying left ventricular wall was also injured, mitral valve incompetence resulted. These animal studies and clinical experience in man suggest that mitral regurgitation in ischemic heart disease is the result of extensive ischemia or infarction of the papillary muscle and the underlying ventricular wall, as seen diagrammatically in Figure 9–16C.

In rare instances, mitral regurgitation develops acutely during the early phase of recovery from myocardial infarction as a result of rupture of a papillary muscle. When the entire muscle body ruptures, the resultant regurgitation is of severe proportions and pulmonary edema, shock, and death occur rapidly in nearly all instances. Immediate support of the circulation and replacement of the mitral valve is now possible and will undoubtedly result in a few survivals in this group of patients. At times, only one or two heads of the papillary muscle with their attached chordae tendineae rupture. In these instances, the regurgitation which results is less severe, and survival with or without surgical treatment may be possible.

Rupture of the Interventricular Septum

The development of an interventricular septal defect is an unusual and serious complication of acute myocardial infarction. In most such cases there is the sudden development of a systolic murmur associated with heart failure and often systemic arterial hypotension. Septal rupture usually occurs during the first six days following myocardial infarction in patients who have extensive transmural infarction of the anterior or posterior wall which also involves the interventricular septum. The prognosis in these patients remains poor despite attempts at surgical repair because of the extensive degree of myocardial damage which is usually present.

Ventricular Aneurysms

Angiocardiographic studies have shown that small areas of the left ventricular wall which bulge paradoxically with ventricular systole are common in patients who have had a transmural myocardial infarction. Large ventricular aneurysms which are apparent on simple chest x-ray and fluoroscopy are less common and probably occur in 3 to 10 per cent of patients who survive transmural myocardial infarction. Large ventricular aneurysms have a profound effect on left ventricular dynamics because as they expand with systole they accept a volume load from the contractile portion of the ventricle. However, the volume load is rarely marked and does not approach the levels of volume load observed in patients with moderate or severe aortic or mitral valve insufficiency. Patients with large ventricular aneurysms usually develop congestive heart failure probably as a result of the loss of a substantial portion of contractile muscle as well as the mechanical effects of the aneurysm. Since most ventricular aneurysms are lined with mural thrombi they are also associated with an increased incidence of systemic embolization. In addition, recurrent ventricular arrhythmias are common in these patients. Surgical resection of large ventricular aneurysms is indicated for heart failure which is resistant to medical treatment and in patients who have had systemic embolization which cannot be controlled with anticoagulants. Occasionally, aneurysms have been resected for recurrent episodes of ventricular tachycardia with apparent success. The risk and success of aneurysm resection depends upon the functional capacity of the remaining myocardium.

VALVULAR HEART DISEASE

Diseases of various types affect the cardiac valves and result in valvular stenosis, regurgitation, or a combination of these lesions. Rheumatic endocarditis remains the main cause of chronic valvular deformity and resultant dysfunction despite the reduction in the incidence of rheumatic fever which has occurred since the introduction of effective antibiotics in Western countries. Rheumatic fever and especially virulent forms of rheumatic valvular disease continue to be a major health problem in the developing countries. In recent years there has been an increasing appreciation of other etiologic factors responsible for valvular heart disease. It is now known, for example, that many cases of isolated aortic stenosis result from congenital bicuspid malformations of the valve. Many causes of pure mitral regurgitation are also recognized, including congenital abnormalities, dysfunction and rupture of the papillary muscles, rupture of chordae tendineae, mitral annular dilatation, myxomatous degeneration of the valve leaflets, and prolapse of the mitral valve. Bacterial endocarditis continues to be an important cause of mitral, aortic, and tricuspid valve destruction, although changes in the clinical and bacteriologic picture have resulted from the widespread use of antibiotics.

Mitral Stenosis

Mitral stenosis for practical purposes is due to rheumatic heart disease, although a congenital form of the disease and obstruction of the valve orifice due to left atrial myxoma do occur. The valve becomes thickened and there is fusion of the valve commissures. Calcification of the valve leaflets and mitral annulus is often present. The chordae tendineae are thickened, shortened, and fused to a variable degree. Generally, the valve orifice will be reduced to 1.2 cm.^{2} or less in cross-sectional area before significant symptoms develop. The major effect of mitral valve obstruction is a chronic increase in left atrial and pulmonary venous pressure. This increased pressure is transmitted back to the pulmonary capillaries and pulmonary artery. There is resultant interstitial edema and marked thickening of the alveolar walls. The small muscular pulmonary arteries and arterioles develop marked muscular hypertrophy and there is reduction in the lumen of these vessels. As one would suspect from these anatomic changes in severe mitral stenosis there may be elevation of pulmonary artery pressure which is greater than can be accounted for by the elevation in pulmonary venous and left atrial pressure, indicating increased resistance across the pulmonary vasculature. This increased pulmonary vascular resistance may at times rise to systemic levels with resultant severe pulmonary artery hypertension.

The major symptom in mitral stenosis is exertional dyspnea. As the disease advances, dyspnea at rest and marked fatigue develop. Right heart failure and functional tricuspid regurgitation often develop and peripheral edema and ascites may then become prominent.

The lungs in mitral stenosis become fibrotic and noncompliant. There is abnormal distribution of alveolar perfusion and ventilation which results in functional shunting of blood through the lungs. The upper lobes have increased perfusion whereas flow to the bases is reduced. This feature of mitral stenosis can often be appreciated on chest x-rays.

Despite the marked anatomic changes which occur in the lungs of patients with severe mitral stenosis, the pulmonary artery hypertension and increased pulmonary vascular resistance are reversible following surgery which successfully relieves mitral valve obstruction. Recent studies in patients immediately following mitral valve replacement have shown that the pulmonary artery pressure and calculated pulmonary vascular resistance fall rapidly within the first few days following valve replacement. Studies done several weeks later indicate that further reduction in vascular resistance occurs with time. The reversibility of pulmonary vascular resistance in mitral stenosis is in contrast to the irreversible nature of the high pulmonary vascular resistance which develops in some patients with congenital heart disease with left-to-right shunts.

The left atrium in mitral stenosis becomes increased in volume and the atrial wall becomes hypertrophied. In a recent study of 25 patients, atrial volume ranged from 44 to 288 ml. per M.^{2}, the average volume being more than three times the normal value. Occasional patients have been seen who have giant left atria, but marked left atrial enlargement is usually associated with mitral regurgitation. The maximum volume of the atrium is not linearly related to the severity of mitral stenosis, since other factors such as the duration of disease and the severity of rheumatic involvement of the atrial myocardium are factors in determining atrial volume. As long as sinus rhythm persists, atrial contraction plays an important role in forcing blood through the obstructed mitral orifice into the left ventricle. Unfortunately, the majority of patients with mitral stenosis eventually develop atrial fibrillation. Presumably this is the result of chronic atrial hypertension and dilatation, although the exact mechanisms are not clear. Atrial fibrillation has three deleterious effects: (1) it reduces left ventricular filling; (2) it usually results in an increase in heart rate, with resultant decrease in the diastolic portion of the cardiac cycle; and (3) it allows stagnation of blood in the dilated left atrium and its appendage. For cardiac output to be maintained in the face of atrial fibrillation left atrial pressure must increase to compensate for loss of atrial contraction and reduced diastolic filling time. This increase in atrial pressure may result in the development of pulmonary edema. The stagnation of blood in the atrium sets the stage for the development of left atrial thrombi which then often embolize with devastating consequences. Control of the heart rate in patients with atrial fibrillation and anticoagulant therapy are, therefore, major therapeutic measures in this disease.

Mitral stenosis is unique among acquired disease of the left side of the heart because it protects rather than stresses the left ventricle. Studies of the left ventricle indicate that in the majority of cases the ventricular volume and mass are normal. In an occasional advanced case, however, actual atrophy of the ventricular myocardium may occur. Despite normal diastolic volume, the left ventricular stroke volume is often reduced. This combination of reduced stroke volume and normal diastolic volume results in a reduced ejection fraction in about one third of patients with mitral stenosis, with half of these having an ejection fraction below 40 per cent. It is not clear at this time whether this reduced ejection fraction is indicative of myocardial dysfunction or whether it is merely an expression of reduced filling volume and pressure (preload).

Right ventricular hypertrophy accompanies the development of pulmonary hypertension in patients with mitral stenosis. Since the right ventricle is unaccustomed to developing high pressures, it often dilates and functional tricuspid regurgitation frequently occurs. Venous hypertension, congestive hepatomegaly, peripheral edema, and ascites then follow. Sustained pulmonary hypertension occasionally causes dilatation of the pulmonary artery and annulus of the pulmonary valve, with resultant pulmonary valvular insufficiency. Since associated aortic valve insufficiency is commonly present in patients with mitral stenosis, the differentiation of aortic from pulmonary valve insufficiency requires cardiac catheterization and angiocardiography. Both tricuspid and pulmonary valve insufficiency can be expected to become less prominent or disappear entirely following successful valve repair or replacement.

Since mitral stenosis commonly occurs in young women, the disease is often complicated by pregnancy. During pregnancy, there is an increase in both blood volume and cardiac output. Although these changes may be accommodated by patients with other types of heart disease of modest severity, they are poorly tolerated by the patient with mitral stenosis. Not uncommonly, in fact, the first symptoms of heart disease leading to the diagnosis of mitral stenosis occur during pregnancy. Reducing activity and the control of blood volume with low-sodium diet and diuretics are generally successful in bringing these patients through pregnancy and delivery. Occasionally, these measures are not adequate and mitral commissurotomy is required during the second trimester.

Surgical Considerations. Mitral commissurotomy can be performed with or without the aid of cardiopulmonary bypass. This operation, as it is performed today, is highly successful in the majority of cases in relieving mitral valve obstruction at least temporarily. The operation can be carried out with low mortality (1 to 4 per cent) in functional class II and III patients, but carries a considerably higher mortality in class IV patients. Most cardiac surgery centers therefore recommend that this operation be carried out on patients with mitral stenosis when they become significantly disabled by symptoms of their disease. It is best to operate on patients well before they have developed severe limitation, since the operative mortality increases greatly and the benefits of surgery are reduced. If valve replacement is contemplated because of heavy valve calcification and/or associated mitral regurgitation, surgery should be delayed longer, since operative mortality is greater and long-term results are less favorable with this procedure.

Mitral Regurgitation

Mitral regurgitation may occur as a "pure" lesion or may be associated with mitral stenosis. When it is associated with stenosis it is nearly always due to rheumatic heart disease, whereas "pure" mitral regurgitation may be the result of many different diseases.

Pure mitral regurgitation resulting from papillary muscle dysfunction and papillary muscle rupture has been discussed in the section on ischemic heart disease, since these abnormalities are usually the result of this disease. Other causes of mitral regurgitation are ruptured chordae tendineae, mitral annular dilatation and displacement of the papillary muscle due to ventricular dilatation, dysfunction of the mitral valve apparatus due to endocardial fibrosis, and postrheumatic deformity of the valve. Congenital clefts of the mitral valve occur and are often associated with atrial septal defects of the primum type. Myxomatous degeneration of the valve leaflets also occurs. Occasionally, mild mitral regurgitation may be present without apparent cause.

In the past, mitral regurgitation was thought to be a benign condition. Although considerable mitral regurgitation may be well tolerated for years, there is no question that it can cause left ventricular failure and death. The hemodynamics of left ventricular ejection are greatly altered in mitral regurgitation. Normally during the isovolumic phase of systole the myocardial fibers develop tension without shortening. When the intracavitary pressure reaches the pressure in the aorta the aortic valve opens and ejection occurs. In the presence of mitral regurgitation, the isovolumic phase of systole is greatly shortened, or eliminated, since ejection into the left atrium occurs as soon as left ventricular pressure exceeds left atrial pressure.

Angiocardiographic studies of patients with pure mitral regurgitation have shown that there is left ventricular dilatation which is linearly related to the severity of valvular regurgitation. There is also left ventricular hypertrophy, although this is less than that seen with aortic regurgitation of similar magnitude. The systolic ejection fraction is generally in the normal range in patients with mitral regurgitation of rheumatic etiology but is nearly always depressed when regurgitation is due to ischemic heart disease or congestive cardiomyopathy. Chronic mitral regurgitation is frequently present in idiopathic hypertrophic subaortic stenosis but is usually of mild to moderate severity and results from displacement of the papillary muscles by the distorted hypertrophied ventricle rather than from disease of the mitral leaflets or annulus. The left ventricle has a normal or increased ejection fraction in contrast to the depressed ejection fraction seen with other types of cardiomyopathy.

The left atrium is always enlarged in patients with chronic mitral regurgitation and is generally larger than in patients with mitral stenosis as shown in Table 9–3. In a small number of cases it reaches giant proportions (greater than 300 ml. per M.^{2}). The maximum atrial volume is a poor guide to the severity of mitral regurgitation, but the change in atrial volume during the cardiac cycle is increased in mitral regurgitation and has been shown to be related to the severity of regurgitation. The large cyclic change in atrial volume is not dependent upon atrial contraction, since it occurs passively early in diastole. Only the small increment of left atrial emptying which results from atrial contraction is lost when atrial fibrillation develops in these patients.

Pulmonary artery pressure is variable in mitral regurgitation and is dependent upon the severity of valvular regurgitation and more importantly upon the compliance of the left atrium and the pulmonary venous bed. Most often left atrial volume is moderately increased and the atrial wall relatively stiff, so that there is a large systolic pulse pressure or "V" wave seen in the left atrial pressure tracing. This large "V" wave plus a variable increase in pulmonary vascular resistance results in elevation of the pulmonary artery and right ventricular pressure. In some cases of chronic mitral regurgitation, however, the left atrium is unusually large and distensible. This large baglike structure absorbs the regurgitant volume from the left ventricle with little increase in pressure. In these circumstances, severe mitral regurgitation may be present with normal pulmonary artery pressure. When mitral regurgitation develops acutely such as occurs with ruptured chordae tendineae, a small noncompliant left atrium is suddenly subjected to a large pressure and volume load. The left atrial "V" wave may be extremely high (in the range of 60 to 80 mm. Hg) and pulmonary artery pressure is likewise greatly elevated. This combination of events often results in the sudden onset of pulmonary edema.

Surgical treatment of pure mitral regurgitation requires cardiopulmonary bypass with open repair of the valve or prosthetic replacement. Valve clefts and fenestrations may be repaired directly or patched with pericardium or fabric. Best results are obtained when the valve is normal and the annulus is enlarged or when there is chordal rupture. When there is considerable loss of valve substance or the valve is thickened and inflexible, replacement is required.

Combined Mitral Stenosis and Regurgitation

Rheumatic involvement of the mitral valve frequently distorts the leaflets and supporting structures so that a combination of stenosis and regurgitation results. Scarring is usually severe in these cases and heavy calcification is frequently present. The symptoms and clinical features will depend upon whether stenosis or regurgitation is the dominant hemodynamic lesion.

Abnormalities in atrial and ventricular function and anatomy are generally midway between those seen in either pure stenosis or regurgitation alone. Quantitation of the severity of regurgitation in a series of these patients showed that regurgitation flows of more than 5.0 liters per min. per M.^{2} occurred only when valve stenosis was absent.

The presence of both stenosis and regurgitation is of therapeutic importance because surgical treatment usually requires valve replacement, with its attendant mortality and postoperative morbidity. These cases should therefore be treated with conservative medical management until they reach functional class III status.

TABLE 9–3 LEFT ATRIAL VOLUME IN MITRAL VALVE DISEASE

	Number of Cases	Mean	1 SD	Range of Volume
Maximum LA Volume (ml./M.^{2})				
Normal	22	35	9	22–50
Mitral Stenosis	25	117	57	44–288
Mitral Stenosis and Regurgitation	27	180	106	84–596
Mitral Regurgitation	27	183	116	63–547
LA Volume Change (ml./M.^{2})				
Normal	22	18	7.4	5–30
Mitral Stenosis	25	14	9	1–45
Mitral Stenosis and Regurgitation	26	23	11	4–50
Mitral Regurgitation	27	46	27	12–124

By permission of the American Heart Association, Inc.

AORTIC VALVE DISEASE

Aortic stenosis is most often the result of rheumatic endocarditis and is frequently associated with mitral valve disease. When aortic stenosis occurs as an isolated lesion and there is no history of prior rheumatic fever the disease is likely to be the result of a congenital malformation of the valve. It is now known from autopsy studies that bicuspid and other abnormalities of the aortic valve are common congenital cardiac abnormalities. It is the gradual thickening, fibrosis, and calcification of these abnormal valves which eventually result in isolated calcific aortic stenosis in middle and later life.

Aortic stenosis in its pure form uncomplicated by a valvular incompetence presents a systolic pressure load on the left ventricle. This pressure load develops gradually as the valve stenosis becomes more severe and ventricular hypertrophy progresses at a rate adequate to maintain normal cardiac output. Severe aortic valve obstruction may be present for a prolonged period during which time the patient remains asymptomatic. Eventually, owing to either further valve narrowing or decrease in myocardial performance, the cardiac output cannot increase adequately to meet the demand of exercise. The patient then develops exertional dyspnea and may also experience angina pectoris, lightheadedness, or actual syncope. Finally, with further deterioration in myocardial function, congestive heart failure develops.

Evaluation of patients who have exertional lightheadedness or syncope has shown that hypotension develops with physical exertion and at that time symptoms appear. This hypotension which occurs with upright exercise is the result of limited ability to increase cardiac output. The available blood flow is preferentially shunted to the low resistance bed of the working leg muscles, with resulting hypotension and cerebral ischemia. The same phenomenon can be observed in patients with tight mitral stenosis, although syncope is uncommon.

Angina pectoris often occurs in patients with aortic stenosis. Since aortic stenosis occurs most commonly in middle-aged men, associated atherosclerotic heart disease may be the cause of the anginal syndrome. When aortic obstruction is severe, however, angina pectoris frequently occurs in the presence of normal coronary arteries. Angina results from inadequate oxygen supply to the myocardium. In aortic stenosis this is due to a combination of factors including increased myocardial oxygen consumption resulting from increased pressure work, left ventricular hypertrophy, and reduced coronary artery perfusion pressure. The reduction in coronary perfusion pressure occurs because of low aortic root pressure and elevated left ventricular chamber pressure during systole and to some extent in the later portion of diastole.

When syncope and/or angina are present in a patient with aortic stenosis there is a high risk of sudden death which often is associated with physical exertion. It is probable that this is secondary to exertional hypotension resulting in reduced coronary arterial blood flow, myocardial ischemia, and the development of ventricular fibrillation. Patients with tight aortic stenosis and symptoms of angina pectoris and/or syncope require urgent evaluation and surgical correction.

Myocardial Function in Aortic Stenosis

Prior to the onset of myocardial failure the left ventricle responds to a pressure load by hypertrophy without chamber dilatation. The left ventricle in aortic stenosis therefore has normal volume and hypertrophy of the left ventricular myocardium, including the wall, trabeculae, and papillary muscles. Ventricular ejection fraction is usually maintained in the normal range. The left ventricular systolic pressure may be as high as 300 mm. Hg, although it is usually in the range of 200 mm. Hg. This results in a large pressure gradient across the stenotic valve. The aortic pressure is low, has a small pulse pressure, and is slow rising with an anacrotic notch.

Despite a normal end-diastolic volume and ejection fraction, the filling pressure may be significantly elevated before the onset of congestive heart failure. This is the result of vigorous left atrial contraction ejecting blood into the thick-walled noncompliant left ventricle. The elevation of end-diastolic pressure is, therefore, a poor indication of left ventricular myocardial failure in these patients.

In patients with aortic stenosis who have developed congestive heart failure the left ventricle often shows moderate chamber dilatation, reduced stroke volume, reduced ejection fraction, and marked elevation in left ventricular end-diastolic pressure. As the myocardium progressively weakens, the pressure generated in the chamber is reduced and the flow and pressure gradient across the valve fall. If only the pressure gradient is measured during cardiac catheterization and the flow and valve orifice are not determined, the severity of valve stenosis may not be appreciated.

Treatment of Aortic Stenosis. Once severe aortic stenosis has resulted in significant dyspnea, angina, syncope, or congestive heart failure, surgical treatment for relief of aortic valve obstruction must be considered, since medical treatment has only a minor supporting role to play. In an occasional case it may be possible to relieve the stenosis by plastic repair of the valve but the vast majority of cases require valve replacement.

The evaluation of patients by quantitative angiocardiographic techniques before and after surgery indicates that there is a reduction in left ventricular systolic pressure work, a decrease in end-diastolic pressure, and little change in end-diastolic volume. Figure 9–17 presents the pressure-volume diagram in a patient with aortic stenosis without myocardial failure before and following successful homograft aortic valve replacement. The difference in the area enclosed by the two loops represents the reduction in pressure-volume work following surgery. The end-diastolic volume is unchanged despite a fall in the diastolic pressure. Studies of left ventricular mass before and one year following surgery suggest that myocardial hypertrophy regresses, at least to some extent, following successful surgical treatment.

Aortic Regurgitation

Unlike aortic stenosis, aortic regurgitation is a disease of many causes, rheumatic heart disease being the major one. Other causes include luetic aortitis, congenital malformations of the aortic valve often associated with a high ventricular septal defect, Marfan's syndrome with ascending aortic dissection, aneurysm with aortic annular dilatation and cusp rupture secondary to chest wall trauma. When bacterial endocarditis involves the aortic valve severe regurgitation often results. Hypertension of a severe degree occasionally causes mild aortic regurgitation which is reversible when the blood pressure is lowered.

Aortic regurgitation, when severe, places a large volume load on the left ventricle. Since the large stroke volume is ejected into the high resistance systemic circulation a component of pressure overload also occurs in this disease in contrast to the pure volume overload seen in mitral regurgitation. The stroke volume is greatly increased and its forceful ejection from the ventricle results in a wide pulse pressure and often in an elevation in aortic systolic pressure. The leaking aortic valve results in retrograde flow in the aorta during diastole and a fall in aortic diastolic pressure. The impressive peripheral vascular findings in this disease, which include pistol-shot pulses, pulsating capillaries in the nail beds, and systolic head bobbing, are expressions of the widened arterial pulse pressure or the retrograde diastolic flow in the large arteries.

The clinical course of patients with chronic aortic regurgitation is usually a long one, with many years of hemodynamically significant regurgitation tolerated without symptoms. When congestive heart failure finally develops, the downhill course is rapid.

Left ventricular enlargement is a major feature of this disease with both hypertrophy of the myocardium and an increased chamber volume. As in mitral regurgitation, the ventricular diastolic

Figure 9–17 Left ventricular pressure-volume diagrams constructed from cardiac catheterization and angiocardiographic data acquired before and after successful aortic valve replacement for severe aortic stenosis. The area beneath the systolic portion of each loop represents the pressure-volume systolic stroke work of the left ventricle. Preoperatively, systolic work was 226 gram-meters per beat; following aortic valve replacement, systolic work fell to 114 gram-meters per beat. The shaded area indicates the reduction in work as a result of surgery. (Adapted from Kennedy, J. W., Twiss, R. D., Blackmon, J. R., and Merendino, K. A.: Hemodynamic studies one year after homograft aortic valve replacement. Circulation, Suppl. II to Vols. 37 and 38, p. 110, 1968. By permission of the American Heart Association, Inc.)

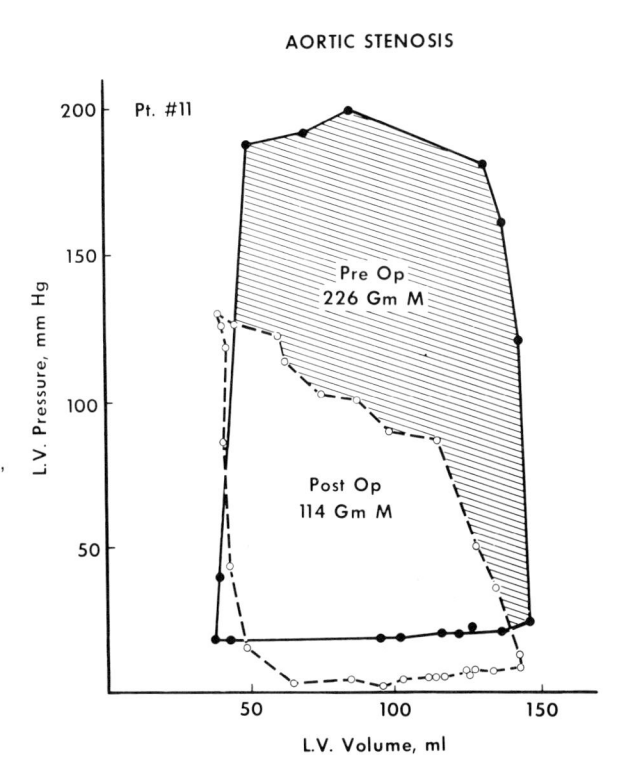

volume is increased in direct proportion to the volume of regurgitation and in extreme cases may reach nearly 800 ml. (Fig. 9–18). The total left ventricular stroke volume is greatly increased, with the forward or systemic stroke volume remaining in the normal range until left ventricular failure develops. Total left ventricular stroke volume including forward and regurgitant fractions may reach 300 ml. or more, with total output approaching 30 liters per minute. This level of ventricular output occasionally seen in these patients at rest is about the same as that achieved by a well-trained healthy young man during maximum exercise. The limits of left ventricular output, therefore, seem to be quite similar in health and in the individual with a compensated left ventricle and severe aortic regurgitation. However, the large minute outputs observed with aortic valve insufficiency are primarily a result of the large stroke volume, whereas the increased outputs observed with exercise are primarily achieved by an increased heart rate. With aortic regurgitation, left ventricular mass may be very large, approaching 1000 grams in severe cases, and averaged 425 grams in 38 cases studied by quantitative angiocardiography. This condition produces the largest left ventricles seen in clinical medicine.

Left ventricular filling pressure is dependent upon the severity of aortic regurgitation, the left ventricular myocardial compliance, and the heart rate. When aortic regurgitation is very severe, the pressures in the aorta and left ventricle may equilibrate during the end of diastole usually at a level of 30 to 40 mm. Hg. This is most likely to occur if the patient has bradycardia. In Figure 9–19, the left ventricular and aortic pressures are seen in a man with severe aortic regurgitation and sinus bradycardia at a rate of 54 per minute. At end-diastole, the pressure in the aorta is 48 mm. Hg and 35 mm. Hg in the left ventricle. Following right atrial pacing at a rate of 82 per minute, the end-diastolic pressure in the aorta became normal at 75 mm. Hg and fell to 10 mm. Hg in the left ventricle. This change in heart rate also resulted in a reduced left ventricular end-diastolic volume and regurgitant flow per beat but no significant change in the volume of aortic regurgitation per minute. This effect of heart rate on ventricular filling pressure accounts for the fact that some patients with aortic regurgitation have dyspnea and angina at rest but have few exercise limitations.

Angina is relatively common in aortic regurgitation, although not as frequent as in aortic stenosis. Left ventricular oxygen consumption is increased in aortic regurgitation because of the associated pressure-volume overload and the ventricular hypertrophy. In addition, the pressure gradient between the aortic root and the intramyocardial and subendocardial coronary vessels is reduced as a result of low aortic diastolic pressure and elevated left ventricular filling pressure. The occurrence of angina pectoris is therefore easily explained in this disease. When aortic regurgitation occurs in middle age, coronary atherosclerosis is also likely to be a contributing factor as a cause of angina, especially when aortic regurgitation is not severe. Patients with leutic aortitis may get calcification and obstruction of one or both of the coronary ostia, which will account for an occasional case of angina in this form of the disease.

When congestive heart failure develops in patients with aortic regurgitation there is either further dilatation of the ventricle, decrease in the total left ventricular stroke volume, or both, so that the ejection fraction falls, the ventricular filling pressure increases, and pulmonary vascular congestion develops. With marked left ventricular dilatation, functional mitral regurgitation occurs owing to enlargement of the mitral annulus or displacement or excessive lengthening of the papillary muscles. The development of mitral regurgitation results in a further decrease of forward output and this combination of valvular defects is poorly tolerated.

Bacterial endocarditis of the aortic valve often results in the sudden development of severe aortic regurgitation due to fenestration, tearing, or rupture of one or more valve cusps. The sudden

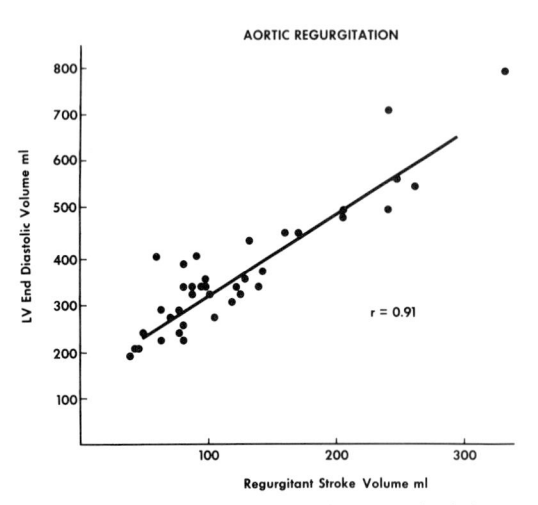

Figure 9–18 The relationship between the left ventricular end-diastolic volume and the regurgitant stroke volume in 38 patients with pure aortic regurgitation. There is a linear relationship between the severity of regurgitation and the ventricular end-diastolic volume. (From Kennedy, J. W., Twiss, R. D., Blackmon, J. R., and Dodge, H. T.: Quantitative angiocardiography, III. Relationship of left ventricular pressure, volume and mass in aortic valve disease. Circulation. 38:838. 1968. By permission of The American Heart Association, Inc.)

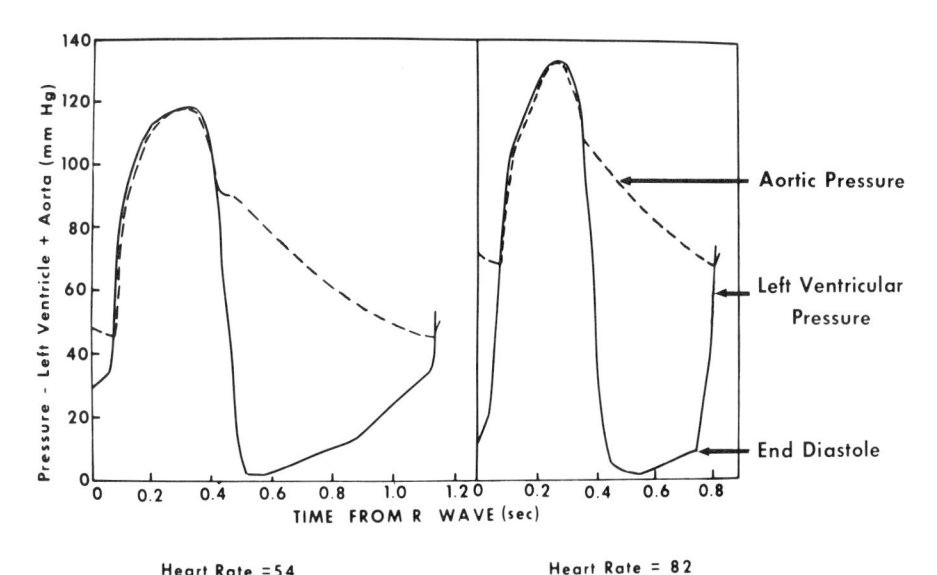

Figure 9-19 Left ventricular and aortic pressure in a patient with severe aortic regurgitation and sinus bradycardia heart rate 54 (left panel) and during right atrial pacing at heart rate 82 (right panel). With pacing, the aortic pressure during diastole has increased, whereas the left ventricular end-diastolic pressure has decreased to a normal level. (From Judge, T. P., Kennedy, J. W., Bennett, L. J., et al.: The quantitative hemodynamic effects of heart rate in aortic regurgitation. Circulation, 44:355, 1971.)

pressure-volume overload imposed upon the normal left ventricle is poorly tolerated and there is extreme elevation of ventricular filling pressure and acute dilatation of the chamber. Pulmonary edema may develop suddenly and immediate surgery is required as a life-saving measure. If the patient survives without surgical treatment, the left ventricle gradually dilates and the myocardium hypertrophies as the left ventricle adjusts to the chronic pressure-volume overload.

Treatment of Aortic Regurgitation. Medical treatment is useful in controlling congestive heart failure. In patients with severe sinus bradycardia or in those with chronic heart block implantation of an artificial pacemaker may result in relief of symptoms. The primary form of treatment is valve repair or replacement. Patients should be disabled by symptoms before valve replacement is recommended. Risk of surgery in aortic regurgitation varies with the cause of the disease, age of the patient, and myocardial function. In good-risk patients without myocardial failure the surgical mortality is in the range of 5 per cent—somewhat lower than the risk in patients with aortic stenosis.

Studies of patients before and after successful valve replacement for severe aortic regurgitation indicate that the end-diastolic volume is greatly reduced following surgery, although it may not return completely to normal. The filling pressure and pressure-volume work are also decreased toward normal. When ventricular myocardial function is depressed prior to surgery it appears to remain abnormal in many patients following surgical correction, suggesting that when better surgical therapy is available valve replacement should be performed at an earlier stage of their disease.

Combined Aortic Stenosis and Regurgitation

The combination of aortic stenosis and regurgitation results from thickened deformed valve leaflets which cannot open or close properly. The disease is most often due to rheumatic endocarditis but also is the frequent result of a congenitally malformed valve. The clinical and hemodynamic pictures are dependent upon whether stenosis or regurgitation is the predominant lesion. Very severe aortic regurgitation does not occur in the presence of significant valve obstruction, so that the marked peripheral vascular signs of aortic regurgitation are less prominent or absent. Surgical treatment is indicated when the patient is disabled by symptoms, and valve replacement is nearly always required.

Combined Aortic and Mitral Valve Disease

When disease of both the mitral and aortic valves is present, one lesion may alter the effects of the other and the overall hemodynamic picture. The most detrimental combination of valve lesions is aortic stenosis and mitral regurgitation because aortic valve obstruction increases the severity of mitral regurgitation and decreases systemic flow. When both aortic and mitral stenosis occur together the left ventricle is protected from pressure load by limited filling and may fail to undergo the usual hypertrophy. Because of decreased flow, the murmurs of both lesions will be diminished, particularly that of aortic stenosis, and the diagnosis may be difficult to make at the bedside. Proper surgical treatment requires that obstruction at both valves be relieved.

In patients with valvular heart disease, tricuspid valve disease is usually associated with mitral valve disease. Tricuspid regurgitation is most often functional and secondary to pulmonary hypertension and right ventricular dilatation. Such functional tricuspid regurgitation usually regresses when mitral valve disease has been adequately treated surgically and there is no residual left ventricular failure to elevate pulmonary vascular pressures. Occasionally, the tricuspid valve is structurally abnormal owing to involvement by the rheumatic process with organic tricuspid stenosis, tricuspid regurgitation, or both. In this situation, the tricuspid valve may require valvuloplasty or replacement. Other types of tricuspid valve disease include congenital tricuspid stenosis and atresia, Ebstein's anomaly of the tricuspid valve, and tricuspid valve insufficiency from endocardial fibrosis of the right heart as observed in the carcinoid syndrome.

THE CARDIOMYOPATHIES

The term cardiomyopathy is used to refer to a group of diseases which involve the myocardium directly. The term primary myocardial disease has been used to refer to the subgroup of cardiomyopathies which are idiopathic and the term secondary myocardial disease used to designate the group in which causative factors are known. Although there is no uniform agreement on terminology, Fowler has suggested that cardiomyopathy is a satisfactory term for this entire group of diseases. Further classification into idiopathic and secondary cardiomyopathy seems sensible and should avoid confusion. A classification from Fowler is given in Table 9–4. The list of secondary cardiomyopathies is long but the number of cases represented by that group is quite small, being less than 25 per cent in the experience of most cardiology services.

The true incidence of the various cardiomyopathies is not well known because of the tendency to diagnose ischemic heart disease when obvious congenital and rheumatic heart disease are not present. When carefully looked for, various types of cardiomyopathy are frequently recognized. It must be remembered that the specific incidence will vary considerably depending upon the particular population of patients concerned. It is known that idiopathic cardiomyopathy is more frequent among indigent patient populations than in individuals from higher socio-economic groups. Recent animal ex-

TABLE 9–4 CLASSIFICATION OF CARDIOMYOPATHIES

Idiopathic Cardiomyopathy
  Nonobstructive cardiomyopathy
    Alcoholic cardiomyopathy
    Postinfectious cardiomyopathy (when infectious agent cannot be identified)
    Familial cardiomyopathy
    Peripartal cardiomyopathy
    Cardiomyopathy without identifiable antecedent illness
  Obstructive cardiomyopathy
    Familial
    Nonfamilial

Secondary Cardiomyopathy
  Myocarditis
    Viral: Coxsackie B, Coxsackie A, echo virus, influenza virus, infectious mononucleosis
    Rheumatic
    Septic (including bacterial endocarditis)
    Diphtheritic
    Syphilitic
    Chagas' disease
    Trichinosis
    Allergic
    Toxic
    Uremic
    Toxoplasmic
  Neuromuscular and neurologic disorders
    Progressive muscular dystrophy; pseudohypertrophic and facioscapulohumeral muscular dystrophy
    Friedreich's ataxia
    Myotonic muscular dystrophy
  Connective tissue diseases: rheumatoid disease, dermatomyositis, scleroderma, disseminated lupus erythematosus
  Mucopolysaccharidosis (e.g., Hurler's syndrome, Hunter's syndrome)
  Sarcoidosis
  Amyloid disease
  Primary and metastatic tumors
  Metabolic disorders
    Glycogen storage disease
    Nutritional deficiency
      Beriberi
      Kwashiorkor
    Thyrotoxicosis
    Myxedema
    Hemochromatosis
    Nutritional cirrhosis

From Fowler, N. O.: Progr. Cardiovasc. Dis., *14*:113–128, 1971. By permission of Grune and Stratton, Inc.

periments suggest that exercise in the face of active myocarditis due to virus infection or Chagas' disease is associated with an increase in myocardial damage. Nutritional deficiency has a similar detrimental influence. These studies offer a possible explanation for the high incidence of these diseases in indigent populations.

Idiopathic Cardiomyopathy

There are two general categories of diseases in the idiopathic group—obstructive and nonobstructive. The obstructive cardiomyopathies are very different from the nonobstructive in their hemodynamic manifestations and will be discussed first.

Obstructive Cardiomyopathies. The obstructive cardiomyopathies, known as idiopathic hypertrophic subaortic stenosis (IHSS), have been well studied since the classic report of Braunwald and colleagues in the early 1960s. The unusual dynamic character of the obstruction has been defined and rational methods of medical and surgical treatment have been developed. A familial incidence has been recognized in about 30 per cent of cases, but the etiology remains obscure.

This disease has been recognized from infancy to old age but is usually seen in young adults. It is manifest by palpitations, angina, or effort or postexertional syncope and is associated with a high incidence of sudden death. Symptoms of pulmonary congestion and congestive heart failure develop late in the disease. Physical examination reveals a systolic ejection murmur at the lower left sternal border and an intact aortic second sound. There is an associated murmur of mitral insufficiency in about 50 per cent of cases. The ejection murmur increases in intensity with standing, during the Valsalva maneuver, or following the administration of amyl nitrite or nitroglycerin. The beat following a premature contraction is characterized by an increase in the systolic pressure gradient and in the intensity of the ejection murmur and by a reduced arterial pulse pressure. Treatment with digitalis may cause an increase in the murmur and a worsening of symptoms and is contraindicated in this disease. Hemodynamic studies reveal a pressure gradient between the left ventricular inflow tract and outflow tract. The pressure gradient is increased by the drugs and maneuvers noted above and is often decreased by the administration of a beta blocking drug such as propranolol.

Left ventricular angiocardiography usually reveals generalized left ventricular hypertrophy with marked hypertrophy of the papillary muscles. The basal portion of the interventricular septum is greatly hypertrophied, although this may be difficult to appreciate by angiography. The end-diastolic volume of the left ventricle is usually normal but the end-systolic volume is smaller than normal with almost complete obliteration of the apical portion of the ventricle, which may appear as a finger-shaped cavity. Quantitative angiocardiographic evaluation reveals an increased ejection fraction and marked increase in left ventricular mass. The coronary arteries often appear to be extremely large.

Left ventricular end-diastolic pressure is usually elevated and may be extremely high while left ventricular dp/dt is elevated as well. The high filling pressure in combination with an elevated ejection fraction and LV dp/dt suggest that the myocardium is noncompliant but retains normal or has increased contractility.

Surgical exploration reveals a normal aortic valve and localized hypertrophy of the basal portion of the interventicular septum just below the aortic valve. This area of the septum may be very fibrotic and there may be considerable thickening of the endocardium. It appears, therefore, that outflow obstruction develops in this disease because the anterior leaflet of the mitral valve is pulled into apposition with the hypertrophied interventricular septum during systole. The actual site of obstruction is often difficult to visualize by angiography.

From the above description it can be appreciated that conditions which reduce end-diastolic volume or increase the contractile state of the left ventricle will tend to increase the subvalvular pressure gradient. These include inotropic drugs such as isoproterenol and digitalis glycosides, reduced venous return to the left heart as induced by postural changes, the Valsalva maneuver or loss of blood volume, and reduced left ventricular afterload as induced with nitroglycerin or amyl nitrite. Beta blocking drugs are specific for this disease in that they can be shown to reduce or eliminate the outflow obstruction in many of these cases. When severe obstruction is present that does not respond to beta blockade, surgical treatment with excision of the hypertrophied muscle of the outflow tract may be beneficial.

Nonobstructive Cardiomyopathies. The majority of idiopathic cardiomyopathies are of the nonobstructive type. In the United States they are found most often in patients with high alcohol consumption or in the immediate pre- or postpartum periods. Although alcohol administration has been shown to reduce ventricular contractility, the actual etiologic role of alcohol in the production of chronic progressive cardiomyopathy is not known. Peripartum cardiomyopathy is also not well understood, although it is most common in poorly nourished individuals, suggesting the importance of nutritional factors.

In years past, it was thought that most cases of chronic heart disease were either of valvular etiology or due to chronic myocarditis. When the high incidence of ischemic heart disease in Western countries became appreciated, chronic myocarditis became an unusual diagnosis. Although there are well-documented cases of acute viral or bacterial myocarditis having progressed to produce chronic myocardial failure, in general there is complete recovery. In fact, it is extremely unusual to see patients with cardiomyopathy in whom one can obtain a history suggesting an etiology of infectious disease. Therefore, although the concept that chronic cardiomyopathy is due to either prior or continuing low-grade myocarditis is appealing, there is little evidence to support this view.

Most patients with nonobstructive cardiomyopathy present with symptoms and signs of heart failure, but occasionally arrhythmias are the presenting complaint. Chest pain is unusual. The heart is large and all four chambers are frequently involved. Auscultation reveals a prominent atrial and/or ventricular gallop sound and there may be no murmur. When a murmur is present it is due to functional mitral and/or tricuspid regurgitation.

Cardiac catheterization usually reveals elevated atrial pressures with large "a" waves. The end-diastolic pressure is elevated in both ventricles and the pulmonary artery pressure is elevated secondary to the elevation of the left heart filling pressure. The cardiac output is low and the arteriovenous oxygen difference may be greatly elevated. Left ventricular dp/dt is depressed.

Angiocardiography reveals dilated cardiac chambers. The left ventricle has an increased diastolic volume and poor stroke volume, yielding a low ejection fraction, usually below 40 per cent. In severe cases, the ejection fraction may be as low as 10 per cent. The papillary muscles are not prominent but the left ventricular free wall is generally hypertrophied to a modest degree. Left ventricular mass is elevated and is generally equal to the diastolic volume of the left ventricle, yielding a left ventricular mass to end-diastolic volume ratio of about one.

Occasionally, there is a restrictive hemodynamic pattern seen in these patients with marked elevation in venous pressure and high plateau diastolic pressures seen in all cardiac chambers as is found in constrictive pericarditis. At times, it may be difficult to distinguish this disease from constrictive pericarditis without the aid of pericardial and myocardial biopsy. The restrictive form of the disease is seen most often in patients who either have myocardial infiltration with amyloid or hemochromatosis or have marked thickening and fibrosis of the endocardium. A form of extreme endomyocardial fibrosis is prevalent among natives of Uganda. In this condition, there is dense fibrosis of endocardium and myocardium with involvement of the papillary muscles resulting in mitral regurgitation. The etiology of this disease remains obscure.

Secondary Cardiomyopathies

Cardiomyopathy may be associated with a large number of specific disease entities as shown in Table 9–4. Myocardial involvement as is seen with most of these diseases has hemodynamic features similar to those observed with the nonobstructive cardiomyopathies described above. There is loss of myocardial contractile force with ventricular dilatation, high filling pressure, low ejection fraction, and low cardiac output. When there is myocardial infiltration there is a tendency toward reduced myocardial compliance and a restrictive filling pattern. Exceptions are the cardiomyopathies associated with thyrotoxicosis and beriberi, in which cardiac output is elevated.

Specific cardiomyopathies are associated with certain neuromuscular diseases including Friedreich's ataxia and the muscular dystrophies. In Friedreich's ataxia there is progressive myocardial fibrosis and obliterative disease of the small coronary arteries which is not due to atherosclerosis. The basis for the relationship between the neuromuscular disease and the cardiomyopathy is not apparent at this time.

Unfortunately, the majority of patients with cardiomyopathy represent difficult therapeutic problems. Cardiomyopathies due to specific infections can be treated and those due to a specific nutritional or metabolic abnormality may also be treated specifically. Patients with obstructive cardiomyopathy often respond favorably to therapy with drugs or surgery, although such therapy does not affect the fundamental basis for the disease. The majority of patients with the nonobstructive types of cardiomyopathy will have a favorable clinical response to nonspecific measures such as bed rest, digitalis, and diuretics. Not infrequently, the response is dramatic and clinical improvement continues for a number of years. However, these diseases are progressive, and response to therapy is less satisfactory with advancement of disease.

PERICARDIAL DISEASE

The pericardium, a fibrous sac surrounding the heart, consists of an outer parietal and inner visceral portion lined by a serous surface and normally contains a small amount of serous fluid. It has been demonstrated to have a function in limiting acute dilatation of the heart and possibly serves to isolate the heart from the lungs and to inhibit the spread of infection from the lungs to the heart. These functions do not seem to be very important in that surgical removal of the pericardium is unassociated with abnormalities of heart function, although there may be some increase in the size of the cardiac silhouette on x-ray examination. Disease of the pericardium is manifest through pain, pericardial effusion, or pericardial constriction of the heart.

Pericardial pain is associated with inflammation or other conditions which irritate the pericardium. The most common cause of pericardial pain is acute pericarditis, but pain also occurs with irritation from leakage of blood into the pericardium, as may be associated with trauma, perforation of the heart, or dissecting aneurysm. The pain is substernal or precordial in location and, in contrast to the pain accompanying myocardial infarction, is accentuated by respiratory movements and occasionally by swallowing. The patient is often more comfortable when sitting and leaning forward. The pain may radiate to the neck, left shoulder, arm, or back. Studies have demonstrated that pain sensation arises from the inferior portion of the parietal pericardium and is transmitted via the phrenic nerves. However, pericardial pain has been relieved by stellate ganglion block, suggesting that at least some pericardial pain fibers travel with the sympathetic nerves.

Pericarditis

The most frequent cause of acute pericarditis is so-called acute idiopathic or nonspecific pericarditis. Pericarditis also occurs in association with a large number of other diseases and conditions which include myocardial infarction, postmyocardial infarction and post-thoracotomy syndrome; specific bacterial, viral, and fungal infections; neoplasms; uremia; certain drug sensitivity reactions; and connective tissue disorders such as rheumatic fever and lupus erythematosus. The pain is often severe and may simulate the pain of myocardial infarction. Inflammatory disease of the pericardium is usually accompanied by systemic signs associated with inflammation such as fever and leukocytosis. On auscultation there is usually a pericardial friction rub, which is a scratchy type sound, often with three separate components associated with atrial systole, ventricular systole, and ventricular diastole. There are often electrocardiographic changes which are characterized by an ST current of injury directed downward and to the left in the direction of the cardiac apex, probably a result of diffuse epicardial injury. Over a period of days, and as the ST subsides, the T wave characteristically becomes abnormal and directed up toward the right shoulder, away from the cardiac apex. Pericarditis is usually associated with pericardial effusion, which is manifest as an increase in the size of the heart on x-ray examination and occasionally by evidence of pericardial tamponade.

Pericardial Effusion

Whether pericardial effusion is associated with pericardial tamponade depends on the rate and volume of fluid accumulation within the pericardium. Acute effusions and/or bleeding of 200 to 300 ml. within the pericardium may result in tamponade. When pericardial fluid accumulates slowly, the pericardial sac enlarges, so that more than a liter may be present with no evidence of tamponade.

Large pericardial effusions are usually observed with the more chronic forms of pericarditis and, in contrast to acute pericarditis, pain is little or absent. Pericardial effusion is also common in myxedema and congestive heart failure. The pressure-volume characteristics of the pericardium are such that substantial amounts of fluid may accumulate with little increase in pressure. However, a volume is reached at which pressure begins to rise rapidly with further small increases in volume.

On examination, the patient with pericardial effusion characteristically shows an increase in the area of cardiac dullness to percussion with a quiet precordium and distant heart sounds. The cardiac silhouette is enlarged, often with a water-bottle type configuration. Low voltage is often present in the electrocardiogram.

With pericardial tamponade there is interference with diastolic filling of the heart, resulting in an elevated filling pressure. A characteristic hemodynamic feature of pericardial tamponade is elevation of right and left atrial pressure and the diastolic pressure in the right and left ventricles to similar levels, as is observed in constrictive pericarditis (Fig. 9–20). This feature is often helpful in differentiating pericardial tamponade from left ventricular failure which is associated with higher filling pressures on the left side of the heart. Dyspnea is usually present, but orthopnea absent unless tamponade is severe. Arterial hypotension also occurs with severe tamponade.

Pulsus paradoxicus is a classic finding in pericardial tamponade and is recognized by a rise and fall of systemic systolic arterial pressure of more than 8 to 10 mm. Hg in the recumbent subject during quiet respiration. There have been a number of explanations for this phenomenon. It appears to be related to increased filling of the right heart with reduced filling of the left heart during inspiration. Because in pericardial tamponade there is a restriction of diastolic volume of the entire heart, an increase in diastolic volume of the right ventricle, as occurs during inspiration, must be associated with a reduced diastolic volume of the left heart. An increased pulmonary blood volume is also suggested as contributing to reduced filling of the left ventricle during inspiration. It should be appreciated that pulsus paradoxicus is not a specific finding for pericardial tamponade but also may occur with any condition associated with larger than normal respiratory changes of intrathoracic pressure and with heart failure.

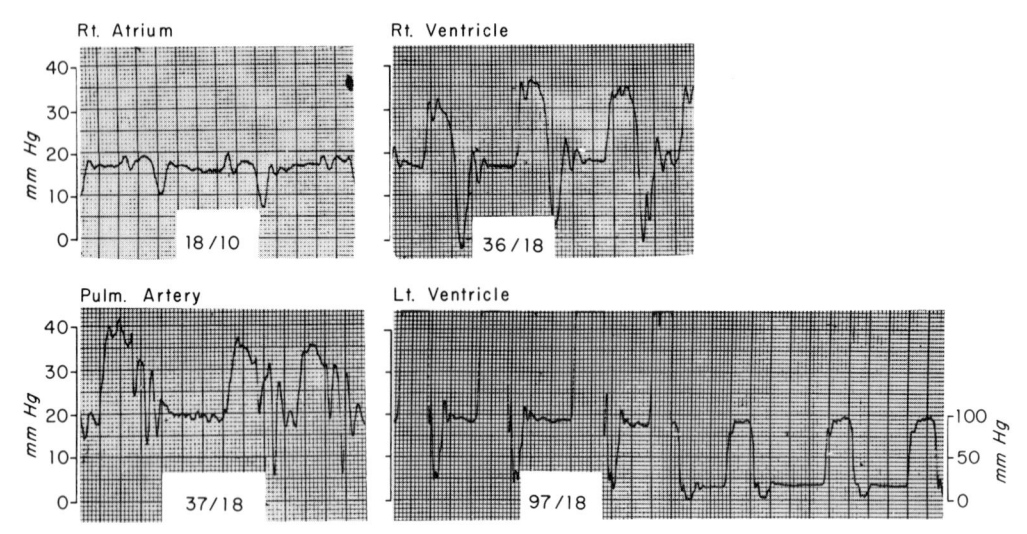

Figure 9-20 Pressures from a patient with constrictive pericarditis. The similarity of pressures during diastole in the right atrium, pulmonary artery, and right and left ventricles is shown. Both right and left ventricular diastolic pressures show a characteristic early diastolic dip followed by a diastolic plateau.

The differentiation of pericardial effusion and tamponade from generalized cardiac enlargement is a rather common clinical problem. Demonstration of pericardial fluid by echocardiography or of a wide margin between the cardiac chamber and the external surface of the cardiac shadow by a radioisotope technique, by angiocardiography, or by filming following the introduction of carbon dioxide into the venous circulation is often helpful. The demonstration of fluid by pericardiocentesis, of course, establishes the diagnosis of pericardial effusion. Examination of the fluid may also be helpful in establishing an etiologic basis for pericardial effusion and pericarditis.

The treatment for pericardial tamponade is removal of pericardial fluid. This results in a prompt relief of symptoms due to the tamponade.

Constrictive Pericarditis

Constrictive pericarditis occurs when pericardial fibrosis and thickening result in restriction of diastolic feeling of the heart. In this condition the visceral and parietal layers of the pericardium are adherent and may be greatly thickened and densely fibrotic with areas of calcification. Pericardial constriction is known to occur with or following infection of the pericardium with tuberculosis, pyogenic organisms, certain viral diseases, and with acute idiopathic pericarditis. It also occurs with neoplastic involvement of the pericardium, with certain connective tissue disorders such as lupus erythematosus, following radiation therapy, and following hemopericardium from a variety of causes. However, in most patients it is not possible to establish a cause.

The laboratory and clinical findings are consequences of the restricted diastolic filling which results in venous pressure elevation. Because the entire heart is encased in this sac, filling pressures are usually elevated to similar levels on the two sides of the heart, so that right and left atrial, right and left ventricular diastolic, pulmonary wedge, and pulmonary artery diastolic pressures are nearly equal. This is illustrated in Figure 9-20. Other features of the pressure tracings characteristic of constrictive pericarditis are as follows: (1) a rapid fall of ventricular pressure in early diastole resulting in an early diastolic dip followed by a flat diastolic plateau (see right and left ventricular pressures in Figure 9-20); (2) a rapid descent of right atrial pressure with the onset of ventricular filling (y descent) which often results in a right atrial pressure curve that has a "w" or "m" configuration. Right ventricular and pulmonary artery systolic pressures are usually only modestly elevated, with the right ventricular diastolic pressure one third or more of the systolic pressure, also as shown in Figure 9-20. These pressure findings are not absolutely diagnostic of constrictive pericarditis and occasionally occur with chronic myocardial failure and fibrosis. However, with left ventricular failure the filling pressure is usually higher on the left side of the heart and right ventricular and pulmonary artery systolic pressures are usually higher than is observed with constrictive pericarditis. Stroke volume is small, but, unless constriction is severe, the cardiac index is only slightly reduced and increases with exercise through an increase in heart rate. The cardiac chamber volumes are characteristically normal or reduced. A thickened wall of the heart due to pericardial thickening can usually be demonstrated by angiocardiography or by positioning a cardiac catheter against the wall of the right atrium at the time of cardiac catheterization, so that the distance from the endocardium to the external surface of the right atrium can be visualized.

Patients with constrictive pericarditis may have an elevated venous pressure for long periods prior to the development of other symptoms or signs such as edema and exertional dyspnea. Edema often appears as ascites and in longstanding cases may be complicated by cardiac cirrhosis of the liver. Weeping of plasma with plasma proteins into the gastrointestinal tract as a result of venous pressure elevation may contribute to hypoproteinemia which is observed in severe cases of long duration. In spite of an elevated venous pressure and edema, orthopnea is usually absent and pulmonary edema is unusual.

On examination, patients with constrictive pericarditis have findings associated with an elevated systemic venous pressure and peripheral edema. Pleural effusion is often present. The area of cardiac dullness and the cardiac silhouette on x-ray examination is of normal size or only moderately enlarged. Heart sounds may be distant, and a pericardial knock sound in early diastole resembling a third heart sound is often present. A paradoxical pulse is occasionally observed. The electrocardiogram commonly has low voltage and flat or abnormally directed T waves. Atrial fibrillation is present in approximately one third of patients. On chest x-ray or fluoroscopic examination approximately 50 per cent of patients with constrictive pericarditis have pericardial calcification.

In patients with constrictive pericarditis and edema, symptomatic improvement is observed following diuresis induced by one of the diuretic drugs. However, surgical removal of the constricting pericardium is the definitive therapy. Unfortunately, pericardiectomy for constrictive pericarditis is associated with a significant mortality, which is in the range of 5 to 10 per cent, and occasionally with incomplete relief or recurrence of constriction.

REFERENCES

GENERAL

Conn, H. L., and Horwitz, O.: Cardiac and Vascular Diseases. Philadelphia, Lea and Febiger, 1971.

Friedberg, C. K.: Diseases of the Heart. 3rd ed. Philadelphia, W. B. Saunders Co., 1966.

Hurst, J. W., and Logue, R. B.: The Heart. 2nd ed. New York, McGraw-Hill Book Co., 1970.

Zimmerman, H. A.: Intravascular Catheterization. 2nd ed. Springfield, Illinois, Charles C Thomas, 1966.

CARDIAC OUTPUT, PRESSURE MEASUREMENTS, AND CARDIAC CATHETERIZATION

Barratt-Boyes, B. G., and Wood, E. H.: Cardiac output and related measurements and pressure values in the right heart and associated vessels, together with an analysis of the hemodynamic response to the inhalation of high oxygen mixtures in healthy subjects. J. Lab. Clin. Med., 51:72, 1958.

Brandfonbrener, M., Landowne, M., and Shock, N. W.: Changes in cardiac output with age. Circulation, 12:557, 1955.

Burch, G. E., and DePasquale, N. P.: Cardiac performance in relation to cardiac output and blood volume. Amer. J. Cardiol., 14:784, 1964.

Donald, K. W., Bishop, J. M., and Wade, O. L.: Effect of nursing positions on cardiac output of man with a note on the repeatability of measurements of cardiac output by the direct Fick method and with data on subjects with normal cardiovascular system. Clin. Sci., 12:199, 1953.

Dow, P.: Estimations of cardiac output and central blood volume by dye dilution. Physiol. Rev., 36:77, 1956.

Fegler, G.: The reliability of the thermo-dilution method for determination of the cardiac output and the blood flow in central veins. Quart. J. Exp. Physiol., 42:254, 1957.

Fry, D. L., Noble, F. W., and Mallos, A. J.: An evaluation of modern pressure recording systems. Circ. Res., 5:40, 1957.

Gorlin, R., and Gorlin, S. G.: Hydraulic formula for calculation of the area of the stenotic mitral valve, other cardiac valves and central circulatory shunts. Amer. Heart J., 1:41, 1951.

Hamilton, W. F., Riley, R. L., Attah, A. M., Cournand, A., Fowell, D. M., Himmelstein, R. P., Wheeler, N. C., and Witham, A. C.: Comparison of Fick and dye injection methods of measuring cardiac output in man. Amer. J. Physiol., 153:309, 1948.

Kinsmann, J. M., More, J. W., and Hamilton, W. F.: Studies on the circulation. Injection method; physical and mathematical considerations. Amer. J. Physiol., 89:322, 1929.

Mandel, D.: A Practice of Cardiac Catheterization. Chapter 13. Oxford and Edinburgh, Blackwell Scientific Publications, 1968.

Reeves, J. T., Grover, R. F., Filley, G. F., and Blount, S. G., Jr.: Cardiac output in normal resting man. J. Appl. Physiol., 16:276, 1961.

Samet, P., Bernstein, W. H., and Levine, S.: Transseptal left heart dynamics in 32 normal subjects. Dis. Chest, 47:633, 1965.

Selzer, A., and Sudrann, R. B.: Reliability of the determination of cardiac output in man by means of the Fick principle. Circ. Res., 6:485, 1958.

Shapiro, G. G., and Kravetz, L. J.: Damped and undamped frequency responses of underdamped catheter manometer systems. Amer. Heart J., 80:226, 1970.

Stewart, G. N.: Researches on the circulation time and on the influences which affect it. J. Physiol., 22:169, 1887.

Swan, H. J., Marcus, H. S., and Allen, H. N.: Cardiac flow, volumes and pressure. In Conn, H. L., and Horwitz, O. (Eds.): Cardiac and Vascular Diseases. Philadelphia, Lea and Febiger, 1971, pp. 54–73.

Thomassen, B.: Cardiac output in normal subjects under standard basal conditions. The repeatability of measurements by the Fick method. Scand. J. Clin. Lab. Invest., 9:365, 1957.

Visscher, M. B., and Johnson, J. A.: The Fick principle: Analysis of potential errors in its conventional application. J. Appl. Physiol., 5:635, 1953.

Wade, O. L., and Bishop, J. M.: Cardiac Output and Regional Blood Flow. Philadelphia, F. A. Davis Co., 1962.

Yanof, H. M., Rosen, A. L., McDonald, N. M., and McDonald, D. A.: A critical study of the response of manometers to forced oscillations. Phys. Med. Biol., 8:407, 1963.

LEFT VENTRICULAR VOLUME AND MASS

Bartle, S. H., and Sanmarco, M. E.: Comparison of angiocardiographic and thermal washout techniques for left ventricular volume measurement. Amer. J. Cardiol., 18:235, 1966.

Bove, A. A., and Lynch, P. R.: Measurement of canine left ventricular performance by cineradiography of the heart. J. Appl. Physiol., 29:877, 1970.

Bristow, J. D., Van Zee, B. E., and Judkins, M. P.: Systolic and diastolic abnormalities of the left ventricle in coronary artery disease. Circulation, 42:219, 1970.

Bunnell, I. L., Grant, C., and Greene, D. G.: Left ventricular function derived from the pressure-volume diagram. Amer. J. Med., 39:881, 1965.

Burns, J. W., Covell, J. W., Myers, R., and Ross, J., Jr.: Comparison of directly measured left ventricular wall stress and stress calculated from geometric reference figures. Circ. Res., 28:611, 1971.

Davila, J. C., and Sanmarco, M. E.: An analysis of the fit of mathematical models applicable to the measurement of left ventricular volume. Amer. J. Cardiol., 18:31, 1966.

Dodge, H. T.: Determination of left ventricular volume and mass. Radiol. Clin. N. Amer., 9:459, 1971.

Dodge, H. T., and Baxley, W. A.: Left ventricular volume and mass and their significance in heart disease. Amer. J. Cardiol., 23:528, 1969.

Dodge, H. T., Hay, R. E., and Sandler, H.: An angiocardiographic method for directly determining left ventricular stroke volume in man. Circ. Res., 11:739, 1962.

Dodge, H. T., Sandler, H., Ballew, D. W., and Lord, J. D., Jr.: The use of biplane angiocardiography for the measurement of left ventricular volume in man. Amer. Heart J., 60:762, 1960.

Dodge, H. T., Sandler, H., Baxley, W. A., and Hawley, R. R.: Usefulness and limitations of radiographic methods for determining left ventricular volume. Amer. J. Cardiol., 18:10, 1966.

Falsetti, H. J., Mates, R. E., Greene, D. G., and Bunnell, I. L.: V_{max} as an index of contractile state in man. Circulation, 43:323, 1971.

Gault, J. H., Covell, J. W., Braunwald, E., and Ross, J., Jr.: Left ventricular performance following correction of free aortic regurgitation. Circulation, 42:773, 1970.

Gault, J. H., Ross, J., Jr., and Braunwald, E.: Contractile state of the left ventricle in man. Circ. Res., 22:451, 1958.

Graham, T. P., Jr., Jarmakani, M. M., Canent, R. V., Capp, M. P., and Spach, M. S.: Characterization of left heart volumes and mass in normal children and in infants with intrinsic myocardial disease. Circulation, 38:826, 1968.

Graham, T. P., Jr., Jarmakani, M. M., Canent, R. V., Jr., and Morrow, M. N.: Left heart volume estimation in infancy and childhood. Circulation, 43:895, 1971.

Grant, C., Greene, D. G., and Bunnell, I. L.: Left ventricular enlargement and hypertrophy. Amer. J. Med., 39:895, 1965.

Greene, D. G., Carlisle, R., Grant, C., and Bunnell, I. L.: Estimation of left ventricular volume by one-plane cineangiography. Circulation, 35:61, 1967.

Holt, J. P.: Estimation of the residual volume of the ventricle of the dog heart by two indicator dilution techniques. Circ. Res., 4:187, 1956.

Hood, W. P., Jr., Rackley, C. E., and Rolett, E. L.: Wall stress in the normal and hypertrophied human left ventricle. Amer. J. Cardiol., 22:550, 1968.

Hood, W. P., Jr., Thomson, W. J., Rackley, C. E., and Rolett, E. L.: Comparison of calculations of left ventricular wall stress in man from thin-walled and thick-walled ellipsoidal models. Circ. Res., 24:575, 1969.

Hugenholtz, P. G., Kaplan, E., and Hull, E.: Determination of left ventricular wall thickness by angiocardiography. Amer. Heart J., 78:513, 1969.

Hugenholtz, P. G., Wagner, H. R., and Sandler, H.: The in-vivo determination of left ventricular volume: comparison of the fiberoptic-indicator dilution and the angiocardiographic methods. Circulation, 37:489, 1968.

Jarmakani, M. M., Graham, T. P., Jr., Canent, R. V., and Capp, M. P.: The effect of corrective surgery on left heart volume and mass in children with ventricular septal defect. Amer. J. Cardiol., 27:254, 1971.

Jarmakani, M. M., Graham, T. P., Jr., Canent, R. V., Spach, M. S., and Capp, M. P.: Effect of site of shunt on left heart-volume characteristics in children with ventricular septal defect and patent ductus arteriosus. Circulation, 40:411, 1969.

Karliner, J. S., Gault, J. H., Eckberg, D., Mullins, C. B., and Ross, J., Jr.: Mean velocity of fiber shortening. A simplified measure of left ventricular myocardial contractility. Circulation, 44:323, 1971.

Kasser, I. S., and Kennedy, J. W.: Measurement of left ventricular volumes in man by single plan cineangiocardiography. Invest. Radiol., 4:83, 1969.

Kennedy, J. W., Baxley, W. A., Figley, M. M., Dodge, H. T., and Blackmon, J. R.: Quantitative angiocardiography. The normal left ventricle in man. Circulation, 34:272, 1966.

Levine, J. H., McIntyre, K. M., Lipana, J. G., and Bing, O. H. L.: Force velocity relations in failing and nonfailing hearts of subjects with aortic stenosis. Amer. J. Med. Sci., 259:79, 1970.

Mason, D. T., Spann, J. F., Jr., and Zelis, R.: Quantification of the contractile state of the intact left ventricle. Maximal velocity of contractile element shortening determined by the instantaneous relation between the rate of pressure rise and pressure in the left ventricle during isovolumic systole. Amer. J. Cardiol., 26:248, 1970.

Mirsky, I.: Left ventricular stresses in the intact human heart. Biophys. J., 9:189, 1969.

Rackley, C. E., Dear, H. D., Baxley, W. A., Jones, W. F., and Dodge, H. T.: Left ventricular chamber volume, mass and function in severe coronary artery disease. Circulation, 41:605, 1970.

Rackley, C. E., Dodge, H. T., Coble, Y. D., Jr., and Hay, R. E.: A method for determining left ventricular mass in man. Circulation, 29:666, 1964.

Rapaport, E., Wiegand, B. D., and Bristow, J. D.: Estimation of left ventricular residual volume in the dog by a thermodilution method. Circ. Res., 11:803, 1962.

Ross, J., Jr., and Sobel, B. E.: Regulation of cardiac contraction. Ann. Rev. Physiol., 34:47, 1972.

Ross, J., Jr., Sonnenblick, E. H., Taylor, R. R., Spotnitz, H. M., and Covell, J. W.: Diastolic geometry and sarcomere lengths in the chronically dilated canine left ventricle. Circ. Res., 28:49, 1971.

Sandler, H., Dodge, H. T., Hay, R. E., and Rackley, C. E.: Quantitation of valvular insufficiency in man by angiocardiography. Amer. Heart J., 65:501, 1963.

Sandler, H., and Dodge, H. T.: Left ventricular tension and stress in man. Circ. Res., 13:91, 1963.

Sandler, H., and Dodge, H. T.: The use of single plane angiocardiograms for the calculation of left ventricular volume in man. Amer. Heart J., 75:325, 1968.

Swan, H. J. C., and Beck, W.: Ventricular non-mixing as a source of error in the estimation of ventricular volume by the indicator-dilution method. Circ. Res., 8:989, 1960.

Taylor, R. R., Covell, J. W., and Ross, J., Jr.: Left ventricular function in experimental aorto-caval fistula with circulatory congestion and fluid retention. J. Clin. Invest., 47:1333, 1968.

Turina, M., Bussmann, W. D., and Krayenbuhl, H. P.: Contractility of the hypertrophied canine heart in chronic volume overload. Cardiovasc. Res., 3:486, 1969.

Urschel, C. W., Covell, J. W., Sonnenblick, E. H., Ross, J., Jr., and Braunwald, E.: Myocardial mechanics in aortic and mitral valvular regurgitation. The concept of instantaneous impedance as a determinant of the performance of the intact heart. J. Clin. Invest., 47:867, 1968.

Hemodynamics of Heart Failure

Baxley, W. A., Jones, W. B., and Dodge, H. T.: Left ventricular anatomical and functional abnormalities in chronic postinfarction heart failure. Ann. Intern. Med., 74:499, 1971.

Braunwald, E., Frahm, C. J., and Ross, J., Jr.: Studies on Starling's law of the heart. V. Left ventricular function in man. J. Clin. Invest., 40:1882, 1961.

Braunwald, E., Ross, J., Jr., and Sonnenblick, E. H.: Mechanism of contraction of the normal and failing heart. New Eng. J. Med., 277:794, 853, 910, 962, 1012; 1967.

Cohn, J. N., Khatri, I. M., and Hamosh, P.: Diagnostic and therapeutic value of bedside monitoring of left ventricular pressure. Amer. J. Cardiol., 23:107, 1969.

Dodge, H. T., and Baxley, W. A.: Hemodynamic aspects of heart failure. Amer. J. Cardiol., 22:24, 1968.

Patterson, S. W., Piper, H., and Starling, E. H.: The regulation of the heart beat. J. Physiol., 48:465, 1914.

Rapaport, E., and Scheinman, M.: Rationale and limitations of hemodynamic measurements in patients with acute infarction. Mod. Concepts Cardiovasc. Dis., 38:55, 1969.

Russell, R. O., Jr., Porter, C. M., Frimer, M., and Dodge, H. T.: Left ventricular power in man. Amer. Heart J., 81:799, 1971.

Russell, R. O., Jr., Rackley, C. E., Pombo, J., Hunt, D., Potanin, C., and Dodge, H. T.: Effects of increasing left ventricular filling pressure in patients with acute myocardial infarction. J. Clin. Invest., 49:1539, 1970.

Sarnoff, S. J., and Bergland, E.: Ventricular function. I. Starling's law of the heart studied by means of simultaneous right and left ventricular function curves in the dog. Circulation, 9:706, 1954.

ISCHEMIC HEART DISEASE

Barnard, P. M., and Kennedy, J. H.: Postinfarctional ventricular septal defect. Circulation, 32:76, 1965.

Bashour, F. A.: Mitral regurgitation following myocardial infarction. The syndrome of papillary mitral regurgitation. Dis. Chest, 48:113, 1965.

Baxley, W. A., Jones, W. B., and Dodge, H. T.: Left ventricular anatomical and functional abnormalities in chronic postinfarction heart failure. Ann. Intern. Med., 74:499, 1971.

Bristow, J. D., Bruce, E. V., and Judkins, M. P.: Systolic and diastolic abnormalities of the left ventricle in coronary artery disease. Studies in patients with little or no enlargement of ventricular volume. Circulation, 42:219, 1970.

Burch, G. E., DePasquale, N. P., and Phillips, J. H.: The syndrome of papillary muscle dysfunction. Amer. Heart J., 75:399, 1968.

Daggett, W. M., Burwell, L. R., Lawson, D. W., and Austen, W. G.: Resection of acute ventricular aneurysm and ruptured interventricular septum after myocardial infarction. New Eng. J. Med., 283:1507, 1970.

Effler, D. B., Favaloro, R. G., Groves, L. K., and Loop, F. D.: The simple approach to direct coronary artery surgery. J. Thorac. Cardiovasc. Surg., 62:503, 1971.

Effler, D. B., Groves, L. K., and Favaloro, R.: Surgical repair of ventricular aneurysm. Dis. Chest, 48:37, 1965.

Falsetti, H. L., Geraci, A. R., Bunnell, I. L., Greene, D. G., and Grant, C.: Function of left ventricle and extent of coronary lesions: failure of correlation in cineangiographic studies. Chest, 59:610, 1971.

Hamilton, G. H., Murray, J. A., and Kennedy, J. W.: Quantitative angiocardiography in ischemic heart disease. The spectrum of abnormal left ventricular function and the role of abnormally contracting segments. Circulation, 45:1065, 1972.

Herman, M. V., Heinle, R. A., Klein, M. D., and Gorlin, R.: Localized disorders in myocardial contraction. New Eng. J. Med., 277:222, 1967.

Miller, G. E., Cohn, K. E., Kerth, W. J., Selzer, A., and Gerbode, F.: Experimental papillary muscle infarction. J. Thorac. Cardiovasc. Surg., 56:611, 1968.

Rackley, C. E., Dear, H. D., Baxley, W. A., Jones, W. B., and Dodge, H. T.: Left ventricular chamber volume, mass and function in severe coronary artery disease. Circulation, 41:605, 1970.

Schrinert, G., Falsetti, H. L., Bunnell, I. L., Dean, D. C., Gage, A. A., Grant, C., and Green, D. G.: Excision of akinetic left ventricular wall of intractable heart failure. Ann. Intern. Med., 70:437, 1969.

Selzer, A., Gerbode, F., and Kerth, W. J.: Clinical hemodynamic and surgical considerations of rupture of the ventricular septum after myocardial infarction. Amer. Heart J., 78:598, 1969.

Stinson, E. B., Becker, J., and Shumway, N. E.: Successful repair of postinfarction ventricular septal defect and biventricular aneurysm. J. Thorac. Cardiovasc. Surg., 58:20, 1969.

Swithinbank, J. M.: Perforation of the interventricular septum in myocardial infarction. Brit. Heart J., 21:562, 1959.

MITRAL VALVE DISEASE

Arvidsson, H.: Angiocardiographic observations in mitral valve disease, with special reference to the volume variations in the left atrium. Acta Radiol., Suppl. 158, p. 1, 1958.

Blackmon, J. R., Rowell, L. B., Kennedy, J. W., Twiss, R. D., and Conn, R. D.: Physiologic significance of maximal oxygen intake in "pure" mitral stenosis. Circulation, 36:497, 1967.

Braunwald, E.: Mitral regurgitation: physiological, clinical and surgical considerations. New Eng. J. Med., 281:425, 1969.

Braunwald, E., and Awe, W. C.: Syndrome of severe mitral regurgitation and normal left atrial pressure. Circulation, 27:29, 1963.

Braunwald, E., Braunwald, N. S., Ross, J., Jr., and Morrow, A. G.: Effects of mitral valve replacement on the pulmonary vascular dynamics of patients with pulmonary hypertension. New Eng. J. Med., 273:509, 1965.

Dalen, J. E., Matloff, J. M., Evans, G. L., Hoppin, F. G., Bhardnaj, P., Harken, D. E., and Dexter, L.: Early reduction in pulmonary vascular resistance after mitral valve replacement. New Eng. J. Med., 277:387, 1967.

DeSanctis, R. W., Dean, D. C., and Bland, E. F.: Extreme left atrial enlargement. Circulation, 29:14, 1964.

Ellis, L. B., and Harken, D. E.: Closed valvuloplasty for mitral stenosis. New Eng. J. Med., 270:643, 1964.

Friedberg, C. K.: Diseases of the Heart. 3rd ed. Chapter 27. Philadelphia, W. B. Saunders Co., 1966.

Friedman, W. F., and Braunwald, E.: Alterations in regional pulmonary blood flow in mitral valve disease studies by radioisotope scanning. Circulation, 24:363, 1966.

Gerami, S., Messmer, B. J., Hallman, G. L., and Cooley, D. A.: Open mitral commissurotomy, results of 100 conservative cases. J. Thorac. Cardiovasc. Surg., 62:366, 1971.

Hawley, R. R., Dodge, H. T., and Graham, T. P.: Left atrial volume and volume changes in heart disease. Circulation, 34:989, 1966.

Hessel, E. A., Kennedy, J. W., and Merendino, K. A.: A reappraisal of nonprosthetic reconstructive surgery for mitral regurgitation based on an analysis of early and late results. J. Thorac. Cardiovasc. Surg., 52:193, 1966.

Kennedy, J. W., Yarnall, S. R., Murray, J. A., and Figley, M. M.: Quantitative angiocardiography: IV. Relationships of left atrial and ventricular pressure and volume in mitral valve disease. Circulation, 41:817, 1970.

Manhas, D. R., Hessel, E. A., Winterscheid, L. C., Dillard, D. H., and Merendino, K. A.: Repair of mitral incompetence secondary to ruptured chordae tendineae. Circulation, 43:688, 1971.

Merendino, K. A., Thomas, G. I., Jesseph, J. E., Herron, P. W., Winterscheid, L. C., and Vetto, R. R.: The open correction of rheumatic mitral regurgitation and/or stenosis: with special reference to regurgitation treated by posteromedial annuloplasty utilizing a pump oxygenator. Ann. Surg., 150:5, 1959.

Oleson, K. H.: The natural history of 271 patients with mitral stenosis under medical treatment. Brit. Heart J., 27:349, 1962.

Osmundson, P. J., Callahan, J. A., and Edward, J. E.: Ruptured mitral chordae tendineae. Circulation, 23:42, 1961.

Roberts, W. C., Braunwald, E., and Morrow, A. G.: Acute severe mitral regurgitation secondary to ruptured chordae tendineae: clinical, hemodynamic and pathologic considerations. Circulation, 33:58, 1966.

Row, J. C., Bland, E. F., Sprague, H. B., and White, P. D.: The course of mitral stenosis without surgery. Ann. Intern. Med., 52:741, 1960.

Sanders, C. A., Armstrong, P. W., Willerson, J. T., and Dinsmore, R. E.: Etiology and differential diagnosis of acute mitral regurgitation. Prog. Cardiovasc. Dis., 14:129, 1971.

Sanders, C. A., Scannell, J. G., Hawthorne, J. W., and Austen, W. G.: Severe mitral regurgitation secondary to ruptured chordae tendineae. Circulation, 31:506, 1965.

AORTIC VALVE DISEASE

Anderson, F. L., Tsagaris, T. J., Tikoff, G., Thorne, J. L., Schmidt, A. M., and Kuida, H.: Hemodynamic effects of exercise in patients with aortic stenosis. Amer. J. Med., 46:872, 1969.

Angell, W. W., Stenson, E. B., Ibur, A. B., and Shumway, W. E.: Multiple valve replacement with fresh aortic homograft. J. Thorac. Cardiovasc. Surg., 56:323, 1968.

Barratt-Boyes, B. G., and Roche, A. H. G.: A review of aortic valve homografts over a six and one-half year period. Ann. Surg., 170:483, 1969.

Duvoisin, G. E., Wallace, R. B., Ellis, F. H., Anderson, M. W.,

and McGoon, D. C.: Late result of cardiac valve replacement. Circulation (Suppl. II), 37–38:1175, 1968.
Glancy, D. L., and Epstein, S. E.: Differential diagnosis of type and severity of obstruction to left ventricular outflow. Prog. Cardiovasc. Dis., 14:153, 1971.
Judge, T. P., Kennedy, J. W., Bennett, L. J., Wills, R. E., Murray, J. A., and Blackmon, J. R.: The quantitative hemodynamic effects of heart rate in aortic regurgitation. Circulation, 44:355, 1971.
Kennedy, J. W., Twiss, R. D., Blackmon, J. R., and Dodge, H. T.: Quantitative angiocardiography: III. Relationships of left ventricular pressure, volume and mass in aortic valve disease. Circulation, 38:838, 1968.
Morrow, A. G., Roberts, W. C., Ross, J., et al.: Obstruction to left ventricular outflow. NIH Clinical Staff Conference. Ann. Intern. Med., 69:1285, 1968.
Najafi, H.: Aortic insufficiency. Clinical manifestations and surgical treatment. Amer. Heart J., 82:120, 1971.
Roberts, W. C.: The structure of the aortic valve in clinically isolated aortic stenosis. Circulation, 42:91, 1970.
Rotman, M., Morris, J. J., Behar, V. S., Peter, R. H., and Kong, Y.: Aortic valve disease – comparison of types and their medical and surgical management. Amer. J. Med., 51:241, 1971.
Segal, J., Harvey, W. P., and Hufnagel, C.: A clinical study of 100 cases of severe aortic insufficiency. Amer. J. Med., 21:200, 1956.
Shean, F. C., Austen, W. G., Buckley, M. J., Mundth, E. D., Scanwell, J. G., and Daggett, W. M.: Survival after Starr-Edwards aortic valve replacement. Circulation, 44:1, 1971.
Spangnuolo, M., Kloth, H., Taranta, A., Doyle, E., and Pasternack, B.: Natural history of rheumatic aortic regurgitation: criteria predictive of death, congestive heart failure and angina in young patients. Circulation, 44:368, 1971.
Wagner, H. R., Hugenhaltz, P. G., and Sandler, H.: Congenital aortic stenosis, compensating mechanisms in pure pressure overload. Circulation (Suppl. VI), 37–38:199, 1968.

THE CARDIOMYOPATHIES

Abelmann, W. H.: Experimental infection with *trypanosoma cruzi* (Chagas' disease). A model of acute and chronic myocardiopathy. Ann. N. Y. Acad. Sci., 153:137, 1969.
Adalman, A. G., McLoughlin, M. J., Merquis, Y., Auger, P., and Wigle, E. D.: Left ventricular cineangiographic observations in muscular subaortic stenosis. Amer. J. Cardiol., 24:689, 1969.
Akbarian, M., Yankopoulos, N. A., and Abelmann, W. H.: Hemodynamic studies in beriberi heart disease. Amer. J. Med., 41:197, 1966.
Alexander, C. S.: Idiopathic heart disease. I. Analysis of 100 cases with special reference to chronic alcoholism. Amer. J. Med., 41:213, 1966.
Alexander, C. S.: Idiopathic heart disease. II. Electron microscopic examination of myocardial biopsy specimens in alcoholic heart disease. Amer. J. Med., 41:229, 1966.
Bashour, F. A., McConnell, T., Skinner, W., and Hanson, M.: Myocardial sarcoidosis. Dis. Chest, 53:413, 1968.
Braunwald, E., Lambrew, C. T., Rockoff, S. D., Ross, J., Jr., and Morrow, A. G.: Idiopathic hypertrophic subaortic stenosis. I. A description of the disease based upon an analysis of 64 patients. Circulation, 30:3, 119; 1964.
Burch, G. E., and DePasquale, N.: Alcoholic cardiomyopathy. A review. Amer. J. Cardiol., 23:723, 1969.
Burch, G. E., and Giles, T. D.: Alcoholic cardiomyopathy. Concept of the disease and its treatment. Amer. J. Med., 50:141, 1971.
Chambers, R. J., Beck, W., and Schrire, V.: Ventricular dynamics in Bantu cardiomyopathy. Amer. Heart J., 78:493, 1969.
Fowler, N. O.: Differential diagnosis of cardiomyopathies. Progr. Cardiovasc. Dis., 14:133, 1971.
Frank, S., and Braunwald, E.: Idiopathic hypertrophic subaortic stenosis. Clinical analysis of 126 patients with emphasis on natural history. Circulation, 37:759, 1968.
Goodwin, J. F.: Congestive and hypertrophic cardiomyopathies. Lancet, 1:731, 1970.
Hamby, R. I.: Primary myocardial disease. A prospective clinical and hemodynamic evaluation in 100 patients. Medicine, 49:55, 1970.
James, T. N.: Observations on the cardiovascular involvement including the cardiac conduction system in progressive muscular dystrophy. Amer. Heart J., 63:48, 1962.
Lerner, A. M.: Virus myopericarditis. Ann. Intern. Med., 59:1068, 1968.
Mattingly, T. W.: The clinical and hemodynamic features of primary myocardial disease. Trans. Amer. Clin. Climat. Assoc., 70:132, 1958.
Mitchell, J. A., and Cohen, L. S.: Alcohol and the heart. Current Concepts Cardiov. Dis., 39:109, 1970.
Perloff, J. K., deLeon, A. C., Jr., and O'Doherty, D.: The cardiomyopathy of progressive muscular dystrophy. Circulation, 33:625, 1966.
Perloff, J. K., Lindgren, K. M., and Groves, B. M.: Uncommon or commonly unrecognized causes of heart failure. Progr. Cardiovasc. Dis., 12:409, 1970.
Popp, R. L., and Harrison, D. C.: Ultrasound in the diagnosis and evaluation of therapy of idiopathic hypertrophic subaortic stenosis. Circulation, 40:905, 1969.
Shaw, P. M., Gramiak, R., Kramer, D. H., and Yu, P. N.: Determinants of atrial and ventricular gallop sounds in primary myocardial disease. New Eng. J. Med., 278:753, 1968.
Wagner, P.: Beriberi heart disease. Physiologic data and difficulties in diagnosis. Amer. Heart J., 69:200, 1965.

PERICARDIAL DISEASE

Berglund, E., Sarnoff, S. J., and Isaacs, J. P.: Ventricular function: Role of the pericardium in regulation of cardiovascular hemodynamics. Circ. Res., 3:133, 1955.
Bradley, E. C.: Acute benign pericarditis. Amer. Heart J., 67:121, 1964.
Capps, J. A.: Pain from the pleura and pericardium. J. Nerv. Ment. Dis., 23:263, 1943.
Conn, H. L., Jr., and Horwitz, O. (Eds.): Cardiac and Vascular Diseases. Philadelphia, Lea and Febiger, 1971, p. 1326.
Cooley, J. C., Clagett, O. T., and Kirklin, J. W.: Surgical aspects of chronic constrictive pericarditis. A review of 72 operative cases. Ann. Surg., 147:488, 1958.
Dalton, J. C., Pearson, R. J., and White, P. D.: Constrictive pericarditis. A review and long-term follow-up of 78 cases. Ann. Intern. Med., 45:445, 1956.
Dressler, W.: The post-myocardial infarction syndrome. Arch. Intern. Med., 103:28, 1959.
Drusin, L. M.: Post-pericardiotomy syndrome: A six year epidemiologic study. New Eng. J. Med., 272:597, 1965.
Effer, D. B.: Chronic constrictive pericarditis treated with pericardiectomy. Amer. J. Cardiol., 7:62, 1961.
Engle, M. A., and Ito, T.: The postpericardiotomy syndrome. Amer. J. Cardiol., 7:73, 1961.
Gimlette, T. M. D.: Constrictive pericarditis. Brit. Heart J., 21:9, 1959.
Guntheroth, W. G., Morgan, B. C., and Mullins, G. H.: Effect of respiration on venous return and stroke volume in cardiac tamponade. Circ. Res., 20:381, 1967.
Harrison, E. C., Crawford, D. W., and Lau, F. Y. K.: Sequential left ventricular function studies before and after pericardiectomy for constrictive pericarditis. Amer. J. Cardiol., 26:319, 1970.
Harvey, W. P.: Auscultatory findings in diseases of the pericardium. Amer. J. Cardiol., 7:15, 1961.
Hurst, J. W., and Logue, R. B.: The Heart Arteries and Veins. New York, McGraw-Hill Book Co., 1970, p. 1254.
McKusich, V. A.: Chronic constrictive pericarditis. Some clinical and laboratory observations. Bull. Hopkins Hosp., 90:3, 1952.
Portal, R. W., Besterman, E. M. M., Chambers, R. J., Sellors, T. H., and Somerville, W.: Prognosis after operation for constrictive pericarditis. Brit. Med. J., 1:563, 1966.
Shobetai, R., Fowler, N. O., Fenton, J. C., and Masangkay, M.: Pulsus paradoxus. J. Clin. Invest., 44:1882, 1965.
Weissbein, A., and Heller, F. N.: A method of treatment for pericardial pain. Circulation, 24:607, 1961.
Wood, P.: Chronic constrictive pericarditis. Amer. J. Cardiol., 7:48, 1961.
Yu, P. N. G., Lovejoy, F. W., Jr., Joos, H. A., Nye, R. E., Jr., and Mahoney, E. B.: Right auricular and ventricular pressure patterns in constrictive pericarditis. Circulation, 7:102, 1953.

CHAPTER 10

CONGESTIVE HEART FAILURE

H. J. C. SWAN
WILLIAM W. PARMLEY

INTRODUCTION

The general term congestive heart failure is used to designate a common series of syndromes seen in the clinical practice of medicine. These syndromes consist of the symptoms and physical signs associated with (1) failure of the left ventricle as a pump, (2) failure of the right ventricle as a pump, (3) pulmonary venous hypertension, and (4) systemic venous hypertension. Although these factors may be present alone or in combination in a given patient, and are frequently interrelated from the standpoint of mechanism, it is relevant to separate the general mechanics and consequences of failure of the left ventricle as a pump from those of failure of the right ventricle as a pump. For example, the usual consequences of failure of the left ventricle as a pump are an increase in pulmonary venous pressure with the associated symptoms of dyspnea and the findings of rales in the lung fields or of pleural effusion. However, pulmonary congestion and edema may also be a consequence of alteration of pulmonary capillary permeability by the direct effects of toxic gases or of central nervous system damage. The symptoms associated with failure of the right ventricle usually include ankle edema, abdominal swelling, and right subcostal pain which may be accompanied by the findings of peripheral edema, an enlarged liver, ascites, and increased jugular venous pulsation and pressure. Systemic venous congestion with the symptoms and signs of right heart failure may be due to failure of the right ventricle associated with chronic obstructive lung disease in association with normal left ventricular function or indeed might occur in the absence of primary disease of the heart itself as a consequence of primary pericardial disease with or without effusion.

DEFINITION OF HEART FAILURE

Perhaps it is appropriate to consider initially a rather broad physiologic definition of heart failure rather than the more specific clinical syndromes. Warren and Stead indicated that heart failure is that state which results from the inability of the heart to pump sufficient blood to the body tissues to meet ordinary metabolic demands. Indeed, when the heart is unable to meet the normal resting metabolic needs of the body tissue, ventricular stroke volume is usually profoundly decreased. Minor or moderate depressions of ventricular performance do not usually result in this alteration because compensating mechanisms become operative. One of the primary compensatory mechanisms available to the body to improve cardiac performance is to increase the heart rate and thus the frequency of emptying of the left ventricle. In the majority of mammalian species in which cardiac output increases under conditions of increased demand, the principal mechanism operates by increasing heart rate with a relatively unchanged level of stroke volume.

Using the current convention for the expression of flow values in the cardiovascular system in terms of body surface area (B.S.A.), the normal stroke volume in a younger subject averages approximately 60 ml. per beat per M.^{2} At a rate of 60 beats per minute, this results in a cardiac output of 3.6 L. per min. per M.^{2}, and during severe exercise at a heart rate of 180 beats per minute, a cardiac index of 10.8 L. per min. per M.^{2} may be achieved in the absence of any changes in stroke volume. While small changes in stroke volume do occur, this is a secondary mechanism in the control of cardiac output. In patients with seriously reduced cardiac performance, one of the principal hemodynamic alterations is that the left ventricle may eject as little as 20 ml. per beat per M.^{2} or one third of normal stroke volume. However, a sinus tachycardia at a rate of 120 beats per minute will result in a cardiac index of 2.4 L. per min. per M.^{2}, which is usually adequate to meet resting metabolic needs.

In addition, partly as a consequence of the reduction in total cardiac output and the associated reduction of renal blood flow, the circulating blood volume increases. This, along with other factors, results in an enhanced filling pressure in the chambers of both right and left ventricles. An increased filling pressure results in a larger end-diastolic volume with a greater degree of fiber stretch. Thus, the performance of the heart may be enhanced secondarily for any given level of intrinsic contractile state by a greater fiber stretch—an additional mechanism to improve the function of the heart as a pump. However, as a consequence of the increased left ventricular diastolic pressure, there is increased pressure upstream in the left atrium and therefore in the pulmonary veins and capillaries which is transmitted into the pulmonary arteries. This results in an increase in pulmonary artery systolic, mean, and diastolic pressures. Hence, the right ventricle must do more work and progressively encounters greater difficulty in overcoming its outflow resistance, and a similar process of failure affects the right ventricle with the manifestations of systemic venous congestion. As a result, the common sequence of clinical congestive heart failure is a reduced left ventricular stroke volume accompanied by tachycardia and an increased left ventricular filling pressure, which tend to partly restore cardiac output and hence tissue perfusion but with an increase in myocardial oxygen needs, which are a direct function of both heart rate and left ventricular filling pressure (preload).

However, an important penalty for this compensation is the congestive changes in the lungs with increases in pulmonary arterial pressure and increased systemic venous pressure with congestive changes and edema. As a further generalization, it should be recognized that neither ventricle of the heart in the nonhypertrophied state is able to sustain significant acute increases in afterload.

This chapter will consider the general and specific mechanisms underlying failure of the heart as a pump with particular reference to the field of ischemic heart disease, in which important new information is developing. The content is also related to our current ability to alter systematically the physiologic determinants of myocardial performance and thus to place the treatment of heart failure on a more rational and hence more effective basis.

NORMAL CARDIAC PERFORMANCE

It is necessary to review briefly certain characteristics of cardiac performance in the normal heart for a comparative background. During ventricular contraction, in association with shortening of the myocardial sarcomere, the volume and the shape of both ventricles alter. The principal shortening occurs in the free wall of each cardiac chamber, with lesser degrees of shortening occurring in the ventricular septum and in the base to apex dimension. The right and left ventricles differ in their geometric contraction characteristics. The right ventricle ejects its content by approximating the free wall to the right ventricular aspect of the ventricular septum. In contrast, the thicker-walled left ventricle contracts in a more circumferential manner, changing from an ellipsoid configuration during diastole to a narrow truncated cone during systole. This change in ventricular volumes between systole and diastole is the process by means of which blood is expelled from the ventricle. Since ventricular volumes are frequently dramatically altered in patients with heart failure, quantitative emphasis will be placed on the consideration of ventricular volumes and their change. Data pertaining to the accompaniments of normal cardiac function are included in Table 10–1.

Left Ventricular Ejection

The following pertains to the ejection characteristics of the left ventricle. The normal left ventricle has a volume of approximately 90 ml. per M.^{2} at end diastole (EDV). During contraction it ejects approximately two thirds of its content or 60 ml. per M.^{2} into the aorta—the stroke volume (SV)—and at end systole it contains a residual volume of 30 ml. per M.^{2} (ESV). As a convenient measure of the pumping function of the left ventricle, the ratio of ejected or stroke volume to the

TABLE 10–1 NORMAL VALUES FOR CARDIAC PERFORMANCE AT REST

Cardiac index (L./min./M.^{2})	3.6
Heart rate (beats/min.)	60
Stroke index (ml./M.^{2})	60
Stroke work index (gm.-meters/M.^{2})	60
End-diastolic volume (ml./M.^{2})	90
End-systolic volume (ml./M.^{2})	30
Ejection fraction	0.67
LV end-diastolic pressure (mm. Hg)	<12
LV max dp/dt (mm. Hg/sec.)	1500
Segmental wall motion (% inward movement)	
Apical	30%
Anterior	50%
Inferior	40%

end-diastolic volume—the ejection fraction (EF)—may be readily calculated. EF = SV/EDV. Utilizing the above data, the normal ejection fraction is approximately 0.66 and may vary from 0.60 to approximately 0.78. Deviations outside this range are usually abnormal. Note that this expression (EF) of ventricular performance will take into account abnormal valve leakage as well as the magnitude of forward blood flow. Thus, it is possible to describe the performance of the ventricle in patients with valvar incompetence in terms of the magnitude and proportion of volume ejected during ventricular contraction. Since EDV − ESV = Total volume ejected, regurgitant volume (RV) is equal to (EDV − ESV) − SV, where SV = forward stroke volume.

The ejection fraction must not be confused with measures of the contractile state of the myocardium. Although it is possible to determine the instantaneous rate of volume change and thus arrive at an interpretation of ventricular function more closely related to the rate of sarcomere shortening, the ejection fraction accounts for only the ability of the heart to discharge its contents without relation to the time course or energetics of that process. The ejection fraction is one practically useful measure of pump function in the description of the heart in normal and abnormal states. Although the contractile state is usually depressed when the EF is reduced, normal values for EF may be found in the presence of a reduced contractile state, particularly when afterload falls.

Ventricular Contraction Patterns

Contraction of the ventricular wall is essentially a uniform process in the normal heart. The different elements and regions of the ventricular wall are displaced over a basically similar time course, occurring simultaneously for practical purposes over the whole mass of ventricular muscle. Normal end-systolic contraction, expressed as 1 minus the ratio of the end-systolic diameter to end-diastolic diameter for anterior, inferior, and apical segments, is given in Table 10–1. In the presence of certain abnormalities of intraventricular conduction, myocardial disease, or sequential underperfusion of the ventricle, this synchronous contraction may not be maintained. Under such circumstances, specific elements of the myocardium may contract at a time later than the normally contracting myocardium, may not contract at all, and, under certain circumstances, may actually bulge or paradox during contraction of the remainder of the ventricle (Fig. 10–1). Each of these abnormalities of ventricular wall motion is mechanically inefficient and metabolically costly to the ventricle.

In addition to the process of contraction, the cardiac ventricles also are subjected to geometric changes associated with ventricular filling. Following ventricular systole, the sarcomeres of the myocardium lengthen to their resting position, thus markedly reducing the tension in the myocardial wall. This reduction in tension immediately results in passive changes in the internal dimensions of the ventricular cavity, particularly associated with the tendency of connective tissue and supportive elements to return to a position of least energy. This may result in diastolic suction when, following relaxation of the contractile elements, the heart develops a negative intracavity pressure and tends to "suck" blood into its cavity. However, this mechanism plays a small part in filling of the ventricles, which is accomplished from the atria and great veins by reason of a slightly positive pressure within the vascular system relative to that external to the ventricle. The passive pressure-volume curve—representative of ventricular compliance—is concave to its pressure axis, so that blood is accepted in relatively large volumes from a low end-systolic volume, with very little change in filling pressure

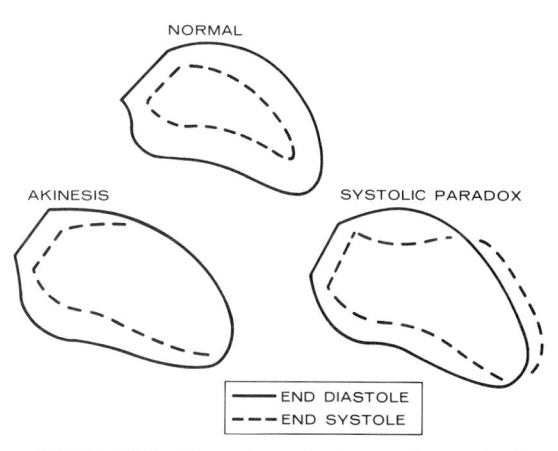

Figure 10–1 Normal and abnormal ventricular contraction patterns. The ventricular contours are shown as might be seen in a cineangiogram obtained in the right anterior-oblique projection. The solid line indicates the contour of the ventricular chamber at end diastole, and the dotted line indicates the position of the ventricular wall at end systole. Normally, the inward movement of the ventricular wall is uniform, involving all portions of the ventricle to approximately the same degree. In patients with diffuse cardiac disease, there is failure of contraction in all dimensions. In patients with localized cardiac disease, as shown in the two lower figures, there may be failure of movement of the affected portion of the ventricular wall, which is either scarred or stiffened (left). In certain instances the affected area may actually bulge during systole (right), providing not only a failure of contribution to contraction but a fundamental mechanical disadvantage.

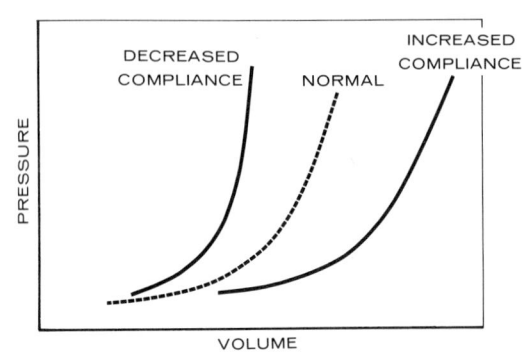

Figure 10–2 Passive pressure-volume relationship of the ventricles. The dotted line in the center indicates the general relationship between pressure and volume. As volume is increased initially, there is but a small rise in pressure. As volume increase continues, the rise in pressure is greater. Each of the solid lines indicates the alteration in pressure-volume relationships in decreased compliance (left) and increased compliance (right). This can be considered as a greater or lesser degree of stiffness of the ventricle in relation to the filling volume. Ventricular compliance is a dynamic phenomenon, and this property can change rapidly.

(Fig. 10–2). However, if filling is prolonged, the pressure will rise at an increasingly rapid level as the stiffer part of the ventricular pressure-volume curve is reached. Little attention has been paid to the passive pressure-volume relationships of the ventricle, yet they are all important in the concepts of heart failure. In normal human cardiac dynamics, the end-systolic volume of 30 ml. per $M.^2$ is achieved at a filling pressure of between 0 and 3 mm. Hg. Addition of 60 ml. per $M.^2$ (equivalent to the succeeding stroke volume) results in an increase in intraventricular pressure to between 8 and 12 mm. Hg at end diastole.

Thus, it is possible to describe the complete cardiac cycle in volumetric and pressure terms (Fig. 10–3). If we commence our consideration at the beginning of systole with an end-diastolic pressure of 12 mm. Hg and an end-diastolic volume of 90 ml. per $M.^2$, the intramyocardial tension rapidly increases until the intraventricular pressure equals that in the aortic root. No net volume change occurs, although a slight distortion of the ventricular wall accompanies the movement of the mitral valve leaflets posterior into the left atrium. When the pressure in the ventricle reaches and exceeds that in the aortic root, ejection commences. In the normal heart, between one half and two thirds of the stroke volume is discharged from the ventricle during the first third of systole, while the flow into the aorta during the last third of systole is between 10 and 20 per cent of the total. The rate of change of dimension and volume follow a similar time course. For this reason, the normal heart has considerable adaptability at high heart rates and even with considerable shortening of the duration of ventricular systole is still able to eject a great part of its content. However, when failure of the heart as a pump supervenes, the proportionate ejection of blood from the ventricle is more evenly distributed across the duration of ventricular systole, and the reserve capabilities of the ventricle are thus curtailed.

At the end of ventricular systole, the volume content of the ventricle has been reduced by the stroke volume and has returned to its end-systolic volume of 30 ml. per $M.^2$ Following reduction of intramyocardial tension as a result of sarcomere relaxation, the pressure in the ventricle drops to between 0 and 3 mm. Hg. At this point, the pressure in the atrium is sufficient to open the atrioventricular valve and allow for the maximal rate of filling of the ventricle, which in the normal heart follows a similar time course as systole. Thus, approximately half of ventricular filling occurs in the first third of ventricular diastole, with a barely measurable increase in intraventricular pressure. The volume rate of filling of the ventricle is progressively reduced as ventricular pressure rises according to the passive compliance characteristics of the myocardial wall until end diastole, at which time atrial contraction adds a final increment of stroke volume to the ventricle. When atrial contraction has been com-

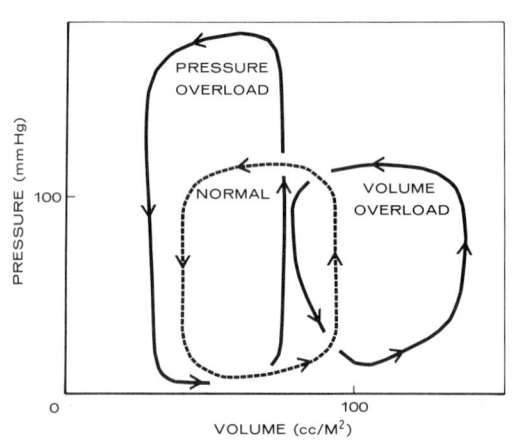

Figure 10–3 Pressure-volume relationships for the normal and abnormal ventricle. The dotted line indicates the normal pressure-volume loop (see text for details). However, greater work is performed in the generation of pressure for ejection of blood from the ventricle. In the presence of volume overload, there is an increase in all dimensions of the ventricle, so that the end-diastolic volume is substantively increased. The volume ejected is also increased, and the end-systolic volume is greater than normal in proportion to the magnitude of volume overload and the degree of compensation of the ventricle.

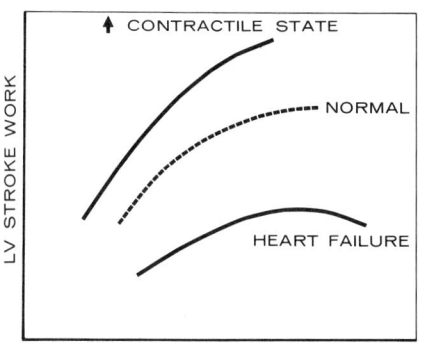

CONGESTIVE HEART FAILURE

Figure 10-4 The relationship between left ventricular performance and left ventricular filling pressure (Frank-Starling relationship). Normally, an increased end-diastolic pressure is accompanied by a substantive increase in performance (dotted line). In the presence of an enhanced contractile state in the same heart, the levels of performance are proportionately greater. In the presence of heart failure, the performance is less and when a critical level of diastolic pressure is reached, further increments of pressure are associated with an actual reduction in performance.

pleted, and the atrioventricular valves have commenced to float into their presystolic position, ventricular systole commences, and the cycle is repeated. The contraction pattern of the free wall of the ventricle is fundamentally uniform, with the greatest degree of shortening in the free wall and the least degree of shortening in the long axis and septal dimensions.

In addition, mechanisms of fundamental importance in the control and modification of normal or abnormal cardiac function include the tripartite relation between function and contractile state and presystolic fiber length—the Frank-Starling relationship (Fig. 10-4). The importance of these factors in the normal heart has already received consideration and will be discussed only in the context of heart failure per se. However, a central theme of critical importance in heart failure is a consideration of the factors which control myocardial oxygen consumption.

MYOCARDIAL OXYGEN CONSUMPTION

Since the report of Evans and Matsuoka in 1915, it has been generally appreciated that myocardial oxygen uptake is directly related to mean arterial pressure but is affected much less by changes in cardiac output. This generalization that pressure-work is much more costly than flow-work has been the framework upon which most of the subsequent studies of oxygen consumption have been performed. Furthermore, this concept has direct relevance to the pathophysiology of congestive heart failure and its effective therapy.

Fundamental studies over the past few years by Sarnoff, Sonnenblick, Braunwald and associates have greatly enhanced our appreciation of the quantitative aspects of myocardial oxygen consumption. The important determinants of myocardial oxygen consumption are listed in Table 10-2 and are divided for convenience into those of major and minor importance. The subsequent discussion will focus on the relative importance of each of these determinants. The oxygen consumption of the beating heart ranges from about 8 to 15 ml. per min. per 100 grams myocardium, while the oxygen consumption of the noncontracting heart is approximately 2 ml. per min. per 100 grams. Thus, the basal requirements for oxygen are approximately 20 per cent of the total needs and are required for the normal metabolic processes in the myocardium which are not associated with contraction.

Tension-Time Index

The initial observations that pressure-work was a major determinant of oxygen consumption were extended by Sarnoff and associates, who demonstrated under carefully controlled conditions in the dog that there was a close relationship between the product of developed intraventricular pressure and the time for which it was maintained and the measured myocardial oxygen consumption. This concept of a "tension-time index" has been of fundamental importance in relating the alterations in oxygen consumption that occur with changes in intraventricular pressure. Subsequently, the importance of wall tension rather than intraventricular pressure was emphasized. Since wall tension, according to the Laplace relation, is a direct function of the radius and intraventricular pressure, wall tension will be increased at the same intraventricular pressure if the heart dilates. Thus, in the enlarged failing heart, wall tension will be increased and

TABLE 10-2 MYOCARDIAL OXYGEN CONSUMPTION

Major Determinants:
  Heart rate
  Tension development
  Contractile state
  Basal
Minor Determinants:
  Activation
  Depolarization
  Direct metabolic effect of catecholamines

Figure 10–5 Relation of cardiac size to wall stress and to myocardial oxygen consumption. In heart failure, the end-diastolic volume (related to radius) is increased. Even when the wall thickness and internal pressure remain unchanged, the wall stress is increased in accordance with the law of Laplace. Hence, the myocardial oxygen consumption is increased.

VENTRICULAR PRESSURE, —— P : SAME
RADIUS, —— R : INCREASED
WALL THICKNESS, —— h : SAME OR DECREASED
WALL STRESS, —— S : INCREASED
MYOCARDIAL O$_2$ CONSUMPTION, MVO$_2$: INCREASED

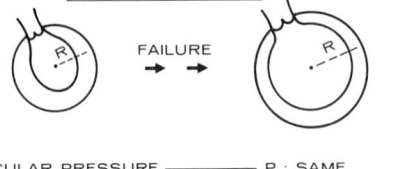

STRESS (S) = PR/2h

myocardial oxygen consumption augmented, although there may be no change in ventricular pressure (Fig. 10–5). This fact further emphasizes the therapeutic importance of reducing the size of the failing heart. This may be accomplished by a reduction of circulating blood volume with diuretics or by inotropic stimulation as with digitalis, which can empty the ventricle more effectively and thus reduce the intraventricular volume.

Despite the obvious importance of the tension-time index as a determinant of myocardial oxygen consumption, it was observed in conscious dogs that myocardial oxygen consumption correlated poorly with the tension-time index during exercise or sympathetic stimulation. Similarly, the administration of inotropic agents, such as isoproterenol, often produced little change or even a decrease in the tension-time index, while oxygen consumption was greatly augmented. In a series of studies by Sonnenblick and associates, it became apparent that the velocity of contraction of the myocardium (as an index of the contractile state of the heart) was also a major determinant of myocardial oxygen consumption. Thus, when the tension-time index was maintained relatively constant, oxygen consumption was greatly augmented by changes in contractile state produced by paired electrical stimulation, norepinephrine, or an increase in calcium concentration. At the present time, therefore, it would appear that any intervention which increases the contractility of the myocardium will also increase myocardial oxygen consumption.

Initially, however, this fact did not appear compatible with data which showed that digitalis glycosides did not increase myocardial oxygen consumption, despite an increase in contractile state. This apparent discrepancy was resolved by Covell and associates, who noted that when digitalis was given to the nonfailing heart, there was little or no change in end-diastolic volume, whereas myocardial oxygen consumption was increased. When digitalis was given to the failing heart, however, oxygen consumption was essentially unchanged. This occurred because of a reduction in ventricular volume which reduced wall stress according to the Laplace relation. Thus, the increase in oxygen consumption produced by the positive inotropic effects of digitalis was offset by the decrease in oxygen consumption produced by a reduction in heart size and myocardial wall tension.

The minor determinants of myocardial oxygen consumption listed in Table 10–2 are of much less importance. For example, it has been estimated that the depolarization process requires only about 0.04 ml. oxygen per min. per 100 grams when the heart is stimulated at a frequency of approximately 100 beats per minute. This amounts to approximately 0.5 per cent of the total oxygen consumed by the normal working heart. The direct metabolic effect of catecholamines on the nonbeating heart was determined by administering isoproterenol to the arrested canine heart. The subsequent increase in basal oxygen consumption was relatively minor, being of the order of 5 to 10 per cent of that occurring when the same hearts were contracting.

PERFORMANCE OF THE HEART AS A MUSCLE

The performance of the heart *as a pump* is usually designated in terms of pressure and flow. Since the performance of the heart *as a muscle* is generally designated in terms of shortening and wall stress, the relationship between intraventricular pressure and wall stress is of importance. From the Laplace relation (T = PR), it is apparent that the wall tension (T) is dependent not only on intraventricular pressure but also on the size of the heart, or more specifically on the radius of curvature and thickness of the particular portion of the wall under consideration. Since the normal left ventricle approximates a truncated ellipsoid, there are at least two radii of curvature at any point on the wall which help determine the stress existing at that point on the ventricle. No attempt will be made in this discussion to present complex formulas which adapt the Laplace relation to an ellipsoid ventricle. Rather, the purpose here is to identify those factors of importance. Thus, if one assumes the heart to be a simple sphere with radius, R, and wall thickness, h, a simplified version of the Laplace formula states that wall stress, S, is related to pressure, P, by the formula $S = PR/2h$ (Fig. 10-5).

This relationship is exemplified in the variation of wall thickness in the normal left ventricle. For example, the apex of the left ventricle has a relatively thin wall, as compared to the free lateral wall. This occurs because the radius of curvature of the apex is proportionately shorter, so that less muscle mass is needed in order to maintain a constant relationship between wall stress and intraventricular pressure. In the free lateral wall of the ventricle, the radius of curvature is greater, and thus a thicker wall is needed in order to maintain the appropriate relationship between wall stress and intraventricular pressure.

Ventricular Hypertrophy

The Laplace relationship is also fundamental to the understanding of the pathophysiology of various forms of heart disease. For example, when a heart undergoes hypertrophy secondary to arterial hypertension, the necessity to produce an increased intraventricular pressure is met by thickening of the wall. From the Laplace relationship, it should be noted that if intraventricular pressure and wall thickness increase proportionately (at a constant radius), wall stress will tend to remain the same. It has been noted in experimental models of hypertrophy, however, that hypertrophied muscle may actually generate less force per cross-sectional area than normal muscle. If this is the case, wall thickness must increase proportionately more than intraventricular pressure in order to generate the appropriate pressure.

The Laplace relation also offers some explanation as to why the left ventricle may hypertrophy, although there is no increase in arterial pressure. When heart failure and cardiac dilatation occur, there is increased wall stress in the free wall of the left ventricle, although there may be no change in intraventricular pressure. This increase in both diastolic and systolic wall stress serves as a stimulus to hypertrophy, without an increase in arterial systolic pressure. A mandatory consequence of cardiac dilatation is also an increase in myocardial oxygen needs. Additionally, there may be nonreversible structural changes in chronic dilatation, such as fiber slippage, increased connective tissue content, and so on, which explain the failure of the heart to again return to its original size after the causative factors are removed.

For example, in patients with aortic insufficiency who undergo aortic valve replacement, those patients whose hearts return toward normal size also have an improvement in cardiac function, while those patients whose hearts remain enlarged (presumably because of irreversible structural changes) have little improvement in cardiac function. Although heart size may increase to enormous proportions following dilatation, there is no concomitant increase in sarcomere length. Instead, sarcomere lengths tend to remain close to their optimum length of 2.2 microns. This presumably can occur because of fiber slippage, which allows the heart to expand considerably, but keeps sarcomeres at a reasonably optimal length. In patients with cardiac dilatation, a beneficial therapeutic intervention generally tends to reduce heart size, with a concomitant reduction in oxygen consumption. This effect is most often produced by salt restriction or diuretics, which reduce intravascular volume, and/or by digitalis, which increases contractile force and allows the heart to empty more completely and return to a smaller size.

It is appropriate now to examine the specific functional aspects of the heart in "failure." As stated in the introduction, for the purposes of this discussion, failure of the left ventricle as a pump means that it is unable to sustain the metabolic needs of the body under ordinary circumstances. Every heart can be subjected to a level of stress at which cardiac insufficiency can occur. A combination of cardiac pacing and alpha constrictor drugs such as angiotensin would be able to increase ventricular afterload and the frequency of cardiac contraction to such a degree that even the most healthy heart would be unable to sustain this workload. Since an older person or a deconditioned younger one may develop dyspnea at low workloads, cardiac insufficiency must be considered in relation to the imposed workload. For example, acute, severe ("malignant") hypertension will produce evidence of failure in a heart with normal myocardium and normal coronary arteries. Relief of the hypertension with appropriate drugs will permit the heart to function normally. Cardiac failure is the term usually applied to an inadequacy of blood flow to sustain the metabolic requirements of the body in the resting state at the optimal level of tissue oxygen tension. When the volume of blood delivered to the tissues of the body is decreased by reason of cardiac disease, a first-order compensatory mechanism available to the body tissues is their ability to extract a greater quantity of oxygen from the available blood flow. Thus, in spite of a reduced cardiac output, sufficient oxygen can be supplied to the tissues to meet resting metabolic needs. However, any increase in oxygen demand cannot be met at optimal levels of oxygen tension, and either local metabolic acidosis occurs or, more commonly, oxygen need is reduced by limitation of activity.

CORONARY CIRCULATION

One organ system deserving particular consideration is the coronary circulation. In the absence of occlusive disease of the epicardial coronary arteries, the coronary circulation is autoregulatory. It appears to function at an abnormally low P_{O_2} (20 to 23 mm. Hg), and there is a very effective extraction of oxygen from the incoming arterial blood. The coronary blood flow varies directly and almost linearly with myocardial oxygen consumption, since there is no reserve available to cardiac muscle by any further widening of the arterial venous oxygen difference. The thermo-dilution method of Ganz permits the study of rapid changes in the coronary circulation in man, and, in particular, the response to acute intervention. In subjects with normal coronary vessels, the mean coronary sinus blood flow was 122 ml. per min. — values similar to those reported for other methods. Blood flow in patients with epicardial occlusive coronary artery disease was not different at rest. However, during activity, normal subjects can increase coronary blood flow to a much greater degree. Although drugs, heart rate, and cardiac arrhythmias cause important changes, the highest resting levels and the greatest increases in coronary blood flow have been determined in subjects in whom a pressure load either existed or was imposed on the left ventricle. In heart failure, coronary blood flow is usually normal.

COMMON UNDERLYING MECHANISMS IN CLINICAL CARDIAC FAILURE (TABLE 10–3)

Increased Metabolic Demands

If the metabolic demand of the body is such that normal tissue metabolism cannot proceed without an increased blood flow, "heart failure" may be said to be present, in spite of a normal ejection fraction, normal stroke volume, and normal cardiac work. The recognized causes include, as an example, severe anemia, in which the quantity of oxygen delivered to the tissues is compromised by the quantity of hemoglobin available in the bloodstream. Since the body tissues require a relatively constant oxygen delivery, the cardiac output must increase in a direct relationship to the reduction in hemoglobin. When hemoglobin levels of 5 grams per 100 ml. or less are present, the cardiac output increases to values of 10 to 14 L. per min. to maintain tissue oxygen needs. This stress, which increases both cardiac frequency and stroke volume, may produce severe alterations of left ventricular filling pressure and signs of pulmonary congestion. Other examples of high output failure are severe fevers, beriberi, Paget's disease, and arteriovenous fistulas, by way of which large quantities of blood may pass directly from the arterial bed to the venous circulation without participating in metabolic exchange at a tissue level. In thyrotoxicosis, there is an increased metabolic demand at the tissue level, but also a direct cardiac effect.

Large left-to-right shunts may occur within the heart itself in certain forms of congenital heart disease. These include interatrial communications, ventricular septal defect, aorticopulmonary window, and patent ductus arteriosus. Since the vascular resistance in the pulmonary circulation is normally much less than in the systemic circulation, relatively large volumes of blood may flow into the lungs and not participate in systemic tissue perfusion. Although heart failure may occur in young patients with ventricular septal defect or patent ductus arteriosus, these common lesions are usually sustained for many years without the development of heart failure. This is due to a peculiar autoregulatory mechanism by means of which a reduction in systemic vascular resistance will deviate more of output of the left ventricle to the systemic circulation during times of increased systemic metabolic need, without an additional increase in cardiac work.

Mechanical lesions which increase left ventricular work include coarctation of the aorta,

TABLE 10–3 FACTORS IN THE CAUSATION OF HEART FAILURE

A. Increased metabolic (output) demand
  1. Anemia, thyrotoxicosis, fever, beriberi
  2. A-V fistula, Paget's disease, left-to-right shunts
B. Increased left ventricular work
  1. Coarctation of aorta, aortic stenosis, subaortic stenosis
  2. Hypertension: primary, secondary
C. Compromised ventricular contraction
  1. Pericarditis, endomyocardial fibrosis
  2. Cardiomyopathies: infiltrative, idiopathic
D. Coronary artery disease
  1. Ischemia, infarction
  2. Fibrosis, scar, aneurysm
E. Disorders of filling
  1. Mitral, tricuspid stenosis
  2. Pericardial disease, cardiac tamponade
F. Volume overload
  1. Aortic incompetence, mitral incompetence
  2. Transfusion
G. Intrinsic depression of contractile state
  1. Acute myocarditis
  2. Cardiomyopathy
H. Arrhythmias
  1. Tachyrhythmias — sinus, atrial, nodal, ventricular
  2. Bradyrhythmias — sinus, partial, complete A-V block

aortic stenosis (supravalvar, valvar, and subvalvar), hypertrophic subaortic stenosis, and systemic hypertension. Although hypertension is fundamentally a disease of the systemic arterial bed, its consequences upon the heart are highly significant and it is one of the two most common causes of heart failure. Hypertension imposes a workload which is usually, but not always, gradual in development and allows for compensatory hypertrophy to take place. Although the cardiac ventricles are effective and adaptable volume pumps, continued increases in afterload present even the hypertrophied heart with a formidable burden. In the presence of compromised coronary circulation due to obstructive atherosclerosis, the more moderate degrees of afterload increase may not be tolerated and heart failure develops.

Mechanical Lesions Compromising Ventricular Contraction

These lesions include adherent pericardium, constrictive pericarditis, infiltrative cardiomyopathies, primary myocardiopathies, familial cardiomyopathy, and the multiple forms of endocardial and endomyocardial fibrosis. In these disease states, there is a major increase in the viscous resistance within the ventricular wall. The tension developed by contraction must overcome this additional burden before appropriate changes in ventricular geometry can result in expulsion of blood from the left ventricle.

Coronary Artery Disease

The commonest cause of left ventricular dysfunction is the reduction of blood flow to areas of the myocardium consequent upon occlusive coronary vascular disease. Atherosclerotic vascular disease may affect one or all of the epicardial arteries, but the intramyocardial vessels are usually spared. As a consequence, there is a limitation of blood flow to the myocardium and ischemia results.

If this is due to a lesion in the larger coronary vessels (proximal occlusive disease), heart failure may occur owing to the nonfunction of a large number of contractile elements. Other effects of coronary atherosclerosis include myocardial infarction, large scar formation, and patchy areas of localized intramyocardial fibrosis, associated with focal infarction, arrhythmias, and depression of ventricular function. This disease process, the commonest form of heart disease afflicting Western man, is characterized by chest pain of cardiac origin—angina pectoris—which is usually stress-related. This symptom is caused by myocardial ischemia, which also results in transient depression of ventricular function toward, if not reaching, those levels of performance considered ordinarily to be heart failure. Patients with coronary artery disease who ultimately exhibit chronic heart failure have, in addition to myocardial ischemia, severe focal or general destruction of myocardium characterized by previous myocardial infarction. Occasionally, patients who are relatively insensitive to cardiac pain under conditions of appropriate stress can exhibit severe primary depression of cardiac function with pulmonary edema and without previous myocardial damage.

Disorders of Ventricular Filling

The primary cause of inadequate left ventricular filling is stenotic disease of the mitral valve. This condition per se does not produce left ventricular failure. However, long-standing "pure" mitral stenosis will result in changes in the geometry and distensibility characteristics, in the submitral valve structures, and in the left ventricle. There is stiffening in the submitral endocardium and a "small" left ventricular cavity, with markedly decreased compliance characteristics.

Volume Overload Associated With Valvar Incompetence

In the presence of incompetence of the aortic or mitral valve, the left ventricle is called upon to discharge a volume equivalent to the sum of that needed by the body tissues and, in addition, that which regurgitates through the incompetent valve. The autoregulatory characteristics of the systemic arterial bed, in which a demand for increased blood flow results in a reduction in peripheral resistance, automatically result in a relative increase in forward cardiac output proportionate to shunt or regurgitant flow. Then, relatively large volumes can be handled by the left ventricle, provided that the demand is not acute and that the contractile state of the myocardium remains adequate. If the mechanical burden increases acutely or gradually, a state is reached in which even a hypertrophied heart with normal contractility is unable to perform adequately, and forward blood flow declines. Not infrequently, the mechanical lesion may worsen (increasing regurgitation) or the contractile state may become depressed.

Intrinsic Depression of Myocardial Contractile State

It has been difficult to prove a functional deficit of chemical substrate or sarcomere function in cases of heart failure. Nevertheless, conditions such as acute myocarditis, cardiomyopathy, and heart failure of old age may be associated with insignificant demonstrable disease. The nature of spontaneous remission as well as the responses to inotropic agents indicates, however, that a true depression of contractile state may be the primary factor occasionally, and a phenomenon secondary to other factors frequently.

Primary Arrhythmias

Severe tachy- or bradyrhythmias may in themselves cause cardiac failure. Also, uncoordinated ventricular activity and loss of atrial contraction are of major significance, particularly when ventricular compliance is decreased.

Multiple Factors

Anemia and congenital heart disease, valvular and coronary disease, underline the interrelation of multiple factors as causes of heart failure. The significant issue here is a comprehension of the adequacy of the heart to sustain its function and to recognize the additive nature of adverse factors as each reaches a critical value. Thus, a young patient may tolerate aortic valve stenosis for many years only to succumb to a small myocardial infarction, which may itself result in minimal symptoms. A patient with mild mitral stenosis will exhibit heart failure on the first attack of atrial fibrillation with a rapid ventricular response.

BIOCHEMICAL AND MECHANICAL ALTERATIONS IN HEART FAILURE

The myocardium is dependent almost exclusively on aerobic metabolism and cannot develop any appreciable oxygen debt as can skeletal muscle. Because of its large number of mitochondria, the heart is fundamentally suited to function in an aerobic manner. Normally, the myocardium can adapt itself to a wide number of substrates and is capable of utilizing almost all nutritional substances which come to it via the coronary circulation. These include glucose, pyruvate, lactate, free and esterified fatty acids, acetate, ketone bodies, and amino acids. Thus, in a postprandial state, the myocardium uses primarily glucose, lactate, and pyruvate, with a respiratory quotient approaching 1.0. During fasting conditions, the arterial concentrations of free fatty acids and ketones are much higher, and the heart will utilize these substrates with a reduction in the respiratory quotient toward 0.8. When glucose is metabolized via the glycolytic and citric acid cycles, 36 of the 38 moles of ATP formed per mole of glucose oxidized are produced as a result of aerobic mitochondrial activity. This emphasizes the importance of aerobic oxidation of glucose in terms of energy production in the form of ATP.

When any portion of myocardium becomes anaerobic, lactate is produced locally, and this has been used, for example, as an indication of ischemia during cardiac catheterization. Normally, uptake of lactate from the arterial blood by the normal myocardium is greater than 10 per cent. With the onset of ischemia, however, tissue lactate is formed as the end product of glycolysis and cannot be metabolized further because of ischemic depression of the citric acid cycle. This results in a level of coronary venous lactate which is higher than in arterial blood; that is, lactate is produced by the myocardium. Lactate production demonstrated by arteriovenous measurements across the heart is typical of the regional ischemia associated with coronary artery disease.

Hypertrophy

One of the compensatory mechanisms available to the heart as it begins to fail is the ability to hypertrophy. The increased mass of hypertrophied myocardium can produce greater pressure and restore the ability of the heart to function as a pump. Several studies of the mechanics of hypertrophied muscle have suggested, however, that this muscle is not normal and is functioning at a lower level of contractility than normal cardiac muscle. Similarly, failing myocardium in various experimental studies has also been shown to have an apparent decrease in contractile state. Table 10-4 lists some of the factors that have been studied in hypertrophy and heart failure which bear a relationship to the depressed function of the myocardium.

Mechanical Factors

In several animal models it has been noted that failing heart muscle has a decreased ability to

TABLE 10-4 THE FAILING MYOCARDIUM

A. Mechanical Alterations
  1. Decrease in force development/cross-sectional area
  2. Decrease in maximum rate of force development
  3. Decrease in velocity of shortening
B. Biochemical Alterations
  1. Catecholamines
    a. Reduced tissue content
    b. Reduced synthesis (tyrosine hydroxylase)
  2. Biochemical
    a. Reduced actomyosin-ATPase
    b. Increased hydroxyproline (hypertrophy)
    c. No reduction in ATP
    d. Decreased calcium binding by sarcoplasmic reticulum
    e. Decreased adenyl cyclase activity
  3. Exogenous
    a. Increased cortisol, catecholamines, and free fatty acids
    b. ? Myocardial depressant factor in shock

shorten with a normal velocity. Since the shortening velocity at zero load (Vmax) has been used as an index of contractile state (see Chapter 8), this decrease in velocity of shortening suggests a decrease in the contractile state of the failing muscle. Furthermore, the muscle is unable to develop the same force per unit mass as normal muscle and has a reduced maximum rate of force development.

Biochemical Factors

Numerous studies have been carried out to investigate the potential reasons for these findings. For example, tissue catecholamines are reduced in the failing myocardium, suggesting that there has been an increased excretion rate by augmented sympathetic tone in an attempt to maintain compensation. This is not responsible for the decrease in contractile state, however, since contractile state is not affected by depletion of catecholamines by either reserpinization or denervation. Additional studies in failing heart muscle have noted that there is a reduction in activity of the enzyme tyrosine hydroxylase, which is in the synthetic pathway of norepinephrine in the myocardium. Thus, there may be not only an increased excretion of norepinephrine but a decreased rate of synthesis to help account for the depletion of tissue catecholamines. It also has been noted that during the process of hypertrophy there is an increased collagen content of the myocardium, as manifested by an increased hydroxyproline concentration. Whether or not this collagen tissue interferes with the process of contraction is not clear. Even if one corrects contractile measurements for this dilution of normal cardiac tissue by connective tissue, the remaining myocardium still appears to be functioning at a reduced level of contractile state.

Actomyosin-ATPase

One biochemical alteration of considerable importance in the failing heart is a reduction in actomyosin-ATPase activity. This enzyme is intimately associated with the myosin filament and actin-myosin cross bridges and is responsible for splitting the ATP which provides the energy for contraction. Previous studies by Barany have demonstrated that actomyosin-ATPase activity in a wide variety of species is closely related to contractile state, as measured by Vmax, the maximal velocity of shortening at zero load. Thus, there is a mechanical-biochemical correlation in failing heart muscle in that both velocity of muscular contraction and baseline actomyosin-ATPase activity are reduced. ATP serves as the immediate source of high-energy phosphate bonds for the process of contraction, although creatinine phosphate also contains high-energy bonds.

In order for this latter energy to be utilized, however, there must be an interchange between creatinine phosphate and ADP to form ATP, which is the final source of energy for cardiac contraction. Studies in failing heart muscle have suggested that the levels of ATP are not reduced in the failing myocardium, so that a reduction in energy supply does not appear to be the reason for a decrease in contractile state.

It has also been noted that there is decreased binding of calcium by the sarcoplasmic reticulum in the failing myocardium. Calcium is the initiator of cardiac contraction by binding with troponin and releasing troponin's inhibition of the interaction of actin and myosin. The reduced ability of the sarcoplasmic reticulum to bind calcium might lead to reduced stores of calcium in the myocardium. Theoretically, this might produce a decreased availability of calcium to the myoplasm and a consequent decrease to contractile state.

In guinea pigs with inherited cardiomyopathy, it has also been noted that adenyl cyclase activity is decreased. This enzyme is intimately associated with the actions of the catecholamines via the beta-adrenergic pathway. Catecholamines, such as norepinephrine, stimulate adenyl cyclase activity and convert ATP to cyclic AMP. Cyclic AMP in turn activates phosphorylase activity and promotes glycogenolysis, making more glucose available for the glycolytic cycle. In some additional way, as yet undefined, cyclic AMP also produces an increase in contractile state. This reduction in adenyl cyclase activity, however, does not appear to be the mechanism responsible for the decrease in contractile state, since the level of this enzyme can vary considerably (depending on the catecholamine content of the myocardium) without affecting basal levels of contraction.

Exogenous Factors

Several exogenous factors have important effects on cardiac function during heart failure. For example, circulating myocardial depressant factor has been identified in animal models in shock, which is released or activated by substances released from the splanchnic circulation. Although this isolated factor has been demonstrated to produce depression of cardiac function in isolated tissue, its function in the intact circulation is uncertain, since there is a concomitant increase in circulating catecholamines, which increase the contractile state of the myocardium. This catecholamine response is apparently part of the overall response of the body to the stress associated with heart failure and also includes elevations of cortisol and free fatty acids. Of some interest is the potential role of increased levels of catecholamines and free fatty acids in producing arrhythmias in the setting of acute heart failure, particularly acute myocardial infarction. Whether the elevation of these substances is responsible for the arrhythmias observed or merely reflects the serious nature of the underlying heart disease is not yet clear.

In summary, although there are several biochemical alterations of importance in the failing heart, it is not yet clear whether these various abnormalities are merely associated with or in some way are responsible for the decreased contractility of the failing heart.

RENAL PHYSIOLOGY IN CONGESTIVE HEART FAILURE*

Renal mechanisms are intimately involved in the retention of fluid and electrolytes and the subsequent peripheral edema which accompanies congestive heart failure. The basic response of the kidney to a fall in cardiac output is retention of salt and water. This receptor response apparently has difficulty in discriminating between a true fall in plasma volume, such as might occur with blood loss or fluid depletion, and a fall in effective circulating volume, which is caused by a depression of cardiac function. The stimulus for retention of salt and water, however, will persist until adequate cardiac output is restored. This results in an increase in extracellular fluid volume, in total body water, and in total exchangeable sodium and chloride. Aldosterone secretion and the concentration of antidiuretic hormone are also increased.

Normally, about 98 per cent of the sodium filtered by the glomerulus is reabsorbed by the tubular system. The great bulk of this is reabsorbed in the proximal tubules. A smaller amount is absorbed in the collecting duct and the ascending loop of Henle, while the remainder, which is not excreted in the urine, is reabsorbed in the distal tubule by ion exchange with hydrogen or potassium. This mechanism is the principal means for excretion of potassium ion. Under the influence of enhanced aldosterone, total exchangeable potassium in the body may actually be reduced owing to this reabsorption of sodium in the distal tubule.

The rate of sodium excretion is determined by the balance between glomerular filtration and tubular reabsorption. In congestive heart failure, the glomerular filtration rate is commonly reduced to at least one half the normal rate. However, there appears to be increased tubular reabsorption of sodium, suggesting that this latter factor is the most significant cause of sodium accumulation, whereas the fall in glomerular filtration rate is only a contributory factor. Although it is not the exclusive factor, the role of aldosterone in this regard appears to be of primary importance in producing the retention of sodium ions. The sequence of events in this series apparently includes the release of renin from the renal afferent arterioles and juxtaglomerular cells, which transforms angiotensin to a decapeptide, angiotensin I. A plasma-converting enzyme converts this material to an octapeptide, angiotensin II, which is the immediate factor stimulating the secretion of aldosterone by the zona glomerulosa of the adrenal cortex. Presumably, decreased pressure or volume in the afferent arterioles is the signal mechanism which activates this system. The retention of sodium, therefore, is accompanied by the retention of water and expansion of the circulating blood volume. This in turn leads to filtration of the retained fluid as edema into tissue spaces and occasionally as pleural or peritoneal effusions.

Associated with this retention of fluid is also a decrease in free water clearance. Therefore, patients who have a continued large intake of water will be unable to clear this water through their kidneys and may develop dilutional hyponatremia. Thus, in severe heart failure, it is clear that therapy must include not only a restriction of salt intake but also some limited restriction of fluid intake, together with appropriate diuretics. Because of the propensity for potassium loss with increased aldosterone secretion and the administration of certain diuretics such as the thiazides, it is often important to provide oral potassium supplementation, particularly in patients who are digitalized. Alternatively, the use of aldosterone antagonists in addition to other diuretics may maintain reasonable potassium balance.

CONTROL OF PERIPHERAL CIRCULATION

In the normal circulation at rest, the total blood flow is divided in a relatively constant proportion among the different organ systems of the body (Table 10–5). Skeletal muscle and the splanchnic and renal beds each receive approximately 20 per cent of the total cardiac output. The cerebral circulation and blood flow through the skin each account for a further 10 per cent of total blood flow. The coronary vascular system receives 4 per cent of the total cardiac output. During activity the cerebral blood flow remains relatively constant. Flow in other segments of the circulation alters in accord with metabolic demand. Thus, during exercise, skeletal muscle blood flow increases promptly and may account for more than 50 per cent of the total cardiac output. At the same time, there is a major increase

---

*See also Chapter 14.

TABLE 10-5 REGIONAL DISTRIBUTION OF CARDIAC OUTPUT

	Normal		Cardiac Failure	
	Rest	Exercise	Rest	Exercise
Cardiac Output (L./min./M.^{2})	3.0	6.0	1.5	2.3
Blood Flows (% of cardiac output)				
Muscle	20	50	36	60
Splanchnic	25	12	25	10
Renal	20	9	10	4
Cerebral	12	6	12	12
Coronary	4	4	9	10
Skin	9	15	3	1
Blood Flows (absolute values in ml./min./M.^{2})				
Muscle	600	3000	540	1380
Renal	600	540	150	92
Coronary	120	240	135	230

From Mason, D. T.: Mod. Conc. Cardiovasc. Dis., *36*: 25, 1967. By permission of The American Heart Association, Inc.

in skin blood flow, presumably to facilitate the loss of metabolic heat from the body. While the proportion of blood flow passing to the other circulatory elements is decreased, the absolute level of blood flow is still maintained.

In skeletal muscle, the arterioles are under essentially local control. The local vascular resistance is determined by the relative degree of vasodilatation resulting from the production of metabolites in skeletal muscle. When the muscle is relatively inactive, the production of metabolites is low and the "net" vascular tone remains high. As metabolic products are formed and their concentration rises, vasodilatation occurs, which has the autoregulatory effect of enhancing the removal of these substances with a tendency to restore the previous level of vasomotor tone. In addition, skeletal muscle is under modest degrees of autonomic control. The circulation in the skin is principally regulated by the autonomic nervous system. Vasodilatation occurs by reason of release of constrictor tone centrally mediated. This appears to be predominantly a heat regulatory mechanism.

Heart Failure

In heart failure, however, there is a reduction in total cardiac output at rest, and there is a failure to increase cardiac output proportionate with activity. Hence, there is a redistribution of the absolute magnitude of organ blood flow in this state, which is further accentuated during exercise. In patients with borderline cardiac compensation of heart failure, the coronary blood flow is preserved. In fact, the coronary blood flow may be much greater proportionate to cardiac output in patients with heart failure than in patients with normally compensated circulations. Relatively speaking, there is a diminution in renal blood flow and, to a lesser extent, in splanchnic blood flow. The skeletal muscles retain their usual proportion of blood flow (Table 10-5).

During activity, there is a pronounced alteration in the distribution of blood flow. Cerebral blood flow is maintained, but there is a marked reduction in blood flow to the splanchnic and renal beds. Within the limits of total cardiac output, blood flow to actively exercising skeletal muscle increases. This, however, is strictly limited by the availability of blood flow. In contrast, normal skin blood flow is not increased in heart failure, owing to sustained vasoconstriction. Vascular reactivity is profoundly altered in heart failure. First, there is an increased resting peripheral resistance throughout the organ systems, both collectively and individually. Thus, the balance between the concentration of dilating metabolites and the vascular tone in skeletal muscle is substantially altered so that a greater concentration is necessary to sustain a given level of vasodilation. This may also be seen in the responses of skeletal muscle and skin to reactive hyperemia. In such instances, the magnitude of dilatation is greatly reduced. In addition, there is an abnormal response to ordinary autonomic reflexes. The vasodilatation in the skin is significantly reduced following heating, and responses to such mechanisms as acute tilting or the Valsalva maneuver are altered. In a normal subject, there is a significant and transient overshoot in arterial blood pressure following the Valsalva maneuver. This overshoot is absent in patients with heart failure, suggesting that the peripheral vascular tone is already high and is not particularly modified during the Valsalva maneuver, nor is stroke volume substantially increased. Heart failure is characterized by an increase in sympathetic vascular tone, which is in direct proportion to the severity of the failure.

One particular syndrome characterizing the failing heart is worthy of note. In the shock state, peripheral vascular responses may be grossly abnormal. Initially there is a marked increase in peripheral vascular resistance in such patients, although occasionally, reduced peripheral vascular resistance and reflex vasodilation due to stimulation of cardiac receptors have been described. However, in the presence of prolonged and severe hypoxia with resulting lactic acidemia and acidosis, a specific paralysis of peripheral vessels occurs. In the shock syndrome, the ability of skeletal muscle vessels to dilate is almost completely abolished. The reactive hyperemic response is negligible in spite of the fact that presumably high levels of vasodilating substances are present in both the resting as well as the exercising muscle.

HEART FAILURE IN ISCHEMIC HEART DISEASE AND ACUTE MYOCARDIAL INFARCTION

Occlusive coronary artery disease is a special disorder of cardiac function which warrants separate consideration from a practical as well as a pathophysiologic standpoint. The processes of atherosclerosis result in the formation of obstructive lesions in the coronary vascular tree which, because of either degree or location, may substantially interfere with the magnitude of coronary blood flow. When the myocardial oxygen demand of the tissue in the distribution of each vessel exceeds the capacity of the restricted arterial bed to supply it with oxygenated blood, ischemic changes result. These changes are usually characterized by the development of chest pain of cardiac origin—angina pectoris—but this is a variable symptom. It is now clear that patients with coronary artery disease and angina pectoris have significant but reversible ventricular dysfunction due to ischemia alone. When the degree of ischemia is extremely severe or the vessel is acutely and completely blocked, major changes occur, both in the structure of the myocardium and in ventricular function. The dynamic nature of this process is shown in Figure 10–6. Patients with acute myocardial infarction are usually classified as being (1) uncomplicated, (2) uncomplicated apart from transient cardiac arrhythmias, (3) exhibiting heart failure of mild degree, (4) exhibiting heart failure of moderate degree, and (5) exhibiting cardiogenic shock. This classification is not always entirely precise, since a true reduction of cardiac performance is not always coincidental with the signs and symptoms of pulmonary venous congestion, which are the usual clinical hallmarks of the diagnosis of heart failure (Fig. 10–7). Thus, the measured values for cardiac performance may show the cardiac output, stroke volume, and stroke work to be normal or even increased in a given patient; may be reduced moderately to levels consistent with normal cardiac performance; or may be reduced profoundly. Indices of ventricular contractile state (Vmax, max dp/dt) show the same variability. The disease dominantly affects the left ventricle; isolated disease of the right ventricle is rare.

Left ventricular filling pressure may be normal, but it is frequently increased. The level of left ventricular filling pressure or pulmonary venous and distending pressure correlates with the presence of increased vascular markings of the lungs on chest x-ray, clinical signs of pulmonary venous congestion, and clinical signs of enhanced filling pressure—third and fourth heart sounds (Fig. 10–8). However, the relationship of cardiac performance to filling pressure is poor, in that patients may have normal cardiac performance with low or high ventricular filling pressures and reduced cardiac performance with low or high ventricular filling pressure.

The time course of changes in these hemodynamics is somewhat variable. Left ventricular filling pressure usually decreases in 2 to 4 days to normal levels, irrespective of whether the cardiac output has been normal or moderately decreased. Pulmonary congesting pressure—pulmonary venous pressure—falls spontaneously without any treatment or with diuretics, which initially act by enhancing venous capacitance and then have a later (½ hour) effect on salt and water excretion.

In myocardial infarction, agents such as digitalis or the catecholamines do not exhibit a powerful inotropic effect. In patients with normal or increased cardiac output there is a small increase in cardiac output or stroke work of approximately 10 to 15 per cent. On the contrary, in patients with severe depression of cardiac function, this does not take place. Hence, patients who are severely ill and who require the use of cardiac stimulators do not respond favorably to inotropic agents. This may be due to total failure of the infarcted or ischemic tissue to respond, while the normal myocardium is already maximally active. A wide variety of effects appear to result from myocardial infarction (Fig. 10–7). In a small infarct, there are few contractile elements that are rendered inactive. In addition, acute myocardial ischemia and/or infarction appears to mediate strong sympathetic activity. Therefore, certain

Figure 10–6 Dynamic representation of the changes in the function of myocardium in coronary heart disease. There is a reversible relation between healthy and ischemic myocardium determined by the level of cardiac metabolism. The reaction becomes irreversible when ischemic tissue passes into the infarcted state and undergoes necrosis and healing in the form of fibrosis or scar. The contractile state is reduced to a varying degree (frequently severely) in ischemia and of course is absent in infarcted or scarred myocardium. The compliant state of myocardium may be decreased during ischemia (ventricular stiffening) and may be normal or increased in infarcted myocardium. Following healing, myocardial scars are noncompliant and extremely stiff, with a minimal mechanical disadvantage.

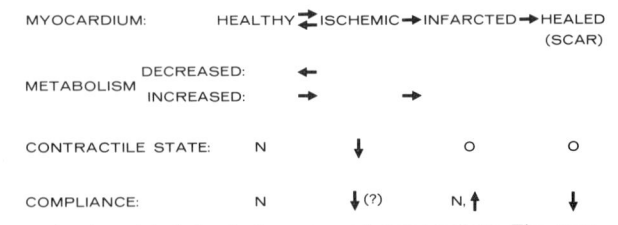

MYOCARDIUM:	HEALTHY ⇌ ISCHEMIC → INFARCTED → HEALED (SCAR)
METABOLISM: DECREASED	←
METABOLISM: INCREASED	→ →
CONTRACTILE STATE:	N ↓ 0 0
COMPLIANCE:	N ↓(?) N,↑ ↓

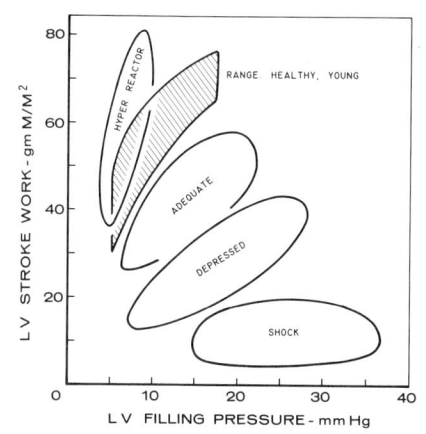

Figure 10-7 Relation of ventricular performance to filling pressure in patients with coronary heart disease and myocardial infarction. A wide spectrum of ventricular response exists. Certain patients may exhibit normal performance characteristics or performance characteristics which are inappropriately enhanced for the sedated, resting individual. Differing degrees of depression of ventricular performance exist that are related dominantly to the magnitude and location of the infarcted-ischemic tissue and the presence of additional mechanical lesions such as mitral valve incompetence. Patients with profound depression of ventricular function usually exhibit the shock state and experience a very high mortality.

patients in the ischemic-infarction syndrome exhibit tachycardia or hypertension in the presence of a normal or increased cardiac output. A second group of patients have an infarct of medium size. In this instance more contractile elements have been rendered ineffective and the cardiac output is usually more depressed. However, the diastolic compliant state of the ventricle is variable. In many patients there is good evidence that the ventricle is stiff and may be exhibiting ischemic contracture. This diastolic stiffness also appears to have a time course similar to that of the change in diastolic filling pressure, so that in 2 to 5 days diastolic pressure has declined and the characteristics of diastolic stiffness have disappeared. The presence of a loud fourth heart sound in the majority of patients with acute myocardial infarction and the typical configuration of the left ventricular pressure pulse render an increased diastolic stiffness likely.

If the infarct is large, many contractile elements are rendered nonfunctional, and the ejection fraction (EF) is proportionately reduced (Fig. 10-9). Not infrequently, additional mechanical lesions are present. Of these, perhaps the most important is paradox of the area of the myocardial infarct. If the infarct does not stiffen (decreased ventricular compliance), it distends as intraventricular pressure rises (Fig. 10-10). The work performed by the normally contracting elements is therefore wasted in the distention of the infarct. In addition, mitral insufficiency due to chronic papillary muscle dysfunction or new and recent as a consequence of ventricular dilatation or papillary muscle abnormality can add to the burden of the already disordered ventricle. In the same way as ventricular paradox, mitral insufficiency or intraventricular flow can acutely and profoundly depress cardiac pump function. In this regard, a soft systolic murmur at the apex of the heart in patients with acute myocardial infarction should never be regarded as an innocent, inconsequential sign. It may be evidence of mitral insufficiency of only moderate magnitude, but of a degree sufficient to account for a substantial proportion of the reduced cardiac output. In certain instances the mitral insufficiency may be completely silent, with the murmur returning only as cardiac compensation is partly restored.

The most profound form of depression of cardiac function results in a clinical syndrome known as *shock*. Shock may be associated with a number of causes, including acute infection, acute loss of blood volume, and acute profound destruction of myocardial elements. The reduction of approximately 40 per cent of the contractile elements in the myocardium causes a fall in cardiac performance to the order of magnitude seen in patients in or close to cardiogenic shock. If, however, additional mechanical lesions are

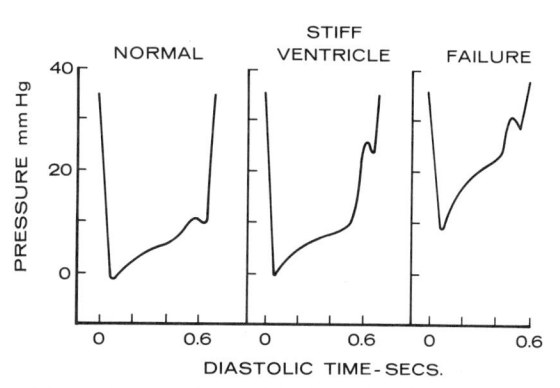

Figure 10-8 Left ventricular diastolic pressure pulses in patients with and without heart disease. In each instance ventricular systole is excluded and the tracing represents only the events in diastole. Note (left) the early diastolic pressure approaching zero with an "a" wave of approximately 10 mm. Hg in magnitude. In acute myocardial infarction the early diastolic contour of the pressure pulse remains unchanged, but there is an "a" wave of large magnitude, possibly owing to an increased ventricular stiffness and, therefore, a shift to the left of the diastolic pressure-volume relation. In the right panel is a tracing of a patient with chronic congestive heart failure and elevated early diastolic as well as late diastolic and "a" wave pressures.

288 CARDIORENAL AND RESPIRATORY SYSTEMS

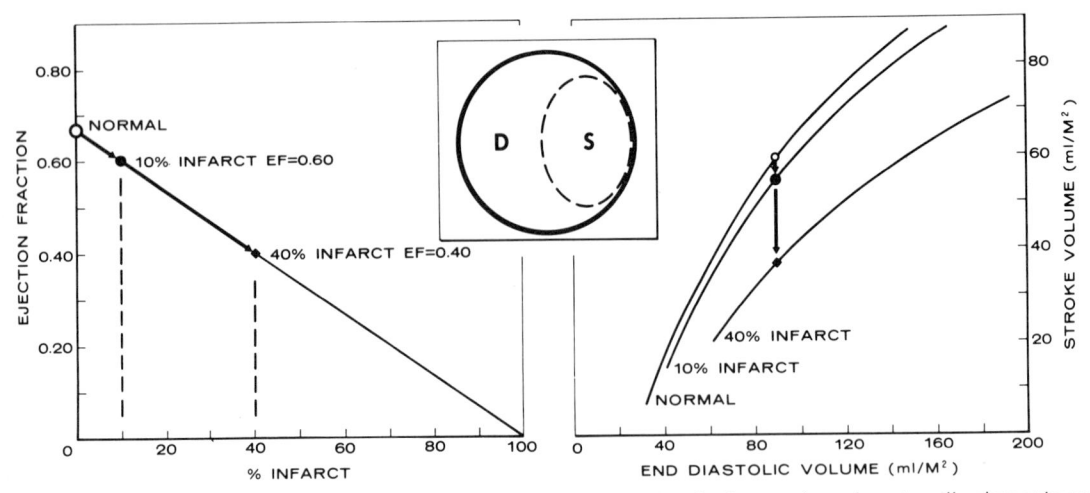

Figure 10-9 Diagrammatic representation of the effect of reduction in the number of contractile elements activated during ventricular systole. In myocardial ischemia or infarction, as the contractile units are rendered nonfunctional the overall performance of the ventricle falls. This is expressed in the left panel as the ejection fraction, or the portion of ventricular content expelled during systole, and on the right panel as isopleths of stroke volume as a function of end-diastolic volume. Note that obligatory reductions in stroke volume must occur as a function of the increasing magnitude of cardiac muscle involved. Further, the ventricle cannot dilate rapidly to compensate for this loss.

present, these effects are additive to the factors depressing the circulatory state and result in a sufficient depression of cardiac function to cause shock in spite of the presence of an infarct of lesser size.

It has been found that patients exhibiting the shock state do indeed fall into appropriate pathophysiologic groupings. The younger patients with a first infarction who progress rapidly through their illness and die in cardiogenic shock have large myocardial infarcts, usually resulting from an acute anterolateral or anteroseptal infarction consequent on a major occlusion in the left coronary arterial system. This amounts to approximately 55 per cent of all patients. Another 15 to 20 per cent of patients have an additional definable mechanical lesion such as those indicated above, while the balance of approximately 30 per

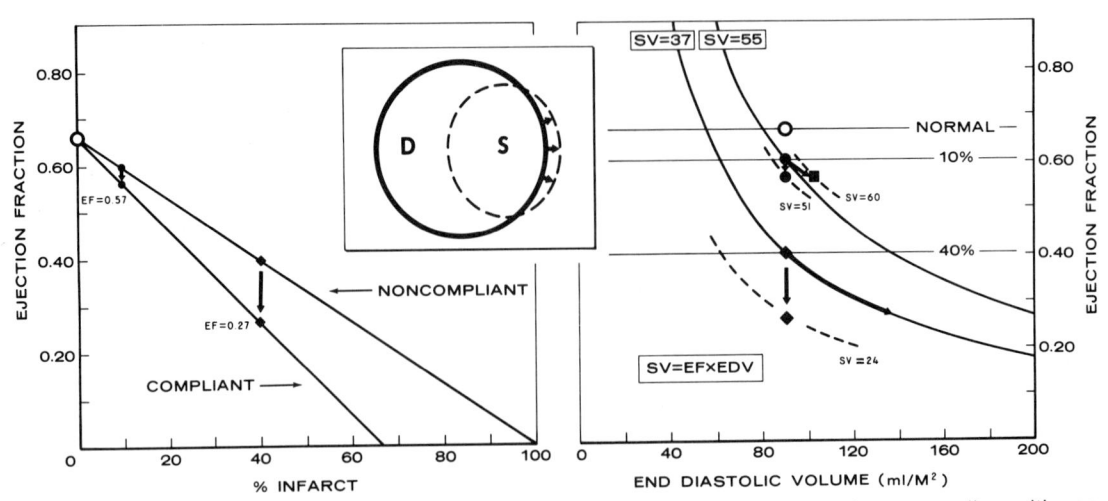

Figure 10-10 Ventricular performance as a consequence of substitution of contracting myocardium with noncontracting but compliant elements. In this instance the nonfunctional fibers elongate and the ventricle distends as a consequence of the rise in intraventricular pressure occasioned by contraction of the healthy elements. The mechanical disadvantage is evident (see Figure 10-9 for comparison).

cent of cases have end-stage heart disease. In these latter cases, the imposition of new small myocardial infarction upon chronic heart disease is sufficient to depress function so that an adequate performance can no longer be maintained.

SYMPTOMS AND SIGNS OF HEART FAILURE

We shall relate the symptoms and signs of heart failure to the four subsystems previously introduced, that is, the left ventricle, the right ventricle, the pulmonary venous circulation, and the systemic venous circulation.

Left Ventricular Failure

The principal symptom associated with failure of the left ventricle as a pump consists of those complaints related to reduced organ perfusion (Table 10-6). Weakness, easy fatigability, and extreme weakness of the musculoskeletal system are characteristic. Dyspnea is principally due to the associated pulmonary venous congestion. The extremities are frequently cool and pale. At times there is mental forgetfulness, and if the condition is prolonged and severe, there is ultimately evidence of dysfunction in many organ systems, including the gut, kidney, and liver. Severe peripheral cyanosis and indeed gangrene may occur in profound chronic heart failure. The signs include tachycardia, with a heart rate exceeding 100 beats per min., and a slight reduction in blood pressure. The pulse pressure is usually narrowed. Cardiomegaly may be present, owing to the nature of the underlying disease, but the heart size may be normal. The first sound is usually muffled and less distinctive than normal. If diastolic blood pressure is diminished, the second heart sound at the pulmonary and aortic areas is reduced. Diagnostic physical findings in significant heart failure include the presence of third and fourth heart sounds (Fig. 10-8). These sounds relate to heightened filling pressure in the left ventricle: the former is associated with a rapid filling of an already partially filled ventricle at the beginning of atrial emptying; the latter is associated with an enhanced rate of pressure rise in the ventricle at end diastole. If a murmur is present, it is usually related to the underlying disease but is reduced in intensity. In heart failure, the diastolic murmur of mitral stenosis may be totally absent. In like manner, in acute myocardial infarction a systolic murmur associated with papillary muscle disease may not be apparent but will be detected as cardiac function improves. The apex beat is usually diffuse and rather weak, with or without associated abnormal pulsation. The carotid pulse may be slow in its upstroke, although this is not a consistent finding.

Right Ventricular Failure

Right ventricular dysfunction may be associated with dyspnea, as in patients with acute pulmonary embolization. More importantly, there is moderate fatigue, which is not so severe as that associated with comparable degrees of left heart failure. Frequently, a right ventricular lift and an accentuated second heart sound at the pulmonary area may be evidence of the presence of concomitant pulmonary hypertension. Occasionally, a pulmonary diastolic murmur is heard, owing to the presence of extremely severe pulmonary hypertension. The second sound of the pulmonary area may also be widely split (Table 10-6).

Pulmonary Venous Congestion

The principal symptom of pulmonary venous congestion is dyspnea, as occurs following exer-

TABLE 10-6 PRINCIPAL CLINICAL SYMPTOMS AND PHYSICAL SIGNS OF RIGHT AND LEFT HEART FAILURE

	Left Heart Failure	*Right Heart Failure*
Symptoms	Fatigue, weakness	Weight gain
	Obtundation	Ankle swelling, pigmentation
	Cyanosis	Abdominal distention
	Exertion dyspnea	Subcostal pain
	Cough	Neck pulsations
	Orthopnea, paroxysmal nocturnal dyspnea	Jaundice
	Anorexia	
	Diaphoresis	
Signs	Tachycardia	Edema, ascites
	Apex diffuse	Increased 2nd sound (second component) of pulmonary area
	First sound ↓	
	Third and fourth sounds present	Left parasternal lift
	Moist rales, pleural effusion	Increased jugular venous pressure

tion in patients with a serious degree of heart failure. If the precipitating cause is acute, as with rupture of a cardiac valve, sudden severe shortness of breath may rapidly disable the patient. Orthopnea exists when the patient is unable to lie flat and is due to a high level of pulmonary venous pressure. Paroxysmal nocturnal dyspnea is usually not associated with severe elevation of pulmonary venous pressure but occurs when a patient with more moderate elevations sleeps flat, allowing a slow accumulation of fluid throughout the interstitial spaces of the lungs. When this reaches a critical value, it is necessary for the patient to assume the upright posture, so that redistribution of interstitial and alveolar fluid can allow effective respiration to be restored. Acute pulmonary edema is associated with a very rapid development of severe dyspnea, even with the patient in the upright position. It may be associated with the production of frothy bright red sputum. The patient will (naturally) be extremely apprehensive. On examination, patients with overt heart failure will be found to exhibit an increase in the frequency and depth of breathing. On auscultation of the chest, the findings are dependent on the degree of pulmonary venous hypertension. Patients with mild heart failure may have relatively few rales at both bases. In patients with acute pulmonary edema, it is possible to identify rales up to the thoracic apex. Unequal distribution of rales in the right and left chest is a frequent finding. Pleural effusion is often an accompaniment and may be so small as to be detectable only by chest x-ray, usually involving the right thoracic cavity. X-rays of the chest reveal several changes which relate to the severity of the heart failure. In the mildest examples, there are increased vascular markings in the lower lobe pulmonary veins. As the pulmonary congestion becomes more severe, the upper pulmonary veins become more prominent, while the lower lobe veins actually appear to become smaller. Hilar congestion and interstitial edema are followed by generalized edema, with a ground-glass appearance across the thorax. Pleural effusions may be noted as indicated above, in the right or left chest cavities or bilaterally.

Systemic Venous Congestion

The principal symptoms relate to swelling of the ankles and dependent parts, abdominal swelling, and subcostal pain. The neck veins may be distended and pulsatile. On examination, edema may be identified and abdominal swelling found associated with ascites or a large and tender liver. The liver may pulsate in the presence of tricuspid incompetence. Neck veins are frequently distended with a high venous pressure, so that even with the patient sitting at 45 to 60 degrees from the horizontal, the neck veins remain filled. In the presence of tricuspid incompetence, venous pulsation characterized by "a" and "v" waves may be identified.

PHYSIOLOGIC PRINCIPLES IN THE THERAPY OF HEART FAILURE

Effective therapy implies an adjustment of the environment or creation of a milieu that will favorably influence the cardiac state. Hence, rational treatment depends on the effectiveness of an action to reverse altered physiology.

The principles in the management of heart failure are to reduce cardiac demand, improve cardiac performance, maximize the rate and completeness of healing, and reverse associated disorders of organ function and fluid balance. It is not our purpose to discuss the mode of action or practical uses of inotropic or diuretic drugs or other conventional therapeutic modalities, or the mechanical benefits consequent on successful surgical treatment of congenital or valvar disease.

Alterations of Preload, Afterload, and Contractile State

It is convenient to think of the mechanical function of the heart in terms of its three principal determinants, i.e., preload, afterload, and contractile state (Table 10–7). *Preload* refers to initial and diastolic fiber length. Thus, changes in preload describe the Starling function curve. In the intact heart, preload is often considered in terms of either end-diastolic pressure or end-diastolic volume.

Since patients with power failure may have either high or low filling pressure, it is important to optimize the filling pressure to the most beneficial place on the Starling curve. Studies in patients with acute myocardial infarction, for example, have shown that a pulmonary capillary wedge pressure of approximately 15 to 18 mm. Hg provides the optimum cardiac performance, as measured by stroke volume or stroke work. Higher values of left ventricular filling pressure

TABLE 10–7 EFFECTS OF ALTERATIONS IN PRELOAD, AFTERLOAD, AND CONTRACTILE STATE ON STROKE VOLUME

	Preload (LVEDP)	Afterload (Arterial Pressure)	Contractile State
Increase in S.V.	↑	↓	↑
Decrease in S.V.	↓	↑	↓

do not augment stroke volume any further, and lower values of filling pressure may reduce stroke volume by the Starling mechanism. Furthermore, high levels of filling pressure may lead to pulmonary congestion, increased work of breathing, and increased myocardial oxygen consumption due to cardiac dilatation and the Laplace relation. These factors emphasize the importance of optimizing the left ventricular filling pressure in patients with cardiac failure.

Afterload refers to the load against which the heart must work. It is convenient to think of afterload as aortic pressure, although in reality the afterload corresponds to wall stress, which is related to pressure by the Laplace relationship. Of importance is the fact that changes in afterload may affect cardiac performance at a given preload. For example, if afterload is abruptly increased, there will be a corresponding reduction in stroke volume, with subsequent compensatory mechanisms tending to return toward normal. Similarly, if there is a corresponding reduction in afterload, there is an initial increase in stroke volume. This latter fact is receiving considerable attention recently in patients with severe heart failure and elevated filling pressure. Such patients are being treated with such drugs as Regitine, nitroprusside, or nitroglycerin to reduce arterial pressure and systemic vascular resistance. This therapy is very beneficial in many patients in that it produces an increase in cardiac output and a reduction in left ventricular filling pressure, in association with a fall in systemic vascular resistance and arterial pressure. The fall in left ventricular filling pressure is probably due to both venodilation, with a reduction in venous return, and more complete systolic emptying as a result of a reduction in afterload.

One group of patients who might especially benefit from a reduction of afterload are those patients with acute myocardial infarction and a hypertensive reaction. Reduction of blood pressure would markedly reduce oxygen needs of the heart and might limit the size of the infarct by reducing the surrounding ischemic zone. Reduction of the afterload has also been shown to be effective in patients with heart failure associated with severe mitral regurgitation. A fall in afterload reduces the regurgitant fraction and increases forward flow and cardiac output. It should be noted, however, that reduction of afterload also reduces diastolic filling pressure, which is the coronary perfusing pressure. Too great a reduction of arterial pressure, therefore, may be deleterious by reason of a concomitant reduction of coronary blood flow.

The third determinant of mechanical performance, *contractile state,* refers to the ability of the heart to alter its contractile force at a given preload and afterload in respose to such factors as intrinsic catecholamine stimulation; circulating catecholamines; or exogenous interventions such as digitalis, norepinephrine, isoproterenol, paired electrical stimulation, and so on. In chronic heart failure, the use of digitalis to increase contractile force, improve systolic emptying, and reduce heart size is accepted as having beneficial effects on the circulation. In the case of acute power failure due to acute myocardial infarction, however, it is unclear what the potential role of these positive inotropic agents is. The effects of drugs such as digitalis, isoproterenol, and norepinephrine are relatively slight in this setting and may even be deleterious, owing to their propensity to produce arrhythmias and the obligatory increase in myocardial oxygen needs because of the increase in contractile state. The general lack of response to positive inotropic agents in acute power failure following infarction may be related to the fact that much of the myocardium is nonresponsive (infarcted) and therefore is unable to increase its contractile state. In addition, the normally responsive myocardium is already maximally stimulated by intrinsic sympathetic tone or circulating catecholamines. Studies of myocardial mechanics have shown that there is a ceiling of contractility; if reached by using one agent, this ceiling cannot be exceeded even though another potent inotropic agent is added. Therefore, the relative lack of response of patients with power failure following myocardial infarction to all inotropic agents may be due to these factors and suggests that these agents may have limited value in this particular setting. Of equal or greater importance may be the correction of such factors as anoxia, arrhythmias, acidosis, and relative hypovolemia.

A knowledge of the factors which determine myocardial oxygen consumption is of importance in several clinical settings. For example, in coronary artery disease with a fixed proximal stenosis of a major vessel it would appear that a potent inotropic agent might be deleterious, since it would increase oxygen consumption by increasing contractile state, while the coronary circulation would be unable concomitantly to increase coronary flow because of the fixed proximal obstruction. This imbalance between oxygen supply and demand might produce or worsen ischemia and angina pectoris. In certain circumstances, however, it has been noted that digitalis will alleviate angina pectoris when given to some patients with ventricular failure. The reason for this observation apparently relates to the fact that when heart size is decreased by digitalis the decrease in myocardial oxygen consumption then offsets the increase in oxygen consumption associated with the increase in contractility produced by digitalis. Since digitalis has only modest inotropic effects, however, this beneficial effect on angina is not observed with other more potent inotropic agents such as isoproterenol.

A further point of clinical importance relates to the use of beta-adrenergic blockers such as propranolol in the treatment of angina pectoris. Such drugs may improve angina by decreasing oxygen consumption. For example, propranolol blocks neural sympathetic tone to the heart and, in addition, blocks the effects of circulating catecholamines, thus reducing oxygen consumption by preventing the increase in contractile state produced by these interventions. Furthermore, propranolol also has a direct depressive effect on the contractile state of the myocardium, which may further decrease oxygen needs. Because of these combined effects, propranolol and similar drugs may improve the relationship between oxygen supply and demand and decrease the frequency and severity of angina pectoris. It should also be noted, however, that when propranolol is given to patients with heart failure, it may worsen the congestive failure. This occurs because propranolol blocks sympathetic tone and the influence of circulating catecholamines, which may be needed to support the cardiovascular system. If propranolol increases congestive heart failure and produces further cardiac dilatation, myocardial wall tension will be increased by the Laplace relation, with a possible increase in myocardial oxygen consumption. Thus, although propranolol may favorably influence the relationship of oxygen supply and demand in a patient with angina pectoris and a small heart, it may actually aggravate angina pectoris in a patient in whom further cardiac dilatation occurs. Thus, the effects of any particular drug on angina pectoris must be evaluated in terms of its effects on heart rate, arterial pressure, contractile state, and cardiac size.

The concept of angina pectoris reflecting an imbalance between oxygen supply and demand has additional clinical implications. For example, in patients with aortic stenosis, large pressure gradients across the aortic valve, and a thick-walled ventricle, the symptoms of angina pectoris can occur, despite normal coronary arteries. This is not surprising when we consider the tremendous increase in oxygen cost produced by the level of systolic pressure in the ventricle and the hypertrophied myocardium. In a similar way, the relief of angina pectoris by nitroglycerin reflects a better balance between oxygen supply and demand, which is unrelated to any direct effect on the coronary arteries. Thus, the reduction in venous return by peripheral venodilation reduces end-diastolic volume and wall stress by the Laplace relation. Similarly, a reduction in arterial pressure by arterial vasodilation reduces the tension-time index. Both effects, therefore, reduce myocardial wall stress and oxygen consumption and are beneficial in relieving angina pectoris.

The importance of myocardial oxygen consumption has also recently been emphasized in the setting of acute myocardial infarction. In established infarction, there is a central zone of dead tissue which is surrounded by a zone of ischemic muscle with a marginal blood supply and oxygen delivery. The potential viability of this area, therefore, is critically dependent on the balance between oxygen supply and demand. Thus, the importance of maintaining coronary perfusion pressure has been emphasized in that it tends to reduce the surrounding area of ischemia as monitored by direct ST segment mapping of the ventricular epicardium in dogs. On the other hand, the use of inotropic agents which increase contractile state tends to enlarge the surrounding area of ischemia by increasing the need for oxygen. The desire to minimize the area of infarction by protecting this zone of ischemic muscle is receiving increasing attention in consideration of various modes of therapy for acute myocardial infarction.

MECHANICAL CIRCULATORY ASSIST

When one considers the management of cardiac decompensation, it is logical to examine the possibility of adding to the circulating bloodstream energy other than that provided by the contracting left ventricle. With this objective in mind, recent attention has been paid to the possibility of total or partial circulatory support by artificial mechanical devices.

Total cardiac replacement by an auxiliary heart has been attempted in a few patients. In most of these endeavors, the cardiac chambers themselves have not been removed but have been used in a nonfunctional manner as part of the conduit traversed by blood to an auxiliary ventricle, either in a portion of the arterial system or between the apex of the left ventricle and the aorta. These devices have sustained the circulation for short periods of time. They require the provision of an external power source with an appropriate transcutaneous connection to the working pump. In addition, the technical problems associated with insertion and vascular connections and the formation of thrombi on the surfaces in contact with flowing blood have not yet been satisfactorily resolved. In the relatively short duration of total cardiac function thus far attempted in man no limitation seems to be imposed by the strength-durability characteristics of the materials utilized.

An artificial heart powered by an atomic energy source appears to be feasible in the future. Prototype heart pumps have been used for relatively long periods in calves. An atomic power source would allow total implantation, probably within the abdomen, and the problems of radiation shielding and heat dissipation are solvable.

It is predicted that such devices will be developed within the next decade with approximately a 10-year life, determined by the stress-strain characteristics of the pump materials. There is no foreseeable limitation imposed by the energy source.

Temporary circulatory assist implies that fundamental abnormal processes may be reversible if the cardiovascular system is supported for a finite period of time, or until more definitive forms of therapy can be undertaken. Circulatory support for hours, or even several days, is now feasible and has been utilized in human patients. However, it has been found that in many instances the degree of myocardial damage which has caused the need for circulatory support is so great as to preclude long-term survival. Hence, many patients must be subjected subsequently to procedures to correct mechanically disadvantageous cardiac lesions or to provide cardiac revascularization by means of aorta-coronary artery anastomosis.

The use of the heart-lung bypass machine conventionally employed in cardiovascular surgery has been suggested for the temporary support of the circulation. Although this is feasible for periods of approximately 3 hours, the oxygenators do not allow prolonged total support of the circulation. Newly developed membrane oxygenators apparently more adequately preserve the structure of the formed elements in the blood and do not lead to thrombus formation. With these devices, total circulatory support has been undertaken for 24 to 60 hours in a small number of patients. As an extension of this principle, total support of the circulation utilizing the patient's lung as the oxygenator has been proposed. However, there are significant technical difficulties in recovering the oxygenated blood effectively from the left atrium or in the procedures necessary to totally empty the ventricle.

Mechanical counterpulsation refers to a form of partial mechanical support of the circulation. It is well known that when the heart exhibits failure, it is an extremely poor pressure pump, but it is less disabled than a volume pump. Therefore, reduction of the opening pressure at the aortic valve and a reduction of blood pressure during ventricular systole favor the more complete emptying of the left ventricle. Although this can be accomplished by the reduction of peripheral vascular resistance by spinal anesthesia or dilating drugs, it is done so at the expense of coronary perfusion, since a sustained pressure greater than 60 mm. Hg is probably needed during diastole to maintain coronary perfusion. Hence, the most favorable circumstance would be a fundamental reversal of the normal sequence of the cardiac cycle, that is, a fall in aortic pressure during ventricular systole and a rise in pressure during ventricular diastole. A number of procedures have been employed to accomplish these ends. Of these, the best known is accomplished by insertion into the descending thoracic aorta of a sausage-shaped 30-ml. balloon, supported by a rigid catheter. The balloon is connected to a source of compressed helium which is allowed access to the balloon via a control valve synchronized with the cardiac cycle. Thus, just before or at the time of ventricular systole, the balloon is evacuated of gas and hence the volume in the aorta is acutely reduced by approximately 30 ml. Consequently, there is a brisk fall in aortic pressure, so that ventricular ejection occurs at a point earlier in the cardiac cycle and at a much lower pressure level. When cardiac ejection is complete and the aortic valve closes, the balloon is reinflated, adding a volume equivalent to 30 ml. to the aortic content, thus raising the intra-aortic pressure. These events are indicated diagrammatically in Figure 10–11. Coronary perfusion pressure is increased during ventricular diastole, while the stimulus to myocardial oxygen consumption is diminished because isometric contraction is shortened and maximal left ventricular wall tension is decreased.

Usually within 10 to 15 minutes after its initiation, this form of circulatory support can reverse profound depression of cardiovascular pump function. There is a prompt improvement in cardiac output, reduction in filling pressure, improved organ perfusion, and reversal of metabolic alterations. However, this technique necessitates surgical insertion of the balloon into the vascular system, a precise synchronization of the electrical action of the heart with the inflation and deflation sequences, and an experienced team of investigators and clinicians to manage other aspects of patient care.

Figure 10–11 The mechanical consequences of counterpulsation. This diagram represents aortic and left ventricular pressure pulses (left panel) and the changes consequent upon counterpulsation (right panel). During counterpulsation the pressure in the aorta during the isometric phase of ventricular contraction suddenly falls. Hence, the aortic valve can open at a lower pressure and early in the cardiac cycle. This may favorably influence the level of myocardial oxygen consumption. Since the aortic capacitance has been increased (see text) the absolute magnitude of pressure generated during ventricular systole is reduced. When the aortic valve closes, aortic pressure is artificially increased by the counter-pulsation device, thus providing a higher head of pressure for the maintenance of coronary arterial blood flow.

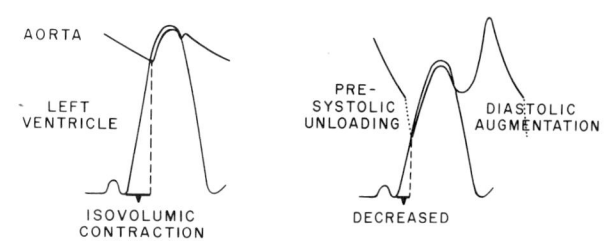

REFERENCES

Braunwald, E.: The determinants of myocardial oxygen consumption. Thirteenth Bowditch Lecture. The Physiologist, *12*:65, 1969.

Braunwald, E., Chidsey, C. A., Pool, P. E., et al.: Clinical Staff Conference. Congestive heart failure: Biochemical and physiological considerations. Ann. Intern. Med., *64*:904, 1966.

Braunwald, E., Ross, J., and Sonnenblick, E. H.: Mechanisms of contraction of the normal and failing heart. Boston, Little, Brown and Co., 1968.

Dodge, H. T., and Baxley, W. A.: Hemodynamic aspects of heart failure. Amer. J. Cardiol., *22*:24, 1968.

Friedberg, C. K. (Ed.): Congestive Heart Failure. New York, Grune and Stratton, 1970, pp. 1–70, 97–171, 195–288.

Ganz, W., Tamura, K., Marcus, H. S., et al.: Measurement of coronary sinus blood flow by continuous thermodilution in man. Circulation, *44*:181, 1971.

Herman, M. V., and Gorlin, R.: Implications of left ventricular asynergy. Amer. J. Cardiol., *23*:538, 1969.

Katz, A. M., and Brady, A. J.: Mechanical and biochemical correlates of cardiac contraction (I and II). Modern Conc. Cardiovasc. Dis., *40*:39 and *40*:45, 1971.

Maroko, P. R., Kjekshus, J. K., Sobel, B. E., et al.: Factors influencing infarct size following experimental coronary artery occlusions. Circulation, *43*:67, 1971.

Mason, D. T.: Control of the peripheral circulation in health and disease. Modern Conc. Cardiovasc. Dis., *36*:25, 1967.

Spann, J. F., Jr., Mason, D. T., and Zelis, R.: Recent advances in the understanding of congestive heart failure. Modern Conc. Cardiovasc. Dis., *39*:73, 1970.

Swan, H. J. C., Forrester, J. S., Diamond, G., et al.: The hemodynamic basis of shock and acute myocardial infarction: a conceptual model. Circulation, *45*:1097, 1972.

CHAPTER 11

HEART SOUNDS, MURMURS, AND PRECORDIAL MOVEMENTS*†

JOHN F. STAPLETON
W. PROCTOR HARVEY

During each cardiac cycle the heart generates many vibrations which are transmitted through surrounding tissues to the chest wall. These arise from the contractile and expansile movements of the cardiac chambers, from valvular opening and closure, from tissue motion caused by blood flow, and from the bloodstream itself.

Vibrations having low frequency (0 to 30 cycles per second) cause subaudible chest wall pulsations which can be palpated when sufficiently forceful. Vibrations having higher frequency (30 to 500 cycles per second) enter the range of human audibility and can be heard at the chest surface when sufficiently loud. Such audible vibrations are called heart sounds when brief and murmurs when sustained. Figure 11-1 illustrates the sensitivity of the human ear to cardiovascular sound.

---

*Supported in part by U. S. Public Health grants, The Benjamin May Memorial Fund, and Metropolitan Heart Guild.
†We wish to express our appreciation to Mr. Bernard Salb and Mrs. Gail Maume for their assistance in preparing this chapter.

HEART SOUNDS AND MURMURS

The first heart sound (S1) occurs as the ventricles start to contract. The major vibrations which make up this sound commence 0.04 to 0.06 second after the onset of the electrocardiographic QRS (Fig. 11-2), about 0.02 second after beginning systolic pressure rise within the left ventricle. Minor vibrations coinciding with the earliest ventricular contractile movement precede the initial major component of the first sound. The main vibrations last 0.04 to 0.08 second and are sometimes followed by further small vibrations lasting another 0.01 to 0.02 second.

The exact genesis of the first sound is not known with certainty. Most authorities agree that movements of the mitral and tricuspid valve structures at the time of closure cause the major vibrations of the first sound. The small initial vibrations are attributed to myocardial contraction, the small terminal vibrations to semilunar valve opening and great vessel movement.

The first sound usually presents as a single

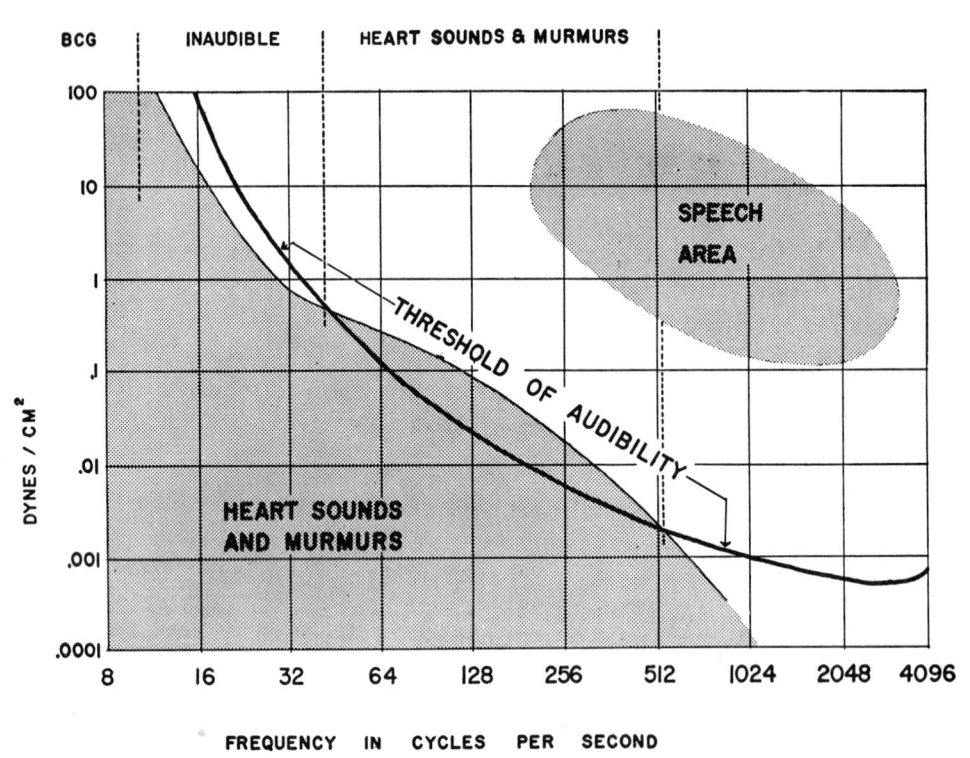

Figure 11-1 The graph illustrates the frequency spectrum of human hearing. Note that only a small component of total cardiac sound can be detected by the human ear. (By permission from Butterworth, J. S., Chassin, M. R., and McGrath, R.: Cardiac Auscultation Including Audiovisual Principles. 2nd ed. New York, Grune and Stratton, 1960.)

sound at the cardiac apex, where it is loudest; it frequently splits into two distinct elements along the mid and lower left sternal border. When split, the initial component derives from mitral valve closure (M1), while the second component arises from tricuspid valve closure (T1). The tricuspid vibrations are usually localized to the left parasternal area, whereas the louder mitral component has a wider distribution over the precordium (Fig. 11-3). When the sound of tricuspid closure does extend to the apex, it is normally fainter than the apical mitral component. When T1 is louder than M1 at the apex, abnormally forceful tricuspid closure is present, such as commonly occurs with atrial septal defect.

The P-R interval of the electrocardiogram relates to the intensity of the first heart sound. Short P-R intervals (0.10 to 0.13) intensify the first sound, while longer intervals (0.20 to 0.24) diminish it. When P-R extends beyond 0.24 to 0.26, its influence on the first sound is less predictable. The first sound–P-R relationship is explained by the proximity of ventricular systole to atrial systole. When the ventricle contracts while still distended by atrial systole (short P-R interval), it generates greater force and more vigorously shuts the mitral valve. When the ventricle contracts after the distending effect of atrial systole has subsided (long P-R interval), it contracts less forcefully.

Conditions which increase the force of ventricular contractions usually increase the intensity of the first sound. Such conditions include thyrotoxicosis, severe anemia, exercise, excitement, and stimulatory drugs such as epinephrine. Mitral stenosis, by stiffening the mitral leaflets, causes a loud and often high-pitched first sound. Conditions which diminish cardiac function, such as myocardial infarction or myxedema, tend to soften the first sound, irrespective of the P-R interval.

Delayed onset of the first sound characterizes mitral stenosis, which impairs leaflet mobility and elevates left atrial pressure. The delay can be detected by measuring the interval between the onset of QRS on the electrocardiogram and the onset of the first major vibrations of the first sound as recorded on a phonocardiogram. This measurement correlates with the severity of mitral obstruction. Systemic hypertension also can cause slightly delayed onset of the first heart sound.

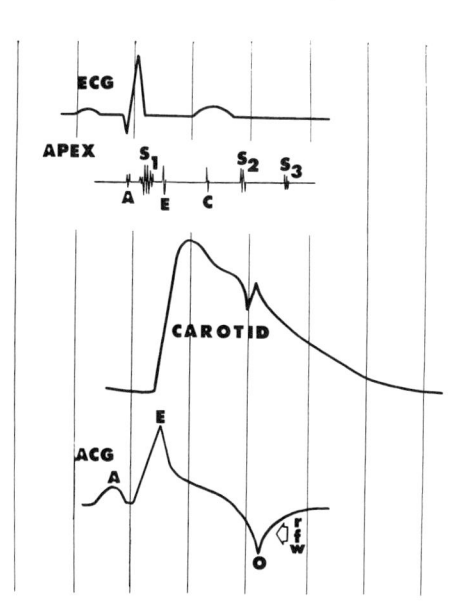

Figure 11-2 Heart sounds heard at the apex correlated with the electrocardiogram (ECG), carotid artery pulse tracing (CAROTID), and apex cardiogram (ACG).

Sound tracing: A, atrial sound or S4 (left atrial); S1, first heart sound; E, aortic ejection sound; C, systolic click; S2, second heart sound; S3, ventricular filling sound.

Apex cardiogram (ACG): E, Peak of apical impulse; O, beginning of ventricular rapid filling (rfw).

Closure of the semilunar valves causes a second heart sound (S2), which signifies the end of systole. This sound occurs when aortic and pulmonary pressures exceed the declining pressures of the relaxing ventricles and cause the aortic and pulmonary valves to shut. Normally the second sound splits into two distinct components, the first due to aortic valve closure, followed by the second due to pulmonary valve closure. The aortic component (A2) can normally be heard all over the precordium, being maximal in the aortic area. The pulmonary component (P2) is usually loudest in the pulmonary area (Fig. 11-4) but often extends to the tricuspid region (Fig. 11-5). Hence, splitting of the second sound is best heard over the pulmonary area and along the mid left sternal border (Figs. 11-4 and 11-5). Aortic closure usually causes a louder tone than pulmonary closure, even in the pulmonary region; however, in some young individuals P2 may normally exceed A2 in the pulmonary region.

Inspiration augments venous return to the chest and increases blood flow into the right heart, requiring longer right ventricular emptying time. Right ventricular systole, therefore, lengthens slightly during inspiration, delaying pulmonary valve closure. At the same time, inspiration expands the pulmonary vascular bed and pulmonary blood volume, reducing flow to the left heart and shortening left ventricular systole, with resultant earlier aortic valve closure (Fig. 11-3).

Inspiratory splitting of the second sound, described by Potain in 1866, has been reemphasized by Leatham. Complete right bundle branch block, by retarding right ventricular depolarization, delays pulmonary valve closure, resulting in wide splitting of the second sound even during expiration; inspiration further widens the split. Conversely, conditions which prolong or delay left ventricular systole may cause A2 to follow P2. When this occurs splitting increases with expiration and narrows with inspiration, a finding called paradoxical or reversed splitting of the second sound (Fig. 11-6). Complete left bundle branch block commonly causes this phenomenon by impeding left ventricular depolarization and so delaying aortic closure. Severe aortic stenosis occasionally prolongs left ventricular ejection sufficiently to cause paradoxical splitting. Right ventricular pacing and right ventricular extrasystoles simulate left bundle branch block by depolarizing the right ventricle before the left, causing reversed splitting of S2. Other infrequent causes of reversed splitting include patent ductus arteriosus, angina pectoris, myocardial infarction, and, rarely, systemic hypertension.

In uncomplicated atrial septal defect with significant left-to-right shunt, right ventricular volume and pulmonary flow change little during the respiratory cycle, since flow across the atrial defect adjusts inversely to respiratory variations of systemic venous return so as to maintain constant total flow into the right atrium. A2 and P2 remain clearly separate during both inspiration and expiration, exhibiting little or no respiratory variation (Fig. 11-7). This phenomenon, known as fixed splitting, characterizes left-to-right shunting of blood at the atrial level and is a valuable diagnostic sign, although occasional patients with atrial septal defects may present normal splitting of S2 (Levine and Harvey).

Pulmonary or systemic hypertension produces forceful closure of the pulmonary or aortic valve. Loud A2 or P2 often accompanies aortic or pulmonary hypertension. The accentuated P2 of pulmonary hypertension is sometimes palpable, if sought. The hyperactive circulation of thyrotoxicosis or severe anemia also intensifies the second sound; however, these disorders increase the first heart sound, unlike hypertension, which selectively augments the second sound. Impaired mobility of a semilunar valve will diminish its closure sound. The aortic second sound of calcific aortic stenosis is usually faint or even absent, whereas congenital aortic stenosis with its supple valve structure usually gives rise to a normal or increased closure sound. Severe pulmonary stenosis greatly diminishes (and delays) P2 (Fig. 11-

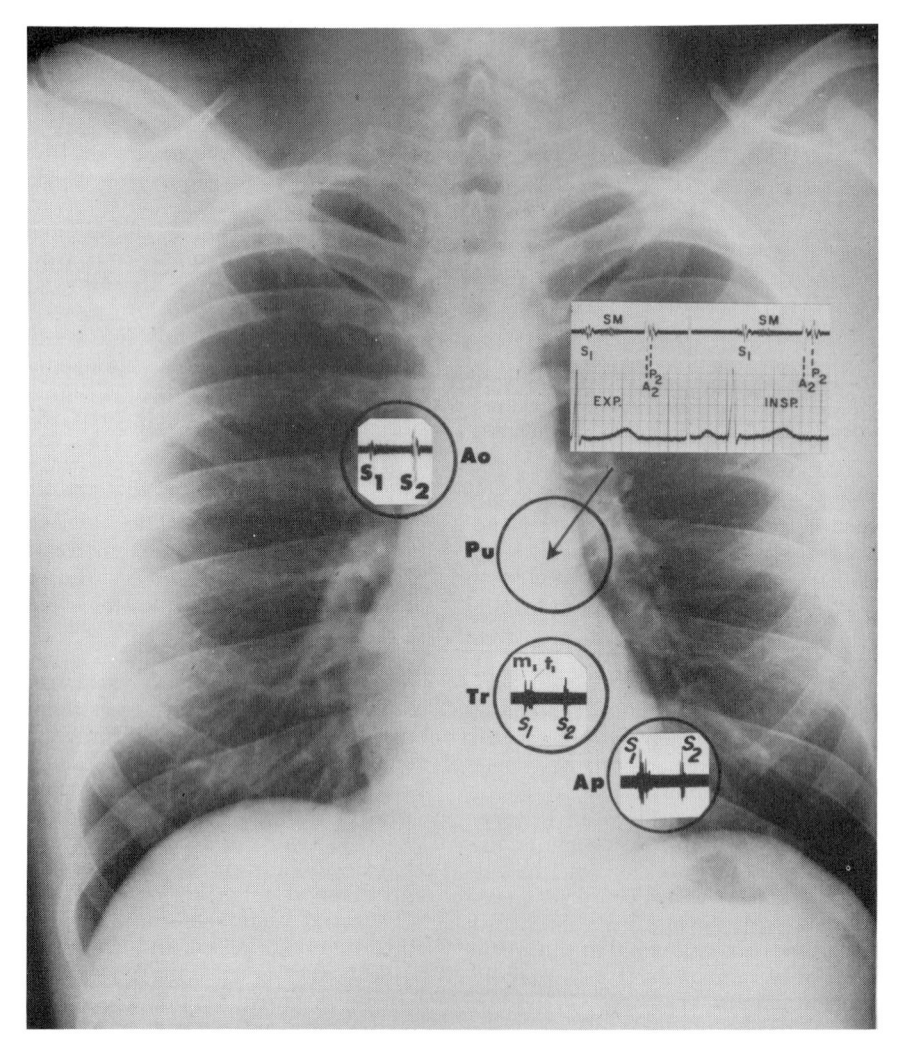

Figure 11-3 Heart sounds as heard over different valve areas. *Ao,* aortic area: Here the first sound *(S1)* is faint and the second sound *(S2)* is loud and single. *Pu,* pulmonary area: Here S1 is reduced and S2 is loud and split into two components, *A2* (aortic closure) and *P2* (pulmonary closure). The split S2 widens with inspiration and narrows with expiration. *Tr,* tricuspid area: S1 splits into two components, *M1* (mitral closure) and *T1* (tricuspid closure). *Ap,* apex: S1 is loud with faint before and after vibrations. S2 is single and less intense than S1, at the apex. *SM,* systolic murmur; *INSP,* inspiration; *EXP,* expiration.

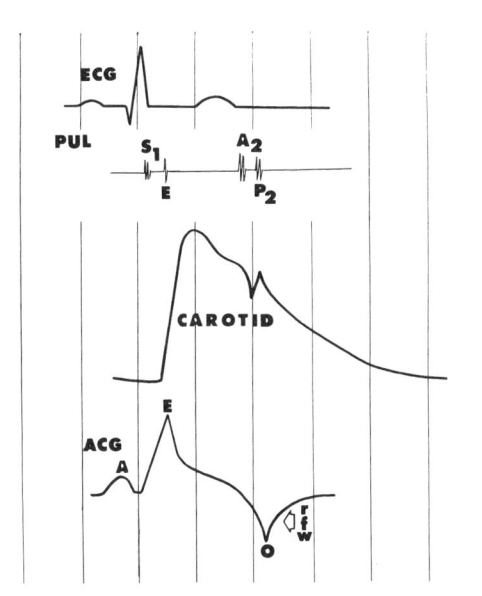

Figure 11-4 Heart sounds heard over the pulmonary area *(PUL)* correlated with the electrocardiogram *(ECG)*, carotid artery pulse tracing *(CAROTID)*, and apex cardiogram *(ACG)*.

Sound tracing: *S1*, first heart sound; *E*, pulmonary ejection sound; *A2*, aortic valve closure sound; *P2*, pulmonary valve closure sound.

Apex cardiogram (ACG): *E*, Peak of apical impulse; *O*, beginning of ventricular rapid filling *(rfw)*.

Another extra heart sound may occur during atrial systole. This sound, known as the atrial or fourth heart sound (S4), relates to the increment of ventricular filling caused by atrial contraction; it probably arises from movement of the atrioventricular valve structure caused by sudden ventricular distention. Atrial sounds may be heard in apparently healthy individuals, particularly in the older age groups. When atrioventricular block separates atrial from ventricular contraction, atrial sounds frequently become audible.

Left atrial sounds begin about 0.17 second (range: 0.14 to 0.24) after the onset of the electrocardiographic P, coinciding with the peak of the precordial atrial movement. The sound is low pitched, apical, and usually faint. Its closeness to the first sound may simulate wide splitting of the first sound. When prominent, the sound can be heard medial to the apex, sometimes extending to the sternal border. Right atrial sounds begin about 0.12 second (range: 0.09 to 0.16) after the onset of P and are low pitched, usually faint, and best heard over the tricuspid area (Weitzman). Faint vibrations often can be recorded preceding an audible atrial sound; these vibrations, usually inaudible, probably arise from myocardial contraction.

10), whereas mild pulmonary stenosis does so only slightly.

Posterior location of the pulmonary valve, as in certain congenital defects, may also diminish or even abolish P2.

Most children and many young adults have a normal third heart sound (S3) in early diastole. This sound coincides with the rapid filling phase of left ventricular diastole and is variously known as a physiologic third sound, a ventricular filling sound, or simply S3. Its genesis is unclear; there is reason to suspect transient vibrations of the mitral valve structure as rapid filling suddenly dilates the left ventricle. The third heart sound is low pitched, best heard at the apex, and usually faint, although occasionally this sound is prominent and may have after-vibrations which extend its duration. Although a third sound during left ventricular rapid filling is physiologic during childhood and youth, this sound in middle life and beyond denotes cardiac dysfunction, usually myocardial failure. It is an early and subtle sign of cardiac decompensation, having great diagnostic and prognostic value. Its detection often requires deliberate listening in a quiet room. Occasionally, regurgitant disease of the aortic or mitral valve so exaggerates ventricular filling that it generates a third sound.

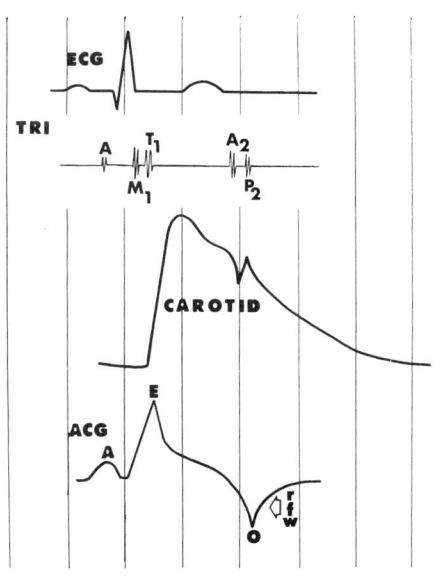

Figure 11-5 Heart sounds heard over the tricuspid region *(TRI)* correlated with the electrocardiogram *(ECG)*, carotid artery pulse tracing *(CAROTID)*, and apex cardiogram *(ACG)*.

Sounding tracing: *A*, atrial sound or S4 (right atrial); *M1*, mitral valve closure sound; *T1*, tricuspid valve closure sound; *A2*, aortic valve closure sound; *P2*, Pulmonary valve closure sound.

Apex cardiogram (ACG): *E*, peak of apical impulse; *O*, beginning of ventricular rapid filling *(rfw)*.

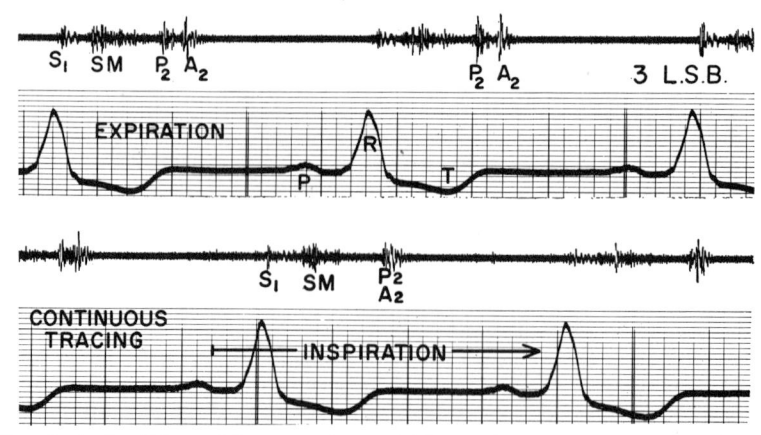

Figure 11-6 Paradoxical splitting of the second sound. The aortic valve closure sound (A2) follows the pulmonary valve closure sound (P2). Inspiration delays P2, narrowing the split. Compare with Figure 11-3, which illustrates normal inspiratory separation of A2 and P2. S1, first heart sound. SM, systolic murmur. (Reproduced from Levine, S. A., and Harvey, W. P.: Clinical Auscultation of the Heart. 2nd ed. Philadelphia, W. B. Saunders Co., 1959.)

Atrial sounds are likely to appear whenever there is increased resistance to ventricular filling. Various myocardial diseases increase resistance to ventricular filling by reducing myocardial compliance and thereby cause atrial sounds. Intrinsic cardiomyopathies frequently cause atrial sounds; the concentric hypertrophy of aortic stenosis and systemic hypertension also stiffens the ventricular wall, leading to vigorous atrial contraction. Atrial sounds regularly accompany these diseases. Acute myocardial infarction often causes high diastolic ventricular filling pressure, low ventricular compliance, and atrioventricular block; hence, atrial sounds appear in most patients with acute myocardial infarction and often persist after the acute stage.

When atrial and ventricular diastolic sounds result from heart disease, the term "gallop rhythm" is often applied, because these extra sounds impart the cadence of a cantering horse to the heart rhythm—particularly when the ventricular rate is rapid. Thus, the atrial and ventricular sounds of heart disease are usually called gallop sounds. A patient with cardiac failure may have a ventricular (or third sound) gallop or an atrial (or fourth sound) gallop or both. When tachycardia is present, a diastolic gallop sound may be difficult to classify. When slowing occurs, identification can be made by noting a constant relationship of the ventricular gallop to the second sound and a constant relationship of the atrial gallop to the electrocardiographic P and, usually, to the first sound (Fig. 11-8).

Atrial and ventricular sounds frequently coexist. When close together, this combination of sounds may resemble a short, low-pitched rumbling murmur. When diastole so shortens that these sounds fuse, a single sound may result, known as a summation gallop sound.

Patients with constrictive pericarditis often present an extra sound in early diastole which coincides with the sudden arrest of the expanding ventricle as the constricting pericardium abruptly halts diastolic filling.

A third sound often follows closely upon the second sound in mitral stenosis. Known as the

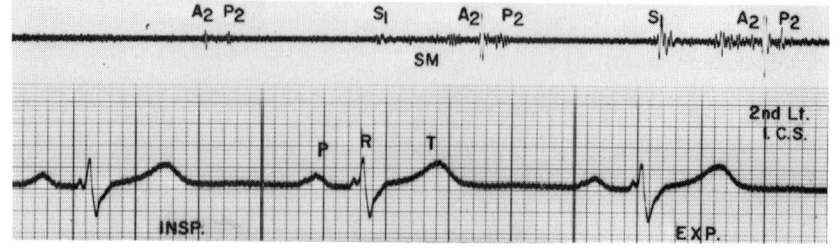

Figure 11-7 Fixed splitting of the second sound. Widely split second sound without significant respiratory variation of the interval between aortic closure (A2) and pulmonary closure (P2). This finding characterizes most individuals with atrial septal defect. S1, first heart sound; SM, systolic murmur.

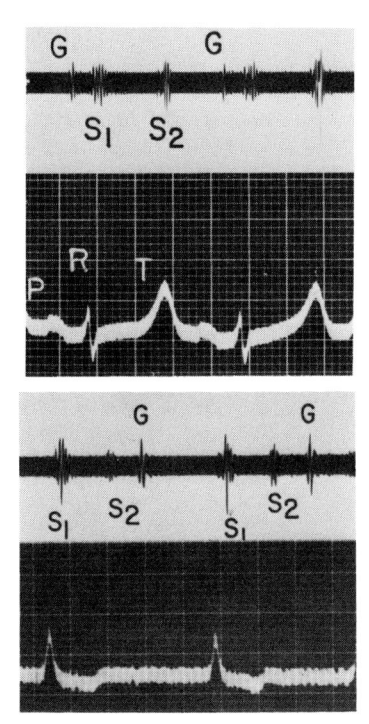

Figure 11-8 Upper panel displays a gallop sound (G) related to atrial systole. This sound is known as an atrial gallop or as an atrial sound or as a fourth heart sound (S4). S1, first heart sound; S2, second heart sound.

Lower panel displays a gallop sound (G) related to ventricular rapid filling. This sound is known as a ventricular filling sound or as a ventricular gallop or as a third heart sound (S3). S1, first heart sound; S2, second heart sound.

opening snap, it probably derives from the suddenly arrested descent of the stiffened mitral valve which occurs as the valve opens in early diastole. This sound signifies the end of isovolumetric relaxation; it is usually high pitched and is best heard at the apex but can transmit widely. It follows the aortic closure sound by 0.06 to 0.12 second. This measurement, which can readily be made with a phonocardiogram and approximated by careful auscultation, correlates with the severity of mitral obstruction—the shorter A2—opening snap periods corresponding to higher grades of stenosis. This interval varies with heart rate, since shorter cycle lengths are associated with higher left atrial pressure and earlier mitral valve opening. When mitral stenosis greatly reduces valve mobility as with dense calcification, the mitral opening snap may become fainter and occasionally disappears. Valve rigidity also frequently diminishes the intensity of the first sound.

Extra heart sounds also occur during systole. Patients with congenital aortic or pulmonary stenosis often have an early systolic sound which closely follows the first sound. Known as an aortic or pulmonary ejection sound, it signifies the end of isovolumetric contraction, coinciding with the maximum excursion of the deformed semilunar valve and initiating ejection. Aortic ejection sounds are best heard in the aortic area (Fig. 11-10) and at the apex (Fig. 11-2). Pulmonary ejection sounds are best heard in the pulmonary area (Fig. 11-5) and characteristically diminish with inspiration; they are generally faint or absent at the apex. Ejection sounds often occur with pulmonary or systemic hypertension or with abnormal dilatation of the ascending aorta or pulmonary artery; these ejection sounds may coincide with sudden distention of the great vessel wall, having a vascular rather than valvular sound source. Thus, an aortic ejection sound may be heard over the aortic and apical areas with coarctation of the aorta.

Other sounds may also occur during systolic ejection; such sounds are frequently brief, high pitched, and therefore called clicks. The "midsystolic click" is a commonly used expression denoting the approximate timing of such sounds (Figs. 11-2 and 11-9). Angiograms of patients with this finding usually demonstrate one or both mitral leaflets to be so copious that they prolapse into the left atrium during late systole, permitting regurgitation; the posterior leaflet is most commonly involved. The click coincides with maximum leaflet excursion and probably arises from the suddenly arrested motion of the affected leaflet(s) and chordae tendineae.

Audible vibrations which persist beyond the brief acoustic impact of a discrete heart sound constitute a heart *murmur;* a murmur is a rapid succession of heart sounds. Most investigators have attributed murmurs to blood flow through irregular or narrowed orifices or through dilated segments of major arteries, through abnormal intracardiac and arteriovenous communications, or backward through incompetent valves. Murmurs also can arise from rapid blood flow through normal structures. The actual genesis of murmur vibrations has not been established with certainty. There are two sources of sound which account for the many varieties of murmurs: the bloodstream itself and solid structures which are caused to vibrate by flowing blood. Murmurs arising from the blood itself are thought to derive from vortex (eddy) formation or from turbulence created as blood flows through varying orifices, chambers, and tubes at varying rates. Murmurs arising from solid structures usually represent the vibrations of heart valves or other cardiac or vascular tissue set into motion by the bloodstream.

Murmurs are classified according to timing,

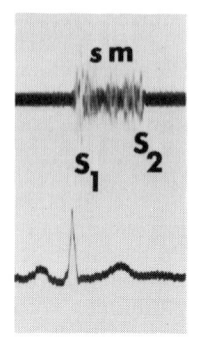

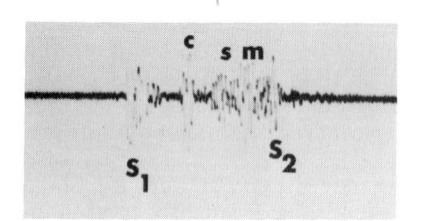

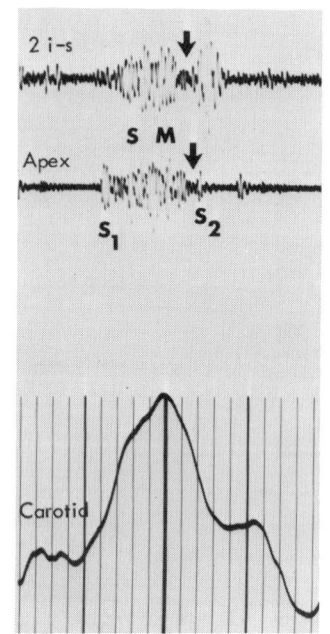

Figure 11-9 Upper left panel displays the holosystolic murmur of severe mitral regurgitation. The murmur *(SM)* extends from the first sound *(S1)* to the second sound *(S2).*

Lower left panel displays the late systolic murmur *(SM)* of mitral regurgitation due to prolapse of posterior mitral leaflet. *S1,* first sound; *S2,* second sound; *C,* systolic click; *SM,* systolic murmur.

Vertical panel on right displays the systolic murmur *(SM)* of acute mitral regurgitation due to rupture of chordae tendineae. Note rapid decline of systolic vibrations in late systole (arrows). Upper sound tracing recorded in aortic area *(2 i-s);* lower sound tracing recorded over the cardiac apex. *S1,* first heart sound; *S2,* second heart sound.

location, and loudness. Most murmurs are either systolic or diastolic; occasional murmurs which continue throughout systole and diastole are called continuous murmurs. The examiner may categorize loudness according to six grades of intensity. Grade I describes a murmur so soft that intent listening is required over several cardiac cycles. A Grade II murmur is also faint but audible immediately upon listening. Grades III and IV represent increasing loudness. Grade VI murmurs are so loud as to be audible through the stethoscope head held just off the chest wall. A Grade V murmur is very loud but cannot be heard off the chest. Grade IV, V, and VI murmurs cause palpable chest wall vibrations, felt by the hand as a gentle, throbbing sensation resembling the purr of a cat. This finding, known as a *thrill,* occurs where the murmur is loudest and represents the tactile counterpart of a loud murmur. The significance of a thrill is that of the underlying murmur.

The examiner localizes the murmur according to the area of maximal intensity. Thus, he may record a Grade III apical systolic murmur or a Grade II pulmonary diastolic murmur or a Grade VI aortic systolic murmur. Many murmurs have special pitch characteristics which merit description. Thus, diastolic flow across a stenotic mitral valve causes low-pitched vibrations usually described as a "rumble." A high-pitched murmur is often called a "blow" or "blowing murmur." Another category, the musical murmur, includes many curious harmonic patterns colorfully labeled as "sea gull," "cooing dove," "twanging string," and other epithets. The musical tonality derives from a single predominating frequency which usually arises from a vibrating structure within the heart, such as a perforated valve cusp or ruptured chordae tendineae.

Expert auscultation refines timing beyond the simple designation of systolic, diastolic, or continuous. A murmur may extend throughout systole or may be limited to early or late systole. A murmur may steadily intensify (crescendo), may steadily decline (decrescendo), or may have a midway loudness peak. Such variations often have meaning and should be noted. The term holosystolic signifies vibrations which commence with the first heart sound and cease at the second heart sound. A holosystolic murmur invariably indicates systolic regurgitation through the mitral or tricuspid valve or through a ventricular septal defect. Holosystolic murmurs are often called regurgitant murmurs. These murmurs are holosystolic because left ventricular pressure exceeds left atrial pressure throughout systole (mitral regurgitation) or because right ventricular pressure exceeds right atrial pressure throughout systole (tricuspid regurgitation) or because left ventricular pressure exceeds right ventricular pressure throughout systole (ventricular septal defect).

The systolic murmur of significant mitral regurgitation is typically a holosystolic murmur, heard best at the cardiac apex (Fig. 11-9). Mitral regurgitation most commonly results from the leaflet distortion caused by rheumatic fever. Fusion of the cusps and shortening and fusion of the chordae tendineae prevent normal valve closure and permit leakage into the atrium. Left ventricular dilatation of any cause may displace the papillary muscles and dilate the mitral annulus, disrupting normal valve closure. Left atrial enlargement itself may further impede closure by exerting traction on the mitral annulus. Other causes of mitral regurgitation recognized with increasing frequency are papillary muscle dysfunction, ruptured chordae tendineae, calcified mitral annulus fibrosus, myxomatous mitral cusps, bacterial endocarditis, endocardial fibroelastosis, and various congenital anomalies.

Mitral regurgitation does not always lead to a holosystolic murmur. Acute mitral regurgitation often causes a murmur which is loud in early and midsystole but subsides before the second sound. The tense left atrial wall of sudden mitral incompetence does not dilate in response to overfilling; instead, mounting left atrial pressure develops during ventricular systole until atrial pressure exceeds the declining pressure of late ventricular systole, thereby reducing regurgitation and its resultant murmur in late systole (Fig. 11-9). This murmur often transmits well to the cardiac base.

A systolic murmur confined to late systole characterizes mitral incompetence caused by leaflet prolapse. This has been termed the late apical systolic murmur. It is frequently preceded by one or more systolic clicks as described previously (Fig. 11-9).

The systolic murmur of tricuspid regurgitation is maximum in the fourth left interspace at the lower sternal edge. It may be holosystolic but sometimes fades out in the latter half of systole. It is often faint and easily overlooked. The murmur usually becomes louder during inspiration. This important characteristic results from the increased right ventricular filling caused by inspiration. Respiratory change can be subtle, requiring careful listening. Tricuspid regurgitation may result from leaflet deformity due to rheumatic fever. It is peculiarly common in heroin addicts, resulting from tricuspid bacterial endocarditis in these individuals. Tricuspid regurgitation frequently accompanies severe right ventricular hypertension of any cause, since dilatation of the right ventricle may displace the papillary muscles and dilate the tricuspid ring to such an extent that normal valve closure is not possible.

Blood flow across an irregular or stenotic semilunar valve causes a systolic murmur which commences after the first sound, increases to a peak in the middle third of systole, and then declines in late systole, ceasing before closure of the affected pulmonary or aortic valve. Sound tracings reveal a diamond shape; this acoustic pattern has been termed an ejection murmur. Such murmurs are often harsh and loud, radiate widely, and may be associated with decreased intensity of A2 or P2 when valvular stenosis reduces leaflet mobility (Fig. 11-10).

Murmurs of aortic and pulmonary stenosis are generally loudest in the aortic or pulmonary areas of the chest wall, respectively. Good transmission to the clavicles and neck characterizes the murmurs of semilunar valve stenosis, although in older patients with aortic stenosis, particularly those with an emphysematous chest, the aortic murmur may be loudest at the apex.

Some ejection murmurs relate to high velocity of blood flow through a normal semilunar valve. Such murmurs are common in conditions such as thyrotoxicosis, pregnancy, fever, excitement, and other states which increase stroke volume. Murmurs like these, which do not arise from structural alteration within the heart, are called innocent ("functional") murmurs in contrast to those arising from anatomic defects, which are called organic murmurs.

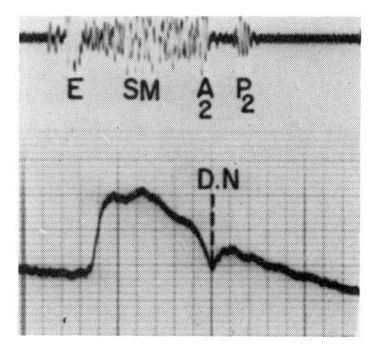

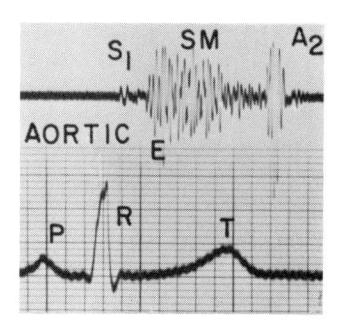

Figure 11-10 Upper panel displays the ejection systole murmur of pulmonary valve stenosis. Note the pulmonary ejection sound *(E)* which initiates the diamond-contoured murmur which subsides before a late and softened pulmonary closure sound *(P2)*. *A2,* aortic closure sound; *SM,* systolic murmur; *DN,* dicrotic incisura.

Lower panel displays the systolic ejection murmur of aortic stenosis. This murmur begins after S1, has midsystolic peak, and then declines before aortic closure *(A2)*. *E,* aortic ejection sound; *SM,* systolic murmur; *S1,* first heart sound.

Another variety of innocent murmur is that which arises in healthy individuals who have no evidence of increased cardiac output or other circulatory alteration. They are most common in children but are also frequently encountered in the adult. The usual murmur is early to midsystolic, of Grade I or II intensity, occasionally Grade III. It is most common in the lower, left parasternal region or in the pulmonary area. Innocent murmurs are seldom loudest at the apex. The genesis of these murmurs is not known, though some appear to arise from high-velocity blood flow through the main pulmonary artery.

Many systolic murmurs are innocent; most diastolic murmurs are organic. Abnormal vibrations during diastole usually result from regurgitation through an incompetent aortic or pulmonary valve or from stenosis of the mitral or tricuspid valve. Incompetence of a semilunar valve leads to a high-pitched decrescendo murmur, commencing with A2 or P2 and subsiding in mid or late diastole (Fig. 11–11). Incompetence of the aortic valve results from the leaflet thickening and fusion of rheumatic fever; from dilatation of the aortic valve ring and separation of cusps associated with syphilis or ankylosing (rheumatoid) spondylitis; from cusp perforation or laceration due to bacterial endocarditis or injury; from cusp prolapse due to dissecting aneurysm or due to loss of supporting septal tissue with certain ventricular septal defects; or from poor apposition of congenital bicuspid leaflets. All these anatomic deformities permit regurgitation when aortic pressure exceeds ventricular pressure during diastole. This pressure differential is highest in early diastole and declines as aortic pressure declines, hence the decrescendo pattern of murmur intensity.

Pulmonary valve insufficiency most commonly results from marked pulmonary arterial hypertension. Elevated pulmonary artery diastolic pressure may dilate the pulmonary valve ring sufficiently to prevent complete cusp apposition. A high-pitched, usually soft, decrescendo murmur is heard in the pulmonary region. Rarely, congenital deformity of the pulmonary leaflets permits regurgitation. Here the pulmonary artery pressure is normal, and the diastolic pressure gradient across the valve is small. The murmur may be similar to that caused by pulmonary hypertension but in some patients it is short, is medium to low pitched, and does not commence promptly with P2 but develops in early diastole, separated from P2 by a brief pause (Fig. 11–11).

The low-pitched apical diastolic murmur or rumble of mitral stenosis is separated from the second sound by a brief interval (0.06 to 0.12 second) which corresponds to left ventricular isovolumetric relaxation period. The rumble begins when the mitral valve opens and blood flows through the obstructed orifice at greater than normal velocity. The murmur usually commences with the mitral opening snap sound. As the pressure gradient between atrium and ventricle subsides in mid and late diastole, the rumble diminishes. If atrial systole, by raising left atrial pressure and/or by constricting the mitral orifice, increases the gradient, the murmur will accentuate just before the first sound, creating a crescendo rumble terminating in the exaggerated first sound of mitral stenosis (Fig. 11–11). This atrial systolic component of the murmur disappears when atrial fibrillation develops.

Tricuspid stenosis causes a diastolic murmur that is similar in timing to the rumble of mitral stenosis but usually subsides earlier in diastole, often without presystolic accentuation. This is probably because the gradient across the stenotic tricuspid valve is generally smaller than that across the stenotic mitral valve and also because the P-R interval is often prolonged, thereby lengthening the time between atrial and ventricular systole. This murmur is maximal along the lower, left parasternal region. It characteristically accentuates with inspiration. This interesting diagnostic feature relates to increased venous return to the right atrium and greater flow through the tricuspid valve as inspiration lowers intrathoracic pressure, thereby facilitating venous flow into the chest.

One of the most striking cardiac murmurs is that caused by patent ductus arteriosus and other arteriovenous communications. Since arterial pressure exceeds venous pressure throughout the cardiac cycle, such murmurs are continuous, waxing and waning as pressure gradients and flow velocity wax and wane. The murmur may be high pitched but often contains loud vibrations of medium and low frequency. When this is so, the murmur has a characteristic musical cadence which has earned the descriptive label of "machinery murmur." The murmur of patent ductus arteriosus peaks in late systole and early diastole, enveloping S2. This contour relates to the larger pressure gradient at this time between upper descending aorta and main pulmonary trunk. These murmurs must be distinguished from "to-and-fro" systolic and diastolic murmur of aortic stenosis and regurgitation or of ventricular septal defect and aortic regurgitation which do not envelope S2 as does the continuous murmur of patent ductus arteriosus (Fig. 11–12).

Pericarditis causes a characteristic rough, scraping sound called a pericardial friction rub. The inflamed pericardial and epicardial surfaces move against each other to create this sound. Since the rub relates to movement, it occurs with three major outward movements of the cardiac cycle—atrial systole, early ventricular systole, and rapid ventricular diastolic filling. Therefore,

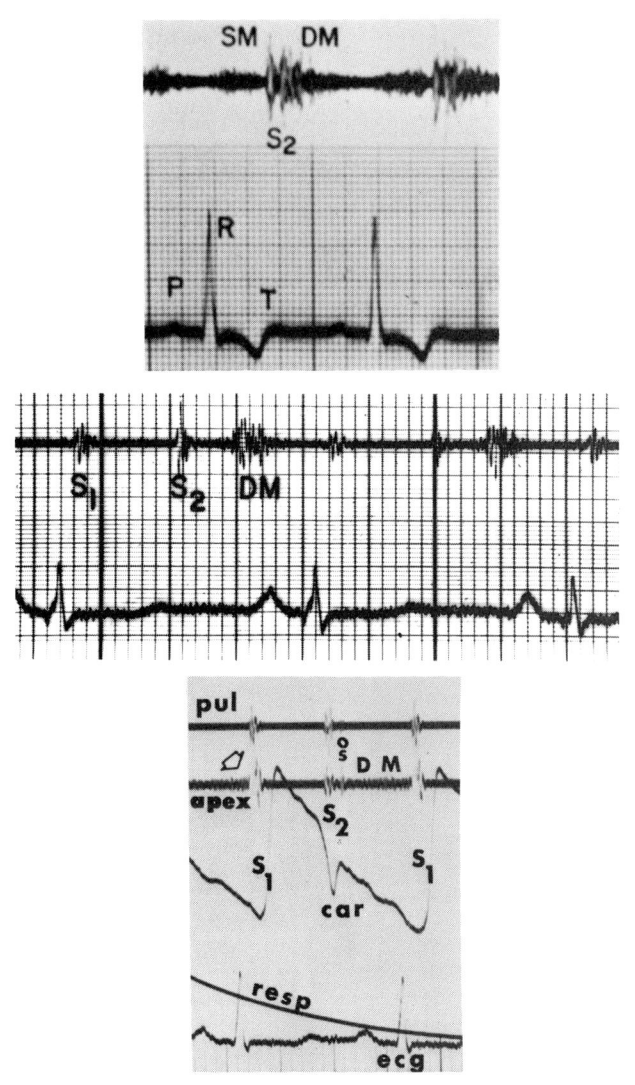

Figure 11–11 Upper panel displays the decrescendo diastolic murmur *(DM)* of aortic regurgitation which begins at aortic closure *(S2)* and fades out in late diastole. Most patients with significant aortic regurgitation have a systolic ejection murmur in the aortic region as shown here *(SM)*.

Middle panel displays the short, early diastolic murmur *(DM)* of congenital pulmonary regurgitation. Note the brief pause between the second heart sound *(S2)* and the onset of this diamond-contoured murmur which subsides quickly as pulmonary artery and right ventricular pressure equalize in mid-diastole. S1, first heart sound. (By permission from Collins, N., Braunwald, E., and Morrow, A.: Amer. J. Med., 28:159, 1960).

Lower panel depicts the rumbling diastolic murmur *(DM)* of mitral stenosis which begins after opening snap *(OS)* which is present in the pulmonary area *(pul)* as well as at the apex. The murmur accentuates with atrial systole (arrow). *Car,* carotid pulse; *resp,* respiration; *ecg,* electrocardiogram.

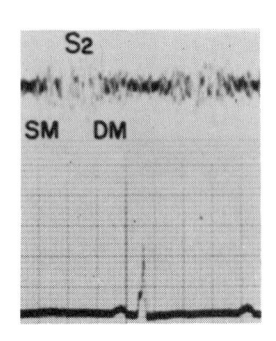

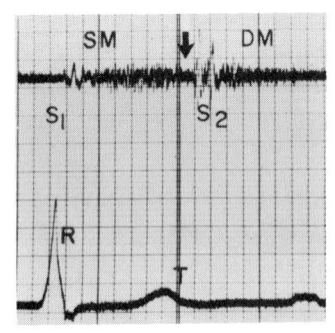

Figure 11-12 Upper panel displays the continuous murmur of patent ductus arteriosus which persists throughout the cardiac cycle, reaching its peak in late systole and early diastole, forming an envelope about the second sound *(S2)*. *SM*, systolic component of murmur; *DM*, diastolic component of murmur. Contrast this murmur with the to-and-fro stystolic *(SM)* and diastolic *(DM)* murmurs of ventricular septal defect and aortic regurgitation seen in the lower panel. Note declining late systolic vibrations (arrow) in contrast to the late systolic crescendo of the continuous murmur.

the typical friction rub will often have three discrete, high-pitched grating noises corresponding to the cardiac movements described (Fig. 11-13). Frequently, only two components can be heard, as when atrial fibrillation eliminates atrial systole; rarely, only a single rub is present.

The sounds are usually maximal over the lower left parasternal area and often have to be sought intently, with the stethoscope diaphragm pressed firmly against the skin. A typical three-component pericardial friction rub is a highly specific and therefore valuable finding which indicates the presence of some form of pericarditis. A two-component rub is also important evidence of pericardial disease but a single rubbing sound does not reliably implicate the pericardium, since an occasional cardiac murmur has a similar scratchy or grating quality. The pericarditis is nearly always acute, though chronic pericardial disease, such as a calcified plaque, may rarely account for a pericardial rub.

PRECORDIAL MOVEMENTS

Four major pulsations dominate the precordial movement pattern. These are (1) a brief, small outward thrust coinciding with atrial contraction; (2) a larger, brisk outward movement which starts during isovolumetric contraction and is followed quickly by (3) a steep, inward movement as systolic ejection begins; and (4) an outward movement then develops in early diastole which corresponds to ventricular filling. This last movement ascends at first rapidly, then more slowly, to a diastolic plateau which precedes the next atrial systole.

Improved recording techniques and hemodynamic correlation have led to better understanding of chest wall motion. The most prevalent method of recording these movements is apex cardiography. According to this technique, a funnel or cup pickup is held to the precordium over the cardiac apex; chest wall displacement causes this device to transmit impulses to a transducer recording system (Fig. 11-14). The pulsations are so inscribed that upward deflections indicate outward movements and downward deflections represent inward movements. The apex cardiograph best records localized impulses, since diffuse pulsations which move the pickup device as a whole do not adequately register. For this reason, recordings are usually made with the patient turned on his left side so as to exaggerate the cardiac apex impulse.

Figure 11-14 depicts a normal apex cardiogram. Note the four major movements just described: a small atrial thrust, labeled A, is followed by a steep upward deflection corresponding to beginning ventricular contraction. Systolic ejection starts at E, whereupon the tracing descends, at first steeply but then more slowly, leveling off in late systole. The curve descends abruptly again in early diastole to a nadir labeled 0. At this point, the mitral valve opens and rapid diastolic filling begins, causing a steeply ascending deflection followed by a more gradual ascent during slow ventricular filling until atrial systole starts another cardiac cycle.

Another recording system less commonly used, but more precise, is kinetocardiography. This technique differs from apex cardiography in that the pickup device is held to the chest wall by an external supporting clamp (Fig. 11-15). This instrument can detect displacement, whether diffuse or localized, small or large. Tracings are obtained from many different precordial sites. The standard kinetocardiogram contains leads from all the precordial electrocardiographic positions,

HEART SOUNDS, MURMURS, AND PRECORDIAL MOVEMENTS 307

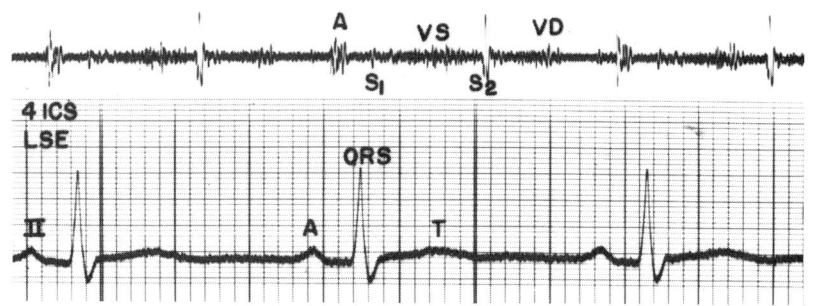

Figure 11-13 The typical pericardial friction rub has three components corresponding to the three major movements of the cardiac cycle: atrial systole (A), ventricular systole (VS), and early diastolic filling (VD). 4ICS/LSE, fourth intercostal space, left sternal edge. S1, First heart sound; S2, second heart sound.

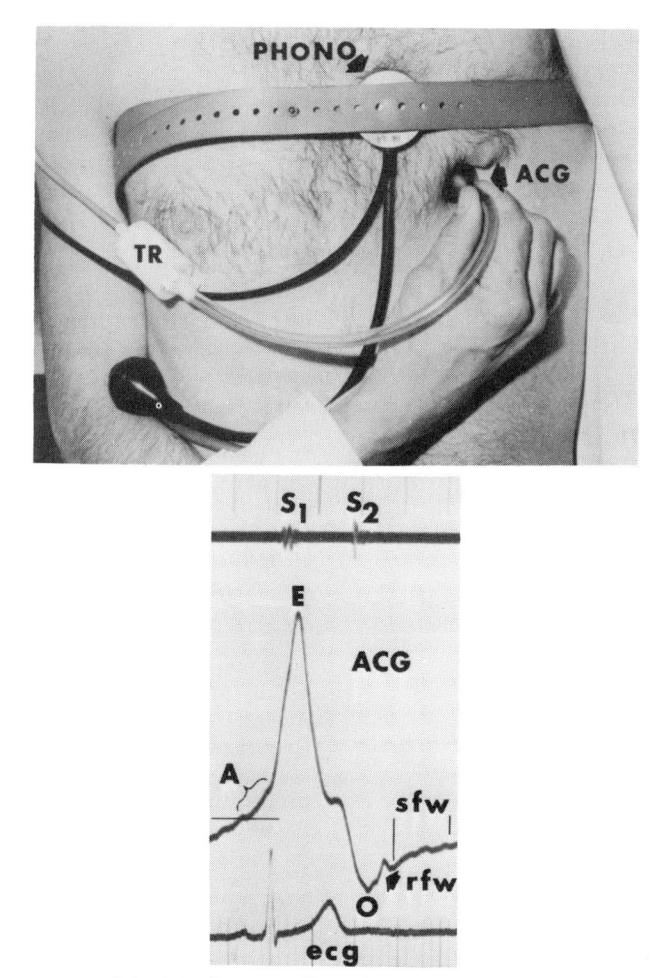

Figure 11-14 The upper panel depicts the recording of an apex cardiogram by means of a funnel which is hand-held over the apex and which transmits the increased air pressure caused by displacement to a transducer and graphic recorder. *Phono*, phonocardiographic microphone; *ACG*, apex cardiographic funnel pickup; *TR*, transducer.

The lower panel displays the apex cardiogram *(ACG)* of a healthy young male adult. Note the four major precordial movements: (1) Atrial contraction *(A);* (2) early systolic outward thrust peaking at E; (3) steep downward deflection following E, representing systolic retraction. The nadir of the systolic inward movement, labeled O, approximates atrioventricular valve opening. (4) Outward diastolic movement to the presystolic baseline, commencing at O, with the brisk upward deflection of rapid ventricular filling *(rfw)* followed by the more gradual ascending deflection of slow ventricular filling *(sfw)*.

each lead being labeled K instead of the electrocardiographic V. Figure 11–15 displays a kinetocardiogram recorded from the apex (K4). The four major movements are again readily seen, the contour differing somewhat from the apex cardiogram.

Aside from these two recording methods, there are other techniques, such as impulse cardiography, which yield useful information when properly interpreted.

Numerous physiologic studies of intracardiac pressure and flow as well as bidimensional angiocardiography have clarified the cardiac events which cause precordial pulsations. Normally only the ventricles contact the chest wall, the right ventricle underlying the lower, left parasternal area while the left ventricle relates to the lateral precordium at the cardiac apex. The right ventricle, therefore, is the anterior ventricle which accounts for most of the anterior surface of the heart.

During atrial systole the ventricles move slightly forward, causing a diffuse outward precordial movement which is not normally palpable but is readily recorded. As systolic contraction begins, a brief outward thrust occurs which can be recorded across the precordium and which is often palpable in the fourth or fifth left intercostal space within 10 cm. of the midsternal line. This movement represents the apical impulse or point of maximum impulse (PMI). It corresponds anatomically to the anteroseptal region of the left ventricle above the actual apex. The apex impulse begins during isovolumetric contraction when the left ventricular base begins to descend, the heart rotates slightly counterclockwise, and the apex thrusts against the chest wall. The impulse rises briskly to a peak which coincides with the onset of left ventricular ejection. At this instant the outward thrust quickly retracts; during the remainder of systole the apex tracing registers sustained retraction. This inward component of the systolic precordial movement sequence is larger and more prolonged than the apical impulse, yet is less easily appreciated. Systolic retraction is diffuse; it can be detected sometimes by observing the motion of an unheld stethoscope head resting on the left parasternal precordium during held expiration. As ventricular contraction ceases, the atrioventricular valves open, ventricular rapid filling begins, and the retracted precordium returns to its pre-atrial systolic baseline, at first swiftly, then more slowly. This movement can usually be recorded but is not normally seen or felt.

Increased left ventricular volume due to hypertrophy and/or dilatation affects the location, amplitude, duration, and area of the apical impulse. Normally, in the supine posture, this impulse occupies an area less than 3 cm. in diameter and is confined to one interspace. Increased area often indicates underlying cardiac disease but may represent normal heart action in young, slender individuals, particularly when the anteroposterior chest diameter is narrowed by sternal depression,

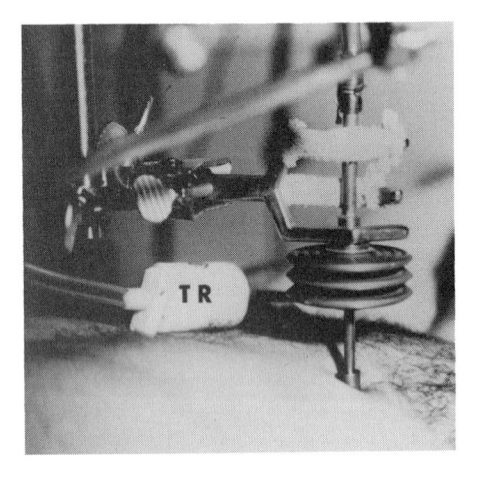

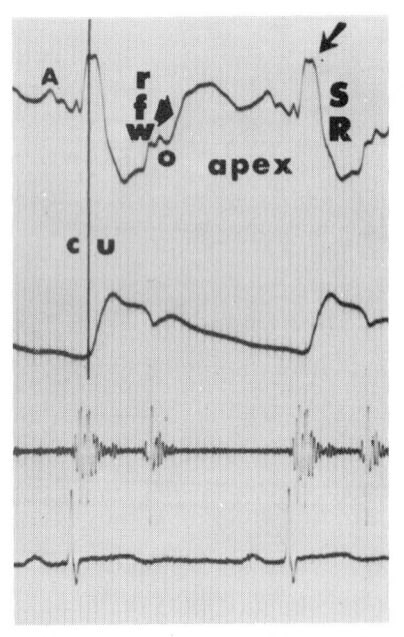

Figure 11–15 The upper panel depicts the recording of a kinetocardiogram with a flexible metal bellows probe held to the chest wall by external support. Air pressure changes within the bellows—as caused by chest wall displacement—are transmitted to a transducer (TR) and graphic recorder.

The lower panel displays a normal apex kinetocardiogram recorded with carotid pulse, heart sound, and electrocardiographic tracings. Note the four major movements: Atrial (A), apical impulse (arrow), systolic retraction (SR), and early diastolic filling (rfw). CU, carotid upstroke; O, beginning of ventricular filling.

Figure 11-16 Apex impulse tracing (kinetocardiogram) of a patient with severe aortic regurgitation and congestive heart failure. Note the pronounced, sustained outward systolic movement, preceded by a smaller outward thrust corresponding to atrial systole (A).

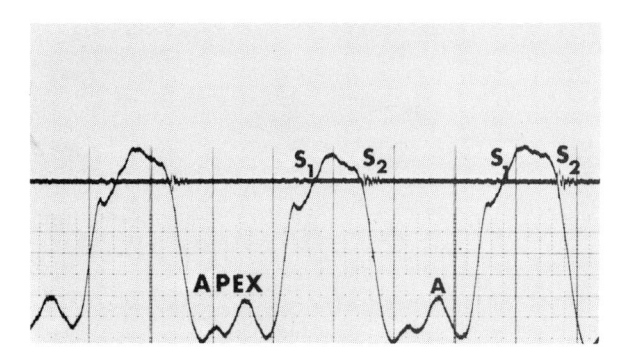

by straightening of the thoracic spine, or by simple disproportion between the lateral and anteroposterior chest dimensions which places the heart closer than usual to the anterior chest wall.

It is difficult to establish normal values for amplitude of chest wall pulsations. Most recording techniques do not accurately quantitate movements, though some investigators have developed measurable values which are useful when properly interpreted. Every physician must determine for himself what constitutes normal amplitude by palpating many normal patients and developing a "feel" for the average apical impulse. Abnormal amplitude often indicates underlying heart disease but may occur in patients with normal hearts and overactive circulation due to thyrotoxicosis, severe anemia, or other extracardiac causes of high cardiac output. Increased outward excursion of the apical impulse also may occur in young patients with slender chest configuration, especially if anteroposterior diameter is narrow.

Left ventricular hypertrophy and dilatation of any cause can heighten the amplitude and extend the area of apical impulse and may also displace it leftward. Conditions which greatly increase left ventricular diastolic volume such as severe aortic or mitral regurgitation cause the most marked displacement of the apical impulse. Conditions which elevate left ventricular systolic pressure such as aortic stenosis or hypertension do not increase total left ventricular volume as much as the regurgitant disorders just cited. Hence, leftward displacement of the apical impulse is found later in pressure overloading than in volume overloading conditions.

The normal apex impulse is a quick, early systolic thrust. Prolongation of this movement is an important and sensitive indication of abnormality. Impulse duration is easily measured on recordings and readily appreciated on palpation, especially if the examiner auscultates at the same time. Abnormally sustained outward movement correlates better with early left ventricular hypertrophy than does any other impulse characteristic and sometimes better than does the electrocardiogram or x-ray. Prolongation of the apical impulse is a more specific abnormality than increased amplitude or area, since there is little overlap with the normal brief impulse. Moreover, the patient with sustained systolic outward movement often has reduced stroke volume and ejection fraction as compared to the patient with abnormally heightened but unsustained apical impulse who usually has normal stroke volume and ejection fraction. Thus, the prolonged apical impulse is not only a more specific but often a more serious finding. Figure 11–16 displays the sustained outward apex movement of a patient with advanced left ventricular hypertrophy and dilatation (cf. Figure 11–15).

Mitral regurgitation may cause a characteristic precordial movement pattern. Initially this lesion can cause leftward displacement of a localized pulsation which may evolve, with increasing duration and severity of disease, into a diffuse, systolic impulse, extending from apex to sternum owing to medial rotation of the anterior left ventricular wall. A prominent late systolic outward movement especially characterizes mitral regurgitation. This pulsation is maximal over the lower sternum and left parasternal region and peaks just after the second heart sound (Fig. 11–17). It relates to forward thrust of the ventricles caused by filling of the distended left atrium, which probably impinges on the vertebral column, thereby moving the heart forward. When this movement coexists with the apical impulse of left ventricular hypertrophy, the asynchronous timing of the two movements can be readily appreciated by simultaneous palpation with both hands.

Since the right ventricle underlies the midprecordium, conditions enlarging this ventricle affect chest wall pulsation in this area. Volume overloading conditions such as atrial septal defect cause brisk, diffuse early systolic outward movement of the lower left parasternal area, with

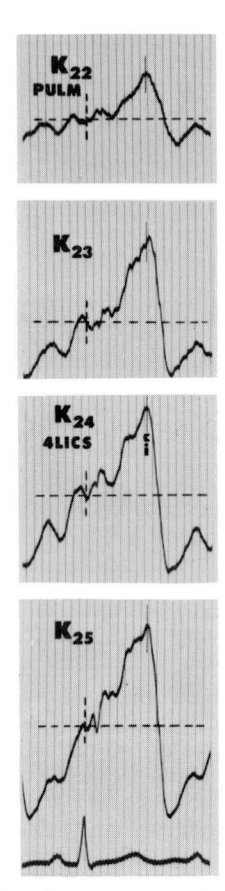

Figure 11–17 Movement tracings (kinetocardiogram) recorded along the left sternal border of a patient with severe mitral regurgitation. A prominent late systolic outward thrust is present from the pulmonary area *(K22)* to the fifth left interspace *(K25)*. This results from forward displacement of the ventricles owing to late systolic distention of the dilated left atrium. *C1*, carotid incisura. Vertical dotted line represents peak of R of electrocardiogram. Horizontal dotted line represents baseline of kinetocardiogram. (By permission from Stapleton, J., and Groves, B.: Amer. Heart J., *81*:409, 1971. Copyright 1971, American Medical Association.)

rapid decline in late systole. Pressure overloading disorders such as pulmonary stenosis give rise to more sustained, diffuse systolic outward movement, often extending from sternum to apex. Mitral stenosis with pulmonary hypertension causes a more medial systolic movement; the maximal thrust is often sternal.

Transmural myocardial infarction frequently causes abnormally sustained systolic outward movement, usually of the midprecordium or apex but occasionally of the sternal or even epigastric areas. This impulse, commonly called a systolic "bulge," relates to the failure of infarcted myocardium to contract normally. Sometimes this expansile movement derives from an anatomic ventricular aneurysm; more often the bulge correlates with contraction failure of infarcted tissue in the absence of true aneurysm. This movement pattern may characterize old or recent myocardial infarction and may occur transiently during angina pectoris.

Cardiomyopathies can also lead to precordial movement abnormalities which typify enlargement of either ventricle or both. Combined hypertrophy can be suspected when abnormal apical and lower left parasternal systolic outward movements are separated by a zone of quiescence or even systolic retraction.

Atrial systole, when exaggerated, may sufficiently amplify atrial chest wall pulsations so as to render them palpable. This occurs when resistance to ventricular filling is high, as with the concentric hypertrophy of aortic or pulmonary or of systemic or pulmonary hypertension. The altered myocardial compliance of myocardiopathies or myocardial infarction also may lead to palpable presystolic impulses. Atrial sounds usually accompany atrial movements. Since atrial hypertrophy often coexists with ventricular hypertrophy, palpable atrial movement is frequently associated with the lifting thrust of ventricular enlargement. The examiner then feels a double or bifid impulse. Such double pulsations are common in clinical practice.

Important pulsations may also occur during diastolic filling. A loud ventricular gallop sound may be associated with a simultaneous brief precordial thrust which corresponds to an exaggerated diastolic rapid filling wave. Thus, the examiner may see, feel, and hear the vibrations of the ventricular gallop phenomenon. Atrial and ventricular rapid filling movements are exaggerated in the left lateral recumbent posture. Palpation in this posture will sometimes detect pulsations not felt with the patient supine.

Constrictive pericarditis and restrictive cardiomyopathy may cause a vigorous, outward impulse in early diastole which is easily mistaken for the movement of ventricular hypertrophy unless the physician carefully times his palpation. This movement corresponds to the sudden arrest of rapid early diastolic filling by restricting pericardium or myocardium.

Careful auscultation and palpation of cardiac vibrations will yield many valuable diagnostic and prognostic clues without patient discomfort and at minimal cost. The examination requires only a few moments of intent observation and knowledge of fundamental normal and abnormal findings. As with other sources of evaluative information, the physician must fit auscultatory and palpatory findings into the total clinical context.

REFERENCES

Conn, R. D., and Cole, J. S.: The cardiac apex impulse. Ann. Intern. Med., *75*:185, 1971.

Craige, E., and Millward, D. K.: Diastolic and continuous murmurs. Progr. Cardiovasc. Dis., *14*:38, 1971.

Davie, J. C., Langley, J. O., Dodson, W. H., and Eddleman, E. E.: Clinical and kinetocardiographic studies of paradoxical precordial motion. Amer. Heart J., *63*:775, 1962.

Deliyannis, A. A., Gillam, P. M. S., Mounsey, J. P. D., and Steiner, R. E.: The cardiac impulse and the motion of the heart. Brit. Heart J., *26*:396, 1964.

Eddleman, E. E., and Thomas, H. D.: The recognition and differentiation of right ventricular pressure and flow loads. Amer. J. Cardiol., *4*:652, 1959.

Harvey, W. P., and Stapleton, J. F.: Clinical aspects of gallop rhythm with particular reference to diastolic gallops. Circulation, *18*:1017, 1958.

Heintzen, P.: The genesis of the normally split first heart sound. Amer. Heart J., *62*:332, 1961.

Leatham, A.: Systolic murmurs. Circulation, *17*:601, 1958.

Leatham, A., and Towers, M.: Splitting of the second heart sound. Brit. Heart J., *12*:575, 1951.

Levine, S. A., and Harvey, W. P.: Clinical Auscultation of the Heart. 2nd ed. Philadelphia, W. B. Saunders Co., 1958.

McCall, B. W., and Price, J. L.: Movement of the mitral valve cusps in relation to first heart sound and opening snap in patients with mitral stenosis. Brit. Heart J., *29*:417, 1967.

McDonald, I. G.: The shape and movements of the human left ventricle during systole. Amer. J. Cardiol., *26*:221, 1970.

McKusick, V. A. (Ed.): Symposium on Cardiovascular Sound. Circulation, *16*:270, 1957.

Reddy, P. S., Shaver, J. A., and Leonard, J. J.: Cardiac systolic murmurs: Pathophysiology and differential diagnosis. Progr. Cardiovasc. Dis., *14*:1, 1971.

Ronan, J. A., Steelman, R. B., DeLeon, A. C., Waters, T. J., Perloff, J. K., and Harvey, W. P.: The clinical diagnosis of acute severe mitral insufficiency. Amer. J. Cardiol., *27*:284, 1971.

Sutton, G. C., and Craige, E.: Quantitation of precordial movement. Circulation, *35*:476, 1967.

Sutton, G. C., Taylor, A. P., and Craige, E.: Relationship between quantitated precordial movement and left ventricular function. Circulation, *61*:179, 1970.

Tantouzas, P., and Shillingford, J.: Impulse cardiogram in early diagnosis of left ventricular dysfunction in hypertension. Brit. Heart J., *31*:97, 1969.

Weitzman, D.: The mechanism and significance of the auricular sound. Brit. Heart J., *17*:70, 1955.

CHAPTER 12

THE ELECTRO-CARDIOGRAM

J. A. ABILDSKOV

INTRODUCTION

The electrocardiogram is a record of electrical phenomena which occur in the heart and result in an electrical field distributed throughout the body. The usual electrocardiographic examination for medical diagnostic purposes is carried out with electrodes located at multiple sites on the body surface. When two electrodes are connected by a conductor, current flows in the conductor and a suitable instrument placed in this current path records evidence of the potential difference between the electrode sites. Such instruments are designated electrocardiographs and the electrode arrangement constitutes an electrocardiographic lead. The electrocardiograph furnishes records in which deflections are calibrated in terms of voltage on the vertical axis and time is represented on the horizontal axis. The conventional electrocardiogram is thus a Cartesian coordinate graph in which voltage variations are plotted against time, as illustrated in Figure 12-1. Many other displays of the same data are possible, one of which has been designated the vectorcardiogram, also illustrated in Figure 12-1. In that display, voltage variations from one set of electrodes are plotted against those from another electrode combination rather than against time as in the electrocardiogram. It should be recognized that different displays of data from particular electrode combinations involve the same information from the body surface, but the accessibility of particular items of this information varies with the display. Thus, the relation of voltage to time is clearly evident in the electrocardiogram but not in the vectorcardiogram. In the vectorcardiogram, however, the relation of voltage variations from one set of electrodes to those in another electrode set is precisely indicated. The precision of this relation in the vectorcardiogram when it is recorded from a cathode ray oscilloscope is difficult to achieve even with simultaneously recorded electrocardiographic leads and is impossible to establish with non-simultaneous leads.

The time-based electrocardiogram is the most widely used and widely useful examination of cardiac electrical activity for medical diagnostic purposes. The vectorcardiogram has more limited diagnostic utility and is less often employed, while the many other possible displays of electrical events in the heart are still less frequently used. The discussion to follow will concern the time-based electrocardiogram unless otherwise specified.

As it is used at present, electrocardiographic examination is a major diagnostic method. Certain abnormalities of waveform are the best available clinical evidence of myocardial infarction. Other abnormalities, although often less specific, are useful evidence of a variety of cardiac and extracardiac states ranging from cardiac enlargement and myocardial ischemia to electrolyte and neurologic disorders. The electrocardiogram is the most certain means of identifying the cardiac rhythm at the time of examination and of detecting changes of rhythm when the record is continuously monitored. The ease and almost risk-free nature of electrocardiographic examination enhance its medical usefulness.

The present role of the electrocardiogram in medical diagnosis has been achieved in two ways. One of these has been the empiric correlation of electrocardiographic findings with particular states, the nature of which has been established by other clinical or by pathologic observations. This is the most certain means of establishing the diagnostic utility of particular electrocar-

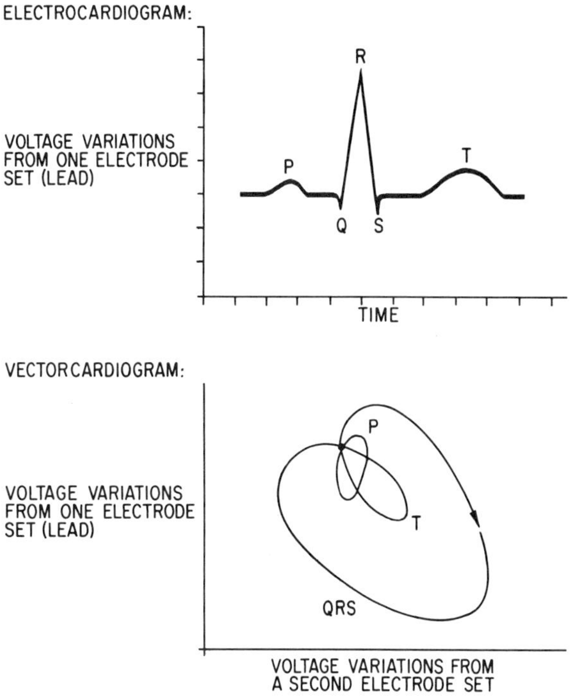

Figure 12-1 The electrocardiogram and vectorcardiogram. Both records reflect potential differences between electrode combinations. In the electrocardiogram these potential differences are recorded as voltage vs. time. The vectorcardiogram presents voltage variations from one electrode set, constituting a lead, vs. voltage variations from another lead.

diographic findings, and findings for which the diagnostic significance is suspected on other grounds must still be subjected to the actual test of diagnostic success or failure in patients.

The other means by which the diagnostic role of the electrocardiogram has been established is that of defining the physiologic basis of the record in normal and abnormal states. Increasing knowledge of the pertinent physiologic mechanisms has increased the degree to which electrocardiographic findings can be explained in these terms. Such explanation of electrocardiographic findings on the basis of their physiologic mechanism is unquestionably desirable for teaching purposes and is the appropriate subject for this text on pathologic physiology. This approach is also likely to be the major means by which further improvements in electrocardiographic diagnoses are achieved, and understanding of the physiologic mechanisms will be the best preparation for the utilization of these improvements.

The material to follow has been organized into seven sections. The first of these describes the *total system* involved in electrocardiography. The various components of the electrocardiographic system are not equally well understood or equally important to diagnostic electrocardiography. This section will therefore specify those components of the total system for which the roles are most fully defined and application of which to diagnostic electrocardiography is most important.

The second section presents a brief description of *electrocardiographic leads,* including those which constitute the present routine electrocardiographic examination. This is an extremely complex subject and detailed consideration is not appropriate in this text. The section will be largely limited to those items which must be appreciated in order for subsequent sections of this text to be understood. These items include description of the electrocardiogram in terms of the electrical axis.

The third section will consider the cardiac basis of the electrocardiogram in general terms applicable to both atrial and ventricular muscle and to the specialized conduction system. The description in this section of the relation between cardiac events and the waveform of the body surface electrocardiogram is, in the author's opinion, the most useful approach to employing the electrocardiogram in medical diagnosis that is available at present.

In the fourth and fifth sections, the relation of cardiac events during *excitation* to electrocardiographic waveform will be specifically applied to *atria* and *ventricles,* and the process of *atrial recovery* will be considered briefly.

Ventricular recovery and its electrocardiographic expressions in the ST-T deflection will be considered in the sixth section. The discussion will emphasize similarities between the cardiac state during recovery and that during excitation and will attempt to elucidate the physiologic basis of the ST-T deflection and QRS complex in the same terms.

The seventh and last section will concern *pathologic states* and their electrocardiographic manifestations using the same terms employed in previous sections to explain the normal electrocardiogram. The pathologic states considered in this section have been chosen as examples and are only a few of those in which the electrocardiogram has diagnostic utility. Texts of medicine, cardiology, and clinical electrocardiography which describe the diagnostic range of the electrocardiogram are available. The purpose of this text is to describe physiologic mechanisms and this is done through the use of selected examples of pathologic states.

THE ELECTROCARDIOGRAPHIC SYSTEM

The total system involved in electrocardiography is illustrated in diagrammatic form in Figure 12-2. The major component of the system is the heart, which is the site of origin of events reflected in the electrocardiogram. As the generator of the electrocardiogram, the heart can be considered at the level of intra- and extracellular ion relations ln the resting and excited states. The generator can also be considered at the level of the cell membrane across which ion concentration gradients exist and ion movements occur. At still another level, the generator can be considered at the cellular level in terms of the transmembrane action potential. Finally, the generator can be considered at the organ level, at which the gross sequence of electrical events during excitation and recovery can be described.

At present, the most useful level at which to consider the physiologic basis of the body surface electrocardiogram is the gross sequence of electrical events together with certain information from the transmembrane action potential. It is at these levels that the cardiac basis of the electrocardiogram will be described in the next section.

Extracardiac components of the electrocardiographic system include a complex, three-dimensional conductive medium. This medium consists of tissues with different conductive properties and the geometrically complex and variable boundaries of the body. These portions of the electrocardiographic system undoubtedly influence the body surface electrocardiogram, and the degree and nature of their influence has and continues to be the subject of intensive study. At present, however, the role of these factors has not been sufficiently well defined that they can be usefully considered in routine diagnostic electrocardiography. Further definition of the role of nonuniform conductive properties and complex boundary conditions can be expected to refine electrocardiographic diagnosis in the future, however.

The remaining portions of the electrocardiographic system are the electrodes with which potentials on the body surface are sampled, the combinations of electrodes which constitute "leads," and the instruments with which potentials are displayed and/or recorded.

ELECTROCARDIOGRAPHIC LEADS

The combination of a minimum of two electrodes in contact with the body and connected to

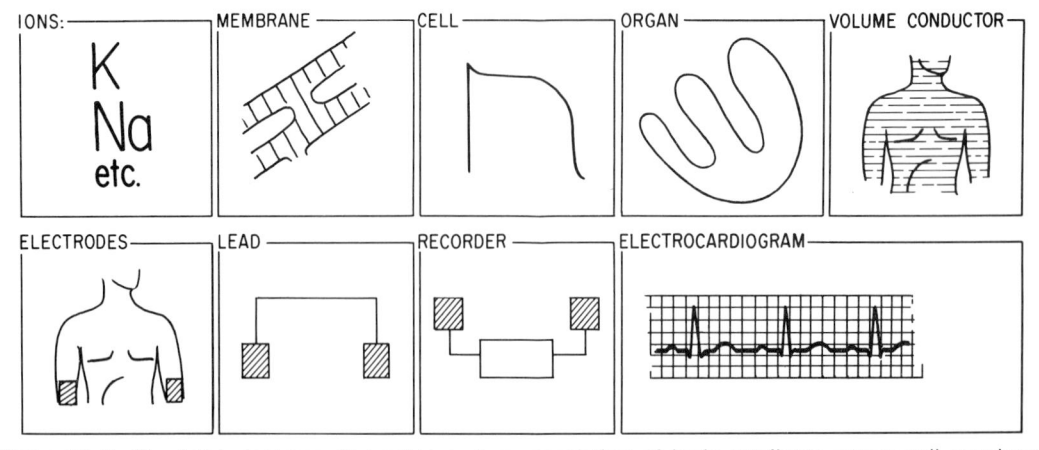

Figure 12-2 The total electrocardiographic system, consisting of ionic gradients across cell membranes, cellular events reflected by the transmembrane action potential, the sequence of electrical events at the organ level, and extracardiac portions of the system, including the conducting medium, recorder, and records.

provide a path for current flow between them constitutes an electrocardiographic lead. The term "lead" is also generally used to refer to the actual electrocardiogram recorded from an electrode combination. The waveform in the electrocardiogram is a description of potential differences at the electrodes constituting the lead as they vary with time. Electrocardiographic examination usually consists of obtaining electrocardiograms from multiple electrode sites. The examination considered to be routine at present includes nine electrode sites with twelve leads consisting of various combinations of these electrodes. Electrodes on the right and left arms and left leg and at six specified sites on the precordium are employed. Leads are designated as standard, precordial, and unipolar limb leads.

The standard lead designated as I consists of right and left arm electrodes, with the polarity of the recording system so arranged that an upright deflection in the recording occurs when the left arm potential is positive with respect to the right arm. Standard leads II and III consist of electrodes on the right arm and left leg and on the left arm and left leg, respectively, both arranged to yield an upright deflection when the left leg potential is positive with respect to the arm.

Precordial leads consist of six electrodes at specified sites on the anterior and left lateral thorax, and a central terminal to which right and left arm and left leg electrodes are all connected. These leads are designated V_1 through V_6 and each consists of a precordial electrode and the central terminal, with the polarity arranged to result in an upward deflection when the precordial electrode is positive with respect to the central terminal.

The remaining three "unipolar" limb leads consist of electrodes on the arms and the left leg, each of which is combined with a modified central terminal to which the other two limb electrodes are connected. The polarity of these leads is so arranged that an upward deflection results when the single limb electrode is positive with respect to the modified central terminal. Leads recorded with the modified central terminal yield larger deflections than would occur with a terminal to which all three limb electrodes were connected and are designated as augmented leads and by the symbols aV_L, aV_R, and aV_F for the three unipolar limb leads. It should be noted that the term "unipolar" lead is a misnomer, since a complete circuit is required to record an electrocardiogram. The term is applied to leads in which one side of the circuit is connected to all three limb electrodes in the case of precordial leads, or to two of these in the case of augmented limb leads. It is applied because potential variations at the central terminal, although neither zero nor negligible, are small, and potential variations at the precordial or limb location of the other electrode are chiefly responsible for the electrocardiographic waveform. Examples of standard, precordial, and unipolar limb leads are shown in Figure 12-3.

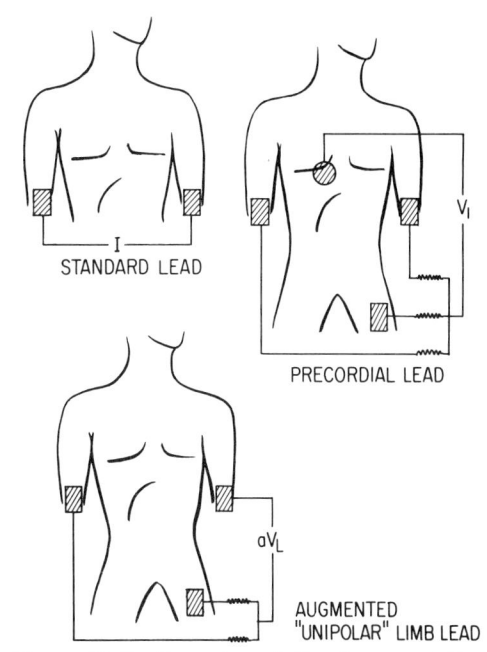

Figure 12-3 Examples of the three varieties of leads employed in the usual 12-lead electrocardiographic examination.

The electrode sites used in the routine 12-lead electrocardiographic examination have been selected according to a combination of technical considerations such as ease and reproducibility of electrode placement; theoretical considerations, including design of the central terminal; empiric evidence of their diagnostic merit; and informed intuition. It is unlikely that they constitute the optimum possible electrocardiographic examination. They do, however, furnish a large amount of diagnostically useful information, and this is the standard by which possible future modifications must be evaluated.

One of the fundamental problems of diagnostic electrocardiography can be appreciated by realizing that a pattern of potential variation due to cardiac electrical events exists at all points on the body surface. This pattern can be defined by recording from extremely large numbers of electrode sites and determining the potential distribution at multiple moments during the cardiac cycle. These patterns constitute virtually all the electrocardiographic information present on the body surface, but sampling from such large numbers of electrodes presents major technical problems. Research is in progress in this area using computer techniques to display the data as isopotential maps at frequent intervals during the cardiac cycle. These studies have definitely demonstrated diagnostically useful information beyond that furnished by the present routine electrocardiographic examination, and this is an extremely promising area for improved electrocardiographic diagnosis in the future. Improved automated methods may make examinations with large numbers of electrodes practical or it may be possible to identify limited numbers of electrode sites which furnish all or most of the diagnostic information possible from body surface electrocardiograms.

Electrode arrangements or systems designated as vectorcardiographic or orthogonal lead systems are in actual clinical use, usually for the purpose of recording vectorcardiograms with the cathode ray oscilloscope or collecting electrocardiographic data for programs of computer analysis. These systems consist of multiple electrodes which in various combinations and with the contribution of individual electrodes weighted by resistor networks yield effects of cardiac electrical activity on three mutually perpendicular axes, namely, horizontal (X), vertical (Y), and anteroposterior (Z) axes. These systems have been designed on the basis of the dimensions and geometry of the human thorax and position of the heart within the thorax. Some of the systems also include qualitative consideration of the nonuniform conductive properties of the body. Evidence has been obtained that the three leads from such electrode systems contain most of the information furnished by the routine 12-lead examination. In addition, there is evidence that the range of normal variability of such leads is less than that of the 12-lead examination. Despite such findings, which suggest that a simpler examination may provide an equal, or nearly equal, amount of diagnostic information and with less normal variability and may be more sensitive to abnormalities, these leads are not extensively employed. The major deterrents to their widespread use have probably been the extensive experience and familiarity with 12-lead examination, the relative lack of standards for interpretation of orthogonal leads, and particularly the lack of convincing evidence that their actual diagnostic merit is substantially greater than the 12-lead examination now in use.

Electrical Axis

Certain features of the electrocardiogram can be conveniently described as the "electrical axis." This description is usually applied to the QRS complex, but there is no inherent reason why it cannot be used to describe other electrocardiographic deflections. In essence, the description consists of relating features in one electrocardiographic lead to those in one or more additional leads. A deflection in one lead can be specified as having a particular amplitude and a positive or negative polarity. As one which can be specified by two terms, this is a scalar quantity, and individual ECG leads are often referred to as "scalar leads." If the relation of one lead to another is known, the magnitude and polarity of electrocardiographic deflections in both may be specified by a single vector quantity which has the additional feature of a specific direction. An example is shown in Figure 12–4. The peak deflection in two leads is illustrated, together with the geometric relation assumed to exist between these levels. The vector shown identifies the deflection in lead I as positive and having an amplitude of four

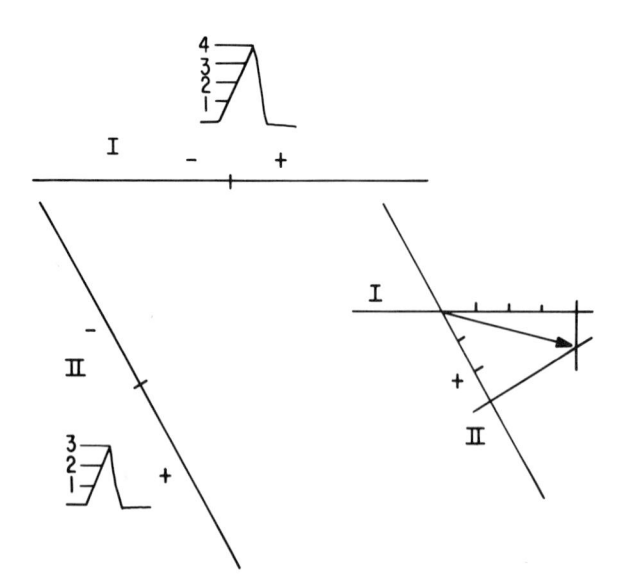

Figure 12–4 The electrical axis. In this description of electrocardiographic features the geometric relation of the leads must be known or assumed. Here, leads I and II are assumed to form sides of an equilateral triangle. The peak QRS deflection in each is indicated, and these values have been employed to plot a vector. In the portion of the illustration showing this vector, the midpoint of the leads has been superimposed.

units, while that in lead II is also positive and has a magnitude of three units. The term for this vector as usually employed in diagnostic electrocardiography is "electrical axis."

This description of electrocardiographic deflections may be applied to the instantaneous deflection in two simultaneous leads and then constitutes the "instantaneous axis." A number of successive instantaneous axes during the QRS complex would have their termini located on the QRS loop of the vectorcardiogram. An axis can also be plotted using the area of deflections. The axis plotted from QRS area in two leads is properly referred to as the mean electrical axis of the QRS. In actual routine interpretation of electrocardiograms an approximation of the mean axis is usually employed. The algebraic sum of peak deflections in a lead is determined and used with a similar sum from another lead to determine the vector which identifies these quantities in the leads being considered.

THE CARDIAC BASIS OF THE ELECTROCARDIOGRAM

As stated earlier, the most useful level at which to consider the physiologic basis of the electrocardiogram is the gross sequence of electrical events on the organ level together with certain information provided by the cellular transmembrane action potential. At the gross level, the cardiac state reflected by an electrocardiographic deflection at a given moment is that of a boundary between areas in different electrical states. When the heart is uniformly in the resting state, no such boundaries exist and the isoelectric reference line of the electrocardiogram is established. When excitation is in progress, one or more boundaries exist between excited muscle and that still in the resting state. The varying size and geometry of boundaries during atrial excitation determine the form of the P wave and those during ventricular excitation determine the QRS complex waveform. After excitation in ventricular muscle there is a period during which the electrical state changes slowly, as reflected by the plateau of the transmembrane action potential. During this period all ventricular muscle is in the same or near-same electrical state, and the isoelectric or nearly isoelectric ST segment of the electrocardiogram reflects this condition. As more rapid changes in electrical state occur during the downstroke of the transmembrane action potential, boundaries of potential difference appear between areas in which the stage of recovery differs from that in an adjacent area.

One of the fundamental and most useful relations in electrocardiography is that between a boundary of potential difference in the heart and the potential at recording electrodes on the body surface. Potential at a recording electrode is influenced by the distance of the recording electrode from the boundary, the magnitude of potential difference across the boundary, and the geometry of the boundary. Figure 12–5 diagrams a closed boundary of potential difference in excitable tissue. If the boundary illustrated is considered to be an excitation front, the magnitude of potential difference across the boundary will be that between excited and resting tissue and will be related to the height of the transmembrane action potential upstroke. Tissue on the excited side of the boundary will have a potential related to the end of the upstroke of the transmembrane action potential while tissue not yet excited will be at resting membrane potential level. The polarity of potential difference will be negative in excited tissue and positive in resting tissue. When the boundary is closed as illustrated, potential differences in all directions are present and the electrocardiographic effects of one segment of the boundary are canceled by effects of an opposing portion of the boundary. A closed boundary of potential difference will not be expressed by an electrocardiographic deflection, regardless of the dimensions of the boundary and regardless of the magnitude of potential difference across the boundary. The foregoing is true of closed boundaries, regardless of their shape, and is true of three-dimensional boundaries as well as those located in a single plane.

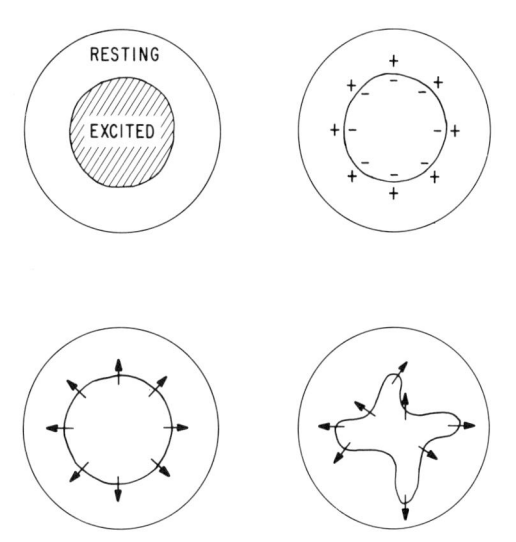

Figure 12–5 Diagrammatic representation of boundaries of potential difference. As described in the text, closed boundaries will not be expressed as electrocardiographic deflections.

It is extremely important that the implications of this relation for diagnostic electrocardiography be appreciated. It should be evident, for example, that the size of electrocardiographic deflections is unlikely to have a simple and direct relation to heart size. It should also be evident that the size of a myocardial infarct or other destructive lesion will not necessarily be proportional to the magnitude of electrocardiographic alterations produced by the lesion. It should further be evident from the relation described that the electrocardiographic effect of a given unclosed boundary will be related to the degree by which it fails to be a closed boundary. A boundary with uncanceled portions is shown in Figure 12-6. The boundary shown can be closed by the line ab and the length of this line will be related to uncanceled portions of the boundary and to the magnitude of electrocardiographic effects of the boundary. In relating boundaries of potential difference to the electrocardiogram it is convenient to employ vectors as shown in the figure. A vector directed toward the positive side of the boundary, perpendicular to the line closing the boundary and having a magnitude equal or proportional to the closing line, indicates the polarity and magnitude of the electrocardiographic deflection in a particular lead by its projection on the lead axis. If the boundary has spatial form it cannot be closed by a line, and the electrocardiographic effect will be related to the area of the surface necessary to close the boundary.

Although the cardiac events responsible for electrocardiographic deflections during excitation and recovery are similar in that both consist of boundaries of potential difference between areas in different electrical states, they differ in significant ways. These differences in the cardiac states of activation and recovery will be introduced here and further explained in a subsequent section. One of the differences between excitation and recovery is the greater time required for the latter process. In individual cells, excitation occurs during the upstroke of the transmembrane action potential and requires only 1 or 2 milliseconds for completion. Recovery as reflected by the transmembrane action potential downstroke begins immediately after excitation but, because of the special features of cardiac recovery reflected by the plateau of the action potential, excited tissue remains at a potential level near that of the peak upstroke during the normal propagation of excitation. These events make it possible to regard excitation as a moving boundary of potential difference. If sequential boundaries are considered, the electrocardiographic effects of later boundaries can be considered without reference to those of earlier boundaries.

Because of the substantially longer time required for recovery, the potential difference boundaries which exist during that process cannot be related to the electrocardiogram in the same manner as excitation. When potential differences arise between two areas which have reached different stages of recovery, the resulting boundary continues to exist until recovery is complete in both areas. During this time, additional boundaries between other areas which reach different stages of recovery are established and also remain present until recovery is complete in the areas involved. The cardiac state responsible for the ST-T deflection of the electrocardiogram cannot therefore be considered as a moving boundary of potential difference, but must be considered as one in which multiple boundaries coexist. Potential differences across these boundaries vary according to the stage of recovery reached on the two sides of each boundary. The relations between each boundary of potential difference during recovery and an electrocardiographic lead are similar to those during excitation. The electrocardiographic expressions of both are related to the magnitude of potential difference across the boundary, polarity of this difference, and the quantity necessary to close the boundary which defines the uncanceled portion of the boundary.

ATRIAL EXCITATION AND THE P WAVE

Normal cardiac excitation begins in the right atrium, specifically in the specialized tissue con-

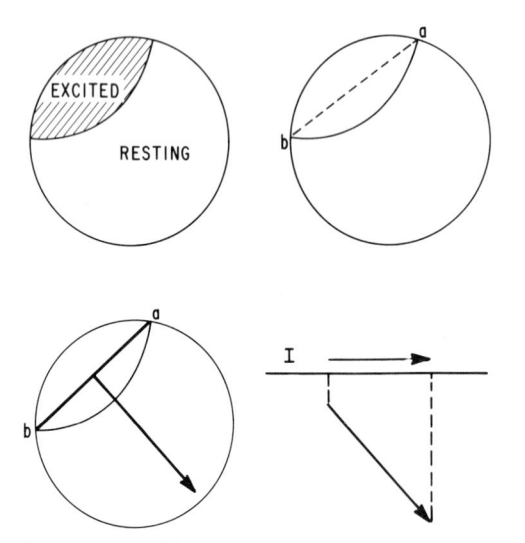

Figure 12-6 Diagrammatic representation of an unclosed boundary of potential difference. The electrocardiographic expression of such a boundary will be related to the quantity necessary to close the boundary. This quantity is the line ab in the example shown. The electrocardiographic effect of such a boundary is conveniently obtained by constructing a vector perpendicular to the closing line, with a magnitude equal or proportional to the line and projecting the vector on lead axes.

stituting the sino-atrial node. This structure is located near the junction of atrium and superior vena cava. According to James, the human sino-atrial node is approximately $2 \times 5 \times 15$ mm. in size and is pierced by a central artery which provides the arterial supply of the node and a large area of surrounding atrial myocardium.

On the cellular level, excitation consists of a sudden increase in membrane permeability to sodium, probably due to inactivation of mechanisms which normally extrude sodium from cells during the resting state. The property of automaticity or pacemaker activity normally exhibited by the sino-atrial node consists of slow diastolic depolarization in which the potential difference between interior and exterior of the pacemaking cell declines to a critical point. At the threshold value of membrane potential, the rapid changes of membrane potential characteristic of excitation occur in the pacemaker cell. Propagation of excitation to surrounding cells occurs as a result of local current flow between excited and nonexcited cells. This acts as a depolarizing current in the same manner as current supplied from an external stimulus source.

The property of automaticity is not restricted to the sino-atrial node, and other portions of the specialized conduction system are also capable of pacemaker activity. Normally, however, slow diastolic depolarization occurs at a higher rate in the sino-atrial node than in other sites also capable of pacemaker activity. The normal sequence of atrial excitation during sinus rhythm is determined by the exact pacemaker site within the sino-atrial node and by the atrial properties which determine the velocity of propagation.

In addition to the sino-atrial node, other sites in both right and left atria have been demonstrated to be capable of pacemaker function. It is not yet clear how frequently or under what conditions these areas are likely to initiate the cardiac rhythm, but the wide variability of P waveform may be partially due to such extra sinus node origins of supraventricular rhythm.

In the thin-walled atria, activation sequence in the endocardial epicardial dimension is not a significant factor in determining P waveform, and atrial activation can be considered a surface phenomenon. It has usually been considered an atrial property that activation spreads with uniform velocity from the pacemaker site. There is, however, both anatomic and functional evidence of specialized preferential conduction paths. Anatomic evidence of three paths containing specialized fibers in direct continuity and extending from the sino-atrial to atrioventricular node and to the left atrium has been reported. Physiologic evidence of such paths, including the effect of localized lesions on P waveform, has also been reported. Conflicting physiologic findings have also been reported, however, ranging from evidence of simple radial spread of excitation with uniform velocity to evidence that excitation spreads in broad areas corresponding to gross anatomic landmarks. These areas are reported to form separate inputs to the AV node but without evidence of narrow specialized internodal tracts.

Whether atrial excitation is propagated uniformly or via specialized tracts, the physiologic basis of many features of normal and abnormal P waves can be reasonably well explained. Even uniform propagation of excitation would result in geometrically complex boundaries of potential difference in the anatomically complex atria. The location of the sino-atrial node determines some of the major features of atrial excitation sequence and P waveform. The normal pacemaker has a superior and slightly posterior location within the right atrium; thus, the overall direction of atrial excitation is obliged to be leftward, downward, and slightly anteriorly. This results in upright P waves in leads I, II, and aV$_F$ and usually in all precordial leads. The relation of the overall direction of atrial excitation to the standard leads is illustrated diagrammatically in Figure 12–7. As shown in that figure, the normal P wave amplitude in lead II is likely to be larger than that in lead I, while lead III may show isoelectric P waves or waves of either polarity with only minor differences in the geometric relation of atrial excitation to that lead axis.

The relation of sequential boundaries of potential difference during atrial excitation to electrocardiographic leads I and II is illustrated in Figure 12–8. It should be noted that the time of onset of the P deflection differs in this example. The first boundary is so located that it produces

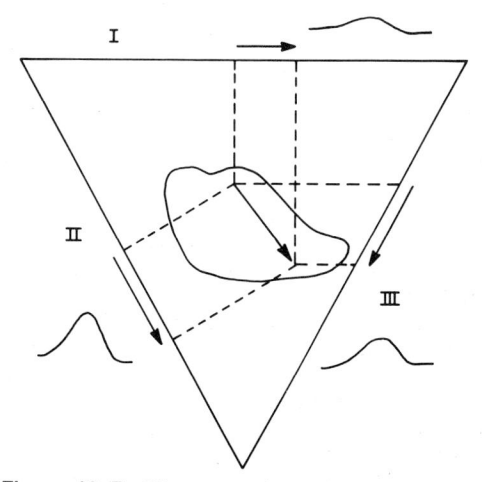

Figure 12–7 Diagrammatic representation of the atria and standard electrocardiographic leads. The average direction of spread of atrial excitation is indicated by the vector and the usual normal relation of P wave amplitude in the standard leads is shown.

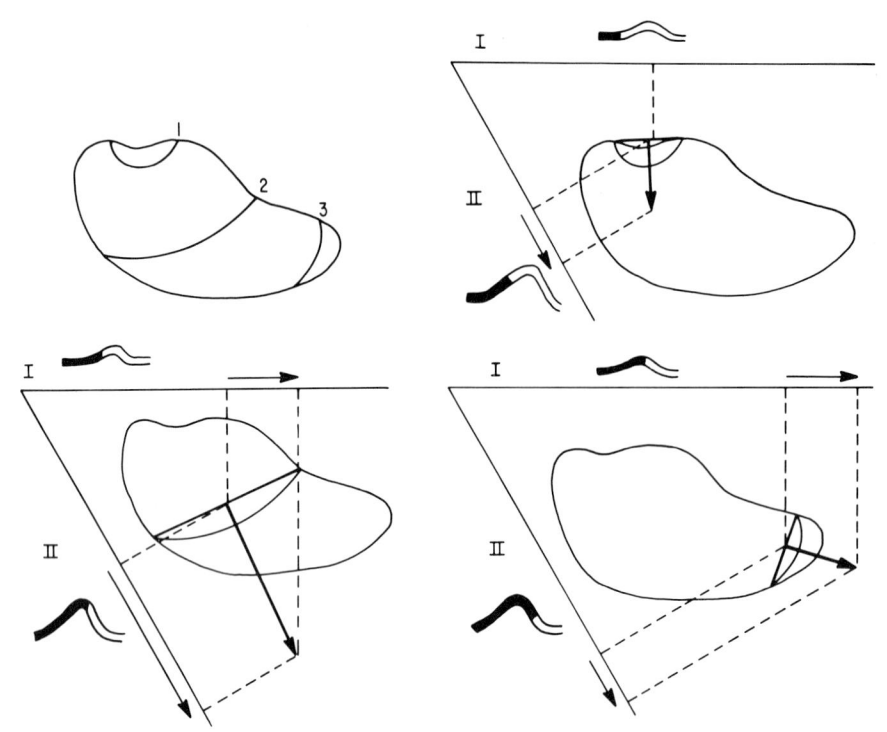

Figure 12-8 Diagrammatic representation of the atria and three sequential excitation boundaries. The electrocardiographic expressions of these boundaries on leads I and II are illustrated.

no effect in lead I but results in a deflection in lead II. This illustrates that the duration of the P wave in any one lead is not necessarily indicative of the total time required for atrial excitation. Similar considerations apply to other electrocardiographic deflections and the actual duration of the cardiac process which they reflect.

Atrial repolarization results in an electrocardiographic deflection, usually designated the Ta wave, whose peak amplitude is smaller and duration is longer than the P wave. The Ta wave is responsible for the level of the P-R segment in relation to the isoelectric interval of the electrocardiogram. The wave also extends into and modifies the form of the QRS complex and the level of the ST segment. Although the Ta deflection has not been extensively studied, it is usually of opposite polarity to the P wave it follows and its area is approximately equal to that of the P wave. At present, the major diagnostic significance of the Ta wave concerns its influence on ST segment level. When large upright P waves are present in a given lead, the Ta deflection can be expected to be proportional and may result in ST segment depression in that lead. Such ST segment depression is not the result of ventricular abnormalities but may be erroneously attributed to these if the effects of atrial repolarization on ST segment level are not appreciated. The Ta wave and its effect on ST segment level is illustrated diagrammatically in Figure 12-9. P wave amplitude and area are often increased with increases in heart rate, and the resulting increase in amplitude and area of the Ta deflection may result in ST segment displacement. Diagnostic errors are therefore especially likely in postexercise electrocardiograms in which ST segment displacement is a frequent manifestation of ischemic heart disease. The tachycardia produced by exercise may result in increased amplitude of the P waves, which are then followed by larger Ta waves superimposed on and displacing the ST segment.

VENTRICULAR EXCITATION AND THE QRS COMPLEX

Normal cardiac excitation originating in the sino-atrial node and spreading through the atria is delivered to the atrioventricular junctional tissues and via these to the specialized intraventricular conduction system. Major components of the junctional and intraventricular conduction system are the atriventricular node, bundle of His, right and left bundle branches, and the subendocardial Purkinje network. Activation of junctional and intraventricular conduction systems is not expressed as a distinct deflection in

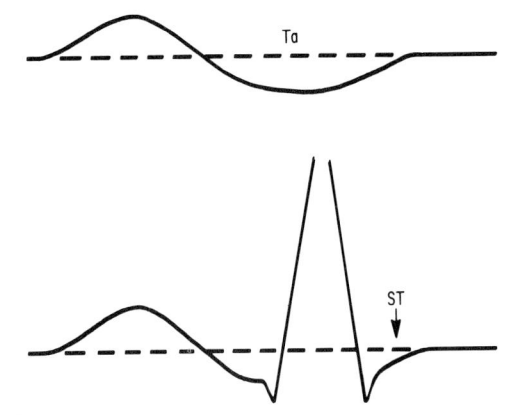

Figure 12-9 Diagrammatic representation of the P and Ta wave and the influence of the latter on ST segment level.

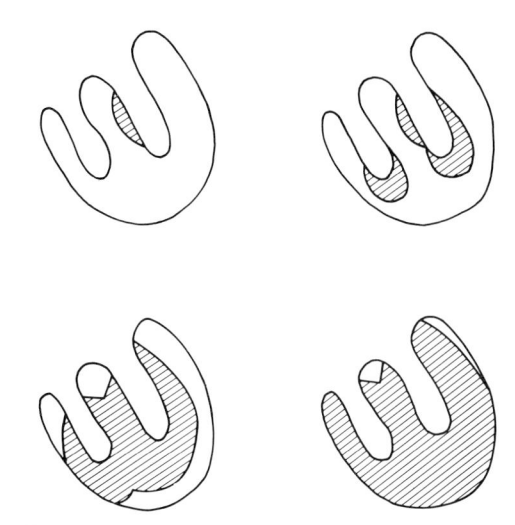

Figure 12-10 Representation of some of the major features of the normal ventricular activation sequence.

the body surface electrocardiogram and normally occurs during the P-R segment of that record. Catheter-mounted intracardiac electrodes positioned near portions of the junctional and specialized intraventricular conduction system show evidence of excitation in these structures and are providing valuable data concerning normal cardiac physiology, drug effects, and, in some cases, diagnostically useful information concerning cardiac rhythm.

The QRS complex reflects excitation in ventricular muscle after the process has reached that level via the Purkinje network. The pattern or sequence of ventricular activation has been defined in considerable detail in the hearts of several species, including man. The time of activation of multiple small areas has been determined, and the major features of the activation sequence so demonstrated account for the principal features of the QRS complex.

Figure 12-10 illustrates diagrammatically some of the major features of ventricular activation order. Excitation of ventricular muscle occurs first on the left side of the interventricular septum in approximately its midportion. The process continues to spread in this area and next appears on the endocardial surfaces of both right and left ventricles near their apices. Excitation then spreads from these three zones from endocardium toward epicardium and from apex toward base in the free ventricular walls and from both right and left, although chiefly from the left, in the interventricular septum. Activation of the thick basal portion of the left ventricular wall and activation of the superior portion of the interventricular septum are the latest events during ventricular excitation.

The relation of boundaries representative of the normal ventricular activation sequence to some leads of the routine electrocardiogram is illustrated diagrammatically in Figure 12-11. As described in previous sections, the electrocardiographic effects of each boundary are related to the quantity necessary to close the boundary and the magnitude of potential difference across the boundary. It is probable that the latter quantity is equal, or nearly so, for all normal activation boundaries, so that the relative size of closing boundaries is directly related to electrocardiographic effects. Early activation in the left side of the interventricular septum results in a boundary of potential difference with the negative side on the left. This is reasonably consistently expressed in the normal electrocardiogram by negative deflections in leads having one electrode on the left (I, aV_L, V_5 and V_6) and polarity so arranged that an upward deflection occurs when the left electrode is positive with respect to the other electrode involved in each lead. Since the negative deflection in these leads is the initial portion of the QRS complex, it constitutes a Q wave. In contrast, precordial lead V_1, in which one electrode is located to the right of the chest midline and has a polarity such that an upward deflection occurs when that electrode is positive with respect to the central terminal which is the other connection of that lead, reflects early septal activation as an R wave. In a similar fashion the other boundaries illustrated in Figure 12-11 account for R waves in leads I and V_6 and S waves in V_1 as well as major features of the QRS complex in other leads not illustrated.

Cardiac events responsible for late portions of the QRS complex include activation of the basal portion of the left ventricular wall and of the upper portion of the interventricular septum. The latter event is variable and sometimes occurs in a rightward direction, resulting in a late negative deflection or S wave in lead I and other leads with

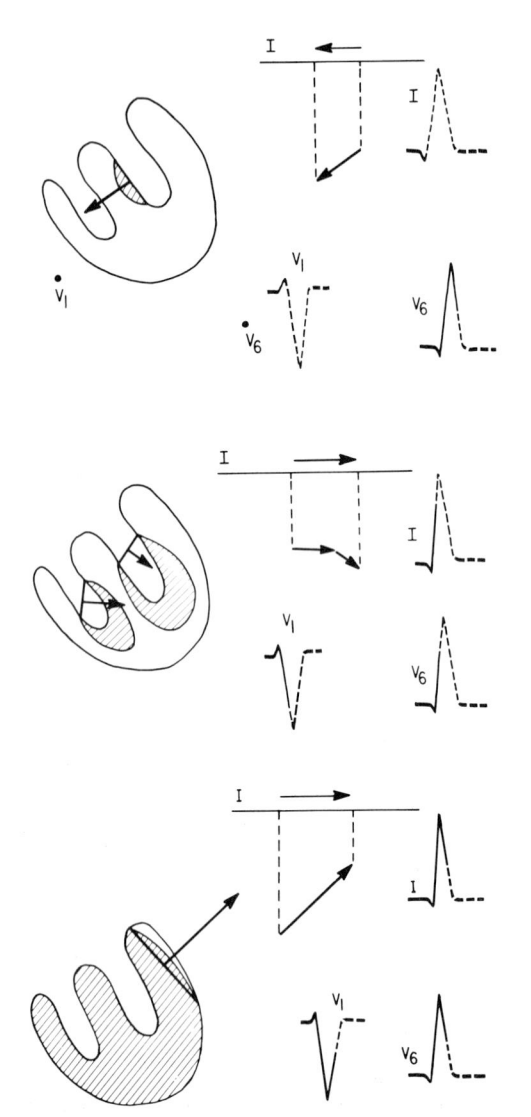

Figure 12–11 The relation of some major features of ventricular activation sequence to electrocardiographic deflections in leads I, V_1, and V_6.

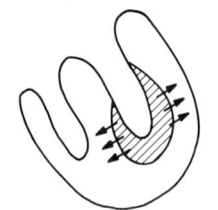

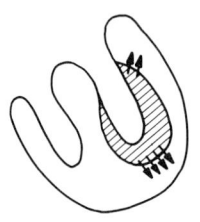

Figure 12–12 Illustration of the cancellation of electrocardiographic effects of portions of a representative boundary during ventricular activation. As shown in the diagram on the left, some portions of the boundary constitute equal and oppositely directed potential differences and cancel each other's electrocardiographic expression. Only those portions of the boundary indicated in the diagram on the right which do not have opposing portions result in electrocardiographic deflections.

comparison to the boundaries themselves. Theoretical, experimental, and clinical estimates of the degree to which events during normal ventricular excitation cancel their electrocardiographic effects suggest that 70 to 90 per cent of the ventricular mass is excited without contributing to the body surface electrocardiogram. This is illustrated in Figure 12–12 with a boundary characteristic of left ventricular activation during the midportion of the QRS complex. Such considerations indicate that large destructive lesions may have only minor electrocardiographic effects when they involve areas whose excitation is not normally expressed in the electrocardiogram. They further suggest that small lesions appropriately located in areas whose normal excitation is expressed in the QRS waveform with only a small degree of cancellation may have marked effects on that form.

VENTRICULAR REPOLARIZATION AND THE ST-T DEFLECTION

The cardiac state responsible for the ST-T deflection is similar to that responsible for the QRS complex in certain respects, but there are also important differences. Both excitation and recovery result in states in which boundaries of potential difference exist between cardiac areas in different physiologic states. In the case of excitation these boundaries are located between areas of excited and resting muscle. During recovery, boundaries are located between areas which have reached different stages of repolarization. If particular excitation and recovery boundaries are considered, their electrocardiographic effects are determined by the same factors. In both cases, the geometry of the boundary and its relation to the electrocardiographic lead under consideration are determinants of the electrocardiographic effect. A closed boundary between areas in different stages

an electrode on the left side. Absence of S waves in these leads is a normal variant, however.

One of the informative relations between cardiac events during ventricular excitation and the electrocardiogram is the degree to which the events cancel their electrocardiographic expression. The degree to which this occurs normally is a useful insight into the diagnostic limits of electrocardiography. A totally closed boundary, as previously described, has no expression in the electrocardiogram and can be said to be 100 per cent canceled. Actual boundaries during ventricular excitation are not usually completely closed but during much of the normal process the quantity necessary to close boundaries is small in of recovery is similar to a closed excitation boundary in having no electrocardiographic expression. The effect of both excitation and recovery boundaries is related to the degree to which they fail to be closed and thereby fail to cancel their electrocardiographic effects.

Both excitation and recovery boundaries produce electrocardiographic effects related to the magnitude of potential difference across the boundary. In the case of excitation boundaries, this value is the potential difference between excited and resting muscle and is related to the height of the transmembrane action potential upstroke. During recovery, the potential difference across a particular boundary is determined by the stage of recovery present on the two sides of the boundary as reflected by the relative height of action potential downstrokes and is always a fraction of the potential difference between excited and resting tissue. Potential differences at any one time during recovery are therefore smaller than the potential difference across activation boundaries. The difference across activation boundaries represents the maximal difference in potential between fully excited and resting muscle, while the potential difference at a given moment during recovery is some portion of that between fully excited and resting levels. Another difference in the cardiac states of excitation and recovery is that potential difference across recovery boundaries varies with time in relation to variations in the relative height of transmembrane action potential downstrokes on the two sides of the boundary. In addition, there is a marked difference in the length of time during which activation and recovery boundaries persist. Activation of individual cells is accomplished during 1 or 2 milliseconds as the action potential upstroke occurs, and individual activation boundaries persist only that length of time. Successive activation boundaries separated by more than that amount of time can be considered individually. The first produces an electrocardiographic effect and then disappears by the time the second boundary comes into existence and produces its electrocardiographic result. This is equivalent to considering activation as a process in which boundaries of potential difference move within cardiac muscle. In contrast, recovery in individual cells requires a considerably longer time, and a given boundary between areas recovering at different rates continues to exist until the repolarization process is complete on both sides of the boundary. During this time, additional boundaries between other cardiac areas with different recovery rates are established. At a given moment during repolarization, the cardiac source of the ST-T deflection may thus be multiple boundaries of potential difference which are widely distributed in ventricular muscle.

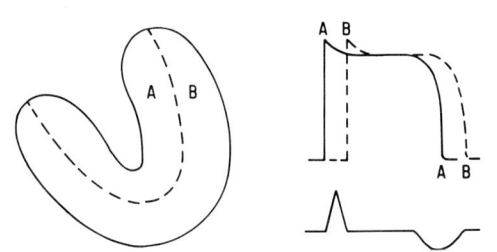

Figure 12–13 Relations between the cardiac state of recovery and the ST-T deflection. In this figure, ventricular muscle is illustrated as two groups of fibers with an excitation sequence such that fiber group A is excited first. The transmembrane action potentials for fiber groups A and B are shown, and the interval between upstrokes A and B represents the QRS interval. The interval in which action potentials A and B are both at the plateau level represents the ST segment portion of the electrocardiogram, and the onset to completion of rapid downstrokes corresponds to the T wave. Action potentials of the same form and duration for the two fiber groups are shown and, as illustrated, result in QRS and T deflections of opposite polarity.

To illustrate some of the relations between the cardiac state of recovery and the ST-T deflection it is helpful to consider a simplified activation sequence and organization of recovery properties. As illustrated in Figure 12–13, consider ventricular muscle as two groups of fibers, with all those in each group activated simultaneously and having particular recovery properties. The activation sequence can then be described as excitation of area A, followed by excitation of area B. This sequence of activation is illustrated in the figure by the upstrokes of action potentials designated A and B. In the interval between upstrokes A and B, a boundary of potential difference between cardiac areas A and B exists, and the magnitude of potential difference across this boundary is related to the height of the action potential upstroke in area A. After area B has also been excited and during the action potential plateau in both areas there is no potential difference between them. During the downstroke of the action potential, however, potential differences again exist between cardiac areas A and B. At any moment the magnitude of this difference is a fraction of that between fully excited and resting muscle.

Figure 12–13 can also be used to illustrate the relation of QRS and T wave polarity. An electrocardiographic lead has been arranged so that the potential difference between cardiac areas A and B results in an upward deflection when A is in the excited and B in the resting state. As shown in the figure, that polarity of potential difference is represented by the action potential from area A being located above that from area B. If action potentials are of equal duration, as shown in the figure, the action potential from area A will be completed before that from area B. During the downstroke of these action potentials the polarity of potential differences between cardiac areas A and B will be opposite that which existed during excitation. This state will result in a T wave of opposite polarity to the QRS deflection.

One of the major features of the normal electrocardiogram is a T wave with the same polarity as the major QRS deflection in most leads and under most circumstances. This suggests action potentials are of nonuniform duration and is, in fact, compatible with an inverse sequence of activation and of recovery. Actual physiologic data concerning the normal recovery sequence is difficult to obtain and is limited, but that which is available is compatible with such an inverse excitation and recovery sequence in ventricular muscle. Subendocardial muscle is excited early during ventricular excitation but has been demonstrated to have a longer refractory period and longer action potential downstroke than subepicardial muscle. Limited data suggest that an apex to base gradient of recovery properties also exists and apical muscle which is normally excited earlier than that at the ventricular base has the longer recovery time. The physiologic mechanism or mechanisms responsible for these normal variations in recovery properties have not been established. Variations in tension to which fibers are subjected, temperature differences, and other mechanisms have been suspected. Whatever the responsible mechanisms are, the normal recovery properties are such that they tend to equalize actual recovery times following a normal sequence of ventricular excitation. This probably has protective functions in that inequalities of recovery time have been strongly implicated in the mechanism of cardiac arrhythmias.

PATHOLOGIC STATES

The physiologic basis of electrocardiographic abnormalities in certain pathologic states will be considered in this section. The pathologic states to be considered have been selected on the basis of their diagnostic importance and because understanding of the mechanisms by which they modify the electrocardiogram is sufficiently complete to make these mechanisms diagnostically useful.

Atrial Enlargement

The physiologic basis of electrocardiographic features associated with atrial enlargement can be qualitatively appreciated even with simplifying assumptions concerning atrial anatomy and activation order. A diagrammatic representation of the atria and a simple radial excitation spread is illustrated in Figure 12-14, together with P waves in the standard electrocardiographic leads. A representation of left atrial enlargement is also shown and, as illustrated, results in several suc-

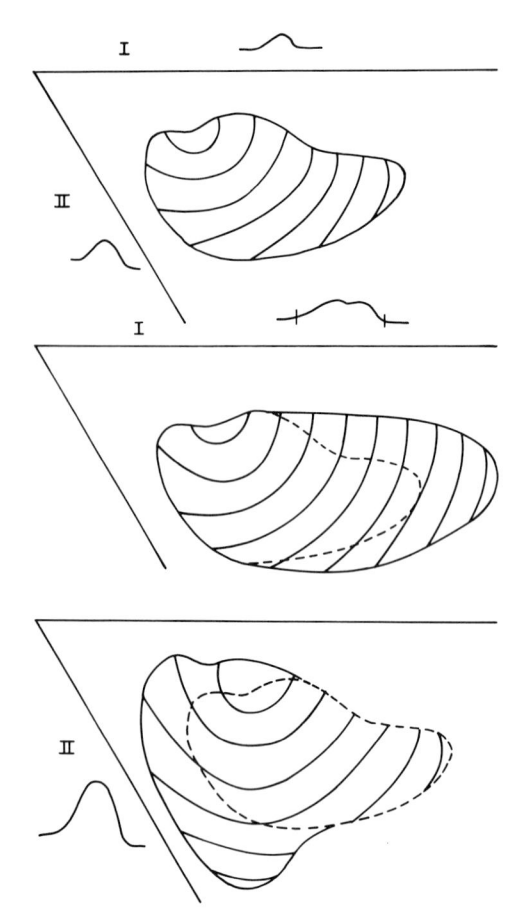

Figure 12–14 Diagrammatic representation of excitation in normal atria and in the states of left and right atrial enlargement. As illustrated, left atrial enlargement results in several successive fronts that are of similar geometry and are so oriented that a flat-topped or notched P wave in lead I results. Right atrial enlargement results in excitation boundaries directed roughly parallel to the axis of standard lead II and results in high P waves in that lead.

cessive excitation boundaries of nearly equal length and approximately the same relation to standard electrocardiographic leads. Potential differences across these boundaries are oriented roughly parallel to the left-right axis of the body, so that the most characteristic evidences of left atrial enlargement are likely to occur in lead I. In that lead the greater time necessary for completion of excitation is evidenced by prolongation of the P wave, and the nearly identical successive boundaries characteristically result in a flat-topped or notched P wave.

Right atrial enlargement is also diagrammatically illustrated in Figure 12–14. As illustrated, activation boundaries extended into the enlarged atrium result in greater potential differences in the vertical axis of the body which are reflected by abnormally high and often peaked P waves in lead II and lead aV_F. Larger than normal P waves often occur in lead I as well but are less characteristic of right atrial enlargement than those in leads II and aV_F.

Myocardial Infarction

Recognition of this frequent and significant lesion is one of the major areas of clinical utility of the electrocardiogram. Positive electrocardiographic findings are the best available evidence of this lesion and the physiologic mechanisms of these are sufficiently well defined to explain the findings in a useful fashion. Alterations of the waveform of the ventricular complex are the major electrocardiographic manifestations of myocardial infarction; and all portions of this complex, including QRS, ST, and T deflections, may be changed.

The QRS alterations are most specific and provide evidence of the location as well as the presence of infarction. Two major mechanisms operate to alter the QRS complex. One of these is the simple loss of excitable tissue which during its activation contributed to QRS complex waveform prior to infarction. The second mechanism is alteration of the excitation sequence in ventricular muscle not actually involved by the infarct.

The loss of ventricular muscle which during its excitation previously contributed to the form of the QRS complex is the mechanism responsible for the most characteristic and diagnostically useful evidence of the presence and location of myocardial infarction. This mechanism is illustrated in Figure 12–15. Under the heading of "normal" in that figure, an activation boundary is shown on a diagrammatic ventricular section. As illustrated, the uncanceled portion of the boundary results in a positive deflection in lead I. In the diagram headed "infarction," loss of excitable tissue in the lateral left ventricular wall is illustrated, together with the remaining portion of the excitation boundary previously illustrated. The uncanceled portion of the remaining boundary now results in a negative deflection in lead I. This is the general mechanism by which myocardial infarction results in Q waves in leads in which normal ventricular activation is represented by upward deflections. The leads in which Q deflections occur are dependent on the location of infarction. As illustrated, lateral wall infarction may result in Q waves in lead I which are actually the result of activation in ventricular muscle not involved in the infarct. Similarly, lateral wall lesions may produce Q waves in lead aV_L and precordial leads V_5 and V_6. A similar mechanism accounts for Q waves in leads II, III, and aV_F with inferior wall location of infarction and leads V_1 through V_4 with anterior wall infarcts. Posterior wall infarcts are also reflected by QRS alterations in precordial leads V_1 through V_4, but the changes consist of increased amplitude of R waves, since normal activation in the posterior wall is reflected by downward deflections in these leads and destruction of part of that wall leaves anteriorly directed activation unopposed.

The portion of the QRS complex in which changes due to the loss of excitable tissue occur depends on the location of the infarct with respect to the normal ventricular activation sequence. Abnormally deep or wide Q waves in leads normally containing an R wave reflect an infarct or portion of an infarct involving areas normally activated during early portions of the QRS complex. Subendocardial and intramural lesions or the subendocardial and intramural portions of transmural lesions are thus most likely to produce pathologic Q waves, which are the most definitive electrocardiographic evidence of infarction. Destructive lesions in this location are also more likely to produce marked QRS alterations than similar lesions located in subepicardial areas. Early activation boundaries in subendocardial and intramural regions surround the ventricular cavities and include portions with potential differences oriented in multiple directions. When tissue loss removes a portion of such a boundary having a particular potential difference direction, portions of the boundary with potential differences in other directions determine QRS form which is often markedly different after infarction. Subepicardial lesions alter activation fronts in which potential differences are largely present in a particular direction. Removal of part of such a boundary can be expected to alter late portions

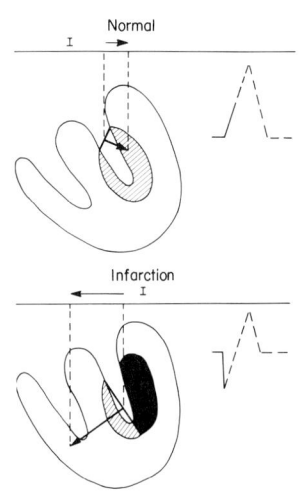

Figure 12–15 The mechanism of alteration of the QRS complex by loss of excitable tissue in myocardial infarction. In the upper diagram a representative excitation boundary in the left ventricle is shown and, as illustrated, is responsible for an upward deflection in lead I. The lower diagram shows part of the same boundary remaining after tissue loss indicated by the solid area. As shown, the remaining portion of the boundary results in a Q wave in lead I.

of the QRS complex, but the direction of the boundary before and after such a destructive lesion is likely to be similar. The presence of subepicardial destructive lesions is thus likely to alter the detailed form of the QRS complex, but changes will be small compared to those associated with lesions in other locations. Actual myocardial infarcts are often transmural, or nearly so, but transmural involvement is not a necessity for diagnostically significant alterations of the QRS complex.

It should be clearly recognized that pathologic Q waves do not occur with all infarcts or with all infarct locations. These waves have special diagnostic significance because they represent a marked deviation from normal QRS waveform and do not overlap the range of normal variation of that waveform. Less marked QRS waveform changes may be expected with infarcts of particular size and in particular locations. For example, a lateral wall infarct may reduce the amplitude of R waves in leads I, aV_L, V_5, and V_6 but fail to produce Q waves if the size or location of the lesion is appropriate. Such a QRS waveform may not lie outside the range of normal variation and is less useful diagnostically than the more marked change to a pathologic Q wave.

The second factor which may alter QRS waveform with myocardial infarction is altered excitation squence in ventricular muscle other than that destroyed by infarction. This mechanism is sometimes titled peri-infarction block and that term will be employed in this text, although the term has also been used with a more limited meaning. Whatever terminology is employed, a destructive myocardial lesion may alter activation sequence in remaining excitable muscle by affecting the spread of excitation in that muscle. Specialized conduction fibers may be interrupted by the lesion, so that areas normally excited via these fibers must be activated by other routes. Even without interruption of specialized fibers, the route of normal activation to a particular area through ventricular muscle may include the area of the destructive lesion, and other paths bypassing the lesion are then taken by the excitation process.

Alterations of the QRS complex by the mechanism of peri-infarction block mainly occur in mid and terminal portions of the complex. In actual diagnostic use it is difficult to distinguish such alterations from ones due to tissue loss in areas normally excited during these portions of the QRS complex. Only if the destructive lesion is known to be restricted to areas normally activated during early portions of the QRS complex can alterations of later QRS deflections be attributed to peri-infarction block with certainty. Since this information is not available ante mortem, the QRS alterations due to peri-infarction block are considerably less helpful diagnostically than those due to tissue loss. In addition, QRS alterations by mechanism of peri-infarction block of necessity involve later portions of the QRS complex, which has a wider range of normal variability than initial deflections, so that changes in the late QRS may not be recognizable unless a pre-infarction electrocardiogram is available.

QRS changes due to loss of excitable tissue are likely to be systematic, particularly when areas normally excited during early portions of the ventricular activation process are involved. At this time during the activation process, excitation is spreading in multiple directions and the localized loss of excitable tissue is likely to leave excitation fronts directed away from the area of lesion. In a similar manner, there is at least a tendency for QRS alterations due to peri-infarction block to be systematic. In this case, however, the muscle near the destructive lesion is likely to be the area in which activation sequence is most markedly altered and the spread of excitation into this region is thus directed toward the lesion. These systematic features of QRS alteration by tissue loss and peri-infarction block may be visualized by an electrocardiographic lead containing an R and S wave during normal excitation. Destruction of excitable tissue during early portions of ventricular activation may alter the initial QRS deflection by changing it from an R to a Q deflection, while the mechanism of peri-infarction block may alter the terminal QRS in an opposite direction, changing the S wave to an R deflection.

ST segments and T waves are also likely to be altered by acute infarction and to change serially over a period of weeks or months. In old infarction, T wave abnormalities often persist, and ST segment displacement may persist in instances of ventricular aneurysm. The physiologic mechanism of both ST segment displacement and T wave abnormalities includes alteration of the duration and form of intracellular action potentials. An additional mechanism, namely reduced resting membrane potential, is also involved in ST segment displacement during acute infarction. Figure 12–16 illustrates the relation of action potential form to the electrocardiogram at various stages of myocardial infarction. For the purposes of this text, the heart may again be considered as consisting of two populations of cells with different intrinsic recovery properties. The normal state in which the area activated earliest is represented by the action potential of longest duration is illustrated. The area represented by action potential B is excited at a later time but completes the recovery process first. As illustrated, potential differences between these areas during the plateau characteristic of cardiac muscle are small and the ST segment is near isoelectric. The polarity of potential differences between the two areas is the same during excitation and recovery, so that a lead reflecting an upright QRS complex also reflects an upright T wave.

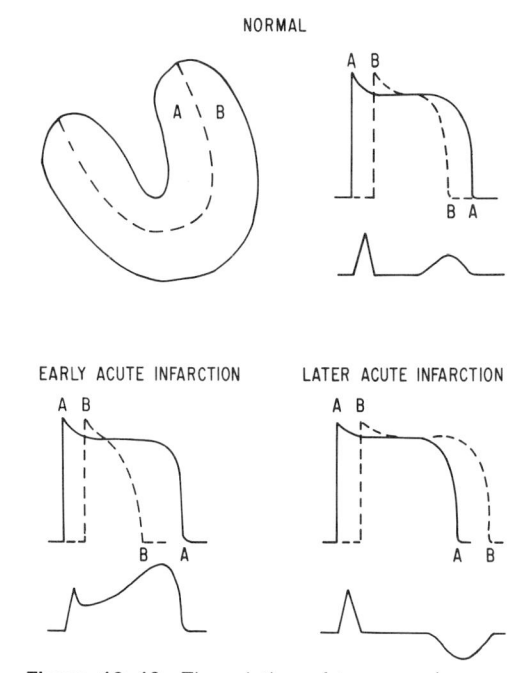

Figure 12-16 The relation of transmembrane action potential alterations by myocardial infarction to ST-T abnormalities. The normal state in which ventricular areas activated early have shorter action potentials and in which QRS and T deflections have the same polarity is illustrated in the upper portion of the figure. Early acute infarction results in reduced action potential duration, and ST displacement due to loss of the action potential plateau and increased T wave amplitude due to shorter action potential duration result. In later stages of infarction, action potential duration in ischemic tissue is prolonged and T wave inversion occurs, as illustrated in the lower right portion of the figure.

Acute ischemia shortens the duration of the transmembrane action potential and increases the slope of that portion of the record normally represented by a plateau. The mechanism of these action potential changes is not certain, but it is most likely that they are the result of local hyperkalemia due to potassium release from injured cells. As illustrated under the heading of "early acute infarction," such alterations are associated with ST segment displacement and increased amplitude of the T waves but with normal polarity of the latter deflection.

Later in the course of acute infarction, ischemic cells exhibit prolonged recovery time. As illustrated, this produces a state in which the polarities of potential differences during excitation and recovery differ from each other and the polarities of QRS and T deflections therefore differ, the latter being abnormal. ST segment displacement decreases as cells recover and action potentials exhibit a more nearly normal plateau, or as injured cells become inexcitable.

Intraventricular Conduction Disorders

Abnormalities in the delivery of excitation to ventricular muscle by the intraventricular portion of the specialized conduction system result in abnormal atrioventricular relations or abnormalities of the QRS complex waveform. Abnormal atrioventricular relations occur with conduction disorders in the junctional tissues, including atrioventricular node and bundle of His, or bilaterally in more distal portions of the intraventricular conduction system and range from prolonged conduction time, resulting in a prolonged P-R interval in the electrocardiogram, to total failure of conduction, resulting in independent cardiac rhythms in the atria and ventricles, with the electrocardiogram showing unrelated P waves and QRST complexes.

Abnormalities of conduction in the specialized conduction system below the level of bifurcation of the bundle of His into right and left bundle branches result in abnormalities of QRS waveform. Some of these abnormalities have considerable diagnostic utility and they can only be recognized by electrocardiographic examination.

The physiologic basis of the distinctive QRS waveform associated with complete failure of conduction through the left bundle branch is shown in Figure 12-17. Ventricular excitation reaches ventricular muscle exclusively via the right bundle branch, and its spread through ventricular muscle necessarily occurs in a right-to-left direction. Leads in which one of the electrodes is located on the left side of the body and which result in an upward deflection when that electrode is positive with respect to the other electrode involved in the lead thus show exclusively positive QRS deflections. Leads I, aV_L, V_5, and V_6 of the 12-lead electrocardiogram have this characteristic in left bundle branch block. In addition, most leads will reflect the abnormally long time required for the completion of ventricular activation by prolongation of the QRS complex. Normal ventricular activation delivered via both right and left bundle branches spreads simultaneously in right and left ventricles and determines the normal QRS duration. When bundle branch block is present and activation is delivered only via the functioning branch, an abnormally long time is required for completion of activation in the contralateral ventricle. A QRS duration of 0.12 second or more is usually considered the most useful index of complete bundle branch block.

The physiologic basis of QRS form in right bundle branch block is illustrated in Figure 12-18. As with left bundle branch block, the QRS duration is prolonged. In right bundle branch block, however, excitation occurs normally in the left ventricle. Early left septal activation may therefore give rise to a small Q wave in leads I, aV_L, V_5, and V_6 as in the normal state. This is followed by normal left ventricular activation proceeding leftward in the free left ventricular wall and rightward in the interventricular septum. As illustrated, this combination of events gives rise to an R wave in lead I and similarly oriented leads. After completion of left ventricular activation including activation of the interventricular septum, activation of the free right ventricular wall takes place and results in an S wave in leads I, aV_L, V_5, and V_6. This deflection together with the prolonged QRS duration constitute characteristic electrocardiographic features of right bundle branch block. In addition, the anterior location of the free right ventricular wall results in additional major electrocardiographic evidence of right bundle branch block. The late activation of this structure is proceeding anteriorly as well as to the right and results in prominent late R waves in one or more of the precordial leads V_1 through V_3. These deflections are preceded by normal R and S waves in these leads and are therefore designated as R prime waves.

The T waves associated with bundle branch block are influenced by the abnormal ventricular activation sequence as well as by the intrinsic recovery characteristics of ventricular muscle. The gross abnormalities of activation sequence and QRS form in these states also result in gross alterations of T waveform, even if ventricular recovery characteristics are normal. In general, the recovery sequence alterations secondary to activation sequence abnormalities in bundle branch block tend to produce QRS and T complexes of opposite polarity, even if intrinsic recovery properties remain the same. The clinical significance of bundle branch blocks is an appropriate subject for texts of diagnostic electrocardiography and cardiology. As previously mentioned, however, the recognition of these

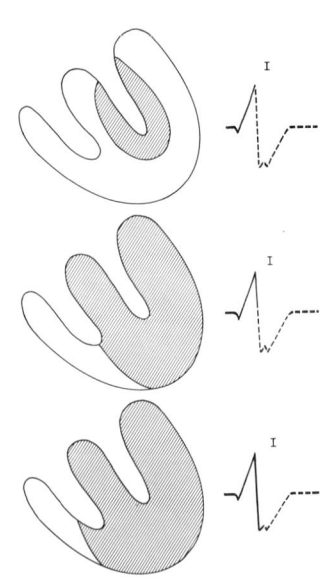

Figure 12–18 Ventricular activation sequence and QRS waveform in lead I in complete right bundle branch block.

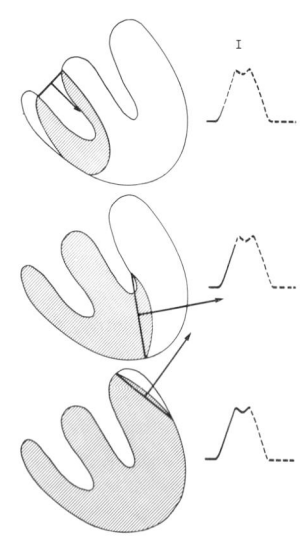

Figure 12–17 Ventricular activation sequence and QRS waveform in lead I in complete left bundle branch block.

states can only be accomplished by electrocardiographic means.

In addition to block at the level of major right and left bundle branches, other abnormalities of intraventricular conduction occur. Slower than normal conduction can occur under appropriate circumstances at any level in the heart, and in the case of the intraventricular conduction system distal to bifurcation of the bundle of His such conduction can alter QRS form in fashions which resemble bundle branch block but are less marked.

Furthermore, conduction defects may occur at sites more distal than the major bundle branches. Evidence has been reported that the left bundle branch consists of two major subdivisions, one of which is distributed to anterosuperior and the other to posteroinferior left ventricular muscle. Classification of electrocardiograms on the basis of findings to be expected with block of each of these has been proposed under the titles of anterosuperior and posteroinferior left hemiblock. Anatomic evidence for distinct subdivisions of the left bundle is conflicting, but classification of electrocardiograms as evidencing hemiblock is being widely employed. The major criterion proposed for recognition of these entities is the electrical axis of the QRS with anterosuperior hemiblock resulting in left axis deviation and posteroinferior block resulting in right axis deviation. Axis deviation compatible with these entities is often associated with right bundle branch block, and the presence of this conduction defect is compatible with the view that the axis deviation is also the result of a conduction disorder.

CHAPTER 13

ARRHYTHMIAS— MECHANISMS AND PATHOGENESIS

YOSHIO WATANABE
LEONARD S. DREIFUS

Both clinical and electrophysiologic studies have suggested certain basic concepts in the genesis of cardiac arrhythmias. For clinical purposes, classification of cardiac arrhythmias is usually based on the origin of impulses (supraventricular or ventricular) and their mode of appearance (premature systole, tachycardia, flutter, fibrillation, and so on). From the electrophysiologic standpoint, on the other hand, genesis of cardiac arrhythmias is often divided into (1) disturbances of impulse formation, (2) disturbances of conduction, and (3) a combination of both (Table 13–1).

AUTOMATICITY

Automaticity is the most fundamental mechanism of impulse formation, and either its enhancement or depression could result in various arrhythmias of clinical significance. In Figure 13–1, transmembrane potentials of the S-A nodal and His-Purkinje fibers are schematically shown to illustrate electrophysiologic characteristics of automatic fibers. Following full repolarization, the S-A nodal fibers show progressive decrease in the negative membrane potential. When this diastolic (or phase 4) depolarization reaches the level of threshold potential, a smooth transition to the more rapid depolarization of phase 0 occurs and a new impulse is formed (the second beat). Although similar diastolic depolarization could start almost simultaneously in other specialized cardiac tissues, including the His-Purkinje system, the slope of phase 4 depolarization is usually less steep than in the sinus node.

As a result, these fibers are depolarized by a propagated S-A nodal impulse before their own threshold potential is reached, and the sinus node assumes the role of pacemaker of the heart. Two

TABLE 13–1 CLASSIFICATION OF CARDIAC ARRHYTHMIAS

I. Disturbances of impulse formation
  A. Automaticity
    1. Physiologic alterations
    2. Enhanced automaticity
    3. Depressed automaticity
  B. Other mechanisms of impulse formation
    1. Oscillation
    2. Afterpotentials
    3. Local potential difference
      a. Asynchronous repolarization
      b. Partial depolarization
II. Disturbances of impulse conduction
  A. Simple conduction block
    1. Refractory tissue
      a. Dissimilar action potential duration and excitability between fiber types
      b. Interference of two impulses
    2. Decremental conduction
    3. Inhomogeneous conduction
  B. Unidirectional block and re-entry
    1. Unidirectional block and re-entry in the A-V junction
    2. Local block and microre-entry
III. Combined disturbances of impulse formation and conduction
  A. Parasystole
  B. Ectopic rhythms with exit block
IV. Fibrillation

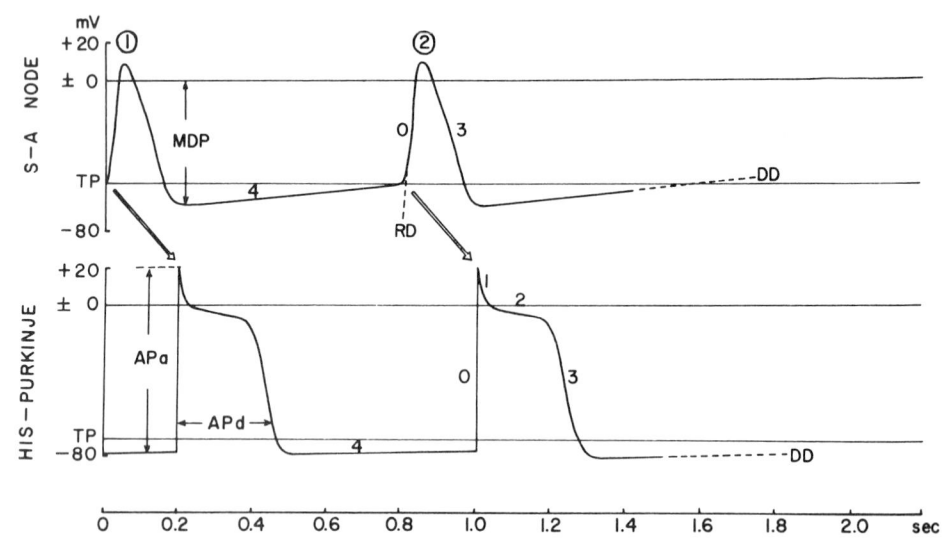

Figure 13–1 Transmembrane potentials of the S-A nodal and the His-Purkinje fibers are schematically shown. The slope of diastolic depolarization *(DD)* is steeper and the threshold potential *(TP)* is attained earlier in the S-A nodal fiber than in the His-Purkinje fiber. Thus, the His-Purkinje system is discharged by propagated sinus impulse (arrows). Note differences in the action potential amplitude *(APa)*, the action potential duration *(APd)*, the rate of phase 0 depolarization *(RD)*, and the time course of repolarization (phases 1, 2, and 3) between the two fiber types. *MDP*, maximal diastolic potential. (Reproduced with permission from Watanabe, Y., and Dreifus, L. S.: Amer. Heart J., *76*:114, 1968.)

major factors which modify the cycle length of an automatic fiber are (1) the slope of diastolic depolarization and (2) the difference between the threshold potential and the maximal diastolic potential attained at the end of repolarization (Fig. 13-1). From the above discussion, however, it becomes readily apparent that the site of impulse formation is determined by the relative rapidity with which phase 4 depolarization brings the membrane potential to the threshold level in different fiber groups. This is illustrated in Figures 13-2 and 13-3.

Figure 13-2A shows that when a second sinus impulse fails to reach the His-Purkinje system owing to S-A or A-V conduction block (blocked arrow), or when the sinus rate is markedly slowed by vagal stimulation (with increased maximal diastolic potential and decreased slope of phase 4 deploarization as shown by the dotted line), diastolic depolarization of the His-Purkinje fiber could now proceed until it attains the threshold potential. An impulse thus formed would prevent prolonged periods of ventricular asystole. This is called an escape beat. A clinical electrocardiogram reproduced in Figure 13-2B illustrates such an example. In both leads AVR and AVF of this record, the first P wave is conducted to the ventricles with a prolonged P-R interval of 0.30 second, while the second P wave is blocked. Thus, there is second-degree A-V block. The pause due to this dropped beat is terminated by a QRS superimposed on the next P wave of sinus origin. This escape beat probably results from automaticity in the A-V junctional fibers, since the QRS configuration suggests the A-V node as the most likely site of conduction block.

On the other hand, if the slope of diastolic depolarization in automatic fibers outside the S-A node becomes abnormally steep, these fibers may eventually take over the control of the atrial and/or ventricular excitation. Figure 13-3A illustrates that an enhanced automaticity in the His-Purkinje system would cause a more rapid impulse formation than that in the sinus node. In Figure 13-3B, there is sinus tachycardia at the rate of 110 beats per min. However, the ventricles are predominantly controlled by an accelerated ectopic pacemaker at the rate of 130 beats per min. Although definite proof in these clinical cases is lacking, it is likely that many instances of self-sustaining ectopic tachycardia result from increased automaticity as schematically shown in Figure 13-3A. Several clinical factors known to produce ventricular arrhythmias have been shown experimentally to enhance automaticity in the His-Purkinje system. These factors include lowered extracellular potassium concentration, cardiac glycosides, and catecholamines.

Under certain clinical conditions, depression rather than enhancement of automaticity engenders serious disturbances of cardiac rhythmicity, especially when associated with disorders of im-

Figure 13–2 *A,* Schematic diagram illustrating the mechanism of escape beat. When a second sinus impulse fails to reach the His-Purkinje system (or the A-V junctional fibers) as a result of S-A or A-V conduction block (blocked arrow), or when the sinus rate is markedly slowed by vagal stimulation or other factors (dotted line), diastolic depolarization of the A-V junctional or His-Purkinje fibers could proceed to attain the threshold potential and cause an escape beat. Note a smoother transition from phase 4 to phase 0 and a slightly reduced rate of phase 0 depolarization, with spontaneous discharge of the His-Purkinje system. *B,* A clinical example of A-V junctional escape in the presence of second-degree A-V block. See description in text. (Reproduced with permission from Watanabe, Y.: Wiederbeleb. Organersatz u. Intensivmed. [in press].)

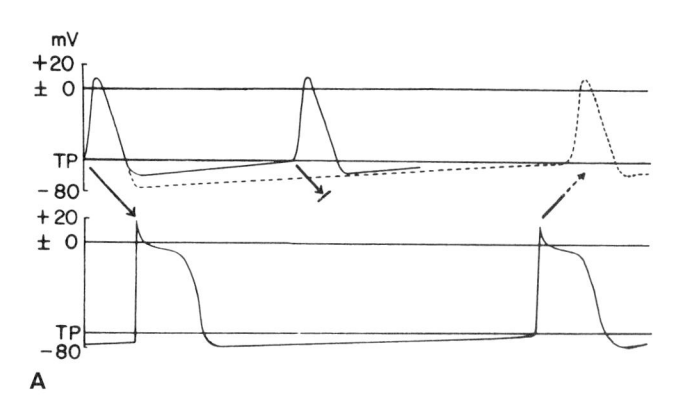

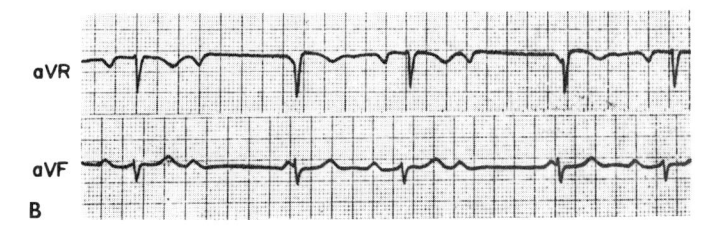

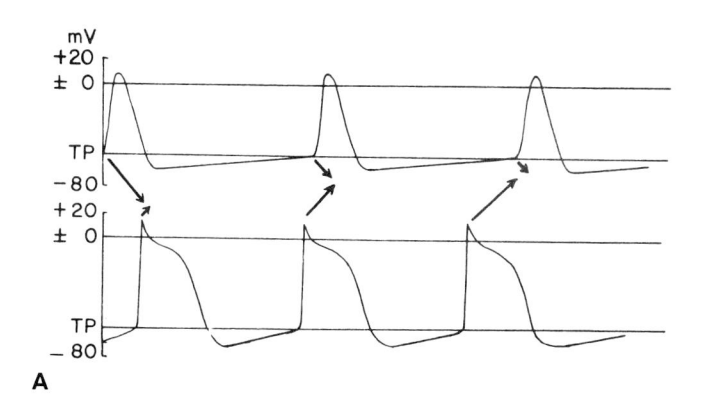

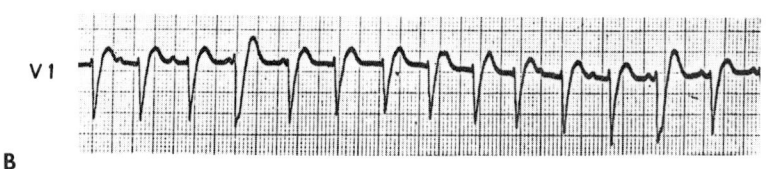

Figure 13–3 *A,* Diagram similar to Figures 13–1 and 13–2 illustrates an accelerated impulse formation in the His-Purkinje system. The sinus node is discharging at a normal rate. However, the His-Purkinje fiber generates its own impulses before a propagated sinus impulse arrives at this region, because of an enhanced automaticity (increased phase 4 depolarization). Interference (or collision) of the two independently formed impulses may occur at different levels within the A-V transmission system (arrows). *B,* A clinical example of A-V junctional tachycardia. The R-R intervals are shorter than the P-P intervals, and A-V dissociation is present. (Reproduced with permission from Watanabe, Y.: Wiederbeleb. Organersatz u. Intensivmed. [in press].)

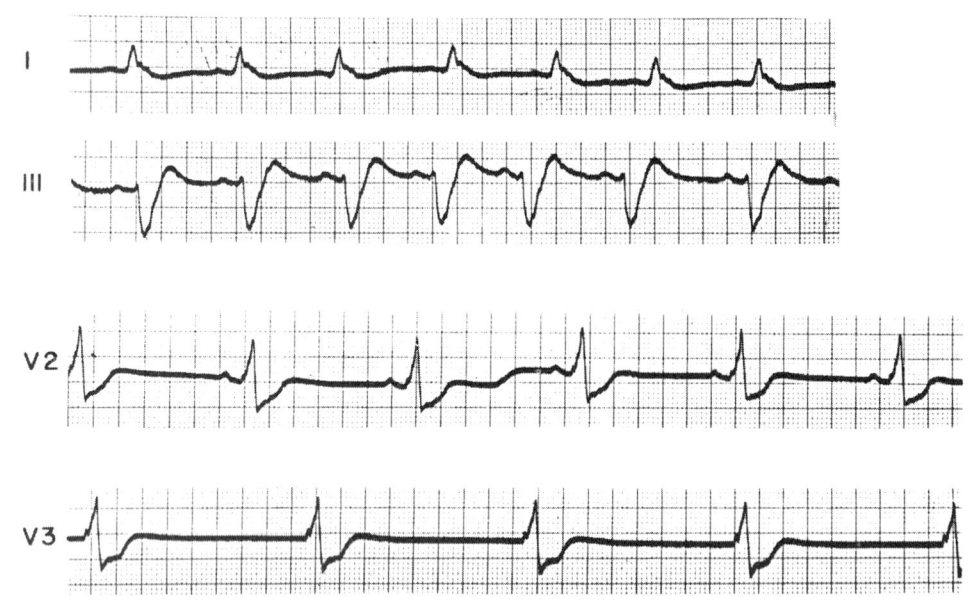

Figure 13-4 An electrocardiogram showing so-called downward displacement of the pacemaker. See text for discussion. (Reproduced with permission from Watanabe, Y.: Wiederbeleb. Organersatz u. Intensivmed. [in press].)

pulse conduction. Some statistics suggest that ventricular standstill occurs more frequently than ventricular fibrillation as an initial mechanism of sudden cardiac death following myocardial infarction. The electrocardiogram reproduced in Figure 13-4 was obtained during a sequential recording of the 12 leads. Leads I and III showed a sinus rhythm at an average rate of 70 beats per min. Marked widening of the QRS complexes indicated intraventricular conduction disturbances, probably involving both of the two fascicles of the left bundle branch system. In lead V_2, the sinus rate has slowed to 45 beats per min., suggesting decreased automaticity in the S-A node. Lead V_3 revealed no sinus activity, and an A-V junctional rhythm appeared to be present at the rate of 33 beats per min. Cardiac arrest soon followed this recording. Such "downward displacement of pacemaker" leading to ventricular standstill most likely resulted from depression of automaticity in all the specialized tissues.

SIMPLE CONDUCTION BLOCK

Of the various mechanisms causing failure of impulse propagation, the one most classically invoked is the presence of refractory tissue ahead of the advancing wave of excitation. This condition may occur at a junction of two fiber groups with dissimilar excitability or duration of refractoriness. It has been demonstrated that the action potential duration becomes progressively prolonged from the atrial fibers through the AN, N, and NH regions of the A-V node, His bundle, bundle branches, and to the more peripheral Purkinje fibers (Fig. 13-5). Thus, at any junction of two specialized conducting tissues, the distal fibers usually have a longer effective refractory period and may fail to respond to high frequency of the proximal fibers (Fig. 13-6). Failure of A-V conduction in the presence of extremely rapid atrial rhythm (e.g., atrial flutter) or of an early atrial premature systole may occur on this basis. Complete failure of propagation of a premature atrial impulse at the level of the right bundle branch, where the action potential duration is significantly longer than in the left bundle branch or in the more proximal fiber, has been demonstrated. A new concept of the "gate" mechanism in peripheral Purkinje fibers, where the duration of refractoriness is the longest, undoubtedly emerged from the above observations and may prove valuable in explaining certain ventricular arrhythmias.

More specifically, failure of impulse propagation in either the sino-atrial (S-A) or the atrioventricular (A-V) transmission can produce varieties of clinical arrhythmias. There are numerous factors which affect propagation of cardiac impulses, particularly in depressed tissue. Only several major mechanisms are herein discussed. In Figure 13-7A, transmembrane potentials were recorded from an atrial fiber bordering the A-V node in an isolated, perfused rabbit heart (middle record marked A). A bipolar surface electrogram recorded from the region of the sinus node (S-A) shows 1:1 response to the driving stimuli at the rate of 130 beats per min. However, the transmembrane recording shows one propagated action potential followed by two local responses. These local responses are obviously ineffective and are not conducted through the A-V node to the ventricles. This, then, is considered an example of either S-A or intra-atrial block. Figure 13-7B illustrates a clinical counterpart of such experimental records. In lead I, two sinus beats are followed by a long pause, with a P-P interval almost equaling two sinus cycles. This suggests a 2:1 S-A conduction. A series of five sinus beats then follows, with sinus arrhythmia. Periods of 2:1 and 3:1 S-A response are again seen in lead II.

It has been suggested that different excitability of S-A nodal vs. ordinary atrial fibers could cause failure of propagation of the sinus impulses. However, observations on experimental "S-A block" revealed that the blocked sinus impulses did spread partially into the atrial tissue but with a decreased rate and amplitude of phase 0 depolarization. The efficacy of stimuli in exciting the adjacent atrial fibers appeared progressively decreased in the course of propagation until only a local response was recorded (Fig. 13-7). Thus, the term decremental conduction seems to describe more adequately the mechanism of intra-atrial (or so-called S-A) block.

Such decremental conduction is likely to develop in the presence of a lower level of membrane potential and a slower rate of phase 0 depolarization. These conditions can be seen in any type of fiber showing either incomplete repolarization (during the relative refractory period), significant diastolic depolarization, or partial depolarization caused by various pathophysiologic factors. Since the fibers in the N region of the A-V node show the above characteristics even under physiologic conditions, decremental conduction is more commonly seen in this tissue than in other portions of the A-V transmission system. Many factors known to impair A-V conduction such as acetylcholine, cardiac glycosides, lowered potassium concentration, or ischemia enhance the degree of decrement and usually cause failure of propagation within the A-V node. However, there are other factors which depress conduction in the atrial as well as His-Purkinje fibers, and multiple levels of block can sometimes be observed.

Normally, successful conduction through the A-V nodal tissue occurs with rather synchronous activation of fibers in the AN and the N regions and a smooth excitation front invading the NH region. When the rate of depolarization is decreased and conduction further slowed, particularly in the critical N region of the A-V node, the spread of excitation in this region becomes inhomogeneous. Such inhomogeneity of conduction could manifest itself as two or more functionally separate portions of tissue, some of which show a relatively rapid conduction. Increasing decrement in all portions or in the slower conducting portions alone can cause further fractionation of the wave front, leading to the failure of propagation. Intranodal conduction block, including the instances with classic Wenckebach periodicity, can be explained on this basis.

The above concept was supported by Janse, who demonstrated that an atrial wave front coming from the interatrial septum excited the atrial margin of the A-V node asynchronously, resulting in inhomogeneous conduction and functional

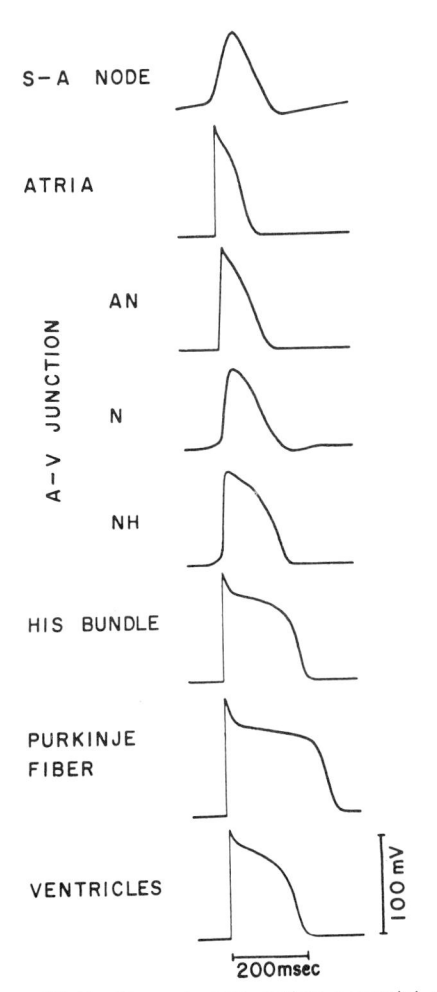

Figure 13-5 Characteristic action potential configurations in various fiber types. The action potential duration is progressively prolonged from the atria to the peripheral Purkinje fiber. (Reproduced with permission from Watanabe, Y., and Dreifus, L. S.: Amer. Heart J., 76:114, 1968.)

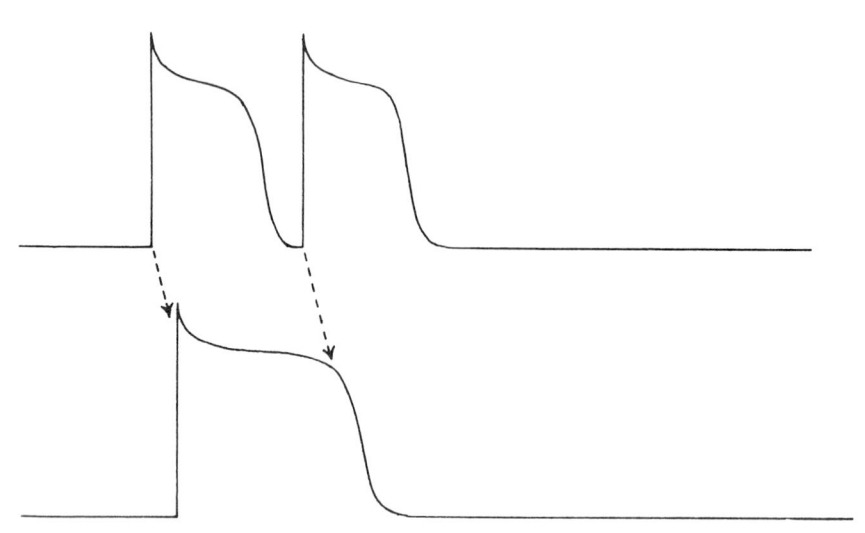

Figure 13-6 Relationship of the refractory period to nonconducted premature systoles. The upper tracing shows an atrial beat which is conducted to the ventricles (Purkinje fiber). The second beat is premature and is not conducted as it arrives at the Purkinje fiber in the absolute refractory period (phase 2). The longer action potential duration in more distal portions of the A-V transmission system prevents ventricular conduction of early premature beats on this basis, and block is not required to explain nonconducted premature beats. (Reproduced with permission from Dreifus, L. S., Watanabe, Y., and Beyer, B.: Ann. N. Y. Acad. Sci., 167:950, 1969.)

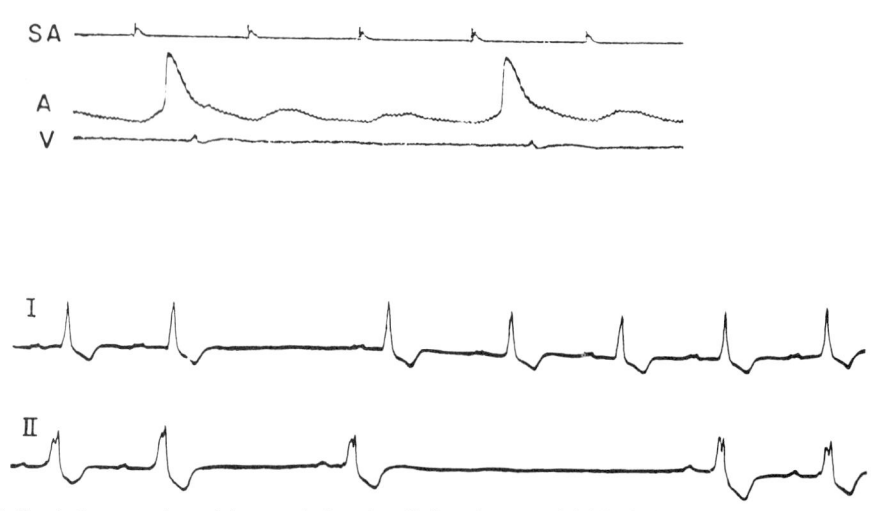

Figure 13-7 A, An experimental record showing S-A or intra-atrial block. Note a decreased rate of phase 0 depolarization in propagated response and two successive local responses recorded from an atrial fiber adjacent to the A-V node. B, An electrocardiographic example of S-A block. Periods of 2:1 and 3:1 S-A conduction are easily identified, although there is some sinus arrhythmia. (Reproduced with permission from Watanabe, Y.: Wiederbeleb. Organersatz u. Intensivmed. [in press].)

longitudinal dissociation within the node. Possible importance of this mechanism in the presence of atrial fibrillation was also pointed out.

On the other hand, if the more rapidly conducting portions are selectively depressed by either a forward or retrograde impulse, slower spread of excitation in this portion may result in a synchronized or smoother wave front. Then, an unexpected, successful A-V or V-A transmission in the presence of advanced degrees of block may ensue. This phenomenon has been described as a variety of supernormal A-V or V-A conduction (Fig. 13–8).

Within recent years an abundance of information has become available concerning the pathology, electrophysiology, anatomy, and clinical significance of disturbances of A-V conduction. Electrophysiologic techniques using ultramicroelectrodes have demonstrated the complex nature of atrioventricular conduction and the precise behavior of the three electrophysiologic regions (AN, N, and NH) of the atrioventricular node. More recently, Sherlag et al., using a percutaneous electrocatheter technique, introduced the method of recording His bundle electrograms in man. These studies as well as the flurry of reports in the past few years have confirmed many important concepts that had been previously described by Wenckebach, Mobitz, Katz and Pick, Scherf, and others. Mobitz conveniently classified second-degree A-V block into two varieties. Type I is associated with a progressive increase in the P-R interval before the dropped QRS complex. This type of A-V conduction had been originally described by Wenckebach and is now often referred to as the Wenckebach phenomenon (Fig. 13–9). In contrast, Type II shows a constant P-R interval before the blocked QRS complex (Fig. 13–10). However, both ultramicroelectrode and His bundle electrographic techniques have shown the complex nature of A-V conduction, with multiple levels of delays contributing to the behavior of the P-R interval. Furthermore, it has become abundantly clear that the site of block, i.e., within the node or in the subjunctional regions and fascicles of the bundle branch system, largely determines the prognosis. More specifically, second-degree block associated with QRS durations of less than 0.12 second suggests block within the A-V node, while QRS durations of 0.12 second or greater indicate block in the subjunctional regions. Although there are occasional exceptions to this concept, the clinical importance of A-V block largely rests on the site of A-V block rather than on the behavior of the P-R interval.

A majority of the patients with second-degree block associated with wide QRS complexes (subjunctional block) are symptomatic and require cardiac pacemakers, whereas those with second-degree block and narrow QRS complexes demonstrate only a transient block, i.e., due to an acute myocardial infarction or digitalis excess, and these patients are rarely symptomatic and seldom require permanent cardiac pacemakers.

Finally, the importance of the nature of A-V conduction is brought into sharp focus when one attempts to understand the precise localization of the pharmacologic action of antiarrhythmic and cardiotonic agents. Digitalis, acetylcholine, and low potassium concentration appear to slow intranodal conduction, while procainamide, quinidine, propranolol, potassium salts, and lidocaine slow conduction above the A-V node and in the subjunctional region. The great success of controlling the ventricular rate in the presence of atrial fibrillation and flutter by the combined use of digitalis and propranolol has matured from these concepts and probably represents the most significant use of propranolol as an antiarrhythmic agent. Hence, modern consideration of the varieties of A-V block is predicated on the precise identification of the site of conduction delay, since prognosis and therapy must follow on this basis.

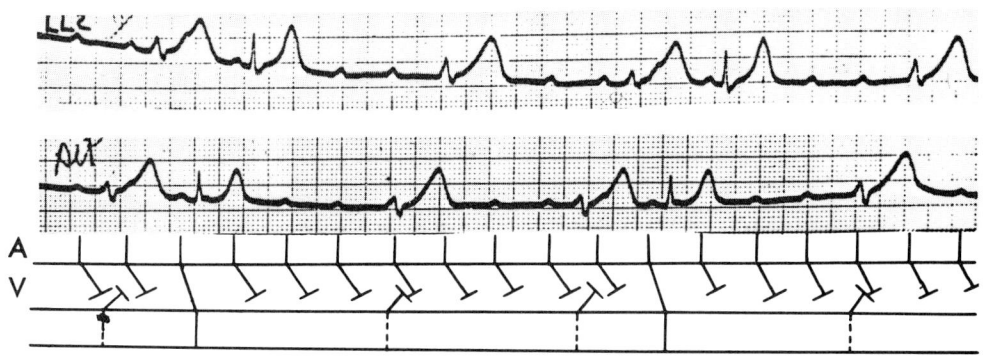

Figure 13–8 So-called supernormal conduction. As seen in the ladder diagram, forward conduction occurs only after 0.58 second of attempted retrograde conduction from the ventricular pacemaker. All other atrial beats are blocked.

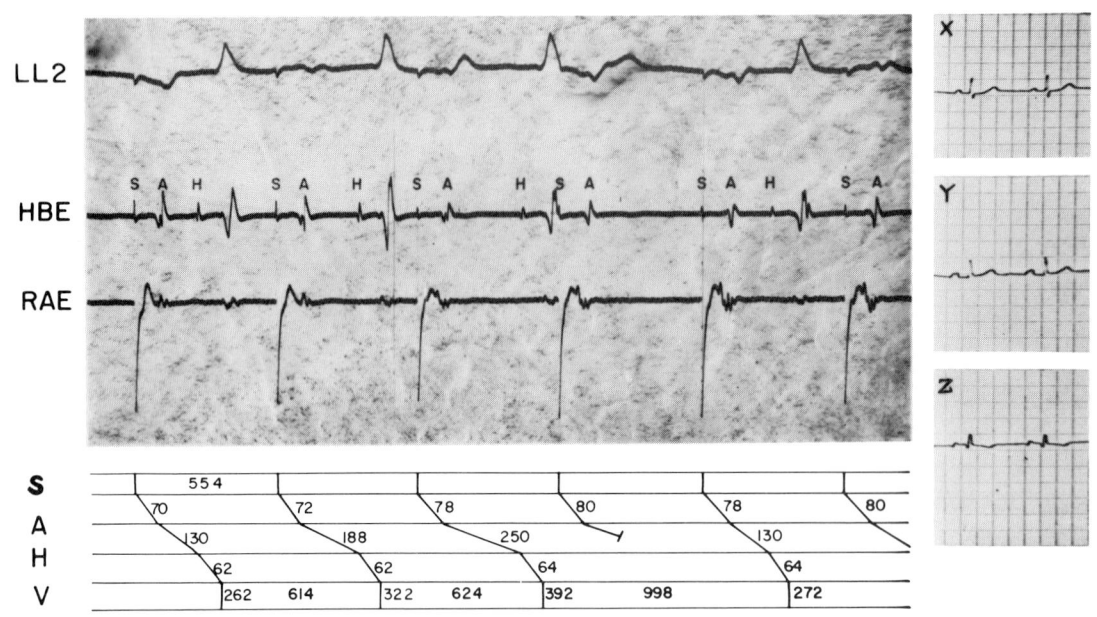

Figure 13-9 Second-degree block (Type I). The A-H interval increases from 130 msec. to 250 msec. before conduction fails above His bundle. The QRS complex is narrow, and block is within the A-V node. *A-H*, atrial-His bundle interval; *H-V*, His bundle-ventricular interval; *HBE*, His bundle electrogram; *H*, His spike. (Reproduced with permission from Dreifus, L. S., Watanabe, Y., Haiat, R., and Kimbiris, D.: Amer. J. Cardiol., *28*:371, 1971.)

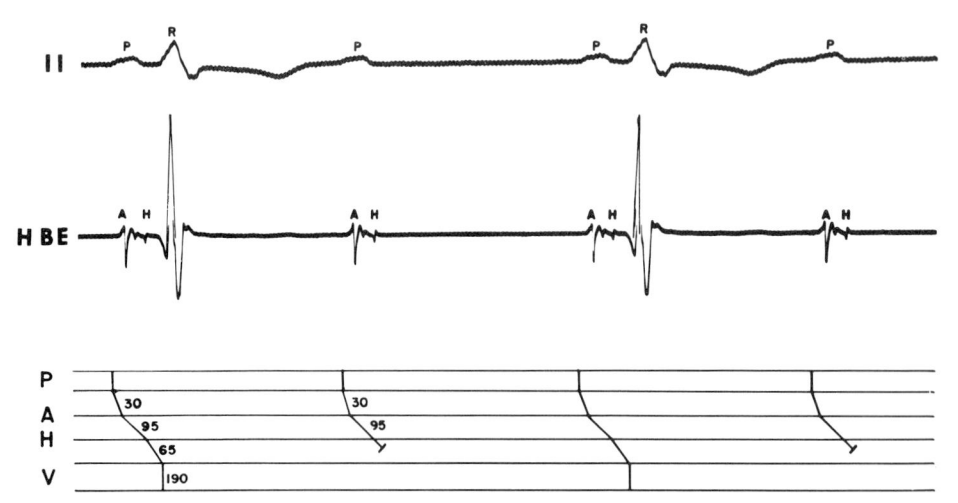

Figure 13-10 Second-degree block (Type II). Both A-H and H-V times are prolonged in the conducted beats. Block occurs below His bundle, most likely in the fascicles of the bundle branches. QRS is wide. Localization of the precise region of conduction failure can not be made by His bundle recordings. (Reproduced with permission from Dreifus, L. S., Watanabe, Y., Haiat, R., and Kimbiris, D.: Amer. J. Cardiol., *28*:371, 1971.)

UNIDIRECTIONAL BLOCK AND RE-ENTRY

This type of conduction disturbance can be divided into two categories which have different clinical implications. The first, unidirectional block and re-entry within the A-V junction, is responsible for the production of reciprocal beating and other arrhythmias. The second, local block and microre-entry, may play an important role in the genesis of coupled premature systoles, ectopic tachycardias, and atrial or ventricular fibrillation.

The mechanism of reciprocal rhythm has been explained either by functional longitudinal dissociation in some portions of the A-V conducting system or by possible dual pathways. Anatomically, the A-V node shows a complex network in which the length and diameter of the fibers are quite variable. This suggests numerous interconnections between fibers with different conductivity. Slow conduction velocity in this tissue could then cause an irregular wave front of excitation, which is less effective in depolarizing the more distal fibers. Once such inhomogeneity of intranodal conduction reaches a certain degree, functional longitudinal dissociation may develop, with areas of unidirectional block and re-entry (Fig. 13-11). Observations by other investigators also suggest functional dissociation of the A-V junctional tissues as the cause of reciprocal beating. A possible example of repetitive reciprocation in an isolated rabbit heart is shown in Figure 13-12A. In this figure, transmembrane potentials from an N fiber (upright polarity) and a proximal NH fiber (reversed polarity) were recorded with atrial (A) and ventricular (V) electrograms. Following successful conduction of two atrial impulses to the ventricles with a normal sequence of nodal activation, a premature action potential appears in the NH fiber. This is followed by rapid succession of N and NH action potentials, with corresponding atrial and ventricular excitation. Although the configuration of N potentials may first suggest an increased automaticity in this area, the presence of an NH action potential heralding a series of repetitive firing makes re-entry movement a more likely mechanism. A similar but shorter sequence of events is again seen toward the end of this record. Figure 13-12B illustrates a possible clinical counterpart of such rhythm disturbances. The conducted sinus beats show a slight prolongation of the P-R interval, while the QRS complexes suggest a minor conduction delay in the left bundle branch system. Following the second QRS of sinus origin, a premature P wave appears on the downstroke of the T wave, initiating a series of seven ventricular complexes at the rate of 175 beats per min. P waves are identified between these QRS complexes, with almost fixed time relationships with the latter. Thus, this electrocardiogram most likely represents an example of reciprocal tachycardia. Many cases of so-called supraventricular tachycardia are now considered to result from a similar mechanism.

In contrast to functional longitudinal dissociation as discussed above, local block with microre-entry may be diagrammatically illustrated as in Figure 13-13. The term microre-entry implies a small geometric arrangement of the re-entry pathway. When an impulse spreads from point A, excitation proceeds normally in pathway AB, while propagation becomes slower and may finally be blocked in the depressed tissue X. The excitation front invading X from the opposite direction (C) may, however, be successful in traversing this depressed area and re-excite the

Figure 13-11 *a*, pathway of re-excitation in the presence of sinus beats. The numbers below individual fiber sites represent the time of activation with reference to the atrial electrogram. The figures in parentheses show the time of the second action potential peak caused by re-excitation. Tapering of arrows indicates decremental conduction. The At-V interval is 117 msec., as shown at the bottom of the map. *b*, Diagrammatic representation of re-excitation in fibers located in the right side of the A-V node. Open circle at SA shows estimated time of S-A nodal discharge. Dotted line between fiber A5 and the turning point indicates conduction block. (Reproduced with permission from Watanabe, Y., and Dreifus, L. S.: Amer. Heart J., *70*:505, 1965. Copyright 1965, American Medical Association.)

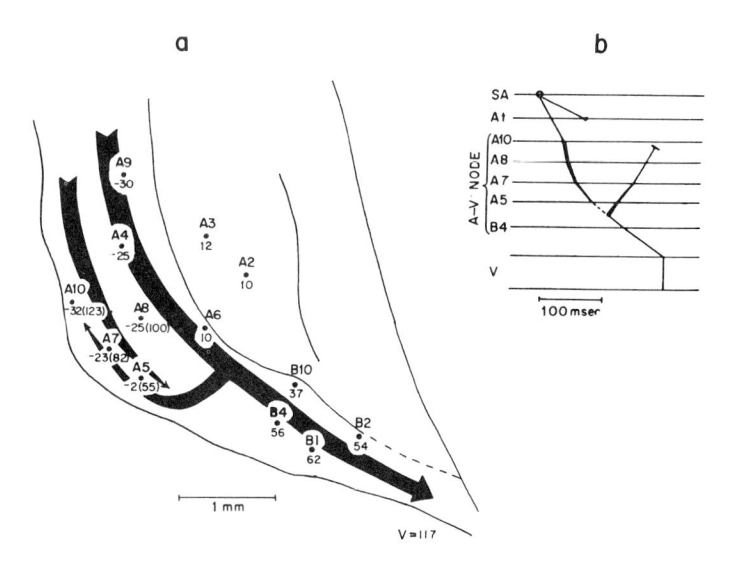

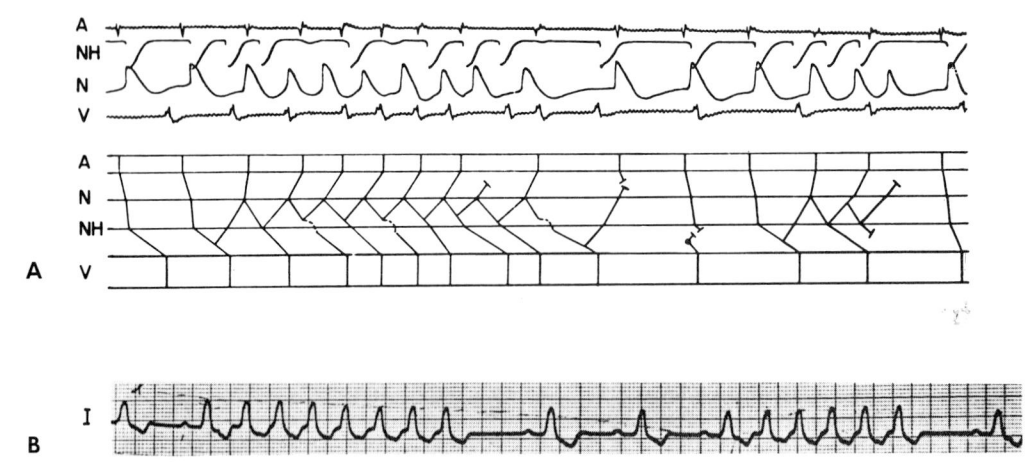

Figure 13-12 *A,* An experimental record showing possible repetitive re-entry within the A-V junction causing tachycardia in an isolated rabbit heart. Transmembrane potentials from an N (true nodal) and an NH fiber are shown with atrial and ventricular electrograms. Action potentials of the NH fiber are recorded with reversed polarity. The ladder diagram indicates possible sequence of excitation. Note that this particular NH fiber does not always participate in forward transmission of impulses. See text for further discussion. *B,* Possible clinical counterpart of the experimental record. The first premature P wave heralding the period of tachycardia may be an atrial premature systole arising in the atrial tissue, although it may already have resulted from the reciprocal movement within the A-V junction. (Reproduced with permission from Watanabe, Y.: Wiederbeleb. Organersatz u. Intensivmed. [in press].)

originally depolarized fibers in pathway AB. Re-entry circuit is thus formed. The mechanism which prevents forward transmission of an impulse but permits subsequent retrograde conduction through the region X is most likely dissimilar degrees of decrement depending on the direction of transmission (unidirectional block). A longer duration of refractoriness in this region, although less likely, may not be ruled out as an alternative mechanism.

Within the ventricular tissues, such an anatomic arrangement of fibers can actually be found between peripheral branches of the Purkinje system and the ventricular myocardium. Two explanations have been offered for the genesis of unidirectional block in the Purkinje-ventricular junction: (1) The supply of one terminal branch of Purkinje system to a greater number of ventricular fibers may result in summation or convergence of impulses when excitation spreads from ventricular to Purkinje fibers, while the opposite will hold in Purkinje-ventricular transmission. (2) Certain factors (e.g., cardiac glycosides) could decrease the resting potential and depress conduction in Purkinje fibers before any significant alterations of the ventricular action potentials are produced. Hence, some Purkinje fibers may fail to participate in ventricular excitation when the ventricular fibers still show normal excitability and conductivity. Recent observations further suggest that unidirectional block and re-entry may develop within the Purkinje system alone, when a branch of Purkinje fibers is selectively depressed.

In these models of re-entry at any portions of the myocardium, re-excitation of some fibers may cause either a single premature systole or repetitive extrasystoles leading to ectopic tachycardia. This mechanism has classically been invoked in

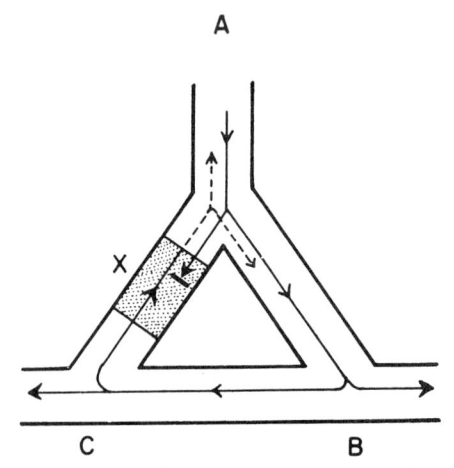

Figure 13-13 Schematic representation of re-entry movement involving anatomically separate pathways. See discussion in text. (Reproduced with permission from Watanabe, Y., and Dreifus, L. S.: Amer. Heart J., 76:114, 1968.)

explaining those premature systoles "coupled" to an initiating beat, although its direct demonstration in clinical arrhythmias is almost prohibitively difficult. There is indirect evidence that re-excitation of the ventricular tissues does not occur until most Purkinje fibers are sufficiently repolarized. Hence, the Purkinje system may be a necessary component in the re-entry circuit in a majority of cases. However, it must be re-emphasized that the mechanism of coupled extrasystoles requires further extensive studies.

COMBINED DISTURBANCES OF IMPULSE FORMATION AND CONDUCTION

Certain cardiac arrhythmias result from combined disturbances of impulse formation and conduction in a localized region of the myocardium. Ectopic rhythms with exit block and parasystole are two such examples.

Clinically, exit block from an ectopic pacemaker is most commonly observed in the presence of accelerated A-V nodal rhythms, although occasional examples of atrial or ventricular tachycardia with exit block have been reported. Our previous studies demonstrated exit block from a pacemaker located in a specific region of the A-V junction. In those instances, the cause of block could be attributed to a small action potential amplitude with a slow rate of phase 0 depolarization, a mechanism favoring decremental conduction.

Regarding the electrophysiologic mechanisms of parasystole, two theories have been proposed. The first theory postulates a high inherent frequency of discharge (often 300 beats per min. or higher) at the site of impulse formation, which keeps the pacemaker refractory to the invading impulses of the dominant rhythm. According to this concept, certain degrees of exit block must be present in cases of parasystole with slower rate. Then, the distinction between parasystole and ectopic tachycardia with exit block would be difficult, although the basic mechanisms of these two rhythm disturbances may well be similar.

The second theory invokes so-called protection (or entrance) block surrounding an ectopic pacemaker, which must have the characteristics of unidirectional block. It has been suggested that increased automaticity in a group of specialized fibers may create an ectopic pacemaker but, at the same time, may make propagation of impulses through this region difficult, since the membrane potential is significantly reduced owing to diastolic depolarization. The mechanism of parasystole could thus be explained on one basis. Perhaps in keeping with this concept is the observation that, in cases with intraventricular conduction delay, the parasystolic beats appeared to originate from the region of blocked bundle or fascicle. One such example is shown in Figure 13–14.

In this electrocardiogram, the presence of ventricular parasystole is easily established by (1) wide variation of the coupling intervals with examples of ventricular fusion, and (2) simple mathematical relationship between the interectopic intervals. The sinus beats show left bundle branch system block, with a QRS duration of 0.12 second. In contrast, the parasystolic beats have a configuration compatible with right bundle branch block plus left posterior division block. Hence, the site of parasystolic impulse formation appears to be within (or close to) the left bundle branch system where conduction delay is present. Fusion of the sinus and the ectopic impulses thus results in a narrower QRS complex (e.g., beat 8 in lead III and beat 4 in lead V_1). The relationship between the shortest coupling intervals at which propagation occurred and the Q-aU intervals in similar cases also suggested proximity of the parasystolic pacemaker to the site of conduction block. Therefore, at least in these instances, the theory of protection block may better explain the mechanisms of parasystole, although a parasystolic focus with rapid impulse formation is by no means ruled out.

FIBRILLATION

It is readily understood that fibrillation may not represent an isolated electrophysiologic entity, but may result from combinations of various mechanisms discussed above. It also appears reasonable that the mechanisms which initiate the fibrillatory state and those sustaining this arrhythmia are not necessarily identical. Regarding the initiating mechanisms, several classic theories have been developed: (1) unifocal impulse formation; (2) multifocal impulse formation; and (3) re-entry. Combination of (1) or (2) and (3) is also possible.

The theory of unifocal impulse formation invokes a rapid firing of a pacemaker from a single ectopic focus. Observation of an extreme tachysystole (up to 3000 beats per min.) at the site of electrical stimulation during the onset of atrial fibrillation may support such a concept. It has been argued that, with a high frequency of stimulation, some fibers fail to respond to every impulse and islands of refractory tissue cause an irregular spread of excitation. Indeed, this mode of initiation is quite possible. However, once irregular spread of excitation is invoked, it automatically implies local conduction disturbances, and the probability of microre-entry is inescapable. On the other hand, multifocal impulse formation would easily account for the fractionation of excitation, since different portions of the myocardium

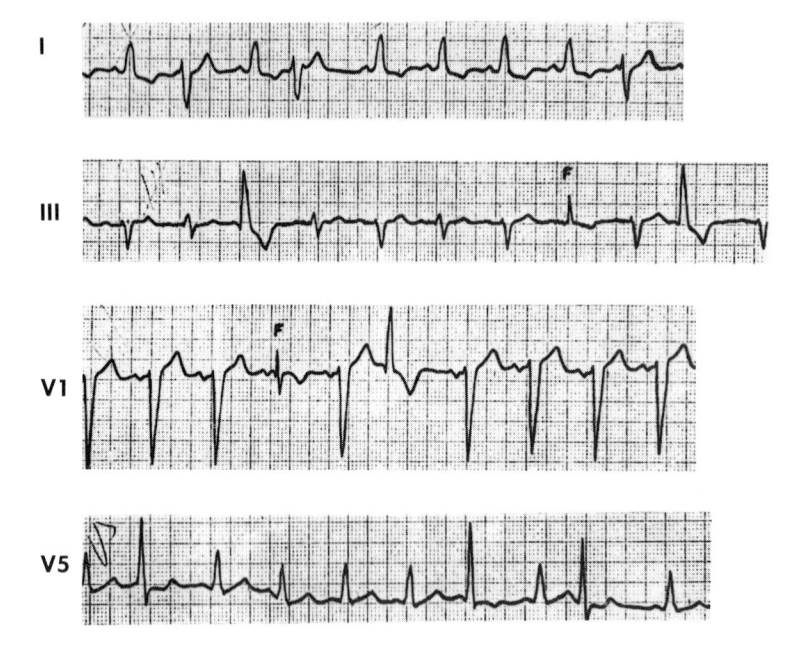

Figure 13-14 An example of ventricular parasystole in the presence of intraventricular conduction disturbances. The sinus beats show a left bundle branch block configuration, while the parasystolic beats have a contour compatible with right bundle branch block and possibly left posterior division block. (Reproduced with permission from Watanabe, Y.: Amer. Heart J., *81*:451, 1971.)

may respond to numerous, independently formed impulses from those foci. An objection to this theory, however, is based on both a rapid onset of fibrillation by a single, early extrasystole and an abrupt, spontaneous termination of fibrillation seen in some instances. Simultaneous development or cessation of all impulse formation in numerous foci is unlikely. From these considerations, the third theory invoking local conduction disturbances with possible microre-entry, or combination of this mechanism with disturbances of impulse formation, appears to give the most plausible explanation, at least for the maintenance and probably also for the initiation of fibrillatory movements.

In both clinical and experimental fibrillation, two modes of initiation have been identified. The first (type A) is characterized by rapid onset of fibrillation with one or two premature systoles early in the repolarization phase of a previous excitation, while type B shows a gradual development of disorganized excitation after a sustained period of tachycardia (Fig. 13-15). In type A, a very early premature systole falling in the vulnerable period produces varying degrees of incomplete depolarization in different fibers, possibly owing to variations of the duration of refractoriness. Local conduction block is thus prevalent, and slow, irregular spread of excitation with multiple regions of microre-entry causes asynchrony between fibers. A clinical example of type A is shown at the top of Figure 13-15. Fibrillation may be initiated by a ventricular premature systole with a long coupling interval, or even by an idioventricular escape beat. However, these initiating beats are usually followed by one or more subsequent beats with progressively shorter coupling intervals. These beats in turn produce a similar sequence of electrophysiologic events, as in the typical example of type A.

On the other hand, gradual transition from tachycardia to fibrillation in type B is usually preceded by (1) the development of prominent electrical alternation of some fibers, accompanied by further decrease in the rate of depolarization in the majority of fibers; and (2) fluctuation of the relative timing of depolarization in individual fibers (Fig. 13-15). The first observation suggests the development of local block, and the second implies variation in the spread of excitation from beat to beat. Here again, numerous areas of microre-entry may readily be expected. Nevertheless, it is of no importance whether ventricular inhomogeneity is manifested by early premature systoles or by gradual deterioration of the electrophysiologic events following sustained tachycardia. Variation in the action potential duration with the development of local block and irregular spread of excitation appeared always to herald the onset of fibrillation.

In addition to these observations during the onset of fibrillation, studies on the mode of termination of fibrillation may also provide some information on the mechanisms of this arrhythmia. The record shown in Figure 13-16 was obtained in an isolated, perfused rabbit heart during spontaneous termination of ventricular fibrillation. Transmembrane potentials from two ventricular fibers (1 and 2) were recorded together with a ventricular electrogram (EG). Irregular and

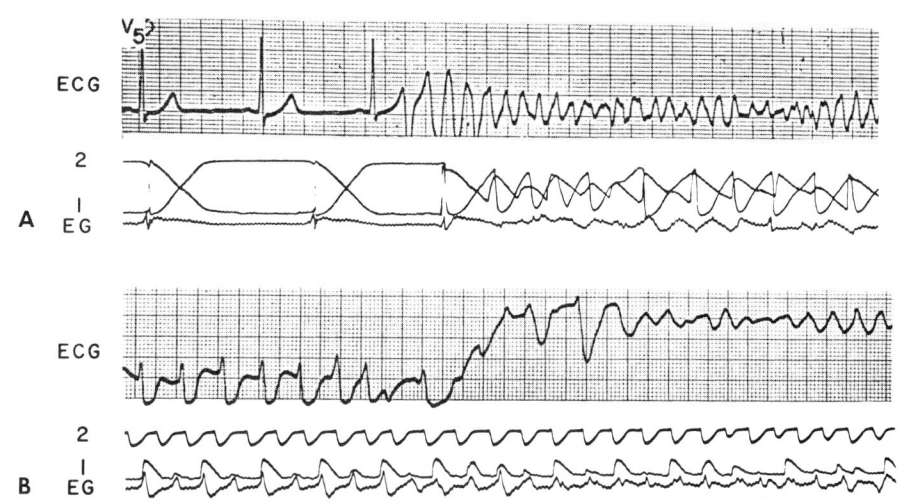

Figure 13-15 *A*, Type A of the initiation of ventricular fibrillation. A ventricular premature systole with a short coupling interval causes rapid disorganization of excitation in both clinical electrocardiogram (top) and experimental record (bottom). In the latter, upright *(1)* and inverted *(2)* action potentials of two adjacent ventricular fibers are shown together with a ventricular electrogram *(EG)*. *B*, Type B of the onset of fibrillation. Sustained period of ventricular tachycardia is followed by a gradual transition into fibrillation in clinical and experimental records. (Reproduced with permission from Watanabe, Y., and Dreifus, L. S.: Amer. Heart J., 76:114, 1968.)

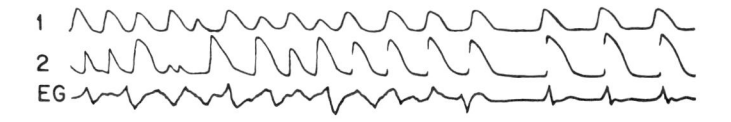

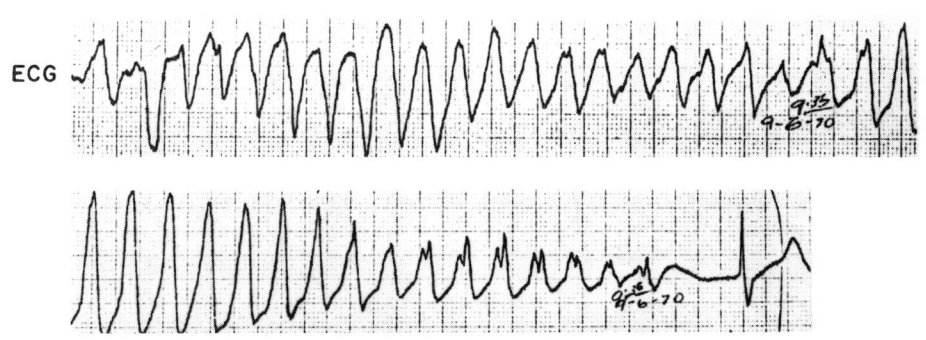

Figure 13-16 *A*, Spontaneous termination of ventricular fibrillation in an isolated, perfused rabbit heart. Transmembrane potentials from two ventricular fibers and a ventricular electrogram are shown. *B*, A clinical electrocardiogram showing similar spontaneous termination of ventricular fibrillation in a hypokalemic patient. (Courtesy of R. Summer, M.D.) (Reproduced with permission from Watanabe, Y.: Wiederbeleb. Organersatz u. Intensivmed. [in press].)

asynchronous depolarization of these two fibers (several millimeters apart), with variation in the amplitude and duration of the action potentials, is characteristic of fibrillation (toward the left). In the middle of the record, several action potentials appear which are relatively regular in timing and configuration and show a higher rate of phase 0 depolarization as well as smaller time difference between fibers 1 and 2. The last one of these action potentials is associated with a slightly more discrete ventricular deflection and is followed by a pause with isoelectric baseline in the electrogram. An apparently supraventricular mechanism is then re-established (toward the right). Such sequence of events prior to the termination of fibrillatory movements may suggest gradual reorganization of the ventricular excitation fronts with increased synchronization of cellular depolarization, possibly owing to a gradual decrease in the number of micro-re-entry circuits. Finally, when all re-entry pathways are abolished, a more uniform recovery of the ventricular tissue will enable the supraventricular impulses to resume the control of ventricular excitation. It may also be argued that similar examples of ventricular fibrillation which show spontaneous reversion to a regular rhythm (Fig. 13–16B) may have a lesser degree of disorganization of excitation than the common variety requiring electric defibrillation.

Slow ventricular tachycardia or idioventricular tachycardia has been usually considered a benign dysrhythmia. However, the appearance of these slow ventricular mechanisms in the presence of a long Q-Tc interval may define a potentially dangerous combination of events. As seen in Figure 13–17, a repetitive ventricular mechanism results from a ventricular premature systole which interrupts the T wave. Usual antiarrhythmic agents such as procainamide or quinidine may further prolong the Q-Tc interval and aggravate this mechanism. As shown in the last strip, cardiac pacing will inhibit the ectopic ventricular focus until ischemia regresses and the Q-Tc interval shortens.

However, the above experimental and clinical observations (Fig. 13–16A and B) are not incompatible with the theory of unifocal impulse formation, as long as its association with re-entry movements is postulated. Indeed, relatively regular undulations seen in Figure 13–16B may suggest such combination of mechanism. Furthermore, during our studies on antifibrillatory action of antiarrhythmic agents, it has oc-

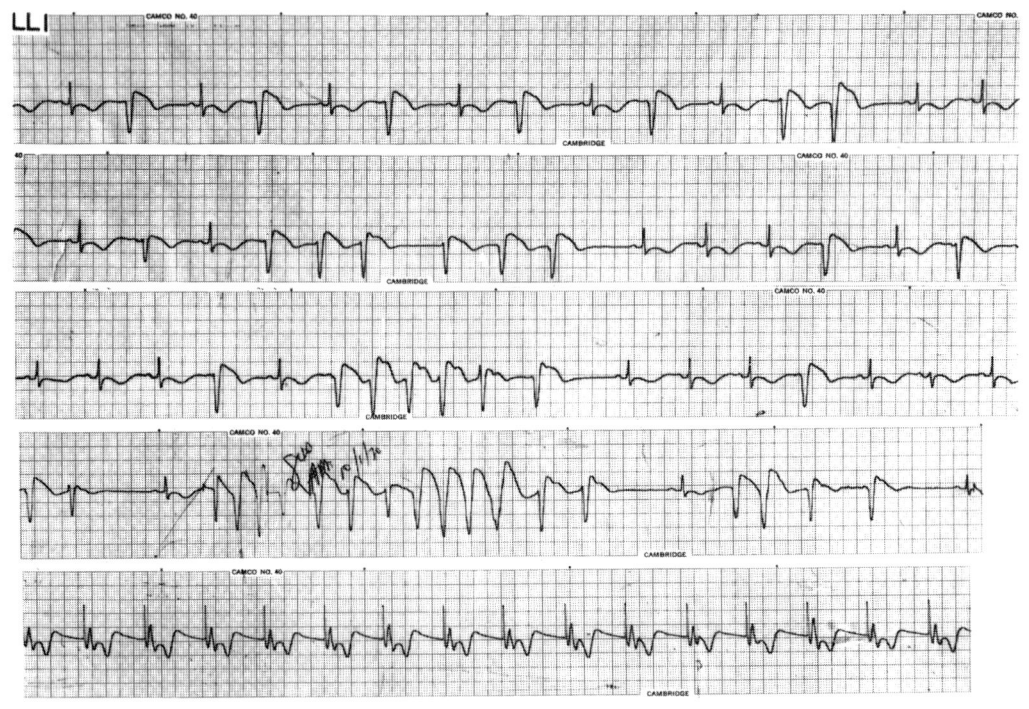

Figure 13–17 "Slow" ventricular tachycardia. In the upper three strips of lead I, groups of ventricular premature systoles suggest a slow ventricular tachycardia. In the fourth strip, the ventricular rate is more rapid after the first ventricular ectopic beat bisects the T wave. Ventricular arrhythmias associated with prolonged Q-Tc intervals do not usually respond to usual antiarrhythmic therapy. Last strip, arrhythmia controlled by ventricular overdrive by a transvenous pacemaker.

casionally been observed that an established ventricular fibrillation may change into what appears to be ventricular tachycardia, which either reverts to normal sinus rhythm or is sustained without resulting in defibrillation. Thus, the possible role of ectopic impulse formation cannot be ruled out as a mechanism of initiating fibrillation, although microre-entry still appears a more likely mechanism for its maintenance.

In conclusion, current concepts on the genesis of cardiac arrhythmias have been reviewed in terms of cellular electrophysiology. Of the various disturbances of impulse formation and conduction, the following five mechanisms were discussed: (1) automaticity, (2) simple conduction block, (3) unidirectional block and re-entry, (4) combined disturbances of impulse formation and conduction, and (5) fibrillation. Appropriate clinical examples were presented to illustrate possible manifestations of these mechanisms, and certain supporting evidence was sought in electrocardiographic observations. Although significant progress has been made in recent years in our understanding of the genesis of arrhythmias, many problems still await extensive studies, both clinically and experimentally.

REFERENCES

Coraboeuf, E., DeLoze, C., and Boistel, J.: Action de la digitale sur les potentiels de membrane et d'action du tissu conducteur du coeur de chien étudiée à l'aide de microélectrodes intracellulaires. C. R. Soc. Biol., *147*:1169, 1953.

Cranefield, P. F., Hoffman, B. F., and Paes de Carvalho, A.: Effects of acetylcholine on single fibers of A-V node. Circ. Res., *7*:19, 1959.

Cranefield, P. F., Klein, H. O., and Hoffman, B. F.: Conduction of the cardiac impulse. I. Delay, block, and one-way block in depressed Purkinje fibers. Circ. Res., *28*:199, 1971.

Cranefield, P. F., Klein, H. O., and Hoffman, B. F.: Conduction of the cardiac impulse. I. Delay, block, and one-way block in depressed Purkinje fibers. Circ. Res., *28*:199, 1971.

Dreifus, L. S., and Watanabe, Y.: Localization and significance of atrioventricular block. Amer. Heart J., *82*:435, 1971.

Dreifus, L. S., Watanabe, Y., Haiat, R., and Kimbiris, D.: Atrioventricular block. Amer. J. Cardiol., *28*:371, 1971.

Dudel, J., and Trautwein, W.: Elektrophysiologische Messungen zur Strophanthinwirkung am Herzmuskel. Arch. Exp. Path. Pharmakol., *232*:393, 1958.

Gettes, L. S., and Yoshonis, K. F.: Rapidly recurring supraventricular tachycardia. A manifestation of reciprocating tachycardia and an indication for propranolol therapy. Circulation, *44*:689, 1970.

Haiat, R., Dreifus, L. S., and Watanabe, Y.: Fate of A-V block: An electrocardiographic study. In Han, J. (Ed.): Symposium on Cardiac Arrhythmias. Springfield, Illinois, Charles C Thomas, Publishers, 1972.

Hellerstein, H. K., and Turrell, D. J.: Mode of death in coronary artery disease. Electrocardiographic and clinicopathological correlation. In Surawicz, B., and Pellegrino, E. D. (Eds.): Sudden Cardiac Death. New York, Grune and Stratton, 1964, p. 17.

Hogancamp, E. E., Kardesch, M., Danforth, W. H., and Bing, R. J.: Transmembrane electrical potentials in ventricular tachycardia and fibrillation. Amer. Heart J., *57*:214, 1959.

Hoffman, B. F.: Physiologic basis of disturbances of cardiac rhythm and conduction. Progr. Cardiovasc. Dis., *2*:319, 1959.

Hoffman, B. F.: The electrophysiology of heart muscle and the genesis of arrhythmias. In Dreifus, L. S., and Likoff, W. (Eds.): Mechanisms and Therapy of Cardiac Arrhythmias. New York, Grune and Stratton, 1966, p. 27.

Hoffman, B. F., and Cranefield, P. F.: Electrophysiology of the Heart. New York, McGraw-Hill Book Co., Inc., 1960.

Hoffman, B. F., and Cranefield, P. F.: The physiological basis of cardiac arrhythmias. Amer. J. Med., *37*:670, 1964.

Hoffman, B. F., Moore, E. N., Stuckey, J. H., and Cranefield, P. F.: Functional properties of the atrioventricular conduction system. Circ. Res., *13*:308, 1963.

Hoffman, B. F., Paes de Carvalho, A., DeMello, W. C., and Cranefield, P. F.: Electrical activity of single fibers of atrioventricular node. Circ. Res., *7*:11, 1959.

Hoffman, B. F., and Suckling, E. E.: Effects of several cations on transmembrane potentials of cardiac muscle. Amer. J. Physiol., *186*:317, 1956.

Janse, M. J.: Influence of the direction of the atrial wave front on A-V nodal transmission in isolated hearts of rabbits. Circ. Res., *25*:439, 1969.

Janse, M. J., Van Capelle, F. J. L., Freud, G. E., and Durrer, D.: Circus movement within the A-V node as a basis for supraventricular tachycardia as shown by multiple microelectrode recording in the isolated rabbit heart. Circ. Res., *28*:403, 1971.

Katz, L. N.: Electrocardiography. Philadelphia, Lea and Febiger, Inc., 1941, p. 729.

Katz, L. N., and Pick, A.: Clinical electrocardiography. Part 1, The arrhythmias. Philadelphia, Lea and Febiger, 1965.

Kaufman, R., and Rothberger, C. J.: Beitrag zur Kenntnis der Entstehungsweise der extrasystolischen Allorhythmien. Z. Ges. Exp. Med., *5*:349, 1917.

Kistin, A. D.: Mechanisms determining reciprocal rhythm initiated by ventricular extrasystoles. Multiple pathways of conduction. Amer. J. Cardiol., *3*:365, 1959.

Matsuda, K., Hoshi, T., and Kameyama, S.: Action of acetycholine and adrenaline upon membrane potential of atrioventricular node (Tawara). Tohoku J. Exp. Med., *68*:16, 1958.

Mendez, C., and Moe, G. K.: Demonstration of a dual A-V nodal conduction system in the isolated rabbit heart. Circ. Res., *19*:378, 1966.

Mobitz, W.: Über die unvollständige Störung der Erregungüberleitung zwischen Vorhof und Kammer des menschlichen Herzens. Z. Ges. Exp. Med., *41*:180, 1924.

Mobitz, W.: Über den partiellen Herzblock. Z. Klin. Med., *107*:449, 1928.

Moe, G. K., and Abildskov, J. A.: Atrial fibrillation as a self-sustaining arrhythmia independent of focal discharge. Amer. Heart J., *58*:59, 1959.

Moe, G. K., and Mendez, R.: The action of several cardiac glycosides on conduction velocity and ventricular excitability in the dog heart. Circulation, *4*:729, 1951.

Moe, G. K., Preston, J. B., and Burlington, H.: Physiologic evidence for dual A-V transmission system. Circ. Res., *4*:357, 1956.

Moore, E. N.: Microelectrode studies on concealment of multiple premature atrial responses. Circ. Res., *18*:660, 1966.

Moore, E. N., Morse, H. T., and Price, H. L.: Cardiac arrhythmias produced by catecholamines in anesthetized dogs. Circ. Res., *15*:77, 1964.

Myerberg, R. J., Gelband, H., and Hoffman, B. F.: Functional characteristics of the gating mechanism in the canine A-V conducting system. Circ. Res., *28*:136, 1971.

Paes de Carvalho, A.: Cellular electrophysiology of atrial specialized tissues. In Paes de Carvalho, A., DeMello, W. C., and Hoffman, B. F. (Eds.): The Specialized Tissues of the Heart. Amsterdam, Elsevier, 1962, p. 115.

Paes de Carvalho, A.: Excitation of the atrioventricular node during normal rhythm. Effects of acetycholine. *In* Dreifus, L. S., and Likoff, W. (Eds.): Mechanisms and Therapy of Cardiac Arrhythmias. New York, Grune and Stratton, 1966, p. 341.

Pamintuan, J. C., Dreifus, L. S., and Watanabe, Y.: Comparative mechanisms of antiarrhythmic agents. Amer. J. Cardiol., *26*:512, 1970.

Pick, A., Langendorf, R., and Katz, L. N.: A-V nodal tachycardia with block. Circulation, *24*:12, 1961.

Rosenbaum, M. B.: Classification of ventricular extrasystoles according to form. J. Electrocardiol., *2*:289, 1969.

Rosenbaum, M. B., Elizari, M. V., and Lazzari, J. O.: The Hemiblocks: New Concept of Intraventricular Conduction Based on Human Anatomical, Physiological and Clinical Studies. Oldsmar, Florida, Tampa Tracings, 1970.

Sano, T., Iida, Y., and Yamagishi, S.: Changes in the spread of excitation from the sinus node induced by alterations in extracellular potassium. *In* Sano, T., Mizuhira, V., and Matsuda, K. (Eds.): Electrophysiology and Ultrastructure of the Heart. Tokyo, Bunkodo, 1967, p. 127.

Sano, T., and Scher, A. M.: Multiple recording during electrically induced atrial fibrillation. Circ. Res., *14*:117, 1964.

Scherf, D.: Zur Entstehungsweise der Extrasystolen und der extrasystolischen Allorhythmien. Z. Ges. Exp. Med., *51*:816, 1926.

Scherf, D.: The mechanism of flutter and fibrillation. Amer. Heart J., *71*:273, 1966.

Scherf, D., and Bornemann, C.: Parasystole with a rapid ventricular center. Amer. Heart J., *66*:320, 1961.

Scherf, D., and Schott, A.: Extrasystoles and Allied Arrhythmias. New York, Grune and Stratton, 1953.

Scherf, D., and Shookhoff, C.: Reitzleitungsstörungen im Bündel. II. Mitteilung. Wien. Arch. Inn. Med., *11*:425, 1925.

Scherf, D., and Shookhoff, C.: Experimentelle Untersuchungen über die "Umkehr-Extrasystole." Wien Arch. Inn. Med., *12*:501, 1926.

Schmitt, F. O., and Erlanger, J.: Directional differences in the conduction of impulse through heart muscle and their possible relation to extrasystolic und fibrillatory contractions. Amer. J. Physiol., *87*:326, 1928.

Sherlag, B. J., and Lau, S. H.: Catheter techniques for recording His bundle activity in man. Circulation, *39*:13, 1969.

Singer, D. H., Lazzara, R., and Hoffman, B. F.: Interrelationships between automaticity and conduction in Purkinje fibers. Circ. Res., *21*:537, 1967.

Trautwein, W.: Generation and conduction of impulses in the heart as affected by drugs. Pharmacol. Rev., *15*:277, 1963.

Truex, R. C.: Anatomical consideration of human atrioventricular junction. *In* Dreifus, L. S., and Likoff, W. (Eds.): Mechanisms and Therapy of Cardiac Arrhythmias. New York, Grune and Stratton, 1966, p. 333.

VanDam, R. T., Moore, E. N., and Hoffman, B. F.: Initiation and conduction of impulses in partially depolarized cardiac fibers. Amer. J. Physiol., *204*:1133, 1963.

Vassalle, M., Karis, J., and Hoffman, B. F.: Toxic effects of ouabain on Purkinje fibers and ventricular muscle fibers. Amer. J. Physiol., *203*:433, 1962.

Watanabe, Y.: Atrioventricular block. Saishin Igaku, *25*:799, 1970. (In Japanese.)

Watanabe, Y.: Reassessment of parasystole. Amer. Heart J., *82*:451, 1971.

Watanabe, Y.: Coupling interval of ventricular premature systoles as related to the U waves. In preparation.

Watanabe, Y., and Dreifus, L. S.: Inhomogeneous conduction in the A-V node: A model for re-entry. Amer. Heart J., *70*:505, 1965.

Watanabe, Y., and Dreifus, L. S.: Electrophysiological effects of digitalis on A-V transmission. Amer. J. Physiol., *211*:1461, 1966.

Watanabe, Y., and Dreifus, L. S.: Mechanisms of supernormal A-V conduction. Fed. Proc., *25*:635, 1966.

Watanabe, Y., and Dreifus, L. S.: Mechanisms of ventricular fibrillation. Jap. Heart J., *7*:110, 1966.

Watanabe, Y., and Dreifus, L. S.: Interactions of quinidine and potassium on atrioventricular transmission. Circ. Res., *20*:434, 1967.

Watanabe, Y., and Dreifus, L. S.: Second-degree atrioventricular block. Cardiovasc. Res., *1*:150, 1967.

Watanabe, Y., and Dreifus, L. S.: Newer concepts in the genesis of cardiac arrhythmias. Amer. Heart J., *76*:114, 1968.

Watanabe, Y., and Dreifus, L. S.: Sites of impulse formation within the atrioventricular junction of the rabbit. Circ. Res., *22*:717, 1968.

Watanabe, Y., and Dreifus, L. S.: Effects of coronary flow on atrioventricular conduction. Fed. Proc., *29*:588(Abs.), 1970.

Watanabe, Y., and Dreifus, L. S.: Interactions of lanatoside C and potassium on atrioventricular conduction in rabbits. Circ. Res., *27*:931, 1970.

Watanabe, Y., and Dreifus, L. S.: Antifibrillatory action of antiarrhythmic agents. Fed. Proc., *30*:554(Abs.), 1971.

Watanabe, Y., and Dreifus, L. S.: Factors determining atrioventricular conduction. In preparation.

Watanabe, Y., and Dreifus, L. S.: Levels of concealment in second-degree and advanced second-degree A-V block. Amer. Heart J., *84*:330, 1972.

Watanabe, Y., Dreifus, L. S., and Likoff, W.: Electrophysiologic antagonism and synergism of potassium and antiarrhythmic agents. Amer. J. Cardiol., *12*:702, 1963.

Weidmann, S.: Elektrophysiologie der Herzmuskelfaser. Bern, Hans Hubert, 1956.

Wenckebach, K. F.: Zur Analyse des unregelmässigen Pulses. Z. Klin. Med., *37*:475, 1899.

Wenckebach, K. F., and Winterberg, H.: Die unregelmässige Herztätigkeit. Leipzig, Engelmann, 1927.

Wiggers, C. J., and Wegira, R.: Ventricular fibrillation due to a single localized induction and condenser shocks applied during the vulnerable phase of ventricular systole. Amer. J. Physiol., *128*:500, 1940.

CHAPTER 14

RENAL DISEASE: WATER AND ELECTROLYTE BALANCE

JOHN M. WELLER

The primary excretory function of the kidney is to maintain the volume and composition of body fluids constant by formation of urine of appropriately varied composition. This complex process depends on vascular and tubular receptor and effector sites that recognize and respond to neural and humoral mediators. The best characterized endocrine function is the renal-adrenal, renin-aldosterone interplay concerned with regulation of sodium output, defense of arterial pressure, and, abnormally, "renal" hypertension. A second function is renal formation of erythropoietin, which stimulates red blood cell formation. These endocrine functions assume importance in disease.

RENAL EXCRETORY FUNCTIONS

Renal Blood Flow

The blood volume of the kidneys is about 20 per cent of their weight, which is only 0.5 per cent of body weight. Perfusion with blood is large and very rapid, since it amounts to about 1 liter per minute or 20 per cent of the cardiac output. Clearly, renal blood flow exceeds metabolic need; it is directed primarily toward excretion, so that renal arteriovenous O_2 difference is small, i.e., 1.7 ml. per 100 ml. as compared with mixed venous blood at 4 to 6 ml. Most of the kidneys' 20 ml. per minute of resting O_2 consumption is spent in providing energy for reabsorption of sodium.

Blood enters the kidney through major arteries that form the interlobar and then arcuate or arciform arteries. The subterminal interlobular arteries run from these at right angles toward the cortex and give rise to afferent arterioles, each of which supplies a glomerulus, branching to form the glomerular capillary loops which segregate into five to eight lobules, then fusing to form the efferent arteriole. Outer cortical efferents rapidly divide into anastomosing peritubular capillary plexuses which lead to venules. In the juxtamedullary nephrons, small peritubular plexuses are also formed which differ from those of outer cortical nephrons in that they also give rise to long looped vessels (vasa recta) that dip down into the medulla. The tubules of many outer cortical nephrons are short; some have longer loops of Henle that reach down with these vessels into the outer medulla, and some (about one in eight in man) have very long loops that enter the inner medulla and return in association with the vasa recta.

This unique arrangement of vessels has several important concomitants. One is that the rate of renal blood flow is relatively constant over a wide range of arterial pressure (e.g., 80 to 200 mm. Hg mean). The autonomy or autoregulation of the renal circulation is at least partly myogenic, i.e., afferent vessels constrict during a rise and dilate during a fall in arterial pressure. Autoregulation is primarily a cortical function, whereas medullary flow is relatively small (cortex ca. 4.7, outer medulla 1.3, inner medulla 0.17 ml. per gm. per minute) and passive. Some degree of plasma skimming occurs, since medullary blood is cell poor. The vasa recta also seem relatively protein permeable, since medullary interstitial fluid is albumin rich.

The juxtaglomerular apparatus (JGA) is composed of juxtaglomerular cells derived from the afferent glomerular arteriole and macula densa cells from the early distal tubule. The juxtaglomerular cells arise by differentiation of the media of afferent arterioles, just before they enter the glomerulus, into a mass of swollen, afibrillar and granular "myoepithelioid" cells that form pillows (polkissen) at the glomerular pole. They also have been known as "Goormaghtigh bodies," since he first postulated their endocrine function. These may be pressure-sensing sites of renin secretion. They also respond to changes in sodium balance by changes in granule content (renin?). Serum sodium concentration physiologically varies over a narrow range and it is unlikely that the polkissen can sense these small changes. Closely applied to the juxtaglomerular cells is a differentiated set of distal convoluted tubule cells, the macula densa, which is in a position to sense changes in sodium composition of distal tubular fluid. The two areas form the juxtaglomerular apparatus, which may be a mechanism of self-regulation of arterial pressure, extracellular fluid volume, and sodium output that operates through secretion of renin and changes in secretion rate of aldosterone.

Glomerular Filtration

The liter of blood that perfuses the kidneys each minute contains about 600 ml. of plasma. More than 90 per cent of this perfuses glomeruli and peritubular structures and contributes to excretory functions. As indicated, some deep glomeruli may be relatively plasma rich and some peripheral glomeruli plasma poor, with proportionate differences in rates of ultrafiltration. Inequalities among nephrons occur in other respects, and function tests show diversities in the normal nephron population. It is therefore an oversimplification to consider renal function as merely an average of the sum of identical activities of 1.5 million glomeruli of each kidney. With this reservation, it is a useful visualization didactically. Thus, since the overall percentage of plasma water filtered off is 20 per cent, or about 120 ml. per minute, this represents an average glomerular filtration rate.

The relationship between glomerular function and structure was first described by Bowman more than a century ago: "It would indeed be difficult to conceive a disposition of parts more calculated to favor the escape of water from the body, than that of the malpighian body. A large artery (the interlobular) breaks up in a very direct manner into a number of small branches (afferent arterioles) each of which suddenly opens into an assemblage of vessels (the glomerular capillaries) of far greater aggregate capacity than itself, and from which there is but one narrow exit (the efferent arterioles)."

The complexity of glomerular structure is shown by electron microscopy (Fig. 14–1). The glomerulus normally contains only two types of cells, endothelial and epithelial, which establish three ultramicroscopic layers of capillary wall. The inner layer, formed by nuclei and spreading cytoplasm of endothelial cells, is a membrane which seems to be coarsely fenestrated with pores that retain cells but not plasma. This, the *lamina fenestrata*, is closely applied to a continuous,

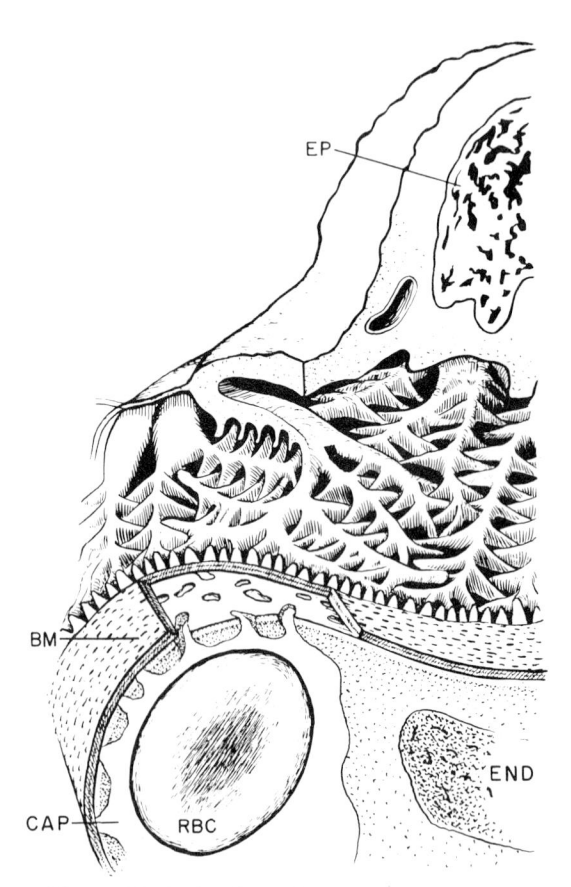

Figure 14–1 A schematic view, based on electron microscopy, of a portion of a glomerulus. In the upper right is the nucleus of an epithelial cell *(EP)*, or podocyte. The foot processes of this cell and its neighbor extend out, like tentacles of an octopus, with their feet, the pedicles, resting tightly upon the basement membrane *(BM)*. The basement membrane is shown cut away, revealing the fenestrated cytoplasmic investment of the endothelial cell *(END)*, which is closely applied to the basement membrane and lines the lumen of the glomerular capillary *(CAP)*, which contains a red blood cell *(RBC)*.

structureless layer of mucoprotein which is the ultimate filtering membrane and represents a specialized and unusually retentive capillary basement membrane. Applied to the outer face of this are epithelial cells. These are large cells arranged like interdigitating octopuses. Their cytoplasmic arms carry ribbed or footlike processes called *pedicles*, which give the cells their name of *podocytes* (foot-bearing cells). The slits between the points of contact of these feet are about 80 Å wide, so that they would retain most hemoglobin molecules. They communicate with each other under the podocytes' arms, or *trabeculae*, forming spaces that are ultimately continuous with the glomerular space. There is therefore no true intercapillary space and what the light microscope indicates as basement membrane is a complex composed principally of lamina densa and pedicles. A cluster of mesangial cells at the root of the lobule seems not to enter into filtration.

The rate of glomerular filtration tends, as a rule, to be more constant than renal blood flow. Falls or rises in renal blood (or plasma) flow are apparently associated with reciprocal changes in transglomerular resistance which depend on relationships between afferent and efferent arteriolar constriction. Thus, renal hyperemia consequent to a pyrogenic reaction may double renal blood flow; however, filtration rate may be unchanged or even decreased, apparently because efferent arteriolar vasodilation has reduced glomerular filtration pressure, so that the plasma fraction filtered diminishes from about 20 to 10 per cent. Contrariwise, a decrease in renal blood flow, such as occurs in congestive heart failure, is associated with an increased filtered or "filtration" fraction consequent to increased intraglomerular pressure. This pressure is normally very high, some 65 mm. Hg, as compared to that in capillaries elsewhere in the body. Apparently glomerular capillaries are able to sustain this and also to maintain a very high relative degree of protein impermeability by reason of their supporting lamina densa and its enveloping podocytes. Net or effective filtration pressure is normally about 40 mm. Hg (hydrostatic minus plasma colloid osmotic pressure of some 25 mm. Hg). Variables other than hydrostatic and colloid osmotic pressure that may affect filtration are renal intratubular and intrapelvic pressures, interstitial pressure, and, to a small degree, venous pressure. The last, at least in arcuate veins of the dog, is as high as 20 mm. Hg. Diseases such as glomerulonephritis that affect the filtering membrane impair both filtration and protein impermeability.

Proximal Tubule

Even the most primitive kidneys have proximal tubules. Their structure under the electron microscope is nearly as surprising as that of the glomerulus. The light microscopist's brush border is seen as bundles of microvilli that lead into little intracellular pools formed by invaginations of cell membrane that are notably rich in alkaline phosphatase, with most of the energy enzyme-rich mitochondria packed into the bases of the cells. It is evident that the microvilli enormously increase the absorbing surface. The size and chemistry of the mitochondria accord with the relatively high metabolic activity of the cells, while their basal infoldings must facilitate transfer of substances into or out of the capillary blood. Many of these transfers involve "active transport," a term that implies movement of a substance against a concentration or electrochemical gradient. This transport may be either reabsorptive, from lumen to capillary, or excretory, from capillary to lumen. In both cases, energy sources of active transport systems involve resynthesis of ATP, and materials that stimulate this (e.g., thyroxine) enhance and those that interfere (e.g., dinitrophenol) suppress these transport systems. Compounds subject to active transport apparently pass through cells in some conjugated form, so that agents that interfere with specific conjugases (e.g., Benemid, in the case of uric acid reabsorption and of secretion of substances such as para-aminohippuric acid, or PAH) also suppress transport. The processes are visualized in terms of (1) entry of the compound X into the tubule cell from lumen (reabsorption) or interstitial fluid (secretion); (2) coupling or conjugation with transfer substance Y, of which there may be more than one compound or one step; (3) movement through the cytoplasm; and (4) decomposition of compound XY, with regeneration of Y, which then moves to cycle in transport; with (5) discharge of free X into tubular or capillary fluid. Saturation of the medium with compound X and determination of the maximum rate of transport thereof is a measure of the amount of available Y (or of coenzymes) and is therefore an index of mass of tubular cells (Tm).

A substance may be completely or incompletely reabsorbed or secreted. Glucose is normally completely absorbed. Phosphate, some amino acids, sulfate, uric and ascorbic acids are not. Some of the seeming vagaries of potassium, phosphate, and urate excretion are attributable to three-phase (filtration, reabsorption, and secretion) systems. These reabsorptions are sometimes associated. For example, saturation of glucose transport impairs phosphate reabsorption. Others, such as those of different groups of amino acids, are quite distinct in their energy sources and limits. Application of the concept of Tm to problems of glycosuria is shown in Figure 14–2. However, it should be noted that, while some renal glycosurics show low overall glucose Tm's, others do not and are apparently glycosuric be-

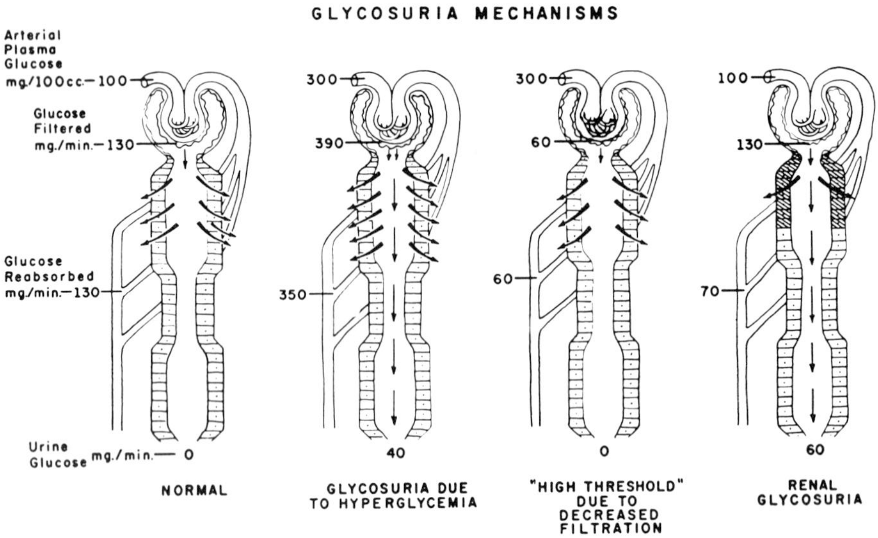

Figure 14–2 Glycosuria. Mechanisms of normal glucose retention (normoglycemia, total reabsorption indicated by arrows, and no glycosuria); of glycosuria due to hyperglycemia (increased arterial glucose, fully loaded reabsorptive mechanism, excess excreted, i.e., indicated as 350 mg. per minute [390 mg. filtered, −40 mg. excreted]); of a "high renal threshold" due to decreased functioning glomerular surface, as in glomerulosclerosis, with filtration rate reduced to 20 mg. per minute, so that glucose load filtered from plasma of 300 mg. per 100 ml. is 300/100×20=60 mg. per minute; and, lastly, of typical familial renal glycosuria with deficient proximal tubular system for glucose reabsorption, so that Tm=70 mg. per minute.

cause of inequalities in glucose reabsorptive capacities of individuals nephrons. The Fanconi syndrome and its variants, as well as the renal injury that occurs in Wilson's disease (poisoning of proximal tubules by copper), are defects of proximal tubular function manifested as phosphaturia, aminoaciduria, uricosuria, and glycosuria.

Secretory systems of the proximal tubule account for excretion of a variety of organic acids, many of them derivatives of hippuric acid. The same transport system carries penicillin, Diodrast, acetylated sulfonamides, and phenosulfonphthalein (PSP). A distinct system transports certain organic bases, notably N-1-methylnicotinamide. As with tubular reabsorption, maximum rates of tubular secretion (Tm's) can be measured by saturating the transport system with a substance X, typically PAH, and measuring this function as total amount in urine less amount filtered per unit time.

Some of the droplets and granules that appear in proximal tubules under the electron microscope represent macromolecular substances in the course of transport or cellular digestion. This process is quite distinct from micromolecular reabsorption. The mass capacity of these systems is very small and a sufficient overload results in retention of aggregates of the compound (e.g., protein) or its product (e.g., in the case of a lipoprotein, lipid). The phenomenon is of most significance in relation to proteinuria (Fig. 14–3).

Retentive as it is, some serum protein, principally albumin, escapes through the glomerular filter and is taken up in this manner from tubule fluid, so that urine is normally protein free, or nearly so. Sufficient tubular injury may paralyze this system and establish proteinuria of tubular origin. However, most proteinurias probably originate in transglomerular leak of protein into tubular fluid as a result of functional or structural damage that disorganizes podocyte function and/or structure of the lamina densa. One sequel to such proteinuria is the appearance of lipid droplets in tubule cells. This may give the kidney the appearance of being fatty and was formerly interpreted as a "degenerative" change. Actually, fatty tubules occur normally in some species, such as cats, and, in the case of most proteinurias, they are more indicative of cellular surfeit than of damage.

Loop of Henle

Animals that have to retain water according to need have a hairpin loop of tubule leading back to the distal convolution. This loop structure was once thought to have some association with water conservation. Since it could not be assumed that antidiuretic hormone (ADH) could act here, the significance of its morphology was not appreciated. Most (80 to 85 per cent) salt and water is reabsorbed in the proximal tubule iso-osmotically

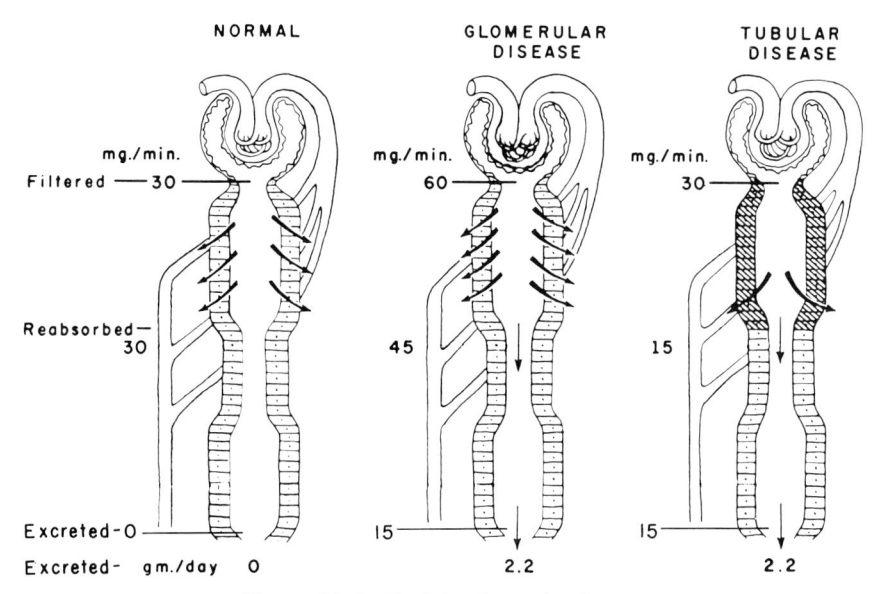

Figure 14-3 Proteinuria mechanisms.

and by "obligatory" (independent of extrarenal controls) reabsorption of sodium, with chloride and water following. Hence, the descending limbs of the loops receive a fluid with an osmolality of about 300 mOsm. in a total volume of about 20 ml. per minute.

The countercurrent concept, developed by chemists Hargitay and Kuhn and physiologist Wirz, and elaborated by others and by evidence from tubular punctures, is based primarily on the facts that renal interstitial and intraluminal fluids (during antidiuresis) increase in osmolality and in sodium, chloride, and urea concentrations as the loops dip into the medulla, while intraluminal and interstitial osmolalities diminish as the ascending limb returns to the cortex, where it delivers hypotonic fluid into the distal tubule. The engineering principle is similar to that of various cooling and heating devices. In the case of the loop, the function is described as a countercurrent osmotic multiplier. This requires a hairpin structure in osmotic equilibrium with interstitial fluid and with each side of the loop, in which one side (ascending limb) extracts sodium from tubular fluid, driving it into interstitial fluid and the descending limb. Water impermeability of the ascending limb allows the tubular fluid to become progressively more dilute. The vasa recta, similarly looped, but lacking active transport, remove fluid and salt from the concentrated interstitial fluid by functioning as slowly flowing countercurrent exchange systems.

The postulate that concentration is achieved by active transport of water has been abandoned. All that need be supposed is that distal and collecting tubules are poorly permeable to water in the absence of ADH, although facultatively responsive to hormonal and metabolic regulation of sodium reabsorption. When ADH is present, the permeability of these structures increases, and they come into osmotic equilibrium with their hypertonic surroundings. The result is formation of a small volume of hypertonic urine, the vasa recta returning conserved water to the body. This clarifies the manner in which urea, a highly diffusible solute, participates in enhancing water conservation. Urea, present in high concentration in medullary interstitial fluid and, by equilibration, in collecting tubules, increases the osmotic "ceiling" without imposing a transcellular osmotic gradient. Lack of urea, and not renal damage, explains the low concentrating power found in patients on protein-deficient diets. This synopsis, even with the aid of Figure 14-4, should be supplemented by references which develop principles in more detail.

The countercurrent concept bears on the mechanism by which partial ligation of a renal artery (a procedure that tends to decrease filtration and blood flow relative to tubular mass) results in formation of a small volume of hypertonic, sodium-poor urine, even in the absence of ADH. Decreased filtration load promotes greater fractional sodium reabsorption by the intact proximal tubule system. Decreased blood flow in the vasa recta permits a very high buildup of osmotic concentration in the medullary interstitial fluid. Then, if one assumes some water permeability of distal and collecting tubules, equilibration between tubular and interstitial fluids reduces volume and increases osmolality. Predominance of renal injury in medulla and collecting ducts

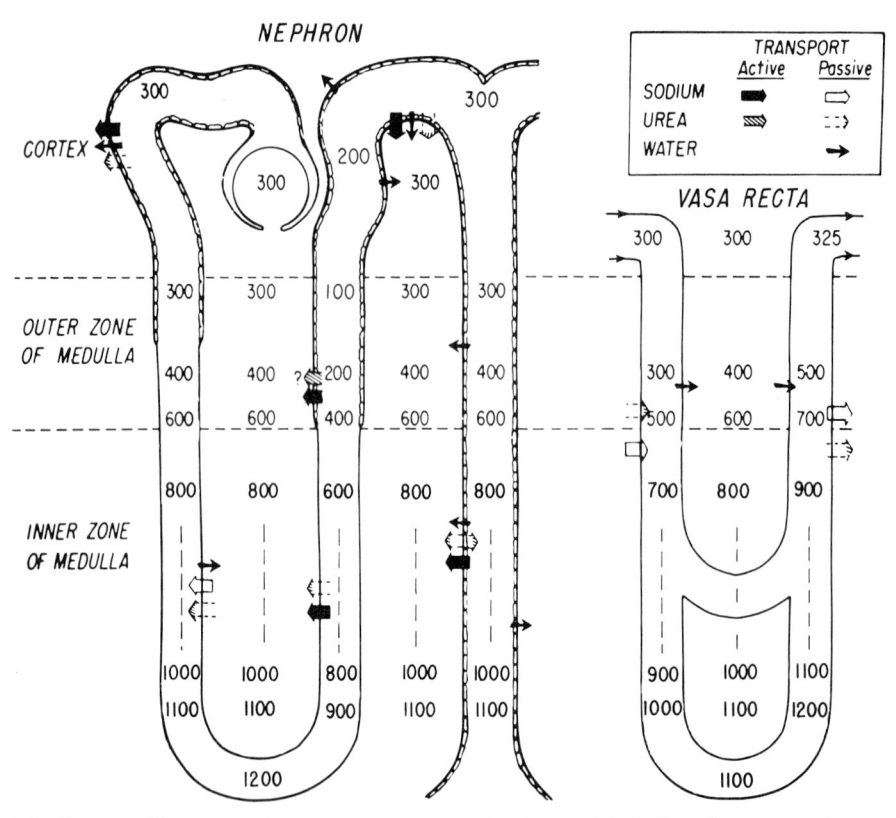

Figure 14-4 Diagram illustrating the countercurrent mechanism as it is believed to operate in a nephron with a long loop and in the vasa recta. Numbers represent hypothetical osmolality values. No quantitative significance is attached to the numbers of arrows and only net movements are indicated. As is the case with the vascular loops, all loops of Henle do not reach the tip of the papilla and hence the fluid in them does not become as concentrated as the final urine, but only as concentrated as the medullary interstitial fluid at the same level. (Courtesy of Dr. C. W. Gottschalk and the publishers of Circulation and the American Journal of Physiology.)

rather than cortex may explain why many patients with pyelonephritis show impairment of concentrating power out of proportion to other tests of excretory function. Similarly, the inability to form concentrated urine found in patients with nephrocalcinosis and hypercalcemia may be explained from the locale of their lesions. Unless it can be assumed that there may occur a state in which distal and collecting tubular segments cannot increase basic water permeability, even in the absence of lesions by electron microscopy, the mechanism of the rare, familial, "Pitressin-resistant" form of diabetes insipidus is unexplained, as is also the nature of the defect that impairs concentrating function but not water reabsorption during osmotic diuresis in sickle cell anemia.

Ion Exchange: Acidification

These processes are primarily functions of the distal tubule. Actually, ion transport, which in the proximal tubule is substantially active sodium transport, probably sets up the electrochemical milieu which allows for hydrogen ion secretion. However, it is in the distal tubule that the fluid actually may become acid. Here, too, potassium and ammonium ions may be secreted. The tubular reabsorption of bicarbonate is normally set as if its threshold were reached at a serum bicarbonate level of about 28 mEq. per liter.

The basic chemical exchanges are schematized in Table 14–1. Two of the major reactions are dependent on the integrity of the carbonic anhydrase system. These provide hydrogen ion for bicarbonate reabsorption and also for formation of titratable acid (NaH_2PO_4). These reactions are deficient in renal tubular acidoses, are suppressed by carbonic anhydrase inhibitors (e.g., sulfanilamide, acetazolamide), and are impaired in potassium deficiency. The reactions making for ammonia secretion are not affected by these enzyme inhibitors or by potassium deficiency

TABLE 14-1 SODIUM CONSERVATION BY ACIDIFICATION AND AMMONIA SECRETION

(a) Cell	(b) Transfer Product	(c) Lumen	(d) Transfer Product	(e) Cell	(f) Blood
A. Carbonic anhydrase dependent					
1. $CO_2 + H_2O$		$Na \cdot HCO_3$		$H_2O + CO_2$	
$H \cdot HCO_3$	H^+	$H \cdot HCO_3$	Na	$H \cdot HCO_3$	
		$CO_2 + H_2O$	CO_2	$NaHCO_3$	$NaHCO_3$
		H_2O			
2. $CO_2 + H_2O$	H^+	Na_2HPO_4		$H \cdot HCO_3$	
$H \cdot HCO_3$		NaH_2PO_4	Na	$NaHCO_3$	$NaHCO_3$
B. Ammonia formation					
Glutamine (glutaminase)		$H^+, NaCl$			
	NH_3	NH_4^+		$H \cdot CO_3$	
Amino acids (amine oxidase)	NH_3	NH_4Cl	Na	$NaHCO_3$	$NaHCO_3$
					$NaCl$

Reactions are listed in sequence of (*a*) intracellular reaction, (*b*) transcellular transfer, (*c*) luminal reaction, (*d*) transfer, and (*e*) cellular reaction with (*f*) final exchange into blood.

(which seems to stimulate this process), but usually are impaired in the acidosis of chronic renal failure. Hydrogen ion secretion is the immediate line of renal defense of blood pH. It can lower urinary pH to about 4.5, a level at which hydrogen ion may substitute for sodium ion of some weak acids, so that organic acids begin to appear in the urine. The basic stimulus to hydrogen ion secretion is determined by the carbon dioxide tension or pH within the tubule cell. Hence, metabolic acidosis is an instant stimulus to secretion of hydrogen ion, whereas alkalosis normally instantly suppresses this function and, with it, reabsorption of bicarbonate. Actually, since the net residue from food is acid, the urine is normally acid and the serum bicarbonate level nearer 25 than 28 mEq. per liter. The ammonia mechanism is a less immediate line of defense; it is capable of stimulation by acidosis of a few days' duration. Hence, agents intended to act by acidifying the urine, such as ammonium chloride, or by carbonic anhydrase inhibition, are most effective when administered only for 2 to 3 days at a time.

Potassium. Potassium ions form a significant fraction of the solute mixture only in the distal tubule. In general, as sodium ions are reabsorbed, either potassium or hydrogen ions are secreted. A direct exchange of ions appears unlikely, since these processes seem to occur at different locations. Nonetheless, impairment or deficiency of the carbonic anhydrase system results in urine rich in sodium and potassium, but low in hydrogen. Similarly, organic acid excess, as in diabetic acidosis, may deplete the body of sodium and potassium once the capacity for acidification of the urine is exceeded.

The association is the more complex because intracellular potassium is intimately related to carbon dioxide tension and pH in the cell. Provision of excess potassium leads to the formation of a potassium-rich, hydrogen-poor urine, even though extracellular bicarbonate level decreases to the point of acidosis. Again, deficit of potassium tends (initially at least) toward formation of acid urine, even though the systemic state is one of alkalosis and chloride deficiency. A further complication arises from the role of adrenal hormones, notably aldosterone, which act to promote distal sodium reabsorption at the expense of potassium loss. Further, whereas the several mechanisms that contribute to avid sodium retention in the face of a deficit act rapidly and effectively, those that would make for potassium retention (presumably by suppressing its cellular secretion) are less prompt and intense. Indeed, they may be less than ineffective, since the conditions that make for potassium deficit often stimulate adrenal secretions that make for potassium loss.

Hence, syndromes of potassium deficit are relatively common, whereas noteworthy potassium retention occurs only in severe renal failure. The potassium deficiency syndromes occur (1) in diarrheal states; (2) with prolonged vomiting or gastric suction; (3) with massive diuresis or glycosuria; (4) in the renal tubular acidoses, including those resulting from carbonic anhydrase-suppressing agents; and (5) in adrenal hypercorticoidism, viz., often in Cushing's syndrome and in primary aldosteronism. If the deficiency is sufficiently severe, functional and structural renal effects ensue. The structural lesion is substantially one of tubular cell vacuolation. Functional effects are impairment of PAH transport and extraction and polyuria with Pitressin-resistant isosthenuria, relieved by providing enough potassium and, in some cases, by restricting sodium. In primary aldosteronism the urine is frequently slightly alkaline and potassium rich. Indeed, the finding of these urinary signs in a patient with hypertension suggests the likelihood of primary aldosteronism. Lesser degrees of potassium deficit may be encountered in patients with severe, especially malignant, hypertension. These patients may develop alkalosis and/or hypokalemia and show definite aldosterone oversecretion in the absence of sodium lack, volume deficit, or congestive heart failure.

Diuresis and Diuretics

Normally, diuresis and antidiuresis depend on excretion of more or less water, according to needs imposed by solute load and water availability. The ultimate determinant of decreased water output is secretion of ADH in response to increases of body fluid osmolality of as little as 2 per cent. Intracerebral osmoreceptors respond to such changes by stimulating the hypophyseal-hypothalamic area to discharge impulses that initiate this secretion. A secretion of only 0.2 milliunit per kg. body weight per hour establishes an adequate physiologic antidiuretic state. Secretion normally is inhibited by decreased osmolality of body fluid or by ethyl alcohol. Normally, the receptors can be stimulated by a sharp upward shift in osmolality (Hickey-Hare test). They can also be stimulated by emotion, nicotine, and acetylcholine in the absence of osmotic changes. Furthermore, volume receptors probably located in the atria may modify ADH output. As stated above, the ultimate effect of secreted ADH is exerted by increasing the permeability of collecting tubules to water.

Both ADH and aldosterone secretion seem to be stimulated in edematous states, including congestive heart failure and the nephrotic syndrome. Diabetes insipidus may reflect injury to the ADH secretory system or to the hypophyseal-hypothalamic nuclei. Deficiency of ADH secretion also may be associated with impairment of osmoreceptor function, with resultant insensitivity of the thirst mechanism and establishment of a hyperosmolar state.

Today the common meaning of the word diuresis is increased urine flow. In its present sense, there are two major physiologic mechanisms of diuresis—water diuresis and osmotic diuresis. A third mechanism may operate when discharge of both salt and water is accelerated by an increase in extracellular fluid volume. The urine formed in water diuresis is hypotonic with reference to plasma; that formed in osmotic diuresis is hypertonic over a wide range and, other things being equal, that formed during discharge of extracellular fluid tends to be isotonic and, of course, sodium rich.

Water diuresis is due to ADH inhibition, physiologically by water loading or pharmacologically by alcohol. However, in edematous states such as congestive heart failure excess water may not be excreted and, when acutely retained, leads to water intoxication. Hence, what is usually a reasonable provision of water to such patients may not be desirable and marked restriction of water administration may be necessary.

Osmotic diuresis is characterized by formation of urine whose osmolality decreases asymptotically toward the isohydric line as the volume flow increases. Anything that contributes to osmotic load (urinary osmolal concentration times volume) is an osmotic diuretic, since its excretion carries with it some water. Typical osmotic diuretics are small molecular substances (urea, mannitol, and excessive amounts of glucose) that are incompletely reabsorbed by the tubules. Because they persist in tubular fluid they osmotically hold water, increasing flow rate from proximal tubules into loops, through which flow is thereby increased. Increased loop flow decreases the efficiency of the loop as an osmotic multiplier and dilutes medullary interstitial fluid, so that even in the presence of an excess of ADH, urine concentration falls. During water deprivation and in subjects on diets adequate in protein (to provide urea) and NaCl, maximum medullary and urinary osmolality is about 1200 mOsm. per kg. water, i.e., $U_{Osm}/P_{Osm} > 3$. As urine concentration falls during osmotic diuresis and solute excretion increases, net reabsorption of solute-free water ("free water") is increased and reaches a maximum of about 5 ml. per minute. This limit is expressed as $Tm^c_{H_2O}$; it is calculated as the osmolal clearance (C_{Osm}) less urine flow (V). At high rates of flow and osmotic load it describes an upper limit of water reabsorption, much as $Tm_{Glucose}$ describes glucose reabsorption.

A side-effect of osmotic diuresis is the washout of increased amounts of NaCl, and the urine formed at high rates of osmotic diuresis can be regarded as very similar to proximal tubular effluent. At such forced rates of flow, tubules dilate, fluid movement is accelerated, and medullary blood flow increases. Possibly all these factors, as well as dilution effects on electrolyte concentration gradients, tend to interfere with electrolyte reabsorption.

In some cases (urea, mannitol, water) classification of the mechanism of action of diuretic drugs is easy. But the actions of most diuretics in clinical use may involve osmotic and transport mechanisms and also hemodynamic changes that are complex. Table 14–2 presents a classification that may be useful.

Within the physiologic group, colloids are indeed active under normal conditions; however, they are most diuretic when they correct hypovolemia, thereby restoring plasma volume, cardiac

TABLE 14–2 FUNCTIONAL CLASSIFICATION OF DIURETIC AGENTS

A. Physiologic
  1. Those that increase filtered Na and/or Cl loads
     a. Colloids: albumin, dextran, and so on
     b. Cardiac glycosides: (only in congestive heart failure)
     c. Afferent vasodilators: aminophylline
     d. Acidifying agents: NH_4Cl
  2. Those that impair Na and/or Cl reabsorption
     a. Aldosterone antisecretory agents: amphenone (experimentally only)
     b. Aldosterone antagonists: spironolactones, prednisone(?)
     c. Agents that increase flow rate or impair ion gradients in distal tubule: water, osmotic diuretics (urea, mannitol)
B. Pharmacologic
  1. Those that specifically impair Na and/or Cl transport
     a. Xanthines: caffeine, theophylline
     b. Aminouracils: aminoisometridine
     c. Mercurial diuretics
     d. Thiazide diuretics
     e. Triamterene
     f. Ethacrynic acid
     g. Furosemide
  2. Those that interfere with HCO_3 transport
     a. Carbonic anhydrase inhibitors: sulfanilamide, acetazolamide

Modified from Pitts, R. F.: The Physiological Basis of Diuretic Therapy. Springfield, Illinois, Charles C Thomas, 1959.

output, filtration, and urine flow while also suppressing stimuli from "volume-receptors" that make for salt and water retention. They pay a modest dividend in promoting loss of NaCl; passage of some smaller molecules of the colloid into tubular fluid may add a slight osmotic effect. Although digitalis glycosides certainly alter cellular ion fluxes and thereby may have some direct renal action, it is not a primary therapeutic mechanism. They are effective diuretics only in those conditions in which they restore renal circulation by enhancing efficiency of cardiac action, i.e., in heart failure. Acidifying agents provide excess chloride ions that trap sodium as the limit of urinary acidification is reached. They are useful as adjuncts to mercurials; diuretic activity of organic mercurials is suppressed in an alkaline medium and enhanced in an acid. They have the disadvantage that they cause acidosis, with the result that renal sodium loss decreases as ammonia production increases.

Amphenone is of experimental interest only, being very toxic. The aldosterone antagonists of the spironolactone group apparently act by competing with aldosterone for receptor sites. They are most useful as adjuncts to other diuretics, since they inhibit the action of excess aldosterone secretion and thereby suppress the tendency to potassium loss. However, they may cause severe hyperkalemia. Triamterene has a similar net, albeit nonendocrine, effect. Diuretic activities of the corticosteroids and their derivatives, such as prednisone, are complex. In part there may be suppression of aldosterone and of other adrenal hormones. In adrenal insufficiency at least, the effect is largely hemodynamic and possibly also one of altered membrane permeability that increases water output.

The largest innovation in the field of diuretics was the advent of chlorothiazide and its congeners. The parent drug shares properties of a carbonic anhydrase inhibitor and a salt-with-water eliminating (saluretic) diuretic, like the mercurials. Mercurials complex with sulfhydryl-rich enzymes, possibly Na-K-activated, Mg-dependent, ouabain-inhibited, "membrane ATPase," that provide some of the energy for sodium reabsorptive transport, primarily in the proximal tubule. Impairment of sodium reabsorption at this level has the net effect of an osmotic diuretic. The prototype substance among the carbonic anhydrase inhibitors, acetazolamide, impairs reabsorption of sodium, potassium, and bicarbonate, tending thereby to provoke a metabolic hyperchloremic acidosis, and has not been a satisfactory agent in heart failure. Chlorothiazide suppresses proximal and distal sodium reabsorption, apparently by a mechanism distinct from that of mercurials, to which its effect may therefore be additive. It has the disadvantage that it tends to promote hypokalemia and metabolic alkalosis, while its proximal tubular action also impairs excretion (promotes reabsorption?) of urate, leading to hyperuricemia and sometimes gout. Its derivatives, beginning with hydrochlorothiazide, are in general more active, weight for weight.

Two much more potent diuretic agents are ethacrynic acid, a phenoxyacetic acid derivative, and furosemide, a benzothiadiazine analogue having a furfuryl group substituted on the amino nitrogen of the anthranilic acid. Both appear to act by blocking renal tubular sodium reabsorption, especially in the ascending limb of the loop of Henle, and promote intense, brief diuresis. These very useful drugs are so potent that excessive administration can bring about diastrous sodium, chloride, and water loss.

Diuretic therapy of hypertension on a large scale is relatively new, although it was shown many years ago that sufficient dosage with mercurials might have the same effect as prolonged, severe restriction of dietary sodium. The thiazide drugs have been used widely, both alone and in association with other antihypertensive drugs. Saluresis, however accomplished, assuming a reasonably limited sodium intake, has the same net effect as sodium restriction and greatly enhances the antihypertensive effect of other drugs. The first result is that sufficient saluresis depletes plasma volume. The hypertensive patient's response to this is increased vasomotor tone. If, concurrently, he is receiving a drug that impairs ability to increase vasomotor tone, blood pressure decreases, particularly when standing. Later in the course of thiazide therapy other poorly defined mechanisms participate in maintaining lower pressure levels.

TESTS OF EXCRETORY FUNCTIONS

The tests of excretory functions are either (1) qualitative or semiquantitative or (2) quantitative.

Qualitative and semiquantitative tests include (1) detection and estimation of proteinuria; (2) estimates and descriptions of urinary sediment, either crystalline or organized (red blood cells, white cells, and casts); and (3) estimation of renal excretory function from determinations of blood creatinine or urea.

The tests which quantitatively measure excretory functions are (1) tests of excretion rates (e.g., phenolsulfonphthalein test), (2) clearance tests, and (3) tests of water reabsorption. (4) Quantitative measurements of urinary protein and sediment may be included in this category. The quantitative tests of renal function are only a little more complicated to perform and usually much easier to interpret than qualitative or semiquantitative procedures. Mean normal values for these measurements of renal function are given in Table 14-3.

Tests of Rate of Excretion

The most commonly used test of excretory rate depends on measurement of percentile excretion of 6 mg. of intravenously injected phenolsulfonphthalein. This dye is excreted almost entirely by the same tubular mechanism as is Diodrast, hippuran, and PAH, all of which block its excretion, as does probenecid (Benemid). The rate at which it appears in urine depends on (1) the rate of renal blood flow, (2) the percentage of dye removed from blood during one renal circulation (normally about 50 per cent), and (3) the rate at which fluid moves down the renal tubules, through the pelvis and ureter to the bladder. Severe renal disease impairs both renal blood flow and tubular secretion and thus reduces excretion of dye. Obstructive uropathies slow the rate of movement of tubular fluid and urine and, in obstructions below the renal pelvis, dilute the excreted dye in the hydronephrotic accumulation of urine. Oliguria also tends to slow the rate of dye excretion.

Normally, 30 per cent of the injected dye is excreted in 15 minutes after intravenous injection. Slower excretion reflects delay in the urinary tract or renal damage. In the proved absence of obstructive uropathy or extreme oliguria, a decreased excretion of dye in urine collected in 15 minutes indicates a reduction of renal blood flow. Because it is more easily seen through the cystoscope than phenolsulfonphthalein, indigo carmine is used as a semiquantitative test of excretion time (blood to bladder) in urologic practice.

The rate of appearance and depth of shadow seen during intravenous urography are other indices of excretory rate. Two radiopaque substances used in this procedure (hippuran and

TABLE 14-3 APPROXIMATE AVERAGE VALUES FOR VARIOUS MEASURES OF RENAL FUNCTION IN NORMAL ADULTS

Test		Mean
Effective renal blood flow	Men	1150 ml./1.73 sq. m./min.
	Women	950 ml./1.73 sq. m./min.
Effective renal plasma flow (Diodrast, PAH clearance)	Men	700 ml./1.73 sq. m./min.
	Women	600 ml./1.73 sq. m./min.
Glomerular filtration rate (inulin, mannitol clearance)	Men	130 ml./1.73 sq. m./min.
	Women	115 ml./1.73 sq. m./min.
PAH (Tm_{PAH})	Men	80 mg./1.73 sq. m./min.
	Women	70 mg./1.73 sq. m./min.
Tubular reabsorptive capacity, glucose	Men	375 mg./1.73 sq. m./min.
	Women	300 mg./1.73 sq. m./min.
Creatinine clearance (12 or 24 hr. collection)	Men	170 L./24 hours
	Women	150 L./24 hours
Phenolsulfonphthalein excretion (6 mg. injection, I.V.) 15 min.		30% excreted
Radio-iodo-hippurate 20 min.		$64 \pm 8.6\%$ excreted
Urinary concentration (Fishberg)		1.023 sp. gr. or greater.
		U_{Osm}/P_{Osm} about 2.8

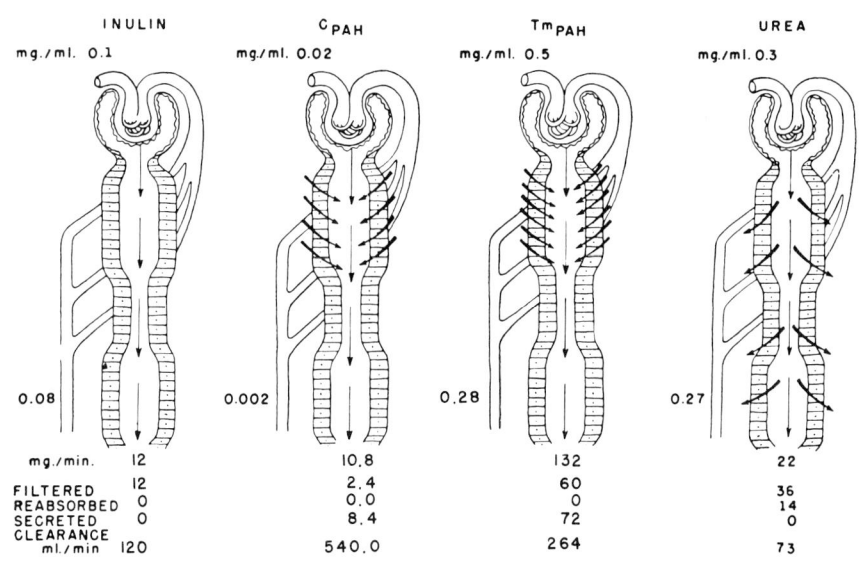

Figure 14–5 Schematic representation of examples of clearance mechanisms and measurement for inulin (arrows indicate filtration alone), for PAH (arrows indicate filtration and secretion) at low and high (Tm measurement) plasma concentrations, and for urea (arrows indicate filtration and reabsorption primarily by diffusion). In each case the value recorded in milligrams per minute is UV (urinary concentration × rate of urine flow) and that indicated opposite the afferent arteriole is plasma concentration P, so that clearance is UV/P. The numerals at the end of the schematic peritubular capillary plexus indicate estimated renal venous plasma concentrations.

Diodrast) at low plasma concentrations are excreted almost entirely by tubular secretion; another (Neo-iopax) is excreted largely by glomerular filtration. While the degree of radiopacity of the pyelographic shadow and the time of its appearance vary with renal excretory function, the shadow will also depend on the degree to which the dye is diluted. The estimate of function provided by this method is useful secondary information. It should not be referred to as dye "clearance," since it does not correspond to quantitative clearance tests.

Related to the above is the "radioisotope renogram." This procedure consists of plotting graphically radioactivity over the two kidneys for 10, 15, or 20 minutes after injection of a radioactively iodinated, renally excreted agent. The graphs show an initial "vascular spike," representing inflow of the tag in a bolus of blood into the kidney and great vessels, followed by a slow rise, representing tubular uptake and secretory activity, and subsequently a fall as urine flows out of the kidney more rapidly than dye is being stored. Abnormalities may be detected in the "vascular" phase, representing decreased inflow of blood, the tubular phase of accumulation (suppressed in severe renal disease), or the outflow phase, absent or impaired in hydronephrosis. It seems to be useful in screening for renal abnormalities, including renal arterial occlusive disease.

Although not truly a test of renal excretory function, renal scintiscans utilizing a mercurial diuretic tagged with ^{197}Hg are easy to perform and may be useful for delineating the size and approximate position of the kidneys and detecting renal vascular abnormalities or space-occupying lesions.

Clearance Tests

The concept of renal clearance began with D. D. Van Slyke as a way of expressing the amount of a substance that seemed to be wholly extracted or "cleared" from blood in one minute's time. Clearance is, in effect, the *least* volume of blood or plasma that contains enough of a substance to account for the amount of that substance present in one minute's urine. It is a calculated, not a real, volume. The concept is schematized in Figure 14–5 in terms of inulin, a levulose polymer that is small enough to be freely filterable but too large and inert to be actively or passively reabsorbed, secreted, or metabolized. Inulin clearance is therefore equal to the rate of glomerular filtration. This discovery was one of the first great contributions Homer Smith made to renal physiology. It provided a base point around which to describe excretory (secretory) and reabsorptive functions. Thus, the clearance of PAH at low plasma levels is much greater than that of inulin, because nearly all the PAH (90+ per cent rather than 20 per cent as is the case with inulin) is extracted from plasma in one renal passage. PAH clearance is nearly equal to renal plasma flow and is accepted as indicative of plasma flow to excretory tissues or "effective renal plasma flow." At high plasma concentrations PAH clearance is "self-suppressed" by saturation of the transfer system—a phenomenon that cannot occur with inulin, which is excreted purely by filtration. Such saturation enables measurement of Tm_{PAH}. Clearance of urea is less than that of inulin because, while it is filtered, it is also reabsorbed, apparently by diffusion, and in some species may also be subject to tubular excretion. A clearance less than that of inulin does not establish the absence of secretion. This is notably the case with potassium. Most filtered potassium is reabsorbed, since nearly all that appears in urine is secreted. As indicated, the same is true of urate.

Measurement of inulin and PAH clearance remains substantially an investigative procedure. Conventional methods require steady intravenous infusion, repeated plasma sampling, and collections of urine by catheterization and bladder washing. This last imposes some risk of urinary tract infection; the risk is diminished by instillation of 0.1 gm. neomycin into the bladder at the time the catheter is withdrawn.

For these reasons two clearance tests are in clinical use. One is the measurement of urea clearance. Changes in urea reabsorption, complicated perhaps by "wash-out" of medullary urea, tend to make the results of this test uncertain at low or rising rates of urine flow. However, at a stable or slowly falling urine flow somewhat in excess of 2 ml. per minute, urea reabsorption is nearly constant at about 40 per cent of that filtered, and urea clearance is normally about 75 ml. per minute and bears a fairly reproducible relation to glomerular filtration rate. The test requires no injection and the laboratory techniques are in common use. It is therefore adapted to routine clinical studies, provided that sufficient care is taken to maintain urine flow by adequate prehydration, to enforce recumbency during the test period, and to forbid smoking.

The second test, used more often, is measurement of endogenous creatinine clearance, usually over fairly long periods of urine collection of 12 or 24 hours. Again, no injection is required and the chemical procedures are familiar. Excretion rate is independent of urine flow, which is an advantage. From technical and nursing aspects, it is easier to perform than the urea clearance test. The normal creatinine clearance is approximately 120 ml. per minute or 180 L. per 24 hours.

Water Tests

Those in common use, the concentration-dilution tests, are aimed at detecting abnormalities in the renal tubular mechanisms responsible for altering the osmolality of tubular fluid by reabsorption or excretion of osmotically unobligated "free water." Other tests, which measure diuretic responses to standard water or salt loads, are directed usually at possible abnormalities of extrarenal (pituitary, adrenal, or circulatory) regulatory mechanisms.

The concentration-dilution tests measure the degree to which tubular cells bring about differences in osmotic concentrations between the glomerular filtrate and urine. Dilution tests are little used. They consist of measuring the ability to achieve a lower specific gravity after a standard water load. The range of measurement is smaller and the influence of extrarenal factors (adrenal, pituitary, hepatic, intestinal, cardiac, hemic) is large.

Concentration tests measure the ability of the kidney to form urine of high osmolar concentration in response to ADH stimulation. ADH stimulation is elicited by endogenous release under the stimulus of water deprivation, or by giving ADH by injection of Pituitrin or vasopressin. The simplest of these tests is that of Fishberg. Hourly urine specimens are collected during continuance of nocturnal water deprivation begun 12 hours before. One of the specimens should yield a specific gravity greater than 1.023. The osmolality of urine which is achieved on a concentration test should be at least 850 mOsm. per kg. water, i.e., U/P osmolal ratio should be 2.9 or more.

Substitution of Pituitrin or vasopressin for water deprivation is used to speed the test and to provide a standard stimulus which is independent of the patient's interpretation of water deprivation. The test is done by measuring specific gravities or osmolalities of specimens collected at intervals after subcutaneous injection of 10 pressor units of pituitary extract. However, the test has the disadvantage that it requires injection of a substance which is sometimes uncomfortable and occasionally lethal. Furthermore, the amount injected is very large as compared with the calculated maximum physiologic rate of ADH release.

The nature of either concentration or dilution tests is that they measure variance from a baseline specific gravity of 1.010, which represents excretion of a urine which is only slightly hypertonic to a protein-free plasma filtrate (specific gravity 1.008). In the common forms of renal disease the ability to concentrate or dilute the urine becomes considerably diminished when the glomerular filtration rate is about 30 per cent of normal. Beyond this degree of renal damage the progress of renal failure must be measured by other means.

It is important to recognize that even at a stage of "fixed" specific gravity there may be no real concentrating defect in the remaining nephrons. They may be responding perfectly to the osmotic diuresis elicited by azotemia, which increases solute (nonprotein nitrogen) concentration in the glomerular filtrate. This follows from the nature of osmotic diuresis, in which the urine tends to an osmolar concentration of 300 mOsm. per kg. water as solute load increases, even in the presence of maximally effective water-reabsorbing mechanisms. This fact has other implications. Thus, it has been assumed that excretion of urine of specific gravity of 1.010 (about 300 mOsm. per kg. water) implies that the tubules are doing a minimum of osmotic work and that they are called upon to do more osmotic work when the urine is either very dilute or very concentrated. From this it has been argued that protein should be restricted in the presence of renal disease, because excretion of urea requires the kidney to do osmotic work. Without prejudice to other unrelated, perhaps sufficient reasons which might justify protein restriction, this rationalization is unjustified. Urea excretion is passive once arterial pressure has forced urea through the glomerulus. Furthermore, from what is known of the many mechanisms of active transport which operate in urine formation, it follows that the only condition in which the kidney would do a clear minimum of osmotic work would be one in which it excreted unmodified glomerular filtrate.

The concentration tests remain as useful indices of renal function which reflect defects in water reabsorption in the nephrons in response to an osmotic load. They have value primarily in the detection of early renal disease. In the presence of any considerable azotemia they are essentially uninformative and the imposition of hydropenia may be harmful to the patient. It is essential to a proper concentration test that the conditions be such as to provide reasonable standardization of solute load and water deficit, so that the volume of fluid which the tubule is called upon to concentrate is small and relatively constant, and the ADH stimulus maximal. The tests are therefore subject to artifacts, such as prior restriction of protein, which diminishes medullary hyperosmolality, and receding edema, which unpredictably adds isotonic fluid to the urine.

Measurements of osmolality by the freezing point method are convenient and much more accurate than the rough equivalent provided by measurement of urine specific gravity. Furthermore, osmolality is of much greater physiologic significance than is specific gravity, since it directly evaluates the amount of osmotic work done by the renal tubular cells when compared with simultaneous plasma (or serum) osmolality. In hospitals, cost of the apparatus should not be a determinant in view of the significant results obtained. The relationship between urine osmolality and specific gravity of patients with hypertension on a normal mixed diet is shown in Figure 14-6. The slope changes during sodium restriction.

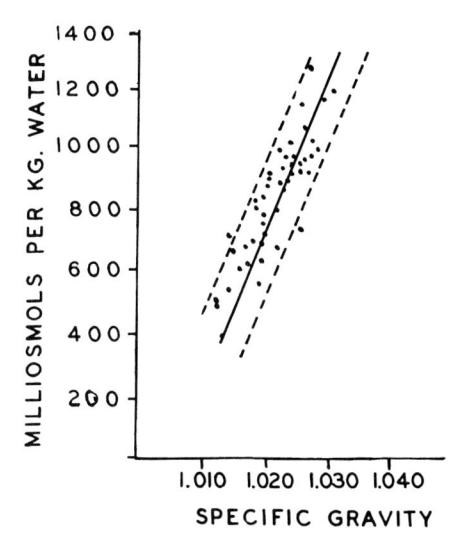

Figure 14-6 Graph of the relationship between urine osmolality and specific gravity. (Adapted from Dustan, H. P., and Corcoran, A. C.: Med. Clin. N. Amer., 39:947, 1955.)

RENAL ENDOCRINE FUNCTIONS

Pressor-Antipressor Function

Bright suggested in 1827 an association between albuminuric renal disease and increased arterial pressure. Goldblatt showed that hypertension of varying severity could be produced by partial, permanent compression of the renal artery. The stimulus to hypertension is apparently a change in the character, possibly in the distribution, but not necessarily in the total volume, of the renal blood flow. Hence, excretory function may be normal or nearly so during persistence of severe hypertension. Alternatively excretory function can be unilaterally abolished and the kidney can still serve as a cause of rapidly fatal renovascular hypertension. Thus, excretory and pressor functions of the kidney can be completely disassociated.

The mechanisms of renovascular hypertension involve liberation of a proteolytic enzyme, renin, which seems to be present in or near the cells of the juxtaglomerular body. Renin then acts on a globulin (renin substrate, angiotensinogen) of hepatic origin, present in plasma in very low concentrations. This highly specific reaction releases a polypeptide, known as angiotensin. This material, as it is split off from renin substrate, is a 10-amino-acid polypeptide which is vasoinactive (angiotensin I). Splitting off of two amino acids converts this (a converting enzyme is present in plasma) to angiotensin II, which is weight for weight more vasoconstrictor than anything known. This product is dissipated by more or less nonspecific peptic enzymes grouped as angiotensinases. Angiotensin is carried in the blood to the adrenal cortex where it stimulates the output of aldosterone. Aldosterone in turn circulates back to the kidney where it promotes renal tubular reabsorption of sodium. Renin is also released on quiet standing, during plasma volume depletion, and in congestive heart failure.

Hypertension also appears in animals that have been bilaterally nephrectomized and kept alive by dialysis. This is "renoprival" hypertension and, at first glance, would seem wholly distinct from renal hypertension. However, it points to an antipressor function of the kidneys. Such an antipressor effect of a normal kidney can be demonstrated by placing the kidney into the circulation of an animal with either renal or renoprival hypertension. Still, the vascular volume and sodium dependence of "renoprival hypertension" emphasize the importance of these factors.

Erythropoietin

Another endocrine function of the kidney is the formation of a substance that has to do with red cell formation. Clinically, the lack of formation of erythropoietin accounts for the anemias of patients with severe renal damage and, when produced in excess, for the polycythemias that have been described in patients with hypernephroma and with renal cysts. (See Ch. 22.)

CLINICAL MANIFESTATIONS OF RENAL DISEASE

The clinical manifestations of kidney disease can be conveniently grouped as (1) proteinuria and the organized sediment (hematuria, pyuria, and cylindruria); (2) isosthenuria, oliguria, and anuria; (3) renal edema and the nephrotic syndrome; (4) renal hypertension and hypertensive disease; and (5) excretory failure and uremia.

Proteinuria

Urine protein estimations are usually semiquantitative (e.g., heat and acetic acid). Urine protein test strips facilitate estimates and are fairly quantitative. Quantitative measurement (e.g., Shevky-Stafford) of proteinuria per unit time (usually 24 hours) is much more interpretable.

The protein content of normal urine is small and, by specific measurement, appears to be about 50 mg. daily. Proteinuria in excess of 150 mg. daily is presumed to be abnormal and of renal origin. As a guide, in the heat and acetic acid test, "trace" should correspond to about 0.3 to 0.5 gm. protein per liter, + to 0.5 to 1, ++ to 1 to 3, +++ to 3 to 8, and ++++ (boils solid) to 10 gm. or more per liter of urine.

The mechanisms of proteinuria were illustrated in Figure 14–3. It is due either to a capillary leak greater than the presumed maximum of 30 mg. per 100 ml. of glomerular filtrate which the tubules can normally absorb or to diminished proximal tubular reabsorptive capacity.

Thus visualized, proteinurias are preglomerular, glomerular, or tubular in origin.

Preglomerular. A normally retentive glomerulus permits the escape of circulating colloids of low molecular size. The comparatively large hemoglobin molecule (molecular weight 68,800) can pass through about 12 per cent of the glomerular surface (inulin through 100 per cent). The relatively greater glomerular permeability of hemoglobin as compared to albumin (molecular weight 72,000) presumably reflects differences in shape and charge of the molecules. With hemoglobin, the amount which will appear in urine depends in part on the amount which the tubules can reabsorb. Hemoglobin, which is normally of constant molecular size, shows a "threshold" at about 100 mg. per 100 ml. of plasma, which at normal rates of filtration reflects tubular absorption of about 20 mg. per 100 ml. of filtrate. Demonstration of haptoglobulin binding of hemoglobin may require revision of this estimate. The excretion of abnormal amounts of a circulating protein of somewhat smaller size occurs in the case of Bence Jones proteinuria. Bence Jones protein is formed in excess by the proliferating plasma cells in certain patients having multiple myeloma. It is unique in that it precipitates between 45° and 60° C. as urine is heated, then becomes soluble as the urine is heated further to boiling, but reprecipitates with cooling between 60° and 45° C. It has been shown that Bence Jones protein consists of light (L) polypeptide chains having molecular weights of about 22,000 for the monomer and 44,000 for the dimer, in which pairs of light chains are linked by intermolecular disulfide bonds (see p. 99). Light chains isolated from myeloma protein and light chains from normal human immunoglobulin of the IgG class (7S γ_2-globulin) appear to be identical with those of Bence Jones protein and show similar reversible thermosolubility properties. Indeed, from both urine and plasma of normal individuals low molecular weight globulins have been isolated which resemble the light chains of normal IgG human globulin, i.e., they appear to be the normal counterparts of Bence Jones protein. In renal amyloidosis, light chains accumulate in the glomerular tufts and peritubular areas.

Thus, the variables which determine "renal threshold" in preglomerular proteinuria are (1) the size, shape, and charge of the abnormal plasma protein; (2) the rate of glomerular filtration; and (3) tubular capacity for protein pinocytosis; while (4) glomerular permeability is assumed to be normal and constant.

Glomerular. The "pore" concept of the glomerulus supposes that the surface is interrupted by "pores" of varying size, few of which are large enough to permit the passage of albumin molecules, while perhaps 20 per cent of the surface is permeable to a small molecule like myoglobin (molecular weight 16,400). Glomerular proteinuria would then arise from the creation of pores of abnormal size. Such can be visualized as occurring in damaged glomeruli in hypertensive or primary glomerular disease. Glomerular origin of proteinuria in malignant hypertension is suggested by the fact that arterial pressure—a large factor in determining increased intraglomerular pressure—is a partial determinant of the rate of this form of proteinuria. Furthermore, in the nephrotic syndrome measurements of albumin clearance show that the filtrate contains more than 30 mg. of protein per 100 ml., presumably because of increased capillary leak. Electron microscopy has been particularly informative in glomerular disease. Acute glomerulonephritis is associated with intense endothelial cell proliferation and, apparently as a consequence, with formation of irregular, thickened bands of lamina densa in bars and strands, with monocytic aggregation. In contrast, in idiopathic nephrosis the endothelial cells and lamina seem relatively intact, but there is swelling and disorganization of the pedicles of podocytes. Presumably, the variations in interpedicle slits determine proteinuria in the latter, and the changes in lamina densa account for hematuria and proteinuria in the former.

The common association of increased capillary leak with a diminished or damaged surface is, at first glance, paradoxical. However, the physical factors of pressure and permeability which determine filtration of water and dissolved substances up to the size of inulin through a normally retentive glomerular surface are basically different from these which would permit a leak of occasional protein molecules through a focus of diminished retentiveness. They are qualitatively distinct and quantitatively of widely different orders. Thus, at a plasma albumin concentration of 4 gm. per 100 ml., proteinuria of 20 gm. daily represents a plasma albumin clearance of 0.5 liter daily, while filtration rate is 360 times greater. This reflects the common situation in which glomerular disease diminishes filtration rate by decreasing average permeability, while it is accompanied by proteinuria as a result of focal capillary lesions which here and there increase porosity.

Because glomerular proteinuria is due to abnormal spans of porosity, the glomerulus still shows differential retentiveness of larger molecules, and the bulk of the proteinuria consists of serum albumin molecules, while the larger globulins are retained. The amounts of globulin which enter the urine vary from case to case, and because the composition of urinary protein is thus variable, the term "proteinuria" is preferred to the common term "albuminuria."

Tubular. Proteinuria of tubular origin results from diminished capacity of renal tubular cells to take up and digest protein. This impairment may be due to structural or functional damage of essential cellular mechanisms. Clearly, when cellular mechanisms of protein ingestion are fully occupied in digestion, capacity for further uptake of protein must suffer. Consequently, glomerular or preglomerular proteinurias have an associated tubular component. This is most apparent in the case of hemoglobin. In rats, injected bovine albumin passes through the glomerulus and is subject to cellular ingestion; during this time the "renal threshold" for injected hemoglobin is decreased because of decreased tubular absorption. Prolonged hemoglobinuria is associated with a decrease in the "renal threshold" for hemoglobin and with albuminuria because of decreased tubular reabsorption of both hemoglobin and the albumin of normal glomerular filtrate. The initial proteinuria of mercury bichloride or bichromate poisoning reflects tubular injury. Possibly some of the proteinuria which occurs during renal ischemia is due to functional impairment of these mechanisms, although such situations are associated with hemodynamic changes which could of themselves alter glomerular porosity. Thus, proteinuria primarily of tubular origin is probably uncommon and usually inconsequential. There seem to occur cases of "familial proteinuria" that may be tubular, but these must be rare and this diagnosis should be cautiously reserved.

Clinical Considerations. Most proteinurias are evidences of glomerular damage, primary or secondary, structural or functional; some reflect the presence of abnormal circulating proteins, and a few are primarily tubular. Altered tubular mechanisms contribute to the extent of preglomerular or glomerular proteinurias, which they may augment by rejection of albumin which would be normally absorbed.

Thus considered, proteinurias are either inconstant or constant. The inconstant proteinurias are occasional, postural or orthostatic, and exertional. The association of proteinuria with severe exercise in normal people is usually obvious. Proteinuria which is demonstrably occasional and transient may be due to some hemodynamic change, such as the proteinuria which may be associated with a cold pressor test or with emotional disturbance or central nervous injury, or to transient change in glomerular porosity occasioned by allergy, fever, or infection.

Orthostatic proteinuria is a poor term. Most proteinurias are either increased or even made overt by standing and exercise. The condition usually is seen in normal, spare, adolescent males, is benign and recoverable, and is important only as a source of disqualification for military service or life insurance. The condition is detected by having the patient void a timed urine specimen one hour after going to bed. He should void again on waking, while still in bed; he is then placed in exaggerated lordosis by putting small pillows under the small of his back for 30 minutes, when he collects another specimen. The proteinuria will thus be established as constant (present in the three specimens), related to the erect posture primarily (specimen one), or related to lordosis (specimen three) by quantitative measurement in grams per hour. Proteinuria, regardless of its cause, usually will be accentuated by the erect posture.

More significant among the inconstant proteinurias are the bursts of protein excretion that occur in some patients with essential hypertension, since these often mark eruptions of nephrosclerotic activity, and the exercise proteinuria that occurs in congestive heart failure. Both presumably reflect renal ischemia, which, in heart failure, is primarily functional.

The constant proteinurias are of more concern, since they are the rule in patients with renal disease. As noted, these are usually intensified by the factors which, of themselves, result in inconstant proteinuria. Thus, during recovery from acute glomerulonephritis, orthostatic proteinuria not increased during lordosis is not uncommon, and as suggested, the proteinuria of severe hypertension is partly a function of the blood pressure level. In general, the presence of constant proteinuria is presumptive evidence of a glomerular lesion which has created foci of increased porosity. Its significance depends on its cause and, to some extent, on its degree. Large, constant proteinurias are usually associated with the nephrotic syndrome.

The Organized Sediment

The principal elements are casts and red and white blood cells. The customary method of examination and characterization in "units per high-power field" (observed with various objectives and oculars from drops of sediment of great or little thickness, obtained with more or less dilution by random observation of a casual sample of urine, uncontrolled in time of collection and of uncertain vintage) leaves almost everything to be desired. However, it enjoys wide application and is inexpensive. The urine of healthy people may contain red blood cells, white cells, and casts in considerable numbers in a 24-hour period.

A quantitative technique established by Addis is to do counts on aliquots from a 10 ml. portion of freshly voided 3-hour morning urine collected during the last 3 hours of a 15-hour period of fluid deprivation. This is centrifuged at 1600 revolutions a minute for 10 minutes in an Addis sediment tube. The sediment is suspended evenly in a given volume of supernatant and a drop of the mixed suspension is placed under the cover slip on each side of a standard hemocytometer slide. Casts are searched for under low power with reduced illumination in the 0.9 sq. mm. of each side, and cells are counted under high power in the central 0.1 sq. mm. of each side. The results are expressed in units per 12 or 24 hours.

Casts. Casts are literally coagulated protein casts of the tubule lumen in which they were formed. Hence, proteinuria is a usual primary condition of cast formation. Casts are formed in distal tubules and collecting ducts. This localization is determined in part by the concentration and acidification of urine in these sites. By definition, globulins require some minimum salt concentration to be maintained in solution; consequently, globulins tend more than albumin to precipitate out in casts, and those globulins of very low isoelectric point and high precipitability, such as form in myeloma, precipitate out even in the proximal tubules, where hydrogen ion concentration is low and the tubule fluid is still isotonic. Hemoglobin and myoglobin are similarly precipitable; pigment casts due to one or the other occur in a wide variety of conditions that cause acute renal failure, such as "acute tubular necrosis." In its initial phases one usually finds large or small amounts of circulating hemoglobin or myoglobin, and decreased renal blood flow, filtration rate, and urine flow. In some situations, as after a large mismatched transfusion or in black-water fever or severe myoglobinuria, obstruction and tubular damage (liberated ferriheme or ferric ion?) by the pigment have been postulated as etiologic factors. However, in most of these conditions the main event is renal ischemia, and tubular necrosis is primarily ischemic. Pigment casts merely mark the kidney as one which has been subject to these abnormalities during hemoglobinemia or myoglobin release.

The noncellular casts are classified as hyaline, finely and coarsely granular, waxy, fatty, and pigmented. The distinction between hyaline and finely granular casts depends largely on the conditions of their precipitation, granularity being more evident when the urine is more acid. McQueen has shown that the matrix of hyaline casts is composed of Tamm-Horsfall urinary mucoprotein. Fluorescent antibody techniques suggest that cast granules are aggregates of serum proteins. The "granules" of some granular casts may represent the remnants of degenerate cells. Some coarsely granular materials are accumulations of lipid in which the presence of cholesterol may be identified with the polarizing microscope. Such casts are common in the nephrotic syndrome. The nature of "waxy" casts is obscure. Possibly they represent lipoproteins which have not yet separated. Pigmented casts either are common types of casts colored with bilirubin or are composed of heme pigment. Casts of heme pigment are usually dense and short. Their granularity sometimes gives the impression that they are composed of degenerate red blood cell aggregates.

Cellular casts are casts in which red blood cells, white blood cells, or renal epithelial cells have adhered in the cast of the renal tubule, so that they testify to the presence of cellular exudation in nephrons. Lastly, renal failure casts are distinguished by great breadth and comparatively short length. They are formed in the terminal collecting ducts. Cast formation can hardly occur in this position, where the flow of urine is normally rapid, unless flow has been slowed. Such slowing is most commonly the result of death or disability of the majority of nephrons that lead from the lobule into the duct in which the cast is formed. Consequently, their presence in urine is evidence of severe structural loss.

Red Blood Cells. Red blood cells may be liberated in either the upper or lower urinary tract. The simple three-glass voiding test is commonly used to establish the source as urethral, vesical, or prostatic. Ureteral catheterization may determine whether prevesical bleeding is due to unilateral or bilateral lesions of the upper tract. Supportive diagnostic evidence is of course obtained from the history and clinical features, from tests of renal function, and from intravenous and retrograde urography.

Typically, hematuria due to lesions of the upper tract is characterized by an even suspension of the red blood cells in the urine, so that the urine may become smoky and brownish because of the suspended cells in which some red hemoglobin has been changed to bronze methemoglobin. Such gross hematuria is easily differentiated from hemoglobinuria and myoglobinuria, in which heme pigments are in solution, by centrifuging the urine and examining the sediment. Hematuria which is less severe may be diagnosed either chemically or microscopically. Chemical procedures are superficially attractive because they seem convenient and quantitative. Actually, results cannot be easily evaluated because of interference with the benzidine reaction by vitamin C and other constituents of urinary sediment. Microscopy is more accurate. The result it yields may be "semiquantitative" (cells per high-power field) or quantitative. Though the method of choice is the Addis count of the sediment, especially when hematuria is scant and its detection significant, this is usually not done because of the time required.

Hematuria of prevesical origin is evidence of a lesion in the ureter, renal pelvis, tubule system, or glomerular apparatus. The presence of red cell casts is presumptive evidence that the lesion involves the renal parenchyma. The causative lesions may be functional, as in the hematurias which may result from renal vasoconstriction, whether from effort, extrarenal trauma, injection of epinephrine, or congestion—as in congestive heart failure—or they may be due to temporarily increased vascular permeability, as from injection of histamine, or to vigorous treatment with heparin. So-called essential hematuria is believed to be due to anomalies of the submucosal venules of the renal papillae. Transient bleeding may be caused by trauma to renal parenchyma or tubular mucosa (renal rupture, crystalluria, lithuria). The remaining causes of hematuria are various forms of vascular damage, either primary, as in hypertensive arteriolar disease, glomerulonephritis, polyarteritis, and so forth, or parenchymal diseases, as in pyelonephritis, renal tuberculosis, sickle cell disease, renal infarction, and neoplasia.

The degree of hematuria is an index of the activity of the underlying lesion in "medical" types of renal disease. Thus, the severe inflammatory glomerular change in acute hemorrhagic glomerulonephritis is characterized by gross hematuria. The attenuated exudative lesions of chronic glomerulonephritis cause persistent microscopic hematuria and pyuria; exacerbations and remissions can be estimated from the counts of the urinary sediment. Similarly, the slow course of occlusive renal microvascular disease in essential hypertension causes at most only a slight and persistent increase in the sediment count, while the acute necrotizing arteriolar lesions of malignant hypertension may lead to gross urinary bleeding. The lesions in these conditions are glomerular or preglomerular, and hematuria is nearly always bilateral, since they occur equally in both kidneys. In contrast, unilateral hematuria is prima facie evidence for the presence of a unilateral postglomerular lesion which may be as benign as "essential" hematuria or as ominous as chronic pyelonephritis, renal tuberculosis, or carcinoma. In "malignant hypertension" it suggests unilateral main renal artery occlusive disease with contralateral necrotizing or malignant nephrosclerosis.

White Blood Cells. The conditions which lead to the appearance of abnormal numbers of white blood cells in bladder urine differ from those which cause hematuria in that they are all exudative. Localization of the lesion is carried out in the same manner as with hematuria, and, as with the latter, the presence of casts in which the cells are adherent is presumptive evidence of a parenchymatous focus.

The most common cause is infection, although the sterile exudates and degenerative changes of chronic glomerulonephritis or other destructive renal lesions, as well as most other types of interstitial nephritis, also may lead to increased numbers of white blood cells in the urine. The small number of white cells which may be present in normal urine are presumably derived from ameboid wandering of leukocytes through the mucosa of the urinary epithelium and are principally polymorphonuclear leukocytes. The significance of pyuria must be evaluated almost entirely from the accompanying clinical and urinary abnormalities.

Enzymes

Acute renal injuries may be associated with increased output of enzymes of renal origin, many of them in cellular debris. X-irradiation of the kidney provokes a large increase in alkaline phosphatase in urine, with concurrent depletion from tubular cells. Estimates of lactic dehydrogenase in the urine of patients with chronic renal disease suggest an association with the disease process. However, such tests are still in the exploratory phase.

Hyposthenuria, Oliguria, and Anuria

Hyposthenuria signifies inability to form hypertonic urine. It is either neurogenic (hypothalamico-hypophyseal) or renal. Renal hyposthenuria results from suppression or permanent loss of distal and collecting tubular ability to concentrate maximally hypotonic tubular fluid as it is delivered from the loop of Henle. A major defect occurs in sicklemia and is attributable to occlusion of medullary vessels and/or ischemia due to sickling therein, with resultant increased medullary blood viscosity. In hypertensive renal disease some of the defect seems to result from ischemia created by reversible vasoconstriction, and is to this degree recoverable. However, major defects in concentrating power usually are associated with irrevocable loss of nephrons. In hypertension, increased intraglomerular pressure tends to maintain filtration rate at levels high in relation to renal blood flow and may increase relative medullary blood flow and thus impair concentration more than filtration. Hence, in this condition, a concentration test of renal function is commonly a more sensitive clinical index of the presence and extent of incipient renal damage than is the urea clearance, which depends on filtration rate. Reduction of concentrating power in hypertensive disease is sometimes much greater than would be estimated from other indices of functional capacity, such as excretory Tm_{PAH}.

Azotemia also results in excretion of urine which tends to be isotonic, but, in this case, the mechanism is one of osmotic diuresis, and concentrating power may be quite normal in residual nephrons.

Symptomatically, hyposthenuria results in nocturnal formation of a large volume of urine of low specific gravity, i.e., nocturia. It is important to remember that nocturia has other causes. It may be habitual and reflect an insomniac's loss of the normal rhythm of concentration and osmolal excretion. More significantly, it may be an early sign of congestive heart failure. In this latter situation, as in famine edema, latent edema accumulates hypostatically during the day and is discharged during the night. Exercise and insomnia lead the patient in a truly vicious cycle.

Another consequence of hyposthenuria is that the minimal urinary volume required for excretion of the urinary osmotic load is increased. A normal person can excrete some 35 gm. of urinary solid in a 24-hour volume of about 500 ml. at a specific gravity of about 1.028, while a patient with hyposthenuria may require three times as much water to excrete the same metabolic load. Failure to provide for this minimal volume results in azotemia and uncomfortable dehydration and, in the presence of advanced renal disease, may precipitate uremia. The summation of true hyposthenuria with azotemic diuresis is dramatically demonstrated in the severe diuresis which may occur during recovery from acute tubular necrosis. Azotemia accumulated during the anuric phase contributes the osmotic diuresis, and tubular injury causes impairment of concentrating power. The result is a urine flow which may reach levels of several liters daily but in which tolerance to excess fluid loads may be poor and pulmonary edema easily precipitated.

Anuria is failure to form urine, whereas oliguria is failure to form urine in amounts sufficient to meet metabolic demand. The daily urine volume at which oliguria begins is therefore a function of concentrating power and solute load and varies from 400 to about 1500 ml. per day. Anuria due to renal lesions begins or terminates in oliguria, so that the two may be regarded as one.

Oliguria may be (1) extrarenal, as in dehydration, cardiac failure, arterial hypotension, or painful stimulation; (2) renal, as the result of damage or loss of renal tissue; or (3) obstructive. The obstructive anurias may be intrarenal, from obstruction of renal tubules and collecting ducts, or due to extrinsic or intrinsic obstruction of the lower urinary tract.

A clue to the mechanism primarily at fault is given by the osmolality (or specific gravity). From this aspect, oliguria may be considered either hypersthenuric or hyposthenuric. In hypersthenuric oliguria the volume of urine formed is inadequate, and the osmolality (or specific gravity) is high, i.e., above 600 mOsm. per kg. water (or more than 1.023), whereas it is only approximately 300 mOsm. per kg. water (or about 1.010) in hyposthenuric oliguria.

Hypersthenuric oliguria can result from inadequate intake or excessive loss of water or from a decrease of glomerular filtration which does not otherwise severely affect tubular function. Such a decrease in glomerular filtration may result from decreased arterial pressure, renal blood flow, and filtration, i.e., from circulatory failure or from diffuse glomerular lesions.

In contrast, hyposthenuric oliguria is an indication that the primary lesion is one which injures or destroys the concentrating power of the renal tubules. Such injury may result from an extrarenal cause, as when in prolonged shock there results renal anoxia, or it may be due to tubular damage by toxins or tubular loss from disease, or to blockage of either intrarenal or extrarenal origin. Thus, parenchymal damage is the rule in hyposthenuric oliguria.

More than one mechanism can participate in causing urinary suppression, and, once the injury has been done, the clinical course may be indistinguishable. This is the case in "acute tubular necrosis." The causes of this condition range from trauma (burns, battle wounds, hypotension, crush injury, obstetric accident) through mismatched transfusions, other acute hemolytic states, some infections, notably Far Eastern hemorrhagic fever, and a variety of intoxications (mercury bichloride, ethylene glycol, carbon tetrachloride, and sulfonamides). Studies indicate that the basic renal injury is intense cortical ischemia. This injury is followed by regeneration of the necrotic tubular epithelium. However, loss of continuity of the basement membrane at the sites of tubulorrhexis may interfere with orderly re-formation of a functioning nephron. When the renal cortical blood flow gradually returns, the tubular fluid again begins to appear as urine. However, the damage to the renal tubules is such that there ensues a hyposthenuric state with osmotic diuresis which is also complicated by inability of the kidney to regulate the output of electrolytes. This diuretic phase subsides over several days or even weeks (hemorrhagic fever) until, at the end of 6 or 12 months, functional recovery usually is nearly complete.

Acute renal failure uncomplicated by major trauma or infection is usually recoverable. Renal failure complicated by major wounds and infections imposes a heavy mortality (about 50 per cent) under the best available conditions, including dialysis.

Edema of Renal Origin

In the restricted sense of this discussion, edema of renal origin is taken to mean edema which is part of the natural evolution of renal disease. It includes the edema of acute glomerulonephritis, that of eclamptogenic toxemia of pregnancy, and the nephrotic syndrome.

Edema in Acute Nephritis and Eclamptogenic Toxemia. The clinical features of acute glomerulonephritis and severe toxemia of pregnancy are strikingly similar, and it seems likely that some of the underlying mechanisms are identical. Edema in these conditions begins in a sudden increase in interstitial fluid and plasma volumes with rapid gain in body weight. Clinically, the edema is "rubbery" and is characteristically evident in the loose subcutaneous tissues around the eyes. The hypervolemia often mimics congestive heart failure.

Two mechanisms seem principally at fault. One is a decrease in glomerular filtration, the result of glomerular exudation and, to some degree, of afferent renal vasoconstriction. This change is not associated with equivalent tubular damage, and, at least in the early stages of these diseases, renal blood flow is well maintained or even increased. The result of this disparate renal change is glomerulotubular imbalance. The amount of sodium filtered is decreased. The still intact renal tubular structure reabsorbs sodium and water at approximately a normal absolute rate. This results in hypersthenuric oliguria, with retention of sodium and water.

The distribution and character of the edema in toxemia of pregnancy indicate that another mechanism plays some part in localizing the fluid accumulations. The occurrence of signs of generalized damage to small vessels, as in the retina, brain, and heart, suggests that the second factor in the edema is exudative, probably as a result of severe subcutaneous arteriolar constriction with capillary stasis and widespread microvascular thromboses.

Hypoproteinemia is usually a minor factor in this form of edema. It is not present at the onset of acute glomerulonephritis, and is only somewhat more common in women with eclamptogenic toxemias, probably because so many of them are poorly nourished, than in those who go through pregnancy without edema. However, hypoproteinemia with nephrotic edema may rapidly supervene if glomerular damage persists in acute glomerulonephritis.

The Nephrotic Syndrome. The "nephrotic syndrome" denotes a state characterized by edema, which is accompanied by profuse proteinuria and hypoproteinemia with lipemia, usually measured as hypercholesterolemia. The edema is most obvious in dependent subcutaneous tissues. It often gives rise to ascites and pleural effusions. It may extend to the submucosa of the intestines, where it can be demonstrated radiologically. Plasma volume is frequently decreased. The edema does not involve significantly the liver, brain, or heart.

The nephrotic syndrome in the adult is often the first sign of glomerulonephritis of insidious onset (pathologically chronic membranous glomerulonephritis). In contrast, the nephrotic syndrome is uncommon in renal disease due to hypertensive arteriolosclerosis and in chronic pyelonephritis. It is characteristic of diabetic intercapillary glomerulosclerosis, in which it persists during uremia. It is not uncommon in the "lupus kidney" of systemic lupus erythematosus. Most of the aspects of the nephrotic syndrome appear in the late stage of renal amyloidosis. Finally, it may be the solitary manifestation of an entity called idiopathic nephrosis, which seems to be frequently a recoverable disorder of podocytes which is more common in childhood.

The principal cause of edema in the nephrotic syndrome is sodium retention associated with secondary hyperaldosteronism. This in turn arises from the decrease in plasma protein content which results in increased filtration into and decreased reabsorption of fluid from tissue spaces so far as it decreases plasma colloid osmotic pressure. The osmotic activity of the albumin fraction is roughly four times that of the globulin, so that hypoalbuminemia is a major cause of hypoproteinemic edema, and the primary mechanism is a net continuing increase in formation of interstitial fluid at the relative and dynamic expense of plasma volume. It is this decrease in plasma volume which is the stimulus for sodium retention. The onset of edema therefore shows no correlation with total plasma globulin content, which, in this condition, tends to remain constant or is often slightly increased. Actually, gamma globulin is typically low and the lipoprotein beta globulin is increased. Edema appears in most adults at plasma albumin concentrations of about 2.5 gm. per 100 ml. This critical level is 0.5 to 1.0 gm. lower in children, who have better tissue elasticity and perhaps lymph flow, than in adults.

It is tempting to attribute the hypoproteinemia to a negative protein balance due to urinary loss of protein. Undoubtedly, this is an important mechanism, for the loss of 10 gm. of protein in the urine daily is roughly equivalent to the drainage of the albumin from more than 200 ml. of plasma. It is likely that a loss of this kind may surpass the possibilities of protein regeneration in some circumstances. The apparent limiting factors in regeneration are (1) protein intake and (2) protein synthesis, especially the synthesis of albumin. The intake of protein in such cases is unfortunately too often limited by the thoughtless prescription of a low-protein diet. It is furthered by anorexia. This is probably the result of edema of the stomach and small bowel, which tends toward a vicious cycle of edema and protein lack. The dietary factor is therefore important and deserving of early correction by the provision of a diet rich in good biological protein calculated to give the nonazotemic patient a maintenance intake of at least 1 gm. per kg. body weight daily of protein plus whatever is needed to supplement urinary loss. It is characteristic in the idiopathic nephrotic syndrome that the hypoalbuminemia tends to be unchanged for long periods until some factor, such as mild infection, alters the homeostasis and is followed by inexplicable loss of edema and increase in plasma protein content. Such is the case of the child who responds favorably to steroid administration. Proteinuria in some patients, especially in those with chronic glomerulonephritis, need not be severe (less than 5 gm. daily, whereas edema and hypoproteinemia may be as extensive as in patients whose proteinuria is marked.

However the hypoalbuminemia may originate, the question arises as to the usefulness of intravenous replacement by transfusion of blood or albumin. Plasma volume is usually decreased. Anemia is not the important factor, so that transfusion of whole blood is not required. Transfusion of plasma or, more specifically, of albumin would seem to be the principal need. Unfortunately, such transfusion can hardly repair the enormous deficit of circulating albumin and, in practice, the albumin administered is rapidly excreted, so that there is no lasting change in plasma protein concentration. Colloid infusions, however, tend temporarily to mobilize water from the tissues and dilute plasma electrolytes and thus stimulate water loss in the urine. Such loss is beneficial and clinically indicated insofar as it relieves edema which has become a hazard or nuisance.

The edema of the nephrotic syndrome results from sodium retention by the renal tubular cells because of the secondary hyperaldosteronism and is therefore advantageously treated by sodium restriction with careful use of agents such as spironolactone or triamterene combined with other diuretic agents. Figure 14–7 schematizes the sequence of altered mechanisms which enter into the nephrotic state.

The mechanism of lipemia in the nephrotic syndrome is still obscure. It is not due to deficient thyroid function and it is not an ineffective homeostatic compensation for lowered colloid osmotic pressure. Rather, it may represent the response to renal reabsorption into the blood of nearly all the lipid from the protein which appears in the tubular fluid. Proteinuric urine contains very little lipid. Possibly cells that are protein-stuffed can still hydrolyze lipoproteins and take up the lipid moiety, hence, in part, their fatty appearance and Bright's "large white" and greasy kidney. Another cause of the visible lipemia is deficiency in albumin which normally serves as a free fatty acid carrier.

The tendency of patients with massive proteinuria to excrete significant amounts of complement has been noted. This, along with the general low level of nutrition, may explain the tendency to infection in nephrosis. Another possible explanation of the low serum complement

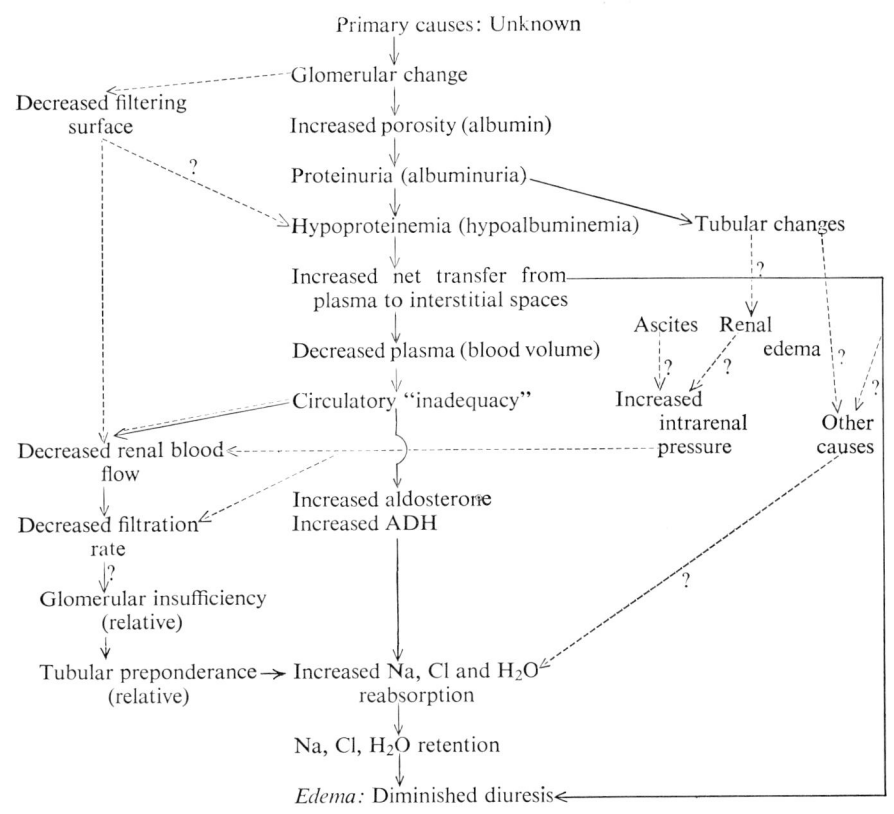

Figure 14-7 Summary of sequential changes in the nephrotic syndrome. (Modified from Eder, H. A., Lauson, H. D., Chinard, F. P., Greif, R. L., Cotzias, G. C., and Van Slyke, D. D.: J. Clin. Invest., *33*:636, 1954.) Solid lines connect processes occurring in established sequence indicated by arrows; dashed lines connect processes which are speculative or of irregular occurrence (e.g., some patients show minimal glomerular lesions and maintain high rates of glomerular filtration).

concentration in patients with chronic glomerulonephritis is that the continuing antigen-antibody reaction which characterizes the disease binds the available complement as it is formed. Especially common, although easily controlled by antibacterials and antibiotics, are erysipeloid infections of the edematous skin of the abdomen, scrotum, and face.

Treatment of nephrotic syndrome with ACTH and/or corticosteroids has now roughly a 20-year background of experience. As with steroid therapy generally (Addison's disease is an exception), the treatment is wholly empirical. The aim is to precipitate diuresis and remission. The same rationale supports the use of newer immunosuppressive agents. The net experience is that corticosteroids will induce diuresis in many children and some adults with the idiopathic nephrotic syndrome, and the diuresis is often associated with diminished proteinuria and relief of hypoproteinemia which, in some cases, is apparently complete and prolonged. The disadvantage of prolonged steroid therapy arises from its many serious side-effects and complications.

However, even when prolonged treatment is duly carried out, a disappointingly large proportion of patients follow the slow, relentless progression into chronic renal failure of chronic glomerulonephritis.

FUNCTIONAL PATTERNS IN RENAL DISEASE

Essential Hypertension

The earliest change in function in essential hypertension is really no change at all. Plasma flow, filtration rate, tubular excretory and reabsorptive capacities, as well as protein and sediment tests, are all normal, because there has occurred an increase in afferent, presumably arteriolar, resistance that maintains a normal intraglomerular pressure and rate of blood flow in the face of increased arterial pressure. Persistence or increased severity of the hypertensive state intensifies this change, increasing afferent resistance in part by causing arteriolosclerosis. Whether by release of renin from stretched "J-G" bodies and formation of angiotensin or otherwise, there also occurs an increase in efferent resistance and intraglomerular pressure. Increased vascular resistance depresses blood flow and increased intraglomerular pressure increases the filtered fraction (filtration fraction = filtration rate/plasma flow) and results in glomerular injury that causes minor proteinuria and cylindruria, although filtration rate is well maintained. Levels of Tm_{PAH} tend to fluctuate downward at this stage, but to a lesser degree than plasma flow. Glucose reabsorption is well maintained, but concentration tests often show some impairment. Administration of a load of hypertonic NaCl solution intravenously results in a more rapid saluresis than occurs in normal persons. Increasing severity of the hypertension tends to speed the rate of these changes, so that the syndrome of malignant hypertension intensifies all these alterations and, if untreated, results in more or less rapidly progressive renal functional deterioration in which proteinuria is the rule and bursts of gross as well as continuing microscopic hematuria are common.

Adequate control of moderately severe and severe hypertension tends to stabilize renal function and prevent further deterioration. A few patients show very distinct improvement. A few others, after a period of stabilization, slowly progress into renal failure, apparently as the result of fibrous hyperplasia of larger renal arteries. The nephrosclerosis that has occurred causes profound changes in architecture of many nephrons, with formation of irregularities and dilatations that provide foci of potential stasis. It is therefore not surprising that patients who have these renal lesions show an increased rate of pyelonephritis in the absence of detectable obstruction in the lower urinary tract. In brief, pyelonephritis may be primary in hypertension, but it seems to be more often secondary. Hence, urine cultures and sediment counts should be done in follow-up visits as well as at the first examination of all hypertensive patients who show signs of renal disease. Lastly, it should be noted that functional changes in patients with essential hypertension are equal and symmetrical in the two kidneys.

Renal Hypertensions

Renal Arterial Occlusion. The advent of aortography and renal angiography led to recognition of occlusive lesions of renal arteries as causes of hypertension. The condition is more common than pheochromocytoma and is often as remediable. Lesions may affect main or branch (segmental) arteries and may be unilateral or bilateral; they range from atheromatous plaques or emboli to fibrous hyperplasia in secondary and smaller branches and "fibromuscular" hyperplasia of main and major arteries. Patients, often with pre-existing hypertension, may suddenly develop hypertension or an exacerbation thereof, as the result of atheromatous occlusion, sometimes with a history of recent flank pain, and occasionally presenting murmurs or thrills over the loins or upper abdomen. Changes in intravenous urograms may not always be recognizable. The radioisotope renogram has, perhaps, its best use in screening such patients for subsequent anatomic diagnosis by aortography.

The "Howard test" consists of demonstrating that ureteral urine from one side has a considerably lower volume and sodium content (and higher osmolality) than urine from the other. Such a change occurs when there is partial occlusion of one main renal artery. If the lesion is in a branch artery, depending on the mass of kidney affected, there results some depression of plasma flow and filtration rate, but without noteworthy differences in sodium concentration or osmolality, so that the functional pattern resembles that found in many patients with bilateral chronic pyelonephritis and is not diagnostic.

The plasma renin activity of peripheral venous blood, or better yet, the differential activities of specimens from each renal vein, is more predictive of surgical cure of renal artery occlusive disease and avoids the morbidity associated with the Howard test.

Pyelonephritis. Chronic pyelonephritis is common. In Brod's study (1956), it was recognized in 6 per cent of routine autopsies but was not diagnosed clinically and was not associated with lower urinary tract obstruction in two thirds of cases. It was associated with hypertension in one third of those with and two thirds of those without recognized obstructive lesions.

The renal functional pattern is overall depression of plasma flow, filtration rate, and tubular excretory and reabsorptive capacities, commonly with a disproportionate decrease in renal tubular concentrating ability. Proteinuria is usually less than 2 gm. per 24 hours. One kidney is commonly affected more than the other. A noteworthy addition to diagnosis is the quantitative culture, obtained on clean-voided urine without catheterization. Other elements in diagnosis are repeated sediment counts, with demonstration of abnormal viable (vital-staining) leukocytes by the Sternheimer-Malbin technique.

Glomerulonephritis. The basic glomerular changes are cellular proliferation, basement membrane disorganization, and, ultimately, fibrous replacement with atrophy of the rest of the nephron. Acute glomerulonephritis may be associated with an increase in renal plasma flow. However, both acute and chronic lesions result in disproportionate depression of filtration rate and decrease in filtration fraction. Concentrating power is impaired in proportion to overall functional loss.

The glomerular lesion results in proteinuria which may be very great and commonly exceeds levels found in both severe hypertension and chronic pyelonephritis. With this is associated hematuria and increased sediment counts of white and renal epithelial cells that tend to be persistent, rather than episodic as in pyelonephritis. The lesion in the idiopathic nephrotic syndrome is a disorganization of podocyte structure and function, which makes for massive proteinuria, without major changes in urine sediment or severe depression of filtering ability, which is sometimes increased. This lesion is reversible, but the condition may continue into renal failure. Other primary glomerular diseases (systemic lupus erythematosus, intercapillary glomerulosclerosis, and so on) yield functional patterns substantially indistinguishable from that of chronic glomerulonephritis and also tend to be associated with a nephrotic state and hypoproteinemia.

Tubular Dysfunctions

Man, more than other species, is prone to hereditary tubular dysfunctions, most of them familial, which may affect single or multiple reabsorptive or excretory functions. Renal glycosuria is one of these. Cases have been reported in which, as in the Dalmatian dog, there is hypouricemia due to impaired urate reabsorption. Nephrogenic diabetes insipidus is a disorder of "porosity" of distal and collecting tubules that makes them unresponsive to ADH. Study of these more or less "isolated" functional defects has clarified knowledge of some tubular functions. In the case of cystinuria—presumed to be a defect of systemic cystine metabolism—renal studies have shown that there is absence of tubular reabsorption of one set of amino acids, viz., cystine, lysine, arginine, and ornithine.

Many of the tubular defects are multiple and sometimes partial, as in the Fanconi syndrome, and several are associated with skeletal lesions, usually with increased phosphate clearance. The number and variety prevents adequate review. This, and more, is provided in Stanbury, Wyngaarten and Fredrickson (see references). However, the Lignac-Debré-de Toni-Fanconi series, with phosphaturia, glycosuria, and aminoaciduria, requires special mention because some are acquired lesions resulting from heavy metal (lead, copper in Wilson's disease) or myeloma. (A similar acquired tubular disorder with associated severe renal tubular acidosis occurs following ingestion of degraded tetracycline.) The hereditary type is either infantile, appearing about the fifth month and associated with cystinosis, or adult, without cystinosis. Sometimes the full series of defects is absent. Thus, there may be phosphaturia with "vitamin D-resistant rickets" and moderate aminoaciduria, but no glycosuria. In what seems to be a milder expression of the same defect, the skeletal lesions may not appear until adult life, as after pregnancy, when they may respond to dihydrotachysterol or other vitamin D-like agents and there is no aminoaciduria or glycosuria.

Renal tubular acidosis of hereditary origin is more common than any of these. It is often associated with renal lithiasis, nephrocalcinosis, and/or remediable metabolic and skeletal defects. The basic abnormality is inability to acidify urine and retain bicarbonate. Secondarily, ammonia formation is reduced. The nature of the defect is not entirely clear, although it is apparently not a selective deficiency of the carbonic anhydrase system. Children seem often to "grow out of it." Inability to retain one anion, bicarbonate, is countered by increased reabsorption of the other major anion, chloride, with resultant hyperchloremic metabolic acidosis. Sodium is lost in excess, and the condition may be complicated by secondary hyperaldosteronism, which adds to the already high rate of potassium loss and results in potassium defect. A decreased urinary concentration of citrate, which normally serves as a chelating and solubilizing anion, in the presence of hypercalciuria (calcium loss is increased with that of other cations), makes for deposition of calcium phosphate in the alkaline medium of tubules and collecting ducts and for renal lithiasis and nephrocalcinosis. Meanwhile, the calcium deficit leads to skeletal lesions. Treatment is by replacement with sodium bicarbonate or citrate, potassium, and, in patients with skeletal lesions, calcium and/or vitamin D.

Renal Failure; Uremia

Deterioration of renal function advances through a stage in which changes in body chemistry are not demonstrable except after stress or during a test of renal function. As this state persists, evidence of generalized metabolic disturbance may appear in the form of resistant anemia, anorexia, and fatigability. In renal failure the patient's economy is in a precarious balance which unusual stress, easily tolerable when renal function is normal, may seriously disturb. Ultimately, the loss of function is lethal even when the patient is protected from situations of special strain.

Uremia is the clinical syndrome which indicates that renal failure has changed the chemistry of the body so seriously as to disable normal functions. Its presence is demonstrated by a combination of clinical and chemical evidence. The symptoms of uremia are weakness, headache, somnolence, apathy and confusion, twitching, convulsions, pruritus, nausea, vomiting, dyspnea, stomatitis, and diarrhea. The resistant anemia invariably present is primarily the result of a reduction in erythropoietin stimulation of the bone marrow, but shortening of red cell survival time is also demonstrable. There is often an associated hemorrhagic diathesis, frequently related to a defect in platelets, which leads to epistaxis, bruising, and melena. Unexplained fibrinous pericarditis occurs in most cases of terminal renal failure and occasionally may be accompanied by significant pericardial effusion. The uremic state may be associated with hypertension and related extrarenal vascular injury, so that to the symptoms of renal failure are added those of cardiac and cerebral damage. This is almost characteristic of the uremia of malignant hypertension. In uremia, congestive heart failure is a common complication and usually is due to overhydration.

Renal Failure and Its Treatment. The consequence of decreased glomerular filtration is that at some point, usually when about 60 per cent of normal function is lost, there develops significant retention in the blood of substances normally excreted by filtration. This change is manifested in elevated blood nonprotein nitrogen and its constituents, urea and creatinine. Decreased tubular reabsorption in some patients results in loss of major electrolytes and water. Such a salt-losing tendency is most commonly seen in chronic pyelonephritis. Failure of tubular secretion is principally reflected in loss of ability to excrete hydrogen ions and to form ammonia, i.e., metabolic acidosis.

ACUTE RENAL FAILURE. The nature of the predominant changes in body fluids which result from renal failure depends largely on the rate at which function is lost and on the volume of urine which is formed. Most renal failures of sudden onset (acute renal failure) result in oliguria or anuria. The predominant change is therefore retention of electrolytes and water which are normally excreted. Such renal failure results in azotemia which may be severe. The cause of death is most commonly infection, but it is very often due to cardiac arrest by potassium poisoning. Such death is sudden and usually occurs about the end of the first week of anuria, unless tissue damage is extensive, in which case it may appear very early.

The importance of potassium intoxication and nitrogenous accumulation is shown by the fact that survival time in anuric rats is inversely proportional to their intakes of potassium and protein. In burns and after crushing injuries to muscles, potassium intoxication is unusually severe because mobilization of tissue fluid releases large amounts of potassium into the circulation. In some of these cases, sodium loss (burns, vomiting) further aggravates the ionic imbalance.

Accumulation of potassium in plasma results in characteristic electrocardiographic changes. First the T waves increase in vertical amplitude, their base is narrowed and the pattern peaked. This is followed by an increase in R and S waves, then by atrioventricular and intraventricular block. The next striking change consists of a loss of P waves. This is followed by depression of the ST segment (obliteration of the segment with the T wave originating from the S wave) and then, finally, by a spread of QRS and T waves into a smooth biphasic curve. T wave elevation commonly occurs in man when plasma potassium reaches about 7 mEq. per liter. P waves disappear at about 9 mEq. per liter, and spread of the QRS complex and death follow at levels of about 10 mEq. per liter. However, the toxic myocardial effects of potassium vary with the balance of other ions, notably Na^+, H^+, and Ca^{++}, so that there is no exact correlation between serum potassium level and the electrocardiographic changes.

Hyperkalemia is countered in several ways. Treatment which is immediately suppressive consists of giving intravenously hypertonic sodium chloride, bicarbonate or lactate, or calcium gluconate. Somewhat slower in action but more prolonged in duration is the administration of glucose (10 to 40 per cent with insulin) by intravenous drip, with the aim of depositing potassium with glycogen intracellularly. More lasting relief is obtained by removal of excess potassium, either by dialysis (peritoneal or blood) or by oral or rectal administration of a cationic resin in the sodium cycle usually with a demulcent such as sorbitol.

Practical hemodialysis had to await the availability of cellophane tubing and heparin, and peritoneal dialysis the antibiotics. Both are now well established in the management of acute renal failure. The procedures consist of dialysis against an isotonic electrolyte solution to which glucose is added. The aim is to restore electrolyte and fluid balance and to remove the accumulated nonprotein nitrogen constituents of the blood.

It is most important in the management of acute renal failure to recognize that these patients cannot excrete water and that they must inevitably drown in any large excess. This is especially the case in post-traumatic or postinfectional failure, in which provision of endogenous water of oxidation by accelerated catabolism may decrease water needs well below amounts estimated from external balance.

CHRONIC RENAL FAILURE. In chronic renal disease the urine volume is usually adequate until shortly before death. Hyperkalemia is not as significant as in acute renal failure. Indeed, in chronic renal failure the mechanism of potassium excretion, inadequately balanced by concurrent hydrogen ion formation, may be so active as to cause actual depletion of potassium.

Muscular twitching and convulsions are thought by some clinicians to be caused by a decrease in the ionized calcium of blood due to renal retention of phosphate. But the relation of symptoms to plasma calcium is tenuous, and it has been suggested that the defect in calcium is in the nervous system itself. Observations in nephrectomized dogs indicate that the onset of twitching is more closely related to increased inorganic phosphate in cerebrospinal fluid than to the increase in plasma. Intravenous administration of calcium tends to relieve twitching. Oral dosage with aluminum hydroxide tends to relieve the hypocalcemia by causing fecal excretion of insoluble aluminum phosphate, thereby lowering serum phosphate levels.

The defect in calcium metabolism extends much further and reaches earlier into the course of renal failure. The depression of ionized calcium secondary to renal retention of phosphate acts as a stimulus to parathyroid hyperplasia, which is manifested functionally and structurally. Functionally, it results in decalcification. This, in the ages of bony growth, accounts in part for some of the syndromes of renal rickets. In adults the bony changes may not be obvious, although areas of decalcification are commonly found in the vertebrae. The result of this hyperfunction is that the clinical and chemical patterns of renal failure with secondary hyperparathyroidism are confusingly similar to that of primary hyperparathyroidism which has resulted in renal failure.

Vomiting, anorexia, and apathy tend to occur early in uremia, often preceding other serious disturbances. They result in undernutrition with loss of weight. In some patients the loss of weight and strength seems to precede other manifestations of renal failure. Apathy and depression in patients and increased blood phenols are certainly associated phenomena, but a definite correlation cannot be established. Guanidinosuccinic acid also has been implicated as a uremic toxin.

Stomatitis, diarrhea, and pruritus are common in uremia when blood urea is greatly elevated. It has been suggested that these are due to liberation of ammonia from the action of oral, intestinal, or cutaneous bacterial ureases on the elevated urea content of saliva, intestinal fluid, and sweat. Such liberation accounts for the ammoniacal odor of the breath of such patients, which, since it is distasteful, may be relieved by a mouthwash containing sodium acid phosphate.

The plasma electrolyte pattern in chronic renal failure is subject to wide variations. Typically, there are increases in plasma SO_4 and PO_4 and, to a lesser extent, of potassium. The loss of sodium and bicarbonate in urine due to failure of reabsorption and diminished H^+ and NH_4^+ excretion tends to deplete plasma sodium, decrease extracellular fluid volume, and lead to acidosis with decrease in plasma bicarbonate.

In patients whose renal function is normal or nearly so, deficits in sodium chloride and bicarbonate can be rapidly repaired by administration of solutions of sodium chloride, depending on the kidney to partition out the excess chloride from the salt, so that sodium bicarbonate is restored to plasma and chloride is excreted. Such dependence is unwise in renal failure. The situation is met by careful intravenous administration of these salts, apportioning them roughly as two volumes of 0.9 per cent NaCl to one volume of 1.3 per cent $NaHCO_3$.

When acidosis is the predominant feature, with resultant dyspnea and discomfort, the administration of alkali is the most urgent need. It is met by infusion of $NaHCO_3$. The amount given in grams is calculated as 0.3 times body weight in kilograms times the deficit in plasma bicarbonate in milliequivalents per liter times 0.084 (times 0.112 when sodium lactate is used instead of bicarbonate). Overzealous administration of alkali may cause tetany due to a reduction in the level of the ionized serum calcium as the blood pH is raised. After correction of acidosis, treatment is completed by administration of sodium chloride solution in an amount sufficient to correct the weight deficit. Patients in chronic renal failure who have polyuria and a salt-losing tendency can be kept in relative comfort for long periods by oral maintenance doses of sodium chloride and sodium bicarbonate. Failure to give such attention in chronic renal failure hastens uremia as a result of oligemia.

The treatment of uremia therefore consists in remedying as best one can the deficits which nature has imposed on the patient. The polyuria of chronic renal disease is treated by administration of adequate volumes of water, with thirst providing the physiologic criterion. Salt restriction, practiced during the nephrotic phase, is substituted by judicious replacement of the salt lost as the result of tubular insufficiency. The deficit of sodium and tendency to acidosis consequent to deficient H^+ excretion and NH_4^+ formation are treated by administration of bicarbonate, either as such or as sodium lactate. Extrarenal excretion of phosphate is accelerated by oral administration of aluminum hydroxide. Uremic osteomalacia may respond to vitamin D, which should be given cautiously and is inappropriate if osteitis fibrosa cystica is present. Potassium intake should be reduced in cases in which potassium is retained.

In chronic renal failure, as in acute, reversible failure, provision of a diet rich in nonprotein calories tends to reduce protein catabolism and alleviate uremia. Special efforts should be made to devise palatable diets high in fat and carbohydrate. Limitation of protein intake to 0.5 gm. per kg. body weight per day, or less, diminishes the accumulation of retained products of protein metabolism. The protein supplied should be of high biological value. Transfusions are only useful in the treatment of the anemia of renal failure if they actually relieve symptoms that are due to the anemia. They should be given with care, since they may precipitate heart failure. It is preferable to give only the red cells. Lastly, anabolic androgen-like substances may be helpful.

In chronic renal disease, there occur hypertrophy of remaining nephrons, especially of their proximal tubules, and osmotic diuresis, which helps to maintain the total amount of urea excreted. Further alterations are decreased relative reabsorption of sodium and potassium, parathyroid hyperplasia, and slowed water diuresis. Conceivably, hypertension and anemia could be considered useful adaptations, since hypertension tends to maintain filtration rate by pressure, and anemia does the same by increasing the volume of plasma per unit blood flow. As stated by Platt, "our concept of renal failure should not be one of disordered function, but rather one of extremely efficient function by a renal remnant too small for its task." This is a good philosophy on which to base our approach to a process in which our present knowledge only permits us to assist rather than contend with nature.

When chronic renal insufficiency is of sufficient degree as to impair the patient's ability to function, other modalities of therapy must be utilized. These include intermittent peritoneal dialysis, chronic hemodialysis either in a center or at home, and renal transplantation utilizing kidneys obtained from either relatives or cadavers. By these means it frequently is possible to extend the useful life of these patients.

REFERENCES

Addis, T.: Glomerular Nephritis, Diagnosis and Treatment. New York, Macmillan Co., 1952.

Black, D. A. K. (Ed.): Renal Disease. Philadelphia, F. A. Davis Co., 1962.

Brod, J., Prat, V., and Dejhar, R.: Early functional diagnosis of chronic pyelonephritis with remarks on the pathogenesis of the pyelonephritic contracted kidney. In Quinn, E. L., and Kass, E. H. (Eds.): Biology of Pyelonephritis (Henry Ford Hospital Symposium). Boston, Little, Brown and Co., 1959.

Corcoran, A. C.: Renal circulation in hypertension. Med. Clin. N. Amer., 45:301, 1961.

Dustan, H. P., Corcoran, A. C., and Page, I. H.: Separate renal functions in patients with renal arterial disease, pyelonephritis and essential hypertension. Circulation, 23:34, 1961.

Earley, L. E.: Diuretics. New Eng. J. Med., 276:966;1023, 1967.

Gottschalk, C. W.: Osmotic concentration and dilution of urine. Amer. J. Med., 36:670, 1964.

Kleeman, C. R., and Fichman, M. P.: The clinical physiology of water metabolism. New Eng. J. Med., 277:1300, 1967.

Laragh, J. H., Ulick, S., Januszewicz, V., DeMing, Q. B., Kelly, W. G., and Lieberman, S.: Aldosterone secretion and primary and malignant hypertension. J. Clin. Invest., 39:1091, 1960.

McQueen, E. G.: Composition of urinary casts. Lancet, 1:397, 1966.

Merrill, J. P., and Hampers, C. L.: Uremia. New Eng. J. Med., 282:953;1014, 1970.

Morris, R. C.: Renal tubular acidosis—Mechanisms, classification and implications. New Eng. J. Med., 281:1405, 1969.

Pitts, R. F.: The Physiological Basis of Diuretic Therapy. Springfield, Illinois, Charles C Thomas, 1959.

Pitts, R. F.: Physiology of the Kidney and Body Fluids. 2nd. ed. Chicago, Year Book Medical Publishers, 1968.

Rutecki, G. J., Goldsmith, C., and Schreiner, G. F.: Characterization of proteins in urinary casts. New Eng. J. Med., 284:1050, 1971.

Smith, H. W.: Principles of Renal Physiology. New York, Oxford University Press, 1956.

Stanbury, J. B., Wyngaarden, J. B., and Fredrickson, D. S. (Eds.): The Metabolic Basis of Inherited Disease. 3rd ed. New York, McGraw-Hill Book Co., 1972.

Strauss, M. B., and Welt, L. G.: Diseases of the Kidney. 2nd ed. Boston, Little, Brown and Co., 1971.

Welt, L. G., Black, H. R., and Krueger, K. K. (Eds.): Symposium on Uremic Toxins. Arch. Intern. Med., 126:773, 1970.

Wesson, L. G., Jr.: Physiology of the Human Kidney, New York, Grune and Stratton, 1969.

CHAPTER 15

PULMONARY VENTILATION AND BLOOD GAS EXCHANGE

ROBERT E. FORSTER

INTRODUCTION

The incidence of lung disease continues to rise with the Gross National Product, and knowledge of the deranged mechanisms will become increasingly valuable to the practitioner. In the past decade there has been a remarkable increase in the quality and availability of apparatus for pulmonary function testing in clinical medical practice, but understanding of the basic physiologic principles has not kept pace.

This chapter is intended to describe in concise and simplified form the disturbances of the physiologic mechanisms of pulmonary exchange which occur in disease. It is not intended to provide the details of pulmonary function tests, on the one hand, or a description of diseases of the lungs, on the other.

It is useful to subdivide function of the lung into the following areas: *Mechanics,* involving the action of the lungs and thorax in pumping gas into and out of the alveoli; *diffusion,* or the exchange of gases between alveolar air and the capillary blood; *circulation,* including the maintenance of pulmonary capillary blood flow, carrying oxygenated blood to the rest of the body; *distribution,* involving the delivery of fresh inspired gas and capillary blood to each alveolus in the same proportion; and *control* of respiration, which modulates the mechanical factors so as to produce the desired alveolar ventilation and arterial CO_2 and O_2 tensions. When the clinician is faced with a disturbance of ventilation, the same approach is helpful in determining the physiologic derangement present.

MECHANICS OF BREATHING

The movements of gas into and out of the alveoli and the associated changes of lung volume are all explicable by physical laws. Today there is a large literature on this subject, much of it extremely complex and not directly related to the practice of medicine. At the same time, the more simple measurements of pulmonary mechanics are easily made and can detect the primary disturbance of lung function in the vast majority of patients.

Lung Volumes,[1] *or Static Mechanics*

The anatomic relations of the diaphragm, chest wall, and lungs at the end of a normal expiration are diagramed and defined in Figure

---

[1] Lung volumes are customarily expressed in liters (or ml.) of gas saturated with water vapor at the patient's body temperature and at the actual atmospheric pressure. This is symbolized as BTPS standing for *B*ody *T*emperature and *P*ressure, *S*aturated with water vapor. Using these determinative conditions the lung volumes represent the actual volumes of the organ in space, rather than a measure of the gas contained, and can be directly compared among patients at various atmospheric pressures and different body temperatures.

Pressures are expressed in cm. of water because in general the water manometer, a simple, reliable instrument, is used to make, or as a reference for, actual measurements. The mercury manometer is not sensitive enough; 1 mm. Hg equals 1.35 cm. water, and one atmosphere, 760 mm. Hg, equals 1026 cm. water, approximated as 1000 cm. water. Pressures are measured in reference to atmospheric and are actually differences. For example, an intrapleural pressure of −2 cm. water means a pressure 2 cm. less than atmospheric, or at sea level, a total absolute pressure of 1024 cm. water.

The numerical values of ventilatory measurements, when given, pertain to a 30-year-old male, 6 feet tall, weighing 170 pounds. In general, pulmonary ventilatory measurements vary with body size, particularly height, age, and sex.

371

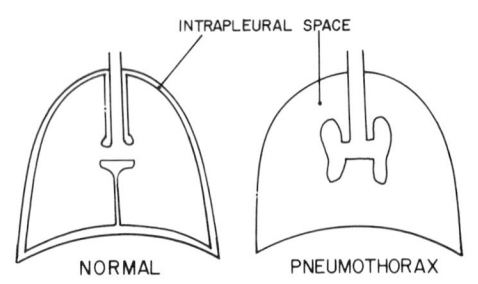

Figure 15-1 Relationship of lungs, thoracic cage, and intrapleural pressure. The diagram on the left represents the situation at the end of a normal expiration, a balance between the tendency of the lung to collapse and of the cage to expand. On the right, the introduction of air into the pleural space (pneumothorax) causes the lungs to decrease in volume and the chest cage to increase in volume.

15-1. The pressure in the pleural space compared to atmospheric pressure is called *intrapleural pressure*. It is sometimes also called the *intrathoracic pressure* because the thoracic contents, heart, great vessels, and esophagus all lie between the parietal pleura and the thoracic cage and are therefore subject to the *intrapleural pressure* (hereafter abbreviated as IPP). IPP is less than atmospheric, and generally varies from -5 to -8 cm. water during normal tidal breathing (Fig. 15-2). When there is no air flowing, alveolar pressure equals atmospheric pressure, and the pressure difference across the lungs equals IPP.[2] At the end of a normal expiration, there is minimal effort or tone of the respiratory muscles. The lungs have a tendency to collapse; if they are out of the chest, their elasticity causes them to empty to about 700 ml. The thoracic cage has a tendency to expand; if the pleural space is open to the atmosphere, the thorax will enlarge. The end expiratory (*functional residual capacity* or FRC) level is the most reproducible volume of the lungs because the tendency of the chest wall to expand is just balanced by the tendency of the lungs to collapse in the absence of respiratory muscle activity. The intrapleural pressure at this point is about -5 cm. water.

When the individual inspires, the diaphragmatic and intercostal muscles contract, tending to expand the rib cage and increase thoracic volume. The intrapleural pressure becomes more negative, producing a larger pressure gradient across the lungs, which expands them. In order to expire passively, the normal mechanism, the patient relaxes his diaphragmatic and intercostal muscles allowing the elasticity of the lungs to decrease the volume of the thoracic cage-lung combination.

The visceral and parietal pleurae can slide over each other, permitting gross movements of the lung parenchyma in relation to the chest wall and diaphragm, but still maintaining thoracic cage and lung volumes equal. This is the body's means of providing minimal friction between sliding surfaces, as in tendon bursae. There is a small fluid volume present in the pleural space in health, estimated at 25 ml., sufficient to make a lubricant film 20 microns thick over the entire surface. The fact that the total dissolved gas partial pressure in venous blood is much less than atmospheric prevents the formation of an air space (pneumothorax) between the pleurae under normal conditions and causes any pneumothorax to resorb if formed (see discussion of blood gases). If gas is introduced into the pleural space, it causes the chest volume to increase and the lung volume to decrease; these changes are about equal in absolute magnitude. Therefore, as the chest physician has known for many years, the lung collapses only 0.5 ml. for each 1.0 ml. of pneumothorax produced.

Tidal volume, normally about 500 ml., is primarily of importance because it is one of the determinants of *minute volume,* the volume of gas pumped into and out of the upper airways per minute.

Tidal volume × Respiratory frequency =
Minute volume   (1)

Thus, tidal volume per se is not of as much clinical concern as the minute volume; in fact, it is the *alveolar ventilation,* the volume[3] of fresh inspired air reaching the alveoli per minute, which is the functionally important gas flow. Abnormalities of tidal volume and minute ventilation will be discussed later.

Vital capacity, the volume of a forced expiration following a maximal inspiration, is the oldest pulmonary function measurement, having been described by Hutchinson in the early 19th century. It requires only a spirometer, and an enormous number of measurements have been collected with it. At this point we will consider only gas volume, not the rate at which it is expelled. The greatest difficulty one has in interpreting a vital capacity measurement is to es-

---

[2] One can consider IPP either a negative pressure outside the lungs or a positive pressure of the same absolute value inside the lungs.

[3] The body normally produces a smaller volume of CO_2 per minute than the volume of O_2 it consumes. This means that the respiratory quotient, CO_2 elimination/O_2 absorption, is less than one. The minute volume exhaled is slightly less than the minute volume inhaled. However, this difference is about 1 per cent and for most purposes can be neglected. This also means the partial pressure of N_2 in the alveoli is greater than that in wet ambient air.

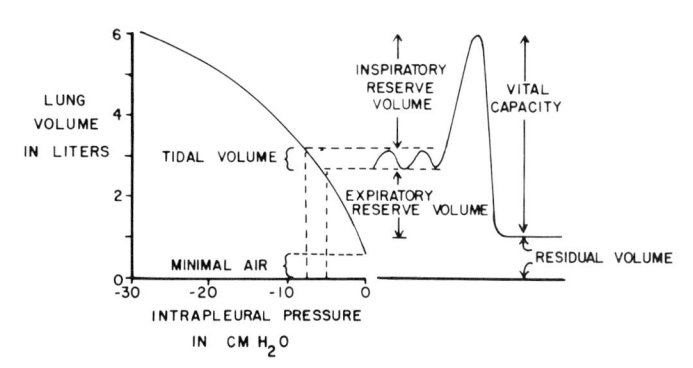

Figure 15-2 On the right is a spirometric tracing of lung volumes. *Tidal volume* (V_T) is the volume of gas inspired, or expired, during a single respiratory cycle, normally under steady-state conditions (500 ml. in this example). *Inspiratory reserve volume* (IRV, 3100 ml.) is the maximum volume of gas that can be inspired from the end of a normal tidal inspiration. *Expiratory reserve volume* (ERV, 1200 ml.) is the maximum volume of gas that can be expired from the end of a normal tidal expiration, the resting end expiratory volume. *Vital capacity* (VC, 4800 ml.) is the maximal volume of gas that can be forced *out* of the lungs by voluntary effort following a maximal inspiration. *Residual volume* (RV, 1200 ml.) is the total volume of gas in the lungs at the end of a maximal voluntary expiration. This is the smallest lung volume a patient can achieve. *Minimal air* is the volume of air that remains in the lungs when there is no difference in pressure between the inside and the outside of the lungs. It can only be reached by opening the chest.

Not shown in the diagram are the following: *Inspiratory capacity* (IC, 3100 ml.) is the maximal volume of gas that can be inspired from the resting end expiratory level. *Total lung capacity* (TLC, 6000 ml.) is the total volume of gas contained in the lung at the end of a maximal inspiration. It equals vital capacity (VC) plus the residual volume (RV). *Functional residual capacity* (FRC, 2400 ml.) is the volume of gas in the lungs at the end of a normal tidal expiration. It equals the expiratory reserve volume (ERV) plus the residual volume (RV).

On the left, the volume of gas in the lung is plotted against the intrapleural pressure. Since the intrapleural pressure is the pressure within the pleural space minus atmospheric pressure, it represents the pressure across the lungs and is more negative outside. These data can be obtained in a patient by measuring changes in esophageal pressure, which equal changes in intrapleural pressure and are independent of the compliance of the chest cage. The slope of the curve is the *lung compliance* and is numerically equal to 0.1 L. per cm. water over the region of normal tidal breathing.

---

timate the value that is normal for that individual. The vital capacity of a healthy individual increases with indices of body frame size, such as height, particularly stem height, rather than weight; decreases with increasing age; and is lower in women than men. Unfortunately, the variation is so great that the best predicted value may still be in error ± 20 per cent for the individual. Thus, one cannot consider a vital capacity reduced unless it is more than 20 per cent less than the predicted value. On the other hand, repeated measurements in the same patient agree to within 200 ml. Therefore the vital capacity is more useful clinically in following changes in lung volume, such as those resulting from treatment of congestive heart failure or asthma.

Only a reduced vital capacity is of clinical importance, and this can result from the following:

1. *Decreased lung gas volume,* produced by space-occupying lesions, such as tumors, atelectasis, pleural effusion, pneumothorax, fibrosis, and decreases in chest cage volume from surgery or kyphoscoliosis.

2. *Decreased ability to inspire or expire maximally.* This could be produced by a decreased muscular force, as from lack of cooperation or pain, or neurologic or muscular disease. It could also be produced by increased resistance to movement of the chest cage, as in arthritis or in the presence of a cast, or of the lungs, as with pleural thickening or bronchial asthma. In the case of severe airway obstruction, the patient may not be able to hold his breath long enough to expire completely.

The resting *end expiratory volume,* the FRC, is the position at which the tendency of the lung to collapse is exactly equaled by the elastic and muscular forces of the chest cage causing it to expand. Although it is the most stable and reproducible lung volume, it is affected by many physiologic factors such as body position, anxiety, pregnancy, and reciprocal changes in *inspiratory reserve* and *expiratory reserve,* which are of little clinical significance.

On the other hand, *residual volume,* RV, must be known to obtain the *total lung capacity,* TLC. In addition, it has intrinsic clinical value because it changes markedly in disease. The residual volume is the air that cannot be expelled from the lungs by a maximal voluntary effort. It will increase (a) if the force required to decrease lung volume becomes greater or (b) if the voluntary expiratory muscular force decreases. The former will occur if the elasticity of the lungs themselves is reduced, as in emphysema, because the tendency of the chest wall to expand will cause the lung volume to be greater for the same expiratory muscular effort. If the chest wall becomes stiffer, as in osteoarthritis or pleural thickening, more effort will be required to expire. The voluntary muscular effort exerted will decrease (b) if there is pain on movement, neuromuscular weakness, or lack of patient cooperation. RV can be increased in the presence of airway obstruction simply because the patient may not have the strength to force the gas out of his lungs before he is driven to take another breath. However, usually RV is increased in chronic obstructive disease because of air trapping; that is, as lung volume decreases with expiration, the finer airways collapse, preventing further gas outflow. RV/TLC in healthy young adults is generally less than 35 per cent. RV/TLC increases with age, so that a value for the ratio over 35 per cent does not of itself make a diagnosis of emphysema as has been stated by some.

RV cannot be measured by spirometry alone, but must be obtained from indirect measurements.[4] Usually the lung volume actually measured is the *functional residual capacity* because it is more reproducible than the RV. Expiratory reserve is then measured carefully on a spirometer and subtracted from FRC to obtain RV.

Total lung capacity, TLC, is obtained by adding RV to vital capacity (VC), and will clearly be altered by the same mechanisms which alter RV and VC. TLC will be decreased when lung parenchymal volume is decreased, as in fibrosis, atelectasis, and space-occupying tumors, and when the patient cannot expand his chest wall normally because of decreased muscular force or increased lung and chest wall stiffness. TLC will be increased whenever lung elasticity is decreased, the most common cause of which is emphysema, or when an increased expiratory resistance chronically impedes lung emptying.

Lung volumes may be considered in the same way as lung anatomy. They may change with disease and give the physician pertinent information, but because they are relatively easy to measure, they are often overemphasized. It is extremely important to realize that the volume of the lung has little importance in gas exchange. It is the alveolar ventilation and lung capillary blood flow which are the determinant factors. However, changes in lung volume may indicate changes in the lung parenchyma associated with disease.

Compliance of the lung is the change in lung volume per change in pressure across the lung, normally about 200 ml. per cm. water in the adult. It is an index of distensibility of the lung and gives a measure of the force needed to expand the lung with respiration. The individual normally has to increase his negative intrapleural pressure by $500/200 = 2.5$ cm. water to produce a change of volume of 500 ml. (A larger pressure has to be developed to overcome airway resistance *during* the actual change in volume.) Compliance is a very useful concept clinically because it gives a measure of the changes in lung elasticity with disease. A decrease in compliance of the lung means the lung has become stiffer, as in fibrosis, pulmonary edema, or pleural thickening. In these conditions, compliance can become as little as 10 ml. per cm. water. Compliance can become greater when the lung becomes more distensible, as it does in emphysema, presumably from loss of elastic tissue. The compliance of the normal lung is larger the greater the lung volume; a change of 1 cm. water in intrapleural pressure will cause a much greater change in the volume of an adult lung than it will in an infant's lung.

Lung compliance, which equals the slope of a graph of lung volume vs. intrapleural pressure (Fig. 15-2), is conveniently measured with a spirometer and an esophageal balloon on the end of a fine plastic tube. This is feasible in most patients and does not require cooperation. Changes in intra-esophageal pressure are equal to changes in intrapleural pressure.

---

[4]Methods of measuring RV include
(a) having the patient wash out all the N_2 in his lungs with O_2, collecting the expirate in a bag, analyzing for N_2, and calculating the original volume of gas containing 80 per cent N_2 in the lung.
(b) having the patient rebreathe in a closed external spirometric circuit of known volume containing a predetermined concentration of a chemically inert insoluble gas such as helium until the concentration of helium becomes the same in the external circuit and in the alveolar gas. Then:

$$\frac{\text{Final He \%}}{\text{Initial He \%}} = \frac{\text{Volume closed circuit}}{\text{Volume lung + Volume closed circuit}}$$

from which the original lung volume can be calculated.
(c) having patient perform respiratory maneuvers in a body plethysmograph. Then:

$$\frac{\text{Change in lung volume (measured by plethysmograph)}}{\text{Lung gas volume}} = \frac{\text{Change in gas pressure in the lungs, measured at mouth}}{\text{Total atmospheric pressure}}$$

From this, lung gas volume can be calculated.

It is technically difficult to obtain a true estimate of the compliance of the chest wall (and for that matter, of the chest wall and lung), because this requires that the respiratory muscles be completely inactive during measurement. Apparently the patient cannot be counted on to achieve this voluntarily and muscle paralysis or anesthesia is necessary. Thus, although measurements of compliance of the thorax would be helpful in assessing pathologic changes in the chest wall, at present these data are not available.

Tissue-Gas Surface Tension in the Lung. There is a surface tension at the tissue-gas boundary which tends to collapse the alveoli, and which increases the force required to expand the lung (decreases the compliance). This can be demonstrated by filling the lungs of an animal with saline, and then determining the pressure needed to expand them. They distend more easily (compliance increases), from which we conclude that the saline-lung tissue interface has less surface tension than the air-lung tissue interface. This normally existing surface tension in the lung must be much less than the surface tension of water in air, because if it were not, we can calculate that an alveolar pressure of over 60 cm. water would be required to keep the lung open at FRC, whereas in actuality, only 2 to 4 cm. water pressure are required.

A material, possibly dipalmitoyl lecithin complexed with protein, can be extracted from minced normal lung or from saline washings of normal lung which markedly decreases the air surface tension of water or saline as measured in a Langmuir trough or with a Wilhelmy balance. The amount of this extractible material present in lungs is decreased in premature infants as compared to full-term infants and in adults. It is decreased transiently following ligation of the pulmonary artery and in several other abnormal conditions of the lung. It has been hypothesized that this in-vitro surfactant material is produced and secreted onto the surface of the alveoli. According to the hypothesis, if its quantity, or effectiveness, is decreased, the function of the lung is impaired. This idea has led to much fruitful experimental work, but final judgment must be reserved at this time.

Air Flow in the Lung: Dynamic Mechanics

Although the lung volumes do change with disease and are important and useful for diagnosis, pulmonary gas exchange does not depend on these volumes over a wide range of values. The functional importance of the mechanics of the lung is in the production of the minute ventilation. On inspiration, the intercostal muscles and diaphragm increase thoracic volume, leading to a decrease in alveolar pressure and producing a flow along the respiratory tract from the mouth to the alveoli. Similarly, during expiration, the elastic recoil of the chest cage-lung combination plus any muscular effort causes an increase in alveolar gas pressure which produces a flow from the alveoli to the mouth. In either case, the rate of flow increases with the magnitude of the pressure gradient. The movement of gas through the airways is opposed by the frictional drag of the gas on the walls, of eddies and of the viscosity of the gas itself. This is known as the *airway resistance*, analogous to the electrical resistance in Ohm's Law and the peripheral vascular resistance of the blood. Pressure, air flow, and airway resistance are related as shown in the formula below. Normal values are about 1.5 cm. water (L./sec.).

Airflow corresponds to current, pressure difference to voltage difference, and airway resistance to electrical resistance. This relationship is only linear to any extent when the air flow is laminar or of the Poiseuille type, in which each particle of gas moves in a straight line through the airways. This condition is present only when there are no branches, bends, or changes in cross section or shape of the bronchial tree. Clearly, this is hardly true anywhere in the lung, but perhaps surprisingly, the relation holds well in practice. When the airflow becomes turbulent, as it may in the larger airways at high flow rates, air velocity becomes proportional to the square, or a higher power, of the driving pressure. However, for clinical purposes this can be ignored.

The concept of airway resistance is extremely useful clinically. Airway obstruction is a major cause of decreased alveolar ventilation, and airway resistance can increase many-fold in asthma and emphysema. At the same time the airway is extremely sensitive to inhalation of pollutants and irritants (when measured in the body plethysmograph) at concentrations that are not detectable subjectively.

Airway resistance depends on the following factors:

1. *Number of patent airways to the alveoli.* When these are decreased by destruction of part of the lung, as with tumors, tuberculosis, or atelectasis, it takes a higher driving gradient of pressure from alveoli to mouth to produce the same flow.

$$\text{Air flow in L./sec} = \frac{(\text{Alveolar pressure} - \text{Mouth pressure})(\text{in cm. water})}{\text{Airway resistance (in cm. water/L./sec.)}} \qquad (2)$$

2. *Cross-sectional area of the airways.* According to the Poiseuille relationship for viscous flow, airway resistance should decrease as the fourth power of the effective radius of the airways. This makes the resistance to airflow at each level of the airway extremely sensitive to slight changes in radius. Changes in the cross-sectional area of the airways can occur because of the following: (a) Contraction of the smooth muscle in the bronchioles and bronchi. Although this is a probable mechanism of obstruction in asthma and possibly other clinical conditions, the extent of its contribution has not been proved. (b) Edema of the tissues of the airways. (c) Secretion into the lumen, or plugging. This is an important factor in asthma in which mucous plugs are frequently found.

3. *Collapse of the airways.* This is an extremely important mechanism and is responsible for the increased expiratory resistance in the majority of patients with obstructive disease. On expiration, both the elastic recoil of the lung-thoracic cage and any muscular effort, indicated by the arrows in Figure 15–3, increase alveolar gas pressure, which produces a gradient from alveolus to mouth and causes expiration. However, the increase in alveolar pressure not only is transmitted through all lung alveoli but also presses on the exterior of the bronchioles and bronchi. If this external luminal pressure becomes greater than the pressure of gas in the lumen and the transmural pressure that can be withstood by the structure of the wall itself, the airway will collapse. This mechanism on a grosser scale causes the bulging of the membranous portion of the trachea and bronchi into the lumen that can be seen with a bronchoscope during forced expiration, even in healthy patients. Airway pressure at a given point will drop below alveolar pressure during expiration because there must be a pressure gradient to overcome the resistance between the alveolus and the point in the bronchiole. This difference will be greater the higher the flow rate and the larger the airway resistance. In healthy individuals the expiratory flow rate eventually reaches a plateau as expiratory effort is increased, and further effort has little effect. This is because intraluminal pressure has fallen far enough below the general lung pressure (alveolar pressure) to cause collapse of the bronchiole walls and prevent further increase in flow rate. A Venturi effect of the flowing gas contributes to this collapse.

The wall of the bronchiole has intrinsic stiffness which must be overcome before it collapses. In addition, stiffening is produced by pull on the outside of the airways from tension in the lung parenchyma. This pull increases as lung volume increases. Therefore, the larger the lung volume, the greater the pressure across the walls of the

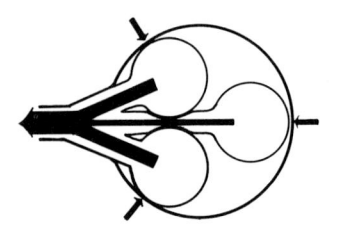

RAPID EXPIRATION NORMAL

Figure 15–3 Mechanism of dynamic airway collapse. Expiratory force, represented by the arrows, is exerted on the lung by the diaphragm and muscles of the thorax, and compresses the gas in all the alveoli. The increased pressure, distributed through the lung, is also applied to the outside of the airways leading from the alveoli. The pressure in the airway lumen must be lower than that in the alveolus to cause gas flow. Thus, the pressure outside the airway can often be greater than the pressure inside by an amount sufficient to overcome the structural resistance of the tissue, leading to narrowing of the diameter, as illustrated, or even collapse.

airways that is required to collapse them. The larger the lung volume, the greater the caliber of the airways and thus the lower their flow resistance. In chronic lung disease there is damage to these tissues from either repeated infection or repeated mechanical trauma from coughing. Thus, the airways collapse and limit expiratory flow at much lower flow velocities. It is important to recognize that airway collapse is a normal phenomenon which is exaggerated in many lung diseases. Even in a healthy young individual some bronchioles shut when lung volume is reduced during expiration to 5 to 10 per cent of vital capacity (designated "closing volume"). This *closing volume* increases with age, approximating end expiratory volume (FRC) at 65 years of age.

The airways do not collapse during inspiration. In this case the most positive pressure is atmospheric, at the mouth. The most negative pressure is in the alveoli, is transmitted throughout the lung, and surrounds the airways. While the pressure in the lumen will be lower than atmospheric during inspiratory gas flow, it will be greater than alveolar, and therefore greater than the pressure surrounding the airway. This transmural pressure will tend to increase airway caliber, instead of collapsing the airway, as occurs during expiration. A forced inspiration will make the net expanding force greater, further lowering airway resistance.

Airway resistance decreases with increased lung volume in normal patients; with expansion of the lung the parenchymal stresses tend to open up the airways, increasing the average radius of the lumen. Airway resistance is lower in larger individuals. Adults and children produce approximately the same cyclic changes in alveolar pressure with breathing, but the minute ventilation in the adult is greater.

How is Obstruction Measured for Clinical Purposes?

The most widely used tests for the presence of obstruction are based on a forced expiration of the vital capacity recorded on a spirometer, which is a ubiquitous instrument in the clinic. It is obvious from the spirometric tracings in Figure 15-4 of a forced expiration of a healthy individual and of a patient with obstructive disease that the latter expires much more slowly. This rate of expiration is greater the greater the alveolar pressure developed by the respiratory muscles and the lower the airway resistance. Although the strength and efficacy of the expiratory effort vary among patients, it appears that these variations are not as great as the variation in airway resistance with disease. Therefore, for practical purposes a decrease in the rate of the forced vital capacity can be taken as an increase in airway resistance, unless there is some clear indication of decreased respiratory effort, as through lack of motivation or muscular weakness.

It is generally impractical simply to produce a spirometric tracing in answer to inquiries as to whether a patient has obstructive disease. Therefore, different indices have been chosen in attempts to represent the important characteristics of the spirometric tracing in a single number, and several of the more common indices are mentioned below. However, the clinician should remember the common origin of these measurements which are highly informative in the majority of patients with chest disease.

Timed vital capacity is the volume of gas that can be expired in a standard time, usually 1, 2, or 3 seconds. This provides the same information as would the measurement of average expiratory flow rate over the same period. The values are often presented as the *fraction of the vital capacity* expired in the given time; for example, 83 per cent of the vital capacity can normally be expired in 1 second. While this is a convenient and simple method of expressing the results, it can mislead the physician because the patient's vital capacity may be grossly reduced, as in pulmonary fibrosis. Thus, although the patient may be able to expire a normal fraction of this vital capacity in 1 second, the absolute amount of gas he can expire is reduced.

Maximal expiratory flow rate is the average rate of flow between 200 and 1200 ml. of expiration and should be from 400 to 600 L. per min. in adults. The first 200 ml. of expirate may come from the mouth and/or compression of the airways, particularly in obstructive disease, and therefore is not included.

Maximal midexpiratory flow rate is the average flow rate during the expiration of the middle 50 per cent of the vital capacity and should be 4 to 5 L. per min.

Maximal voluntary ventilation (MVV), also termed *maximum breathing capacity* (MBC), is the maximal volume of gas (inspiring air) that a patient can expire over a fixed period, usually 15 seconds, choosing his own rate and tidal volume. This is about 100 L. per min. for an adult male. MVV is decreased in obstructive disease, but can also be decreased for reasons other than a higher

Figure 15-4 Superimposed tracings of a forced vital capacity maneuver in a normal healthy adult with a vital capacity of 4000 ml. and a patient with severe emphysema with a vital capacity of only 1730 ml. The normal individual expired 83 per cent of his VC in 1 second, while the patient with emphysema expired only 47 per cent of his VC in 1 second, even though his VC was less than half that of the normal.

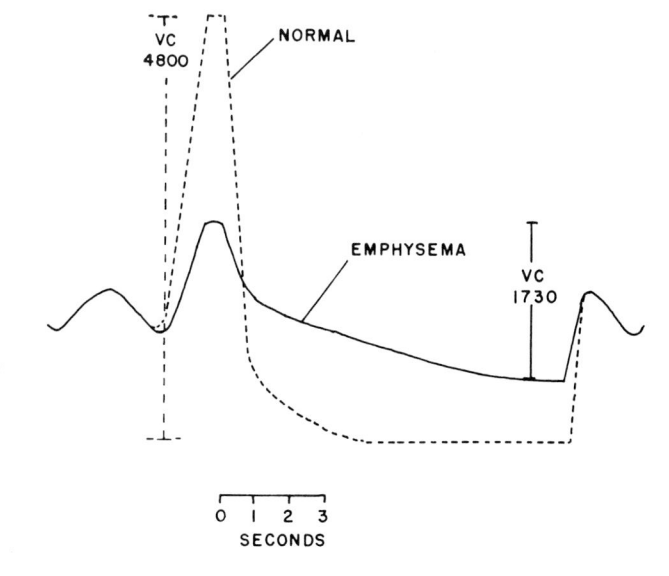

airway resistance, such as lower muscular strength. The test demands considerable exertion, which can rule it out for some patients, and since other tests give the same or more information, it is not always needed. A patient does not use or need all his vital capacity in performing the MVV measurement, so that even in the presence of a reduced vital capacity, such as in pulmonary fibrosis, he may have normal MVV.

Airway resistance, which is the most exact measurement of airway obstruction, can be obtained with more sophisticated techniques, but in general the additional effort required does not produce a corresponding increase in clinically useful information. The calculation of airway resistance requires simultaneous measurement of air flow and alveolar pressure (see Equation 2). The latter is the more difficult to obtain, requiring a body plethysmograph, or esophageal pressure measurements plus corrections for lung elastic pressure.

In normal adults the air flow resistance of the small bronchi (2 to 5 mm. in diameter) plus that of the bronchioles (0.1 to 1.0 mm. in diameter) is 0.5 cm. water per L. per sec., about half the total resistance of the airway from the mouth to the ultimate alveolus of 1 cm. water per L. per sec. The other half of the total resistance, 0.5 cm. water per L. per sec, is produced by air flow through the oro- and nasopharynx, larynx, trachea, and large bronchi. The unobstructed nose has an airway resistance about two and a half times the total resistance breathing through the mouth, that is, 2.5 cm. water per L. per sec. When the nasal passages are obstructed by congestion, the resistance will be many times greater.

Although the air flow resistance of the bronchioles is normally only about 15 per cent of the total resistance breathing through the mouth, it is markedly increased in emphysema and chronic obstructive disease of the lungs and is a major site of obstruction. In these conditions the decrease in the elastic forces of the lung parenchyma decreases the caliber of the smaller airways, and collapse of the airways occurs much more easily. In asthma, the major site of the airway resistance is in the smaller bronchi rather than in the bronchioles. Even large increases in bronchiolar airway resistance cannot be detected by measuring lung airway resistance, because they represent such a small fraction of the total. Therefore, the early stages of bronchiolar disease are difficult to diagnose. However, bronchiolar disease increases lung *closing volume,* which can be measured conveniently.

In children, the bronchioles normally provide about one third of the total airway resistance, a larger fraction than in adults. Therefore, when the child gets bronchiolitis, the interference with respiration is more marked and wheezing is common.

Normally the vocal cords are separated and the epiglottal valve opened during inspiration and expiration, offering minimal resistance to air flow. Edema, spasm, or paralysis of the cords can increase air resistance of the larynx acutely, to the extent of requiring tracheotomy for survival.

Work of Breathing. It requires energy to pump the minute ventilation into and out of the lungs. This energy is supplied by the diaphragm, intercostals, and accessory muscles of respiration. Normally these muscles do most or all of their work during inspiration, overcoming the elastic force of the lung and thoracic cage as well as the viscous resistance of gas flow through the bronchial tree. During expiration the elastic recoil of the lung and thoracic cage exerts a force tending to return the lungs to resting end expiratory level (FRC), so that no muscular effort is normally needed. During a forced expiration or in disease in which expiratory resistance is increased, muscular effort is required.

In general the work of breathing is about 5 per cent of the resting metabolic rate. It is difficult to measure because we cannot easily determine the energy needed to expand the thoracic cage. In contrast with the lungs, the compliance of the chest wall is difficult to determine because we can never be sure that the thoracic muscles are not exerting some force. The compliance of the thoracic cage has been determined during muscle paralysis with drugs, but this is not a useful technique for most patients.

Cough. This maneuver frequently accompanies pulmonary disease. It is produced by closing the glottis, making a forced expiratory effort, and then suddenly opening the glottis, releasing the pent-up alveolar gas. It is generally an involuntary reflex, sometimes a series of uninterrupted efforts, triggered by the stimulation of nerve endings in the larger bronchi, presumably designed to clear the airways. However, the movement of the mucus sheet lining the bronchial tree, impelled by the ciliary beat, is much more important and effective in cleansing the airways. Moreover, it is likely that cough itself leads to parenchymal damage by the following mechanism. During the forced expiratory effort against the closed glottis (Valsalva), gas pressure increases markedly in all alveoli, often to remarkable levels (over 100 mm. Hg). When the glottis is now suddenly opened, the pressure falls first in those alveoli with airways having the lowest resistance. This can leave the intra-alveolar pressure dangerously high in those alveoli out of which the gas has not been able to flow as rapidly. The relative pressure difference across the walls of these disadvantaged alveoli may reach levels high enough (over 40 mm. Hg) to rupture them. It is more likely that this situation will develop in already diseased lungs.

Cough can produce deleterious effects by another mechanism as well. During the Valsalva effort, aortic blood pressure first rises by an increment approximating the change in intraalveolar pressure, high enough to precipitate cerebrovascular accidents, for example. The venous return to the heart is blocked by the continued high intrathoracic pressure, so that cardiac output falls, particularly if the cough is prolonged. This can lead to marked syncope and even to myocardial infarction.

Blood O_2 and CO_2

Before considering the forms in which O_2 and CO_2 are carried in the blood it is necessary to discuss the meaning of the *partial pressure* of a dissolved gas in liquid, because an understanding of this is fundamental to the effective application of arterial blood O_2 and CO_2 measurements to the management of a patient.

Let us expose a few ml. of saline in a tonometer at 37° C. to a gas mixture containing 14 per cent O_2 and the remainder N_2. The partial pressure of O_2, symbolized as Po_2, in the gas will be 14/100 (760 mm. Hg − 47 mm. Hg) = 100 mm. Hg. Gases are analyzed dry and thus it is necessary to reduce the total barometric pressure, 760 mm. Hg, by the vapor pressure of water at 37° C., namely 47 mm. Hg, to obtain the total pressure of dry gas in the mixture.

We now rotate the tonometer in a water bath until diffusion equilibrium has been reached between the gas and the saline. This means that the partial pressure of O_2, Po_2, is the same in the fluid and in the gas, namely, 100 mm. Hg. Po_2 of the fluid is also called its O_2 *tension* in the fluid. The O_2 concentration, on the other hand, the physically dissolved O_2 in ml. per 100 ml., is equal to the Po_2 times the solubility (see formula below). The solubility factor, 0.003 ml. per 100 ml. per mm. Hg is experimentally determined.

We can remove the fluid from the tonometer in a syringe, taking care not to expose it to air. Its Po_2 is still 100 mm. Hg, even though there is now no gas phase. This is, of course, the situation in the blood. The sum of the partial pressures of the gases dissoved in blood does not have to equal atmospheric pressure, although that in arterial blood, which has just equilibrated with alveolar gas in the lung, does. The sum of the partial pressures of dissolved gases in venous blood is significantly less than atmospheric, the exact value depending on conditions.

Blood O_2. We can replace the saline in the tonometer with whole blood and repeat the equilibration procedure. Again, the final Po_2 will be 100 mm. Hg and the concentration of O_2 physically dissolved in both plasma and cell water will be 0.3 ml. per 100 ml. The presence of the hemoglobin does not alter this.

In addition, there will be O_2 reversibly bound to the hemoglobin as oxyhemoglobin (HbO_2), 1.34 ml. O_2 per gram of hemoglobin. The concentration of HbO_2 is defined as the ml. of O_2 gas (STPD)/100 ml. bound. The maximum HbO_2 concentration that can be carried by the blood, determined by equilibrating the blood with air at room temperature, is known as the *blood O_2 capacity*. The normal blood hemoglobin concentration is 15 grams per 100 ml., so that the blood O_2 capacity is 1.34 × 15 = 20 ml./100 ml. If there is a hemoglobin pigment present which does not bind O_2, such as CO hemoglobin or methemoglobin, the total hemoglobin concentration, determined spectrophotometrically as cyanmethemoglobin, may be normal, but the O_2 capacity will be reduced.

When normal whole blood is equilibrated at 37° C. with gas mixtures containing a partial pressure of CO_2 (Pco_2) of 40 mm. Hg, at Po_2 up to 150 mm. Hg, the HbO_2 concentration varies in an S-shaped fashion (Fig. 15-5) with Po_2. It is more convenient to graph the ratio HbO_2 concentration/O_2 capacity, which is called O_2 saturation, than HbO_2 concentration in ml. O_2 (STPD) per 100 ml. blood itself. HbO_2 saturation does not vary with changes in blood hemoglobin concentration and is usually expressed in percentage.

Several important chemical factors can shift the position of the HbO_2 equilibrium curve to the right or left by uniformly expanding or shrinking the curve parallel to the abscissa. Thus the "shape" of the curve remains the same. A shift of the equilibrium curve to the right means that a greater Po_2 is required for a given HbO_2 per cent saturation; in other words, the affinity of O_2 for hemoglobin has decreased. A shift to the left is an increase in affinity. It is useful to indicate the position of the curve by stating the Po_2 at 50 per cent HbO_2 saturation, namely, the P_{50}. An increased P_{50} means a shift to the right and a decreased affinity means a shift of the equilibrium curve to the left. While a decreased P_{50} might be considered an advantage to the patient because it increases the HbO_2 saturation at the same Po_2 in the lungs, it is generally detrimental to the delivery of O_2 to the tissues. This is because O_2 requires a Po_2 gradient to diffuse from the

---

Dissolved O_2 concentration in ml./100 ml. = 0.003 × 100 = 0.3 ml./100 ml. (3)

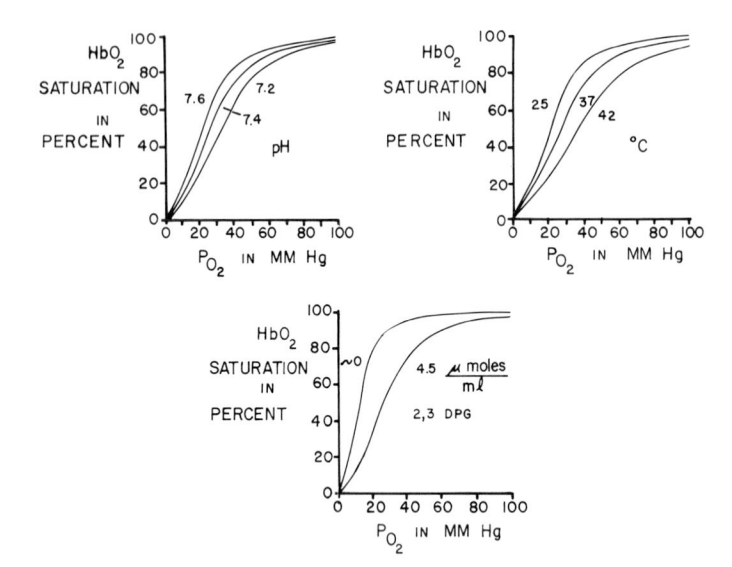

Figure 15-5 Oxygen-hemoglobin equilibrium curves for normal whole blood in which HbO_2 in per cent saturation is plotted against oxygen partial pressure, Po_2, in mm. Hg. The graph in upper left demonstrates the effect of plasma pH (Bohr effect). Temperature was 37° C. Pco_2 was varied to alter the pH to the values indicated on the graph. The graph in the upper right demonstrates the effect of temperature. Plasma pH was 7.4. Temperature was varied 5° above and below the control value at 37° C. The lower graph demonstrates the effect of changing 2,3-diphosphoglycerate concentration (2,3-DPG) in the cell. The concentration of 2,3-DPG is indicated on the figure in micromoles of the compound per ml. cells; 4.5 is normal. pH was 7.4; temperature was 37° C.

capillary blood to the mitochondria. When the HbO_2 equilibrium curve shifts to the left, the capillary blood Po_2 has to fall to a much lower level in order to release the same amount of O_2 in the tissue capillaries. Obviously, this hampers the delivery of O_2 to the tissues from the capillary blood.

As pH decreases, or [H⁺] increases, in the red cell, the HbO_2 equilibrium curve shifts to the right. This phenomenon is known as the Bohr shift. An increase in pH causes a shift to the left. It is the pH inside the red cell that is important, not that in the plasma. However, for general clinical purposes, the difference between plasma and intracellular pH may be considered constant. Intercellular pH is 0.2 to 0.3 units lower.

An increase in Pco_2 causes a right-shift in the equilibrium curve by increasing intracellular [H⁺] secondary to the hydration of CO_2. CO_2 also causes a right-shift by reacting with the terminal valine NH_2 groups on the globin chains of the hemoglobin to form hemoglobin-carbamate. This last specifically decreases the O_2 affinity of the hemoglobin.

In the peripheral tissues, when CO_2 and acid are added to the capillary blood, the resulting shift of the equilibrium curve to the right facilitates the removal of O_2 from the hemoglobin.

DPG (2,3 diphosphoglycerate), which makes up most of the phosphate in the red cell, binds to hemoglobin and decreases its affinity for O_2 (Fig. 15-5). Other phosphates, such as ATP, will also do this to varying degrees. It is extremely important to appreciate that this decrease in O_2 affinity for hemoglobin *increases* capillary Po_2 for the same tissue O_2 consumption and blood flow. A chronic reduction in tissue Po_2, such as occurs in residence at high altitude, chronic obstructive lung disease, or anemia, increases red-cell DPG by influencing the glycolytic metabolism of the cell, and it is reasonable to assume that this is an adaptive phenomenon to maintain normal tissue Po_2 in disease states.

CO has an affinity for hemoglobin about 250 times that of O_2, forming a relatively stable compound, carboxyhemoglobin, that does not dissociate significantly during a passage through the lung or tissue capillaries. Therefore, the fraction of the blood hemoglobin bound to CO is functionally ineffective. In addition, the remaining hemoglobin available for transport of oxygen has an increased O_2 affinity, tending to decrease tissue capillary Po_2 and hinder oxygen unloading in the tissues.

A decrease in temperature of the blood increases the O_2 affinity of hemoglobin (Fig. 15-5). Thus, in the cold, although the extremities may be pink because of the high HbO_2 saturation in the capillaries and dermal venous plexus, the tissues may not be able to maintain a normal Po_2. This can be of concern in artificial hypothermia.

If a patient is placed in a hyperbaric chamber and the inspired Po_2 is gradually increased, the concentration of dissolved O_2 in the arterial blood will increase proportionally, as long as the alveolar Po_2 continues to rise. For example, if a patient breathes approximately 100 per cent O_2 at 2 atmospheres total pressure (1520 mm. Hg), the arterial blood will have a Po_2 of 1430 mm. Hg (there will be 40 mm. Hg Pco_2 and 47 mm. Hg water vapor in the alveoli). Therefore, the dissolved O_2 in the blood will be 4.3 ml. per 100 ml., enough to supply a major part of the body's needs without considering the O_2 bound to the hemoglobin. In contrast, the HbO_2 concentration will rise to equal the capacity, 20 ml. per 100 ml., but will rise no further as inspired Po_2 is increased.

Blood CO_2. The CO_2 equilibration curve for whole blood is shown in Figure 15-6, which is a graph of total blood CO_2 in ml. (STPD) per 100 ml.[5] blood versus Pco_2 in mm. Hg at 37° C. These graphs were obtained by equilibrating normal whole blood with gas mixtures containing partial pressures of CO_2 from 10 to 60 mm. Hg in a tonometer and measuring the total CO_2 content in the blood sample. There are two striking differences between this figure and the blood oxygen equilibrium curve (Fig. 15-7). Over the normal range of blood Pco_2, from 47 mm. Hg in venous blood to 40 in arterial blood, the slope of the equilibration curve is nearly linear, not markedly curved as for HbO_2, and the total CO_2 content is about twice the total O_2 content.

CO_2 is carried in the blood in three forms (see Table 15-1). First is the dissolved CO_2. This is proportional to Pco_2 just as in the case of dissolved O_2, but the solubility factor is twenty times greater, 0.0645 ml. per 100 ml. per mm. Hg. Thus, in normal arterial blood with a Pco_2 of 40 mm. Hg the dissolved CO_2 equals $0.0645 \times 40 = 2.58$ ml. per 100 ml. This is only 5 per cent of the total CO_2 in the arterial blood. Changes in dissolved CO_2 account for only 7 per cent of the total difference in CO_2 content across the lungs. The arterial Pco_2 is extremely important as an index of alveolar ventilation, rising immediately upon hypoventilation and falling with hyperventilation.

Dissolved CO_2 reacts with water to form carbonic acid, which immediately ionizes to H^+ and HCO_3^-. Thus

$$CO_2 + H_2O \rightarrow H_2CO_3 \rightleftharpoons H^+ + HCO_3^- \quad (4)$$

The concentration of H_2CO_3 is about 1/800 of the concentration of dissolved CO_2 and can be neglected. The *blood bicarbonate*, on the other hand, is large, representing about 90 per cent of the total CO_2 in blood. The change in blood HCO_3^- concentration represents 63 per cent of the arteriovenous CO_2 content difference.

CO_2 also reacts with the NH_2 groups on the end of the globin chains to form *hemoglobin carbamate*. The total amount of hemoglobin carbamate in arterial blood is small, but over half is lost in passage through the lungs, contributing about a third of the total CO_2 transported.

---

[5] CO_2 can also be given in millimoles per L. CO_2 content in millimoles per liter = CO_2 content in ml. per 100 ml. $\times 1/2.24$.

If we combine the two reaction steps in Equation 4 in one equilibrium constant, we obtain

$$K' = \frac{[H^+][HCO_3^-]}{[CO_2]} \quad (5)$$

This can be transformed into the Henderson-Hasselbalch equation by taking the logarithm and substituting pH for $-\log_{10} H^+$ and pK' for $-\log_{10} K'$. Thus

$$pH = pK' + \log_{10}[HCO_3^-]/[CO_2] \quad (6)$$

This can also be expressed in terms of Pco_2, which is more useful for the chest physician.

$$pH = pK' + \log_{10}[HCO_3^-]/(Pco_2 \times \text{solubility}) \quad (7)$$

This extremely useful relation permits the calculation of pH from the dissolved CO_2 concentration, or Pco_2, and the bicarbonate concentration.[6] It is the ratio $[HCO_3^-]/[CO_2]$ which determined the pH, and not the absolute values of the concentrations.

The data in Figure 15-6 and Table 15-1 refer to whole blood. The Pco_2 and the dissolved CO_2 are the same in the water of the cells and plasma. However, the bicarbonate concentration of the plasma is greater than that of the red cells because of the negative charges on the hemoglobin which cause the intracellular region to have a negative electric potential with respect to the

---

[6] Normally, $[HCO_3]/[CO_2] = 20/1$. Therefore, pH = $6.1 + \log_{10}(20/1) = 6.1 + 1.3 = 7.4$.

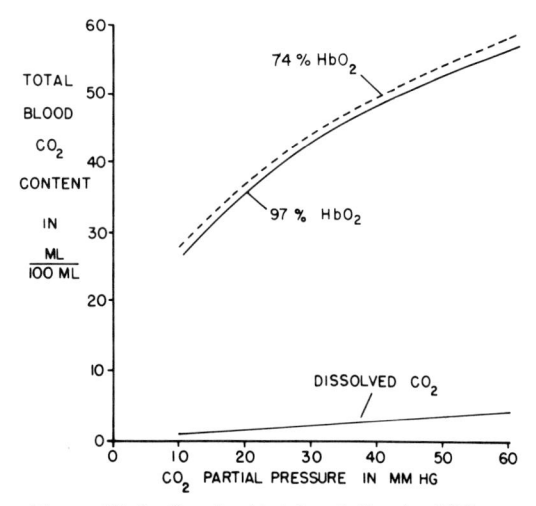

Figure 15-6 Graph of total and dissolved CO_2 content at 37° C. against CO_2 partial pressure for normal blood with Hb saturation of 97 per cent (solid line) and 74 per cent (dotted line).

TABLE 15–1 O_2 AND CO_2 IN ARTERIAL AND MIXED VENOUS BLOOD

	Arterial Blood	Mixed Venous Blood	O_2 or CO_2 Arteriovenous Difference
O_2 partial pressure (Po_2)	95	40	+55.0 mm. Hg
Total O_2 content	19.7	15.1	+4.6 ml./100 ml.
O_2 dissolved	0.30	0.12	+0.18 ml./100 ml.
O_2 combined with Hb (HbO_2)	19.4	15.0	+4.4 ml./100 ml.
O_2 combined with Hb as saturation	97	74	+23%
CO_2 partial pressure (Pco_2)	40	45	−5 mm. Hg
Total CO_2 content	48.20	51.90	−3.70 ml./100 ml.
CO_2 dissolved	2.58	2.84	−0.26 ml./100 ml.
HCO_3^-	43.70	46.04	−2.34 ml./100 ml.
Carbamino CO_2	2.92	4.02	−1.10 ml./100 ml.
pH	7.41	7.39	−0.02 ml./100 ml.

The following normal values were assumed: pulmonary blood flow = 5400 ml./min.; O_2 consumption = 250 ml./min.; CO_2 production = 200 ml./min.; blood O_2 capacity = 20 ml./100 ml.; and hematocrit = 45 per cent.

plasma. Similarly, the [H$^+$] of the cell interior is more than that of the plasma.

Most of the CO_2 removed from the blood in the lungs comes from HCO_3^-. While the reaction of H$^+$ and HCO_3^- to form H_2CO_3 is instantaneous, the uncatalyzed dehydration of H_2CO_3 to form CO_2 is slow, requiring 5 to 10 seconds for completion. Since blood only remains in the lung capillaries 0.3 to 1.0 sec., this means that the CO_2 would not be released rapidly enough if it were not for the presence of the enzyme carbonic anhydrase in the red cells in a concentration high enough to increase the rate of the dehydration of carbonic acid about 10,000 times. This also means that almost all the CO_2 formed from HCO_3^- in the lungs appears inside the red cell and much of the HCO_3^- consumed in the process must eventually come from the plasma, diffusing across the cell membrane in exchange for Cl$^-$ ion. This is known as the chloride or Hamburger shift. The whole process is fast enough to produce chemical equilibrium among alveolar Pco_2, blood Pco_2 and [H$^+$] and [HCO_3^-] in the red cell during one transit through the pulmonary capillary bed.

If the carbonic anhydrase is inhibited, as by acetazolamide, the blood HCO_3^- cannot be hydrated fast enough to form sufficient CO_2 in the capillaries, and CO_2 elimination is hindered.

In order to determine the ventilatory efficiency of a patient's lung, it is ultimately necessary to measure arterial Po_2 and Pco_2. Diffusion exchange of gas occurs in the lung because of a partial pressure gradient and equilibrium is complete when the partial pressure is equal in alveolar gas and arterial blood (see section on Diffusion). Fortunately, electrodes are available commercially for this purpose and are widely used in general hospital practice. The blood sampled should be arterial, because passage through any tissues will alter the blood Pco_2 and Po_2.

The sum of the partial pressures of the dissolved gases in venous blood is *less* than atmospheric, which causes any closed gas pocket in the body to be absorbed. Arterial blood is approximately equilibrated with alveolar gas, and therefore the sum of the gas partial pressures in it approaches atmospheric. In mixed venous blood, for example, the Po_2 has fallen 55 mm. Hg while the Pco_2 has risen only 5 mm. Hg, leaving a deficit of 50 mm. Hg (see Table 15–1). If there is a pneumothorax, the pressure in it will approximate atmospheric.[7] This pressure will be about 40 mm. Hg greater than the sum of the gas pressures in venous blood. This 40 mm. Hg pressure difference will cause the pneumothorax eventually to be absorbed by the venous blood. If the patient is given 100 per cent O_2 to breathe, the nitrogen will be washed out of his lungs and the arterial Po_2 will approach 700 mm. Hg. The mixed venous Pco_2 will still be 45 mm. Hg and the mixed venous Po_2 will rise to only 50 or 60 mm. Hg. Therefore, there will be approximately a *600 mm. Hg pressure difference* between gas in the pneumothorax and venous blood, increasing the rate of gas absorption by about 10-fold. Breathing 100 per cent O_2 does increase the rate of absorption of any gas space in the body, be it the middle ear, pneumothorax, or intestinal gas.

---

[7] Precisely, the total pressure in the pneumothorax will equal intrapleural pressure, which will be only about 5 mm. Hg less than atmospheric.

$$\text{O}_2 \text{ exchange (in ml./min.)} = \frac{\text{D}_\text{L} \text{ (in ml.)}}{\text{min.} \times \text{mm. Hg}} (\text{Alveolar Po}_2 - \text{Average capillary Po}_2) \text{ (in mm. Hg)} \quad (8)$$

DIFFUSION OF GASES IN THE LUNG

The actual exchange of gases in the lungs takes place by diffusion between the alveolar gas and capillary blood. The movement of each gas occurs at a rate which is proportional to the difference between its partial pressure in the alveolar air and its average partial pressure in the capillary blood (see formula above). O_2 exchange, under steady-state conditions, equals metabolic rate. The constant of proportionality, D_L, is known as the *diffusing capacity of the lung*. Its normal value for O_2 in adults is from 25 to 35 ml. per min. per mm. Hg. Its value decreases with (a) decreasing total capillary surface area; (b) decreasing diffusivity or solubility of O_2 or the particular gas of interest in the alveolar membrane (the alveolar membrane consists of the capillary endothelial cell, the capillary basement membrane, the interstitial space, the alveolar basement membrane, and the alveolar epithelium); (c) decreasing average capillary blood volume; and (d) increasing thickness of the alveolar membrane.

Pulmonary capillary blood normally enters the alveolus with a Po_2 of 40 mm. Hg, compared to 100 mm. Hg in the alveolar gas, and rises to within less than 1 mm. Hg of alveolar Po_2 by the end of the capillary. Although the hemoglobin represents a large sink for oxygen in the blood, the diffusing capacity for oxygen is normally large enough to exchange sufficient oxygen to produce near equilibration in one passage through lung capillaries.

CO has approximately 250 times as great an affinity for hemoglobin as does oxygen. When a low (<1 per cent) concentration of CO is inspired, there is an enormous sink for it in the hemoglobin. The amount of CO that can diffuse into the blood during a single capillary transit is only a few hundredths of the amount needed to produce equilibrium between alveolar Pco and capillary blood Pco. Thus, there is essentially no progress toward the equilibration of CO in the lungs. Because the blood Pco and HbCO inside the red cell does not rise significantly, it can be neglected, and the diffusing capacity of the lung for CO becomes

$$\text{D}_{\text{L}_\text{CO}} = \text{CO exchange/alveolar Pco} \quad (9)$$

The fact that we can neglect the erythrocyte Pco has made the use of CO for the measurement of D_L nearly universal. The only alternative gas is O_2, and because the capillary Po_2 rises during transit to approach equilibrium[8] with alveolar gas, the estimation of mean capillary Po_2 is extremely difficult and inaccurate. $\text{D}_{\text{L}_{\text{O}_2}}$ is proportional to $\text{D}_{\text{L}_\text{CO}}$, the proportionality taking into account the differences in solubility, diffusivity, and chemical reaction rates. Thus, for clinical purposes the measurement with CO is equally as useful as a measurement of $\text{D}_{\text{L}_{\text{O}_2}}$ would be. CO is also a "physiologic" gas, because it is always present in the blood, being produced at the rate of 0.4 ml. per hour in the catabolism of heme.

There are several techniques for the measurement of $\text{D}_{\text{L}_\text{CO}}$ in wide use. The *steady-state* $\text{D}_{\text{L}_\text{CO}}$ is obtained by having the patient breathe a gas mixture containing a low concentration of CO for several minutes. The CO uptake is calculated from the difference between the amount of CO inspired and that expired. Alveolar Pco can be obtained from collection of a sample of expired alveolar gas. *Single-breath* or *breath-holding* $\text{D}_{\text{L}_\text{CO}}$ is obtained by having the patient make a single inspiration of a gas mixture containing CO, holding this breath for 10 seconds, and then expiring an alveolar gas sample which is collected and analyzed. CO uptake is calculated from the change in alveolar CO concentration over the 10 seconds, multiplied by the alveolar gas volume. Alveolar Pco is also obtained from the expired sample.

It has been found experimentally that during the uptake of CO in the lung at a normal alveolar Po_2, 100 mm. Hg, plasma Pco, as contrasted to intracellular Pco, is not zero. This occurs because, in spite of the small size of the red cells, the rate of chemical reaction of CO with hemoglobin occurring simultaneously with diffusion through the very high intracellular concentration of the protein is too slow to bind the gas as rapidly as it enters the plasma. Another way of looking at it is to consider that there are two resistances opposing the diffusion of CO from alveolar gas to its final combination with the hemoglobin molecule. One is the diffusion resistance of the alveolar membrane, consisting of endothelium, basement membrane, and epithelium. The second is the resistance to the uptake of CO by the red cells in the alveolar capillary

---

[8] A stable isotope of oxygen, $^{18}\text{O}^{16}\text{O}$, can be used to circumvent this problem because it is not completely equilibrated between alveolar gas and capillary blood at the end of transit. However, this technique is complicated and requires the use of a mass spectrometer, so that the use of CO remains the method of choice.

bed at any time. With an alveolar Po_2 of 100 mm. Hg, about half the diffusion resistance to CO uptake is in the alveolar membrane and half in the red cells themselves. Thus, the overall diffusing capacity of the lung, D_L, has two subdivisions: the *diffusing capacity* of the *membrane*, D_M, in ml. CO diffusing per min. per mm. Hg of Pco difference between alveolar gas and blood plasma, and the *diffusing capacity* of the *red cells* themselves, in ml. CO diffusing into the cells per min. per mm. Hg of Pco difference between the plasma outside the cells and the cell interior. The diffusing capacity of the cells is customarily expressed as the volume of blood in the pulmonary capillary bed (V_C) times the rate of CO uptake by one ml. of this blood per mm. Hg of Pco in the plasma (θ).

Raising alveolar Po_2 leads to a decrease in the diffusing capacity of the red cells for CO because the actual chemical combination of CO with hemoglobin can take place only when a bond to an iron atom is free. As Po_2 rises, the saturation of HbO_2 increases and the number of uncombined bonds that are free at any instant falls, decreasing the rate of formation of carbon-monoxyhemoglobin. In symbols, θ falls as Po_2 rises; the higher the alveolar Po_2, the lower the $D_{L_{CO}}$. This must be taken into account during interpretation of measurements of $D_{L_{CO}}$ in patients. Breathing 80 per cent O_2 or more, the resistance to CO uptake presented by the red cells increases to such an extent that the resistance to gaseous diffusion across the alveolar membrane can be neglected. Therefore, the diffusing capacity of the lung for CO becomes equal to the diffusing capacity of the red cells, so that

$$D_{L_{CO}} = \theta V_C \tag{10}$$

θ can be obtained from in-vitro measurements using rapid-reaction apparatus. It decreases with increasing Po_2 and rises proportionally to hematocrit, so that these factors must be specified. Using measurements of $D_{L_{CO}}$ at high alveolar Po_2, the pulmonary capillary blood volume, V_C, can be obtained with Equation 10. V_C is normally from 60 to 100 ml., a relatively small portion of the 500 to 1000 ml. in the lesser circulation.

CO_2 has a solubility in water about 20 times that of CO and O_2, so that its diffusing capacity will be that much greater than that of O_2. Since the capillary blood Po_2 is largely equilibrated with alveolar gas at the end of capillary transit, Pco_2 will certainly be the same in blood at the end of the capillary and alveolar gas, even in pathologic conditions, provided that only the alveolus is aerated at all. A patient would perish from arterial anoxemia long before his diffusing capacity decreased sufficiently to produce a CO_2 diffusing gradient between alveolar gas and blood at the end of the alveolar capillaries. This is an extremely important point for the chest physician, because it is a necessary condition in the use of arterial Pco_2 as a measure of alveolar ventilation.

The greater an individual's body size, the greater his pulmonary diffusing capacity. This is necessitated by the increase of oxygen consumption with body size. With exercise, $D_{L_{CO}}$ and pulmonary blood flow increase, although mean pulmonary arterial pressure does not rise significantly until the blood flow has increased more than twofold. This indicates that the pulmonary vascular bed has large reserves. Because of this, destruction of a portion of the total lung capillary bed may not lead to a significant reduction of $D_{L_{CO}}$, at least at rest, because other capillaries open up to replace those lost.

A syndrome, *alveolar-capillary block*, has been described in which the primary dysfunction is a decrease in the diffusing capacity of the lung, producing arterial hypoxemia in spite of relatively normal alveolar ventilation. This fits the clinical concept of pulmonary fibroses such as scleroderma, berylliosis, and sarcoidosis. It has turned out that there is also a considerable element of uneven alveolar ventilation/capillary blood flow in these patients. On reconsideration, this is eminently reasonable because an alveolus with extreme reduction in diffusing capacity becomes, in effect, a venous-arterial shunt across the lungs.

The term *pulmonary edema*, as generally used, includes both (a) thickening of the space between the endothelium and epithelium in the alveolar membrane with edema fluid and (b) filling of the alveolar space with edema fluid. The former produces only minimal lowering of D_M with slight reduction of arterial Po_2. Arterial Pco_2 is normal because diffusing capacity for CO_2, although also reduced slightly below normal, is about 20 times greater than that for O_2. When the alveolus is filled with fluid, it is not aerated at all, and resembles a shunt; neither O_2 nor CO_2 are exchanged. Thus, in pulmonary edema an alveolus is either functionally near-normal or obliterated, and the physiologic abnormality is uneven alveolar ventilation/capillary blood flow.

$D_{L_{CO}}$ is decreased in anemia because of the decrease in the number of red cells in the alveolar capillaries at any time, but it is not decreased sufficiently to lower arterial Po_2 significantly.

In emphysema the single-breath $D_{L_{CO}}$ is normal or slightly decreased. On the other hand, the steady-state $D_{L_{CO}}$ is reduced so predictably that this test is often used to diagnose the condition. The apparently contradictory results of the two methods occur because the steady-state method is reduced in the presence of uneven distribution of alveolar ventilation/capillary blood flow, which is a hallmark of emphysema. The single-breath test is relatively uninfluenced by distribution abnormalities. The failure of single-breath $D_{L_{CO}}$ to decrease in emphysema renders suspect the historic hypothesis that the basic pathologic process is the destruction of the capillary bed.

In asthma, $D_{L_{CO}}$ is relatively normal, an important point in differentiating this condition from the chronic obstructive conditions.

PULMONARY CIRCULATION

As the simplified diagram in Figure 15-7 shows, under normal conditions the entire cardiac output flows through the pulmonary capillary bed. However, the vascular resistance in the lung is much less than that of the periphery, so that the pressure in pulmonary artery is much less than that in the aorta.

The hemodynamics of the pulmonary circulation are complicated because the vascular resistance is influenced by three extravascular pressures:

1. *Atmospheric pressure.* The fine alveolar capillaries, which contain no muscle or supporting structures are surrounded by alveolar pressure, which will always be within several mm. Hg of atmospheric pressure, provided that the glottis is open. If the blood pressure within the capillaries becomes less than alveolar pressure (minus surface-tension forces), the vessels will collapse.

2. *Intrapleural pressure.* The great vessels and right and left heart are surrounded by intrapleural, also sometimes called intrathoracic, pressure. Thus, as intrapleural pressure falls in relation to ambient pressure with inspiration, pressure in the right and left sides of the heart also falls.

3. *Pressure in the abdominal cavity.* This pressure surrounds the inferior vena cava. When it increases, as from constriction of the abdominal and diaphragmatic musculature, an increased pressure gradient is produced from abdomen to thorax, and venous return rises. During Valsalva maneuver, or cough, the respiratory muscles and diaphragm contract against a closed glottis, raising the intra-alveolar as well as intrapleural pressure with respect to ambient. The normal pressure gradient from abdominal vena cava and neck veins to the right heart is decreased in magnitude and the return of blood to the heart is reduced, leading to a decrease in cardiac output and eventual fall in peripheral blood pressure.

The pressure inside the lung capillaries is about 10 mm. Hg above the right auricular pressure. However, the apex of the lung is about 15 cm. above the right auricle in the upright position. The hydrostatic pressure of a 15-cm. column of blood equals 11 mm. Hg, for the density of mercury is 13.7 times that of blood. Right auricular pressure is the accepted reference blood pressure, but since it is within the intrapleural region, it will be lower than atmospheric by an amount equal to the intrapleural pressure. Assuming an intrapleural pressure of −5 cm. water, which approximates −3 mm. Hg, the average pressure in the pulmonary capillaries at the apex of the lung will be 10 − 11 − 3 = −4 mm. Hg, 4 mm. Hg less than the pressure in the alveoli, causing them to collapse. When the lung volume increases, the intrapleural pressure around the heart will fall, lowering the capillary pressure even further with respect to atmospheric. Although the numbers are only approximate, this means the blood flow through the apical capillaries will be less than that through the bases. During exercise, with increased pulmonary blood flow, or when there is vascular congestion in the lung capillary bed, as in mitral stenosis, the higher pressures tend to keep the apical capillaries open.

Control of Pulmonary Circulation

Although there are sympathetic and parasympathetic nerves to the vasculature of the lung, their influence on the pulmonary circulation is equivocal. In general it is concluded that sympathetic stimulation leads to constriction and parasympathetic stimulation to vasodilation, based in part on analogy with the measured, but weak vasoconstriction produced by epinephrine and norepinephrine and the vasodilation produced by intra-arterial acetylcholine. The most important chemical factor affecting the pulmonary circulation is hypoxia, which causes vasoconstriction through an unknown mechanism. Young healthy individuals living at high altitude

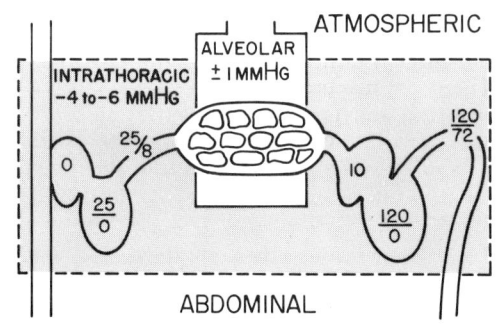

Figure 15-7 Schematic diagram of the pressure relationships of the pulmonary circulation. The shaded area indicates those parts of the circulation exposed to intrapleural pressure. The numbers give typical systolic/diastolic pressures in mm. Hg with reference to the right auricular pressure as zero. In reference to atmospheric pressure, the right auricular pressure (range −3 to −5 cm. H$_2$O) falls several mm. Hg during inspiration and rises again with expiration. Note that the pressure surrounding the capillary bed is approximately atmospheric, regardless of lung volume.

have remarkably high pulmonary artery pressures which fall to normal levels when arterial Po_2 is raised. In general, diseases accompanied by arterial hypoxia show increased pulmonary arterial pressure, presumably on the same basis.

NONUNIFORM ALVEOLAR VENTILATION/CAPILLARY BLOOD FLOW

The Pco_2 and Po_2 of each alveolus in the lung is determined by the ratio of the fresh inspired gas reaching it, that is, its alveolar ventilation, to the blood flow through its capillary bed. An alveolus which is relatively hyperventilated, which means its alveolar ventilation/capillary blood flow is high, will have a decreased Pco_2 and an increased Po_2. Conversely, a relatively hypoventilated alveolus, one with a decreased alveolar ventilation/capillary blood flow, will have an increased Pco_2 and a decreased Po_2. The value of either alveolar capillary blood flow or alveolar ventilation alone does not necessarily affect the alveolar Po_2 or Pco_2. An alveolus with a decreased alveolar ventilation can have a normal arterial Pco_2 and Po_2 if capillary blood flow is decreased in the same proportion and there exist mechanisms controlling local blood flow and ventilation to perform this regulation. The ideal situation is for the alveolar ventilation/capillary blood flow to be the same in each alveolus. This comes close to being realized in the normal healthy lung of a person lying down. However, in the upright position, capillary blood flow tends to be lower in the apices and greater in the bases for reasons discussed in the section on Pulmonary Circulation. On the other hand, minute ventilation tends to be higher in the apices and lower in the bases; one important cause for this is that the weight of the lung makes inflation of an alveolus in the basal region more difficult. The net result is a high alveolar ventilation/capillary blood flow in the apices, with a corresponding decrease in Pco_2 and rise in Po_2. The reverse is true for the bases. The local mechanisms for control of airway resistance and capillary blood flow act to reduce the nonuniformity.

In many lung diseases this delicate adjustment is deranged, such as by destruction of some capillaries or local increases in airway resistance. This results in an increased arterial Pco_2 and a decreased arterial Po_2, even though the total lung minute ventilation and total capillary blood flow are normal. One can say that nonuniformity of alveolar ventilation/capillary blood flow produces an inefficiency of ventilation. This has a greater effect in decreasing arterial Po_2 than in increasing arterial Pco_2, because of the different shapes of the blood O_2 and CO_2 equilibrium curves. Let us suppose a patient's lung has one portion which is hyperventilated and one which is hypoventilated in relation to capillary blood flow. Considering first the case of CO_2, the hyperventilated region will have an alveolar Pco_2 less than 40 mm. Hg (see Figure 15–6) and the hypoventilated region will have a Pco_2 greater than 40 mm. Hg. The blood draining the hyperventilated alveoli will have a CO_2 content less than normal, that is, less than 47 ml. per 100 ml., and that draining the hypoventilated alveoli will have a CO_2 content greater than 47 ml. per 100 ml. The mixture of these venous bloods in the arteries will have a CO_2 content approximating 47 ml. per 100 ml., giving an arterial Pco_2 of about 40 mm. Hg. The hyperventilated region can compensate, at least in large part, for the hypoventilated region.

In the case of O_2 (see Figure 15–5), the hyperventilated alveoli will have a Po_2 greater than the normal value of 100 mm. Hg, but this will not elevate the HbO_2 saturation at the end of the capillaries much over the normal value of 97 per cent because of the bend in the HbO_2 equilibrium curve. On the other hand, the hypoventilated alveoli will have a Po_2 less than 100 mm. Hg and the blood draining these alveoli will have a HbO_2 saturation less than 97 per cent. Thus, the mixed blood in the peripheral arteries will have a saturation less than 97 per cent and the arterial Po_2 will be significantly less than 100 mm. Hg. Even though the total minute ventilation, total pulmonary capillary blood flow, and pulmonary diffusing capacity are all normal, uneven distribution of alveolar ventilation/capillary blood flow leads to a decreased arterial Po_2. Arterial Pco_2 is theoretically also increased but to a much lesser degree, often insignificantly.

For these same reasons in clinical conditions with markedly uneven alveolar ventilation/capillary blood flow, particularly emphysema, arterial Po_2 is decreased, while arterial Pco_2 is relatively normal, rising only later in the disease when the nonuniformity becomes extreme.

There is no practical, sensitive method of measuring uneven alveolar ventilation/capillary blood flow clinically, but there are methods available[9] for the determination of the distribu-

---

[9] Examples of these methods are the *single-breath N_2 test* for the uneven distribution of inspired gas, in which the patient inspires a large volume of O_2 and then expires while a meter follows the concentration of N_2 in the breath. Normally, this N_2 concentration reaches a plateau in the expired alveolar gas. If uneven distribution of inspired gas is present, this plateau shows a marked upward slope. The expired N_2 concentration shows an additional abrupt rise when lung volume reaches *closing* volume and some bronchioles shut. The rate of N_2 washout while breathing O_2 or the rate of equilibration of alveolar gas with helium in an external rebreathing circuit also give indices of unevenness of inspired gas.

$$\text{Alveolar ventilation} = \text{Respiratory frequency} \times (\text{Tidal volume} - \text{Dead space volume}) \quad (11)$$

tion of inspired gas with respect to *alveolar volume* throughout the lung. The presence of severely uneven distribution of inspired gas indicates a breakdown in lung architecture, which has been reliably found to associate with uneven alveolar ventilation/capillary blood flow in chronic pulmonary disease states. It is for this practical reason that tests of distribution of inspired gas are considered diagnostic of nonuniformity of alveolar ventilation/capillary blood flow.

Alveolar Ventilation

It is not the minute ventilation, which is the volume of gas moving in and out of the mouth per minute, that is important as far as the respiratory gas exchange in the lung is concerned, but the volume of fresh inspired gas that reaches the alveoli. The inspired gas that passes the lips does not immediately enter the alveoli to exchange with pulmonary capillary blood, but must first flow through the pharynx, larynx, trachea, bronchi, and bronchioles where no significant gas exchange with blood occurs. The total volume of the conducting airways is known as the *anatomical respiratory dead space*[10]; the adjective "dead" is fitting because an equivalent volume of inspired air is lost or "dead" as far as ventilation of the alveoli is concerned. The adjective "anatomical" indicates that it applies to true geometric volume of the airways.

The size of the anatomical dead space of a normal individual in ml. is approximately numerically equal to his weight in pounds. A 150-lb. man has a dead space of 150 ml. At the start of inspiration, the dead space is filled with expired alveolar gas remaining from the preceding breath. After 500 ml. has been inspired, the volume of the alveoli will have increased 500 ml., but 150 ml. of this will be previously expired gas that was in the dead space. Only 500 ml. − 150 ml. = 350 ml. would be fresh inspired gas (see formula above).

---

[10]It must be distinguished from the effective or "physiologic dead space," discussed in the section on uneven distribution.

Alveolar ventilation is given in ml. per min., frequency in breaths per min., and volumes in ml. This is a very practical and useful equation, permitting the physician to calculate the volume flow of minute ventilation needed for a patient if the dead space is known. For a given minute ventilation, which equals frequency × tidal volume, alveolar ventilation is greater if tidal volume is large and rate is slow, because dead space volume is constant. For example, if the patient referred to above has a respiratory frequency of 15 breaths per min., the minute ventilation is 15 × 500 = 7500 ml./min. Alveolar ventilation will be 15 × (500 − 150) = 5250 ml./min. If the patient reduces his rate to 10 breaths per min. and increases his tidal volume to 750 ml., the minute ventilation will remain at 7500 ml. per min., but alveolar ventilation will become 10 × (1750 − 150) = 6000 ml./min. Since the goal of the ventilation is to aerate the alveoli, this represents an improvement of 750 ml. per min., for the same minute ventilation.

Alveolar Ventilation Defined by Arterial P_{CO_2}. Possibly the most helpful, in many patients the only, approach to an estimate of alveolar ventilation is by means of the arterial P_{CO_2}. The basis for the method is as follows: CO_2 in ml. per min. eliminated by the lungs must equal alveolar ventilation × the fractional concentration of CO_2 in alveolar gas. This is so because alveolar ventilation is the volume flow of gas out of the alveoli that leaves the mouth and because there is no CO_2 in the inspired gas. Arterial P_{CO_2} is in equilibrium with alveolar gas, even in severe lung disease, as discussed in the section on Diffusion. Therefore, we can substitute arterial $P_{CO_2}/760$ mm. Hg for the fractional CO_2 concentration in the alveolar gas. Under steady-state conditions, the CO_2 eliminated from the mouth equals the metabolic rate (see formula below). The metabolic rate of a patient is independent of the function of the lungs (except for the slight work of breathing) and is determined by those factors that control tissue metabolism such as bodily activity and work, body temperature, and level of thyroid hormone. The variation in metabolic rate among patients is small, because measurements are generally made at rest. As a practical matter, the magnitude of arterial P_{CO_2}

$$\text{Metabolic } CO_2 \text{ production} = \text{Alveolar ventilation} \times \frac{\text{Arterial } P_{CO_2}}{760} \quad (12)$$

depends only on pulmonary function, including the control of respiration. Thus, an increased arterial Pco_2 (normally 40 mm. Hg) means a decrease in alveolar ventilation (hypoventilation). A decrease in arterial Pco_2 indicates increased alveolar ventilation (hyperventilation). Today, arterial blood can be obtained with ease and Pco_2 determined with an electrode on several ml. of blood. Therefore the measurement is available in most patients and is of tremendous clinical utility.

Abnormalities of Alveolar Ventilation. A decrease in alveolar ventilation causes CO_2 retention. It can be produced by several mechanisms, the most obvious of which is a decrease in minute ventilation. The lower minute ventilation can result from abnormalities such as muscle weakness in myasthenia gravis, neurologic disease as in poliomyelitis, damage to the ventilatory regulatory system from damage to the central nervous system in a cerebral accident, and central depression from pharmacologic agents as in general anesthesia or intoxication.

Another mechanism is an increase in physiologic dead space, the most common cause of which is uneven alveolar ventilation/capillary blood flow as seen in emphysema. Anatomical dead space can be increased artificially, as it is when respiratory tubing is connected to the airway. It can be decreased by tracheostomy, which is sometimes done surgically to increase alveolar ventilation in patients with CO_2 retention. Alveolar ventilation is also decreased if respiratory rate rises and minute ventilation and dead space volume remain constant. Under these conditions, tidal volume is reduced and the constant dead space represents a larger fraction of the minute ventilation (see Equation 11).

CONTROL OF RESPIRATION

The major center of integrated respiration is in the medulla oblongata above the obex. Minute ventilation is normally regulated by the arterial Pco_2 and is extremely sensitive to changes in this value; an increase of 1 mm. Hg in arterial Pco_2 increases minute ventilation 2.5 L. per min. This effect is produced by Pco_2 sensors in the medulla, although the peripheral chemoreceptors, the aortic and carotid bodies, contribute.

Minute ventilation also increases when arterial Po_2 decreases but far larger changes in Po_2 are required as compared to those in Pco_2. For example, the arterial Po_2 has to fall from a normal value of 100 mm. Hg to about 70 mm. Hg before a reliable increase in steady-state minute ventilation occurs. The influence of decreased arterial Po_2 on minute ventilation is exerted through the peripheral chemoreceptors. A decreased arterial Po_2 depresses rather than stimulates the medullary respiratory center.

A decrease in arterial pH stimulates minute ventilation. This can be seen in diabetic acidosis, in which the arterial Pco_2 is reduced, arterial Po_2 is slightly increased, and arterial pH is reduced. Only the decreased arterial pH among these three factors could be causing the *increase* in minute ventilation. It is difficult to separate the effects of an increased Pco_2 and a decreased pH, since one will rapidly produce the other in the blood or other body tissues.

An increase in cerebrospinal fluid Pco_2 or a decrease in its pH stimulates respiration by acting upon superficial regions of the medullary center which are bathed in the fluid. This is not an important mechanism for rapid readjustments because the chemical composition of the CSF changes slowly as compared to that of arterial blood, but it is important for slow adaptations such as that of living at high altitude. There is an active transport mechanism between the CSF and blood which regulates CSF bicarbonate concentration to maintain normal pH.

The CO_2-sensitive medullary center is depressed by analgesics, sedatives, and anesthesia as well as lowered arterial Po_2. On the other hand, the peripheral chemoreceptors are rugged, relatively uninfluenced by drugs, and stimulated, not depressed, by anoxia.

The rhythmicity of respiration is produced by the medullary center and ceases if this part of the brain stem is destroyed. However, this rhythm resides in the myriad interneuronal connections rather than in the individual cells themselves. This is contrasted with the heart, in which each cell is inherently rhythmic, although at different rates.

Afferent vagal impulses from endings in the lung and airways modulate the respiratory movements. It is important for the surgeon to leave these fibers intact in the course of any surgical procedure, such as gastric vagotomy. Sensory afferents produce an expulsive cough when the surface of the upper airway is stimulated. These particular endings do not extend much further into the lung than the carina, so that large foreign bodies can lodge below this level and give no sign of their presence.

The minute ventilation can be altered by volition, within limits. The length of time a patient can hold his breath, the *breath-holding time*, increases with increasing initial alveolar Po_2 and decreasing alveolar Pco_2 and if movements of the lungs and chest wall are possible (breathing a gas mixture of the same composition as alveolar gas, so that there is no change in alveolar Po_2 or Pco_2). It is not a good test of pulmonary function or athletic ability. Under various circumstances, an individual can hold his breath long enough to produce anoxic damage and unconsciousness. Breath-holding while swimming under water is particularly hazardous because the individual commonly hyperventilates before submerging. This reduces the usual stimulus to respiration from alveolar P_{CO_2} and enables the swimmer to hold his breath to a much lower alveolar P_{O_2}. Movement of the chest accompanying swimming as well as the expiration of small amounts of lung gas reduces the normal inspiratory stimulation from the nerve endings of the lungs and thorax. Thus, the respiratory drive depends predominantly on the alveolar P_{O_2} which may fall so low as to produce unconsciousness from anoxia before the swimmer is compelled to surface and inspire. If he is swimming at any depth, the hydrostatic pressure on his chest and on the gas in his lungs as he rises to the surface decreases, reducing the alveolar P_{O_2} as well. Swimmers all too frequently have amnesia for the period after they have swum under water, or, if they are unfortunate, pass out and drown while floating on the surface.

Ventilation is accomplished by a control system involving negative feedback. The peripheral chemoreceptors and medulla sense an increase in arterial P_{CO_2}, which is integrated along with all the other information concerning the state of respiration. The respiratory center then sends out nervous impulses to the lower neurons of the respiratory muscles, and minute ventilation increases, lowering arterial P_{CO_2} toward normal. This system acts as a whole, and special efforts have to be made to determine the function of the different components. A patient with increased arterial P_{CO_2} does not necessarily have a depressed respiratory center; he could also have increased airway resistance or muscular paralysis, requiring a greater number of nervous impulses to the muscles to produce a normal amount of respiratory effort, which in turn requires a high P_{CO_2}.

In exercise in a normal individual, arterial P_{CO_2} and P_{O_2} are maintained so close to resting levels in spite of the increase in CO_2 production that it is not clear what has caused the large increase in ventilation. There are numerous explanations, such as the stimulation caused by afferents from muscles and joints, but we do not have a wholly satisfactory answer. The *maximal voluntary ventilation* (or MVV) is normally greater than the peak ventilation during exercise. Thus, there is a reserve ventilation which is not used.

Minute ventilation decreases during sleep; arterial P_{CO_2} rises. This presumably results from a general reduction in tonic impulses on the respiratory center. Patients whose alveolar ventilation is already marginal when they are awake may become critically hypoventilated when they are asleep, lowering arterial P_{O_2} and raising arterial P_{CO_2}. The administration of sedatives or even analgesics at bedtime exacerbates this situation.

In patients with chronic CO_2 retention and increased arterial P_{CO_2}, the minute ventilation becomes less sensitive than normal to the level of the P_{CO_2}, and these patients react as if the level of arterial P_{O_2} acting through the chemoreceptors had become the dominant control of ventilation. If one of these patients is now given a high concentration of oxygen to breathe, the respiratory drive is reduced and arterial P_{CO_2} rises, even to the point of coma, convulsions, and death. The patient should not be denied oxygen, which can be life-sustaining, but he should be carefully observed to be sure he maintains an adequate minute ventilation.

Cyclically varying minute ventilation, such as Cheyne-Stokes breathing, may be seen, particularly with central nervous system damage. Although the exact alteration in the normal control system is not known, it is possible to imitate the phenomenon in animals by introducing a delay in blood flow from the lungs to the chemoreceptors and medullary respiratory center.

There is no clinically useful drug which stimulates minute ventilation specifically. Those which are widely employed, such as caffeine and amphetamine, are generally central nervous system stimulants. Progesterone may be an exception. It increases ventilation, accounting for the lower arterial P_{CO_2} in pregnancy. The mechanism is unknown. Salicylates produce a chemical acidosis which stimulates respiration nonspecifically, but in addition the drug stimulates respiration directly. The result is that in salicylate intoxication, ventilation is stimulated to such a degree that blood pH becomes alkaline in spite of a metabolic acidosis, offering a confusing picture to the physician.

Stress or anxiety can produce a hyperventilation through the higher central nervous centers. This lowers arterial P_{CO_2}, which reduces cerebral blood flow, which in turn causes dizziness, producing more anxiety. The vicious cycle can end in tetany and convulsions, particularly in neurotic patients.

Abnormalities of Respiration

Anoxia. Anoxia means a lack of oxygen, assumedly at the tissue level, although the term is vague in current context. Anoxia of a tissue cell can be caused by the following:

1. *Decreased arterial* P_{O_2}. This has been called anoxemic anoxia. It could result from any of the causes listed in Table 15-2, decreased inspired P_{O_2}, decreased alveolar ventilation, uneven distribution of alveolar ventilation/capillary blood flow, or a right-to-left shunt.

2. *Decreased capacity of the blood for oxygen (anemic anoxia).* Anemia, COHb, methemoglobi-

nemia, or abnormal types of hemoglobin (hemoglobin M) could produce this.

3. *Reduced blood flow to the tissue (stagnant anoxia)*.

4. *Shift in the oxygen-hemoglobin equilibrium curve to the left.* Because oxygen can move only by diffusion during the last part of its journey to the cytochromes, that is, from the capillary to the mitochondria, P_{O_2} in the capillary blood is the ultimate determinant of the oxygen supply to the tissues. Even when tissue oxygen consumption is not elevated and capillary blood flow, arterial P_{O_2}, and arterial HbO_2 concentration are normal, if the affinity of hemoglobin for oxygen is increased (decreased P_{50}) the capillary venous blood P_{O_2} will have to decrease below normal in order for the amount of oxygen required by the tissue to be extracted from the blood. This reduces the P_{O_2} at the mitochondria and can cause it to fall low enough to produce local anoxia of the cell.

5. *Inhibition of the cytochromes in the cell (histotoxic anoxia).* Cyanide poisoning produces this type of anoxia.

Cyanosis. Cyanosis means blueness of the skin and is interpreted clinically as an indication of the presence of an abnormal amount of deoxygenated hemoglobin in the blood. However, it is not a sensitive index of arterial unsaturation. The average clinician cannot recognize cyanosis until the arterial HbO_2 saturation is less than 85 per cent saturated, corresponding to an arterial P_{O_2} of about 50 mm. Hg, which is grossly reduced. The color of the skin depends more on the color of the blood in the venous plexus of the skin than on that in the arterial side; thus, a slow circulation can lead to local cyanosis even with a normal arterial HbO_2 saturation. Anemia reduces the amount of deoxygenated hemoglobin in the blood at the same P_{O_2}, and thus may conceal the presence of a considerable reduction in HbO_2 saturation.

Dyspnea. Dyspnea, which means difficult breathing, is a subjective symptom and is for practical purposes a translation of "shortness of breath." It can be present even though arterial P_{O_2} and P_{CO_2} are within normal limits. Probably the mechanical difficulty of breathing is the most important factor in producing the sensation in a patient. Numerous theories have been proposed to explain dyspnea, generally relating it to an increased mechanical effort of breathing, but none are completely satisfactory and it remains a subjective symptom.

Acid-Base Disturbances.[11] The lungs excrete about 13,000 mEq. per day of acid (as carbonic acid) and can alter this rate immediately following a change in alveolar ventilation. The kidney normally excretes less than one eleventh as much acid per day in the form of nonvolatile acids (fixed acids) but requires minutes to change this rate. On the other hand, the lungs cannot excrete any fixed acids or electrolytes, which all must leave through the kidney. *Acidosis* is defined as a decrease in plasma pH below the normal range of around 7.4; *alkalosis* is defined as an increase in plasma pH above this range.

ACIDOSIS. Probably the most common blood disturbance of ventilatory origin is *respiratory acidosis*. This results from a decreased alveolar ventilation, also called alveolar hypoventilation, which will increase arterial P_{CO_2} in a second, leading to the formation of additional H^+ and HCO_3^-. The buffers in the blood, mainly hemoglobin and phosphates, bind much of the H^+ produced, but there will still be a net reduction in plasma pH. If the hypoventilation is maintained, extravascular tissues buffer H^+ in addition to that bound in the blood, reducing the increment in H^+ concentration. Referring to the Henderson-Hasselbalch equation, P_{CO_2} and dissolved CO_2 concentration will increase more than HCO_3^- concentration, reducing the logarithmic term and lowering pH. After a matter of minutes, the kidneys will start compensating for the acidosis by excreting more acid, freeing additional Na^+ to form more $NaHCO_3$, which tends to return the plasma pH toward normal. The end result is *chronic respiratory acidosis*, which is common in emphysema and other obstructive diseases. It is characterized by an acid pH, increased P_{CO_2}, and increased HCO_3^- concentration of arterial plasma. Acidosis also results from increased formation, or retention, of nonvolatile acids, such as phosphoric, lactic, and keto-acids in the body. These *fixed acids* displace HCO_3^- from the blood and decrease plasma pH, producing a *metabolic acidosis*. The decrease in arterial pH stimulates respiration per se, leading to a decrease in arterial P_{CO_2} below the normal 40 mm. Hg, which tends to raise pH again toward normal. Thus, metabolic acidosis classically has a decreased plasma pH, a decreased plasma HCO_3^- concentration, and a decreased P_{CO_2} in the arterial blood.

ALKALOSIS. Alkalosis is defined as an increase in plasma pH above the normal 7.4. Hyperventilation leads immediately to a decreased arterial P_{CO_2} and a lowering of blood CO_2 content. Equal amounts of H^+ and HCO_3^- are consumed in the formation of expired CO_2. Because the concentration of H^+ is about 10^{-5} that of HCO_3^-, this decreases plasma H^+ concentration proportionally far more than it decreases plasma HCO_3^- concentration. Therefore, pH increases and HCO_3^- decreases. Just as in the case of hypoventilation, extravascular tissues buffer the pH

---

[11]This is not intended as a complete discussion of blood acid-base, but only of salient points particularly related to ventilation abnormalities. The reader is referred to Chapter 32 for a more detailed discussion.

changes in the blood, if the hyperventilation is maintained, attenuating the rise in plasma pH. The kidney retains acid in an effort to compensate for the rise in arterial pH as well. Thus, in respiratory alkalosis there is a primary decrease in arterial Pco_2, a rise in arterial pH, and a fall in blood HCO_3^- concentration. A metabolic *alkalosis* can also occur from loss of H^+ via routes other than the lung. An example is excessive vomiting with loss of HCl from the stomach. Plasma pH rises above 7.4, and for the same alveolar ventilation, that is, the same arterial Pco_2, blood HCO_3^- concentration rises. However, the increased alkalinity of the blood acts on the respiratory control system to reduce alveolar ventilation and raise arterial Pco_2, reducing plasma pH toward 7.4. Thus, in metabolic alkalosis arterial pH is increased and blood HCO_3^- concentration is increased, as is arterial Pco_2.

The situation in an actual patient is often a combination of metabolic and respiratory disturbances, distorted by the body's compensatory responses and by therapy, and is therefore much more complicated than this very brief outline indicates.

The physician cannot tell from knowledge of blood CO_2 content or blood bicarbonate concentration alone what the acid-base disturbance is. Blood CO_2 content is increased in respiratory acidosis but is also increased in metabolic alkalosis. Blood CO_2 content is decreased in respiratory alkalosis but is also decreased in metabolic acidosis. It is necessary to know the three variables in the Henderson-Hasselbalch equation in order to be able to determine a patient's acid-base status, that is, arterial plasma HCO_3^- concentration, pH, and Pco_2. Only two of the three need be measured; the third is thereupon calculable. In the past, blood total CO_2 and pH have been the measurements generally obtained, but with the present availability of Pco_2 and pH electrodes, it has become more common to make these measurements instead. The arterial Pco_2 has the intrinsic advantage that in addition to the information it provides about acid-base status, it is the best estimate of alveolar ventilation.

Causes of Abnormalities of Arterial Po_2 and Pco_2

Table 15-2 summarizes the effects of different functional abnormalities of the lung on arterial Pco_2 and Po_2. A decreased inspired Po_2 leads to a decreased arterial Po_2, which in turn causes hyperventilation because of stimulation of the chemoreceptors (carotid and aortic bodies) which lowers arterial Pco_2 secondarily. A decreased alveolar ventilation, whether from decreased minute ventilation or increased dead space volume, will lead to an increased arterial Pco_2 and a decreased arterial Po_2. A reduced pulmonary diffusing capacity will tend to decrease arterial Po_2, more markedly in exercise, but will leave arterial Pco_2 normal, or slightly decreased as a secondary result of respiratory stimulation. Uneven alveolar ventilation/capillary blood flow will reduce arterial Po_2 but leave arterial Pco_2 normal. As the disease progresses, the unevenness of distribution will become more severe and the arterial Po_2 will drop further and eventually the arterial Pco_2 will rise.

The effect of a right-to-left shunt across the lung is similar to that of uneven alveolar ventilation/capillary blood flow, in that the effect on arterial Po_2 is much more severe than that on arterial Pco_2. However, it is possible to distinguish between these two dysfunctions by having the patient breathe 100 per cent oxygen long enough to wash out the N_2 in the lungs. There is almost no difference between alveolar and arterial Po_2 under these circumstances in the presence of uneven distribution, but if there is a true shunt, the arterial Po_2 will be strikingly

TABLE 15-2 FACTORS ALTERING ARTERIAL Po_2 AND ARTERIAL Pco_2

	Arterial Po_2	Arterial Pco_2
↓ Inspired O_2 concentration or high altitude	↓	↑
↓ Alveolar ventilation (hypoventilated)	↓	↑
↑ Alveolar ventilation (hyperventilated)	↑	↓
Uneven $\dfrac{\text{Alveolar ventilation}}{\text{Capillary blood flow}}$	↓↓	↑
↓ Diffusing capacity of lung	↓	No effect
Right-to-left shunt across lung (Breathing air)	↓	↑
(Breathing 100% O_2)	↓↓↓	↑

less than alveolar P_{O_2}. Under these conditions each alveolus will have a partial pressure of water of 47 mm. Hg; a partial pressure of CO_2 which will vary with the alveolar ventilation/capillary blood flow, but cannot be greater than mixed venous P_{CO_2}, about 50 mm. Hg; and a partial pressure of O_2. Since the total must equal atmospheric, the P_{O_2} in any alveolus will be in the range from 580 to 613 mm. Hg. An alveolar P_{O_2} this great will saturate the hemoglobin with oxygen early in the passage of the blood through the capillary bed and will then rapidly raise the blood P_{O_2} to equal alveolar, because the oxygen is now acting like an inert gas (see discussion on Diffusion). Thus, the blood leaving each alveolus will have a P_{O_2} from 580 to 613 mm. Hg. Only if there is a shunt across the pulmonary capillary bed can arterial blood have a P_{O_2} significantly less than this.

High Altitude.
The removal of an individual to a higher altitude reduces the inspired P_{O_2}, leading immediately to a decreased arterial P_{O_2} and stimulation of the aortic and carotid bodies. This produces an increase in minute ventilation, which in turn lowers arterial P_{CO_2} and increases arterial pH, tending to reduce minute ventilation acting through the medullary respiratory center. In a matter of minutes to hours the decreased arterial P_{CO_2} leads to a decreased cerebrospinal (CSF) fluid P_{CO_2}, raising CSF pH (see the Henderson-Hasselbalch equation). This acts to lower minute ventilation through the chemosensitive regions on the surface of the medulla. If the individual remains at high altitude, a series of compensatory changes takes place. The concentration of bicarbonate in the CSF is decreased by active transport into the blood, lowering the CSF pH and increasing minute ventilation. Red blood cell 2,3-diphosphoglycerate (2,3-DPG) increases, shifting the HbO_2 equilibrium curve to the right (a decreased affinity) and improving the delivery of O_2 from the capillary bed to the tissues in the periphery. The decreased arterial P_{O_2} produces an increased excretion of erythropoietin from the kidney, leading to an increased formation of red cells. The kidney also compensates for the increased arterial pH by excreting an alkaline urine and Na^+, to reduce plasma bicarbonate concentration.

The decreased arterial P_{O_2} tends to increase pulmonary arterial resistance. Apparently healthy adults may develop acute pulmonary edema with right but not left ventricular failure. The pathogenesis of this syndrome is unclear.

Oxygen Toxicity.
Although oxygen is essential for life, there is a growing realization that having a patient breathe an oxygen-enriched atmosphere is not without some hazard. The most obvious site of toxic effects is in the lungs. Breathing 100 per cent O_2 for as little as 12 hours produces irritation of the airways and lungs and reduces the vital capacity. Longer exposures produced capillary congestion, edema, and thickening of the alveolar membrane. The exposure of infants to increased P_{O_2} has been incriminated as the cause of retrolental fibroplasia. The retina is peculiarly sensitive to oxygen in many species. Recently, breathing oxygen has been shown to produce damage to the alveolar parenchyma in infants, so that increased inspired oxygen should only be administered to infants if their arterial P_{O_2} is known to be low.

Breathing 100 per cent oxygen at greater than 3 atmospheres produces so-called "oxygen toxicity," with restlessness, convulsions, unconsciousness, and death. The situation is reversible if the inspired P_{O_2} is immediately reduced. This great an inspired P_{O_2} is seen only in pressure chambers or in underwater swimming. The mechanism, or mechanisms, by which oxygen produces its toxic effects is not known. If high O_2 pressures are inspired by a patient with a right-to-left shunt across the lungs, arterial blood P_{O_2} does not rise as high as in a normal subject and no acute signs of "oxygen toxicity" develop, indicating that it is the arterial P_{O_2} and not the alveolar P_{O_2} that is important in CNS toxicity.

The rate of a chemical reaction is proportional to the effective concentrations of the reactants. In the case of O_2 consumption in tissues, one would therefore expect it to increase with increased inspired O_2. Such is apparently not the case. Human oxygen consumption does not vary significantly as inspired P_{O_2} increases from the lowest safe level (around 50 mm. Hg) to over 2000 mm. Hg. The oxygen consumption of mitochondria and even of the electron transport particle, that unit of the mitochondrion which contains the respiratory enzymes, is independent of P_{O_2} from less than 1 mm. Hg to nearly 2000 mm. Hg. This represents a molecular mechanism of chemical control which is not understood at present.

REFERENCES

Bates, D. V., Macklem, P. T., and Christie, R. V.: Respiratory Function in Disease. 2nd ed. Philadelphia, W. B. Saunders Co., 1971.

Comroe, J. H., Jr., Forster, R. E., II, DuBois, A. B., Briscoe, W. A., and Carlsen, E.: The Lung, Clinical Physiology and Pulmonary Function Tests. 2nd ed. Chicago, Year Book Medical Publishers, 1962.

Comroe, J. H., Jr.: Physiology of Respiration, Chicago, Year Book Medical Publishers, 1965.

Davenport, H. W.: The ABC of Acid-Base Chemistry. 5th ed. Chicago, University of Chicago Press, 1969.

Fenn, W. O., and Rahn, H. (Eds.): Handbook of Physiology. Vol. II. Section 3, Respiration. Washington, D.C., American Physiological Society, 1965.

CHAPTER 16

PROTECTIVE MECHANISMS OF THE LUNGS; PULMONARY DISEASE; PLEURAL DISEASE

JOHN H. KILLOUGH

INTRODUCTION

For the lungs to perform their basic function as a membrane for two-way gaseous exchange between the external and internal environments, it is necessary that they be in constant contact with air. Thus, the lungs are exposed to air which may contain dust, bacteria, fungi, viruses, and various other noxious agents. For defense against these potentially harmful materials the lungs possess a complex of protective mechanisms. Disruption of these mechanisms by internal changes or overwhelming onslaught from without accounts for many pulmonary diseases. To understand these disease processes, some knowledge of the structure and function of the various elements of the respiratory system is necessary.

Although the respiratory tract is divided arbitrarily into upper and lower portions, it functions as a physiologic unit directed toward the cleansing, warming, and humidification of ventilated air, and gaseous exchange. From the nasopharynx to the alveoli there are many gross and microscopic changes in structure which reflect these different physiologic functions.

Nasopharynx

Air entering the upper passage is grossly filtered by hairs in the nose and further filtered, warmed, and humidified as it comes in contact with the moist mucous membranes of the turbinates. At sites where air currents strike the membrane, cilia are present which beat in a coordinated fashion, so that particles are swept toward areas where they can be expectorated, swallowed, or expelled by nose blowing. Absorption from the olfactory area occurs rather freely; thus, various allergens and infectious agents as well as medications may enter at this level.

Trachea and Bronchi

The trachea branches into the right and left bronchi, and this pattern of dichotomous division is repeated with decreasing cross-sectional diameters to the level of the respiratory bronchioles. Here the branching becomes much more extensive and gives rise to alveolar ducts, alveolar sacs, and alveoli.

Structurally, the trachea and bronchi contain more or less the same elements, although there are important quantitative variations. They have been divided into layers on cross section: the epithelial, the subepithelial, the muscular, and the adventitial layers. The first three layers are most important in terms of protective mechanisms and diseases and will be briefly described.

The *epithelial layer* consists of ciliated columnar cells, among which are interspersed goblet cells. This pattern persists throughout the trachea and bronchi until bronchioles are reached which are 0.4 mm. in diameter. Here the goblet cells disappear and the cilia-bearing cells become cuboidal and interspersed with nonciliated cuboidal cells. Finally, in smaller bronchioles the ciliated cells disappear altogether.

Sensory fibers of the trigeminal, glossopharyngeal, and vagal nerves are present at various levels in the mucous membranes of the pharynx, larynx, trachea, and bronchi. Stimulation of these fibers by irritating substances results in cough. At present it is not known whether ciliary action is under nervous control; however, it is quite evident that the activity of the cilia is coordinated by some means.

The *subepithelial layer* lies between the basement membrane upon which the epithelial cells rest and the muscular layer. It is composed largely of connective tissue elements, arterioles, venules, and capillaries of the bronchial vasculature. There are also fibers of the vagi and sympathetics distributed to the blood vessels. The lymphatic vascular system is found in this layer and it should be appreciated that it represents one of the most extensive in the body. The lymphatic capillaries do not extend to the alveoli but appear at the level of the alveolar ducts. From Miller's diagrams it is evident that the lymphatics form a plexus about the arteries and the airways and anastomose at the level of the alveolar ducts, with a somewhat separate system about the pulmonary veins. Lymph flow in the periarterial and peribronchial vessels is believed to be centrifugal, whereas the flow in the perivenous vessels is centripetal and into the hilar lymph glands. Peripheral connections are made with the lymphatic plexus in the pleura. The pleural lymphatics form a set which unites into a variable number of trunks and drains into lymph nodes at the hilum. One of the peculiarities of the pulmonary lymphatic system is that nearly all the lymph from both lungs drains into the right lymphatic duct. Only lymph from the left upper lobe drains into the thoracic duct. There are, however, frequent connections between the two sides, so that this separation is not entirely complete. These patterns are of importance in the understanding of metastatic spread of infection and malignant disease. As in other parts of the body, lymph flow is dependent upon the movement of tissues. In the central portions of the lung, movement is restricted by large vascular and bronchial structures, with resultant sluggish lymph flow. As a consequence, in certain disease states accompanied by pulmonary edema, the edema, as revealed radiographically, may be more marked centrally and in a "butterfly" arrangement.

The *muscular layer*, composed entirely of smooth muscle, is so extensive that it is said to be impossible to cut through a cubic millimeter of lung without encountering muscle. It extends from the trachea to the alveoli, where occasional delicate muscle fibers have been identified in the walls. The helical turns of crisscrossing muscle fibers are almost circular in the larger bronchi but the turns become steeper peripherally. This more or less circular arrangement of the muscle fibers provides efficiency in constriction as well as strength against high intraluminal pressures. Innervation of the musculature is via the vagi and sympathetics, which, by their activity, may produce constriction and relaxation, respectively. However, it is most likely that the changes in bronchial diameter during normal respiration are a passive phenomenon without an element of alternating vagal and sympathetic activity. Beneath the smooth muscle are the longitudinal elastic fibers which passively resist the expansion of inspiration and by elasticity alone bring the airways back to their resting length on expiration.

The submucosal glands which extend throughout the three outer layers produce a mucoprotein secretion of varying viscosity. Secretion occurs on vagal stimulation, but the effect is largely a quantitative rather than a qualitative one.

Cartilage, which at first is regularly disposed and almost surrounds the trachea and large bronchi, eventually becomes fragmented into irregular plaques, and in bronchioles disappears altogether. Where cartilaginous support is absent, the encircling muscle fibers can produce maximal constriction.

Alveoli

The respiratory bronchiole divides twice, giving rise to three orders of respiratory bronchioles. The third order then divides into two alveolar ducts, which in turn divide five to eight times and terminate as alveolar sacs. There are occasional small projecting spaces called alveoli on the walls of the first-order respiratory bronchioles. With continued branching, the frequency of these alveoli increases markedly until at the level of the alveolar sacs the walls are beset solidly with alveoli. The walls of the alveoli consist of a moist surface (see Surfactant, p. 396), a thin alveolar epithelium which is one cell thick, a narrow "basement membrane," and the underlying capillary membrane. Through these tissues, gaseous diffusion occurs between the air and the blood. Various mononuclear cells are found on and within these thin structures as histiocytes, fibroblasts, and undifferentiated mesenchymal cells. Some of these cells may become active phagocytes to remove offensive matter which, by damaging the alveolar epithelium, would interfere with the essential process of gaseous diffusion.

Minute openings called alveolar pores exist between adjacent alveoli, and considerably larger epithelium-lined communications exist between bronchioles and alveolar sacs. These two types of communications are of importance, for they permit the direct passage of air from alveolus to alveolus and bronchioles to alveolar sac. This situation is referred to as collateral ventilation, since alveoli may continue to be ventilated in the presence of obstruction of their normal ventilatory pathways.

PROTECTIVE MECHANISMS

The protective mechanisms of the lung are directed toward maintaining the integrity of the alveoli, their blood supply, and ventilation. This requires the cleansing, humidification, and temperature regulation of relatively large volumes of air. The size of the task is impressive when one realizes that air contains bacteria, fungi, viruses, and many other forms of particulate matter which are potentially damaging to the 70 or 80 sq. m. of alveolar surface area. Air that seems clean may contain as many as 3 million particles per cubic foot, whereas visibly dusty air may contain over 100 million particles per cubic foot. The efficiency of these protective mechanisms is evident from the fact that the alveoli are maintained essentially sterile and free of foreign matter in the presence of these agents and a necessary basal alveolar ventilation of approximately 4 liters each minute.

A large portion of the cleansing of air, humidification, and temperature adjustment occurs in the nose. From the moment air enters the nose, the processes for removing particulate matter are at work. Larger material is immediately trapped by hairs in the nose and those particles getting past this gross filter still may be removed in the nose by coming in contact with the moist turbinates. If this happens, the particles are swept away by cilia for elimination by swallowing or nose blowing.

In the trachea and bronchi the process becomes somewhat more elaborate. Mucus, produced by the goblet cells and mucous glands, enters the lumen of the bronchi and forms a continuous, moist, sticky surface. Beneath the surface lies the ciliated epithelium. The wavelike movements of the cilia are coordinated in such a way as to move the mucus sheet upward at a rate of 2 centimeters or so each minute. Thus, a tubular "conveyer belt" is provided which continuously moves upward in the normal individual and is being replenished continuously throughout the airways from the level of the alveolar ducts on up. The ciliated epithelium is interrupted only by stratified squamous epithelium over the vocal cords, but recurs again above them. It is believed that the mucus sheet is drawn uninterrupted over the vocal cords through its cohesive and elastic properties. Airways are somewhat tortuous, and, where particles impinge upon the walls, they adhere and are swept out of the respiratory tract. As will be noted in the subsequent discussion of lung disorders, there are many factors which alter the efficiency of this self-cleansing mechanism. For example, cold air, sedatives, anesthetics, tobacco smoke, systemic alcohol, sulfur dioxide, and possibly high concentrations of oxygen may depress ciliary action; ciliary efficiency may be disrupted seriously by dry air and various drugs which render the mucus sheet too viscous for efficient ciliary action. Even here there is considerable latitude, for as much as 50 per cent of the water may be removed from mucus before there is a great increase in its consistency.

The movement of the mucus sheet and the expelling of foreign matter are assisted to some extent by changes in the diameter of airways on inspiration and expiration. Bronchi have been observed to widen and elongate on inspiration and narrow and shorten on expiration. The narrowing on expiration increases the rate of air flow considerably and therefore has a tendency to blow out mucus and other intraluminal matter.

Normally, the cleansing secretions of the lung are handled entirely by ciliary action with some assistance from the expulsive forces of quiet respiration. However, when bronchial or tracheal secretions become slightly excessive, acceleration of the expiratory air flow by clearing of the throat may be necessary to clear the nonciliated vocal cords. If this is ineffective, a more forceful mechanism, the cough, may be called forth to blast the secretions upward. The cough reflex is initiated by stimulation of afferent nerve endings in the laryngeal, tracheal, or bronchial mucosa. The act itself can be divided into three parts. First, there is a deep inspiration, followed immediately by closure of the glottis. Second, with the glottis still closed, positive pressure develops in the thorax by contraction of muscles of the chest and the abdominal wall. Lastly, the glottis is suddenly opened and the air under pressure is rapidly expelled. If the offending substance is eliminated, or if it is moved upward to an insensitive area, coughing ceases. There may, however, be continuous paroxysms of coughing which move the offensive matter little by little until it is eliminated or until the cough reflex is suppressed by medication.

In addition to the cleansing action of the mucus sheet and the expulsive forces of normal respiration and coughing, peristaltic movements in the finer bronchi probably assist in eliminating secretions. Jarre and Di Rienzo, in separate studies using radiopaque material, have demonstrated peristalsis in the bronchi of man. It is believed that the peristaltic waves assist in moving foreign material to larger airways where coughing may be more effective.

Up to this point the mechanisms of defense that have been described are the ones which are at work in the airways lined with a ciliated epithelium and coated with a moving mucus sheet. However, some respired matter may penetrate beyond these barriers. Very small particles, 10 microns or less in diameter, are respirable, and after inhalation can be found rather uniformly deposited over the alveolar walls. Heppleston has observed this in coalminers who have died very shortly after exposure in dusty mines. Disposal of foreign material at this level of the respiratory tree is quite different from what has been described thus far. It depends upon phagocytosis and, from the observations of Heppleston, must occur rapidly. If the ingested material is bacterial, it may be destroyed within the phagocyte. If, as in the case of various dusts, it is resistant to digestion, the phagocyte moves upward to an alveolar duct. This is the level of termination of both the ciliated epithelium and the lymphatic system. Disposition may then be accomplished by ciliary action sweeping the phagocyte upward, or the cell may enter the lymphatic vessels and arrive in nearby lymphoid collections or hilar lymph nodes. Some of the variations in this process of removing dust particles are discussed in the section on Pneumoconiosis.

The mechanisms which trap inspired dry material are not as successful against liquids or even insoluble material suspended in a liquid. For example, Barclay found in his experimental studies that finely powdered lead-glass insufflated into lungs did not reach the alveoli and frequently was eliminated from the larger airways within a matter of hours. Yet, the same material suspended in a liquid reached the alveoli and might still be visible on roentgenography for weeks. The significance of this observation to patients with sinusitis, bronchitis, and other morbid conditions characterized by excessive pulmonary secretions is quite obvious.

The inhalation of irritating fumes may elicit reflex constriction of the bronchioles. This is similar to the response in asthma, and although it may be looked upon as a mechanism for protecting the alveoli, it is a two-edged sword. If the irritation is long maintained, as in the case of industrial fumes, it can produce bronchitis and asthmatic symptoms. Voluntary breath-holding or limitation of ventilation as an obvious defense against inhalation of noxious material can be effective for only short periods of time.

Defensive mechanisms can be active to extremes which are disadvantageous. The dry cough which does not become productive even when expectorants are employed may be exhausting to the patient and accomplish nothing toward removing the irritative focus. Occasionally, the cough reflex has been incriminated in the spread of infection from one area of the lung to another. The risk of spreading infection which is inherent in excessive liquid secretions has been alluded to above. In general, however, the effectiveness of the self-cleansing mechanisms of the lungs is quite impressive when one considers how much extraneous material must be removed even from air that seems to be clean.

For many years it has been known that the alpha-1-globulin fraction of serum contains a factor which inhibits the activity of proteolytic enzymes. More recently this factor has been designated as alpha-1-antitrypsin and recognized as the chief biological substance responsible for the alpha-1-globulin band on electrophoresis. The biological function of this antitrypsin is not well understood at the present, but the possibility of it having a role in protecting the lungs has been suggested.

The lysis of inflammatory exudate by the proteolytic enzymes of macrophages and granulocytes is an important supplement to cough and mucociliary action in clearing the lungs of inflammatory products. However, it is postulated that the released leukocytic enzymes, if uncontrolled, could lead to the excessive destruction of pulmonary tissue. The role, then, of alpha-1-antitrypsin might be in inhibiting excessive proteases and thus protecting the lung. Whether this is the biological function of antitrypsin is not proved, but it is recognized that abnormally low concentrations of antitrypsin are associated with "hereditary" emphysema.

Maintenance of the integrity of alveoli depends on defense mechanisms not only against foreign matter but also against the tendency of surface tension of the moist lining to collapse the alveoli. Patency of alveoli is accomplished in part by negative intrathoracic pressure and supporting tissues; however, these alone do not prevent collapse under certain pathologic conditions. The relationship between pressure (P) within a sphere, tension (T) in the wall, and the radius (r) of the sphere is expressed in the Laplace equation, $P = \frac{2T}{r}$. A moist sphere such as an alveolus with airway connections to the atmosphere would tend increasingly to collapse as the radius diminished were it not for the presence of a "surfactant system" which adjusts surface tension in relation to radius. Normally there is believed to be a complex mixutre of lipids, protein, and carbohydrates—the surface-active system—lining the alveolus. This surface-active material, or surfactant, reduces surface tension as the surface area of alveoli decreases. By thus varying the surface tension of the alveolar wall (in relation to radius), the right side of the equation $\left(\frac{2T}{r}\right)$ is maintained relatively constant, so that an antiatelectatic effect is produced. The exact site of surfactant production is unresolved; however, the larger cells of the alveolar epithelium are suspect.

Additional physiologic functions of surfactant are postulated as protecting the integrity of the alveolus. By maintaining a lower surface tension, and thus a lower tension on the alveolar wall, the capillary hydrostatic pressure is augmented to a lesser degree than would otherwise be the case. This diminishes the tendency of hydrostatic pressure to move fluid into the alveoli. Another characteristic of surface-active agents, the spreading tendency, may be important in moving bacteria, cellular debris, and foreign particles to phagocytic alveolar macrophages. This is a physical phenomenon in which a surfactant tends to move from areas of high concentration and a low surface tension to areas of low concentration and a high surface tension.

PULMONARY DISEASE

A virulent infectious organism introduced into the respiratory tract in one individual may result in progressive disease. In another, the organism may obtain a temporary foothold only to be eliminated later or held in a quiescent state, though still alive. In still another, the infectious agent may be eliminated promptly without any measurable effect on the host. Thus, there are varying degrees of effectiveness of the protective mechanisms. Pulmonary disease, whether infectious or not, may be looked upon as the result of the disruption or undesirable response of one or more of these mechanisms. The pulmonary protective mechanisms probably are modified by many factors, including heredity, age, sex, nutritional status, environment, and ill-defined fluctuations in individual resistance to disease. It must be remembered that very little information is available concerning the physiologic effects of these factors. The bodily defenses are many and varied so that the failure of one mechanism is generally compensated for by other processes. As a consequence, many pulmonary disorders are reversible, and on recovery the functional status of the lungs is little or none the worse for the experience.

In the consideration of pulmonary disorders, it is desirable to interpret the pathologic alterations in terms of effects on physiologic processes. Thus, pulmonary disease should be considered in the light of the various components of pulmonary function that are discussed in the preceding chapter. When doing this, however, it must be remembered that a patient may have pulmonary disease without significant deviation from normal in functional studies. This may be due to the statistical range of normal values, limited extent of the pathologic process, or the inherent inaccuracies of testing techniques.

Asthma

Bronchial asthma is characterized by diffuse airway obstruction which is largely at the bronchiolar level (see p. 396). Hypersensitivity to inhaled extrinsic allergens or to intrinsic infectious agents of the respiratory tract are believed, in the majority of patients, to initiate the pathophysiologic changes. However, once the asthmatic reaction pattern is established, psychophysiologic reactions, smoke, fumes, physical exertion, and changes in the temperature or humidity to the air may precipitate attacks.

The obstructive characteristics of asthma arise mainly from two physical changes in the airways which increase the resistance of gas flow: irregularities of the walls and narrowing of the lumina. Slight irregularities in larger airways such as the bronchi increase the resistance to flow by producing turbulence. The physical accompaniment of this is audible wheezing. In smaller airways, turbulence, if it occurs at all, is less important, and viscosity of the air becomes dominant because of the extreme degrees of bronchiolar narrowing.

The narrowing is brought on by at least three factors. One is the inflammatory reaction with its accompanying vascular engorgement, edema, leukocytic infiltration, and eventual fibroblastic proliferation. Another is the excessive, tenacious secretions produced by the hyperactive mucous glands. This sticky material adheres, narrows, blocks, and produces irregularities and increased thickness in the walls of the bronchi and bronchioles. Lastly, there is constriction of smooth muscle in the bronchial walls.

The mechanism which initiates these narrowing processes is not known. Acetylcholine, which may be produced by the antigen-antibody reaction, is known to simulate asthmatic attacks by causing the production of excessive mucus and bronchial constriction. Histamine or a histamine-like compound also can cause edema of mucous membranes and smooth muscle spasm. Serotonin has a similar action. Each of these substances may produce an asthmatic attack in an asthmatic subject, but no one substance has been clearly incriminated as a factor in the pathogenesis of bronchial asthma.

The ventilatory alterations of bronchial asthma are those of bronchiolar obstruction and as such are not diagnostic for asthma alone, but occur with any process obstructing small airways. Diffusing capacity, however, remains relatively normal in uncomplicated asthma. The primary value of function tests is that they are objective and allow better evaluation of the disability as well as the results of therapy. In the early stages there is a high degree of reversibility of the changes in bronchial asthma, and the lungs may be normal between paroxysms. This is the chief point of functional differentiation from emphysema, which is characterized by relative irreversibility. As paroxysms of asthma are repeated over and over again, the narrowing of airways may become persistent. There is disruption of alveolar walls, and the pulmonary-cardiac abnormalities become indistinguishable from those of obstructive emphysema. Thus, the pathophysiologic changes described in the section on emphysema are applicable in various degree to bronchial asthma.

Emphysema

Obstructive pulmonary emphysema is a pathologic entity characterized by obstructive phenomena at the level of the smaller bronchioles. As such it is clearly distinguished from compensatory emphysema and the normal aging lung, conditions which lack the obstructive element. Etiologic factors are not sharply defined. In more than 60 per cent of patients, obstructive emphysema is accompanied or preceded by chronic bronchitis. The etiology of that disease is unclear, but the continued accumulation of data incriminates irritants such as cigarette smoke and air pollutants as well as repeated bouts of respiratory tract infection. An interesting fact is that cigarette smoke lowers the surface tension of lung extracts. This might contribute, if true in vivo, to the pathogenesis of emphysema by promoting the hyperinflation of alveoli. Cigarette smoke, which is ciliatoxic and inhibits the phagocytic activities of macrophages, may also contribute by diminishing the protection from foreign matter. Other factors cited are pneumoconiosis, sarcoidosis, bronchiectasis, mucoviscidosis, and tuberculosis. An etiologic role for bronchial asthma is highly questionable. Since 1963, when a deficiency of alpha-1-antitrypsin in the serum was first noted to be associated with obstructive pulmonary emphysema in certain patients, there have been many reports of "familial" or "hereditary" emphysema. Reliable figures on incidence are not available but current estimates are that from 1 to 10 per cent of patients with emphysema have the homozygous antitrypsin deficiency.

The initial pathophysiologic lesion in obstructive emphysema is unknown. An interesting speculation is based on the fact that an appropriate stress from continuing irritants or infections leads to an outpouring of macrophages. This might in turn lead to increased amounts of protease released by these cells which would not only overcome the reduced concentration of alpha-1-antitrypsin in the person with the hereditary antitrypsin deficiency but also overcome normal levels of the antienzyme. The excess concentrations of enzyme would in turn lead to tissue damage.

Concomitants of tissue damage are edema, exudate, hyperactivity of the muscular layers and, in time, fibrosis. Each of these by narrowing pulmonary airways, particularly at the bronchiolar level, may cause air trapping in the alveoli. There are several factors which facilitate the passage of air beyond the partial obstruction in inspiration yet do not assist in its egress on expiration. One of these is the fact that airways are wider on inspiration than on expiration. Thus, an obstruction which is of minor significance on inspiration may increase to a serious degree on expiration. If the narrowing is further increased, the discrepancy between the forces of inspiration and those of expiration comes into play. Air is taken into the lungs by the powerful contraction of the diaphragm supplemented by the levator muscles of the ribs which enlarge the diameter of the thorax. Forces of expiration consist of fiberelastic recoil of the lungs, the use of depressor muscles of the ribs, relaxation of the diaphragm, and contraction of the abdominal muscles so as to force the diaphragm up. From the studies of von Neergaard, it is clear that the surface tension of the air-liquid interface of the approximately 300 million alveoli is also a significant contributory factor in expiration. These combined forces do not approximate those of inspiration; thus, with airway narrowing, air can be forcibly pulled into the alveoli but expiration is less effective in discharging it. Even with complete obstruction, the alveoli distal to the obstruction may receive air via collateral pathways from alveoli which are normally aerated. These pathways also narrow on expiration, and, in addition, this collateral ventilation is tortuous, so that air trapping is continued. On expiration, and particularly when expiration is forced, there is a sharp, abnormal rise in pressure in the areas of trapped air, leading to compression and further narrowing of adjacent bronchi and bronchioles. All these processes lead to an increasing accumulation of air and a rising pressure beyond the obstruction. Eventually, distention becomes so great that there is disruption of alveolar walls and the encircling mesh of musculo-elastic tissues about the smaller airways. Paroxysms of coughing increase the intrapulmonary pressures still further and contribute to the hyperinflation.

With repetition of acute exacerbations of the underlying disease there may be excessive amounts of tenacious mucus or mucopurulent secretion, hypertrophy and spasm of bronchial muscle, and permanent thickening of the mucosa. Each of these, by interfering with mechanisms such as ciliary action, cough, and collateral ventilation, serves to increase the obstructive process and trapping of air in the lungs. When the lungs enlarge, their bases push the diaphragm downward toward its position of maximal inspiration so that its excursion becomes less and less. As distention continues, the intrapleural pressure becomes less negative and, during expiration, actually may be 1 or 2 cm. of water pressure above atmospheric, so that when the sternum is removed at autopsy, the lungs balloon out of the thoracic cavity. With increasing intrapleural pressure, the ribs elevate, the chest becomes barrel-shaped, and the diaphragm flattens. This is the position of full inspiration; hence, the ability to inspire additional air and maintain effective ventilation is markedly impaired. An improvement in ventilation might be anticipated if the diaphragm could be returned to a more normal position on expiration—the rationale behind the use of emphysema belts, breathing exercises, and pneumoperitoneum.

In obstructive emphysema, as during acute attacks of asthma, the timed vital capacity is reduced and the total lung volume is increased. This is the result of expiratory air trapping beyond narrow airways, producing an increase in the residual volume. As noted previously, rapid expiration increases the obstructive element and augments air trapping still further. Under these circumstances, therefore, the vital capacity varies with the speed of expiration—hence, the importance of the timed vital capacity as a measure of obstruction. The midexpiratory flow rate and maximal breathing capacity are reduced and the work of breathing is increased.

The physiologic and pathologic changes are not uniform throughout the lungs; some areas are better ventilated than others. The effect of this variation is that inspiratory and expiratory gaseous mixing is poor or absent in some regions and relatively better in others. Venous blood passing through poorly ventilated regions with impaired mixing of gases is exposed to a low pressure of oxygen and a high pressure of carbon dioxide. If this defect is pronounced, there will be a fall in the oxygen saturation of arterial blood and a rise in the partial pressure of carbon dioxide. Contributing to the fall in oxygen saturation is a reduction of diffusing capacity. This reduction is due to a disruption of normal alveolar architecture and a decrease in the functioning capillary bed, both of which decrease the effective surface area for diffusion.

In advanced obstructive emphysema, cyanosis and respiratory acidosis develop, and the same may occur in acute asthmatic attacks if the attack continues long enough. With severe respiratory acidosis the medullary respiratory centers lose their sensitivity to the normal carbon dioxide stimulus for respiration. In this circumstance, hypoxia provides the respiratory drive. If this is not recognized and high concentrations of oxygen are given to relieve cyanosis without mechanical aids to respiration, the termination may be fatal.

Several factors operate to produce pulmonary hypertension, viz., destruction of interalveolar septa, which diminishes the area of the capillary bed; vasoconstriction due to hypoxia; increased viscosity of blood due to secondary polycythemia; and hypervolemia and high intra-alveolar pressure coincident to air trapping which squeezes small pulmonary vessels. With hypoxia the cardiac output is normal or somewhat elevated. The combination of relatively normal cardiac output and increased pulmonary vascular resistance increases right heart work and leads to the development of cor pulmonale. If the process continues, cardiac failure follows. Elevated intrapleural pressure and prolonged expiration add to the elevation of systemic venous pressure by impeding venous return to the heart.

The *aging lung* is characterized by minimal functional changes. In the absence of complicating pulmonary disease, vital capacity is slightly reduced, residual lung volume is increased, maximal breathing capacity may be reduced by half, and there is a mild increase in airway resistance. These changes apparently are related to a reduction of pulmonary elasticity and are not inconsistent with decreased elasticity in other tissues. Arterial oxygen and carbon dioxide values remain within the limits of normal.

The term "senile emphysema" has fallen into disrepute. It has been used in the past to describe a form of nonobstructive pulmonary overdistention secondary to kyphotic distortion. In aging, the collapse of vertebrae or changes in the intervertebral discs produce rotation of the ribs, so that the sternum is pushed forward and the chest becomes barrel-shaped. The lungs accommodate to the expanding chest but the functional changes remain minimal and are indistinguishable from those of the normal aging lung.

Compensatory emphysema is a nonobstructive panacinar dilatation called forth by a decrease in volume of lung parenchyma, most commonly from atelectasis, surgical resection, or fibrosis. The remaining pulmonary tissues overdistend to fill the available space and, to this extent, compensate for the loss. If the diseased pulmonary segment becomes functional again, the emphysema may disappear. But, if the emphysema persists, as after pneumonectomy, there is a gradual loss of pulmonary elasticity with some associated functional impairment.

Interstitial emphysema occurs when air from ruptured alveoli or bronchi enters the interstitial tissues of the lung and dissects along the peribronchial and perivascular sheaths into the mediastinum. From here it may enter the pleural space or travel to the subcutaneous tissues of the suprasternal notch and extend over the neck, face, arms, and trunk. Pain which may simulate angina pectoris often heralds the onset of interstitial emphysema. If the volume of air is large and if it is under pressure, it may interfere with venous return to the heart and be associated with dyspnea and cyanosis. Most commonly interstitial emphysema occurs in association with trauma, surgery, asthma, obstructive pulmonary processes, and pulmonary infections.

Hypersensitivity Pneumonitis

There are several clinical entities of interstitial pneumonitis which are recognized as hypersensitivity reactions to organic dusts inhaled during certain activities of man. Pigeon-breeder's disease, farmer's lung, bagassosis, sequoiosis, and maple-bark disease are those recognized thus far. The hypersensitivity reaction results in a sarcoid-like granulomatous reaction with associated interstitial plasma cells, lymphocytes, areas of focal histiocytosis, and multinucleated giant cells. Alveolar walls and bronchioles are involved in the process. Precipitating antibodies to the appropriate inciting antigen generally are demonstrable. The chief pulmonary functional defect is a low diffusing capacity which correlates with the alveolar and bronchiolar involvement. However, low compliance and a disturbed ventilation-perfusion relationship are also noted in some patients. A few studies seem to suggest that prolonged exposure to the offending antigen in some patients leads to airway obstruction, although in most patients there is no obstructive element. On removal of the offending agent, there is an impressive abatement of the various symptoms and laboratory abnormalities.

Eosinophilic Pulmonary Infiltration (Loeffler's Syndrome)

Eosinophilia associated with transient, migratory, and symptomless roentgenographic shadows was described first by Loeffler in 1932. Subsequently, he suggested that an allergic mechanism might be responsible, and this seems compatible with later opinions. The meager amount of autopsy material indicates that the lesion is a pneumonitis composed largely of aggregates of eosinophils together with histiocytes and giant cells in a background of edema fluid. Eosinophils are predominant in both the interstitial and alveolar exudates and in the sputum. The size of the lesions is such that significant alterations in pulmonary function have not been described. Similar areas of eosinophilic pulmonary infiltrates with systemic eosinophilia have been reported in bronchial asthma, helminthiasis, chronic brucellosis, tuberculosis, tropical eosinophilia, coccidioidomycosis, drug sensitivities, chemical sensitivities, and polyarteritis nodosa.

Pulmonary Alveolar Proteinosis

This chronic disease of the lungs, characterized by the deposition of eosinophilic material in alveoli, was described first by Rosen, Castleman, and Liebow in 1958. To date, the etiology remains unknown. Certain histologic similarities to pneumocystis infection have led to intensive but unsuccessful searches for this parasite. Efforts to isolate other infectious agents or to identify an inhalant or aspirant common to all cases have also been unsuccessful. The suggestion that the disease may be due to an excess of pulmonary surfactant remains speculative.

In the early stages of pulmonary alveolar proteinosis, septal cells in the walls of alveoli increase in both size and number. Increasing further, they may line the alveoli, project into the lumina, slough, disintegrate, and give rise to PAS-positive granular and floccular material with numerous small acicular spaces. Continuation of this sequence leads to the filling of the alveoli and distal air spaces, including respiratory bronchioles. In these areas of consolidation there is a striking absence of cellular infiltration into the interalveolar septa and there is no evidence of vascular congestion. The ultimate histologic fate is not clearly defined, although it is known from clinical studies that regression may occur. Biopsy studies of areas believed to have been involved previously have shown slight interstitial fibrosis of questionable significance and some residual granularity of the alveolar lining cells.

In this disease, although the distal parenchyma is not normal and air containing, there is no primary involvement of the airways. Hence, spirographic studies show no evidence of obstruction to air flow. There is, however, filling of alveoli by "proteinaceous" material and replacement of functioning lung volume by consolidation. As a consequence of this, there is a restrictive pattern of ventilation with a decrease in vital capacity. The patient may complain of dyspnea and there may even be objective hyperventilation at rest. Inspiration of high concentrations of oxygen does not relieve the hyperventilation, although it does decrease any arterial unsaturation which may be present. As in many other forms of diffuse lung disease, the hyperventilation is believed to be due to an alteration in the proprioceptive reflex mechanism within the diseased lung.

The increase in size and number of alveolar septal cells and the early partial coating of alveoli with eosinophilic material interferes with the diffusion of oxygen across the alveolar-capillary membrane. This does not permit full saturation of hemoglobin passing such alveoli and results in various degrees of arterial unsaturation and its clinical manifestation, cyanosis. Further arterial oxygen unsaturation is caused by venous blood passing through the intact vasculature of consolidated alveoli which contain no air at all. Thus, the pathophysiology of pulmonary alveolar proteinosis is a consequence of a ventilation-perfusion inbalance. There is no evidence of impaired carbon dioxide excretion. If clinical improvement occurs, the oxygenation of blood may return to normal.

From clinical studies thus far published, patients with pulmonary alveolar proteinosis seem unusually susceptible to superimposed infections. In the presence of pulmonary insufficiency, such infections, even though minor in extent, may lead to death. Those who have died without recognized infection showed progressive respiratory failure in the form of dyspnea and cyanosis.

Hyaline Membrane Disease

One of the causes of the respiratory distress syndrome of infancy is hyaline membrane disease, a diagnosis that can be established with certainty only on necropsy. The characteristic findings are dilation of respiratory bronchioles and of alveolar ducts as well as extensive alveolar collapse and hyaline membranes. Functionally, there is diminished lung volume, reduced compliance, arterial oxygen desaturation, right-to-left vascular shunts, increased physiologic dead space, respiratory and metabolic acidosis, decreased cardiac output, and decreased effective pulmonary blood flow. Although the pathophysiology of hyaline membrane disease is not established in each patient as attributable to a deficiency or absence of surfactant, it is evident that in most such patients there is an absence of the material. However, surfactant has been found in certain infants who had hyaline membrane disease. It is postulated that infants may be born with an immature mechanism for producing surfactant and although they have a hyaline membrane and the associated symptoms, the mechanism may mature so that surfactant is produced 5 to 15 days after birth. Thus, at death both the hyaline membrane and surfactant may be present. As for the hyaline membrane itself, it appears to consist of plasma from alveolar capillaries and possibly fibrin. The absence of the action of surfactant in reducing surface tension would result in transmitting the surface tension of the alveoli to the alveolar walls and thus would augment the capillary hydrostatic pressure and in this manner move fluid into the alveoli. The tissue asphyxia would add to the tendency to plasma loss and the membrane would be created. The collapse of the alveoli themselves would be governed by the theorem of Laplace, as discussed in the section on Protective Mechanisms.

Congenital Cystic Disease

Although it is difficult in a given case to be certain that a cystic pulmonary lesion did not develop after birth, there is little doubt as to the existence of true congenital cysts. It is believed that if intrauterine lung development is arrested at an early stage, a large solitary cyst may be formed; whereas, if the arrest occurs later, multiple cysts may result. The cysts, as observed in the patient, may be walled off and filled with serous fluid or they may be partly or entirely air-containing if there are communications to functioning bronchi. The lining epithelium of the cyst may be invested partially with cartilage and smooth muscle. Other cysts may be thin-walled and lined by a flattened epithelium.

There is a great tendency for these lesions to become infected, because bacteria gaining access to cysts cannot be removed by normal mechanisms. The absence of any connections to an airway or the inadequate size where a connection does exist prevents drainage of infected material and elimination by ciliary action and coughing. In those cysts connected to airways, infection, mucus accumulation, and the valvelike mechanism from changes in duct sizes on inspiration and expiration cause air trapping.

Pulmonary Embolism

The pulmonary vascular tree is an efficient filter which can remove emboli of neoplastic cells, bacteria, blood clots, fat globules, air, and the debris of amniotic fluid. Frequently overlooked is the fact that pulmonary infarction is not an invariable accompaniment of embolism. Pulmonary embolism alone is much more common than pulmonary infarction. The collateral bronchial circulation is, in many cases, adequate to maintain viability of the area involved. In the presence of conditions such as diminished ventilation, pulmonary infection, or cardiac disease which tend to produce vascular stasis, an embolus is much more likely to produce frank infarction.

Embolic obstruction leads to hyperemia and edema, which, if some of the above conditions are present, will progress in about 24 hours to infarction with alveolar wall necrosis and hemorrhage into the alveoli and associated bronchi. This gives rise to the so-called meaty sputum which contains dark red clots. Within two weeks, fibroblastic proliferation is in progress and the end result is a contracted scar which may not be visible on roentgenographic examination.

The severity of response to embolism is a function of the previous cardiovascular status and the subsequent degree of blood pressure elevation in the pulmonary arterial tree. In general terms, the obstruction of a small pulmonary artery may be silent, whereas occlusion of the main trunk of the pulmonary artery is followed by cessation of cardiac output, gasping respirations, and death. Between these extremes is a spectrum of variations in the pathophysiologic response.

If the vascular bed obstructed is of intermediate size, the systemic blood pressure falls suddenly and there is a concomitant rise in the pulmonary artery pressure, the right ventricular end-diastolic pressure, and the venous pressure. The mechanism or mechanisms producing the pulmonary hypertension continue to be a source of considerable controversy. Experimental studies in animals indicate that embolus-particle size is important. Emboli lodging at the precapillary level elicit hypertension by vasoconstriction, whereas emboli trapped in muscular and larger elastic arteries produce hypertension by mechanical blockage. Clinical data seem to be compatible with this concept of particle size. Pulmonary hypertension in some patients is demonstrated as being based on mechanical obstruction; in others, the hypertension is secondary to vasoconstriction; and in a third group there is a combination of obstruction and vasoconstriction.

With embolism there is a sudden onset of dyspnea which has been explained variously as a consequence of anoxia and reflexes from stimulation of receptors in the pulmonary artery. Tachycardia occurs as a response to the fall in systemic blood pressures, anoxia, and apprehension. Cyanosis is a manifestation of arterial unsaturation rather than the stasis cyanosis seen after myocardial infarction. This unsaturation may be the result of shunting through normal arteriovenous anastomoses and a decreased area of functional pulmonary capillaries, producing in turn a decreased diffusing capacity of the lung. Pulmonary embolism per se is generally not accompanied by fever and leukocytosis; however, both may occur as a consequence of an underlying infection or pulmonary infarction with the embolism. When cough occurs, it is probably in response to the inflammation of bronchial mucosa within the area of infarction. With involvement of the visceral pleura by infarction there is frequently pleuritic pain, but there may also be substernal discomfort reminiscent of myocardial ischemia. This discomfort may be attributable to the mechanical block of pulmonary arteries reducing, in turn, the cardiac output and coronary blood flow. Distention of the right cardiac chambers may also impede coronary flow by interfering with coronary venous return. Since pulmonary hypertension of other types has been noted to produce similar pain, it is also possible that some of the pain may result directly from distention of the pulmonary arteries.

One consequence of pulmonary embolism is that alveoli may continue to be ventilated although there is no capillary circulation. In the absence of effective circulation, the CO_2 tension in these alveoli will fall to very low levels instead of remaining approximately equal to the CO_2 tension of arterial blood, as in the normal state. On the basis of this, it was thought that a pulmonary embolus could be detected and quantitated on the basis of a comparison of arterial CO_2 and mixed expired alveolar CO_2. In practice this has not been too successful for three reasons: first, any pulmonary disease such as obstructive emphysema which alters ventilation-perfusion relationships may give similar results; second, when an area of lung loses its circulation, there is, in fact, reduction of ventilation of the area; and third, the effects of smaller emboli are not detected. In the presence of obstruction of large areas of the pulmonary bed or with the use of differential bronchospirometry, the theory has some practical application.

Pneumoconiosis

If large airborne particles are inhaled, they impinge upon the walls of the tortuous airways and are either swept out in the mucus sheet by ciliary action or expelled by the cough mechanism. However, if the particles are small, less than 10 microns in diameter, they are respirable and, as such, a portion of them will reach the alveoli and become scattered evenly over the walls. With surprising rapidity these particles are engulfed by phagocytes and transported toward the respiratory bronchioles. Even in normal lungs this is a relatively inefficient process, and silting up of these dust cells occurs in the respiratory bronchioles. Thus, not all the material reaches the continuous layer of ciliated epithelium which could expel the dust from the lung. Those cells which do not progress up the bronchial tree enter the interstitial tissues. Furthermore, some of the dust cells take a short cut via interstitial routes, arriving in the walls of other alveoli, or they aggregate about venules. The possibility that some dust particles enter the interstitial tissues without previous phagocytosis is not ruled out.

Once within the interstitial tissues, the dust particles may remain in situ or enter the lymphatics lying in relation to the airways, arteries, and veins. Much of this dust is arrested in foci of lymphoid collections at the divisions of the airways or vessels, while the remainder is carried to the tracheobronchial and hilar lymph nodes. In many instances, more distant lymph nodes such as those in the supraclavicular area also contain the inspired particles. There is no clear-cut evidence that phagocytes have any destructive action on the contained inorganic particles. Apparently, they act merely as vehicles to free the alveoli from foreign matter.

As dust particles arrive within the pulmonary tissues, a foreign-body type of response is elicited. Reticulum cells are transformed into fibroblasts and there is a deposition of fibrous tissue. When this reaction occurs about small bronchioles, there is impairment of air flow at the site, distortion and disruption of alveoli, the development of focal emphysema, and a sequence of events similar to that in obstructive emphysema. In advanced pneumoconiosis in which conglomerate lesions appear, there will be a decrease in lung volume in such areas from scarring and a compensatory emphysema in other areas. If the process is extensive, not only is the ventilatory function affected but there is disruption of the pulmonary capillary bed. Fibrosis occurring within the lymphatics impedes lymph flow, so that the irritating dust and phagocytes escape into the areolar tissue about the blood vessels. In this position, further fibrosis, with the added element of decreased capillary bed, contributes to the development of pulmonary arterial hypertension. In time this may eventuate in cor pulmonale and right heart failure. The obstruction of the lymphatics is possibly related to the known susceptibility of these patients to superimposed pulmonary infections. The severe ventilatory disturbances are those found in emphysema and fibrosis. In a given patient the changes may be predominantly those of emphysema or fibrosis, or a combination of the two. The decreases in arterial blood oxygen saturation are due primarily to poorly ventilated or nonventilated alveoli which are perfused with blood. This, in effect, is a right-to-left shunt of blood and, if severe, will be attended by cyanosis, secondary polycythemia, and clubbing of the fingers.

Each type of dust invokes a particular response, and there is considerable variation in the pathologic characteristics and the attendant physiologic alterations. In general, carbon particles cause only mild changes in the lymphatic vessels and nodes with which they come in contact; silica produces intense fibrosis; and asbestos, diffuse fibrosis. The sputum produced in pneumoconiosis can be revealing. With anthracosis it may be black with carbon. In asbestosis, asbestos bodies may be found. Chronic infection is a common complication of the pneumoconioses, and the mucopurulent sputum produced is suggestive of tuberculosis. The possibility of superimposed tuberculosis always must be considered, for it is a frequent secondary invader, particularly in silicosis and anthracosilicosis. In asbestosis, bronchogenic carcinoma and, less frequently, mesothelioma must be considered as possible complications.

Pulmonary Fibrosis

Pulmonary fibrosis is not an etiologic entity, but it may occur as a consequence of tuberculosis, scleroderma, sarcoidosis, roentgen irradiation of the lungs, the inhalation of various noxious dusts and fumes, the Hamman-Rich syndrome, the administration of a number of drugs, various degrees of pulmonary venous obstruction, aspiration pneumonia, the organization of inflammatory exudates of pneumonia, as well as a familial variety which is hereditary. Systemic symptoms in this group of diseases vary widely and are generally characteristic of the particular clinical entity, but the pulmonary manifestations may be strikingly similar. The spectrum of pulmonary signs and symptoms varies from none at all in the earlier stages to cough, mucopurulent sputum, chest pain, cyanosis, clubbing of the digits, severe dyspnea, weight loss, and fatigue. As fibrosis progresses, pulmonary hypertension, cor pulmonale, and cardiac failure ensue. The common denominator pathologically is interstitial fibrosis, which may be localized, as in the case of irradiation pneumonitis following therapy for cancer of the breast, or diffuse, as in many of the other diseases. When the lesions are small, there may be no detectable alteration of pulmonary function. However, if the lesions become diffuse and the fibrosis becomes extensive, the lung will lose its elastic distensibility and there will be a decrease in total lung capacity, vital capacity, and residual volume. The dyspnea reflects the poor compliance and results in a concomitant increase in the work of breathing. If the fibrosis is not evenly distributed throughout the lungs, compensatory emphysema develops in the uninvolved tissue. An element of airway obstruction may also be present from fibrosis about bronchioles. Frequently, the fibrosis disturbs the relationship between the air-containing alveoli and the alveolar capillaries so as to impair gaseous diffusion. If extensive, this results in chronic hypoxemia, hyperventilation, and lowered Pco_2. These may be the predominant aberrations of pulmonary physiology in the Hamman-Rich syndrome, miliary tuberculosis, sarcoidosis, scleroderma, beryllium granulomatosis, and certain neoplasms with lymphangitic spread in the lungs.

Atelectasis

A bronchus may become obstructed either by an intraluminal mass or by external pressure so that the passage of air beyond is prevented. When obstruction occurs and is complete, gas in the segment supplied by the bronchus is absorbed into the bloodstream, leaving the lung airless and collapsed. Secondary to the collapse, there is a decrease of surfactant activity in the affected area of the lung. Although not known with certainty, the decrease of surfactant in atelectasis may be related to its short half-life (14 hours) and the fact that normal ventilation is required for its constant replenishment. Adjacent normal lung retains normal activity of the antiatelectic surfactant.

Depending upon the size of the atelectatic area, various aberrations in pulmonary function may be observed. The vital capacity is reduced through the absolute reduction in functioning lung tissue. Arterial oxygen saturation is reduced owing to the passage of desaturated venous blood through alveolar capillaries which are no longer in contact with air. Pulmonary elasticity is reduced. If the collapsed volume of lung is large, these physiologic changes are manifested as dyspnea and cyanosis. Fever is usual and is due either to the process initiating the atelectasis or to bacteria already present in the bronchi or introduced from aspiration, bloodstream, or lymphatics. In most cases, antibody and leukocytic activity controls the infective agents, but at times pulmonary abscess or chronic bronchiectasis may develop in the affected area. If infection does not intervene, restoration of normal function may occur after removal of the obstruction, even though atelectasis has been long persistent.

A type of atelectasis which is not obstructive may occur in the presence of processes which decrease the effective intrathoracic space. This is commonly observed in patients with sizable pleural effusions or pneumothorax and may also be noted with the high diaphragm and retracted intercostal spaces of patients with respiratory paralysis. The atelectasis is a consequence of compression from outside the lung and represents an adjustment to a new intrathoracic volume. Among the terms used for this entity are adjustment atelectasis, compression atelectasis, and disc, or platelike, atelectasis.

Atelectasis in association with pneumonia may occur as a consequence of obstruction of airways by viscid bronchial secretions, inflammatory exudate, or edema. It also may occur in the absence of obstruction and in any stage of the disease, including even convalescence. The mechanism is not entirely clarified. There is evidence that smooth muscle elements extend as far distal as alveolar walls. It is postulated that these muscular elements are under autonomic control and might under certain circumstances give rise to "contraction atelectasis." There is also a decrease in surfactant activity in infected portions of lungs and contiguous areas which might contribute to pulmonary collapse.

At birth, various degrees of atelectasis might well be anticipated, since intrauterine life is essentially aquatic. A certain amount of physiologic atelectasis exists in the normal full-term infant but generally disappears during his first week of life (see Hyaline Membrane Disease, p. 401).

In children, atelectasis has no predilection for a particular area, presumably because all the bronchi are narrow. Adults, however, are particularly vulnerable to obstruction of the right middle lobe. This fact led E. A. Graham to coin the term "middle lobe syndrome." Since the etiologic factors are many, this unusual susceptibility would seem to be on an anatomic basis. The middle lobe bronchus is not only relatively narrow but also more compressible by virtue of the acute angle that it forms with the main bronchus. Brock has emphasized that this situation is made more precarious by the fact that the bronchus is surrounded closely by lymph nodes draining not only the middle lobe but also the lower lobe. Thus, infection in any part of these two lobes may produce sufficient lymphadenopathy to be obstructive.

Atelectasis as a postoperative complication is attributed to bronchial obstruction from retained secretions. Many of the processes which normally protect the bronchi from occlusion by secretions are rendered ineffective by surgery. Anesthesia, narcotics, pain, and fear of damage to the wound interfere with the expulsion of secretions by eliminating or making ineffective the cough reflex and by diminishing the tidal volume and associated bronchial movements. Also, as shown by Brock, lying on one side for long periods of time allows secretions to gravitate to the dependent lung segments. Aggravating each of these deficiencies is the increased viscosity of the sputum as a consequence of drugs administered for premedication, anesthesia, and postoperative pain. Not only is the sputum so sticky that it is difficult to move by coughing, but this same viscid characteristic impairs the movement of the cilia, which are otherwise unchanged. Consideration of these various surgical effects on the pulmonary protective mechanisms provides the rationale for effective therapy of atelectasis—thinning of the sputum, restoration of the cough, changing body positions, alleviation of pain on respiration, and increasing the depth of respiration.

Tumor of the Lung

The respiratory symptoms of tumor of the lung are largely manifestations of partial or complete mechanical obstruction of an airway. Intraluminal tumors obstruct by direct growth into a bronchus, whereas parenchymal tumors produce similar effects through external pressure on the airways. As the tumor enlarges, asthmatic type breathing or stridor may be observed over the area of one lung or lobe in approximately 10 per cent of the cases. Since bronchi enlarge on inspiration and narrow on expiration, there may be localized emphysema beyond the tumor. This can be demonstrated often if roentgenograms are taken in both full inspiration and full expiration. Cough is an early symptom which is difficult to evaluate, since most of these patients are heavy smokers and chronic cough is such a prevalent symptom in this group. However, as ulceration occurs the sputum changes and there may be blood streaking or frank hemoptysis. Drainage from the bronchus is impaired and secondary infection appears. The sputum becomes more abundant and is mucoid or mucopurulent. Pneumonia may develop and respond to antibiotics, only to recur again. Lung abscess, either distal to the obstructing lesion or within the necrotic tumor, is relatively common. With complete obstruction there is atelectasis. All these symptoms are predominantly attributable to mechanical effects of the tumor and are not indicative of its origin or cell type, benign or malignant.

As the malignant tumor spreads to the pleura, or as a consequence of pneumonia, there is pleuritis with pain and effusion. Extension to the mediastinum may produce back pain and obstruction to the superior vena cava. Rarely, a primary or metastatic carcinoma in the lungs may have a lymphangitic spread throughout the lungs. Pulmonary hypertrophic osteoarthropathy, which may resemble rheumatoid arthritis, is said to occur in approximately 10 per cent of malignant lung tumors.

Pulmonary Infections

The remarkable effectiveness of protective mechanisms of the lung maintains the alveoli essentially free of particulate matter such as dust and bacteria. This is in striking contrast to the upper respiratory tract, where there is a wide variety of bacteria which, if permitted to travel downward into the alveoli, would produce serious disease. However, like all defensive mechanisms, those of the lung are not perfect, and infectious disease of the lung still ranks high among infections as a cause of death.

Consideration of the fact that mechanisms are in action to remove particles from the air from the moment it enters the nares until the time it reaches the alveoli would suggest that the major onslaught would be in the trachea and bronchi. Experimentally, this theory is supported by the radiologic studies of Jarre, in which opaque dusts insufflated into lungs did not appear to enter the alveoli, although bronchi were rendered opaque. Clinically, it is supported by the fact that the majority of respiratory tract infections actually are limited to the trachea and bronchi. Ordinarily, the mucus lining of the bronchi and trachea is being constantly swept upward for elimination of foreign material deposited on it from ventilation. When the foreign material is irritating and produces inflammation of the larger airways, the cough mechanism and orally directed peristaltic waves help to move the mucus sheet more rapidly. Yet this constant cleansing action is not impregnable. During sleep, for example, defenses are lowered and septic material from the nose and pharynx, particularly if it is abundant, gravitates readily into the lungs. Other factors which must be taken into consideration when there is a breakdown of protective mechanisms are the virulence of organisms inhaled, the dosage of the infectious material, and variation in the patient's native resistance to pathogenic organisms. Once an organism invades and produces an inflammatory reaction, secondary defenses involving phagotcytes and antibodies, still assisted by the expulsive mechanisms, are manifested.

Acute Tracheitis and Bronchitis

The inflammatory reaction may be a consequence of infectious diseases such as influenza or pertussis, drainage from suppurative sinusitis, allergies, dust, or chemical irritants. Among the latter, excessive cigarette smoking and atmospheric pollution are relatively common. Treatment is directed toward assisting the normal protective mechanisms. Termination of exposure to dust or chemical irritants; thinning of secretions with expectorants, steam, or aerosols; antihistaminics for allergy; and correctly directed antibiotic or chemotherapeutic agents for infections are used as indicated in a given situation. Occasionally, bronchodilators are useful when there is a bronchospastic element. If the cough is excessive or nonproductive, it may be desirable to suppress this reflex to avoid undue exhaustion of the patient.

Chronic Bronchitis

When the etiologic factors considered in the section on acute tracheitis and bronchitis are constant or frequently repeated, so that the bronchial inflammation cannot be completely eliminated, chronic bronchitis is said to exist. In the British Isles, chronic bronchitis as a reported cause of death is exceeded only by heart disease, cerebrovascular accidents, and carcinoma. By contrast, chronic bronchitis is not a frequently appearing diagnosis on death certificates in the United States. The difference in incidence may be in part real, but it is certainly in part a matter of definition. Gaensler and Lindgren in the United States reinvestigated the medical histories of their patients who had been given a diagnosis of chronic obstructive emphysema on the basis of pulmonary function tests. They found that 68 per cent of their patients with the physiologic alterations of obstructive emphysema met the British criteria for chronic bronchitis. Patients with chronic bronchitis had a progressive increase of a productive cough, worse in the mornings and in cold or inclement weather, and, ultimately, dyspnea. In patients who had a productive cough with chronic obstructive emphysema, the dyspnea antedated the cough. This study suggests that chronic bronchitis is an important etiologic factor in most of the patients presenting with obstructive emphysema.

The etiologic relationship of chronic bronchitis to obstructive emphysema emphasizes the need for more serious regard of "bronchial troubles." Chronic bronchitis may lead to rigidity and thickening of the bronchial mucosa from vasodilation, congestion, and edema. There is infiltration of the mucosa by lymphocytes and polymorphonuclear cells and there may be an increase in the tonicity of the bronchial musculature. Mucous glands are enlarged and the excessive secretion interferes with ciliary activity, as does tobacco smoke, so that the cough mechanism must assist in the expulsion of mucus. The pathologic changes also involve the smaller bronchi and bronchioles.

Thickening of the bronchial mucosa, excessive mucus secretion, and increased tone of the bronchial musculature first slow the rate of maximal expiratory air flow and subsequently that of maximal inspiratory flow. Initially there is a normal total lung capacity, normal vasculature by x-ray examination, and a normal diffusing capacity. However, as the disorder continues, the results of functional pulmonary tests may become those of obstructive emphysema.

Treatment is directed along physiologic lines of assisting the normal pulmonary defenses: antibiotics for infectious elements; removal from exposure to airborne irritants; thinning of secretions with expectorants and aerosols; and treatment for allergy, if such is present. Histologic examination of the secretion is of considerable value in establishing the type of bronchitis.

Lung Abscess

Aspiration of infectious material from the upper air passages is probably the most common cause of lung abscess. When dental or surgical procedures on the mouth or surgical procedures on the paranasal sinuses are performed under general anesthesia, the incidence of acute pulmonary abscess is relatively high. Blood clots and other material, along with organisms from the mouth, are inhaled into the lungs at a time when the cough reflex is depressed by general anesthetics and sedatives. Simultaneously, viscosity of the bronchial secretions is increased, as a consequence of premedication, anesthesia, and dehydration, rendering ciliary action ineffective. With the inactivation of these mechanisms for clearing foreign material and the presence of a culture medium in the form of blood, the groundwork is laid for bacterial multiplication and abscess formation. The anatomic distribution of these bronchogenic abscesses has been presented admirably by Brock.

All pulmonary abscesses, however, are not sequels to *aspiration* of infectious material. Bronchogenic mechanisms such as strictures and tumors may disrupt the processes which normally remove foreign material from the lower respiratory tract. Abscesses may arise from hematogenous spread of organisms in septicemias and in septic pulmonary infarcts. Even aseptic infarcts, by devitalizing pulmonary parenchyma may precipitate abscess formation. Necrotizing pneumonitis caused by Friedländer's bacillus, staphylococci, streptococci, mixed flora, and poorly drained bronchogenic cysts may also overwhelm local defenses. It is rare for a simple pneumococcal pneumonia to progress to abscess formation. Infrequently, pulmonary abscess may result from transdiaphragmatic spread of infectious material. Amebic hepatic abscess is generally considered in this situation if the abscess is in the base of the right lung, but this same route may be taken by any subdiaphragmatic abscess. Progress of the infection is usually slow enough to allow symphysis of the pleura, so that the lung is invaded without empyema occurring first.

In most cases of simple abscess the defense mechanisms discussed in the section on Pneumonia, when aided by antibacterial agents, bronchoscopy, and postural drainagé, will be adequate. The abscess wall collapses, fibrosis occurs, and the end result may be a scar which is invisible on roentgenography. The chronic abscess with a thick fibrous wall which will not collapse even on adequate bronchial drainage is seen less frequently than in the past—even in tuberculosis—because of earlier diagnosis and effective antibiotic agents.

Bronchiectasis

Prolonged bronchial obstruction, whether by tumor, foreign body, viscid mucous, scar, or lymphadenopathy, and parenchymal disease with infection are the two chief pathogenic factors in bronchiectasis. Among the most frequently cited parenchymal diseases are pulmonary atelectasis, chronic bronchial infection with parenchymal scarring, pneumonitis, and pulmonary fibrosis. Although the pathogenesis varies somewhat, each of these is characterized by some reduction in air-containing lung and concomitant traction on bronchial walls. This traction combined with weakening of the bronchial walls by infection results in dilatation or bronchiectasis. When the parenchymal infection is reversible and of short duration, so is the bronchiectasis. Pneumonia and atelectasis are notable examples of this type of clinically reversible bronchiectasis. However, when the bronchial obstruction is prolonged and complicated by infection, bronchiectasis results. Thus, infection complicating obstruction from tenacious mucus in mucoviscidosis, lymphadenopathy in the middle lobe syndrome, or healing with fibrosis in tuberculosis may progress to bronchiectasis. There is also a congenital form in which embryologic development is arrested after the outgrowth of bronchial buds but before there is differentiation into alveolar tissue. This is more frequently referred to as congenital cystic disease. Another congenital defect, intralobar bronchopulmonary sequestration with aberrant systemic arterial supply is also generally complicated by persistent infection and bronchiectasis.

In the diseases mentioned there is a relative lack of aerated alveoli distal to the bronchiectasis. As a consequence, the current of air generated in coughing is inadequate to expel secretions from the bronchi. Thus, secretions tend to stagnate and become secondarily infected because the weakened cough mechanism cannot eliminate completely the dependent secretions. The accumulated secretions destroy much of the bronchial wall, including cilia and muscle, if the disease is long continued. Large anastomotic communications develop between the bronchial and pulmonary vasculature and may give rise to hemoptysis. Since the bronchiectatic lung is often functionless in terms of gaseous exchange, these segments may constitute a considerable area of arteriovenous shunting. It is therefore not surprising that pulmonary osteoarthropathy is a frequent finding. So-called dry bronchiectasis does exist as a clinical entity, but it is confined most commonly to the upper lobes where gravitational drainage exists.

Pneumonia

When an acute infectious process involves the alveoli, pneumonia results. The route of transport of the infectious agent to the alveoli varies somewhat with the organism, being via the airways, blood vessels, or lymphatics.

The pattern of response to a particular organism has a tendency to be characteristic. For example, the pneumococcus and Friedländer's bacillus tend to elicit a lobar type of consolidation, whereas the streptococcus is more apt to lead to bronchopneumonia and the staphylococcus to abscess formation. With earlier etiologic diagnosis and specific treatment this anatomic differentiation has lost much of its diagnostic significance, and infections are frequently arrested at the stage of scattered consolidation, resulting in bronchopneumonia.

Among the bacterial pneumonias, the pathogenesis of pneumococcal pneumonia has been the most extensively studied. The current concept is that the pneumococci reach the alveoli via the airway in droplets of mucus or saliva. Because of gravity and the absence of acute angles of the bronchi leading to the right lower and left lower lobes, these areas are the most frequently involved. Once established in the alveolus, the pneumococcus elicits an acute outpouring of edema fluid with neutrophilic leukocytes and small numbers of erythrocytes. This fluid constitutes not only a favorable culture medium for the organisms but also the vehicle for spread. With respiration and coughing this watery exudate laden with bacteria is carried via the smaller air passages and collateral pathways to adjacent areas. As the lesion enlarges it may be divided into three zones. The peripheral zone consists largely of bacteria floating in edema fluid and represents the advancing wave of infection. Beneath this there is an area of leukocytes, fibrin, and bacteria where phagocytosis is occurring. In the central zone the infection is under control and advanced consolidation is present. The alveoli contain many leukocytes, but there is a relative absence of bacteria. It is in this inner zone that resolution first appears.

With increasing numbers of leukocytes and the appearance of macrophages, the outer zone is invaded by the phagocytes and the lesion ceases to progress in size. When, or whether, this occurs is a function of many factors, including the dose, virulence, and rate of multiplication of the infecting bacteria, antibody formation, and the general health of the patient.

In the early stages, when the infection is spreading rapidly, bacteremia is commonly observed. However, it may occur at any stage should the defense mechanisms of the host be overwhelmed. When bacteremia occurs it is believed that the organisms gain access to the bloodstream via the lymphatics. The consequence of bacteremia may be metastatic lesions such as meningitis, bacterial endocarditis, peritonitis, and arthritis.

The development of antibodies such as precipitins, lysins, and opsonins constitutes an important aspect of host defense. Before the development of chemotherapeutic and antibiotic agents, type-specific antipneumococcus serum was an important agent in therapy. This serum is thought to be effective largely by its enhancement of phagocytosis. Pneumococci in the presence of opsonins tend to agglutinate, presumably through altered surface tension, and agglutinated organisms are more readily ingested by phagocytes.

By the time of crisis, living bacteria have been disposed of and the temperature falls to normal. Consolidation is still present but liquefaction sets in rapidly and the debris is removed largely via the lymphatics but in part by coughing and ciliary activity. Complete resolution may be delayed for several weeks, particularly in older individuals, but in the absence of complications proceeds in most patients with striking rapidity. Rarely, the process is not completely resolved and the involved area is replaced by fibrous tissue. Lung abscess is an extremely rare complication of pneumococcal pneumonia, apparently because there is little or no necrosis of lung tissue. The pleura is involved in most instances and small pleural effusions occur. If there is delay in the initiation of specific therapy, an empyema may develop.

Systemic manifestations depend upon the characteristics of the organism, the host, and the degree of impairment of lung function. Fever and cyanosis, if the process is extensive, are constant. At the outset of lobar pneumonia and throughout bronchopneumonia, cyanosis is due to imperfect oxygenation of the blood which passes through the affected lobes. As a consequence of consolidation of alveoli and obstruction of airways, the venous blood is not exposed to high levels of oxygen and, in effect, venous blood is shunted through these areas into the pulmonary veins and systemic circulation. When consolidation of one lobe is complete, cyanosis improves somewhat, since all the alveoli have lost their function and there is a decrease in pulmonary blood flow to the lobe.

When pain occurs in pneumonia, it is indicative of involvement of the parietal pleura. The localization of pain by the patient is generally accurate because the impulse travels over fibers of the corresponding spinal nerves. The pulmonary parenchyma and the visceral pleura are themselves devoid of pain fibers. When the diaphragmatic pleura is involved, pain may be referred less accurately to the abdomen and simulate acute disorders for which surgery is indicated. Similarly, as a consequence of the cervical origin of the phrenic nerves, pain of diaphragmatic pleuritis may be experienced in the shoulder region.

Pneumonia also is associated with many viral and rickettsial infections such as influenza, parainfluenza, measles, mumps, chickenpox, respiratory syncytial virus, adenovirus and several related viruses, psittacosis, and *Coxiella burnetii* (Q fever). *Mycoplasma pneumoniae* (Eaton agent), which is a pleuropneumonia-like organism (PPLO), has been identified as the cause of primary atypical pneumonia (PAP) in from 10 to 85 per cent of cases. Adenovirus also has been frequently identified in civilian and military populations as an agent in PAP. "Primary atypical pneumonia" was coined to describe a clinical syndrome, not an etiologic entity. Now that approximately 50 per cent of acute viral lower respiratory tract infections can be identified etiologically, several authorities have suggested that the term be dropped.

Lipoid Pneumonia

Certain oils, particularly mineral oil and vitamin oils, when introduced into the lungs, produce an acute pneumonitis which may progress to fibrosis. Access to the airways is through the use of oily nasal drops or sprays, forceful administration of oily preparations to crying infants, defective swallowing mechanisms, or the aspiration of oily laxatives taken at bedtime.

The lesion produced is an organizing bronchopneumonia with an abundance of macrophages and desquamated alveolar lining cells. In time it may progress to fibrosis with obliteration of the pulmonary vasculature and contraction of the area, producing bronchial distortion and even bronchiectasis. If the involvement is extensive, there may be some reduction in the vital capacity. Oil is partly ingested by macrophages and carried off into the lymphatics and partly eliminated in sputum. When the latter occurs, the etiology of the pneumonitis may be established by cytologic and histochemical studies of 24-hour sputum specimens. The clinical spectrum varies from asymptomatic to simulation of most of the usual pulmonary diseases, including carcinoma.

Aspiration Pneumonia

Although not invariably true, aspiration generally occurs when the patient's state of consciousness is depressed. The more commonly associated conditions are the administration of an anesthetic agent or debilitation, stroke, brain tumor, drugs, and alcoholic intoxication. Each of these conditions may either depress or eliminate the normal protective mechanism of reflex glottic closure associated with vomiting and swallowing. When large solids are aspirated, bronchi may be occluded, with consequent distal pulmonary collapse, mediastinal shift, cyanosis, dyspnea, tachypnea, and tachycardia. The pathophysiologic mechanisms are those discussed in the section on Atelectasis.

The most virulent form of aspiration pneumonia results from the aspiration of acidic gastric fluid. When the pH of the aspirate is below 2.5 and the volume is sufficiently large, the mortality is high—over 70 per cent in some reports. The pathologic manifestations vary from acute inflammatory reaction, with the destruction of epithelium, hemorrhage, and an outpouring of plasma-like fluid, to near complete pulmonary parenchymal destruction. Data on the pathophysiology of the acute process in man are not available and must be inferred from animal studies. Initially, there is acute intense bronchospasm, a brief period of apnea, followed by shallow tachypnea, a prompt rise in pulmonary artery pressure, and a fall to shock levels of the systemic blood pressure. The pressures return to normal levels within an hour but later may fall again until death occurs. Bloody froth appears as a consequence of hemorrhage and the outpouring of plasma-like fluid. The net result is an increasing hematocrit and a fall in plasma volume. There is a fall in blood pH and evidence of significant right-to-left shunting of blood in the lungs. With severe injury the arterial blood pH falls and there is an increase in Pco_2. With minimal injury, the blood gas changes are those of hyperventilation, i.e., a rise in pH and a fall in Pco_2. With survival, the sequelae may be those of interstitial pulmonary fibrosis.

Tuberculosis

In primary pulmonary tuberculosis, the bacilli are inhaled and arrive at the alveoli in the same manner as other small particulate matter. Because ventilation is greater in the lower two thirds of the lungs, most bacilli and consequent primary lesions occur in this area, where, depending upon the number of organisms, their virulence and the native resistance of the host, there may be little prompt reaction or the formation of a relatively acute inflammatory exudate. The latter develops into a patch of bronchopneumonia with bacillary proliferation, neutrophils, and other inflammatory changes which are not unique to tuberculosis. However, whatever the initial reaction, tuberculous necrosis occurs with a surrounding zone of tuberculous granulation tissue consisting of blood vessels, lymphocytes, epithelioid and Langhans' cells, and collagen fibrils. Bacilli become scarce in the areas of necrosis for reasons that are not understood, although it has been suggested that caseation itself may be the defense mechanism. With the development of adequate acquired resistance the lesions become quiescent with the formation of a hyalinized connective tissue capsule from the zone of granulation and a consequent reduction in the size of the lesion. The caseous material may be resorbed, inspissated, calcified, or subsequently liquefied. Bacilli in such a primary lesion may be completely eliminated or they may remain quiescent but virulent for years.

Simultaneous with the development of the pulmonary lesion, bacilli appear in the hilar lymph nodes. Although these areas of involvement are larger than those in the pulmonary parenchyma, the progressive anatomic changes are similar. If the hilar lesion and the pulmonary parenchymal lesion both become calcified, a Ghon complex is formed.

It is believed that, in the evolution of the primary lesion, bacilli reach the blood stream either directly from the parenchyma or via the hilar lymph nodes and thoracic duct into the subclavian vein. Generally, the seeding is slight, the lesion is minute, and the end result is encapsulation, calcification, or complete absorption. Infrequently, persistent, viable bacilli in these extrapulmonary sites later may give rise to progressive disease in the organ in which they are situated. Tissues with a high oxygen tension constitute a preferential site for the bacilli to proliferate, hence the prime frequency of pulmonary infections with a lesser tendency to metastatic lesions of the kidney, brain, and the epiphyses of bones before maturation.

Postprimary adult tuberculosis occurs in many patients despite the defense mechanisms of specific immunity and the walling-off of necrotic lesions. In the past this has been called reinfection tuberculosis, largely because it may become evident many years after the primary infection; however, from epidemiologic data it is now believed that the "reinfection" is largely endogenous in origin. This is true in nations such as the United States where the annual tuberculin-reaction conversion is low, but it is not necessarily true in developing nations where the high endemnicity of tuberculosis suggests that reinfection from exogenous sources is still the predominant process.

For reasons that are not understood, softening and liquefaction occurs in the necrotic foci of some patients. As noted previously, bacilli are scarce in areas of necrosis, but concomitant with liquefaction they multiply and may reach large numbers. With rupture of the softened lesion into a bronchus, discharged infectious material is washed through previously uninfected airways establishing a mechanism for further spread and repetition of the sequence of caseation and cavitation. The cavitary lesions are prolific sources of bacilli, since the establishment of an airway connection makes growth-promoting oxygen available.

The gross mechanisms of defense are evident from the preceding accounts of primary and postprimary tuberculosis. As in other infectious processes, it is an inflammatory reaction with exudation, phagocytosis, fibrosis, and walling-off of the involved area. There are, however, unique characteristics of tuberculosis and the host response which make it inadvisable, if not impossible, to make dogmatic statements regarding other protective mechanisms. The mechanism of variation of racial resistance, for example, is not understood, although it is an evident fact. White adults respond to the presence of tubercle bacilli by inhibiting their multiplication and spread by marked reparative fibrosis. Negroes of all age groups and white children are deficient in these responses and, hence, less well protected. Hereditary constitutional characteristics, age, and sex are factors influencing the course of tuberculosis in the individual; yet the role of these parameters in causing fluctuations in the level of resistance to infection is not understood. Although antibodies develop in response to the tuberculous focus, their role in acquired resistance is not yet clear. Still, acquired resistance can be demonstrated in experimental animals and there is indirect evidence for its occurrence in man. In 1886, Marfan observed that individuals who had healed cervical adenitis before puberty subsequently did not develop pulmonary tuberculosis as frequently as others. This "Law of Marfan" has been held to be true even in African natives who are highly susceptible to tuberculosis. Rich has indicated the important role of mononuclear phagocytes in ingesting free bacilli as well as dead ploymorphonuclear cells with their contained bacilli. In the susceptible host, bacilli may not only survive but also multiply within the monocytes. Yet, once resistance is acquired through infection, not only do these mononuclear phagocytes continue to ingest bacilli but in addition they then inhibit multiplication and increase the rate of destruction of bacilli.

When tuberculin is injected into a person who has never had a tuberculous infection, the material is harmless and no significant reaction occurs. When injected into the skin of a person who has or has had a tuberculous infection, the tuberculin causes a sterile inflammatory reaction. Using a pure culture of tubercle bacilli rather than tuberculin, Koch observed this altered reactivity in infected guinea pigs, and subsequently the altered reaction to reinfection has been referred to as the "Koch phenomenon." This hypersensitiveness has been a source of considerable controversy. Some investigators have considered it an important protective mechanism, since acceleration and augmentation of the inflammatory response occur in response to tubercle bacilli in the hypersensitive organism. This response and the concomitantly accelerated tubercle formation are believed to represent an acceleration of the normal body defense. Others have regarded hypersensitivity as undesirable because of the associated necrosis of connective tissue, epithelium, blood vessels, and even the inflammatory cells themselves. In considering this problem, Rich comes to the conclusion that acquired resistance and hypersensitivity are separate phenomena and that hypersensitivity is at times decidedly deleterious and at other times is neither deleterious nor beneficial. This role of hypersensitivity as an advantageous defense mechanism remains an unsettled question and it is even doubted by many that it in any way participates in the development of acquired immunity.

From the standpoint of systemic symptoms the presence or absence of hypersensitivity is important. The very hypersensitive patient with a focus producing tuberculoprotein may have malaise, fever, headache, anorexia, and the other constitutional symptoms of tuberculosis. But another individual who is anergic may have a more extensive process with active bacilli and yet fail to develop any appreciable systemic response. The experimental counterpart of this is the desensitized tuberculous animal that will tolerate enormous doses of tuberculin which would be fatal to a hypersensitive but similarly infected animal.

The tendency of postprimary adult tuberculosis to localize in the posterior portions of the upper lobes is well recognized, but the mechanism of the localization has not been defined clearly. Various theories have been proposed based upon diminished respiratory movement in the apices, direct retrograde spread from cervical lymphatics, streaming of blood flow to the lungs so that blood from the superior vena cava flows preferentially to the apices, and relative anemia of the apices due to man's erect posture. There is now increasing evidence that the hydrostatic effect of gravity diminishes circulation to the apical areas of the lung. It is postulated that there is also a decreased transport of humoral factors and possibly a decrease in lymph flow. All these factors might contribute to increased susceptibility to infection in the apices.

The functional alterations in advanced pulmonary tuberculosis are secondary to parenchymal infiltration, loss of lung substance, fibrosis and pleural disease. Infiltrations result in destruction of alveoli and localized stiffening of the lung. The loss of lung substance in itself is infrequently serious owing to the large pulmonary reserve. The normal minute ventilation is of the order of 5 liters and this can be increased, on demand, to as much as 150 liters. However, the loss may be critical when combined with extensive fibrosis of the lung parenchyma and pleura, resulting in increased lung stiffness (loss of compliance) and slowing of both inspiration and expiration, defects in gas mixing, and compensatory emphysema. Pulmonary function tests reveal these pathologic changes as decreases in vital capacity, an increase in dead space, an increase in the ratio of the residual air to total lung capacity, and a decrease in arterial oxygen saturation on exercise. Although cor pulmonale is less common in tuberculosis than in chronic bronchitis and emphysema, it does occur in long-standing cases as a consequence of extensive vascular destruction from inflammation and fibrosis and increased shunting of blood from the bronchial arteries into the pulmonary veins.

In recent years it has become evident that mycobacteria other than *M. tuberculosis* and *M. bovis* may produce human pulmonary disease. These strains, such as *M. kansasii* and *M. intracellularis* (Battey mycobacteria), are generally referred to as "atypical" mycobacteria. Early skepticism as to their pathogenicity was based on the lack of virulence for guinea pigs. Repeated recovery in culture from sputa and tissue specimens in the absence of other organisms has been convincing evidence of their primary role in certain cases. Although pulmonary disease caused by these unclassified mycobacteria is uncommon, it is now evident that the disease produced is indistinguishable from tuberculosis, both clinically and pathologically. Although not yet demonstrated, it is supposed that the pathologic physiology will closely resemble that of tuberculosis.

Fungus Infections

There are many systemic mycoses which at times involve pulmonary tissues. Among the more important are histoplasmosis and coccidioidomycosis. Others, less frequently encountered, are actinomycosis, nocardiosis, cryptococcosis, candidiasis, blastomycosis, aspergillosis, geotrichosis, and mucormycosis. These various mycoses may occur as independent infections, but it is not unusual for them to appear as complications in the terminal stages of diseases such as the lymphomas, leukemia, and cancer. Candidiasis if often reported as a complication of broad-spectrum antibiotic therapy and mucormycosis as a complication of uncontrolled diabetes mellitus.

As a group, the fungi are poor antigens, and they do little to stimulate resistance mechanisms. In some, the response is more reminiscent of that to a foreign body than to a living infectious agent. Like the tubercle bacillus, fungi have a tendency to elicit hypersensitivity in the patient, and it is believed that the necrosis of tissue and abscess formation are consequences of this.

Clubbing of Fingers and Toes

The bizarre phenomenon of clubbing is associated with pulmonary neoplasms and various chronic disorders of the lung, as well as chronic disorders of the heart, gastrointestinal tract, liver, thyroid, and parathyroids and subacute bacterial endocarditis. In its more advanced stages, clubbing may be associated with periostitis and synovitis in the triad referred to as hypertrophic osteoarthropathy. The sequence, however, may be reversed so that the osteoarthropathy precedes the clubbing, and at times the manifestations may be unilateral or unidigital. There are also two hereditary-familial conditions, congenital clubbing and idiopathic hypertrophic osteoarthropathy, which are of little clinical significance except that their presence may be interpreted incorrectly.

Clubbing is a process of soft tissue proliferation at the base of the nail which elevates the nail root. The bony aspect is a proliferative periostitis which most commonly involves the distal portion of long bones of the forearms and legs and metacrapals and metatarsals. When joints are involved, there is osteoporosis, chronic synovitis, and nonspecific changes in the cartilage.

The pathogenesis is not clearly understood. Increased peripheral blood flow is a constant feature in the acquired form, but the flow is believed to be largely through dilated arteriovenous anastomoses. Limitation to fingers, toes, and occasionally the nose is attributed to the fact that these areas are endowed richly with arteriovenous anastomoses. Various hypotheses as to how clubbing is brought about have included endocrine imbalance, reduced oxygen tension of the blood, and reflex circulatory changes mediated through efferent nerves of the lung. Hall has postulated that digital clubbing may be the result of long-term action of a vasoactive substance on the arteriovenous anastomoses. On the basis of experimental studies he suggests the substance to be reduced ferritin which has not been oxidized by circulation through normal lung tissue. At present, however, one need not assume that there is a single cause of clubbing.

PLEURAL DISORDERS

The pleura is a thin, serous membrane. It is composed of an outer mesothelial layer, which rests on an avascular elastic layer and an areolar layer, consisting of elastic and collagenous fibers, blood vessels, lymph vessels, and nerves. The blood vessels of the visceral pleura are derived from the bronchial artery and, after breaking up into capillaries, reunite into branches of the pulmonary vein. The lymphatics drain into the hilar lymph nodes.

Since the relationship of the pleura to the subpleural alveoli is an intimate one, disorders involving these alveoli are readily reflected in pleural disease. This is well illustrated by the pleurisy and serous exudate which occur as a result of a small tuberculous focus in the lung. Cardiac decompensation, trauma to the thoracic duct, or any generalized disease affecting blood vessels or lymphatics also may lead to the appearance of fluid in the pleural space. Pleural effusion associated with the ascites of hepatic cirrhosis or solid ovarian tumors is occasionally observed. Examination of such fluid for its physical, chemical, and cellular characteristics is a useful clinical procedure.

Although there are various means of driving fluid into the pleural space, there are probably only two defense mechanisms for its subsequent removal. In those circumstances in which the protein concentration of the fluid is low, the resorption is probably at the venous end of the pleural blood capillaries. This is a consequence of the colloidal osmotic pressure of the blood plasma. However, in the presence of fluid of high protein content, the hydrostatic effect is nullified and the absorption of fluid, as well as of any particulate matter, is through pleural lymphatics.

Tumors of the Pleura

The true, primary pleural origin of tumors which are found in the pleura is under considerable question. In a given case it is extremely difficult to rule out the possibility of a primary pulmonary origin with growth of secondary lesions in the pleura. The localized tumors have the characteristics of lipomas, fibromas, fibrosarcomas, and differentiated neural tissue. As a group, they are slow-growing and may reach huge size without evidence of metastases. The only diffuse tumor is the mesothelioma, and it may involve the entire pleural surface. Whether metastases of this neoplasm ever extend beyond mediastinal lymph nodes is open to question, but the clinical course may nevertheless be rapidly downhill. The symptoms of pain, dyspnea, and cyanosis associated with pleural tumors are due to the interference with ventilation from the space occupied by the tumor, stiffening of the lung, and the accompanying effusion. Clubbing of the fingers may occur. Cytologic examination of the massive serous or serosanguineous fluid may be diagnostic.

Pleuritis

Inflammatory reaction of the pleura is almost always a consequence of spread of infection from contiguous structures. Thus, the primary site may be within the lungs, mediastinum, chest wall, diaphragm, or subdiaphragmatic area. Pulmonary infarctions, neoplasms, and systemic diseases such as the so-called collagen diseases are at times the causes of pleurisy. The early reaction to insult is erythema and edema of the pleura, followed promptly by the exudation of cellular elements and fibrin deposition. As the inflammatory reaction involves the parietal pleura and as the rough fibrinous surface stimulates parietal pain receptors during respiration, the symptoms and signs of pleurisy are evident. The pain of diaphragmatic pleuritis may be referred to the abdomen or the shoulder area, whereas involvement of the parietal pleura of the chest wall is rather accurately localized by the patient. Partial relief is obtained by voluntary and involuntary splinting which, by decreasing the amplitude of pleural excursions, reduces the stimulation of parietal pleural nerves. This limitation of tidal ventilation is partially compensated for by an increase in the rate of respiration. The clinical manifestation is tachypnea and the patient may complain of dyspnea if he resorts to any exertion. A friction rub may be audible over the area of disease. Pleural pain is absent in interlobar pleurisy, and any symptoms produced are those of the primary lesion or those of decreased lung volume should the effusion be very large.

If the disease progresses from the stage of dry pleurisy, an exudate which is usually serofibrinous is produced and this may become frankly purulent. As fluid separates the inflamed pleural surfaces, there will be alleviation of the acute pleuritic pain and the appearance of a more generalized chest pain. With large effusions, dyspnea is largely a consequence of volume displacement and reduced vital capacity.

Protective mechanisms brought into play are those that deal with the pulmonary problem precipitating the pleuritis, as well as absorption of fluid through the pleural capillaries and lymphatics and formation of adhesions that tend to seal the pleural surfaces together and wall off the process. The latter is readily induced, particularly when pulmonary movement is retarded, as it normally is at the apices.

At times the needle aspiration of pleural fluids is attended by symptoms of dizziness and faintness, even in the absence of pain. This is attributable to a fall in blood pressure, and its degree is a rough function of the volume aspirated and the rate of removal. Infrequently, the reaction to thoracentesis may be more serious and has even been reported to be a cause of death. Capps and Lewis studied this phenomenon in dogs and demonstrated that the aspiration of fluid with stimulation of the visceral pleura in the presence of inflammation is attended by a much greater risk than in the absence of inflammation. Their studies indicated that two different reflex mechanisms are involved. One is cardio-inhibitory, with slowing of the cardiac rate and usually slowing of respiration. This type of reflex is infrequently fatal. The other reflex is of the vasomotor type and is characterized by a rapid fall in blood pressure and more frequent termination in death unless therapy is directed toward the restoration of arteriolar tone.

Empyema

In thoracic empyema the pleural surfaces are abscess walls which are thickened, inflamed, and granular. Initially, there is an acute pleuritis which may be a consequence of pulmonary infection, surgery, trauma, or extension of an infection from the subdiaphragmatic area, mediastinum, or esophagus. When the origin is neither traumatic nor iatrogenic, the infectious agent most generally reaches the pleural space by direct extension from the lung, by rupture of a subpleural abscess, by lymphatic drainage into an effusion, or by septic embolization. Once the organism is established, an inflammatory exudate appears and the previously glistening pleural surface becomes a dull, thickened, granulating surface and pyogenic membrane. Further progress results in fibrous bands crisscrossing the empyema space and loculation of the exudate so that complete removal by thoracentesis is not possible. The wall of the empyema becomes organized into elastic fibrous tissue which may, as in tuberculosis empyema, effectively limit the infection and lead to quiescence for years.

If the empyema is small, the only alteration in pulmonary function may be a decrease in the excursions of the diaphragm and ribs. This is secondary to pain and reduces the vital capacity and maximal breathing capacity. If the empyema is large, the lung is compressed and the mediastinum is shifted toward the opposite lung, decreasing its volume also. The total pulmonary volume is reduced, vital capacity decreases, and pulmonary blood flow diminishes. Reduced oxygenation of the blood is generally evident. Although the loss of volume may not be great, the development of a nonelastic fibrous peel over the pleurae will reduce ventilatory function by mechanically limiting changes in volume. With maturation of the fibrous tissue, contraction occurs, which may reduce the lung volume severely by pulling the mediastinum toward the affected side and elevating and fixing the diaphragm. Particularly when this develops in early life, there may be a deforming scoliosis. With the decrease in volume on the side of disease, there is an absolute increase in volume in the normal hemithorax which results in compensatory emphysema.

The principles of management are directed toward the elimination of the infection by use of appropriate antibiotics, aspiration of the exudate, and enzymatic debridement if the purulent exudate is thick. If this is delayed or unsuccessful, surgical drainage of the abscess or decortication of the fibrous peel will be required to restore more normal pulmonary function. It has been observed repeatedly that bacteria may occur in pleural effusions and be eliminated by host defenses so that empyema does not develop. This situation, however, is a risky one, because if empyema does develop, the defense mechanisms walling off the empyema may in themselves result in crippling pulmonary disease.

Epidemic Pleurodynia

Epidemic pleurodynia, or Bornholm disease, is an acute febrile illness due to Coxsackie virus, Group B. In experimental animals the typical lesion in striated muscle resembles Zenker's hyaline degeneration. In man, the histologic changes are unknown because the illness is self-limited and followed by complete recovery. There may be severe pain and tenderness of muscles in the trunk and extremities, suggesting that the basic lesion is perhaps a myositis which also involves the diaphragm. Pleuritis, pleural effusion, exanthems, orchitis, diarrhea, hepatitis, meningitis, and pulmonary infiltrations have been noted. There are no significant alterations in pulmonary function. Recovery is characterized by a rise in specific neutralizing antibodies.

Pneumothorax

Pneumothorax occurs when air enters the pleural space. If entry of the air is via the bronchial tree, the condition is termed closed pneumothorax, and if via the thoracic wall, open pneumothorax. The latter is a consequence of trauma, whereas the causes of closed pneumothorax are many. Most commonly, closed pneumothorax is a consequence of the rupture of emphysematous blebs, but there are other entities occasionally incriminated: abscess, staphylococcal infections, tuberculosis, various forms of pulmonary fibrosis, and, rarely malignant disease.

The physiologic complications are related to the loss of or, at least, decrease in normal intrapleural negative pressure, which in turn interferes with the return of venous blood to the heart. If there is a valvelike mechanism at the site of the tear in the visceral pleura, a tension pneumothorax with pressures many times atmospheric may be obtained. Valsalva maneuvers associated with sneezing or coughing continue to force air into the pleural space. The lung first collapses with the loss of negative pressure and eventually is compressed toward the mediastinum. This structure may be forced toward the opposite side, resulting in partial compression of the intact lung, and the diaphragm may be forced downward. Dyspnea and cyanosis may occur as a consequence of pain, impairment of the volume of ventilation, and the passage of blood through nonaerated lung.

The vast majority of pneumothoraces are simple in that the pressures developed are not strikingly elevated and the process does not proceed beyond partial collapse. The pleural opening closes spontaneously and the healthy pleura absorbs the air within a matter of a few weeks. Complications such as tension pneumothroax, hemopneumothorax, bilateral spontaneous pneumothroax, and infectious processes require intervention to remove air, halt bleeding, and eradicate infection.

REFERENCES

Altschule, M. D.: Physiology in Diseases of the Heart and Lungs. Cambridge, Harvard University Press, 1949.

Barclay, A. E., Franklin, K. J., and Macbeth, R. G.: Roentgenographic studies of the excretion of dusts from the lungs. Amer. J. Roentgenol., *39*:673, 1938.

Basch, F. P., Holinger, P., and Poncher, H. G.: Physical and chemical properties of sputum. II. Influence of drugs, steam, carbon dioxide and oxygen. Amer. J. Dis. Child., *62*:1149, 1941.

Bates, D. V.: Chronic bronchitis and emphysema. New Eng. J. Med., *278*:546, 600; 1968.

Blanshard, G.: Sputum viscosity and postoperative pulmonary atelectasis. Dis. Chest, *37*:75, 1960.

Brock, R. C.: The Anatomy of the Bronchial Tree with Special Reference to the Surgery of Lung Abscess. London, Oxford University Press, 1954.

Cameron, J. L., Anderson, R.P., and Zuidema, G. D.: Aspiration pneumonia, A clinical and experimental review. J. Surg. Res., *7*:44, 1967.

Canetti, G.: Pathogenesis of tuberculosis in man. Ann. N. Y. Acad. Sci., *154*:13, 1968.

Capps, J. A., and Lewis, D. D.: Observations upon certain blood-pressure-lowering reflexes that arise from irritation of the inflamed pleura. Amer. J. Med. Sci., *134*:868, 1907.

Cherniack, N. S., and Carton, R. W.: Factors associated with respiratory insufficiency in bronchiectasis. Amer. J. Med., *41*:562, 1966.

Cohen, H. J., Merigan, T. C., Kosek, J. C., and Eldridge, F.: Sequoiosis. A granulomatous pneumonitis associated with redwood sawdust inhalation. Amer. J. Med., *43*:785, 1967.

Comroe, J. H., Jr., Forster, R. E., II, Dubois, A. B., Briscoe, W. A., and Carlsen, E.: The Lung. Clinical Physiology and Pulmonary Function Tests. Chicago, Year Book Medical Publishers, 1962.

Corssen, G.: Changing concepts of the mechanism of pulmonary atelectasis. J.A.M.A., *183*:314, 1963.

Cudkowicz, L., and Armstrong, J. B.: The bronchial arteries in pulmonary emphysema. Thorax, *8*:46, 1953.

Dickson, J. A., Clagett, O. T., and McDonald, J. R.: Cystic disease of the lungs and its relationship to bronchiectatic cavities. J. Thoracic Surg., *15*:196, 1946.

Di Rienzo, S.: Radiologic Exploration of the Bronchus. Springfield, Illinois, Charles C Thomas, 1949.

Drinker, C. K.: The Clinical Physiology of the Lungs. Springfield, Illinois, Charles C Thomas, 1954.

Ellis, F. H., Jr., and Carr, D. T.: The problem of spontaneous pneumothorax. Med. Clin. N. Amer., 38:1065, 1954.

Emanuel, D. A., Wenzel, F. J., and Lawton, B. R.: Pneumonitis due to *Cryptostroma corticale* (Maple-bark disease). New Eng. J. Med., 274:1413, 1966.

Fleischner, F. G.: The pathogenesis of bronchiectasis. Radiology, 53:818, 1949.

Fraimow, W., Cathcart, R. T., and Taylor, R. C.: Physiologic and clinical aspects of pulmonary alveolar proteinosis. Ann. Intern. Med., 52:1177, 1960.

Golden, A.: Pathologic anatomy of "atypical pneumonia, etiology undetermined." Acute interstitial pneumonitis. Arch. Path., 38:187, 1944.

Gordon, R. B., Lennette, E. H., and Sandrock, R. S.: The varied clinical manifestations of Coxsackie virus infections. Arch. Intern. Med., 103:63, 1959.

Hall, G. H.: The cause of digital clubbing. Testing a new hypothesis. Lancet, 1:750, 1959.

Hamman, L., and Rich, A. R.: Acute diffuse intersitital fibrosis of the lungs. Bull. Johns Hopkins Hosp., 74:117, 1944.

Hauser, T. E., and Steer, A.: Lymphangitic carcinomatosis of the lungs: Six case reports and a review of the literature. Ann. Intern. Med., 34:881, 1951.

Head, J. R.: Cystic disease of the lung with emphasis on emphysematous blebs and bullae. Amer. J. Surg., 89:1019, 1955.

Heppleston, A. G.: The pathogenesis of simple pneumoconiosis in coal workers. J. Path. Bact., 67:51, 1954.

Jarre, H. A.: Roentgenologic studies on physiologic motor phenomena. Radiology, 15:377, 1930.

Kilburn, K. H.: Cilia and mucus transport as determinants of the response of lung to air pollutants. Arch. Environ. Health, 14:77, 1967.

Klosk, E., Bernstein, A., and Parsonnet, A. E.: Cystic disease of the lung. Ann. Intern. Med., 24:217, 1946.

Krahl, V. E.: Anatomy of the mammalian lung. *In* Fenn, W., and Rahn, H. (Eds.): Handbook of Physiology. Vol. I. Washington, D.C., American Physiological Society, 1964, p. 213.

Lewis, P. A., and Sanderson, E. S.: The histological expression of the natural resistance of rabbits to infection with human type tubercle bacilli. J. Exper. Med., 45:291, 1947.

Lieberman, J.: A unified concept and critical review of pulmonary hyaline membrane formation. Amer. J. Med., 35:443, 1963.

Liebow, A. A.: Atlas of Tumor Pathology. Tumors of the lower respiratory tract. Washington, D.C., Armed Forces Institute of Pathology, 1952.

Loeffler, W.: Zur Differential-Diagnosis der Lungeninfiltrierungen. II. Über fluchtige Succendan-Infiltrate (mit Eosinophilie). Beitr. Klin. Erforsch. Tuberk., 79:368, 1932.

Macklin, C. C.: The dynamic bronchial tree. Amer. Rev. Tuberc., 25:393, 1932.

Mallory, T. B.: The pathogenesis of bronchiectasis. New Eng. J. Med., 237:795, 1947.

Mayer, E., and Rappaport, I.: Developmental origin of cystic, bronchiectatic and emphysematous changes in the lungs. A new concept. Dis. Chest, 21:146, 1952.

McIntyre, K. M., and Sasahara, A. A.: The hemodynamic response to pulmonary embolism in patients with prior cardiopulmonary disease. Amer. J. Cardiol., 28:288, 1971.

McLaughlin, R. F., and Tueller, E. E.: Anatomic and histologic changes of early emphysema. Chest, 59:592, 1971.

Michelson, A. L., and Lowell, F. C.: Blood acetylcholine in bronchial asthma. J. Lab. Clin. Med., 47:119, 1956.

Miller, W. S.: The Lung. Springfield, Illinois, Charles C Thomas, 1947.

Mittman, C., Lieberman, J., Marasso, F., and Miranda, A.: Smoking and chronic obstructive lung disease in alpha-1-antitrypsin deficiency. Chest, 60:214, 1971.

Morgan, T. E.: Pulmonary surfactant. New Eng. J. Med., 284:1185, 1971.

Morrow, P. E., Gibb, F. R., and Gozioglu, K. M.: A study of particulate clearance from the lung. Amer. Rev. Resp. Dis., 96:1209, 1967.

Motley, H. L.: Pulmonary function impairment in pneumoconioses. J.A.M.A., 172:1591, 1960.

Negus, V. E.: The action of cilia and the effect of drugs on their activity. J. Laryng. Otolaryng., 49:571, 1934.

Norris, R. F., and Tyson, R. M.: The pathogenesis of congenital polycystic lung and its correlation with polycystic disease of other epithelial organs. Amer. J. Path., 23:1075, 1947.

Proetz, A. W.: Essays on the Applied Physiology of the Nose. St. Louis, Annals Publishing Co., 1941.

Reynolds, E. O. R., Robertson, N. R. C., and Wigglesworth, J. S.: Hyaline membrane disease, respiratory distress, and surfactant deficiency. Pediatrics, 42:758, 1968.

Rich, A. R.: The Pathogenesis of Tuberculosis. Springfield, Illinois, Charles C Thomas, 1951.

Robertson, O. H.: Phagocytosis of foreign material in the lung. Physiol. Rev., 21:112, 1942.

Rococeanu, S. F., Mendlowitz, M., Suck, A. F., Wolf, R. L., and Naftchi, N. E.: Digital capillary blood flow in clubbing. Ann. Intern. Med., 75:933, 1971.

Rosen, S. H., Castleman, B., and Liebow, A. A.: Pulmonary alveolar proteinosis. New Eng. J. Med., 258:1123, 1958.

Sasahara, A. A.: Pulmonary vascular responses to thromboembolism. Mod. Conc. Cardiovasc. Dis., 36:55, 1967.

Schlueter, D. P., Fink, J. N., and Sosman, A. J.: Pulmonary function in pigeon breeder's disease. A hypersensitivity pneumonitis. Ann. Intern. Med., 70:457, 1969.

Sladen, A., Zanca, P., and Hadnott, W. H.: Aspiration pneumonitis—The sequelae. Chest, 59:448, 1971.

Sodeman, W. A., and Stuart, B. M.: Lipoid pneumonia in adults. Ann. Intern. Med., 24:241, 1946.

Sosman, A. J., Schlueter, D. P., Fink, J. N., and Barboriak, J. J.: Hypersensitivity to wood dust. New Eng. J. Med., 281:977, 1969.

Steinberg, I.: Lipoid pneumonia associated with paresophageal hernia. Angiocardiographic study of a case. Dis. Chest, 37:157, 1960.

Stevens, P. M., Hnilica, V. S., Johnson, P. C., and Bell, R. L.: Pathophysiology of hereditary emphysema. Ann. Intern. Med., 74:672, 1971.

Stewart, P. B.: The rate of formation and lymphatic removal of fluid in pleural effusions. J. Clin. Invest., 42:258, 1963.

Sturm, A.: Der Lungenkrampf (Kontraktionsatelektase durch Pulmonalen Spasmus). Deutsch. Med. Wschr., 71:201, 1946.

Sutnick, A. I., and Soloff, L. A.: Atelectasis with pneumonia. A pathophysiologic study. Ann. Intern. Med., 60:39, 1964.

Vogl, A., Blumenfeld, S., and Gutner, L. B.: Diagnostic significance of pulmonary hypertropic osteoarthropathy. Amer. J. Med., 18:51, 1955.

von Meyenburg, H.: Eosinophilic pulmonary infiltration: Pathologic anatomy and pathogenesis. Schweiz. Med. Wschr., 72:809, 1942.

von Neergaard, K.: Neue Auffassungen über einen Grundbegriff der Atemmechanik, abhängig von der Oberflächenspannung in den Alveolen. Z. Ges. Exp. Med., 66:373, 1929.

West, J. B., Holland, R. A. B., Dollery, C. T., and Mathews, C. M. E.: Interpretation of radioactive gas clearance rates in the lung. J. Appl. Physiol., 17:14, 1962.

Wood, W. B., Jr.: Studies on the mechanism of recovery in pneumococcal pneumonia. I. The action of type specific antibody upon the pulmonary lesion of experimental pneumonia. J. Exp. Med., 73:201, 1941.

Woods, W. B., Jr., Smith, M. R., and Watson, B.: Studies on the mechanism of recovery from pneumonia. The mechanism of phagocytosis in the absence of antibody. J. Exp. Med., 84:355, 1946.

Yoo, O. H., and Ting, E. Y.: The effects of pleural effusion on pulmonary function. Amer. Rev. Resp. Dis., 89:55, 1964.

Zimmerman, L. E.: Fatal fungus infections complicating other diseases. Amer. J. Clin. Path., 25:46, 1955.

Zohman, L. R., and Williams, M. H., Jr.: Cardiopulmonary function in pulmonary fibrosis. Amer. Rev. Resp. Dis., 80:700, 1959.

SECTION III

RHEUMATOLOGY, ALLERGY, INFECTIOUS DISEASE, AND HEMATOLOGY

CHAPTER 17 RHEUMATIC DISEASES

WILLIAM D. ROBINSON

The rheumatic diseases are grouped together, not because of a common etiology or pathogenesis, but because they produce symptoms in and impairment of function of the musculoskeletal system. The musculoskeletal system can be visualized as a highly integrated apparatus consisting of (1) the bones which provide the skeletal supports of the body, (2) the joints between the osseous structures which permit mobility while maintaining the capacity for stability, and (3) the neuromuscular apparatus for moving or stabilizing the supporting structures as needed. This chapter will be concerned primarily with the articulations and with the disturbances in function of the musculoskeletal system produced by diseases of the joints and closely related structures. It will also deal with closely related diseases.

The joints and the tendinous structures which transmit the motivating forces to permit smooth and efficient motion represent specialized forms of connective tissue. Basic information regarding the structure and function of connective tissues is needed for an understanding of normal function of these structures and the alteration produced by disease.

STRUCTURE AND FUNCTION OF CONNECTIVE TISSUES

It is no longer possible to regard connective tissue as an inert stuffing material, supporting and binding together the parenchymatous, neural, and vascular structures of multicellular organisms. As a result of the studies of numerous investigators, there has emerged a concept emphasizing the complex and dynamic state of these tissues, their importance in maintaining the physiologic integrity of the musculoskeletal system, and the significance of pathologic alterations in diseases of the connective tissues. The several types of connective tissues which differentiate from the mesenchyme include loose (areolar) connective tissue, dense fibroelastic connective tissue, reticular, adipose and elastic connective tissue, as well as bone, cartilage, and synovium.

Connective tissue can be regarded as composed of *cellular* and intercellular elements, with the intercellular components consisting of an *amorphous ground substance* interlaced with extracellular *fibrillar* materials. The proportion of these three constituents varies greatly with anatomic location and functional requirements: tendons and fascia are largely fibrillar, Wharton's jelly of the umbilical cord is predominantly ground substance, and cartilage and synovium are relatively rich in cells.

Connective tissue has the obvious important function of mechanical support and protection. In addition, it is essential for the smooth transmission of mechanical energy derived from muscle contraction to move the organism or its parts, facilitated by lubrication from ground substance components located in the gliding planes of joints, bursae, and tendon sheaths. Since connective tissue is everywhere interposed between capillaries and cellular structure, it has an important transport function, influencing the passage of essential nutrients to the cells and the return of metabolic wastes to the circulation. Particularly noteworthy is the remarkable potential of connective tissue in the process of anatomic repair. Following tissue injury, cellular components usually neutralize or destroy noxious agents, remove debris, and produce a framework of fibers and ground substance which bridges the anatomic defect and frequently restores functional capacity.

Connective Tissue Cells

The cellular elements of connective tissue control the formation, maintenance, and breakdown of the extracellular components. Primordial mesenchymal cells, located around the adventitia of vessel elements traversing the connective tissue, may differentiate to become macrophages, mast cells, plasma cells, lymphocytes, and fibroblasts. Macrophages and fibroblasts appear to be capable of mitotic division and are not dependent on a "stem cell" for their perpetuation. Tissue macrophages, widely distributed throughout the connective tissue, serve a scavenger role, ingesting foreign substances and removing debris. Tissue mast cells, also diffusely distributed, may be present in significant numbers in certain tissues. They represent 3 per cent of the cells in the superficial aspect of the synovial membrane. Their role in the physiology of connective tissue is not clear; they contain heparin, histamine, and 5-hydroxytryptamine. Plasma cells, lymphocytes, and eosinophils, undoubtedly to some extent derived from the bloodstream, are sparsely and irregularly distributed throughout connective tissue.

Fibroblasts are responsible for the formation and maintenance of fibrous and fibroelastic connective tissues. Specialized variants of fibroblasts—the chondrocytes, osteocytes, and synoviocytes—are credited with the formation of cartilage, bone, and the synovial fluid, respectively. The fibroblast appears as a stellate or spindle-shaped cell with a large pale nucleus and faintly staining cytoplasm under conventional light microscopy. By histochemical methods the cytoplasm has been demonstrated to contain cytoplasmic particles identified as ribonucleic acid, glycogen, and acid phosphatase; a number of oxidative enzymes have also been found. By tissue culture it has been convincingly demonstrated that the fibroblast synthesizes the acid mucopolysaccharides of the ground substance. In addition, the fibroblast produces collagen, which is first detectable in aggregated form outside of, but close to, the cell periphery.

Fibrillar Components

Three types of intercellular fibers can be distinguished by staining techniques and light microscopy. The most abundant is collagen, composing one third of total body protein. With conventional histologic techniques this appears as wavy bundles of fibers with the smallest units appearing to be nonbranching fibers with a uniform diameter of 0.3 to 0.5 microns. Under the electron microscope these fibers appear to be made up of submicroscopic fibrils with a characteristic periodic banding measuring 640 Å. Physical properties of collagen include a tendency to swell in dilute acetic acid and the formation of solutions with heat-dependent viscosity. Warming a solution of collagen converts it to gelatin, with an irreversible fall in viscosity. Physical-chemical and x-ray diffraction measurements indicate that the collagen macromolecule consists of three polypeptide chains wound around each other in an extended helical pattern and has a molecular weight of about 300,000. On chemical analysis, it is found that glycine (30 per cent), hydroxyproline (13 per cent), and proline (16 per cent) make up more than one half the macromolecule. Such hydroxyproline content is unique in mammalian proteins and is regarded as the "chemical fingerprint" of the collagen family. About 0.6 per cent of collagen is hexose, apparently covalently linked to the polypeptides at the hydroxylysine sites.

Detailed studies permit visualization of the biosynthesis of collagen in the following sequence. Polypeptide synthesis takes place on polyribosomal aggregates of the endoplasmic reticulum of the fibroblasts. This newly formed "tropocollagen" serves as substrate for a post-ribosomal hydroxylation reaction which converts many proline and lysine residues to hydroxyproline and hydroxylysine, forming molecules resembling the polypeptide chains. Extracellular aggregation of these chains into tropocollagen particles, measuring 2000 to 3000 Å in length and 15 Å in width, may result from the steric configuration of the polypeptide chains, although a role for mucopolysaccharides and glycoproteins in the ground substance cannot be excluded. This tropocollagen is the stage at which the first submicroscopic structural characteristics are detectable, and at this point the collagen triple helix can be demonstrated. The stability of the triple helix is attributed to the development of covalent hydrogen bonding both within and between the polypeptide chains. These tropocollagen super-helices then aggregate to form the collagen fibril with its characteristic periodic banding.

Some indication of the metabolic activity of collagen has been obtained by turnover studies using ^{14}C-labeled glycine. Three fractions are recognized: a neutral salt or alkali soluble fraction, a citric acid soluble fraction, and an insoluble fraction which constitutes by far the largest proportion of the collagen mass. The neutral salt or alkali soluble fraction, which presumably contains the tropocollagen, has a turnover rate in the range of that shown by plasma proteins. Except in rapidly growing animals, this fraction is small and probably represents the precursor of mature insoluble collagen. The insoluble collagen has a very slow rate of turnover, indicating that fibrous collagen is metabolically relatively inert. The acid soluble fraction also shows a slow turnover rate but is believed to be less highly cross-linked than the insoluble material.

Enzymes capable of degrading collagen (collagenases) have been demonstrated in living cells in regions of active collagen resorption, such as the tail fin of the tadpole during metamorphosis, the involuting uterus, and in bone undergoing remodeling. They are also found in polymorphonuclear leukocytes and in rheumatoid synovial tissue. Collagen degraded by collagenase is susceptible to further degradation by less specific proteases.

The second type of intercellular fibers, reticulin, is widely distributed through the body, especially around blood and lymph vessels, nerves, and muscle fibers; in basement membranes; and in the lymphoid organs. Under the light microscope they appear smaller than collagen fibers and frequently branch. They are distinguished by their affinity for silver stains and intense staining by PAS procedures. A relationship to collagen is indicated by similar 640 Å periodic banding under the electron microscope, a similar amino acid pattern, and comparable susceptibility to enzymatic degradation. However, reticulin has a higher carbohydrate content (4 per cent) and fatty acids account for about 11 per cent of the dry weight of reticulin.

Elastic fibers, the third type of intercellular fibers, quite clearly differ from collagen. With appropriate stains, they appear under the microscope as curling, branching, refractile fibers or fenestrated sheets. Electron microscopy shows no periodic banding and the x-ray diffraction pattern is unlike that which characterizes the collagen family. Amino acid analysis shows very little hydroxyproline. The source of elastic fibers has not been identified, although both fibroblasts and muscle cells have been suggested. Elastic fibers do not have the tensile strength of collagen fibers, but they have a greater capacity to return to their previous fiber length after removal of a distorting force.

Ground Substance

The cellular and fibrillar components of connective tissue are embedded in an amorphous sol-gel continuum known as ground substance. In routine histologic preparations much of the ground substance is leached out, leaving empty spaces between cells and fibers. By special fixation and appropriate histochemical procedures a dramatic staining of ground substance is produced. Information concerning its chemical composition is limited and much remains to be learned about variations with anatomic location and alterations with aging and in disease states. It is clear that this optically structureless sol-gel is an aqueous solution of electrolytes, proteins, highly polymerized carbohydrate substances known as mucopolysaccharides, combinations of amino acids and carbohydrate substances known as glycoproteins and mucoproteins, and lipids.

By extraction procedures the proteins of ground substance have been characterized as quite distinct in amino acid content from the fibrillar proteins, and as closely resembling plasma proteins in electrophoretic properties. The glycoprotein content of connective tissue is somewhat higher than in plasma, and there is evidence that at least some of these glycoproteins are synthesized by connective tissue cells.

Acid mucopolysaccharides (glycosaminoglycans), the most intensively studied components of ground substance, have the capacity to bind water and ions and are chiefly responsible for the viscosity of ground substance. They consist of high molecular weight polymers of carbohydrate, often associated with protein but separable from it by mild chemical methods. Recent evidence indicates that the molecular structure is a protein core with the carbohydrate chains radiating in a perpendicular manner at regular intervals. The polysaccharide portion is characteristically a large polymer of a disaccharide unit, usually containing a hexosamine and a hexuronic moiety linked by a glycosidic bond. The nature of the hexosamine and hexuronic acid varies with different types of connective tissues and with anatomic location. Table 17–1 records the composition of the carbohydrate component of some important mucopolysaccharides found in man and other mammals.

The anatomic distribution of these mucopolysaccharides may have considerable functional significance. Synovial fluid and vitreous humor contain only hyaluronic acid. Cartilage ground substance contains chondroitin sulfate A and C. The major mucopolysaccharide in adult bone is chondroitin sulfate A. Mixtures of the chondroitin sulfates and hyaluronic acid occur in diverse tissues such as umbilical cord, skin, tendon, heart valve, and aorta. Heparitin sulfate, a family of compounds with variable acetyl and sulfate ratios, has been isolated from aorta, lung, liver, and amyloid tissue. It is also excreted in large amounts in the urine by some patients with a hereditary disease of connective tissue, Hurler's syndrome. Heparin can be isolated from lung and aorta as well as liver. Keratosulfate has been identified in cornea, nucleus pulposus, aging cartilage, and growing bone. Chondroitin has been found only in the cornea.

Many investigators have contributed to an understanding of the enzymatic pathways by which the biosynthesis of repeating disaccharide units of the mucopolysaccharide chains is accomplished and some indication of the mechanism of linkage of these chains to the protein core is emerging. Tissue culture and isotope studies indicate that connective tissue cells from many sources synthesize glycosaminoglycans locally from simple precursors, including glucose. Cultures of human synovial tissue synthesize hyaluronic acid from

TABLE 17-1 COMPOSITION OF CARBOHYDRATE COMPONENT OF SOME IMPORTANT MAMMALIAN MUCOPOLYSACCHARIDES

Glycosaminoglycan	Hexosamine	Hexuronic Acid	Hexose	Sulfate
Hyaluronic acid	N-Acetyl-D-glucosamine	D-glucuronic acid	——	——
Chondroitin-4-sulfate (Chondroitin sulfate B)	N-acetyl-D-galactosamine	D-glucuronic acid	——	+
Dermatan-4-sulfate (Chondroitin sulfate B)	N-acetyl-D-galactosamine	L-iduronic acid (D-glucuronic acid, 5 to 15%)	——	+
Chondroitin-6-sulfate (Chondroitin sulfate C)	N-acetyl-D-galactosamine	D-glucuronic acid	——	+
Heparin	D-glucosamine	D-glucuronic acid (L-iduronic acid, trace)	——	+
Chondroitin	N-acetyl-D-galactosamine	D-glucuronic acid	——	?
Heparitin sulfate	D-glucosamine (acetyl)*	D-glucuronic acid	——	+*
Keratosulfate	N-acetyl-D-glucosamine	——	D-galactose	+

*The acetyl and sulfate content of heparitin sulfate varies in different preparations. Expressed as a molar ratio in relation to hexosamine, acetyl varies from 0.4 to 1.0 and sulfate varies from 0.6 to 1.8.

the components of a chemically defined medium. Turnover rates determined with isotopes indicate that the mucopolysaccharides of connective tissue are continuously in active flux, in contrast to the relatively static collagen. The half-life of hyaluronic acid is 2 to 4 days, and that of chondroitin sulfate, 7 to 10 days.

Enzymes capable of degrading the polysaccharide components are widely distributed in nature. Hyaluronidase acts by depolymerizing the glycosaminoglycan chains to shorter oligosaccharides. The viscosity of synovial fluid is reduced to that of water after the action of this enzyme. But the physical properties of at least some of the protein-polysaccharide complexes are dependent on an intact protein core as well as the polymerization of the carbohydrate component. When the protein component of such a complex found in cartilage (chondromucoprotein in a complex with chondroitin sulfate) is disrupted in vitro by papain, a fall in viscosity ensues. Intravenous administration of papain to rabbits leads to a loss of sulfated mucopolysaccharide from cartilage and to collapse of some cartilaginous structures.

Formation of Connective Tissue

An orderly sequence of connective tissue formation has been demonstrated in the healing wound and in the response stimulated by the implantation of polyvinyl sponges. Such studies frequently combine histochemical and analytical chemical techniques. The connective tissue defect is promptly flooded with plasma proteins and leukocytes from the circulatory system. Early in the reparative phase there is an impressive increase in the number of cells. This active proliferation of connective tissue cells is accompanied by a striking change in the tinctorial properties of the ground substance, characterized by prominent metachromatic staining that indicates high local concentrations of acid mucopolysaccharides. Soon fine intercellular reticular fibers, more likely small collagen fibers than true reticulin, can be detected. As the repair continues, the fibers become more numerous and individually larger, the cellular elements decrease in size and number, and the metachromatic hue of the ground substance subsides. Chemical analyses along the time course of this process show the hexosamine content (from glycoproteins and mucopolysaccharides) to peak in the first few days and then fall steadily, while hydroxyproline (an index of collagen content) rises steadily.

Information concerning factors which regulate the formation and maintenance of connective tissue in health and disease may be of fundamental importance; as yet, such information is fragmentary. There is evidence that aging, nutritional factors, and hormonal influences may be significant. In polyvinyl sponge granulomas the proportion of total protein represented by collagen increases with aging, as does the lipid content. Most studies of costal cartilage and intervertebral discs show a decrease in water content with increasing age, but such change in articular cartilage is less convincing. Analyses of human costal cartilage show that, whereas the predominant mucopolysaccharide of neonatal cartilage is chondroitin sulfate, the relative amount of keratosulfate increases with age as the proportion of chondroitin sulfate falls. In human aortic tissue the relative amounts of hyaluronate and chondroitin sulfate C decrease with aging while heparitin sulfate and chondroitin sulfate B increase.

Protein depletion prior to wounding is known to retard healing and decrease wound tensile strength. The granulation tissue in healing wounds of protein-depleted animals contains decreased amounts of hexosamine and hydroxyproline, suggesting that fibroblastic synthesis of both ground substance and collagen has been retarded. Ascorbic acid deficiency in guinea pigs and in man results in the failure to form collagen fibers, probably owing to the inability to hydroxylate proline to hydroproline. Correction of the vitamin C deficiency is followed within hours by the appearance of collagen fibers.

The effect of adrenal glucocorticoids on connective tissue has been extensively studied. An excess of hydrocortisone will interfere with wound healing and the formation of granulation tissue, reduce the cellularity and thickness of skin following local application, reduce the ratio of hexosamine to collagen in rat connective tissue, suppress the uptake of labeled sulfate into the sulfated mucopolysaccharide of rodents, and suppress both oxidative and glycolytic metabolism of rheumatoid synovium in vitro. Cell culture studies show that near physiologic concentrations of hydrocortisone induce multiple effects on human fibroblasts, including accelerated mitosis, suppression of collagen deposition, and depression of the specific rate of hyaluronate synthesis.

Quite recently, a "connective tissue activating peptide," which markedly stimulates the glycolysis of synovial cells in culture and increases the formation of hyaluronic acid by 10 to 40 times over the basal rate, has been demonstrated in a variety of mammalian cells, including leukocytes and connective tissue cells. In experimental granulomas, an early peak in the activating polypeptide corresponds to the time of maximal elaboration of hyaluronate into the ground substance.

STRUCTURE AND FUNCTION OF JOINTS

Simple gliding joints (diarthroses) consist of two bone ends covered by articular hyaline cartilage and held together by a sleeve of white fibrous connective tissue—the joint capsule. The inner layers of this capsule consist of specialized connective tissue cells—the synovium or synovialis. Within the joint space is a small amount of synovial fluid (Fig. 17–1). In the human embryo, the future joint can be identified by the fifth to seventh week as a remnant of mesenchyme interposed between two chondrogenous zones. Later, the center of this zone appears to liquefy, owing to elaboration of soluble ground substance, and the mesenchyme appears to retract peripherally

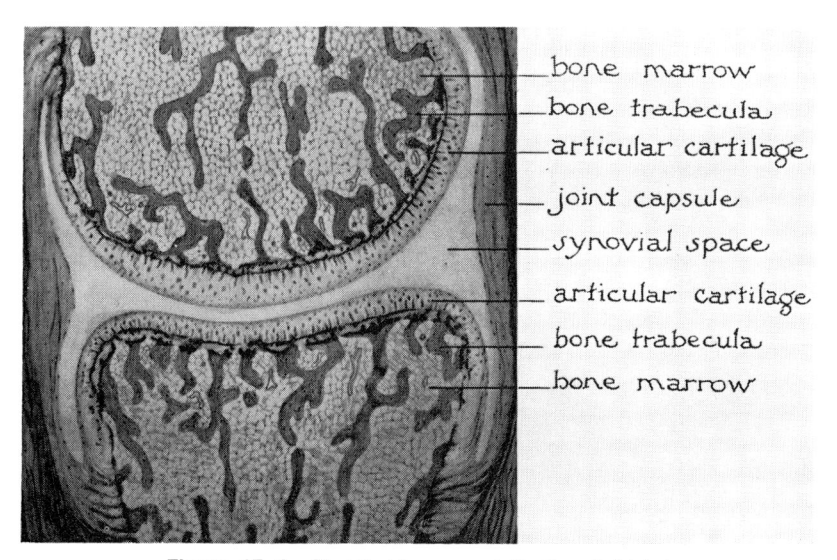

Figure 17–1 Sketch of a normal diarthrodial joint.

and to produce large numbers of closely packed fibrils. This is the future joint cavity, and its lining is the embryonic equivalent of the synovium.

Joint Capsule

The joint capsule consists largely of fibrous collagenous tissue with few elastic fibers. It is reinforced in areas by ligaments. It blends with periosteum of the bone shaft above and below the joint, and with tendinous and ligamentous periarticular structures. Stability and normal movement of the joints require that the relationships of the articulating bones maintain a normal alignment. This is accomplished to some extent by the anatomic configuration of the articulating surfaces ("congruity"), by the slight negative pressure in the joint cavity (-2 to -12 cm. water), and by the molecular cohesive properties of the synovial fluid. But the most important stabilization is provided by the strong fibrous outer part of the joint capsule and its reinforcing ligaments. When the joint capsule is weakened, joint stability and function are threatened or destroyed. The collagenous layers determine the mechanical properties of the joint capsule. It has very little elasticity, but its resistance to a stretching force is 30 times that of a sheet of pure rubber of equal thickness. Like tendinous connective tissue it has a high resistance to tear. The pliability of the synovium helps it to withstand the stresses of joint motion.

The blood vessels which supply the joint usually arise in common with those supplying adjacent bone and form a prominent arterial circle around the joint. Those that supply the joint ultimately pass into a rich capillary network which is prominent in the cellular and areolar areas of the synovium.

Articular nerves carry fibers from several spinal nerves and may supply more than one joint. They contain sensory fibers and autonomic fibers. The branches are widely distributed to joint capsule, ligaments, and synovium. The larger sensory fibers form proprioceptive endings in the capsule and ligaments which are very sensitive to position and motion. They play an important role in reflex control of posture, locomotion, and kinesthetic sensation. The smaller sensory fibers form pain endings in the capsule and ligaments and along the blood vessels. Twisting and stretching are the most effective pain stimuli to the joint capsule. Joint pain is perceived as diffuse and poorly localized; when severe, it may be felt distally over most of the extremity. Like visceral pain, it may be referred to another anatomic location. Joint pain not uncommonly leads to reflex contraction of adjacent muscles, which may take the form of a protective spasm.

Articular Cartilage

Cartilage is tough, resilient connective tissue consisting of cells and fibers embedded in a firm gel-like matrix which is largely made up of chondroitin A and C complexed with protein. Since the collagen fibers have nearly the same refractive index as the matrix, they are not visualized by conventional light microscopy. With polarized light the fibers are seen to be arranged so as to provide optimal resilience (Fig. 17-2). They extend as a looping curve resembling a croquet wicket with the ends anchored in the deeper calcium-rich zone of cartilage adjacent to the underlying bone. In relation to the cartilage surface this provides a surface zone of closely packed fibers parallel to the surface, an intermediate zone where the fibers are tangential, and a deeper zone where the direction is perpendicular to the surface. This arrangement permits the cartilage to expand laterally and diminish in thickness when pressure is exerted on the cartilage surface, and to rebound when the pressure is relieved (Fig. 17-3). This capacity of the cartilage mass to change in shape under pressure provides a cushioning effect protecting the subchondral bone and is the major method of buffering the blows and jolts received by the skeleton. The surface arrangement of the fibers assists the cartilage in providing a smooth gliding surface for the opposing bone ends. Under frequent intermittent pressures cartilage continues to be elastic. But with continuous compression its expansile power is

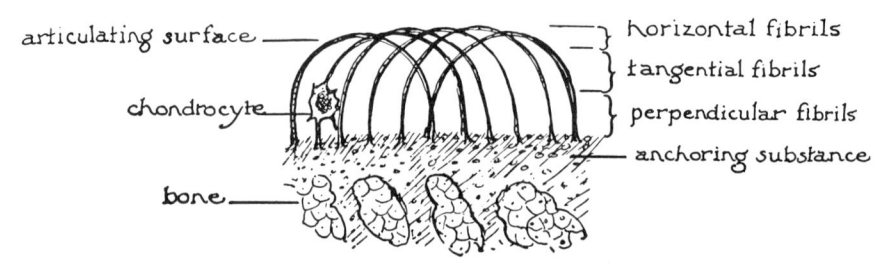

Figure 17-2 Sketch showing arrangement of collagen fibrils in articular cartilage as seen with polarized light. Note the three zones of fibrils aligned in horizontal, tangential, and radial positions.

Figure 17-3 Alterations in configuration of articular cartilage in response to pressure applied to cartilage surface (arrow). The fibrils flatten and separate more widely (broken lines). When pressure is relieved, the fibrils quickly resume the original high-arched resting shape (solid lines).

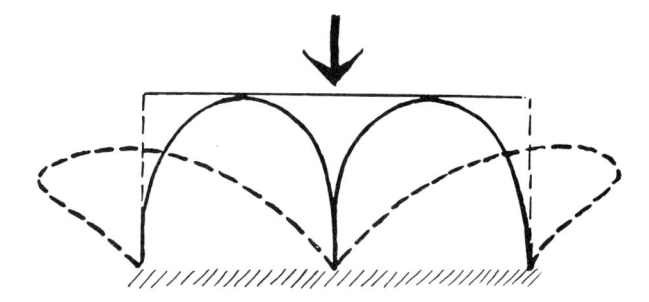

decreased and the time for recovery becomes longer. Elasticity is also reduced as water content decreases.

Articular cartilage has no blood supply. It receives most of its nourishment from the synovial fluid, probably augmented by the pumping action of intermittent compression and decompression. Some nutrition may be derived from diffusion from vessels in the underlying subchondral bone or subsynovial vessels located at the junction of the capsule and cartilage at the periphery of the joint.

Articular cartilage contains relatively few cells; therefore, the rate of respiration is relatively low. However, the rate of metabolism per cartilage cell is in the range exhibited by other connective tissues. New cartilage is formed interstitially by chondrocytes which are most numerous in the deeper layers of the cartilage. The cells of adult articular cartilage have usually lost the power of mitotic division. Consequently, the ability of this tissue to repair itself or to regenerate after injury is distinctly limited. Nevertheless, there is evidence that in normal use some replacement of articular cartilage may occur, and that opposition of articular surfaces is necessary for maintenance of cartilage integrity. Reaction to injury depends on the depth of the damage to the cartilage. Superficial cuts show little or no reaction. Peripheral lesions reaching the joint capsule or central lesions extending to the subchondral bone are promptly filled with fibrous tissue.

The Synovium

Synovial tissue, a vascular connective tissue basically similar to connective tissue elsewhere in the body, lines the inner surface of the joint capsule but does not cover the articular cartilage. It consists of cells, fibers, and ground substance. The cells near the surface have long cytoplasmic processes which overlap and intertwine. They may be one to several layers thick, forming a relatively smooth surface from which villi, folds, and fat pads may project into the joint cavity. Tissue deep to the surface may be fibrous, fatty, or areolar. The surface cells do not form a complete lining, so that intercellular material may be directly adjacent to the synovial space. Thus, the joint cavity is not a body cavity like the pleura, pericardium, and peritoneum. It is specialized connective tissue space.

The synovium is richly supplied with blood vessels, lymph vessels, and some nerve fibers. The capillary network and lymphatic network are adjacent to the joint cavity, and diffusion takes place readily between these vessels and the joint cavity. Most substances in the bloodstream easily enter the joint cavity, and many substances injected into the joint cavity readily enter the blood. The size and configuration of large molecules appear to influence the ease with which they may pass. Colloidal solutions, fine suspensions, and proteins, when injected into the joint cavity, enter into the subsynovial tissue and are removed chiefly by the lymphatics. Large particles are removed with difficulty and leave the joint by way of the lymphatics after phagocytosis. Motion of the joint definitely facilitates removal of materials injected into the joint cavity by both vascular and lymphatic routes.

Since the synovium is quite cellular and has an excellent blood supply, it is not surprising that it has a very good capacity for regeneration. After surgical removal, it will be formed again either from remnants of synovial tissue or from the joint capsule.

Synovial Fluid

The fluid within the joint cavity is highly viscous and sticky, resembling egg white in consistency. It is slightly alkaline and ranges from colorless to deep yellow. It contains relatively few cells (see Table 17-2), predominantly mononuclear cells derived from the synovium. Normal fluid is 95 per cent water and has a specific gravity around 1.010. In normal joints the amount of synovial fluid present is small; one can expect to aspirate only 1 to 3 ml. of fluid from a normal knee.

The relative viscosity of normal joint fluid ranges from 50 to 200 or more times that of water. This viscosity is due to the hyaluronic acid content which averages 3.5 mg. per gram of fluid.

TABLE 17-2 CHARACTERISTICS OF SYNOVIAL FLUID IN NORMAL JOINTS AND IN COMMON FORMS OF ARTHRITIS

		Appearance	Viscosity	Mucin Clot	Cell Count (per mm.³)	Crystals	"R.A." Cells*	Bacteria (on stain or culture)
Group I Noninflammatory	Normal	Straw colored, clear	High	Good	±200 WBC 20% PMN	0	0	0
	Traumatic Arthritis	Yellow to bloody, often turbid	High	Good	±2000 WBC 30% PMN Many RBC	0	0	0
	Osteoarthritis	Yellow, clear	High	Good	±1000 WBC 15-25% PMN	0	0	0
Group II Inflammatory	Rheumatoid Arthritis	Yellow to greenish, cloudy	Low	Fair to poor	15,000 to 40,000 WBC 60-90% PMN	Occasionally cholesterol	+	0
	Rheumatic Fever	Yellow, slightly cloudy	Low	Good	10,000 to 12,000 WBC ±50% PMN	0	0 or +	0
	Systemic Lupus Erythematosus	Straw colored, slightly cloudy	High	Good	±5000 WBC 10-15% PMN	0	0 or +	0
	Gout	Yellow to milky, cloudy	Low	Fair to poor	10,000 to 15,000 WBC 60-70% PMN	Urate +	0	0
	Pseudogout	Yellow, clear to slightly cloudy	Low	Fair to poor	1000 to 5000 WBC 25-50% PMN	Calcium pyrophosphate +	0	0
Group III Septic	Tuberculous Arthritis	Yellow, cloudy	Low	Poor	±25,000 WBC 50-60% PMN	0	0	+
	Septic Arthritis	Grayish or bloody, turbid to purulent	Low	Poor	80,000 to 200,000 WBC 75-90% PMN	0	0	+

*"R.A." cells—Inclusion-bearing cells, not morphologically specific, but most frequently found in large numbers in rheumatoid arthritis.

The viscosity increases exponentially with increases in concentration of hyaluronic acid and is also clearly related to the degree of polymerization of this polysaccharide. The viscosity of hyaluronic acid is due to the complex, highly asymmetric long-chain structure of the high molecular weight mucopolysaccharide. This structure confers the property of binding large amounts of water to form a viscous sol. Thus, the joint fluid is provided with high viscosity with negligible osmotic properties. A protein solution with comparable viscosity would produce an osmotic pressure far beyond the physiologic range.

In joint fluid, the hyaluronic acid is conjugated with but easily separated from a protein core; the protein content is less than 2 per cent of the total complex. This mucoprotein forms a clotted precipitate when treated with dilute acids, forming what is called *mucin*. The characteristics of the mucin clot formed on addition of dilute acetic acid provide a crude index of the degree of polymerization of the hyaluronic acid. In normal joint fluids, a tight adherent clot is formed. Such good mucin clot formation is also seen in fluids from traumatized joints, in degenerative joint disease, and in most types of acute inflammatory arthritis. In more chronic types of inflammatory joint disease this "mucin clot test" produces a flocculent, loosely adherent precipitate or even a powdery precipitate (Table 17-2).

The electrolyte content of joint fluid is comparable to that of the blood plasma. The amount of nonprotein nitrogenous substances and uric acid is usually slightly lower than in plasma. The glucose content varies with the level in the plasma, with changes in joint fluid sugar lagging slightly behind fluctuations in blood sugar. The total protein content is lower than plasma, ranging from 1 to 2 grams per 100 ml. In normal joint fluids the protein is largely albumin, with albumin-to-globulin ratios as high as 20:1. This is attributed to the smaller size of the albumin molecule.

Thus, synovial fluid, aside from its hyaluronic acid content, can be considered as a dialysate of plasma. Just as the joint cavity can be considered a specialized connective tissue space structurally and functionally, the synovial fluid can be visualized as a specialized type of ground substance, composed of a dialysate of plasma to which the synovial cells have added a characteristic mucopolysaccharide.

Joints as Functional Units

The structure of joints appears to be well adapted to serve the primary purposes of bearing weight and providing motion. Stability with motion is afforded by the fibrous joint capsule, ligaments and tendons, and muscle tone. The elasticity of articular cartilage permits adaptation to changing pressures and buffers impacts to which skeleton is subjected. Viscous synovial fluid forms a strong fluid interface with the cartilage surface, so that motion can occur with negligible friction.

Joint lubrication is so extremely efficient that the coefficient of friction is less than that of ice sliding on ice. The rheologic properties of synovial fluid contribute to this end. Since the viscosity of synovial fluid is non-Newtonian in character, it offers high resistance to static pressures, while at the same time providing lowered resistance to the increasing rates of shear encountered in joint motion. Joint lubrication is usually considered to be an example of fluid film or "floating" lubrication. Since the articular surfaces do not fit perfectly throughout the whole range of motion, this incongruity permits the development of wedge-shaped spaces filled with synovial fluid. The intra-articular pressure increases during motion, and it is greatest where the articular cartilages are closest together. Since this pressure is great enough to keep the articular surfaces apart, the intervening film of synovial fluid, rather than the bearing surfaces, takes up the effects of friction. In many joints, intra-articular fibrous and fibrocartilaginous structures such as menisci and discs, as well as fat pads and synovial folds, aid in distributing the synovial fluid. In the joints, this classic concept of hydrodynamic lubrication must be modified to take into consideration the fact that synovial fluid is absorbed by articular cartilage and oozes from the cartilaginous surfaces under pressure. This provides an element of boundary lubrication where the moving surfaces are separated by a layer of lubricant which is adherent to or incorporated into the surface and need be only a few molecules thick.

Like all moving mechanical systems, the human joint wears with time. Some wear and tear is inevitable with normal activity. The most evident result is wearing away of the articular cartilage to some degree. Articular cartilage is subjected to wear and tear unequaled by any other tissue except the skin. Since articular cartilage has no blood supply and since adult cartilage cells have largely lost the power of mitosis, the potential for regeneration of cartilage is slight.

In contrast, the highly vascular and cell-rich synovium has great capacity for regeneration. But alterations in the synovium can result in modifications in exchange equilibria between plasma and synovial fluid and changes in the characteristics of the mucoprotein of synovial fluid. Since the articular cartilage is dependent primarily on the synovial fluid for its nutrients, sooner or later the cartilage can be expected to reflect the results of functional aberrations of the synovialis.

FUNDAMENTAL PATHOLOGIC CHANGES OF JOINT DISEASE

Virtually all forms of joint disease can be understood in terms of two pathologic processes—degeneration and inflammation. Degenerative changes are dependent primarily on the limited capacity of articular cartilage to repair itself. Inflammation may be predominantly exudative or predominantly proliferative, or a combination of the two. It is not surprising that both degenerative and inflammatory changes can often be seen in the same joint. Cartilage which has been damaged as a result of inflammation is rendered more vulnerable to subsequent degenerative changes. In older persons, degenerative changes which have developed over the years do not render the joint immune to superimposed inflammation.

Degenerative Joint Changes

Much of the knowledge of the sequence of degenerative changes has been obtained from studies of the normal aging process in the joints. Bennett, Waine, and Bauer reported the gross and microscopic appearance of 63 knee joints obtained postmortem or following amputation and covering a wide age span. Abnormality of articular structure was first seen in the second decade and increased with advancing age. The first changes appear in the articular cartilage and show a predilection for those areas which are subjected to weight-bearing or shearing pressures. These are seen as localized areas of softening of the cartilage associated with a fine velvety disruption of the surface. In these areas, dehiscence of the cartilage occurs along the planes of the collagen fibers. The most superficial dehiscences are oriented parallel to the surface and, when confined to the tangential layers at the surface, produce "flaking." As the dehiscences proceed to the deeper layers they arch downward in a more vertical direction, producing "fibrillation" of the cartilage. A change in the ground substance in these areas of cartilage is indicated by decrease in metachromatic staining and more conspicuous

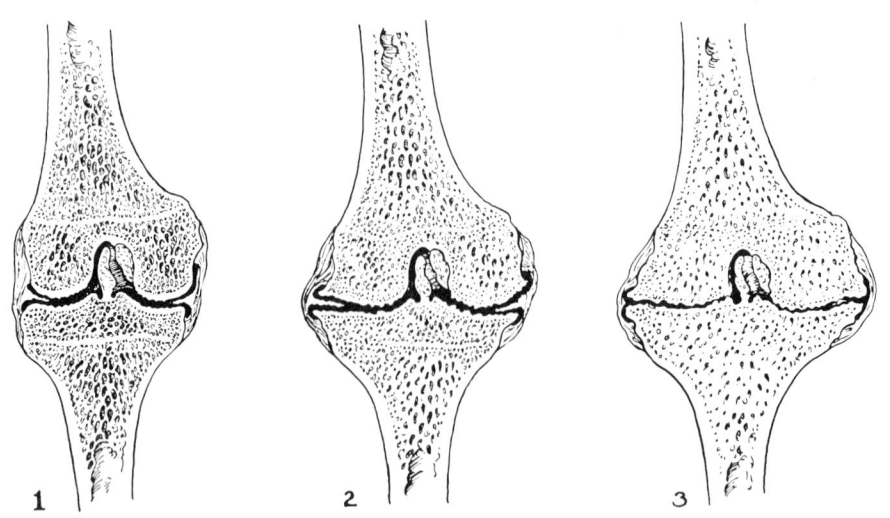

Figure 17-4 Sketches showing progression of joint abnormalities in degenerative joint disease: (1) early degenerative changes in the cartilages; (2) more extensive cartilage degeneration, with development of marginal osteophytes; (3) late stage, with almost complete loss of articular cartilages, extensive hypertrophic spur formation at joint margins, and irregularity and eburnation of subchondral bone.

fibrillar elements—the "unmasking" of the collagen fibrils. Chemical studies show a decrease in the chondroitin sulfate content relative to the collagen in such areas.

With abrasion of the fibrillated cartilage, clefts and fissures develop, followed by erosion and progressive denudation of the underlying bony cortex. Associated with this progressive wearing away of the cartilage is new bone formation in two separate locations relative to the joint surface: (1) exophytic growth at the margins of the articular cartilage and (2) in the marrow and cortex of the subchondral bone immediately underlying the articular cartilage (Fig. 17-4). The marginal osteophytes develop at the periphery of the articular cartilage where the joint capsule blends with the periosteum covering the shaft of the bone. They may extend into the joint cavity and tend to develop within capsular and ligamentous attachments to the joint margins, generally growing in a direction governed by the lines of mechanical forces exerted on the area. Such marginal bony lipping may be seen in the knee joint as early as the fourth decade of life. The osteophyte consists largely of bone which merges imperceptibly with the cortical and cancellous structure of subchondral bone. Proliferation of bone in the subchondral area results in increased density of the bony structure underlying the cartilage. It is most marked in areas that have been denuded of their covering of cartilage. Here the exposed bone becomes dense and hardened and takes on a highly eburnated appearance.

The synovial tissue itself is largely unaffected in degenerative joint disease. Some thickening and hypertrophy of the villous processes may occur. Synovitis occurs rarely and is usually due to mechanical irritation. The joint cavity is not obliterated and ankylosis does not develop.

Because of the development of marginal osteophytes and sclerosis of subchondral bone, degenerative joint disease is called *osteoarthritis* or *hypertrophic arthritis*. There is difference of opinion as to whether the disease represents an exaggeration of the normal process of aging, or whether other additional pathologic processes are operating. Predisposing factors may be grouped as (1) those which influence the integrity of the articular cartilage and (2) those which accentuate or accelerate normal wear and tear.

Genetic influences may be important determinants of the resistance of cartilage to wear and tear. Stecher demonstrated a hereditary pattern in the occurrence of *Heberden's nodes*, osteophytes which form at the base of the distal phalanges of the fingers and which are more common in women than in men. *Acromegaly*, in which there is excessive proliferation of cartilage, is associated with osteoarthritis with an unusual degree of bony overgrowth. In ochronosis which complicates alkaptonuria an abnormal pigment discolors articular cartilage and intervertebral discs, with gross alterations of their physical properties; this is often associated with unusually severe degenerative arthritis. A disease of growing children characterized by defective growth and maturation of the epiphyses results, despite the age of the patient, in joint changes indistinguishable from osteoarthritis. This disorder, known as Kaschin-Beck disease, is seen in Manchuria and eastern Siberia and is clearly of nutritional origin. In *hemophilia,* repeated hemorrhage into the joint leads to deposition of hemosiderin in the articular cartilage and eventually results in severe degenerative arthritis. These rare forms of degenerative joint disease suggest that extreme endocrine, metabolic, and dietary influences may alter the integrity of articular cartilage and predispose to the development of osteoarthritis. Whether more subtle influences of the same nature are operative in the more common types of degenerative joint disease is as yet in the realm of speculation.

It is much easier to document the role of predisposing factors which accentuate or accelerate the wear and tear on the joints. *Secondary osteoarthritis* can result from excessive or abnormal stresses and strains related to postural or orthopedic abnormalities. A variety of structural abnormalities of the hip joint in childhood such as congenital dysplasia, Legg-Perthes' disease, slipped femoral epiphysis, and congenital coxa vara lead to premature osteoarthritic degeneration. It may be a late result of trauma to the joint structures or of chronic irritation produced by derangement of internal joint structures—for example, a torn semilunar cartilage in the knee. It may appear in joints previously damaged by other types of arthritis.

The clinical features of osteoarthritis are readily explained by the underlying pathologic changes in the joint. It affects chiefly older individuals and characteristically involves weight-bearing joints. It is a localized disease of the joints and is not accompanied by systemic symptoms. The most common complaint is an aching pain which occurs on use, is rarely intense, and is relieved by rest. Stiffness after sitting is noted particularly with the first few motions involving use of the part. Such stiffness is dissipated rapidly and rarely persists more than a few minutes. Objectively, the joints may appear normal, but bony enlargements may be felt around the joint margins. Occasionally these are tender. Crepitus, creaking, or grating on motion can usually be detected. Increase in synovial fluid is uncommon; when it does occur—usually in the knees—it subsides within a day or two after elimination of weight bearing. The range of motion is usually only slightly impaired except in osteoarthritis of the hip. The roentgenographic features of osteoarthritis are decrease in thickness of articular cartilage (erroneously termed "loss of joint space"), formation of intra-articular and marginal osteophytes ("lipping"), and increased density of the subchondral bone. In advanced disease there may be crumbling and remodeling of the subchondral bone.

Neurologic disorders which result in loss of proprioceptive and pain sensation may be complicated by *neuropathic joint disease,* which has many features of osteoarthritis. Deprived of its protective reflexes the joint is subject to severe and cumulative injury. There is relaxation of supporting structures with chronic instability of the joint. The degenerative changes progress rapidly and cartilage damage is extensive. With relative absence of pain, continued use results in extensive damage to cartilage and subchondral bone. These structures fragment, leaving loose bodies of cartilage and bone free in the joint cavity. These loose bodies and the extensive erosion of bone irritate the synovium, with a resulting proliferative synovitis and persistent joint effusion. Subluxations and dislocations are common, as are intra-articular and juxta-articular fractures. The degenerative changes are accompanied by exuberant overgrowth of bone. The characteristic clinical features are the relative absence of pain and remarkable hypermotility of the affected joint. Radiographic features are the combination of extensive destructive and hypertrophic changes.

Classically, neuropathic joints occur as a complication of tabes dorsalis ("Charcot's joints"). Syringomyelia and spinal cord degeneration accompanying diabetes and pernicious anemia may also be the basis. Usually one joint only is affected—most often the hip, knee, ankle, midtarsal joints, and the lumbar and the lower spine. In syringomyelia, joints in the upper extremity may be involved.

Effects of Trauma

The simplest type of joint abnormality is that which results from injury. The trauma may be slight and cause only a strain on the fibrous capsule or ligaments. The response of edema and congestion produces swelling around the joint, with pain and stiffness from stimulation of the nerve endings which are abundant in the periarticular tissues. Since the tissues affected have a good blood supply, healing is usually rapid and complete. With more severe trauma, the synovium may be injured, followed by traumatic synovitis and effusion within the joint cavity. In the absence of repeated trauma, such sterile inflammation persists for a relatively short time and recovery is usually complete. More severe trauma can damage the cartilage and, at times, the underlying bone and may provoke changes in the dynamics of the joint which, after a period of time, result in post-traumatic degenerative changes. If the injury is to the cartilage located centrally in the joint, little regeneration takes place and the irregularity of the joint surface places a strain on the periarticular structures at the joint margins, stimulating proliferation of bone. If the injury is at the articular margin of the cartilage, abnormal bone formation may develop rapidly. The late changes resulting from severe joint trauma are those of osteoarthritis, with rapidity of development determined by severity and location of the damage to joint structures.

Joint Inflammation—Synovitis

Inflammation can be visualized as a progressive impairment of the microcirculation of a tissue, initiated by a variety of agents and mediated by mechanisms that are incompletely characterized. The classic manifestations of heat, redness, swelling, pain, and impaired function correlate with alterations in the microcirculation, dominantly increased local blood flow, and increased vascular permeability ("leaks"). Since the vascular and lymphatic supply to the joint is predominantly in and just beneath the synovium, it is this tissue which is initially and principally involved in joint inflammation.

In acute synovitis, exudative inflammation predominates. The joint is swollen, warm, tender to touch, and painful to move. Redness and heat over the joint vary with the type and severity of inflammation. The joint capsule is distended by an outpouring of synovial fluid with an increased content of inflammatory cells, nearly always polymorphonuclear neutrophils. Microscopically, the venules and capillaries of the synovium are dilated; the synovium and subsynovial tissues are edematous and infiltrated to a varying degree with inflammatory cells. Some types of arthritis such as the synovitis of serum sickness and acute rheumatic fever, which are self-limited and subside without residual joint damage, can be regarded as examples of purely exudative inflammation of the synovium.

However, in the more chronic forms of arthritis, the proliferative phase of inflammation develops and may dominate the pathologic and clinical features of the disease. Rheumatoid arthritis is the prototype of such combined exudative and proliferative inflammation, with extensive formation of granulation tissue accounting for the joint destruction and disability (Fig. 17–5). The synovium is swollen and deep red in color and there is hypertrophy of the villous processes. There is reduplication of the synovial lining cells and proliferation of fibroblasts. The inflammatory cells are chiefly lymphocytes and may appear in a follicle-like arrangement. The fibroblastic and angioblastic proliferation forms granulation tissue which replaces the synovium and invades the joint capsule and periarticular structures. Particularly significant is the invasion of the interior of the joint by a reddish, roughened, tongue-like protrusion of granulation tissue, growing over the articular cartilage from the joint margins (pannus formation).

By lysis of cartilage ground substance and fibers, interference with nutrition of the cartilage, and actual invasion, this inflammatory tissue slowly destroys the articular cartilage. It may join with similar granulation tissue arising from subchondral marrow. The capsular inflammation and proliferative granulation tissue tend to persist and to progress slowly, with remissions and exacerbations leading to cumulative damage to cartilage and subchondral bone. This damage, consequences of the original inflammation, accounts for the deformities and crippling that characterize the later stages of rheumatoid arthritis. In these later stages the evidences of exudative inflammation usually lessen and may appear to subside completely. The granulation tissue becomes primary fibrous and is converted to a dense scar. This tough fibrous scar limits or prevents joint motion (fibrous ankylosis). On occasions, this scar becomes calcified and is converted to osseous tissue (bony ankylosis).

Alterations in Joint Fluid Produced by Disease

It is to be expected that changes in the permeability of the synovial tissues and vessels will be reflected by changes in the joint fluid. The increased permeability accompanying inflammation permits more ready passage into the joint cavity of water, electrolytes, and easily diffusible colloids. The passage of protein molecules is enhanced, and the increase in total protein content of the joint fluid is proportional to the intensity of the inflammation. The proportion of globulin increases with lowering of the ratio of albumin to globulin. This increased permeability also accounts for the presence of fibrinogen, immune globulins, leukocytes, and proteins with enzymatic activity in the joint fluid during inflammation. The glucose content tends to decrease as the leukocyte content increases, and is characteristically low or absent in septic joints. This is attributed to the increased glycolytic activity of the leukocytes and synovial cells.

The viscosity of joint fluid is reduced in inflammatory disease, particularly in rheumatoid arthritis. This is explained in part by a decrease in concentration of hyaluronate; however, since the volume of joint fluid is increased severalfold, the total amount of hyaluronate is considerably greater than in the normal joint. Some of the decrease in viscosity is also due to the presence of less highly polymerized molecules of hyaluronate, which is also evidenced by deterioration of the mucin clot produced by the addition of dilute acetic acid. These changes are usually considered to reflect alterations in metabolic activity of synovial cells during inflammation, a concept supported by the observation that rheumatoid synovial cells in culture produce larger amounts of less highly polymerized hyaluronate as compared

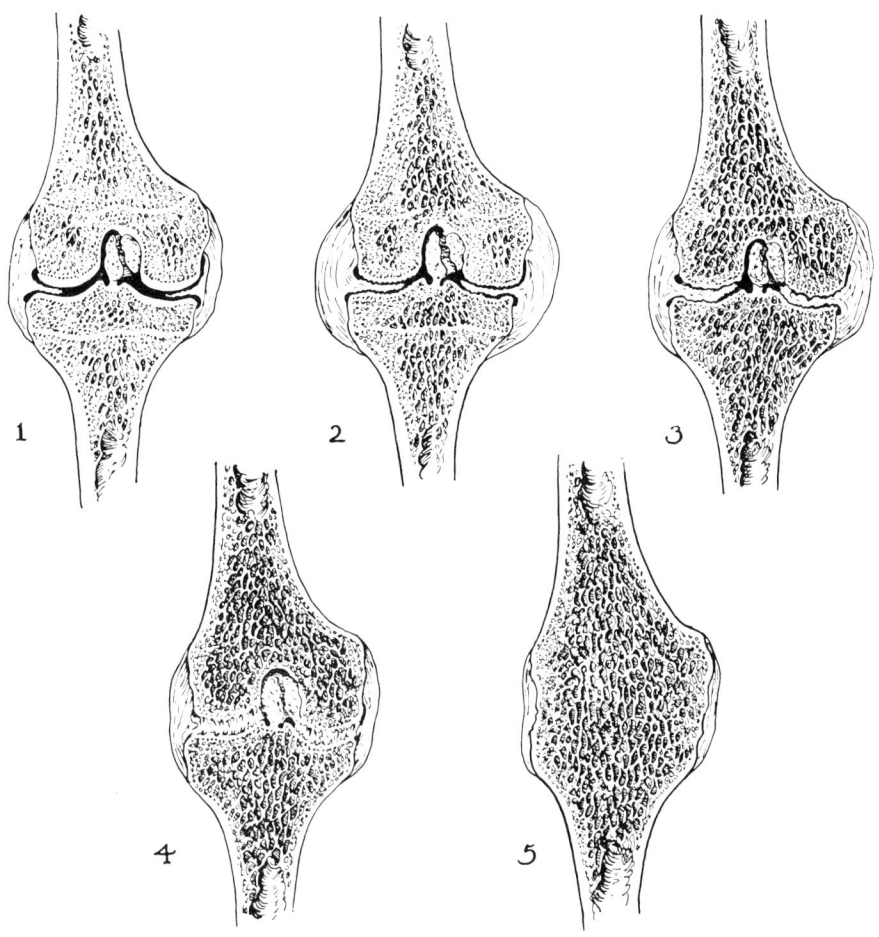

Figure 17–5 Sketches showing joint disease in rheumatoid arthritis: (1) Inflammation of joint capsule with synovitis and early proliferative changes; (2) progression of proliferative inflammation with pannus formation, beginning cartilage destruction, and mild osteoporosis; (3) more advanced synovitis with extensive pannus formation, severe cartilage destruction, and marked osteoporosis; (4) late stage, with fibrous ankylosis and inflammation less active; (5) bony ankylosis.

with synovial cell cultures from noninflamed joints. The possibility of degradation by enzymes released from leukocytes and synovial lining cells into the synovial fluid cannot be ruled out.

The characteristic changes in the synovial fluid in the more common forms of arthritis are listed in Table 17-2. As an aid in differential diagnosis, examination of the synovial fluid by simple methods is of greatest help in differentiating noninflammatory from inflammatory synovial effusions, in the detection of septic arthritis, and in the demonstrations of characteristic crystals in gout and pseudogout. Effusions in traumatic and degenerative joint disease are relatively clear, do not clot, and characteristically show only a modest increase in number of white blood cells. Viscosity is well maintained and the mucin clot is firm, ropy, and nonfriable. Inflammatory fluids are more turbid, may clot on standing owing to the presence of fibrinogen, and usually contain more than 5,000 leukocytes per mm.[3] and may range as high as 60,000 to 80,000 in chronic inflammation. The leukocytes are predominantly polymorphonuclear neutrophils. Varying degrees of deterioration in viscosity and characteristics of the mucin clot reflect alterations in the hyaluronate. In septic joints the fluid is turbid to frankly purulent, the leukocyte count is 80,000 to 200,000 per mm.[3], almost all of which are polymorphonuclear leukocytes, and the responsible microorganism may be demonstrated by direct staining or by culture.

PATHOGENESIS OF JOINT INFLAMMATION

Extensive investigation is beginning to elucidate the physiologic and biochemical mechanisms by which inflammation is produced. Since the joint in an extremity is a well-demarcated tissue space which can be sampled easily and repeatedly by needle aspiration or biopsy, studies of joint inflammation have contributed significantly to concepts relating inflammatory mechanisms to human disease. Present knowledge permits only what must be regarded as an oversimplified and incomplete concept of the mechanisms and mediators of the changes in the microcirculation which is the "final common pathway" of inflammatory damage. Factors which have been considered mediators of the microcirculatory effects can be conveniently grouped under headings of small molecular mediators, plasma factors, leukocyte factors, immune mechanisms, and tissue necrosis, with full appreciation of the interplay between such factors and others yet to be identified.

The role of *immune mechanisms* in producing tissue damage and inflammation is covered in Chapter 4. The biological activities of complement may be of particular significance in rheumatic disease.

Plasma factors implicated in inflammatory reactions include Hageman factor, the kininogen system, and the fibrinogen and plasminogen systems. Each of the systems involves specific substrates, enzyme activators, cofactors, and inhibitors.

Small molecular mediators include histamine, the kinin peptides, serotonin, and the catecholamines. These chemicals, produced by body cells, have profound effects on the microcirculation in extremely small concentrations. In model systems, injections of histamines, bradykinin, and serotonin produce only an immediate and transient effect on the microcirculation. Whether such substances serve only to initiate the inflammatory response or whether continued production of them may sustain the inflammation is not clear. Kinin peptides in synovial fluids from inflamed knees have been demonstrated by bioassay.

Among leukocyte factors, the concept of *lysosomes* has attracted much attention in recent years. This concept, originated by DeDuve, visualizes many types of cells to contain small lipid bags of hydrolytic enzymes active against a variety of substrates. These enzymes are active only when leaks develop in the wall of the sacs that contain them. Once released, the enzymes all have optimal activity at an acid pH. The key to the lysosome is its lipid wall, which can be either stabilized or weakened by a number of exogenous factors. The lipid walls can be disrupted by mechanical means, by chemical means, and by enzymes. They may be stabilized by compounds such as corticosteroids, cholesterol, and chloroquine.

It is convenient to measure the activity of one or more of these enzymes as an index of lysosomal disruption; acid phosphatase and beta glucuronidase are most often measured. Acid phosphatase can also be identified by the Gomori reaction in histochemical and electron microscope preparations, a technique useful in defining the location of this enzyme in cells and tissues. It is of interest that acid phosphatase has been demonstrated in the cytoplasm of proliferating fibroblasts. Both acid phosphatase and beta glucuronidase have been found in the synovial fluid from inflamed joints, with levels paralleling the number of polymorphonuclear leukocytes.

While lysosomes are found in many types of cells, the polymorphonuclear leukocytes are particularly rich in them, and they constitute the familiar neutrophilic granules seen with the Wright's stain. Three mechanisms of disruption of the lysosomes of these cells have been described. (1) During phagocytosis of particulate matter the cell membrane invaginates to surround the ingested particle, forming an autophagic vacuole; the lipid wall of the lysosome fuses with the vacuole and discharges the hydrolytic enzymes into the vacuole. Leukocytes exuding in response to particulate matter such as bacteria and crystals die in a few hours. (2) Certain bacterial exotoxins, such as streptolysin O and S, can rupture lysosomes within the cytoplasm of the leukocyte, resulting in rapid death of the cell. This phenomenon has led some workers to refer to lysosomes as "suicide bags." (3) A staphylococcal exotoxin, "leukocidin," causes the granules to swell into vesicles, some of which fuse with the cell membrane and rupture to the outside. The end result in each case is a degranulated leukocyte showing the nuclear and cytoplasmic changes of cell death, and nearly every exudate rich in polymorphonuclear leukocytes has shown elevation of the activity of those enzymes which serve as an index of lysosomal disruption.

The interrelations among these various factors and their relative importance in producing the microcirculatory alterations characteristic of inflammation are not well understood at the present time. Nevertheless, it is possible to examine these mechanisms as they apply to the various types of inflammatory joint disease. Much of the remainder of this chapter represents an attempt to do this.

SPECIFIC INFECTIOUS ARTHRITIS

Almost every type of microorganism can infect joint tissues and cause inflammation. Rarely, the entry to the joint is directly by laceration or by extension of infection from contiguous bone.

Usually the infection is carried by the bloodstream, with initial localization of the microorganism in the synovial and subsynovial tissues. The inflammatory reaction in the joint has the same characteristics as that provoked by the particular microorganism in other body tissues.

Bacteria most commonly responsible for purulent inflammation of the joint are staphylococcus, streptococcus, gonococcus, meningococcus, and pneumococcus. Infection by these organisms in their more usual habitat may be evident but at times must be searched for carefully. The large joints, such as the hip, knee, or shoulder, are most commonly affected, although any articulation, either spinal or peripheral, can be involved. The process usually involves only one or a few joints, although with gonococcal or meningococcal infection there may be an early migratory phase with pain in several joints before the bacteria settle down to provoke a true septic arthritis. The inflammation is dominated by the purulent exudate, and the "leukocyte factors" are undoubtedly principally responsible for the intensity of the inflammatory reaction. These factors also account for the rapid destruction of articular cartilage which accompanies the presence of pus in the joint cavity. Proteolytic and other hydrolytic enzyme activity can be demonstrated in leukocyte autolysates, and purulent synovial fluids containing 110,000 or more leukocytes per mm.^{3} are capable of digesting small pieces of cartilage, whereas synovial fluid with leukocyte counts of 6,000 to 20,000 are not. If septic arthritis is not recognized promptly and treated with appropriate antibiotics, extensive joint destruction may occur. Also, the natural repair of joint tissue which has harbored prolonged purulent inflammation results in granulation tissue with ensuing scar formation, and fibrous ankylosis may result.

Tuberculous infection usually involves only one joint, provoking a slowly progressive low-grade synovitis dominated by the granuloma formation and proliferative inflammation characteristic of the response to the tubercle bacillus. Doughy swelling of the joint with slight to imperceptible increase in local heat may be present, owing to the thickened synovium rather than increase in synovial fluid. The tuberculous synovitis forms a pannus of granulation tissue which tends to spread over and destroy the cartilage and also infiltrates under the cartilage, resorbing the bony articular cortex and the lower layers of the cartilage. In some cases this results in detachment of the articular cartilage. Since the synovial fluid in tuberculous arthritis is not rich in proteolytic and other hydrolytic enzymes, such loosened cartilage may persist for months but is eventually destroyed. Early destruction of periarticular bone is one of the roentgenographic features of tuberculous arthritis. An exception is the knee joint, where tuberculous synovitis of low grade may persist for months or years with little discomfort and little bone destruction. However, in almost all cases the joint tuberculosis should be regarded as involving synovium, cartilage, and bone. The tuberculous process may extend into periarticular tissues, producing a "cold abscess" about the joint, or it may travel between muscle and fascial planes and drain to the exterior through sinus tracts.

Mycotic infections of the joint, which develop in the disseminated granulomatous phase of coccidioidomycosis, histoplasmosis, blastomycosis, cryptococcosis, and actinomycosis, provoke an inflammatory reaction which has many of the clinical, radiographic, and pathologic features of tuberculous arthritis.

CRYSTAL-INDUCED SYNOVITIS

Acute Gouty Arthritis

The rediscovery in 1960 of the vital role of urate crystals in the acute gouty attack has stimulated extensive studies of mechanisms involved in acute joint inflammation. Crystals of sodium urate were demonstrated to be a constant finding in synovial fluid of patients with gout and to be uniformly absent from nongouty fluids. The presence of such crystals within leukocytes is characteristic of acute gouty inflammation. The crystals are seen in wet preparations as short rod shapes with rounded ends, or as needle-like. Under polarized light they show a strong negative birefringence, which is definitive. Injection of urate crystals into the joints or subcutaneously into experimental animals or human subjects (both normal and gouty) produces an acute inflammatory response, whereas amorphous urates produce only a mild response, and urates in solution produce no response. Other crystalline substances of similar configuration produce a similar inflammatory reaction, indicating that the phenomenon is dependent on the physical rather than the chemical nature of the crystal. In man the inflammatory response strikingly resembles the acute gouty attack.

It has been convincingly demonstrated that this inflammatory response requires leukocytes. Dogs rendered profoundly leukopenic by prior administration of vinblastin or by the use of specific antileukocyte serum displayed suppression of the inflammatory response to intra-articular injection of urate crystals. The ability to respond was restored when the injected joint was perfused by blood from a normal animal. Following intra-articular injection of microcrystalline urate, the joint pressure increases and the pH of the synovial fluid falls, owing to a rise in the concentration of lactic acid resulting from increased metabolic activity of the leukocytes. The crystals are phagocytized and either destroyed by uricolytic enzymes of the leukocytes or released if the leukocyte ruptures and may be reingested by others. The concentration of kinin-like peptides in the synovial fluid rises during the crystal-induced inflammation as it does in spontaneous attacks of gout.

Such observations support the concept of the pathogenesis of acute gouty arthritis illustrated in Figure 17-6. The initial event is precipitation or release of urate crystals locally. The presence of even a few crystals in supersaturated body fluids promotes further crystallization. The crystals provoke a polymorphonuclear leukocyte response. These leukocytes phagocytose the urate crystals; accompanying phagocytosis, leukocyte metabolic activity increases, and lactic acid production increases, producing a lowering of local pH. Because urate solubility decreases at a more acid pH, this change tends to promote further precipitation of urate crystals and a self-perpetuating cycle is produced. Colchicine, the drug which for centuries has been the classic and highly specific treatment for the acute gouty attack, appears to interrupt this cycle by a direct effect upon the leukocyte, with inhibition of its metabolic and biological activity.

This system has also permitted study of possible mediators of the inflammatory response. Considerable evidence has accumulated to support the role of kinin polypeptides in this response. It has been demonstrated that urate crystals are capable of activating Hageman factor (factor XII). In addition to its role in initiating coagulation, Hageman factor has the ability to activate kallikrein, the enzyme regulating the formation of bradykinin from kininogen. It has been established that Hageman factor is present in normal synovial fluid and that kinins are present in the synovial fluid in acute gout (and in other inflammatory joint diseases), decreasing in concentration as the inflammation subsides. There is evidence that Hageman factor (and urate crystals without the intervention of Hageman factor) can activate C'1-esterase; this in turn promotes activation of complement components which produce increased vascular permeability, phagocytosis, and chemotaxis. The leukocytes may also significantly contribute to the production of kinins. Alternatively, or in addition, they may contribute to the inflammatory process by release of lysosomal enzymes.

Gout is fundamentally a disorder of purine metabolism, usually genetically determined but sometimes acquired, characterized by persistent elevation of urate in the plasma. Discussion of the mechanisms responsible for this hyperuricemia is beyond the scope of this chapter. Clinically it is manifested by recurrent attacks of a charac-

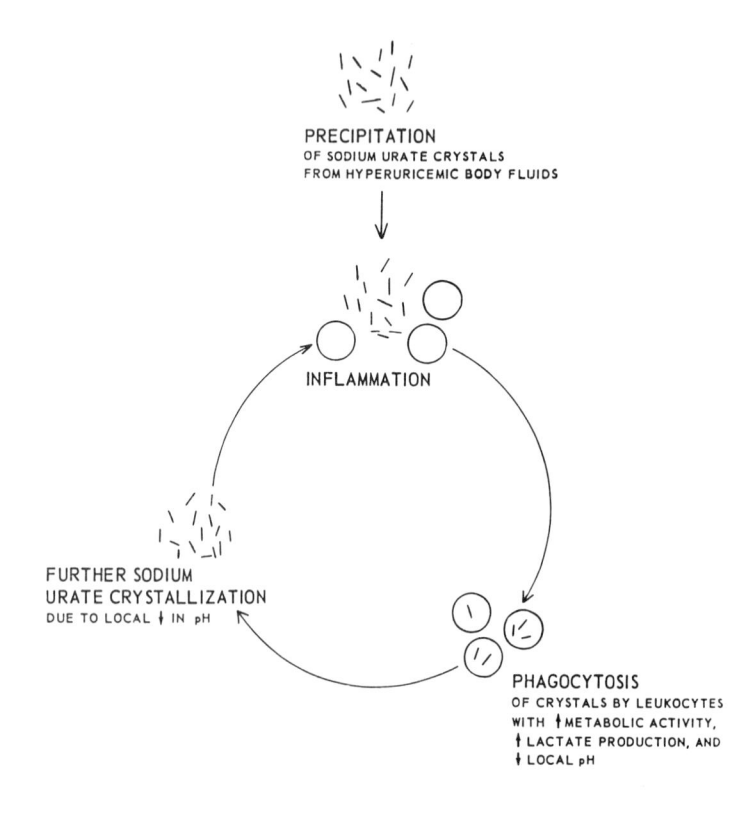

Figure 17-6 Concept of pathogenesis of acute gouty arthritis as a self-propagating inflammatory reaction. (From Seegmiller, J. E., and Howell, R. R.: Arthritis Rheum., 5:616, 1962.)

teristic type of acute arthritis, by depositions of sodium urate monohydrate in and around joints of the extremities and by renal disease which may include deposits of urate crystals in the kidney and formation of urate calculi. The clinical manifestations are ultimately dependent on the fact that, even in normal humans, uric acid is present in concentrations near the limit of its solubility in body fluids.

Acute attacks of gout are characterized by abrupt onset and extremely severe inflammation which may easily be mistaken for a septic joint. Although the victim of this disease may be totally incapacitated, the synovitis subsides in several days to a week or two, with complete resolution of the inflammation and restoration of normal joint function. The concepts outlined above provide an explanation for many features of the acute episodes, including the abruptness of onset, the severity of the synovitis, and the intermittent pattern of attacks. However, the events leading to the initial crystallization of sodium urate from the supersaturated fluid are poorly understood. Furthermore, these concepts do not clarify how and why the untreated attack resolves spontaneously.

Chronic Gouty Arthritis

In gout, urates tend to deposit in cartilage, epiphyseal bone, periarticular structures, and the kidneys. Such deposits may form visible tophi and may be responsible for permanent joint damage or chronicity of symptoms. Such urate deposition is dependent on the height of the serum uric acid concentration, the severity of the renal involvement, and the duration of the disease. Tophi are seen most often in patients who have had gout for 6 to 10 years or more. Lowering of the serum urate concentration with appropriate medication can prevent urate deposition and can actually lead to disappearance of tophi that have previously developed.

Deposition of urates produces a local necrosis and (unless the tissue is avascular) an ensuing foreign-body reaction with proliferation of granulation tissue. In the joint, synovial proliferation with pannus formation may develop, producing chronic synovitis with capsular fibrous thickening. Deposits of urate on the surface of the articular cartilage are often present with associated cartilaginous degeneration and accelerated appearance of degenerative joint changes. Destruction of subchondral bone with depositions of urate in the marrow results in the punched-out lesions of bone commonly seen in roentgenograms of gouty patients. These marrow tophi often communicate with the urate crust on the articular surface through erosions and defects in the articular cartilage.

Pseudogout

When, stimulated by the findings in gout, microscopic examination of wet preparations of synovial fluid by compensated polarized light was applied to examination of many synovial fluids, nonurate crystals were discovered in the joint fluids of patients whose clinical diseases had many features of gout. The crystals appear as rodlike or rhomboid forms with sharp corners, and under polarized light they demonstrate weakly positive birefringence. By x-ray diffraction these crystals were identified as calcium pyrophosphate dihydrate. Fluids removed from acutely inflamed joints with pseudogout invariably showed such crystals within polymorphonuclear leukocytes, indicating that they had been phagocytosed. Crystals with morphologic features identical to the natural crystals were synthesized. Injection of synthetic or natural crystals into human and canine joints was followed by acute inflammation associated with phagocytosis of the crystals by polymorphonuclear and mononuclear leukocytes. The inflammation was related in severity to the dose of crystals injected and was completely reversible. Although the details of mediation of the inflammation in this condition have not been studied as completely as in gout, there seems to be little question that this condition is another example of crystal-induced synovitis.

As this disease was recognized, it soon became apparent that it was associated with miliary calcium deposits in fibrocartilaginous structures, articular cartilage, ligaments, and joint capsule which can be seen on roentgenograms (chondrocalcinosis). These punctate and linear densities are seen most frequently in the menisci of the knee; other fibrocartilaginous structures calcified in this fashion are the articular discs of the distal radio-ulnar articulation, the symphysis pubis, the glenoid and acetabular labra, and the annulus fibrosus of the intervertebral discs. Calcification in the hyaline articular cartilage appears as a midzonal radiopaque line paralleling the contour of the underlying bone. Calcification may also be seen in the articular capsules of the larger joints. The deposits visualized radiographically have been studied in 3 patients at necropsy and have been convincingly demonstrated to be calcium pyrophosphate dihydrate crystals.

The clinical pattern of the arthritis ranges from intermittent acute attacks with complete remission between attacks, to clusters of almost continuous acute episodes in a number of joints, to a chronic progressive arthritis with superimposed acute episodes. Synovial biopsy shows inflammatory and reparative changes consistent with the clinical appearance of the joint. Some patients show only a chronic progressive arthritis without acute episodes; in such patients often the crystals cannot be demonstrated in the synovial fluid. Some patients with chondrocalcinosis are completely asymptomatic, and many patients will show calcific deposits in the tissues of joints which have never been the site of acute or chronic inflammation.

The mechanism for deposition of the calcium pyrophosphate crystals in cartilage and periarticular structures is unknown. Undoubtedly, local tissue changes must be favorable for the physical-chemical formation of the crystals. Aside from the occasional patient with hyperparathyroidism, serum values for calcium and phosphorus are normal.

Calcareous Tendinitis (With Subacromial Bursitis)

Inflammatory involvement of tendons and contiguous bursae associated with deposition of calcium in and about the tendon is presumably another example of crystal-induced inflammation. This occurs commonly around the shoulder, with calcium deposition in one or more of the tendons in the rotator cuff, notably the supraspinatus tendon. Such deposits, visualized radiographically, are the most frequent abnormality encountered in acutely and subacutely painful shoulder. However, similar calcifications are found in many asymptomatic patients. The deposition of calcium is believed to be associated with degenerative changes in the tendon, perhaps related to wear and tear. As long as the calcium is confined to the relatively avascular fibrous tendon, it excites little or no reaction. But with encroachment into more vascular areas, a severe acute inflammatory reaction with hyperemia and edema is aroused. In the shoulder, the floor of the subacromial bursa forms part of the sheath for the supraspinatus tendon. Fluid collects within the tendon sheath and bursa and produces pressure, pain, and muscle spasm.

The nature of the calcium deposit in calcareous tendinitis and the characteristics of the inflammatory response have not been well studied. The inflammation is self-limited, and subsidence may be accelerated by removal of the calcium by needle aspiration or by the injection of antiinflammatory agents. Often, as a result of the hyperemia of the inflammation, the calcium densities seen radiographically may appear to be resorbed.

IMMUNOLOGICALLY MEDIATED INFLAMMATION

As experimental immunologic observations have been correlated with clinical experience, a workable system of general classification of the immunologic reactions producing tissue injury has emerged. As proposed by Gell and Coombs, the system is based on four general types of reactions. Those of principal interest in rheumatic diseases are types II, III, and IV, or a combination thereof. Type II reactions (complement-dependent cytotoxic reactions) are dependent on the interaction of antibody with cell-bound antigen, with consequent activation of the complement system to produce cell damage or lysis. Type III reactions (immune-complex reactions) are mediated by the deposition of soluble antigen-antibody complex at a reaction site. Following complex formation, complement fixation occurs, with sequential activation of the complicated complement system accounting for the biological alterations of the reaction. Among the diverse biological consequences of the interaction of antigen, antibody, and the complement system are activation of the kallikrein-kinin system, the attraction of polymorphonuclear leukocytes, and increase in capillary permeability. The kinin peptides induce vasodilatation, pain, and increased vascular permeability. The infiltrating leukocytes have been shown to ingest complexes, then to degranulate and release their lysosomal enzymes, which in turn act as even more powerful chemotactic agents and mediators of increased permeability.

Type IV reactions (delayed or cellular reactions) depend on the interaction of specifically sensitized small lymphocytes with the antigen. Developmentally, these small lymphocytes with the capacity for immunologic memory appear to be thymus-dependent. A brief and undoubtedly oversimplified summary of the mechanism of this type of delayed reaction is as follows. Contact of these small lymphocytes with antigen leads to blast transformation and biosynthetic events producing a "sensitized lymphocyte." Cell-free extracts of disrupted leukocytes from individuals displaying delayed hypersensitivity are capable of transferring this capacity to sensitize the small lymphocyte (transfer factor). Upon recurrent contact with the antigen, these sensitized lymphocytes can recruit other mononuclear cells to the reaction site by the elaboration of "migration inhibiting factor." Cytolysis of antigen-bearing cells may then result from adherence of sensitized cells and elaboration of lytic substances. Under the microscope the delayed or cellular reaction may show variable accumulation of fluid and polymorphonuclear leukocytes for the first 24 hours but thereafter is dominated by mononuclear cells, predominantly macrophages and monocytes with occasional small lymphocytes. The macrophages may coalesce to form giant cells. In severe reactions, necrosis in the central portion of the lesion may develop.

Serum Sickness

The basic mechanism of serum sickness is a type III antigen-antibody interaction. In studies with suitably tagged foreign protein, the concentration of circulating antigen shows a gradual decrease for 10 to 14 days. This corresponds to the latent period between introduction of the foreign protein and the appearance of symptoms, a period of development of the immune response. Circulating antibody is not easily detected at this time because of the formation of soluble complexes with the circulating antigen. This is indicated by a sudden drop in the level of circulating antigen, and onset of the inflammatory lesions corresponds to the appearance of circulating soluble immune complexes. The disease continues until antibody is entirely removed from the circulation. Antibodies to the foreign protein are easily demonstrated in the patient's serum during convalescence and for long periods of time thereafter. Readministration of the foreign antigen leads to prompt formation of antibodies and immune complexes and recurrence of the clinical disorder.

In experimental animals, localization of immune complexes containing antigen, antibody, and complement has been demonstrated in the endothelium of vessels of several organs. In synovial tissue this immune complex deposition leads to inflammatory infiltration, edema, and fibrinoid necrosis.

Clinically, serum sickness is characterized by fever, arthralgia, skin eruptions, and edema. Objective evidence of synovitis may be present. It is a self-limited disease, the manifestations usually subsiding in 1 to 3 weeks. With the advent of antimicrobial therapy the use of serum for the treatment of bacterial infection has declined markedly. At the present time the most common cause of serum sickness is an administered drug, most often an antibiotic.

Rheumatic Fever

Rheumatic fever is an uncommon but by no means rare sequel to an upper respiratory tract infection caused by Group A hemolytic streptococci. Although most, if not all, serologic M types of Group A streptococcal infections of the pharynx can lead to rheumatic fever, only 3 per cent or less of all patients who do not receive adequate antimicrobial treatment for streptococcal infection will develop subsequent rheumatic fever. There is a latent period of 1 to 4 weeks between the streptococcal infection and the appearance of signs and symptoms. Multiple focal aseptic inflammatory lesions are the basis of the acute manifestations. These include migratory arthritis, carditis, chorea, skin lesions, and subcutaneous nodules. The acute disease is of limited duration, but the carditis can lead to permanent valvular damage.

The arthritis in rheumatic fever is characterized by an inflammation which develops and subsides in the joints first affected, only to occur in other joints which were initially spared ("migratory polyarthritis"). The inflammation can be mild, with only vague discomfort in the region, but is often severe, with acutely inflamed red swollen joints which are very painful to touch or on attempted motion. The fluid in such joints is turbid and contains inflammatory leukocytes (Table 17–2) but is sterile on bacteriologic culture.

An immunologic mechanism in the production of at least the acute inflammatory lesions in rheumatic fever is inferred rather than established. Such a mechanism is strongly suggested in the production of the synovitis by the intriguing parallelism between the latent period of serum sickness and rheumatic fever and by the fact that the inflammation in both conditions is self-limited, subsiding completely and without residual joint damage. Antibodies to numerous components of the streptococcus appear in the circulation of patients during pharyngeal infection by this organism, whether or not they subsequently develop rheumatic fever. Therefore, an increase in the titer of antistreptococcal antibodies is evidence of a recent streptococcal infection and is not diagnostic of rheumatic fever. Most but not all of those who develop rheumatic fever have a higher antibody response which may persist longer than in those who do not develop this complication after streptococcal pharyngitis.

The mechanism for production of the carditis and the late valvular lesions is not clear. Autologous antibodies that react with mammalian muscle including myocardial elements occur in the sera of patients with rheumatic fever in concentrations greater than those in the sera of patients who do not develop this complication. This autologous antibody cross-reacts with a streptococcal antigen. The source of the antigenic stimulus for this antibody and the role which it plays in the pathogenesis of the disease remain to be determined.

Rheumatoid Arthritis

Much evidence has accumulated in recent years implicating immunologic mechanisms in the pathogenesis of rheumatoid arthritis. This dates from the identification over 20 years ago of the presence of autologous immune globulins ("rheumatoid factor") in the serum of most patients with rheumatoid arthritis. This immune globulin has the characteristics of an antibody to normal human gamma globulin. Later, the presence of complexes of this antigen and antibody in the leukocytes of rheumatoid synovial fluid was demonstrated. In the past few years, impressive evidence for activation of the complement system in rheumatoid synovial fluid has emerged.

It has long been recognized that the sera of

some patients with rheumatoid arthritis could cause the agglutination of a number of different particles. These included certain strains of streptococci and staphylococci, collodion particles, and various erythrocytes, such as those of sheep coated with subagglutinating quantities of rabbit antiserum. It was then found that the particle involved was nonspecific, and that the essential reaction was between the gamma globulin coating the particle and a factor in rheumatoid serum. It was shown that tanned sheep erythrocytes and inert particles such as latex or bentonite, when coated with gamma globulin, are agglutinated by rheumatoid sera.

The factor responsible for these reactions was identified as euglobulin, with the electrophoretic properties of gamma globulin and a sedimentation constant in the ultracentrifuge of a macroglobulin (19S). It is frequently found in serum in a complex with 7S gamma globulin. Thus, classic rheumatoid factor was defined as IgM with antibody binding sites directed toward determinants of IgG. Later, globulins of the IgG (and possibly IgA) classes were found to have anti-IgG activity, and polymorphism among the rheumatoid factors is well established. Rheumatoid factors react most avidly with IgG which has been partly denatured or aggregated, presumably owing to exposure of additional binding sites by the alteration in molecular configuration. Immunofluorescent studies indicate that rheumatoid factor is produced by lymphoid tissues in the "large pale cells" in the germinal centers of lymph nodes and in plasma cells surrounding the germinal centers. The same distribution of staining is seen in the lymphoid nodules within the synovial membrane of rheumatoid joints.

As this information developed there was difficulty in visualizing the way in which rheumatoid factor was involved in producing the pathologic lesions and clinical manifestations of rheumatoid arthritis. Rheumatoid factor cannot be detected in some 30 per cent of patients who meet the criteria for the diagnosis of rheumatoid arthritis ("seronegative" rheumatoid arthritis). It has been found in high titers in other disorders without arthritis and in some normal subjects. In short-term studies, infusion of serum containing high titers of rheumatoid factor did not induce the disease in normal recipients.

By 1965, several observers using phase contrast microscopy for examination of wet film preparations of synovial fluid had demonstrated the presence of particulate inclusions in the cytoplasm of leukocytes in a high proportion of rheumatoid synovial fluids. Rheumatoid factor was released when these leukocytes were disrupted. Determinants of both IgG and rheumatoid factor were identified in these cytoplasmic particles by immunofluorescent techniques. This finding was not restricted to rheumatoid arthritis, being seen at times in other forms of inflammatory synovitis. IgM globulins were more frequently found in seropositive patients with rheumatoid arthritis, and some of these inclusion bodies were shown to contain certain components of complement. Rheumatoid synovial fluid was found to contain both kinin polypeptides and lysosomal enzymes. Phagocytosis of the rheumatoid factor-IgG complex by leukocytes with release of lysosomal enzymes was demonstrated by in-vitro studies. Injection of autologous IgG into inactive or clinically uninvolved joints of patients with rheumatoid arthritis produced inflammation in some, but not all, patients studied.

Immunofluorescence studies demonstrated certain components of complement in tissue sections of rheumatoid synovium along with deposits of immunoglobulins. Although the serum level of complement in patients with rheumatoid arthritis is in the normal range, the complement activity of the synovial fluid usually is definitely lower in rheumatoid fluids as compared with other joint effusions. This lowered complement activity is most consistently found in the fluids from seropositive patients. Such determinations first were done in terms of total hemolytic complement activities (CH50). As the 12 serum proteins constituting the complement system (nine "components" and three "inhibitors" or "inactivators") were identified, methods became available for quantitative studies of the sequential activation of this complicated system. Austen and colleagues have recently applied such methods to measure the activities of the first four components of the complement sequence in synovial fluids from patients with seropositive or seronegative rheumatoid arthritis or osteoarthritis. Certain of the fluids from seropositive patients demonstrated marked reduction in activity of the first component (C1). Although depressed activities of C1 were not uniformly found, there was ample evidence of activation of this component in the striking reduction in the second (C2) and fourth (C4) components. These two components are the natural substrates for activated C1 ($\overline{C1}$). There was also reduction of the third component (C3), indicating generation of C3 convertase by the action of $\overline{C1}$ on C4 and C2. Taken together, these alterations in complement component activities are consistent with the intrasynovial activation of the complement system in rheumatoid synovial fluids by an immune complex or its equivalent. Although such evidence for complement activation was most impressive in fluids from seropositive patients, borderline reductions in activities of the C2 and C4 components suggest that activation of C1 also occurs in fluids from seronegative patients.

Such observations have led to the concept that immune complexes activate the complement system within the joint, with the biological con-

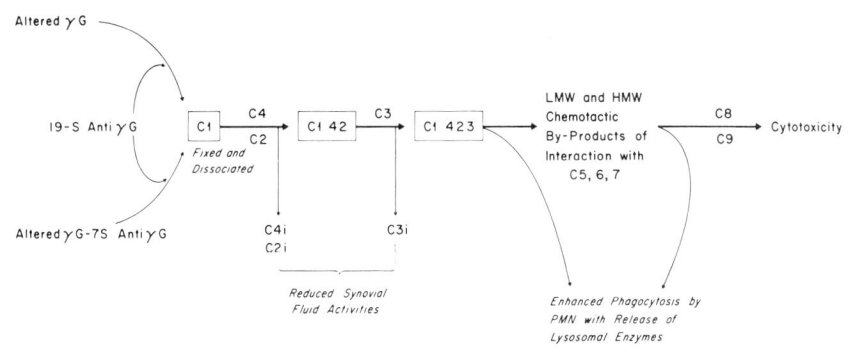

Figure 17-7 Possible pathways by which complement activation occurs in rheumatoid arthritis, and biological consequences. (From Austen, K. F.: Trans. Assoc. Amer. Physicians, 83:61, 1970.)

sequences leading to the inflammatory process (Fig. 17-7). The role of rheumatoid factor of the 7S class (7S-anti-IgG) may be particularly important in activating the complement system. Complexes of IgG–7S-anti-IgG are demonstrable in rheumatoid synovial fluid, and the extent of complement depletion can be correlated with the quantities of these complexes contained in the fluid. There is evidence that the presence of 19S (IgM) rheumatoid factor may greatly augment the activating effects of these complexes. This would account for the fact that the most profound alterations in the complement system are observed in synovial fluids from seropositive patients.

It is clear that several steps remain obscure in the elucidation of a completely satisfactory immunologic explanation of rheumatoid arthritis. The nature of the original antigenic stimulus remains unknown. If the rheumatoid factors are antibodies, presumably IgG should be the antigen. Several observations suggest that some alteration in the molecular configuration of IgG is required to provide such antigenic properties. There are few clues to the nature of such alterations or the mechanisms which could produce them.

In contrast to some of the other immunologically mediated forms of arthritis, rheumatoid synovitis is characterized by fluctuating but continuing inflammatory activity with predominance of the proliferative and granulomatous reaction. The basis for this chronicity is not easily explained. There may well be continuing release of biologically active substances by the mechanisms outlined above, but the process may also be perpetuated by other means. Castor, using synovial cell culture, has demonstrated several differences in the biological activity of fibroblasts from rheumatoid synovium as compared to normals. These "abnormalities" are reproducible on successive subculture. Comparable "abnormalities" in the biological activity of normal fibroblasts in culture result from the addition of small amounts of "connective tissue activating peptide," which is widely distributed in mammalian cells. Substantial amounts of this peptide can be extracted from leukocytes and from the granulation tissue of rheumatoid joints.

Rheumatoid arthritis, however, is not just a localized disease of the joints. It is a systemic disease, and constitutional manifestations such as ease of fatigue, weight loss, weakness, and at times fever and anemia are common. The outstanding characteristic is a chronic proliferative synovitis in multiple joints with a predilection for smaller joints such as the proximal interphalangeal, the metacarpal-phalangeal, and the metatarsal-phalangeal and a tendency for symmetrical distribution of the joint involvement once the disease has become established. Yet inflammatory lesions are seen throughout the connective tissues of the body. Both the constitutional symptoms and the inflammatory activity are subject to fluctuations in severity, with a strong tendency to remission and exacerbations without apparent reason.

Prominent among the extra-articular manifestations is the rheumatoid nodule. These nodules occur in 20 to 30 per cent of patients at some time during the course of their disease. These are granulomas with a characteristic microscopic appearance (Fig. 17-8). They are most common over bony prominences and often are attached to the articular capsule or to bursae, but they may be attached to the periosteum, lie loose in the subcutaneous tissue, or involve the deeper layers of the skin. They may persist for months or years. Such nodules are occasionally seen in pleura and pulmonary tissue, and actually have been found in virtually every connective tissue structure throughout the body. In addition, focal collections of mononuclear cells, predominantly lymphocytes, occur around the vessels in the connective tissue between bundles of skeletal muscle and in the connective tissue sheaths of peripheral nerves. Although not specific for rheumatoid arthritis, they are more numerous and are found in

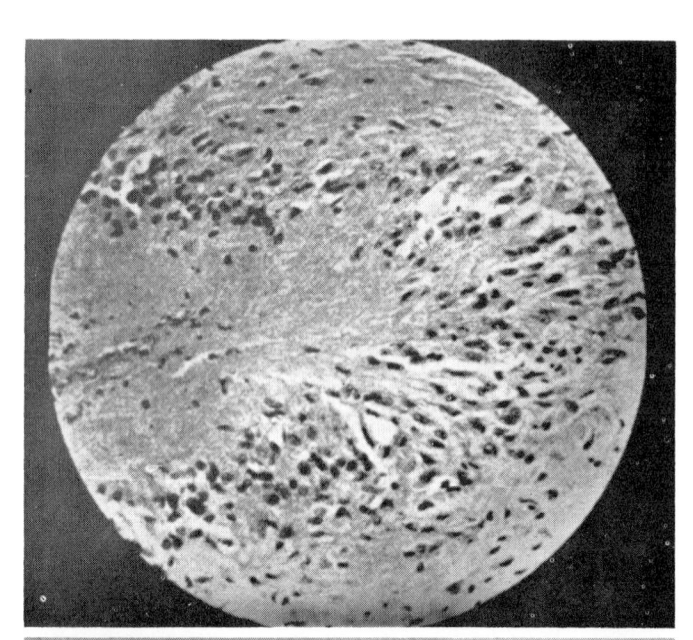

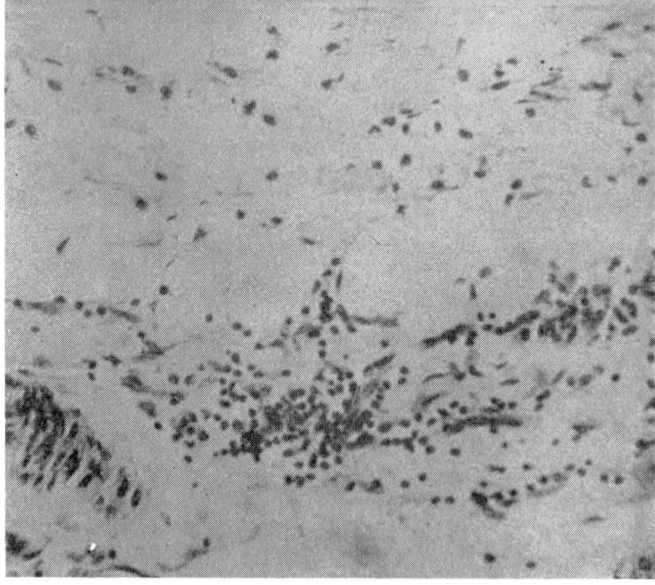

Figure 17–8 Extra-articular inflammatory lesions in rheumatoid arthritis. *Upper,* subcutaneous rheumatoid nodule. Note the central zone of fibrinoid necrosis, the middle palisading zone of epithelioid cells, and the outer fibrous zone. *Lower,* microscopic aggregates of inflammatory cells, largely lymphocytes, in perineurium. (Ragan, C., and Tyson, T. L.: Amer. J. Med., Vol. *1*:252, 1946.)

a higher percentage of patients with this disease. Vasculitis may be found in about 15 per cent of patients with rheumatoid arthritis, and an arteritis, at times difficult to distinguish from polyarteritis nodosa, is occasionally encountered in severe cases. The pathogenesis of these extra-articular lesions remains obscure. It may be significant that more than 95 per cent of patients with nodules are seropositive for rheumatoid factor, and that patients with the severe complications of rheumatoid arthritis usually have uncommonly high titers for rheumatoid factor in their circulating blood.

Systemic Lupus Erythematosus

Systemic lupus erythematosus (SLE) is a chronic disease affecting connective tissue, cells, and many organ systems, either individually or in various combinations. The clinical course may be fulminating or indolent but usually is characterized by periods of remission and exacerbations. Typically, patients with this disease manifest a host of immune phenomena, with circulating antibodies to their own cells, cell constituents, and proteins. Among these, particular significance is usually attributed to antibodies to nuclear materials. These antinuclear antibodies are responsible for the LE cell phenomenon—an in-vitro "happening" dependent on the traumatization of some leukocytes with release of nuclear material, then the binding of the antibodies to nuclear material, and the subsequent phagocytosis of this complex by white blood cells, usually polymorphonuclear neutrophils. Soon after the initial description of this phenomenon by Hargraves and associates, the responsible factor in serum of patients with SLE was identified as belonging to the 7S gamma class of immunoglobulins (IgG), which was detectable because of its unusual affinity for whole nuclei or for nucleoprotein. There is ample evidence for fixation of complement when the LE factor becomes associated with whole nuclei or nucleoprotein. In addition to or even in the absence of antibodies directed against nucleoprotein, some patients with SLE have circulating antibodies specific for the deoxyribonucleic acid (DNA) moiety of nucleoprotein. Less common are antibodies directed against glycoprotein, histone, and nucleolar components of nuclear materials.

Clinically, SLE has a bewildering array of acute and chronic manifestations. Nearly all patients have constitutional symptoms, ranging from malaise and weight loss to high fever and prostration in fulminating cases. Ninety per cent will have joint and muscle pain, and of these about half will have objective evidence of synovitis. Most characteristic is episodic inflammatory arthritis, especially of joints around the hands and feet, which develops rapidly and persists for only a few days. Although more persistent synovitis can occur, major joint swelling, capsular thickening, development of deformities, and ankylosis are uncommon. A variety of skin and mucous membrane lesions occur, especially in skin areas exposed to the sun. The classic erythematous "butterfly rash" on both cheeks and over the bridge of the nose is seen in less than half the patients. Involvement of serosal surfaces with pleuritis, pericarditis, or, less often, peritonitis may dominate the clinical picture. There may be pulmonary infiltrates. The myocardium and endocardium can be involved as well as the pericardium. Depression of one or more of the formed elements in the blood with anemia, neutropenia, or thrombocytopenia is common. The Coombs' antiglobulin test is frequently positive. Involvement of the central nervous system may be reflected in organic neurologic disturbances or psychiatric syndromes, and peripheral neuropathy is not uncommon. Renal involvement occurs in about half of patients with SLE, presenting as either nephritis or the nephrotic syndrome. SLE is frequently the explanation for false positive serologic reactions for syphilis. Rarely do all these manifestations occur at the same time in any one patient, but they may present simultaneously in various combinations. When it is possible to follow patients with SLE over long periods of time the sequential development of these varied manifestations is impressive. Such acute episodes, dominated at one time by one manifestation and later by another, are often separated by months or years of apparent good health.

The pathologic changes of SLE, even in organs and tissues known to be clinically involved, are often minor when examined by usual histologic techniques. Vasculitis and fibrinoid deposition are the most common findings in inflammatory sites such as pleura, pericardium, synovium, skin lesions, and in Libman-Sacks nonbacterial verrucous endocarditis. Vasculitis can involve venules, capillaries and arterioles, and occasionally arteries. Fibrinoid is an amorphous eosinophilic material deposited along tissue fibers and in blood vessels. By immunofluorescent methods fibrin and serum proteins, including immunoglobulins, complement, and DNA, have been detected in fibrinoid. These may represent deposits of immune complexes. The only in-vivo analogue of the LE cell is the "hematoxylin body," a rounded hematoxylin-stained mass, roughly the size of nuclei, occasionally seen in areas of inflammation.

Renal involvement in SLE is of special interest. From a practical point of view, progressive impairment of renal function terminating in uremia is a common cause of death in this disease. The renal involvement also provides the best insight into immunologic mechanisms which appear to be important in the pathogenesis of SLE. The renal lesions may vary from mild to severe. The mildest form consists of deposits of immunoglobulins (chiefly IgG) and complement (especially C3) in the mesangium and along the glomerular basement membrane, without any other apparent abnormality. The most common renal lesion is focal glomerulitis with fibrinoid change, focal thickening of basement membrane, and slight increase in cellularity. In SLE glomerulonephritis these lesions are more generalized and severe, with a mixture of proliferative and membranous changes and hypercellularity leading to crescent formation. Some kidneys show only a diffuse membranous glomerulonephritis with considerable thickening of the glomerular basement but little hypercellularity.

It is in SLE nephritis that the most definite changes in the immune mechanisms have been noted. The LE cell phenomenon and the titer of antibody to nucleoprotein do not fluctuate closely with clinical activity of the disease or with the presence or absence of renal involvement. However, the titers of antibodies to DNA are characteristically higher during periods of clinical activity, especially nephritis, than during remissions. Minute amounts of DNA have been demonstrated in serum at the same time that anti-DNA antibodies are present. Markedly decreased levels of circulating complement are seen primarily in active lupus glomerulitis. This can be measured as whole complement (CH_{50}) or complement components (C3 and C4). Less impressive decreases in complement levels occur at some time during the course of SLE in 95 per cent of patients. These low levels are evidence of in-vivo activation of the complement system and fixation of complement components by circulating immune complexes.

The demonstration of these immunologic phenomena has led to the concept that these antibodies with determinants directed against the patient's own cells, cell constituents, and proteins are "autoantibodies," and that SLE, rheumatoid arthritis, and related diseases are "autoimmune" diseases. In this discussion, these terms have been deliberately avoided, since they imply a degree of certainty which is not warranted by present knowledge. The nature of the antigenic stimulus remains a mystery. A viral etiology for SLE has long been suspected. This possibility has received added impetus by the recent detection, under the electron microscope, of cytoplasmic microtubules in the glomerular endothelium of patients with this disease. Although not specific or pathognomonic for SLE, such virus-like particles are demonstrable very frequently in the kidneys and other tissues of patients with the disease, and their recognition has some diagnostic value. However, these particles may represent ultrastructural manifestations of endothelial cell injury due either to secondary imposition of a viral infection in a more vulnerable host or tissue or to some other deleterious mechanism.

OTHER CONNECTIVE TISSUE DISEASES

Other diseases often grouped together with rheumatoid arthritis, rheumatic fever, and SLE under the heading of connective tissue diseases ("collagen diseases") are progressive systemic sclerosis, polymyositis, and polyarteritis nodosa. These diseases of unknown etiology are grouped together because of common or overlapping clinical and histopathologic features. The common histologic features are widespread inflammatory damage to connective tissues and blood vessels, often associated with deposition of fibrinoid material. Clinical findings which justify a common grouping include the occurrence of major features of more than one entity in the same patient; sequential transitions between one entity and another in the same patient; suggestions of familial aggregation of more than one disease; and serologic abnormalities which predominate in one entity but have an appreciable incidence in others. For example, approximately 15 per cent of patients with rheumatoid arthritis have positive tests for antinuclear antibodies, while 15 to 20 per cent of patients with SLE have positive serologic reactions for rheumatoid factor.

Progressive systemic sclerosis (scleroderma) was first recognized as a disease of the skin characterized by dermal fibrosis and fixation of the skin to underlying structures. Later, involvement of visceral organs (notably gastrointestinal tract, lungs, kidney, and heart) were recognized as part of the same process. The pathologic lesions are essentially those of mild to moderate inflammation followed by excessive laying down of collagen in both appropriate and inappropriate sites, with ensuing fibrosis. There is no evidence of a qualitative abnormality in this excessive collagen. About 40 per cent of patients with progressive systemic sclerosis have circulating antinuclear antibodies, usually of the type directed against the glycoprotein component of nuclear material rather than against nucleoprotein. Also in contrast to patients with SLE, immunochemical analysis of the fibrinoid vascular lesions in systemic sclerosis has not demonstrated deposition of immunoglobulins or complement. Rheumatoid factor is present in 20 to 40 per cent of patients with systemic sclerosis.

Polymyositis (also termed dermatomyositis if there is an associated dermatitis) is a less common disease in which weakness of skeletal muscle is the outstanding clinical feature. Although inflammatory degenerative and regenerative changes are seen in the muscle, inflammation and pain are rarely prominent among the clinical manifestations. Aside from dysphagia due to involvement of muscle in the pharynx and upper third of the esophagus, visceral involvement is rare. Occasionally, patients show features of both polymyositis and systemic sclerosis. Overlapping with features of rheumatoid arthritis and SLE also occurs at times. The muscle biopsy may show edema and inflammatory cells, particularly around blood vessels in the connective tissue between muscle fibers, with degeneration of muscle fibers and phagocytosis of remnants of muscle necrosis. Other features include evidence of efforts at muscle regeneration, non-necrotizing perivasculitis, and interstitial fibrosis.

Evidence of muscle involvement can be documented by electromyographic abnormalities and by characteristic biochemical changes. Release of several enzymes normally found in muscle is reflected by elevated serum levels of creatinine phosphokinase, aldolases, transaminases, and lactic dehydrogenases. There is usually creatinuria. An immunologic mechanism has been suggested by the association of malignant disease in 15 to 20 per cent of adults with polymyositis, but attempts to demonstrate antibodies to the patient's own tumor have rarely been successful. About 5 per cent of patients with polymyositis exhibit the LE cell phenomenon; frequency of positive tests for rheumatoid factor has ranged from 10 to 50 per cent in various series.

Polyarteritis Nodosa (Periarteritis Nodosa)

The term polyarteritis is applied to a disease characterized pathologically by inflammation and fibrinoid necrosis of medium-sized or small arteries. The widespread distribution of these arterial lesions produces a diversity of clinical manifestations which depend on the particular organ system which has suffered impairment of its arterial supply. Common presentations include renal disease, hypertension, abdominal symptoms which may simulate conditions requiring emergency surgery, coronary artery disease, cerebrovascular disease, peripheral neuritis, and fever of unknown origin with weight loss. A majority of patients complain of migratory muscle and joint aching, but true synovitis is uncommon.

The pathologic lesions typically involve one or more segments of small or medium-sized arteries with necrosis, fibrinoid change, and infiltration with polymorphonuclear neutrophils and varying numbers of eosinophils. The media is involved with extension to the intima and adventitia. Weakening of the arterial wall may lead to dissection or aneurysmal dilation with rupture and hemorrhage. As the areas of fibrinoid necrosis are replaced by cellular granulation tissue, proliferation of the intima may lead to thrombosis with arterial occlusion and infarction. As the involved segment is finally replaced by scar tissue the periarterial fibrosis may be sufficient to produce gross nodules and partial vascular occlusion. Characteristically, both fresh and healing inflammatory lesions are found together in an individual case.

No clear line of demarcation can be drawn between the pathologic lesions of polyarteritis and other types of systemic necrotizing angiitis, including those which may be associated with any of the other connective tissue diseases. Necrotizing vascular lesions resembling those of human polyarteritis can be produced in rabbits by repeated injections of foreign protein. Indeed, it was from such studies that the current understanding of the mechanism of serum sickness and the concept of the type III immunologic reaction developed. But as yet no characteristic immunologic abnormality has been defined for the human disease. There is a very low incidence of positive tests for either rheumatoid factor or antinuclear antibodies in patients with polyarteritis. Some pathologists distinguish the angiitis related to hypersensitivity to serum and drugs from classic polyarteritis on the basis of inflammatory and necrotic changes in arterioles and venules (which are characteristically spared in classic polyarteritis); the development of changes first in the intima and then by extension involving the entire vessel wall; the relatively uniform character of the lesions at any particular evolutionary stage; and the frequent involvement of pulmonary vessels. It seems reasonable to conclude that several entities associated with necrosis and inflammation of arteries cannot yet be clearly distinguished, and that they may well be produced by diverse mechanisms.

NONARTICULAR RHEUMATISM

In addition to the diseases which affect the joints themselves, discomfort and dysfunction of the musculoskeletal system can be caused by disorders of the muscles which move the joints, by neurologic diseases, and by circulatory disturbances. Pain and interference with joint function can also be produced by disorders in periarticular connective tissue structures such as tendons, tendon sheaths, bursae, and fascia; these are termed nonarticular rheumatism.

Inflammation of tendon sheaths (tenosynovitis) and bursae can result from specific infections, with or without accompanying joint involvement. Sterile inflammation of these structures occurs in rheumatoid arthritis, gout, and systemic lupus erythematosus; it may also develop as a local disturbance without other disease. Bursitis around the shoulder has been discussed under the heading of calcareous tendinitis. Inflammation of bursae located around the elbows, knees, ischial tuberosities, hips, and Achilles' tendons can cause similar pain and interference with function of the adjacent joint, although seldom as troublesome as that produced by bursitis around the shoulder. Tenosynovitis may interfere with free motion of the enclosed tendon, impairing motion of the joint moved by the tendon. The sheaths of the flexor tendons of the fingers are common sites of such inflammation, with fibrous tissue reaction leading to adhesive tenosynovitis, so that if the finger is flexed, it cannot be extended without assistance ("trigger finger"). In some cases, inflammation of the flexor tendon sheaths and palmar fascia may result in adhesions so strong that the fingers become fixed in a partially flexed position. A fibroblastic reaction in the palmar fascia may cause adhesions with contractures resulting in flexion deformities of the fourth and fifth fingers (Dupuytren's contracture).

Primary fibrositis is the term applied to a symptom complex characterized by generalized or localized muscle stiffness and discomfort, particularly after rest, made worse by cold and usually alleviated by heat, massage, and exercise. It is also called "muscular rheumatism." It may occur in acute attacks, accounting for the "stiff neck" or low back pain of "lumbago," which nearly everyone experiences at some time in life. It may also occur in more chronic forms, involving many structures at one time, or it may migrate from one part to another. Although the name fibrositis implies an inflammation of fibrous tissue, biopsies have failed to show histologic abnormalities in either connective tissue or muscle. The symptom complex is presumed to be an expression of localized biochemical disturbances in the muscle or connective tissue.

Like any other system in the body, the musculoskeletal system may serve as the means of somatic expression of psychiatric disorders. Such expression is more common in psychoneurosis than in psychosis, although complaints referred to the musculoskeletal system are not uncommon in depression. Such manifestations are sometimes termed "psychogenic rheumatism."

REFERENCES

Structure and Function of Connective Tissue

Asboe-Hanson, G. (Ed.): Connective Tissue in Health and Disease. Copenhagen, Munksgard, 1954.
Castor, C. W.: Study of connective tissue. *In* Hollander, J. L. (Ed.): Arthritis and Allied Conditions. Philadelphia, Lea and Febiger, 1966.
Castor, C. W.: Connective tissue activation. I. Nature, specificity, measurement and distribution of connective tissue activating peptide. Arthritis Rheum., *14*:41, 1971.
Castor, C. W., and Fries, F. F.: Composition and function of human synovial connective tissue cells measured *in vitro*. J. Lab. Clin. Med., *57*:394, 1961.
Edwards, L. C., and Dunphy, J. E.: Wound healing. I. Injury and normal repair. II. Injury and abnormal repair. New Eng. J. Med., *259*:224, 275; 1958.
Gould, B. S., and Woessner, J. F.: Biosynthesis of collagen, influence of ascorbic acid on proline, hydroxyproline, glycine and collagen content of regenerating guinea pig skin. J. Biol. Chem., *226*:289, 1957.
Harris, E. D., Jr., Evanson, J. M., DiBona, D. R., and Krane, S. M.: Collagenase and rheumatoid arthritis. Arthritis Rheum., *13*:83, 1970.
Kao, K. T., Boucek, R. J., and Noble, N. L.: Protein composition of sponge-biopsy connective tissue with special regard to biospy-tissue age. J. Geront., *12*:153, 1957.
McCluskey, R. T., and Thomas, L.: Removal of cartilage matrix, in vivo, by papain; identification of crystalline papain protease as cause of the phenomenon. J. Exp. Med., *108*:371, 1958.
Meyer, K., Davidson, E., Linker, A., and Hoffman, P.: The acid mucopolysaccharides of connective tissue. Biochim. Biophys. Acta, *21*:506, 1956.
Rosenberg, E. L., Hellman, W., and Kleinschmidt, A. K.: Macromolecular models of protein polysaccharides from bovine nasal cartilage based on electron microscopic studies. J. Biol. Chem., *245*:4123, 1970.
Shatton, J., and Schubert, M.: Isolation of mucoprotein from nasal cartilage. J. Biol. Chem., *211*:565, 1954.
Slack, H. G. B.: Some notes on composition and metabolism of connective tissue. Amer. J. Med., *26*:113, 1959.

Structure and Function of Joints

Barnett, C. H., and Cobbold, A. F.: Lubrication within living joints. J. Bone Joint Surg., *44B*:662, 1962.
Castor, C. W.: Microscopic structure of human synovial tissue. Arthritis Rheum., *3*:140, 1960.
Davies, D. V., and Edwards, D. A. W.: Blood supply of synovial membrane and intra-articular structures. Ann. Roy. Coll. Surg., *2*:142, 1948.
Gardner, E.: Physiology of movable joints. Physiol. Rev., *30*:127, 1950.
Gardner, E.: Structure and function of joints. *In* Hollander, J. L. (Ed.): Arthritis and Allied Conditions. Philadelphia, Lea and Febiger, 1972.

Pathologic Changes of Joint Disease

Bennett, G. A., Waine, H., and Bauer, W.: Changes in the knee joint at various ages, with particular reference to the development of degenerative joint disease. New York, Commonwealth Fund, 1942.

Jessar, R. A.: The synovial fluid. *In* Hollander, J. L. (Ed.): Arthritis and Allied Conditions. Philadelphia, Lea and Febiger, 1972.

Pinals, R. S.: Traumatic arthritis and allied conditions. *In* Hollander, J. L. (Ed.): Arthritis and Allied Conditions. Philadelphia, Lea and Febiger, 1972.

Ropes, M. W., and Bauer, W.: Synovial Fluid Changes in Joint Disease. Cambridge, Harvard University Press, 1953.

Sokoloff, L.: Pathology and pathogenesis of Osteoarthritis. *In* Hollander, J. L. (Ed.): Arthritis and Allied Conditions. Philadelphia, Lea and Febiger, 1972.

Sokoloff, L.: Pathology of rheumatoid arthritis. *In* Hollander, J. L. (Ed.): Arthritis and Allied Conditions. Philadelphia, Lea and Febiger, 1972.

Stecher, R. M.: Hereditary factors in arthritis. Med. Clin. N. Amer., *39*:499, 1955.

PATHOGENESIS OF JOINT INFLAMMATION

Coleman, R. W., Mason, J. W., and Sherry, S.: The kallikreinogen-kallikreinin enzyme systems of human plasma. Assay of components and observations in disease states. Ann. Intern. Med., *71*:763, 1969.

DeDuve, C.: The lysosome. Sci. Amer., *208*:64, 1963.

DeReuck, A. V. S., and Cameron, M. P. (Eds.): Lysosomes. Boston, Little, Brown and Co., 1964.

Kellermeyer, R. W., and Graham, R. C., Jr.: Kinins – possible physiologic and pathologic roles in man. New Eng. J. Med., *279*:754, 802, 859; 1968.

Kulka, J. P.: Microcirculatory impairment. *In* Spector, W. B. (Ed.): The Acute Inflammatory Response. Ann. N.Y. Acad. Sci., *116*:1018, 1964.

Melmon, K. L., Webster, M. E., Goldfinger, S. E., and Seegmiller, J. E.: Presence of kinins in inflammatory synovial effusions from arthritides of varying etiologies. Arthritis Rheum., *10*:13, 1967.

Thomas, L., Uhr, J. W., and Grant, L. (Eds.): Injury, Inflammation and Immunity. Baltimore, Williams and Wilkins Co., 1964.

Weissmann, G.: Lysosomes. Blood, *24*:594, 1964.

Willoughby, D. A., Coot, A., and Turk, J. L.: Complement in acute inflammation. J. Path., *97*:295, 1969.

SPECIFIC INFECTIOUS ARTHRITIS

Clark, G. M.: Tuberculous arthritis. *In* Hollander, J. L. (Ed.): Arthritis and Allied Conditions. Philadelphia, Lea and Febiger, 1972.

Pinals, R. S., and Ropes, M. W.: Meningococcal arthritis. Arthritis Rheum. *7*:241, 1964.

Sharp, J. T.: Gonococcal arthritis. *In* Hollander, J. L. (Ed.): Arthritis and Allied Conditions. Philadelphia, Lea and Febiger, 1972.

Wright, V.: Arthritis associated with venereal disease. Comparative study of gonococcal arthritis and Reiter's syndrome. Ann. Rheum. Dis., *22*:77, 1963.

CRYSTAL-INDUCED SYNOVITIS

Kellermeyer, R. W., and Breckenridge, R. T.: The inflammatory process in acute gouty arthritis. I. Activation of Hageman factor by sodium urate crystals. J. Lab. Clin. Med., *65*:307, 1965; II. The presence of Hageman factor and plasma thromboplastin antecedent in synovial fluid. J. Lab. Clin. Med., *67*:455, 1966.

McCarty, D. J., Jr.: Pseudogout; articular chondrocalcinosis. *In* Hollander, J. L. (Ed.): Arthritis and Allied Conditions. Philadelphia, Lea and Febiger, 1972.

McCarty, D. J., Jr., and Hollander, J. L.: Identification of urate crystals in gouty synovial fluid. Ann. Intern. Med., *54*:452, 1961.

Moscowitz, R. W., and Katz, D.: Chondrocalcinosis and chondrocalsynovitis (pseudogout syndromes). Analysis of 24 cases. Amer. J. Med., *43*:322, 1967.

Naff, G. B., and Byers, P. H.: Possible implication of complement in acute gout. J. Clin. Invest., *49*:1099, 1967.

Phelps, P., and McCarty, D. J., Jr.: Crystal induced inflammation in canine joints. II. Importance of polymorphonuclear leukocytes. J. Exp. Med., *124*:115, 1966.

Seegmiller, J. E.: The acute attack of gouty arthritis. Arthritis Rheum., *8*:714, 1965.

Seegmiller, J. E., and Howell, R. R.: The old and new concepts of acute gouty arthritis. Arthritis Rheum., *5*:616, 1962.

IMMUNOLOGICALLY MEDIATED INFLAMMATION

Adams, D. D.: Theory of pathogenesis of rheumatic fever, glomerulonephritis, and other autoimmune diseases triggered by infection. Clin. Exp. Immun., *5*:105, 1969.

Austen, K. F.: Inborn and acquired abnormalities of the complement system of man. Trans. Assoc. Amer. Physicians, *83*:49, 1970.

Bloom, B. R., and Bennet, B.: Migration inhibitory factor associated with delayed hypersensitivity in man. J. Immunol., *104*:95, 1970.

Castor, C. W.: Connective tissue activation. II. Abnormalities of cultured rheumatoid cells. Arthritis Rheum., *14*:55, 1971.

Christian, C. L.: Immune complex disease. New Eng. J. Med., *274*:606, 1966.

Dixon, F. J.: Experimental serum sickness. *In* Samter, M. (Ed.): Immunological Diseases. Boston, Little, Brown and Co., 1965.

Gell, P. G. H., and Coombs, R. R. A. (Eds.) Clinical Aspects of Immunology. 2nd ed. Philadelphia, F. A. Davis Co., 1969.

Germuth, F. G.: Comparative histologic and immunologic study in rabbits of induced hypersensitivity of serum sickness type. J. Exp. Med., *97*:257, 1953.

Hargraves, M. M.: The L.E. cell phenomenon. Advances Intern. Med., *6*:133, 1954.

Hollander, J. L., McCarty, D. J., Jr., Astorga, G., and Castro-Murrilo, E.: Studies on the pathogenesis of rheumatoid inflammation. I. The "R.A." cell and a working hypothesis. Ann. Intern. Med., *62*:271, 1965.

Kunkel, H. G.: Immunologic aspects of connective tissue disorders. Fed. Proc., *23*:623, 1964.

Lakin, J. D.: Classification of hypersensitivity reactions. *In* Patterson, R. (Ed.): Allergic Diseases. Philadelphia, J. B. Lippincott and Company, 1972.

Lawrence, H. S.: Transfer factor. Advances Immun., *11*:195, 1969.

Mellors, R. C., Heimer, R., Corcos, J., and Korngold, L.: Cellular origin of rheumatoid factor. J. Exp. Med., *110*:875, 1959.

Pekin, T. J., and Zvaifler, N. J.: Hemolytic complement in synovial fluid. J. Clin. Invest., *43*:1372, 1964.

Pollack, V. E., and Pirani, C. L.: Renal histologic findings in SLE. Mayo Clin. Proc., *46*:630, 1969.

Ruddy, S., and Austen, F. K.: The complement system in rheumatoid arthritis. Arthritis Rheum., *13*:713, 1970.

Sliwinski, A. J., and Zvaifler, N. J.: In vivo synthesis of IgG by the rheumatoid synovium. J. Lab. Clin. Med., *76*:304, 1970.

Schur, P. H., and Sandson, J.: Immunological factors and clinical activity in lupus erythematosus. New Eng. J. Med., *278*:533, 1968.

Tisher, C. C., Kelso, H. B., Robinson, R. R., Gunnels, J. C., and Burkholder, P. M.: Intraendothelial inclusions in kidneys of patients with systemic lupus erythematosus. Ann. Intern. Med., *75*:537, 1971.

Weissmann, G.: Lysosomes and joint disease. Arthritis Rheum., *9*:834, 1968.

Winchester, R. J., Agnello, V., and Kunkel, H. G.: The joint fluid and gamma globulin complexes and their relationship to intra-articular complement diminution. Ann. N.Y. Acad. Sci., *168*:195, 1969.

Zvaifler, N. J.: Breakdown products of C3 in human synovial fluids. J. Clin. Invest., *48*:1532, 1969.

Zvaifler, N. J.: Further speculation on the pathogenesis of joint inflammation in rheumatoid arthritis. Arthritis Rheum., *13*:895, 1970.

Other Connective Tissue Diseases

Austen, K. F.: Connective tissue diseases ("collagen diseases") other than rheumatoid arthritis. Introduction. *In* Beeson, P. B., and McDermott, W. (Eds.): Textbook of Medicine. 13th ed. Philadelphia, W. B. Saunders Co., 1971.

Austen, K. F.: Periarteritis nodosa (Polyarteritis nodosa). *In* Beeson, P. B., and McDermott, W. (Eds.): Textbook of Medicine. 13th ed. Philadelphia, W. B. Saunders Co., 1971.

D'Angelo, W. A., Fries, J. F., Masi, A. T., and Shulman, L. E.: Pathologic observations in systemic sclerosis (scleroderma). Amer. J. Med., *46*:428, 1969.

Pearson, C. M.: Polymyositis. *In* Milhorat, A. T. (Ed.): Explanatory Concepts of Muscular Dystrophy and Related Disorders. Amsterdam, Excerpta Medica Foundation, 1967.

Rodnan, G. P.: Progressive systemic sclerosis (diffuse scleroderma). *In* Samter, M., and Alexander, H. L. (Eds.): Immunological Diseases. Boston, Little, Brown and Co., 1965.

Nonarticular Rheumatism

Graham, W.: Fibrositis and non-articular rheumatism. Physiotherapy Rev., *35*:128, 1955.

Weiss, E.: Psychogenic rheumatism. Med. Clin. N. Amer., *39*:601, 1955.

CHAPTER 18

ALLERGY: ITS NATURE AND RELATIONSHIP TO OTHER IMMUNOLOGICALLY INDUCED DISEASE STATES

HERBERT C. MANSMANN

INTRODUCTION

The context of the concept of allergy has been changing rapidly during the last decade; yet, unfortunately, in many ways it has extended much beyond that which was originally described, intended, or probably conceived. When von Pirquet in 1906 suggested the use of the word *allergy,* he originally intended its use to mean a "changed reactivity" of the tissues to repeated exposure to foreign antigenic materials, both infectious and noninfectious. Through the years, loose interpretations by physicians and the lay public have led to a broadening of its application, in spite of an obvious need, based on both human experiences and human and animal experiments, either to restrict its use very narrowly to mean reagin-mediated reactions or at least to reserve the term for tissue reactions resulting from only immunologically induced mechanisms. Allergy and immunology are related yet distinctly different when one considers the total implications of each subject. The current interpretation is that while immunology is a major essence of reagin-mediated allergic reactions, clinical syndromes usually due to allergy can be mimicked or complicated by other immunologically induced tissue reactions, in addition to a very broad spectrum of mechanisms that may involve one or more anatomic, pathologic, physiologic, biochemical, pharmacologic, or genetic abnormalities. For example, idiosyncratic drug reactions, which are pharmacogenetically determined abnormal responses, and toxic drug reactions must be differentiated from each other, as well as from immunologically induced phenomena with similar, if not identical, clinical manifestations.

The use of the broadened interpretation of the word allergy appears to be a philosophical error for several reasons. First, this "changed reactivity" occurs in the form of at least three immunologically induced tissue reactions in nearly everyone, or the individual is unlikely to survive. Thus, the word allergy in the immunologic sense has lost much of its intended discriminating qualities. Second, the word allergy is also often used to signify hypersensitivity, which clearly involves a quantitative state that is only relative at best. Even hypersensitivity requires a more precise definition. Third, the word allergy generates a considerable number of emotional responses varying from hilarious laughter because of an embarrassing contact dermatitis to tragic grief because of an anaphylactic death. Although they are due to totally different mechanisms, these two diseases are often mistreated because of this lack of differentiation. Knowledge of the exact mechanisms should result in a more appropriate and specific choice of medications to prevent or modify manifested disease. Even between these extremes of emotional responses, there exist significant emotional reactions, both within and outside the medical profession, that are fundamentally due to acquired biases based primarily upon therapeutic failures. These failures often result from the expectation that a specific agent or modality of therapy can do something it is absolutely not capable of doing. Yet, this is understandable, because the serious student of medicine who is required to solve these clinical problems daily cannot but be confused by the numerous contradictory reports that result from the lack of precise identification of *all* the mechanisms operative in each individual patient in most studies reported. This bias in these physicians can change only when the clinician significantly increases his own data base and learns the *why* and *how* of the management of these patients. In order to accomplish this, he needs more precise definitions. Although complicated, these mechanisms are rapidly being separated because there is exponentially growing scientific information.

This chapter should be read in conjunction with Chapters 4 and 5 and those reference lists on Immunobiology as a starting point to understand the immune response. It is essential to understand the following clinical interpretations of the biochemistry and the evolving pharmacologic modifications of immune tissue reactions.

These immune reactions may result in significant serious pathophysiologic changes if they occur in vital areas of the affected organs. However, they may cause only minimal physiologic derangements in most tissues, especially if they are uncomplicated single reactions. Unfortunately, by the time the patient requires and then seeks medical attention, the reaction often is already complicated.

Fundamental to the resolution of many of these clinical problems is the need for a rather comprehensive understanding of the total person, in addition to the allergic or immune mechanism involved in initiating or complicating tissue damage. Most of these symptoms are subject to recurrence if the etiologic factors are not eliminated. Thus, the physician needs to know the genetic nature of his patient; his occupation and life style; his physiologic response to various physical, chemical, and biological stimuli; and his pharmacogenetic nature, as well as his psychosocial behavior patterns. These factors will significantly modify the clinical diagnosis and the ultimate prognosis. An early aggressive approach to the individual patient's medical needs as well as his physical, emotional, and social needs should make him least likely to develop permanent pathologic tissue changes with ultimate dysfunction, especially in the case of the reagin-mediated allergic syndrome of bronchial asthma.

THE NATURE OF ATOPIC SENSITIZATION

The clustering of the major reagin-mediated syndromes—that is, seasonal and nonseasonal allergic rhinitis (hay fever), bronchial asthma, and atopic dermatitis (infantile eczema)—in the immediate family of a human propositus with one of these disorders caused Coca and Cooke in 1923 to classify these allergic diseases as manifestations of *atopy*. They emphasized the role of heredity in the demonstration of the presence of atopic reaginic antibody, which was capable of passively sensitizing the skin of a nonallergic recipient (Prausnitz-Küstner reaction), as well as the occurrence of symptoms upon natural re-exposure to the specific allergen. The four hallmarks of atopy—its presence only in man, its familial incidence, its association with a reaginic antibody (IgE), and its apparent spontaneous occurrence in the absence of any known sensitizing events—have not stood the tests of time and increased scientific knowledge. Although atopic tissue reactions associated with IgE type of antibodies have been demonstrated to occur spontaneously after natural exposure to many allergens, as well as following specific immunization in several species of animals, including man, there appear to be other poorly understood host factors, strongly genetically determined, that predispose certain persons to the familial incidence of manifestations of disease after previous sensitization and upon subsequent exposure to allergen. Thus, certain families appear to possess an atopic diathesis that predisposes them to the likelihood of manifesting reagin-mediated immediate-type allergic diseases. Those without this diathesis do not manifest illness even though they appear to have a sufficient quantity of specific reagins and have the same environmental exposure to specific allergens as those that do become ill. There are currently no data about qualitative differences of IgE antibodies from different individuals. Yet, the difference may be at the receptor sites of the peripheral basophils for the Fc portion of the antibody molecule, since the basophils from one third of nonatopic individuals do not bind reaginic antibody in passive in-vitro sensitization experiments. However, there are also other explanations for this difference.

Those with an atopic diathesis have also recently been identified by their enhanced nasal transmucosal permeability to inhaled immunogens, that is, antigens that induce immune components. Both a highly purified protein and polysaccharide usually exclusively induced the formation of reaginic antibodies in greater frequency in atopic rather than nonatopic persons. In addition, it should be noted that many allergic diseases are also associated with and can be precipitated by transmucosal exposure to allergens, either by natural exposure or by clinical laboratory challenges.

Even though there is currently no sine qua non method of confirming the atopic diathesis, new methods of evaluating these disease states are evolving. For example, allergic asthmatic patients' sera have a mean concentration of IgE six times that of sera from nonallergic (intrinsic) asthmatics, while sera from those patients with atopic dermatitis have the largest amount of IgE. Moreover, the serum IgE concentration of patients with pollen allergy increases from their preseasonal level following seasonal inhaled pollen exposure. The normal concentration of IgE is 0.1 to 0.4 μg. per ml, as determined by use of anti-IgE sera made in animals. The importance of this quantitative difference in atopic individuals needs additional evaluation. Yet, it is tempting to consider these situations as truly being states of increased sensitivity or hypersensitivity.

There are at least two additional phenomena that appear to be hallmarks of atopic diathesis. The first is the relationship of the autonomic imbalance, noted primarily in asthma, which is probably associated with a beta-adrenergic blockade. The second consideration is the role of enhancement of tissue reactivity associated with the "priming effect" which follows repeated allergen nasal challenges. Both these conditions will be discussed later.

IMMUNOLOGICALLY INDUCED TISSUE REACTIONS

Localized immunologically induced tissue responses are the prototypes of immune mechanisms causing diseases which affect the various organ systems. The humoral and cellular components of three distinct reactions have been extensively investigated. Table 18–1 summarizes the important differences among these reactions.

Allergen-Reagin Reactions

Allergens are immunogens that induce the production of specific reaginic antibodies which belong to the IgE class of immunoglobulins. The allergen then functions like most antigens in its ability to combine with its specific antibody combining sites. Since purified immunogens, and hence allergens and antigens, possess a broad mosaic of antigenic determinants and since many immunogens are part of a bacterium, virus, pollen grain, or mold spore, the immune "chemical recognition" system is stimulated by a multimolecular mixture of polydeterminant immunogens derived from the various constituent proteins, carbohydrates, lipids, and nucleic acids. It is known that the same substances can induce IgE, IgM, IgG, and IgA antibodies in addition to cellular immunity. It is not known whether the antigenic and the allergenic determinants are identical, although one might expect them to be different in most instances because of the polydeterminant nature of immunogens.

Reaginic antibody has historically been called skin-sensitizing antibody because of the ability to demonstrate its active or passive presence in the skin by direct skin testing. However, this antibody has the capacity to fix to mast cells in

TABLE 18–1 TYPES OF IMMUNOLOGICALLY INDUCED TISSUE REACTIONS

Types of Reactions	Skin Test as Prototype	Time in Hours	Induced Immune Component	Chemical Mediators	Cellular Response
Reagin-Mediated	Wheal and flare	0.01 to 0.4	IgE*	Histamine SRS-A ECF-A	Eosinophils
IgG-Mediated	Arthus reaction	4 to 6	IgG* +C'	PMN-CF	Polymorpho-nuclear
Cell-Mediated	Tuberculin reaction	24 to 28	Small* lymphocyte (Transfer Factor*)	MIF	S. lymphocytes and macrophages
Mixed	←——————————one or all of above——————————→				

*Transfers susceptibility to nonimmunized (sensitized) recipients.

many organs and to circulating basophils, and therefore should be called tissue-sensitizing. Although no one knows for sure the role of IgE in normal man, it is likely that its function is to enhance local immunity by reacting with bacterial cell wall determinants to cause histamine release, which results in increased vascular permeability. Thus, it likely acts also as a reaginic antibody. In vitro, the exposure of this antibody to a temperature of 56° C. for 4 hours changes the Fc portion of the molecule, so that it loses its tissue-sensitizing capacity, while the antibody combining sites retain their capacity to react with the allergenic determinants.

A typical allergen-reagin reaction can be elicited by introducing into the superficial skin by prick, scratch, or intradermal injection, a dilute solution of allergen. The manifestation is an immediate urticarial lesion, referred to as a wheal and flare reaction. The reaction can occur in seconds, but usually develops over a period of 3 to 5 minutes, reaches its peak at 20 to 30 minutes, and disappears in one hour. Histologically, the tissue shows eosinophilic infiltration for over 48 hours. Certain allergens in exquisitely sensitive individuals will evoke a reaction even upon contact with intact skin and also in less sensitive persons upon contact with conjunctiva or nasal, bronchial, or gastrointestinal mucosae. Sera from allergic patients contain unbound reagin, and whole blood also contains reagin bound to basophils. Serum has the ability to sensitize passively circulating basophils as well as mast cells in various tissues, including human lung fragments. These variants of the Prausnitz-Küstner reaction, that is, the passive sensitization of normal skin with reagin, lend themselves to excellent in-vitro methods to study the biochemistry of and the pharmacologic modification of reagin-mediated immediate-type allergic diseases.

Turnover studies of IgE myeloma protein in normal subjects have been performed. The average serum half-life was 2.3 days, whereas the half-life of IgG is 25 days. While the half-life of IgG injected into human skin is approximately 2 days, IgE has an initial diffusion of all but 1 to 5 per cent of the dose at the same rate as IgG for 3 to 4 days. However, the remainder of the IgE has a half-life of 8.5 to 14 days. Moreover, the half-life of reaginic antibodies in sensitized skin sites is 13 days.

By the fluorescent antibody technique, plasma cells producing IgE have been found in tonsil and adenoid tissue, the greatest number after recurrent infection, and in the nasal, bronchial, tracheal, and gastrointestinal mucosae. In addition, IgE, as well as specific reaginic antibody, has been isolated from nasal secretions and bronchial sputa. It is very likely that the local production and local fixation of reaginic antibody play an important role in the manifestations of allergic diseases.

In-Vitro Allergen-Reagin Reactions

Allergen challenge of basophils or human lung fragments sensitized with reaginic antibody results in an allergen-reagin interaction on the cell membrane, which initiates a sequence of events resulting in the noncytotoxic release of chemical mediators. First, to become sensitized the cell membrane must fix two molecules of antibody at their Fc end. Then, allergen, in the absence of calcium, will activate the cells as the first stage of histamine release, the activation stage. The resuspension of the sensitized activated cells in allergen-free calcium-containing solution causes the cells to release histamine, hence the histamine release (second) stage. The intracellular events that lead to the release of histamine or slow-reacting substance of anaphylaxis (SRS-A) are currently unknown. While many substances that increase intracellular cyclic $3',5'$-adenosine monophosphate (cyclic AMP) will also inhibit histamine release, there is no evidence to date that an allergen-induced decrease in cyclic AMP causes histamine release.

Inhibition of histamine release has been found to occur solely or predominantly in the first stage, and is believed to be mediated by an increase in cyclic AMP. Both basophils and lung tissue mast cells are under such control. Catecholamines, epinephrine, and isoproterenol stimulate membrane-bound adenyl cyclase, which promotes the conversion of adenosine triphosphate (ATP) to cyclic AMP, the "second messenger" system. Cyclic AMP influences various physiologic responses, depending upon the cell stimulated. In the case of basophils and mast cells an increase in cyclic AMP results in the inhibition of histamine and SRS-A release, whereas in the case of the thyroid and adrenal cortex an increase in cyclic AMP results in an increase of thyroid hormone release and steroidogenesis, respectively. Cytoplasmic phosphodiesterase catabolizes cyclic AMP to 5'-AMP, and this conversion is inhibited by methylxanthines.

In-vitro experiments in different laboratories have shown that catecholamines and methylxanthines both inhibit histamine and SRS-A release from both basophils and lung tissue mast cells. Moreover, there is a synergistic effect noted when these drugs are used together. Propranolol, a beta-adrenergic blocker, prevents the catecholamines from inhibiting histamine release. While the prostaglandins PGE_1 and PGE_2 are potent enhancers of adenyl cyclase activity, propranolol does not block the inhibition of histamine release by these substances. In addition, propranolol does not block the inhibition of histamine release in a feedback situation in which histamine, another adenyl cyclase activator, inhibits the first stage response. Interestingly, the basophil histamine receptor site is not blocked by a 100-fold greater concentration of the three different antihistamines so far reported. In addition, exogenous dibutyryl cyclic AMP also inhibits histamine release in this system.

The human lung fragment model used in allergen-reagin interaction has resulted in the demonstration of three chemical mediators, that is, histamine, SRS-A, and eosinophil chemotactic factor of anaphylaxis (ECF-A). These are believed to be major producers of an increase in airway resistance seen in reagin-mediated bronchial asthma. Histamine release results in mucosal edema by causing an increase in vascular permeability, in addition to an early and short-lived smooth muscle constriction and an increase in exocrine gland secretion. SRS-A contracts smooth muscle more slowly than does histamine or acetylcholine; yet, it produces a prolonged contraction and also potentiates the effect of histamine. There also appears to be a permeability-enhancing activity of SRS-A which might be operative in these diseased lungs. The documentation of the allergen-reagin release of ECF-A seems to explain the observations of the accumulation of eosinophils in allergic tissue. The exact function of the eosinophil in the tissue needs additional investigation.

There are additional mediators that, at least superficially, appear to be candidates for producers of immune tissue damage. Although serotonin and the kinins are active agents in species other than man, they cannot currently be implicated in reagin-mediated bronchial asthma. As mentioned before, prostaglandins PGE_1 and PGE_2 inhibit histamine release from human basophils. Moreover, an aerosol of PGE_1 causes an improvement in flow rates and lung volumes of asthmatic patients. Yet, PGF_{2a} is known to contract human bronchial smooth muscle. The role of this complex group of compounds is not yet established in either asthma or other immunologically induced tissue reactions.

Antigen-IgG Antibody Reactions

The Arthus reaction has been most completely studied. It requires relatively large quantities of both antigen and antibody. There is preliminary direct and indirect evidence that an allergen-reagin reaction must occur initially to cause an increase in capillary permeability to permit sufficient IgG and polymorphonuclear leukocytes to accumulate and to produce the lesion. This reaction slowly reaches its maximum intensity in 4 to 6 hours and usually subsides between 12 and 24 hours. These lesions, when studied immunohistochemically, contain antigen, IgG antibodies, and complement. Whenever this occurs in an airway, there is an increase in airway resistance, because of mucosal inflammation.

Whenever this type of reaction occurs systemically, immune complex disease may occur. The antibodies (Ab) react with antigen (An) to form soluble macromolecules ($AbAn_2$ or Ab_2An_3) or insoluble precipitates (Ab_3An to Ab_5An_2) in liquid (intravascular) or semisolid (tissue) media. Serum-sickness types of disease occur when large quantities of an immunogen remain in the circulation during the period of antibody synthesis. At first, circulating soluble macromolecules are formed; as more antibodies are made, precipitates are formed, which result in coarse, irregular, granular depositions in the walls of small blood vessels. Antigen, IgG, and complement have been demonstrated in the arteritis lesions by immunochemical methods. This manifestation of illness is dependent upon the amount of circulating antigen that remains for 7 to 10 days. Small quantities will result in subclinical tissue damage. Large quantities, or a replicating antigen such as a virus, might cause a severe life-threatening generalized vasculitis, including serum-sickness type of glomerulonephritis. This reaction has been described in the bronchial tissue of some asthmatics. Interestingly, in some cases the predominant immunoglobulin was IgM, while several specimens also contained IgA aggregates. Thus, these immune tissue reactions can complicate allergen-reagin reactions. Clinically, this is also the immune mechanism of pulmonary aspergillosis. Precipitins to the fungus *Aspergillus fumigatus* have been reported in 7 per cent of sera from asthmatics.

Cell-Mediated Reactions

Many immunogens sensitize thymus-dependent small lymphocytes. Upon subsequent exposure, a tissue reaction develops over a period of 6 to 8 hours, reaching a maximum at 24 to 48 hours, in which a small number of sensitized lymphocytes accumulate and release migratory inhibitor factor (MIF). MIF is responsible for the local accumulation of macrophages. The tuberculin skin reaction is the classic model of cell-mediated reactions, also called delayed hypersensitivity reactions, and this type of reaction can be elicited by the injection of tuberculin into most tissues of sensitized animals. The predominant histologic picture is that of perivascular mononuclear cellular infiltration, provided that a minimal amount of antigen has been injected. If the reaction is severe with necrosis, polymorphonuclear cells become prominent. It takes approximately 500 times more antigen to elicit a delayed hypersensitivity skin reaction than it takes of allergen to elicit a wheal and flare reaction. Because of this dose difference and the possibility of inducing an anaphylactic reaction, most reagin-mediated diseases have not been adequately evaluated for the simultaneous presence of allergen-reagin and delayed hypersensitivity reactions.

CONCEPTUAL EVOLUTION FOR IMMUNOLOGICALLY INDUCED DISEASES

A conceptual model of the evolution of chronic disease resulting from recurrent immune tissue damage is graphically illustrated in Figure 18–1. The severity of the disease follows a normal distribution curve and becomes worse as the duration increases, as the attacks or symptom periods become more frequent, or if complications develop. Most family physicians see the complete spectrum of disease, whereas hospital physicians often see only those patients with more severe symptoms, usually the therapeutic failures. Patients can be grouped by frequency of symptomatic periods. Moreover, as symptoms continue unabated, the emotional reaction to chronic illness becomes more apparent, while the reagin-mediated allergic components become more obscure. Since most allergic diseases are both reversible and preventable, and since individual patients can have less frequent symptomatic periods when properly managed clinically, therapeutic goals should be set with these factors in mind.

Part of the evolution of chronic manifestation of disease is the development of a nasal mucosa tissue "priming effect," which follows daily single allergen exposure for a week. The primed tissue then has a heightened reactivity to lower doses of the same and *also* to unrelated allergens to which the patient is known to be allergic. These observations help explain some of the variation of symptoms often seen in cases in which at one time a large dose of allergen produces little or no symptoms, while at other times, such as after priming, a low dose exposure results in severe symptoms. Much could be learned if this same effect could be demonstrated in other tissues, especially in the bronchial mucosa. Also, one cannot but wonder whether acute or chronic infection or diseases such as cystic fibrosis do not also predis-

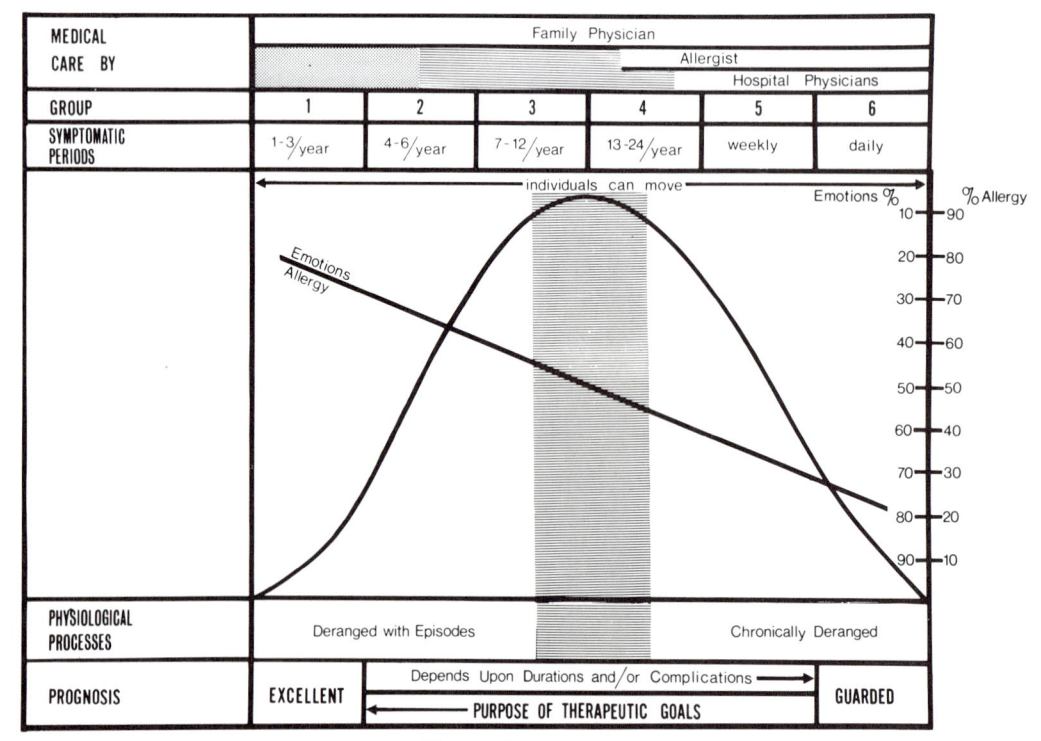

A CONCEPTUAL EVOLUTION FOR IMMUNOLOGICALLY INDUCED DISEASE

MEDICAL CARE BY	Family Physician					
				Allergist		
					Hospital Physicians	
GROUP	1	2	3	4	5	6
SYMPTOMATIC PERIODS	1-3/year	4-6/year	7-12/year	13-24/year	weekly	daily
PHYSIOLOGICAL PROCESSES	Deranged with Episodes				Chronically Deranged	
PROGNOSIS	EXCELLENT	Depends Upon Durations and/or Complications →				GUARDED
		← PURPOSE OF THERAPEUTIC GOALS				

Figure 18–1

pose the mucosa to defects which set the stage for similarly heightened reactivity.

THE NATURE OF IMMUNOTHERAPY

Aside from a complete immunologic rest by the elimination of allergen from the body for a prolonged period of time, the only available method that offers the patient any hope of changing his basic reactivity to unavoidable inhalant allergens is hyposensitization, now referred to as immunotherapy. Originally, this was thought to be desensitization, in that all existing reaginic antibodies were completely neutralized by the injection of an excess of allergen. Although theoretically possible, this would require a great deal of allergen, which could hardly neutralize tissue-fixed reagin without producing mediator release and severe symptoms. Moreover, since reagin is constantly being made, it would require constant neutralization.

During the course of immunotherapy, there is an increase in concentration of a heat-stable, allergen-neutralizing antibody of the IgG type. This antibody competes for allergen and thus protects reagin-sensitized cells from allergen challenge. This has been well documented by the in-vitro histamine release model using circulating basophils. Some patients develop more than a 20-fold increase in IgG blocking antibody, in addition to a decrease in leukocyte sensitivity to specific allergen. Clinically, immunotherapy, if successful, must be maintained for at least 2 years after the last allergic symptoms are noted. The evaluation of this therapy in individual patients is currently purely subjective and objective data are necessary. Ideally, a quantitative inhalation challenge of both primed and unprimed mucosa during symptom-free seasons could answer the question of efficiency; yet, to evaluate this therapy fairly it must be used only when reagin-mediated disease has been documented and remains uncomplicated. For example, it has been demonstrated clinically that a few chronically ill reagin-mediated asthmatic patients develop acute symptoms 6 to 12 hours after an injection, even with a very dilute concentration of allergen. If this had been due to allergen-reagin interaction, the symptoms would have occurred within a half hour. Sera from such reacting patients frequently contain sufficient specific IgG antibodies to form a precipitin line in a semisolid medium (agar), whereas patients who do not get sick and, indeed, are clinically improving with immunotherapy do not have enough IgG antibodies to form a precipitin line. Thus, it can be postulated that the original reagin-mediated bronchial asthma was complicated by trace amounts of the injected allergen reaching the bronchial tissue via the bloodstream. Its antigenic determinants react with IgG antibodies to cause an immune tissue reaction that results in an increase in airway resistance.

AUTONOMIC IMBALANCE IN ALLERGY

Any reconsideration of the nature of atopic diathesis will probably require an explanation for accumulating evidence that a common final pathway exists and accounts for the manifested illness resulting from a wide variety of physiologic, biochemical, pharmacologic, immunologic, and psychological abnormal disease states. While the initial disease mechanism may set the stage, initiate a sequence of events, be recurrently stimulating tissue damage, or be complicated by one or more concurrently present different disease mechanisms, the final clinical picture appears to be a single disease. A typical example is the clinical syndrome called bronchial asthma. Recently, the treatment of status asthmaticus has become rather stereotyped, regardless of the cause, and the great majority of patients respond even if in respiratory failure. Yet, the long-term management of a patient with chronic asthma necessitates the utilization of rather specific measures, depending upon the underlying disease mechanism. Asthma could have immunologic or nonimmunologic features. The presence of reagin-mediated allergic reactions would be an adequate initiating cause, and in some cases even the total cause, but not an exclusive explanation. The presence of an autonomic imbalance could produce and explain a common final pathway. In some or all patients it could be an inherited congenital defect, a spontaneously acquired phenomenon, or an induced or conditioned response.

Beta-Adrenergic Blockade Theory

There appears to exist a diminished sensitivity of the beta-adrenergic receptors of bronchial smooth muscle, mucous glands, mucosal blood vessels, nasal mucosa, skin, antibody-forming cells, eosinophils, lymphocytes, and leukocytes. Evidence suggests that the beta-adrenergic receptor site is or is closely associated with the cellular membrane-bound enzyme, adenyl cyclase. When stimulated, this enzyme converts ATP to cyclic AMP, which in bronchial smooth muscle results in relaxation. Therefore, the autonomic nervous system beta receptors inhibit constriction, while the alpha receptors have excitatory effects. Moreover, by the use of pharmacologic blockers of beta receptors, it appears that only beta$_2$ stimulation results in bronchodilatation.

A number of studies of asthmatic patients, undifferentiated, suggest that beta-adrenergic blockade is present in much the same way as when normal subjects are given a beta-adrenergic blocker, such as propranolol. The following examples of this response may be cited to illustrate this point. (1) Beta receptor stimulation with isoproterenol and epinephrine results in a smaller rise in blood glucose, lactate, and pyruvate concentrations. (2) The characteristic eosinophilic response to epinephrine is reduced. (3) There is less isoproterenol-induced suppression of phytohemagglutinin-induced DNA synthesis in peripheral lymphocytes. (4) Leukocyte membrane adenyl cyclase activity is decreased, resulting in a decreased production of cyclic AMP. Therefore, a major deficit of those with atopic diathesis—those patients likely to have bronchial asthma, hay fever, and atopic dermatitis—is an imbalance in the autonomic nervous system through an inability to counteract a normal or heightened cholinergic response with an intact beta-adrenergic system.

Cholinergic Participation

The neurotransmitter released by cholinergic neurons is acetylcholine, which in bronchial homeostasis maintains bronchoconstriction. Moreover, the asthmatic patient has marked bronchial hyperreactivity to acetylcholine and methylcholine inhalation. Extremely small amounts induce objective evidence of increased airway resistance. This reaction is prevented by pretreatment with atropine or treated after it occurs with the beta-adrenergic stimulator isoproterenol. Some patients with hay fever and atopic dermatitis, without previous asthma, respond to methylcholine with an increase in airway resistance.

Alpha-Adrenergic Participation

Membrane-bound ATPase appears to be involved in alpha-adrenergic activity. While the bronchial smooth muscle has a predominance of beta receptors, there is evidence that some alpha receptors are also present. Alpha receptor stimulation results in smooth muscle constriction. In severe asthma with beta-adrenergic blockade, the worsening of the attack by an injection of epinephrine, which contains both alpha and beta stimulators, may be due to alpha-stimulated constriction in the absence of beta-induced relaxation.

Unfortunately, this system has been neglected experimentally. However, a recent report showed that the leukocyte membrane ATPase activity was elevated in asthmatics. This causes ATP to be shunted away from cyclic AMP production as ADP is produced instead. Thus, there is a decrease in second messenger, cyclic AMP function, which protects cells from allergen-reagin histamine release and also results in bronchial smooth muscle relaxation.

In conclusion, the experimental evidence of the interaction of these three components of the autonomic nervous system, including the generalized cellular phenomena, will require frequent review by clinicians to provide their patients with current therapy. For example, the effects of the leukocyte adenyl cyclase and ATPase abnormalities noted above are both reversed with systemic treatment with corticosteroids. The exact mechanisms are not yet clear. However, in-vitro hydrocortisone depressed ATPase and phosphodiesterase activity. Moreover, as mentioned before, the exact origin of these defects needs investigation starting in utero.

REAGIN-MEDIATED DISEASES IN MAN

Although there are many manifestations of allergic diseases, the author has elected to discuss only two to illustrate typical examples of the problems encountered.

Anaphylaxis

Anaphylactic reactions may be both local and systemic. Local anaphylaxis is another term for the immediate wheal and flare reactions that can be elicited by a wide variety of inhalant, ingestant, and drug allergens in sensitive persons. Many cases of urticaria and angioedema are also examples of local anaphylaxis. Systemic anaphylaxis is characterized by reversible or irreversible peripheral vascular collapse, with or without preceding respiratory distress. Itching, diffuse erythema, abdominal and uterine cramps, vomiting and/or diarrhea may be present. The acute severe respiratory distress is often due to acute obstructive laryngeal edema with or without acute obstructive lower airway edema and bronchospasm leading to severe hyperinflation of the lungs. Patients with only central cardiac arrhythmia or profound circulatory collapse have no significant postmortem findings.

In cases of cold urticaria the allergen is thought to be a tissue protein that has the ability to change its physical structure at lower temperatures. It is reagin-mediated, usually IgE, but an IgM reagin has been described in this disorder, as sera from such patients passively sensitize the skin of nonreactive persons, yet the application of ice causes the recipient of the serum to provide the allergen. Although this allergen-reagin reaction likely releases histamine, which can produce the above symptoms, the role of the kinin system requires investigation. The kinins are known to increase in the serum of some animals during anaphylaxis and they produce vasodilatation and an increase in vascular permeability. Before it can be accepted that the kinin system is actively involved in human anaphylaxis, it will be necessary to develop techniques to study the specific activation of kallikrein, the utilization of kininogen, and the formation of bradykinin. To date, only the decrease in serum kininogen level has been seen in one patient during anaphylaxis. The level returned to normal afterward. Moreover, cyproheptadine is believed to be primarily a blocker of kinin effect rather than a simple antihistamine.

Since all patients with cold urticaria can develop anaphylactic shock when exposed to sudden changes in environmental temperature, they must be warned of this possibility, because it may be fatal. This is especially true of diving into cool water. Cyproheptadine has been shown to prevent such a reaction, yet any drug's effectiveness should be verified for its ability to suppress the critical response following the application of an ice cube to the skin for three minutes.

Human anaphylaxis due to aggregated antigen-IgG antibody has not been documented, although it is theoretically possible. However, the absolute assurance that reagin was not also involved will be difficult to prove. In experimental animals, antigen-IgG antibody complexes formed in vitro will produce shock, and IgG antibodies passively sensitize animals to systemic shock with specific antigen.

Bronchial Asthma

In 1968, the writer formulated and published the following definition of bronchial asthma:

"Bronchial asthma is a form of pulmonary functional derangement resulting from reversible obstructive hyperinflation of both lungs throughout. It is characterized clinically by paroxysmal episodes of cough and dyspnea, accompanied by a prolonged expiratory phase with wheezing. Such attacks, at least in the early stage, are typically relieved by sympathomimetic drugs. Spontaneous remission may occur. This complex syndrome may be acute or chronic; acute superimposed on chronic; mild or severe; seasonal or perennial; of single, multiple, or unknown etiology; simple or complicated; symptomatic or asymptomatic; and reversible or irreversible. It often precedes, occurs with, and is intensified by chronic bronchitis."

The writer now believes that the words "bronchial asthma" in the above definition should be replaced by the words reversible obstructive airway disease (ROAD), which may be intermittent (acute) or continuous (chronic). Since there are several subclassifications of ROAD, this symptom complex is analogous to chronic obstructive lung disease (COLD) with its subclassifications. While ROAD represents a constellation of subjective symptoms and objective signs, often indistinguishable from patient to patient due to the airway's ability to react through a final common pathway, the primary mechanisms will occasionally be different (see Table 18–2). It is to be anticipated that in the future the availability of drugs to prevent the formation, storage, release, or action of each mediator will continue to require identification of the mechanism in order to prevent illness. The treatment of the established increased airway resistance, while necessary, will be to alleviate symptoms and will be less specific. Such episodes must be considered to be due to multifactorial inducers within each mechanism, in addition to a change in mechanism. One betrays his own bias by constantly trying to ascribe these illnesses to only one process such as to allergy, acute or chronic infections, exertion, environmental physical changes, nonspecific irritants, psychogenic factors, or obstructive lung disease. Although any of these factors may be acting alone or in combination, the fact remains that whatever the precipitating factor may be, it is not necessarily the same in each episode.

Acute bronchitis is probably the most common ROAD. Yet, reagin-mediated asthma is by far the most common ROAD between the ages of 2 and 40, while nonreagin-mediated asthma is most common in those less than 2 and over 40 years of age. The next most common ROAD is probably chronic bronchitis. Bronchiolitis is rather common in the young infant.

The physiologic derangements of the lungs that result from changes in caliber of the airways are best explained through pulmonary physiology. The tidal volume must provide oxygen and eliminate carbon dioxide in order to maintain alveolar ventilation. The patency, resistance, and compliance of the airways play important roles. In ROAD there are often pathologic lesions that interfere with these properties of the airways. As the lumina get smaller, segmental atelectasis develops and alveolar ventilation decreases. Alveolar capillary perfusion continues and arteriovenous pulmonary shunting goes from a normal of 7 per cent to a mean of 17.3 per cent when radiographic evidence of atelectasis is seen. This is due to perfusion of nonventilated alveoli. This rapidly leads to carbon dioxide accumulation and the resultant respiratory acidosis. Once respiratory insufficiency develops, aggressive respiratory care is indicated. These events are the end result of the common final pathway and can occur in most of the patients with ROAD, if supportive therapy is delayed.

TABLE 18–2 REVERSIBLE OBSTRUCTIVE AIRWAY DISEASE

Pathophysiological Reactions Leading to Increased Airway Resistance

Proposed Classification Based on Mechanism	Bronchoconstriction Primary	Bronchoconstriction Secondary	Inflammatory Cell Response Eosinophils	Inflammatory Cell Response Polymorphonuclear	Inflammatory Cell Response Mononuclear	Tissue Edema	Mucus Hypersecretion	Synonyms Often Used
I. *Immunologically Induced*								
1. Reagin-Mediated Bronchial Asthma	+	−	Predominate	Usually none	Occasional	Marked	Markedly increased	Type I reaction; Allergic, atopic, extrinsic, and noninfectious asthma; Immediate hypersensitivity
2. IgG-Mediated Disease	±	+	Some	Predominate	Rare	Moderate	Moderately increased	Type III reaction; Immune complex disease; Late-onset asthma; Intermediate hypersensitivity
3. Cell-Mediated Disease	−	+	Rare	Occasional	Predominate	Slight	Slightly increased	Type IV reaction; Delayed hypersensitivity; Bacterial allergy; may be intrinsic, idiopathic, and infectious asthma
4. Mixed Immunologic Disease	±	±	Many	Many	Many	Present	Increased	Same as 1, 2, and 3
II. *Infection-Induced*								

TABLE 18–2 *continued on opposite page.*

5. Bacterial Infection						
a. Acute bronchitis	−	Some	Predominate	Rare	Moderate	Moderately increased	Could be same as 1, 2, and 3
b. Chronic bronchitis	−	Some	Many	Many	Moderate	Moderately increased	Could be same as 1, 2, and 3
c. Bronchiectasis	−	Some	Some	Some	Moderate	Moderately increased	Could be same as 1, 2, and 3
6. Viral Infection						
a. Bronchiolitis	±	Some	Some	Predominate	Moderate	Moderately increased	Could be same as 1, 2, and 3
b. Acute bronchitis	−	Some	Rare	Predominate	Moderate	Moderately increased	Could be same as 1, 2, and 3
c. Chronic bronchitis	−	Some	Rare	Predominate	Moderate	Moderately increased	Could be same as 1, 2, and 3
III. Idiopathic						
7. Autonomic Imbalance	+	Many	Rare	Rare	Moderate	Moderate	May be associated with all, especially intrinsic
8. Aspirin Triad	±	Predominate	Some	Some	Moderate	Moderately increased	Same as 1, 2, and 3
9. Exercise-Induced	±	?	?	?	?	?	Probably associated with all
10. Emotion-Induced	−	?	?	?	?	?	May be associated with all

REFERENCES

THE NATURE OF ATOPIC SENSITIZATION
Berg, T., and Johansson, S. G. O.: IgE concentration in children with atopic diseases. Int. Arch. Allerg., *36*:219, 1969.

Coca, A. F., and Cooke, R. A.: On the classification of the phenomena of hypersensitiveness. J. Immun., *8*:163, 1923.

Ellis, E. F.: Immunological basis of atopic disease. Advances Pediat., *16*:65, 1969.

Hilman, B. C.: The allergic child. Ann. Allerg., *25*:620, 1967.

Osler, A. G., Lichtenstein, L. M., and Levy, D. A.: *In vitro* studies of human reaginic antibodies. Advances Immun., *8*:183, 1968.

Salvaggio, J. B., Castro-Murillio, E., and Kundur, V.: Immunologic response of atopic and normal individuals to keyhole limpet hemocyanin. J. Allerg., *44*:344, 1969.

Salvaggio, J. B., Cavanaugh, J. J. A., Lowell, F. C., and Leskowitz, S.: A comparison of the immunologic responses of normal and atopic individuals to intranasally administered antigen. J. Allerg., *35*:62, 1964.

Salvaggio, J., Kayman, H., and Leskowitz, S.: Immunologic responses of atopic and normal individuals to aerosolized dextran. J. Allerg., *38*:31, 1966.

Sly, R. M., and Heimlich, E. M.: Physiologic abnormalities in the atopic state: A review. Ann. Allerg., *25*:192, 1967.

Stanworth, D. R.: Reaginic antibodies. Advances Immun., *3*:181, 1963.

IMMUNOLOGICALLY INDUCED TISSUE REACTIONS
Austen, K. F.: Histamine and other mediators of allergic reactions. *In* Samter, M. (Ed.): Immunological Diseases. 2nd ed. Boston, Little, Brown and Co., 1971, p. 332.

Becker, E. L.: Nature and classification of immediate-type allergic reactions. Advances Immun., *13*:267, 1971.

Butcher, R. W., and Hittelman, K. J.: The metabolism of cyclic AMP and its role in cell function. *In* Austen, K. F., and Becker, E. L. (Eds.): Biochemistry of the Acute Allergic Reactions. Second International Symposium. Oxford, Blackwell Scientific Publications, 1971, p. 141.

Callerame, M. L., Condemi, J. J., Bohrod, M. G., and Vaughan, J. H.: Immunologic reactions of bronchial tissue in asthma. New Eng. J. Med., *284*:459, 1971.

Ishizaka, K., and Ishizaka, T.: IgE immunoglobulins of human and monkey. *In* Austen, K. F., and Becker, E. L. (Eds.): Biochemistry of the Acute Allergic Reactions. Second International Symposium. Oxford, Blackwell Scientific Publications, 1971, p. 13.

Kay, A. B., and Austen, K. F.: The IgE-mediated release of an eosinophil leukocyte chemotactic factor from human lung. J. Immun., *107*:899, 1971.

Lichtenstein, L. M., and Bourne, H. R.: Inhibition of allergic histamine release by histamine and other agents which stimulate adenyl cyclase. *In* Austen, K. F., and Becker, E. L. (Eds.): Biochemistry of the Acute Allergic Reactions. Second International Symposium. Oxford, Blackwell Scientific Publications, 1971, p. 161.

Lichtenstein, L. M., and Norman, P. S.: Human allergic reactions. Editorial, Amer. J. Med., *46*:163, 1969.

Orange, R. P., Kaliner, M. A., and Austen, K. F.: The immunological release of histamine and slow-reacting substance of anaphylaxis from human lung. III. Biochemical control mechanisms involved in the immunological release of the chemical mediators. *In* Austen, K. F., and Becker, E. L. (Eds.): Biochemistry of the Acute Allergic Reactions. Second International Symposium. Oxford, Blackwell Scientific Publications, 1971, p. 189.

CONCEPTUAL EVOLUTION FOR IMMUNOLOGICALLY INDUCED DISEASES
Connell, J. T.: Quantitative intranasal pollen challenge. II. Effect of daily pollen challenge, environmental pollen exposure and placebo challenge on the nasal membrane. J. Allerg., *41*:123, 1968.

Mansmann, H. C., Jr.: The evolution and modification of intractable bronchial asthma. *In* Pulmonary Care in the 1970's, Hahnemann Medical College Symposium, 1973, in press.

THE NATURE OF IMMUNOTHERAPY
Bush, A. M., and Bryant, D. J.: Precipitating antibodies in asthma: A preliminary communication. New Zeal. Med. J., *72*:28, 1970.

Colldahl, H.: The importance of inhalation tests in the etiological diagnosis of allergic diseases of the bronchi and in the evaluation of the effects of specific hyposensitization treatment. Acta Allerg., *22(Suppl. 8)*:7, 1967.

Johnstone, D. E., and Dutton, A.: The value of hyposensitization therapy for bronchial asthma in children. A fourteen-year study. Pediatrics, *42*:793, 1968.

Lowell, F. C., and Franklin, W.: A "double-blind" study of the effectiveness and specificity of injection therapy in ragweed hayfever. New Eng. J. Med., *273*:675, 1965.

Osler, A. G., Lichtenstein, L. M., and Levy, D. A.: *In vitro* studies of human reaginic allergy. Advances Immun., *8*:183, 1968.

Sadan, N., Rhyne, M. B., Mellits, E. D., Goldstein, E. A., Levy, D. A., and Lichtenstein, L. M.: Immunotherapy of pollinosis in children. New Eng. J. Med., *280*:623, 1969.

AUTONOMIC IMBALANCE IN ALLERGY
Middleton, E., Jr.: Autonomic imbalance in asthma with special reference to beta adrenergic blockade. Advances Intern. Med., *18*:177, 1972.

Parker, C. D., Bilbo, R. E., and Reed, C. E.: Methacholine aerosol as test for bronchial asthma. Arch. Intern. Med., *115*:452, 1965.

Reed, C. E.: Beta adrenergic blockade, bronchial asthma and atopy. J. Allerg., *42*:238, 1968.

Szentivanyi, A.: The beta adrenergic theory of the atopic abnormality in bronchial asthma. J. Allerg., *42*:203, 1968.

REAGIN-MEDIATED DISEASES IN MAN
Becker, E. L., and Austen, K. F.: Anaphylaxis. *In* Miescher, P. A., and Mueller-Eberhard, H. J. (Eds.): Textbook of Immunopathology. Vol. 1. New York, Grune and Stratton, 1968, p. 76.

Irvin, W. S., Johnson, P. K., Creger, W. P., Danliker, W. B., and Feigen, G. A.: Antibodies and vasoactive compounds in a case of anaphylactic shock to penicillin. Ann. Intern. Med., in press.

Itkin, I. H.: Study and management of severe asthma. Geriatrics, *18*:696, 1963.

James, L. P., and Austen, K. F.: Fatal systemic anaphylaxis in man. New Eng. J. Med., *270*:597, 1964.

Mansmann, H. C., Jr.: Management of the child with bronchial asthma. Pathologic, physiologic and pharmacologic problems. Pediat. Clin. N. Amer., *15*:357, 1968.

Reversible airway disease (formerly called asthma). 15th Aspen Emphysema Conference, Suppl. to Chest, 1973, in press.

Toogood, J. H.: Physiologic and pharmacologic basis of treatment in respiratory allergy. Mod. Treatm., *3*:816, 1966.

Tooley, W. H., DeMuth, G., and Nadel, J. A.: The reversibility of obstructive changes in severe childhood asthma. J. Pediat., *66*:517, 1965.

Wanderer, A. A., and Ellis, E. F.: Treatment of cold urticaria with cyproheptadine. J. Allerg. Clin. Immun., *48*:366, 1971.

Wanderer, A. A., Maselli, R., Ellis, E. F., and Ishizaka, K.: Immunologic characterization of serum factors responsible for cold urticaria. J. Allerg. Clin. Immun., *48*:13, 1971.

Wilhelm, D. L.: Kinins in human disease. Ann. Rev. Med., *22*:63, 1971.

Zweiman, B.: Diagnostic procedures in atopic patients. *In* Montagna, W., and Billingham, R. E. (Eds.): Advances in Biology of Skin. Vol. XI, Immunology and the Skin. New York, Appleton-Century-Crofts, 1971, p. 123.

CHAPTER 19 PATHOGENIC PROPERTIES OF INVADING MICROORGANISMS

LOUIS WEINSTEIN
MORTON N. SWARTZ

INTRODUCTION

Although the terms "health" and "disease" are mutually exclusive, "health" and "infection" are not. For example, within a few days of birth an infant is "infected" with a variety of bacteria and remains so infected throughout his lifetime. Thus, bacterial (and viral) colonization of body surfaces and the intestinal tract is the early and inevitable consequence of the ubiquitous distribution of microorganisms in man's surroundings. A delicate but peaceful balance is ordinarily maintained between the host and his normal flora through the operation of a variety of natural antibacterial defenses. These serve to limit the flora to areas where it may be tolerated safely such as the surfaces of the upper respiratory tract, the skin, and the intestinal tract. However, there are two ways in which microorganisms may gain access to tissues not normally colonized: (1) The intrinsic pathogenicity of the organism may be such that it is capable of breaching the natural protective physical or biochemical barriers. *Streptococcus pyogenes* (Group A streptococci) is an example of a bacterial species with such potential. (2) Natural defenses may be sufficiently compromised (trauma, immunosuppression, phagocytic malfunction, etc.) to allow commensal organisms to enter tissues not normally infected and to produce disease. This situation has become increasingly familiar during the past several decades as advances in the treatment of a variety of diseases have been won at the price of decreasing the host's natural resistance to invasive infection by elements of his own flora. Such infections have been designated "opportunistic." In this setting, ordinarily bland organisms such as *Staphylococcus epidermidis, Serratia, Herellea,* and so on may produce life-threatening invasive infection.

Whatever the mechanism of microbial invasion, once invasion has taken place the clinical manifestations of the infection are the result of the interaction of several major factors: (1) the intrinsic virulence of the microorganisms, (2) the nature of the host response to infection, and (3) specific anatomic features at the site of infection. The role of these factors in the pathophysiology of the infectious process and thus in the development of characteristic signs and symptoms will be the theme of this and the succeeding chapters in this section. An attempt will be made not to be encyclopedic but rather to examine some of the important examples of the aforementioned interactions. Since the presentation of most infections is that of involvement of a specific organ, and since this is necessarily the focus of the clinician's initial attention, considerable emphasis will be given to the particular pathophysiologic features of infection at specific sites such as the heart, central nervous system, skeletal system, and so on.

BASIC MECHANISMS OF PATHOGENICITY

Bacteria produce disease by either (1) the elaboration of toxins or (2) the invasion of tissues. The pathogenicity of certain bacterial species appears to reside exclusively in their ability to elaborate a potent toxin (e.g., *Clostridium tetani,* the causative organism in tetanus), while that of other species appears to be due to bacterial multiplication and invasiveness alone (e.g., *Diplococcus pneumoniae*). However, the combination of invasive and toxigenic potential accounts for the pathogenicity of many other species (e.g., *Streptococcus pyogenes*).

TOXIN PRODUCTION

There are two major types of bacterial toxins: *exotoxins* and *endotoxins.* The former are produced within the interior of the cell and appear in filtrates of growing cultures and in infected tissues. Some exotoxins diffuse readily through the bacterial cell wall and appear in greatest concentration in culture filtrates toward the end of the logarithmic phase of growth (e.g., alpha toxin of *Clostridium perfringens*). Others, sometimes designated "protoplasmic toxins," do not diffuse through the cell wall as easily and do not appear in appreciable amounts in culture fluid until the cells have autolyzed (e.g., tetanus and botulinum toxins). Those toxins that have been purified thus far appear to be proteins. In contrast, endotoxins are lipopolysaccharides of the cell wall of many gram-negative bacteria and are released into culture media only on autolysis or disruption of the organisms. In the case of several of the potent bacterial exotoxins, rather specific mechanisms of action have been elucidated at both the gross physiologic and subcellular levels. Although endotoxins have been studied extensively and although a variety of consequences of their administration have been demonstrated, their exact role in human disease is less specific and remains unclear.

EXOTOXINS

The number of bacterial exotoxins that have been reasonably well characterized is now rather extensive. Most of these, but not all, are produced by gram-positive bacteria, and they are listed in Table 19–1. No attempt is made here to provide a complete catalogue. In several instances, a given organism produces a variety of toxic products but only an illustrative example of clear clinical import is listed. Thus, *Clostridium perfringens* produces, in addition to the α toxin (lecithinase), κ toxin (collagenase) and λ toxin (protease), and so on. A variety of exotoxins similar to those produced by *Cl. perfringens* are produced by other clostridial species. Very recent additions to the

TABLE 19–1 SOME TOXIGENIC BACTERIA AND THEIR EXOTOXINS

Bacterial Species	Disease	Toxin	Mechanism of Action
Corynebacterium diphtheriae	Diphtheria	Diphtheria toxin	Neurotoxic; generally cytotoxic
Clostridium tetani	Tetanus	Tetanus toxin	Neurotoxic (spastic)
Clostridium botulinum	Botulism	Botulinum toxin (5 immunologic types)	Neurotoxic (paralytic)
Clostridium perfringens	Gas gangrene; bacteremia	Alpha toxin	Lecithinase (necrotizing, leukotoxic, hemolytic)
Streptococcus pyogenes (Group A streptococcus)	Pyogenic infections; scarlet fever	Streptolysin 0 and DPNase Erythrogenic toxin	Leukotoxic (?) Vascular dilatation and injury
Staphylococcus aureus	Pyogenic infections; food poisoning	Alpha toxin Leukocidin Enterotoxin "Exfoliatin"	Necrotizing Leukotoxic (?) Enterotoxic (vomiting; diarrhea) Exfoliation
Bacillus anthracis	Anthrax	Lethal toxin	Lethal; edema production
Pasteurella pestis	Plague	Plague toxin	Necrotizing (?); vascular injury causing shock
Vibrio cholerae	Cholera	Cholera enterotoxin	Intestinal loss of water and electrolytes
E. coli (enteropathic serotypes)	Gastroenteritis	*E. coli* enterotoxin	Intestinal loss of water and electrolytes
Shigella	Gastroenteritis	Shigella enterotoxin	Intestinal loss of water and electrolytes

list of toxigenic bacteria include enteropathic strains of *E. coli* and certain enteropathic strains of *Shigella*. In the case of certain exotoxins, the altered physiology they produce is now understandable at a subcellular or molecular level (diphtheria toxin, α toxin of *Clostridium perfringens*, *Vibrio cholerae* enterotoxin); in other instances, the biochemical lesion is not as clearly understood but the cellular localization of the toxin and the ensuing functional alterations have been reasonably well characterized (botulinum and tetanus toxins). On the basis of their mechanisms of action, certain of the exotoxins can be characterized as *general cytotoxins, neurotoxins,* or *enterotoxins.*

General Cytotoxins

Diphtheria Toxin. The variety of clinical manifestations which may develop in the course of diphtheria are directly due to the production of toxin at the site of the pharyngeal (or rarely cutaneous) infection. The hallmark of the disease, the gray faucial membrane, is due to the local effect of the potent necrotizing exotoxin and the inflammatory response of the body. This membrane may progress downward and involve the larynx and trachea, causing airway obstruction. Absorption of exotoxin into the general circulation may lead to abnormalities in many distant organ systems.

Cardiac involvement (in the second week or later) occurs in about two thirds of patients with diphtheria, as judged by electrocardiographic observations. Frank myocarditis is seen in 10 to 25 per cent of patients. Conduction abnormalities, are prominent features: bundle branch block (commonly), complete heart block, sinus tachycardia, auricular fibrillation, increased ventricular irritability or ventricular tachycardia and fibrillation. Congestive heart failure and cardiogenic shock may occur owing to the toxic myocarditis and are ominous developments. Diffuse involvement of the myocardium with granular and hyaline myofiber degeneration, mononuclear cell infiltration, and scarring has been found on pathologic examination of the heart in fatal cases. These findings are consistent with the expected effects of a potent cytotoxin (see below).

Nervous system complications occur in about 10 per cent of patients with diphtheria. Post diphtheritic paralysis affects cranial and peripheral nerves. In severe cases, paralysis of the soft palate may appear early (first 1 to 2 weeks) and is probably due to the direct action of the toxin on the pharyngeal motor nerve endings. More commonly, neuritis involving cranial nerves III, VI, VII, IX, and X, or peripheral nerves occurs in the second to sixth week. Motor loss is the predominant feature. A late (2 to 3 months) form of peripheral neuritis, initially characterized by symmetrically distributed sensory loss and identical to the Guillain-Barré syndrome, also may occur. Very rarely diphtheria is associated with encephalitis.

Hepatitis and nephritis are occasionally seen in diphtheria and are probably due to effects of the toxin. Necrosis, fatty infiltration, and cellular degeneration are demonstrable histologically in the liver, kidney, and adrenal glands.

Clinical evidence suggests that a variety of types of body cells are injured by diphtheria toxin. The work of Pappenheimer and his colleagues on the molecular basis of the action of diphtheria toxin is in keeping with these observations. The toxin interferes with mammalian cell protein synthesis, a process common to all cells of the body. Diphtheria toxin at a concentration of approximately 1 microgram per ml. completely suppresses protein synthesis when added to HeLa cells or to cell cultures derived from animal species that are sensitive in vivo to the toxin. In cell-free systems from mammalian sources, the toxin promptly inhibits the incorporation of amino acids into protein in the presence of the cofactor nicotinamide adenine dinucleotide (NAD). Transfer of amino acids from aminoacyl-tRNA to the growing polypeptide chains on the polyribosomes is blocked. This inhibition of polypeptide chain elongation is the result of the specific inactivation of transferase II, a soluble protein required for the guanosine triphosphate (GTP)-dependent translocation of peptidyl transfer RNA from the aminoacyl ("A") site to the peptidyl ("P") site on the ribosome (Figs. 19–1 and 19–2). An inactive adenine diphosphate ribosyl (ADPR) derivative of transferase II is formed in a reaction catalyzed by diphtheria toxin:

$$NAD^+ + \text{transferase II (active)} \xrightleftharpoons{\text{Diphtheria toxin}} \text{ADP-ribosyl transferase II (inactive)} + \text{nicotinamide} + H^+$$

The effect of toxin can also be demonstrated in cell-free extracts prepared from a diphtheria-toxin-susceptible species such as the guinea pig. Relatively small amounts of toxin (less than 25 M.L.D.) administered parenterally render inactive the "soluble enzyme fraction" (transferase), prepared from heart and skeletal muscle, that is an essential component of the in-vitro protein synthesizing system. Polyribosomes prepared from intoxicated guinea pigs function normally in in-vitro protein synthesis, provided that the "soluble enzyme fraction" is obtained from animals that have not been treated with toxin.

The toxin is extremely potent. Only a few molecules located in the cell membrane of a HeLa cell in the presence of the internal NAD concentration are capable of converting the entire cell content of free transferase II to its inactive ADP-

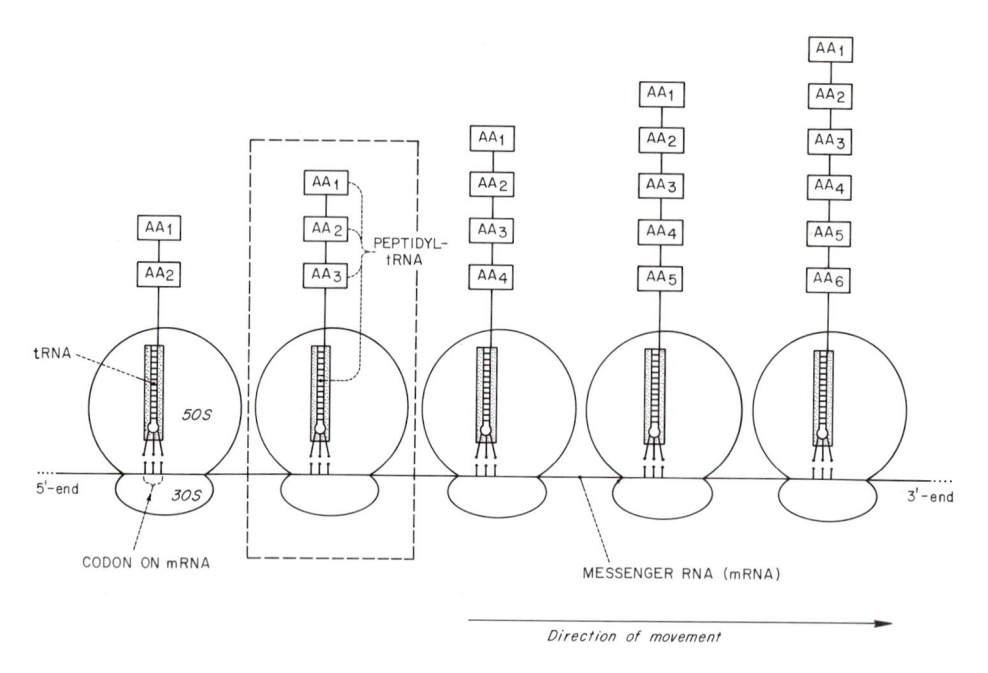

Figure 19–1 Polypeptide synthesis on polyribosome. Schematic representation showing polypeptide chain elongation during movement of the ribosomes (made up of 30S and 50S subunits) along the messenger RNA (mRNA) molecule. Five ribosomes are shown bound to the mRNA. Initiation of protein synthesis begins at the 5' end of the mRNA and polypeptide chain elongation proceeds on each ribosome as it moves toward the 3' end of the mRNA. The ribosomes shown on the right of the diagram (toward the 3' end of the mRNA) bear the longer polypeptide chains. The tRNA molecule is shown in a specific site (darkened area) on each ribosome, positioned in relation to the codon on the mRNA by its complementary codon (anticodon). The tRNA serves as an "adapter" to which an amino acid is attached, so that the latter can be adapted to the triplet-based (nucleotide) genetic code. When an incoming amino acid is added to the initiating aminoacyl-tRNA, the latter is converted to a peptidyl tRNA. The initial amino acid is designated as AA_1. Subsequent amino acids added to the nascent polypeptide chains are designated AA_2, AA_3, and so on. Because each of the five ribosomes above are traveling down the same mRNA molecule, the same five polypeptide chains will ultimately be made. The detailed steps involved in the addition of a single amino acid to form the peptidyl-tRNA shown in the boxed area in the figure are illustrated in Figure 19–2. The molecular site of action of diphtheria toxin is located there.

ribosyl derivative. In vivo, certain tissues, such as the heart and skeletal muscle, are particularly sensitive to small amounts of toxin. The inhibition of protein synthesis in subcellular components is consistent with the clinical and pathologic findings. Since the turnover rate of protein in muscle is slow, the toxin may inhibit synthesis at a functionally critical site (the S-A node or conduction system) or of specific enzymes involved in maintaining normal cardiac function. In vitro, the direct addition of diphtheria toxin to brain and liver tissue extracts of the susceptible guinea pig inhibits polypeptide synthesis. However, the protein-synthesizing ability of the in-vitro system prepared from brain tissues of intoxicated guinea pigs is not significantly impaired. This is in contrast to the aforementioned results with heart and skeletal muscle. The reason for this apparent difference is obscure. It would be informative to study the protein-synthesizing system in peripheral nerves, since the major impact of diphtheria toxin is registered there rather than in the brain. Nonetheless, the available body of evidence is sufficient to strongly suggest that diphtheria toxin acts in the susceptible animal in a manner analogous to its action in cell cultures and in cell-free systems, namely, by inactivation of transferase II.

Clostridium Perfringens Toxins. *Clostridium perfringens* is an obligate anaerobe normally inhabiting the lower gastrointestinal tract of man. Wound contamination with this organism is very common; however, significant infection is very rare. Clostridial infections are not due to uniquely pathogenic strains but rather to local circumstances such as low oxidation-reduction potential, ischemia, and necrosis that are favorable for multiplication. The critical pathogenetic step which transforms the relatively mild gas-forming infection (anaerobic cellulitis) into the devastating, rapidly advancing anaerobic myositis ("gas gangrene") capable of involving healthy muscle is as yet unknown. Several of the exotoxins, such as κ toxin and λ toxin, produced

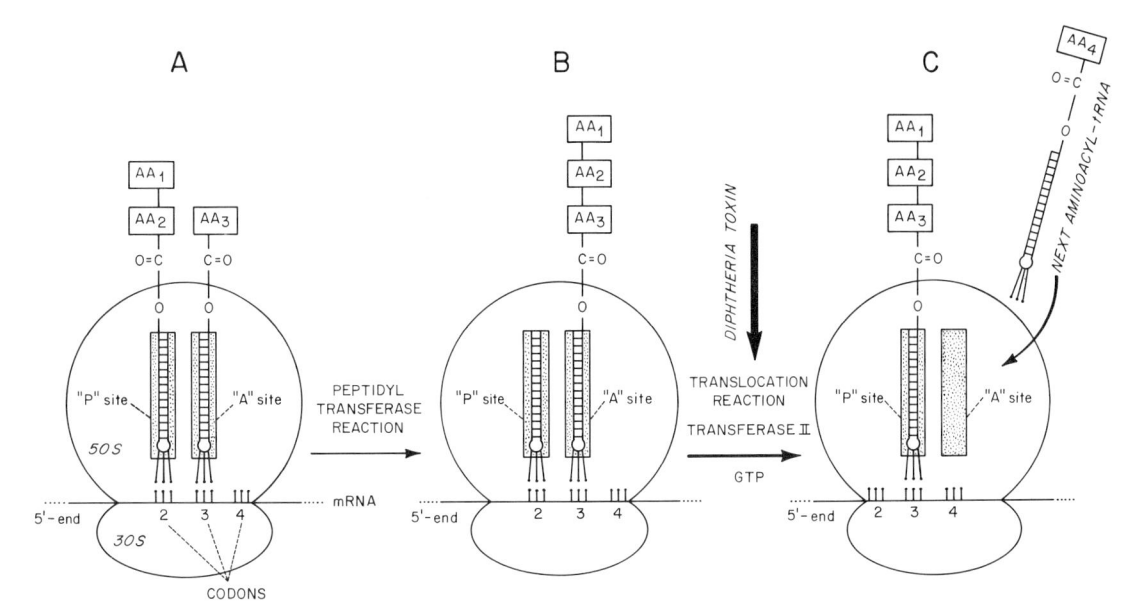

Figure 19-2 Schematic view of the individual steps involved in polypeptide chain elongation on an individual ribosome.

A, A ribosome (made up of its 50S and 30S subunits) is shown bound to a segment of mRNA. Two sites (aminoacyl or "A"; peptidyl or "P") are shown on the ribosome. The incoming aminoacyl-tRNA (bearing AA₃) is bound to the "A" site, positioned in accordance with the complementary nucleotide sequence it bears to the next codon (codon 3) of the mRNA. The "P" site is occupied by a peptidyl-tRNA (in this case bearing the two amino acids, AA₁ and AA₂).

B, The addition of AA₃ to the growing polypeptide chain involves peptide bond formation between the amino group of AA₃ and the esterified carboxyl group of AA₂ of the peptidyl-tRNA. This reaction is catalyzed by the enzyme peptidyl transferase, a part of the 50S subunit of the ribosome. As a result of this reaction, AA₁ and AA₂ are displaced from their tRNA in the "P" site to the tRNA in the "A" site, forming a new, elongated peptidyl-tRNA. The tRNA portion of the peptidyl-tRNA formerly in the "P" site (tRNA-AA₂-AA₁) remains (without its amino acid charge) bound to the "P" site.

C, The next step in polypeptide chain elongation is the translocation reaction, a complex step involving a specific protein (transferase II in mammalian cell systems) and the ribonucleoside triphosphate GTP. This reaction involves the physical movement of peptidyl-tRNA (tRNA-AA₃-AA₂-AA₁) from the "A" site to the "P" site, with resulting displacement of the empty (uncharged) tRNA from the latter site. This is shown in Section C of the figure. As a result of this movement, the "A" site is now open and available to receive a new incoming aminoacyl-tRNA coded for by codon 4. The cycle can then be repeated. Diphtheria toxin acts to inhibit the transferase II-requiring translocation reaction by causing the adenosine diphosphate ribosylation of the protein (see text).

by the organisms may contribute to the rapid advance of the highly lethal infection through their collagenolytic and proteolytic activities respectively. However, it is important to recognize that the mere fact of production of these toxins is not sufficient evidence to establish their role in the pathogenesis of the infection. The alpha toxin, or lecithinase, of *Cl. perfringens* has been implicated in both the local tissue necrosis and toxemic features of gas gangrene. However, it should be noted that some strains of *Cl. perfringens* isolated from severe gas gangrene have been poor producers of alpha toxin. Furthermore, specific antitoxin to the lecithinase will not protect against the development of gas gangrene, not stop its spread, and not alleviate the toxemia and shock which are features of this disease. The interaction of alpha toxin or other extracellular enzymes with injured muscle is thought by some to be the source of the as yet unidentified toxic factor in gas gangrene. Although the direct role of alpha toxin has been somewhat de-emphasized in the foregoing discussion, it should be appreciated that it is nonetheless an extremely potent and lethal product. Intravenous administration in experimental animals produces fever, hypotension, intravascular hemolysis, jaundice, hemoglobinuria, renal shutdown, and death. The clinical counterpart with the identical constellation of findings develops in the course of high-grade *Cl. perfringens* bacteremia. This does not occur ordinarily in gas gangrene but is a fairly common complication of clostridial infection of the uterus following a septic abortion. The lethal effects of the lecithinase are due to splitting of lecithin (Fig. 19-3) which is present in the membranes of

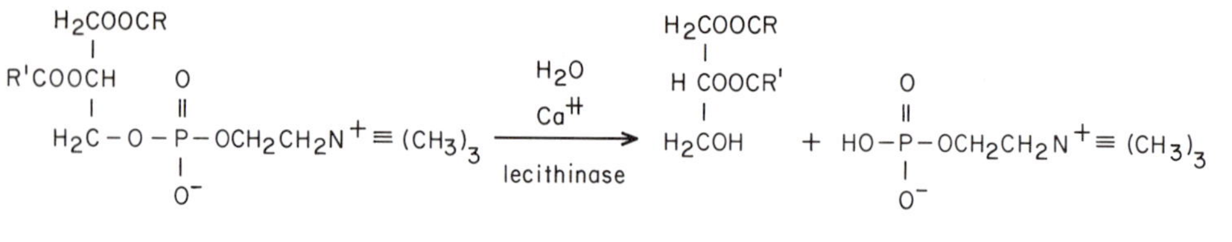

Figure 19-3 Action of *Cl. perfringens* lecithinase (α toxin) on lecithin. Cleavage of the bond between the phosphoric acid and glycerol moieties yields a diglyceride and phosphorylcholine. R and R' represent fatty acids esterified with glycerol.

a variety of cells in the body. These cells include erythrocytes, which are hemolyzed by this enzyme; leukocytes are probably similarly injured, accounting for the paucity of these cells in the exudate of gas gangrene.

Neurotoxins

Tetanus Toxin. Tetanus is an intoxication with the exotoxin of *Clostridium tetani* and is characterized by intense, severe muscle spasms. The toxin, known as tetanospasmin, is one of the most potent bacterial toxins known. Spores of the etiologic agent, *Clostridium tetani,* are introduced by contamination of a wound. The wound may be an extensive laceration, gun shot or puncture wound, or a very trivial lesion into which spores of the organism have been introduced. The mere presence of *Cl. tetani* in a wound does not mean that tetanus will develop. Transformation of the spores into toxin-producing vegetative forms requires a lower oxidation-reduction potential than is present in normal tissues. Necrotic tissue produced by the trauma or by invasion by pyogenic bacteria simultaneously present and the introduction of foreign material can lower the reduction-oxidation potential sufficiently to allow this to occur. There is little or no capacity of the organism to invade tissues, and often the wound hardly appears to be infected. All the clinical manifestations of the disease are due to the physiologic changes produced by the toxin in the nervous system—spinal cord, brain stem, and sympathetic nervous system. Toxin introduced into muscle spreads centrally along motor nerves and up the spinal cord. Toxin may also be spread via the bloodstream, and this route may be the more important one in generalized tetanus. Despite the violent and widely distributed symptoms of the disease, no lesions are detectable in the nervous system (or other tissues), even with the electron microscope.

The major clinical manifestation of tetanus is muscular rigidity. This may be mild in "local tetanus," in which rigidity affects only one limb or one group of muscles (the site of injury) and usually occurs in patients with a limited degree of immunity. More often, the initiating injury is followed within a matter of days by local muscular spasm about the wound and then trismus. Stiffness of the facial muscles may produce a bizarre sneering expression *(risus sardonicus)*. Stiffness of the back, neck, and abdomen may become marked enough to produce pain as a prominent symptom. Dysphagia and hydrophobia are due to spasm of the pharyngeal and glottal muscles. With the progression of generalized tetanus, opisthotonos and violent spasmodic contractions of the neck, trunk, and limb muscles occur. Despite the severity of such manifestations the sensorium is still clear. Sudden stimuli (noise, bright light, an injection) may precipitate a generalized tonic convulsion, with accompanying spasm of the larynx and respiratory muscles, resulting in respiratory arrest. Thus, afferent stimuli appear to produce an exaggerated effect. This suggests that the toxin produces its characteristic effects by disturbing the normal regulation of the reflex arc. Reciprocal innervation is abolished and as a result both the stimulated muscle groups and the opposing groups contract simultaneously. This produces the characteristic muscular spasm. The particular features of this spasm are determined in each area by the relative bulk (strength) of the opposing muscle groups. Thus, since the masseters are stronger than the opposing mylohyoid and digastricus muscles, trismus results. The masseters generally show greater sensitivity to tetanus toxin than the muscles of the extremities. It has been suggested that this is because the masseters are normally maintained in a state of partial contraction when man is awake. In the lower extremities the strength of the extensor groups exceeds that of the flexors, and the predominant posture in tetanus is that of extension at the hips and knees.

The neurophysiology of the action of tetanus toxin now seems reasonably clear, particularly as a result of the studies of Sir John Eccles. The main impact of the toxin is on the spinal cord.

Grossly, the effects of the toxin are very similar to those of strychnine. The toxin does not act on reflex arcs which include only sensory and motor neurons (two-neuron or monosynaptic reflexes). It profoundly affects the more complex reflexes (polysynaptic reflexes that involve interneurons), blocking the normal postsynaptic inhibition of spinal motorneurons that results from afferent impulses. This action of the toxin in selectively blocking inhibitory synapses in the central nervous system results in multiplication of excitatory impulses which run in unchecked fashion and are not coordinated by inhibitory mechanisms. This produces the muscular spasms (tetanic seizures) characteristic of tetanus.

In the normal resting state, muscle tone is maintained by the constant mild tension of opposing muscle groups. Thus, motion at the elbow is controlled by two sets of muscles—the extensor (triceps) and the flexor (biceps). When the biceps contracts slightly, the triceps is stretched, activating stretch-sensitive receptors. These, in turn, send afferent impulses to the spinal cord, where they stimulate the motor neurons and cause contraction of the triceps opposing the stretch. The stretch reflex thus plays an important role in maintaining postural tone. However, for proper functioning of the elbow joint, for example, it is essential that the biceps not be opposed too vigorously by the triceps. Otherwise, the forearm would be locked into spasm by the action of the opposing muscles, and voluntary movement would be impossible. Therefore, the afferent impulse that causes the activation of the biceps must facilitate relaxation of the triceps. This inhibition is effected in the spinal cord by branching of the axon carrying the afferent impulse. One branch excites the biceps and the other excites the internuncial neuron ("inhibitory cell") to release an inhibitory transmitter (Fig. 19-4). This inhibitory transmitter in turn acts on the anterior horn cells innervating the triceps, thus opposing the action of the excitatory transmitter released there from the stretch-sensitive afferent nerve. The net result is that triceps motor neurons are not excited and the triceps does not contract; the biceps is then able to flex the forearm unhindered. Tetanus toxin acts in the spinal cord to disrupt this balanced reciprocity by suppressing the normal inhibition through the internuncial connections. The toxin appears either to reduce the amount of inhibitory transmitter (? glycine or a "glycine-like" amino acid) available for release or to block its release. As a result, in the absence of inhibition the normal stretch reflex of the triceps is unopposed, and when the biceps contracts, the antagonist muscle, the triceps, does likewise, locking the forearm in spasm.

An unusual form of tetanus results from action of the toxin primarily on the motor innervation

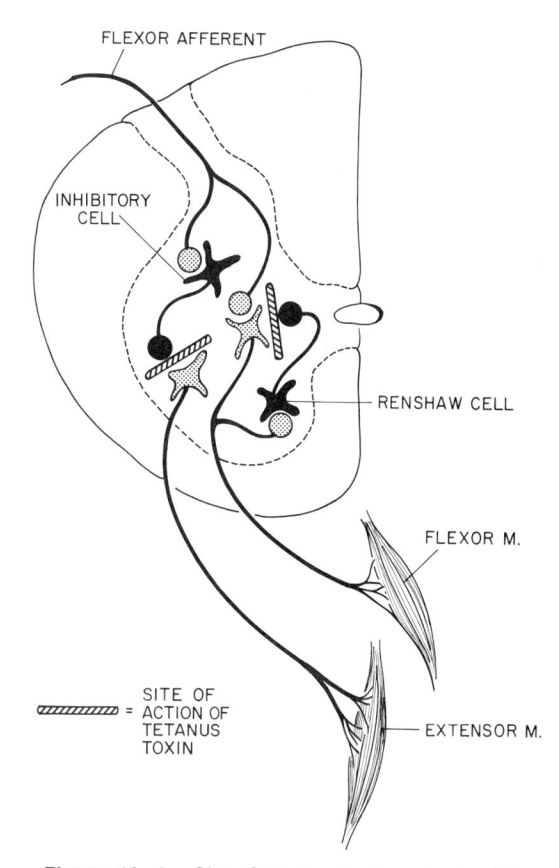

Figure 19-4 Site of action of tetanus toxin. Schematically shown are neural connections involved in controlling the action of opposing flexor and extensor muscle groups such as the biceps and triceps. Contraction of the biceps normally stretches the triceps, activating receptors which pass to the spinal cord (this afferent is not shown on the illustration) and stimulating the motor innervation of the triceps. Another afferent to the biceps is shown which synapses with an inhibitory cell ("interneuron"). The latter releases an inhibitory transmitter, preventing the stretch-induced excitation of the triceps. Also shown is a second inhibitory pathway, involving an axon collateral from the flexor motor neuron extending to a Renshaw cell. This cell, in turn, synapses with the flexor motor neuron, producing postsynaptic inhibition, controlling the stimulation of flexor contraction. Tetanus toxin appears to act by blocking both of the above inhibitory pathways in the spinal cord.

(in the brain stem) of the facial, glossal, pharyngeal, jaw, and ocular muscles. Whether the toxin reaches these areas by the neural or hematogenous route is not clear. This form of tetanus is known as "cephalic tetanus." It occurs when the spores of *Cl. tetani* are introduced into wounds involving the eye, during tonsilloadenoidectomy, during the course of chronic otitis media, or following trauma to the head or neck.

In this form of tetanus the affected muscles appear to be paralyzed, especially those involving facial and ocular movements. The apparent facial palsy in reality is a pseudoparalysis. Hypertonia involves all the muscles supplied by the facial motor neurons, and voluntary movements are prevented. Although "cephalic tetanus" may be the only clinical presentation, it is important to emphasize the fact that generalized disease may develop subsequently.

Overactivity of the sympathetic nervous system has been observed in patients with severe tetanus, suggesting that tetanus toxin may also directly affect this portion of the nervous system. Among the manifestations that may develop, in any combination, are labile hypertension, tachycardia, peripheral vasoconstriction, irregularities of cardiac rhythm, profuse sweating, increased respiratory rate, increase in the urinary excretion of catecholamines, and, in some instances, during the late stage of the disease, hypotension. These manifestations do not appear to be related to hypoxia secondary to involvement of the innervation of the muscles of respiration or to pulmonary infection. Such evidences of sympathetic overactivity are not generally observed in other paralyzed patients treated in identical fashions to support respiration and maintain adequate oxygenation.

"Localized tetanus" is an unusual clinical form of tetanus in which intermittent twitching and spasm of muscles occur in a circumscribed area of the body, with or without a known wound or injury in that area. Stiffness of the muscles in the involved area, usually a limb, may be the initial symptom. The manifestations may persist over several weeks or months restricted to the initial area of involvement, or the process may progress to generalized tetanus within a few days. Although it was originally believed that this form of tetanus was due to the local action of the toxin on muscle near the site of injury, it is now thought that the manifestations of this form of tetanus are also due to suppression of spinal inhibitory mechanisms. Toxin reaching the spinal cord either by passage along regional nerves or by hematogenous spread (as seems more likely) produces an increased central excitatory state. This, however, is so slight in localized tetanus as to be inapparent if it were not for the increased afferent inflow from the periphery provided by the local skin and muscular lesion at the site of trauma.

The pathophysiology of the action of tetanus toxin at the molecular level is unknown. However, Van Heyningen has demonstrated that the site of toxin binding in nervous tissue is the synaptic membrane of the nerve endings. The chemical substance binding the toxin is a ganglioside, a compound containing fatty acid, sphingosine, and several sugars. The role of toxin binding in clinical tetanus is not clear; there is no detectable change in the ganglioside molecule where the toxin is bound. Binding may not be an essential feature of the action of toxin but may simply be a means of channeling this toxin to the central nervous system.

Botulinum Toxin. Botulism is an intoxication with the exotoxin of *Clostridium botulinum* and is characterized by profound weakness of both skeletal and smooth muscle. The disease results from the ingestion of food (canned meats and vegetables, packaged fish, sausages) in which the organism has grown under anaerobic conditions and elaborated its potent exotoxin. There is absolutely no invasive potential to the organism itself and all the clinical manifestations are due solely to the toxin. The toxin is heat labile; cooking at boiling temperature for a few minutes destroys it. Clinical symptoms usually develop 18 to 36 hours after ingestion of contaminated food. The cranial nerves are involved earliest, resulting in paresis of accommodation, diplopia due to weakness of the external ocular muscles, dysphagia, difficulty talking, and weakness of the jaw muscles. Subsequently, the muscles of the trunk and limbs become weak. The deep tendon reflexes remain normal; sensory abnormalities are absent.

Like tetanus toxin, botulinum toxin is extremely potent yet produces no apparent structural damage. There is no evidence of involvement of the central nervous system. In contrast to the diffuse muscular overactivity of tetanus, the characteristic feature of botulism is a flaccid weakness; this is not due to any loss of contractile power of the muscles themselves, since they respond normally to direct electrical stimulation. Burgen, Dickens, and Zatman have reported that the toxin acts at the neuromuscular junctions, preventing release of acetylcholine, the excitatory transmitter. They noted that the quantity of acetylcholine liberated by stimulation of phrenic nerve-diaphragm preparations of rats was very much smaller in the presence of botulinum toxin than in control preparations. Thus, excitatory impulses are blocked between the efferent nerve endings and the muscle; this leads to flaccid weakness.

Enterotoxins

Cholera Enterotoxin. Cholera, an infection due to *Vibrio cholerae*, is characterized by dramatic and devastating diarrhea, resulting in enormous fluid and electrolyte losses. It occurs endemically and epidemically in Asia but recently has spread to Africa and southern Europe. The disease is usually transmitted by contaminated water but occasionally by fruits or vegetables contaminated with human feces. Its onset is sudden and the course is, as a rule, fulminant. Chills and fever are not prominent features; the body temperature may, in fact, be depressed. Abdominal pain and vomiting may accompany the initial diarrhea. Later, however, the striking feature of the disease is the prodigious fluid loss from the intestine. This may exceed one liter of fluid per hour. The "rice water" stool is watery, odorless, and mucoid. The various clinical manifestations that develop later are secondary to the severe degree of dehydration and the loss of electrolytes. These include hypotension and shock, metabolic acidosis, muscle cramps, stupor and coma, hypokalemic flaccid paralysis, acute tubular necrosis, and, occasionally, myocardial infarction.

The primary pathophysiologic disturbance in cholera is severe loss of fluid and electrolytes from the small intestine. These changes occur in the absence of any invasion of the intestinal mucosa by the organisms or a significant inflammatory response. The initial outpouring of large volumes of fluid into the lumen of the intestine occurs at a time when there is no disruption of the intestinal mucosa. Denudation of the mucosa is a late phenomenon and is secondary to severe hypovolemia in the end stages of cholera. The only histologic changes noted consistently in early human cases and in the experimental animal (rabbit) are mild hyperemia of the mucosal capillaries and edema of the tunica propria of the small intestine.

The fluid lost from the intestine is isotonic and has a low protein content similar to that found in the intestinal fluid of normal persons. The bicarbonate concentration of this fluid is about twice and the potassium concentration about four times that of normal plasma. All the clinical manifestations of the disease can be corrected by prompt intravenous administration of appropriate fluid and electrolytes.

Recent studies of the effects of cholera enterotoxin indicate that it produces increased fluid and electrolyte movement across the small intestine from plasma to the gut lumen. This could be due to either increased filtration of electrolytes from intestinal capillaries across the mucosal cells, or to active secretion of one or more electrolytes by the epithelial lining cells. Present evidence suggests that the former is not the case. For example, decreasing the mesenteric blood flow in the dog by as much as 70 per cent does not reduce the rate of fluid production by intestinal loops treated with cholera enterotoxin. Even more telling evidence against the filtration hypothesis is provided by the examination of the intestinal clearance of mannitol and sodium in patients with acute cholera. Gordon has demonstrated that the clearance of intravenously administered ^{14}C mannitol is only 25 per cent of the clearance of sodium, indicating less resistance to the flow of sodium than of mannitol.

Considerable insight into electrolyte movement across the normal and cholera enterotoxin-treated intestine has been provided by study of the isolated rabbit ileal mucosa. Normally, the net secretory flux of HCO_3^- balances the net absorptive flux of Cl^-. There is also a net absorptive flux of Na^+, and this can be increased by the addition of glucose to the solution on the luminal side of the isolated ileum. (This experimental observation has a very important therapeutic implication. Indeed, orally administered glucose-containing solutions can reduce considerably the electrolyte loss of patients with the disease.) The addition of cholera enterotoxin to the musocal side of such an in-vitro preparation produces distinct changes after a latent period of about an hour. These consist of (1) complete disappearance of the net absorptive flux of Na^+ and (2) reversal of the direction of chloride transport, the net absorptive flux being replaced by a net secretory flux. The HCO_3^- net secretory flux remains unchanged. *Thus, the effect of enterotoxin on solute transport consists of stimulation of chloride secretion and inhibition of sodium absorption.* The toxin-induced secretion of anion would then cause isosmotic accumulation of water. Fluid pouring into the intestine in the cholera patient, or in the rabbit ileal loop, is indeed isotonic. Large losses of HCO_3^- occur when the reabsorptive capacity of the colon for diarrheal fluid is exceeded. The same mechanism may be responsible for substantial losses of potassium.

Cyclic AMP (3',5'-AMP), when applied to the isolated rabbit ileal mucosa preparation, produces changes in ion flux similar to those produced by cholera enterotoxin. This suggests that the cholera enterotoxin-induced fluid and electrolyte loss may be mediated by cyclic 3',5'-AMP. There is a large body of circumstantial evidence in support of this concept: (1) Adenyl cyclase, the enzyme involved in the synthesis of 3',5'-AMP from ATP, is demonstrable in the mucosa at all levels of the small intestine but is present in highest concentration in the duodenum. Outpouring of fluid and solute in response to cholera enterotoxin occurs at all levels of the small bowel; the highest rate of secretion is in the duodenum. (2) Theophylline, an inhibitor of the phosphodiesterase that normally breaks down 3',5'-AMP to 5'-AMP, produces effects similar to those of cholera enterotoxin: infusion of theophylline into the superior mesenteric artery of dogs produces fluid and solute secretion into the small intestine comparable to that produced by cholera enterotoxin, and theophylline produces alterations of ion flux similar to those produced by cholera enterotoxin on the isolated rabbit ileal mucosa. (3) Cholera enterotoxin increases the adenyl cyclase activity of membranes prepared from rabbit small intestine. (4) 3',5'-AMP levels in intestinal mucosa are increased several fold after preincubation with the toxin either in vitro (membrane preparations) or in vivo (intact mucosal cell in the experimental animal). The addition of enterotoxin to disrupted cell preparations does not increase the adenyl cyclase activity. This suggests that enterotoxin must be converted to some active intermediate by a membrane-bound enzyme in order to effect a change in the adenyl cyclase system.

Several other acute infectious diarrheal diseases of man may be produced by a mechanism identical to that operative in cholera. These are disorders in which bacterial invasion of the bowel wall does not take place, but in which exotoxins may have a major pathogenetic role. These include the gastroenteritides due to enteropathic strains of *E. coli*, Shigella, and *Clostridium perfringens*. Extracellular products of these organisms have been shown experimentally to stimulate small intestinal fluid secretion. It is very possible that these bacterial toxins (and also staphylococcal enterotoxin, the cause of "staphylococcal food poisoning") have a common mode of action involving intestinal adenyl cyclase stimulation.

ENDOTOXINS

Bacterial endotoxins are integral parts of the bacterial cell wall and are released only upon disruption of the bacterial cell. Endotoxins differ in a variety of ways from bacterial exotoxins: (1) Endotoxins are particulate macromolecules. Although originally isolated as phospholipid-polysaccharide-protein complexes, their biological activity resides in an extractable lipopolysaccharide fraction. Their toxicity appears to reside predominantly in the phospholipid component; the major antigenic determinants are in the polysaccharide fraction. On the other hand, bacterial exotoxins are proteins, usually of relatively small size (M.W. 50,000 to 100,000, occasionally as large as 1,000,000). (2) True endotoxins are found predominantly, if not exclusively, in gram-negative bacteria. In contrast, exotoxins are produced by many types of bacteria, most frequently by gram-positive bacilli. (3) Endotoxins are less potent by at least several orders of magnitude than most exotoxins. (4) Endotoxins from a variety of bacterial species elicit the same responses after parenteral administration, even though the intrinsic pathogenicity of the organism from which they were derived shows considerable differences. (5) Endotoxins are relatively heat-stable, unlike bacterial protein exotoxins (with the exception of the enterotoxin of *Staphylococcus aureus*). (6) Bacterial endotoxins are much more varied in their activity and less specific in their cytotoxic actions. Thus, no effects of endotoxin can compare with the exquisite selective neurotropism of the toxins of *Cl. tetani* and *Cl. botulinum*.

Endotoxins have been identified in *E. coli*, Salmonella, Shigella, *Vibrio cholerae*, Brucella, *Neisseria gonorrhoeae*, *Neisseria meningitidis*, and other gram-negative organisms. When injected intravenously in experimental animals, they produce a variety of biological effects. These include fever, diarrhea, hypotension, shock, transient leukopenia followed by leukocytosis, hyperglycemia, abortion, capillary hemorrhages, diffuse intravascular coagulation, altered resistance to bacterial infections, and the Shwartzman phenomenon. Despite this large number of physiologic derangements produced by endotoxins, their role in the clinical features of illnesses due to gram-negative bacteria remains speculative. Tolerance, or refractoriness to the pyrogenic and other biological effects of endotoxin, develops on repeated injection. The state appears to be independent of the development of demonstrable circulating antibody, since it subsides after 1 to 2 weeks following a course of repeated injections, whereas active immunity persists much longer. Tolerance results from an increased clearance of injected endotoxin by cells of the reticuloendothelial system (RES); it can be prevented by prior injection of particulate material (Thorotrast, India ink) which is readily taken up by the RES, resulting in "blockade" of its ability to clear subsequently injected endotoxin. It has been suggested that circulating endotoxin plays an important role in sustained gram-negative infection and that the development of tolerance is an important aspect of recovery from the illness. Tolerance to endotoxin is not a feature of infections of man produced by gram-negative bacteria (brucellosis, typhoid, tularemia). There is, in fact, an enhanced reactivity to its effects. Indeed, in experimental typhoid fever an enhanced pyrogenic response to injected endotoxin can be elicited from late in the incubation period through the early phase of convalescence. As the convalescent phase progresses, tolerance to the pyrogenic effects of endotoxin develops. Tolerance to endotoxin, induced in man by daily injections, disappears during the active stage of typhoid fever and reappears when chemotherapy has produced a favorable response.

Biological Effects

1. *Fever* is produced by the intravenous injection of endotoxin in most laboratory animals and man. The febrile response occurs in humans after a lag period which may be as long as 90 minutes. Clearer understanding of the febrile response to endotoxin has come from the animal studies of Atkins and Wood. Immediately following the injection of endotoxin, blood was found to contain a weak pyrogen which had all the properties of the originally injected material. This then disappeared from the blood, which became nonpyrogenic; 90 to 120 minutes after the endotoxin injection a second pyrogen appeared in the circu-

lation. The properties of this substance differed in many ways from those of endotoxin and appeared to be identical with those of pyrogenic material ("endogenous pyrogen") isolated from polymorphonuclear leukocytes (see Chapter 20). The marked neutropenia produced by the injection of endotoxin has been presumed to be evidence of direct damage to leukocytes by this macromolecule. Release of the leukocytic pyrogen from the injured neutrophils is the most likely cause of the later fever. The nonidentity of leukocytic pyrogen and endotoxin has been demonstrated in several ways. Leukocytic pyrogen is active in animals previously rendered tolerant to the pyrogenic effects of bacterial endotoxin. Unlike endotoxin, leukocytic pyrogen produces a single febrile peak after a very brief lag period when injected into animals.

2. *Granulocytopenia* appears promptly after intravenous injection of endotoxin, persists for 3 to 6 hours, and is followed by a marked leukocytosis. The short period of granulocytopenia is associated with impairment of leukocytic migration into areas of active inflammation. Granulocytopenia develops as neutrophils shift from the circulating pool to the marginal one, as a result of increased adherence of leukocytes to the vascular endothelium, particularly in the lung.

3. *Hypotension and shock* are produced in animals by the injection of large doses of endotoxin. Species difference among animals with regard to the pattern of vascular response to this substance has been a source of confusion in attempts to understand the pathophysiology of endotoxic shock and to relate the circulatory changes in bacteremia due to gram-negative organisms in man to "endotoxic shock." For example, in the dog the early systemic hypotension that develops after injection of endotoxin stems from a decreased cardiac output. This follows a marked decrease in venous return that is due primarily to pooling in the portal system secondary to constriction of hepatic veins produced by release of histamine. Recovery from the initial hypotension occurs within a few minutes. A second fall in blood pressure occurs in 1 to 2 hours; this is more gradual, and spontaneous recovery is not usual. There is gradual slowing of blood flow in the microcirculation and vasospasm of arterioles and venules. Decreased perfusion of many organs ensues, with the greatest effects occurring in the renal and splanchnic circulation. Catecholamines are released and produce an increase in total peripheral arterial resistance. When endotoxin shock has gone on for several hours in the dog the process becomes irreversible. This stage is featured by arteriolar and capillary dilatation, venular contraction, stasis, and morphologic evidences of damage to capillaries and veins (hemorrhage and edema, especially of the intestine). In contrast to the response to endotoxin in the dog, the circulatory changes in man are less clear and well-defined. The cause of the circulatory changes occurring in patients with sepsis due to gram-negative bacteria is uncertain. Many of the features may be attributed to the bacteremia itself or to endotoxemia alone. The very recent development of a test for the detection of endotoxin (Limulus test) in blood may shed some light on this problem. Preliminary data suggest that hypotension and death occur twice as frequently in patients with demonstrable endotoxemia ($\pm$ bacteremia) as in patients in whom gram-negative bacteria alone are present in the blood.

4. *Coagulation* may be profoundly altered following injection of endotoxin into experimental animals. The changes in hemostasis are biphasic. After a lag period there is a hypercoagulable state (associated with an increased amount of circulatory fibrinogen), followed in a matter of hours by a prolonged hypocoagulable period. The latter is characterized by depletion of plasma fibrinogen, thrombocytopenia, and other changes associated with intravascular clotting. In-vitro studies of human and animal plasma suggest that endotoxin initiates intravascular clotting by activating Factor XII (Hageman factor) which appears to be capable of activating plasma prekallikrein to the active protease kallikrein. This in turn releases bradykinin (an extremely powerful vasodepressor) from its inactive plasma precursor kininogen. Bradykinin, with its ability to increase vascular permeability and its vasodepressor effects, may be responsible for many of the circulatory effects of septic shock. Thus, it is likely that the same site of endotoxin action (activation of Factor XII) may initiate both the coagulation and hemodynamic alterations associated in some instances with shock.

5. The *Shwartzman phenomenon* is a peculiar toxic reaction observed in rabbits following two injections of endotoxin. Two types of this phenomenon have been described. The *local Schwartzman* reaction consists of gross hemorrhage and necrosis in the skin. It occurs after an initial *cutaneous* injection of endotoxin (or endotoxin-containing bacteria), which is then followed in some hours by an *intravenous* injection of endotoxin. The initial ("preparatory") and second ("eliciting") injections may utilize endotoxin from different bacterial species. Nonbacterial materials such as washed antigen-antibody precipitates may be employed for the "eliciting" reaction. Polymorphonuclear leukocyte "cuffing" develops about the small veins at the skin site following the "preparatory" injection. Peripheral vasoconstriction, particularly at the prepared skin site is produced by the intravenous injection. Leukocyte-platelet thrombi develop and occlude capillaries and small veins resulting in necrosis of vessel walls and secondary hemorrhage.

The *generalized Shwartzman reaction* develops when both the "preparatory" and "eliciting" injections of endotoxin are given intravenously approximately 24 hours apart. The typical histologic lesion that develops is characterized by deposition of fibrinoid material within capillaries. This occurs most dramatically in the kidney and produces bilateral renal cortical necrosis. The histologic findings appear to be the result of disseminated intravascular coagulation. Polymorphonuclear leukocytes are essential to the development of the Shwartzman phenomenon; the prior induction of leukopenia will prevent both the localized and generalized forms of the reaction. Although it is tempting to ascribe the characteristic hemorrhagic necrotic skin lesions of meningococcemia to this mechanism, convincing proof that the Shwartzman reaction occurs during disease in man is still lacking.

INVASION OF TISSUES

Local Effects

Most infectious agents produce demonstrable damage to host cells in the area immediately surrounding their site of invasion. In many instances, this is due primarily to multiplication of the infecting agent (usually bacteria or fungi) or to its growth (parasites). Among the invasive bacteria, *D. pneumoniae* (pneumococcus) is an example of an agent the pathogenicity of which appears to be solely related to its capacity to multiply rapidly and successfully in the susceptible host. No toxins capable of producing local or distant effects have been demonstrated in infections produced by this organism. The essential ingredient in its pathogenicity is the antiphagocytic activity of its capsular polysaccharide. Thus, smooth encapsulated strains are capable of resisting surface phagocytosis, the first line of host defense, prior to the appearance of specific antibody. Pneumococci invading the lung are thus capable of extensive multiplication and of eliciting marked edema and inflammatory response in the alveoli. The extensive lobar involvement that occurs is responsible for the characteristic dyspnea and tachypnea due to both arterial oxygen undersaturation (secondary to continued perfusion of the poorly ventilated area of lung) and splinting of the chest (secondary to spread of the bacterial inflammation to the pleural surface with its attendant pain). Rarely, the unrestrained growth of pneumococci may be so extensive that frank tissue destruction and abscess formation occur. This is almost invariably due, when present, to type 3 pneumococci, strains which, because they produce unusually abundant capsular material, are almost totally insulated from surface phagocytosis.

Localized pyogenic foci (abscesses) due to a large variety of bacteria may develop almost anywhere in the body and increase in size sufficiently to produce obstructive or pressure phenomena. However, when they occur in the central nervous system their effects may be most dramatic because of their anatomic location and the lack of elasticity of the surrounding structures. Thus, an abscess in the cerebrum or cerebellum can produce marked neurologic deficit by two mechanisms: neuronal destruction by the invading microorganisms, and swelling of surrounding brain tissue due to edema and the inflammatory response. The abscess may be well walled-off by a thick capsule, and there may be little or no fever or other manifestations of infection. The clinical picture may then mimic that of an enlarging cerebral mass lesion such as a brain tumor. Manifestations of increased intracranial pressure such as headache, papilledema, and sixth and third cranial nerve palsies may dominate the clinical picture. If untreated, the lesion may go on to cause herniation of the temporal lobe and midbrain compression, or it may rupture into the ventricular system and cause fulminating meningitis. A temporal lobe lesion that may present in a similar way may occasionally be seen in viral infection of the central nervous system, especially encephalitis due to *Herpes hominis*.

The dramatic mass effects of infection are particularly prominent in certain parasitic infestations. Heavy loads of adult Ascaris may produce abdominal pain and even intestinal obstruction. Migration of these worms into the biliary tree may produce obstruction and ascending cholangitis. Cysticercosis represents the invasion of various tissues by the larval form of the pork tapeworm, *Cysticercus cellulosae*. The brain is most commonly involved. The parasitic cyst surrounded by a thick capsule can mimic a neoplasm and cause seizures, personality changes, long tract signs, or increased intracranial pressure. The larvae of *Toxocara canis* may migrate in man to a variety of organs such as liver, lung, or eye. In the ocular form, a space-occupying granulomatous mass resembling a retinoblastoma may develop and distort the retina.

Effects of Widespread Dissemination of Infection

Bacteremia may result when initial host defenses are insufficient to contain the invading microorganism locally. Thus, *Staphylococcus aureus* bacteremia following an initial skin or other focus of infection may produce abscess formation in distant organs such as kidney, bone, and brain. The symptoms and signs of the infection that develops in this situation are related to dysfunction of the particular organ involved. A transient bacteremia may become high grade and continuous when staphylococcal infection is superimposed on a previously damaged (or entirely normal) heart valve to produce acute bacterial endocarditis (see Chapter 21). Rarely, the density of staphylococci in the blood may be sufficiently high as to be visible in Gram-stained smears of a "buffy-coat" preparation of venous blood. The nature of the factors that contribute to staphylococcal pathogenicity is unclear. Clinical isolates do not appear to contain an antiphagocytic capsule component.

Another organism that, in the setting of nosocomial infection, is notoriously capable of producing abscesses in multiple organs following bacteremia is *Pseudomonas aeruginosa*. It is an aggressive secondary invader in open wounds, in decubiti, at the sites of foreign bodies (e.g., indwelling venous catheters), and particularly in extensive third-degree thermal burns. It is an opportunist par excellence in patients suffering from complicated, debilitating illness, in premature or malnourished infants, in individuals whose normal bacterial flora has been altered by prior antibiotic therapy, and in persons with neoplastic disease (especially leukemia) whose antibacterial defenses are compromised by deficiencies of circulating and/or cellular immunity or by defective circulating granulocytes. Invasion of the bloodstream by *P. aeruginosa*, unlike that due to *S. aureus*, is frequently followed by the development of widespread bacterial vasculitis. Growth of the organism in the walls of small and medium-sized arteries leads to thrombosis and septic infarction in many organs. Nodular, necrotic septic lesions occur, particularly in lung, kidney, heart, and brain. Unusual but characteristic bullous, hemorrhagic, and necrotic lesions of a similar pathogenesis may develop in the skin. Involvement of the lung results in pneumonia characterized by multiple nodular areas of consolidation which may rapidly undergo abscess formation. Dyspnea, pleuritic pain, and hemoptysis are prominent clinical manifestations. Involvement of the heart may lead to endocarditis, myocardial infarction secondary to coronary artery occlusion by the arteritis, or pericarditis, as a result of spread of infection to the pericardial sac by the bacteremic route or by contiguity from a septic myocardial infarct. The cellular or extracellular factors involved in the invasive propensity of *P. aeruginosa* in the compromised host have not been characterized. The role of the extracellular proteases produced by the organism in the pathogenesis of the arteritis is not clear.

Widespread dissemination of infection leading to involvement of multiple organs is not restricted exclusively to bacterial disease. Although viral infections often demonstrate rather remarkable tropism for specific organs (poliomyelitis for anterior horn cells, infectious hepatitis for the hepatocytes, influenza for respiratory epithelial cells), certain viruses may, under special circumstances, proliferate in many organs and produce tissue damage. Thus, *Herpes hominis* infection in the neonate may eventuate in viremia which is followed by invasion of multiple sites. Destruction of cells of the skin, brain, liver, lung, and adrenal glands may occur as a result and contribute to the usually lethal outcome. Overt, clinically evident pneumonia, encephalitis, and hepatitis may dominate the picture.

Widespread involvement of organs may also occur in protozoan disease such as malaria. In infection due to *Plasmodium vivax*, up to 2 per cent of erythrocytes may be parasitized; in disease produced by *P. malariae*, such involvement usually does not exceed 1 per cent. *P. falciparum* has the greatest invasive propensity of the three major species of malarial parasites and may parasitize as many as 10 per cent of the red blood cells of a patient. The consequences of such marked multiplication may be extensive and produce a variety of organ dysfunctions secondary to circulatory changes. Hemolysis produced by red cell rupture at the time of schizogony leads to the rapid development of severe anemia. Evidence suggests that the hemolysis in malaria is related to the loss of erythrocyte membrane function. This appears to be the consequence of the usurpation by the parasite of the metabolic machinery of the red cell needed for the maintenance of the membrane. Further, hemolysis may be related to splenic removal of parasitic inclusions from the erythrocytes ("pitting") as they pass between the walls of splenic sinusoids. The red cells that survive this procedure re-enter the circulation as spherocytes. Some of these spherocytes are damaged in the process and subsequently exhibit a shortened survival in the circulation. Capillary distention and blockage by parasitized red cells result in anoxia that may produce irreversible damage in brain, liver, and kidneys. Pulmonary edema may develop as a consequence of cerebral, pulmonary, and cardiovascular injury in patients with acute falciparum malaria.

COMBINATION OF TOXIN PRODUCTION AND INVASIVENESS AS BASIS OF PATHOGENICITY

The clinical manifestations of certain infections are due exclusively to the effects of potent exotoxins in the absence of bacterial invasion (tetanus, botulism). The primary features of other infectious processes, on the basis of current evidence, appear to be related almost exclusively to the local or disseminated proliferation of the invading microorganism itself. A third class of infectious diseases is one in which clinical manifestations appear to be related both to the activity of exotoxin and to the multiplication of and invasion by bacteria. Three different diseases produced by three distinct bacterial species serve as examples of this type of infection.

Scarlet fever is a syndrome characterized by a localized infection, usually of the pharynx but occurring anywhere in the body, accompanied by a toxic rash. The eruption is produced by an erythrogenic toxin elaborated by the organisms at their site of multiplication and absorbed into the bloodstream. This toxin is produced by the majority of strains of Group A and by occasional strains of Group C and G streptococci. Its production is related to the presence of a temperate bacteriophage in the streptococcus, a phenomenon very similar to that involving diphtheria toxin elaboration by lysogenic strains of *Corynebacterium diphtheriae*.

The signs and symptoms of scarlet fever consist of two groups: (1) The *local manifestations of infection* in the pharynx are the result of the inflammatory reaction and response of the lymphoid tissues to bacterial invasion. These account for the redness of the pharyngeal mucosa, the development of soft, yellow exudate that fills the crypts of the tonsils and may overflow onto the pharynx and over the uvula, the edema and enlargement of lymphoid tissues including those of the posterior pharynx. In an occasional patient with streptococcal tonsillitis, bacteremia may develop as a complication. Although an abundance of extracellular products are produced by Group A streptococci and although it is tempting to assign them a role in the invasiveness of the organism (e.g., streptolysin O and DPNase are leukotoxic; hyaluronidase may assist in breaking down tissue barriers; streptokinase is fibrinolytic and might account for lack of localization of many streptococcal infections), there is no clear evidence to establish such a role. (2) *The manifestations of scarlet fever due to the erythrogenic toxin* are a characteristic skin eruption and various peripheral signs. This agent acts primarily on the capillary bed to produce dilatation, congestion, and increased fragility.

The typical scarlatiniform eruption, a punctate rash superimposed on an erythematous base, the bleeding lines (Pastia's lines), the suggestive early "strawberry" and later "raspberry" tongue, the increased excretion of red blood cells in the urine, and the swelling of the hands and feet that may be present at the onset of the disease are all due to activity of erythrogenic toxin in the vascular bed. The generalized abdominal pain, nausea, and vomiting that may be early features have a similar pathogenesis. The diffuse erythema of the skin is related to the dilatation of the capillaries; the punctate erythematous lesions are manifestations of the same effect on the tufts of blood vessels in the dermal papillae, causing them to be raised and somewhat darker than the surrounding skin. Histologic study reveals dilatation of small blood vessels which are surrounded by an accumulation of neutrophilic exudate. When injected into the skin of normal nonimmune subjects, purified erythrogenic toxin produces a localized area of erythema (Dick test). The action of the toxin on the capillary tuft in the papillae may be sufficiently intense to cause increased fragility and the appearance of petechiae. The effect of the toxin on the integrity of the capillary vasculature is readily shown by the occurrence of "bleeding lines" and hematuria. Because of increased fragility, vessels in skin folds (e.g., inguinal, axillary, and antebrachial areas), which are subjected to considerable movement and minor trauma, rupture and produce linear extravasations of blood (Pastia's lines). The renal glomerular capillaries are also injured by the toxin and leak small numbers of red cells in the urine early in the disease and for as long as a week.

The changes in the tongue characteristic of scarlet fever are also due to the effects of the erythrogenic toxin on the capillary bed of this organ. The "strawberry" tongue, present at the onset of the disease, is not pathognomonic of scarlet fever. It represents the early effect of toxin on the capillaries in the lingual papillae, which become enlarged, reddened, and protrude through the white coat on the surface of the tongue, giving the appearance of an unripe strawberry. The "raspberry" tongue appears after 3 to 4 days and is much more characteristic of the disease. It is the result of continued activity of the toxin on the blood vessels, which are now diffusely dilated, accounting for the deep red color of the tongue after the coat has been shed. Because of the greater number of capillaries in the lingual papillae, these become large and deeper in color than the the surrounding tissue, standing out as strikingly elevated structures.

Within a week or so, desquamation of the skin and tongue begins. This represents shedding of superficial dermal and lingual layers of these organs that have borne the brunt of the activity of the erythrogenic toxin and have eventually been destroyed. This leads to separation of large patches of skin from the hands and feet, "brawny" desquamation on the trunk, and loss of lingual papillae (to such an extent that the surface of the tongue becomes quite smooth).

The diffuse abdominal pain, nausea, and vomiting that often characterize severe scarlet fever are probably the result of the effects of erythrogenic toxin on the capillary vasculature of the intestinal tract as well as on the lymphoid tissues in the intestinal wall and mesenteric nodes. The fact that lymph nodes may be affected by erythrogenic toxin in the absence of bacteremia is strongly suggested by the presence of generalized lymphadenopathy in most cases and splenomegaly in about 10 per cent of patients.

Jaundice, accompanied by evidence of dysfunction of the liver, may be a feature of severe scarlet fever and is probably due to a toxic hepatitis produced by the erythrogenic toxin.

When scarlet fever is severe, it is not uncommon for patients to complain of arthralgia and to exhibit a considerable degree of swelling of the hands and feet. Since these findings appear during the first one or two days of the disease, it is clear that they are not manifestations of rheumatic fever but are manifestations of the activity of erythrogenic toxin on blood vessels, resulting in the development of edema. An unusual feature of the early stage of scarlet fever is the presence of meningeal irritation, with stiff neck and back and positive Kernig and Brudzinski signs. Examination of the cerebrospinal fluid discloses a pleocytosis (up to 1000 cells per mm.^{3}, practically all of which are lymphocytes), a moderate increase in the concentration of protein, and a normal content of sugar. This is the "serous meningitis" of scarlet fever and has been considered to be due to the effect of the erythrogenic toxin or other extracellular products of *Streptococcus pyogenes.*

Toxic epidermal necrolysis (Lyell's disease or "scalded-skin" syndrome) is a dramatic and serious skin disease, usually occurring in infancy. It is characterized by tenderness of the skin and striking erythema, followed by desquamation in sheets over most of the body. This disorder has been associated with the presence on the epidermis of large numbers of *S. aureus* of phage group II. Some, but not all, such strains produce a protein ("exfoliatin") capable of causing exfoliation in neonatal mice; this is presumed to be the agent responsible for the scalded-skin syndrome in infants. This toxin is separate and distinct from the alpha and delta toxins of the organism. It has been proposed that the rare case of scarlatiniform eruption associated with some infections due to *S. aureus* is a somewhat different clinical manifestation of the same etiology. However, in this case the initiating staphylococcal infection is not necessarily in the skin itself.

Anthrax is a disease in which bacterial multiplication and dissemination and toxin production in vivo proceed pari passu. Recent evidence has suggested a predominant role for a toxin in the pathophysiologic changes that occur in the lethal form of the disease. Anthrax is an infection, primarily of animals, caused by *Bacillus anthracis*. It is occasionally transmitted to man by exposure to animal products (wool, bone, etc.). The commonest manifestation of the disease in man is a necrotic skin or mucous membrane ulcer ("malignant pustule") surrounded by a wide zone of gelatinous edema. Dissemination of infection from the original focus may occur via the bloodstream and may lead to the development of a hemorrhagic mediastinitis or hemorrhagic meningitis. Following inhalation of anthrax spores, a fulminant form of the disease may occur, characterized by a hemorrhagic mediastinitis and meningitis. When dissemination of the infection occurs, blood cultures are usually positive. The bacteremia is often high grade and it may be possible to identify the bacilli on stained smears of centrifuged sediment of blood. No quantitative data are available on the number of organisms per milliliter of blood in man. However, in the experimental animal, 10^8 to 10^9 organisms per ml. of blood may be found terminally. Although it was originally thought that death was due to widespread capillary blockage produced by the large number of bacilli in the circulation, this hypothesis is no longer accepted.

A toxin has recently been demonstrated in the edema fluid of the anthrax lesion and in the plasma of animals dying of anthrax. This substance appears to be made up of a complex of three serologically distinct components: an *edema-producing factor*, a *protective antigen*, and a *lethal factor*. The level of the toxin in the blood roughly parallels the degree of bacteremia. The most recent experimental evidence strongly suggests that the exotoxin contributes significantly to the pathophysiology of the infection. Purified anthrax toxin complex is lethal for several animal species. Its main effect is to increase vascular permeability; this may account for the gelatinous edema about the local lesion and the terminal pulmonary edema in fatal disease in experimental animals. The molecular mechanism of action of the toxic moiety is unknown. It is now generally believed that death from anthrax is due to the effects of this toxin.

REFERENCES

General Cytotoxins

Bornstein, D. L., Weinberg, A. N., Swartz, M. N., and Kunz, L. J.: Anaerobic Infections: Review of current experience. Medicine, *43*:207, 1964.

Bowman, C. G., and Bonventre, P. F.: Studies on the mode of action of diphtheria toxin III. Effect on subcellular components of protein synthesis from the tissues of intoxicated guinea pigs and rats. J. Exp. Med., *131*:659, 1970.

Collier, R. J.: Effect of diphtheria toxin on protein synthesis: Inactivation of one of the transfer factors. J. Molec. Biol., *25*:83, 1967.

Collier, R. J., and Pappenheimer, A. M.: Studies on the mode of action of diphtheria toxin II. Effect of toxin on amino acid incorporation in cell-free systems. J. Exp. Med., *120*:1019, 1964.

Davis, B. D., et al.: Anaerobic spore-forming bacilli. *In:* Microbiology. New York, Hoeber Medical Division of Harper and Row, 1967.

Gill, D. M., Pappenheimer, A. M., Brown, R., and Kurnick, J. T.: Studies on the mode of action of diphtheria toxin. J. Exp. Med., *129*:1, 1969.

Honjo, T., Nishizuka, Y., Kato, I., and Hayaishi, O.: Adenosine diphosphate ribosylation of aminoacyl transferase II and

inhibition of protein synthesis by diphtheria toxin. J. Biol. Chem., 246:4251, 1951.
Lehninger, A. L.: Ribosomes and protein synthesis. *In:* Biochemistry – The Molecular Basis of Cell Structure and Function. New York, Worth Publishers, Inc., 1970.
MacLennan, J. D.: The histotoxic clostridial infections of man. Bact. Rev., 26:177, 1962.
Pappenheimer, A. M., and Brown, R.: Studies on the mode of action of diphtheria toxin VI. Site of the action of toxin in living cells. J. Exp. Med., 127:1073, 1968.

NEUROTOXINS
Burgen, A. S. V., Dickens, F., and Zatman, L. J.: The action of botulinum toxin on the neuromuscular junction. J. Physiol., 109:10, 1948.
Eccles, J. C.: The Physiology of Synapses. Berlin, Springer-Verlag Publishers, 1964.
Koenig, M. G., Spickard, A., Cardella, M. A., and Rogers, D. E.: Clinical and Laboratory Observations of Type E Botulism in Man, Medicine, 43:517, 1964.
Prys-Roberts, C., Kerr, J. H., Corbett, J. L., Crampton Smith, A., and Spalding, J. M. K.: Treatment of sympathetic overactivity in tetanus. Lancet, 1:542, 1969.
Struppler, A., Struppler, E., and Adams, R. D.: Local tetanus in man. Arch. Neurol., 8:162, 1963.
Wright, G. P.: The Neurotoxins of *Clostridium botulinum* and *Clostridium tetani.* Pharmacol. Rev., 7:413, 1955.
Zacks, S. I., and Sheff, M. F.: Tetanism: Pathobiological aspects of the action of tetanal toxin in the nervous system and skeletal muscle. Neurosciences Res., 3:209, 1970.

ENTEROTOXINS
Field, M.: Intestinal secretion: Effect of cyclic AMP and its role in cholera. New Eng. J. Med., 284:1137, 1971.
Gordon, R. S.: Moderator-Combined Clinical Staff Conference at the National Institutes of Health. Ann. Intern. Med., 64:1328, 1966.
Keusch, G. T., Grady, G. F., Mata, L. J., and McIver, J.: The pathogenesis of Shigella diarrhea I. Enterotoxin production by *Shigella dysenteriae* I. J. Clin. Invest., 51:1212, 1972.
Kimberg, D. V., Field, M., Johnson, J., Henderson, A., and Gershon, E.: Stimulation of intestinal mucosal adenyl cyclase by cholera enterotoxin and prostaglandins. J. Clin. Invest., 50:1218, 1971.
Pierce, N. F., Greenough, W. B., III, and Carpenter, C. C. J.: *Vibrio cholerae* enterotoxin and its mode of action. Bact. Rev., 35:1, 1971.

ENDOTOXINS
Cluff, L. E.: Effects of Endotoxins on Susceptibility to Infections. J. Infect. Dis., 122:205, 1970.
Greisman, S. E., Hornick, R. B., Carozza, F. A., and Woodward, T. E.: The role of endotoxin during typhoid fever and tularemia in man. I. Acquisition of tolerance to endotoxin. II. Altered cardiovascular responses to catecholamines. III. Hyperreactivity to endotoxin during infection. J. Clin. Invest., 42:1064, 1963, and 43:986, 1774, 1964.
Landy, M., and Braun, W., (Eds.): Bacterial Endotoxins. New Brunswick, Institute of Microbiology, Rutgers University, 1964.
Nowatny, A. (Ed.): Symposium on Molecular Biology of Gram-Negative Bacterial Lipopolysaccharides. Ann. N.Y. Acad. Sci., 133:277, 1966.
Thomas, L.: The physiologic disturbances produced by endotoxins. Ann. Rev. Physiol., 16:467, 1954.
Zweifach, B. W., and Janoff, A.: Bacterial endotoxemia. Ann. Rev. Med., 16:201, 1965.

INVASIVE INFECTIONS
Brooks, M. H., Malloy, J. P., Bartelloni, P. J., Tigertt, W. D., Sheehy, T. W., and Barry, K. G.: Pathophysiology of acute falciparum malaria. I. Correlation of clinical and biochemical abnormalities. Amer. J. Med., 43:735, 1967.
Conrad, M. E.: Pathophysiology of malaria. Ann. Intern. Med., 70:134, 1969.
Lincoln, R. E., and Fish, D. C.: Anthrax toxin. *In* Montie, T. C., Kadis, S., and Ajl, S. J. (Eds.): Microbial Toxins. Vol. III. New York, Academic Press, 1970.
Melish, M. E., Glasgow, L. A., and Turner, M. D.: The staphylococcal scalded-skin syndrome: Isolation and partial purification of the new exfoliative toxin. J. Infect. Dis., 125:129, 1972.
Neva, F. A., Sheagren, J. N., Shulman, N. R., and Canfield, C. J.: Malaria: Host defense mechanisms and complications. Combined Clinical Staff Conference of the National Institutes of Health. Ann. Intern. Med., 73:295, 1970.
Nungester, W. J.: Proceedings of the Conference on Progress in the Understanding of Anthrax. Fed. Proc., 26:1491, 1967.
Rabin, E. R., Graver, C. D., Vogel, E. H., Finkelstein, R. A., and Tumbusch, W. A.: Fatal Pseudomonas infection in burned patients: A clinical, bacteriologic, and anatomic study. New Eng. J. Med., 265:1225, 1961.
Rogers, D. E.: The current problem of staphylococcal infections. Ann. Intern. Med., 45:748, 1956.
Wood, W. B., Jr.: Studies on the cellular immunology of acute bacterial infections. The Harvey Lectures, Series *XLVII*:72, 1951–52.

CHAPTER 20   HOST RESPONSES TO INFECTION

LOUIS WEINSTEIN
MORTON N. SWARTZ

INTRODUCTION

The host response to an invading microorganism may be varied in nature, in extent, and in pathophysiologic consequences.

1. *In some circumstances the response may be minimal.* The majority of individuals exposed to *Mycobacterium tuberculosis* do not develop symptomatic pulmonary involvement or manifestations of disseminated infection. The host response is sufficient to contain the infectious process without progression to overt clinical disease. The only evidence that infection has taken place is the development of delayed hypersensitivity to antigens of *M. tuberculosis* (O.T. or P.P.D.) as indicated by positive skin tests. A similar situation prevails in certain areas of the western United States where a fungus, *Coccidioides immitis,* is present in the soil; the majority of the population in such areas are infected with the organism (positive skin reactions) but do not develop an identifiable illness.

2. *In other circumstances the response of the host may be significant but the major impact of the infection is the result of the invasive properties and/or toxigenicity of the organism.* Examples of such infections (anthrax, cholera, streptococcal and staphylococcal sepsis) have been discussed in Chapter 19.

3. *In another group of infectious processes, the host response may be so exaggerated and troublesome, or so specific in nature, that it alone induces pathophysiologic consequences of considerable magnitude.* These responses may then account for various disorders that dominate the clinical picture. The invasive or toxin-producing phase of the infection may never develop, or if it does, it is concluded by the time symptoms become manifest. The signs and symptoms due to the host response become paramount or, in effect, constitute the entire clinical illness itself. It is this third category of infection that is the focus for discussion in this chapter. A variety of general responses may be elicited by most infections. Some, such as fever, are so common as to be considered a hallmark of this kind of disease. Others, such as disseminated intravascular clotting, are relatively uncommon but are being recognized more and more frequently as the laboratory criteria for their diagnosis have been clarified.

GENERAL HOST RESPONSES

Fever

Fever is an almost universal response of warm-blooded animals to infection. The normal oral body temperature is 98.6° F. (37° C.). However, this represents a mean value derived from studies of large numbers of normal people, and the "normal" for occasional individuals may deviate from this value by as much as 0.5 to 1.0° F. During the course of the day body temperature varies over a range of 0.5 to 2.0° F., the low point occurring in the early morning hours during sleep and the peak being reached late in the afternoon. In addition to disease, a variety of physiologic and environmental factors may transiently elevate the temperature by temporarily overwhelming the mechanism available for heat loss. For example, in very warm weather the temperature may rise 0.5° to 1.0° F. Similarly, after vigorous exercise or a hot shower even greater increases may occur. Commencing at the time of ovulation and persisting during the second half of the menstrual cycle, a more prolonged physiologic rise in morning temperature (0.50 to 0.75° F.) occurs and continues until the onset of menstruation. Such elevations are minor and, in most instances, only transitory. The term fever is commonly reserved for more sustained elevations of greater magnitude occurring in the course of disease.

The role of fever as a potential defense mechanism is obscure. There is as yet no clear evidence that a rise in body temperature confers a selective advantage to the host over the invading microorganism. However, this may be the case in a few infections. The optimal temperature for the retention of the infectivity of *Treponema pallidum* in vitro is 34° to 35° C. Higher temperatures are progressively more unfavorable for the spirochete. It is not unreasonable to suggest that this sensitivity to temperature is involved in the predilection of this organism for the skin. In addition, the occasional favorable response of certain forms of syphilis subjected to fever therapy in the pre-antibiotic era may be accounted for on this basis. Although fever is usually associated with infection, this is by no means an exclusive relationship. Thus, it may be a manifestation of neoplastic disease (e.g., lymphoma), noninfectious inflammatory disorders (e.g., vasculitis, rheumatoid arthritis, ulcerative colitis, regional enteritis), or excess catabolism in certain metabolic states (e.g., pheochromocytoma, thyrotoxicosis). On the other hand, severe infection may exist without eliciting hyperpyrexia. Hypothermia (accompanying hypotension) may be present in the course of overwhelming infections. The presence of certain metabolic abnormalities (myxedema, uremia) may completely quench the usual febrile response to infection.

Normal Thermoregulation. Normal body temperature is the result of a delicately maintained balance between heat production and heat loss. In the resting state, the major sites of heat production, under normal circumstances, are the liver and skeletal muscles; during exercise or in disease-associated febrile states the latter is the major site. Loss of heat takes place at the surface of the body (skin and lungs) through radiation, convection, and vaporization. The primary mechanisms by which control of temperature is maintained involve the nervous system. Generation of heat is produced through the somatic motor efferents (shivering); conservation or loss of heat is achieved through the control, by the autonomic nervous system, of cutaneous blood supply (loss of heat) and sudomotor activity (sweating). The central guidance for these efferent connections is the thermoregulatory center in the anterior hypothalamus. It responds to stimuli from two sources: (a) the superficial thermoreceptors of the skin that respond to changes in surface temperature and (b) the deep thermoreceptors located in or near the hypothalamus that respond to slight changes in the temperature of the blood perfusing this part of the central nervous system. The thermoregulatory center in the hypothalamus operates as a thermostat, with a "set point" at 98.6° F., and responds to superficial and deep stimuli from external heat load (e.g., high environmental temperature) by initiating loss of heat via sweating and vasodilatation.

Thermoregulation in Febrile Disease States. An endogenous febrile reaction consists of four phases which are fairly sharply defined and which follow in regular sequence; these are (1) prodrome, (2) chill, (3) flush, and (4) defervescence. During the prodrome, there are only nonspecific complaints such as fleeting aches and pains, mild headache, nausea, and malaise; the circulation through the skin is normal. The initial discernible event in the chill phase is cutaneous vasoconstriction—the patient complains of being cold, and often covers up with more bedclothes. He becomes increasingly pale and the extremities appear somewhat cyanotic. The skin is cool and dry, except perhaps for a little perspiration of the forehead or upper lip. This phase lasts approximately 1½ hours. These changes suggest that during the early phases of a febrile illness the hypothalamic thermostat responds as though its "set point" had been raised to a new higher maintenance level. If the decrease in surface temperature due to reduced blood flow is of sufficient magnitude, the superficial cutaneous thermoreceptors are triggered. Feedback from the latter to the hypothalamus reflexively produces increased muscular activity in the form of shivering or, when this is maximal, a shaking chill. Production of heat is markedly increased by this muscular activity. During the chill phase the low skin temperature makes the patient feel cold even though the rectal temperature is rising. In fact, since the most severe chills are associated with the most marked rises in rectal temperature, patients feel coldest when they are storing the most heat. The patient continues to feel cold; a disproportion between internal and cutaneous temperatures may be responsible in part for the sensation of cold. The clinical and physiologic manifestations of chills may be precipitated or aggravated by exposure to cold when the subject is in the chill phase of a febrile reaction.

The effectiveness of shivering as a means of increasing heat production for the maintenance of the body heat balance can be gauged in a quantitative way. Thus, in an experiment in a calorimeter at 23° C. reported by Hardy, production of heat prior to a chill was 63 kcal. over an hour, and heat loss was 87 kcal. In the next half hour, during a chill, the rate of heat production was 164 kcal. per hour and heat loss was 116 kcal. per hour. Shivering is a more efficient means of increasing body temperature than exercise because loss of heat can be minimized by reducing the body surface area (site of convection loss) by curling up and by maintaining some degree of insulation by simultaneous vasoconstriction.

As the temperature of the skin rises with prolonged shivering, a sensation of warmth develops, and the shivering ceases. Cutaneous vasodilatation proceeds rapidly and the flush phase begins. The increased flow of blood in the skin causes an increase in the rate of heat loss, balancing the abnormally high level of heat production. As a result, body temperature remains poised at the newly established higher level. When the skin temperature reaches about 34° C., sweating occurs and marks the defervescent phase of the febrile response. Stimulation of the sweat glands is produced by efferent impulses from the hypothalamus, stimulated itself both by afferent impulses from the skin and by the elevated temperature of the blood flowing through the brain.

As already suggested, deviations of body temperature from the "set point" initiate mechanisms that tend to restore body temperature to the programed level. Fever appears to represent, in essence, a rise in the "set point." In keeping with this is the observation of Cooper and coworkers that in man, when body temperature is elevated but stable, the skin vasomotor responses to a heat load are normal. In a normal subject infused with endogenous pyrogen (see below), prepared by pre-incubation of the subject's blood with bacterial endotoxin, an abrupt rise in temperature ensues and reaches its peak in about an hour. This is associated with marked cutaneous vasoconstriction, myalgias, and chills. Following this, there is a stable period (several hours) in which the peak temperature level is maintained. An additional heat load (generated by immersion of an arm in warm water) during the phase of rising temperature causes no cutaneous vasodilatation measured in the other hand. In contrast, immersion during the stable phase at the peak temperature produces a transient rise in oral temperature with increased elimination of heat in the other hand. The elevation of temperature required to induce vasodilatation is very small (0.10 to 0.15° C.) in contrast to the increase (1.70° C.) induced by the administration of pyrogen. These observations are compatible with the view that fever represents an alteration in the level at which the thermostat is set, and that, at this new setting, thermostatic control is as well exercised as at the former lower setting.

A variety of pathophysiologic changes involving the cardiorespiratory system accompany the febrile state. Changes in respiration may be prominent. In the chill phase, respiratory rate and minute volume increase and the tidal volume decreases. There may be a small decrease in arterial Po_2 due to rapid shallow breathing, but respiratory alkalosis is the more common finding. The increased respiratory activity during fever serves to eliminate some of the heat. The stimulus for this is thought to be the increased temperature of the blood supplying the respiratory center; accumulation of carbon dioxide in the respiratory center as a result of decreased cerebral blood flow during the chill phase may also play a role.

Cardiac output differs in the different phases of the febrile state. With severe chills a considerable decrease in cardiac output may occur, resulting in hypotension. During the flush phase, the cardiac output is increased in excess of the rise in oxygen consumption. During defervescence, cardiac output and oxygen consumption return toward normal. During the febrile period, the pulse rate in man roughly parallels the temperature; a rise of 9 beats per minute occurs for each degree Fahrenheit increase in rectal temperature. However, the pulse rate is a poor indicator of changes in cardiac output during fever, since it often increases disproportionately and may rise when the cardiac output falls.

Mediators of Fever. The well-known clinical association of fever with inflammatory processes led to an early examination of purulent exudates for materials capable of evoking a febrile response in experimental animals. The results of such studies were obscured by the probable presence, in the soluble fractions of the exudates, of endotoxin, a pyrogenic lipopolysaccharide from the cell envelopes of contaminating gram-negative bacilli. In 1948, Beeson, employing procedures to exclude endotoxins, was able to extract from granulocytes a fever-producing material that he termed *endogenous pyrogen* (E.P.). Since then this substance has been the subject of considerable interest and study by many investigators. Most of the current knowledge concerning E.P. has been derived from investigations of experimental fever in animal models. When rabbits are given injections of endotoxin (typhoid vaccine) intravenously, fever develops and lasts for 5 to 8 hours. Serum obtained at intervals during the febrile period elicits a febrile response when injected into normal animals. Except for the serum obtained early in the experiment, the development of fever in the recipient animal is not due to carry-over of endotoxin, since elevation of temperature is produced in endotoxin-refractory (tolerant) animals as well. Thus, the febrile response is induced by another pyrogenic material which appears to have properties indistinguishable from the pyrogen obtained from granulocytes.

The granulocyte pyrogen (E.P.) is released from exudate neutrophils incubated in isotonic saline. This in-vitro system has been the major source for isolation and purification of the pyrogen. Leukocytes from circulating blood rather than exudates are less capable of releasing E.P. when incubated with 0.15 M NaCl. However, leukocytes from blood are better producers of E.P. than those from exudates, when exposed to endotoxin in vitro. Little if any active E.P. is present in exudate or blood granulocytes. Incubation of the former with saline or of the latter with endotoxin causes apparent conversion of an inactive precursor molecule to an active pyrogen during its release from the cell. Purification of pyrogen from rabbit exudate has reached the stage at which injection of as little as 30 to 50 nanograms produces fever in a rabbit. It has been characterized as a heat-labile (56° C.) protein with a molecular weight of 10,000 to 20,000 (small amounts of carbohydrate or lipid may be present also).

Sources of Endogenous Pyrogen. The prominent role of granulocytes in the production of E.P. is suggested by the association of an initial leukopenia (mainly granulocytic) with the experimental fever induced by endotoxin. Animals in which leukopenia has been induced by nitrogen mustard respond to endotoxin with less fever and less circulating E.P. than normal ones.

The stimulus for the release of E.P. from circulating granulocytes in vivo or in vitro is not restricted to endotoxin. Intravenous injection of various bacteria or viruses in normal or specifically sensitized rabbits has been followed by fever and the appearance of demonstrable E.P. in the circulation. Release of E.P. from suspensions of rabbit granulocytes occurs when they have been incubated in vitro with bacteria, viruses, tuberculin, or antigen-antibody complexes. Successful phagocytosis appears to be an important feature of the bacteria-induced E.P. release.

Granulocytes are not the only cells capable of releasing E.P. That there are other sources of endogenous pyrogen has been suggested by the common occurrence of fever in patients with marked and prolonged agranulocytosis. Monocytes and macrophages have recently been shown to be sources of E.P. Alveolar macrophages obtained from the lungs of rabbits sensitized to tuberculin by intravenous injection of BCG release abundant E.P. when incubated with tuberculin in vitro. This finding may provide an explanation for the fever occurring in diseases like tuberculosis in which mononuclear cells are histologically the major element. Kupffer's cells of the liver, but not hepatocytes, produce E.P. in vitro when activated by endotoxin, bacterial phagocytosis, or tuberculin. The common functional characteristic of all cell types capable of E.P. production is their ability to carry out phagocytosis. Lymphocytes from human blood in contrast to monocytes and macrophages, do not release pyrogen in vitro when subjected to a variety of stimuli. Nonetheless, lymphocytes may have a somewhat indirect role as activators of the febrile state in diseases in which delayed hypersensitivity is a prominent feature. Lymphocytes of rabbits sensitized to a foreign protein, when exposed to that specific antigen in vitro release a nonpyrogenic substance that stimulates blood leukocytes to release E.P.

Site of Action of Endogenous Pyrogen. The introduction of endotoxin or any of many other activators of E.P. in a susceptible animal or man appears to set off the following sequence of events in which E.P. is the final common pathway (see formula below). The central site of action of E.P. has been demonstrated in rabbits. When this substance is infused slowly into the carotid artery to perfuse the brain directly, a more rapid and greater febrile response is generated than when it is given intravenously. In contrast, the degree of fever produced by endotoxin is the same when given by either route. These observations are consistent with the concept that E.P. acts directly on the hypothalamus, and that endotoxin activates circulating leukocytes to release E.P. Direct perfusion of the anterior hypothalamus of rabbits with extremely small amounts of E.P. via microcannulas causes an immediate rise in body temperature.

Mechanism of Fever Production During Overt Infections. Crucial to the definition of the role of E.P. in fever production is the demonstration of its presence in some common infectious processes. In experimental pneumococcal peritonitis produced in rabbits, the substance is present in the peritoneal cavity in the early stages of infection; it is detectable in thoracic-duct lymph and in blood later in the course of the fever. When the infection is controlled by therapy with penicillin, fever subsides and E.P. can no longer be demonstrated.

The possible role of continuing endotoxemia from *Salmonella typhosa* in typhoid fever has been studied by Greisman et al. in human volunteers. Endotoxin tolerance, induced immediately before or during experimental typhoid fever, did not inhibit the febrile course or toxemia characteristic of the disease. This appeared to eliminate continuing circulating of endotoxin as responsible for the sustained fever in this infection. Thus, it seems likely that in this disease persistence of

---

Endotoxin (or similar activator) ⟶ Cell Injury (granulocytes, monocytes, macrophages) ⟶ Endogenous Pyrogen Activation and Release ⟶ Stimulation of Hypothalamic Thermoregulatory Centers ⟶ Fever

fever is due to the production of E.P. by phagocytes in areas of inflammation.

Headache

Headache is a common symptom of systemic infection and is usually associated with fever. We are concerned here only with elevations of temperature unrelated to specific infections of the central nervous system such as meningitis or brain abscess. The febrile headache is usually throbbing in character at the onset of the febrile reaction and then becomes a deep dull ache of varying severity. It is usually generalized but may be predominantly in the frontotemporal, occipital, or suboccipital areas. It is aggravated by bodily movement. Several mechanisms may be active in the pathogenesis of headache occurring in the course of fever related to infection. First, there may be microscopic evidence of central nervous system inflammation without obvious meningeal signs. Thus, an occasional patient with mumps and a more severe than usual headache will have a small (but abnormal) number of lymphocytes in the cerebrospinal fluid. In most other infections in which febrile headaches occur, however, there is no evidence of active infection of the central nervous system or its linings. Such headaches may be a particularly prominent feature of influenza, typhoid fever, typhus and other rickettsial diseases, mycoplasma pneumonia, and infectious mononucleosis. It usually parallels the fever but may precede or outlast it.

The pain-sensitive structures in the central nervous system are the dural sinuses and their principal branches, the arteries in the dura and the areas immediately surrounding them, and the large intracranial arteries. It seems reasonable to suggest that disturbance of one or more of these structures during infection is responsible for febrile headaches.

Present evidence strongly suggests that pyrexial headaches result from stretching of sensitive structures about the intracranial arteries due to dilatation of these vessels. Sutherland and Wolff have reported that after intravenous administration of typhoid vaccine an increased amplitude of pulsations of the cerebrospinal fluid preceded the onset of headache, the severity of which closely paralleled the magnitude of the oscillations which occurred synchronously with the pulse. In addition, a direct relation was noted between the intensity of the headache and the amplitude of pulsations in the temporal artery. Direct visualization of pial vessels through skull windows in experimental animals has shown that intravenous administration of typhoid vaccine is followed by cerebral vasodilatation. The immediate factor(s) directly responsible for the cerebral vasodilatation is unknown at present. It is of interest that the headache following injection of histamine is similar in character, and that dilatation of intracranial arteries is the basis of the pain.

It appears reasonable to consider the following sequence of events in the development of the headache produced by infections in which direct invasion of the central nervous system is not a feature: Phagocytosis of the infecting agent ⟶ Activation of granulocyte or mononuclear pyrogen (E.P.) ⟶ Action of E.P. on the thermoregulatory center, generating a febrile response ⟶ Cerebral vasodilatation mediated in some way directly by E.P. or through alterations secondary to the E.P.-induced fever.

Hypotension and Shock

Shock associated with bacteremia is the major cause of mortality in infections otherwise amenable to antibiotic therapy. Although gram-negative bacteria are the most frequent offending organisms, the syndrome may develop in the course of disease produced by viruses, fungi, and rickettsiae. Shock in bacteremia is not due simply to endotoxin. The pathophysiology of septic shock is still poorly understood. It was formerly believed that the fundamental problem was a low pressure state due to loss or paralysis of vasomotor tone. Thus, treatment in the past was directed at restoration of circulating blood volume and correction of defective vasomotor tone by administration of vasopressor agents. The more recent concept of the mechanism of septic shock is that it is due to redistribution of blood within the vascular bed in a manner precluding maintenance of an adequate circulating blood volume. Tissue ischemia and anoxia are a consequence of this pooling and lead to decreased renal function, myocardial failure, lactic acidemia, and ultimately to cell death.

Two types of septic shock have been defined on the basis of hemodynamic considerations:

(1) *Shock With High (or Normal) Cardiac Output:* Cardiac output is normal or increased, the circulation time is slow, and total peripheral vascular resistance is reduced. It has been suggested that this form of shock is associated with the opening of multiple arteriovenous shunts in the pulmonary and splanchnic areas. This is the syndrome that has been labeled "warm shock"; it occurs commonly in association with sepsis. Unfortunately, one cannot reliably predict the true hemodynamic state based on the presence of a warm flushed appearance. An intense degree of peripheral vasoconstriction and reduced tissue perfusion due to increased sympathetic activity may be present early during hyperdynamic or high output shock or may occur later.

(2) *Shock With Reduced Cardiac Output:* Cardiac output is usually markedly reduced, circulation time is markedly prolonged, and the total peripheral vascular resistance is normal or increased. Patients are pale, with cold, clammy

extremities and peripheral cyanosis due to vasoconstriction.

Initially, most patients with bacteremia who develop hypotension appear to be warm and dry, with an increased cardiac output and decreased peripheral resistance. Adrenergic effects are not prominent at this stage. There is an increased circulatory demand which cannot be met. As a result, hypoxia, oliguria, and alterations in the sensorium occur. As septic shock progresses, cardiac output is reduced and an adrenergic response may dominate the picture. Decline in renal perfusion results in reduction of urine output. Peripheral blood flow is markedly diminished. The extremities are cold and clammy. As tissue hypoxia increases, serum lactic acid levels rise, and blood pH and bicarbonate fall. If the shock is of severe degree and persists for a protracted period, the picture of "shock lung" develops. Patients in whom prolonged septic shock has been reversed may nevertheless die from acute respiratory insufficiency as a result of this type of pulmonary difficulty. Persistence of shock leads to intense vasoconstriction of both the arterial and venous sides of the microcirculation. Eventually the precapillary arterial vasoconstriction diminishes without a concomitant decrease on the venous side. A consequence of this is a high degree of congestion in the pulmonary capillary bed. Hypoxia and lactic acidosis intensify. Congestion and edema, hemorrhage, and capillary thrombi are the characteristic changes in the lung.

Other Circulatory Changes

The elevation of body temperature accompanying infection is usually associated with a proportional increase in heart rate. Relative bradycardia is seen during infections due to gram-negative bacilli (e.g., typhoid fever, tularemia). Endotoxin has been suggested as the element inducing this peculiar response. The definition of the actual microbial component inducing the response seems more complex than this, however, since relative bradycardia is also observed in viral diseases (dengue, yellow fever), mycoplasma infections (primary atypical pneumonia), and during illness due to Bedsoniae (psittacosis). Bradycardia (accompanied by hypertension) may be present in infections of the central nervous system (meningitis, subdural empyema, brain abscess, and encephalitis) as a consequence of increased intracranial pressure.

Reversible Alterations of Sensorium—Confusion, Delirium, Stupor, and Coma

Alterations of sensorium occur in many infectious diseases in the absence of cerebral invasion by the attacking microorganism or of histologic evidence of inflammatory brain disease. Stupor and coma are usually more evident and more severe in systemic infections in which high fever and hypotension are prominent features. However, such changes may occur in the absence of hypotension or extreme hyperthermia. They are usually reversible and disappear when the infection is brought under control. The usual sequence involves a progressive change from a state of drowsiness and confusion to stupor and finally coma. The pathophysiologic alterations producing these changes are not well understood.

In the presence of severe hypotension (systolic level below 70 to 75 mm. Hg), the cerebral metabolic rate is reduced as a result of decreased blood flow to the brain. This may account for the stupor or coma often seen in septic shock. Extremes of hyperthermia (106° F. or higher) or hypothermia (below 97° F.) may develop during bacteremia or septic shock and are thought to induce coma by altering neuronal metabolism nonspecifically. Hyperthermia due to any cause may initiate a convulsion (febrile seizure) in infants and young children presumably through temporary alterations in cerebral cortical function. Alterations in sensorium that occur in some bacterial infections are thought to be due to "toxins" elaborated by the organisms. However, such toxins have not been identified or isolated and their role remains hypothetical. Cerebral metabolic rate is reduced while blood flow remains normal in the course of coma associated with some systemic infections.

A severe and extreme example of alteration of cerebral function during the course of infection is *acute toxic encephalopathy*. This syndrome occurs during or following bacterial or viral disease. It is characterized by fever, confusion, stupor, and coma. Generalized convulsive seizures are prominent and, unlike simple febrile convulsions, are recurrent. Focal disease of the cerebrum or brain stem is absent. Although bacterial "toxins" have been proposed as the cause of the cerebral changes, no clear-cut substantiating evidence is available. There does not appear to be a close correlation between the severity of the initiating infection and the degree of neurologic dysfunction. Contributing factors initiating the process may be fever, hypoxia, and cerebral edema secondary to water intoxication.

Skin Reactions in Disseminated Infection

Skin eruptions of differing morphology are frequently associated with systemic bacterial or viral infections. The cutaneous changes may be produced in several different ways: (1) Bacteremic or viremic spread to the skin, with local proliferation of the organism (subcutaneous abscesses in *S. aureus* bacteremia, cutaneous vesicles in disseminated *Herpes simplex* infection of infants). (2) Development of a cutaneous vasculitis. The etiologic agent (bacteria or virus) may or may not be found in the vessel wall or surrounding dermis. (3) The damaging effect of antigen-antibody complexes on the skin, or possibly by the development of delayed hypersensitivity to the infecting agent. Staphylococcal infections are an example of bacteremic skin lesions due to direct invasion of the skin. Frank, fluctuant subcutaneous abscesses, nodular subcutaneous lesions, pustules, and purulent purpura (a small area of hemorrhage with a white purulent center) may be present. *S. aureus* can be demonstrated without any difficulty in any of these lesions. Vasculitis involving small blood vessels of the skin may occur in the absence of demonstrable localization of bacteria. The macular, papular, nodular, and petechial lesions of chronic meningococcemia are examples of this phenomenon. The painful, nodular pretibial lesions of erythema nodosum exhibit a prominent element of vasculitis, but the instigating organism in certain cases is located at a distance from the subcutaneous lesions (e.g., streptococcal pharyngitis). Vasculitis of the skin may also be associated with direct invasion of the vessel wall by bacteria. A characteristic example of this is the widespread involvement of blood vessels that occurs in the course of Pseudomonas bacteremia. Bullous, hemorrhagic, and necrotic skin lesions develop as a result of intramural bacterial proliferation which leads to occlusion of vessels by fibrin thrombi.

Immunologic factors may play a role in the production of the skin lesions in certain systemic infections, particularly in the case of some viral exanthems. Measles is a good example of this. The pathogenesis of the rash in this disease is not clearly established. It could be produced by direct viral invasion of the epidermal and vascular endothelial cells or the result of damage induced locally by a virus-antibody complex. There is some evidence in support of the latter concept. The time of appearance of the rash coincides with the appearance of circulating antibody. Another intriguing bit of evidence is the absence of rash in some children, usually those with leukemia, who develop chronic measles with giant cell pneumonia but do not produce specific antibody. The use of inactivated measles virus vaccine has suggested an altered cutaneous reactivity in the host. Individuals previously immunized with this agent develop an atypical measles syndrome characterized by unusual skin lesions (petechiae, purpura, urticaria, or vesicles superimposed on a maculopapular rash) following exposure several years later to the natural disease. Local reactions, consisting of erythema and vesicle formation, have developed at the site of live measles vaccine injection in patients who had previously received inactivated measles vaccine. Little is known of the exact basis of these reactions. It is of interest in this regard, however, that a high incidence of delayed hypersensitivity to antigens in inactivated measles vaccine has been demonstrated in recipients of the killed vaccine.

Hematologic Changes

A variety of alterations of blood elements occur during the course of human infectious diseases. They are common; the magnitude of the changes is usually minor and contributes little to the overall symptomatology or clinical findings. On occasion, however, they may be so profound as to completely dominate the clinical picture or to influence significantly the host response to the infection. The roles of the neutrophil in phagocytosis and bacterial killing as well as in producing leukocytic pyrogen establish its importance in the initial host response to infection.

Changes in Circulating Neutrophils. Most infections due to pyogenic bacteria are accompanied by a polymorphonuclear leukocytosis. A relation between this response and the inflammatory reaction at the site of the infectious process has been inferred from the known phagocytic function of these cells and their presence in abundance in the early stages of inflammation. The best insights into the dynamics of the neutrophil response to infection have evolved from studies of neutrophil kinetics employing radioactive isotopic techniques.

Polymorphonuclear leukocytes are produced continuously in the bone marrow through the differentiation of precursor myeloid cells. Upon maturation, the granulocytes enter the marrow storage pool, one of several "pools" in the body. From the *marrow pool* they are discharged into the circulation, where they enter either the *circulating granulocyte pool* (CGP) or the *marginal granulocyte pool* (MGP). The former is made up of actively circulating cells, whereas the latter consists of granulocytes which are sequestered or "marginated" in various capillary beds. Prompt increases in numbers of circulating granulocytes that result from exercise or injection of catecholamines involve movement of the marginated leukocytes into the circulating pool. The size of the CGP depends on three concurrent processes: (1) rate of release from marrow, (2) proportion of granulocytes held in MGP, and (3) rate of loss of granulocytes into tissues.

It has been difficult to study leukokinetics in acute infections of man because patients are not seen until disease is well established and treatment initiated. However, acute infections have been studied in experimental animals (pneumococcal pneumonia in the dog) and have provided valuable insights into the kinetics of the response. The sequence of events that takes place is as follows: (1) Infection produces an increased demand for migration of granulocytes from the CGP. (2) Egress from the blood is via diapedesis from the MGP; an increase in the size of this pool is required for this. However, migration from the MGP to the tissues is a one-way street; there is no evidence that the granulocytes re-enter the circulation from infected areas. (3) The marrow responds to the foregoing with acceleration of the rate of release of cells from the marrow storage pool. This might involve a feedback loop mediated by a serum factor. Also contributing to the marrow response is a subsequent wave of differentiation down the myeloid pathway to the granulocyte level. (4) Enlargement of the CGP occurs only after the acceleration of release from the marrow storage pool has exceeded the enhanced rate of movement from the blood into the tissues. Within 4 hours of inoculation of pneumococci, an accelerated rate of release of neutrophils from bone marrow to blood, as indicated by an increase in the ratio of band forms to segmented forms, can be observed. This can sometimes be detected before there is an increase in the numbers of circulating neutrophils in venous blood. This lag period before the rise in neutrophil count appears to be the result of restoration of the MGP before the CGP.

An occasional patient with severe pneumococcal pneumonia will develop severe neutropenia. When this same response occurs in the experimental animal, it is associated with an acceleration of marrow neutrophil release and a marked increase in the ratio of band to segmented forms. Neutropenia in this situation stems from inability of the marrow to replenish the accelerated cell loss to the sites of tissue inflammation. Data from kinetic studies with labeled cells as well as examination of marrow (loss of mature neutrophils) suggest exhaustion of the marrow granulocyte pool. There is no evidence that infection blocks release of neutrophils from the marrow. The well-known poor prognosis of such severe pneumococcal (and other bacterial) infections is more readily understandable if the mechanism of the neutropenia is depletion of the marrow granulocyte reserve.

In certain bacterial infections, particularly typhoid fever, leukopenia is a common finding. The basis for this phenomenon is not known. However, it is of interest that a similar blood picture features the initial response in rabbits and man to the injection of gram-negative bacilli or of bacterial endotoxin. This occurs at the time of the chill and is followed by leukocytosis in 1/2 to 4 hours. The initial leukopenia is due to enlargement of the MGP before that of the CGP. The subsequent leukocytosis is secondary to release of cells from both the MGP and the marrow storage pool.

Anemia of Infection. Anemia is a common feature of chronic infections but may occasionally complicate acute ones. In the latter case, the anemia is usually hemolytic. High-grade bacteremia with *Clostridium perfringens* may produce massive intravascular destruction of erythrocytes, with shock and anuria. The production by this organism of a lecithinase (α toxin) which acts on the membranes of red cells and causes their lysis is the basis for the hemolytic anemia of clostridial bacteremia (see Chapter 19). Primary atypical pneumonia due to *Mycoplasma pneumoniae* is, on rare occasions, complicated by severe hemolysis presumably related to the development of autoantibodies, the cold agglutinins. In patients with congenital deficiency of the erythrocyte enzyme glucose-6-phosphate dehydrogenase (G6PD), episodes of hemolysis may be precipitated by a variety of infections. Bacterial infections (pneumonia) and viral infections (infectious hepatitis) have been associated with hemolytic episodes. Accumulation of metabolites capable of oxidizing glutathione, and thus decreasing the concentration of the reduced form of this compound, has been suggested as the basis for the hemolysis. However, direct exposure of G6PD-deficient erythrocytes to influenza virus produces increased hemolysis; this suggests a direct effect on the red cell rather than an indirect one due to toxic metabolites produced in the host.

The anemia associated with chronic infections is usually normocytic and normochromic but may be normocytic and hypochromic. The infectious process is usually of many weeks' duration, since the life span of the normal erythrocyte is 120 days. Anemia is common in cases of subacute bacterial endocarditis, tuberculosis, brucellosis, and chronic pulmonary infections such as lung abscess and empyema. A decrease in serum iron, serum iron-binding capacity, and saturation of transferrin with iron are the biochemical changes characteristic of this type of anemia. Ferrokinetic and erythrokinetic studies have revealed the following: (1) A rapid rate of clearance of injected iron from the plasma. (2) Normal or only moderately increased erythropoiesis. (3) Mildly shortened erythrocyte survival. The latter finding suggests a *hemolytic process*, yet the usual evidences of increased blood destruction (increased serum bilirubin and urobilinogen excretion) are not present. (4) Increased iron stores in bone marrow and reticuloendothelial system (RES). The reason for this avidity of the RES for iron is unclear. The serum transferrin levels are low and its turnover rate is increased, findings thought to be due to increased catabolism and decreased synthesis of transferrin.

The pathophysiologic basis for the anemia of infection is not clear. The defect may be in erythropoietin production (the bone marrow has more than enough potential for the replacement of the red cells lost as a result of the shortened red cell survival), RES function, transferrin metabolism, or a combination of these factors. The manner in which bacterial products or the inflammatory response affects any or all of these targets remains a mystery.

Coagulation Defects. Isolated thrombocytopenia may develop during the course of some acute gram-positive and gram-negative bacterial infections. It may also appear immediately before, during, or after some systemic viral diseases such as measles. During bacteremia and viremia, platelets tend to adhere to each other and the vascular endothelium; this probably accounts for their depletion. This adherence may be due to the action of bacterial toxins or other products on the platelet. For example, staphylococcal alpha toxin causes agglutination and lysis of rabbit platelets in vitro. The extent of thrombocytopenia may be sufficient to cause bleeding, usually in the form of petechiae and purpura. Bone marrow depression secondary to the infection may also contribute to the thrombocytopenia in a lesser degree.

A more profound coagulation defect, *disseminated intravascular coagulation* (DIC), may occur as a complication of infections with a variety of agents: gram-positive organisms (Group A and Group B streptococci, Pneumococcus, *S. aureus, Clostridium perfringens*); gram-negative bacteria (Meningococcus, *E. coli,* Proteus, Pseudomonas, etc.); viruses (varicella, variola, rubella, rubeola, hemorrhagic fevers, etc.); rickettsiae (*Rickettsia rickettsii* of Rocky Mountain Spotted Fever); protozoa (malaria, *Leishmania donovani* of kalaazar). DIC is a distinct clinical entity in which the clinical manifestations are fever, petechial or purpuric eruption, hypotension, and a widespread hemorrhagic diathesis. Renal failure is usually evident secondary to hypotension or occasionally, to renal cortical necrosis. Histologically, there is evidence of fibrin deposition in blood vessels of various organs, particularly in the capillaries and venules of the skin. The basic pathophysiology of DIC involves a host response to an underlying illness (many processes other than infection may also trigger this response) that sets off a generalized activation of the normal clotting mechanism. As a result of systemic infection, endothelial damage and inflammation of blood vessel walls occur. The subsequent depletion of fibrinogen and other clotting components and the ensuing clinical bleeding diathesis are the results of two fundamental processes: (1) activation, by endothelial damage, of the coagulation sequence, leading to the generation of thrombin; and (2) activation of the natural defense of the body (fibrinolytic system) against widespread clotting initiated by uncontrolled thrombin production.

The current state of knowledge suggests that the following sequence of events is involved in the coagulation aspect of DIC. The initiating event is a vascular injury such as occurs in meningococcemia, Rocky Mountain Spotted Fever, and so on. This can activate the clotting mechanism in three ways:

1. *Activation of the Intrinsic Clotting System:* Loss of integrity of the vascular endothelium exposes the circulating blood to collagen, which converts Factor XII (Hageman factor) from an inert precursor to its enzymatically active form, which then initiates the intrinsic clotting cascade (Fig. 20-1) by converting Factor XI, plasma thromboplastin antecedent (PTA), from the precursor to the active form. Activated Factor XI then activates Factor IX [Christmas factor or plasma thromboplastin component (PTC)]. Activated Factor IX forms a complex with Factor VIII (antihemophilic factor) and with platelet phospholipids (platelet Factor III). This complex then activates Factor X (Stuart factor). Activated Factor X, in the presence of platelet phospholipids and Factor V (proaccelerin), forms a complex which converts prothrombin (Factor II) into thrombin. Thrombin then transforms soluble fibrinogen (Factor I) to the still soluble fibrin monomer. The latter then polymerizes and is converted to the stable insoluble fibrin polymer by the action of Factor XIII (fibrin stabilizing factor). Factor XIII exists as an inert precursor and must be activated by thrombin before it can act on the fibrin polymer. In addition to converting fibrinogen to fibrin and to activating Factor XIII, thrombin also enhances the activities of both the activated Factor IX-Factor VIII-phospholipid complex and the activated Factor X-Factor V-phospholipid complex, thus accelerating its own formation.

2. *Activation of the Extrinsic Clotting System:* Vascular injury secondary to infection releases tissue thromboplastin (probably from the walls of blood vessels) which interacts with calcium and Factor VII (serum prothrombin conversion accelerator) to form a complex capable of activating Factor X. At this point the extrinsic clotting system joins the intrinsic system, and the steps leading to the formation of fibrin are identical.

3. *Activation of the Plasma Kallikrein System:* Shock may occur during the course of infections with a wide variety of organisms. However, shock per se, regardless of its cause, can induce intravascular coagulation. Endothelial damage due to infection or due to endotoxin is capable of activating Factor XII (Fig. 20-2). Activated Factor XII or its derivatives are able to activate plasma prekallikrein to the active enzyme kallikrein. This results in elaboration of bradykinin, a highly potent vasodepressor, from its precursor plasma kininogen. Thus, the same trigger point, Factor XII activation, appears capable of initiating both activation of the coagulation pathway directly and bacteremic shock via the kallikrein-kinin system. Once developed, shock itself may elicit further intravascular coagulation. In keeping with this interrelation is the clinical observation that DIC commonly occurs in patients with

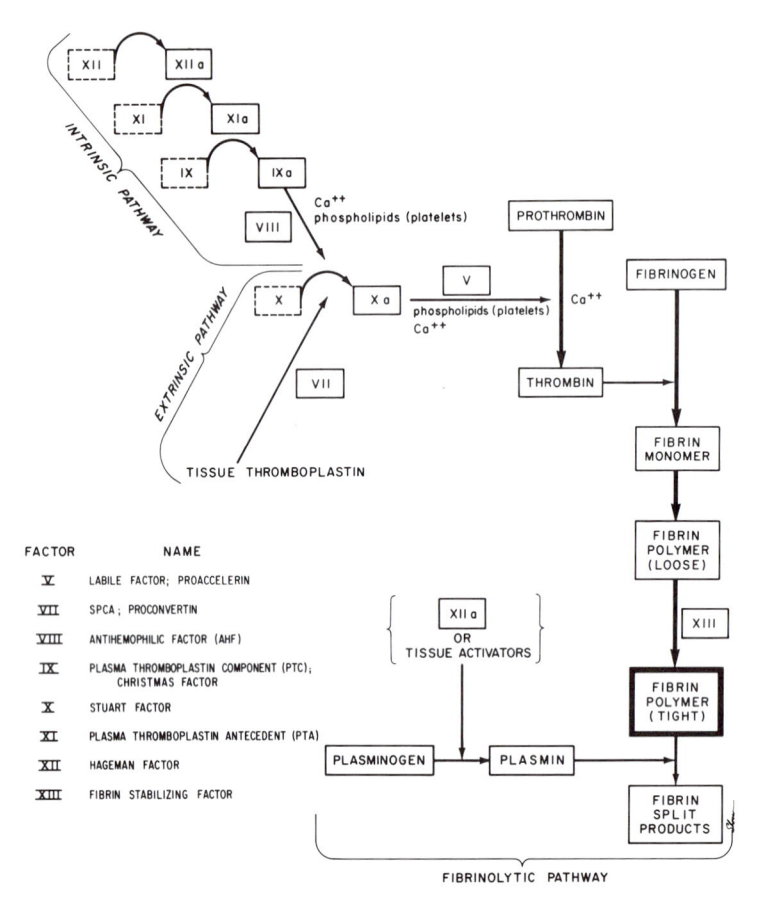

Figure 20–1 Coagulation cascade and fibrinolytic pathway. Clotting factors in ⌐ ¬ represent inert precursor forms of the factors. Clotting factors with subscript *a* in ☐ represent activated forms of the factors. *Intrinsic pathway* for prothrombin conversion to thrombin is initiated by conversion of Hageman factor to its activated form. Cascade follows, in which various clotting factors are sequentially converted from their precursor form to their active form. Activated Factor X with Factor V, platelet phospholipids, and Ca^{++} forms a *prothrombin converting principle,* which liberates thrombin from its precursor, prothrombin. Once thrombin forms, it converts fibrinogen to the fibrin monomer, which after several steps becomes a tight fibrin polymer (clot). *Extrinsic pathway* is initiated by tissue thromboplastins (present in many tissues, particularly blood vessel walls, lung, and brain) which interact with Factor VII, calcium ions, Factor X, and Factor V to form the prothrombin converting principle. This then converts prothrombin to thrombin.

The *fibrinolytic pathway* is initiated by the conversion of the inactive proteolytic enzyme plasminogen, present in all body fluids, to its active form, plasmin. This conversion is activated by either Factor XIIa or by activators present in tissues and vascular endothelium. Plasmin then cleaves fibrin, releasing fibrin split products.

Figure 20-2 Pathogenesis of disseminated intravascular coagulation (DIC). The chain of events initiated by bacteremia is shown schematically. Vascular injury has a central role. It causes activation of Factor XII, release of tissue thromboplastins (TPL), and aggregation of platelets. All three then initiate activation of clotting factors, XIIa by the intrinsic pathway and TPL and platelet aggregation by the extrinsic pathway. Thrombin generation and fibrinogen conversion to fibrin occur intravascularly.

Activation of Factor XII contributes to intravascular coagulation by another mechanism as well. Factor XIIa (activated factor XII) interacts with the kallikrein-kinin system, converting prekallikrein (kallikreinogen) to its active form kallikrein. Plasma kallikrein, in turn, acts on its major substrate, bradykininogen, releasing the nonapeptide bradykinin, a powerful vasodilator. Hypotension and shock develop as a result of the activity of bradykinin. The effect of these circulatory changes is to decrease the hepatic clearance rate of activated clotting factors and to induce additional intravascular clotting. Hypotension induced directly as a result of bacteremia by mechanisms other than the kinin pathway similarly decreases hepatic processing of clotting factors and enhances intravascular coagulation.

Activation of Factor XII has a third major effect, one related to its role in the activation of plasminogen to plasmin. Plasmin furthers the incoagulability of blood in DIC by attacking fibrinogen and fibrin to produce split products which inhibit thrombin and fibrin polymerization.

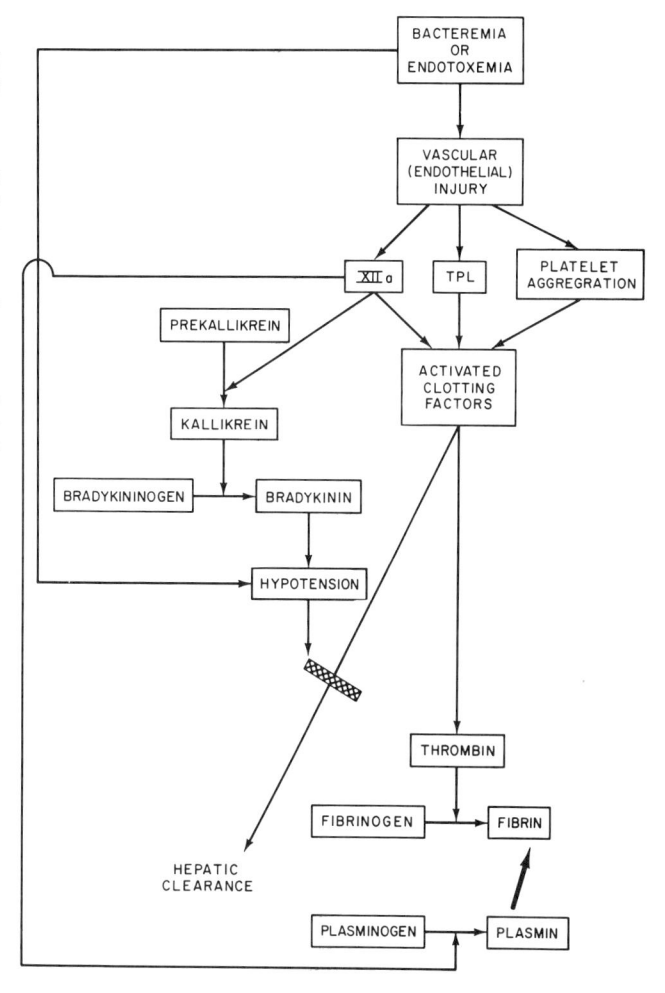

bacteremia and hypotension, but does not develop when infection is unaccompanied by hypotension. However, it is still not clear whether the intravascular coagulation appears first and causes shock and hypoxia, or vice versa.

Once thrombin has been generated in the circulation in the coagulation process, several mechanisms come into play to limit its unimpeded action. One is its rapid removal by adsorption to the newly formed fibrin gel and another is its slow inactivation by a serum factor, antithrombin III. The most important mechanism for interfering with the action of thrombin involves plasmin (fibrinolysin), which destroys fibrinogen, the substrate for thrombin. Plasmin is a potent but relatively nonspecific proteolytic enzyme which degrades many proteins, including fibrinogen. Activation of the plasmin system involves cleavage of an inert circulating protein, plasminogen, by activated Factor XII. This results in the conversion of plasminogen to the active enzyme plasmin, which then acts on fibrinogen to degrade it into a series of large and small fragments. It also digests fibrin; this results in the production of polypeptides (fibrin split products). A potent anticoagulant activity is produced when fibrinogen is cleaved by plasmin. The anticoagulants are two large fragments of fibrinogen which act as (1) competitive inhibitors of fibrinogen for thrombin and (2) blockers of the formation of a tight fibrin gel by forming incoagulable complexes with fibrin monomers.

The inappropriate and extensive clotting process proceeds at an accelerated rate in DIC. Fibrin deposition extends throughout the vascular tree causing local tissue necrosis and more extensive organ damage. Soon, hemorrhage becomes a major clinical feature as blood coagulation factors are depleted (II, V, VII, fibrinogen) and fibrin can no longer be formed. Aggravating the coagulation picture is the activation of the fibrinolytic system. Five major events are involved to produce the net result—incoagulable blood: (1) Depletion, during coagulation, of blood clotting components; (2) depletion of fibrinogen by the intravascular clotting; (3) plasmin-mediated digestion of fibrinogen and possibly Factors V and VIII; (4) suppression of thrombin action by the split products of fibrinogen and fibrin; and (5) inhibition of fibrin polymerization by the split products of fibrinogen and fibrin.

Treatment of DIC is aimed at control of the underlying infection with the appropriate antibiotic, and interruption of the clotting process with a potent anticoagulant, heparin.

SPECIAL HOST RESPONSES

Eosinophilia

Eosinophilia is observed frequently in patients with certain parasitic infestations, in the recovery phase of certain infections, as well as in a variety of other disorders such as allergies, dermatoses, polyarteritis nodosa, and some neoplastic diseases. The function of the eosinophil is unknown, but accumulating evidence suggests that eosinophilia is mediated by immune processes. The circulating eosinophil is believed to be an end-cell. Its maturation takes place in the bone marrow, where it enters a reserve pool several orders of magnitude larger than the total of circulating eosinophils. Upon release from the marrow it circulates for only a few hours in the blood before migrating into tissue sites where it dies or is extruded from a mucosal surface.

Most of the present knowledge of eosinophilia has been obtained during studies of parasitic infection in the rat with *Trichinella spiralis* by Beeson and his coworkers. Intact *T. spiralis* larvae, administered either orally or intravenously, induce an eosinophilic response in rats after a latent period. Similar to the induction of a secondary immune response, rechallenge with *T. spiralis* larvae produces an even greater increase in the number of eosinophils. The eosinophilia appears to be the result of interaction between intact parasites and host cells, particularly after intravenous administration which leads to trapping of larvae in the lungs and causes an acute inflammatory reaction. This does not occur if the parasites are homogenized before they are infused intravenously. The degree of production of antibodies to larval extracts does not appear to correlate well with the magnitude of the eosinophil response.

Production of eosinophils by the bone marrow appears to consist of an inductive and a proliferative phase. Induction lasts for about 24 hours after intravenous injection of *T. spiralis*; it is during this phase that the capacity for "memory" of the stimulus is registered. Induction is suppressed by antilymphocyte serum. A 16- to 64-fold increase in formation of eosinophils occurs during the proliferative phase which cannot be blocked by antilymphocyte serum but is inhibited by cytotoxic drugs such as methotrexate and cyclophosphamide.

A role for the lymphocyte in the inductive phase of eosinophilia is suggested by the fact that depletion of the pool of recirculating lymphocytes by a variety of procedures (neonatal thymectomy, antilymphocyte serum, prolonged thoracic duct drainage) reduces the eosinophilic response to trichinosis. More direct evidence of a role for the lymphocyte in inducing an eosinophilic response is provided by the results of studies of lymphocyte transfer. Transfer of the eosinophilic response from infected donors into normal syngeneic recipients has been effected with thoracic duct lymphocytes (after oral infection) and with buffy-coat cells (from donors infected intravenously). The thymus-processed (T) lymphocytes appear to be the ones mainly involved. They are the cells principally affected by antilymphocyte serum and they make up the major part of the thoracic duct lymphocyte population.

Antigen-antibody complexes have long been associated with the development of eosinophilia. However, the reason for their activation only by certain types of immune response remains obscure. Available evidence suggests that eosinophilia is neither dependent on nor a consequence of the induction of antibodies to Trichinella larvae.

Lymphocytosis

An absolute lymphocytosis of great magnitude and consisting of mature lymphocytes is characteristic of two infectious diseases: pertussis and infectious lymphocytosis (an unusual viral disease of children). Lymphocytosis featured primarily by atypical lymphocytes ("viral cells") develops in other diseases such as infectious mononucleosis and infectious hepatitis. The basis for this change in lymphocyte structure and the specific stimuli inducing lymphocytosis in the course of these infectious disorders are unknown. It is of interest, in this regard, that injection of killed virulent *Bordetella pertussis* in laboratory animals induces a hyperleukocytosis and a hyperlymphocytosis.

Alterations Due to the Immune Response of the Host

One of the major defenses of the host against bacterial and viral disease is the mounting of an antibody response. This may be of great importance in the complement-dependent bactericidal reaction against gram-negative bacilli, and in the phagocytosis and intracellular killing, by polymorphonuclear leukocytes, of various species of bacteria and viruses. The presence of specific circulating antibody also provides protection against reinfection on re-exposure to the same microorganism. The role of type-specific antibody to the pneumococcal capsular polysaccharide in the response of the host to pneumococcal infection (pneumonia) was manifest, during the pre-antibiotic era, in the dramatic clinical improvement that occurred coincident with the appearance of circulating antibody. The development of an immune response against an invading organism is, however, not invariably a salutary event. Occasionally, this may result in injury to the host and the appearance of overt clinical disease. Several examples will be cited here to illustrate this phenomenon, but no attempt will be made to be encyclopedic.

Immune Complex Diseases. Circulating antigen-antibody complexes contribute to the pathophysiology and pathology of at least several human diseases such as acute poststreptococcal glomerulonephritis and viral hepatitis.

Poststreptococcal glomerulonephritis appears to be primarily an immunologic disorder in which antigen-antibody complexes are produced and subsequently trapped in or adjacent to the glomerular capillary walls. Evidence for this is the following: (1) The appearance of the disease after a latent period following streptococcal infection. (2) The high titers of antibodies to streptococcal products present in the sera of patients. (3) The involvement of only certain type-specific strains of Group A streptococci in outbreaks of acute glomerulonephritis. (4) The reduction of complement levels in the sera of patients. (5) The presence of granular and lumpy deposits of complement and bound gamma globulin in the glomerular capillary walls and near the renal basement membrane. These deposits are similar to those observed on electron microscopy and by immunofluorescence in experimentally induced immune complex glomerulonephritis. (6) Demonstration of streptococcal antigen (cell wall rather than cell membrane in origin) in the glomeruli. However, the presence of streptococcal antigen in the nodular, gamma globulin and complement-containing deposits in the kidney must be proved by elution techniques. (7) Development of a possible laboratory model in the rat of experimental poststreptococcal glomerulonephritis. This involves intraperitoneal implantation of millipore chambers containing Group A streptococci. Proteinuria develops a short time after the appearance of type-specific antibodies in the serum and simultaneous with the demonstration of bound gamma globulin, complement, and streptococcal M-protein in the region of the glomerular basement membrane.

The circulating soluble immune complexes appear capable of mediating immunologic injury following deposition on the glomerular basement membrane through activation of complement and stimulation of an inflammatory response consisting of polymorphonuclear leukocytes. This glomerular inflammation accounts for many of the clinical manifestations of acute glomerulonephritis such as hematuria, proteinuria, edema, hypertension, and azotemia.

Circulating immune complexes appear to be involved in the pathogenesis of the glomerulonephritis that occurs in other infections such as bacterial endocarditis, quartan malaria, infected ventriculo-atrial shunt pathways, and possibly secondary syphilis. With the exception of secondary syphilis, the feature common to these disorders is a chronic relapsing course. Instances of diffuse glomerulonephritis as a complication of bacterial endocarditis due to a variety of organisms have been reported. These include *Streptococcus viridans, Staphylococcus aureus, Staphylococcus epidermidis,* and Group G streptococcus.

Antibody-Induced Agglutination and Hemolysis of Erythrocytes. Cold agglutinins develop in 50 per cent or more of individuals with primary atypical pneumonia due to *Mycoplasma pneumoniae*. They may also appear in high titer in patients with the protozoan disease trypanosomiasis. Although the incidence of these antibodies in mycoplasma pneumonia is high, acute hemolytic anemia develops only rarely, most often toward the end of the second week of illness and is featured by fever, prostration, and hypotension. The latter, or less commonly hemoglobinemia and hemoglobinuria, may lead to renal failure.

Amyloid Disease. A variety of chronic infectious diseases may be complicated by the development of amyloidosis. These include tuberculosis, leprosy, chronic osteomyelitis, and chronic bronchiectasis. The clinical manifestations and pathophysiologic consequences depend on the major sites of deposition of the amyloid. The kidneys, spleen, liver, and adrenal glands are most commonly affected, but the nervous system, gastrointestinal tract, blood vessels, and heart may be damaged as well. Deposition in the kidney is usually manifest by proteinuria and the nephrotic syndrome and may lead to progressive renal insufficiency. Nervous system amyloidosis is characterized by a peripheral combined sensory-motor polyneuropathy involving the distal extremities initially. Involvement of the heart usually occurs in the older age group and its clinical correlates include myocardial failure, conduction disturbances, coronary artery insufficiency, and restrictive cardiomyopathy presenting a clinical picture of chronic constrictive pericarditis.

Recent studies have established that in many, if not all instances, amyloidosis consists of the deposition in various organs of specific fragments of immunoglobulins. The insolubility of partially purified amyloid fibrils had raised some question as to the relation of amyloid to the immunoglobulins and presented problems in its further purification. However, it has recently been possible to solubilize these fibrils in 6 M guanidine in the presence of a reducing agent and to analyze their composition. Most amyloid fibrils are made up of the amino-terminal variable portion of the kappa or lambda light chain of immunoglobulin molecules as determined by amino acid sequencing studies. Further support for the immunoglobulin origin of amyloid fibrils is derived from the in-vitro conversion, by proteolytic digestion, of a soluble light chain (Bence Jones protein), with production of insoluble fibrils having the staining properties of amyloid and a partial amino acid sequence derived from the amino-terminal variable region of the Bence Jones protein.

The mechanism of formation and the specific localizations in tissues of amyloid are not clearly understood. It has been reported that Bence Jones proteins from patients with amyloidosis have a greater tendency to bind to kidney, liver, and heart muscle than those from individuals with myeloma uncomplicated by amyloidosis. The possible route for generation of the amyloid fibril is unclear. It has been suggested that antigen-antibody complexes may be processed by macrophages and the immunoglobulin degraded in such a manner as to produce fibrils which are then deposited in the macrophage-rich organs such as liver and spleen. It has also been postulated that free whole immunoglobulins (as in chronic infections) or free light chains (as in myeloma) circulating in increased concentrations may be the immediate source of the fibrils in the vascular system.

Unusual Responses of the Host to Viral Disease

Hypersensitivity Induced by Viral Agents—Postinfectious Encephalomyelitides. Demyelinating encephalitis occasionally follows some viral infections, particularly measles, vaccinia, rubella, and varicella. The disorder occurs most commonly on the fourth or fifth day after the rash, but may develop earlier or later. The histologic pattern is that of a lymphoplasmacytic infiltration of the adventitia of cerebral blood vessels with microglial proliferation in the perivascular spaces. Distinctive perivenous demyelinization is a prominent feature. The infecting virus has not been isolated from the brain or spinal cord of patients with this disease. However, it is important to note that in a few cases of measles encephalitis, cytoplasmic and nuclear inclusion bodies as well as small multinuclear giant cells have been found in brain tissue.

Similar histologic lesions are observed in the brain and spinal cord of laboratory animals in which experimental allergic encephalomyelitis has been produced by a single injection of brain or spinal cord tissue suspended in Freund's adjuvant. The immunologic basis of this disease is suggested by several features: (1) It occurs 9 days or more following the injection; there is a shorter latent period when animals that have recovered are re-injected, as would be expected in a secondary response. (2) The inciting ingredient is specific, namely, myelin-containing tissues. (3) The pathologic changes are distinctive and are limited, for the most part, to the white matter. (4) Brain-reactive antibodies are demonstrable in serum, and lymphoid cells cause cytopathic effects on myelinated brain tissue and glial cells in tissue culture. Although antibodies are present in serum the lesions appear to be due to the cellular type of immunity as judged by (a) a delayed type skin response to intradermal injection of myelinated tissue in affected animals and (b) transfer of the disease from affected animals by lymphocytes but not by serum. The neurologic signs are extremely varied, reflecting the patchy distribution of the lesions; they may include pyramidal tract involvement, akinetic mutism, cortical blindness, cerebellar ataxia, choreiform movements, and so on.

It is tempting to relate the experimental disease to the naturally occurring encephalomyelitis that develops following viral infections. However, this is still hypothetical; the lesions of the experimental and natural disease are not absolutely identical.

Chronic Viral Infections of the Central Nervous System. There are four known chronic viral infections ("slow virus" diseases) of man: subacute sclerosing panencephalitis (SSPE), kuru, Creutzfeldt-Jacob disease, and progressive multifocal leukoencephalopathy. Common to all these are an incubation period of many months to years and a clinical course of prolonged motor and mental deterioration. The unusual features may be related primarily either to unique properties of the virus or to an unusual host response to a typical viral agent. The agents of kuru and Creutzfeldt-Jacob disease have been transmitted to chimpanzees but have not been cultivated in tissue culture, and thus are not yet well characterized. However, the agent of SSPE has been identified as the measles virus in tissue culture. This disease is uncommon (1 case per million population in the United States), with the onset in childhood. Clinically, it is characterized by progressive motor and mental dysfunction with myoclonic movements. Extremely high levels of measles antibody are present in the spinal fluid and blood. SSPE (measles) viruses have been isolated from lymph nodes as well as from the brains of patients with the disease, suggesting that the infection may be a disseminated one. These viruses have biological properties that are more characteristic of the laboratory-adapted vaccine strains of measles than of isolates of the wild virus. It has been suggested that these features may be the result of defective viral replication in nondividing neurons. Another, perhaps more appealing, suggestion is that the disease represents an unusual host response to the virus, one characterized by a specific defect in cellular immunity to the agent of measles.

Metabolic Alterations in Infection

A variety of metabolic changes accompany systemic infection. Some may be the direct result of the activity of the infecting agent, some may represent the consequences of epiphenomena such as fever and infection-induced glucocorticoid and aldosterone excess, and others may be related to specific organ dysfunction due to localization of the infectious process (e.g., hepatitis or pyelonephritis). The sorting out of the contributions to the overall picture by each of these elements has not thus far been achieved.

Changes in electrolyte metabolism have been described in a variety of infectious diseases due to extracellular and intracellular agents. Increased urinary losses of sodium and chloride occur in the immediately prefebrile and early symptomatic periods. This may be due to increased renal perfusion and sodium delivery to renal tubules secondary to increased cardiac output early in the febrile phase. Poor dietary intake, vomiting, diarrhea, and sweating may contribute to electrolyte loss. In sum, these factors probably account for the hyponatremia and hypochloridemia observed at the height of symptoms. The initial heightened urinary sodium and chloride loss is followed by renal retention of sodium coincident with increasing compensatory aldosterone excretion.

In chronic infections involving the lung (slowly resolving pneumonias, pulmonary tuberculosis) and central nervous system infections (tuberculous meningitis), water retention and hyponatremia may develop secondary to inappropriate antidiuretic hormone activity (ADH). The role of hyponatremia in the symptoms of acute infections is not established but it may contribute to the asthenia and malaise that commonly occur.

The most obvious metabolic consequences of acute infection are catabolic. A negative nitrogen balance occurs regularly during infections but does not begin until after the onset of symptoms. It is usually paralleled by potassium losses. The role of these catabolic changes in the not infrequent occurrence of the troublesome and prolonged postinfectious asthenia is still speculative.

Alterations in whole blood amino acid concentrations have been observed during the course of a variety of experimentally induced infections in man. An increase in the total amino acid concentration occurs during the incubation period of typhoid fever. This is followed by a decrease in amino acid concentrations, accompanying the development of overt clinical illness. It is not clear whether these alterations are the direct effect of the infectious agent on host amino acid metabolism, or the consequence of a nonspecific host response to stress mediated by adrenocorticosteroids. No clinical manifestations have been directly attributable to these biochemical changes.

Marked elevations in the concentrations of total serum lipids have occurred in patients with severe infections, particularly bacteremia, due to gram-negative bacilli. The lipid pattern consists of a predominant increase in free fatty acids, accompanied by lesser increases in triglycerides and phospholipids. In contrast, similar changes in serum lipids have not been observed in severe infections caused by gram-positive cocci. In experimental animals injection of endotoxin has produced hyperlipidemia, and this component of gram-negative bacilli may be responsible for the changes in lipids during bacterial infections.

REFERENCES

Fever

Altschule, M. D., and Freedberg, A. S.: Circulation and respiration in fever. Medicine, 24:403, 1945.
Atkins, E.: Pathogenesis of fever. Physiol. Rev., 40:580, 1960.
Atkins, E., and Bodel, P.: Fever. New Eng. J. Med., 286:27, 1972.
Bennett, I. L., Jr., and Beeson, P. B.: The properties and biological effects of bacterial pyrogens. Medicine, 29:365, 1950.
Cooper, K. E.: Temperature regulation and the hypothalamus. Brit. Med. Bull., 22:238, 1966.
Cooper, K. E., Cranston, W. I., and Snell, E. S.: Temperature regulation during fever in man. Clin. Sci., 27:345, 1964.
Greisman, S. E., Hornick, R. B., Carozza, F. A., and Woodward, T. E.: The role of endotoxin during typhoid fever and tularemia in man. I. Acquisition of tolerance to endotoxin. II. Altered cardiovascular responses to catecholamines. III. Hyperreactivity to endotoxin during infection. J. Clin. Invest., 42:1064, 1963; 43:986, 1774, 1964.
Hardy, J. D.: Physiology of temperature regulation. Physiol. Rev., 41:521, 1961.
Hornick, R. B., Greisman, S. E., Woodward, T. E., et al.: Typhoid fever: Pathogenesis and immunologic control. New Eng. J. Med., 283:686, 739; 1970.
Wood, W. B., Jr.: Studies on the cause of fever. New Eng. J. Med., 258:1023, 1958.
Wood, W. B., Jr.: The pathogenesis of fever. In Mudd, S. (Ed.): Infectious Agents and Host Reactions. Philadelphia, W. B. Saunders Co., 1970.

Headache Associated With Fever

Scott, R. B., and Warin, R. P.: Observations on the headache accompanying fever. Clin. Sci., 6:51, 1948.
Sutherland, A. M., and Wolff, H. G.: Experimental studies on headache: Further analysis of the mechanism of headache in migraine, hypertension, and fever therapy. Arch. Neurol. Psychiat., 44:929, 1940.
Wolff, H. G.: Headache and Other Head Pain. New York, Oxford University Press, 1963.

Septic Shock

Gilbert, R. P.: Mechanisms of the hemodynamic effects of endotoxin. Physiol. Rev., 40:245, 1960.

Hershey, S. G. (Ed.): Shock. Boston, Little, Brown, and Co., 1964.

MacLean, L. D.: Patterns of septic shock in man: A detailed study of 56 patients. Ann. Surg., 166:543, 1967.

Mills, L. C., and Moyer, J. H. (Eds.): Shock and Hypotension: Pathogenesis and Treatment (The 12th Hahnemann Symposium). New York, Grune and Stratton, 1965.

Udhoji, V. N., and Weil, M. H.: Hemodynamic and metabolic studies on shock associated with bacteremia. Ann. Intern. Med., 62:966, 1965.

ALTERATIONS OF SENSORIUM

Lyon, G. Dodge, P. R., and Adams, R. D.: The Acute Encephalopathies of Obscure Origin in Infants and Children. Brain, 84:680, 1961.

HEMATOLOGIC CHANGES

Basten, A., and Beeson, P. B.: Mechanism of eosinophilia. II. Role of the lymphocyte. J. Exp. Med., 131:1288, 1970.

Basten, A., Boyer, M. H., and Beeson, P. B.: Mechanism of eosinophilia. I. Factors affecting the eosinophil response of rats to *Trichinella spiralis*. J. Exp. Med., 131:1271, 1970.

Cartwright, G. E., and Wintrobe, M. M.: The anemia of infection XVII. A review. In Dock, W., and Snapper, I.: Advances in Internal Medicine. Vol. V. Chicago, Year Book Medical Publishers, Inc., 1952, p. 165.

Colman, R. W., Girey, G. J. D., Zacest, R., and Talamo, R. C.: The human plasma kallikrein-kinin system. Progr. Hemat., VII:255, 1971.

Corrigan, J. J., Ray, W. L., and May, N.: Changes in the blood coagulation system associated with septicemia. New Eng. J. Med., 279:851, 1968.

Deykin, D.: Thrombogenesis. New Eng. J. Med., 276:622, 1967.

Marsh, J. C., Boggs, D. R., Cartwright, G. E., and Wintrobe, M. M.: Neutrophile kinetics in acute infection. J. Clin. Invest., 46:1943, 1967.

Rodriguez-Erdmann, F.: Bleeding due to increased intravascular blood coagulation. New Eng. J. Med., 273:1370, 1965.

Wilhelm, D. L.: Kinins in human disease. Ann. Rev. Med., 22:63, 1971.

MISCELLANEOUS

Beisel, W. R., Sawyer, W. D., Ryll, E. D., and Crozier, D.: Metabolic effects of intracellular infections in man. Ann. Int. Med., 67:744, 1967.

Feigin, R. D., Klainer, A. S., Beisel, W. R., and Hornick, R. B.: Blood amino acids in experimentally induced typhoid fever. New Eng. J. Med., 278:293, 1968.

Gallin, J. I., Kaye, D., and O'Leary, W. M.: Serum lipids in infection. New Eng. J. Med., 281:1081, 1969.

Glenner, G. G., Ein, D., and Terry, W. D.: The immunoglobulin origin of amyloid. Amer. J. Med., 52:141, 1972.

Gutman, R. A., Striker, G. E., Gilliland, B. C., and Cutler, R. E.: The immune complex glomerulonephritis of bacterial endocarditis. Medicine, 51:1, 1972.

Lennette, E. H., Magoffin, R. L., and Freeman, J. M.: Immunologic evidence of measles virus as an etiologic agent in subacute sclerosing panencephalitis. Neurology, 18:21, 1968.

Miller, H. G., Stanton, J. B., and Gibbons, J. L.: Para-infectious encephalomyelitis and related syndromes. Quart. J. Med., 25:427, 1956.

Payne, F. E., Baublis, J. V., and Itabashi, H. H.: Isolation of measles virus from cell cultures of brain from a patient with subacute sclerosing panencephalitis. New Eng. J. Med., 28:585, 1969.

Swartz, M. N., and Weinberg, A. N.: Infections due to gram-positive bacteria. Gram-negative coccal and bacillary infections. In Fitzgerald, T. B.: Dermatology in General Medicine. New York, McGraw-Hill Book Co., 1971.

Zabriskie, J. B.: The role of streptococci in human glomerulonephritis. J. Exp. Med., 134:180, 1971.

CHAPTER 21
PATHOPHYSIOLOGIC CHANGES DUE TO LOCALIZATION OF INFECTIONS IN SPECIFIC ORGANS

LOUIS WEINSTEIN
MORTON N. SWARTZ

The major impact of a number of human infections is directly related to the specific anatomic site of disease, and the pathophysiologic abnormalities that develop are due primarily to dysfunction of the single or principal organ involved. In some instances, a wide variety of organisms are capable of localizing at the same site, where they produce roughly similar pathophysiologic changes (e.g., infective endocarditis due to any of a number of bacterial and mycotic species). In others, a specific discrete site may be involved by only a very limited group of infectious agents (e.g., involvement of the motor neurons of the spinal cord in disease due to poliomyelitis or Coxsackie viruses).

The pathophysiology of many of the common infectious diseases represents, in effect, the changes due to dysfunction of a particular organ. These are little different from those that might be induced in the same area by noninfectious processes. Thus, the abnormalities that develop in viral hepatitis have much in common with those that appear in acute alcoholic hepatitis. This is also true for chronic pyelonephritis and chronic renal disease due to other causes such as hypertension and chronic glomerulonephritis. The cardiovascular alterations associated with myocarditis are much the same whether it is due to viral infection or alcoholic cardiomyopathy. Likewise, the dramatic circulatory consequences of cardiac tamponade are similar whether this is the result of viral or tuberculous pericarditis on the one hand, or pericardial invasion by a neoplastic process on the other. The pathophysiology of these and many other infectious diseases is considered in sections devoted to organ-system physiology elsewhere in this book. The focus in this chapter is on selected organ involvement in which the pathophysiologic changes, although reflecting primarily organ dysfunction, are quite uniquely produced by infectious agents. Emphasis is put on a limited number of illustrative examples rather than on a comprehensive listing of infectious diseases appropriate to this category.

The characteristic pathophysiologic changes to be considered may be centered about one organ primarily (e.g., osteomyelitis) or the ramifications may be broad, involving many other organs in a specific fashion (e.g., infective endocarditis, syphilis with its multiple stages).

INFECTIONS WITH PATHOPHYSIOLOGIC CONSEQUENCES IN MULTIPLE ORGAN SYSTEMS

Infective Endocarditis

Although this infection involves primarily the heart valves or mural endocardium, the peripheral changes secondary to bland (or septic) emboli, associated vasculitis, or antigen-antibody complexes may be so striking as to become preeminent. Thus, neurologic dysfunction, skin and joint changes, or renal failure may dominate the picture and draw attention to organs other than the heart.

Pathogenesis of Endocarditis. The pathophysiologic processes involved in the development of subacute bacterial endocarditis are strikingly different from those operative in the development of the acute form of the disease. Four mechanisms are responsible for the initiation of the subacute infection: (1) a previously damaged cardiac valve, or a hemodynamic situation in which a "jet effect" is produced by blood flowing from an area of high pressure to one of relatively low pressure, as in mitral insufficiency or ventricular septal defect; (2) a sterile platelet-fibrin thrombus; (3) bacteremia (often transient); and (4) a high titer of agglutinating antibody for the infecting organism. As blood flows over a valve leaflet that has been distorted by acquired heart disease such as acute rheumatic fever, or malformed because of a congenital defect, a "whipping" effect is produced, inducing platelet deposition. Platelet aggregation occurs, initiating coagulation factor activation and local fibrin formation. A platelet-fibrin thrombus is thus deposited at the site of the deformity on the valvular surface. The valvular defect responsible for this phenomenon is occasionally of insufficient magnitude to cause enough turbulence of flow to produce a murmur. Although transient bacteremias probably occur very frequently in man, they are usually without clinical significance, even in the individual with abnormal cardiac valves on which sterile platelet-fibrin thrombi may be situated. In most instances, the failure of implantation of organisms on such a valve is related to the small number of bacteria in the circulation at any given time. A factor that possibly plays an important role in the development of valvular infection is the level of circulating antibody, especially agglutinins. These may result in conglutination of a sufficiently large number of bacterial cells to allow their successful multiplication, and the establishment of infection within the platelet-fibrin thrombus. This phenomenon may be of particular importance in the pathogenesis of subacute endocarditis because of the relatively low invasive capacity of the bacterial species usually involved.

The pathophysiologic changes involved in the development of acute bacterial endocarditis are, in most respects, quite different. In at least 50 to 60 per cent of cases of acute endocarditis, previously normal valves are the site of infection. It appears, therefore, that the presence of a sterile platelet-fibrin thrombus is unnecessary in the pathogenesis of this form of the disease. Because the organisms responsible for this type of infection (*Staphylococcus aureus*, pneumococci, meningococci, gonococci, *Streptococcus pyogenes,* and *Haemophilus influenzae*) are highly invasive, only small numbers are required to establish infection. Thus, the only requirement for the establishment of acute endocarditis is bacteremia due to an invasive organism. It should be pointed out, however, that in the instances in which underlying valvular damage, either acquired or congenital, is present, sterile platelet-fibrin thrombi may develop and facilitate the initiation of this type of infection. The exact mechanism by which "pathogenic" bacteria invade normal valve leaflets is unknown. Although small blood vessels have been suggested as the route by which organisms reach and invade a normal valve in the course of bacteremia, there is little or no anatomic evidence to support this hypothesis. In fact, most observers have failed to demonstrate a distinct blood supply in the leaflets of undamaged valves. In a great many cases of subacute bacterial endocarditis, the bacteremia responsible for the infection originates not from an infectious process, but from trauma to an area where the causative organisms normally reside as components of the indigenous flora (e.g., the teeth, urinary tract, and intestine). This is in sharp contrast to acute infective endocarditides, in which the inducing bacteremia has its origin in an active infection at a site remote from the heart.

Support for the concept that nonbacterial thrombotic endocarditis is the initial lesion that is converted to subacute bacterial endocarditis comes from studies of an experimental model of this disease by Durack and Beeson. In this model, nonbacterial thrombotic endocarditis is produced by insertion of a polyethylene catheter into the right side of the heart of a rabbit. Subsequent intravenous injection of *Streptococcus viridans* results in adherence of the bacteria to the vegetation, where they multiply rapidly and serve as a source of continuing bacteremia. Microcolonies appear beneath and within a superficial layer of material that appears to be fibrin.

Pathophysiology of the Clinical Features of Endocarditis. Four mechanisms are responsible for the clinical features of infective endocarditis: (1) the infectious process on the involved valve; (2) the occurrence of emboli; (3) metastatic infection; and (4) the development of abnormal globulins and clinical manifestations of hypersensitivity, including vasculitis. All these are not found in every patient. There are also striking qualitative and quantitative differences in their roles in the acute and subacute forms of the disease.

THE INFECTIOUS PROCESS ON THE INVOLVED HEART VALVE. The striking differences in the clinical course of subacute and acute endocarditis can be related almost entirely to the patho-anatomic and pathophysiologic changes induced at the primary site of infection, the heart valve. Microscopic study of the lesions in subacute bacterial endocarditis reveals evidence of both slowly progressive activity and early or complete healing. Neutrophils, lymphocytes, plasma cells, and Anitschkow cells compose the cellular infiltrate. The impression is one of simultaneous slow destruction and healing, with the latter not quite "catching up" with the former. In contrast to this are the anatomic changes characteristic of acute endocarditis. Grossly, the vegetations on the involved valve surface are often larger, softer, and more friable than the smaller, harder thrombi observed in the subacute infection. In the more fulminant forms or when the lesion has been present for some time, a variety of destructive changes may occur in proximity to the valvular vegetation. Tears, aneurysms, and/or perforation of one or several cusps of the aortic valve may take place during the course of active infective endocarditis. Eversion or extreme distortion of the aortic valve cusps may occur in some instances after bacteriologic cure has been achieved. Free aortic regurgitation is produced, and marked acute left ventricular failure ensues. Some similarly destructive changes may involve the mitral valve and produce rupture of the chordae tendinae or of a head of a papillary muscle. Catastrophic mitral regurgitation with a loud, harsh systolic murmur then develops, accompanied by sudden dyspnea and attacks of acute pulmonary edema.

A mycotic aneurysm of the sinus of Valsalva may develop in the course of acute or subacute bacterial endocarditis involving the aortic valve. The aneurysm occasionally enlarges by burrowing through the commissure into the wall of the ventricle and there forms an abscess, destroying myocardial fibers. The aneurysmal sac may even dissect upward between the right and left atria. Rupture of the aneurysm into the right atrium may take place and be followed by the development of a roaring continuous murmur and acute congestive failure. Infection of the aortic valve may also burrow into the root of the aorta, and the inflammation may extend to the pericardial wedge between the aorta and pulmonary artery, producing "pericarditis."

Infection involving the mitral valve may burrow into the mitral annulus and even become superimposed on degenerative calcification of the mitral annulus.

Myocardial abscesses may develop not only by extension from valvular vegetations but also as a result of seeding of the coronary circulation with organisms from the vegetations on the aortic valve, or as a consequence of septic embolization. Hectic fevers with or without positive blood cultures (while the patient is receiving antibiotic therapy) and rapidly progressive left-sided heart failure are prominent features. Myocardial abscesses in a strategic location in the septum may cause striking changes in conduction. Infection that involves this area may have (1) spread down the septum from the aortic valve to the A-V bundle, causing disruption of A-V conduction; (2) spread from the mitral valve through the annulus to the region of the A-V bundle or node; or (3) reached the septum by embolization through the coronary circulation. Such lesions may produce a variety of cardiac arrhythmias including bundle branch block, nonparoxysmal junctional tachycardia, and complete heart block. Rupture of the septum secondary to a myocardial abscess occurs very rarely and is characterized by the abrupt appearance of a pansystolic murmur and thrill, as well as rapidly developing cardiac failure.

The constitutional reaction to the valvular infection is manifested by elevated temperature, rigors and generalized malaise; it is, in general, less intense in subacute than in acute endocarditis. Although the level of fever may be the same in either type of disease, it is lower, as a rule, in the chronic form and may never exceed 100 to 101° F.; in about 5 per cent of cases, particularly in patients with azotemia, it may be absent entirely. In contrast, the temperature is very often high in the acute disease and commonly reaches 103 to 104° F. or more. Although rigors may occur at the beginning or during the course of untreated subacute bacterial endocarditis, they are more frequently present in acute endocarditis. Anemia is usually present in both types of disease and may develop quite rapidly in the absence of overt intravascular hemolysis; it is usually the anemia of infection (see Chapter 20).

A changing murmur has been considered a common and characteristic feature of subacute endocarditis. However, broad experience has made it clear that this is rarely the case when *Streptococcus viridans*, the usual cause of this disease, is involved. In contrast, murmurs often undergo rapid and striking changes in intensity and quality in patients with acute valvular infections. This is due to several factors: (1) decrease or increase in size of the relatively soft valvular thrombi, (2) tears or fenestration of valve leaflets, (3) rupture of chordae tendineae or papillary muscles, (4) perforation of the ventricular septum, or (5) development of an aneurysm in an aortic cusp or in the sinus of Valsalva. Of great importance is the fact that murmurs may be absent in patients with subacute bacterial endocarditis, even when the disease has been present for some weeks. Also, about one third of patients with *acute* valvular infections involving the left side of the heart, or patients with right-sided endocarditis (commonly acute) may have no detectable murmurs early in the course of the disease.

Valvular infection due to the enterococcus occupies a clinical position between that produced by *S. aureus* (acute) and *S. viridans* (subacute). Distant septic complications may develop but are most uncommon in endocarditis due to *S. viridans.*

Although the white blood count may be elevated (10,000 to 20,000 per mm.^{3}), it is commonly not increased in patients with subacute bacterial endocarditis. Indeed, the presence of a leukocytosis usually suggests the occurrence of embolic complications or an infecting organism other than *S. viridans* (e.g., enterococcus). Leukocytosis is common in the acute type of disease; however, the number of white cells in the peripheral blood may be normal or even strikingly decreased.

The interval between the onset of infection and the establishment of the diagnosis, as well as the duration of disease in untreated patients with endocarditis is directly related to the character of the valvular lesion. The progression of the infectious process in the acute form is so rapid that severe constitutional manifestations force the patient to seek early medical attention. If undetected, and therefore untreated, death may occur in one or two weeks as the result of marked destruction of the involved valve, multiple metastatic infections, or embolization to a vital area. The course of subacute endocarditis is strikingly different. In this, the symptoms of infection are often very insidious in onset, mainly low-grade fever and slowly developing anemia. The patient's only complaints may be loss of appetite, increasing fatigue, weight loss or night sweats, symptoms which both he and his physician may fail to associate with potentially serious disease. The interval between the onset of symptoms and definitive diagnosis in 100 cases of subacute bacterial endocarditis was about 3.5 months. Life expectancy after development of this disease is usually rather long, even in the absence of antimicrobial therapy, unless rupture of a mycotic aneurysm or lethal embolization occurs. The chronicity of the disease reflects the slow progress of the pathologic process on the infected valve. Survival for 3 to 6 months is common. It may be even longer (over one year) when *Staphylococcus epidermidis* is the responsible organism.

EMBOLIC PHENOMENA. Embolic episodes are common in both acute and subacute bacterial endocarditis. Although they occur most often when infection is still present, they may supervene at any time in the course of the disease, even well into convalescence when the active process has been eliminated. Almost any organ may be the site for embolic deposition. However, the kidneys, heart, brain, spleen, and eyes are more frequently involved than other organs. The areas of resulting infarction may be solitary and large, or multiple and quite small; the clinical manifestations that develop as well as the risk of death depend on the organ involved and the extent of damage. Although emboli in both acute and subacute endocarditis usually contain organisms early in the course of infection, there is a striking difference in the changes that develop at the sites of deposition. The areas of infarction that occur in the subacute disease are, as a rule, sterile. Thus, in subacute endocarditis one observes the paradox of an infected embolus producing a bland infarct. In contrast, infarcts that develop in the course of acute valvular infections, especially those caused by *S. aureus*, rapidly suppurate. Emboli that occur in patients with mycotic endocarditis or atrial myxoma tend to be large. Occlusion of major vessels should, therefore, suggest the presence of these diseases rather than the commoner bacterial infections of valves.

Myocardial infarction secondary to coronary embolization may occur in the course of bacterial endocarditis. Pericarditis may result from extension of the area of infarction to the pericardial surface. Although this is the basis of the pericardial involvement in some patients with endocarditis it is not the only cause for pericardial inflammation in this setting. Other causes include myocardial abscess, erosion of a mycotic aneurysm of the sinus of Valsalva, extension of aortic valve infection into the pericardial wedge between the root of the aorta and the pulmonary artery, uremia, bacteremic spread of infection to the pericardium, and reactivation of acute rheumatic fever.

METASTATIC INFECTIONS. One of the most striking differences between subacute and acute bacterial endocarditis is the high frequency with which metastatic infection occurs in the latter. Infarcts in subacute infection usually do not become infected. This may be attributed to several factors: (1) the invasive capacity of the organisms involved is relatively low, (2) the number of organisms present in the embolus is insufficient to establish metastatic infection, and (3) a high titer of specific antibody results in killing of the few bacteria that are deposited at the local site. Thus, while infarction of the kidneys, heart, and brain occurs in patients with subacute bacterial endocarditis, abscesses in these organs, meningitis, pyelonephritis, or suppurative myocarditis develop only very rarely. However, a sterile meningitis, with the biochemical and cellular characteristics of "aseptic" meningitis, is not an uncommon occurrence in the subacute form of the disease. Mycotic aneurysms of the aorta and its branches that may develop in the course of subacute valvular infection are usually not due to suppuration in and about the vessel walls. In most instances, the vascular necrosis, mural weakening, and aneurysmal dilatation result from sterile occlusion of the vasa vasorum; histologic study of such lesions rarely reveals evidence of active inflammation. Mycotic aneurysms may occur intracranially, particularly in the distribution of the middle cerebral artery. Leakage or rupture of such aneurysms may produce neurologic dysfunction secondary to intracerebral or subarachnoid bleeding. Mycotic aneurysms may also develop in a coronary artery, in the mesenteric arterial tree, or in arteries of the extremities. Because the organisms contained in emboli in acute infective endocarditis are usually highly invasive, they are able to successfully multiply and establish infection in the infarcted areas. Thus, when valvular disease is due to *S. aureus*, multiple abscesses are often detectable, particularly in the kidney and myocardium.

Brain abscesses, often small and multiple may complicate acute endocarditis, particularly when *S. aureus* is the cause. Purulent meningitis may occur also owing to seeding during bacteremia, or it may develop from intraventricular rupture of a cerebral abscess. It is important to recognize that the symptoms of headache, nuchal rigidity, and a mild cerebrospinal fluid pleocytosis during endocarditis do not necessarily represent pyogenic meningitis; they may result from cerebral emboli. Such emboli may involve relatively silent areas of the cortex and produce few if any localizing neurologic findings.

IMMUNOLOGIC ASPECTS AND HYPERSENSITIVITY PHENOMENA. Agglutinating, complement-fixing, and opsonizing antibodies specific for the infecting bacteria in subacute bacterial endocarditis are regularly present. There is an increased level in the serum of both IgG and IgM. Over 50 per cent of patients develop some type of antiglobulin factor. The latex fixation test for rheumatoid factor is positive in about 50 per cent of cases when the disease has been present for 6 weeks or longer. Large amounts of cryoglobulins and macroglobulins may be present. It has been suggested that the articular symptoms, a prominent feature in some patients with subacute endocarditis, are related to the presence of the rheumatoid factor. Arthralgia or florid arthritis may occur early or late in the course of subacute endocarditis. The synovial fluid is usually sterile. Changes in serum globulins are much less marked and less frequently present in the acute endocarditides, because death occurs early if the disease is untreated.

Renal lesions often develop in the course of bacterial endocarditis, particularly the subacute variety. These are of several types: (1) diffuse membranous glomerulonephritis, both acute and subacute, in which immune complexes consisting of antigen, antibody, and complement are deposited as "lumpy-bumpy" aggregates on the glomerular basement membrane (see Chapter 20); (2) renal infarcts, both large and small; and (3) so-called "focal embolic glomerulonephritis," an entity presumed in the past to be the result of multiple small emboli, but now considered to represent some form of hypersensitivity vasculitis. The renal lesions appear to play an important role in death from prolonged and untreated endocarditis. Disease that has persisted for protracted periods may no longer require the active participation of viable bacteria. A "bacteria-free stage" of chronic bacterial endocarditis has been described, the predominant features of which are those of chronic renal failure.

The classic peripheral signs of bacterial endocarditis, originally considered to be of embolic origin, are now thought to represent lesions of allergic vasculitis involving small arteries. Among such signs are *Osler's nodes* (painful and tender bluish-red lesions in the pulp spaces over the terminal phalanges of the fingers or toes); *Janeway's lesions* (nontender, irregular, erythematous or hemorrhagic lesions situated most often in the skin over the thenar and hypothenar eminences of the hands or on the soles of the feet); *Roth's spots* (boat-shaped exudates with a surrounding zone of hemorrhage in the retina); *subungual* or *"splinter"* hemorrhages in the nail beds; and *petechial skin lesions.*

Salmonella Infections (Salmonellosis)

Infections caused by different species of salmonella have in common a number of clinical features such as fever, chills, and diarrhea. However, careful consideration of the pathophysiologic processes involved in the syndromes of "acute gastroenteritis," "enteric fever," and isolated "bacteremia" produced by this group of organisms clearly indicates striking differences that sharply distinguish one disease pattern from another. In fact, these are distinct disorders in most respects, the only common denominator being invasion by salmonella, some species of which are more commonly responsible for certain clinical pictures.

Salmonella Gastroenteritis. A very large number of species of salmonella are capable of producing acute gastroenteritis. This form of infection is usually limited to the intestine. Unlike cholera, this enteritis appears to be related to bacterial invasion of the intestinal mucosa and not to elaboration of a specific enterotoxin. The presence of polymorphonuclear leukocytes in the feces is consistent with an inflammatory reaction in the bowel. Although the stools may be copious and watery in character, there is no evidence that disturbances in the handling of water and electrolytes by the intestine similar to those that occur in cholera are present in salmonella gastroenteritis. Bloodstream invasion is very uncommon except in young infants and elderly individuals. Metastatic infections of the hepatobiliary and other organ systems is also very infrequent. Several abnormal states appear to be of importance in increasing susceptibility to this type of intestinal infection. Among these are *subtotal gastrectomy* (probably related to a decrease in gastric acid production which permits viable organisms to pass through the stomach), *neoplastic diseases, hemoglobinopathies,* the *administration of antimicrobial agents* (related to suppression of competing components of the normal intestinal flora), and the *use of corticosteroids* (possibly due to alteration in immune mechanisms).

Enteric Fever. The enteric fevers include typhoid (*S. typhosa*) and the paratyphoid (*S. paratyphi, S. schottmülleri,* and *S. hirschfeldii*) fevers. A similar clinical picture may be produced occasionally by others of the approximately 1500 salmonella species. The pathogenesis and pathophysiologic phenomena involved in this group of infections are quite distinct and different from those that characterize salmonella gastroenteritis. The enteric fevers are not primary diseases of the intestinal mucosa but rather affect principally the lymphoid tissues in certain areas of the small intestine. The clinical manifestations of dysfunction of the intestine that occur are secondary to this anatomic localization of the infection. The following sequence takes place after ingestion of an inoculum of one of the salmonella species causing enteric fever. Organisms in contaminated water or food pass through the stomach into the small intestines, where they enter the smaller lymphatic channels and are deposited in the lymphoid tissues within the bowel wall. The organisms multiply in the lymph follicles and are often found intracellularly within plasma cells. This intracellular location may be responsible for persistence of infection in the presence of circulating antibodies. A marked macrophage response is induced locally, and a varying degree of necrosis of the nodes occurs. At the end of about 2 weeks, the average length of the incubation period for the enteric fevers, the organisms invade the bloodstream from the lymphatics. At this point clinical manifestations of disease (fever, chills, and other constitutional reactions to infection) appear. The bacteremic phase may, in fact, be made up of two periods, as suggested by studies of experimental typhoid fever in the mouse. The initial bacteremia is a transitory one, rapidly brought to an end by the removal of the bacilli by the reticuloendothelial system, particularly in the liver and spleen. This is followed by a period of very active bacterial proliferation in the reticuloendothelial cells of these organs. A secondary and more intense bacteremia then ensues, resulting in widespread dissemination of the bacteria. The bacteremia usually persists for several days but may last as long as 10 days; during this time salmonella ordinarily cannot be recovered from the feces. However, after this they are demonstrable in fecal cultures. During the bacteremic phase, salmonella reinvade the intestine via the gallbladder and bile ducts. Ulcerations occur in Peyer's patches in the ileum, and salmonella appear in the feces. Because of the location of the collections of lymphoid tissue in the intestinal wall, the ulcerations are not linear but encircle the bowel. The fact that intestinal involvement is secondary to disease in the lymphoid structures is supported by the absence of diarrhea in over half the patients with enteric fevers. The two commonest complications of this type of salmonella infection, intestinal hemorrhage and perforation, are directly related to the active inflammatory and destructive process in the submucosal aggregations of lymphoid cells. Despite the prominent bacteremia, it is uncommon for metastatic infections of various organs to occur in the course of typhoid and paratyphoid fever.

Salmonella Bacteremia. A number of unrelated factors play important roles in the pathogenesis of salmonella bacteremia. Although not known for some, the pathophysiology of others has been partly defined. *Advancing age* appears to predispose to this type of disease. Individuals with *hepatic cirrhosis* are also more prone to develop this syndrome. This may be related to their greater susceptibility to bacteremia in general because of the decreased effectiveness of the liver in removing members of the intestinal microflora from the portal circulation. *Various types of neoplastic disease* predispose to this type of salmonellosis; although not proved, it is likely that this is related to the immunosuppressive effects of certain malignant diseases. The *administration of antimicrobial agents and corticosteroids* may play a role in the pathogenesis of salmonella bacteremia; the former by eradicating competing elements of the normal flora, and the latter by decreasing immunocompetence. A group of disorders characterized by *chronic or acute episodes of hemolysis*—malaria, sickle cell anemia (or other hemoglobinopathies), louse-borne relapsing fever (*Borrelia recurrentis*), and Oroya fever (*Bartonella bacilliformis*)—are associated with a markedly increased risk of intestinal infection and bacteremia due to salmonella. The loading of macrophages with large quantities of hemoglobin breakdown products may make it impossible for these cells, the major defense against salmonella, to ingest and kill the organisms. It has also been suggested that hyperferremia, consequent on acute hemolysis, is responsible for the increased susceptibility to invasion by salmonella. There is some evidence, from animal studies, that hypoferremia may be associated with some increase in resistance to certain infections, whereas excessive levels of iron in the serum may be associated with a decrease in resistance. The association of salmonella osteomyelitis with hemoglobinopathies is well recognized. The microscopic areas of bone infarction that commonly occur in sickle cell anemia appear to serve as a nidus for the engraftment and multiplication of salmonellae that have previously entered the circulation.

One of the most interesting pathophysiologic phenomena that may play a very important role in the pathogenesis of continuing salmonella bacteremia is an *arteriosclerotic aneurysm of the aorta*, or one of its major branches. The aneurysmal sac or the clot may become infected during a transient salmonella bacteremia. This then becomes the site of a bacterial endarteritis, which thereafter is a source for a continuous intense bacteremia. However, in some patients with this syndrome, neither clot nor infection of the aneurysmal wall can be demonstrated. An aortic aneurysm in a rare patient with salmonella infection of a vertebral body may become infected as the result of direct spread of infection to its outer wall from the adjacent area of osteomyelitis. The pathophysiologic changes in salmonella bacteremia consist of three groups of phenomena: (1) those due to the presence of viable gram-negative bacilli in the circulation; (2) those related to circulating endotoxin (myalgias, fever, and even disseminated intravascular coagulation in an occasional patient); and (3) the tendency for metastatic infections to develop. The lungs, meninges, synovial membranes, bones, and endocardium (valvular) are most often involved. The intestine is usually not a site of metastatic infection. However, bacteremia may occur as a complication of salmonella gastroenteritis, particularly in very young and elderly individuals.

Syphilis

Syphilis may involve almost any part of the body, particularly in its late stages, and may produce profound functional changes in many organs. The pathophysiologic phenomena in this disease are the result of inflammatory and vascular changes in organs where *Treponema pallidum*, the etiologic agent, has been deposited during the early phase of invasion of the bloodstream. The changes are conveniently considered under three major groupings: *early, late,* and *congenital* syphilis. The relative impact of the disease on various organ systems depends on the stage of the process; the latter is determined to a large measure by the effectiveness of the immunologic response to the invading spirochete. Certain organs such as the heart and aorta, the central nervous system, and the eye are prominently involved; important functional derangements occur as a result. The natural history of untreated early syphilis, as observed at the turn of this century, suggested that in about two thirds of individuals the disease became latent and produced no major manifestations. However, it was found, 50 to 60 years later, that 10 per cent of these patients had syphilitic cardiovascular disease and another 6.5 per cent had neurosyphilis.

Early Syphilis. The usual portal of entry for *T. pallidum* is skin or mucous membrane. Symptomatic early syphilis is made up of two stages. The initial lesion of *primary syphilis* is a papule which evolves into a painless, eroded or crusted lesion (chancre), usually located on the genitals but occasionally at extragenital sites. The chancre develops 2 to 6 weeks after inoculation of the organism. Painless regional lymphadenopathy appears shortly thereafter. Pathologically, the primary lesion shows a dermal infiltrate (lymphocytes and plasma cells), a proliferation of capillaries, and endarteritis. *T. pallidum* is present in the lesion and in the regional nodes. The chancre, even if untreated, slowly heals over the next 2 to 6 weeks. During the evolution of the primary lesion and extension of infection to regional lymph nodes, the treponemes enter the circulation and are widely disseminated. Metastatic foci develop, particularly in the skin, the mucous membranes, and the nervous system.

Secondary syphilis occurs 5 to 6 weeks after the appearance of the chancre and is a manifestation of treponemal multiplication in metastatic foci. The principal features are a generalized measles-like rash (often accompanied by erosive superficial lesions in the oral, genital, or anal mucous membranes) and generalized lymph node enlargement. The *secondary eruption*, even if untreated, disappears within several weeks; and the treponemes in other foci appear to die out, presumably as a result of the immunologic response of the host. Occasionally, sufficient numbers of the organisms survive to initiate another round of treponemia. This is responsible for one or more recurrent episodes of secondary syphilis (mucocutaneous relapse). Meningitis due to invasion by treponemes is not uncommon in secondary syphilis. In addition to the usual findings common to many types of aseptic meningitis, delirium and seizures occasionally occur. Damage to the third, sixth, seventh, and eighth cranial nerves may develop as a result of reactive fibrosis of the leptomeninges about the base of the brain. Acute hydrocephalus with papilledema may rarely complicate the process. The cerebrospinal fluid shows a pleocytosis of up to 500 cells, predominantly lymphocytes. The duration of the meningitis is usually less than a month. Other areas that may be involved in secondary syphilis are the *eye* (visual loss due to iritis or optic perineuritis secondary to meningitis); *kidney* (interstitial nephritis; nephrotic syndrome due to membranous glomerulonephritis, with proteinuria and edema); *liver* (hepatitis mimicking viral hepatitis in its manifestations); and *bones* (pain and tenderness of long bones due to periostitis).

Late Syphilis. In about one third of patients with untreated early syphilis sufficient immunity does not develop to render the disease asymptomatic (latent) for the remainder of the patient's life. Instead, chronic destructive inflammatory and vascular changes slowly progress over many years and produce late manifestations. These occur principally in the skin and mucous membranes, bones, joints, central nervous system, and heart and great vessels.

The characteristic lesion in late syphilis is the gumma, a granulomatous lesion in which there is coagulation necrosis due to obstructive inflammation of small arteries; treponemes are usually absent.

SKIN AND MUCOUS MEMBRANES. The changes of late syphilis in the skin consist of gross, nodular, ulcerating lesions. Gummas also may occur in the oral mucosa and cause perforation of the palate and destruction of the nasal septum.

SKELETAL SYSTEM. Gummatous periosteal involvement of bones produces pain and swelling, particularly of the tibia and clavicle. Destructive involvement of weight-bearing joints ("Charcot's joints") is not due to invasion of the synovia by treponemes, but rather to the effects of constant trauma on joints lacking pain sensation because of the neurologic changes of syphilis (tabes dorsalis).

CENTRAL NERVOUS SYSTEM. There are five definable patterns of late syphilis of the central nervous system. (1) *Meningovascular syphilis:* This develops a few years after the primary lesion and lacks the usual features of acute bacterial meningitis. The fundamental lesion is an arteritis. The clinical features result from arterial thromboses and fibrosis. A variety of neurologic syndromes may develop, depending on the site of vascular occlusion. These may be located in the cerebral cortex and produce hemiplegia, aphasia, homonymous hemianopia, or seizures. Occlusions of the anterior spinal artery may lead to paraplegia. Other vascular lesions may produce sensory loss and impairment of bowel and bladder function. A mild lymphocytic pleocytosis (up to 100 cells) of the cerebrospinal fluid is common. (2) *Tabes dorsalis:* This occurs 10 to 30 years after the initial infection. Atrophy of the dorsal roots and demyelinization of the sensory fibers that ascend in the posterior columns of the spinal cord are the characteristic pathologic changes. These are produced by the inflammatory arteritis in the meninges, and not by direct invasion of the cord substance by treponemes. As a result of posterior column involvement, position sense is grossly impaired. Patients have difficulty walking, particularly in the dark. Sharp stabbing pain over the extremities or trunk occurs episodically and is due to the changes in the dorsal roots. Involvement of the sacral nerve roots causes impotence, incontinence, and constipation. Atrophy of the optic nerve and changes in function of the pupil (poor responsiveness to light but normal reaction to accommodation—Argyll Robertson pupil) is common. (3) *Primary optic atrophy:* This may occur in the absence of tabes dorsalis. Damage to the optic fibers results from continuous leptomeningitis. This is confirmed by the observation that the outer portions of the optic nerve are first affected, causing impairment of peripheral vision. Subsequent decrease in central visual acuity develops, owing to involvement of the deeper placed fibers in the optic nerve. (4) *General paresis:* This is a very serious form of central nervous system syphilis, involving primarily the cerebral cortex, meninges, and cerebral arteries. Large numbers of *T. pallidum* are found in the cortex, and diffuse neuronal destruction with reactive gliosis is prominent. Atrophy of the frontal and temporal lobes and dilatation of the ventricles are marked. As a result of these extensive pathologic changes in the cerebral cortex, evidence of a wide range of mental and neurologic dysfunction is present. Delusions, hallucinations, hypomania, and paranoia may be prominent. As in tabes dorsalis, patients with paresis may have the Argyll Robertson pupil (irregular miotic pupil responsive to accommodation but not to light). Seizures and strokes secondary to the syphilitic endarteritis are not uncommon. Once developed, general paresis progresses rapidly, with profound mental deterioration followed by physical incapacitation. If untreated, the disease is uniformly fatal. (5) *Gummas of the central nervous system (intracranial or intraspinal):* These are rare and present with manifestations consistent with an expanding lesion, such as a tumor.

CARDIOVASCULAR SYSTEM. Cardiovascular syphilis takes the form of either an aortitis of the ascending aorta, producing the clinical features of aortic insufficiency with left ventricular strain, or an aneurysm of the ascending aorta. Involvement of the coronary ostia in the aortitis may lead to coronary insufficiency. Syphilitic aortic aneurysms cause hoarseness (impingement on the recurrent laryngeal nerve); cough and dyspnea (pressure on the trachea and bronchi); dysphagia (compression of the esophagus); and pain (erosion of ribs, sternum, or vertebrae).

Congenital Syphilis. As a result of treponemia occurring after the fourth month of pregnancy, the fetus becomes extensively infected. The placenta is enlarged and there is extensive proliferation of fibrous connective tissue. Similar fibrotic lesions with mononuclear cell infiltrations are present in many viscera. The most characteristic findings are in the lungs ("pneumonia alba"), which show a marked increase in fibrous tissue and poorly developed alveoli filled with macrophages. Periostitis and osteochondritis are also common.

Late congenital syphilis is a prenatally acquired infection that has been less acute and the clinical manifestations are not evident until the child is over 2 years of age. Osseous changes (saddle nose, saber-shaped tibia from periostitis), synovitis of the knees, dental deformities (upper central incisors), and eighth nerve deafness are usually present. The most common manifestation is interstitial keratitis, an inflammatory process of the cornea complicated by neovascularization, which may progress to blindness. Central nervous system involvement may occur, as in the acquired disease, and result in meningitis, meningovascular disease, juvenile paresis, and, rarely, tabes dorsalis.

INFECTIONS WITH PATHOPHYSIOLOGIC CONSEQUENCES IN A SINGLE ORGAN OR ORGAN SYSTEM

Lobar Pneumonia

The pneumococcus is the commonest cause of lobar pneumonia, but other organisms such as *Klebsiella pneumoniae* may produce a similar lesion. The onset of pneumococcal infection of the lung is usually preceded by a viral upper respiratory tract infection of several days' duration. Aspiration of the infected mucus from the nasopharynx into the distal ramifications of the bronchial tree, usually in the lower lobes, sets up the initial focus of pulmonary infection. The occurrence of such an aspirational event is enhanced by alcoholic intoxication, anesthesia, or depressant drugs, all of which are known to diminish the epiglottal reflex.

Following establishment of infection in the alveoli a characteristic sequence takes place in the evolution of pneumococcal pneumonia. First, bacterial invasion by the encapsulated diplococci evokes an outpouring of edema fluid. This thin fluid serves as a vehicle for carrying the organisms into terminal bronchioles and through the alveolar pores of Kohn into adjoining alveoli. Inspiratory movements aid the rapid spread of infection toward the lung periphery. Polymorphonuclear leukocytes quickly enter the infected area and soon reach sufficient numbers to completely fill the alveoli and produce frank consolidation. At this stage phagocytosis by leukocytes begins to take place even though type-specific opsonizing capsular antibodies have not yet appeared. Such early phagocytosis ("surface phagocytosis") follows the trapping by the leukocytes of pneumococci against alveolar walls or against the surface of other leukocytes. Unspecific heat-labile opsonins (capable of acting on bacteria in general) contribute to the effectiveness of this early phagocytic process and the subsequent destruction of the organisms. After the untreated patient has been ill for some days, monospecific anticapsular antibody appears. By neutralizing the antiphagocytic properties of the capsular polysaccharide, this antibody considerably enhances phagocytosis and intracellular killing. Once most of the organisms have been ingested, macrophages derived from the monocytes of the blood and the lining cells of the alveoli enter the lesion to clear away the bacterial and leukocytic debris.

Although the events described above occur sequentially in a given area of involvement, all are going on simultaneously when the entire spreading lobar process is considered. Three areas of activity are discernible. The peripheral portion of the lesion, the edema zone, is composed of alveoli filled with bacteria and serous fluid containing few if any cells. Inside this is a second zone characterized by the presence of leukocytes and red blood cells which have entered through injured alveolar walls. These two peripheral areas exhibiting edema and hemorrhage together present the gross appearance of "red hepatization." The third or central zone is one in which the alveoli are crowded with polymorphonuclear leukocytes and in which the appearance of macrophages may herald early resolution. This dense consolidation, when viewed in the gross, is the area of "gray hepatization."

The spreading pneumonic process may rapidly involve a whole lobe, extending as far as the pleural surface. Aspiration of infected edema fluid into the bronchial tree may spread the infection to several lobes. The infection may not be contained by the pleural boundaries but may enter the pleural space and produce empyema.

Clinical Manifestations of Pneumonia. A variety of clinical manifestations develop in association with the progression of the histologic changes in the lung. The pathophysiologic basis of the signs and symptoms that characterize this kind of pneumonia is understood to a varying degree.

Cough. This is usually an important feature of the disease. The cough reflex is stimulated by irritation of the lower respiratory tract and by the accumulation of purulent exudate in the bronchial tree. Pink, bloody, or "rusty" sputum is produced by the majority of patients and is the result of the bleeding into alveoli that characterizes the early inflammatory process.

Chill and Fever. The first major symptom of lobar pneumonia is frequently a single shaking chill which is temporally related to the stage of bacterial invasion of the lung. Whether a specific pyrogenic component of the pneumococcus analogous to the endotoxin of gram-negative bacilli is involved in stimulating endogenous leukocytic pyrogen (EP) is not known. Phagocytosis stimulates the production and release of EP and thus may be the responsible mechanism. Bacteremia is present in approximately one third of cases of pneumococcal lobar pneumonia and is usually detectable when patients enter the hospital some time after the chill has occurred.

PLEURITIC PAIN. Severe chest pain occurs in the majority of patients with pneumococcal pneumonia. It often occurs at the onset of the disease and is the result of inflammation of the pleural surface following peripheral extension of the pneumonia. The pain is usually referred directly to the overlying chest wall. However, when the diaphragmatic pleura is involved, it is referred to the shoulder. The discomfort is strikingly accentuated by inspiratory movement; this leads to splinting of the affected side of the chest and rapid, shallow, and grunting respiration.

CYANOSIS. Cyanosis of the lips and nail beds is commonly present, in the absence of shock, in pneumococcal lobar pneumonia. This indicates a significant degree of arterial hypoxemia. Several mechanisms may be involved in the pathogenesis of this phenomenon: (1) *Shunting of blood through consolidated lung tissue.* The extensive exudate that completely fills the alveoli in much of the involved lobe decreases or abolishes effective gas exchange in this area. However, blood flow to the consolidated, poorly aerated lobe continues. Thus, venous blood perfusing the area is not exposed to high oxygen tensions and is, in effect, physiologically shunted into the pulmonary veins, and then to the systemic circulation. (2) *Postpulmonary shunting.* This results from admixture of unsaturated blood that occurs distal to the pulmonary capillaries from such venous channels as thebesian vessels, bronchial veins, and anastomoses between portal vein collaterals and the pulmonary circulation (portopulmonary shunt). (3) *Ventilation-perfusion disturbances in unconsolidated areas of the lung.*

Most of the hypoxia in patients with lobar pneumonia is accounted for by a right-to-left shunt. When the disease is moderately severe, essentially all of the shunt is pulmonary. When it is severe, both pulmonary and postpulmonary shunting is markedly accentuated. The increase in the postpulmonary shunt in severe pneumonia has been attributed to an increase in bronchial circulation. However, a more likely explanation is that the heightened tissue metabolism in the area of infection causes an increase in the observed total shunt (without affecting the pulmonary shunt) by decreasing the oxygen content of pulmonary venous blood. Later in the course of pneumonia (after 4 days) the magnitude of the shunt declines. After 4 days of illness, ventilation-perfusion disturbances begin to contribute relatively more to the observed hypoxia in some instances. This may be due to altered lung mechanics known to be present in acute pneumonia (decrease in lung compliance out of proportion to the amount of lung tissue involved as observed in roentgenogram of the chest). The reason for this increased rigidity of apparently normal parts of the lung may be the reduction of surface activity that has been noted in grossly normal areas from lungs containing lobar consolidations. The causes of hypoxemia in lobar pneumonia clearly appear to depend to some extent on both the severity and the duration of the pulmonary infection.

CIRCULATORY CHANGES. Cardiovascular function may be taxed heavily by the stress of pneumonia. The impact on the heart may be so severe that death results. The adequacy of the circulation and tissue perfusion can be appraised by measurement of the arteriovenous (A-V) oxygen difference. A normal (not exceeding 5.5 vol. %) or narrowed A-V difference is an indication of a physiologically adequate circulation. In the presence of fever, the cardiac output is normally increased in parallel or in excess of the increase in oxygen consumption. The net effect is that the A-V O_2 difference remains normal or is narrowed. In two thirds of patients with pneumonia, tissue perfusion is adequate as judged by evidence of an appropriate circulatory response—an increased cardiac output associated with increased oxygen consumption, and an A-V O_2 difference not in excess of 5.5 vol. %. In the other one third of patients there is an inadequate hemodynamic response, consisting of a relatively low cardiac output that results in a widened A-V O_2 difference. This occurs in patients who have no apparent evidence of preexisting heart disease and whose venous pressure is normal. These individuals also have an abnormally high total peripheral resistance and an increased hematocrit. The hypodynamic state in this group appears to be due principally to depressed myocardial function which returns to normal during convalescence. Relative hypovolemia due to decreased fluid intake, fluid losses secondary to fever, and shifts out of the vascular compartment may also contribute to the lowered cardiac output. The underlying nature of the myocardial dysfunction is unknown. T-wave changes have been reported in the ECG during pneumonia; infiltration of the myocardium with inflammatory cells has been noted in some fatal cases. Whether these represent direct effects of a bacterial product or of hypoxia is not known.

ILEUS. Adynamic ileus and gastric dilatation may be prominent features in pneumococcal pneumonia. They may be of sufficient magnitude to add to the patient's discomfort and interfere with respiration. The cause of the ileus is not established, but it may result from the low O_2 saturation of the blood supplying the bowel.

Complications of Pneumococcal Pneumonia. A variety of complications may occur and produce pathophysiologic consequences depending on their location.

PULMONARY AND PLEURAL INVOLVEMENT. Lung abscess is a rare complication of pneumococcal pneumonia and is almost always due to infection with type III strains. These organisms possess an abundant "slime layer" of antiphagocytic capsular polysaccharide. This interferes with initial surface phagocytosis as a result of which the density of bacteria in the pneumonic focus may reach an extremely high level and produce local necrosis of the lung. Pleural involvement may lead to the development of an effusion or a frank empyema. Fever and evidence of infection will persist if the latter is not properly drained. Compression of the lung may become chronic owing to fibrosis and produce restrictive changes in pulmonary function.

CARDIAC INVOLVEMENT. Purulent pericarditis and acute bacterial endocarditis are the serious cardiac complications of pneumococcal pneumonia and are due to direct bacterial invasion. Pericarditis may produce cardiac tamponade with limitation of venous return and cardiac output as the physiologic consequences of this constrictive process.

MENINGITIS. This complication is the result of bacteremic spread of infection.

ARTHRITIS. This is a suppurative process due to growth of pneumococci in the synovia and extension into the joint space.

PERITONITIS. Although pneumococcal peritonitis may occur in the course of pulmonary infection due to this organism, it is rare. Patients with either postnecrotic hepatic cirrhosis or the nephrotic syndrome are particularly susceptible to the development of peritoneal involvement. The clinical picture is that of a septic process complicated by adynamic ileus.

Interstitial Pneumonia

Interstitial pneumonia is a diffuse inflammatory process of the lung in which the pathologic changes are located mainly in the alveolar walls and, to a varying degree, within the alveoli. There is involvement of the alveolar ducts and bronchioles to a lesser extent. Histologically, there is an extensive interstitial inflammatory infiltration, usually consisting of mononuclear cells, in the walls of alveoli and in the connective tissue septa about the small pulmonary vessels. This process usually accompanies or immediately follows an initial intra-alveolar inflammatory reaction. It may be manifest clinically as an acute process and resolve completely or occasionally lead to severe interstitial fibrosis and run a subacute or chronic course.

A wide range of infectious agents may be involved in the pathogenesis of interstitial pneumonia: (1) viruses, such as influenza, varicella, adenovirus, and *Herpes hominis;* (2) *Mycoplasma pneumoniae* (the cause of the common type of "atypical pneumonia"); (3) *Chlamydia* (psittacosis or ornithosis); (4) *Rickettsia,* principally *Coxiella burnetii* (Q fever); (5) bacteria, primarily *Haemophilus influenzae;* (6) fungi such as *Histoplasma capsulatum;* and (7) protozoa such as *Pneumocystis carinii.* However, a somewhat similar clinical and pathophysiologic picture can also be produced by a variety of noninfectious processes. These include (1) *infiltrative disorders* (sarcoidosis, histiocytosis); (2) *pneumoconioses;* (3) *collagen vascular diseases;* (4) *radiation pneumonitis;* (5) *drug sensitivity* (busulfan, methotrexate); and (6) *unusual pathologic processes of unknown etiology* ("desquamative interstitial pneumonia," "lymphocytic interstitial pneumonia").

Nonproductive cough, fever, and slight shortness of breath are the principal symptoms in mild cases of interstitial pneumonia. Breathing is rapid and shallow, even at rest, in more severe cases. Roentgenographic changes are usually minimal and consist of fine mottling and a reticular pattern. The oxygen saturation of arterial blood may be markedly reduced, and cyanosis, incompletely relieved by oxygen administration, may be present. The Pco_2 of arterial blood is normal or decreased (owing to hyperventilation). The low arterial oxygen tension (Po_2) was originally interpreted to be the result of impairment of diffusion of oxygen through a thickened alveolar membrane ("alveolar-capillary block" syndrome). However, physiologic studies have indicated that it is unlikely that this can account for the observed arterial oxygen unsaturation. A more likely explanation stems from the finding that there are irregularly distributed areas of lung with altered mechanical properties in this disease. Alveoli in such areas of reduced compliance have somewhat decreased ventilation but are still normally perfused. Thus, abnormalities of ventilation-perfusion and ventilation-diffusion ratios result in inadequate oxygenation of blood leaving certain areas of the lung (venous admixture).

Physiologic studies of patients with acute interstitial pneumonias have been very limited. Varicella pneumonia, a disease seen almost exclusively in adults, has been examined more extensively than others. Dyspnea, nonproductive cough, and cyanosis are common features due to pulmonary involvement in patients with extensive and severe chickenpox. Death may occur from respiratory failure. X-ray examination discloses prominent bronchovascular markings and diffuse nodular densities. There is no evidence of obstructive ventilatory difficulty. Increased venous admixture has been found during the acute phase of illness. There may be chronic impairment of gas transfer after resolution of the pneumonia. Scattered, small nodular pulmonary calcifications may develop some time after recovery.

Bacterial Meningitis

The syndrome of uncomplicated bacterial meningitis represents a combination of the *nonspecific manifestations of infection* (fever, malaise, headache), the *signs of meningeal irritation* (stiff neck and back, positive Kernig and Brudzinski signs), and *abnormalities of the spinal fluid* (variable numbers and types of cells, and changes in content of sugar and protein). These alterations are induced by pathophysiologic processes which are, for the most part, well understood.

Manifestations of Infection. As with infections of most types, fever is an almost universal accompaniment of meningitis; chills are often, but not invariably, present. Generalized malaise, often with pain in the muscles and joints, is common. Myalgia appears to be a more prominent feature during the prodromal stages of meningococcal meningitis than during other bacterial meningitides. This may be a manifestation of the accompanying meningococcemia or of endotoxemia.

Manifestations of Meningeal Irritation and Intracranial Infection. The signs of meningeal irritation are produced by the inflammatory reaction about the pain-sensitive spinal roots and nerves. As attempts are made to flex the neck or back or to extend the lower legs on the flexed thighs, traction occurs on the spinal roots and nerves; this produces pain and results in involuntary spasm of the muscles innervated by these nerves. The inability to flex or extend respective muscle groups is responsible for the stiffness of the neck and back and the positive Kernig and Brudzinski signs.

Headache, often extremely severe and "pounding" in character, is the most common symptom of meningitis. Although an increase in intracranial pressure is relatively frequent, the pain in the head is usually not due to this, but appears to be related to distortion of the meningeal vessels which are usually encased in the inflammatory exudate.

A common occurrence in the course of the bacterial meningitides is the development of *cerebral edema.* This may be of a degree severe enough to produce changes in the state of consciousness, confusion, or even localizing neurologic signs. It may develop early during meningitis and may be accentuated by excessive administration of parenteral fluids in the course of treatment. The primary danger is herniation of the temporal lobe or cerebellum with compression of the midbrain at the tentorium, producing respiratory arrest. Removal of cerebrospinal fluid in the presence of heightened intracranial pressure may precipitate herniation. Marked brain swelling is usually reflected clinically by coma, by signs of third nerve dysfunction (irregularity of the size or fixation of the pupils), or by respiratory arrest. Papilledema may occur in various types of meningitis. However, the majority of patients with meningitis and increased CSF pressure do not have papilledema. Elevated CSF pressure in the early stages of bacterial meningitis is, in most instances, due to brain swelling and not to obstructive hydrocephalus or intraspinal block. It is important to remember, however, that meningeal infection may be the consequence of intraventricular leakage of a cerebral abscess, or may be accompanied or complicated by subdural empyema. Both cerebral abscess and subdural empyema are space-occupying lesions which can produce increased intracranial pressure and papilledema. Since their treatment is different from that of meningitis, early diagnosis is essential.

Seizures frequently complicate bacterial meningitis. The incidence is higher in infants. However, convulsions are known to be frequent in young children with fever due to a variety of causes. The seizures associated with meningeal infection may be focal or generalized. A common type of focal episode consists of rhythmic jerkings of the eyes conjugately to one side. Seizures may occur during the peak of the meningitis or may appear for the first time during the second or third week of the disease when evidence of active meningeal infection has all but disappeared. Delayed thrombosis of cortical veins is responsible for late seizure activity; it can also account for seizure activity which develops earlier in the disease. Bacterial cerebritis and brain swelling are other pathologic findings that may be responsible for seizures during the course of meningitis.

Focal cerebral signs, aside from seizures and alterations of consciousness, occur in meningitis infrequently. Focal cerebral signs that appear early are commonly due to cortical necrosis or occlusive vasculitis (usually venous). Among these are hemiparesis, quadriparesis, visual field defects, disorders of conjugate gaze, and dysphasia. Temporary hemiparesis (persisting up to several hours or longer) can occur as a postictal phenomenon, and its significance can be considerably different from that of a true dense hemiplegia. Prominent and persisting focal cerebral signs always raise the spectre of an associated pyogenic process such as brain abscess, subdural empyema, or possible cerebral embolism from bacterial endocarditis.

Cranial nerve dysfunction is not uncommon in bacterial meningitis. Impaired ocular movement (paresis of third or sixth cranial nerve) is the most frequently encountered evidence of such dysfunction. Facial weakness (seventh nerve) and deafness (eighth nerve) are the other principal signs of cranial nerve involvement. In general, dysfunction of the cranial nerves is transient and disappears shortly after recovery from the meningitis. It is generally assumed but not yet proved that damage to these nerves results from their entrapment by the meningeal exudate. Deafness and labyrinthine deficits tend to persist in contrast to the transient character of the disturbance of other cranial nerve functions. This suggests the possibility that damage to the inner ear is the result of the activity of bacteria or their products.

Sterile subdural effusions occur in about 10 per cent of patients under the age of 2 years with bacterial meningitis. They are only rarely reported in children older than this. However, this is misleading, since the usual techniques for diagnosis (transillumination of the skull and subdural taps) cannot be employed in older children or adults. Repeated vomiting, persistence or recurrence of fever, increasing irritability, seizures, fullness of the fontanelle, or increasing cranial circumference have been attributed to subdural effusion when they occur later in the course of meningitis. Transillumination has proved to be a useful means of making the diagnosis. In many infants with meningitis such sterile subdural effusions disappear without the need for subdural tap. Indeed, they may be found (on routine transillumination of infants with meningitis) in the absence of any clinical manifestations attributable to the process. Rarely, subdural effusions are invaded by bacteria as a result of penetration of the arachnoid by the infectious process. The resulting subdural empyema is characterized by high fever, considerable toxicity, and a variety of cortical signs (seizures, hemiplegias, visual field defects). The latter signs are due to (1) inflammation and thrombosis of the cortical veins that run through the subdural space and (2) pressure phenomena secondary to the often large accumulation of pus over one or both cerebral hemispheres.

Abnormalities of Cerebrospinal Fluid. An increase in the number of cells is demonstrable, with very rare exceptions, in patients with bacterial meningitis. Almost without exception, the predominant cell in the early stages of the disease is the neutrophil. In rare instances, mobilization of inflammatory cells into the spinal fluid may not occur, and culture of the spinal fluid may yield organisms that are too few in number to be detectable in stained preparations. Although not frequent, this phenomenon appears to be most common in the early stage of meningococcal infection. This may be due to the fact that insufficient time had elapsed for the developing inflammatory exudate in the meninges to extend into the spinal fluid. Rarely, the cerebrospinal fluid may be strikingly turbid in the absence of cells; the turbidity then is due entirely to large numbers of organisms. The pneumococcus is the usual etiologic agent in these circumstances. In such cases, studies of bone marrow and peripheral blood have revealed no abnormalities; in fact, a leukocytosis with a shift to the left is commonly present. Patients with leukemia may develop meningitis with similar findings; in this instance, the lack of cerebrospinal fluid pleocytosis is attributable to the marked reduction in circulating neutrophils.

The increased content of protein in the spinal fluid in cases of meningitis is the result of leakage of serum proteins, the release from the meninges of the products of inflammation, and the breakdown of leukocytes introduced during the infectious process. The pathophysiologic basis of very high levels of protein (up to 1 gram or more per 100 ml.) in fluid removed from the lumbar sac is intraspinal block, usually complicating more chronic forms of meningitis such as that due to *Mycobacterium tuberculosis;* excessive concentrations in ventricular fluid are suggestive of block in the internal circulation of spinal fluid, most commonly due to obstruction of the sylvian aqueduct.

Reduction of the concentration of glucose in the spinal fluid is usually, but not always, observed in the active, untreated phase of bacterial meningitis. Although levels may be normal in the very early stage of the disease, these decrease, as a rule, as the infection progresses. It must be stressed that the content of glucose in the cerebrospinal fluid in healthy individuals is directly related, except in uncommon instances, to the concentration of glucose in the blood. High blood sugar levels in a patient with diabetes may be accompanied by a normal or elevated concentration in the spinal fluid. In contrast, quite low levels of glucose in the spinal fluid of young infants do not necessarily indicate infection but may reflect hypoglycemia due to vomiting or poor food intake.

Although extensive bacterial multiplication may play some role in the fall in cerebrospinal fluid glucose concentration in certain types of experimentally produced meningitis (pneumococcal) in animals, it is clear that the metabolic demands of the bacteria or of the leukocytes alone do not account for the lowered levels of sugar. The limited surface phagocytosis that occurs in early bacterial meningitis may contribute in a small measure to lowering CSF glucose through augmented glucose utilization, a characteristic of the phagocytic event. However, interference with the transport of glucose from blood to cerebrospinal fluid appears to be the major factor contributing to the lowering of the concentration of sugar in the spinal fluid. Under physiologic conditions the transfer of sugar from blood to spinal fluid is mediated by two processes: simple diffusion and carrier-facilitated diffusion. The facilitated diffusion of glucose from blood to the cerebrospinal fluid and outward diffusion of sugar from spinal fluid to blood are impaired in bacterial meningitis. This may be secondary to alterations in the blood-CSF barrier due to increased metabolism of the cells involved, or due to structural changes produced by the inflammatory process. In addition there may be greater utilization of glucose by the brain in the course of meningeal infection.

An increase in the concentration of cerebrospinal fluid hydrogen ion has been reported in some patients with bacterial meningitis or subarachnoid hemorrhage. The decrease in pH is associated with a rise in the level of lactic acid in the CSF. It has been suggested that some of the changes in respiration and sensorium that occur in the course of bacterial infection of the meninges may result from this. The decreased pH of CSF may stimulate medullary chemoreceptors and induce hyperventilation, an event that occurs occasionally, in severe meningitis. The alkalosis produced by hyperventilation may then reduce cerebral perfusion, and, in this way, exacerbate the acidosis.

The pathophysiologic processes described above are common to practically all the bacterial meningitides. However, each etiologic type of meningeal infection has individual physiologic and anatomic features which may account for some of their special clinical characteristics.

Meningococcal Meningitis. Meningococcal infection may have its sole impact as a meningeal disease. However, there may also be widespread effects on other organ systems. Infection of the upper respiratory tract is the most common form of meningococcal disease in man, but produces few if any symptoms. In a small percentage of these patients, there is a sequential development of clinical manifestations: bacteremia, meningitis, and/or other metastatic localizations. The presence of circulating antibodies specific for the various serologic groups of meningococci (A,B,C,D,X,Y,Z) affords protection against bloodstream invasion.

The occurrence of meningococcal bacteremia (meningococcemia) precedes the development of meningococcal meningitis. The pathophysiologic consequences of meningococcemia vary.

MILD MENINGOCOCCEMIA. The onset is usually acute, with fever, chilliness, myalgias, arthralgias, nausea, and vomiting. Macular skin lesions, particularly on the extremities, are replaced by petechiae and, at times, purpuric lesions. The petechiae that are so common in this disease often contain a bloodless necrotic center surrounded by a small zone of hemorrhage. Meningococci may sometimes be demonstrated in Gram stains or culture of material obtained by needle from the pale center of such lesions. The pathophysiologic basis of the lesions in the skin may be a bacterial vasculitis, an endotoxin-induced Shwartzman-like reaction, or thrombocytopenia secondary to the bacteremia. Meningitis quickly follows the bacteremia in some cases; in others, meningeal infection never develops. Some patients develop meningitis without even exhibiting any manifestations in the skin, despite the presence of organisms in the circulation.

ACUTE FULMINATING MENINGOCOCCEMIA (WATERHOUSE-FRIDERICHSEN SYNDROME). The striking feature of this process is the abruptness of its onset and the rapidity with which it inexorably progresses. Shock, extensive purpura, and rapid death (within 24 hours of the intrusion of meningococci into the bloodstream) are attributable to the overwhelming bacteremia and the effects of endotoxin. Circulatory collapse, coma, and disseminated intravascular coagulation (see Chapter 20) may occur within a few hours of onset of the disease. The coagulopathy is responsible for widespread but patchy gangrene of the skin, digits, ears, and nose that may lead to spontaneous amputation of the involved areas in some instances. Gastrointestinal bleeding may occur secondary to mucosal lesions of the bowel. Bilateral hemorrhages of the adrenal glands are often present in fatal cases. Levels of corticosteroids in the circulation are usually normal or elevated in fulminant meningococcemia. Thus, acute adrenal insufficiency is probably not the major pathophysiologic basis of the shock occurring in this form of disease.

METASTATIC INFECTIONS SECONDARY TO MENINGOCOCCEMIA. The meninges are the commonest sites of metastatic infection in the course of meningococcemia. However, the organisms may be deposited at many other sites. This usually occurs early in the disease and most often coincides with the meningitis. Metastatic infections of joints, endocardium, myocardium, pericardium, eye, testes, and lungs have been recorded.

CHRONIC MENINGOCOCCEMIA. This is a rare syndrome characterized by recurrent episodes of fever, chills, arthralgias (or arthritis), and an erythematous papular rash. These tend to occur at intervals of 48 to 72 hours and last for 1 to 2 days. Blood cultures usually yield meningococci early in the febrile stage. The source of the organisms cannot be defined in every case; in some instances, however, they may be recovered from the upper respiratory tract. Recurrent attacks may go on for weeks to months if treatment is not instituted; meningitis or endocarditis may develop in patients who are not treated.

The clinical characteristics of the meningitis due to *N. meningitidis* are, in general, similar to those present in other types of pyogenic meningeal infections. However, several features are more often associated with disease caused by the meningococcus than with that in which the pneumococcus or *H. influenzae* is involved. Among these are severe agitation, delirium, and maniacal behavior in the early stages of the meningitis; acute brain swelling also appears to be more common and, indeed, may be the pathophysiologic basis of the cerebral signs.

An interesting group of late complications may appear in a small percentage of patients late in the course of meningococcal bacteremia or meningitis. Among these are marked arthralgia or frank arthritis, pericarditis (usually with effusion), and myocarditis (primarily electrocardiographic abnormalities). These usually develop during convalescence and are not prevented or abolished by effective antimicrobial therapy. The synovial or pericardial fluids contain a moderate number of polymorphonuclear leukocytes but are sterile. This process is distinct from the septic arthritis or pericarditis that accompanies or complicates the acute phase of meningococcemia or meningitis. It has been suggested but not proved that these manifestations represent immunologic reactions, involving complexes of meningococcal polysaccharide antigens and antibody deposited in various tissues. Host responses to the antigen-antibody complexes are thought to produce the ensuing sterile inflammation in the involved areas.

Haemophilus influenzae **Meningitis.** The age distribution of *H. influenzae* meningitis is striking, the vast majority of cases occurring between the ages of 6 months and 3 years. The presence of bactericidal antibody appears to be a crucial determinant in this predilection of the young for this disease. Antibody to type B *H. influenzae*, the strain principally responsible for human infection, is transferred across the placenta to the fetus and persists at effective levels until somewhere between the ages of 3 and 6 months. Thereafter, infants are without this protective antibody until they are 3 years of age, when they begin to acquire it as a result of contact or of relatively minor infections. By the time most individuals are 12 to 15 years old they are immune to invasion by the type B organism. This accounts for the relative infrequency of this type of meningitis in otherwise normal adults. However, recent studies indicate an increasing incidence of this infection in the latter age group. This has been associated with an increase in the number of older individuals lacking specific bactericidal antibody, owing to lack of contact with the organism or to very prompt treatment of respiratory infections in the past.

The pathophysiology of meningitis due to *H. influenzae* is, for the most part, similar to that produced by the meningococcus. Bacteremia originating from the respiratory tract occurs frequently in this type of infection but is not necessary for initiation of meningeal infection. Suppurative arthritis is a rare complication. Petechial rashes may develop rarely in patients in whom the organisms have invaded the bloodstream.

Seizures and sterile subdural effusions occur more commonly with meningitis due to *H. influenzae* than with that caused by the meningococcus. This does not stem from a difference in the invasive properties of the organisms but rather from the age distribution of the two types of meningitis. *H. influenzae* meningitis commonly occurs in infants or young children, whereas the peak age incidence of meningococcal meningitis is in older children and young adults. The prominence of seizures in *H. influenzae* meningitis may reflect merely the frequency of "febrile convulsions" in young infants prone to develop this disease. The higher incidence of subdural effusions with *H. influenzae* meningitis may similarly reflect the age distribution of this type of meningitis, and the availability of easy methods of detecting the presence of subdural fluid (transillumination or subdural tap) in children less than 2 years of age.

Pneumococcal Meningitis. Many, but not all, instances of pneumococcal meningitis are secondary to bacteremia. This is particularly so when the source of the organisms is pneumonia. In about 25 per cent of patients, the primary infection involves the middle ear or paranasal sinuses from which it extends to the lining of the central nervous system along venous channels that drain these areas, or the disease reaches the meninges by direct invasion of bone (e.g., the mastoid).

Most instances of recurrent bacterial meningitis are caused by the pneumococcus; as many as 20 episodes have occurred in the same patient. The anatomic basis for this disease is the presence of a cranial lesion that permits communication between the external environment and the meninges. Organisms then can pass directly from the upper respiratory tract, most commonly the nose and its accessory structures, to the central nervous system. The predisposing conditions are usually tears in the dura, fractures of the cribriform plate, nasal meningoceles, and osteomyelitis of the floor of the anterior fossa of the skull.

Meningitis due to the pneumococcus tends to be a more severe disease with a significantly higher mortality than that due to the meningococcus or *H. influenzae*. The exudate tends to be thicker, particularly over the convexity of the brain, in pneumococcal meningitis. Cerebral venous and arterial occlusions leading to hemiplegia or other syndromes appear to be more common in this type of meningeal infection than in the other two types, probably reflecting the effect of the markedly purulent exudate that is often present.

Tuberculous Meningitis. Bacteremia is probably not the immediate predisposing event in tuberculous meningitis. The most likely focus from which *Mycobacterium tuberculosis* reaches the meninges is a preexisting small tuberculoma within the cerebral substance or abutting on the meninges. These lesions usually develop during the course of a transient postprimary tubercle bacillemia. The tuberculoma is quickly walled off by host defenses and then remains quiescent for many years or for the lifetime of the patient; however, in a rare instance, breakdown of the lesion occurs later and leads to spread of organisms to the meninges. Meningitis may develop occasionally as a complication of disseminated (miliary) tuberculosis, particularly in children. Even under these circumstances it is probable that the meningeal infection is not the result of direct implantation of organisms, but is secondary to the development of microscopic tuberculomas within the central nervous system. In support of this is the observation that injection of tubercle bacilli into the carotid arteries of dogs produces tuberculomas of the brain and meninges but not tuberculous meningitis. Overt pulmonary tuberculosis is not a prerequisite for the development of meningitis; infection of the lung is not apparent in about one third of instances of central nervous system disease. Two pathophysiologic features of tuberculous meningitis account for several characteristic aspects of this form of meningitis. These are the basilar location of the inflammatory exudate and the common involvement of blood vessels, particularly in the form of an occlusive arteritis. These are responsible for the frequent development of cranial nerve dysfunction, especially bilateral paralysis of the sixth nerve, and the sudden appearance of signs of vascular thrombosis, including hemiplegia and other manifestations of localized brain or spinal cord damage. Ventricular block or spinal block may occur secondary to the chronic inflammatory process and may lead to obstructive hydrocephalus.

The abnormalities in the spinal fluid in tuberculous meningitis differ from those found in meningitis due to pyogenic bacteria. The cellular response consists predominantly of lymphocytes, whereas in untreated pyogenic meningitis over 80 per cent of the cells are polymorphonuclear leukocytes. While the cell count in meningitis caused by other bacteria is usually between 1,000 and 10,000 per mm.[3], it rarely exceeds 500 per mm.[3] in tuberculous meningitis. The other changes in the spinal fluid in this disease are qualitatively the same as those in the other bacterial meningitides; they are, however, quantitatively different. In contrast to other infections of the meninges, the sugar content of spinal fluid falls much more slowly and the quantity of protein usually increases to appreciably higher levels. Although it was formerly thought that a reduced concentration of chloride in the cerebrospinal fluid was characteristic and even diagnostic of tuberculous meningitis, this is now known not to be the case. Decreased levels of chloride may occur in other types of meningeal infection and are directly related to hypochloremia, a not uncommon phenomenon in this disease due to the loss of chloride from the profuse sweating and vomiting that frequently occur in the early stages of infection. The syndrome of inappropriate antidiuretic hormone secretion, though not common, occurs more frequently in tuberculous than in other types of meningitis, perhaps related to its longer course and the accompanying chronic pulmonary tuberculosis. It may contribute significantly to the low levels of chloride in the serum and spinal fluid.

Serous tuberculous meningitis is an unusual clinical entity that occasionally develops in children with tuberculosis. The clinical features associated with this syndrome are similar to those characteristic of the early stage of infection of the meninges by the tubercle bacillus — fever, apathy, irritability, headache, vomiting, and stiff neck. Cranial nerve abnormalities do not occur. Serous meningitis differs from caseous tuberculous infection in several ways: (1) It may resolve spontaneously in several weeks or less, whereas true tuberculous meningitis is almost invariably fatal without antimicrobial therapy. (2) Tubercle bacilli are not found in the cerebrospinal fluid. (3) Chemical alterations are generally not observed in the CSF: the glucose concentration is normal and the protein level is, at most, only slightly increased. (4) The number of cells, usually predominantly lymphocytes, is sometimes normal, but is frequently increased to as high as 300 per mm.[3]

Serous meningitis is thought to be an inflammatory response of the meninges to the presence of localized adjacent (parameningeal) caseous foci, the result of hematogenous infection. These foci induce a "sympathetic" response in the meninges that is similar to that which occurs in pyogenic intracranial infections (brain abscess, subdural empyema), without creating a diffuse meningitis due to seeding with tubercle bacilli. Another interesting, but unproved, hypothesis for the mechanism of serous meningitis is based on the concept of a tuberculin reaction restricted to the meninges. The setting for this process is thought to be an individual with an "inactive" pulmonary lesion and a quiescent tuberculoma of the meninges. Release of tuberculoprotein into the circulation when the pulmonary process becomes active may initiate a response of delayed hypersensitivity (tuberculin reaction) in the meningeal focus. This results in development of fever, signs of meningeal irritation, and CSF pleocytosis.

Poliomyelitis

Poliomyelitis virus, acquired by a nonimmune person from a patient with active disease or from a healthy carrier, enters the body by the oral route. It multiplies in the oropharynx for a short period, then disappears from this site. At the same time that the virus becomes established in the upper respiratory tract, it also is implanted in the intestine. There it continues to replicate throughout the incubation period and active stage of the disease, and for some time during and after convalescence. From the intestine, the infectious agent invades the regional lymphatic channels;

from there, it reaches the bloodstream. The virus enters the central nervous system at many points by direct passage from capillaries to the motor neurons.

A number of physiologic processes play important roles in determining susceptibility and response to infection by poliomyelitis virus. The mechanism by which these processes operate is obscure in most instances. (1) Age is an important determinant of severity of the disease. Young children with spinal involvement usually have paralysis of one extremity, most commonly a leg. In contrast, a quadriplegia is the most frequent consequence of involvement of the spinal cord in adults. Paralysis of the bladder is about 10 times more common in older individuals than in youngsters. (2) Pregnancy increases the risk of developing poliomyelitis. Women who come in contact with the virus at about the time of ovulation are more prone to infection than if they are exposed at other times in the menstrual cycle. (3) Muscles that have been subjected to trauma or intense exercise may be particularly vulnerable. Muscles that are sites of injection of vaccines, particularly those containing *H. pertussis,* are prone to becoming paralyzed, if immunization is carried out during a period of endemicity of poliomyelitis. (4) Patients who have undergone tonsilloadenoidectomy are much more susceptible to the development of the bulbar form of the disease than those not subjected to this procedure, regardless of when the operation had been performed.

The clinical pictures that characterize poliomyelitis are primarily the direct result of pathophysiologic phenomena involving areas of the nervous system invaded and injured by the virus. The sore throat, often present as a prodromal manifestation of the disease, is due to the growth of and accompanying local inflammatory reaction initiated by the virus. The gastrointestinal manifestations (nausea, vomiting, diarrhea) are related to multiplication of the agent in this area and to its effect on the function of the plexuses of Meissner and Auerbach. The anterior horn cells of the spinal cord are the site of predilection for viral invasion; but this occurs in a scattered ("skip") fashion, with variation in the degree and distribution of neuronal involvement. This is manifested by varying degrees of asymmetrical paresis or paralysis of extremities and of weakness of the muscles of respiration. The neurologic findings are characteristic of a lower motor neuron lesion: flaccid weakness, loss of reflexes, and fasciculation of muscles. Sensory modalities are unimpaired. Alterations in blood pressure, irregularity of cardiac rhythm, variation in skin and muscle temperature, and a variety of skin rashes may be related to invasion of autonomic ganglia by the virus.

When neurons in the medulla are involved, two pathophysiologic consequences are observed. Striking irregularity in the rate and depth of breathing (Biot respiration) is the result of involvement of the respiratory center. As the disease progresses, there are longer periods of apnea until breathing ceases completely. Hiccupping, probably related to irritation of the respiratory center, is often present in the early phase of involvement of this area. Hypoxia, without visible cyanosis, is common and may produce transient elevations of blood pressure. Viral injury to the neurons in the vasomotor center in the medulla is manifested by hypertension initially, followed by fluctuations in the level of blood pressure, and finally by severe hypotension together with the clinical manifestations of shock. Myocarditis is not uncommon in poliomyelitis; it is probably due to direct invasion by the virus. Electrocardiographic abnormalities, mainly T and ST and P-R alterations, are present in from 10 to 20 per cent of cases. Irregularities in cardiac rhythm, including sinus tachycardia or bradycardia, atrial fibrillation, premature ventricular contractions, and ventricular fibrillation, may supervene. Hyperpyrexia, with temperatures of 106° or higher, often develops in the late stages of the type of disease in which the medulla is involved.

The brain may be affected, to a varying degree, by poliomyelitis. Encephalitic manifestations occur as isolated syndromes, or together with bulbar or spinal disease. The diffuse form of encephalitis is featured by confusion, agitation, anxiety, or somnolence. Quivering and jerking of the facial muscles and extremities, flushing of the face, tremor of the hands, and restless movements occur. In focal polioencephalitis, there may be clinical evidence of dysfunction, or the lesions may be silent and demonstrable only at necropsy. Visual-verbal agnosia, myoclonic jerks, grand mal seizures which occasionally persist long after recovery, spastic hemiparesis, ataxia of one arm or leg, and hydrocephalus have been described.

Dysfunction of the peripheral vascular tree may accompany severe poliomyelitis in some cases. This is probably related to invasion of the sympathetic ganglia by the virus. A variety of skin eruptions including miliaria, morbilliform rashes and scarlatiniform eruptions may develop in the severely paralyzed patient; these are usually transient but tend to recur. Abnormalities of sweating are quite common. Autonomic disturbances may be reflected in coldness, pallor, and even cyanosis of the paralyzed limbs. These have been attributed to persisting spasm of the peripheral blood vessels. However, it has been suggested that, while peripheral vasoconstriction is probably a very common phenomenon in chronically paralyzed muscles, angiospasm may not be a feature of the early phase of poliomyelitis. The exact mechanism involved in this phase is not clear.

There is considerable evidence that artificial respiration effected in a tank respirator under negative pressure is physiologically the same as that produced by application of positive pressure to the upper airway. Positive airway and negative intratank pressures produce identical changes in intrapulmonary, intrapleural, intracardiac, and systemic arterial and venous pressures. These result in (1) impairment of the circulation and decrease in cardiac output, (2) increase in cerebral venous and spinal fluid pressures, (3) rise in central venous pressure, (4) loss of blood volume, and (5) increased filling of the venous bed and arteriolar constriction. In the individual who has normal hemodynamics at the time of institution of artificial respiration, compensatory mechanisms tend to counteract these deleterious circulatory effects. Positive pressure applied to the airway results in transmission of a large fraction of the increase to the pleural space, great veins, and right atrium. The elevated pressure in the right atrium produces a momentary decrease in the venous gradient. Although venous return and cardiac output are momentarily decreased, they return to normal rapidly because there is a rise in peripheral venous pressure which reconstitutes the venous gradient and re-establishes venous return. The reconstitution of the venous gradient is dependent upon the existing vascular tone, the capacity for reflex vasoconstriction, and the presence of a normal circulating blood volume. The increase in peripheral venous pressure required to establish the venous gradient causes a rise in capillary filtration pressure; this results in a reduction of the circulating blood volume. When the sympathetic pathways are affected in severe poliomyelitis, re-establishment of the venous gradient after the application of positive pressure to the airway is greatly hindered. Because of this, venous return, cardiac output, and blood pressure fall in direct proportion to the degree of pressure applied. When intense generalized vasoconstriction is present in poliomyelitis because of diffuse involvement of the autonomic nervous system, positive pressure breathing produces a decline in arterial pressure, because the mechanisms responsible for re-establishing the venous gradient are already maximally active. Although this discussion has been limited to the pathophysiologic changes in the circulation that develop when respiratory assistance is required during poliomyelitis, it must be pointed out that similar phenomena are present in other situations which require the use of artificial respiration.

Life-threatening pulmonary edema develops in some individuals with poliomyelitis, especially those who are severely ill because of medullary involvement or because of difficulty in respiration as a result of paralysis of the diaphragm and intercostal muscles. Although the exact mechanisms involved in the pathogenesis of this phenomenon are unknown, several factors that may contribute to its development have been suggested. Among these are hypoxia, oxygen toxicity (overuse of 100 per cent oxygen), constriction of the pulmonary vessels, pulmonary infection, circulatory changes produced by artificial respiration, and myocardial dysfunction.

An interesting and clinically important pathophysiologic phenomenon that develops in practically all patients severely paralyzed by poliomyelitis is mobilization of calcium from the bones. This is responsible for the nephrolithiasis that commonly complicates the prolonged course of illness in these cases. The presence of stones is often the factor responsible for infection of the urinary tract which leads, if untreated, to chronic pyelonephritis and subsequent renal failure. The stones that are formed may be so large as to produce sufficient obstruction to require nephrostomy.

Some of the clinical features of poliomyelitis may have as their basis direct viral involvement of extraneural tissues. Thus, some of the cardiovascular abnormalities are unquestionably related to invasion of the myocardium resulting in interstitial lymphocytic infiltration in most instances or in severe necrosis in others. Generalized lymphadenopathy, a common feature of the disease, is probably due to multiplication of the virus in lymph nodes.

Herpes Zoster

Herpes zoster and varicella are produced by the same virus, and the initial event in the natural history of the herpetic syndrome is an episode of chickenpox at any age, but usually in childhood. It has been proposed (but not proved) that recovery from varicella is sometimes accompanied by passage of the virus from the lesions in the skin and mucous membranes into the sensory nerve endings of these tissues. From here, it is thought, the agent is transported up the sensory fibers to the sensory ganglia, where it may become established in the nuclei of the ganglion cells and remain quiescent for varying periods, often for many years. During this latent period, small quantities of virus might possibly enter the circulation from the ganglia but would be quickly and effectively neutralized by specific antibody. Such periodic intrusions of the virus into the circulation, when they occurred, would be expected to stimulate production of neutralizing antibody.

It appears most likely that activation of the latent varicella-zoster agent is responsible for clinical herpes zoster. In most instances, provoking factors are not readily apparent. However, a variety of disorders which lead to generalized immunosuppression (or drugs such as corticosteroids and cytotoxic agents that produce the same effect) seem to predispose to the development of clinical herpes zoster, presumably by activating the latent virus. Among such diseases are the lymphomas, leukemia (usually lymphatic), and multiple myeloma.

It has been postulated (but not proved) that when antibody levels are reduced, the virus, which has remained latent in the nucleus of sensory ganglia, emerges and travels antidromically down the sensory nerve. In its passage from the ganglia along the sensory nerve it may produce a severe neuritis; this is thought to account for the severe pain commonly present in the pre-eruptive stage (before skin lesions are apparent) of herpes zoster. The virus may travel over only a portion of the length of the nerve and may not reach the skin; the only manifestation in this situation is severe root pain without dermal lesions, so-called *herpes zoster sine eruptione* or *zoster sine herpete*. If, as is the case in most patients, the virus reaches the dermal sensory nerve endings, the typical vesicular eruption develops; the lesions are always in the most precise anatomic relation to the neurons of the sensory ganglia that have been involved or destroyed. Virus is shed from the vesicles and may lead to the development of characteristic varicella if acquired by nonimmune individuals.

Although the spinal ganglia are most frequently involved, others may be the site for presumed long-term residence of the virus. Activation of the virus may produce a variety of syndromes characterized by neurologic dysfunction related to the area affected. The fifth cranial nerve is the apparent pathway for transport of the virus from its ganglion (gasserian). When virus in this location is activated, any one of the three main branches of the fifth nerve may be involved; pain and skin lesions are distributed along the course of the mandibular, maxillary, or ophthalmic divisions. Involvement of the latter (*herpes zoster ophthalmicus*) produces lesions of the cornea; the earliest sign is loss of the corneal reflex. Enlargement of the ipsilateral preauricular lymph nodes and conjunctivitis (Parinaud's syndrome) are common. When the nasociliary branch of the ophthalmic division is affected, the skin lesions usually appear at the end of the nose; other manifestations of this syndrome include conjunctivitis, keratitis, uveitis, and retrobulbar neuritis which may lead to blindness. The geniculate ganglion may be involved (Ramsay Hunt syndrome). In this situation, the skin lesions are present on the pinna, tympanic membrane, or external ear canal. The accompanying neurologic abnormalities are facial palsy alone or together with diminished hearing and tinnitus. If the chorda tympani is involved, there is loss of the sensation of taste over the anterior two thirds of the tongue.

In rare instances, the virus may spread from the posterior to the anterior portion of the spinal cord and lead to paralyses. Paralysis of the muscles of the arms, legs, abdomen, and urinary bladder, as well as of the diaphragm, have been described. On occasion, the lesions of herpes zoster may be diffusely distributed in the skin in a centripetal fashion similar to that of initial episodes of varicella. "Cropping," that is, the continuing appearance of new lesions of varying structure in the same area of skin, as is the case in varicella, does not occur in the disseminated form of herpes zoster. These lesions are practically always painless. This is probably so because only latent virus in the skin (not that in the ganglia) is activated. The appearance of this form of the infection, especially in patients with Hodgkin's disease, is an ominous prognostic sign.

Osteomyelitis

Osteomyelitis may take the form of either an acute or a chronic infection. However, there is no abrupt shift from acute to chronic disease but rather a gradual blending of one into the other. On the basis of the pathogenesis of the lesion, cases of osteomyelitis fall into one or another of three categories: (1) *hematogenous osteomyelitis;* (2) *osteomyelitis secondary to a contiguous focus of infection* (including postoperative wound infections, osteomyelitis in which bacteria have been introduced following a puncture wound, and bone involvement from an adjoining soft tissue focus of infection); and (3) *osteomyelitis associated with peripheral vascular disease.* Osteomyelitis secondary to a contiguous focus of infection is the form of the disease most commmonly seen in large general hospitals.

Hematogenous Osteomyelitis. Acute hematogenous osteomyelitis most frequently involves rapidly growing bone, as evidenced by the fact that over 85 per cent of cases occur in children. There is often a history of antecedent trauma to the area subsequently involved in the septic process. The disease characteristically affects the metaphysis of long bones. The anatomic features of the microvasculature adjacent to the metaphyseal side of the growth plate provide the most satisfactory explanation for the localization of blood-borne bacteria and initiation of infection. The capillary ramifications of the nutrient arteries supplying bone loop sharply just below the epiphyseal growth plates and then enter large sinusoidal veins, where the flow of blood is sluggish (Fig. 21–1). These sinusoidal vessels connect with the venous channels of the medullary cavity. In the experimental animal (and probably also in man) the inability of the metaphysis to handle infection is related to several factors: (1) The afferent loop of the metaphyseal capillary lacks phagocytic lining cells, and the phagocytic cells present in the efferent loop (a sinusoidal structure) are functionally inactive; (2) flow in the descending loops of the metaphyseal capillaries is slower and more turbulent because the descend-

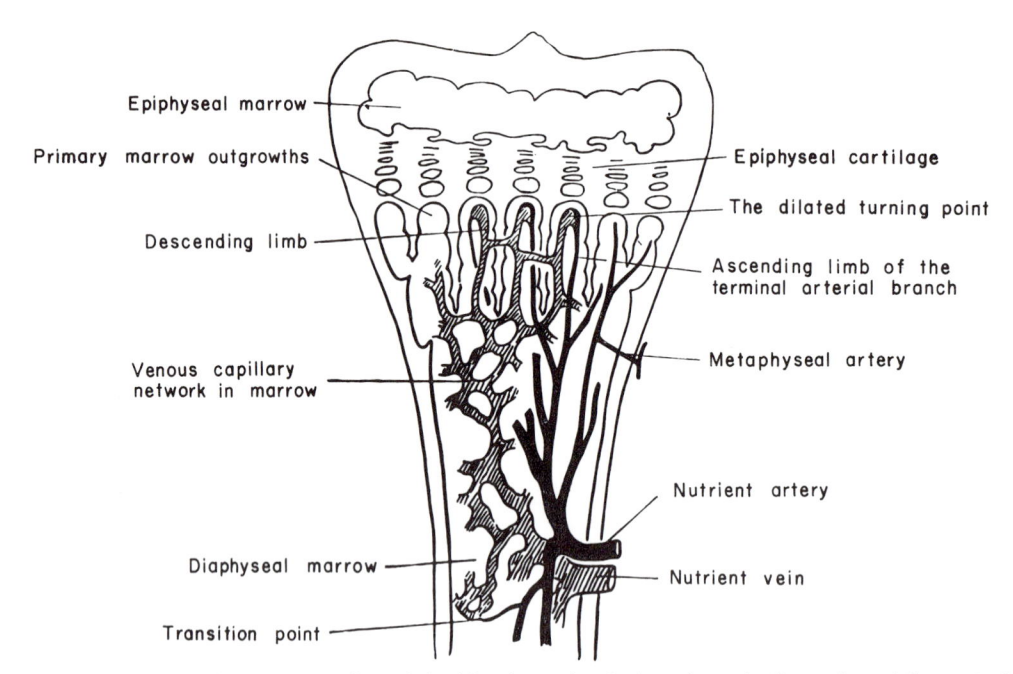

Figure 21-1 Schematic representation of the blood supply of a long bone in the region of the metaphyseal growth plate (epiphyseal cartilage). (From Waldvogel, F. A., Medoff, G., and Swartz, M. N., Osteomyelitis: A Review of Clinical Features, Therapeutic Considerations and Unusual Aspects, 1971. Courtesy of Charles C Thomas, Publisher, Springfield, Illinois.)

ing loops are often multiple and have a diameter 2 to 7 times as great as that of the ascending loops; (3) the capillary loops adjacent to the epiphyseal growth plates are nonanastomosing branches of the nutrient artery, and obstruction (by bacterial growth or microthrombi) would be expected to result in small areas of avascular necrosis, a mechanism conducive to progressive infection.

Once infection has started, the local decrease in pH, the edema, and the accumulation of leukocytes (and possibly their collagenase) all contribute to tissue necrosis and breakdown of bone trabeculae. The infection extends to the neighboring bone through the haversian and Volkmann canals, occludes vascular channels, and causes the death of more osteocytes in the process. Larger segments of bone, deprived of blood supply by this process of vascular compromise, may become separated and form sequestra. These act as foreign bodies, converting the infection into a chronic one and rendering eradication by antibiotic therapy impossible until the devitalized bone is removed. Osteoblastic apposition can take place on smaller pieces of already dead bone, further compounding the problem by burying the infection behind a rampart within which bacteria can multiply uninhibited by circulating bactericidal and phagocytic cells. The suppurative process may also produce a septic thrombophlebitis of the diaphyseal vessels, impairing venous return and increasing the high pressure created within bone. Upon reaching the outer part of the cortex the infection causes an inversion of the slow periosteal blood flow and enters the subperiosteal space. This then may progress to formation of a subperiosteal abscess which is associated with considerable local pain, tenderness, and swelling because of accumulation of pus under pressure. The local presence of heat, pain, and erythema may be so prominent that a subcutaneous abscess is erroneously suspected. Incision and drainage may be carried out in the mistaken belief that the process is a soft tissue infection, when, in fact, the process merely represents extension from a focus of acute osteomyelitis. Subperiosteal infection may induce exuberant circumferential growth of the periosteum (involucrum). Progressive chronic destruction of the cortex is followed by spontaneous pathologic fracture in some instances.

MANIFESTATIONS IN DIFFERENT AGE GROUPS. The clinical course of hematogenous osteomyelitis may vary somewhat, depending on the age of the patient. These differences are related to certain anatomic features and their changes during growth. In the infant below the age of one, infection begins in the metaphyseal sinusoidal veins. However, at this age some patent capillaries still perforate the epiphyseal growth plate, and infection can spread rapidly via this route to the epiphysis. This results in septic arthritis, thrombosis of nutrient vessels, and possible destruction of the epiphyseal growth anlage. Such destruction may result in loss of hip joint function and eventual shortening of the involved leg. *Between the age of one and puberty*, the initial metaphyseal infection is contained by the epiphyseal growth plate and spreads laterally through the paths of least resistance. It commonly perforates the cortex, lifting off the periosteum which is loosely adherent, and produces a subperiosteal collection of pus. The epiphysis in this age group is protected from the spread of infection by the epiphyseal plate, and normal growth is usually not impaired. *In the adult*, because resorption of the growth cartilage has occurred, anastomoses between metaphyseal and epiphyseal blood vessels are re-established and make spread of the infection to the subarticular space a distinct possibility. Subperiosteal abscess formation and extensive periosteal proliferation are unusual in this age group, since the periosteum is firmly attached to the underlying bone.

About one third of patients with acute hematogenous osteomyelitis have demonstrable bacteremia and exhibit a toxic, febrile course. *Staphylococcus aureus* is the most common etiologic agent but other pyogenic gram-positive cocci (pneumococcus, Group A streptococcus) are occasionally implicated. Salmonella infections are a relatively common complication of sickle cell anemia. If salmonella bacteremia occurs in patients with this disease, it is almost always associated with subsequent localization in bone. It has been suggested that the small "bone infarcts" that occur in sickle cell anemia secondary to occlusion of small blood vessels by the deformed red cells are favorable sites for the initiation of infection.

FEATURES DUE TO SPECIFIC SITES OF INVOLVEMENT. Vertebral body involvement in hematogenous osteomyelitis has been seen with increasing frequency in recent years, usually in adults, and often complicating pelvic surgery and urinary tract infections. Infection of the vertebral body spreads readily to adjacent ligaments and adjoining vertebral bodies by anastomosing venous channels. Thus, this type of osteomyelitis frequently involves two adjacent vertebral bodies and the intervening intervertebral disc. Special problems may arise with this type of osteomyelitis because of proximity to the spinal cord. Infection may extend through the thin vertebral periosteum, and pus may accumulate between the periosteum and the dura mater (spinal epidural abscess). Further extension of infection through the dura, either directly or through venous channels, into the subarachnoid space may lead to acute bacterial meningitis. The initial site of bone infection may, not infrequently, fail to produce prominent manifestations. In this situation, the illness is heralded by the sudden onset of the complicating spinal epidural abscess (compressing the spinal cord) or bacterial meningitis. Compression of the cord with resultant paraplegia may result from the epidural extension of the infectious process itself, from secondary vascular impairment with infarction of the cord, or from compression fractures of the involved vertebrae.

The particular anatomic feature of the hip and shoulder joints account for the common occurrence of septic arthritis secondary to osteomyelitis of the femur and humerus in children. Although the epiphyseal plate serves as an effective barrier to the direct extension of infection from the metaphysis to epiphysis (and thence to the joint space) in this age group, an alternative route is available. The synovial capsules in these joints reach beyond the epiphyseal growth plate; thus, infection can rupture through the cortex and spread directly from the metaphyseal focus into the joint.

Osteomyelitis Secondary to a Contiguous Focus of Infection. This type of disease is at present most common after surgical procedures such as open reduction of fractures, craniotomy, and reconstruction of joints severely affected by degenerative arthritis. However, it may follow burns, infection of the ears or paranasal sinuses, animal bites, and infection of soft tissue produced by trauma. Because the route of infection is different than in hematogenous osteomyelitis, metaphyseal localization of the process is much less frequent. In contrast to hematogenous osteomyelitis, which is predominantly a disease of the young, most patients with this form of bone disease are over 50 years old. These infections tend to be chronic, recurrent, and difficult, if not impossible, to eradicate until all foreign bodies (plates, screws, and other orthopedic appliances) have been removed. The most frequent clinical manifestations are local pain and drainage from a sinus tract. *S. aureus* is the organism most commonly involved. However, less invasive bacteria can produce this syndrome when infection of an orthopedic prosthesis takes place. The usual manifestations of acute infection are often absent in this setting. There may be only minimal local erythema and only low-grade fever. Pain and limitation of motion secondary to spasm of muscle due to inflammation in and around bone may be important features. Infection is a major consideration in patients who have continuing pain following reconstructive hip surgery (cup arthroplasty or total hip replacement).

Osteomyelitis Associated With Vascular Insufficiency. The pathogenesis of the process in this situation involves extension of infection to bone secondary to ischemic ulceration of the skin. The toes or the small bones of the feet are almost invariably involved. This is a problem almost always in patients with long-standing diabetes mellitus, occasionally in individuals with severe atherosclerosis, and rarely in persons with vasculitis secondary to a connective tissue disorder. Local symptoms (pain, swelling, erythema) dominate the clinical picture. There are few systemic manifestations of infection.

REFERENCES

INFECTIVE ENDOCARDITIS
Angrist, A. A.: Pathogenesis of bacterial endocarditis. J.A.M.A., *183*:249, 1963.
Durack, D. T., and Beeson, P. B.: Experimental bacterial endocarditis. I. Colonization of a sterile vegetation. Brit. J. Exp. Path., *53*:44, 1972.
Kerr, A., Jr.: Subacute Bacterial Endocarditis. Springfield, Illinois, Charles C Thomas, Publisher, 1955.
Lerner, P. I., and Weinstein, L.: Infective endocarditis in the antibiotic era. New Eng. J. Med., *274*:199, 323, 388; 1966.
Rodbard, S.: Blood velocity and endocarditis. Circulation, *27*:18, 1963.
Ziment, I.: Nervous system complications in bacterial endocarditis. Amer. J. Med., *47*:593, 1969.

SALMONELLA INFECTIONS
Bennett, I. L., Jr., and Hook, E. W.: Infectious diseases (some aspects of salmonellosis). Ann. Rev. Med., *10*:1, 1959.
Black, P. H., Kunz, L. J., and Swartz, M. N.: Salmonellosis—a review of some unusual aspects. New Eng. J. Med., *262*:811, 864, 921; 1960.
Gill, F., Kaye, D., and Hook, W.: The influence of erythrophagocytosis on the interaction of macrophages and salmonella *in vitro.* J. Exp. Med., *124*:173, 1966.
Greisman, S., Hornick, R. B., Carozza, F. A., Jr., and Woodward, T. E.: The role of endotoxin during typhoid fever and tularemia in man. I. Acquisition of tolerance to endotoxin. J. Clin. Invest., *42*:1064, 1963.
Hook, E. W.: Salmonellosis: Certain factors influencing the interaction of salmonella and the host. Bull. N.Y. Acad. Med., *37*:499, 1961.
Kaye, D., and Hook, E. W.: The influence of hemolysis on susceptibility to salmonella infections: Additional observations. J. Immun., *91*:518, 1963.

SYPHILIS
Clark, E. G., and Danbolt, N.: The Oslo study of the natural history of untreated syphilis. J. Chronic. Dis., *2*:311, 1955.
Merritt, H. H., Adams, R. D., and Solomon, H.: Neurosyphilis. New York, Oxford University Press, 1946.
Turner, T. B.: Syphilis and the treponematoses. In Mudd, S. (Ed.): Infectious Agents and Host Reactions. Philadelphia, W. B. Saunders Co., 1970.
Yobs, A., Clark, J. W., Jr., Mothershed, S. E., Bullard, J. C., and Artley, C. W.: Further observations on the persistence of *Treponema pallidum* after treatment in rabbits and humans. Brit. J. Vener. Dis., *44*:116, 1968.

PNEUMONIA
Benson, H., Akbarian, M., Adler, L. A., and Abelmann, W. H.: Hemodynamic effects of pneumonia. I. Normal and hypodynamic responses. J. Clin. Invest., *49*:791, 1970.
Bocles, J. S., Ehrenkranz, N. J., and Marks, A.: Abnormalities of respiratory function in varicella pneumonia. Ann. Intern. Med., *60*:183, 1964.
Davidson, F. F., Glazier, J. B., and Murray, J. F.: The components of the alveolar-arterial oxygen tension difference in normal subjects and in patients with pneumonia and obstructive lung disease. Amer. J. Med., *52*:754, 1972.
Herzog, H., Staub, H., and Richterich, R.: Gas-analytical studies in severe pneumonia. Observations during the 1957 influenza epidemic. Lancet, *1*:593, 1959.
Marshall, R., and Christie, R. V.: The visco-elastic properties of the lungs in acute pneumonia. Clin. Sci., *13*:403, 1954.
Mellemgaard, K.: The mechanism of hypoxemia in lobar pneumonia. Scand. J. Resp. Dis., *48*:109, 1967.
Triebwasser, J. H., Harris, R. E., Bryant, R. E., and Rhoades, E. R.: Varicella Pneumonia in Adults. Report of seven cases and review of the literature. Medicine, *46*:409, 1967.
Wood, W. B., Jr.: Studies on the cellular immunology of acute bacterial infections. The Harvey Lectures, Series *XLVII*:72, 1951–52.

INFECTIONS OF THE CENTRAL NERVOUS SYSTEM
Bodian, D.: Histopathologic basis of clinical findings in poliomyelitis. Amer. J. Med., *6*:563, 1949.
Denny-Brown, D., Adams, R. D., and Fitzgerald, P. J.: Pathologic features of *Herpes zoster.* Arch. Neurol. Psychiat., *51*:216, 1944.
Dodge, P. R., and Swartz, M. N.: Bacterial meningitis. II. Special neurological problems, post meningitic complications and clinicopathological correlations. New Eng. J. Med., *272*:954, 1003; 1965.
Fishman, R. A.: Carrier transport of glucose between blood and cerebrospinal fluid. Amer. J. Physiol., *206*:836, 1964.
Harter, D. H., and Petersdorf, R. G.: A consideration of the pathogenesis of bacterial meningitis: Review of experimental and clinical studies. Yale J. Biol. Med., *32*:280, 1960.
Hope-Simpson, R. E.: The nature of *Herpes zoster.* A long-term study and a new hypothesis. Proc. Roy. Soc. Med., *58*:9, 1965.
Horstmann, D. M., McCollum, R. W., and Mascola, A. D.: Viremia in human poliomyelitis. J. Exp. Med., *99*:355, 1954.
Lincoln, E. M., and Sewell, E. M.: Tuberculosis of the meninges and central nervous system. *In:* Tuberculosis in Children. New York, McGraw-Hill Book Co., 1963.
Miller, L. H., and Brunnel, P. A.: Zoster, reinfection or activation of latent virus? Observations on the antibody response. Amer. J. Med., *49*:480, 1970.
Montani, S., and Perret, C.: Lactic acidosis of the cerebrospinal fluid in bacterial meningitis. Schweiz. Med. Wschr., *94*:1552, 1964.
Petersdorf, R., and Harter, D.: The fall in cerebrospinal fluid sugar in meningitis. Arch. Neurol., *4*:21, 1961.
Swartz, M. N., and Dodge, P. R.: Bacterial meningitis—a review of selected aspects. I. General clinical features, special problems, and unusual meningeal reactions mimicking bacterial meningitis. New Eng. J. Med., *272*:725, 779, 842, 898; 1965.
Weinstein, L.: Cardiovascular disturbances in poliomyelitis. Circulation, *15*:735, 1957.
Weinstein, L.: Influence of age and sex on susceptibility and clinical manifestations in poliomyelitis. New Eng. J. Med., *257*:47, 1957.
Weller, T. H., Witton, H. M., and Bell, E. J.: The etiologic agents of varicella and *Herpes zoster.* Isolation, propagation, and cultural characteristics *in vitro.* J. Exp. Med., *108*:843, 1958.

OSTEOMYELITIS
Collins, D. H.: *In* Dodge, O. G. (Ed.): Pathology of Bone. London, Butterworth, 1966.
Diggs, L. W.: Bone and joint lesions in sickle cell disease. Clin. Orthop., *52*:119, 1967.
Trueta, J.: The three types of acute hematogenous osteomyelitis: a clinical and vascular study. J. Bone Joint Surg., *41B*:671, 1959.
Waldvogel, F. A., Medoff, G., and Swartz, M. N.: Osteomyelitis—clinical features, therapeutic considerations, and unusual aspects. New Eng. J. Med., *282*:198, 260, 316; 1970.

CHAPTER 22
PATHOPHYSIOLOGY OF HEMATOLOGIC DISORDERS

ALLAN J. ERSLEV
THOMAS G. GABUZDA

INTRODUCTION

Hematology is traditionally defined as the study of the formed elements of blood. However, this subspecialty has such close ties with the fluid phase of blood and with the function and kinetics of other organ systems that it has been increasingly difficult to establish its pathophysiologic limits. The erythrocytes need the cooperation of the cardiac output, pulmonary capacity, vascular reactivity, and renal function in order to bring oxygen to the tissues; the granulocytes need a host of supporting plasma factors for their phagocytic mission; the lymphocytes produce and react with gamma globulins; and the thrombocytes can functionally not be separated from the coagulation factors. With this in mind, an attempt will be made here to correlate structure, function, and kinetics of the formed elements of blood with those of other organ systems and with overall human pathophysiology. This correlation and its documentation must of necessity be of an introductory nature, but it is hoped that it will stimulate the reader to seek more in depth information from the many current textbooks and monographs available.

BONE MARROW

The formed elements of blood constitute an organ of considerable size and complexity. On an average this organ measures about 30 ml. per kg. body weight and if the active bone marrow, measuring about 20 ml. per kg. body weight, is added it reaches a size of about twice that of the liver. The addition of spleen, lymph nodes, and reticuloendothelial tissues would further swell the size and importance of the hematologic system. However, the lymphoreticular tissues are treated elsewhere in this book—a somewhat artificial separation, since it seems probable that lymphocytes, both T cells and B cells, and macrophages are in part bone marrow-derived cells. Although the lymphocytes in patients with chronic granulocytic leukemia do not have the characteristic Philadelphia chromosome present in the other bone marrow cells, this presumably does not suggest a fundamental difference but rather suggests an origin of the lymphocytes from a stem cell proximal to the multipotential bone marrow stem cells responsible for the production of erythroid, myeloid, and megakaryocytic cells.

With the exception of lymphocytes, blood cell formation in the normal adult is the exclusive prerogative of bone marrow cavities. Other areas can support hematopoiesis, but the bones appear to provide an optimal environment for differentiation and multiplication of blood cells. Before bone cavities form during the fifth fetal month, blood cell formation takes place first in the yolk sac and then in the liver (Fig. 22-1). During the brief yolk-sac phase the erythrocytes produced are nucleated and contain an embryonic hemoglobin $\alpha_2\epsilon_2$, but the subsequent crops of fetal erythrocytes produced by the liver, spleen, and bone marrow are non-nucleated and contain fetal hemoglobin with $\alpha_2\gamma_2$ polypeptide chains. Although the spleen in the human fetus plays only a brief role in hematopoiesis between the third

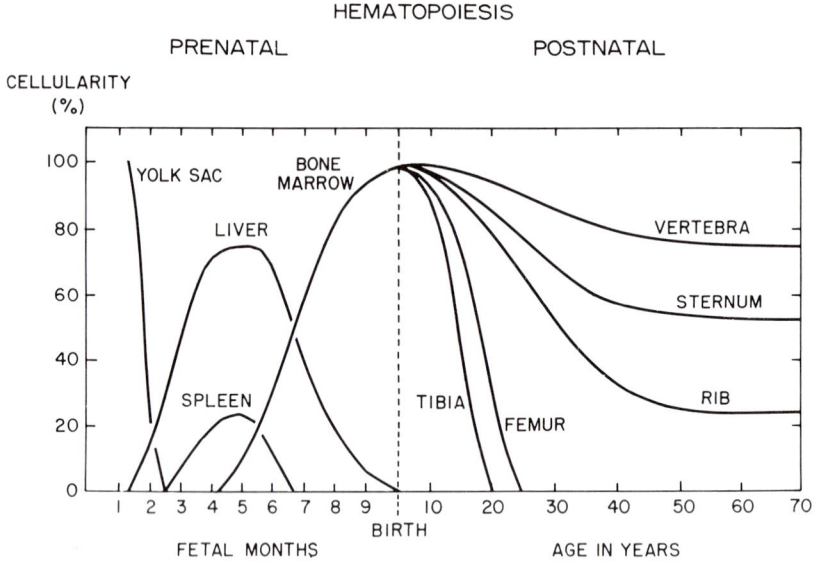

Figure 22-1 Expansion and regression of hematopoietic tissue during fetal and adult life.

and the seventh months, the splenic microcirculation appears to be well suited for blood cell formation, and the spleen serves as the principal back-up organ for the bone marrow. At time of birth the splenic and hepatic phases have ceased, the slow transformation from fetal to adult hemoglobin production is under way, and all bone cavities are actively involved in blood cell formation.

For the first few years of life there is a precarious balance between the need for blood cells of a rapidly growing infant and the available bone marrow space, and reactivation of hepatic and splenic hematopoiesis takes place whenever there is an increased demand for blood cell formation. At about the age of 4 the growth of bone cavities has outstripped the growth of the circulating blood cell mass, and fatty reserve bone marrow becomes noticeable. Fatty replacement occurs first in the diaphysis of the peripheral long bones, then slowly creeps centripetally until at the age of about 18 hematopoietically active bone marrow is found only in the vertebrae, ribs, sternum, skull, and proximal epiphysis of the long bones. This obviously must mean that the available bone marrow space has continued to grow faster than the circulating blood cell mass, since the ratio between progenitor cells in the marrow and mature cells in the circulation is the same at all ages. In support of this assumption are measurements by Hudson which indicate that the volume of bone marrow cavities increases from about 1.5 per cent of body weight at birth to about 4.5 per cent of body weight in the adult, while the blood volume actually decreases from about 8 per cent of body weight at birth to about 7 per cent of body weight in the adult. During adult life the expansion of bone cavities continues, owing to bone resorption, and there is a gradual increase in the amount of fatty tissue present in all bone marrow areas. Because of the abundant bone marrow space, compensatory reactivation of extramedullary sites rarely takes place in later life, even during periods of accelerated hematopoietic activity. When present, extramedullary hematopoiesis often indicates inappropriate rather than compensatory blood formation.

Structurally, the bone marrow consists of a delicate pattern of vessels and nerves, of reticuloendothelial cells, of differentiated and undifferentiated progenitor cells, and of fatty tissue serving as a space-occupying filler. The vascular network consists of arterioles emptying into a complex sinusoidal venous system which drains into a central collecting vein. Blood cell formation takes place outside the sinusoidal system and finished cells have to pass through narrow openings in the endothelial vascular lining in order to enter the circulation (Fig. 22-2). This sievelike barrier may play a role in the erythroblastic nuclear extrusion and may also control the release of newly formed red cells.

Measurements of blood flow and hematopoietic activity have shown a close relationship between cellular production and blood supply, and some interesting experiments by Huggins suggest that this relationship goes in both directions and that induced vascularization is followed by increased hematopoietic activity. Huggins and coworkers implanted the tip of a rat's tail into the abdominal cavity or enclosed it in a heating chamber and found after some weeks that the inactive fatty marrow had become red and hematopoietically active. The conclusion from these experiments was initially that the low peripheral temperature in the long bones impairs blood cell formation and is responsible for the centripetal regression of active marrow in the adult. However, fatty marrow appears in the fingers even before birth and active marrow is found in peripheral epiphyses when more proximal diaphyses are completely inactive. It seems more likely that temperature, among other variables, controls vascularization, which in turn determines the hematopoietic activity. In support of this hypothesis is the observation by Knospe and coworkers that recovery of an irradiated or mechanically injured marrow always is preceded by endothelial regeneration and vascular restoration, and that irreversible endothelial injury leads to local bone marrow aplasia despite the

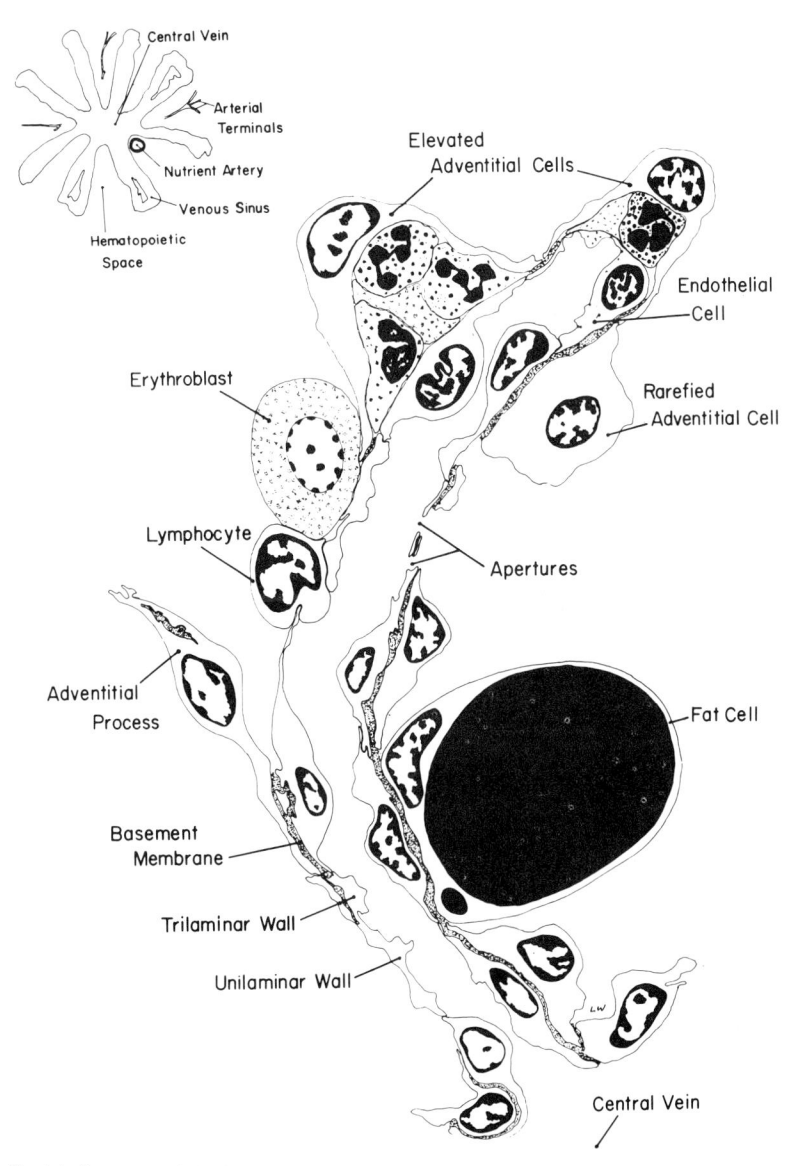

Figure 22-2 Sketch in upper left depicts cross section of bone marrow with spokelike sinusoids draining into a control longitudinal vein. Larger sketch depicts sinusoidal basement membrane covered on both sides by reticular cells acting as phagocytes, as "nurse" cells to hematopoietic elements, and as guards of the fenestrations in the basement membrane. (From Weiss, L.: In Gordon, A. S. (Ed.): Regulation of Hematopoiesis. Vol. 1. New York, Appleton-Century-Crofts, 1970.)

presence of hematopoietic stem cells in other bone marrow areas.

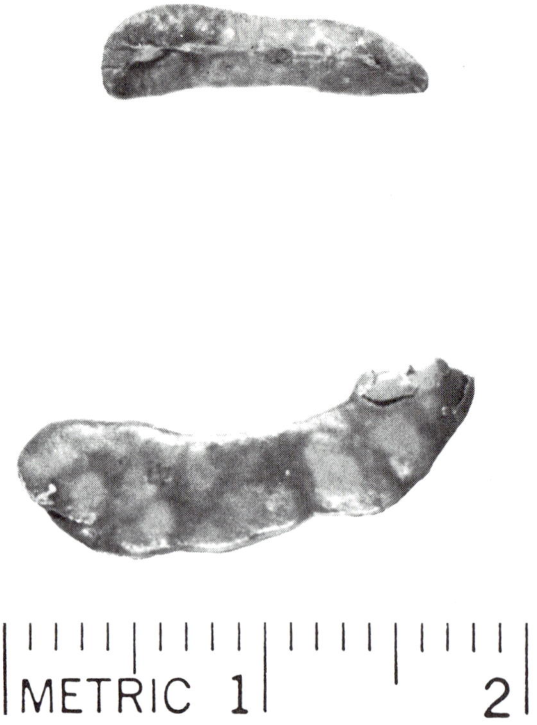

The nervous supply to the bone marrow is quite extensive, as everyone having been exposed to bone marrow aspiration can attest to. Some of the nerves are in close contact with the hematopoietic islands and may sense pressure changes caused by cellular proliferation. If such signals are transmitted to the nerves which are attached to the vessel walls, an autoregulatory system may well exist, adjusting the blood flow to permit undisturbed proliferation and maturation before the cells are released into the circulation.

The fatty tissue which in the adult fills about 50 per cent of the bone cavities probably serves merely as a space-occupying material. Attempts have been made to assign primary regulatory functions to it, but the evidence presented so far has been unimpressive. The remaining 50 per cent of the bone marrow is made up of reticuloendothelial and hematopoietic cells.

As described in the chapter on the spleen and reticuloendothelial tissues, the bone marrow is one of the major lymphoreticuloendothelial organs and is involved in antigen processing, cellular and humoral immunity, and the recognition and removal of senescent cells. The lymphoreticuloendothelial cells may possibly also serve as stem cells for the production of differentiated hematopoietic cells. As described by Boggs and Chervenick, the self-perpetuating hematopoietic stem cell pool is currently believed to consist of multipotential cells and of unipotential cells committed to erythropoiesis, myelopoiesis, or thrombopoiesis. Since administration of tritiated thymidine in doses which will cause radiation-induced "suicide" of all cells actively synthesizing DNA will not destroy multipotential stem cells, it is believed that these cells provide a dormant bone marrow reserve. Under conditions of bone marrow depletion or injury they become activated and enter a regenerative and differentiating cell cycle. Such a sequence of events was first described by Till and McCulloch in their classic observations of the spleens of irradiated mice in which surviving or transplanted marrow attempts to replenish the hematopoietic tissues. Initially, the few available stem cells enter into intense proliferative activity and produce minute clonal colonies of undifferentiated stem cells. After the fifth day, specific differentiation takes place and discrete bone marrow colonies can be observed macroscopically on the surface of the spleen and microscopically in the parenchyma of the spleen and the bone marrow (Fig. 22-3). Since chromosomal studies have shown conclusively that each colony is derived from a single stem cell, it is possible to quantitate the number of multipotential stem cells present initially. In the mouse, it has been estimated that there are about 1 to 3 multipotential stem cells per 1000

Figure 22–3 Each white raised plaque on the surface of the lower mouse spleen contains a colony of bone marrow cells. These colonies were found 7 days after total body radiation immediately followed by a transfusion of bone marrow cells obtained from an isogeneic donor. Each colony is derived from a single sequestered multipotential stem cell. The upper spleen is a normal control.

nucleated bone marrow cells, or about 1 per 100 nucleated red blood cells.

Recent studies by Fliedner and coworkers employing complete cellular labeling with tritiated thymidine have helped in establishing the morphologic identity of the multipotential stem cells. Tritiated thymidine was given continually in small amounts until all bone marrow cells became labeled. After discontinuation of the thymidine administration the label of differentiated hematopoietic cells decreased and disappeared, suggesting rapid cellular turnover, while the label of endothelial cells, reticular cells, and lymphocytes remained unchanged. However, when cellular injury or depletion had caused stem cell activation, the label of small mononuclear-lymphocyte-like cells also decreased, suggesting that these are the cells responsible for cellular renewal and bone marrow regeneration.

Studies on the distribution and composition of bone marrow colonies in the spleen have also provided valuable information about the interrelationship between parenchymal structure and cellular differentiation. Each colony is made up of a mixture of hematopoietic cellular elements, usually with one cell type dominating. Although the specific differentiation probably is determined by humoral stimuli, it has been demonstrated by Trentin that the immediate cellular environment or HIM (hematopoietic inductive microenvironment) modifies the effectiveness of the stimuli. Colonies derived from stem cells lodged on the surface of the spleen are primarily erythroid, while colonies from cells lodged in the center of the spleen or in the bone marrow are primarily myeloid and megakaryocytic. This effect of the microenvironment on cellular differentiation is undoubtedly of major importance for normal hematopoiesis but it is not known whether it is caused by a modification of the activities of stem cells or of differentiated cells.

The unipotential stem cells have been shown by the use of "suicide" techniques to be in active cell cycle and capable of self-renewal for a considerable period of time. However, they need the stimulus of a humoral "poietin" in order to undergo blast transformation and further differentiation. Erythropoietin is known to be the specific "poietin" for stem cells committed to erythropoiesis. Erslev has recently reviewed the mounting evidence for the existence of a leukopoietin and a thrombopoietin responsible for the differentiation of stem cells committed to granulocytopoiesis and thrombopoiesis, respectively.

The mode of action of these poietins is not clear. Kretchmar has suggested that the poietins act by regulating the rate of entry of resting G_0 cells into mitosis (Fig. 22–4). However, it has been shown that the unipotential stem cells are proliferating continuously even in the absence of stimulating poietins. An alternate explanation would be that the poietins act by causing blast transformation and differentiation of newly formed stem cells. In order to accept either explanation the mitotic divisions of the unipotential stem cells must be unequal, with one daughter cell destined to replace the dividing mother cell and the other destined to differentiate or to die (Fig. 22–4). Recent studies, summarized by Craddock and coworkers, provide some support for this latter assumption by showing the presence of very short-lived "lymphocytes" in the bone marrow.

The newly formed proerythroblasts and myeblasts will subsequently undergo three to five mitotic divisions, resulting in an 8- to 32-fold multiplication (Fig. 22–5). The nucleus of the megakaryoblast will undergo the same number of endomitotic divisions, resulting in the formation of a few huge cells with multilobed nuclei. Concomitant with nuclear proliferation the cytoplasm will undergo specific maturation and 3 to 5 days after the initial differentiation the cells are almost completely mature and functional.

The maturing reticulocyte and the maturing granulocytes remain in the bone marrow for some days before they are released into the circulation. The length of this delay appears to be responsive to the immediate needs for circulating blood cells. However, because the circulating granulocyte mass is much smaller than the circulating red cell mass, a premature release of the marrow reserve of maturing cells is of importance only for the functional adjustment of the peripheral granulocyte count. After the release from the bone marrow, the erythrocytes are all in active use in circulating blood, while about 50 per cent of the granulocytes and 30 per cent of the thrombocytes are sequestered in the microvasculature or in the spleen as functional reserves. Figure 22–6 and Table 22–1 give a summary of the cellular mor-

Figure 22–4 Proposed actions of poietins in the differentiation of stem cells. The differentiation of multipotential stem cells to committed unipotential stem cells is believed to be the result of an HIM-induced mitotic division in a dormant G_0 cell (I). The differentiation of committed stem cells by erythropoietin, leukopoietin, or thrombopoietin may also involve the induction of a mitotic division (I). However, since the unipotential stem cells appear to be in a state of continuous proliferation, the poietin may cause differentiation without division (II). In both cases, the mitotic divisions in the stem cell pool must be unequal, with one daughter cell destined to differentiate or die and the other to replace the mother cell.

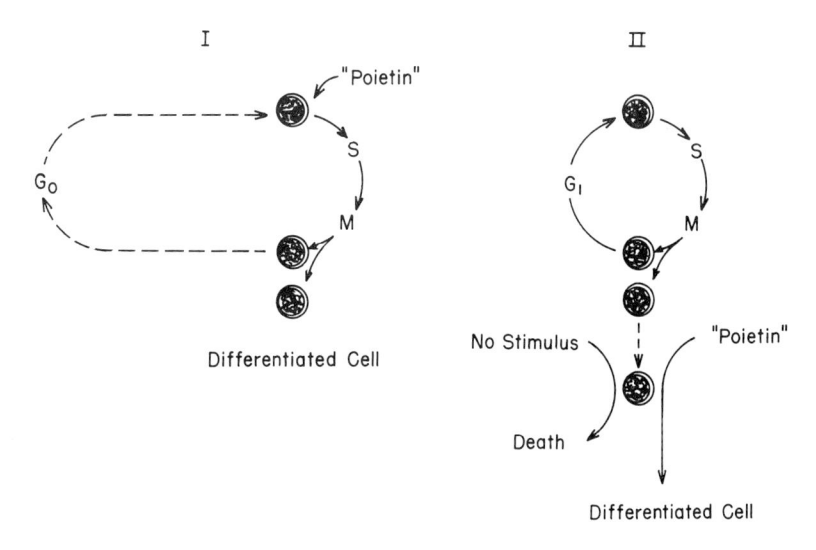

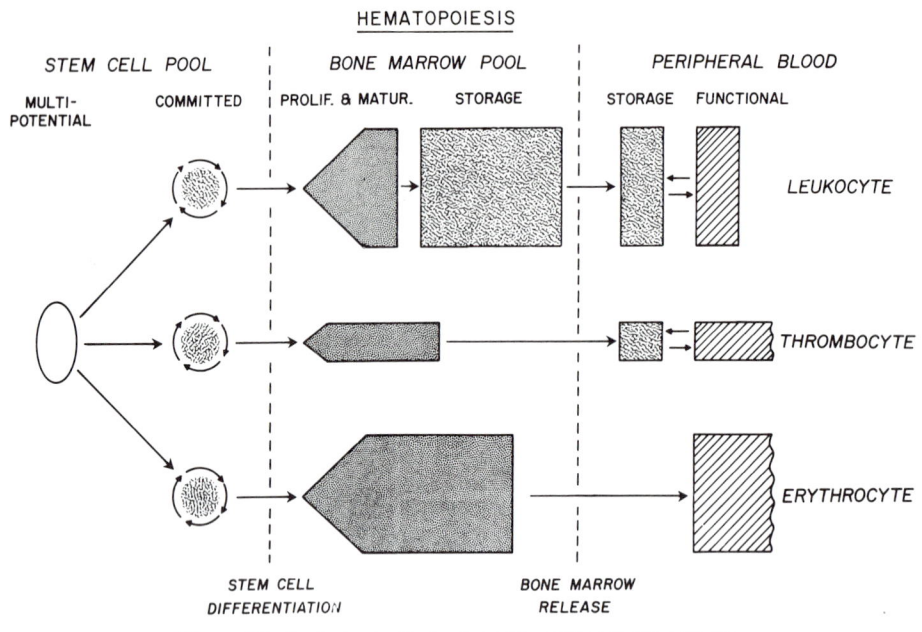

Figure 22-5 A dynamic model of hematopoietic activity.

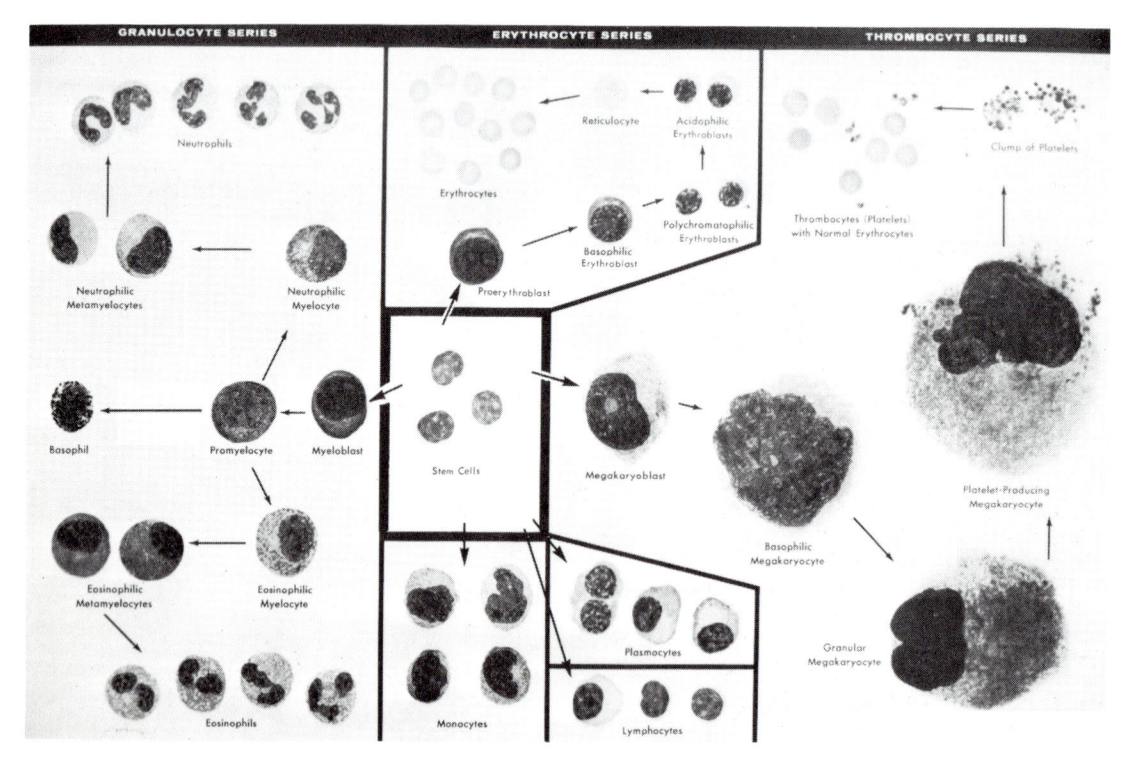

Figure 22-6 Morphologic appearance of hematopoietic cells. (Adapted from chart "Maturation of Human Blood Cells, M4-60" prepared by Eastman Kodak Co., Rochester, N.Y.)

TABLE 22-1 BONE MARROW-DERIVED CELLS

	Number of Cells in 10^9 per kg. Body Weight		
	Erythroid	Myeloid	Megakaryocytic
Proliferating cells	2.0	3.0	0.006
Marrow reserve	8.0	7.5	–
Circulating pool	333.0	0.4	15.0
Circulating reserve	–	0.3	5.0
Daily production and destruction	3.0	1.5	2.5

phology and composition of the hematopoietic tissue. The apparent discrepancy between the 1:1 ratio between erythroid and myeloid cells and the 1:3 ratio found in bone marrow smears is caused by the fact that the bone marrow reticulocytes are included in Table 22-1 but usually not in bone marrow differential counts.

ERYTHROCYTES

STRUCTURE

The ultrastructure of the erythroid cells has by now been so closely correlated with metabolic activities that structure and function cannot be separated and will be dealt with together in this chapter. However, the morphology of blood cells stained with the Romanovsky dyes deserves some separate remarks, since stained blood and bone marrow smears are cornerstones in the clinical management of patients with hematologic disorders.

The earliest nucleated red blood cell, the proerythroblast is a large cell with a diameter of about 20 to 25 μ and a nucleus occupying about three fourths of the cell (Fig. 22-6). The nuclear chromatin, stained dark violet with the usual Wright or Giemsa stain, is finely dispersed, and the nucleus with its one or several nucleoli is clearly separated from the deep-blue cytoplasm by a distinct membrane. The nucleus is usually perfectly round and the cytoplasm devoid of granules. The subsequent proliferation and maturation through the stages of basophilic, polychromatophilic, and orthochromatic erythroblasts are characterized by a stepwise reduction in cellular and nuclear size, by a condensation of the nuclear chromatin into well-defined chunks, and by a dilution of the blue staining cytoplasmic ribosomes with newly synthesized hemoglobin. At the orthochromatic stage, the nucleus has become condensed into a small pyknotic mass and is extruded. Hemoglobin synthesis continues for a few more days until the nucleus-dependent synthetic machinery is exhausted. During this period precipitation and condensation of the remaining basophilic ribosomes with oxidant dyes such as brilliant cresyl blue and methylene blue will result in the characteristic appearance of the reticulocyte on a blood smear. The final transformation of reticulocytes to mature cells is associated with a considerable loss in volume due to cytoplasmic dehydration and loss of cellular membrane.

The mature erythrocyte is a biconcave disc with an average diameter of about 8 μ and a central pallor occupying the middle third of the cell. Owing to a relative excess of surface over volume, the cell is soft and pliable, accounting for the ease with which it can pass through tissue capillaries and splenic fenestrations and diameters considerably less than its own. Its membrane has a remarkable self-healing capacity, and red cell injury may cause the production of viable fragments rather than intravascular hemoglobin leakage. As the cell grows older it becomes slightly more dense, but it maintains its normal pliable biconcave appearance until enzymatic failure leads to rigidity, reticuloendothelial trapping, and destruction.

FUNCTION

Erythroblasts

Erythroblastic function is exclusively inner-directed. Each proerythroblast is programed to undergo 3 to 4 mitotic divisions and to synthesize hemoglobin until its 8 to 16 daughter cells contain about 300 million hemoglobin molecules each. This program has general and special metabolic requirements. The general requirements are common to all actively proliferating cells and include the building blocks and coenzymes needed for cellular construction. The special requirements are those needed for the synthesis of hemoglobin molecules and of enzymes designed to protect the integrity and function of these molecules. The various synthetic functions and their influence on red cell production have been reviewed by Marks and Rifkind and will be described later.

Erythrocytes

The red blood cells are usually considered to be functionally quite unsophisticated, since their only obligations appear to be the transport and protection of the oxygen-carrying pigment, hemoglobin. Nevertheless, the survival of cells containing neither nuclei nor mitochondria for about 4 months in a high oxygen and sodium environment demands the presence of efficient metabolic defenses and long-lived enzymes. The cargo of enzymes provided during the nucleated phase of development has to provide sufficient energy to maintain hemoglobin iron in its active ferrous state; to power the cation pump needed to maintain intracellular sodium and potassium concentrations despite the presence of unfavorable concentration gradients; to keep the sulfhydryl groups of globins, enzymes, and membranes in an active reduced state; and to preserve the integrity of the membrane. The metabolic pathways responsible for maintaining structure and function of the red cells will be described in the section dealing with the pathophysiology of red cell survival.

As mentioned earlier, the raison d'être for the existence of erythroid tissue and circulating red blood cells is the synthesis, transport, and protection of hemoglobin molecules. The significance of the structure of these molecules for respiratory function has been known for many years but has been understood only recently.

The hemoglobin molecule is a tetramer consisting of two α and two β polypeptide chains, each with an attached heme group. The sequential mapping of the 141 amino acids of the α chain and 146 amino acids of the β chain has been of great importance for our identification of abnormal hemoglobins with specific amino acid substitutions. However, normal function of the hemoglobin molecules and the functional impact of such amino acid substitutions was not comprehended until the spatial positioning of the chains and of the individual amino acids had been established. Recent studies initiated by the classic x-ray crystallographic observations by Perutz and coworkers have shown that each of the four chains coils into eight helices (Fig. 22-7), forming an egg-shaped molecule with a central cavity (Fig. 22-8). The polar, hydrophilic amino acid residues cover the surfaces while hydrophobic residues line four superficial pockets, each containing a heme group with its iron positioned between two histidine radicals. The proximal histidine is firmly bound to the ferrous atom while the distal histidine provides a protective and reversible link for deoxygenated iron. In our sequential nomenclature these histidine radicals are far apart (histidine 58 and 87 for α chains and histidine 63 and 92 for β chains) (Fig. 22-7), but spatially they are close together in the well of the heme pockets.

The uptake and delivery of oxygen by the hemoglobin molecules are associated with considerable spatial rearrangement of the hemoglobin molecule, and as Perutz has pointed out, the well-known oxygen dissociation curve can best be explained on the basis of such rearrangement (Fig. 22-9). The oxygen affinity of deoxygenated hemoglobin is low, and it takes a relatively large increase in oxygen tension to attach an oxygen molecule to the first heme group. However, the oxygenation of this heme group causes a widespread molecular displacement, presumably initiated by changes in the distal histidine radical which formerly was linked to the ferrous atom (Fig. 22-8). A sliding motion in the α–β contact area reduces the size of the central cavity and makes the other heme pockets more available, so

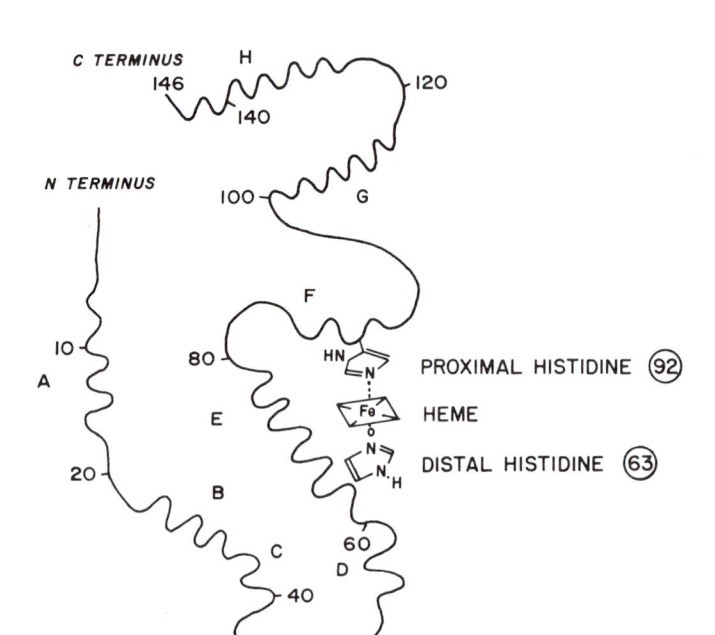

Figure 22-7 Diagram of the β polypeptide chain of hemoglobin with its eight helices (A to H) and the histidine enclosed heme group. (Adapted from Giblett, E. R.: Genetic Markers in Human Blood. Oxford, Blackwell Scientific Publications, 1969, p. 349.)

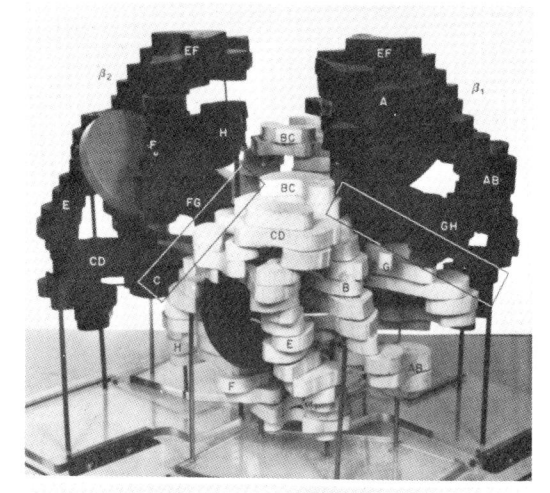

Figure 22-8 Model of the hemoglobin molecule depicting the α–β contact areas and the sliding motions which occur in the transformation from a deoxygenated form with a large central cavity (*top*) to an oxygenated form with a smaller cavity (*bottom*). (From Muirhead, H., et al.: J. Molec. Biol., *13*:646, 1965.)

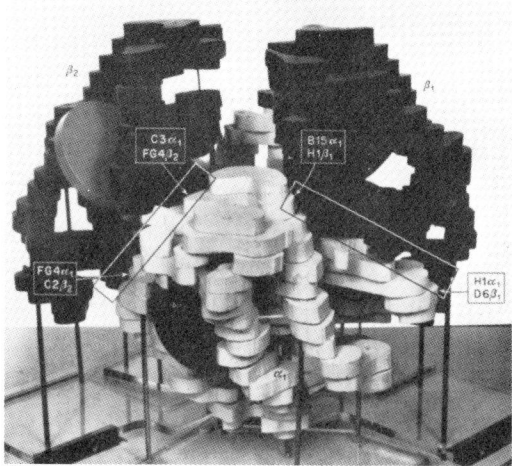

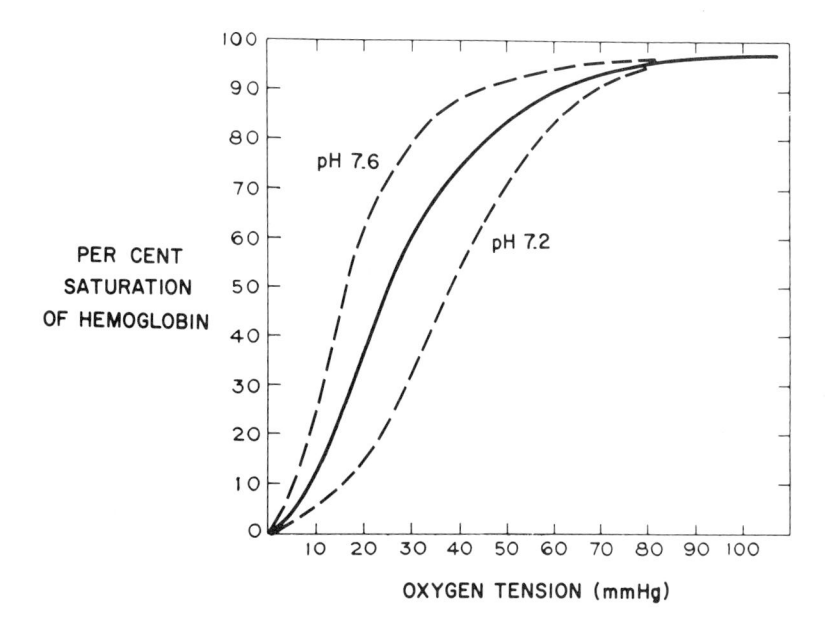

Figure 22-9 Oxygen dissociation curve of normal human blood showing the pH-dependent Bohr shift to the right (acidosis) and left (alkalosis).

that two more oxygen molecules can be attached with only slight additional increases in the oxygen tension. Further molecular rearrangement is finally responsible for the fact that the last heme group has a low oxygen affinity and demands a considerable oxygen pressure to be oxygenated.

The sequential changes in oxygen affinity are reflected in the sigmoid shape of the oxygen dissociation curve and are responsible for the ease with which hemoglobin can be loaded with oxygen in the lungs and unloaded in the tissues. Hemoglobin variants with amino acid substitution in the heme pocket or in the α–β contact area often have altered oxygen dissociation curves. If these substitutions cause a shift to the left in the curve, the oxygen affinity is increased, the tissues become hypoxic, and a compensatory polycythemia ensues. If the substitution causes a shift to the right, the oxygen affinity is decreased and the tissues can be provided with adequate amounts of oxygen at low hemoglobin concentrations. Obviously, if the amino acid substitutions involve the proximal or distal histidine in the heme pockets, much more severe changes will occur, with loss of the oxygen-carrying capacity of the heme pockets involved. The oxygen dissociation curve for hemoglobins made up by like chains such as β^4 in hemoglobin H or γ^4 in hemoglobin Bart are not sigmoid but are shifted far to the left, making these hemoglobin variants useless as oxygen carriers.

It has been known for many years that the shape of the oxygen dissociation curve is dependent on the pH (Fig. 22–9). This so-called Bohr effect is responsible for the fact that the curve is shifted to the right in the acid microenvironment of hypoxic tissues, causing an enhanced capacity to release oxygen where it is most needed. The reason for this favorable shift in the oxygen affinity of hemoglobin is related to the oxygen-dependent acidity of the hemoglobin molecule. Oxyhemoglobin is a stronger acid than deoxyhemoglobin, presumably because of oxygen-dependent ionization of certain histidine radicals. The degree of this ionization is influenced by the pH of the environment and will in turn influence the oxygen affinity.

In addition to the Bohr effect, the oxygen dissociation curve is also responsive to the intracellular concentration of certain organic phosphates. This recent discovery has explained the fact that oxygen affinity can be adapted to compensate for a decreased oxygen supply, such as at high altitudes, or an impaired oxygen supply system, such as in anemia. In both these conditions there is an increase in glycolysis and in the intracellular concentration of 2,3-diphosphoglycerate (2,3-DPG). This phosphate fits into the expanded central cavity of deoxygenated hemoglobin and impedes the transformation of deoxyhemoglobin with a low oxygen affinity to oxyhemoglobin with a high oxygen affinity. The result is that the oxygen dissociation curve shifts to the right, permitting more oxygen to be released at a certain tissue tension of oxygen. The opposite of such a facilitated oxygen unloading occurs in conditions in which the 2,3-DPG concentration is decreased, such as in stored bank blood. Here the shift of the curve is to the left, and the tissues may become hypoxic despite a normal oxygen carrying capacity of the perfusing blood.

The respiratory function of hemoglobin also includes support for carbon dioxide transport from the tissues to the lungs. Carbon dioxide will diffuse into the red cells and catalyzed by carbonic anhydrase becomes transformed into carbonic acid. The hydrogen ions of carbonic acid will be buffered by the relatively alkaline deoxyhemoglobin and the bicarbonate ion diffuses back into plasma. In the pulmonary capillary the same process in reverse will liberate carbon dioxide for pulmonary elimination. In addition to this so-called Bohr effect on carbon dioxide transport, the amino groups of globin form reversible carbamino groups with carbon dioxide and are responsible for about 10 per cent of carbon dioxide transport and excretion.

KINETICS

Self-Renewal and Differentiation

The earliest recognizable erythroid cell is the proerythroblast, but since it is synthesizing and accumulating hemoglobin from the time of its appearance, it cannot maintain itself merely through mitotic division but must be renewed from an earlier undifferentiated stem cell (Fig. 22–10). The existence of such a precursor cell is supported by the fact that nonerythroid cells in an erythropoietically inactive mouse spleen are capable of being transformed into proerythroblasts (Fig. 22–11). The morphologic identity of this precursor cell has not as yet been firmly established, but it probably is a mononuclear lymphoid cell. As described in the bone marrow section, it is replenished from an earlier multipotential stem cell pool, but it is in active cell cycle and capable of some degree of self-renewal. It is solely committed to the erythroid series, and it is generally accepted that the hormone erythropoietin will activate its potential as a proliferating and hemoglobin synthesizing cell and transform it into a proerythroblast.

The mechanism by which erythropoietin induces blast transformation is still obscure. It may directly cause a derepression of the production of a messenger RNA coded for a key enzyme in the synthesis of hemoglobin such as the production of ALA synthetase. It is also possible that it acts in-

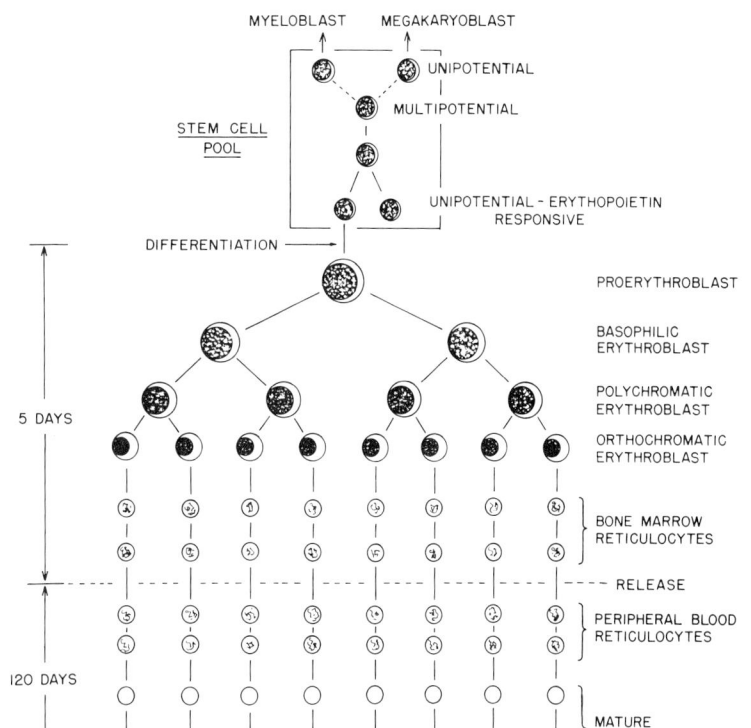

Figure 22-10 A pictorial model of the stem cell compartment and its differentiation to proliferating and maturing erythroid cells.

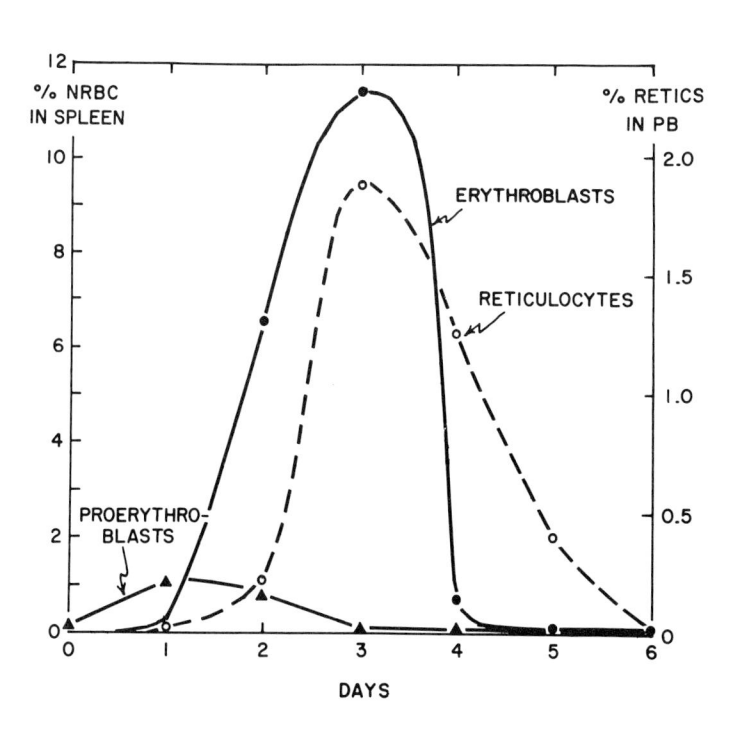

Figure 22-11 Erythropoietic effect of a single injection of erythropoietin on a mouse spleen rendered erythropoietically inactive by prior hypertransfusion. (Redrawn from Filmanowicz, E., and Gurney, C. W.: J. Lab Clin. Med., 57:65, 1961.)

directly on DNA transcription by activating a membrane adenyl cyclase, which in turn increases the production of cyclic AMP, a common second messenger for hormonal action. In either case, the activated cell will differentiate and proliferate according to a preformed program and it is questionable whether erythropoietin plays a role in the subsequent development of nucleated red blood cells.

Multiplication and Maturation

Following erythropoietin-induced blast transformation of the unipotential erythropoietin-sensitive stem cells, the emerging proerythroblast will immediately begin an integrated and controlled process of protoporphyrin production, globin-chain synthesis, iron absorption, and hemoglobin assembly. The newly formed ALA synthetase initiates synthesis of protoporphyrin in the mitochondria by condensing activated glycine and succinic acid to ALA. The final step in the synthetic chain occurs again in the mitochondria and consists of the formation of heme from protoporphyrin and iron. It has been proposed that heme exerts an end-product repression of the formation of ALA synthetase and that this feedback control system also is of importance for the integrated formation of other proteins in the proper proportions (Fig. 22–12). The predominant proteins produced are the alpha and beta chains of normal hemoglobin. Small amounts of gamma and delta chains are also synthesized, as are proteins necessary for the enzymatic generation of ATP, NADH, and NADPH.

Iron necessary for the transformation of protoporphyrin to heme is provided from iron-charged transferrin which becomes attached to specific receptors on the immature red cell membrane. The iron passes through the membrane and is immediately bound to an intracellular carrier protein while the iron-free transferrin is released and reused for shuttling iron from reticuloendothelial to erythroid cells. The intracellular iron is transported to the mitochondria for heme production or temporarily deposited as ferritin complexes in the cytoplasm. The fate of these so-called siderotic granules is not known. They may provide storage iron for further heme production, or they may be extruded and returned to the circulating iron pool.

Although transferrin-mediated delivery presumably provides adequate amounts of iron to the maturing cell, a second supply exists with iron provided by reticulum cells through direct cell-to-cell delivery. Since such an intercellular

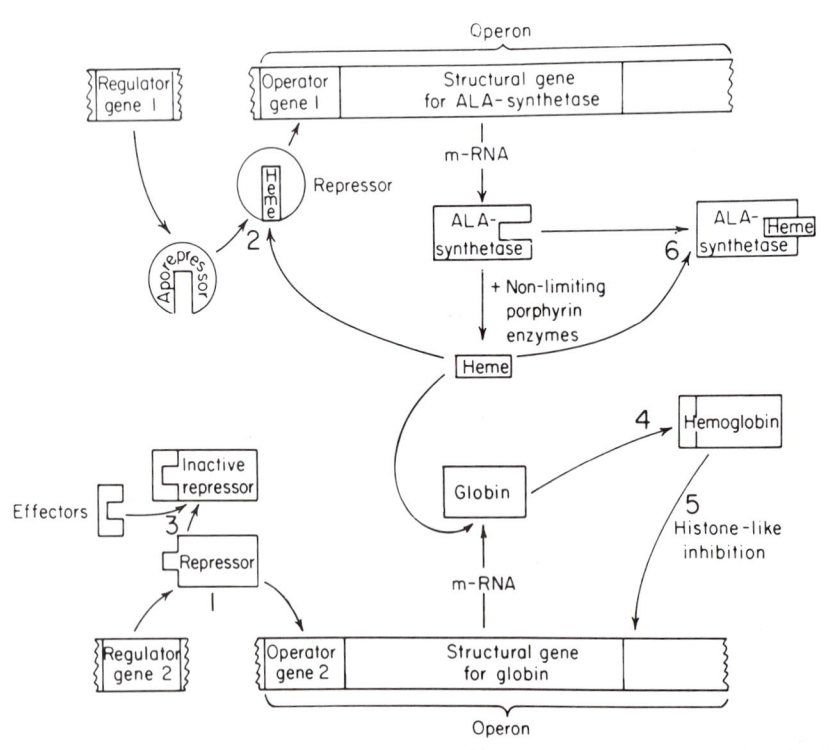

Figure 22–12 Hypothetical control of heme and globin synthesis providing end-product inhibition and coordinated production of heme and globin. (From Granick, S., and Levere, R.: Plenary Session Papers. XIIth Int. Soc. Hematol. Congress, 1968, p. 274.)

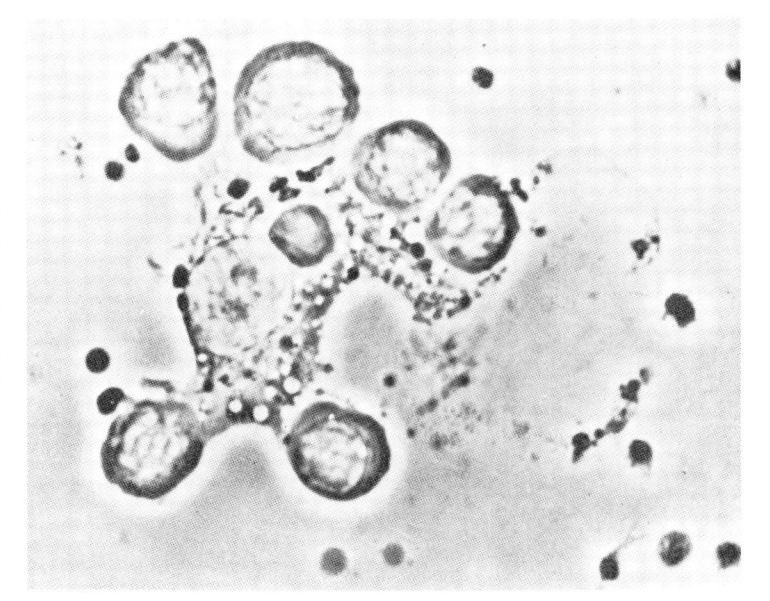

Figure 22–13 Phase contrast picture of a reticuloendothelial cell (nurse-cell) "servicing" attached erythroblasts. (From Lessin, L. S., and Bessis, M.: *In* Williams et al. (Eds.): Hematology. New York, McGraw-Hill Book Co., 1972, p. 62, by permission of Sandoz Ltd., Basel, Switzerland.)

transport system also could facilitate removal or pitting of intracellular iron by the phagocytic RE cells, the exact role played by the RE cells in cellular maturation is not clear. Nevertheless, it seems clear that erythroid development occurs in close physical proximity with RE cells (Fig. 22–13). This proximity is not always apparent from observing regular bone marrow smears, since the cells are torn apart from each other and from the thin, wide-flung cytoplasmic veil of the RE cells. However, biopsy sections and in-vitro bone marrow cultures often show the presence of characteristic erythropoietic islands, each consisting of an RE cell and nucleated red cells at the same stage of maturation. As the cells mature and proliferate, the islands increase in size until they break up and release their finished cellular products, not too dissimilar to the production of platelets from huge megakaryocytes.

Concurrently with the cytoplasmic maturation, the cell will undergo 3 to 4 mitotic divisions, causing a stepwise reduction in volume. Since all nucleated red cells are diploid, the reduction in nuclear size must be caused by a progressive condensation of nuclear protein, a condensation which eventually results in the appearance of a dense pyknotic nucleus incapable of further DNA synthesis. Occasionally in normal bone marrow and frequently in bone marrow from patients with accelerated red cell production the last division may be incomplete, with the production of a cloverleaf nucleus or satellite nuclear pieces, so-called Howell-Jolly bodies. In most non-mammalian species, the condensed nucleus is carried as an inert inclusion by the mature circulating red blood cells. In mammals, however, it is extruded by a process of intracellular demarcation and extracellular pressure. The cell is pitted either when it forces its way into the circulation through narrow endothelial openings in the bone marrow sinusoids or when it passes a similar sievelike hazard in the spleen. The extruded nucleus is surrounded by a thin layer of hemoglobin, and in patients with accelerated red cell formation the breakdown of this hemoglobin may contribute significantly to the concentration of circulating bilirubin.

After the nucleus has been extruded, hemoglobin synthesis continues but at a gradually diminishing rate for another 3 to 4 days. The cells lose membrane receptors for transferrin-iron, the mitochondria diminish in number, and the polyribosomes disaggregate. When the ribosomes finally disappear, the cells no longer show the characteristic staining qualities of a reticulocyte and they have become mature red blood cells. The cells also diminish in size, and the stickiness which characterizes immature red cells is lost. This stickiness may be caused by a coating of transferrin, and the diminishing number of iron receptors could be responsible in part for the loss of cellular cohesion and adhesion and could promote the release of cells into the circulating blood.

According to nuclear size and degree of cytoplasmic maturation, the developing bone marrow cell goes through five stages designated respectively as proerythroblasts, basophilic erythroblasts, polychromatic erythroblasts, orthochromatic erythroblasts, and bone marrow reticulocytes. Since each of the first three stages appears to be separated from the next by a mitotic division, it is possible to estimate their duration or generation time by enumerating mitotic figures. The fraction of cells in mitosis (mitotic index) depends on the duration of the mitosis (about 30 to 60 minutes) and on the generation time:

$$\text{Mitotic Index} = \frac{\text{Number of cells in mitosis}}{\text{Total number of cells}}$$

$$= \frac{\text{Mitotic time}}{\text{Generation time}}$$

The mitotic index has been measured to be about 2.5 per cent for proerythroblasts, 5 per cent for basophilic erythroblasts, and 6 per cent for polychromatic erythroblasts, and the generation times are calculated to be 30 hours, 15 hours, and 13 hours, respectively. Similar generation times have been obtained by using tritiated thymidine to label cells during their synthetic phase (lasting about 6 hours) and by employing radioautography to measure the fraction of cells labeled, the so-called labeling index. Since the orthochromatic erythroblasts and the bone marrow reticulocytes do not synthesize DNA or undergo mitotic divisions, the time spent in each of these stages is estimated from the turnover of appropriately labeled cells and is about 24 hours and 48 hours, respectively. Using a model based on these values (Fig. 22-10) one can estimate that the number of erythropoietic cells in the bone marrow is about 3 per cent of the circulating red cells, or, if the red cell mass is 30 ml. per kg. body weight and the mean red cell volume is $90\mu^3$, about 10×10^9 cells per kg. body weight. More accurate methods for enumeration of erythropoietic bone marrow cells have disclosed very similar values (Table 22-2), a numerical agreement which supports the validity of the model presented in Figure 22-10.

Part of the transformation of nucleated red cells to mature red cells takes place in circulating blood which contains about one half the reticulocyte pool. Under normal conditions, the reticulum persists for about 1 to 2 days, but in patients with accelerated red cell production, reticulocytes are released earlier and stay longer in the blood. As has been emphasized by Hillman and Finch, this has to be taken into account when reticulocytes are used to estimate the rate of red cell production. The earlier release of reticulocytes is also reflected by the fact that these so-called "stress reticulocytes" are larger and more immature than normal circulating reticulocytes and that the bone marrow transit time is shortened. It has been suggested that the early release is caused by a direct action of erythropoietin on the bone marrow release mechanism. However, it could also be due to ecologic crowding of the bone marrow by new erythroid cells derived from an overstimulated stem cell pool.

Regulation

Maturation and proliferation of nucleated red cells proceed at an integrated speed and rate. Changes in the speed of cellular maturation or in the rate of cellular proliferation could influence the total output of red cells from the bone marrow but cannot be solely responsible for the remarkable range of erythropoietic activity. A shortened maturation time or an early release of cells will only augment the circulating red cell mass slightly, and many extra mitotic divisions are needed in order to provide the bone marrow with its capacity to increase its rate of red cell production 5- to 10-fold. Since most studies indicate that an accelerated rate of red cell production is associated with a shortened transit time, it seems most unlikely that added mitotic divisions can be squeezed in. Furthermore, direct measurements of cellular generation times have suggested that the maturation and proliferation of immature red cells proceed at fixed rates independent of the overall erythropoietic activity. Consequently, it seems more likely that the rate of red cell production depends on the number of operational erythropoietic units rather than on the activity within each unit. According to this widely accepted erythropoietic quantum theory, the rate of red cell production is controlled primarily, if not exclusively, by the rate at which stem cells differentiate to proerythroblasts and initiate the formation of an erythropoietic unit.

Under normal steady-state conditions the rate of differentiation provides just enough red cells to replace the daily loss of cells. Maintenance of such a homeostatic balance demands the existence of a feedback system responsive to red cell loss and capable of inducing the necessary adjustment in the production of red cells. Occasionally the reticulocyte count displays the oscillatory pattern which characterizes all feedback control systems (Fig. 22-14), but under normal conditions the system is usually too finely tuned to be noticeable. Under pathologic conditions with in-

TABLE 22-2 ERYTHROID POOLS

Cell Types	Number of Cells in 10^9 per kg. Body Weight
Proerythroblast	0.10
Basophilic erythroblast	0.48
Polychromatophilic erythroblast	1.47
Orthochromatic erythroblast	2.95
Marrow reticulocytes	5.00
Blood reticulocytes	3.30
Mature red blood cells	330.00
Daily production and destruction	3.00

Adapted from Donohue, D. M., et al.: J. Clin. Invest., 37:1571, 1958.

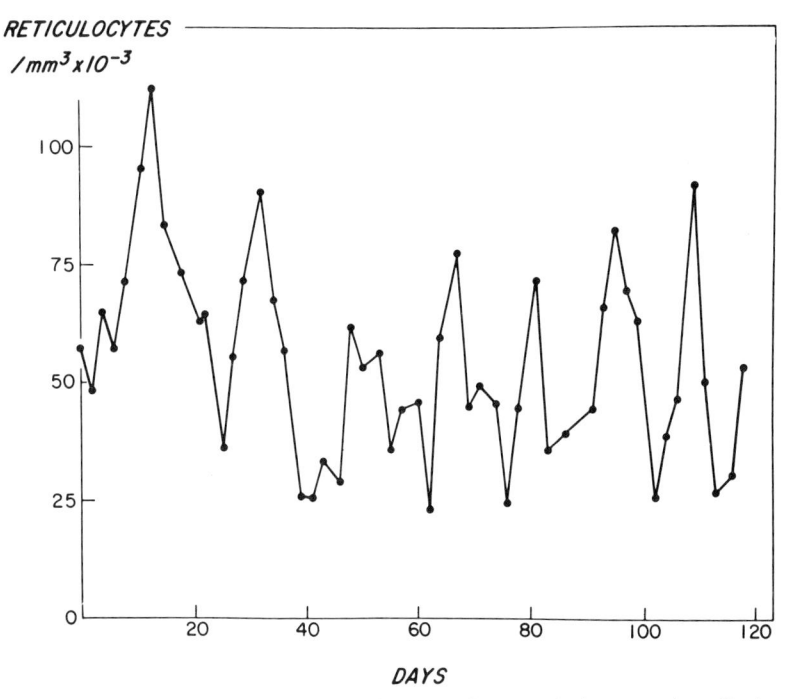

Figure 22-14 Absolute reticulocyte counts of a dog showing regularly spaced oscillations. The period is about 16 days, presumably twice the time from stem cell differentiation to reticulocyte maturation. (Redrawn from Morley, A., and Stohlman, F., Jr.: Science, *165*:1025, 1969.)

creased loss or destruction of red cells the compensatory adjustment in the rate of red cell production becomes evident. The triggering event in the activation of the adjustment must in some way be related to the physical or functional effect of red cell loss, and it has variously been suggested that red cell production is controlled by a device responsive to breakdown products of red cell destruction, to blood viscosity, to red cell volume, or to oxygen transport. Of these possibilities, a responsiveness to oxygen transport is by far the most likely, since oxygen transport is the main function of the red cell mass. Furthermore, numerous studies have shown that a decreased supply of oxygen to the tissues almost invariably is associated with an increased rate of red cell production.

The existence of an erythropoietic feedback system responsive to the tissue tension of oxygen was first suspected by Paul Bert about 100 years ago. After having studied the short-term physiologic effect of varying barometric pressures, he predicted that man living at high altitudes had to be polycythemic in order to survive the effect of low atmospheric oxygen tension. This prediction was soon confirmed by studies of the inhabitants of the high-altitude villages in Peru, and it became accepted that a low arterial oxygen tension stimulates red cell production. Supporting evidence came from the fact that many patients with chronic pulmonary disorders or with right-to-left shunts were polycythemic. Since anemia, despite normal arterial oxygen tension, is also associated with increased red cell production, it was concluded that erythropoietic stimulation is caused by tissue hypoxia due to either a decreased oxygen tension or a decreased oxygen content.

Subsequent observations of the effect of an increased supply of oxygen to the tissues showed that the rate of red cell production is suppressed and that the tissue tension of oxygen apparently influences or controls the full range of red cell production. Direct confirmation of this hypothesis has been difficult to achieve because of our ignorance of the exact cellular location of the oxygen sensor. Measurements of the oxygen tension of subcutaneous tissue have disclosed an inverse relationship between oxygen tension and erythropoietic stimulation (Fig. 22-15). However, the oxygen sensor is probably not located in the subcutaneous tissue, and measurements of the oxygen tension in the kidney, a more likely site, have not been too informative. This may be related to the fact that the oxygen sensor appears not to be responsive directly to the intercellular tissue tension of oxygen, but rather to a component of intracellular oxidative metabolism. Co-

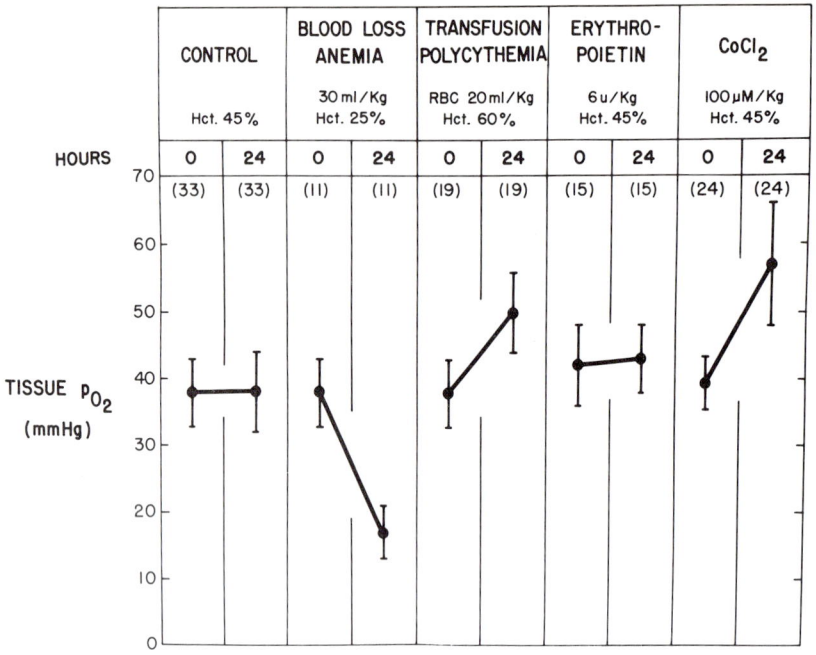

Figure 22-15 Oxygen tension of airpockets introduced subcutaneously in rats. The effects of bleeding, transfusion, erythropoietin, and cobalt on the oxygen tension are given. As expected bleeding causes hypoxia, transfusion causes hyperoxia and erythropoietin has no immediate effect. Cobalt causes tissue hyperoxia, presumably reflecting impaired oxidative utilization because of inhibited cellular oxidative metabolism.

balt chloride administration, for example, causes an accelerated rate of red cell production despite an increase in the tissue tension of oxygen (Fig. 22-15), and the triggering event for the increase in both red cell production and tissue tension of oxygen appears to be impaired intracellular oxidative metabolism and oxygen utilization.

The mechanism which links the oxygen sensor to the bone marrow has recently been clarified and appears to consist of a feedback system mediated in one direction by red cell-bound oxygen and in the opposite direction by erythropoietin, a renal erythropoietic hormone (Fig. 22-16).

The suggestion that tissue hypoxia causes the release of a humoral mediator was given its first solid experimental support in 1950 when Reissmann demonstrated that hypoxia induced in one rat of a parabiotic pair caused increased red cell production in both partners. A few years later an erythropoietic factor was found in the serum of anemic rabbits (Fig. 22-17), and since then this factor, named erythropoietin, has been isolated and partially characterized.

Erythropoietin is a glycoprotein with a molecular weight of about 35.000 and a sialic acid content of about 13 per cent. It is present in both plasma and urine of all mammals tested, and similar substances have been described in birds and fish. It has a biological half-life of about 4 to 6 hours, but its renal clearance is quite low (about 0.5 ml. per min.). Attempts to characterize and purify erythropoietin and to elucidate its site of production have been impeded by our crude and cumbersome assay technique. Agglutination inhibition tests and radioimmunoassays are being

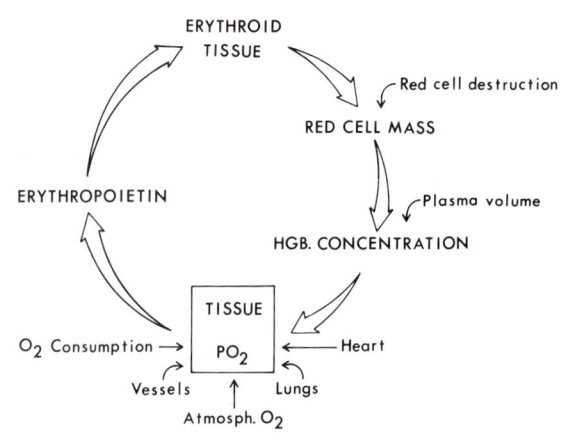

Figure 22-16 The feedback circuit which links red cell production to the tissue tension of oxygen. (From work reviewed by Erslev, A. J.: Medicine, *43*:661, 1969.)

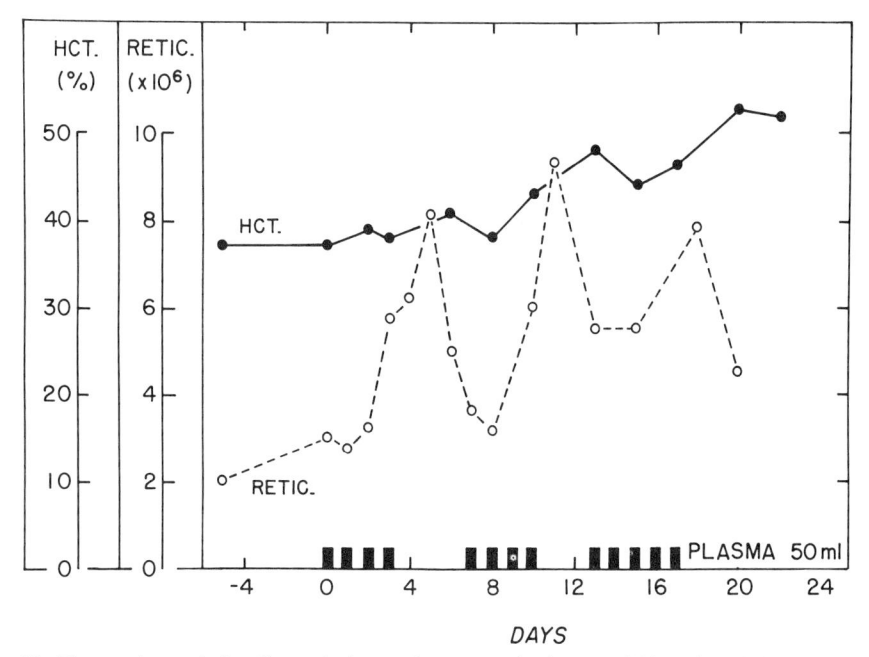

Figure 22-17 The erythropoietic effect of plasma from anemic donor rabbits when infused in large amounts to normal rabbits. (Redrawn from Erslev, A. J.: Blood, 8:349, 1953.)

developed, but the only acceptable technique for measurement at present involves bioassay in mice. This assay utilizes mice in which endogenous erythropoietin production is first abolished by transfusion or by hypoxia-induced polycythemia. The technique is unfortunately not sensitive enough to detect erythropoietin in unconcentrated serum unless the hemoglobin concentration is reduced to less than 9 grams per 100 ml. (Fig. 22-18). However, assay of urine concentrated about 50 times has shown that there is a linear relationship between the 24 hour erythropoietin excretion and the hemoglobin concentration and has also shown that the daily erythropoietin excretion in normal men is about 2 units and in normal women 3 units (Fig. 22-18).

Following the observations by Jacobson and coworkers that the production of erythropoietin ceases after bilateral nephrectomy, it has generally been accepted that erythropoietin has a renal origin. Support for this hypothesis has come from the observation that erythrocytosis occasionally occurs in patients with compromised renal blood supply or with renal ischemia due to space-occupying lesions. Although hypernephromas specifically have been reported to be a source of inappropriate production of erythropoietin, other tumors, as well as cysts or hydronephroses, have been associated with an increased rate of red cell production, and it seems more likely that erythropoietin is released by the compressed normal kidney tissues rather than by the pathologic lesion. Intrarenal injury due to experimental induction of microinfarcts or as a consequence of tissue rejection after kidney transplantation may also lead to overproduction of erythropoietin and erythrocytosis. However, the usual consequence of renal injury and renal failure is impaired erythropoietin production and anemia.

In order for the normal kidney to adjust erythropoietin production to the oxygen requirements of the body it appears that it, in addition to erythropoietin-producing tissue, also must contain an oxygen-sensitive device. The kidneys actually appear to be most unsuited to act as oxygen sensors, since their large blood flow should make them insensitive to small changes in the oxygen carrying capacity of blood. This is especially true for the cortex which, owing to plasma skimming, is perfused by blood with a high hematocrit. However, oxygen is shunted between the descending and ascending capillaries at the base of the medulla, leaving the apex of the medulla relatively hypoxic, and this area could serve as an oxygen-sensing apparatus. The fact that renal cysts made up of dilated tubules occasionally contain erythropoietin would also suggest that the site of the erythropoietin-producing tissue may reside in the medulla. However, studies of the juxtaglomerular apparatus in anemia have suggested that this may be the site of erythropoietin production, a suggestion supported by the fact that fluorescent-tagged antibodies to erythropoietin are attracted to the glomerular

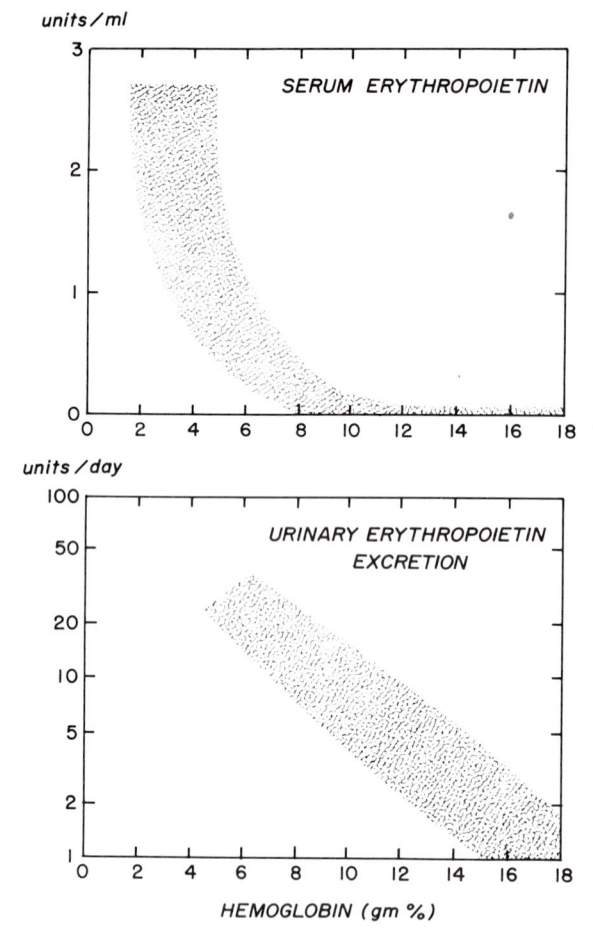

Figure 22–18 The relationship between hematocrit and the content of erythropoietin in plasma (*upper panel*) and the 24 hour excretion of erythropoietin in urine (*lower panel*).

tuft. In order to consolidate some of these observations, it has been proposed that an oxygen sensor in the medulla controls erythropoietin production in the cortex by means of a short-range releasing hormone, but so far such a hormone has not been demonstrated.

The validity of many of these observations and speculations has recently been questioned because studies of renal extracts have disclosed that kidney tissue is not erythropoietically active. A possible explanation for this surprising finding has been provided by Gordon and coworkers. They suggest that the kidney does not produce erythropoietin directly but rather produces an enzyme which is capable of transforming a circulating erythropoietin precursor into the active hormone. Considerable experimental support has been marshalled for the existence of such a renal erythropoietic enzyme, and the hypothesis has received wide acceptance because of its close analogy to the renin-angiotensinogen system and to many other cascade-activation schemes. Unfortunately, only trace amounts of erythropoietin can be generated by mixing the renal erythropoietic enzyme with normal plasma, and alternate explanations for the erythropoietic inactivity of renal homogenate may exist. One of these proposed by Erslev and coworkers is that erythropoietin is inactivated by an erythropoietin inhibitor during the processing of the kidney extract. Such an inhibitor has been demonstrated in crude renal homogenate and in its lipid component. This inhibitor is extremely powerful and could completely conceal the presence of many thousands of units of erythropoietin in kidney tissue. Whether or not this lipid inhibitor plays a physiologic role in the storage and release of erythropoietin is not known, but if erythropoietin is present in the kidneys, in an inactive lipid-bound form, practical recovery will have to await methods for inactivating the inhibitor or breaking the erythropoietin-inhibitor bond.

Recent studies of anephric animals and humans have disclosed that extrarenal erythropoietin production occurs. It amounts to a fraction of what is normally produced but the erythropoietic material produced is immunologically identical to renal erythropoietin. Since its production is enhanced by severe anemia and hypoxia, we are forced to accept the existence of both extrarenal oxygen sensors and erythropoietin-producing cells. Extrarenal erythropoietin production has been described in association with various neoplasms, particularly cerebellar hemangiomas and hepatomas, but the relationship between this inappropriate secretion by neoplastic cells and the slight but appropriate secretion found in anephric mammals is completely unknown.

The action of erythropoietin on red cell precursors is better understood, although the exact target cells have not been morphologically identified or isolated. As outlined in Figure 22–10, the target cells are undoubtedly the unipotential stem cells committed to erythroid development. Stimulating effects on other cell types have been described, but at present such effects appear to be related to increased stem cell activity rather than to a direct action of erythropoietin. Changes in granulocyte and thrombocyte counts are frequently observed under conditions of increased erythropoietin release, but these changes are temporary and may depend on a secondary activation of multipotential cells with either an increased rate of differentiation in all directions or a possible competition by the unipotential stem cell pools for the attention of the multipotent cell compartment. Since an erythropoietin-stimulated bone marrow regularly displays a shortened erythroid transit time with an early release of large immature reticulocytes, a direct effect of erythropoietin on red cell maturation and release has been postulated. However, this effect could also be caused by the rapid growth of the early erythroid cells stressing the physical capacity of bone marrow to provide room for maturing erythroid cells.

Although the capacity of renal hypoxia to generate erythropoietin and in turn to accelerate red cell production explains most clinical and experimental observations on the control of red cell production, the existence of additional regulatory mechanisms has been proposed. The pituitary, hypothalamus, and carotid bodies have all been claimed to be involved in the physiologic regulation of red cell production, but the experimental support for such neuroendocrine control is not convincing. More impressive are reports suggesting that hemolyzed red cells may exert an end product feedback stimulation on red cell production. Because of the high reticulocyte count in hemolytic anemias, it has usually been assumed that these anemias exert a more powerful stimulation on red cell production than similar anemias caused by blood loss. However, the difference in the rate of red cell production between the two kinds of anemia may actually not be as pronounced as suggested by the reticulocyte counts, since hemolysis often causes a selective destruction of old red cells, leaving relatively more reticulocytes in the circulation. Nevertheless, hemolyzed red cells do appear to have some effect on red cell production, mediated either by their iron content or by a "stimulatory" effect on the erythropoietin-producing cells in the kidney.

In summary, it appears that the main, if not only, feedback system regulating red cell production is based on the capacity of the kidneys to sense tissue hypoxia and translate this information into production of erythropoietin. Figure 22–19 shows an updated feedback model which incorporates current concepts of erythropoietin production and action and more recent information about the compensatory adjustments of oxygen transport.

PATHOPHYSIOLOGY

Definition and Classification of Anemias and Polycythemias

The anemias and polycythemias are defined as hematologic disorders with either too few or too many red cells in the circulation. Functionally, the anemias are better characterized by a reduced hemoglobin concentration, since the clinical manifestations depend on the oxygen carrying capacity of blood. The polycythemias, on the other hand, are functionally better characterized by an increased hematocrit, since the clinical

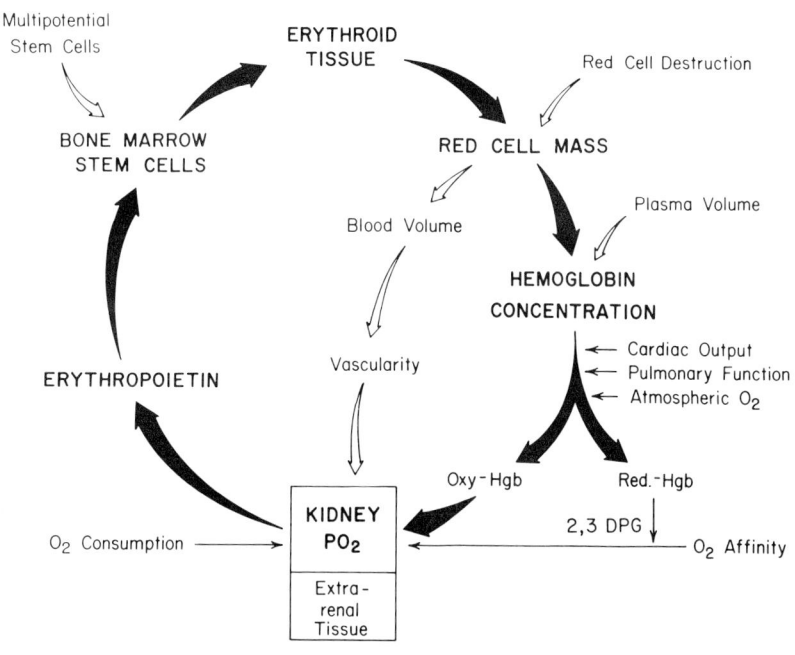

Figure 22–19 A current version of the erythropoietic feedback circuit incorporating oxygen affinity, blood volume, and stem cell pool.

manifestations are not caused by a change in oxygen delivery but rather by hypervolemia and hyperviscosity, both consequences of a high hematocrit.

Based on the size of the red cell mass, both anemias and polycythemias can be classified as either relative, caused by changes in the plasma volume, or absolute, caused by changes in the red cell mass. Strictly speaking, the relative anemias or polycythemias are not primary hematologic disorders. However, from a differential diagnostic point of view they play a considerable role in hematology.

The absolute anemias can further be classified into anemias caused by decreased production or increased destruction (decreased red cell survival), while the absolute polycythemias traditionally are subdivided into primary and secondary polycythemias. In order to emphasize the importance of cellular kinetics and function, the anemias and polycythemias are not kept separate in this chapter but are considered together in the sections dealing with the functional dynamics of various cellular elements (Table 22-3).

General Effects of Anemia

The pathophysiologic effects of a reduced oxygen carrying capacity of blood are all related to tissue hypoxia and to the compensatory mechanisms mobilized to alleviate this hypoxia. Tissue hypoxia occurs when the pressure head of oxygen in the capillaries is too low to provide distant cells with enough oxygen for their metabolic needs. This may happen despite the presence of several times the needed oxygen in the circulating blood. Using approximate figures for a normal adult, the red cell mass has to provide the tissues with about 250 ml. of oxygen per minute to support life. Since the oxygen carrying capacity of normal blood is 15×1.34 ml. or 20 ml. per 100 ml. of blood and the cardiac output is about 5000 ml. per minute, 1000 ml. of oxygen per minute is made available at the tissue level. The extraction of one fourth of this amount will reduce the oxygen tension of 100 mm. Hg in the arterial end of the capillary to 40 mm. Hg in the venous end. This partial extraction will maintain a diffusion pressure throughout the capillaries sufficient to provide all cells within a truncated cone segment with enough oxygen for their metabolism (Fig. 22-20). In anemia, the extraction of the same amount of oxygen would lead to greater hemoglobin desaturation and a lower oxygen tension at the venous end of the capillary. Since this would result in destructive cellular hypoxia or anoxia in the immediate vicinity, compensatory and frequently symptomatic adjustment in the supply of blood and oxygen must be mobilized in order to keep the oxygen gradient almost unchanged.

Decreased Oxygen Affinity. One of the earliest and least traumatic adjustments is a shift in the oxygen dissociation curve to the right, permitting the extraction of increased amounts of oxygen without a decrease in oxygen pressure. As mentioned before, the position of the oxygen dissociation curve is dependent on the intracellular pH. At an acid pH, as experienced in tissues in which incipient hypoxia has led to anaerobic metabolism and lactic acid accumulation, the curve will be shifted to the right. This shift is partly due to the direct effect of protons on the hemoglobin molecule, the so-called Bohr effect (Fig. 22-9), and partly due to a pH-dependent stimulation of red cell glycolysis with accumulation of 2,3-diphosphoglycerate. The 2,3-DPG binds to and stabilizes the hemoglobin molecule in its reduced, low-affinity state and facilitates the unloading of oxygen in the tissues. This change in oxygen affinity plays a substantial role in reducing the ar-

TABLE 22-3 CLASSIFICATION OF ANEMIAS AND POLYCYTHEMIAS

I. Relative
    Anemia of pregnancy
    Stress polycythemia

II. Absolute
  A. *Stem cell disorders*
    Multipotential
      Aplastic anemia
      Polycythemia vera
    Unipotential, erythropoietin sensitive
      Anemia of uremia
      Secondary polycythemia
  B. *Multiplication disorders*
    DNA formation
      B_{12} deficiency
      Folic acid deficiency
  C. *Maturation disorders*
    Iron supply
      Iron deficiency anemia
    Porphyric defects
      Lead poisoning
    Globin defects
      Hemoglobinopathies
      Thalassemia
  D. *Survival disorders*
    Intrinsic hemolysis
      Hereditary spherocytosis
      G-6-PD deficiency
      Hemoglobinopathies
      Paroxysmal nocturnal
        hemoglobinuria
    Extrinsic hemolysis
      March hemoglobinuria
      Microangiopathic hemolytic disease
      Acquired autoimmune hemolytic
        anemia
      Hypersplenism
    Blood loss
      Acute blood loss anemia

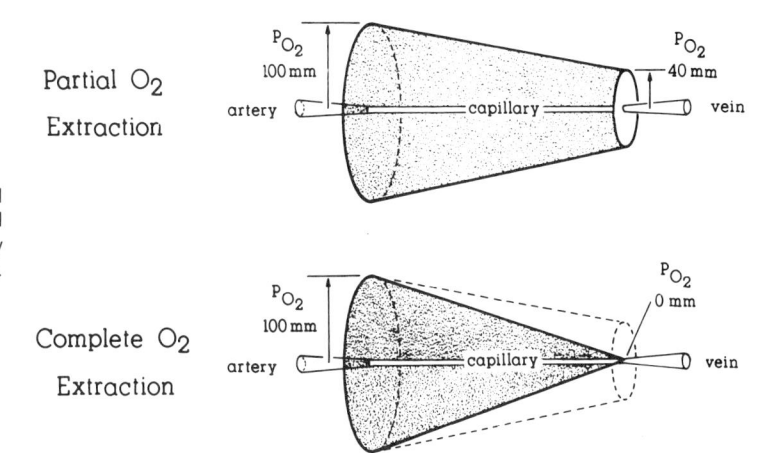

Figure 22-20 A hypothetical model of the tissue cone provided by oxygen when the blood is partially or completely extracted of oxygen.

teriovenous oxygen pressure gradient and in minimizing cellular hypoxia.

Increased Tissue Perfusion. Redistribution of blood from tissues with fairly low oxygen requirements and high blood supply such as skin or kidneys to oxygen-dependent tissues such as brain and myocardium provides an early and efficient protection of these vital tissues. The metabolic price for maintaining a high oxygen tension in some selective organs or tissues appears reasonable. Subcutaneous vasoconstriction and oxygen deprivation are tolerated well, since dermal blood supply is geared more toward temperature regulation than toward oxygen delivery. The same is true for the kidney, in which the blood supply is far in excess of the oxygen requirement. The effect on renal excretory function is relatively minor, since the decrease in blood supply is offset by the increase in "plasma crit" of the perfusing anemic blood.

Increased Cardiac Output. In mild to moderate anemia, the combined effects of decreased oxygen affinity and selective redistribution of blood maintain oxygen pressure at close to normal levels, and these anemias are usually quite asymptomatic. However, with more severe anemias it becomes necessary to increase cardiac output in order to provide the tissues with enough oxygen. Although the low viscosity of anemic blood and the peripheral vasodilation reduce the workload on the heart, the metabolic cost and the wear and tear on the moving part of the cardiac pump make an increase in cardiac output an undesirable device for long-term compensation.

The clinical manifestations of severe anemia are to a great extent caused by the compensatory cardiac overactivity. Pallor is due primarily to dermal vasoconstriction and blood redistribution, but tachycardia and symptoms of decreased cardiac reserve are related to cardiac stress. The characteristic shortness of breath of severe anemia may be a sign of incipient cardiopulmonary failure rather than a manifestation of ventilatory compensation to the anemia. Owing to the almost complete saturation of anemic blood with oxygen in the lungs, a pulmonary compensation would actually be of little practical importance.

Increased Red Cell Production. The most appropriate but also the slowest compensatory device in anemia is an increase in the rate of red cell production. Tissue hypoxia will lead to increased erythropoietin production within 4 to 7 hours, but owing to the time lag from stem cell differentiation to the release of reticulocytes from the bone marrow, a compensatory increase in the number of circulating red cells does not begin until 4 to 5 days later. Increased bone marrow activity may be associated with sternal pain or tenderness, increased erythropoietin titers in serum and urine (Fig. 22-18), and large immature reticulocytes on the blood smear.

These compensatory mechanisms are all designed to keep the capillary oxygen pressure up and the oxygen delivery adequate for the cellular needs. However, a complete rectification of tissue hypoxia cannot occur until the hemoglobin concentration has been restored to normal. Some degree of tissue hypoxia is needed in order to provide a driving force for the various compensatory devices. The symptomatology of such remaining hypoxia is difficult to separate from that of the compensatory mechanisms, but leg cramps, angina pectoris, and light-headedness appear to be caused directly by tissue hypoxia.

General Effects of Polycythemia

The pathophysiologic manifestations of polycythemia, or more correctly of erythrocytosis, are caused by hyperviscosity and hypervolemia associated with an increase in the red cell mass.

Under normal conditions, the red cell mass is maintained carefully at about 30 ml. per kg. body weight, a value which presumably must be considered optimal. The reason for not maintaining a higher red cell mass does not reside in any bone marrow limitation, since a mere doubling of the rate of red cell production would sustain a red cell mass twice normal size. The reason seems to be that an increased red cell mass will be associated with a high viscosity and sluggish flow of circulating blood.

Such sluggish blood flow is responsible in part for the tendency to thrombosis found in patients with polycythemia and would, if not compensated for, result in decreased oxygen flow to the tissues (Fig. 22-21) and obviate any benefits derived from the development of secondary polycythemia. Fortunately, the body compensates for the high viscosity by an increase in blood volume (Fig. 22-22), and the resulting vasodilation will enhance the tissue perfusion with blood and oxygen. Using measurement for cardiac output it can be shown directly that oxygen transport at a given hematocrit is greater in hypervolemic than in normovolemic dogs (Fig. 22-23). Furthermore, the optimum value for oxygen transport, which is about 45 per cent for normovolemic animals, is also increased, facilitating the mutual adjustment between hematocrit, red cell mass, and oxygen transport.

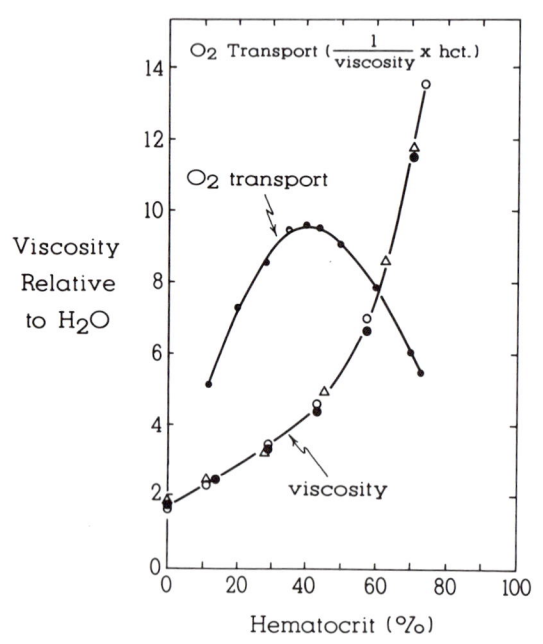

Figure 22-21 Oxygen transport as calculated from blood oxygen carrying capacity (hematocrit) and blood flow (reciprocal of viscosity).

The high blood volume in polycythemia is tolerated quite well, though symptoms such as headache, tinnitus, and dizziness and signs such as nose-bleeding and ruddy cyanosis probably are caused by the vascular dilation needed to accommodate the blood volume. Since the increase in red cell production needed to sustain a polycythemia is quite moderate, clinical or laboratory signs of bone marrow hyperactivity are usually absent. However, a slight increase in bilirubin, uric acid, and lactic dehydrogenase levels may occur, reflecting an increase in the number of red cells destroyed daily.

Stem Cell Disorders

Introduction. Under physiologic conditions, the red cell mass is maintained at an optimal size by appropriate adjustments in the rate of transformation of stem cells to nucleated red blood cells. These adjustments are accomplished by feedback systems, and a disturbance at any point in the circuits of these systems will lead to disordered stem cell function, causing anemia or polycythemia. A disordered function of the multipotential stem cells such as observed in patients with aplastic anemia or polycythemia vera is usually believed to be caused by an intrinsic defect of the stem cell itself. However, very little is known of its regulatory feedback system, and it is possible that cellular dysfunction is secondary to defective feedback signals from the immediate microenvironment.

The feedback system regulating the unipotential erythropoietin-sensitive stem cells is much better understood, and it is now possible to relate various aregenerative anemias or secondary polycythemias to defects in specific key stations in this circuit. The major distinction between regulatory disorders of the multipotential and the unipotential stem cells is that multipotential stem cell disorders are characterized by pancytopenia or pancytosis and unipotential stem cell disorders by erythrocytopenia or erythrocytosis.

Disorders of Multipotential Stem Cells

APLASTIC ANEMIA. Aplastic anemia is a bone marrow disorder characterized by a reduction in the number or function of multipotential stem cells. This reduction leads in turn to a decrease in the volume of active blood-cell–producing bone marrow and to a pancytopenia. The remaining marrow becomes confined to small, often intensely active islands surrounded by fatty tissue. This fatty replacement is the sine qua non of true aplastic anemia.

The clinical manifestations are all directly related to the pancytopenia. The anemia may cause weakness, fatigue, and pallor; the granulocytopenia may cause fever and infections; and the thrombocytopenia may cause hemorrhages, hematomas, or petechiae. Hepatomegaly and splen-

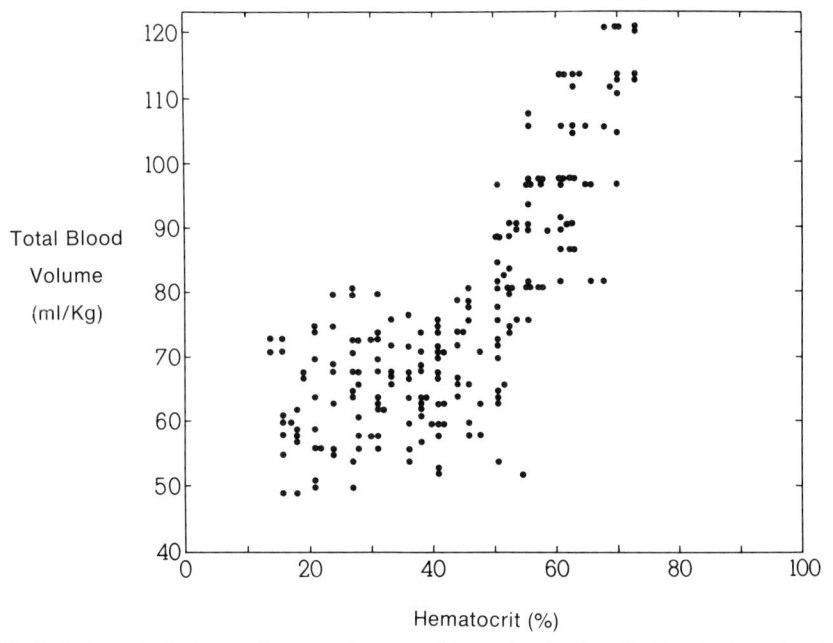

Figure 22-22 Relationship between blood volume and hematocrit. A reduction in hematocrit to about 15 per cent does not cause a significant change in blood volume, but an increase in hematocrit above 50 per cent appears to cause hypervolemia. (Data from Metcalfe, J., et al.: Circ. Res., 25:47, 1969.)

omegaly are unusual findings in the early phase of the disease and their presence should lead to re-examination of the diagnois. However, after prolonged illness, recurrent infections may produce a reactive reticuloendothelial hyperplasia of the spleen, and late transfusion hemosiderosis may lead to hepatomegaly and congestive splenomegaly.

The anemia is often macrocytic, and the reticulocytes are few in number but relatively immature. These findings reflect an accelerated bone marrow transit time and release, possibly caused

Figure 22-23 Calculated in-vivo oxygen transport in normovolemic and hypervolemic conditions. As can be seen, the oxygen transport in hypervolemia is better than that in normovolemic states, even at higher hematocrits. The curves also indicate that the optimal value for oxygen transport is higher at higher blood volumes. (From Murray, J. F., et al.: J. Clin. Invest., 42:1150, 1963, and Thorling, E. B., and Erslev, A. J.: Blood, 31:332, 1968.)

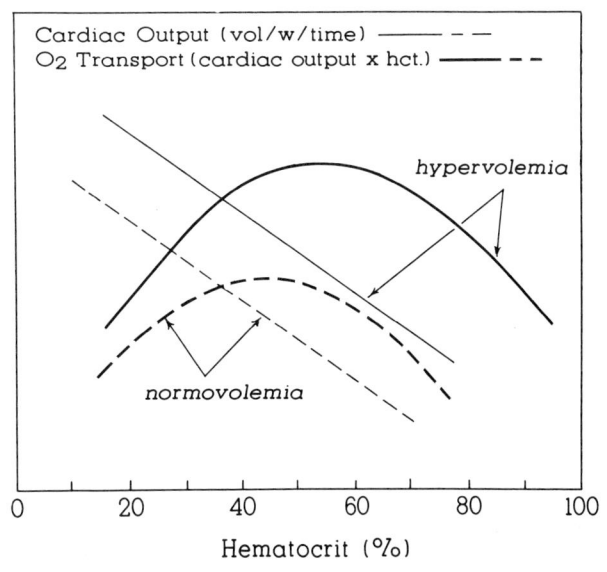

by a high level of erythropoietin or by the crowded environment in the remaining bone marrow islands. Ferrokinetic studies reveal a reduced plasma iron turnover but this reduction may be difficult to appreciate, since the normal baseline value is quite low.

Of greater importance for the demonstration of a reduced rate of red cell production are the iron clearance time and the red cell utilization of iron. The reduced bone marrow mass can clear iron from plasma only slowly, giving extramedullary tissues such as liver or spleen extra time in which to compete with the marrow for circulating radioactive iron. The result is a prolonged iron clearance time and a low red cell iron utilization. This combination is characteristic for all anemias caused by a reduction in erythropoietic tissue and distinguishes them from anemias caused by ineffective red cell production. In the latter anemias, intramedullar destruction of nucleated red cells will also cause a low utilization of radioactive iron, but the iron clearance is short because of an abundance of erythropoietic bone marrow (Fig. 22–24). This distinction is of particular importance in establishing whether pancytopenia is caused by bone marrow hypoplasia or by ineffective cellular production. This latter condition has been called "aplastic anemia with a hyperplastic bone marrow," a term which has caused much confusion with regard to pathogenesis and should be abandoned.

Both plasma iron and erythropoietin concentrations are high in aplastic anemia, probably reflecting decreased utilization by a reduced bone marrow mass. The high plasma iron concentration may cause excessive tissue incorporation of iron and eventually hemosiderosis. Bone marrow preparations disclose many siderotic granules in the reticulum cells, but since maturation of the individual nucleated red cells is normal, siderotic granules in these cells are seen only rarely. The high erythropoietin titer in plasma and urine has made patients with aplastic anemia useful sources for the preparation of erythropoietin concentrates.

In some patients with aplastic anemia, particularly in children, there may be a substantial increase in the production of fetal hemoglobin. This challenging but still unexplained finding is of great potential interest, since it may provide a clue for the mechanism by which gamma chain production can be activated, a mechanism of potential use for patients with sickle cell anemia or Cooley's anemia.

Absolute granulocytopenia is always present in aplastic anemia and its severity will determine to a great extent the immediate prognosis. As a rough guide, an absolute granulocyte count of less than 200 per cu. mm. suggests imminent danger of infectious complications and demands some kind of a sheltered environment. In addition to an absolute granulocytopenia, there is often a reduction in the total number of lymphocytes. The reason for this reduction is not known but the functional significance is apparently of little importance, since immunoglobulin synthesis and delayed sensitivity reactions are usually intact.

Thrombocytopenia with its dramatic and visible hemorrhagic manifestations are also always part of the clinical picture of advanced aplastic anemia. Because of the insidious onset of this

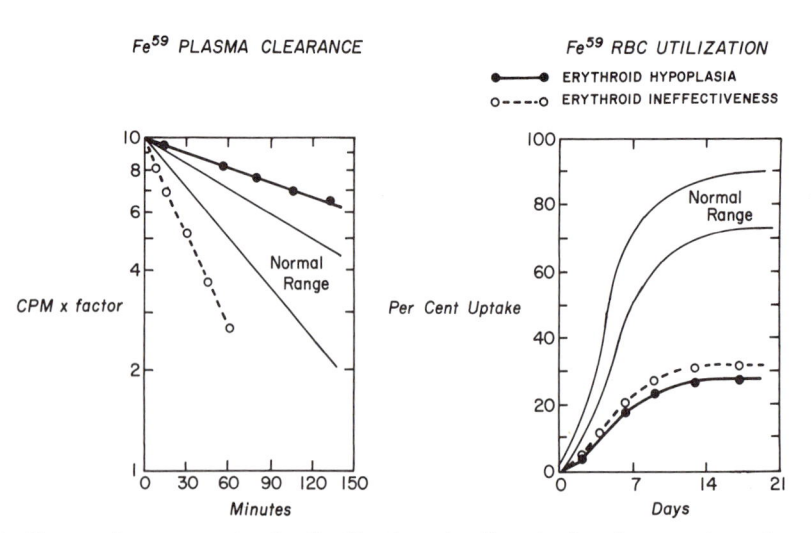

Figure 22–24 Plasma clearance and red cell utilization of radioactive iron in normals, patients with erythroid hypoplasia, and patients with ineffective red cell production.

disease, it is difficult to assess the sequence by which the various cytopenias appear. However, during the recovery phase, thrombocytopoiesis is often the last bone marrow function to recover and many patients may have thrombocytopenia for years after the other cytopenias have been corrected.

Etiology and Pathogenesis (Table 22-4). Numerous drugs, illnesses, and physical agents have the capacity to alter stem cell function presumably by interfering with intracellular metabolism. However, these agents could also alter the stem cell microenvironment, and the relative importance of "seed" and "soil" in the pathogenesis of aplastic anemia is still not resolved. Although statistical and clinical course-effect relationships between a specific agent or event and the development of aplastic anemia can be quite impressive, aplastic anemia is a disease in which the etiology can only be suspected, not established. No in-vitro test system is capable of duplicating the in-vivo events, and in-vivo tests in patients are too potentially dangerous to be justified. This makes the designation of an etiologic agent a question of judgment and clinical experience, hallowed but quite vulnerable criteria. In patients without exposure to a suggestive etiologic agent, the term "idiopathic" is used to conceal our ignorance. Obviously, even in these cases an etiologic agent must exist and may be present among the host of environmental toxins which have become part of our civilized existence.

Drugs and Chemicals. The drugs suspected of being potentially toxic for the hematopoietic stem cells have been listed in booklets published by the American Medical Association in 1965 and 1967

TABLE 22-4 ETIOLOGIC CLASSIFICATION OF APLASTIC ANEMIA

I. Idiopathic
   A. *Constitutional* (Fanconi's anemia)
   B. *Acquired*

II. Secondary
   A. *Chemical and physical agents*
      Drugs
      Nonpharmacologic chemicals
      Radiation
   B. *Infections*
      Viral (Hepatitis)
      Bacterial (Miliary TB)
   C. *Metabolic*
      Pancreatitis
      Pregnancy
   D. *Immunologic*
      Acute immunity
      Graft-vs.-host
   E. *Neoplastic*
      Myelophthisic anemia
   F. *Paroxysmal nocturnal hemoglobinuria*

TABLE 22-5 DRUGS LISTED BY A.M.A. AS BEING ASSOCIATED WITH THE DEVELOPMENT OF APLASTIC ANEMIA IN MORE THAN 5 INSTANCES

	Number of Cases Receiving Drug Alone, or Drug in Combination with Nontoxic Drugs	Number of Cases Receiving Drug in Combination with Potentially Toxic Drug
Acetazolamide	3	7
Chloramphenicol	182	156
Chlordiazepoxide HCl	2	7
Chlorothiazide	2	13
Chlorpheniramine	2	15
Chlorpromazine	3	18
Chlorpropamide	4	2
Colchicine	2	3
Diphenylhydantoin sodium	3	21
Epinephrine	2	4
Gold salts	8	2
Mepazine	4	1
Meprobamate		15
Penicillin	4	91
Phenacetin	3	31
Phenantoin	9	14
Phenylbutazone	18	22
Potassium perchlorate	6	4
Primidone	2	6
Prochlorperazine	1	9
Pyrimethamine	2	3
Quinacrine HCL	3	2
Salicylamide	2	3
Streptomycin		31
Sulfadimethoxine	2	4
Sulfamethoxypyridazine	3	11
Sulfisoxazole	3	30
Sulfonamides	4	17
Tolbutamide	7	5
Trimethadione	2	4

and include about 329 items. Table 22-5 lists those drugs with a strong etiologic relationship to aplastic anemia. It is a difficult list to interpret, since it does not give the actual incidence, the number of cases per number of patients receiving the particular drug. However, it is possible to make a mental adjustment and realize that the incidence of aplastic anemia following treatment with aspirin or penicillin must be much lower than that following treatment with phenantoin, gold salts, or phenylbutazone. Furthermore, the incidence following treatment with the nitrobenzene compound chloramphenicol must be far higher than that following treatment with any other commonly used drug.

Many attempts have been made to relate potential toxicity to the presence of a benzene or nitrobenzene radical in the chemical structure of suspected drugs. Benzene itself is a major bone marrow toxin capable of inducing both aplastic anemia and leukemia, and in addition to chloramphenicol, many benzene-related chemicals such as trinitrotoluene, toluene, and the insecticides lindane and DDT have been strongly suspected of inducing aplastic anemia. However, many drugs without the benzene radical also appear to be toxic to stem cells, and the common denominator may reside in an intermediate metabolic product rather than in the parent molecule.

Because of the high incidence of aplastic anemia in patients receiving chloramphenicol many attempts have been made to clarify the mechanism of the toxic action of this drug on the bone marrow. Although we talk about "high" incidence, it has to be emphasized that only 1 out of 10 to 20,000 treated patients develops aplastic anemia and that prospective metabolic studies are almost impossible. However, mild, reversible bone marrow suppression is observed in many treated patients, a suppression related to drug dosage and length of treatment. Clinically it can easily be recognized by a decrease in reticulocyte counts and an increase in serum iron concentration. Bone marrow examination reveals vacuolization of erythroid cells. After prolonged treatment vacuolization can be observed in other cellular elements as well, and granulocytopenia and thrombocytopenia may ensue. These effects were initially thought to be related to a suppressive action on the ribosomal protein synthesis similar to the action of chloramphenicol on the bacterial cells. However, in-vitro studies of bone marrow suspensions by Yunis and coworkers have suggested that in the mammalian cell chloramphenicol inhibits mitochondrial protein synthesis. Since many consider the mitochondria to be intracellular inclusions of plant origin with independent mechanisms for replication and metabolism, this finding could provide a link between the bacteriostatic and the bone marrow suppressive actions of chloramphenicol.

It is tempting to consider the suppressive action of the bone marrow as an early, still reversible manifestation of a stem cell injury which eventually leads to irreversible aplastic anemia. However, it seems more likely that patients who develop aplastic anemia have an abnormal response to the bone marrow suppressive effect of chloramphenicol. Not only is the regularly occurring suppression readily reversible even after prolonged treatment with large amounts of chloramphenicol, but many patients who develop aplastic anemia do so weeks or months after exposure to relatively small amounts of this drug. It has been proposed that the few unfortunate victims have an underlying genetic or acquired hypersensitivity to chloramphenicol. This could reside in the rate or extent of detoxification of the drug or in a specific stem cell abnormality. In-vitro studies of bone marrow from patients who have recovered from aplastic anemia or from their immediate relatives have suggested a greater than normal susceptibility to the suppressive action of chloramphenicol. However we are still far from having established the pathogenetic mode of action of chloramphenicol or from having learned how to predict individual hypersensitivity to this or to other potentially toxic drugs.

Radiation. Bone marrow suppression is a well-recognized side-effect of the diagnostic and therapeutic use of radiation. Radiation energy, whether mediated by a direct hit of waves or particles or by the production of highly reactive free radicals, is capable of breaking molecular bonds in critical intracellular macromolecules. Although all cells can be injured by radiation energy, organ systems dependent on a rapid cellular turnover of nucleic acids are particularly vulnerable. These systems can be ranked, according to Cronkite and Bond, with regard to radiosensitivity as follows: (1) germinal cells of the testes, (2) hematopoietic cells, (3) intestinal cells, and (4) epidermal basal cells.

Brief exposure to radiation of high energy as in reactor accidents leads to extensive destruction of the bone marrow and intestine, and death is usually caused by acute granulocytopenia and thrombocytopenia and by intestinal ulcerations. If the patient should survive the acute effects the recovery is usually almost complete, since the dormant multipotential stem cells will have sustained very little radiation injury and are capable of bone marrow repopulation. In the aftermath of the atomic attacks on Nagasaki, for example, Kirschbaum and his Japanese coworkers found that aplastic anemia was observed in only a very small number of survivors.

Prolonged exposure to more moderate doses of radiation, on the other hand, may cause chronic bone marrow failure and aplastic anemia. This has been described in patients vigorously treated with external or internal total body radiation and in Martland's famous report on watch-dial painters who accidentally ingested paint containing radium with a long biological half-life. It has also been suspected as a pathogenetic mechanism in aplastic anemia occurring in physicians or radiologists exposed to minimal amounts of radiation for many years, but as is the case for exposure to drugs and chemicals a definite cause-effect relationship can never be firmly established. The reason for defective bone marrow repopulation after chronic radiation exposure may reside in the fact that multipotential stem cells are activated and then share in the radiation injury. An alternate explanation for the development of aplastic anemia after chronic radiation has been provided by Knospe and coworkers and is that radiation-induced damage to the "endothelial stem cells" will change the structural microenvironment of the bone marrow and prevent bone marrow regeneration.

Immunologic Rejection. Aplastic anemia has been associated with a variety of seemingly unrelated diseases. Miliary tuberculosis has always been listed prominently among such disorders, but a critical evaluation of reported cases indicates that this association is rare indeed. Hepatitis with its many immunologic manifestations looms much larger as a possible etiologic event, and aplastic anemia associated with complement-sensitive red cells and nocturnal hemoglobinuria has been described so frequently by Lewis and Dacie in England and Vincent and de Gruchy in Australia that this combination ought to contain some clue to etiology or pathogenesis.

The most reasonable explanation is that an immunologic mechanism underlies the development of aplastic anemia. Support for this hypothesis is that aplastic anemia has been described after the transfusion of whole blood or bone marrow into immunologically deficient children. Miller has suggested that the disease in these unfortunate patients reflects a graft-versus-host, immunologic rejection of either hematopoietic or structural stem cells. The therapeutic implication of such a concept would be to use immunosuppressive drugs, a most difficult decision to make because of the inherent bone marrow suppressive effect of currently used drugs. The effect of prednisone in aplastic anemia has unfortunately been too erratic to be of use in pathogenetic considerations and at present the possibility that aplastic anemia is another "autoimmune" disorder is merely a hypothesis.

Constitution. Fanconi's anemia is a form of aplastic anemia which occurs as an inborn defect associated with other congenital abnormalities such as skin pigmentations, renal hypoplasia, absent thumb or radius, and microcephaly. Multiple abnormalities of the chromosomal pattern of lymphocytes and bone marrow cells have been described, but whether or not the basic disorder resides in the hematopoietic or the structural stem cells is no better known here than in the acquired cases. Of great interest, however, has been the demonstration by Shahidi and Diamond that the hypoplastic bone marrow in Fanconi's anemia appears to be quite responsive to the myelostimulatory effect of androgens. Many patients have been kept alive and well on a maintenance regimen of androgens, and these results have led to a revival of the therapeutic use of androgens in all cases of aplastic anemia. Androgens do enhance erythropoietin release, but this cannot explain their occasional effect on granulocyte and thrombocyte production and, as emphasized by Gardner and coworkers, they must have some direct or indirect action on the hematopoietic or the structural bone marrow stem cells.

The hope that bone marrow transplantation eventually will become the definitive treatment for all cases of aplastic anemia is still held by many but does depend on a final clarification of the pathogenetic mechanism. Is aplastic anemia a disease of the "seed" or the "soil," of hematopoietic or of structural stem cells? If the hematopoietic stem cells are destroyed, the administration of tissue-compatible bone marrow stem cells should induce complete recovery, a result actually achieved by Thomas and coworkers in a few cases of bone marrow transplantation between identical twins and well-matched individuals. If, however, the microenvironment is destroyed, the infusion of bone marrow cells would in most cases be to no avail.

PRIMARY POLYCYTHEMIA. Polycythemia vera is a "myeloproliferative" disorder characterized by an uncontrolled proliferation of erythroid, myeloid, and megakaryocytic bone marrow elements. The proliferation is predominantly erythroid, and the circulating red cell mass is invariably increased during the early part of the disease. The concomitant increase in granulocytes and platelets has led to the assumption that polycythemia vera is caused by an inappropriate activation of multipotential stem cells. However, the unipotential committed stem cells must also be involved in the disease process, since the erythropoietin-sensitive stem cells undergo differentiation despite the fact that the production of erythropoietin is almost completely suppressed.

The cause for this autonomous overactivity of the stem cell pool is unknown, but the existence of a viral-induced polycythemia in mice has raised the possibility that the human disorder also is virus-related. However, as is the case for most neoplastic proliferative disorders, firm evidence for a viral etiology is not available.

The increased rate of red cell production causes a steady rise in red cell blood count and hematocrit. In order to ameliorate the effect of a high hematocrit on blood viscosity, the plasma volume also increases, and the erythrocytosis becomes characterized by an increase in both the red cell mass and the blood volume. This process may be quite slow and may be accomplished by a slight but sustained excess of red cell production over red cell destruction. For example, a mere doubling of the rate of red cell production for a period of 4 months will result in a doubling of the size of the red cell mass. Since the establishment of a clinically recognizable polycythemia may take much longer, it is not surprising that a routine bone marrow examination may not show evidence of much erythroid hyperactivity.

Ferrokinetic studies, measuring total bone marrow activity, are more apt to demonstrate the presence of a slight increase in erythroid bone marrow mass. Such studies also show that the red cell production in patients with polycythemia vera is effective with the release of normal long-lived red blood cells. Because of the increase in the number of erythroid cells in the bone marrow and circulating blood, a greater than normal amount of iron is "trapped" in these cells, and the tissue iron stores may become depleted. This trend is aggravated by the frequent therapeutic use of phlebotomy and by spontaneous nose and gastric bleedings and leads to an iron-deficient erythropoiesis. Fortunately, the production of microcytic and hypochromic cells may be of considerable symptomatic benefit, since the hematocrit and in turn the viscosity will become disproportionately lower than the red cell count.

Most symptoms are related to hypervolemia and hyperviscosity and are alleviated by phlebotomy. They frequently consist merely of nonspecific headaches, dizziness, blurred vision, and a feeling of "fullness in the head." Engorgement of thin-walled vessels may cause nose and gastric bleedings, serving as convenient means for spontaneous bloodletting. However, more serious symptoms may occur if the hyperviscosity causes venous stagnation, thrombosis, and embolization. Such events can cause fatal vascular accidents when they occur in cerebral, coronary, or intestinal veins.

The characteristic splenomegaly found in polycythemia vera may be caused in part by vascular engorgement but is probably more closely related to the development of extramedullary hematopoiesis, especially extramedullary granulocytopoiesis. The granulocyte count in polycythemia vera is regularly increased, although it rarely exceeds 30,000 cells per cu. mm. The cells are usually mature and normally functioning, but more immature myeloid elements may be present. The leukocyte alkaline phosphatase is either normal or high, a finding of uncertain functional significance but of use in distinguishing the granulocytosis of polycythemia vera from the granulocytosis of chronic myeloid leukemia. The granulocytes of polycythemia vera reportedly contain an increased amount of histidine decarboxylase, an enzyme involved in the production of histamine from histidine. Excessive histamine may be responsible for the common complaint of itching, especially following warm baths or showers.

The platelet count is regularly increased, but frequently not as much as would be expected from examining bone marrow specimens. These often reveal sheets of megakaryocytes, a finding which may justify bone marrow aspiration as a differential diagnostic test in the polycythemias. The characteristic tendency of patients with polycythemia vera to develop thrombotic complications is frequently related to the increased platelet count. However, morphologic and functional studies of platelets indicated that they are not quite normal and that despite their increased numbers they may not be responsible for these complications. Actually, studies by Spaet and coworkers on the coagulation process in this disease suggest the presence of impaired hemostasis with poor clot formation rather than hypercoagulability. In evaluating the results from such studies, it is important to realize that the plasma volume is relatively decreased in polycythemic blood and that the amount of available coagulation factors may not be adequate for the establishment of a firm red cell clot.

It is usually not difficult to make a diagnosis of polycythemia vera in patients with full-blown pancytosis and splenomegaly. However, early in the course, polycythemia vera may be more difficult to recognize, and Table 22-6 gives some of the findings of value in the differential diagnosis of various polycythemias. As the disease progresses, patients with polycythemia vera develop specific and characteristic complications not seen in the other polycythemias. The paradoxical occurrence of both thromboses and hemorrhages occurs quite frequently, and cerebral, coronary, mesenteric, or portal thrombosis may cause life-threatening situations in a patient who displays nasal, gastric, or dermal hemorrhages. In a considerable number of patients the disease slowly changes in character, with myelofibrosis and myeloid metaplasia becoming predominant features. These features are the results of excessive fibroblastic activity, an integral part of the general myelostimulatory disease process. The reduction in available bone marrow space and the increase in splenic size will lead first to anemia and eventually to pancytopenia.

Acute myelogenous leukemia develops ultimately in about 10 to 15 per cent of patients with polycythemia vera. The occurrence of this dreaded complication has been reviewed by Modan and Lilienfeld and it seems to be related to the therapeutic use of radioactive phosphorus. Recent reports suggest that the use of so-called

TABLE 22-6 DIFFERENTIAL DIAGNOSIS OF POLYCYTHEMIAS

	Relative Polycythemia	Polycythemia Vera	Secondary Polycythemia
Hematocrit	Increased	Increased	Increased
Red blood cell mass	Normal	Increased	Increased
Erythropoietin	Normal	Decreased	Increased
White blood count	Normal	Increased	Normal
Platelet count	Normal	Increased	Normal
Bone marrow	Normal	Hyperplastic	Erythroid hyperplasia
Spleen	Normal	Enlarged	Normal
Arterial oxygen saturation	Normal	Normal	Decreased
Serum iron	Normal	Decreased	Normal

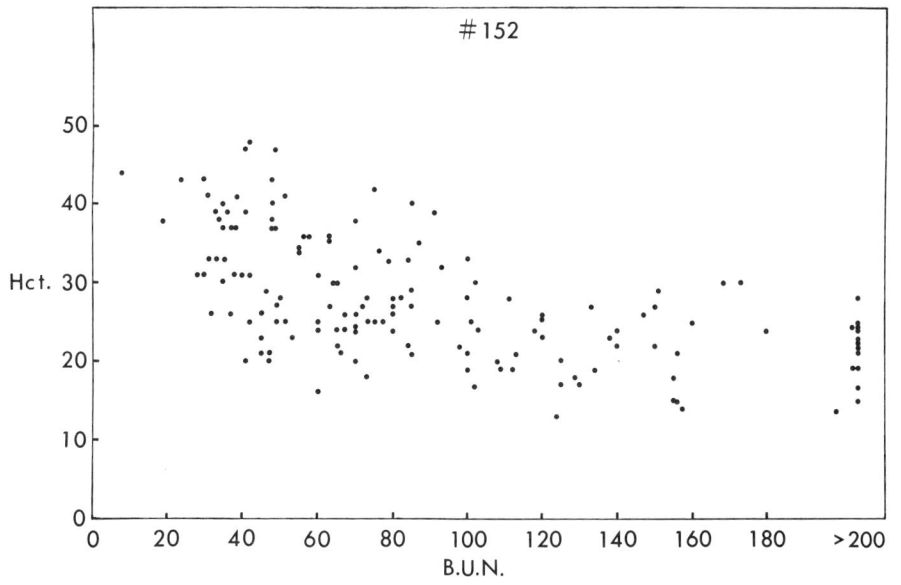

Figure 22-25 Relationship between hematocrit and BUN in 152 patients with various degrees of renal failure and uremia. (From Erslev, A. J.: Arch. Intern. Med., *126*:774–780, 1970. Reprinted from Wesson, L. G. (Ed.): Physiology of the Human Kidney, 1969, by permission of Grune and Stratton, Inc., New York.)

radiomimetic agents such as busulfan also may be followed by the development of acute myelogenous leukemia. Polycythemia vera was the first "neoplastic" disease with a long enough survival to make possible prolonged follow-up studies after the use of myelosuppressive agents. The more recent successes in the treatment of Hodgkin's disease, breast cancer, chronic lymphatic leukemia, and transplantation rejection have permitted similar prolonged follow-ups after the use of other forms of radiation or radiomimetic drugs, and it has become clear that the development of acute myelogenous leukemia is an appreciable therapeutic hazard. So far the therapeutic results have been well worth the risk, but obviously these agents should be used with reluctance and caution.

Disorders of Unipotential Stem Cells. Regulation disorders of the unipotential erythropoietin-sensitive stem cells include common diseases such as the anemia of chronic renal disease and common nondiseases such as high-altitude polycythemia. Using current concepts about the regulation of red cell production it is possible to classify these disorders according to their place in the feedback circuit outlined in Figure 22-19. However, it should be appreciated that the pigeon-holing of a complex disease according to the pathologic condition of a single functional system often becomes quite artificial, and that the classification given in Table 22-6, although useful, is rather single-minded.

RENAL DISEASE. Anemia is a hallmark of chronic renal disease and is roughly proportional to the degree of renal failure as measured by urea or creatine retention. Since the pathogenesis of the anemia and the uremia are related to the failure of many independent functions, it is actually surprising that the proportionality is as good as depicted in Figure 22-25. The two major failing functions are the renal excretory function and the renal endocrine function.

Failure of Renal Excretory Function

HEMOLYSIS. The red cell of patients with uremia frequently shows multiple tiny spicules (Fig. 22-26). The presence of this so-called burring has been related to the accumulation of toxic endproducts in the circulation and has been thought to be responsible for an impaired sodium-potassium pump activity and a shortened red cell life span. However, the relationship between azotemia and red cell life span is not that good (Fig. 22-27), and when hemolysis occurs it is often related more closely to changes in the microvasculature than to the degree of uremia. Indeed, extensive red cell fragmentation and hemolysis can be observed in patients with malignant vascular hypertension or with inflammatory vascular changes (hemolytic uremic syndrome) and with only mildly elevated BUN or creatine concentrations. At present it seems most reasonable to relate the premature destruction of red cells in chronic renal disease to mechanical disruption of metabolically fragile red cells.

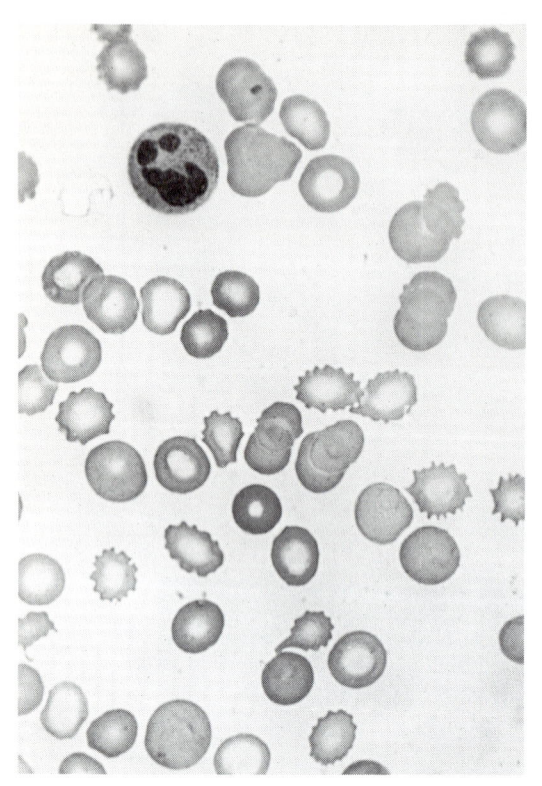

Figure 22-26 Burr cells in smear of blood from patient with severe uremia.

rhage may cause a considerable loss of blood and increase the demands for an accelerated rate of red cell production. The pathogenesis of the bleeding tendency is poorly understood, since thrombocytopenia and coagulation factor deficiency, when present, are rarely severe enough to be responsible for overt blood loss. Recent studies by Horowitz and coworkers, however, suggest that certain retention products may affect normal platelet function and cause an abnormal bleeding time, clot retraction, platelet adhesion, and platelet aggregation. The responsible toxic factor is believed to be a guanidino compound, and intensive dialysis has been found to reduce the bleeding tendency.

RESPONSIVENESS TO ERYTHROPOIETIN. In addition to inadequate production (see later) there is a marked decrease in the bone marrow responsiveness to erythropoietin (Fig. 22-28). The reason is not known, but the degree of responsiveness appears to be related to the severity of uremia. It seems probable that the improvement in erythropoietic function found after intensive dialysis is caused by an increased response to available erythropoietin rather than to an increased production of erythropoietin. Because of this refractory condition, it is anticipated that much more erythropoietin will be needed to abolish the anemia of chronic renal disease than is required for normal erythropoietic maintenance.

Failure of Renal Endocrine Function. The various effects of uremia on the rate of red cell destruction and production result in an increased demand for erythropoietin. This demand could easily be met by a normal but apparently not by an abnormal kidney. Impaired renal tissue is not capable of producing normal quantities of erythropoietin unless stimulated by intense ane-

BLEEDING TENDENCY. As a manifestation of chronic renal disease, purpura is almost as characteristic as pallor. In addition to subcutaneous bleedings, gastrointestinal and uterine hemor-

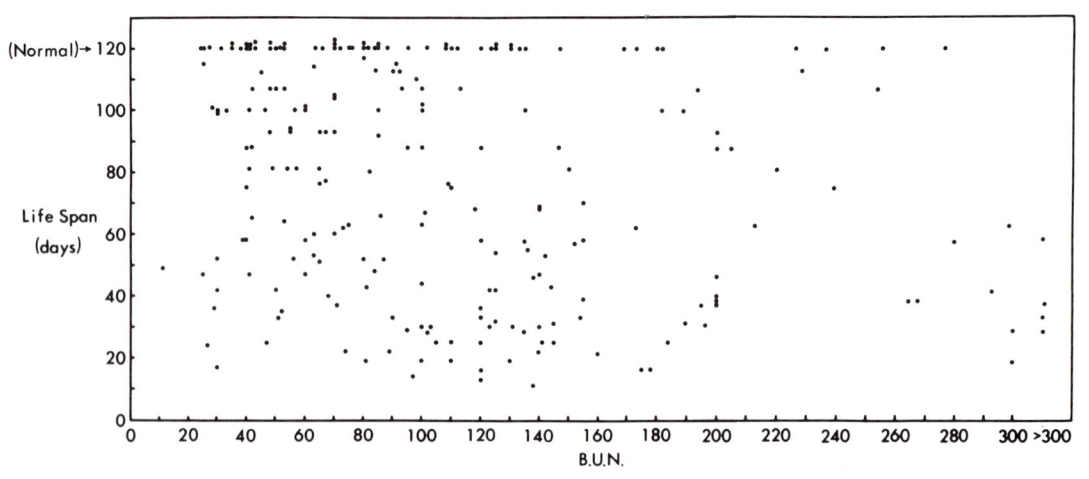

Figure 22-27 Relationship between red cell life span and BUN of 221 patients with various degrees of renal failure and uremia. (From Erslev, A. J.: Arch. Intern. Med., *126*:774, 1970. Copyright 1970, American Medical Association.)

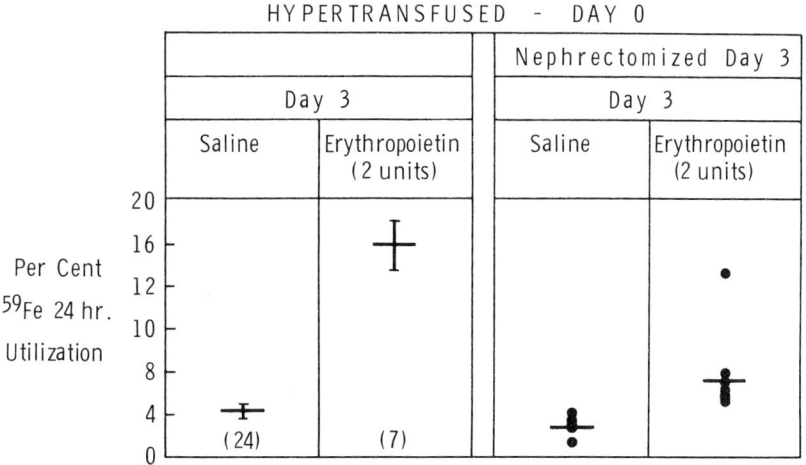

Figure 22-28 Erythropoietic response of normal and nephrectomized, uremic rats to the same amount of erythropoietin.

mic hypoxia, and a balance between the rates of red cell destruction and red cell production is not achieved except at anemic levels. Under conditions of progressive kidney failure, the hypoxic stimulus needed to produce adequate amounts of erythropoietin becomes greater and the anemia more severe. However, there is an apparent limit for the degree of hypoxia needed; even anephric individuals continue to manufacture red blood cells (Fig. 22-29). This residual erythropoietic activity may be generated by the release of extrarenal erythropoietin or may be caused by bone marrow stem cells spontaneously differentiating to proerythroblast at a slow idling rate. In any case, the hemoglobin concentration which can be maintained in anephric patients is usually too low to be compatible with life and has to be augmented by transfusions.

CHRONIC DISORDERS. Although one of the most common of anemias, the anemia of chronic disorders is of relatively little clinical significance, since it is rarely severe enough to cause symptoms or demand active transfusion therapy. On the other hand, it probably has been treated by more unneeded and ineffective hematinics than any other anemia, and the pathogenesis of this refractory anemia is still a fascinating enigma.

During the early part of this century, anemia was an invariable complication of many chronic

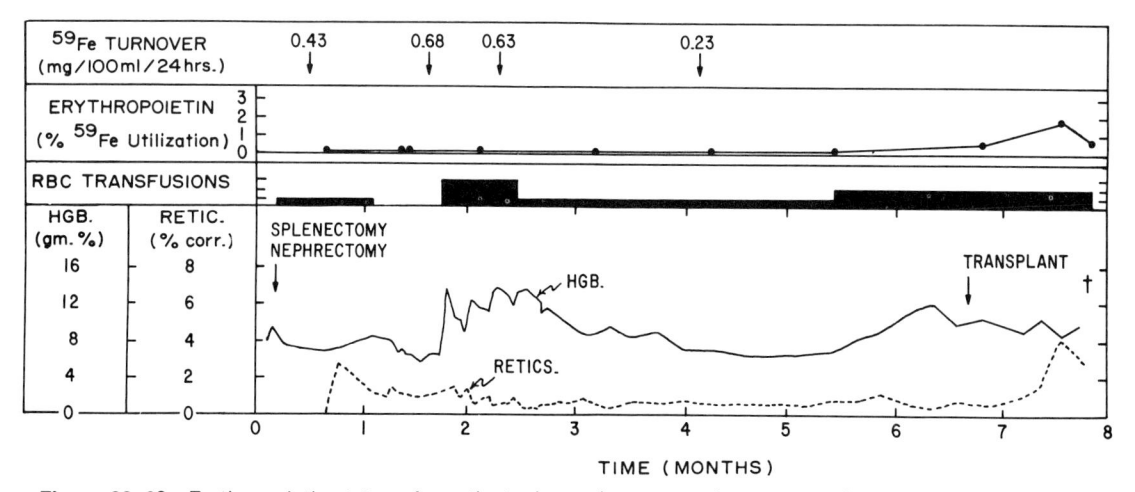

Figure 22-29 Erythropoietic status of a patient who underwent nephrectomy and splenectomy 7 months before a successful kidney transplantation. Although erythropoietin levels were unmeasurable, reticulocytes were produced throughout the anephric period.

debilitating infections, such as tuberculosis, osteomyelitis, or brucellosis, and it was known as anemia of chronic infection. With the change in the ecology of disease, it was realized that a similar anemia also occurred in patients with chronic, noninfectious diseases, such as rheumatoid arthritis, lymphomas, or disseminated carcinomas, and the anemia was given the noncommittal name of anemia of chronic disorders. It is characterized by a moderate reduction in hemoglobin concentration, a reduction in the level of both serum iron and iron-binding capacity, and an increased amount of storage iron in the reticuloendothelial cells of the bone marrow.

The presence of decreased amounts of circulating iron, despite abundant iron stores, is probably caused by a defective iron release mechanism by the reticuloendothelial cells. The erythroid cells in the bone marrow apparently can handle available iron, and the utilization of radioactive iron is normal. However, the reutilization of iron is decreased (Fig. 22–30), indicating that hemoglobin iron, which normally is reutilized after being processed by the reticuloendothelial cells, is trapped in these cells and removed from the dynamic iron economy of the body. This relative iron deficiency is aggravated by a moderate shortening of the red blood cell life span, resulting in a mild anemia. However, it has always been of some concern that the anemia of chronic disorders does not display the morphologic characteristics of an iron deficiency anemia but is usually normocytic and normochromic, as if the basic defect resided in the stem cells. Recent studies by Ward and coworkers have suggested that there may indeed be an element of stem cell failure, since the serum level and the 24 hour excretion of erythropoietin are subnormal (Fig. 22–31). No renal injury or abnormality can be held responsible for this defect, and studies so far have not shown any change in red cell oxygen affinity. Consequently, it is possible that the anemia of chronic disorders may reflect a primary defect in the oxygen sensing device or in the erythropoietin-producing cells. It is hoped that the unraveling of the pathogenesis of the anemia may provide us not only with means to correct the anemia but also with basic knowledge as to the relationship between erythropoietin production and iron metabolism.

Endocrine Disorders

Pituitary and Thyroid Dysfunction. Pituitary and thyroid dysfunction or ablation are characteristically associated with a moderate normochromic, normocytic anemia. Although many attempts have been made to assign a specific erythropoietic effect to the thyroid, pituitary, or hypothalamic secretions, most current studies indicate that the anemia is an appropriate response to a decreased cellular demand for oxygen. The administration of thyroxin, triiodothyronine, or desiccated thyroid will increase this demand, and the rate of red cell production will respond appropriately. It is questionable whether the administration of growth hormone, ACTH, or gonadal hormones are of additional benefit. In many cases

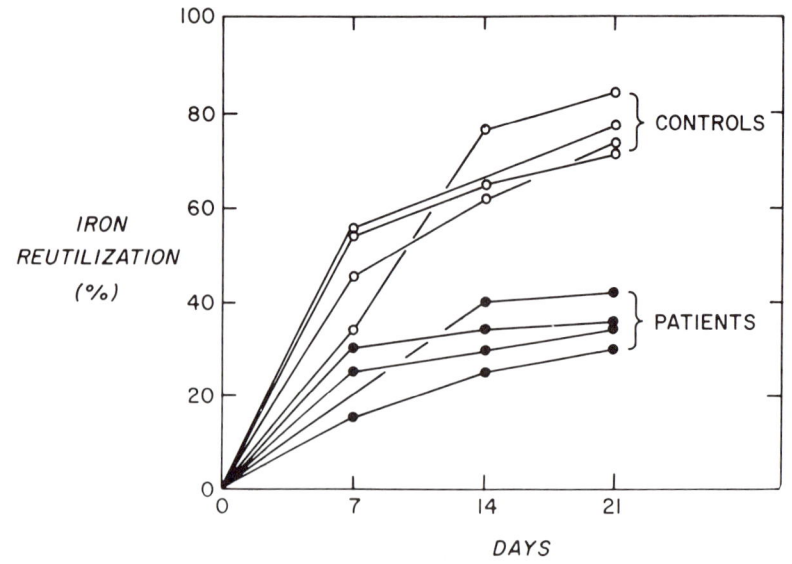

Figure 22–30 Utilization and reutilization of radioactive iron in normal individuals and in patients with anemia of chronic disease. (Redrawn from Haurani, F. I., et al.: J. Lab. Clin. Med., 65:560, 1965.)

Figure 22-31 Relationship between hematocrit and erythropoietin concentration in plasma from patients with anemia of chronic disease and patients with various other anemias. The erythropoietin titers are given in terms of ^{59}Fe uptake of polycythemic mice receiving injections of the plasma. (Data from Ward, H. P., et al.: J. Clin. Invest., 50:332, 1971.)

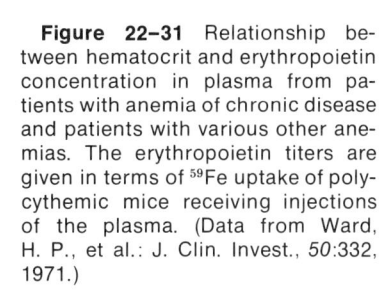

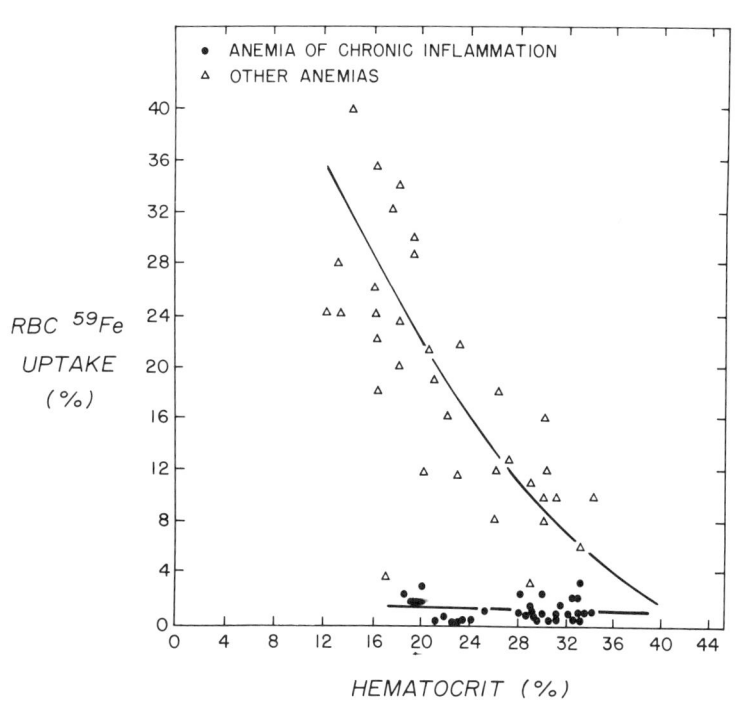

of myxedema or other hypothyroid conditions, the anemia is somewhat atypical because of associated nutritional deficiencies. Malabsorption of B$_{12}$ or folic acid may lead to a megaloblastic, macrocytic blood picture and the frequent uterine bleedings in hypothyroid females may lead to an iron-deficient, microcytic, hypochromic anemia. Even in hypothyroid men, the common achlorhydria may result in malabsorption of iron and an iron deficiency anemia.

Despite the erythropoietic effect of increased oxygen consumption induced by thyroid hormones, patients with hyperthyroidism or thyrotoxicosis are rarely polycythemic. This may be explained by the fact that thyroid hormones also increase cardiac output and tissue perfusion, making an increase in red cell mass less needed. Nevertheless, direct measurements by Muldowney and coworkers of red cell mass and plasma volume suggest that the absence of a high hematocrit in these conditions is caused by a concomitant increase in plasma volume, and that hyperthyroidism will cause true secondary polycythemia as defined by an increased red cell mass.

Gonadal Dysfunction. In normal mature men the hemoglobin concentration is about 1 to 2 grams higher than in normal females, whereas the male hemoglobin concentration in childhood, in advanced age, and in gonadal deficiency states is similar to that of females. This phenomenon has led to the assumption that physiologic excretions of androgens have an erythropoietic effect on the bone marrow. Conversely, it has been postulated that physiologic doses of estrogens cause a slight suppression of red cell production. Many experimental data on castrated animals have been marshalled to support these contentions, but unfortunately many studies were designed to prove rather than to test, and the erythropoietic effects of physiologic doses of gonadal hormones are still not quite clear. More impressive are the data indicating that androgens in pharmacologic doses can stimulate red cell production and even cause full-blown secondary polycythemia (Fig. 22-32). This effect may be mediated by a release of renal erythropoietin or by an enhanced effect of erythropoietin on the bone marrow or by both mechanisms.

Anemia of Pregnancy. Anemia of pregnancy is most often caused by an iron deficiency, and the routine use of iron in prenatal care is definitely in order. However, even under conditions of adequate iron intake, a mild anemia is present during the third trimester in almost all pregnant women. This anemia is normochromic and normocytic and unresponsive to any kind of treatment. Recent measurements of the red cell mass has shown it not to be caused by a lack of red cells but rather by an increase in plasma, a so-called dilution anemia. The red cell mass actually increases by about 20 per cent during pregnancy, but the plasma volume increases even more. The physiologic effect of such an increase in blood vol-

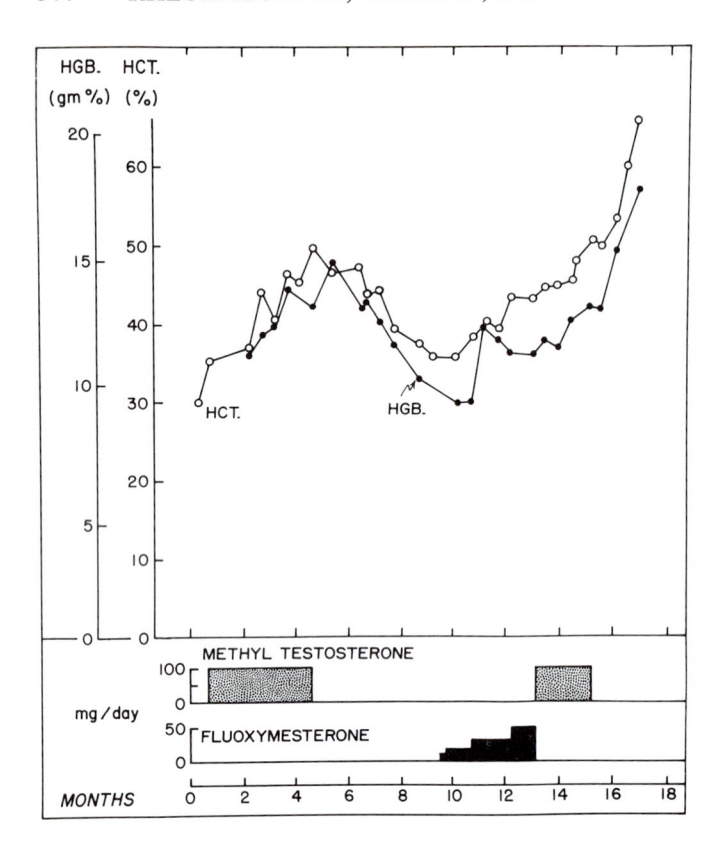

Figure 22-32 Erythropoietic response of a patient with myelofibrosis to various androgen preparations. (Redrawn from Gardner, F. H., and Pringle, J. C., Jr.: New Eng. J. Med., *264*:103, 1961.)

ume is very advantageous for oxygen transport (Fig. 22-23), and despite the moderate decrease in hemoglobin concentration, the pregnant woman and her fetus are undoubtedly well provided with oxygen for their metabolic demands.

IMMUNOLOGIC DYSFUNCTION. Pure red cell aplasia is an unusual but dramatic disease characterized by severe anemia due to the isolated depletion of the erythroid tissue and is believed to be related to an immunologic dysfunction. The production and turnover of erythropoietin appear to be normal but the bone marrow response to this hormone is inadequate, as evidenced by the absence of proerythroblasts and other nucleated red blood cells despite high plasma titers of erythropoietin.

An acute, self-limited form of pure red cell aplasia has been reported following "virus" infections in patients with hereditary spherocytosis or other congenital hemolytic disorders. The predominance of reports dealing with such patients may be due to the fact that a brief period of erythroid aplasia in a patient with a short red cell life span will have a much more noticeable effect on the hemoglobin concentration than the same period of aplasia would have if the red cell life span were normal (Fig. 22-33). Consequently, it is assumed that brief periods of asymptomatic erythroid aplasia may actually be quite common and if properly looked for found in many normals suffering from upper respiratory infections or viral gastroenteritis. The exact pathogenetic mechanism is unknown but it has been proposed that the erythroid cells or their immediate erythropoietin-sensitive progenitors are affected by a viral-related antibody.

Chronic pure red cell aplasia is a far more unusual disorder, but its relationship to thymic tumors has recently caused a flurry of interest regarding its pathogenesis.

Thymomas are present in about 30 to 50 per cent of cases, and although thymectomy is rarely of dramatic benefit, "spontaneous" recoveries have been described in patients who have undergone thymectomy. Since so-called autoimmune disorders are frequently associated with thymus abnormalities, it is of additional pathogenetic importance that prednisone may occasionally cause a striking reticulocyte response (Fig. 22-34) and that remissions may be induced by the therapeutic use of immunosuppressive drugs. Recent studies by Krantz and coworkers have demonstrated antibodies directed against erythroid bone marrow cells in the serum of some patients. These antibodies presumably coat and possibly reject the erythroid cells or the erythro-

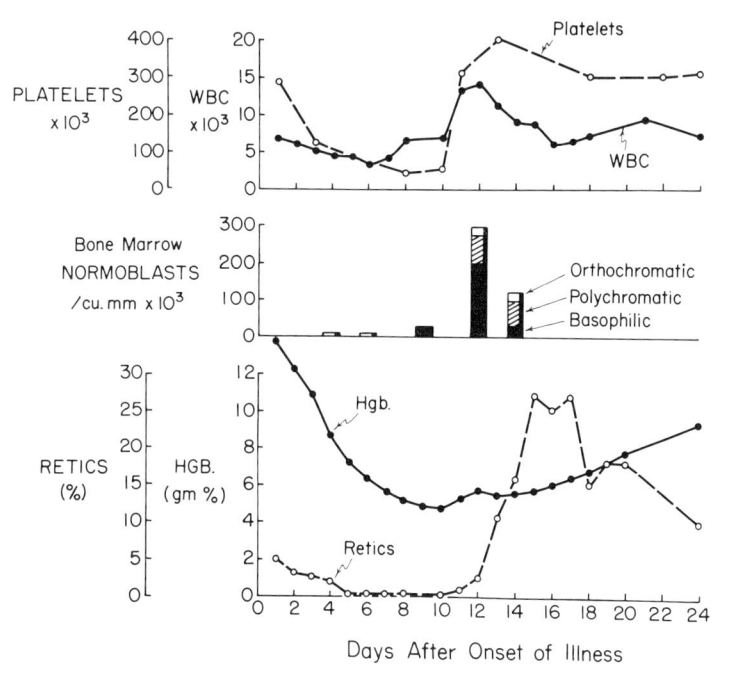

Figure 22-33 Acute aplastic crisis following a brief febrile illness in a patient with hereditary spherocytosis. (Redrawn from Owren, P. A.: Blood, 3:231, 1948.)

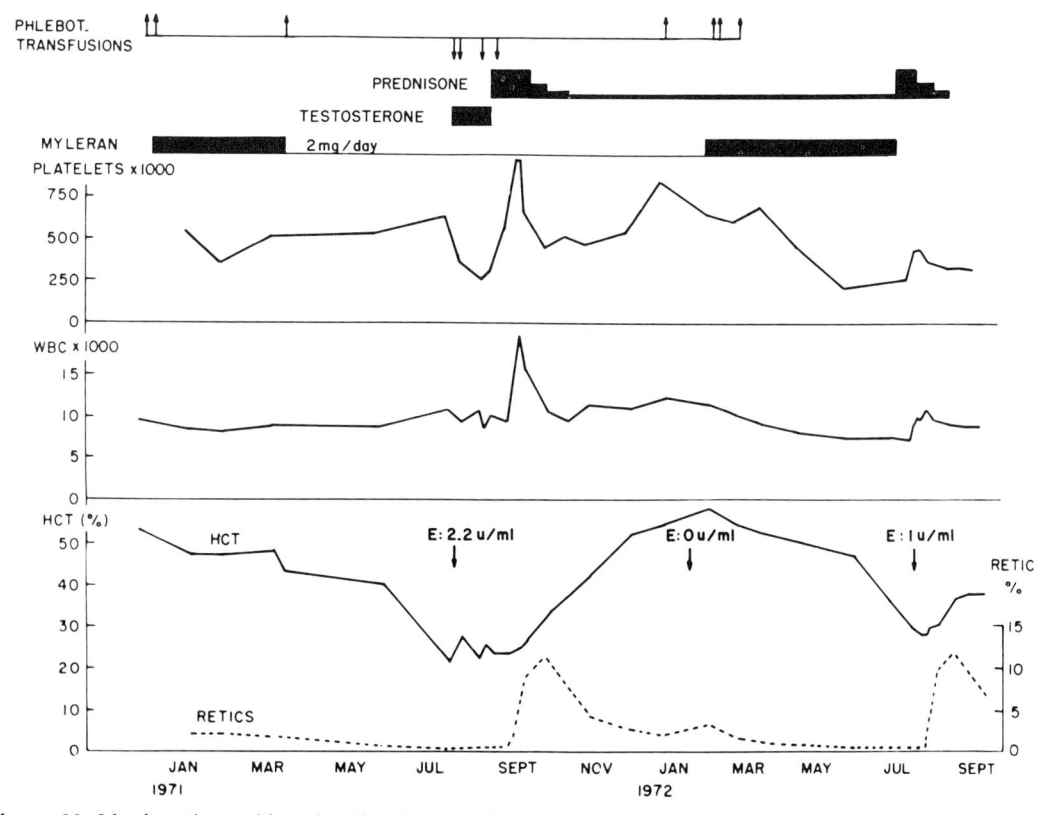

Figure 22-34 A patient with polycythemia vera, disseminated lupus erythematosus, and recurrent bouts of pure red cell aplasia. In each instance prednisone medication caused a striking increase in reticulocytes, followed by a return of the hematocrit to normal or even polycythemic values.

poietin-responsive stem cells, and their presence could explain the development of a pure red cell aplasia. The existence of antibodies directed against erythropoietin has also been reported, but since the erythropoietin titer is usually very high, these reports are difficult to accept. The cause-effect relationship of the autoantibodies to the thymic tumor is not clear, but it has been suggested that the tumor destroys normal thymic function and permits the survival of lymphocytic clones programed to produce autoantibodies. Further studies of this fascinating disease may well lead to concepts of importance for the management not only of patients with pure red cell aplasia but also of patients with other autoimmune diseases.

SECONDARY POLYCYTHEMIA. Secondary polycythemia is a condition characterized by an enhanced, erythropoietin-mediated stimulation of red cell production and an increased red cell mass. In most cases the erythropoietin release is an appropriate response to tissue hypoxia, but in some the release is inappropriate and the resulting erythrocytosis presumably serves no useful function.

Appropriate Secondary Polycythemia

HIGH ALTITUDE. The erythrocytosis experienced by high altitude dwellers is probably the most common of the secondary polycythemias and it must be considered an appropriate physiologic adaptation rather than a pathologic disorder. However, sustained physiologic adaptations are usually achieved at a certain biological cost, and individuals at high altitudes pay for an enhanced oxygen transport by problems related to hypervolemia, hyperviscosity, and hyperventilation.

Most studies of high-altitude polycythemia have been carried out in the small town of Morococha at 15,000 feet in the Peruvian Andes. Only a few precarious settlements exist above this altitude, the highest permanent settlement probably being Aucanguilcha in the Chilean Andes at 17,500 feet. At this level the atmospheric oxygen pressure is not much higher than the mean capillary oxygen pressure at sea level, making it very difficult to provide a downhill gradient for oxygen from air to cells. Above 17,500 feet only short-term sojourns are possible and no one has yet managed to reach the top of the world, Mt. Everest, at 29,000 feet without being sustained by supplemental oxygen (Fig. 22–35).

The ability of the inhabitants of the mining town Morococha to live active, strenuous lives at 15,000 feet is directly related to their adaptable oxygen transport system. The tissue requirements for oxygen are the same as or higher than at sea level, but increased pulmonary function, increased oxygen carrying capacity of blood, increased blood volume, and decreased oxygen affinity of hemoglobin succeed in reducing the oxygen gradient needed to bring oxygen from the air to the tissues (Fig. 22–36). Such a reduction will ensure that the oxygen molecules in the capillaries are under enough pressure for their subsequent diffusion into the tissues.

Sustained hyperventilation causes a reduction in the oxygen gradient between ambient and alveolar air. Because of the inherent effect of dead

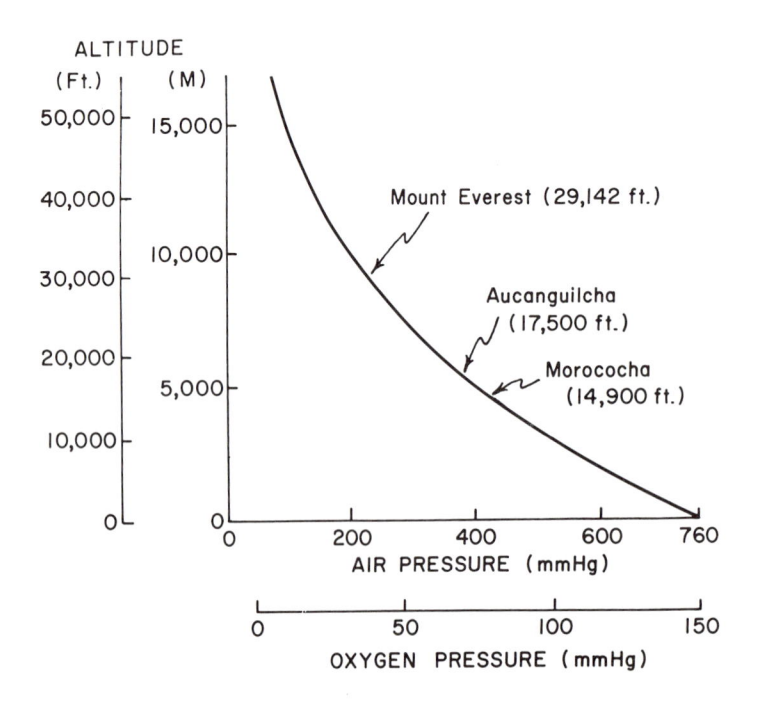

Figure 22–35 The oxygen pressure at altitudes inhabited or visited by man.

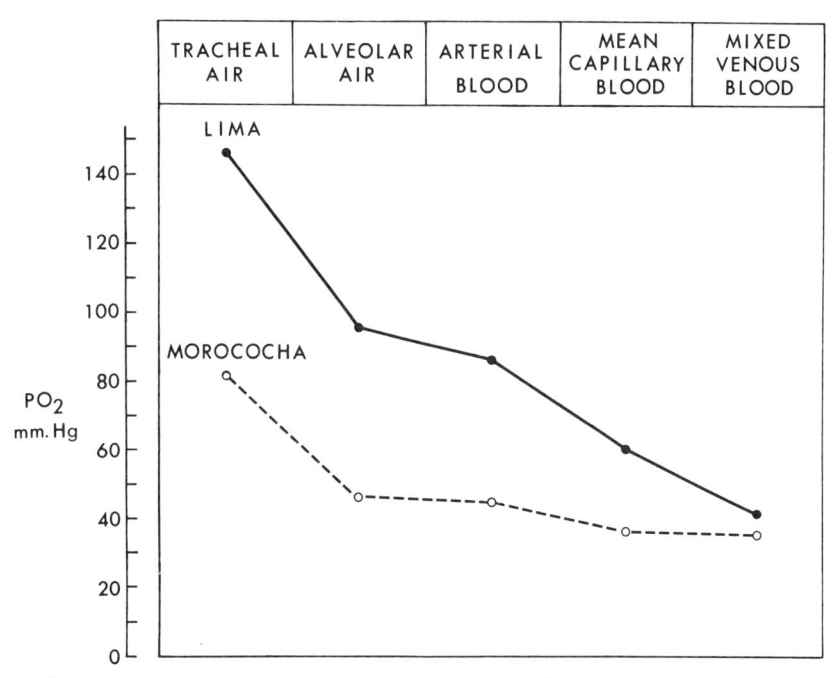

Figure 22–36 The oxygen gradient from lungs to tissues at sea level (Lima) or at 15,000 feet (Morococha). (Redrawn from Hurtado, A.: In Weike, W. H. (Ed.): Physiological Effects of High Altitude. New York, Pergamon Press, 1964.)

space and water vapors, this part of the gradient can be only moderately reduced. However, hyperventilation causes a pulmonary "stretch" with enlargement of the alveolar diffusing area and almost eliminates the alveolar-capillary gradient. The most important reduction occurs in the arterial-venous gradient, permitting unloading of oxygen throughout the length of the capillary at a relatively high pressure. Since the tissue demands for oxygen are not reduced, the maintenance of a shallow gradient demands an increased flow of oxygen-carrying blood through the tissues. Although an increase in cardiac output would accomplish just this, the added workload on a vital organ is unacceptable for chronic adjustments. Of more importance for the maintenance of an increased oxygen flow to the tissues is an increase in the red blood cell count.

Tissue hypoxia will lead to the release of erythropoietin which in turn will increase the rate of red cell production and enhance the oxygen carrying capacity of blood. Furthermore, the increased rate of red cell production will cause an increase in blood volume, with dilatation and opening of vessels, and an increase in tissue perfusion. This dual effect on oxygen flow far outweighs the moderate disadvantages derived from the higher viscosity of circulating blood.

Recent studies have indicated that the oxygen dissociation curve is shifted to the right at high altitudes, thereby permitting the unloading of oxygen under relatively high pressure in the tissue capillaries. Such a shift is undoubtedly of great importance in the initial adaptation to high altitudes, especially since acute hyperventilation alkalosis would tend to eliminate the normal Bohr shift to the right (Fig. 22–9). However, it is less certain whether it plays a significant role in chronic acclimatization. At that point the blood pH is usually normal and, as emphasized by Finch and Lenfant, an excessive shift to the right might significantly reduce the loading of hemoglobin in the lungs, an important consideration when the ambient oxygen pressure is about one half normal. It is of interest that the animals indigenous to high altitudes such as llamas and vicunas have oxygen dissociation curves positioned far to the left, suggesting that the adjustments of the shape of the curve in sustained acclimatization is aimed at improving the loading of oxygen in the lungs rather than at the unloading in the tissues.

The clinical manifestation of chronic high altitude acclimatization is dominated by ruddy cyanosis and physiologic emphysema. The vascular enlargement can be observed readily in the conjunctiva, mucous membrane, and skin and may contribute to the remarkable capacity of Sherpas to walk barefoot and sleep on ice and snow.

The blood studies reveal a normochromic and normocytic erythrocytosis, with increased red cell mass but only borderline increases in granulocyte or platelet counts. The plasma iron concentration is normal in contradistinction to polycythemia vera, in which it is usually low. This may be due merely to blood loss and to therapeutic phlebotomies in polycythemia vera, but it has been suggested that tissue hypoxia as experienced at high altitudes enhances intestinal iron absorption. Erythropoietin titers in plasma and urine are increased, also in contradistinction to polycythemia vera, in which they are extremely low.

It is difficult to evaluate the biological cost of chronic acclimatization to high altitudes, since very few reliable data on the longevity and morbidity of high altitude dwellers exist. However, the compensatory reserves are undoubtedly decreased and the effect of cardiopulmonary disorders must be more serious than at sea level. So-called chronic mountain sickness (Monge's disease) is caused by an acquired refractoriness of the respiratory center leading to relative alveolar hypoventilation and excessive tissue hypoxia. Since this in turn will cause an increase in an already expanded red cell mass and high blood viscosity, cardiovascular decompensation occurs. Therapeutic venesection provides symptomatic relief, but the individuals suffering from Monge's disease usually need to be brought down to sea level for permanent improvement.

PULMONARY DISEASE. Chronic pulmonary disease associated with cyanosis, clubbing, and arterial oxygen unsaturation is only rarely accompanied by an increase in hemoglobin concentration (Fig. 22–37). In some cases a concomitant increase in plasma volume may conceal the effect of an increased red cell mass, but in most cases true secondary polycythemia does not occur. The release of erythropoietin appears to be commensurate to the degree of tissue hypoxia, but for unknown reasons there is an unresponsiveness of the stem cells to this hormone or an impairment in the subsequent proliferation of nucleated red cells.

CARDIOVASCULAR DISEASE. Right-to-left shunt in congenital heart disease is characteristically associated with cyanosis, clubbing, and often extreme secondary appropriate polycythemia. Despite high hematocrit and high viscosity, hyperviscosity symptoms are rarely present, probably owing to the simultaneous increase in total blood volume. Whether or not to perform phlebotomy on blue babies prior to surgery is still an unanswered question, but most surgeons feel more comfortable if the hematocrit is brought down below 60 per cent by judicious phlebotomies. It certainly will provide a little more reserve if fluid intake becomes inadequate.

In acquired heart disease with chronic decompensation, erythrokinetic studies by Chodos and coworkers have shown that a mild increase in red cell production and red cell mass is usually

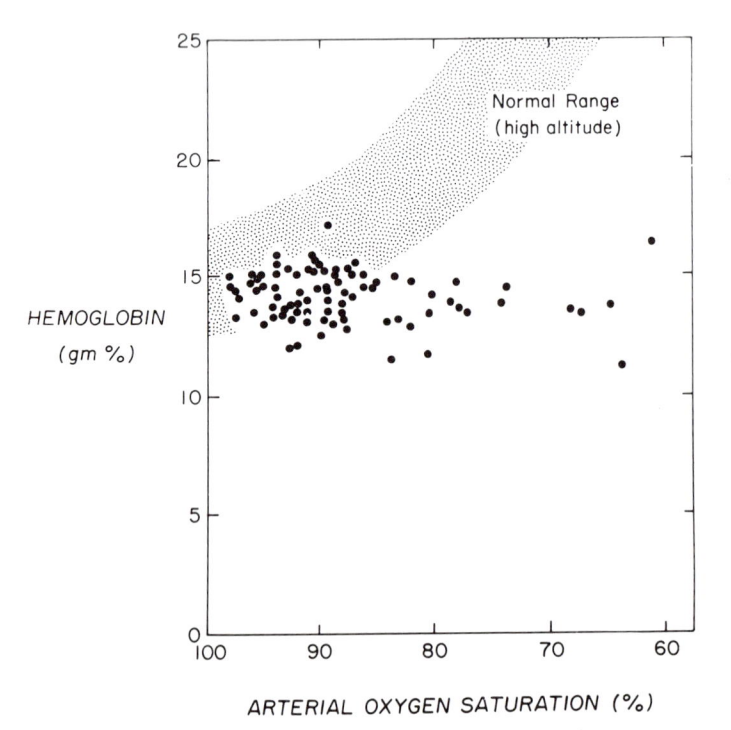

Figure 22–37 Hemoglobin concentrations of patients with various degrees of arterial oxygen desaturation due to chronic pulmonary disease. (Redrawn from Gallo, R. C., et al.: Arch. Intern. Med., *113*:559, 1964. Copyright 1964, American Medical Association.)

present. However, the increased plasma volume prevents an accurate assessment of the size of the red cell mass from hematocrit determinations alone.

ALVEOLAR HYPOVENTILATION. Alveolar hypoventilation, whether related to central or peripheral impairment, causes arterial hypoxemia, cyanosis, and secondary polycythemia. Its two most colorful variants are Monge's chronic mountain sickness (see earlier) and the Pickwickian syndrome. In the latter syndrome, named by Ratto and coworkers, obesity, peripheral hypoventilation, hypercapnia, somnolence and central hypoventilation are involved in a vicious circle leading to the characteristic somnolent cyanosis of Mrs. Wardle's proverbial boy, Joe.

DEFECTIVE OXYGEN TRANSPORT. Secondary polycythemia is occasionally observed in patients with cyanosis due to acquired or congenital methemoglobinemia. However, the erythropoietic response in these patients is caused less by a reduction in oxygen carrying capacity and more by a shift of the oxygen dissociation curve to the left. Cyanosis may be present with as little as 1.5 grams per 100 ml. of methemoglobin in the circulation, an amount which in itself should not result in significant tissue hypoxia. An increase in oxygen affinity is also present in hemoglobin partially combined with carbon monoxide and is probably responsible for the occasional polycythemia observed in patients with chronic carbon monoxide poisoning.

Familial polycythemias have recently been described in a number of individuals with abnormal hemoglobins. In most of these, the amino acid substitution occurs in the contact area between the alpha and beta chains. Such substitutions appear to interfere with the release of oxygen to the tissues, and a compensatory erythrocytosis occurs despite fully oxygen-saturated blood.

DRUG-INDUCED TISSUE HYPOXIA. Although a number of drugs and chemicals can induce histiotoxic anoxia, only cobalt has convincingly been associated with the development of a secondary appropriate polycythemia. Several recent studies have shown that cobalt administration causes the release of erythropoietin, and that this release presumably is related to its inhibitory effect on intracellular oxidative metabolism in the kidneys. Since the histiotoxic anoxia is generalized (Fig. 22-15), the use of cobalt in the treatment of refractory anemias is of little benefit to the patient. His oxygen carrying capacity may increase, but merely enough to counteract the effect of the additional tissue hypoxia induced by cobalt.

Inappropriate Secondary Polycythemia (Table 22-7)

RENAL DISORDERS. A partial obstruction of the renal artery or its tributaries may cause localized renal hypoxia, the stimulus for erythropoietin production. However, an impaired

TABLE 22-7 INAPPROPRIATE SECONDARY POLYCYTHEMIA

Location	Pathologic Condition	Number of Case Reports Until 1972
Kidney		
	Hypernephroma	118
	Other tumors	13
	Hydronephrosis	14
	Cystic disease	35
	Renal artery stenosis	2
	Transplantation rejection	7
	Barter's syndrome	1
Liver		
	Hepatoma	64
Uterus		
	Leiomyoma	24
Cerebellum		
	Hemangioblastoma	50
Adrenal Gland		
	Pheochromocytoma	5

Data from Thorling, E. B.: Scand. J. Haemat., Supple. 17, 1972.

blood supply to the kidneys usually causes structural damage and impaired erythropoietin production, and it is only the rare patient who responds with an increased release of erythropoietin and a secondary polycythemia. It is of potential importance that intrarenal vascular obstruction as observed in transplanted kidneys undergoing rejection will cause the release of erythropoietin. Unfortunately, the current assays are too laborious to permit the erythropoietin titer to be used to monitor patients who have received transplants to detect threatening rejection reaction. However, the appearance of an increased number of nucleated red cells or reticulocytes in the circulating blood may be used as a warning signal.

A more common cause of secondary polycythemia is the presence of space-occupying renal lesions. These lesions can be cysts, either solitary or part of polycystic renal disease, hydronephrosis, or a variety of renal neoplasms. Erythropoietin assays of cyst fluid have disclosed the presence of erythropoietin, and it has been proposed that the tubular lining of cysts is capable of secreting erythropoietin, possibly a reflection on the physiologic role of renal tubules in erythropoietin production. In regard to the neoplasms, assays of tumor extracts, especially extracts of hypernephromas, for erythropoietin have occasionally been positive. However, the fact that so many histologically different lesions can lead to an excessive production of erythropoietin has raised the suspicion that it is not the tumor cells which are engaged in inappropriate erythropoietin production, but it is the adjoining normal parenchyma which secretes this hormone in response to pressure-induced hypoxia.

Successful removal of renal tumors in patients with polycythemia has in many cases resulted in a normalization of the red blood cell count. Subsequent metastases in the opposite kidney have been associated with a recurrence of the polycythemia. However, the important question of whether or not extrarenal metastases can cause polycythemia has still not been answered.

EXTRARENAL DISORDERS. Cerebellar hemangiomas are frequently implicated in the induction of a secondary, inappropriate polycythemia. Cyst fluid from the tumor has, in a few cases, been shown to contain erythropoietic stimulatory material indistinguishable from erythropoietin. However, the proximity of the tumor to the respiratory center and to the hypothalamus has also suggested that central hypoventilation plays a role or that a hypothetical hypothalamic-renal connection is involved. In areas such as Hong Kong with a high incidence of hepatocarcinoma, 10 per cent of afflicted patients develop erythrocytosis. The most favored explanation is that the tumor is responsible for inappropriate secretion of erythropoietin, an explanation supported by direct assays of tumor extracts and by the hypothesis that the liver normally produces a precursor of erythropoietin. The rare polycythemia observed in patients with large uterine myomas may be caused by mechanical interference with renal blood supply. An inappropriate neoplastic production of erythropoietin by these fibrous, differentiated tumors seems unlikely in view of their histologic character. The occasional association between certain endocrine lesions such as Cushing's syndrome and pheochromocytomas is intriguing but has not been too informative. Steroid hormones appear to stimulate bone marrow activity mildly but the relationship between hypertension and erythropoietin is still quite tenuous. Although androgen-producing lesions have not been associated with polycythemia, androgens have empirically been found to be potentially potent stimulators of erythropoiesis. This effect may be mediated via a release of renal erythropoietin, although some data suggest a direct action of androgens on the bone marrow stem cell pool.

Multiplication Disorders

Vitamin B_{12} and Folic Acid. The identification of vitamin B_{12} and folates as important anti-anemia principles ranks among modern medicine's greatest triumphs. The exemplary clinical investigations of Minot and Murphy and of Castle in the 1920s and 1930s have been the source of a steady stream of basic and applied research accomplishments to the present day, the most recent of which has been the description of the synthesis of vitamin B_{12} in the laboratory by Woodward and Eschenmoser (see Maugh reference). These nutritional factors participate as cofactors in a wide variety of biochemical reactions in the body. In some respects their biochemical reactions are interrelated. Their essential role in DNA synthesis explains why deficiencies of either or both lead to "megaloblastic anemia" and to disturbances in cell division not only in the marrow but in other proliferating cell populations, such as the gastrointestinal epithelium (see Sullivan reference). Nervous tissue, which is not in a state of cellular proliferation, has a unique requirement for vitamin B_{12}.

Vitamin B_{12} (molecular weight 1355) is built asymmetrically around cobalt much like heme is built around iron, with its suspension between histidine residues in the "heme pocket." Cobalt, like iron, has six coordinate positions, four of which are bound to nitrogen atoms in a planar tetrapyrrole corrin ring (Fig. 22–38). Below and almost perpendicular to the plane of the corrin ring, a benzimidazole nucleotide occupies the fifth coordinate position, also in a nitrogen linkage. The sixth position is ionic, and in "cyanocobalamin," the parent compound of the family of vitamin B_{12} relatives, it is occupied by cyanide. The presence of the cyanide ligand in this position, however, is an artifact of isolation. The physiologically active coenzyme forms of the vitamin contain either a methyl or a deoxyadenosyl group in this position. Cyanocobalamin, as well as its relative hydroxycobalamin, are readily converted to these active forms within the body (see Silber and Moldow).

The absorption of vitamin B_{12} is dependent upon a unique mechanism unshared by any other essential nutrient (see Corcino and coworkers). The parietal cells of the stomach produce, along with hydrochloric acid, a glycoprotein known as "intrinsic factor" (IF), which tightly and specifically binds B_{12}, the "extrinsic factor," after it has been ingested and is released from complexes in foodstuffs (Fig. 22–39). IF has a molecular weight of 60,000 and binds B_{12} on a mole-for-mole basis. The binding occurs with the benzimidazole nucleotide moiety of B_{12} and is independent of the specific chemical form of the vitamin. Dimers are formed when the vitamin is bound. It then travels down the length of the intestinal tract, protected in the IF complex from the degradative activities of digestive enzymes. Specific receptors on the surface of the microvilli of the terminal ileum take up the IF-B_{12} complex in a process dependent upon a pH of above 6.5 as well as upon divalent

Figure 22-38 Structure of deoxyadenosyl cobalamine, a physiologically active form of vitamin B_{12}. (From Chanarin, I.: The Megaloblastic Anemias. Philadelphia, F. A. Davis Co., 1969, p. 16.)

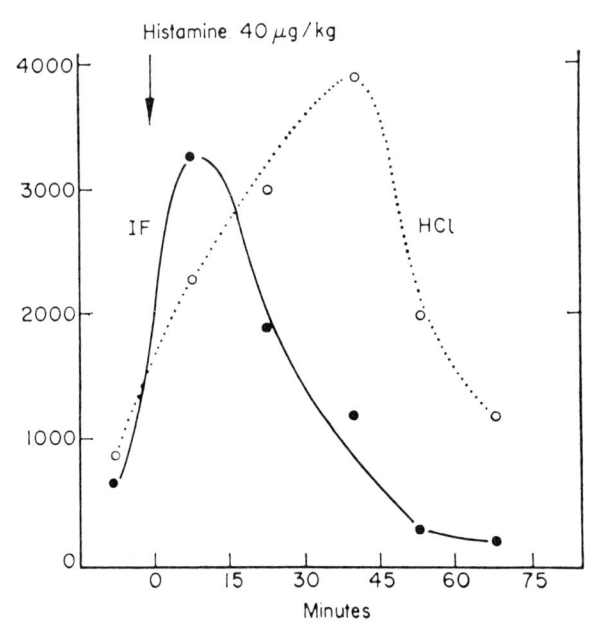

Figure 22-39 Stimulation of gastric secretion of intrinsic factor (IF) and hydrochloric acid by histamine. (Redrawn from Arderman, S., et al.: Brit. Med. J., 2:600, 1964.)

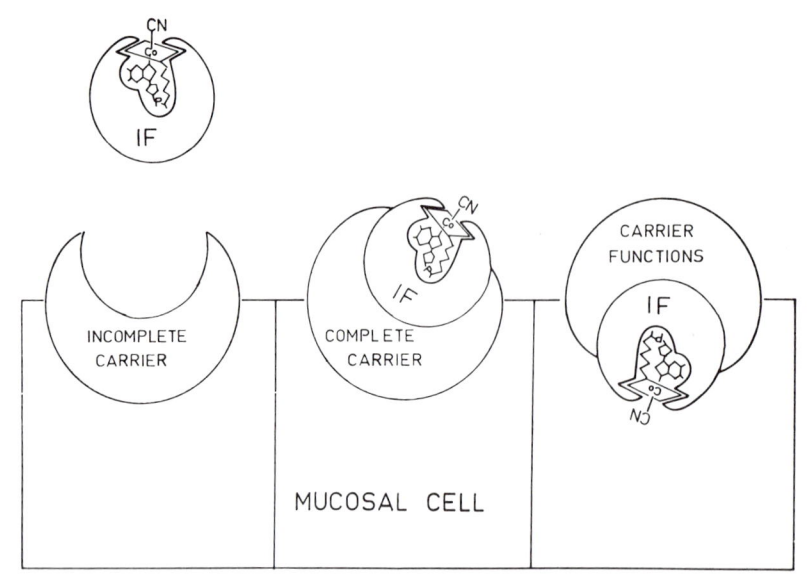

Figure 22-40 Mucosal absorption in the terminal ileum of vitamin B_{12} bound to intrinsic factor. (From Gräsbeck, R.: Scand. J. Clin. Lab. Invest., 19:7 (Suppl. 95.), 1967. Universitetsforlaget, Oslo.)

cations (calcium and/or magnesium) (Fig. 22-40). It is still uncertain whether the entire complex enters the cell or whether IF is released back into the lumen after the vitamin is released.

After a small dose of 1 μg. of B_{12} about 60 to 80 per cent is absorbed. However, the proportion absorbed decreases as the amount of ingested B_{12} increases. About 1 to 5 μg. is absorbed from a dietary intake of 5 to 30 μg. per day. A tiny amount of B_{12}, less than 1 per cent, is absorbed in an IF-independent manner, but this is too small to be of physiologic significance. There is a substantial excretion of B_{12} from the biliary tract into the intestinal lumen, but this is efficiently reabsorbed in an IF-dependent enterohepatic circuit, and thus is not lost to the body economy.

The plasma contains two vitamin B_{12} binding proteins (see Hall reference). The native plasma B_{12} is bound to transcobalamin I, an alpha globulin which may originate from release from certain tissues, most notably granulocytes. Its level, along with that of B_{12}, is markedly elevated in association with extreme elevations in the granulocyte count, as in chronic granulocytic leukemia. Conversely, low levels of both occasionally occur in the presence of severe granulocytopenia. Vitamin B_{12} added to plasma in vitro or in vivo is chiefly bound to transcobalamin II, a transport protein which rapidly yields up the vitamin to tissue depots, especially the liver. Normally, transcobalamin II circulates without significant quantities of bound vitamin. How it picks up the vitamin from the ileal mucosal cell is still not clear.

Folic acid contains one molecule of pteroic acid in combination with one molecule of L-glutamic acid and is thus alternately designated pteroylmonoglutamic acid (Fig. 22-41). The term "folates" refers to a family of related compounds containing variable numbers of glutamic acid residues in a polypeptide linkage involving the gamma glutamyl carboxyl residue. These pteroylpolyglutamates contain up to seven glutamic acid residues and are the natural form in which most food folates occur. They are less well absorbed than the monoglutamate (see Baugh et al. reference). Their absorption is facilitated by the intestinal enzyme "conjugase," which hydrolyzes the glutamyl peptide bonds, reducing the chain length (Fig. 22-42). Folic acid is converted to physiologically active forms within the body by reduction and methylation reactions. The reduction to tetrahydrofolate (FH_4) is accomplished in two steps, involving two hydrogen atoms in each step, by the enzyme dihydrofolate reductase. This enzyme is inhibited by very low concentrations of the antifolate compound, methotrexate, which is the basis of both its chemotherapeutic efficacy in neoplastic conditions and its toxicity to the bone marrow and gastrointestinal epithelium. The methylation of FH_4 involves a number of different points of attachment of the active carbon unit, which itself exists in a variety of forms (methyl, formyl, hydroxymethyl, methylene, methenyl, formimino), giving rise to a large family of biologically active FH_4 derivatives (Fig. 22-41). These "active" folates are not pharmacologically available, with the exception of citro-

Figure 22-41 Structure of folic acid and its derivatives. Tetrahydrofolate is abbreviated here as THF and in the text as FH_4. (From Harris, J. W., and Kellermeyer, R. W.: The Red Cell. Cambridge, Harvard University Press, 1970, p. 395.)

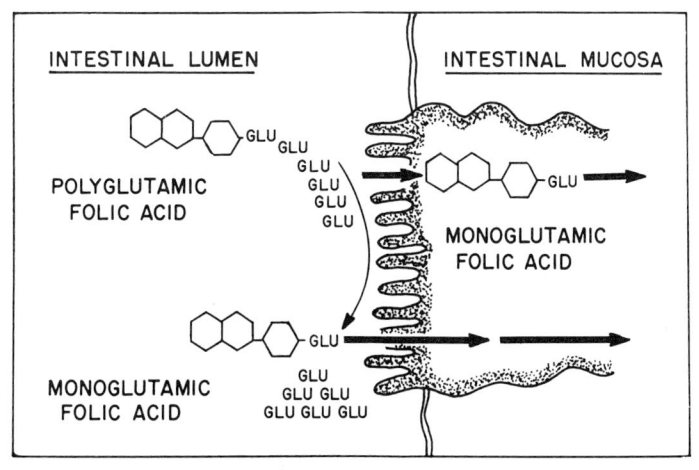

Figure 22-42 Intestinal absorption of the folate derivatives of food. (From Streiff, R. R.: J.A.M.A., 214:105, 1970. Copyright 1970 by the American Medical Association.)

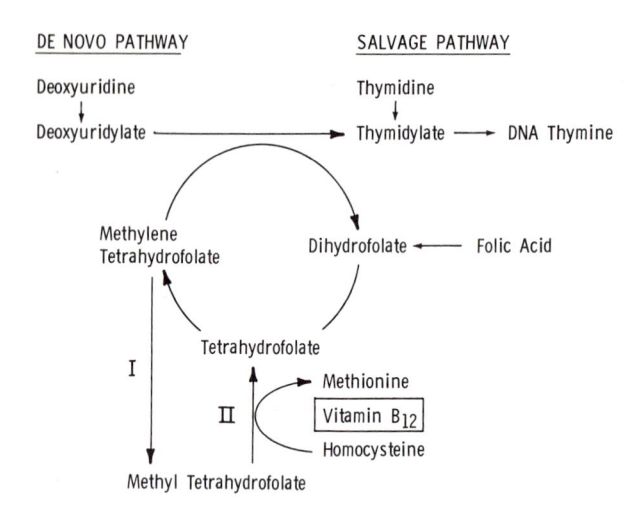

Figure 22-43 Vitamin B_{12}-folate interrelationships. Tetrahydrofolate is abbreviated in the text as FH_4. (Redrawn from Waxman, S., et al.: J. Clin. Invest., 48:284, 1969.)

vorum factor (Leucovorin, folinic acid), the N^5-formyl derivative. This agent is of use as an antidote for methotrexate toxicity, against which folic acid is ineffective.

Although B_{12} and folate participate as active coenzymes in a number of biochemical reactions involving transfer of carbon or hydrogen atoms, their roles in DNA synthesis are of particular interest with respect to the pathogenesis of the megaloblastic anemias. Beck has proposed that deoxyadenosyl cobalamin is a coenzyme in the reduction of oxyribotides to deoxyribotides by the enzyme ribonucleotide reductase. This hypothesis has the attractive feature of explaining why DNA synthesis is impaired while RNA synthesis is spared, but unfortunately the experimental evidence in favor of it has come exclusively from studies on bacterial systems. An alternate "folate trap" hypothesis conceives of closely related but distinctive roles for active folate and cobalamin in hematopoiesis. It states that B_{12} deficiency interferes only indirectly with DNA synthesis by impairing the folate-mediated conversion of uridylate (a precursor only of RNA) to thymidylate (a precursor only of DNA) (Fig. 22–43). In postulated sequence, (1) lack of B_{12} impairs the methylation of homocysteine to methionine, which in turn (2) causes accumulation of N^5-methylFH_4 (the "trap") at the expense of FH_4, and (3) FH_4 (but not N^5-methylFH_4) is required for the formation of N^5,N^{10}-methylene FH_4, which is essential as the cofactor in the conversion of uridylate to thymidylate, and thus also for DNA synthesis.

The biochemical action of B_{12} in the nervous tissue is still controversial, but circumstantial evidence has pointed to its role in propionate metabolism (Fig. 22–44). Deoxyadenosylcobalamin acts as cofactor in the rearrangement of active methylmalonate, formed as a result of carboxylation of propionate, to succinate. Indeed, in-

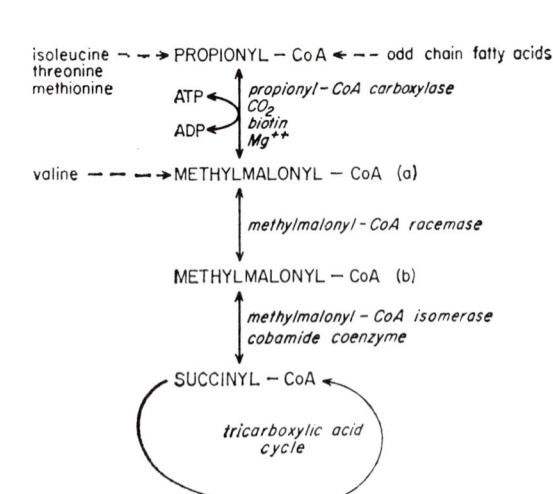

Figure 22-44 The role of vitamin B_{12} in propionate metabolism. The cobamide coenzyme is deoxyadenosyl cobalamin. (From Rosenberg, L. E., et al.: Science, 162:805, 1968. Copyright 1968 by the American Association for the Advancement of Science.)

creased urinary excretion of methylmalonate is a reliable indicator of B_{12} deficiency. An increase in the serum concentration as well as the urinary excretion is also seen in methylmalonic acidemia, a rare inherited defect of B_{12} conversion to its active deoxyadenosyl coenzyme form.

A urinary test for folate deficiency is available. It depends on the requirement for FH_4 in the conversion of histidine to glutamic acid. The block leads to accumulation of urocanic and formiminoglutamic (FIGLU) acids, which are excreted in excess in the urine after a loading dose of histidine.

General Effects of Megaloblastic Anemia. The signs and symptoms are primarily related to the hematopoietic and gastrointestinal systems, although the neurologic system is also affected in B_{12} deficiency. The degree of anemia may be quite profound, but its onset is very slow and as a result it is amazingly well tolerated, unless congestive heart failure or angina pectoris supervenes. The sclerae are often slightly icteric, the tongue is usually atrophic and smooth, and splenomegaly may be present. There may be vague gastrointestinal complaints. The neurologic signs of B_{12} deficiency include a spastic and incoordinate gait, paresthesias, and sometimes mental changes. Increased reflexes, Babinski signs, and loss of position and vibration sense are indicative of posterior and lateral column demyelination (Fig. 22-45). Decreased reflexes and hypesthesia are signs of peripheral neuropathy, and altered behavior and impaired mentation may indicate cerebral involvement.

The deficiency affects all the proliferating hematopoietic elements and therefore pancytopenia is commonly observed, but granulocytopenia and thrombocytopenia are usually not so severe that infectious susceptibility or hemorrhage results.

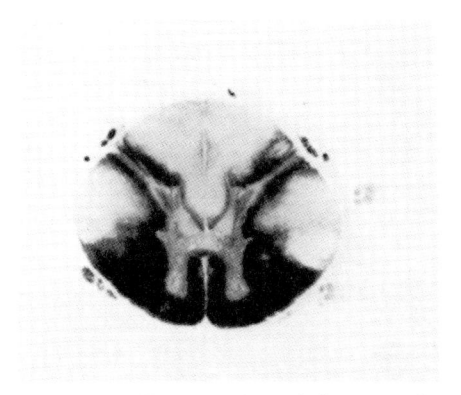

Figure 22-45 Degeneration of the posterior and lateral columns of the spinal cord in vitamin B_{12} deficiency. (From Chanarin, I.: The Megaloblastic Anemias. Philadelphia, F. A. Davis Co., 1969, p. 576.)

The anemia is macrocytic, but wide variations within the cell population of mean erythrocyte volume are characteristic, and indeed some erythrocytes are microcytic. The presence of "macro-ovalocytes" is a particularly valuable morphologic sign. Mature segmented neutrophils have a greater than normal mean number of lobes per nucleus; a few may contain as many as 7 or 8.

When the anemia is severe, megaloblastic erythroid precursors are found in the circulation, and a small proportion of mature erythrocytes contains nuclear remnants (Howell-Jolly bodies, Cabot's rings). The reticulocytes are not increased and polychromasia is not prominent. Distinctive morphologic changes are also seen in the gastrointestinal epithelial cells, but the diagnosis rests upon the finding of "megaloblastic" changes in the bone marrow. This term was originally applied to erythroid precursors only, but today it is used to refer to changes in all three cell lines—granulocytic and megakaryocytic as well as erythroid. The entire erythroid line of maturation is altered to form a "megaloblastic series." There is the appearance of a "maturation arrest" because of the marked shift to the left, with large numbers of early erythroid precursors having intensely basophilic cytoplasm. The arrest in nuclear development is reflected in an abnormally finely divided and open pattern of the nuclear chromatin. Hemoglobin formation proceeds in the cytoplasm, however, and "nuclear-cytoplasmic dissociation" is observed. The entire series is larger than normal, and mature cells emerge as macrocytic erythrocytes. The marrow granulocytic precursors also show distinctive changes, in particular large horseshoe- and C-shaped nuclear forms at the band stage of maturation. The marrow shows a marked overall increase in cellularity.

Why the deficient marrow should react with a hypercellular proliferative response remains unexplained. It is clear, however, that the defect in nuclear development leads to intramedullary destruction of the blood cell precursors. Heme catabolism from the breakdown of erythroid precursors in the marrow is the major factor contributing to the signs of hemolysis—the elevated serum indirect bilirubin, the absence of plasma haptoglobin, and the elevation of serum lactic dehydrogenase to levels rarely seen in the hemolytic anemias. Megaloblastic anemia is a classic example of the pathophysiology of ineffective erythropoiesis. The number of reticulocytes in the peripheral blood is not elevated despite intense erythroid hyperplasia in the marrow. The serum iron concentration is raised, and its rate of clearance from the circulation to the erythroid marrow is increased, with only small amounts appearing over subsequent days in the newly formed erythrocytes (Fig. 22-24). The amount of radioactive label appearing in the "early bilirubin" peak after administration of a tagged heme precursor is markedly increased (Fig. 22-71).

With treatment, the signs promptly revert to normal within several days: the serum iron concentration decreases and its utilization for the production of circulating erythrocytes becomes effective, the jaundice disappears, the elevated serum lactic dehydrogenase falls, and the megaloblastic signs are no longer seen in the marrow. The reticulocyte count becomes elevated within 3 to 4 days, reaches a peak at 7 to 10 days, and then falls (Fig. 22-46). The reticulocyte response is the most reliable early sign of response, and in the more anemic individuals it may peak at 25 to 50 per cent. The anemia is corrected within 12 weeks. The neurologic symptoms of B_{12} lack are reversed, unless they have progressed to an advanced degree of severity. Pharmacologic doses of folic acid will produce a hematologic response in the B_{12}-deficient patient while worsening the neurologic complications. Presumably the folate causes a fall in serum B_{12} level, with a diversion of available B_{12} away from neural to hematopoietic tissue. Large doses of B_{12} will also give a hematologic response in the folate-deficient patient. Response to therapy is specific if the administered dose is limited to the range of the minimal daily requirement, about $1\mu g$. per day of B_{12} or 50 μg. per day of folate.

Vitamin B_{12} Deficiency

DIETARY LACK. Inadequate intake is an exceptionally rare cause of deficiency. B_{12} is present in a wide variety of products of animal origin—meat, fish, eggs, butter, milk, and cheese—and the minimal daily requirement of 1 to 5 μg. is readily met unless a strict vegetarian diet is followed. Even then, the total body stores of 2000 to 5000 μg. are well conserved, with a loss of only 0.1 per cent per day of the total body pool. The B_{12} deficiency is mild even after 10 to 20 years on a rigidly restricted diet.

INTRINSIC FACTOR LACK. The term "pernicious anemia" (PA) no longer seems appropriate, considering the fact that the condition is now effectively cured (see Castle reference). However, its historical roots are deep and there is no inclination to displace it with a new designation. PA should be used exclusively for conditions primarily characterized by a lack of the gastric intrinsic factor.

Congenital PA is a rare autosomal recessive condition which is apparently clinically manifest only in the homozygous state. There is an isolated lack of IF without insufficiency of gastric acid or pepsin. Passively acquired B_{12} stores present at birth are exhausted in two or three years, and anemia then develops.

Adult PA, a disorder of mature and older adults, only rarely affects older children and young adults. Genetic factors still not well defined play some role, since there is a significant intrafamilial occurrence as well as an ethnic predilection for individuals of northern and western European background. The absence of IF in the gastric juice is always found in association with atrophic gastritis, and there is accordingly a lack of gastric acidity and pepsin, even after stim-

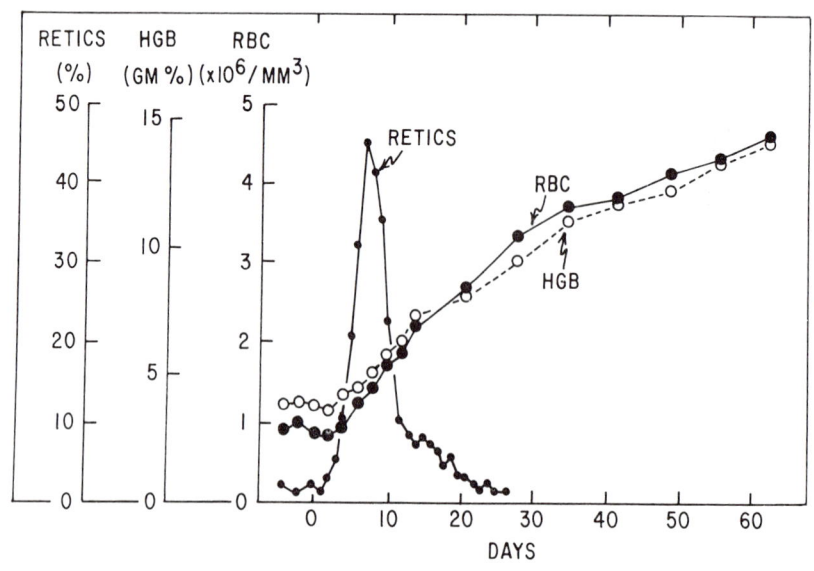

Figure 22-46 Hematologic response to treatment of vitamin B_{12} deficiency in a patient with pernicious anemia. (Redrawn from Castle, W. B., *in* Cecil and Loeb (Eds.): A Textbook of Medicine. Philadelphia, W. B. Saunders Co., 1959, p. 1131.)

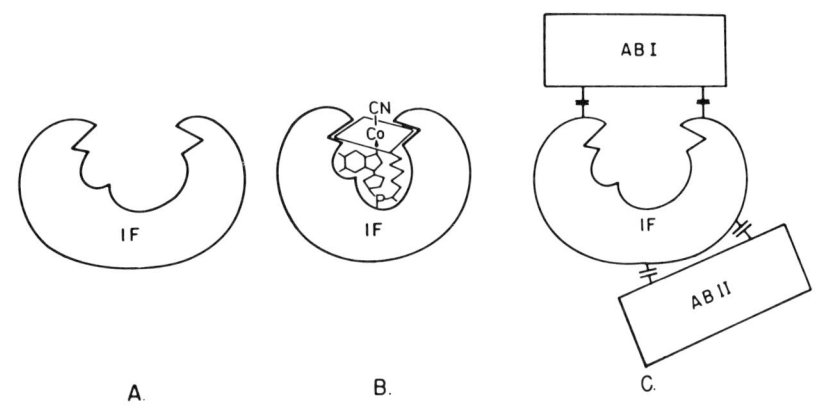

Figure 22-47 Anti-intrinsic factor antibodies of the blocking (AB I) and binding (AB II) types. (From Gräsbeck, R.: Progr. Hemat., 6:233-260, 1969. By permission of Grune and Stratton, Inc., New York.)

ulation with histamine. Atrophic gastritis is not uncommon in the general population, and its incidence increases with age. Why certain affected persons develop pernicious anemia is still uncertain, but the following current evidence supports an autoimmune theory of pathogenesis:

(1) The histologic appearance of lymphocytic infiltration of the gastric mucosa suggests a local immunologic process.

(2) Antibodies which react against the cytoplasm of the gastric parietal cell are present in the serum of 90 per cent of patients with adult PA. A significant incidence of such antibodies is present, however, in patients who do not have PA. These include 60 per cent of all individuals with atrophic gastritis, 30 per cent of blood relatives of PA patients, and slightly less than 10 per cent of a control population. PA patients frequently have serum antibodies directed against parenchymal endocrine glands, most notably the acinar cells of the thyroid. Conversely, patients with primary myxedema and Hashimoto's thyroiditis have a 30 per cent incidence of antiparietal cell serum antibodies and a 12 per cent incidence of coexisting PA.

(3) About three fourths of PA patients have anti-IF antibodies in serum, saliva, and gastric juice. These are much more specific for PA and are rarely found in its absence. These antibodies are polyclonal and may be either IgG or IgA. They apparently react at two different sites on the IF molecule (Fig. 22-47). "Blocking" antibodies prevent the binding of B_{12} to IF, presumably by obstructing the site of attachment. "Binding" antibodies do not interfere with the attachment of B_{12} to IF, but they do impede absorption in the ileum.

Whether these various autoimmune phenomena associated with PA are cause or effect remains uncertain, but the properties of the anti-IF antibodies present in gastric secretions clearly suggest a role in pathogenesis.

Total gastrectomy will predictably produce megaloblastic anemia after 5 or 6 years, but partial gastrectomy in most instances does not deplete IF sufficiently to lead to frank megaloblastosis. With the passage of years, however, an increasing proportion develop low serum B_{12} levels, some of whom have mild megaloblastic changes in the marrow (Fig. 22-48). Iron deficiency is the commonest cause of postgastrectomy anemia, and its presence may mask concomitant megaloblastosis, the signs of which are brought out following iron repletion.

DECREASED ILEAL ABSORPTION. Ablation of the specific site of B_{12} absorption in the terminal ileum by surgical resection or by such diseases as regional ileitis, lymphoma, or tuberculosis leads to B_{12} deficiency without an associated lack of IF or of gastric acid. Certain drugs (neomycin, colchicine, para-amino salicylate) reportedly interfere with B_{12} absorption by mechanisms which remain obscure. The gastrointestinal epithelial changes of tropical sprue are extensive and commonly cause B_{12} deficiency, especially in chronic cases. The megaloblastic alterations of B_{12} or folate deficiency themselves cause sufficient epithelial change to interfere with ileal absorption (see Haurani et al. reference). Indeed, patients with folate deficiency tend to have lower than normal serum concentrations of B_{12}, with spontaneous correction after folate repletion (Fig. 22-49). Poor absorption may also occur consequent to pancreatic insufficiency, presumably because secreted bicarbonate is needed to maintain pH and ionic calcium concentration at optimal values for uptake of the IF-B_{12} complex. Imerslund's syndrome is a rare congenital deficiency of the receptor site in the terminal ileum causing megaloblastic anemia in children. IF

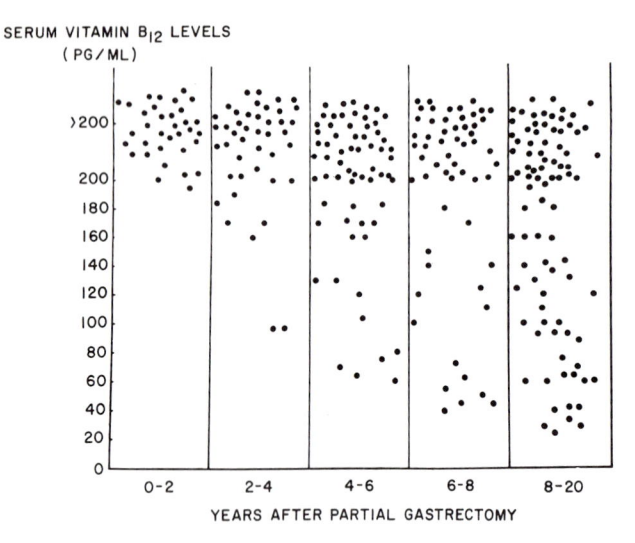

Figure 22-48 Serum vitamin B_{12} levels at various intervals after subtotal gastrectomy. Patients with B_{12} deficiency megaloblastic anemia have values in the range of 0 to 100 pg. per ml. (Redrawn from Hines, J. D., et al.: Amer. J. Med., *43*:555, 1967.)

secretion is normal. Renal structural abnormalities and proteinuria are also commonly present.

DECREASED AVAILABILITY. Decreased serum B_{12} levels and megaloblastic anemia are found in association with anatomic abnormalities of the gastrointestinal tract which lead to stasis and pooling of the luminal contents. Such "blind loop syndromes"—strictures, surgically created bypasses, fistulas, and large diverticula—have in common the presence of bacterial overgrowth along with steatorrhea. The anemia does not respond to orally administered B_{12}, but parenteral replacement is effective. Intrinsic factor is present in normal amounts, indicating that the IF-B_{12} complex is unavailable for absorption in the terminal ileum. The finding that therapy with broad-spectrum antibiotics causes disappearance of the stigmata of B_{12} lack provides strong evidence that bacterial utilization is responsible for the deficiency. A similar mechanism explains the megaloblastic anemia associated with the fish tapeworm (*Diphyllobothrium*

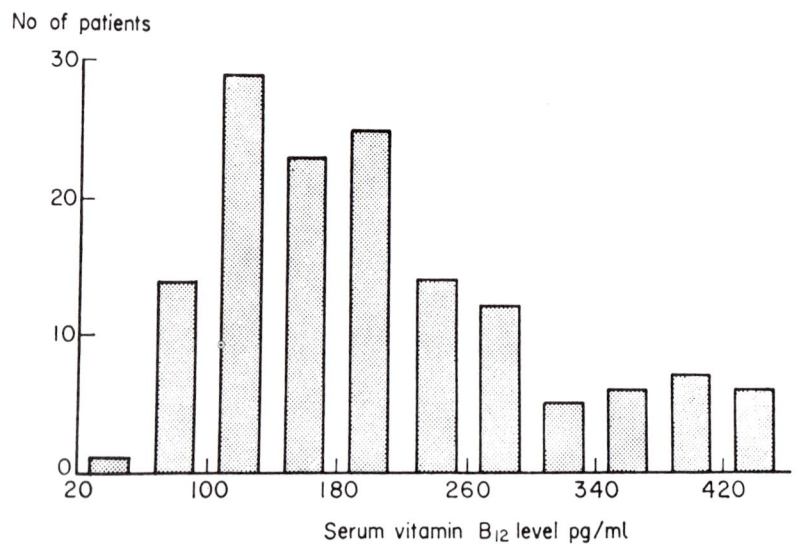

Figure 22-49 Serum vitamin B_{12} levels in patients with megaloblastic anemia due to folate deficiency. The normal range of values is 200 to 800 pg. per ml. (Redrawn from Mollin, D. L., Waters, A. H., and Harriss, E., *in* 2 Europaisches Symposium, Hamburg, 1961 (H. C. Heinrich, Ed.), Stuttgart, Enke. Reprinted in Chanarin, I.: The Megaloblastic Anemias. Philadelphia, F. A. Davis Co., 1969.)

latum). Infestation occurs because of eating improperly cooked fresh-water fish. The worms grow to great lengths in the intestinal tract and effectively compete with the host for available IF-B_{12} complex. The disorder is especially common in Finland.

Folate Deficiency

DIETARY LACK. Poor nutrition—an unusual cause of B_{12} deficiency—frequently gives rise to folate depletion. The elderly recluse, the "tea and toast" faddist, and the alcoholic are prototypes of deficiency in the United States. In other countries, excessive cooking of food, often limited in amount and diversity, destroys labile folates and causes leeching out of the soluble folates in the cooking water. Newborns procure sufficient amounts even from deficient mothers, but develop megaloblastic anemia when they reach the 2-year stage of rapid growth if they are raised on low folate diets, such as goat's milk or boiled milk. Folates are present in many different foodstuffs—leafy green vegetables, fruits, meats, eggs—and food intake must be severely limited in diversity in order to fall short of the minimal daily requirement of 50 µg. Lack of ascorbate, thiamin, and other essential nutrients often coexists. In alcoholics, poor diet is not the only factor, since ethanol seems to interfere with folate absorption, its intermediary metabolism, and its hepatic storage. It also exerts a direct toxic suppression on the bone marrow elements.

The sequence of events after limitation of folate intake has been studied experimentally by Herbert (Fig. 22–50). The serum folate concentration is the most sensitive indicator of deficiency, falling within a month of deficient intake. Red cell folate concentration is more stubbornly defended, but it also falls as megaloblastic anemia appears after 3 to 4 months of deficiency. Folate stores are neither as ample, relative to daily requirement, nor as avidly guarded as B_{12} stores.

The minimal daily requirement of folate increases during pregnancy to about 400 µg. Serum folate levels tend to fall as pregnancy proceeds to term. A diet that maintains body folate in a marginal state of balance will prove inadequate in the face of such an increase in demands, and thus folate deficiency is the commonest cause of megaloblastic anemia of pregnancy. Conditions of increased cellular proliferation, such as hemolytic anemia, as well as thyrotoxicosis also raise the minimal requirement for folate.

MALABSORPTION. "Blind loop syndromes," which bring on B_{12} deficiency because of bacterial utilization, are not associated with folate lack. Possibly bacterial synthesis in the stagnant loop may actually add to the body's supply. On the other hand, gastrointestinal disorders affecting extensive areas of absorptive surface, with attendant malabsorption, frequently lead to folate deficiency. Gluten-sensitive enteropathy (nontropical sprue) most severely affects the upper reaches of the bowel—the duodenum and jejunum—where folate absorption normally is maximal, sparing the terminal ileum along with B_{12} absorption in many instances. In tropical sprue, the involvement extends throughout the gut, affecting B_{12} as well as folate absorption. Folic acid therapy often improves the malabsorption along with the megaloblastic anemia in tropical sprue, but in nontropical sprue improvement in gastrointestinal function is achieved by

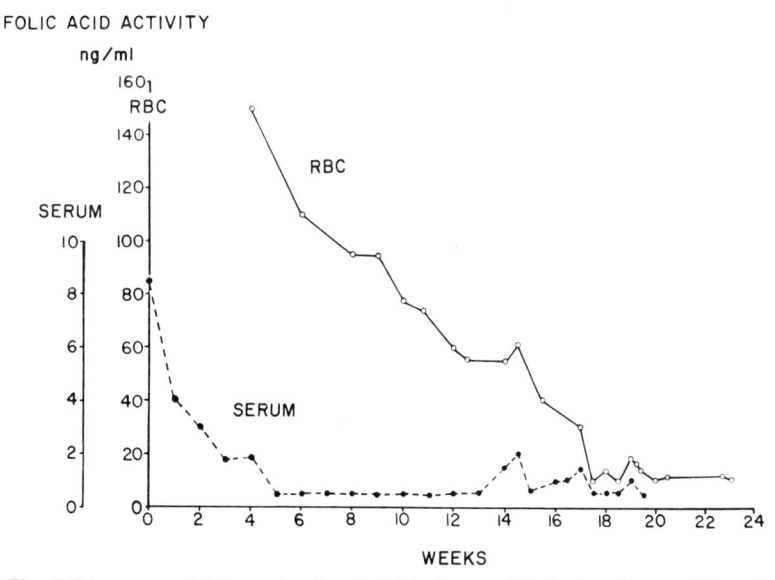

Figure 22–50 The fall in serum folate and red cell folate in a subject placed on a folate-deficient diet. (Redrawn from Herbert, V.: Trans. Amer. Assoc. Physicians, 75:307, 1962.)

eliminating gluten from the diet. Oral therapy with folic acid—the monoglutamate form—is often effective, suggesting that the polyglutamates of food folates are not well hydrolyzed by intestinal conjugase to more readily absorbed less polymerized forms.

Other gastrointestinal disorders with malabsorption are lymphoma, scleroderma, amyloidosis, Whipple's disease, and extensive surgical resection. In addition to deficiencies of folate and/or B_{12}, iron lack is also commonly present in malabsorption syndromes, giving the picture of a combined deficiency anemia.

DRUGS. Patients on diphenylhydantoin therapy have a significant incidence of low serum folate levels and of megaloblastic anemia which responds readily to oral folic acid therapy. The pathogenesis of this adverse drug effect is currently viewed as an inhibition of polyglutamate absorption, possibly through an effect on the intestinal conjugase activity. Estrogenic contraceptives occasionally have a similar side-effect. Although some evidence has been reported suggesting that diphenylhydantoin interferes with folate metabolism, the mechanism of megaloblastic anemia produced by the antimalarial pyrimethamine is more closely akin to that of methotrexate as a competitive inhibitor of folate metabolism.

Miscellaneous Megaloblastic Anemias. Therapy of neoplastic disease often leads to megaloblastic bone marrow and macrocytic red cells. Some of the cytotoxic agents in use which predictably inhibit nucleotide synthesis with secondary megaloblastic change are the antifolates (methotrexate), purine inhibitors (6-mercaptopurine, thioguanine, azathioprine), pyrimidine inhibitors (5-fluorouracil), and pentose analogues (cytosine arabinoside). Primary refractory megaloblastic anemia may represent a nuclear maturation defect of a myeloproliferative syndrome. When such a defect affects both the erythroid and granulocytic precursors, it is known as erythroleukemia (Di Guglielmo syndrome). In some proliferative disorders of the bone marrow, local shortages are brought on by the increased requirements of the abnormal proliferation, causing morphologic signs of deficiency in neighboring cells. Hereditary orotic aciduria is a rare megaloblastic anemia of childhood caused by an inherited block in pyrimidine synthesis.

Maturation Disorders of the Erythrocyte Cytoplasm

Hemoglobin Synthesis. The circulating erythrocyte is the most specialized of the body's cells—95 per cent of its cytoplasm consists of the respiratory pigment hemoglobin packed into the cell interior at a concentration almost five times that of the proteins of the exterior plasma. The formation of hemoglobin begins at the earliest precursor stage of the developing erythroid cell and is completed when the anucleate reticulocyte matures to an erythrocyte. No additional hemoglobin is produced during the 120-day period of the erythrocyte's life span in the circulation. The biosynthesis of hemoglobin is a complex series of distinct but delicately coordinated biochemical events, so well balanced that component parts are brought together assembly-line fashion, without significant shortages or surpluses, to form the completed molecule. Heme is formed in a sequential series of enzymatically controlled reactions. Dissimilar polypeptide globin subunits under separate genetic control are assembled on polyribosomes. The finished molecule has two pairs of such subunits, each linked with its own prosthetic heme group into a tetrameric macromolecule.

General Effects of Disorders of Hemoglobin Synthesis. Deficiency in the quantity of hemoglobin leads to microcytic, hypochromic anemia. The hemoglobin lack comes either from a lack of heme, as in iron deficiency, or from insufficient globin, to which the designation "thalassemia" is given. Qualitative abnormalities of the hemoglobin may alter the internal consistency of the erythrocyte cytoplasm and cause increased cell rigidity which leads to premature destruction and hemolysis. Abnormal hemoglobin oxygen affinity or oxidation state gives rise to cyanosis or erythrocytosis. Many abnormal hemoglobins produce no pathophysiologic abnormality because they function quite normally.

Porphyrins

NORMAL PORPHYRIN SYNTHESIS. Of all the tissues in the body, the erythroid marrow and the liver are by far the most preeminent porphyrin producers. The synthesis is accomplished on mitochondria under the control of preformed enzymes. The initial step requires energy. The brightly colored finished product contains four pyrrole rings connected into a larger cyclic tetrapyrrole structure by methene bridges. Side chains are attached to the ring structure: 4 methyl, 2 vinyl, and 2 propionyl (Fig. 22-51). In the first step, active succinate, obtained chiefly from the tricarboxylic acid cycle, is joined to glycine by delta-aminolevulinic acid synthetase to form delta-aminolevulinic acid (δ-ALA). This enzyme is both rate-limiting and regulatory, being subject to end-product inhibition (Fig. 22-12). Pyridoxal phosphate is required for the activation of glycine. Monopyrrole porphobilinogen rings are then formed by head to tail linkages of two δ-ALA molecules. Four porphobilinogens in turn condense into the cyclic tetrapyrrole structure (Fig. 22-52). The tetrapyrrole, after deamination, undergoes change from uroporphyrinogen (containing 8 carboxyl side chains) to coproporphyrinogen (containing 4 carboxyl side chains) to

Figure 22-51 The structure of heme. (From Harris, J. W., and Kellermeyer, R. W.: The Red Cell. Cambridge, Harvard University Press, 1970, p. 3.)

protoporphyrinogen (containing 2 carboxyl side chains). Progressive decarboxylation is associated with an increased degree of insolubility which to some degree determines fecal as opposed to urinary excretion. The suffix "-ogen" refers to the reduced colorless state in which these derivatives are synthesized. Oxidation to the colored forms follows in the tissues and excreta. The "uro-" and "copro-" intermediates are bridged together by methylene bonds which are oxidized to methene bonds in the protoporphyrins. The tetrapyrroles may occur in isomeric states, depending on the position of the side chains. Four isomers are possible for the "uro-" and "copro-" derivatives, but only the type I and III isomers occur biologically. An isomerase presides over the initial step of tetrapyrrole formation and normally guides the bulk of synthesis toward the family of III isomers, which go on to form protoporphyrin 9, the isomeric precursor of heme. In the final step of heme synthesis, four of the six coordinate positions of ferrous iron are chelated to protoporphyrin 9 by the enzyme heme synthetase (ferrochelatase). The heme produced for combination with globin is chemically identical to that found in cytochromes, myoglobin, and other heme proteins.

GENERAL EFFECTS OF DISORDERS OF PORPHYRIN SYNTHESIS. Overproduction of porphyrin intermediates and/or precursors causes increased urinary and fecal excretion along with tissue accumulation (see Taddeini and Watson reference). The oxidized forms cause red urine and sometimes red staining of the tissues. Absorption of light in the 400 nm. wavelength range is a common property of the porphyrins, and those derivatives which are excited by the absorbed light to emit fluorescence cause photosensitive skin lesions to appear on exposed body surfaces, such as the face and the back of the hands, which are af-

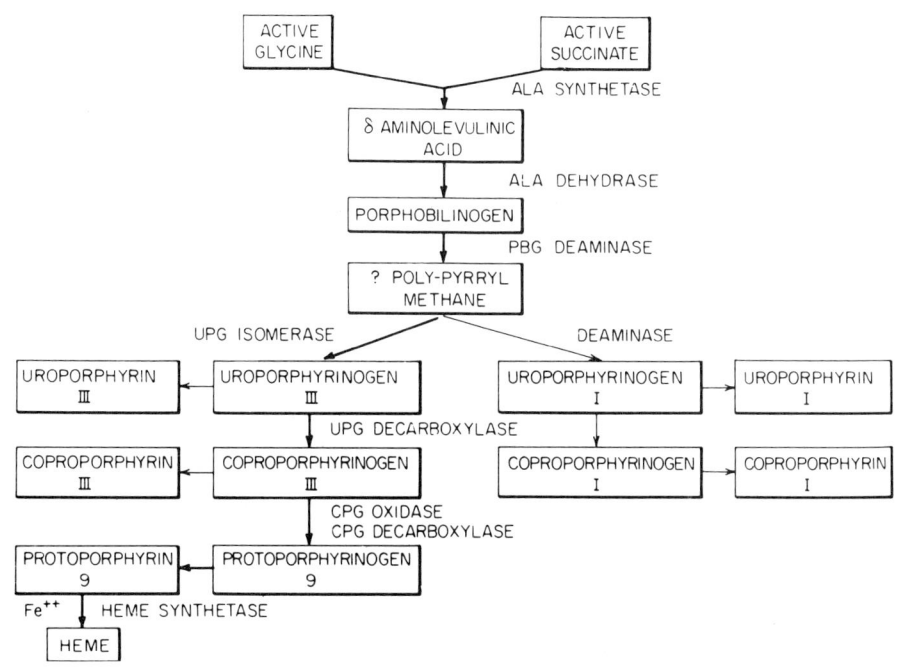

Figure 22-52 The synthesis of heme. (From Harris, J. W., and Kellermeyer, R. W.: The Red Cell. Cambridge, Harvard University Press, 1970, p. 40.)

fected with erythema, edema, itching, blistering, and eventually even scarring and disfigurement. Some porphyrias are predominantly of hepatic pathogenesis and do not affect red cells.

Disorders of Porphyrin Synthesis

Inherited. "Congenital erythropoietic porphyria" is a rare autosomal recessive condition associated with an abnormal isomerization of tetrapyrrole intermediates in such a way that type I isomers are excreted in greater quantity than type III, which normally are the major form. The erythrocytes are not hypochromic, so that sufficient quantities of the III isomers are produced to fulfill the requirements of hemoglobin synthesis. Red staining of tissues and of the urine is prominent, along with the signs of hemolysis and splenomegaly, but photosensitivity is especially severe. Another variety of erythroid type is "erythropoietic protoporphyria," an autosomal dominant condition associated with mild anemia. Protoporphyrin concentration in the erythrocytes is markedly increased along with its excretion in the feces. Photohemolysis is demonstrable in vitro.

The hepatic porphyrias do not produce red cell disturbances. "Acute intermittent porphyria," an autosomal dominant condition which is often "latent," is more correctly described as a porphobilinogenuria, because its pathogenesis rests in defective inhibition of δ-ALA synthetase in the liver, causing overproduction of δ-ALA along with colorless porphobilinogen, which in urine becomes oxidized and colored on standing. Certain drugs, notably barbiturates and estrogens, induce increased δ-ALA synthetase activity in the liver and provoke symptomatic attacks. The pathogenesis of symptoms—attacks of abdominal pain, polyneuropathy, and even behavioral and mental change—is presumably related to tissue accumulation of the precursors, but proof for this mechanism is still pending. Light-sensitive skin eruptions are not found except in a genetic variant referred to as "variegate porphyria." In still another genetic variant fecal coproporphyrin excretion is increased. Porphyria cutanea tarda is presumed to originate from the superimposition of acquired factors—alcoholism and liver disease—upon a latent genetic background, but proof for this is also lacking. The symptoms, in addition to those of the liver disease itself, are those of red urine and photosensitive skin lesions. Urinary uro- and coproporphyrins are increased, along with high concentrations in the hepatic parenchyma, but the porphobilinogen excretion is normal. Increased urine urobilinogen is commensurate with the presence of liver disease.

Acquired. Lead poisoning inhibits heme synthesis at several points, the most prominent of which block δ-ALA dehydrase and heme synthetase mediated reactions. These blocks cause accumulation of δ-ALA in the serum and urine, increased urinary excretion of coproporphyrin III, and high concentrations of free protoporphyrin in the erythrocyte (see Goldberg reference). Increased amounts of hemosiderin and ferritin accumulate in erythroid precursors because of the block in heme synthesis. Polychromasia of circulating erythroid cells is altered to coarse basophilic stippling because of ribosome aggregation. Porphobilinogen excretion is normal or only slightly increased. Mild hypochromic anemia is present in which the erythrocytes have a slightly to moderately shortened life span. Neurologic damage—encephalopathy in the child and peripheral motor neuropathy in the adult—is more serious. Abdominal pain as well as renal disease may also occur. Toxic exposure to hexachlorobenzene is another form of acquired porphyria manifested by photosensitivity and red-colored urine, as described by Schmid.

Iron

NORMAL IRON METABOLISM. Iron, by far the most abundant heavy metal in the body, is used chiefly for hemoglobin synthesis. About 1 mg. is required for each ml. of red cells produced, adding up to a daily need of 20 to 25 mg. for erythropoiesis. Almost all this iron is obtained through recycling and only about 5 per cent, or 1 mg. per day, is newly absorbed to balance losses incurred via fecal and urinary excretion and also in sweat and desquamated skin (see Jacobs reference). The average menstruating female loses about twice this amount and so must absorb more to maintain balance. Menstrual loss of blood, however, is difficult to estimate and varies a great deal from woman to woman.

Absorption by the gastrointestinal epithelial cell is finely tuned to admit just enough iron to cover losses, without permitting either excess or deficiency of body iron to develop. Absorption normally admits about 5 to 10 per cent of a total dietary intake of 10 to 20 mg. per day. The physiologic signal between the size of the body iron supply and the gastrointestinal mucosal cell is still only vaguely understood. The mucosal cell itself appears to act as a "ferrostat" by reflecting within its own cytoplasm the state of the body store of iron. A high concentration of cytoplasmic iron, present presumably almost entirely as ferritin, discourages further uptake at the membrane, while an iron-poor intracellular environment encourages uptake into the cell and then on into the plasma for binding to transferrin (Fig. 22–53). The mucosal epithelial cells are in a constant state of renewal, proliferating from the crypts out toward the tips of the villi, where they are shed into the lumen. Such cellular loss is an auxiliary mechanism for iron excretion in the feces, according to Conrad and Crosby.

The existence of a specialized iron transport protein within the mucosal cell remains open to question. In addition to depleted iron stores, the

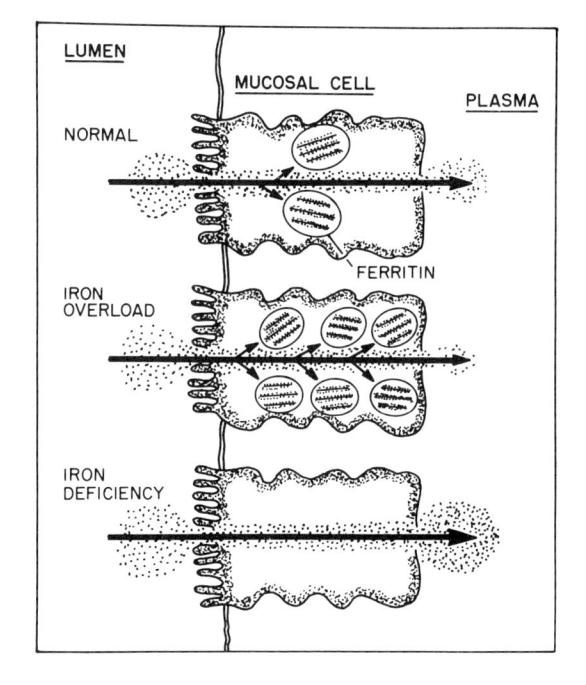

Figure 22-53 Regulation of iron absorption at the intestinal mucosa. (Redrawn from Finch, C. A.: Nutrition Today, Summer, 1969.)

absorption of iron is also increased in response to increased erythropoietic activity.

The barrier to excessive iron absorption set up by the mucosal cell is easily overcome, since increasing amounts of iron presented to the intestinal epithelial surface are met by additional increments of absorbed iron, although the proportion absorbed falls off (Fig. 22-54). The mucosal barrier is temporarily raised, however, by recently ingested iron, which decreases the absorption of a

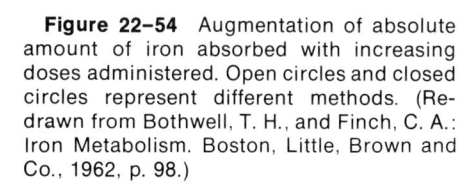

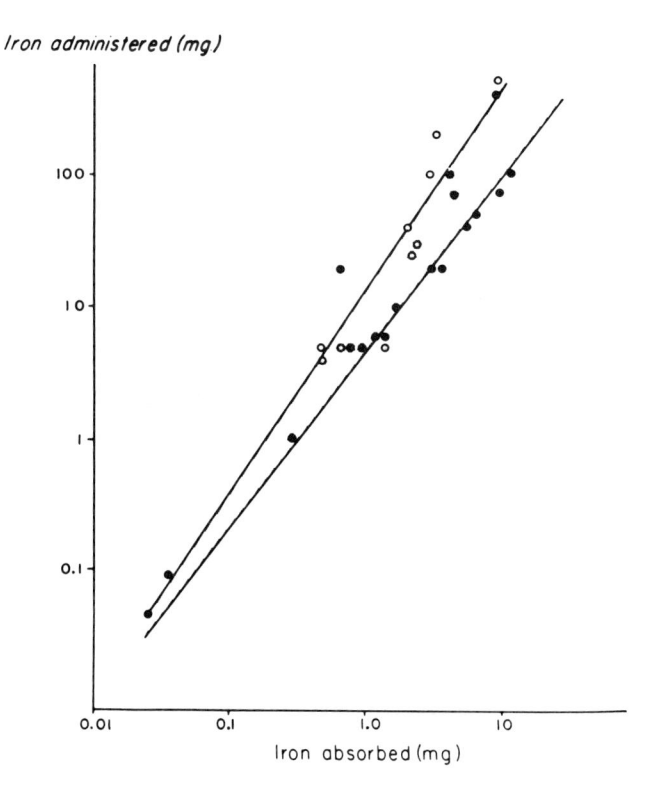

Figure 22-54 Augmentation of absolute amount of iron absorbed with increasing doses administered. Open circles and closed circles represent different methods. (Redrawn from Bothwell, T. H., and Finch, C. A.: Iron Metabolism. Boston, Little, Brown and Co., 1962, p. 98.)

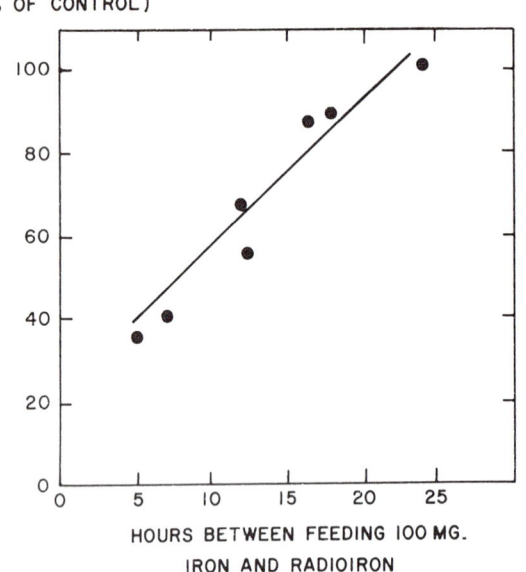

Figure 22-55 The change in absorption of a test dose of radioactive iron at intervals after an initial loading dose of nonradioactive iron. (Redrawn from Stewart, W. B., et al.: J. Exper. Med., 92:375, 1950.)

second dose given several hours later (Fig. 22-55).

The entire gastrointestinal tract has the capacity to absorb iron, but maximal activity is found in the duodenum and upper jejunum, probably because of the presence there of optimal conditions of pH and redox potential. Absorption occurs in the ferrous state, and ferric iron, which forms insoluble hydroxides at neutral and alkaline pH, must first be reduced before it is absorbed, for which an acid gastric juice is indispensable (Fig. 22-56). Chelation with low molecular weight compounds, such as fructose and amino acids, may also promote solubility preparatory to absorption. Whether the gastric juice itself contains special iron-chelating substances of either high or low molecular weight remains somewhat controversial. Dietary constituents such as phosphate and phytate render iron less soluble and thus less available for absorption. The concept that pancreatic insufficiency, by reducing duodenal pH, causes increased iron absorption has been challenged. Food iron, in contrast to the inorganic ferrous form of medicinal iron, occurs as organic complexes, such as ferritin and myoglobin, much of it in the trivalent state. Some of the complexes are broken up and solubilized during acid digestion in the stomach, but the heme iron passes on and is readily absorbed intact into the mucosal epithelial cells, without dependence upon reducing systems and by a mechanism which is distinct from that for inorganic iron (see Weintraub et al. reference). The iron is stripped away from its complex with porphyrin only after cellular uptake. Myoglobin and hemoglobin are better nutritional sources of iron than ferritin and hemosiderin, which are not as well absorbed.

Effete red cells which have lived out their 120-day life span are taken up by the phagocytic re-

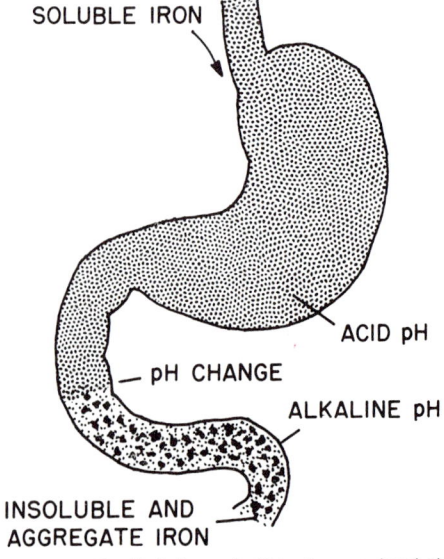

Figure 22-56 Relation of pH to the maximal site of iron absorption in the upper duodenum. (Redrawn from Finch, C. A.: Nutrition Today, Summer, 1969.)

ticuloendothelial cells, chiefly in the spleen, liver, and bone marrow. Inside these phagocytic cells the hemoglobin is broken down into its essential constituents, with an efficient salvage of the iron taken from degraded heme. This salvaged iron is packed in extremely high concentration inside apoferritin protein shells to form molecules of ferritin, each of which may contain up to 2500 atoms of iron, as reviewed by Crichton (Fig. 22-57). Ferritin molecules, in turn, are compressed into still larger amorphous aggregates of insoluble material called hemosiderin, which form granules visible by light microscopy. Thus it is as ferritin and hemosiderin, chiefly in reticuloendothelial cells, that the bulk of the reserve iron is stored. It is from these depots that the iron recycling fulfills the continuing needs of erythropoiesis (Fig. 22-58).

The storage iron most recently obtained from degraded heme is the first to be reutilized for hemoglobin synthesis; the chronologically more archaic iron depots may remain untouched for very long periods of time. In a normal adult with 2500 ml. red cell mass, 2500 mg. of iron circulates as hemoglobin while another 500 to 1500 mg. is present as storage iron. Although the vast bulk of the storage iron is found in reticuloendothelial cells, ferritin is detectable in many of the tissues of the body, including erythroblasts and the intestinal epithelial cells. Other significant pools of body iron are in myoglobin (130 mg.) and a variety of enzymes, such as the cytochromes, catalase, peroxidase, and many others (8 mg.).

Iron is taken from storage depots and transported back to erythroid precursors by a highly specialized plasma protein, transferrin. Stored in ferritin in the trivalent state, the iron is first reduced to the ferrous form for removal from the apoferritin shell, and then it is carried in the ferric state, up to two atoms per molecule of transferrin. The normal concentration of iron in the plasma is about 100 μg. per 100 ml., one third the total binding capacity of available transferrin. The total amount of iron in the transferrin pool, assuming that approximately half of it is intravascular and half extravascular, is about 4 to 5 mg. Although this transferrin-bound iron is only 1 per cent of that in the body, its metabolic rate of turnover is extremely rapid—50 per cent of it is cleared from the intravascular space every 60 to 120 minutes. Transferrin molecules deliver their iron at the surface of the erythroid precursors and return empty to the RE cells to pick up another load.

The rate of disappearance of radioactive iron from the plasma as well as its reappearance in the circulating red cells as newly produced labeled hemoglobin is a convenient method of measuring the functional state of erythropoiesis (see Finch et al. reference) (Fig. 22-24). In hypoplas-

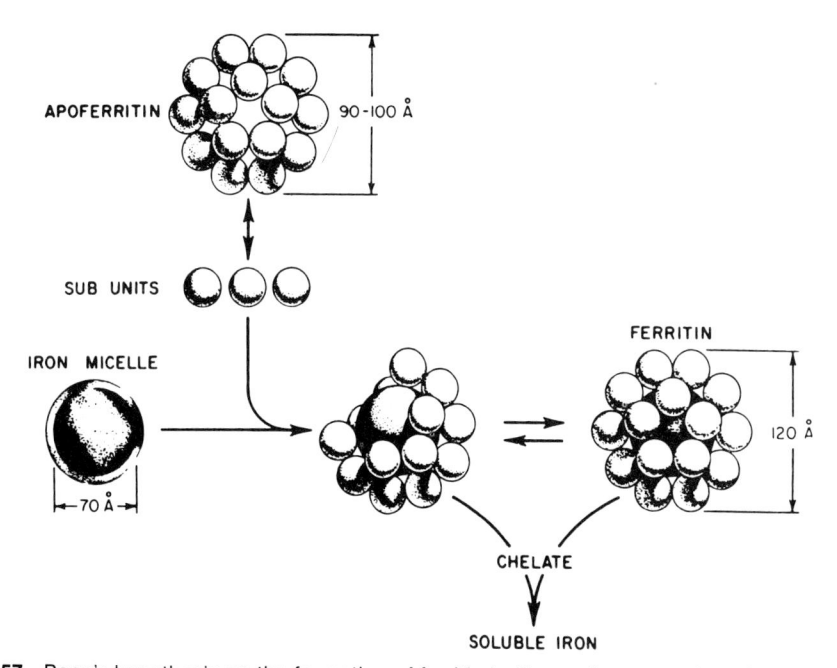

Figure 22-57 Pape's hypothesis on the formation of ferritin by the coalescence of apoferritin subunits around the central iron micelle core. An alternate theory considers that apoferritin subunits are first arranged into a hollow sphere, after which an interior iron micelle forms. (Reprinted from Pape, L., et al.: Biochemistry, 7:606, 1968. Copyright 1968, American Chemical Society. Reprinted by permission of the copyright owner.)

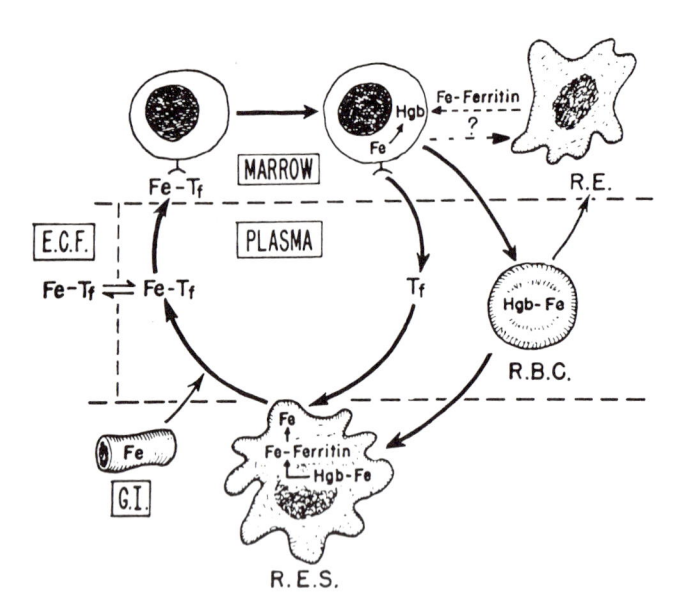

Figure 22-58 Metabolic pathways of iron. *Tf* = transferrin; *ECF* = extracellular fluid. (Redrawn from Katz, J. H.: Scand. J. Haemat., Suppl. 6:15, 1965.)

tic conditions the utilization of iron is depressed, causing a rise in its plasma concentration along with a decrease in the rate at which it is cleared from the normal half-life of 1 to 2 hours to 3 to 4 hours or longer. In iron deficiency the clearance rate is more rapid than normal, as it is in conditions associated with increased proliferation of red cell precursors in the marrow, such as hemolytic anemia. Normally about 70 to 80 per cent of the tracer iron reappears in circulating erythrocytes within 10 days of administration, but this figure may approach zero in the absence of red cell production. The red cell utilization of tracer iron is also depressed in conditions such as thalassemia or megaloblastic anemia, in which the marrow is rich in proliferating erythroid precursor cells and in their requirement for iron, but owing to extensive intramedullary destruction of these cells, little of the radioiron reappears in circulating erythrocytes despite its rapid clearance from the plasma. Pollycove has postulated that a labile pool of storage iron contributes a minor slow component to the plasma radioiron disappearance curve.

IRON LACK

General Effects. The first change in the development of iron deficiency is the loss of storage iron from the macrophages of the spleen, liver, and bone marrow. The evaluation of marrow iron stores is a convenient method of assessing the state of the body iron stores; if they are preserved, iron deficiency can be excluded as a cause of anemia. After the stores of iron are used up, the plasma iron concentration falls, at the same time stimulating an increase in the synthesis of transferrin. The saturation of transferrin with iron thus falls from 30 per cent to values often below 10 per cent (Fig. 22-59). Anemia is the last change to be observed. At first, the erythrocytes may be normocytic and normochromic and show only a few shape changes, but microcytic, hypochromic, more misshapen erythrocytes emerge as significant anemia develops. Even with only a moderate degree of anemia, the deficit in body iron is thus already advanced.

Whether iron deficiency without anemia causes significant symptoms remains a controversial issue. The activities of certain iron-containing enzymes decrease, but this change may not be of pathophysiologic significance. When anemia develops it is often well tolerated, except when there is acute blood loss or cardiovascular limitation. Changes in epithelial tissues complicate more protracted deficiency. There is inversion of the normal curvature of the fingernails ("spooning"), which also become more brittle; hair splits and breaks off; and a smooth red tongue reflects glossitis. Dysphagia with web formation in the upper esophagus rarely complicates iron lack of many years' duration. Atrophic gastritis with anacidity is frequently associated with iron deficiency, whether primarily the result of it (through secondary epithelial changes) or the cause of it (through impaired absorption of food iron) or both is not clear. Infants with iron deficiency anemia frequently have detectable occult blood in the feces without demonstrable gastrointestinal disease, presumably because of mucosal friability secondary to the deficient state. Mucosal changes secondary to iron deficiency in infants reportedly may be of sufficient magnitude to cause malabsorption. A moderately elevated platelet count is often seen in infants with iron deficiency anemia. Thrombocytosis in iron-deficient adults seems to be less prominent and more often explainable on the basis of reactive changes to hemorrhage, tumor, or other underlying disorders.

Pathogenesis. Iron deficiency always arises because of the inability of diet and absorption to keep pace with the increased requirements imposed either by the expansion of the red cell mass or by blood loss. The efficiency of absorption depends not only on the total amount of food iron but also on its form as well as on the dietary content of phosphate and phytate. Habitual eating of laundry starch or of clay is commonly seen among iron-deficient patients of certain population groups. Such materials may have an adverse effect upon iron absorption, but of even greater importance is the fact that among such patients the dietary intake of good sources of iron, such as meat, is also often severely limited. A peculiar craving for ice may develop.

The growth spurt of the 2-year-old and of the adolescent are common times for iron deficiency to appear. The well-nourished milk-fed infant is particularly prone because such a diet, while adequate in calories, is sorely lacking in iron. Iron deficiency is very rare at the time of birth, even if the mother is deficient. However, the rapid growth which follows premature birth requires iron supplementation during the first weeks of life to prevent the development of anemia. During pregnancy, the red cell mass expands by 20 per cent, which may require about 400 mg. of additional iron. The fetus requires about 280 mg., which is lost to the mother along with blood loss at childbirth. The losses of lactation are about equal to those which would have occurred from menstruation (Fig. 22-60).

The proper absorption of food iron being dependent upon a normal gastric milieu, anacidity acquired from either atrophic gastritis or from partial or total gastrectomy very commonly leads to iron deficiency anemia. Billroth type II procedures, which bypass the duodenum, are more commonly associated than those procedures which leave this site of maximal iron absorption intact. Rapid intestinal transit time may limit the time available for absorption. Excessive gastrointestinal blood loss contributes to iron depletion in those clinical situations which require gastric surgery, such as peptic ulcer. Iron lack coexists with other multiple deficiencies in the intestinal malabsorption syndromes, but if the duodenal surface is well preserved, sufficient iron may be absorbed to meet requirements.

Blood loss is the most important factor in the development of iron deficiency. Identification of its origin may bring to light the presence of unsuspected but significant underlying disease,

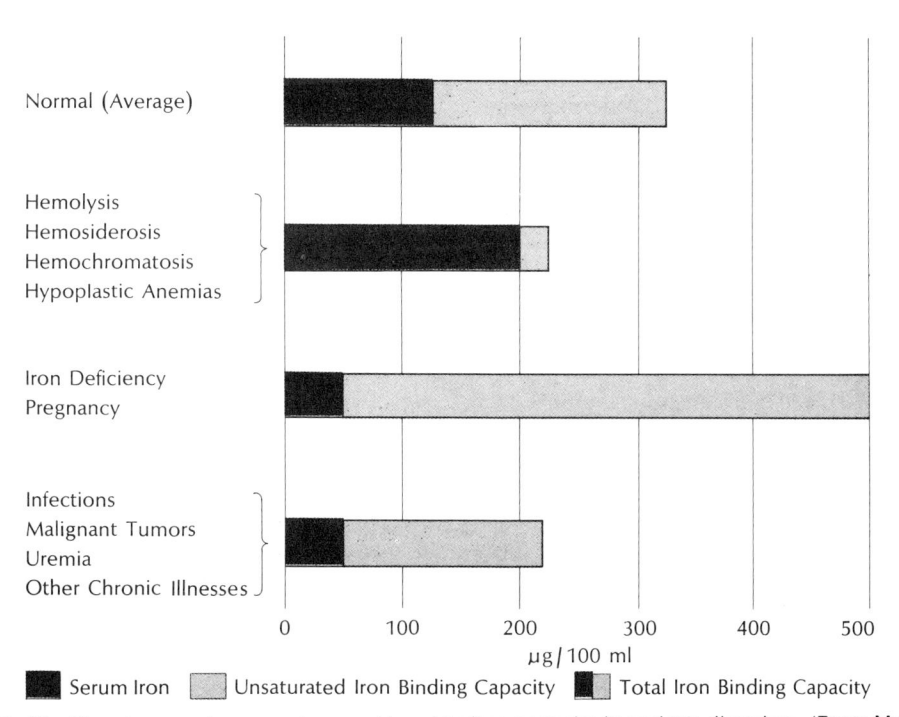

Figure 22-59 The changes in serum iron and iron binding capacity in various disorders. (From McIntyre, P.: Hosp. Pract., March, 1972, p. 101.)

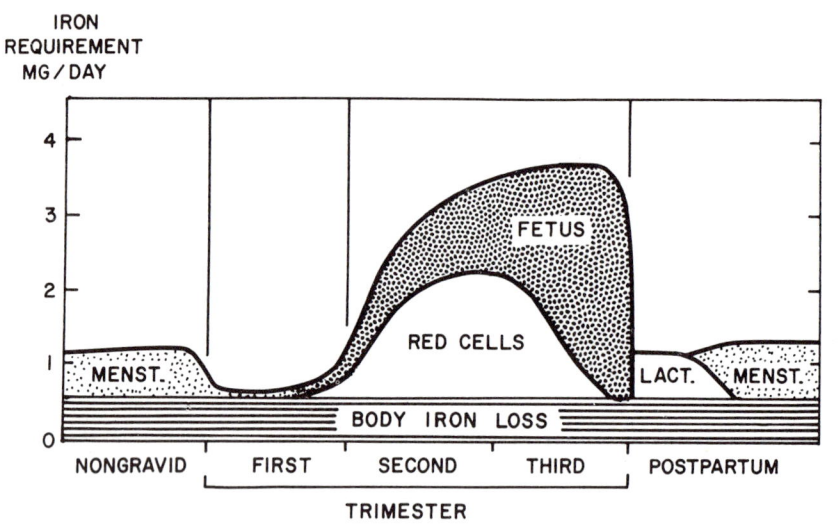

Figure 22-60 The change in iron requirement during pregnancy. (Redrawn from Bothwell, T. H., and Finch, C. A.: Iron Metabolism. Boston, Little, Brown and Co., 1962, p. 309.)

such as carcinoma of the colon. Hiatus hernia, hemorrhagic gastritis, and peptic ulcer disease are particularly frequent causes of upper gastrointestinal bleeding. Chronic aspirin users develop iron deficiency anemia because of increased gastrointestinal blood loss with or without demonstrable underlying disease. Menorrhagia, sometimes associated with such underlying disease as uterine fibroids, is the most frequent cause in premenopausal females. Sources of urinary blood loss include renal tumors as well as the chronic hemoglobinuria and hemosiderinuria associated with chronic intravascular hemolysis. Vasculitis of the pulmonary vessels with chronic hemorrhage into the lungs will cause pulmonary macrophages to become iron-laden in Goodpasture's syndrome. However, iron is not efficiently reutilized from these cells and an iron-deficient bone marrow with microcytic, hypochromic anemia complicates the picture.

IRON EXCESS

General Effects. The accumulation of excessive quantities of iron in the body ultimately originates from increased absorption or from parenteral administration as transfusions or as pharmacologic iron complexes. The capacity of the RE system to gather the extra iron within its protective confines is immense, but ultimately the degree of transferrin saturation rises, its synthesis is inhibited, and the plasma iron concentration approaches 200 µg. per 100 ml. with near 100 per cent saturation of the iron-binding capacity (Fig. 22-59). Under these changed circumstances parenchymal cells are no longer protected from pathologic iron uptake and damage occurs over the years to various organs, especially the liver, heart, and pancreas. The term hemochromatosis is used to describe the disease which thus arises from such chronic iron overexposure. Grayish pigmentation of the skin is caused by deposition of melanin in the deeper layers of the epidermis. Deposits of iron are seen in the glandular structures of the skin.

Acute iron poisoning occurs chiefly in children who accidentally swallow an overdose of iron pills. Nausea, vomiting, and intestinal bleeding is soon followed by vascular collapse and shock, with a high likelihood of a fatal outcome.

Pathogenesis. An increase in the body content of iron in primary hemochromatosis occurs because of an inappropriate and as yet unexplained increase in iron absorption by the intestinal mucosal cells (see Balcerzak et al. reference). Erythrocyte morphology is normal, and erythropoiesis is unaffected. Indeed, anemia is noteworthy for its absence. Although the disorder may run in families, its hereditary nature has been disputed. Excess dietary iron—usually in the form of certain beers and wines with high iron content, food cooked in iron utensils, or medicinal iron—leads to a similar disorder. Instances of apparent primary hemochromatosis which develop in patients with alcoholic cirrhosis are presumably related to the fact that a small proportion of such patients develop increased iron absorption secondary to the liver disease. The pathogenesis of this increase is obscure.

Hemochromatosis also complicates disorders of erythropoiesis in which iron is not properly utilized for hemoglobin formation. The increased iron absorption is apparently related to the hyperplastic, although ineffective, erythropoiesis which characterizes these conditions. Red cell morphology is abnormal. The anemia is of any degree from minimal to severe. An excessive number of hemosiderin granules accumulate in the cytoplasm of erythroid precursor cells as well as in mature erythrocytes, where their presence becomes much more obvious after splenectomy. The term "sideroblast" is applied to any nucleated erythroid precursor which contains stainable iron granules (see Dacie and Mollin). In normal marrow about 25 per cent of erythroid precursors are sideroblasts containing two or three small cytoplasmic granules. The number and size of such iron granules as well as the proportion of erythroid cells containing them increase in a number of states of increased erythropoiesis, including hemolytic anemia and megaloblastic anemia. However, in the marrow of certain iron-loading anemias there are seen a large number of "ringed sideroblasts," erythroid cells in which a necklace of iron granules surrounds the nucleus. To these conditions the term "sideroblastic anemia" is applied. The ringed configuration is presumably related to the fact that the iron accumulation is concentrated on the mitochondria, which cling to the nuclear membranes in the fixed and stained preparations.

The sideroblastic anemias are classified as primary or secondary, hereditary or acquired (see Kushner et al. reference). Hypochromic, small, misshapen erythrocytes are often seen in the midst of a population of normocytic, normochromic cells. Hereditary sex-linked hypochromic anemia is usually first detected in young adult or adolescent males, whereas primary acquired sideroblastic anemia is seen in patients of either sex over the age of 60. Occasionally, with observation the latter condition will ultimately prove to be a secondary variety associated with a myeloproliferative syndrome culminating in acute myelogenous leukemia. The condition can also occur secondary to certain drugs (isoniazid, cycloserine, chloramphenicol), to lead poisoning, or to alcoholic excess, but reversibility averts the development of hemochromatosis. Rare ringed sideroblasts are occasionally seen in the marrow of patients with certain chronic diseases, such as rheumatoid arthritis or carcinoma, but hyperferremia and iron-loading do not complicate the picture.

Some of the sideroblastic anemias are pyridoxine responsive, as described by Harris. The doses required are pharmacologic, and signs of pyridoxine deficiency are absent. Anemia is improved and the serum iron decreases. The response is not complete, although it is generally more satisfactory in the hereditary than in the primary acquired cases. The explanation of responsiveness may reside in a defect in conversion of pyridoxine to its active form, pyridoxal phosphate, which is required for the first step in heme synthesis on the mitochondria, upon which iron accumulates. Recent studies have provided some evidence for superior therapeutic efficacy of pyridoxal phosphate, but it would appear that the entire group of disorders is at present too heterogeneous to be properly analyzed until a more precise biochemical classification is achieved. Indeed, megaloblastic erythropoiesis and macrocytic erythrocytes are also sometimes observed along with a degree of folic acid responsiveness.

Hemochromatosis is a major cause of morbidity and mortality in thalassemia, a primary deficiency of globin synthesis. Erythroid cells are iron-loaded, but ringed sideroblasts are not prominent. Transfusional hemosiderosis contributes to the iron-load in thalassemia major, as well as in any anemia of sufficient severity to require chronic transfusion therapy.

Primary hemochromatosis is treated with removal of iron by repeated phlebotomy over a long period of time, until iron stores become depleted and the serum iron falls. This approach has also been used in hemochromatosis secondary to iron-loading erythrocyte disorders in which the anemia is mild. Iron-chelating agents, such as desferioxamine, have generally not been effective except in the treatment of acute iron poisoning, in which their use can be life-saving.

Globin

NORMAL STRUCTURE AND SYNTHESIS. The primary structure of the globin molecule as well as its production rate are under genetic control. Its specific amino acid sequence is governed by the triplet code of DNA bases passed down in the chromosomes from generation to generation. The rate at which globin polypeptide chains are synthesized is a function of the rate at which the DNA code is transcribed into messenger RNA. The sequence of translational events which follow modifies the production rate of the completed chains. These include the initiation and assembly on, and the release of the polypeptide chains from the messenger RNA-polyribosome complex upon which the amino acids are joined together in proper sequence.

At least five genetic loci direct globin synthesis. The α and β chains of normal adult hemoglobin (Hb A) are produced in matched amounts but under the control of separate genes located far apart from one another, possibly on different chromosomes. The δ chain closely resembles the β chain, to which it is genetically linked on the same chromosome, but it is synthesized at only 1/40 the rate of β chains. Thus the concentration of Hb A_2 ($\alpha_2\delta_2$) in the normal adult is only about 2.5 per cent of the total hemoglobin. The ϵ globin chain is formed during the first trimester of intrauterine development, but since α chain production at this stage of development is in short supply, two embryonic hemoglobins are present: Gower-1 consists of a tetramer of only ϵ chains

(ϵ_4), and Gower-2 has both α and ϵ chains ($\alpha_2\epsilon_2$). Beyond the first trimester α and γ chain synthesis predominate in the formation of fetal hemoglobin, Hb F ($\alpha_2\gamma_2$), which makes up 75 to 90 per cent of the total hemoglobin at birth. Schroeder and coworkers have shown that at least two genetic loci govern the production of different types of γ chains, one with glycine at the 136 position, the other with alanine. Although the synthesis of adult type β chains is begun early in intrauterine development, predominance is not established until its synthetic rate sharply rises in the weeks just preceding birth. Hb A then gradually replaces Hb F in the circulating erythrocytes until the normal adult level of Hb F (< 2 per cent) is attained, usually at about 6 months of age, although slight elevations may persist for two years (Fig. 22–61).

Thanks largely to the work of Perutz, the three-dimensional fine structure of the hemoglobin molecule is rather well understood. The α and β subunits, similar but not identical in size and shape, possess a complementariness of structure which causes them to spontaneously associate with each other and form a dimer which constitutes the basis of both the function of the molecule as an oxygen transporter and its physicochemical stability. Unpaired, the subunits not only are incapable of oxygen transport but are also excessively unstable. The stability of the dimer ($\alpha_1\beta_1$) comes from the extensive area of surface contact between the two subunits, involving 34 amino acid residues. When two dimers come together to form the complete tetrameric configuration, an "asymmetric" contact point forms between the α chain of one dimer and the β chain of the other (Fig. 22–62). This asymmetric ($\alpha_1\beta_2$) contact area is somewhat less extensive, involving only 19 amino acid sites, but this region is important in the regulation of the normal sigmoid shape of the hemoglobin oxygen dissociation curve. It is at this point that the allosteric properties of hemoglobin, as it combines with its substrate oxygen, are modulated. The initial attachment of oxygen to the α chain heme causes its iron to "snap back" as if released from a position under tension. This signal then sends a "shock wave" through the molecule which increases the affinity of the β chain heme groups for oxygen atoms, producing the upward inflection of the oxygen dissociation curve and at the same time causing the β chains to move closer to one another by 7 Å. The β chains shift back apart when oxygen is once again removed (Fig. 22–8). The binding of low molecular weight phosphates, such as 2,3-diphosphoglycerate, takes place in the cleft between the two β chains when they are in the deoxy configuration, thus diminishing the oxygen affinity of the hemoglobin.

The globular subunit, which is divided into eight helical regions designated by the letters A through H, is physiologically submerged in an aqueous medium with which it blends because it carries all its hydrophilic groupings on its exterior surface. These include hydroxyl groups, such as those of serine and threonine, as well as polar carboxyl and amino groups. The molecular interior is arid and is lined with hydrophobic nonpolar groups. Each subunit has its heme group neatly tucked into a "heme pocket" which

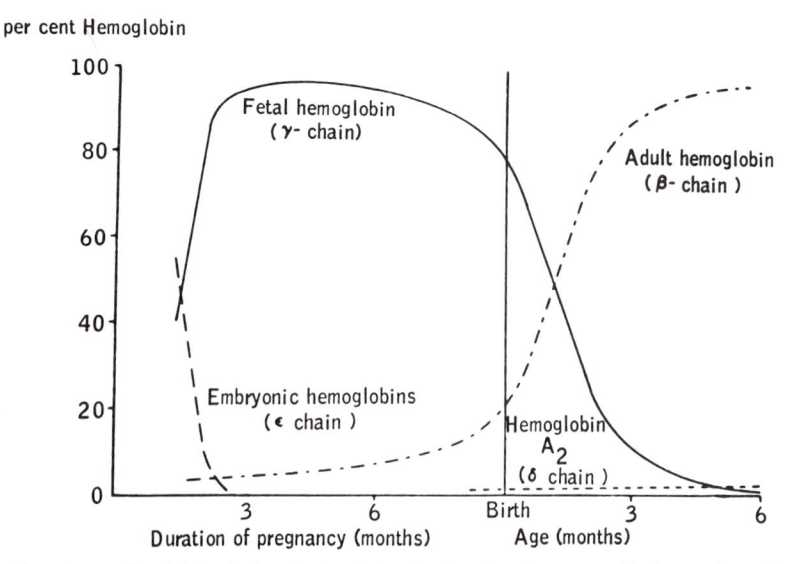

Figure 22–61 The change in globin chains during intrauterine development. (Redrawn from Huehns, E. R., and Shooter, E. M.: J. Med. Genet., 2:48, 1965.)

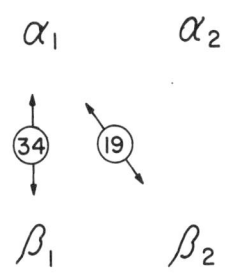

Figure 22-62 The α and β subunit contact regions in the hemoglobin molecule. The numbers of amino acids in the contract regions are indicated. (Redrawn from Weatherall, D. J., and Clegg, J. B.: The Thalassemia Syndromes. Oxford, Blackwell Scientific Publications Ltd., 1972, p. 17.)

dips down from the molecular surface and is also completely lined with hydrophobic groups which exclude water from the region. The heme comes into contact at about 60 atomic sites with the surface of the pocket. The fifth coordinate position of the heme iron is bound to the "proximal histidine" residue (β^{92} and α^{87}). Molecular oxygen is carried between the sixth coordinate position of iron and the "distal histidine" (β^{63} and α^{58}) (Fig. 22-7).

HEMOGLOBINOPATHY DUE TO STRUCTURAL DEFECTS (TABLE 22-8)

Nomenclature. In the years that followed the first description of sickle hemoglobin (Hb S) in 1949 it became evident that the letters in the alphabet would not be sufficient to accommodate names for the large number of mutant hemoglobins being discovered. Family names and then place names were given as trivial expressions, to be followed by a specific designation of the amino acid substitution which characterized the abnormal hemoglobin. For example, "Hb Philly" was first observed in Philadelphia. It has normal α chains, but the β chains are affected by an inherited abnormality of the 35th amino acid from the N-terminal end of the β chains, at which phenylalanine is found in place of tyrosine (Fig. 22-63). This abnormal hemoglobin is thus designated $\alpha_2^A \beta_2^{35\ tyr \rightarrow phe}$. Mutations of the β chain outnumber those of the α chain. Abnormal δ and γ chains have also been discovered. Many abnormal hemoglobins produce no abnormality in erythrocyte appearance or function and are not pathogenetic. Some are harmful only in the homozygous state, while others are lethal in the homozygous state and thus are only observed in heterozygous carriers.

Methemoglobinemia. A substitution of tyrosine for histidine at either the proximal or distal histidine residues of either the α or the β chains locks the heme iron into a trivalent state resistant to the action of the enzyme methemoglobin reductase, which has the responsibility of maintaining the iron atoms of hemoglobin in the ferrous state. The affected heme groups in half the molecule are incapable of oxygen transport while the unaffected pair of hemes retains the ability to combine reversibly with oxygen. In the α chain methemoglobinemias, the normal β partner has a somewhat decreased affinity for oxygen because of the absence of the "signal" which is normally sent across to the β chain from the α when it first combines with oxygen. In the β chain mutants,

TABLE 22-8 SELECTED HEMOGLOBINS — THEIR STRUCTURES AND STRUCTURAL MUTATIONS

Normal Amino Acid Sequence	
HbA	$\alpha_2^A \beta_2^A$
Hb A$_2$	$\alpha_2^A \delta_2$
Hb F	$\alpha_2^A \gamma_2$
Hb H	β_4^A
Hb Bart's	γ_4
Methemoglobinemia	
Hb M Boston	$\alpha^{58\ his \rightarrow tyr} \beta_2^A$
Hb M Iwate	$\alpha^{87\ his \rightarrow tyr} \beta_2^A$
Hb M Saskatoon	$\alpha_2^A \beta_2^{63\ his \rightarrow tyr}$
Hb M Hyde Park	$\alpha_2^A \beta_2^{92\ his \rightarrow tyr}$
Increased Oxygen Affinity with Erythrocytosis	
Hb Chesapeake	$\alpha_2^{92\ arg \rightarrow leu} \beta_2^A$
Hb Rainier	$\alpha_2^A \beta_2^{145\ tyr \rightarrow his}$
Hb Hiroshima	$\alpha_2^A \beta_2^{143\ his \rightarrow asp}$
Decreased Oxygen Affinity with Cyanosis	
Hb Kansas	$\alpha_2^A \beta_2^{102\ asn \rightarrow thr}$
Unstable Hemoglobin with Hemolytic Anemia	
Hb Torino	$\alpha_2^{43\ phe \rightarrow val} \beta_2^A$
Hb Hammersmith	$\alpha_2^A \beta_2^{42\ phe \rightarrow ser}$
Hb Zürich	$\alpha_2^A \beta_2^{63\ his \rightarrow arg}$
Hb Tacoma	$\alpha_2^A \beta_2^{30\ arg \rightarrow ser}$
Hb Philly	$\alpha_2^A \beta_2^{35\ tyr \rightarrow phe}$
Hb Freiburg	$\alpha_2^A \beta_2^{23\ val \rightarrow 0}$
Hb Gun Hill	$\alpha_2^A \beta_2^{93-97 \rightarrow 0}$
Hb Genova	$\alpha_2^A \beta_2^{28\ leu \rightarrow pro}$
Hb Seattle	$\alpha_2^A \beta_2^{76\ ala \rightarrow glu}$
"Exterior" Mutants	
Hb S	$\alpha_2^A \beta_2^{6\ glu \rightarrow val}$
Hb C	$\alpha_2^A \beta_2^{6\ glu \rightarrow lys}$
Hb E	$\alpha_2^A \beta_2^{26\ glu \rightarrow lys}$
Hb C Harlem	$\alpha_2^A \beta_2^{6\ glu \rightarrow val;\ 73\ asp \rightarrow asn}$
Hb Korle-bu	$\alpha_2^A \beta_2^{73\ asp \rightarrow asn}$
Hb G Accra	$\alpha_2^A \beta_2^{79\ asp \rightarrow asn}$
Hb D Punjab	$\alpha_2^A \beta_2^{121\ glu \rightarrow gln}$
Mutants with Low Synthetic Rate	
Hb Lepore	$\alpha_2^A \delta\text{-}\beta_2$ (fusion gene)
Hb Constant Spring	$\alpha_2^{141 \rightarrow 162} \beta_2^A$

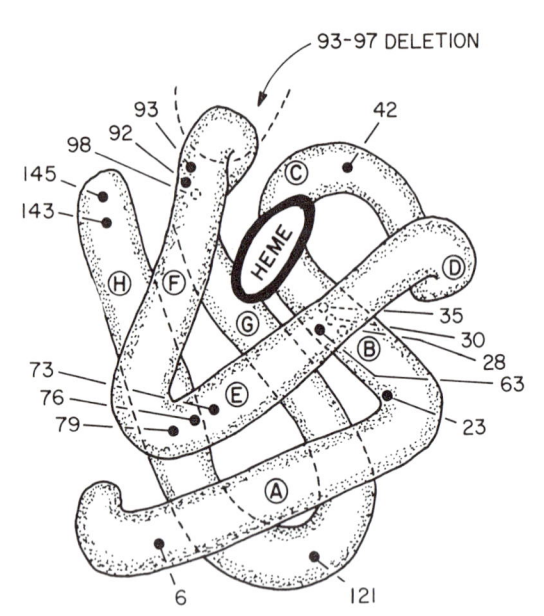

Figure 22-63 The β globin subunit. The numbered positions indicate amino acid sites discussed in the text and in Table 22-8. (Redrawn from Giblett, Genetic Markers in Human Blood. Oxford, Blackwell Scientific Publications Ltd. 1969.)

the oxygen affinity of the unaffected α subunit is more nearly normal. Inheritance is autosomal dominant and homozygosity is apparently lethal, in contrast to inherited deficiency of methemoglobin reductase, which is an autosomal recessive state. The methemoglobinemia of mutant hemoglobins is resistant to therapy while that occurring as a result of deficiency of the enzyme responds to treatment with such reducing agents as methylene blue or ascorbic acid.

High Affinity Hemoglobin With Erythrocytosis. Mutant hemoglobins which raise the hemoglobin oxygen affinity shift the oxygen dissociation curve to the left, impeding oxygen unloading at the tissues (Fig. 22-64). The erythropoietin response evokes a secondary form of polycythemia which is familial and benign and is unassociated with increases in the platelet or leukocyte count. The mutation sites affect either the area of $\alpha_1\beta_2$ subunit contact or the C-terminal ends of the β chains close to the cove where low molecular weight phosphates are bound. Mutants such as Hb Chesapeake, which are located at the $\alpha_1\beta_2$ contact, have a raised oxygen affinity along with a loss in the normal sigmoid contour of the oxygen dissociation curve, but their Bohr effect is preserved. In Hb Hiroshima and Hb Rainier, which affect the C-terminal region of the β subunits, the Bohr effect is impaired. These substitutions presumably raise oxygen affinity by interfering with low molecular weight phosphate binding and allosteric movements.

Low Affinity Hemoglobin With Cyanosis. Hb Kansas is a mutation at the $\alpha_1\beta_2$ contact which causes a lowered oxygen affinity (Fig. 22-64). Cyanosis is reversed if the patient is placed in an atmosphere of sufficiently high partial pressure of oxygen. Compensatory erythropoietic changes result in mild but "physiologic" anemia.

Unstable Hemoglobin With Congenital Heinz Body Hemolytic Anemia. Amino acid replacements which loosen the attachment of heme in its pocket or the dimeric association of the subunits at the $\alpha_1\beta_1$ contact region cause the mutant hemoglobin to be inordinately susceptible to oxidation. Water entry into normally hydrophobic regions is followed by conversion to methemoglobin, by oxidation of the reduced thiol groups of the globin to disulfides with formation of molecular aggregates, and finally by precipitation of the oxidized hemoglobin into insoluble lumps which become attached to the erythrocyte membrane (see Jacob reference). These impede erythrocyte pliability and cause hemolysis. The intact spleen plucks these precipitates from the erythrocytes. After splenectomy, a large proportion of the circulating erythrocytes contain Heinz bodies, the term which is used to describe these intracellular inclusions of precipitated hemoglobin. The replacement of one hydrophobic amino acid for another inside the heme pocket, as in Hb Torino, causes only mild hemolysis, but when a hydrophilic group is placed into the heme pocket lining, as in the case of serine in Hb Hammersmith, heme loss is marked and hemolysis severe. A gross

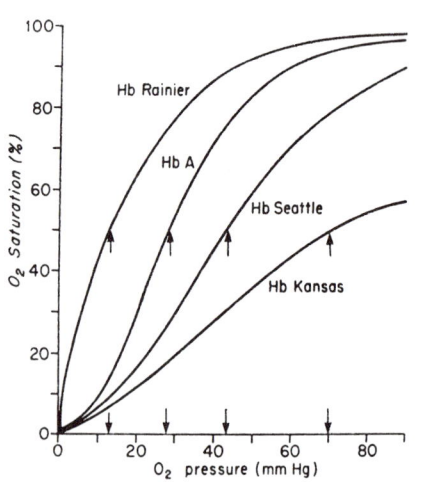

Figure 22-64 Examples of hemoglobins with abnormal oxygen affinity. Arrows indicate P_{50}. (From Stamatoyannopoulos, G., et al.: Ann. Rev. Med., 22:221, 1971.)

deletion of a block of five amino acids adjacent to the proximal histidine residue produces gross molecular distortion with heme-deficient globin subunits and marked hemoglobin instability. Hb Zürich affects the distal histidine residue of the β chain, which is replaced by arginine. The polar group of arginine lies poised just outside the heme pocket and leads to very mild hemolysis unless the patient is given certain "oxidant" drugs, such as sulfonamides, which explosively provoke episodes of severe hemolysis. Hb Philly and Hb Tacoma are unstable because they affect the $\alpha_1\beta_1$ contact area. The globin subunit also cannot bear disruption of its helical regions without suffering molecular instability. The insertion of the hydroxyl group of proline into the B helix of the β chain in Hb Genova breaks up the regular helical structure and causes a gross alteration in molecular configuration with hemolysis.

The oxygen affinity of the unstable hemoglobins may be raised or lowered, with an effect on the level of hemoglobin at which the patient compensates. When the affinity is high, the erythropoietin response is greater and the degree of anemia less than in those mutants with a lowered affinity, in which compensation is achieved at a lower concentration of circulating hemoglobin (see Bellingham and Huehns reference). The severity of the hemolytic process obviously also determines the severity of the anemia.

Exterior Mutants. Mutants placed on the hydrophilic exterior of the molecule do not alter either the oxygen affinity or the oxidative stability of the molecule. Relatively few of the more than 50 variants described in this class of abnormal hemoglobins cause any significant signs. Two major exceptions are the most common structural hemoglobinopathies, Hb S and Hb C. Both these hemoglobins are substituted at the 6 position from the N-terminal end of the β chain, where glutamic acid is replaced by valine in the case of Hb S and by lysine in the case of Hb C. Hb E, prevalent in Southeast Asia, also has a lysine in place of glutamic acid, but the affected site is 26 from the N-terminus of the β chain.

Erythrocytes which contain Hb S undergo jagged distortion of their membranes under reduced partial pressure of oxygen, a phenomenon known as sickling (Fig. 22-65). The sickling is visualized by electron microscopy as a linear molecular stacking of hemoglobin molecules, the filaments intertwining into cable-like structures which undergo cross-branching and arborization. The process is reversible, and as the oxygen tension is raised, the semisolid gelled hemoglobin liquefies once again, and the cell reassumes its normal biconcave shape. The reversibility of the process is a function of the allosteric shift of the β chains, the deoxy configuration causing a "fit" between the β chains of one molecule and the α chains of the next, on to a linear stacking of molecule upon molecule. With reoxygenation, the β chains move closer together and the complementariness between adjacent molecules is broken. The erythrocyte membrane may undergo irreversible deformation, presumably because of ATP depletion. The cell will then remain irreversibly sickled, even though the interior structure of the oxyhemoglobin S is not in the gelled state. These irreversibly sickled erythrocytes are those seen in oxygenated capillary blood films (see Bertles and Milner reference).

The molecular basis of sickling is still not thoroughly understood. Murayama has proposed that the substitution of valine with its hydrophobic side chain in place of glutamic acid with its exterior polar carboxyl group causes, in a sense, an interiorization of a portion of the molecular exterior. He has suggested that a cyclic hydrophobic valine-to-valine bond forms between the 1 and 6 amino acid residues of the β chain of Hb S. This changes the exterior molecular configuration and thus causes a key and lock arrangement between molecules when the β chains are in the deoxy configuration. This hypothesis, however, does not explain the nature of the cross-branching forces which are evident by inspection of sickled hemoglobin under the electron microscope. Electrostatic bonds are also involved, since high NaCl concentration disrupts sickling in solutions of deoxy Hb S. Individuals who inherit an abnormal hemoglobin in addition to Hb S in their erythrocytes provide important clues about the location on the molecular surface where intermolecular contact occurs. Hb C Harlem has two

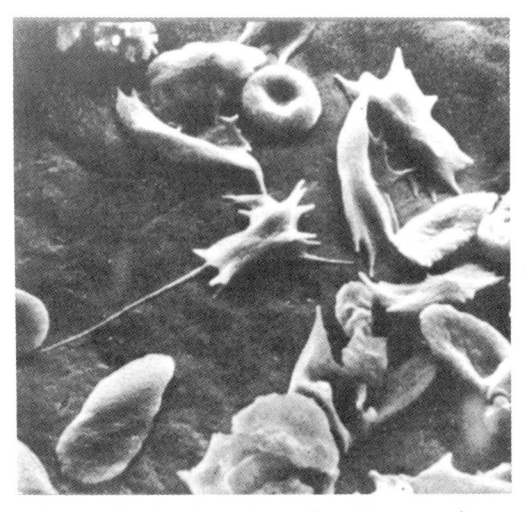

Figure 22-65 Sickled erythrocytes as demonstrated by scanning electron microscopy. (From Jensen, W. N., and Lessin, L. S.: Seminars Hemat., 7:409–426, 1970. By permission of Grune and Stratton, Inc., New York.)

amino acid substitutions in its β chain, one identical to that of Hb S, the other at the 73 position, where an asparagine replaces aspartic acid (see Bookchin et al. reference). Despite the fact that this molecule is more abnormal than Hb S, its presence inhibits the gelation of deoxy Hb S. Subsequently, it was discovered that Hb Korlebu, which affects only the 73 position with the same substitution, has the same property, indicating that this site on the beta chain is of importance in the surface fit of one hemoglobin molecule into the next. The presence of fetal hemoglobin together with Hb S similarly inhibits gelation. Newborn infants do not suffer from sickle cell disease. Symptoms only become manifest as the fetal hemoglobin is replaced by the adult type. Hb F levels are commonly raised in sickle cell anemia to values from 5 to 15 per cent, but the fact that it is heterogeneously distributed among the erythrocytes explains why its level is not related to disease severity. However, those erythrocytes with higher Hb F content do survive longer in the circulation. In the doubly heterozygous condition of hereditary persistence of fetal hemoglobin and sickle trait, erythrocytes uniformly have 20 to 30 per cent Hb F mixed together with Hb S and the result is a benign condition. On the other hand, Hb C rather strongly interacts with Hb S in the gelation and its presence in erythrocytes together with Hb S in equal proportions causes significant in-vivo sickling in the disorder known as Hb SC disease (see Bertles et al. reference). Normal Hb A, which is found in a proportion of about 60:40 relative to that of Hb S in individuals who are carriers of sickle cell trait, also interacts with Hb S in the gelation, but to a much lesser degree. These hemoglobins interact with Hb S in sickling through the formation of hybridized molecules consisting of one Hb S dimer combined with a dimer from the interacting hemoglobin to form the hybrid tetramer.

Heterozygous carriers of the sickle cell trait show no abnormality of erythrocyte morphology, life span, or function, except under certain extenuating circumstances, such as severe hypoxia, or normally in the renal circulation. At the tips of the papillae in the renal medulla a number of factors combine to produce an optimal environment for erythrocyte sickling. The region is hypoxic, acidotic, and has a high salt concentration. Acidosis, by shifting the oxygen dissociation curve to the right, promotes sickling, while alkalosis inhibits it. The gelation of deoxy Hb S is also highly dependent upon the intracellular hemoglobin concentration, which is raised as water moves out of erythrocytes as they move through a hyperosmolar environment. Low molecular weight phosphates (inorganic phosphate as well as 2,3-DPG) also promote sickling by decreasing the oxygen affinity of the hemoglobin.

Sickle cell anemia is usually a severe disease in which erythrocytic sickling causes chronic hemolytic anemia in a setting of vaso-occlusive phenomena which may affect any organ of the body. Periodic bouts of occlusion of the microvasculature in one or several parts of the body cause "painful crises," which at their worst produce prolonged excruciating pain, sometimes associated with fever (see Diggs reference). Major arteries and veins may also suffer occlusion. There is a serious susceptibility to infection. Organ damage is cumulative over the years, and death, if not from infection, may come unannounced from a major occlusion affecting a vital function, or it may come in more chronic fashion from gradual failure of any one of several organs, such as liver, kidney, or heart. The sickle variants, Hb SC disease and Hb S thalassemia, also suffer vaso-occlusive phenomena, but symptoms are usually milder. Carriers of sickle cell trait are asymptomatic except for an incidence of hematuria due to renal infarction.

Vascular changes occur in reaction to erythrocytic sickling. These changes are demonstrable in the kidney and are presumably etiologically related to a renal concentrating defect which cannot be reversed in adults despite exchange transfusion of normal for sickle erythrocytes. Vascular changes are also present in the eye, and retinal aneurysms leading to vitreous hemorrhage cause blindness, a complication particularly associated with Hb SC disease (see Condon and Serjeant reference).

Therapy over the years has been essentially symptomatic. Acidosis is treated, hydration ensured, and occasionally the sickled erythrocytes replaced by normal transfused cells as a temporary expedient. The search for a pharmacologic agent which would prevent sickling has been elusive. Methemoglobin as well as such liganded states of hemoglobin as carboxyhemoglobin and cyanmethemoglobin all assume the oxy configuration and therefore do not sickle (see Bookchin and Nagel reference). Beutler in fact attempted to produce methemoglobinemia as a treatment for sickling, but these altered states of hemoglobin do not function in oxygen transport. More recently it was discovered that treatment of Hb S erythrocytes with cyanate results in a carbamylation of the hemoglobin molecules which not only inhibits sickling but also results in a marked improvement in the life span of the treated erythrocytes (see Gilette et al. reference). Although the spatial alteration of the molecular surface by attachment of the carbamyl groups to free amino groups of globin might offer steric hindrance and thus prevent sickling, the evidence suggests that its mechanism of action may rest solely in the fact that the oxygen affinity of the altered hemoglobin is raised (Fig. 22–66).

Individuals homozygous for Hb C have a mild chronic hemolytic anemia associated with splenomegaly. The pathogenesis of the hemolysis apparently lies in the fact that this abnormal hemoglobin spontaneously crystallizes at a slightly lower concentration than Hb A (see Charache et al. reference). As red cells age in the circulation they undergo a measure of water loss, with concomitant increase in the intracorpuscular concentration of hemoglobin to values approaching 36 grams per 100 ml. Hb A does not begin to crystallize into an insoluble state until its concentration is over 40 grams per 100 ml., but Hb C begins to develop this change in physical state at the values physiologically approached during red cell aging in the circulation. At this point the cell becomes rigid and is subject to entrapment and destruction. The presence of this abnormal hemoglobin within erythrocytes causes a prominent tendency for the central deposition of a mass of hemoglobin into a "target cell" configuration. Intracellular crystals are readily demonstrable in vitro by suspending the erythrocytes in hypertonic saline, which raises intracorpuscular hemoglobin concentration, or in vivo after removal of the spleen. Heterozygotes have fewer target cells and do not show signs of significant hemolysis. The pathogenesis of Hb E disease presumably resembles that of Hb C.

HEMOGLOBINOPATHY DUE TO QUANTITATIVE DEFECTS. The structure-rate hypothesis as conceived by Itano in the 1950s postulated that the structure of an abnormal globin chain was an important factor which determined its synthetic rate. The fact that Hb S was synthesized at a slightly less efficient rate than Hb A provided support for this theory, but subsequent attempts to identify a mutant hemoglobin produced at a very low rate in thalassemic states were not successful, with the exception of two types of rare structural alterations which cause a marked slowing of their synthetic rate. One affects β chain production, and the other α. The first of these, Hb Lepore, is a globin chain which is a hybrid polypeptide consisting of a portion of the δ chain connected to a portion of the β chain to make a completed globin subunit of normal chain length which pairs with α chains in the completed tetrameric hemoglobin molecule. This hybrid globin subunit is the product of a fusion gene which presumably first originated in prior generations by a crossover occurring between homologous chromosomes slightly displaced during synapsis. Several different types of Lepore hemoglobins have been described, differing from one

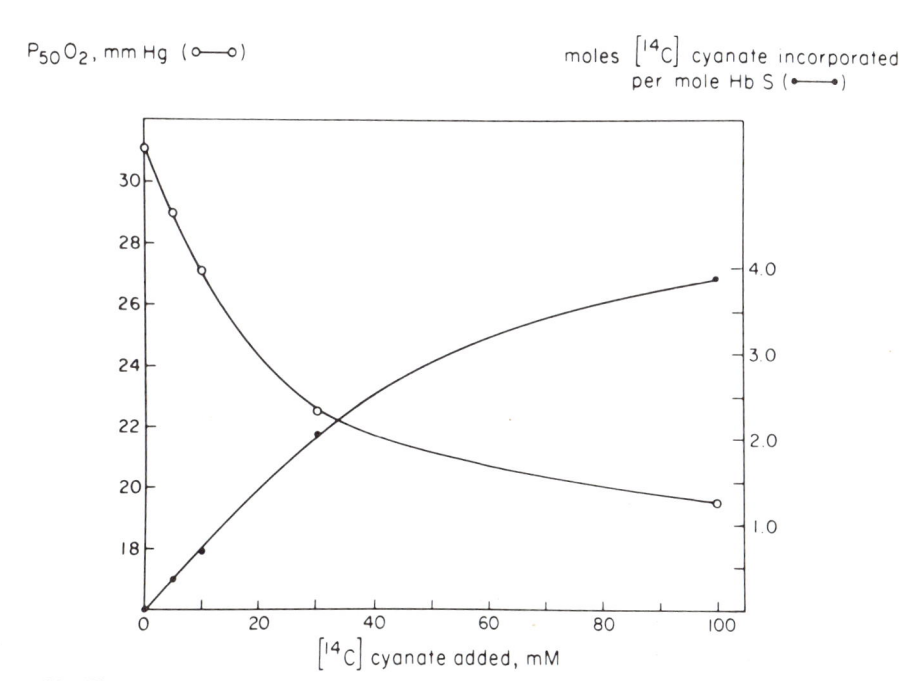

Figure 22–66 The increase in hemoglobin oxygen affinity after treatment of sickle cell anemia erythrocytes with cyanate, a possible mechanism for the inhibition of sickling. (Redrawn from deFuria, F. G., et al.: J. Clin. Invest., 51:566, 1972.)

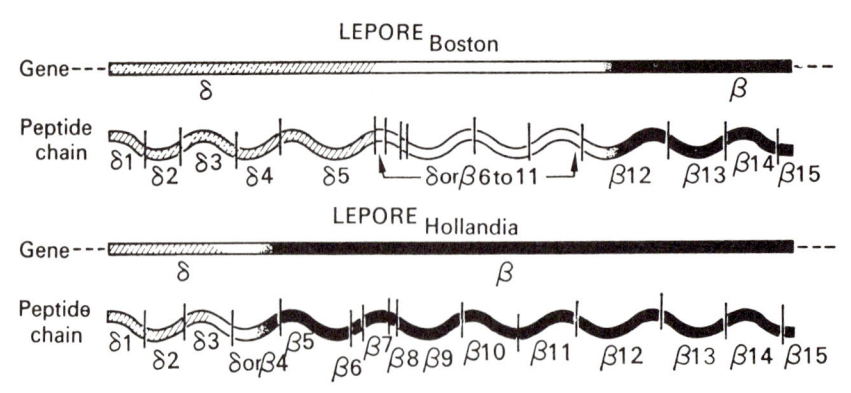

Figure 22-67 Examples of two different types of Lepore hemoglobins. (From Giblett, E. R.: Genetic Markers in Human Blood. Oxford, Blackwell Scientific Publications Ltd., 1969. Reprinted from Baglioni, C.: Proc. Natl. Acad. Sci., *48*:1880, 1962.)

another in the proportion of the molecule which resembles the δ chain (Fig. 22–67). Protein synthesis is normally initiated at the N-terminal end of the molecule, which in the Lepore hemoglobins is always that of the δ portion of the chain, and thus its synthesis takes on the slow character of normal δ chain production. The deficit results in a β-thalassemia syndrome.

Hb Constant Spring, described by Milner and coworkers, is found in trace quantities in association with α-thalassemia states. In contrast to the normal α chain, which has 141 amino acids, this abnormal hemoglobin carries a defect in chain length which causes it to grow to an abnormal length of 162 amino acids, 21 too long. The pathogenetic basis of the defect appears to lie in the fact that at position 142 of the messenger RNA, where the triplet codon normally signals "terminate," a mutation signals instead for the insertion of a specific amino acid. Additional amino acids are then added until the next terminating codon is read from the messenger RNA strand at position 162. The defect in chain termination markedly slows its synthetic rate and causes an α-thalassemia syndrome.

However, these two examples notwithstanding, the basic pathogenesis of most of the thalassemia syndromes is still not understood. The translational aspects of globin chain synthesis, including the function of the initiator factors and of the ribosomes, are normal. Messenger RNA has been isolated from thalassemia erythroid cells and clearly bears the responsibility for the low synthetic rate. Whether the messenger RNA is qualitatively defective in structure and so has an impaired function or whether it is transcribed on the chromosome at an abnormally low rate remains unknown. Any one or combination of the genes directing globin chain synthesis may hypothetically be affected by a thalassemic lesion causing depressed production rates, but only those affecting the α or the β loci are important (see Nathan reference). The degree of depression of globin chain formation may be minimal, moderate, or virtually complete, but it is relatively consistent within the affected members of the same family.

In the heterozygous carrier state one member of the chromosome pair produces globin chains at a normal rate and the clinical condition is asymptomatic. Anemia is minimal or mild, the erythrocytes are microcytic and are often present in greater than normal numbers, and the erythrocyte morphology is abnormal. Some thalassemic carrier states are so minimal that they are completely silent and exhibit no abnormalities whatsoever. The depressed β chain production in the carrier state of β-thalassemia is reflected in an increased proportion of Hb A_2 to approximately twice the normal value, the shortage of β chains altering the ratio of β to δ chain production. About a third also have slight elevations of Hb F to about 2 to 6 per cent of the total hemoglobin. Hb F is more elevated and the Hb A_2 normal in a less common strain of β-thalassemia trait. In carriers of α-thalassemia trait the proportions of Hb A_2 and Hb F are not altered, since these hemoglobins, in common with Hb A, are all affected by the shortage of α chains.

Homozygosity for β-thalassemia (Cooley's anemia) is associated with little or no capacity to produce β chains (and thus Hb A), because both alleles responsible for β chain synthesis are affected. Hb F becomes the major hemoglobin type produced, usually exceeding 50 per cent and often approaching 95 per cent of the total. The Hb A and the Hb F are contained in variable mixtures in the erythrocyte population, the better filled cells containing more Hb F have a more prolonged survival time than the more empty Hb F-poor cells (see Gabuzda et al. reference). The pathogenesis of the severe hemolysis is explained by imbalanced production of α as compared to β chains. The surplus unpaired α chains are exceedingly unstable and precipitate readily within nucleated erythroid precursor cells, causing marked intramedullary destruction, i.e., ineffective erythropoiesis (see Yataganas and Fessas reference). Those cell lines which retain a greater capacity for γ chain production not only are better filled with hemoglobin but also have fewer surplus unpaired α chains and thus are less rapidly hemolyzed. The patients are severely anemic, are transfusion dependent beginning in early childhood, develop massive enlargement of the spleen and of the liver, show prominent signs of extramedullary hematopoiesis, and suffer physical disfigurement because of the bone deformity brought on by the extreme erythroid hyperplasia in the marrow. Iron overload ultimately causes failure of the heart or liver, along with diabetes mellitus. Some apparently homozygous patients have a much milder anemia because one or both of their inherited thalassemic genes are mild or minimal. Patients in such a state, designated as "thalassemia intermedia," are not transfusion dependent but over the years are apt to develop hemochromatosis.

Homozygosity for severe α-thalassemia, so far observed only in Oriental newborns with an erythroblastosis fetalis-like picture, is a lethal condition in which severe anemia is associated with nearly 100 per cent Hb Bart's (γ_4) which lacks α chains and therefore does not function in oxygen transport, its affinity for oxygen being too great. Death thus occurs before or soon after birth (see Lie-Injo reference). A milder form of α-thalassemia in a subject who carries one mild and one severe gene is associated with about 20 per cent Hb Bart's at birth, which is subsequently replaced by its adult counterpart Hb H(β_4), which also cannot function in oxygen transport. Hb H is the product of surplus β chains in the face of a shortage of α chains. Its degree of instability is not as marked as that of unpaired α chains, and it precipitates in more mature circulating erythrocytes, causing hemolytic anemia without the same degree of intramedullary erythroid cell destruction seen in Cooley's anemia (see Gabuzda reference). Newborn heterozygous carriers of α-thalassemia trait have slight increases in Hb Bart's in the cord blood, but this disappears with development, leaving no disturbance in the proportions of Hb A or Hb F in the adult erythrocytes (see Lehmann reference).

HEMOGLOBINOPATHY: POPULATION GENETICS. Inherited abnormalities of globin chain structure or production rate sporadically affect individuals from all population groups, but by far the most frequently affected are those originating from tropical or subtropical regions. Incidence figures are highest in Africa, the Mediterranean Basin, the Near and Middle East, and Southeast Asia. Hb S reaches its highest frequency in Africa, where it affects 20 to 30 per cent or more of the Negro population in regions of West, Central, and East Africa. There is also a significant incidence in the Mediterranean countries and in localized regions of Arabia and India. Hb C has a peak prevalence of 10 to 20 per cent among West African Negroes in the region of Ghana. Hb E attains a comparable frequency in areas of Southeast Asia. The α- and β-thalassemia genes are relatively frequent throughout the entire "hemoglobinopathy belt," but Southeast Asia and regions of Greece and Italy have an especially high incidence.

Red Cell Survival Disorders

General Signs of Hemolysis. After a 4-month trip through the streams and bogs of the circulation, the normal erythrocyte ends its life span and is ingested by the cells of the phagocytic reticuloendothelial system. Its death is heralded by cellular changes of aging: loss of surface membrane, decrease of cell water, and decline in activity of several enzyme systems. Premature disappearance of erythrocytes either by hemorrhagic loss from the circulatory compartment or by hemolysis may lead to anemia. Hemolysis occurs when the cell itself is intrinsically defective or when the milieu in which it is bathed contains noxious factors.

When the life span of the erythrocyte is only slightly shortened, the consequence may not be of significance. On the other hand, in severe hemolytic states a red cell life span of only 1/10 of 1/20 the normal period of 120 days severely strains the capacity of the bone marrow to sustain erythroid cell production at a rate sufficient to maintain a circulating hemoglobin concentration compatible with health. The production of erythroid cells in the marrow is increased to meet the demands of increased erythrocyte turnover. This is reflected in hyperplasia of the erythroid precursor cells. Marrow normally occupied by fat is converted to cellular tissue. The proportion of erythroid to granulocytic precursors is increased. Young reticulocytes and sometimes nucleated erythroid cells are released into the circulation. The bone marrow is able to increase red cell production to a limited degree—about 6 to 8 times the normal rate. Therefore it is possible to compensate for shortened erythrocyte life spans that are 1/6 to 1/8 normal.

The hemolytic state is thus not necessarily associated with severe anemia. Indeed, the term "compensated hemolysis" is used to describe hemolytic states that are not associated with anemia at all. However, it is still not clear how the bone marrow, in the absence of the stimulus of anemic hypoxia, maintains a rate of red cell production high enough to fully compensate for the reduced erythrocyte life span. When production and destruction sets up a new steady-state condition, the red cell mass is reduced and turns over at a faster rate. Limitations upon production may cause anemia even when the degree of erythrocyte hemolysis is moderate. Such limitation occurs secondary to other diseases, such as neoplastic or inflammatory states, or to deficiency of essential nutrients, especially iron and folate. The acute "aplastic crisis" is the most critical imbalance between production and destruction—erythroid precursors suddenly vanish from the marrow, the reticulocyte count drops, and soon after there is a rapid increase in the degree of anemia as the remaining short-lived erythrocytes, no longer being replenished from the marrow, disappear from the circulation. Fortunately, the period of aplasia of red cell formation, probably triggered by a minor infection, is usually short-lived, and recovery is the rule. Similar infections may well arrest erythropoiesis in normal individuals, but during the period of marrow arrest, the fall in blood count is imperceptible because of the characteristic longevity of normal erythrocytes.

In the Wright's stained peripheral blood film, reticulocytes are recognized as polychromatophilic macrocytes. Microspherocytes are small, round, densely stained erythrocytes seen in a variety of hemolytic states. Regular and irregular distortions of the erythrocyte membrane into spurs and burrs and the fracturing of erythrocytes into bits and pieces suggest mechanical or metabolic damage.

The biochemical signs of hemolysis are those of the release and breakdown of the pigment of the red cells. Erythrocyte destruction within the confines of the circulatory system ("intravascular hemolysis") causes leakage of hemoglobin directly into the plasma. Phagocytosis of intact erythrocytes or of erythrocyte fragments releases hemoglobin inside the phagocytic reticuloendothelial cell, where the heme is degraded to bilirubin ("extravascular hemolysis"). Hemolytic states are not exclusively intra- or extravascular, but when extensive cell damage causes the erythrocytes to "fall apart" in the circulation the signs of hemoglobin release into the plasma and urine are marked. Hemoglobin released from erythrocytes into the circulation is first bound to haptoglobin, a plasma protein with alpha-2 electrophoretic mobility (Fig. 22–68). The complex of hemoglobin with haptoglobin is then rapidly cleared from the plasma into the reticuloendothelial system, promptly reducing the plasma concentration of haptoglobin to near absent levels. Thus, a reduction of the plasma haptoglobin concentration (and of the alpha-2 fraction of the serum proteins) is often observed in hemolytic states, regardless of pathogenesis. Haptoglobin concentration, however, is subject to rather pronounced increases secondary to many inflammatory and neoplastic states, and its final level represents a balance between those factors promoting its synthesis and those producing its degradation, such as hemolysis. Haptoglobin normally is capable of binding hemoglobin to the extent of about 100 mg. per 100 ml. plasma. When the haptoglobin binding capacity is exceeded, hemoglobin is lost in the urine. Haptoglobin serves the purpose of conserving iron by preventing its loss in the urine as heme. Oxidized heme, split apart from its globin bond, may also be detected bound to hemopexin, a beta globulin of the plasma, as well as to the albumin (as methemalbumin), giving the plasma a dirty brown color. Heme bound to hemopexin is taken up into the hepatic parenchymal cells.

The detection of free hemoglobin in the plasma and urine indicates that the haptoglobin binding capacity has been exceeded and that the degree of intravascular hemolysis has been extensive. The free plasma hemoglobin, unattached to high molecular weight haptoglobin, is readily filtered through the glomerulus. Some passes through directly to produce urine benzidine positive for the presence of heme pigment. However, hemoglobin is also resorbed into the tubular epithelial cells, where its iron is removed and deposited within

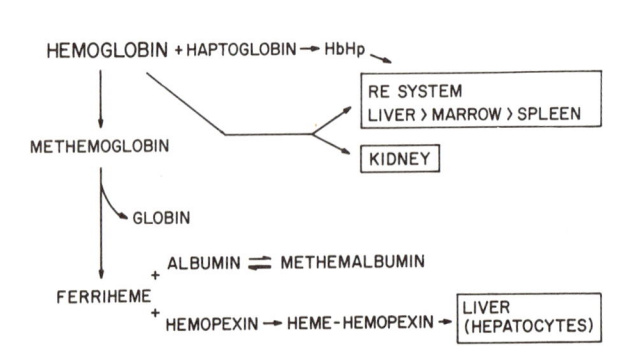

Figure 22–68 The intravascular handling of hemoglobin. (From Bunn, H. F.: Seminars Hemat., 9:3–17, 1972. By permission of Grune and Stratton, Inc., New York.)

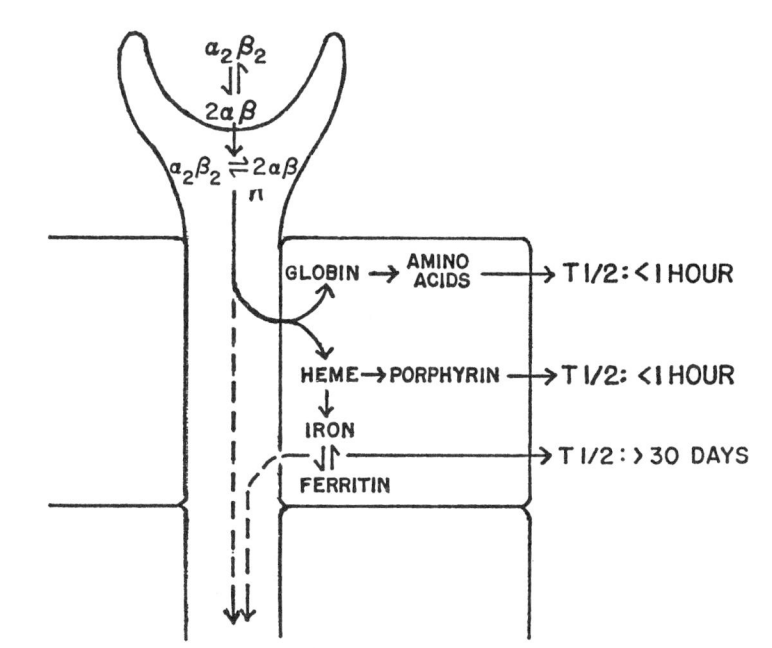

Figure 22-69 The renal handling of hemoglobin. (From Bunn, H. F., and Jandl, J. H.: J. Exper. Med., *129*:925, 1969.)

the cell as ferritin and hemosiderin. These iron-rich proteins are then sloughed with the normal loss of tubular epithelial cells into the urine, where they can be detected in the sediment by the Prussian blue reaction for iron (Fig. 22-69). Hemosiderinuria is a valuable sign that the patient either is suffering from intravascular hemolysis or has recently done so. After recovery from an acute intravascular hemolytic episode, the urine stain for hemosiderin will remain positive for some days after hemoglobinuria has stopped.

Jaundice is a common sign of hemolysis. Often the degree is subclinical and cannot be detected except by chemical measurement of the serum bilirubin concentration. The degree of jaundice is never intense; total serum bilirubin concentrations in excess of 6 mg. per 100 ml. suggest malfunction of the liver or of its biliary drainage system, since the capacity of the normal liver to process bilirubin is immense. Hemolytic jaundice involves primarily elevation of the unconjugated bilirubin (or indirect-reacting fraction). It circulates bound to plasma albumin and therefore is not lost in the urine. After its transport to the liver, bilirubin is processed by the hepatic cells and converted to the water-soluble diglucuronide derivative (direct-reacting, or conjugated), which is the major form excreted in the bile (see Gartner and Arias reference). A portion of this conjugated bilirubin is absorbed and undergoes enterohepatic circulation. Most of it is reduced by colonic bacteria to urobilinogen, which also has an enterohepatic circulation. In hemolysis the output of bile pigments into the intestinal tract is increased in direct proportion to the degree of heme degradation and thus to the extent of the hemolytic process. Measurement of the fecal urobilinogen excretion may be used to quantitate the extent of hemolysis as a function of heme degradation rate, but the procedure is too cumbersome for general use. Urine urobilinogen is likewise increased as a reflection of the increased enterohepatic circulation, but only a small proportion of the total is excreted by this route.

Bilirubin is produced in phagocytic cells throughout the body from degraded heme pigments of a variety of types, chief among which by far is hemoglobin. Phagocytes possess an efficient enzymatic mechanism which rapidly and voraciously strips away the iron for metabolic recycling, digests the globin into its constituent amino acids for re-entry into the body pool, and oxidizes the tetrapyrrol ringed structure of heme into biliverdin. This conversion, mediated by heme oxidase, fractures open one of the four bridges (the alpha methene) that hold together the four pyrrol groups into a ringed tetrapyrrol structure. Carbon monoxide is produced in this reaction and is delivered to the lungs for respiratory excretion, one mole for each mole of heme degraded. Since there is no other source of endogenous carbon monoxide, measurement of its production rate accurately quantitates the catabolism of heme compounds and thus also the rate of hemolysis (Fig. 22-70). Biliverdin, a green pigment, is reduced to bilirubin, which is then transferred from the phagocytic cells to the hepatic parenchymal cells for conjugation.

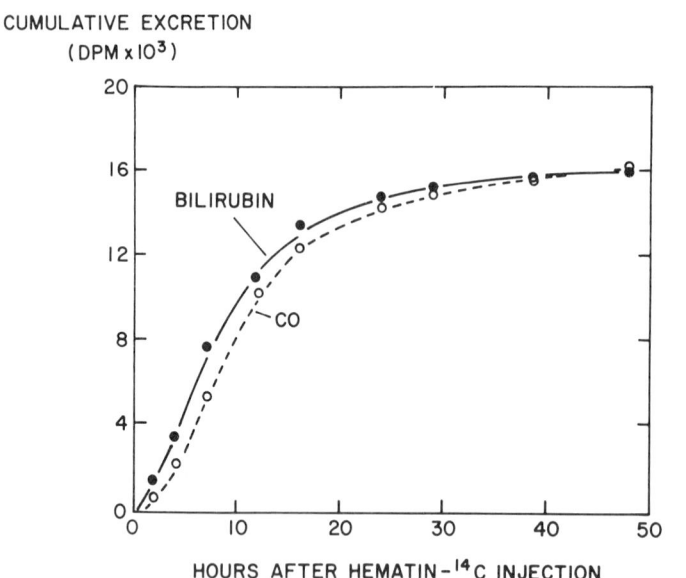

Figure 22-70 Parallel appearance of radioactivity into bilirubin and carbon monoxide after administration of radioactive hematin. (Redrawn from Landaw, S. A., et al.: J. Clin. Invest., 49:914, 1970.)

The load of heme pigments normally presented for degradation comes chiefly from dying senescent erythrocytes, but about 15 per cent is from other sources, some from the liver and some from the bone marrow (Fig. 22–71). The hepatic contribution may be increased in porphyria of hepatic origin or following the administration of certain drugs, as phenobarbital, which stimulate the endoplasmic reticulum along with heme synthesis. The bone marrow also produces heme which never reaches the safe haven of the circulating erythrocyte. This marrow heme, destined for early degradation, consists partly of hemoglobin shrouds which veil normoblast nuclei after their extrusion (Fig. 22–72), partly of defective normoblasts destroyed before they gain access to the circulation as mature erythrocytes, and possibly partly of heme which is never incorporated into hemoglobin but is "shunted" into an early catabolic demise. From the foregoing, it is apparent that hepatic or marrow defects can markedly affect the net pattern of heme degradation. The process of intramedullary hemolysis, i.e., ineffective erythropoiesis, so prominent in megaloblastic anemia and in homozygous β-thalassemia, may be the major contributor to heme catabolism and thus to the increased production of carbon monoxide and bilirubin associated with these disorders.

The measurement of red cell survival time would appear to be the most direct approach to the diagnosis of hemolytic disorders, but this measurement presents a number of difficulties

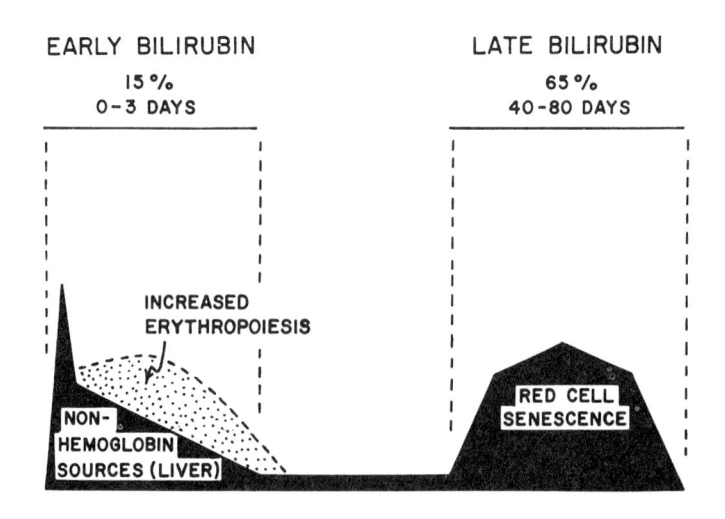

Figure 22-71 The formation of "early" and "late" bilirubin from degraded heme in the rat. (From Robinson, S. H.: Seminars Hemat., 9:43–53, 1972. Reprinted from Stohlman, F. (Jr.): Hemopoietic Cellular Proliferation, 1970, by permission of Grune and Stratton, Inc., New York.)

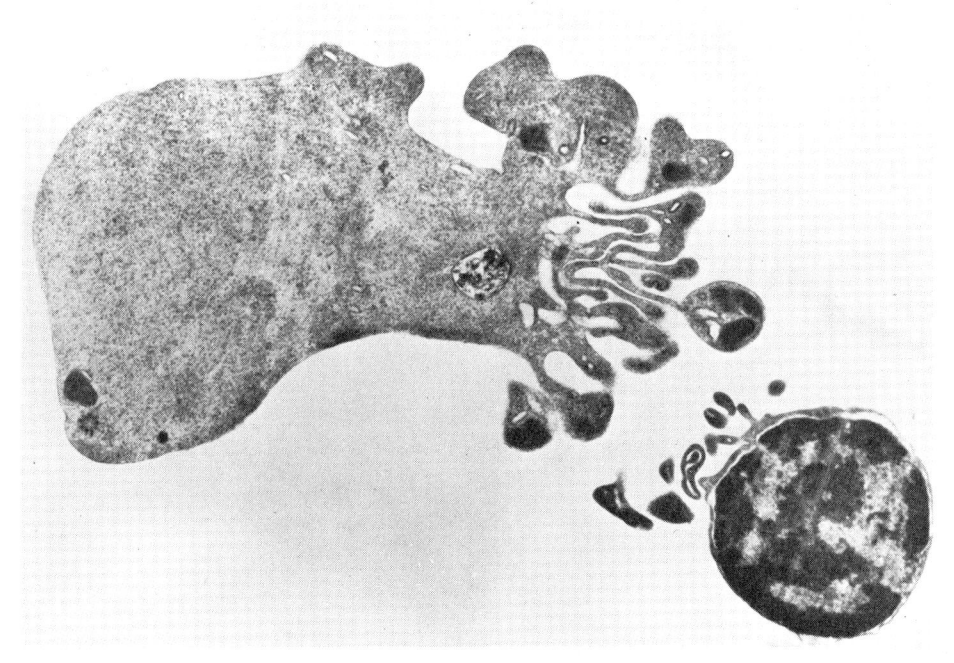

Figure 22-72 The extrusion of a nucleus covered with a shroud of hemoglobin from an erythroid precursor, leaving behind a reticulocyte containing mitochondria and ribosomes. (Reproduced from the Sandoz-Monograph, The Life Cycle of the Erythrocyte. Basel, Switzerland, M. Bessis, 1966.)

from practical as well as theoretical points of view. Not the least of these is the rather long time required, during which the patient should be in the steady state with regard to the maintenance of a constant red cell mass as well as to absence of significant loss of blood by hemorrhage. There are two basic approaches, both of which follow the behavior in the circulation of a tag on the erythrocytes. The first, called the cohort label, employs the use of a radioisotope which is administered and is then incorporated into a cohort of newly formed cells. Examples are isotopes of iron (e.g., ^{59}Fe) and of amino acids (e.g., glycine-2-^{14}C, ^{75}Se selenomethionine). Normally the cohort tag will appear in the peripheral blood erythrocytes and then rise to a plateau in about 10 days. This plateau is maintained until about 100 days, and at 120 days it reaches a maximum rate of decline as the cohort dies off. Mean erythrocyte survival time can be estimated from such curves, but this method is difficult to carry out and may be hampered by reutilization of these biologically active tags.

The second method, the population or random label, uses a nonphysiologic marker of a representative sample of the entire erythrocyte population. The sample should be uniformly tagged without difference or discrimination as to cell age, pathologic state, or any other cell variable, so that when it is reintroduced into the circulation, a clear picture is obtained of the rate of removal of the population of erythrocytes it represents. Normally a fixed number of erythrocytes reaches senescence and dies each day; the tag will represent this by a straight-line decline intercepting zero at 120 days, when the last of the tagged cells will have died off. This is an age-dependent pattern of cell destruction. Many hemolytic states are characterized by random destruction of erythrocytes, without regard to their age. A fixed percentage of the remaining cells are destroyed per day; the tag disappears from the circulation at an exponential rate according to first order kinetics. The time required for disappearance of half the tag (the half-time or T/2) is the most conventional method of expressing erythrocyte survival time as measured with a population label.

No tags are ideal, but two of the best are diisopropylfluorophosphate (DF^{32}P) and sodium chromate (Na$_2^{51}$CrO$_4$). DF^{32}P attaches to red cell cholinesterase to form a tight bond which lasts for the duration of the erythrocyte's life span; its disappearance rate from the circulation yields a value quite close to the true life span, but the method is inconvenient. Na$_2^{51}$CrO$_4$ penetrates the red cell membrane and is reduced to the chromic state, and then the chromium tag forms a chelate with the β chain of hemoglobin. Its bond to proteins is not nearly so tight and it elutes from red cells at a rate of about 1 per cent per day, with significant differences in various disease states. Consequently, its disappearance rate from the circulation does not give a true measure of erythrocyte survival but rather a composite of this function minus the elution rate of the chromium. The normal half-time of ^{51}Cr-labeled erythrocytes is 25 to 35 days, a value considerably shorter than the physiologic half disappearance time of 60 days. Despite these patent disadvantages, ^{51}Cr has practical virtues and has gained widespread acceptance as a convenient method for the clinical assessment of erythrokinetics. As a gamma emitter it is easy to count and permits body surface counting to determine whether or not the spleen is the major site of erythrocyte destruction.

Membrane Function and Energy Metabolism. The biochemistry of the erythrocyte has long been a subject of practical interest in the development of satisfactory methods of preserving shed blood intended for transfusion therapy. This deceptively simple cell has also served as a model system in the basic investigation of glycolysis and of the structure and function of cell membranes. Along with the elucidation of the biochemical clockworks of the erythrocyte has come the definition in precise biochemical terms of a large number of different hemolytic states.

The red cell membrane consists of a protein shell heavily clothed with lipids, chiefly phospholipids and cholesterol (see Cooper, Shohet references). The membrane proteins include the carbohydrate-rich blood group substances, a filamentous structural protein called spectrin, certain enzymes, and other proteins yet to be identified (Fig. 22–73). The membrane maintains a certain excess of surface area which, by dimpling into a biconcave shape, squeezes the hemoglobin into the peripheral ring of the doughnut-like cell. Weed and coworkers have shown that the preservation of this shape depends on energy expenditure. The extent of this surface area is subject to change; it normally decreases as the cell ages. However, mature erythrocytes, no longer able to synthesize lipid, may undergo volume changes through membrane interaction with the external environment. Rapid passive exchange of free cholesterol (but not esterified cholesterol) takes place between the membrane and the plasma. Phospholipid exchange also occurs, but at a much slower rate. The quantity of membrane free cholesterol can be manipulated by varying the free cholesterol content of the surrounding medium (Fig. 22–74). A high level will cause free cholesterol to accumulate in the membrane, thereby increasing its surface area. The increased surface-to-volume ratio confers upon the erythrocytes a greater distensibility in hypotonic media, i.e., their osmotic resistance is increased (Fig. 22–75). The redundant membrane of such cholesterol-replete cells produces a

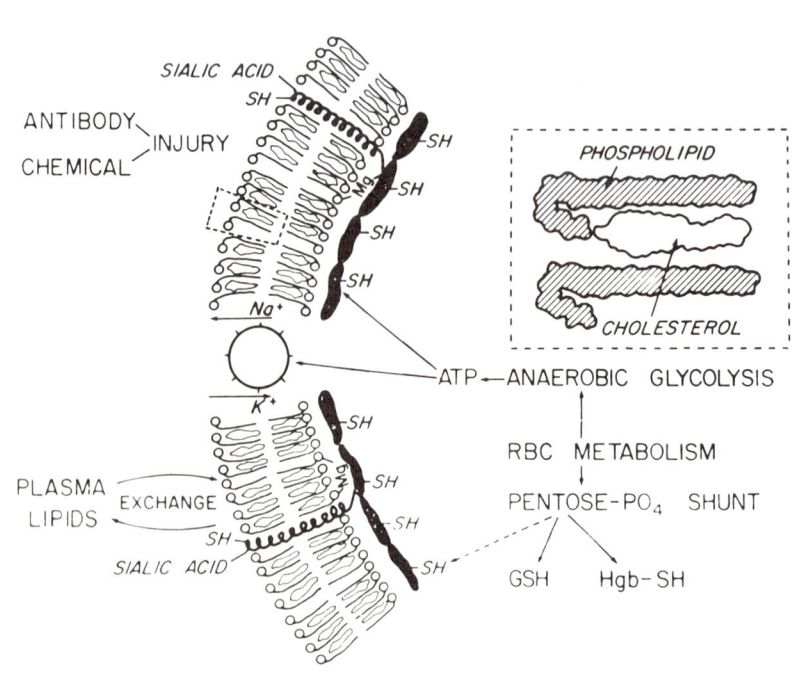

Figure 22–73 Diagrammatic representation of the erythrocyte membrane. (From Weed, R. I., and Reed, C. F.: Amer. J. Med., 41:681, 1966.)

Figure 22-74 The exchange of free cholesterol between serum and the erythrocyte membrane, as represented by parallel changes in red cell cholesterol and osmotic fragility. After initial incubation with free cholesterol-poor serum, heated serum replete with free cholesterol was added. (Redrawn from Cooper, R. A., and Jandl, J. H.: J. Clin. Invest., 48:906, 1969.)

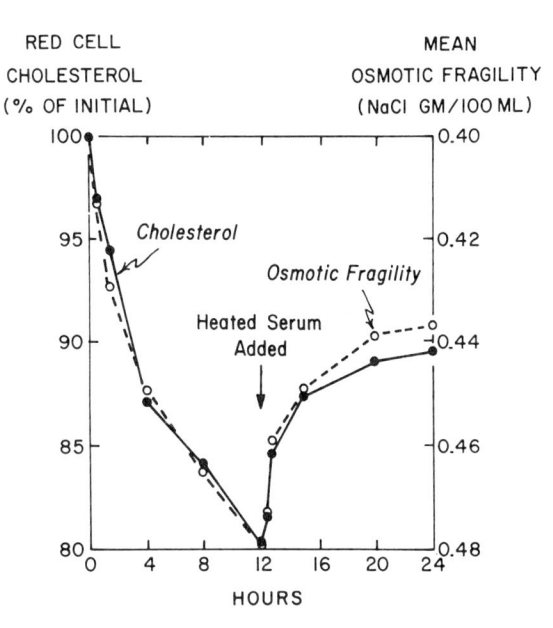

targeted appearance; the area of central pallor has a "bulls-eye" of hemoglobin deposited within. Conversely, suspension of erythrocytes in plasma or serum poor in free cholesterol will cause cholesterol loss from the membrane along with decreased osmotic resistance. Other important factors such as the serum lipoproteins modify the plasma-membrane exchange.

A busy traffic hums through the pores of the erythrocyte membrane. Gas transport is high on the priority list in fulfillment of the cell's chief function. An active uptake of glucose is required to power the metabolic machinery. Of great interest — and still considerably a mystery — is the movement of electrolytes across the membrane (see Nathan and Shohet reference). The pores, seemingly guarded by positively charged sentries (possibly calcium ions), freely allow anions to pass rapidly into the cell. Permeability to cations is quite another matter; cations diffuse across the membrane much more slowly. To oppose this slow, passive diffusion of cations, an active pumping mechanism in the membrane maintains concentration gradients of sodium and potassium.

Figure 22-75 Acquired changes in erythrocyte osmotic fragility due to changes in membrane cholesterol. Normal cells become more resistant when incubated with serum from a patient with obstructive jaundice as compared to normal serum. The osmotic resistance of the patient's erythrocytes, which showed target cell formation, was increased. (Redrawn from Cooper, R. A., and Jandl, J. H.: J. Clin. Invest., 47:809, 1968.)

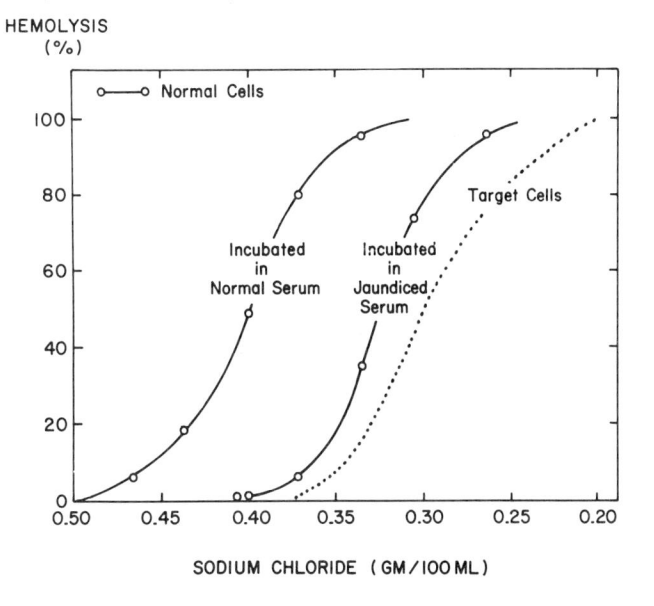

Sodium is actively extruded from the cell against a concentration gradient of 10 mEq. per liter inside the cell to 145 mEq. per liter in the extracellular plasma. Potassium is pumped into the cell against a concentration gradient from 4.5 mEq. per liter in the plasma to 100 mEq. per liter inside the cell. The active transport of cations requires ATP as an energy source; it consumes about 15 per cent of the erythrocyte ATP production. The membrane contains an ATPase to mediate its utilization there. Energy deprivation may therefore lead to a breakdown of the pumping mechanism, with serious consequences to the osmotic equilibrium of the cell.

The erythrocyte is the principal transporter of oxygen as fuel for the entire body. In addition to the high-energy phosphate bonds of ATP, it requires energy to perform biochemical reductions to protect its own parts from oxidative denaturation by this fuel. There are two major reducing systems. One, utilizing NADH, maintains the iron atoms of hemoglobin in the reduced state, a need imposed by the continuous slow conversion of hemoglobin to methemoglobin. The reduction is mediated by an enzyme, methemoglobin reductase (see Jaffé and Hsieh reference). The other reducing system assumes responsibility for maintaining the cell's thiol groups—those of the membrane, the enzymes, and the hemoglobin—in the reduced state. This pathway is mediated through NADPH, which in turn ultimately works through maintaining glutathione in the reduced state.

Glucose is the sole source of energy. The mature erythrocyte consumes 90 per cent of its glucose through the anaerobic Embden-Meyerhof pathway, with conversion to lactate as the end-product and the net production of two moles of ATP and the reduction of two moles of NAD to NADH per mole of glucose (Fig. 22–76). Normally about 10 per cent of the glucose is consumed through the pentose phosphate pathway with the reduction of two moles of NADP to NADPH per mole of glucose. Under the influence of certain redox compounds (for example, methylene blue) the amount of glucose processed through this route is markedly increased, a factor of considerable importance in the pathophysiology of hemolysis in patients lacking key enzymes in this pathway. Reticulocytes possess mitochondria and therefore have an active Krebs cycle for the oxidative metabolism of glucose, but this apparatus is lost as the reticulocyte matures. A third pathway of glucose metabolism in the erythrocyte does not participate in energy generation, but rather sacrifices energy production to the cause of an important adaptive mechanism for changing hemoglobin oxygen affinity (see Brewer and Eaton reference). This pathway (the Rapoport-Luebering shunt), controlled by diphosphoglycerate mutase (DPGM), generates 2,3-DPG, which binds to deoxyhemoglobin and reduces its affinity for oxygen. As more 2,3-DPG becomes bound, the free unbound pool becomes depleted, thus coaxing DPGM into detouring triose intermediates to replenish the pool. This detour costs the cell a loss of 2 moles of ATP per mole of glucose, but this loss does not appear to have any significant effect on fulfilling total energy requirements.

Classification of Hemolytic States. The seeds of premature erythrocyte destruction may lie either within the erythrocyte or outside in a hostile environment. Hemolytic states are thus readily categorized as "intrinsic" or "extrinsic" disorders, although some represent combinations of both. Most intrinsic defects are inherited; most extrinsic disorders are acquired. A classic experimental approach, no longer in common use, applied cross-transfusion techniques between the patient and a normal individual with compatible blood type. Erythrocytes from a patient with an intrinsic defect will exhibit a shortened survival time not only in the patient's own circulation but also in that of the normal recipient. Erythrocytes from a normal subject will survive as well in the patient's circulation as in his own. However, normal compatible erythrocytes will suffer a shortened survival time in the circulation of a patient with an extrinsic hemolytic disorder. Variations of this approach have also been applied to the study of combined disorders. Thus, tagged erythrocytes from a patient with glucose-6-phosphate dehydrogenase deficiency, an intrinsic drug-sensitive state, will survive quite normally in the circulation of a normal compatible recipient until the offending drug is administered, which will cause hemolysis of the tagged abnormal erythrocytes but not of the normal person's own erythrocytes. The interaction of the intrinsically defective red cells of hereditary spherocytosis with the extrinsic splenic environment has been demonstrated by the observation that such erythrocytes, appropriately labeled, will exhibit a shortened survival in the bloodstream of a normal recipient with intact spleen (Fig. 22–77) but a normal survival time in a normal person lacking a spleen.

To establish that a hemolytic state exists, measurements of the reticulocyte count, the conjugated and unconjugated serum bilirubin, the serum haptoglobin, the plasma and urine hemoglobin, and the urine hemosiderin, along with careful morphologic examination of the peripheral blood and bone marrow should indicate its severity and point to the diagnosis. A second echelon of hemolytic tests may then pinpoint the precise cellular or extracellular pathophysiologic condition. These include osmotic fragility measured in a graded series of hypotonic NaCl solutions; the autohemolysis of erythrocytes incubated in vitro under sterile conditions; screening for enzyme defects; hemoglobin analysis; tests for immunologic factors, such as the Coombs' anti-

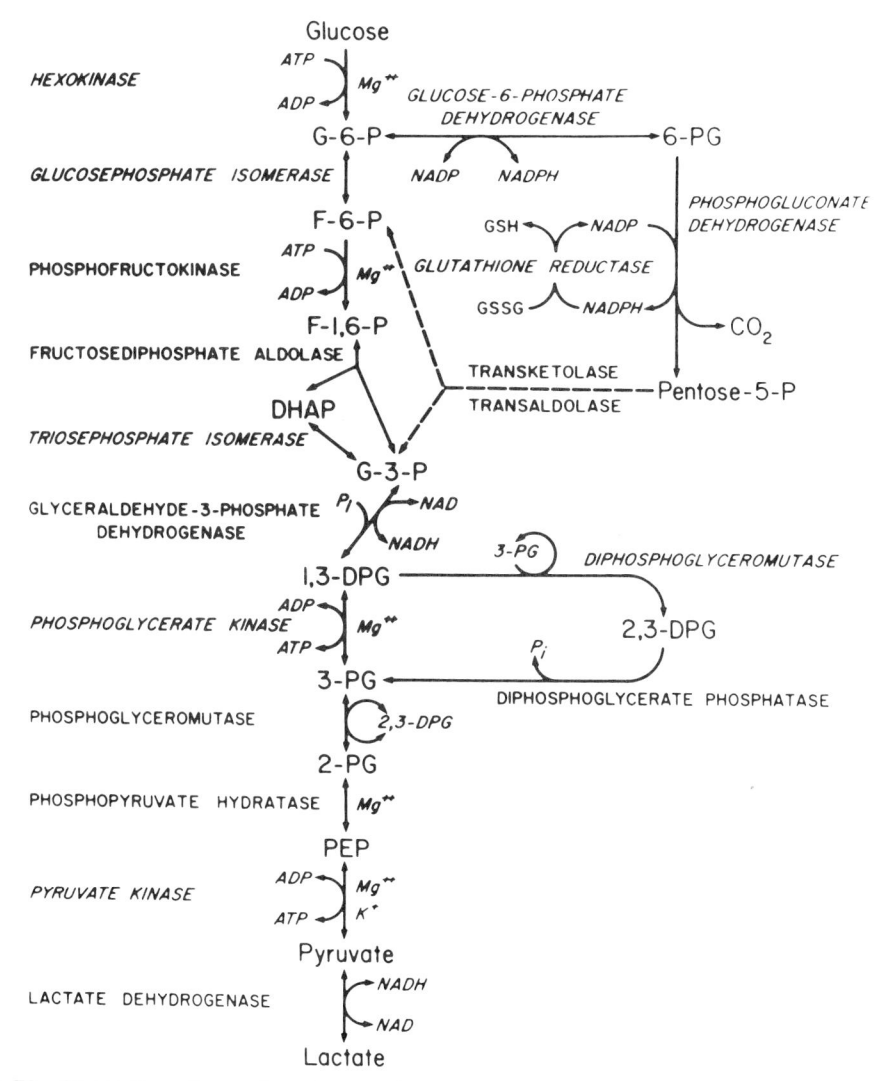

Figure 22-76 Glycolytic pathways in mature erythrocytes. (From Valentine, W. N.: Calif. Med., 108:280, 1968.)

globulin, cold agglutinin, and cold hemolysin tests; and tests for the complement-sensitive erythrocytes of paroxysmal nocturnal hemoglobinuria (sucrose hemolysis and acid hemolysin tests). The morphology of the red cells or the clinical circumstances (such as the fact that the patient has cirrhosis or uremia) may alone readily yield the pathophysiologic classification.

Intrinsic Hemolytic Disorders. *Hereditary spherocytosis* (HS) is generally classified as a red cell membrane defect, but the inherited molecular defect is not known. Its clinical expression is extraordinarily variable. At times it is first discovered incidentally in old age, but at the other extreme it may produce a severe hemolytic syndrome in the neonate or in early childhood. Many adults with HS maintain a state of completely compensated hemolysis. As with any chronic hemolytic disorder, there is a great likelihood that pigment gallstones will eventually develop. The inheritance pattern is autosomal dominant. Spherocytosis is a prominent feature in the peripheral blood film along with polychromasia. Tests for autoimmune disorders are negative. The family study is typically positive. The autohemolysis and osmotic fragility tests, to be described, are abnormal. The enlarged spleen is the site of the premature red cell destruction and its removal predictably restores the erythrocyte life span to almost normal, even though the intrinsic red cell defect remains.

Elegant investigations over the years have

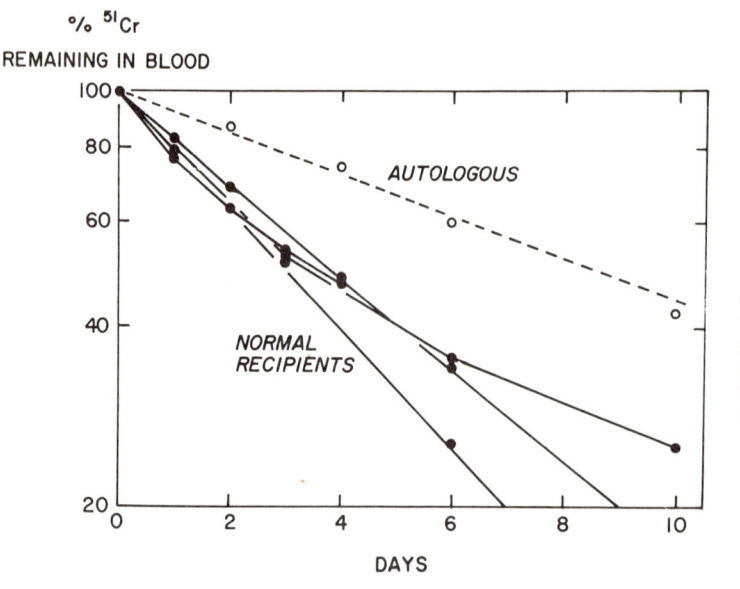

Figure 22-77 The survival of intrinsically defective ^{51}Cr-labeled erythrocytes from a patient with hereditary spherocytosis with intact spleen is even shorter in normal compatible recipients with intact spleen than in the patient. Survival time is normal (half-life equals 25 to 35 days by this method) in the absence of the spleen. (Redrawn from Wiley, J. S.: J. Clin. Invest., *49*:666, 1970.)

elucidated the cellular pathophysiology of HS. The membrane is leaky and allows potassium to escape and sodium to enter the cells at a faster than normal rate. Osmotic balance is maintained at the cost of increased energy expenditure required to increase the pump rate of sodium out of and potassium into the cell, a feat easily accomplished as long as an adequate supply of glucose is available to provide the necessary ATP. The circumstance, however, places the erythrocyte in a precarious state of dependence upon favorable surroundings; it is critically susceptible to glucose deprivation or other limitations on the availability of energy. If osmotic balance of the sodium ion cannot be maintained, water will enter the cell and cause it to swell and become a "macrospherocyte" and possibly eventually to rupture forth its contents.

This inability of the HS erythrocyte to withstand deprivation is demonstrated in the autohemolysis test. Whole blood is incubated at 37° C. under sterile conditions for 48 hours. The available glucose supply is sufficient to keep normal erythrocytes intact; less than 5 per cent will hemolyze. The HS erythrocyte consumes glucose at an increased rate. When the supply runs low, erythrocyte lysis is greatly increased, and 20 to 40 per cent autohemolysis is commonly observed. The addition of supplemental glucose prior to incubation has a salutary effect in reducing the degree of autohemolysis, sometimes to normal levels. Since lysis is produced by the osmotic imbalance between the cell interior and exterior, addition of impenetrable osmotically active agents, such as sucrose or ATP, to the plasma will also reduce autohemolysis.

In addition to increased cation permeability and glucose consumption, the cellular pathophysiology of HS is characterized by the loss of lipid materials from the membrane with a parallel loss of membrane surface area. The reduction in surface area without commensurate volume loss forces the biconcave erythrocytes to change into "microspherocytes"—small cells, densely stained, round, and lacking in central pallor. Since microspherocytes rather than macrospherocytes are the hallmark of this and of other spherocytic hemolytic conditions, the loss of surface is probably the more important pathophysiologic event (Fig. 22-78). The microspherocyte contains its hemoglobin at a higher concentration than normal. Thus, the mean corpuscular hemoglobin concentration (MCHC) in HS frequently is elevated above 36 grams per 100 ml. Spherocytic erythrocytes (whether micro or macro) are exquisitely sensitive to osmotic lysis following suspension in hypotonic solutions of NaCl. Since as spheres they already have the minimum ratio of surface to volume, they can undergo no further volume expansion as water is taken into the cell. As the spherocyte attempts to swell further, the membrane pores distend and offer free permeability to cations soon to be followed by leakage of large molecules. The hemoglobin escapes from the cell interior into the surrounding medium, leaving behind the hollow "ghost."

The osmotic fragility test is always abnormal in HS, although at times it may be necessary to "bring out" the abnormality by first exposing the erythrocytes to glucose deprivation by a 24-hour in-vitro preincubation. The lipid-depleted microspherocytes represent a discrete subpopulation of

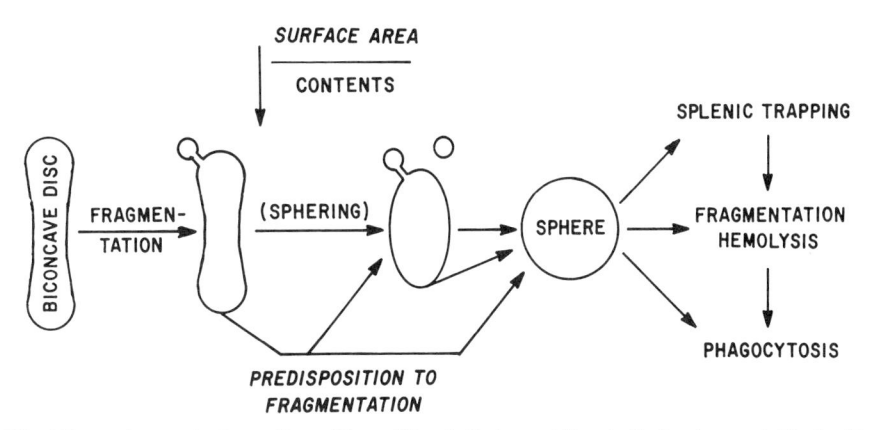

Figure 22–78 Microspherocyte formation. (From Weed, R. I., and Reed, C. F.: Amer. J. Med., 41:681, 1966.)

especially osmotically fragile erythrocytes. These show up in the complete osmotic fragility test as a "fragile tail," some of them lysing even at a slight reduction of the NaCl concentration below 0.85 gram per 100 ml. The remaining nonspherocytic cells may exhibit normal osmotic fragility. But if the blood is incubated for 24 hours before being tested in graded concentrations of saline, the entire cell population will swell somewhat because of the cells' inability to maintain osmotic equilibrium. This limited degree of volume expansion produces spherodicity and increases osmotic susceptibility. Thus, the entire erythrocyte population in HS after 24 hours' incubation will show a marked shift toward increased fragility, much greater than that of normal red cells similarly treated.

Of crucial importance in the pathophysiology of hemolysis in HS is the unhappy interaction between the erythrocyte and the spleen. Removal of the spleen restores red cell life span to normal or near normal; all hemolytic manifestations are brought to a prompt halt, yet the cellular defect, along with the abnormal autohemolysis and osmotic fragility tests, remains. What is so unique about the splenic interior that these erythrocytes find so hostile to longevity? In many respects, the spleen subjects the red cells to the same stresses they undergo during sterile in-vitro incubation. The spleen is an organ of erythrostasis; erythrocytes linger in their passage through the splenic pulp. Plasma skimming concentrates erythrocytes to higher packed cell volumes. The splenic pulp has a lower glucose concentration and a more acid pH than the circulating blood. These factors place limitations upon glycolysis and cause lipid loss from the membrane surface. This damage may not be fatal to the erythrocyte during its first passage through the spleen, but with repeated passages the red cell becomes "conditioned," that is, it loses so much membrane surface area that it becomes a microspherocyte. This ball-like erythrocyte lacks the extreme pliability of the normal biconcave shape and it is finally retained in the filter of the spleen, the 3-micron mesh sieve that fenestrates the walls of the splenic cords and sinuses in the red pulp. The erythrocytes in the splenic cords must squeeze through this meshwork—past quality-conscious macrophages—to gain access into the splenic sinuses and on to drainage into the splenic vein. The small but plump spherocytes traverse this porous barrier with difficulty, if at all, in the meantime suffering the ravages of the splenic environment to the point of outright cell destruction and phagocytosis. No other site in the body possesses such a finely tuned filtering mechanism as the spleen; it places the most stringent limitation upon rigid erythrocytes which cannot easily squeeze and twist through its small orifices (Fig. 22–79).

Hereditary elliptocytosis, an autosomal dominant condition about one fifth as common as HS, is just as obscure in terms of precise molecular genetics. The majority of erythrocytes have an elliptical shape. The diagnosis is clear from inspection of the peripheral blood film alone. Smaller numbers of elliptocytes are often present in the deficiency anemias, thalassemias, myeloproliferative syndromes, and other situations. The defect presumably resides in the membrane, but the pathogenesis of the shape change is not understood. About four fifths of cases exhibit little or no hemolysis. Those with clinical stigmata of hemolysis resemble HS in pathophysiology. Splenomegaly is also present and the hemolysis, as in HS, is corrected by splenectomy.

Paroxysmal nocturnal hemoglobinuria (PNH) is peculiar among the intrinsic red cell disorders in that it is acquired. Despite its rarity it has

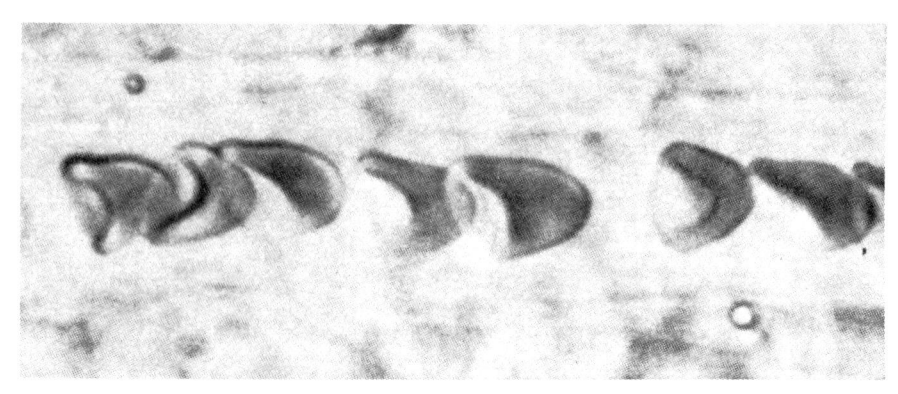

Figure 22-79 The pliability of normal erythrocytes as they move through small capillaries by assuming a parachute configuration. Rigid erythrocytes, such as microspherocytes, sickled erythrocytes, or erythrocytes containing Heinz bodies are subject to entrapment. (From Skalak, R., and Branemark, P. I.: Science, 164:717, 1969. Copyright 1969 by the American Association for the Advancement of Science.)

been intensively investigated, but a precise definition of its molecular basis is still lacking. At present PNH is considered to be an acquired defect of the red cell membrane that renders it pathologically sensitive to destruction by the complement system. This destruction is accomplished without the interposition of the antibodies which usually are required for the initiation of complement-related cell lysis (see Hartmann and Jenkins reference). The onset may be at any age, and the disease usually has a chronic protracted course. Its name is derived from the fact that intravascular hemolysis occurs at night, causing the first voided morning urine to be darkly colored by its hemoglobin content. In many cases, however, the nocturnal character is not prominent. Periods of exacerbation of the hemoglobinuria may follow infections, exercise, surgery, or other physical stresses. The most serious morbidity and mortality stem from a high incidence of intravascular thrombosis, chiefly venous and often involving the mesenteric and portal venous systems. Some patients become dependent on blood transfusion. Fortunately for them, normal compatible erythrocytes survive normally in their circulation.

The etiology of PNH is unknown. It seems to bear an obscure relationship to aplastic anemia, both idiopathic and drug-induced. Interconversions from one syndrome to the other have been well documented. A few patients with PNH have developed acute leukemia, but this is decidedly a rare occurrence. Some exceptional cases of PNH have undergone complete and permanent remission. Along with the anemia and the elevated reticulocyte count and signs of intravascular hemolysis, the white cell and platelet counts are commonly reduced. Thus the disorder is "trilineage."

Although the red cell life span is shortened, the life span of the platelets is normal. Several odd cellular enzyme deficiencies are associated with PNH, including deficiency of granulocyte alkaline phosphatase and erythrocyte acetylcholinesterase, with unknown pathophysiologic significance.

The diagnosis is usually established by a positive stain of the urinary sediment for hemosiderin and a positive sucrose hemolysis test. The hemosiderinuria is a reflection of the predominantly intravascular nature of the hemolysis. Indeed urinary losses of iron, up to 20 mg. per day, frequently lead to iron deficiency, otherwise an uncommon complication of hemolytic anemia. The sucrose hemolysis test relies on the promotion of complement fixation to the PNH erythrocyte under the conditions of lowered ionic strength obtained when the cell-plasma suspension is diluted in an aqueous sucrose solution as described by Jenkins and coworkers. The reason for using sucrose is to maintain osmotic balance, since the erythrocyte membrane is impermeable to it. Another simple screening test is the observation that gross hemolysis is present in the serum surrounding the retracted clot of freshly drawn PNH blood after 2 hours' incubation at 37° C; autologous complement lyses the erythrocytes in vitro. The acid hemolysin (Ham) test utilizes still another property of complement activation, namely, its optimum at an acid pH of about 6.4. PNH erythrocytes suspended in fresh compatible complement-containing serum properly acidified will show lysis, absent when the serum is heated to 56°C. to inactivate complement. The hemolysis may be enhanced by the addition of crude bovine thrombin preparations (Crosby test), possibly because their heterophile antibody content promotes complement fixation.

The pathophysiologic basis of the disorder remains the subject of much speculation. There are two erythrocyte populations, one sensitive and the other insensitive (Fig. 22–80). The sensitive population, perhaps the offspring of stem cells with a somatic mutation or a self-perpetuating drug-induced change, undergoes hemolysis. The insensitive population has a more normal cell life span. Immune cytolysis requires a certain critical density of antibody molecules on the membrane surface to achieve fixation of the first component of complement (C1), followed by complete activation through C9, the last of the sequence, which then erodes huge holes in the membrane sufficiently large to allow hemoglobin to leak out. However, as noted, such antibodies are not thought to be present. Götze and Müller-Eberhard have reported that properdin or similar serum proteins are able to fix C3 directly onto the PNH cell, without the usual prior attachment of C1, C4, and C2. The subsequent progression through to the final C9 step and hemolysis is the same in antibody-coated and PNH erythrocytes. Mengel and coworkers have shown that PNH cells are extraordinarily sensitive to peroxide hemolysis. A variety of chemically treated erythrocytes resemble PNH cells, the closest facsimile being normal erythrocytes treated with sulfhydryl reagents, suggesting that an acquired defect of the membrane protein thiols may be responsible for the development of PNH.

Intrinsic enzyme deficiency of the erythrocytes may cause either overt hemolysis or hemolytic susceptibility under adverse environmental circumstances. Dacie recognized that a group of hereditary hemolytic disorders could be set apart from hereditary spherocytosis, which they otherwise resembled clinically. Their distinguishing features were the presence of few, if any, spherocytes in the peripheral blood and either a less favorable or no response to splenectomy. He also soon recognized that the "hereditary nonspherocytic hemolytic anemias" did not form a homogeneous group, and he classified them as Type I or Type II according to the results of the autohemolysis test. Type I showed a modestly positive test with correction by the addition of glucose. Type II showed marked autohemolysis without correction by the addition of glucose. The subsequent development of methods for the assay of red cell enzymes has led to the discovery of a large number of deficiencies which appear to explain the etiology of many of the hereditary nonspherocytic hemolytic anemias. Hemolysis has been attributed to deficiency of hexokinase, glucose phosphate isomerase, triose phosphate isomerase, diphosphoglyceromutase, phosphoglycerate kinase, glutathione reductase, pyruvate kinase, and glucose-6-phosphate dehydrogenase, among others. Only the two most common—pyruvate kinases and glucose-6-phosphate deficiency—will be discussed here.

Pyruvate kinase deficiency, itself a rare disorder, ranks second only to G-6-PD deficiency in frequency among the red cell enzymopathies. The clinical severity is extremely variable, even within a given family. Inherited as an autosomal recessive, the disorder produces hemolysis only in the homozygous state. The heterozygote is hematologically normal, but demonstrates about half the normal enzyme activity. Most patients have splenomegaly. Splenectomy may produce some improvement if the anemia is severe, but the benefit is not nearly as predictable nor as great as it is in hereditary spherocytosis. The postsplenectomy changes in the peripheral blood also contrast with those in HS. In the latter the reticulocyte count promptly declines to near-normal levels within a week as the hemolysis is halted, while patients with PK deficiency often demonstrate a paradoxical rise in reticulocyte count along with the rise in hemoglobin concentration after splenectomy. This clinical observation has suggested that, as in paroxysmal nocturnal hemoglobinuria, the young erythrocyte population is particularly susceptible to hemolysis. In PK deficiency, the destruction of reticulocytes is in the spleen, whereas in PNH it is primarily intravascular.

Pyruvate kinase stands astride an important ATP generating step, the conversion of phosphoenol pyruvate to pyruvate. Deficiency thus leads to impairment of the erythrocyte's ability to provide an adequate supply of energy in the form of ATP necessary to power the membrane cation

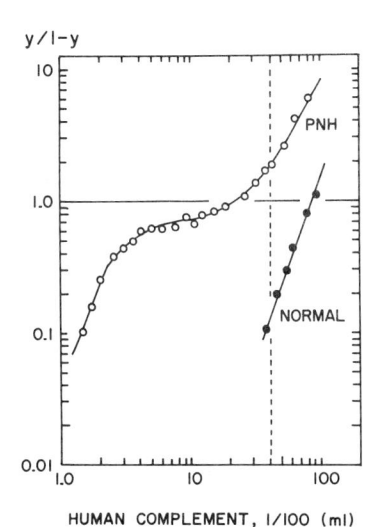

Figure 22–80 Complement sensitivity of normal and PNH erythrocytes. Two cell populations are evident in PNH. Complement concentration is shown on the horizontal axis and the proportion of lysed to unlysed erythrocytes on the vertical. (Redrawn from Rosse, W. F., et al.: J. Exper. Med., *123*:969, 1966.)

pump as well as other glycolytic reactions. PK-deficient erythrocytes exhibit a positive autohemolysis test of the Type II variety; adding glucose does not correct the positive test because of failure to utilize glucose. The reason for the inordinate susceptibility of reticulocytes to PK deficiency is not entirely clear, but their high energy requirement presumably narrows their margin for survival in the circulation of the spleen. Reticulocytes derive their energy primarily through the high ATP generating capacity of the oxidative Krebs cycle, which is lost as the reticulocyte matures. The conditions in the spleen—low glucose concentration, low pH, hemoconcentration, plus the delay of the passage of reticulocytes owing to their excessive stickiness in comparison with mature erythrocytes—all lead to a lower safety factor, especially when the mitochondria are in the process of being lost. Although, as with many enzymes, PK concentrations are higher in young than in old red cells, the activity is not high enough to prevent the cell damage which then subsequently leads to cell destruction in both the liver and spleen.

PK deficiency can be caused by a variety of different molecular defects, as is the rule in hereditary disorders. Some represent qualitative structural defects of the enzyme which lead to low activity; others presumably are a quantitative lack of a structurally normal enzyme. In either circumstance the result is a lack in enzyme function.

Glucose-6-phosphate dehydrogenase (G-6-PD) deficiency is by far the most common red cell enzyme abnormality (see Motulsky reference). A sex-linked condition, it affects 11 per cent of American Negro males. In Mediterranean regions it affects about 1 in 1000, but in certain isolated populations it has higher frequencies, affecting up to 50 per cent of male Kurdish Jews, for example. Over 100 genetic variants have already been discovered. From the clinical point of view, three major categories are recognized:

(1) Chronic hereditary nonspherocytic hemolytic anemia is a rare condition that occurs sporadically among various ethnic groups, including Northern European, and represents a variety of differing molecular genetic defects of the enzyme.

(2) The "Mediterranean" variety is one in which the loss of enzyme activity is profound (about 1 per cent of normal) but does not produce clinically significant hemolysis until the erythrocyte is exposed to an extrinsic stress, usually of an oxidative nature, to which the erythrocyte, unable to regenerate reduced glutathione, cannot respond in self defense. The extrinsic stresses include certain drugs as well as such acquired illness as hepatitis and other infections, acidosis, and uremia. Certain deficient individuals in this group are sensitive to fava beans, a sensitivity which may be so severe that it can lead to fatal hemolysis. Genetic factors apparently set these fava bean-susceptible patients apart from the others (see Stamatoyannopoulos et al. reference).

(3) The "Negro" variety resembles the Mediterranean variety but is less severe, deficient males having about 10 to 15 percent of the normal G-6-PD activity. The affected individual also is hematologically normal until exposed to one of the extrinsic stresses mentioned previously (with the exception of fava beans).

Inheritance is sex-linked, and significant hemolytic episodes are thus observed among affected males and the relatively rare homozygous females. The identification of heterozygous females is not always possible because of the wide range of enzyme levels found in this group, many falling within the normal range. Beutler and coworkers showed that random inactivation of the X chromosome in the female leads to a dual red cell population, some erythrocytes carrying the normal X chromosome and others in the affected heterozygote carrying the G-6-PD-deficient one. Thus, the mean enzyme level in the female will depend upon the relative proportions of normal and deficient erythrocytes. Tests which utilize intact erythrocytes rather than cell lysates may thus be more successful in detecting female heterozygotes.

The two most common types—the "Mediterranean" and the "Negro"—form relatively homogeneous genetic groupings. In the normal Negro population there are two electrophoretic types of G-6-PD which differ in only one amino acid site on the molecule. The faster migrating type is designated A and the slower B. Thus, Negro males possess either A or B (approximately 18 per cent carry A), while the female may be homozygous AA or BB or heterozygous AB. The Negro type of G-6-PD deficiency is a subgroup occurring only among those individuals with the A type of the enzyme. For this reason it has been designated the A⁻ type. Caucasoids, including the Mediterraneans, have only the B type of G-6-PD, and the Mediterranean type of G-6-PD deficiency is called B⁻ (Fig. 22–81).

The clinical severity of the drug-induced hemolysis varies from a clinically inapparent episode to a life-threatening event in an individual who may experience flank and abdominal pains, faintness from shock, and dark-colored urine from massive intravascular hemolysis. The severity depends not only on the genetic type of G-6-PD deficiency but also on the dosage and type of drug. The antimalarials such as primaquine, pamaquine, and quinine are the best known offenders, but sulfonamides, nitrofurans, analgesics, sulfones, and vitamin K derivatives are also significantly frequent. The hemolysis begins within 1 to 3 days of drug exposure, preferentially affecting the more aged erythrocytes because their level of enzyme is lower than that in the young

BA   A−   BA−   B−   B   A

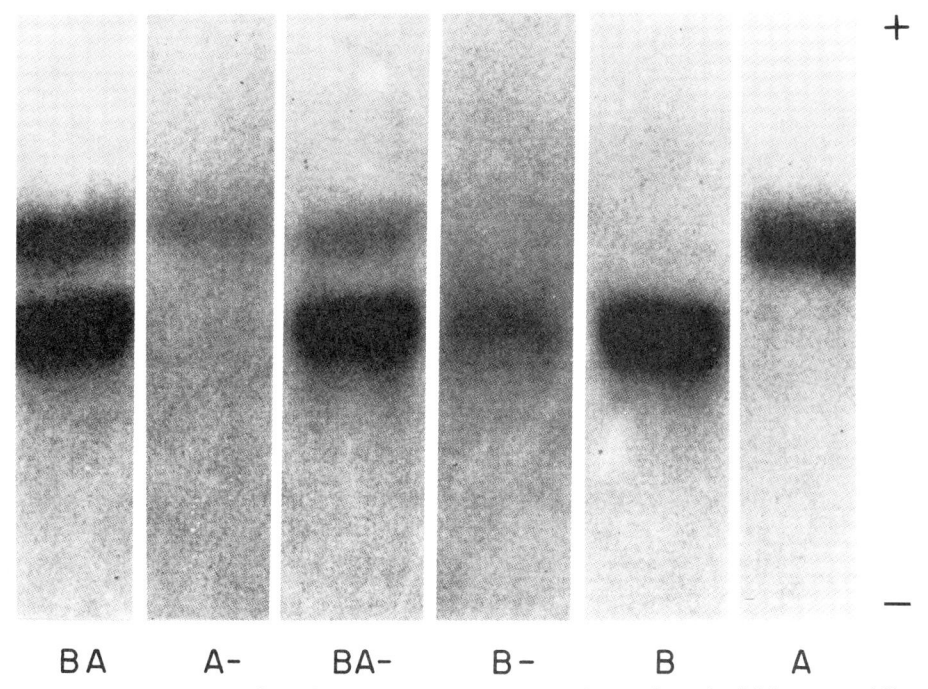

Figure 22–81 Genetic types of G-6-PD deficiency separated by electrophoresis. BA is a normal Negro female heterozygote and BA− is a deficient Negro female heterozygote. The other patterns demonstrate normal and deficient male phenotypes. (From Giblett, E. R.: Genetic Markers in Human Blood. Oxford, Blackwell Scientific Publications Ltd., 1969.)

cells. The initial change is a rapid drop in hemoglobin concentration in the peripheral blood. A reticulocyte elevation is observed 4 to 5 days later. After 7 to 10 days the patient enters into a phase of "drug resistance" during which the anemia becomes less pronounced and the patient appears to develop a tolerance to the drug (Fig. 22–82). The explanation for this apparent tolerance is that the younger erythrocytes have a higher enzyme level than the older ones and thus are somewhat better able to cope with the oxidative stress.

Current thinking attributes the pathogenesis of the drug toxicity to its ability to generate intracellular hydrogen peroxide, which deals an oxidative blow to thiol groups on the membrane and on the hemoglobin molecule. The oxidized thiols form mixed disulfides, causing hemoglobin aggregation with denaturation and then precipitation. The precipitates, so-called "Heinz bodies," can be demonstrated by special vital stains and are usually attached to the inner surface of the red cell membrane (Fig. 22–83). In the normal erythrocyte the pentose phosphate pathway is able to cope with the oxidative challenge by increasing NADP reduction to NADPH, which in turn reduces oxidized glutathione (via glutathione reductase). It is the reduced glutathione which bears the direct brunt of battle by detoxifying hydrogen peroxide (via glutathione peroxidase). In the G-6-PD–deficient erythrocyte the initial step of the pentose phosphate pathway is blocked, rendering it impotent to respond to the oxidative attack.

Direct enzyme assay is commonly used to establish the diagnosis of the G-6-PD–deficient state, but the result is affected by the average age of the red cell population. Thus, immediately following a hemolytic episode the levels may be nearly normal unless a correction is made for the mean cell age by the simultaneous measurement of another nonaffected enzyme such as hexokinase which also has a higher concentration in young than in old red cells. A number of simple screening tests have been devised, two of the more common in clinical use being the methemoglobin reduction test and the fluorescent spot test. The methemoglobin reduction test takes advantage of the fact that methylene blue establishes a redox bridge between the pentose phosphate pathway and methemoglobin reduction with NADPH as hydrogen donor. Intracellular hemoglobin is first converted to methemoglobin by incubation with sodium nitrite. After addition of methylene blue, normal erythrocytes rapidly reduce the methemoglobin and change color from brown to red. G-6-PD–deficient erythrocytes, unable to increase glycolysis through the pentose

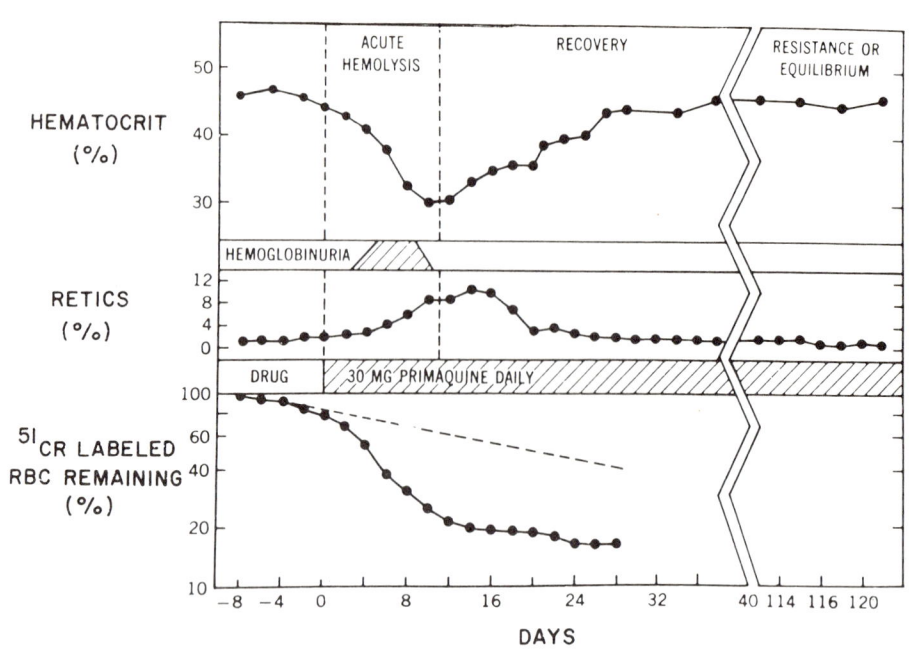

Figure 22-82 Drug-induced hemolysis in a male with G-6-PD deficiency. (Redrawn from Alving, A. S., et al.: Bull. WHO, 22:621, 1960.)

phosphate pathway, remain the chocolate-brown color of methemoglobin. The fluorescent spot test is based on the reduction by lysate of NADP to NADPH, which fluoresces under ultraviolet light. G-6-PD–deficient erythrocytes, unable to accomplish this reduction, fail to produce fluorescence in the spot.

Intrinsic hemolysis may result from the presence of *abnormal hemoglobin*. Some abnormal hemoglobins are so unstable to oxidative stresses that they undergo spontaneous precipitation into insoluble deposits in the red cell, even in the presence of a normal enzymatic machinery. Some are drug sensitive, and in this respect resemble G-6-PD deficiency. The selective destruction of newly formed erythroid cells in homozygous β-thalassemia is reminiscent of a similar preferential susceptibility of young cells in paroxysmal nocturnal hemoglobinuria and in pyruvate kinase deficiency, but the pathogenetic mechanism is quite distinctive for each of these disorders. Sickle cell anemia, the most common of the hemoglobin diseases, results not from oxidative instability but from a physicochemical alteration of the hemoglobin which produces rigid erythrocytes. The final common pathway in the intrinsic hemoglobin disorders is membrane damage and reduction in cell pliability to the point of entrapment and destruction.

Extrinsic Hemolytic Disorders. Hemolytic conditions are caused by a wide variety of extrinsic physical and chemical factors. Extensive burns cause thermal damage to the erythrocyte membrane, with fragmentation, spherocytosis, and acute hemolysis. Acute poisoning (with arsenate or copper, for example) or drowning (with hypotonic hemolysis) are other examples of acute hemolytic syndromes in patients suffering severe medical emergencies. Infections may produce hemolysis indirectly, as in hypersplenism secondary to miliary tuberculosis or subacute bacterial endocarditis, or by a direct attack upon the erythrocyte, as in the case of malaria or bartonellosis, in which the organism invades the erythrocyte, or by *Clostridium welchii* septicemia, in which the organism secretes a phospholipase which attacks the phospholipid backbone of the red cell membrane. The high oxygen tensions used in hyperbaric therapy or in early model space capsules demonstrated that high oxygen tensions cause hemolysis, presumably by peroxidation of membrane lipids. Chemical hemolysis by phenylhydrazine was once used therapeutically to reduce the red cell mass in patients with polycythemia. This agent, still commonly used to produce hemolytic anemia experimentally in animals, has an oxidative effect and causes a "Heinz body anemia" in normal erythrocytes quite similar to that observed in G-6-PD–deficient individuals given drugs to which they are sensitive. The types of extrinsic hemolysis of greatest current interest from the pathogenetic point of view are those caused by mechanical damage and those which are the result of serum factors which may be of either a nonimmune or an immune nature.

Mechanical hemolysis is vividly illustrated by *march hemoglobinuria,* so called because it was observed in soldiers after the exertion of a long march (see Davidson reference). The hemolysis is intravascular but benign and self-limited. The mechanical damage to the red cells occurs during the physical impact of the soles of the feet on hard surfaces. Ingeniously simple experiments have shown that it can be prevented among track athletes by placing shock absorbing material in the footwear or by running on soft grass instead of hard asphalt or concrete. The syndrome has even been seen in karate fighters, the damage in this instance coming from the palms of the hands rather than the soles of the feet.

A more significant form of mechanical hemolysis occurs because of damage to erythrocytes from physical impacts within the confines of the circulation of the heart or of the small arterioles. Modern cardiovascular surgery has contributed an important iatrogenic variety of *"traumatic" hemolysis* due to red cell damage in high pressure streams in the heart after insertion of prosthetic devices (see Marsh and Lewis reference). The hemolysis may be mild or severe and usually indicates an abnormal turbulence of blood and/or an exposed plastic surface not yet covered with endothelium. Examples of underlying causes are a loosened stitch at the base of a valve prosthesis through which a high-pressure jet of blood squirts; a bare Teflon patch in ostium primum repair upon which a regurgitant jet of blood strikes; and "ball variance," a late cause of postoperative hemolysis due to a slow swelling and distortion of the plastic ball, causing inadequate valve closure. Technical improvements such as the use of a metal ball have reduced the frequency of postoperative traumatic hemolysis. Reduction of the red cell life span may indeed precede surgery, usually because of red cell trauma against high pressure in a stenotic aortic valve, but the hemolysis is mild. Cardiac hemolysis is intravascular. When it is severe the loss of iron in the urine from the chronic hemoglobinuria and hemosiderinuria leads to iron deficiency and compromises the ability of the bone marrow to compensate for the reduced red cell life span.

Traumatic cardiac hemolysis has been aptly

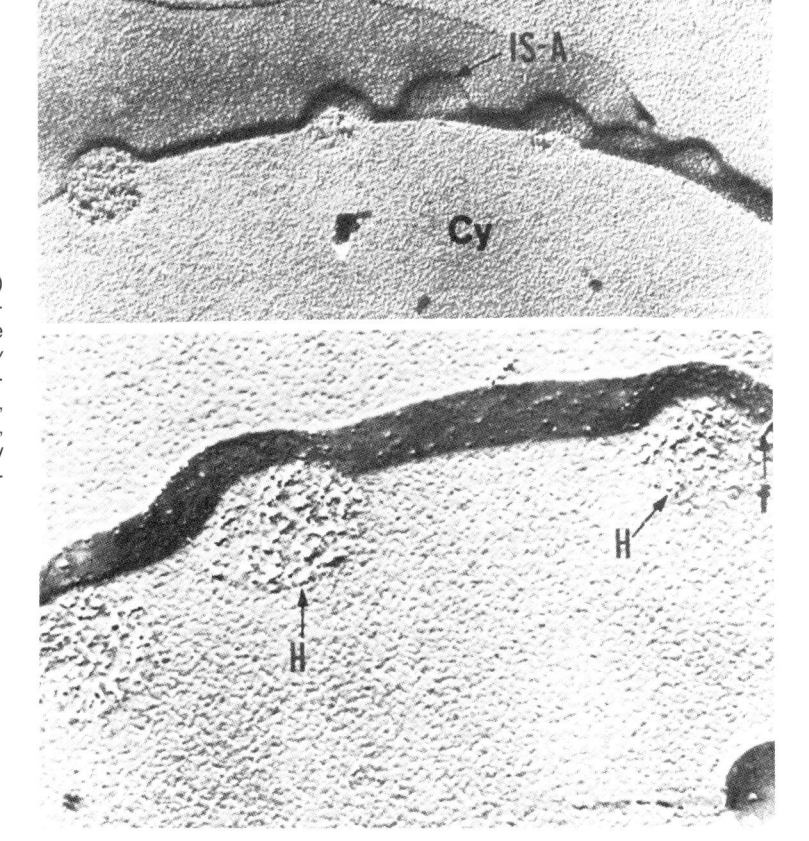

Figure 22–83 Heinz bodies (*H*) attached to the erythrocyte membrane demonstrated by freeze etching electron microscopy. *Cy* = cytoplasm; *IS-A* = intramembrane surface A. (From Lessin, L. S., et al.: Arch. Intern. Med., *129*:306, 1972. Copyright 1972 by the American Medical Association.)

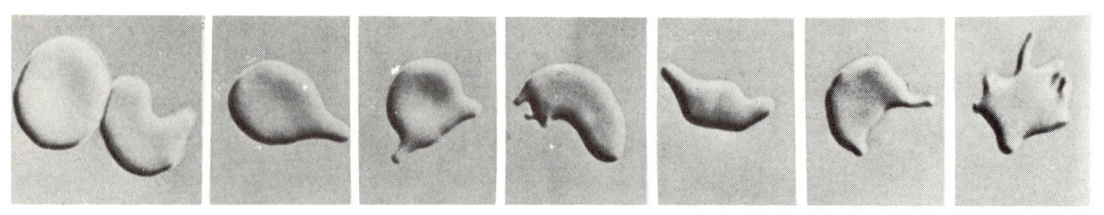

Figure 22-84 Irregular distortion of erythrocytes demonstrated by interference microscopy. (Reproduced from the Sandoz-Monograph, The Life Cycle of the Erythrocyte. Basel, Switzerland, M. Bessis, 1966.)

called the "Waring blender syndrome" because the morphologic alterations of the red cells suggest that they have been chopped by the whirling blades of this kitchen apparatus. They are sheared into bits and pieces, and display pointed and triangular forms, "helmet" shapes, and other distorted contours (Fig. 22-84). Microspherocytes and polychromasia are also present. These morphologic changes are also a characteristic feature of another group of disorders which have in common an occlusive process of the microvasculature and hence have been called by Brain the *"microangiopathic hemolytic anemias."* The fragmentation has been reproduced experimentally in vitro by forcing red cells through a fibrin meshwork and in vivo by inducing intravascular coagulation in animals by injections of endotoxin or thrombin (Fig. 22-85). These experiments presumably are the counterparts of clinical circumstances in which small vessels are occluded by fibrin deposits, such as in the various disseminated intravascular coagulation syndromes, hemolytic uremic syndromes, and thrombotic thrombocytopenic purpura. Fragmentation hemolysis has also been encountered in patients with malignant hypertension and in cases of disseminated carcinoma with vascular occlusive disease from metastasis or fibrin deposition.

Anemia in cirrhosis is the result of a combination of factors—blood loss, iron and/or folate lack, and hypersplenism. Even in the absence of these complicating factors, the erythrocyte life span is slightly to moderately reduced. Macrocytosis is a common feature of hepatocellular disease, often in association with target cells. The increased erythrocyte volume comes from accumulation of excessive lipid in erythrocyte membrane, free cholesterol to a greater degree than phospholipid. The passive exchange between plasma and red cell membrane favors uptake into the latter because the impairment of cholesterol esterification in liver disease leads to a relative increase in plasma free cholesterol at the expense of cholesterol esters. Indeed, inherited deficiency of the cholesterol esterifying enzyme which is also reduced in liver disease, lecithyl cholesterol acyl transferase (LCAT), causes macrocytosis with target cells. This enzyme mediates the transfer of a fatty acid from lecithin to cholesterol, so its lack promotes increases not only in free cholesterol but also in the phospholipid lecithin, which also accumulates to some degree in the erythrocyte membrane. The increased levels of plasma free cholesterol secondary to obstruction of the biliary tract affect erythrocytes in a similar way. Marked hemolysis is not a feature of any of these forms of

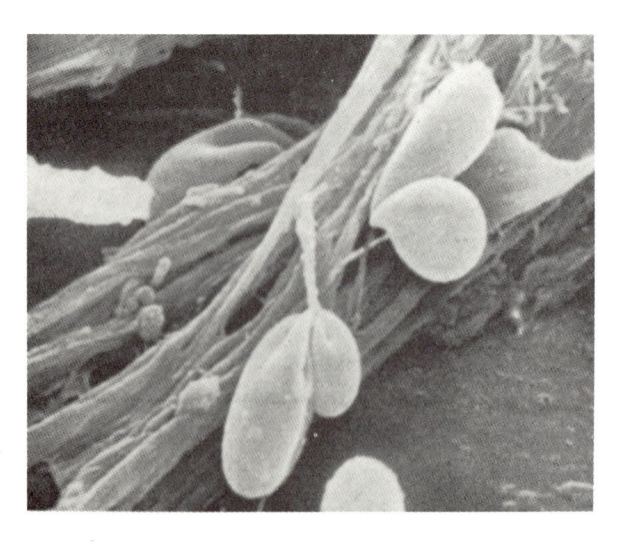

Figure 22-85 Erythrocyte fragmentation on fibrin strands. (From Bull, B. S., and Kuhn, I. N.: Blood, 35:104–111, 1970, by permission of Grune and Stratton, Inc., New York.)

target cell anemia. The *"spur cell" anemia of cirrhosis* is a more severe form of hemolysis. Its name is derived from the pointed thorny projections which protrude from the red cells (Fig. 22-86). This hemolytic disorder is seen in association with severe fulminating hepatocellular disease and is apparently a more extreme form of membrane accumulation of free cholesterol in excess of phospholipid. Abnormal plasma lipoproteins and possibly retained bile acids may also be important in the pathogenesis of spur cell anemia of cirrhosis, but the details of their adverse effects on the erythrocyte membrane are unknown. The spur cells are susceptible to entrapment in the enlarged spleen which commonly is present in cirrhosis. Normal compatible erythrocytes transfused into affected patients soon acquire the membrane defect. Serum from patients with these disorders when added in vitro to normal compatible erythrocytes will produce macrocytosis and targeting or spur cell formation, as the case may be.

Hereditary acanthocytosis is characterized by absence of plasma beta-lipoproteins together with hypolipidemia and abnormal erythrocytes which closely resemble spur cells but which are called "acanthocytes." The degree of hemolysis is mild, however. Acanthocytosis is occasionally seen in individuals after splenectomy who are otherwise hematologically normal. The pathogenesis of the erythrocyte shape change in these disorders remains unexplained. A similar shape change is sometimes seen in association with uremia, but the responsible plasma factors have not yet been identified.

Among the most potent of plasma hemolytic factors are the isoantibodies directed against red cell antigens of the ABO system. These antierythrocyte antibodies are predominantly high molecular weight IgM immunoglobulins and are active in complement fixation and erythrocyte lysis. They readily induce red cell agglutination in vitro at room temperature, even when the cells are in saline suspension. After the transfusion of red cells incompatible in the ABO system, the hemolysis is abrupt, complete, and largely intravascular, with hemoglobinemia and hemoglobinuria. Isoantibodies to blood group substances other than the ABO antigens may be present if the individual has been immunized to the foreign antigen either by previous transfusion or during the course of pregnancy. Immunization due to exposure of the individual to red cells differing, for example, in the Rh complex of red cell surface antigens leads to the formation of antierythrocyte antibodies which are IgG immunoglobulins and do not cause spontaneous agglutination at room temperature. Their activity is maximal at 37° C. The presence of the antibody on the red cell surface is demonstrated by the Coombs' test, in which clumping of the antibody-coated erythrocytes is produced by suspending them in an antiserum containing antibodies to human immunoglobulins (see Rosse reference). Antierythrocyte antibodies of this type are called "warm" antibodies. They have also been called "incomplete" because of the necessity to apply special techniques to demonstrate their presence, in contrast to the saline-active IgM antibodies which are considered "complete." These 7S IgG warm antibodies generally do not fix complement nor do they cause gross agglutination within the circulation. Their presence on the red cell surface can be detected by the macrophages, especially in the splenic bed, and extravascular hemolysis, often predominantly in the spleen, is the result.

When an antibody in the plasma is directed against the individual's own erythrocytes, autoimmune hemolysis may occur (see Dacie and Worlledge). The autoimmune hemolytic anemias are classified according to the nature of the antibody present. The cold hemolytic syndromes are caused by an IgM antibody, often with specificity against the I red cell surface antigen (and occasionally against the i antigen). These antibodies are more active at room temperature than at 37° C. and have maximal activity at 4° C. They are active complement fixers. The warm antibody autoimmune hemolytic anemias are produced by a 7S IgG antibody, usually nonspecific, which has maximal activity at 37° C. and is demonstrated by the Coombs' test. One very rare syndrome,

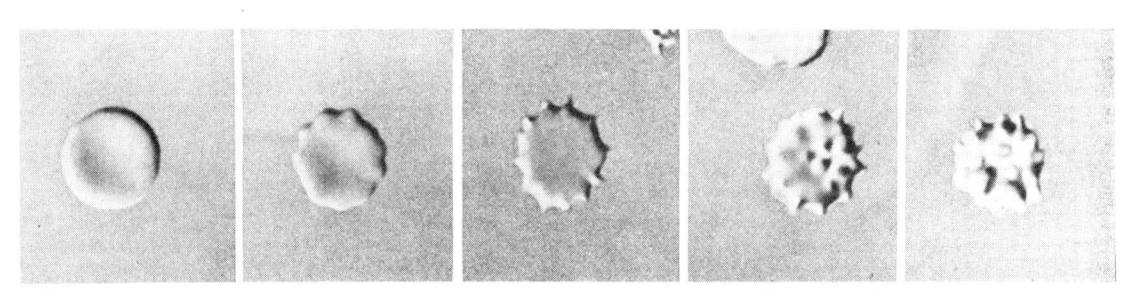

Figure 22-86 Regular distortion of erythrocytes to form acanthocytes. (Reproduced from the Sandoz-Monograph, The Life Cycle of the Erythrocyte. Basel, Switzerland, M. Bessis, 1966.)

paroxysmal cold hemoglobinuria, is associated with a 7S IgG antibody which, contrary to the pattern in most cases, is cold reactive and fixes complement.

The acute form of *cold agglutinin hemolytic anemia* is observed during the recovery phase from certain infections such as mycoplasma pneumonia and infectious mononucleosis. It is usually self-limited; occasionally the course is fulminant and fatal. The chronic variety either is idiopathic or occurs as a "secondary" or "symptomatic" hemolytic process in a patient with some other disorder of the immune system, as discussed later. Areas of the body subject to reduced temperature are those most susceptible, and Raynaud-like phenomena may occur, along with gangrenous lesions of such exposed parts as the nose, ears, or extremities. The degree of hemolysis is often mild in chronic cases. The coated erythrocytes undergo agglutination and in addition complement-induced cell lysis is frequently present. Thus, erythrocyte destruction occurs primarily in the liver or in the circulation rather than in the spleen, and splenectomy is usually not an effective therapeutic choice. The cold agglutinin titer of the patient's serum is often very high (1:10,000 or higher, in contrast to titers up to 1:64 in normal individuals). The cold agglutinin test measures the ability of the patient's serum to agglutinate normal compatible erythrocytes at 4° C., but those sera with the very high titers have a wide "thermal amplitude" and are active at room temperature and even at physiologic temperatures. Thus, a drop of blood from a patient with cold agglutinin hemolytic disease usually will show spontaneous agglutination when placed on a glass microscope slide at room temperature. Such "autoagglutination" is usually significant if it persists after 1:4 dilution of the blood with saline. The autoaglutination phenomenon is usually also evident on inspection of the peripheral blood film. A positive Coombs' test of the "non-gamma" type is often obtained owing to the presence of a complement coating on the erythrocyte surface that remains after the IgM antibody (which initially fixed it to the surface) spontaneously comes off with the warming of the test system to 37° C. In such instances the positive Coombs' test is brought out by "non-gamma" anticomplement antibodies present in the anti human globulin serum.

Paroxysmal cold hemoglobinuria is very rare. The acute hemolytic episodes are provoked by exposure to cold. A significant fraction of cases occur as a complication of syphilis, but most are idiopathic. The signs are those of intravascular hemolysis. The diagnosis is made by finding a positive Donath-Landsteiner test. The 7S IgG antibody attaches to normal compatible erythrocytes at lowered temperatures (4° C). The antibody fixes complement, which does not cause cell lysis at such low temperatures. Then, as the complement-sensitized cells are slowly warmed, complement becomes activated and hemolysis is observed.

The *warm antibody autoimmune hemolytic anemias* are the most common and affect all age groups. The onset of clinical symptoms may be very acute, with fever, weakness, and flank and abdominal pains, or at the other extreme the disorder may be incidentally detected by the discovery of a positive Coombs' test. The peripheral blood film frequently shows large numbers of microspherocytes mixed in with polychromatophilic macrocytes, a picture resembling that seen in hereditary spherocytosis. The autohemolysis test is variable, but when it is positive, the addition of glucose results in no improvement. The osmotic fragility curve may reflect a fragile tail of the osmotically susceptible microspherocyte population. The warm antibody-coated erythrocytes are usually sequestered in a moderately enlarged spleen. Splenectomy is often successful if medical therapy with adrenal corticoids fails to control the hemolysis. The severity of the anemia is related to the density of IgG antibody molecules attached to the erythrocyte membrane surface (Fig. 22–87). Below a certain critical density, the Coombs' test becomes negative, but the life span of the coated erythrocytes still is reduced, indicating that the macrophage in vivo is a more sensitive detector of the antibody coat than the in-vitro Coombs' test. Complement fixation is also related to antibody density on the membrane surface. Two IgG antibodies must have reacted with antigen on the membrane surface and also be placed at a critical distance from each other in order to react with the first component of complement. This critical distance is usually not achieved in the warm antibody hemolytic anemias because the density of antibody molecules on the surface is not great enough. The cold antibody hemolytic anemias are more effective complement fixers because each individual IgM antibody molecule is a polymer consisting of a dense cluster of combining sites which achieve the critical distance required for complement fixation. Since complete engulfment of an antibody-coated cell by phagocytes requires complement, the mechanism of hemolysis in warm antibody hemolytic anemias is different. The antibody coating causes adherence of the erythrocyte to receptors on the surface of the macrophage. During the cell-to-cell contact the macrophage removes small fragments from the erythrocyte membrane (Fig. 22–88). The reduction of erythrocyte membrane lipid and surface area produces a rigid microspherocyte which is then subject to splenic entrapment.

Autoimmune hemolytic disease of the newborn is caused by 7S IgG antibodies which cross the placenta from the maternal circulation. Fortu-

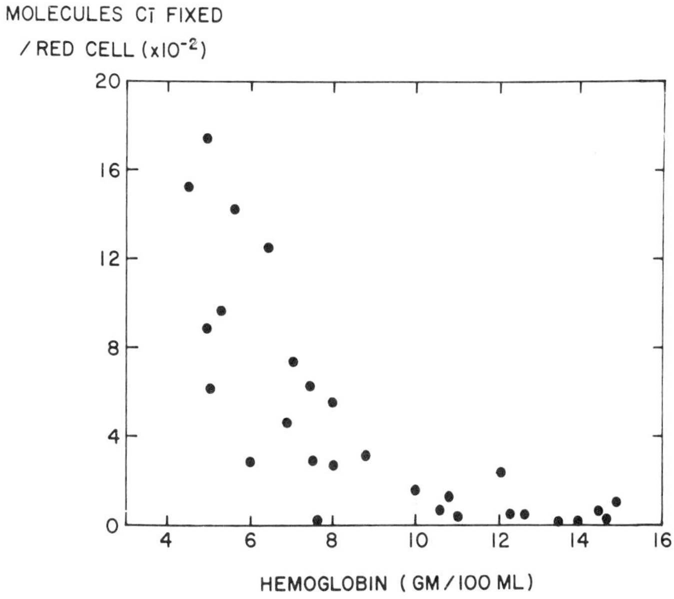

Figure 22-87 The relation between IgG density on the erythrocyte membrane and the degree of anemia in nonsplenectomized patients with warm antibody autoimmune hemolytic anemia. The measurement of membrane antibody density employs a sensitive technique of first reacting the coated erythrocytes with anti-human gamma globulin and then measuring complement fixation on the doubly coated cells. (Redrawn from Rosse, W. F.: J. Clin. Invest., 50:734, 1971.)

nately the IgM isoantibodies of the ABO system are too large to get across the placental barrier. Although 7S antibodies of the ABO system may produce neonatal hemolysis when fetomaternal ABO incompatibility is present, the hemolysis is mild and usually does not require special treatment. Severe hemolysis is usually the consequence of incompatibility within the Rh system

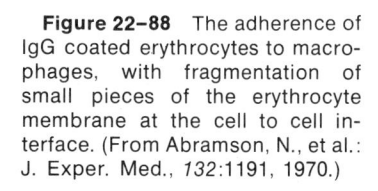

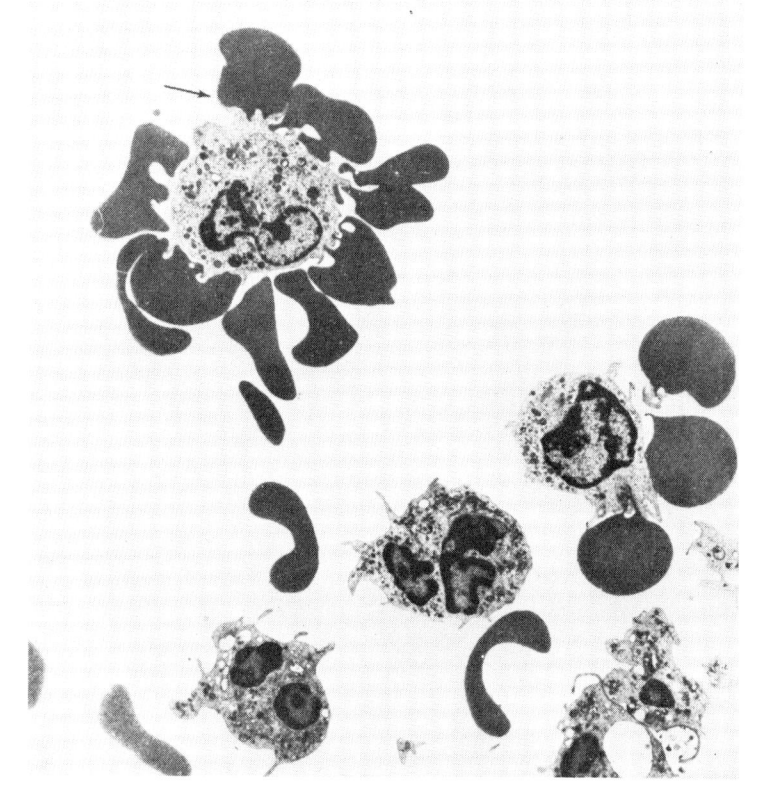

Figure 22-88 The adherence of IgG coated erythrocytes to macrophages, with fragmentation of small pieces of the erythrocyte membrane at the cell to cell interface. (From Abramson, N., et al.: J. Exper. Med., 132:1191, 1970.)

of surface antigens. Antibodies against foreign antigens in the Rh system are raised during pregnancy in response to the hemorrhage of small quantities of fetal blood into the maternal circulation. The presence of fetal erythrocytes in the maternal circulation is readily detected and quantitated by a morphologic slide technique which depends on the resistance of fetal hemoglobin containing erythrocytes to acid elution. Transfusion of blood containing Rh incompatible erythrocytes is another means of causing sensitization.

A number of natural factors operate to reduce the risk of hemolytic disease of the newborn when Rh incompatibility between mother and fetus is present. One protective factor is the necessity for fetomaternal hemorrhage to have previously occurred and to have sensitized the mother. Since fetomaternal hemorrhage usually occurs at the time of delivery, first borns are spared difficulty, only subsequent pregnancies being at risk in those mothers who have previously become sensitized. Another natural protective factor is that coexisting presence of incompatibility within the ABO system prevents maternal sensitization to foreign Rh antigens on the fetal erythrocyte. This phenomenon, called "ABO cancellation" by Clarke, suggested that rapid removal of the fetal erythrocytes along with their foreign Rh antigen from the maternal circulation prevents active immunization.

Following on this hypothesis, the therapeutic use of human gamma globulin preparations, hyperimmune with respect to anti-Rh antibodies, given to mothers at risk immediately after delivery has markedly reduced the incidence of maternal sensitization. The passively administered antibody reacts with the fetal erythrocytes, brings about their rapid removal, and prevents active immunization of the mother. This preventive form of therapy promises to markedly reduce the incidence of erythroblastosis fetalis, previously one of the most serious threats to neonatal health. The major pathophysiologic consequence of this syndrome resides in the toxic effects of the lipid-soluble unconjugated fraction of bilirubin. The immature liver of the newborn has a limited ability to conjugate the bilirubin into a nontoxic water-soluble form. When the binding capacity of the serum albumin for the unconjugated fraction is exceeded, its uptake into lipid nervous tissue causes toxic damage resulting in kernicterus. Therapeutic strategy, directed at preventing the levels of unbound unconjugated bilirubin from reaching toxic proportions, has traditionally been based on exchange transfusion, but recent efforts have explored the use of bilirubin-binding substances, such as albumin; the stimulation of bilirubin-conjugating enzymes by agents such as phenobarbital which are active on the hepatic endoplasmic reticulum; and the exposure of the infant to light, which reduces the serum bilirubin concentration by a mechanism which is still not clearly understood.

The pathogenesis of the autoimmune hemolytic anemias acquired after birth has continued to defy all but hypothetical explanations. Some are associated with infections or with the recovery phase after an infection, as though the antibodies to the infectious agent are attracted by mistake to the erythrocyte. A large proportion of the autoimmune hemolytic anemias are idiopathic and are not associated with any other disease process, but many occur in the context of other disorders of the immune system, such as the lymphoproliferative disorders (especially lymphoma and chronic lymphatic leukemia), "collagen" diseases (especially disseminated lupus erythematosus), ulcerative colitis, or agammaglobulinemia. There is no predictable chronological relationship between the two associated immunologic illnesses, and either one may precede or follow the other with a time gap as long as several years. It appears that the affected individual has a defective system of "immune surveillance" which permits more than one immune disorder to arise in the same patient. Alternately, one immune disorder may give rise to the other.

Observations of the immunohemolytic anemias seen after the administration of certain drugs have given support for the hypothesis that exogenous agents may trigger immunologic disorders (see Croft et al. reference). There are three classes of drug-induced immunohemolytic anemia, but only one of these leads to a truly autoimmune hemolysis:

(1) The "haptene" (or penicillin) type. The serum of the patient contains antipenicillin antibodies of the 7S type. Penicillin, if given in very high doses, is soaked up into the erythrocyte membrane. The antipenicillin antibodies are not directed against red cell antigens but do bind to the penicillin in the membrane, giving rise to a positive "gamma" Coombs' test and to hemolysis.

(2) The "immune complex" (or "innocent bystander") type. IgM antibody is formed to the drug (quinidine, quinine, stibophen) which is presumably associated with an unidentified serum protein as carrier. The antibody then reacts with the antigen to form an immune complex, which attaches to the red cell membrane and fixes complement. The antibody may then be detached, leaving complement behind. The "non-gamma" Coombs' test is positive because of the complement coat. The red cell is considered the innocent bystander. The mechanism is the same as that of quinidine thrombocytopenia, except that the latter is characterized by the production of a 7S IgG antibody.

(3) The true autoimmune (or alpha-methyldopa) type. In a time- and dose-dependent manner, the drug induces the formation of an anti-

body specifically directed against a normal red cell antigen, usually of the Rh complex. The autoimmune state persists for months after discontinuation of the drug, gradually subsiding without additional treatment. This drug-related form of autoimmunity suggests a possible pathogenesis of other types of autoimmune states by undefined exogenous agents.

PHAGOCYTES

STRUCTURE

A recent trend in dynamic morphology has been to separate the leukocytes into two major groups: the phagocytes and the immunocytes. This separation has taxonomic merits and will be followed in this chapter.

The phagocytes can be divided into the granulocytes and the monocyte-macrophages (Fig. 22-6). It appears plausible that these cells have a common precursor, either a stem cell committed to the phagocytic cell lines or a blast cell designated as a myeloblast or a myelomonoblast. This blast cell is smaller, and both nucleus and cytoplasm are less basophilic than those of the proerythroblast. It is distinguished from the lymphoblast in that it has two or more nucleoli and a nucleus with an indistinct nuclear membrane and no perinuclear halo. The pale blue cytoplasm is scant and frequently present only as a faint outline on one side of the nucleus. The subsequent differentiation to granulocytes is heralded by the appearance of coarse granules made up of lysosomes staining blue or violet with Wright's stain. At this promyelocytic stage, the nucleus is still blastic with nucleoli, but at the next stage, the myelocytic stage, the nuclear chromatin becomes clumped and the capacity for mitotic division ceases. New species of lysosomal granules appear, giving the mature granulocytes their characteristic morphologic appearance. The neutrophilic granules are small and pink and contain, among many hydrolytic enzymes, an alkaline phosphatase. The eosinophilic granules are large and round and contain red-staining, basic mucopolysaccharides. The basophilic granules are coarse, often concealing the nucleus and containing histamine, heparin, and acid mucopolysaccharides. The background cytoplasm of all three cell types is pink, and the nucleus becomes lobulated with 2 to 5 distinct lobes connected by thin strands.

The differentiation from myelomonoblast to mature monocytes is undoubtedly also a process of integrated proliferation and maturation, but distinct stages are difficult to recognize. The mature monocyte is a large cell with a diameter of about 20 to 30 microns and a prominent multishaped nucleus. The chromatin structure is less clumped than that of the mature granulocyte or lymphocyte and appears veil-like, with small chromatin particles tied together by fine strands. The cytoplasm is grayish-blue and contains many fine lysosomes stained pink with Wright's stain. Even on fixed smears, the cytoplasm gives an impression of being "free flowing," reflecting active ameboid motions right up to the time the cell becomes permanently fixed to the glass slide. The clear cytoplasmic vacuoles frequently observed may be artifactual and caused by the smearing technique. After the monocyte leaves the circulating blood it is transformed into a lysosome-filled macrophage. Cline has recently reviewed the sequence of this transformation which involves a sudden burst in metabolic activities. Energy production is increased, synthesis of hydrolytic enzymes by the endoplasmic reticulum and their subsequent packing by the Golgi apparatus into lysosomes are enhanced, and the cell enlarges until it has taken on the appearance of the large mobile macrophage found in pulmonary alveoli, peritoneal cavities, and inflammatory exudate. The fixed macrophage in the liver, spleen, and bone marrow appears to exist in a dynamic equilibrium with the mobile macrophage, and the characteristic foreign body giant cell or Langhans cell may represent fusion of a number of mobile macrophages.

FUNCTION

Although the functions of the granulocytes and the monocyte-macrophages overlap, it seems reasonable to suggest that granulocytes function primarily as the first line of defense against microbial organisms, whereas the monocyte-macrophages provide final removal of such organisms and also clear the body of its own aged and damaged cells. In order to accomplish this, the phagocytes have to (1) accumulate in sufficient numbers at the right place, (2) become attached to the foreign or nonviable material, (3) engulf, (4) dissolve, and (5) dispose of this material.

Granulocytes spend less than a day in the circulation before they migrate through the endothelial wall and are disposed of in various tissues. Inflammatory lesions will release specific leukotaxines which increase capillary permeability and induce local migration of the granulocytes. These leukotaxines are poorly defined but, as shown by Ward, Cochrane, and Müller-Eberhard, they may include fragments of the activated complement C3. In addition, transformed lymphocytes release a "migration inhibition factor" which acts as a chemotaxic agent by arresting macrophages at sites of antigen accumulation.

The process responsible for the attachment of granulocytes to antigens also involves activated complement. Specific C3 binding sites are present on the surface of the granulocytes, and these sites provide anchors for the C3 bound to antigen-antibody complexes. However, the mechanism responsible for the attachment of granulocytes to antigens prior to antibody formation or to devitalized cells is still obscure. After the attachment, the membrane responds by pinocytosis, or engulfing the material in toto. Inside the cytoplasm the engulfed material is enveloped by part of the interior interiolized surface membrane and distinct phagosomes are formed. Lysosomal granules become attached and empty their cargo of hydrolytic enzymes into the phagosomes, killing and/or dissolving the engulfed material (Fig. 22–89) and morphologically degranulating the phagocytes. The process of killing involves peroxidation of H_2O_2, which in the presence of iodide derived from tyrosine will destroy the microbial membrane. Subsequent dissolution involves the integrated action of numerous hydrolytic enzymes. The ingestion of foreign or devitalized material is associated with a rapid increase in energy production and the generation of H_2O_2. Since the granulocytes contain only a few mitochondria, the major energy-producing pathway is glycolysis, and phagocytosis appears to stimulate both the Embden-Meyerhof pathway and the hexose monophosphate shunt. It has been proposed that increased demands for ATP energy cause an accumulation of NADH, which in the presence of an oxidase generates H_2O_2. Excess H_2O_2 will in turn oxidize reduced glutathione and stimulate shunt activity (Fig. 22–90).

The final release of the degradation products tends to amplify the inflammatory response. Attached lysosomal enzymes may cause injury to surrounding tissues, endogenous pyrogens cause fever, thromboplastic products may cause fibrin obstruction of vessels, and cationic proteins cause vasodilatation. It has also been postulated that the important process of antigen-induced blast transformation of lymphocytes is dependent on a preliminary processing or digestion of the antigens by the macrophages. However, it is equally possible that the macrophage surface provides sites of attachment for both antigens and lymphocytes, permitting optimal interaction (Fig. 22–91).

The pathophysiologic relationship of eosinophils and basophils to so-called "allergic reactions" is still unexplained. The basophils have been shown to contain sites of attachment for IgE antibody, and their degranulation is associated with the release of histamine. However, the eosinophils, which are much more closely identified with allergy than the basophils, have not as yet been found to interact specifically with antigen-antibody complexes.

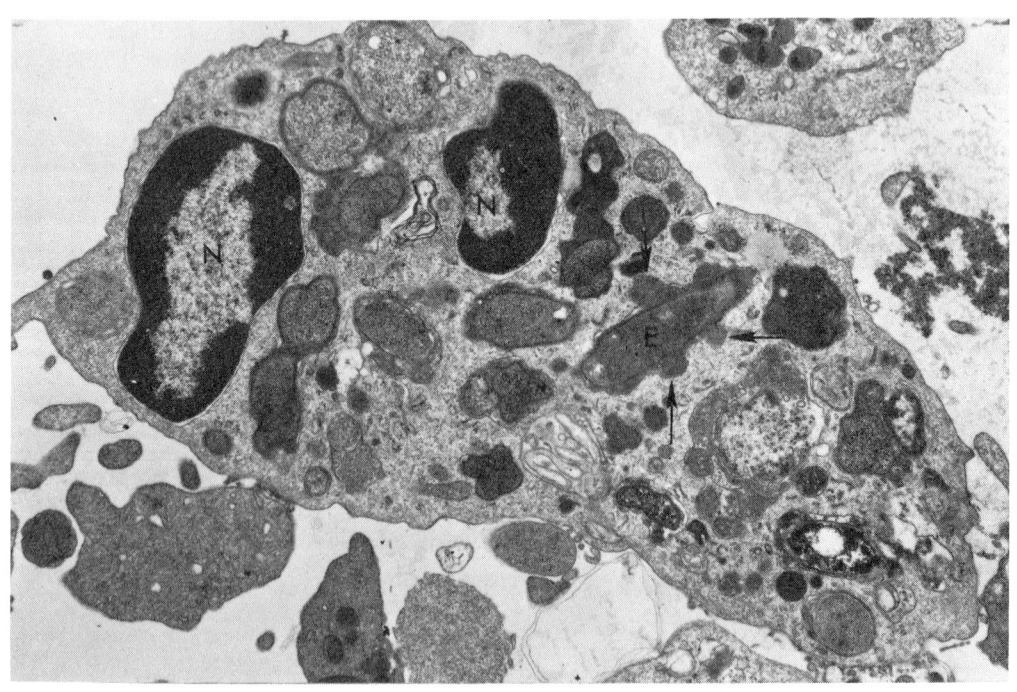

Figure 22-89 Electron microscopic picture of a human granulocyte after phagocytosis of *E. coli* (*E*). Coalescence of lysosomes with the phagocytic vacuoles is seen at arrows. *N* = nucleus. (From Zucker-Franklin, D., Elsbach, E., and Simon, P. J.: Lab. Invest., 25:415, 1971.)

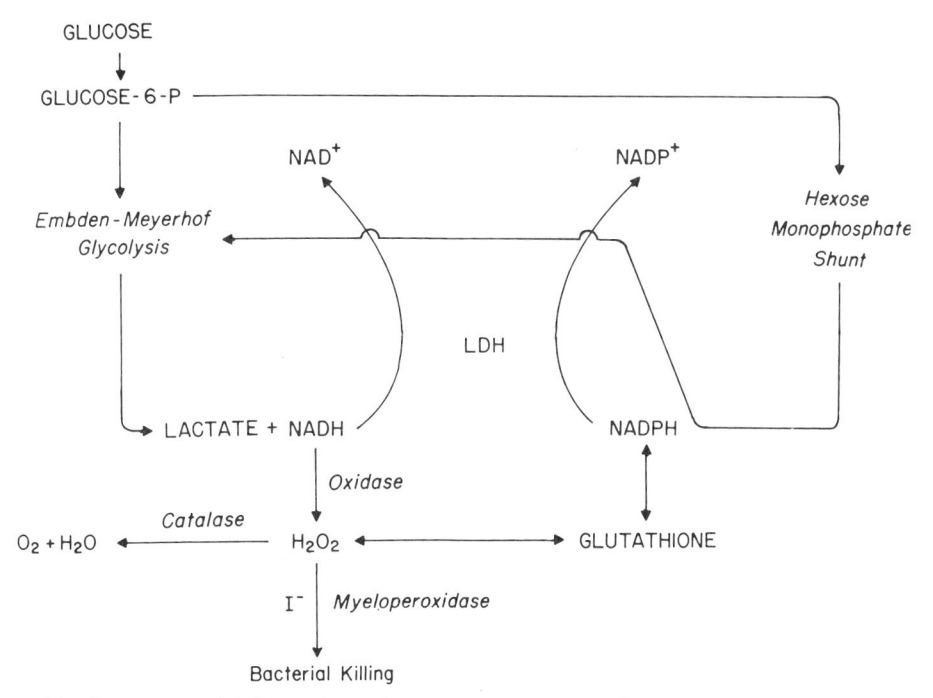

Figure 22-90 Generation of H_2O_2 by the action of an oxidase on NADH from the Embden-Meyerhof glycolytic pathway. The H_2O_2 can be used for bacterial killing and for oxidation of glutathione with activation of the hexose monophosphate shunt. (Adapted from Karnofsky, M. L., et al.: *In* Greenwalt, T. J., and Jamieson, G. A. (Eds.): Formation and Destruction of Blood Cells. Philadelphia, J. B. Lippincott Co., 1970.)

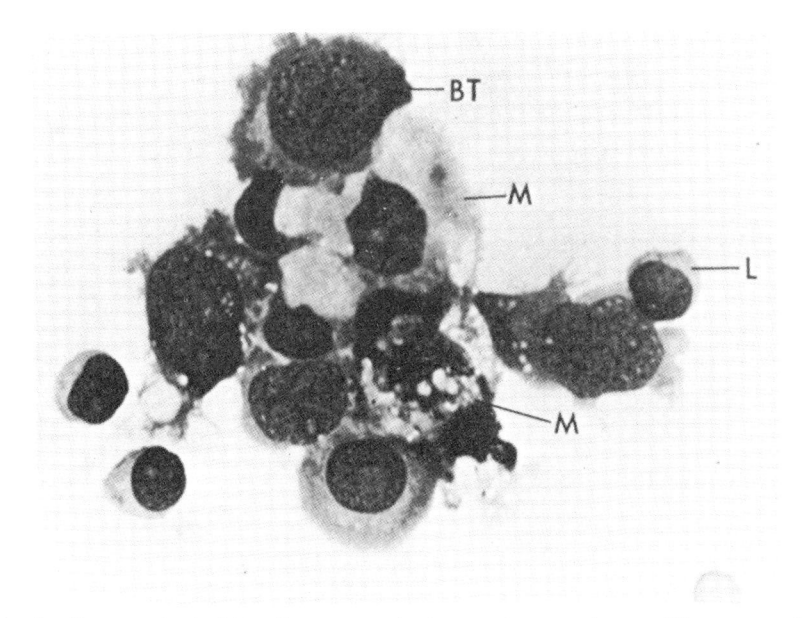

Figure 22-91 An "immunologic island" composed of central macrophages (*M*), surrounding lymphocytes undergoing blast transformation (*BT*) and untransformed lymphocytes (*L*). (From Cline, M. J.: *In* Williams et al. (Eds.): Hematology. New York, McGraw-Hill Book Co., 1972.)

KINETICS

Because of the relatively long tissue phase prior to and following the brief appearance of the granulocyte in the bloodstream, information about the rate and control of production and destruction has been difficult to obtain. Recently, however, reliable labeling techniques have been developed, both cohort labeling of DNA with ^{32}P or with tritiated thymidine and random labeling with radioactive diisopropyl fluorophosphate or with ^{51}Cr. Utilizing such techniques it has been possible to construct a model for granulocyte kinetics not too dissimilar to those models developed for erythrocytes and thrombocytes (Fig. 22-5).

In order to account for granulocyte renewal and control it is almost a necessity to accept the existence of a stem cell precursor pool. As described in the erythrocyte section, this pool is probably divided morphologically or functionally into a multipotential stem cell pool and several unipotential stem cell pools committed to specific cell lines. It is tempting to believe that a humoral factor, akin to erythropoietin, is involved in the differentiation or blast transformation of stem cells committed to the myelomonocytic cell lines. The newly formed myelomonoblasts are programed to divide about 3 to 5 times and simultaneously to mature into myelocytes and metamyelocytes. Warner and Athens have proposed that the final divisions in the myelocytic pool are not predetermined but are actively regulated, and that skipped divisions or additional divisions in this pool may amplify the responsiveness of granulocytic production to peripheral demands. After the myelocytes have become mitotically inactive, maturing cells accumulate as a marrow granulocyte reserve. This reserve is under normal conditions made up by about 5 days' worth of granulocytes. Following their final release from the bone marrow, the granulocytes spend about one day in the bloodstream, establishing two pools of about equal size—a circulating pool and a marginated pool. From the bloodstream they migrate into the tissues in which they will be destroyed either randomly in defense actions or by senescence about 5 to 6 days later (see review by Boggs).

Table 22-9 gives some approximations of the size of the various granulocytic pools. The combined size of the marrow pools is almost 2.5 times that calculated for the nucleated red blood cell pools, despite the fact that the daily production of red cells is about twice the daily production of granulocytes. This, of course, is due to the fact that the marrow contains a large reserve of maturing and mature granulocytes. It is of interest that if the bone marrow reticulocyte pool, which may have a similar reserve function, is added to the nucleated red cell pool, the relationship between erythroid precursor cells in the bone marrow and daily erythrocyte production tends to become similar to the relationship between the granulocytic precursor cells and granulocyte production.

In peripheral blood, the normal granulocyte count should always be considered a range rather than a value. The fluctuating equilibrium between circulating and marginated cells precludes a completely stable granulocyte count and the existence of extensive granulocyte reserves in the bone marrow permits the granulocyte count to adjust acutely to the demands for phagocytic cells.

The exact mechanism regulating granulocyte production is still unknown, although it undoubtedly involves a feedback between circulating granulocytes and the bone marrow. In support of the existence of a feedback mechanism is the observation that the granulocyte count in some patients with depleted bone marrow reserves exhibits an oscillatory pattern and that each period in this pattern is about 11 to 15 days, about twice the length of time it takes for myeloblasts to become mature granulocytes (Fig. 22-92). The reason for not observing such oscillations more often probably is the fact that under normal conditions the large bone marrow reserve pool will dampen or obliterate the amplitude of oscillations.

Various factors have been claimed to be responsible for maintaining the feedback adjustment between the peripheral demands for granulocytes and the bone marrow supply of granulocytes. Several granulocyte-mobilizing factors have been described, including endotoxin, etiocholanolone, Menkin's tissue leukotoxins, and a leukocytosis-mobilizing factor, but, as emphasized by Craddock and coworkers, it seems unlikely that any of these are involved in the physiologic regulation of granulocyte production. Other factors have been claimed to be released by mature circulating granulocytes and to act as inhibitors of mitotic divisions within the myelocyte pool. True leukopoietins acting on the stem cell pool have not been identified for certain, although recent studies of the in-vitro formation of granulocytic colonies on soft agar strongly indicate that col-

TABLE 22-9 MYELOID POOLS

Cell Types	Number of Cells in 10^9 per kg. Body Weight
Proliferating Cells	3.0
Marrow Granulocytic Reserve	7.5
Circulating Granulocytes	0.4
Marginated Granulocytes	0.3
Daily Production and Destruction	1.5

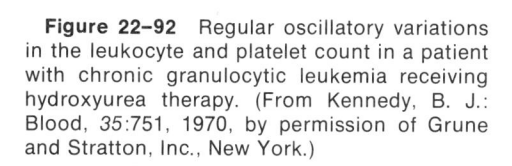

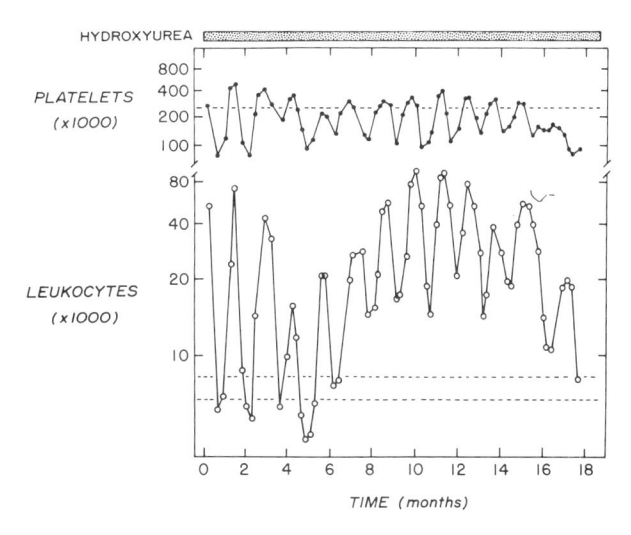

Figure 22-92 Regular oscillatory variations in the leukocyte and platelet count in a patient with chronic granulocytic leukemia receiving hydroxyurea therapy. (From Kennedy, B. J.: Blood, 35:751, 1970, by permission of Grune and Stratton, Inc., New York.)

ony stimulating factors may be present in plasma and urine. Granulocytic colonies appear to originate from single stem cells committed to the myeloid cell line, and Richard and coworkers have shown that the addition of plasma or urine from leukopenic animals or humans will stimulate their formation. These observations make it possible to construct a feedback model for the control of granulocyte production. However, the model outlined in Figure 22-93 is obviously quite hypothetical, since solid experimental data are lacking and it is still unknown how the demand for granulocytes is translated into a feedback stimulus.

The kinetics and regulation of the monocyte-macrophage complex are even less understood than those of the granulocyte complex. The monocytes appear to have a shorter intramedullary life span than the myeloid cells, since they tend to emerge earlier than the granulocytes after a temporary bone marrow suppression. The half-life of the monocyte in the circulation is not known but is probably very short. The extravascular life span after it has been transformed to a macrophage is undoubtedly long and may be counted in months if not years. One study suggests that the fixed tissue macrophages, which traditionally have been thought to originate from endothelial cells, actually originate from mobile macrophages, making it even more difficult to determine the total life span of the monocyte-macrophages.

Figure 22-93 Hypothetical model of a feedback circuit which could account for the physiologic control of the granulocyte count.

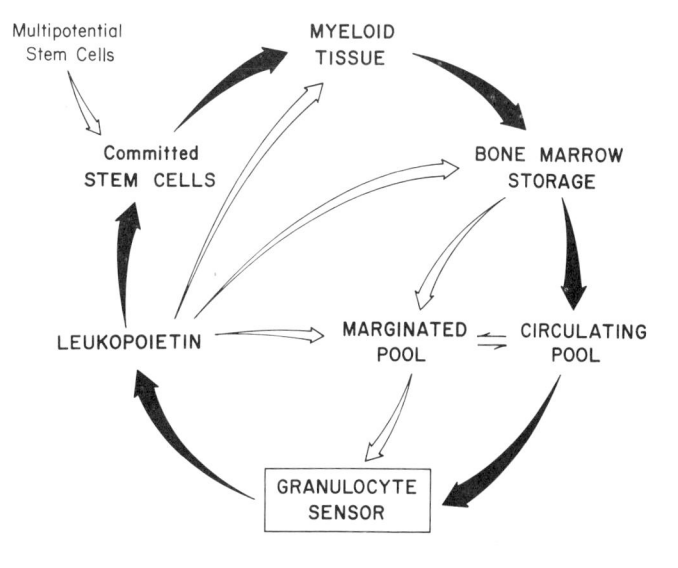

PATHOPHYSIOLOGY

Classification and General Considerations

Disorders of the granulocytes are traditionally classified according to the number of circulating granulocytes into granulocytopenias and granulocytoses. However, a classification based on function and kinetics is of more contemporary importance. Using such criteria, the following classes of disorders can be recognized: quantitative abnormalities, qualitative abnormalities, and myeloproliferative disorders (Table 22-10).

The pathophysiologic effect of quantitative disorders is determined by the size of the actual and potential granulocyte pools. In granulocytopenia the lack of defense against microorganisms and other foreign invaders dominates the clinical picture, whereas in granulocytosis the problems are more subtle. Although much larger and stickier than the red cells, the viscosity of blood with a high granulocyte count is about the same as for normal blood with the same total hematocrit (white plus red cell crit), and hyperviscosity due to granulocytosis is rare. More common is bone tenderness caused by expansion of the bone marrow and uric acid arthropathy or nephropathy caused by destruction of granulocytes. The qualitative disorders are characterized by impaired granulocyte defense despite a normal number of circulating neutrophils. Finally, the clinical manifestations of myeloproliferative disorders are related to the extent and character of cellular proliferation and cellular replacement.

Quantitative Abnormalities

Granulocytopenia. When the absolute granulocyte count is less than 3000 per cu. mm., the term granulocytopenia is used, but even at this level there are adequate numbers of granulocytes for normal defense activities. When the absolute number reaches 1000 per cu. mm., the patient becomes vulnerable to microbial attacks, but serious risks are usually first experienced at absolute counts of less than 500 per cu. mm. When playing this numbers game it is important to take into account the presence of monocytes which, although not as readily phagocytic as granulocytes, do contribute to the defense. The term agranulocytosis is usually reserved for the serious granulocytopenias in which both the marginated pool and the bone marrow reserve have been depleted. A depletion of the marrow reserve leaves the proliferating immature cells as the only myeloid cells present in the marrow and has given rise to the erroneous expression "maturation arrest." The immature cells are not arrested at all, but as soon as they reach maturity they are swept out of the marrow to shore up peripheral defenses.

The granulocytopenias can be caused by decreased production, ineffective production, or increased destruction. Decreased production occurs after exposure to radiation or to radiomimetic drugs. The granulocytopenia is part of a general suppression of cellular proliferation in the bone marrow, but because of the short granulocyte life span and the limited reserves, granulocytopenia is observed earlier than thrombocytopenia or anemia. Pisciotta has described a similar suppressive effect on the bone marrow of certain susceptible individuals by the use of phenothiazine-type drugs. These appear to have a predominant effect on the myeloid cells, with less suppression of the erythroid cells and almost complete sparing of the megakaryocytic elements. In addition to drug-induced bone marrow hypoplasia underproduction of granulocytes has been found to be responsible for a number of hereditary and acquired granulocytopenias. Of special interest is cyclic neutropenia, a disorder in which at regular intervals patients develop granulocytopenia, fever, mouth ulcerations, and infections. The pathogenesis has been linked to hormonal cycles, but recent studies indicated that the recurrent granulocytopenia may be caused by an undampened feedback circuit between the peripheral granulocyte pool and myeloid committed stem cells.

Ineffective granulocytopenia is undoubtedly responsible for the granulocytopenia observed in megaloblastic anemias. Blume and coworkers have suggested that the granulocytopenia observed in Chediak-Higashi's syndrome may also be caused by intramedullary autodestruction by the large abnormal lysosomes which characterize the myeloid cells in this interesting disease.

Increased peripheral destruction is caused by antibody-coating of the granulocytes and/or by

TABLE 22-10 CLASSIFICATION OF GRANULOCYTE DISORDERS

I. *Quantitative Abnormalities*
   Granulocytopenia
   Granulocytosis

II. *Qualitative Abnormalities*
   Defective delivery
   Defective phagocytic activity
   Defective bactericidal activity

III. *Myeloproliferation Disorders*
   Polycythemia vera
   Chronic granulocytic leukemia
   Myelofibrosis
   Thrombocythemia
   Erythroleukemia
   Acute granulocytic leukemia
   Acute myelo-monocytic leukemia

hypersplenism. As in patients with ineffective myelopoiesis the granulocytopenia is associated with a striking myeloid hyperplasia in the bone marrow. Antibody destruction of circulating granulocytes is dramatic but rare. It involves the interaction of a drug hapten such as aminopyrine, phenylbutazone or methyluracil, with a specific antibody and the subsequent attachment of the antigen-antibody complex to granulocytes, the so-called "innocent bystander" concept (Fig. 22-118). These coated granulocytes are then destroyed by the reticuloendothelial system particularly in the spleen. Hypersplenism or splenic neutropenia is observed in conditions without overt antibody production but with splenomegaly. Despite many studies of the pathogenesis of the hypersplenic syndrome we still do not understand why a large spleen should destroy otherwise healthy granulocytes. It may be a question of sequestration rather than destruction similar to hypersplenic thrombocytopenia or it may involve antibodies too few to be detected by current techniques.

Granulocytosis. Granulocytosis is present when the granulocyte count exceeds 10,000 per cu. mm. When the granulocyte count exceeds about 30,000 per cu. mm. the term "leukemoid reaction" is often used. Although a nonleukemic granulocytosis may reach levels of 50,000 per cu. mm. or higher, counts in excess of 100,000 per cu. mm. are extremely rare.

An acute granulocytosis of moderate degree can be caused by a mere shift of granulocytes from the marginal pool and the bone marrow reserve pool into the circulation. It is frequently observed after exposure to acute infections, trauma, and emotional stress or after the administration of epinephrine, cortisone, and endotoxin. Chronic granulocytosis is observed under conditions of sustained overproduction of granulocytes. The most common causes are bacterial infections and tissue injury. Lymphomas and other neoplasias presumably cause granulocytosis by inducing tissue necrosis with the release of hypothetical bone marrow-stimulating substances. Eosinophilic granulocytosis is observed primarily in conditions characterized by the sustained presence of antigen-antibody complexes such as in conditions with chronic parasitic invasion or with dermatologic or allergic manifestations.

Qualitative Abnormalities

A decreased resistance to infection may occur despite normal granulocyte counts if the functional competence of the granulocytes is impaired. In the so-called "lazy leukocyte syndrome" described by Miller, Oski and Harris the granulocytes do not respond appropriately to chemotaxic factors, and the granulocytes fail to accumulate and produce an inflammatory focus. Defective attachment and phagocytosis of foreign bodies are usually caused by impaired antibody production and complement function. Impaired killing of ingested microorganisms causes recurrent and chronic infections and may lead to massive granuloma formation. Despite its rarity, this so-called "chronic granulomatous disease," studied extensively by Holmes and co-workers and by Baehner and Nathan has provided considerable insight into normal and abnormal bactericidal function. Morphologic and metabolic studies have shown that the granulocytes are capable of phagocytosis of microorganisms but incapable of their subsequent killing and disposal. The lysosomes, present in normal number, discharge their enzymatic cargo into the phagosomes, but the enzymes apparently are not bactericidal. The usual acceleration of glycolysis and hexose monophosphate shunt activity does not occur and the production of H_2O_2 is decreased. It has been proposed that in the absence of H_2O_2 the iodination of the microbial membrane cannot take place, and the organisms remain unharmed inside the phagosomes. Support for this hypothesis has been obtained from the fact that some hydrogen peroxide-producing organisms such as lactobacillus are killed by the granulocytes from patients with chronic granulomatous disease, and phagocytosis of latex particles coated with a hydrogen peroxide-producing oxidase will restore killing of simultaneously phagocytized bacteria. Chronic granulomatous disease is inherited as a sex-linked disease; however, although an inherited deficiency of a NADH oxidase could explain both the lack of H_2O_2 production and hexose monophosphate shunt acceleration (Fig. 22-90), such deficiency has not been definitely established.

A distinct disorder of lysosomal morphology is characteristic of the Chediak-Higashi syndrome, in which giant lysosomes can be observed in granulocytes, melanocytes, fibroblasts, and other cellular elements. As suggested by White, the granulocytic lysosome may be responsible for intramedullary autodestruction, ineffective granulopoiesis, and granulocytopenia. Whether phagocytosis and lysosomal killing also are abnormal is not known, since the decreased resistance to infection exhibited by these patients is easily accounted for by their granulocytopenia. The abnormal melanocytic lysosomes may in some way be responsible for the hypopigmentation observed in patients with Chediak-Higashi syndrome and in the closely related lysosomal disorders of the Aleutian mink and the beige mouse.

Myeloproliferative Disorders

In 1951, Dameshek, with characteristic abandon, lumped all the disorders which involve uncontrolled proliferation of bone marrow cells into one syndrome, the myeloproliferative syndrome. Some investigators have objected to this apparent oversimplification of a difficult problem and marshalled impressive evidence for the basic differences among the diseases included. However, so far the similarities are more numerous than the differences and the unified myeloproliferative concept has been useful in our pathophysiologic and clinical approaches to these diseases.

The prototype for the myeloproliferative diseases is polycythemia vera (see page 537), with its uncontrolled proliferation of erythroid, myeloid, and megakaryocytic elements and its frequent termination in myelofibrosis. The cellular proliferation characterizing the other members of the syndrome appears a little more unicellular but shares, to some extent, the effects of an excessive proliferation of the multipotential stem cells.

Chronic Granulocytic Leukemia. This dramatic disease was undoubtedly the disorder observed by Rudolf Virchow in 1845 and reported under the catching title "Weisses Blut" or, in Latin terminology, "leukemia." Even today we occasionally see untreated patients in whom the white cell crit exceeds the red cell crit and the blood appears pale and the bone marrow whitish green as in Virchow's original case.

The characteristic of early chronic granulocytic leukemia is an expansion of all granulocytic pools overflowing into peripheral blood and spleen. Since the proportional sizes of the pools closely approximate those of normal bone marrow, it has been tempting to consider this disease as being caused merely by an impaired cellular control. In polycythemia vera it is assumed that erythroid committed stem cells operate autonomously, without being impeded by the lack of erythropoietin. A similar autonomy of myeloid committed stem cells could conceivably explain the granulocytic overproduction in chronic granulocytic leukemia but it has to be conceded that so far no firm experimental data are available in support of this working hypothesis. It also has to be emphasized that, as with polycythemia vera, the manifestations cannot be explained on the basis of uncontrolled committed stem cell function alone, but most include dysfunction of the multipotential stem cells as well.

In 1960, Nowell and Hungerford described a specific chromosomal abnormality in the myeloid cells of patients with chronic granulocytic leukemia, an abnormality which subsequently has been found to be present in about 90 per cent of cases. It consists of a deletion of part of the long arm of the G chromosome number 21, leaving a tiny chromosome named the Philadelphia chromosome (Ph^1) (Fig. 22–94). This fortunate discovery has been of considerable diagnostic and biological importance. It has separated the classic Ph^1 positive patients from a small subgroup of Ph^1 negative cases with similar physical and laboratory findings but apparently with a more aggressive course and poorer prognosis. It has also established that myeloid, erythroid, and megakaryocytic cells are derived from the same stem cell, since all are Ph^1 positive in chronic granulocytic leukemia, and that the lymphatic cells which always are Ph^1 negative cannot share this common stem cell origin. Since all differentiated bone marrow cells contain the Ph^1 chromosome even during complete and prolonged remissions, the disease process responsible for chronic granulocytic leukemia must in some way have produced irreversible changes in the total bone marrow stem cell population.

The initial expectation that it would be possible to map the gene structure of the deleted arm of the 21 chromosomes by observing which functions of Ph^1 positive cells are absent has unfortunately not been fulfilled. Even the low leukocyte alkaline phosphatase content of leukemic granulocytes cannot definitely be related to the abnormal chromosome. The suspected relationship between the high incidence of leukemia in mongoloid children and their trisomy of the 21 chromosomes is probably not valid, since recent studies by O'Riordan and coworkers indicate that the Ph^1 chromosome is not the same as that which is involved in Down's syndrome. Nevertheless, the finding of a specific and consistent abnormality of a chromosome at the multipotential stem cell level has provided strong evidence in favor of the hypothesis that chronic granulocytic leukemia is caused by a stem cell mutation leading to the unrestrained production of mutant cell clones.

In most patients with chronic granulocytic leukemia there is no inkling as to the character of the insult which has caused such a somatic mutation. In a few cases, however, past exposure to radiation or to drugs suggests a cause-effect relationship. For many years radiation has been recognized to be leukemogenic in certain strains of mice, but its potential for inducing leukemia in humans was not appreciated until the early 1940s. At that time statistical studies of the incidence of leukemia in physicians showed an overall incidence of 1.7 times that in the general population, and more importantly the studies by March indicated that the incidence of leukemia in radiologists was 9 times that of physicians with little personal radiation exposure. This startling finding was accentuated by the finding of a high incidence of leukemia among the Japanese survivors from the atomic bomb explosions in Hiroshima and Nagasaki. Here, as summarized by Bizzozero and coworkers, the incidence of granulocytic leukemia either acute or chronic increased to about 3 times normal during the period from 1946 to 1955 and then slowly returned toward

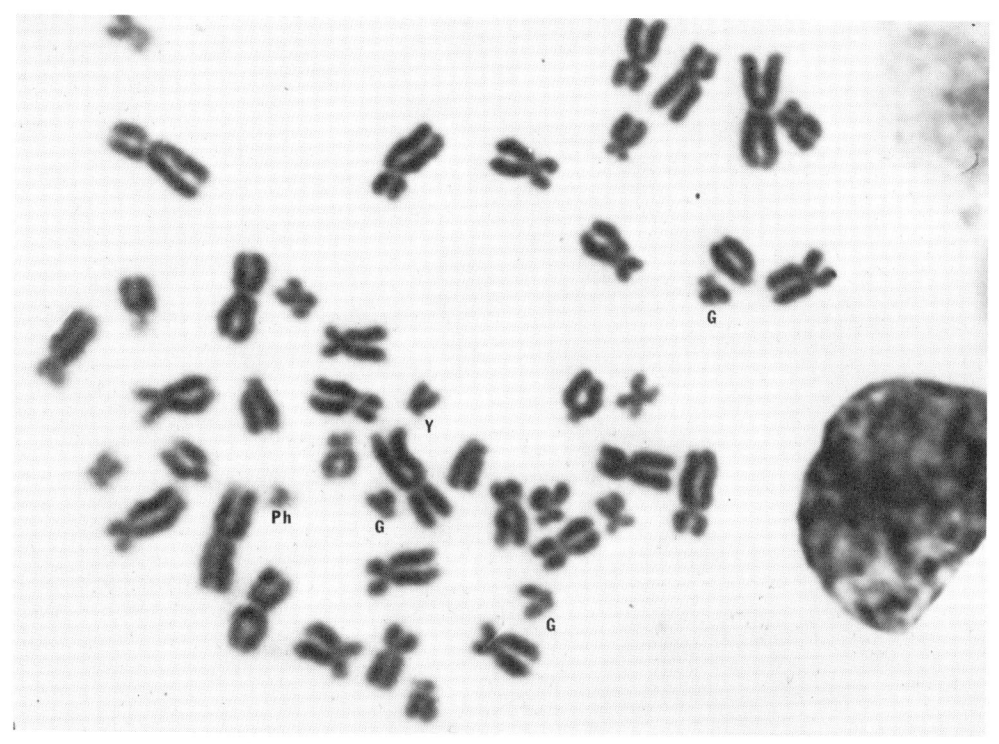

Figure 22–94 Chromosomal pattern of a male (Y chromosome) with chronic granulocytic leukemia (three normal G chromosomes and one tiny Ph¹ chromosome). (Courtesy of Dr. L. Jackson, The Thomas Jefferson University, Philadelphia.)

normal again. Studies of patients receiving therapeutic radiation have indicated that this form of radiation exposure also may be leukemogenic, but at present there are no convincing data showing that diagnostic radiation will cause leukemia. The obvious issue is whether or not the leukemogenic effect of radiation has a threshold. Some feel that any amount of radiation is potentially dangerous and should be avoided at all cost, whereas others feel that the leukemogenic risk of diagnostic radiation or radiation from natural sources or atomic bomb fallout is too small to be of public health concern.

Chemical leukemogens are playing an increasing role in the etiology of granulocytic leukemias. Any chemical interference with DNA replication must be considered potentially leukemogenic, and the widespread and successful use of chemotherapeutic and immunosuppressive agents probably will have to be paid for some years hence by an increased incidence of granulocytic leukemia. So far, most of the cases reported in which drugs are suspected as etiologic agents have been cases of acute rather than chronic granulocytic leukemia.

The clinical and laboratory features of chronic granulocytic leukemia are predominantly caused by the increased body load of myeloid cells. This load may be increased up to 150 times normal and causes bone marrow expansion with sternal tenderness, splenomegaly, and granulocytosis. The nutritional demands made by the overproduction of myeloid cells may cause an increased metabolic rate, with fever and weight loss, and the final breakdown of these cells may cause uricemia, gouty arthritis, and renal stones. The red cell production is usually decreased in unrestrained cases of chronic granulocytic leukemia, probably owing to decreased "Lebensraum" in the marrow. The same may be true for platelet production. When myeloid production has become controlled by adequate therapy the red cell and platelet mass will return to normal and frequently even overshoot, causing erythrocytosis and thrombocytosis. The differential count of the granulocytes of peripheral blood is similar to that of the myeloid cells in normal bone marrow and is distinctly different from that of patients with leukemoid reactions in whom the cells are predominantly mature. These cells also have a normal or high content of alkaline phosphatase, whereas the cells of chronic granulocytic leukemia characteristically have a reduced content. Despite this biochemical abnormality, the phagocytic and bactericidal functions of the leukemic granulocytes appear normal. The number of basophils is usually increased and may even dominate the granulocytic picture, an unexplained but prognostically ominous sign. Serum vitamin B_{12} levels are high as is the concentration of the main B_{12} binder, transcobalamin I. Both appear to be derived from the broken-down granulocytes, but their role in the symptomatology of chronic granulocytic leukemia is unknown.

The treatment of chronic granulocytic leukemia with radiation or suppressive drugs (Table 22-11) is initially very successful, causing an unmaintained remission of often several years' duration. Incipient relapses can usually be recognized by an increase in the granulocyte count and are handled quite easily by the sparing use of myelosuppressive drugs. However, after about 2 to 4 years the differential count and the disease process begin to change character. Myeloblasts appear in the peripheral blood, anemia and thrombocytopenia become evident, the spleen increases in size, the response to treatment becomes increasingly inadequate, and eventually the patient succumbs to the metabolic and cellular effects of an acute refractory leukemia. As in patients with polycythemia vera, the question has been raised as to the pathogenetic role of treatment in the final development of acute leukemia. No definite answer can be given, since in the past patients with untreated chronic granulocytic leukemia usually died from the effects of their chronic leukemia and only a few lived long enough to reach the stage in which contemporary patients develop their blast crisis.

Myelofibrosis. Bone marrow fibrosis with distortion and obliteration of marrow cavities may occur as an independent disease or as a complication of polycythemia vera or chronic granulocytic leukemia. Because of this relationship, myelofibrosis is considered a member of the myeloproliferative family. However, it seems somewhat farfetched to give the proliferation of fibroblasts the same status as the uncontrolled proliferation of blood cell precursors. For once, the fibroblasts do not share the Ph^1 chromosome of the other bone marrow cells. Furthermore, similar fibrotic reactions have been observed in tuberculosis, Hodgkin's disease, and carcinomatosis involving the bone marrow and are presumably reactions to tissue destruction and necrosis.

The characteristic splenomegaly of this disorder is usually believed to be caused by compensatory extramedullary hematopoiesis. However, the adult spleen appears to have lost most of its fetal capacity as a primary hematopoietic organ, and compensatory extramedullary hematopoiesis is rarely found in older people who develop an increased requirement for extra blood cell production. When foci of so-called extramedullary hematopoiesis in the spleen are found, they are probably made up of clones of bone marrow cells originating from immature cells prematurely released from the marrow and trapped in the sinusoids of the spleen. In myelofibrosis, on the other hand, the spleen is packed with hematopoietic tissue. Since this may occur at a time when the bone marrow is only minimally replaced by fibrous tissue and is in no need of supplementary extramedullary support, it seems more likely that the splenomegaly is caused by a pathologic myeloid metaplasia rather than by a physiologic extramedullary hematopoiesis. Foci of myeloid metaplasia are also observed in the liver but rarely anywhere else.

The most striking laboratory finding is an abnormal blood smear. The red blood cells show distorted and fragmented forms, and immature blood cells such as late erythroblasts, metamyelocytes, and myelocytes are present. It is usually assumed but has not been proved that such abnormalities are caused by cells being produced in and released from a microenvironment with less organized and regulated architecture than normal bone marrow. Progressive anemia with low reticulocyte counts is part of the disease, but the platelet count behaves erratically, and thrombocytosis may be as common as thrombocytopenia. It is of interest in this connection that bone marrow biopsies of the fibrous marrow often reveal nests of megakaryocytes, as if these were the most hardy of the hematopoietic elements. When anemia or thrombocytopenia is severe, the question is always raised whether the spleen destroys more cells than it produces. Erythrokinetic studies including organ scanning have been of only limited help in answering this question, and the decision to perform a splenectomy should be made only with great reluctance. The administration of androgens is very popular at present, and striking improvement in the anemia has been observed in some cases (Fig. 22-32). Other

TABLE 22-11 CHEMOTHERAPEUTIC AGENTS CURRENTLY USED IN TREATMENT OF CHRONIC LEUKEMIAS

Drug	Drug Category	Mechanism of Action
Bulsulfan	Sulfonic acid ester	Cross-linkage of DNA
Chlorambucil	Nitrogen mustard	Cross-linkage of DNA
Melphalan	Nitrogen mustard	Cross-linkage of DNA
Cyclophosphamides	Nitrogen mustard	Cross-linkage of DNA
Prednisone	Synthetic adrenocorticosteroid	Lysis of lymphocytes

wise, treatment does not appear to influence the slow but relentless progress of the disease.

Chronic erythroleukemia and essential thrombocythemia are two rare diseases which have been included in the myeloproliferative syndrome. They are characterized by an unrestrained proliferation of erythroid and megakaryocytic elements, respectively. In chronic erythroleukemia, this proliferation is ineffective and the patients are severely anemic. In essential thrombocythemia, large numbers of viable platelets are produced, causing a characteristic but unexplained mixture of bleeding and clotting problems.

Acute Granulocytic Leukemia. Acute granulocytic leukemia is a rapidly progressive disease characterized by the replacement of the bone marrow with immature and undifferentiated granulocytic cells. At present we relate the acute granulocytic leukemia to the myeloproliferative syndrome on the one hand and to acute lymphocytic leukemia on the other, relationships which may be spurious but nevertheless are useful in the clinical approach to this frustrating and discouraging disorder.

About 50 per cent of all leukemias are of the acute variety. There appears to be a slow but definite increase in this percentage, possibly owing to better diagnostic skills, possibly to an increased exposure to leukemogenic agents.

The acute leukemias can be divided into two major groups: the acute granulocytic and the acute lymphocytic. This subdivision of a rapidly progressive and uniformly fatal disease was initially felt to be a wasteful exercise of morphologic hair-splitting. However, at the present we recognize a fundamental difference between these two groups with regard to incidence, etiology, course, and prognosis. Acute granulocytic leukemia is a disease of adulthood, occasionally related to past exposure to radiation or chemicals, frequently with a long preleukemic phase and discouragingly resistant to chemotherapeutic agents. Acute lymphocytic leukemia is the predominant leukemia of childhood, rarely preceded by chemical exposure or preleukemic symptoms and highly responsive to chemotherapeutic agents. Acute granulocytic leukemia can further be subdivided into acute granulocytic, acute promyelocytic, acute myelocytic, acute myelomonocytic, and acute erythrocytic. Acute promyelocytic leukemia is listed as a separate group because leukemias with a predominance of promyelocytes often display the characteristic syndrome of disseminated intravascular coagulation. However, owing to the high content of thromboplastic material in leukocytes, this syndrome has also been described in the other acute leukemias. The acute myelomonocytic designation is of considerable help in leukemias in which the immature cells have features of both myeloblasts and monoblasts, since it prevents the clinicians from getting into futile arguments about morphologic minutiae. The erythrocytic group, the so-called Di Guglielmo's syndrome, is a rare but dramatic acute granulocytic leukemia in which the bone marrow during the early stages is dominated by a profusion of abnormal, often multinucleated but always ineffective erythroblasts (Fig. 22–95).

Various cytochemical techniques have been used to assist in the morphologic differentiation but such methods still belong to the frontier of leukemia research and have little practical relevance today. The important separation of the acute leukemias into granulocytic and lymphocytic types is usually not too difficult for the experienced hematologist relying on blood and bone marrow smears stained by Wright's or Giemsa stain. Occasionally, he is assisted by finding an eosinophilic rod in the cytoplasm of the leukemic blast cells. This so-called Auer rod is probably a giant lysosome and is never present in lymphoblasts, a useful diagnostic tidbit.

The etiology of acute leukemias is not known, but there is mounting evidence for the hypothesis that leukemia is caused by the action of a leukemogenic virus on stem cells rendered susceptible by genetic predisposition or chemical alteration. The presence of a genetic or chromosomal susceptibility is supported by statistical studies which indicate that the chance of developing acute leukemia is about 1 in 5 if one's identical twin has leukemia, 1 in 60 if one's nonidentical twin has leukemia, 1 in 700 if one's sibling has leukemia, and 1 in 3000 if no one else in the family has leukemia (see Zuelzer and Cox). However, these data also tend to rule out an inborn mutation as the sole etiologic mechanism, since only 20 per cent of individuals with a leukemic identical twin develop the disease. Certain chromosomal defects, both congenital and acquired, appear to predispose to acute leukemia. Children with inborn chromosomal defects such as in Down's syndrome, Fanconi's anemia, and Bloom's syndrome all have an increased incidence of acute leukemia, and leukemogenic chemicals or radiation seems generally to have the capacity to cause chromosomal changes. However, the relationship between chromosomal defects and the development of acute leukemia cannot be too direct, since no single unifying chromosomal change has been found among patients with preleukemia or acute leukemia.

The potential leukemogenic effect of ionizing radiation and cytotoxic and immunosuppressive drugs has already been mentioned. Although these agents could cause a chromosomal mutation with the production of autonomous leukemic blast cells the possibility that they provide a latent leukemogenic virus with the opportunity for unchecked multiplication appears equally good.

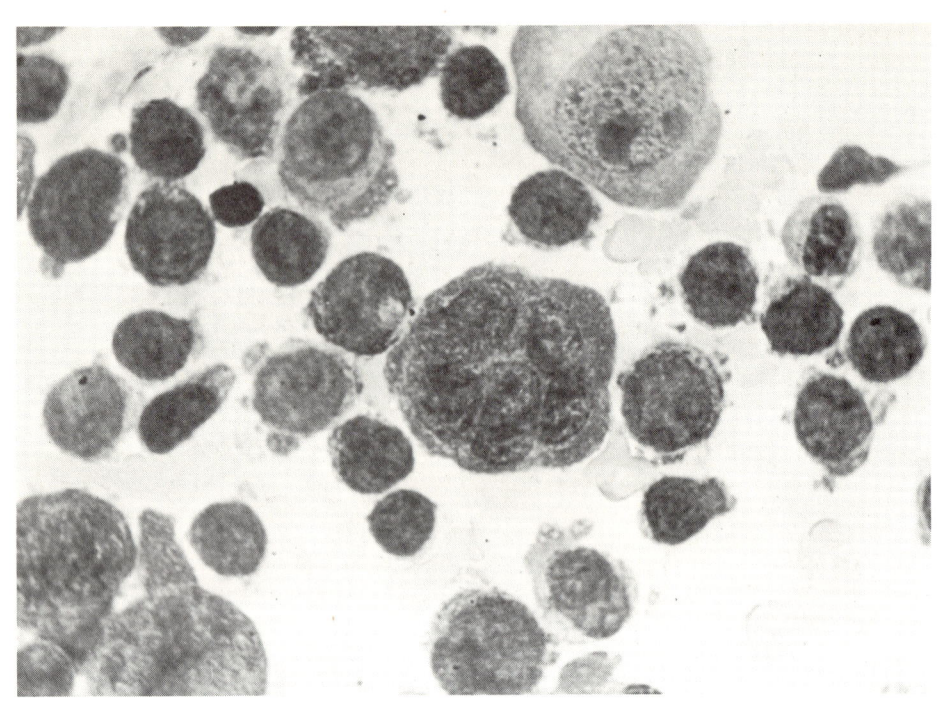

Figure 22-95 Multinucleated erythroblasts in bone marrow from patient with acute granulocytic leukemia of the DiGuglielmo variety.

It has been known for about 65 years that avian leukemia is caused and transmitted by a virus, and studies by Gross 20 years ago provided strong evidence for the existence of a similar etiologic mechanism for murine leukemias. The murine leukemogenic viruses are RNA viruses and their mechanism of replication has recently been clarified by the discovery of a reverse transcriptase, an enzyme capable of incorporating the information coded in viral RNA into DNA of the host. Such an enzyme has been found in human leukemic cells but its presence there is of questionable significance, since it has also been found in human nonleukemic embryonic cells. Direct demonstration of viral particles in and around leukemic cells is difficult to accomplish and, when found, their pathogenic importance is difficult to interpret.

Epidemiologic data suggesting direct transmission of leukemia are sparse, but strong indirect evidence for the presence of an infective agent has recently been provided by Fialkow and coworkers, who reported the course of leukemia in a girl who had received a bone marrow transplant from her brother. After some months the leukemia recurred, but this time the leukemic blast cells were cytogenetically XY cells. This unique case has generated considerable speculation and has even raised the possibility that leukemic relapses after prolonged remission are caused by reinfection rather than by the survival of a few leukemic cells, a most unorthodox view.

The orthodox view of cellular kinetics in acute leukemia is based on data obtained by Skipper and coworkers and suggests that the relapses and remissions of the disease are determined by the size of the leukemic mass. Manifest leukemia with the presence of leukemic cells in the bloodstream and with considerable leukemic bone marrow replacement is present when the leukemic mass is about 1 kg in weight or 10^{12} cells in number. The reduction in mass to about 1 gram will cause a morphologic and symptomatic remission but will still leave about 10^9 leukemic cells at large. Further therapy will reduce the body load and prolong the remission but only total cell kill will provide a cure (Fig. 22-96). This latter assumption is derived from data in rodents in which the transplantation of a single leukemic cell into an inbred recipient will result in leukemia. However, immunologic assistance in an outbred species such as man may make it less mandatory to aim for total cell kill, a goal which probably could not be accomplished without irreparable damage to normal tissues.

By now, it has been shown convincingly that leukemic blast cells do not proliferate as actively as normal bone marrow cells (see review by Killmann). The mitotic index and the tritiated thymidine labeling index are lower for leukemic blast cells than for normal blast cells. Even without the help of sophisticated quantitative techniques it is evident from looking at leukemic bone marrow smears that mitotic figures are relatively rare. This paradox that a rapidly growing tumor such as acute leukemia should consist of sluggishly proliferating cells has been difficult to accept. However, the therapeutic use of cytotoxic agents is based on the fact that normal bone marrow cells recover early, while there is a much more delayed recovery of leukemic blast cells, in other words, leukemic cells must have a longer generation time than normal cells. It is possible that the leukemic cell mass is made up of several cellular populations, with the majority of the cells being inert, long-lived, and slowly proliferating, while a minority have a rapid cellular turnover. It is the activity of this latter population which presumably accounts for the abrupt changes which occur in the bone marrow and peripheral blood during relapse.

The signs and symptoms of acute granulocytic leukemia can usually be attributed to mechanical or metabolic interference with the normal function of a number of organs. The leukemic cells will amass in great numbers in the bone marrow, spleen, liver, lymph node, and blood. Bone marrow function is first and most seriously threatened, presumably because the finite marrow volume precludes compensatory expansion. The liver, spleen, and lymph nodes can expand considerably without functional impairment, but a liver extensively infiltrated with leukemic cells may show signs of failure, an enlarged spleen will cause sequestration and injury to normal blood cells, and lymphatic tissue with architectural displacement may be immunologically less effective.

The effect of leukemic cells on the function of blood is less clear. Whole blood viscosity is probably not changed significantly, since an increase in the white blood cell mass usually is offset by a decrease in the red blood cell mass. Since extensive organ infiltration with mature lymphocytes in chronic lymphocytic leukemia causes only minimal functional organ impairment, it has been proposed that the impairment observed in acute leukemias is caused by leukemic blast cells either competing for essential nutrients or releasing metabolic toxins.

The principal clinical features of acute granulocytic leukemia are caused by bone marrow dysfunction and consist of anemia, hemorrhage, and infection.

Anemia is almost invariably present at the time of diagnosis. Hypersplenic red cell destruction and ineffective erythropoiesis may contribute, but the cause is usually clear-cut—lack of space for the erythroid precursors. The anemia is best managed by judicious transfusions of packed red blood cells.

Hemorrhages and petechiae are most often the features which bring the patient to a physician. With few exceptions they are caused by thrombocytopenia and are ameliorated by transfusion of concentrated platelet preparations. The critical level of platelet count below which spontaneous bleedings occur is hard to define, since the thrombocytopenia is caused by a variable mixture of splenic sequestration and decreased production. In general, platelet counts below 30,000 per cu. mm. should cause concern, and platelet counts below 10,000 per cu. mm. are associated with hemorrhage and petechiae.

Infections and fever are common and are most often caused by granulocytopenic impairment of host defenses. Although it has been claimed that an infection is always present when a leukemic

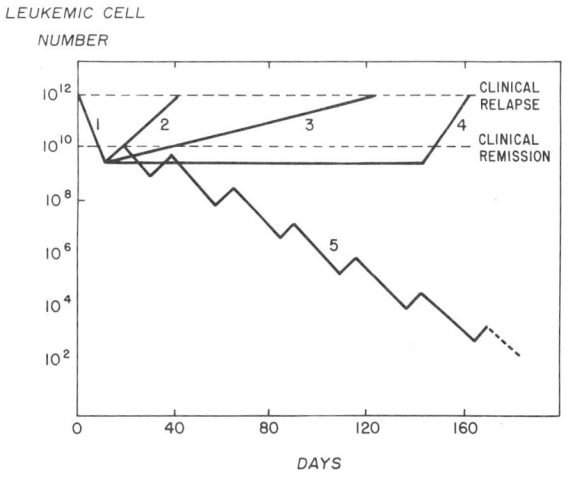

Figure 22-96 Hypothetical relationship between therapy of acute leukemia, leukemic cell number, and remission or relapses. (*1*) the effect of a successful induction therapy on cell count, (*2*) the immediate relapse which occurs after unmaintained therapy, (*3*) the slow relapse after partially effective maintenance therapy, (*4*) the prolonged remission on effective maintenance therapy, and (*5*) the hoped-for effect of repeated course of reinduction therapy on leukemic cell number. (Redrawn from Spiers, A. S. D.: Clin. Haemat., *1*:127, 1972.)

patient develops fever, tissue necrosis and endogenous pyrogens undoubtedly contribute. Nevertheless, fever in a granulocytopenic patient in whom defenses often are reduced even further by steroids and immunosuppressive drugs should always be treated promptly, as if an infection were present. If the fever persists despite the use of effective bactericidal agents and if all cultures are negative, a short symptomatic trial with prednisone may occasionally lead to a gratifying reduction in fever and toxic symptoms (Fig. 22–97). During the last decades important changes have occurred in the ecology of the infecting microorganisms. Bacteria and fungi of low virulence and high antibiotic resistance have emerged as major offenders and contribute to the chilling statistics which show that about 70 per cent of all leukemic patients die from infections. The preventive use of absorbable antibiotics has had little or no effect on infectious morbidity or mortality, but the use of careful reverse isolation techniques, laminar air flow chambers, and nonabsorbable oral antibiotics has been of some help. Complete isolation in life islands tends to isolate patients from good nursing care and compassionate personal attention, and the transfusion of normal granulocytes or granulocytes from patients with chronic granulocytic leukemia has too many intrinsic logistic problems to be of therapeutic importance today.

The triad of anemia, hemorrhage, and infection will respond to effective treatment of the leukemia. Unfortunately, ineffective treatment will aggravate these clinical problems by further re-

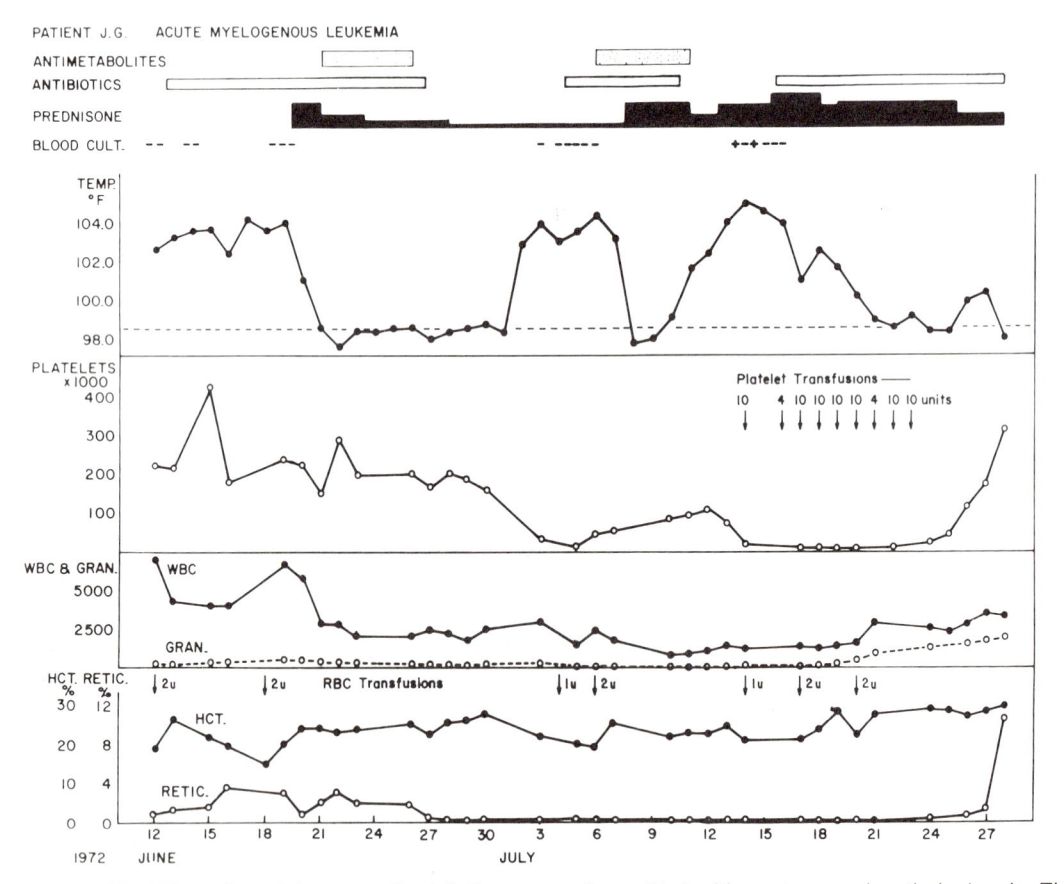

Figure 22–97 Effect of prednisone on the febrile course of a patient with acute granulocytic leukemia. The first febrile episode was associated with negative blood cultures and was unresponsive to antibiotics. Prednisone in the dose of 60 mg. a day resulted in prompt reduction in temperature and great symptomatic impairment. The second febrile episode was also associated with negative blood cultures and prednisone again was effective. However, the fever recurred despite prednisone, and this time the patient was found to have a bloodstream infection, which was promptly managed by appropriate antibiotics.

TABLE 22-12 CHEMOTHERAPEUTIC AGENTS CURRENTLY USED IN TREATMENT OF ACUTE LEUKEMIA

Drug	Drug Category	Mechanisms of Action
Cytosine arabinoside	Pyrimidine antagonist	Inhibition of de-novo synthesis of deoxycytidine riboside and DNA synthesis.
6-Mercaptopurine, thioguanine	Purine antagonists	Inhibition of de-novo synthesis of deoxycytidine riboside and DNA synthesis.
Cyclophosphamide	Polyfunctional alkylating agent	Cross-linkage of DNA.
Prednisone	Synthetic adrenocorticosteroid	Direct lysis of lymphocytes and lymphoblasts. Inhibition of cell cycle. Inhibition of DNA synthesis and/or DNA-directed RNA synthesis.
Vincristine	Alkaloid of periwinkle plant	Metaphase arrest resulting from inhibition of mitotic spindle (microtubule) formation.
Methotrexate	Folic acid antagonist	Inhibition of dihydrofolate reductase. Inhibition of DNA synthesis
L-asparaginase	Enzyme, catalyzing the hydrolysis of L-asparagine	Depletion of exogenous L-asparagine needed for the metabolism of malignant cells incapable of synthesizing this amino acid.
Daunorubicin	Antitumor antibiotic isolated from *Streptomyces peucetius*	Inhibition of DNA synthesis.

ducing bone marrow function, and currently patients die as often from unchecked leukemia as from drug-induced bone marrow failure.

In about 30 per cent of cases, the clinical and laboratory manifestations of acute granulocytic leukemia have been preceded for months and even for years by bone marrow changes which retrospectively can be designated as preleukemia. These involve various degrees of neutropenia and thrombocytopenia and the presence of peculiarly shaped erythrocytes, often associated with ineffective erythropoiesis. When the leukemia first becomes manifest, untreated survival is about 3 to 6 months long, and spontaneous remission exceedingly rare. Modern multi-agent treatment induces a complete remission in about 40 to 50 per cent of patients, but such patients will still have only a median survival of about 1 year. The therapeutic strategy for acute granulocyte leukemia is quite pragmatic, since drugs shown to be effective in animal studies, such as hydroxyurea, are quite ineffective, and drugs shown to be effective in acute lymphatic leukemia, such as vincristine and prednisone, are far less effective in acute granulocytic leukemia. Table 22-12 lists some of the agents used currently in the treatment of acute granulocytic leukemia and their presumed mode of action.

IMMUNOCYTES

STRUCTURE

The immunocytes work together with the phagocytes to maintain the integrity of the whole organism against foreign invaders. With functional responsibilities in such close accord, it is natural that these two families of cells should share many common anatomic sites in the reticuloendothelial system of the body. Lymphatic tissue is found throughout the body and, on cytogenetic grounds, is classified into primary and secondary types. Lymphocytes are first differentiated in the primary lymphatic tissue. They are then sent out to populate the secondary lymphatic tissue, where they function in specific immune responses. The primary lymphoid organs in mammals are the bone marrow and the thymus. The secondary lymphatic organs, consisting of the spleen and the lymph nodes along with subepithelial lymphoid tissue in the gastrointestinal tract, are characterized by a basic arrangement of lymphocytes into follicles with germinal centers. In the marrow the lymphocytes typically are scattered among the other cellular elements; germinal follicles are not seen in either thymus or marrow. A primary lymphoid organ equivalent to the "bursa of Fabricius" in the fowl has been postulated to exist in mammalian species in subepithelial lymphoid tissue of the gut, but whether or not such a "bursa equivalent" truly exists remains an open question (see Abdou and Abdou reference). A circulating pool of lymphocytes is found in the blood, mixed with other cell types, as well as in lymph, which contains few cellular elements other than lymphocytes.

Immunocytes are subclassified morphologically as lymphocytes, plasma cells, and their respective precursor cells. The small lymphocyte, a nondividing cell (which therefore does not take up tritiated thymidine), is about 9 μ in diameter on fixed and stained peripheral blood films. It has a skimpy rim of pale blue homogeneous cytoplasm which may contain a few azurophilic granules. Its nucleus has a chromatin pattern tightly arranged in bluish-purple blocks, often with a small notch or indentation in the nuclear membrane (Fig. 22–98). The large lymphocyte has a more generous rim of cytoplasm which may be more deeply blue. Its nucleus is also larger, with nuclear chromatin blocks spaced somewhat further apart, giving the nucleus a more "loose" appearance. Nucleoli may be seen. Large lymphocytes are proliferating and take up tritiated thymidine into their nuclei. The lymphoblast has a nuclear chromatin pattern which no longer exhibits a blocklike pattern but instead is finely divided, with a "grainy" texture in the midst of which one or two nucleoli are seen. Plasma cells (or "plasmacytes") are recognized in Wright-Giemsa stains by the eccentrically placed nucleus, with densely stained chromatin blocks close together, and a deep blue-green cytoplasm, with a clear zone containing the Golgi apparatus adjacent to one side of the nucleus (Fig. 22–99). The high level of secretory activity of plasma cells is reflected not only by the intense cytoplasmic basophilia but by the frequency of cytoplasmic inclusions (such as grapelike vacuoles or crystalloidal structures). "Proplasmacytes" and "plasmablasts" are progressively less mature plasma cells, with increasing looseness of nuclear chro-

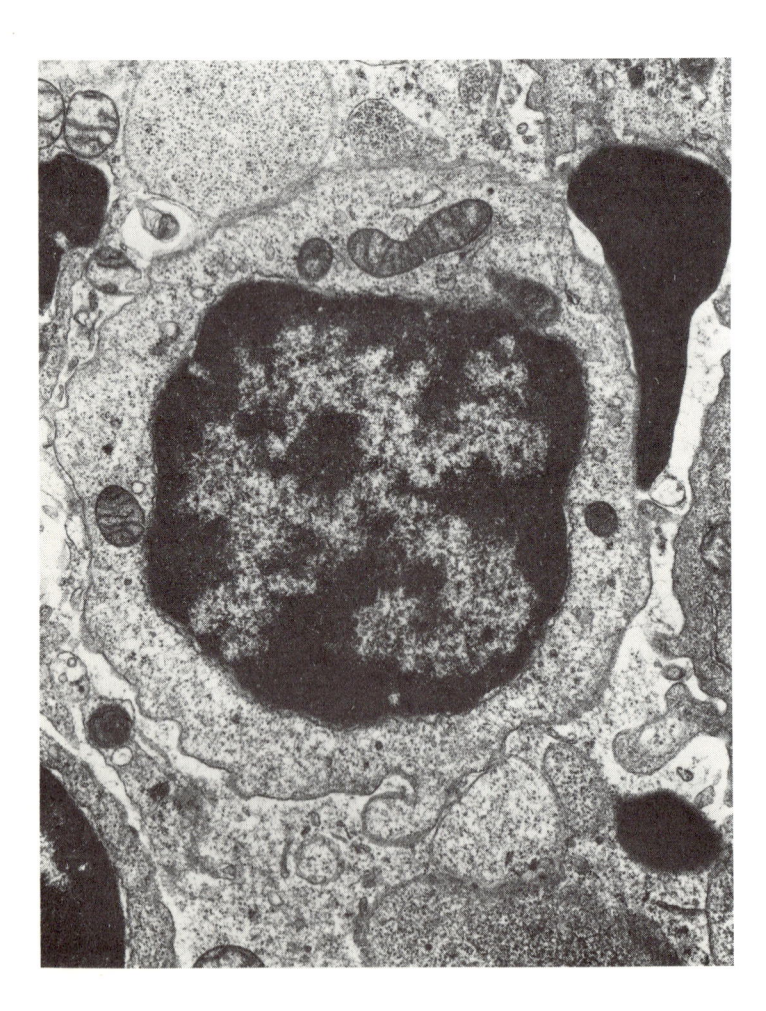

Figure 22–98 Electron microscope picture of a small mature human lymphocyte. Cytoplasm is scanty and contains mitochondria and ribosomes. Chromatin is densely packed into masses in a centrally placed nucleus. (Courtesy of Dr. A. Abraham.)

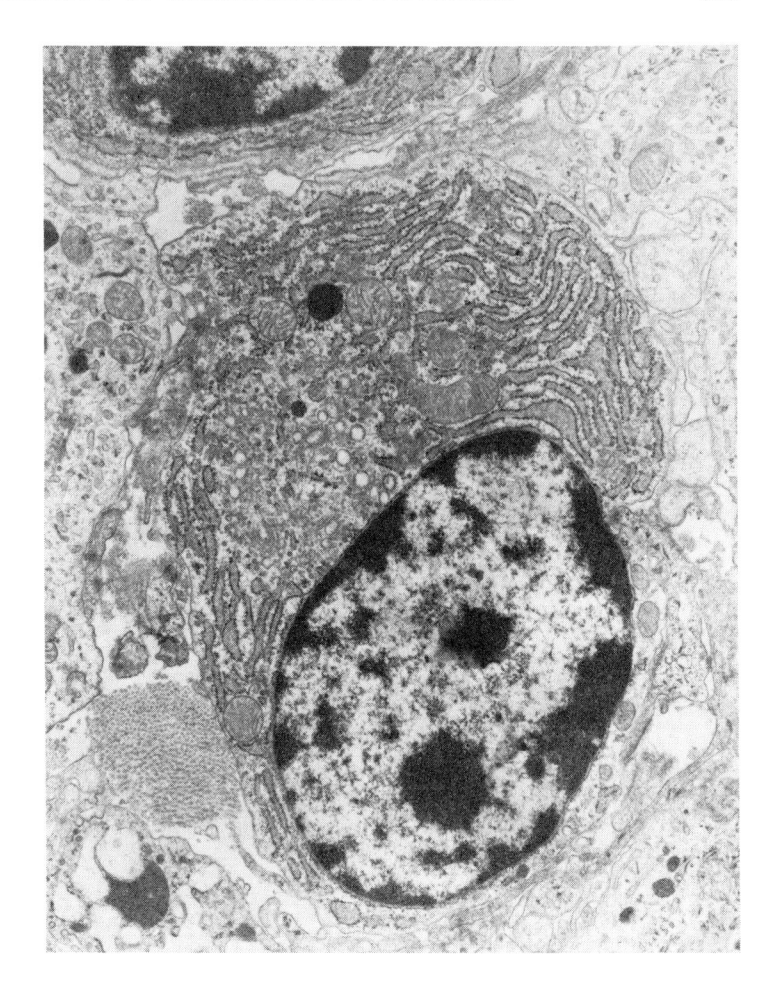

Figure 22-99 Electron microscope picture of a mature human plasma cell. Rough endoplasmic reticulum completely fills the cytoplasm of this immunoglobulin-secreting cell. The nucleus resembles that of the small lymphocyte but assumes an eccentric position. (Courtesy of Dr. A. Abraham.)

matin and prominence of nucleoli as the developmental stage is less mature.

FUNCTION

The primary function of the immunocytes is to give *specificity* to the attack of the warrior phagocytes upon foreign antigenic foes. *Memory* of such specificity is still another responsibility of the immunocyte, so that future defenses against a known antigenic opponent are more easily mustered. To a limited degree immunocytes may themselves participate directly in the attack.

Immune responses are of two types—one is cell borne and mediated by "T" (for thymus-derived) lymphocytes, the other is humoral and mediated by "B" (for "bursa-equivalent" or "bone marrow"-derived) lymphocytes. This functional division of the immunocytes is paralleled by separate developmental lines as well as by separate (although closely intermingled) anatomic sites of distribution.

Cell-mediated immunity is responsible for delayed hypersensitivity, homograft rejection, graft-versus-host reaction, defense against certain intracellular organisms, and possibly even defense against the growth of neoplastic cells in the body. The T lymphocytes mediate immunity but do not have the capacity to secrete circulating antibody. Surface markers have been described which allow them to be distinguished from B lymphocytes. Their anatomic sites of distribution in the lymph nodes are in the deep cortical regions and in the periphery of the germinal follicles (Fig. 22-100). In the spleen they are found in the periarteriolar lymphatic tissue. They also constitute the majority of lymphocytes in the circulating pool of blood and lymph. The population of these specific anatomic sites with T lymphocytes is dependent upon the thymus gland, which in turn is dependent upon the marrow as the source of its stem cells. The thymus may directly "condition" a lymphocytic stem cell derived from the marrow or it may secrete a hormonal substance which conditions marrow lymphocytes at some distance from the thymus to

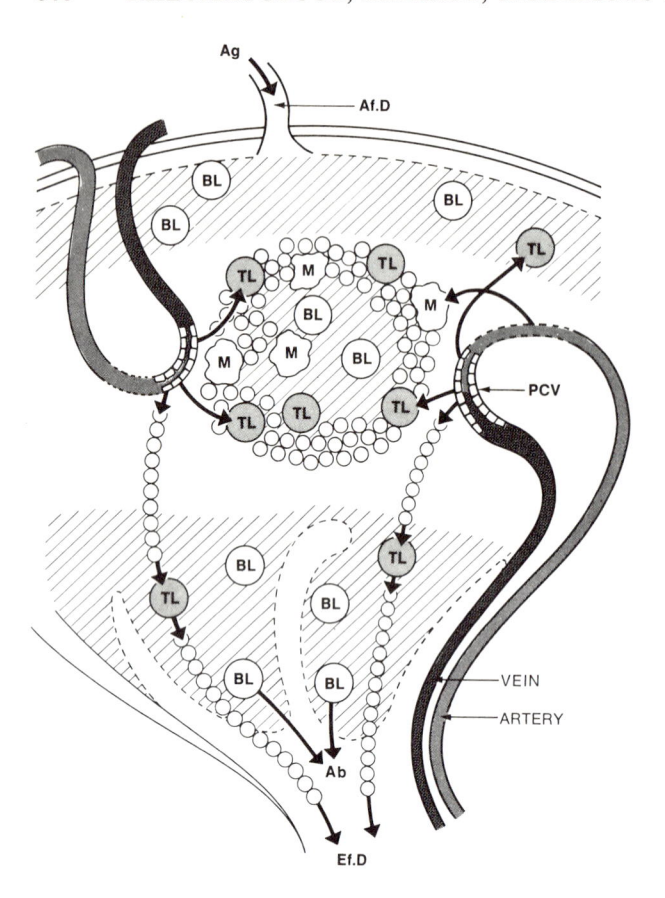

Figure 22-100 Diagram of lymph node. *TL* = T lymphocyte; *BL* = B lymphocyte; *M* = macrophage; *Ag* = antigen; *Ab* = antibody; *Af. D* = afferent lymphatic duct; *Ef. D* = efferent lymphatic duct; *PCV* = post-capillary venule. The cross-hatched zones represent areas populated by B lymphocytes. Areas containing open circles represent T lymphocyte regions. T lymphocytes circulate in close proximity to macrophages, allowing interaction between these cells and specific antigen. (From Craddock, C. G., et al.: New Eng. J. Med., *285*:380, 1971.)

function as T lymphocytes or both mechanisms may prevail.

B lymphocytes, consisting of lymphocytes and plasma cells, occupy the superficial cortical regions, the medullary cords, and the centers of the germinal follicles of the lymph nodes (Fig. 22-100). In the spleen they are found in the red pulp and in the peripheral white pulp. The B lymphocytes form an immobile pool; the majority do not circulate. They are also derived from a bone marrow stem cell but their further development is not dependent upon the thymus.

The cell-mediated immune response differs from that of the humoral response in several important respects. After initial recognition and processing of specific antigen by phagocytes, T lymphocytes are programed in a still unknown manner and become specifically "activated" (Fig. 22-101). This activation causes DNA synthesis, blast transformation, and subsequent cellular proliferation. It also causes the production of nonimmunoglobulin humoral factors (transfer factor, lymphocyte transforming activity), reviewed by David, which further amplify the immune response by recruiting other noncommitted T lymphocytes to become specifically activated and to proliferate. Another humoral substance, macrophage migratory inhibition factor, prevents macrophages from leaving the area, presumably serving the cause of antigen localization and destruction. Most of the activated T lymphocytes serve as "effector" cells by exerting a cytotoxic effect, by complement activation, and by attracting macrophages. Some of the activated T cells produce a population of small nondividing lymphocytes which bear a "memory" of the event. These "memory cells" remain for very long periods of time, possibly even a lifetime, in a resting and nondividing state, ready to resume immediate proliferation upon re-exposure to the specific antigen to rapidly mount a "secondary" immune response. Certain nonspecific mitogens such as phytohemagglutinin cause T lymphocytes to enter DNA synthesis and divide. Whether or not such nonspecific mitogenic reactions play any physiologic role is problematic, but they have been extensively used experimentally.

B lymphocytes must also be specifically programed with information about the specific antigen, and recent evidence suggests that they are somewhat dependent upon T lymphocytes to perform a cooperative role in this process (Fig. 22-102). Possibly the relatively immobile B lymphocytes require the cooperation of the freely circu-

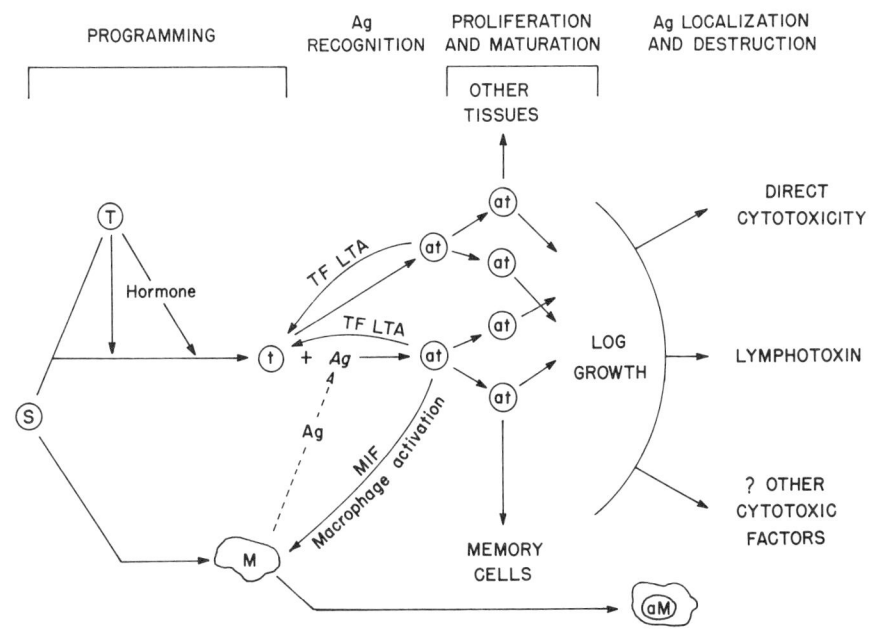

Figure 22–101 Cell-mediated immune response. The marrow stem cell (S) is programed under the influence of the thymus (T) to become a "T" lymphocyte (t). This cell is activated (at) by interaction with antigen (Ag), causing blast transformation followed by proliferation. Nonimmunoglobulin lymphocyte substances are released (TF = transfer factor; LTA = lymphocyte transforming activity; MIF = migratory inhibition factor) which further amplify the proliferative response and immobilize macrophages (M) which become activated (aM) at the site of the immune response. Antigen destruction follows. (From Craddock, C. G., et al.: New Eng. J. Med., 285:382, 1971.)

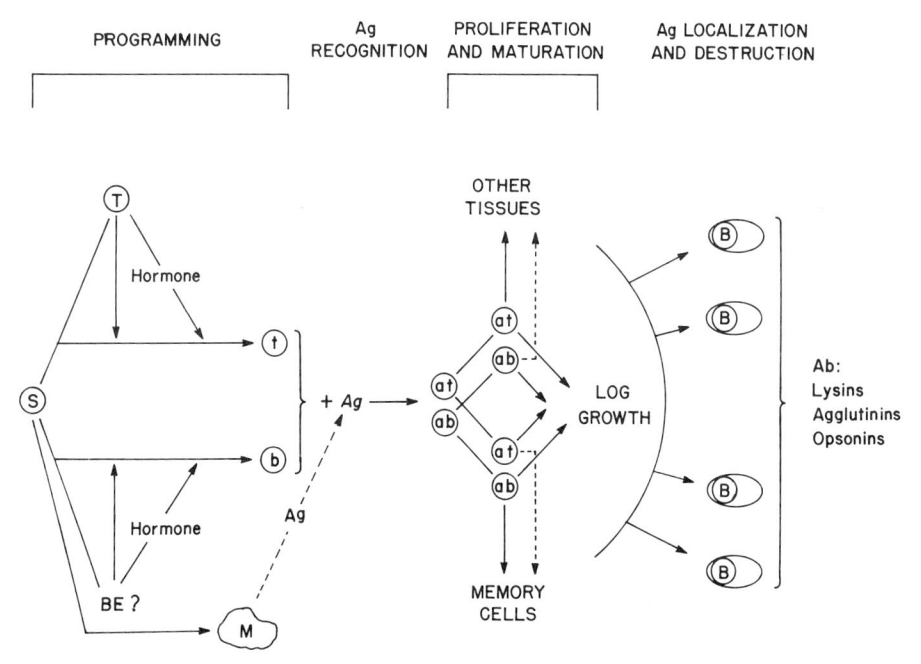

Figure 22–102 Humoral immune response. The marrow stem cell (S) gives rise to the "B" lymphocyte (b), with possible assistance from a "bursa equivalent" (BE) mechanism. Activated "B" lymphocytes (ab) proliferate, interacting with simultaneously proliferating "T" lymphocytes and then maturing to plasma cells (B), which produce antibody (ab). (Other symbols are designated in the legend to Fig. 22–101.) (From Craddock, C. G., et al.: 285:383, 1971.)

lating T cells to achieve rapid widespread activation throughout the body. As the B lymphocytes proliferate and mature to plasmablasts and plasma cells, they commence specific antibody synthesis. The plasma cell represents the most mature form of the activated B lymphocyte and no longer has the capacity to divide. The antibodies produced effect the immune response by virtue of their functional properties as agglutinins, lysins, and opsonins. It is not certain that B lymphocytes have the capacity to develop long-lived "memory" cells.

The secretion of antibodies of great diversity into plasma and extravascular fluids is the special prerogative enjoyed by the B lymphocytes. An understanding of the molecular structure of antibodies is necessary to appreciate how precise specificity yet wide diversity are combined in one family of closely related proteins. The immunoglobulins fall into five families of proteins. IgG immunoglobulins, of molecular weight 160,000 and sedimentation constant 7S, are normally present in serum at a concentration of about 1250 mg. per 100 ml., constituting by far the major type. Their relatively small molecular size permits transport across the placenta. IgA immunoglobulins (normal serum concentration 250 mg. per 100 ml.) are the major type found in body secretions (saliva, tears, colostrum, and gastrointestinal, respiratory, and urinary tract fluids). They form polymers of 9S, 11S, and 13S from the basic unit of 7S. IgM immunoglobulins (normal serum concentration 120 mg. per 100 ml.) are large 19S molecules, also an association of 7S units, especially well suited for agglutination and complement fixation. The other two families of immunoglobulins, IgD and IgE, are present in much lower concentrations, 3 mg. per 100 ml. and 0.03 mg. per 100 ml., respectively. The function of IgD is still unknown. IgE is important in allergic reactions involving the skin, the lungs, and other tissues (Table 22–13).

All the immunoglobulin families have a basic structure in common (Fig. 22–103). This unit consists of two light (or "L") and two heavy (or "H") chains, so termed because of their difference in molecular weight (22,000 as opposed to 52,000).

The two H chains are bound together by a disulfide bridge. Each of the L chains is also bound to an H chain by a disulfide bridge. Hydrogen bonding also helps hold the molecular pieces together. The N-terminal ends of an L and H chain together form the antigen binding site. Since there are two such regions on the molecular surface, the immunoglobulin unit is divalent, i.e., it can combine with two antigen molecules. Univalent antibody can be artificially produced by cleavage of the molecule with papain. Such treatment produces one Fc fragment, which carries the C-terminal ends of both H chains, and two Fab fragments, each of which carries the N terminal of one H and one L chain. The Fab fragments function as univalent antibodies. The molecule contains a variable amount of carbohydrate, which is attached to the H chain.

The amino acid sequence of the H and L chains is governed by the same kinds of genetic controls that govern the structure of other body proteins. The H chains each contain about 450 amino acid residues, and the L chains about 214. About three fourths of the H chain and one half of the L chain are invariant in their amino acid structure. Specificity, however, lies in the remaining one fourth of the H chain and one half of the L chain where regions of the molecule show great variation in amino acid structure which determines their specificity for antigen. These two gene regions have been called "C" (for common) and "V" (for variant).

All the classes of immunoglobulins have the same basic structure of L and H chains. There are only two different types of L chains— κ and λ. Only one type is present in any given molecule, but both types are represented in all immunoglobulin families. Class specificity lies in the type of H chain.

There are four subclasses of IgG H chains ($\gamma 1$, $\gamma 2$, $\gamma 3$, $\gamma 4$). IgA is characterized by α heavy chains and represents polymers of two, three, or four 7S units plus a "secretory piece" which presumably facilitates transport into body secretions. IgM, a pentamer of 7S units, has μ heavy chains (Fig. 22–104). IgA and IgM contain considerably more carbohydrate than IgG.

TABLE 22–13 COMPARISON OF IMMUNOGLOBULIN CLASSES

	Ig	IgA	IgM	IgD	IgE
Serum concentration (mg. per 100 ml.)	1250	250	120	3	0.03
Sedimentation constant S_{20}	6.6S	7S, 9S, 11S, 13S	18S	6.5S	7.9S
Carbohydrate (total %)	2.9	7.5	11.8	?	?
Heavy chains	γ	α	μ	σ	ϵ
Light-chain frequency kappa:lambda ratio	2:1	1:1	3:1	1:4	?

Figure 22-103 Diagram of the structure of the 7S immunoglobulin. C and N represent C-terminal and N-terminal amino acids, respectively. *CHO* = carbohydrate. Disulfide bonds connect the smaller L chains with the larger H chains, and the latter with each other. The interrupted line represents papain cleavage in Fc and Fab fragments. The InV locus at the 191st amino acid residue of the L chain is shown. The cross-hatched areas represent the variable regions, and the clear areas the common regions. (Adapted from Fahey, J. L.: *in* Williams, et al. (Eds.): Hematology. New York, McGraw-Hill Book Co., 1972, p. 795.)

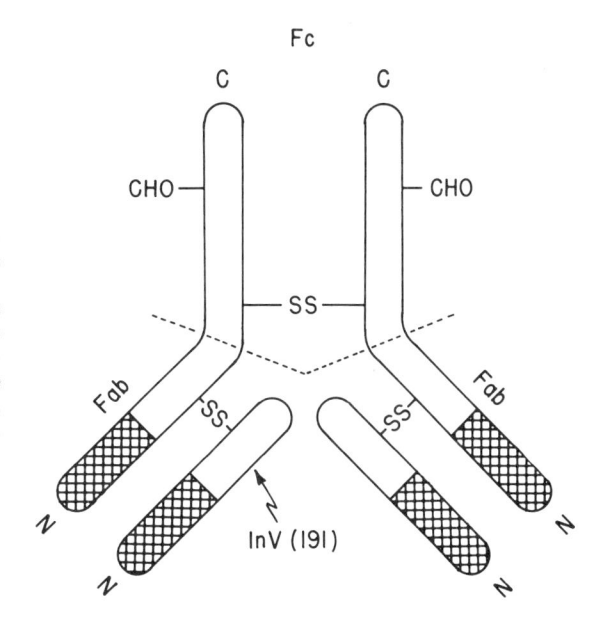

In basic respects the genetic control of immunoglobulin synthesis resembles that of hemoglobin. The major subunits of the molecule—L and H chains of immunoglobulin and α and β chains of hemoglobin—are under the control of gene regions which are separate and independent and yet which must coordinate their efforts in order to produce balanced synthesis of the subunits, thus avoiding shortages or surpluses of unpaired polypeptide chains. The extraordinary molecular diversity of the immunoglobulins, however, is a major point at which genetic control of this system of body proteins differs from all others. The synthesis of a given specific immunoglobulin—including one complete common and variant region each for one H chain and for one L chain—is under the control of one clone of B lymphocytes. The body contains numerous such clones, leading to heterogeneous production of almost countless different immunoglobulin molecules. Both lymphocytes and plasma cells synthesize immunoglobulin, plasma cells producing about two thirds of the IgG. On the other hand, about 90 per cent of IgM is produced by lymphocytes. The gene

Figure 22-104 Assembly of 7S units in higher molecular weight immunoglobulins, IgA (*above*) and IgM, showing "secretory piece" (*SC*) and "joining piece" (*J*). (From Tomasi, T. B.: New Eng. J. Med., 287:501, 1972.)

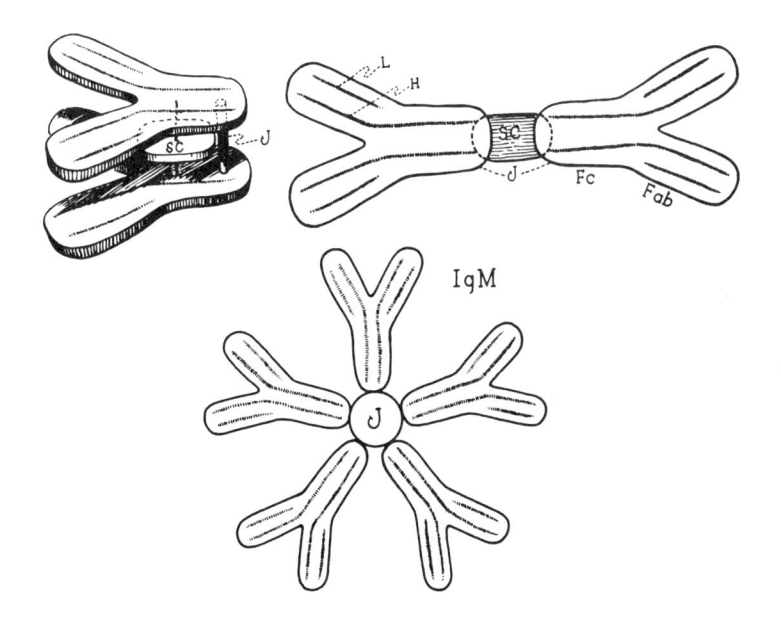

regions controlling the common structural regions of L and H chains are inherited. Inherited amino acid substitutions may affect these common regions. Thus, INV-1 and INV-3 are genetic alleles affecting the κ chain at the 191st amino acid site, where either leucine or valine, respectively, is placed. Precisely how B lymphocytes develop gene regions in different clones to control the variant regions of the L and H chains remains a mystery. A somatic theory postulates that the antigen, after being processed by a macrophage, somehow produces a "reverse flow" of information from RNA to DNA which thus establishes itself as a permanent record in the programed genome of a given clone of B cells. The germ line theory postulates that all genetic information, common as well as variant, is obtained through inheritance.

KINETICS

The differentiation, proliferation, and fate of the body's lymphocytes contrast sharply with those of the other cellular elements of the blood. The maturation and proliferation processes which give rise to a specialized peripheral lymphatic tissue are not accompanied by significant morphologic changes other than that change which sets apart the large proliferating cells from the small nonproliferating cells. The marrow serves as the ultimate source of all lymphocytes and together with the thymus is considered a primary lymphatic structure concerned with the differentiation and proliferation of a peripheral population of mature, specialized lymphocytes in the blood, lymphatics, lymphatic tissue, and spleen. The fully developed red cells, granulocytes, and platelets have a finite life span at the end of which the cell disintegrates. In the case of the peripheral lymphatic tissue, the cells retain the ability to undergo cell division once again by a process of "blastogenesis." The peripheral lymphatic system is also charged with the task of maintaining immunologic memory, which it does by means of a small population of exceedingly long-lived cells which may survive for many years and then once again re-enter cell division upon specific stimulation by antigen. Thus, the cell life span of lymphocytes varies tremendously.

The information which has been obtained about lymphocyte kinetics has relied heavily upon cytologic techniques of DNA labeling by tritiated thymidine. More recently specific membrane markers have been identified to permit T cells and B cells to be distinguished from one another (see Wilson and Nossal reference). Lymphocytes identified by chromosomal markers have also been used.

The lymphocytes in the primary lymphatic tissue—the marrow and the thymus—undergo relatively rapid and continuous proliferation quite independently of specific antigenic stimulation (Fig. 22–105). For decades evidence has been presented for and against the theory that the marrow lymphocytic stem cell is pluripotential and also gives rise to the diverse cells of the myeloid series. However, the fact that the Philadelphia chromosome (Ph^1) is found in the myeloid cell lines—erythroid, megakaryocytic, and granulocytic—but not in lymphocytic argues against the pluripotential nature of this lymphocytic stem cell. Marrow and thymic lymphopoiesis appears to be more active than a fully developed adult's peripheral lymphatic tissue would require for replenishment, and therefore it is reasonable to assume that the bulk of lymphopoiesis in these organs is wasteful, most of the proliferated cells undergoing destruction in order to prevent massive accumulation of unwanted numbers. Relatively few are directed to assume positions in peripheral secondary lymphatic tissue. Under normal conditions, the secondary lymphatic tissue is not actively proliferating, but upon exposure to antigen, specifically stimulated cells undergo rapid division, with germinal centers showing the greatest level of activity.

The bulk of the T lymphocytes of the peripheral lymphatic tissue recirculate. They follow a path from blood to lymph node and spleen to lymphatic channels back to blood. Egress from the blood into the lymphatic tissue occurs through the wall of the postcapillary venule, where the T cells percolate through the periphery of follicles and the deep cortical areas eventually to be collected into the efferent lymphatic (Fig. 22–100). Approximately 10 hours are required for lymphocytes to leave the blood and appear in the thoracic duct. The T cells do not recirculate into the marrow or thymus to any significant degree. This system can be lymphocyte-depleted by means of thoracic duct drainage or extracorporeal irradiation, leaving the T areas of the lymphatic tissue in an empty state. The recirculating population consists of "short-lived" and "long-lived" cells. This conclusion is based on experiments in animals given continuous injections of tritiated thymidine over a period of many months. In rats, about 40 to 45 per cent of small lymphocytes take up label in 5 to 10 days. The labeling index continues to increase thereafter, but even after nine months, about 5 to 10 per cent of the small lymphocytes remain unlabeled. They are considered to be the long-lived memory cells. All large lymphocytes label within three days. The gradual slope of decline of the DNA labeled cells shows a slow replacement rate and a long survival time of most small lymphocytes.

The B cells are largely noncirculating. They maintain a fixed position in the germinal centers, medullary cords, and superficial cortical zones of the secondary lymphatic tissue. Apparently the majority of cells produced are short-lived. Ma-

LYMPHOPOIESIS

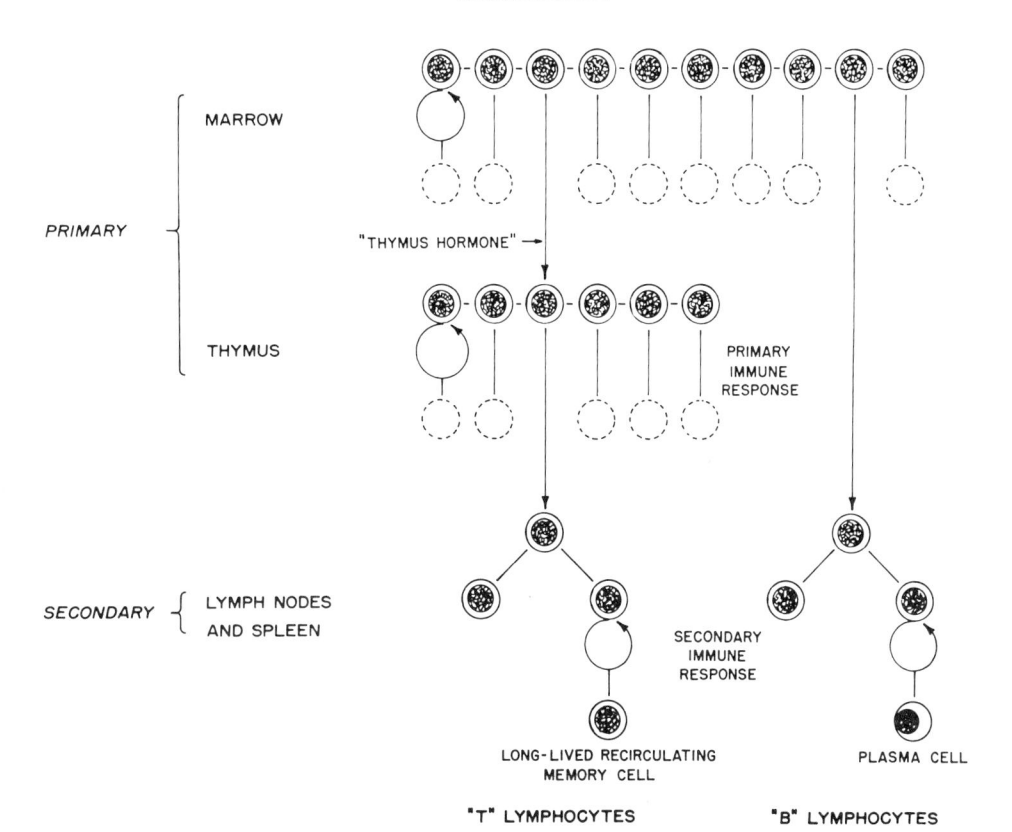

Figure 22-105 Diagram of lymphopoiesis. Interrupted circles represent effete cells in marrow and thymus which do not achieve perpetuity in the second lymphatic tissue. Proliferation takes place in both the primary and secondary tissues, in the latter as a result of specific immune response.

ture plasma cells probably do not survive longer than two or three days. A small proportion of B cells mature in the marrow because a few plasma cells are normally seen there.

PATHOPHYSIOLOGY

Classification and General Considerations

The system of fixed and circulating immunocytes which constitute the secondary lymphatic tissue provides a vital defensive function. Thus, the most common alterations occur in reactive response to the presence of foreign antigens, such as local or systemic infections. The reaction may consist of focal or generalized adenopathy, splenomegaly, the presence of large "young" lymphocytes or plasmacytoid cells in the circulation, or an elevation of the absolute lymphocyte count. Another common reactive change is a generalized increase in all immunoglobulin types.

Neoplastic alterations of the immunocytes represent inappropriate proliferative responses which produce an increase in the number of immunocytes and may be associated with either an increase or a decrease in the concentration of immunoglobulins. These conditions are often associated with functional impairment of cellular or humoral immune mechanisms which, in turn, leads to an abnormal susceptibility to a variety of infections which are often quite different from those commonly observed in patients with an intact immune system (see Levine, Graw, and Young reference). Autoimmune phenomena, such as hemolytic anemia or thrombocytopenia, are also observed in patients with lymphoproliferative disorders. In clinical practice the problem of distinguishing neoplastic from reactive conditions affecting the immune system may be difficult, and judgments must be made with great care because of the vast differences in prognosis and treatment between the two states.

An overall classification of disorders of the immunocytes is summarized in Table 22-14.

TABLE 22-14 CLASSIFICATION OF IMMUNOCYTE DISORDERS

I. *Quantitative Disorders*
    Lymphocytopenia and hypogammaglobulinemia
      Primary
        Congenital
        Acquired
      Secondary
    Lymphocytosis and hypergammaglobulinemia
      reactive
      immunoproliferative
II. *Immunoproliferative Disorders*
    Leukemia
      Chronic lymphatic
      Acute lymphatic
    Lymphoma
      Hodgkin's
      Non-Hodgkin's
        Follicular lymphoma
        Lymphosarcoma
        Reticulum cell sarcoma
    M-component disorders
      Myeloma
      Macroglobulinemia
      Benign monoclonal gammopathy

Quantitative Disorders

Lymphocytopenia and Hypogammaglobulinemia. A reduction in the number of circulating lymphocytes below the normal level of 1000 to 1500 per mm. comes about through either increased loss or decreased production. The alteration represents primarily a change in the T cells, which constitute the majority of circulating lymphocytes. Mechanical loss of lymphocytes can be produced by tapping the circulating stream at the thoracic duct and draining off the lymph. A similar mechanism may explain the lymphocytopenia of intestinal lymphangiectasia and other disorders associated with leakage of lymph into the gastrointestinal tract. Loss of lymphocytes by destruction is a consequence of radiation exposure or adrenal glucocorticoids. Lymphocytes are extraordinarily radiosensitive and a fall in the lymphocyte count of the peripheral blood precedes the decrease in either granulocytes or platelets caused by radiation. Not all lymphocytes are equally susceptible to lysis by glucocorticoids; the short-lived small lymphocyte seems to be more susceptible than the long-lived variety. At any rate, lymphocytopenia is often present in patients during acute stress or therapy with corticoids, as reviewed by Claman.

The immediate source of the circulating lymphocytes is the secondary lymphatic tissue. Ablation of this source by malignant replacement, as in the case of advanced Hodgkin's disease or widespread metastatic carcinoma, or its destruction by irradiation of the lymph node-bearing regions of the body, leads to an inability of these regions to return adequate numbers of lymphocytes into the blood through the lymphatics. Chemotherapeutic alkylating agents will also affect lymphocyte replacement by interfering with the proliferating and the short-lived small lymphocyte pools.

Hypogammaglobulinemia occurs as an acquired or congenital syndrome, but it is not necessarily associated with lymphocytopenia, since the source of immunoglobulins is not T lymphocytes but rather the noncirculating B cells. In infants or children, hypogammaglobulinemia usually represents a congenital immune deficiency. In adults, the condition is acquired either by increased loss in the urine or the gastrointestinal tract as a complication of nephrotic syndromes or protein-losing enteropathy, or by decreased production, usually owing to a lymphoproliferative disorder.

The congenital immune deficiency syndromes of childhood form an array of rare but intriguing conditions upon which much of our understanding of the normal immune mechanism is based. The Bruton type of agammaglobulinemia is a sex-linked developmental defect of the B system of lymphocytes and plasma cells. Those regions of the secondary lymphatic tissue populated by these cells are empty, whereas the thymic-dependent areas remain intact. Circulating lymphocytes are present in normal numbers, but the concentration of immunoglobulins in the plasma is very low. The numerous infections which occur, usually in the sinopulmonary tract, can be prevented by the therapeutic use of gamma globulin injections. The DiGeorge syndrome is a severe developmental defect of the third and fourth pharyngeal pouches with consequent thymic aplasia and a profound lack of the thymic-dependent system of T cells. The corresponding regions of the T system are depleted of lymphocytes, and this is associated with lymphocytopenia but normal plasma immunoglobulin concentrations. Swiss type lymphocytopenic agammaglobulinemia affects both systems of immunocytes and thus would appear to trace its origins back to the common stem cell of origin in the bone marrow. This syndrome may thus conceivably be corrected by successful bone marrow transplantation, whereas thymic transplantation should suffice in the DiGeorge syndrome. Other congenital immune deficiency syndromes have been described, some resembling the Swiss type, others of a more mixed nature, such as Wiskott-Aldrich syndrome and hereditary ataxia telangiectasia. The features of Wiskott-Aldrich syndrome include thrombocytopenia, eczema, and susceptibility to infection associated with impaired ability to form antibody in response to polysaccharide antigens. The level of IgM is low, but IgG is normal and concentrations of IgA are often very high. Death in childhood is the result, owing either to severe infection or to the development of malignant disease, often of a lymphoma-like character. Successful therapy with transfer factor has been reported. In ataxia telangiectasia, the immune deficiency affects IgA and IgE along with qualitative deficiency in cell-mediated response.

The physiologic hypogammaglobulinemia of infancy must be distinguished from the congenital immune deficiency syndromes. Following the gradual disappearance from the infant's circulation of maternal IgG, endogenous synthesis takes over, raising IgG and IgM levels to about three fourths the adult level by one year of age. IgA levels increase more slowly, reaching adult levels by about two years.

Lymphocytosis and Hypergammaglobulinemia. Lymphocytosis is defined as an increase in the absolute lymphocyte count above 4000 per cu. mm. in adults, above 7000 cu. mm. in young children, and above 9000 per cu. mm. in infants. In "relative" lymphocytosis, the proportion of lymphocytes in the peripheral blood is increased because of concomitant granulocytopenia, but the absolute number is not above the normal range.

The leukocyte response evoked by a particular infection varies with the particular organism and also with the stage of the infection. Some infections, mostly viral but including some bacterial, are noted for their ability to evoke a lymphocytic response. Pertussis and acute infectious lymphocytosis are two childhood illnesses with a particularly striking tendency to raise the blood lymphocyte count—predominantly small mature forms—to very high levels in the range of 15,000 to 50,000 per cu. mm., but occasionally to as high as 100,000 per cu. mm.

Infectious mononucleosis is associated with a more modest lymphocytosis, usually not in excess of 20,000 per cu. mm., but there is a greater proportion (usually about 20 per cent of the total) of young and "atypical" forms. These are as large as 15 to 25 microns in diameter, with a generous rim of cytoplasm, often deep blue, foamy, and containing vacuoles, and with an irregular outline which tends to cling to adjacent red cells. The nucleus is also larger, its chromatin clumps are somewhat more widely spaced, and its outline is often indented, irregular, or lobulated into "monocytoid" forms. One or two nucleoli per nucleus are occasionally seen. Infectious mononucleosis, a prevalent disease among young people, is now thought to be caused by the Epstein-Barr virus (see Smith and Bausher reference).

The heterophile antibody test is positive in the great majority of cases, distinguishing this infection from a large number of other infections which may give rise to a similar blood picture, although usually with fewer atypical lymphocytes (see Wood and Frenkel reference). These infections include measles, mumps, adenovirus, viral hepatitis, cytomegalovirus, toxoplasmosis, brucellosis, typhoid fever, *Listeria monocytogenes,* and even tuberculoses. These infectious agents sometimes cause only a relative lymphocytosis, the most prominent change being a reduction in circulating granulocytes. Relative lymphocytosis is also a feature of the very early (usually preclinical) stages of bacterial infection, as granulocytes begin to leave the circulation to go into the infected tissues, or the very late stages of severe and overwhelming bacterial infection after exhaustion of granulocyte reserves. In the latter circumstance, the relative lymphocytosis is an ominous prognostic indicator. As one would predict from the lymphocyte-adrenal relationship, adrenal insufficiency may cause a rise in the blood lymphocytes.

An inappropriate increase in the absolute lymphocyte count, not explainable on the basis of either immunoreactive states or endocrine disease, is indicative of a lymphoproliferative disorder, usually lymphatic leukemia. Small mature lymphocytes predominate in chronic lymphatic leukemia. In the early stages of this disorder the elevation may be slight, but counts are usually in the range of 50,000 to 250,000 per cu. mm. when the diagnosis is first made. A rare patient may reach values as high as 1,000,000 per cu. mm. The leukocytosis of acute lymphatic leukemia is usually lesser in degree. Instead of the small mature lymphocyte, it features immature lymphoblasts.

One of the most important problems in clinical hematologic diagnosis is the distinction between leukemia and "leukemoid" reactions. The clinical course, whether benign and self-limited or persistent or progressive, is one obvious point of difference. The ability to distinguish the morphologic features of leukemic lymphoblasts from the young and atypical lymphocytes found in infectious states is another. The association of anemia, thrombocytopenia, and/or granulocytopenia suggests leukemia, but these findings singly or in combination are sometimes seen in infections. Perhaps the most salient pathophysiologic point of distinction lies in the fact that replacement of the primary lymphatic organ, the bone marrow, is a prominent feature of leukemia. Reactive states cause proliferation mostly in the secondary lymphatic tissue; the reactive young and "atypical" lymphocytes which characterize infectious mononucleosis and other infections therefore do not replace the normal marrow cells to any significant degree. Lymphocytes and plasma cells may increase in the marrow as a reactive change, but they usually are in the range of 15 per cent of the total marrow cells, hardly ever above 30 per cent, and never replace the marrow tissue as leukemic proliferation usually does.

An increase in plasma immunoglobulin concentration above the normal range is a common response not only in many infectious diseases but also in other conditions, such as liver cirrhosis, carcinoma, sarcoidosis, and lupus erythematosus, to name a few. Such responses are polyclonal and affect a variety of immunoglobulins. This is reflected in the serum electrophoretic pattern by a diffuse increase, or "broad-band" hypergammaglobulinemia. Immunoelectrophoretic analysis shows increases in all immunoglobulin families, IgG, IgA, and IgM. In an acute immune response, the increase in IgM occurs first. The finding in a serum electrophoretic pattern of hypergammaglobulinemia due to a narrow dense band in the broad region where the gamma globulins are normally found has a different significance. It is the secretory product of a monoclonal line of B cells producing only one type of immunoglobulin. This narrow band is often referred to as a "spike," but the term "M-component", for monoclonal component, is more appropriate (Fig. 22–106). The presence of an M-component in the serum or urine requires investigation of the patient for a malignant proliferative disorder of the B cells, i.e., myeloma or primary macroglobulinemia. On the other hand, the mere presence of such a component does not by itself establish such a diagnosis.

Qualitative Disorders

There are several points in the immune response at which qualitative defects in lymphocyte function may be the primary factors responsible for a poor immune response. In contrast to the granulocytic series, however, it is difficult to separate functional defects of the lymphocyte from numerical deficiency, since the process of specific activation (with the assistance of modifying factors) sets off a series of cell proliferations of the specifically activated clone. Thus, a qualitative defect at the afferent level of the immune response will be reflected in deficient numbers at the efferent limb.

Malignant transformation of cells in the body is increasingly being viewed as a qualitative breakdown in the function of "surveillance" lymphocytes whose function it is to recognize specific "tumor" antigens on the surface of such cells and to thus bring about their destruction. The association of defective lymphocyte function, on the one hand, with malignant transformation, on the other, in the congenital immune deficiency states is indeed a striking example of a lack of surveillance. In a similar fashion, individuals who are under prolonged immunosuppressive therapy

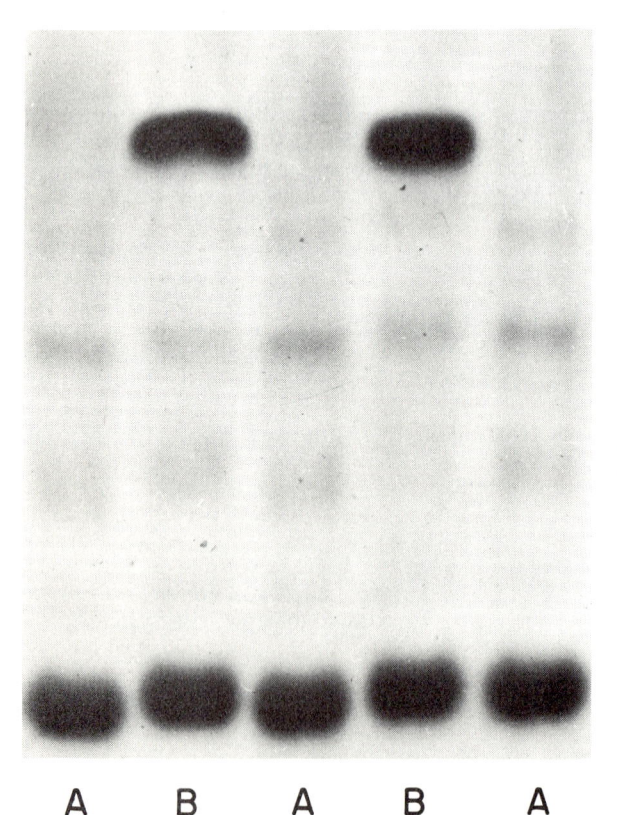

Figure 22–106 Electrophoretic separation of serum proteins on cellulose acetate. A is normal serum. B is abnormal serum containing an M-component located near the cathodal end of the strip in the gamma zone.

also show an increased tendency to develop malignant disease, often a lymphoma. Immune deficiency is a common feature of most of the lymphoproliferative disorders, but whether it precedes the development of the neoplasia or comes as a consequence of it – or both – remains a controversial subject.

Immunoproliferative Disorders

The neoplastic alterations of the lymphoid tissue produce an array of conditions quite distinct from but equally as rich in diversity as the myeloproliferative group of hematologic syndromes. The lymphatic leukemias originate as a disturbance of the primary lymphoid tissue, the bone marrow, with a prominent tendency to infiltrate the circulating bloodstream. The condition spreads to involve lymph nodes, spleen, and indeed many other tissues in the body. The lymphomas are a group of related conditions which affect the secondary lymphatic tissue first with tumor formation which subsequently spreads to the other tissues including the marrow, without much tendency in most cases to release significant numbers of malignant cells into the circulation. The third major group of immunoproliferative conditions, myeloma and primary macroglobulinemia, cause extensive marrow replacement but show little tendency to infiltrate the blood. They do give rise to a high frequency of aberrations of immunoglobulin synthesis.

Chronic lymphatic leukemia increases in frequency with advancing age, whereas acute lymphatic leukemia is mostly a disease of childhood. The terms "chronic" and "acute" were originally descriptive of the clinical courses, but therapeutic advances in the management of the acute variety have narrowed the gap in life expectancy between the two. As a result, the terms are now more indicative of the morphology of the leukemic cell than of the prognosis. The small mature lymphocyte is the hallmark of chronic lymphatic leukemia; the lymphoblast is the sign of the acute variety.

Chronic Lymphatic Leukemia (CLL). Rare in childhood but not uncommon in mature and older adults, two thirds of patients are over the age of 60. There is a 2:1 sex predominance in favor of males. The diagnosis is usually easily made by the observation that large numbers of small mature lymphocytes have accumulated in the blood and bone marrow. In comparison with the normal these lymphocytes are often more friable, have deeper nuclear clefts, and sometimes have more cytoplasm. Immature lymphoid cells are less than 5 per cent of the total. The absolute lymphocyte count in the blood is usually elevated to 10,000 to 150,000 per cu. mm. or even higher at the time of initial diagnosis, although a "subleukemic" (or "aleukemic") variety may be seen in which the cellular infiltration is confined to the marrow. Generalized lymphadenopathy and splenomegaly are common. Lymphocytic infiltration of the liver and of other body tissues increases as the disease progresses. The median life expectancy is about five years, but the clinical course is variable. One fifth of the patients, often those in the somewhat younger age group, are resistant to therapy and die within a year. At the other extreme, one third of patients are still alive after 10 years.

From the pathophysiologic point of view this disorder is better described as an abnormality of cell accumulation rather than one of the cell proliferation. The leukemic cell population is predominantly nondividing and inert. Whether the accumulation represents a breakdown of a normal physiologic mechanism for disposing of those proliferating marrow lymphocytes which are not required for the replenishment of the secondary lymphatic tissue is not known. Immunoglobulins of the IgM type have been detected on the lymphocyte membrane in patients with CLL, suggesting that at least some of these cells may be of B origin. Etiology is obscure, but the rarity of CLL among individuals of Oriental extraction along with a significant occurrence of multiple cases within the families of affected patients suggests that genetic factors are important.

Although years may pass without the occurrence of significant symptoms, many patients have anorexia, fatigue, weight loss, and sweats. Growth of lymphatic tumors may cause mechanical symptoms. Anemia, thrombocytopenia, and granulocytopenia are unfavorable signs and usually indicate impending trouble in any one or a combination of the functions these respective cellular elements fulfill. The most important cause of this cytopenia is the crowding out from the marrow of the normal precursor cells by the closely packed lymphocytes. Massive splenic enlargement may add to the severity of the cytopenia by trapping and sequestering or destroying any one or a combination of the blood cells. About 5 to 10 per cent of patients have an associated Coombs'-positive autoimmune hemolytic anemia, with spherocytosis, reticulocytosis, and erythroid hyperplasia in an otherwise lymphocytic marrow, along with the other usual signs of hemolysis. Death as a result of infectious complications runs high, since the disease fundamentally represents a breakdown in the normal defense mechanism. The susceptibility to infection may stem either from severe neutropenia or from the impediment to the production of circulating antibody. About half the cases show decreased serum immunoglobulin concentrations and about 5 per cent show an M-component in the serum electrophoretic pattern. The abnormal lymphocytes are poorly responsive to mitogenic stimulation with phytohemagglutinin, as would be expected of a B lymphocyte.

The goal of therapy is to relieve symptoms and to improve anemia, thrombocytopenia, or granulocytopenia by reducing the size of the lymphocyte mass. Since cell proliferation is not a prominent feature, chemotherapeutic agents which depend on the DNA synthetic or mitotic phases of cycling cells are not useful. Chemotherapeutic destruction of the lymphocyte mass by alkylating agents (chlorambucil or cyclophosphamide) and adrenal glucocorticoids used singly or in combination are the mainstay of treatment.

Therapy has no doubt decreased morbidity and improved quality of life in CLL, but it seems likely that it has not dramatically increased life expectancy. Although peripheral blood counts often improve, hypogammaglobulinemia is not affected by treatment. The goal is to achieve "control" of the disease rather than "complete remission," as in the acute leukemia, since there is no evidence that added clinical benefit would accrue from the additional therapy that would be necessary.

Acute Lymphatic Leukemia (ALL). Primarily a disease of childhood with peak incidence at the age of four, ALL affects 20- to 30-year-old adults with a frequency about equal to that of acute granulocytic leukemia. Above that age, 90 per cent or more of the acute leukemias are granulocytic. The onset is relatively sudden, with symptoms of anemia, bleeding, or fever. Preleukemic manifestations are absent. Bone pain is not uncommon. The white blood cell count is usually increased, occasionally to values of 100,000 per cu. mm. or higher, with infiltration of the blood with lymphoblasts, but about one third of the cases present with a normal or low white cell count. Anemia and thrombocytopenia are the rule, but immunologic abnormalities are not observed, except inasmuch as they may come later as a result of the immunosuppressive effects of therapy. Intracranial hemorrhage is a life-threatening event, the likelihood of which is increased if severe thrombocytopenia occurs together with extreme elevations of the white cell count. Serum uric acid concentrations often are high, and precautions are necessary to avoid urate nephropathy. Neurologic manifestations due to infiltration of the central nervous system or of peripheral nerves are not uncommon. A slight to moderate degree of lymphadenopathy and hepatomegaly is often present. Many other body tissues also become infiltrated with leukemic cells.

Like CLL, this disease appears to arise in the lymphocytic cells of the primary lymphatic tissue. However, in ALL, slow but unrestrained proliferation of the lymphoblasts crowds out normal blood precursor cells and produces death within a few months from hemorrhage or infection if the condition is not treated. Successful treatment eradicates all visible evidence of malignant tissue and allows the normal marrow cells to repopulate the marrow and to restore peripheral blood counts to normal, a state called "complete remission."

By means of experiments using tritiated thymidine, Mauer and his coworkers in Cincinnati have found that the leukemic cells in patients with ALL do not proliferate in a uniform fashion. There appear to be two pools, one consisting of larger blasts which take up tritiated thymidine and are thus proliferating, while the other is made up of smaller blast cells which do not take up the DNA label and thus are not in a state of proliferation (Fig. 22–107). The cell cycle times of the proliferating leukemic cells generally vary in the range from 3 to 10 days, although some apparently do not divide more often than once every 20 days. The large proliferating blasts predominate in the bone marrow; the small nonproliferating blasts are relatively more frequent in the circulating blood, where they have a relatively short life span with T/2 of about 25 hours. The importance of the nonproliferating pool of leukemic cells lies in its resistance to modalities of therapy which depend on cells being in a state of cycle, i.e., entering phases of DNA synthesis and/or mitosis. These nondividing cells have the capacity to re-enter a proliferative phase after some period of dormancy, suggesting that they may be the bearers of the seeds of relapse, which is such a constant feature of the disease.

Chromosomal abnormalities, usually aneuploidy, are inconstantly present in ALL. They vary from case to case, but seem to remain constant in any given patient throughout the course of the disease. Their relationship to pathogenesis is unknown. Other aspects of cytogenetics and etiology of acute leukemia are discussed in the section on acute granulocytic leukemia.

The following concepts of chemotherapeutic strategy have been developed for the treatment of acute leukemia:

Induction—the initial stage of chemotherapy designed to bring about complete remission in leukemia, i.e., alleviation of the symptoms, restoration of normal blood counts, and a return to a normal bone marrow in which less than 5 per cent of the cells are blasts. In ALL, vincristine and prednisone given together produce complete remission in about 90 per cent of new cases. The two agents act on different phases of the cell cycle, vincristine on the M (mitotic) phase and prednisone chiefly on the G_1 (intermitotic) phase. This example illustrates an important principle which has proved itself in certain other oncologic circumstances, namely, that combinations of agents are more effective and have no more toxicity than when each of the agents is used singly. Meticulous supportive care during induction with such measures as platelet transfusion, protective

Figure 22-107 The labeling of large and small blast cells in a patient with acute leukemia after an injection of tritiated thymidine. The large cells are proliferating and therefore immediately take up the label. Initially, small cells take up no label because they are not dividing. Large blasts, however, become small nondividing blasts, causing a belated appearance of the label in these cells. (Redrawn from Mauer, A. M., et al.: Human Tumor Cell Kinetics. National Cancer Institute Monograph No. 30, p. 71.)

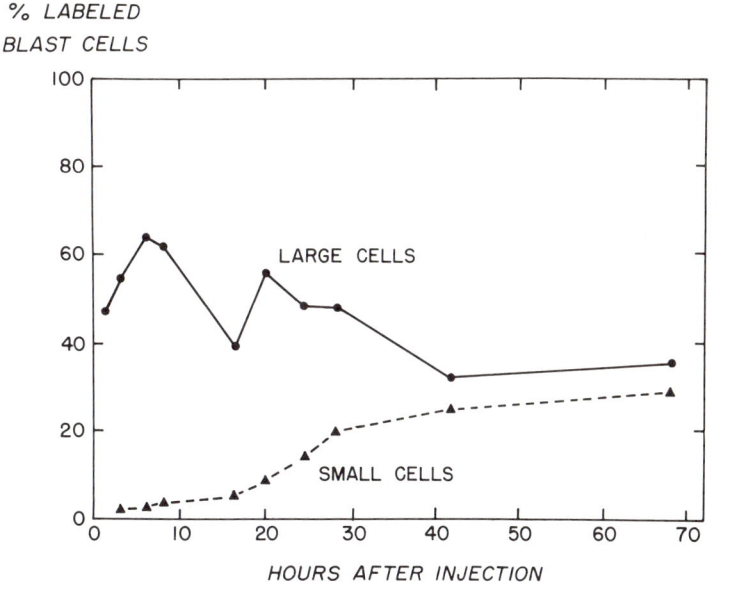

isolation, and the judicious use of antibiotics is important to the attainment of a successful outcome, especially in acute granulocytic leukemia, in which remission is so much more difficult to achieve than in ALL.

Consolidation and Intensification—a relatively intense phase of chemotherapy which may be administered for an arbitrary period of time after the induction of complete remission. The object is to further reduce the number of leukemic cells, already so few that they are clinically inapparent, and thus delay clinical relapse by increasing the number of cell doublings necessary to grow enough leukemic tissue to produce clinical signs and symptoms. During this phase the improved bone marrow function brought about by the remission induction markedly increases the patient's hematologic tolerance to the cytotoxic effects of the chemotherapy.

Maintenance—a prolonged therapeutic effort to maintain the patient in a continuous state of complete remission for as long a time as possible. Without such treatment the remission in ALL lasts only 1 to 4 months. Those patients who relapse sooner after unmaintained remission probably have a shorter leukemic cell cycle time than those who stay in remission longer. Single or multiple agents, given alone or together, continuously, sequentially, or in cycles, have been used. Methotrexate, 6-mercaptopurine, and cyclophosphamide have been particularly useful. Mathé has shown that nonspecific immune stimulation with such agents as BCG vaccine also appears to be effective in maintaining remission.

Reinforcement—the application during the period of maintenance therapy of treatments of the type with which remission was first induced. For example, in ALL, vincristine and prednisone given from time to time during maintenance therapy appear to significantly lengthen remission duration.

Total Therapy—the effort, in addition to all the above stratagems, to eradicate completely hidden nests of leukemic cells which otherwise escape the chemotherapeutic onslaught (see Pinkel reference). The central nervous system is a favorite hideout for such nests, a fact which is amply documented by the 30 to 50 per cent incidence of meningeal leukemia, a complication which almost always arises when the patient is in bone marrow remission. Meningeal leukemia causes symptoms and signs of increased intracranial pressure—headache, nausea and vomiting, and papilledema. Leukemic cells are found in the cerebrospinal fluid along with an elevated pressure, a decreased glucose concentration, and often some elevation of the protein concentration. With the exception of prednisone and the nitrosourea derivatives, chemotherapeutic agents do not readily cross the blood-brain barrier. The response to intrathecal therapy with methotrexate or to irradiation of the craniospinal axis is prompt. Based on the frequency of this complication and on the efficacious nature of the therapy, the most recent addition to the therapeutic strategy in ALL is the prophylactic treatment of this body site, in the hope of eliminating secluded nests of leukemic cells, with either intrathecal chemotherapy or radiation therapy or both.

The development of therapeutic strategy over

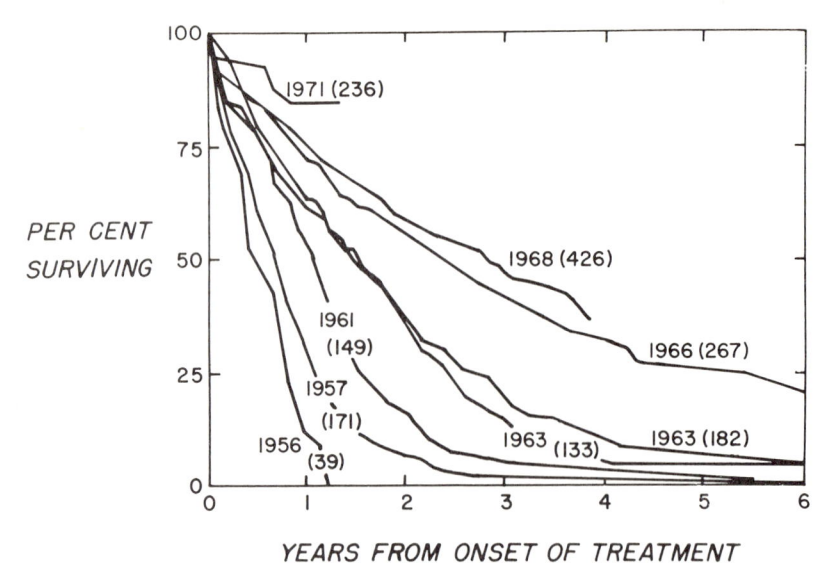

Figure 22-108 Improved survival in acute lymphatic leukemia (patients less than 20 years old) between 1956 and 1971. Improvements in treatment programs have been associated with improved survival. (Data of Acute Leukemia Group B.) (Redrawn from Holland, J. F., and Glidewell, O.: New Eng. J. Med., *287*:770, 1972.)

the years has been paralleled by a progressive increase in life expectancy in children with ALL (Fig. 22-108). In adults with ALL, the results of treatment have not been as good, with the increase in life expectancy having been lengthened from a median of 4 to 6 months to about 18 months.

Malignant Lymphoma, Hodgkin's Type. Noted for its predilection for young adults, Hodgkin's lymphoma makes up about one third of all cases of lymphoma (see Rubin reference). All age groups are affected, a low frequency in childhood rising to about 2.5 cases per 100,000 population in adolescents and young adults. After the age of 50, the frequency increases along with that of other malignant disease. Males predominate 3:2, but females appear to have a better prognosis. In contrast to the other lymphomas, Hodgkin's is more likely to start in the low cervical or supraclavicular lymph nodes and to cause high fever and intense itching. A small percentage of cases arise outside of the lymphatic system. Sometimes it is the cause of fever of unknown origin, even in the absence of apparent external lymphadenopathy.

Often the peripheral blood is entirely normal, but a variety of different changes can be seen. Increases in the granulocyte and platelet counts are not uncommon. Monocytosis and eosinophilia are less frequent. Coombs'-positive acquired hemolytic anemia occurs in occasional patients, but anemia, when it is present, is usually the variety seen with chronic disease. Pancytopenia may be caused by any combination of the factors of bone marrow invasion, hypersplenism, and bone marrow suppression from treatment. One of the most significant findings is absolute lymphocytopenia, a sign of rather advanced involvement of the lymphatic system significantly associated with an impairment of delayed hypersensitivity and other cellular immune responses (see Young et al. reference). The ability to form specific antibody is usually preserved, but the cellular immune defect leads to the occurrence of complicating infections which are often of an unusual nature, such as aspergillosis, moniliasis, and other fungal diseases; *Pneumocystis carinii* infection; and localized or generalized herpes zoster. Rare "epidemics" have suggested that it may be spread as an infectious disease with a low order of contagion, but there is no proof that Hodgkin's disease is caused by an oncogenic infectious agent (see Cole reference).

In contrast to the other lymphomas, Hodgkin's appears to begin in one site and to spread locally from one involved lymph node region to the next nearest group of lymph nodes, accounting for the high cure rate after local treatment and for the better results obtained by "extended field" as compared to "limited field" radiotherapy (Fig. 22-109). The other lymphomas are more likely to be "polycentric" rather than "unicentric" at the time of their origin. With the passage of time, however, the tendency is strong for relentless progression of lymphoma of any type, first within the lymphatic system, and then finally to extralymphatic structures such as liver, bone, lungs, and other organs. The course in any individual patient, however, is sometimes unpredictable.

Histologic classification of lymphoma has been beset by a lack of universally accepted nomenclature. The Lukes-Butler system for Hodgkin's disease has gained a large measure of acceptance, chiefly because it is clinically useful in terms of prognosis and management (Table 22–15). The presence of the Reed-Sternberg cell is a sine qua non for the diagnosis in any of the subgroups. The feature of lymphocytes being preserved or depleted within the lymph node forms the extreme of prognosis. Two intermediate categories, nodular sclerosing and mixed cellularity, have a more favorable and a less favorable outcome, respectively (see Keller et al. reference).

The evaluation by means of physical examination, lymphangiography, and even exploratory laparotomy of the extent of the disease (or "staging") is essential in order to properly design a program of treatment. The stages into which Hodgkin's lymphoma is classified are shown in Figure 22–110. The presence of symptoms increases the probability that the disease is more disseminated. Splenic involvement increases the likelihood that the liver is also involved.

Extended field radiotherapy is the treatment of choice for patients with involvement confined to lymphatic tissue. When extralymphatic structures are involved, chemotherapy is preferred. Combined programs of radiotherapy plus chemotherapy are now under investigation. Although localized palliative radiotherapy is occasionally necessary, the major goal of radiotherapy is the cure of the patient. Chemotherapy has been traditionally considered to offer nothing more than temporary, although often very effective, palliation. Following in the footsteps of the experience gained with acute lymphatic leukemia, the chemotherapy of Hodgkin's disease has recently utilized combinations of agents, rather than single agents, given for a number of months to "induce" remission (see DaVita and Canellos reference). Maintenance therapy appears to be necessary for the most prolonged remissions. The chemotherapeutic agents of greatest value are the alkylating agents (nitrogen mustard, cyclophosphamide, and chlorambucil); the vinca alkaloids (vincristine and vinblastine); the nitrosourea derivatives; procarbazine; and adrenal glucocorticoids. When these principles of chemotherapy are properly applied, as many as 40 per cent of patients with relatively advanced disease are alive and well for five years, a finding that encourages the hope that chemotherapeutic cure may be possible in some cases.

Malignant Lymphoma Other Than Hodgkin's Type. Equally diverse in clinical manifestations and just as obscure etiologically, the non-Hodgkin's lymphomas are sufficiently distinct from the Hodgkin's type that the principles of manage-

Figure 22–109 Survival in patients with localized Hodgkin's disease treated with radical radiation therapy. Most of the deaths and recurrences occurred within 3 years. A similar group of patients not treated radically had a 5-year survival of 35 per cent, but no survivor was free of disease. (Redrawn from Prosnitz, L. R., et al.: Amer. J. Roentgen., 105:618, 1969.)

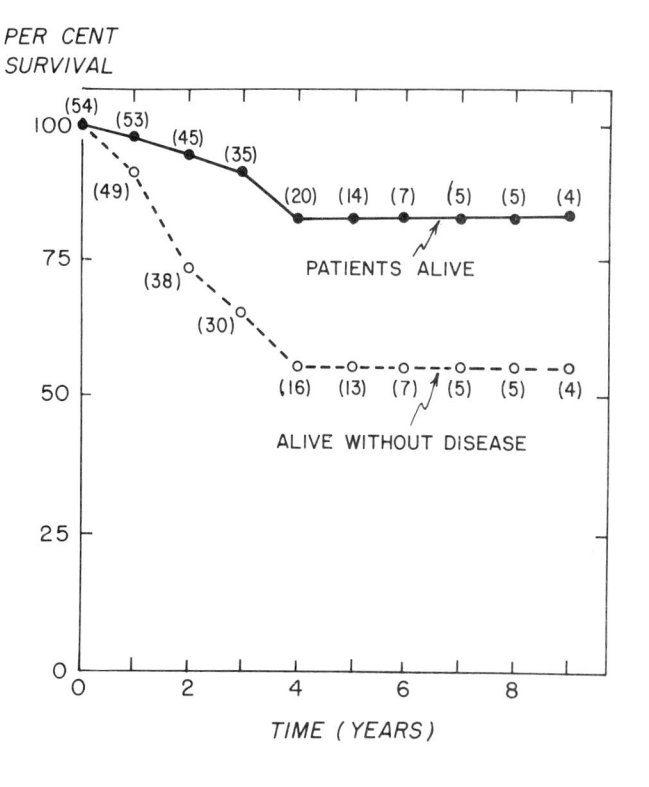

TABLE 22-15 LUKES-BUTLER NOMENCLATURE: HODGKIN'S LYMPHOMA

Subgroup	Median Survival (Years)*	General Histologic Features
Lymphocyte predominant	9.2	Reed-Sternberg cells are seen in the midst of a sea of small mature lymphocytes arranged into a nodular or diffuse pattern.
Nodular sclerosis	4.2	A nodular pattern with the nodules separated by broad fibrous bands containing collagen bundles. The cellular pattern in the nodules may vary considerably, resembling that in any of the other three subgroups.
Mixed cellularity	2.5	A heterogeneous, usually diffuse cellular pattern containing lymphocytes, plasma cells, eosinophils, neutrophils, histiocytes, and fibroblasts, along with Reed-Sternberg cells, sometimes very numerous. Collagen bundles are absent.
Lymphocyte depletion	1.3	Undifferentiated histiocytes (or "reticulum cells") usually predominate in a diffuse pattern; at times Reed-Sternberg cells are very numerous. Fibrous obliteration of the entire lymph node is another variant of this subgroup.

*Lukes, R. J.: J.A.M.A., *222*:1294, 1972.

ment and therapy may differ considerably (see Jones et al. reference). The most important difference is the greater tendency for the disease to be disseminated at the time of initial diagnosis by lymph node biopsy or histologic examination of an adequate piece of tissue from some extranodal site. Indeed, 90 per cent of patients with apparent Stage I or II disease show retroperitoneal node involvement by lymphography. This important point of difference no doubt explains why extended field radiotherapy does not clearly produce better results than more limited fields, as it does in patients with Stage I or II Hodgkin's disease. There is a slight male predominance. Most patients are older than 45 years of age. Systemic symptoms resemble those of Hodgkin's disease, but temperature elevations tend not to run as high. Their presence bears a similar poor prognostic significance.

A time-honored classification much used by clinicians includes three major categories: reticulum cell sarcoma, lymphosarcoma, and giant fol-

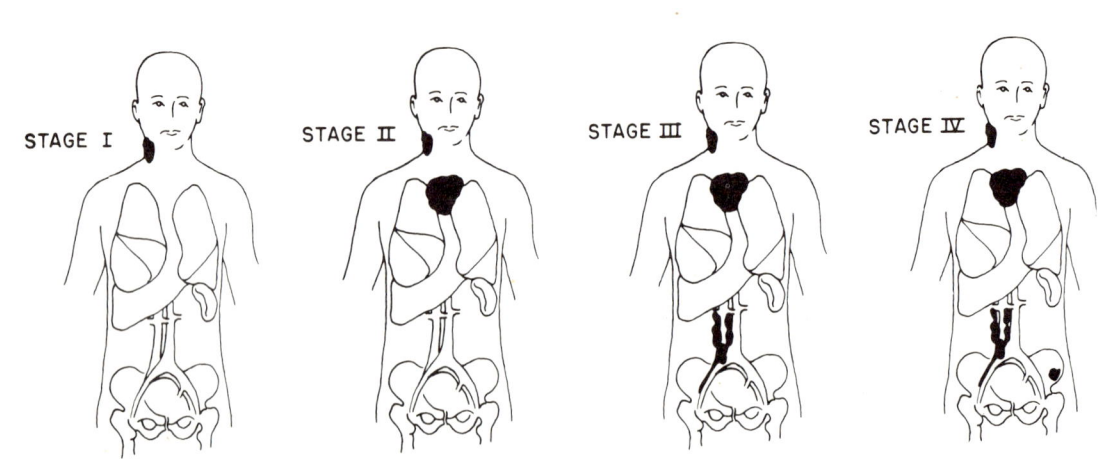

Figure 22-110 Stages of Hodgkin's disease. I to III represent progressively greater degrees of lymphatic involvement, while IV represents spread to extralymphatic structures.

licular lymphoma. This breakdown has been very useful from the clinical point of view because of the prognostic differences between these major groups. However, histologic classification has often proved difficult and even contradictory in some instances. This has been especially true for reticulum cell sarcoma because of the lack of uniform criteria and of a generally accepted nomenclature. The system of Rappaport has gained some measure of acceptance in recent years. This system classifies the overall node architecture as "diffuse" or "nodular" and the predominant cell type as a "well differentiated lymphocyte," a "poorly differentiated lymphocyte," or an "undifferentiated histiocyte." A nodular pattern and a well differentiated cell type are indicators of more favorable prognosis.

A life expectancy of 8 to 10 years is not an unreasonable hope for the majority of patients with giant follicular lymphoma ("lymphocytic, well differentiated, nodular"). The course of this lymphoma, which is the least frequent of the group, may continue to follow a remarkably benign pattern even after the lymphatic system is rather generally involved. Lymph node enlargement may occur in very erratic fashion, first in one body region and then later in another near or distant region. The symptoms are often those of mechanical obstruction or of compression caused by the enlarged lymph nodes. After several years of disease the histologic pattern frequently changes to a less differentiated cytologic type (usually reticulum cell sarcoma). Systemic symptoms intervene, relapses become more frequent, and resistance to treatment increases as the malignant cells spill beyond the confines of the lymphatic system. A fatal outcome is the ultimate rule, despite the initial symptom-free years.

Lymphocytic ("well differentiated, diffuse") and lymphoblastic ("poorly differentiated, diffuse") lymphosarcoma are somewhat less benign, although individual cases may well follow a benign and protracted course. About 50 per cent succumb within two years but 25 per cent are still alive after five years, and a significant number survive well beyond that. Focal or diffuse involvement of the marrow can be demonstrated in about one third of cases. When significant numbers of malignant cells infiltrate the circulating blood, the disorder is called lymphosarcoma cell leukemia, a condition which rather closely resembles chronic lymphatic leukemia. Lymphosarcoma cells have a more immature lacy nuclear chromatin pattern, a folded nucleus, and often irregular cytoplasmic outlines, but the distinction from chronic lymphatic leukemia may be difficult. A lymph node biopsy is not useful in the diagnosis of chronic lymphatic leukemia, but if one is obtained it will show a pattern indistinguishable from that of lymphocytic lymphosarcoma.

Reticulum cell sarcoma ("histiocytic, nodular or diffuse") is the most malignant; 60 to 80 per cent of patients succumb within one year. However, even in this category individual patients not uncommonly defy overall statistics and survive for five years or longer. The tendency for the disease to first become apparent in extranodal sites—especially the gastrointestinal tract and bone—is most striking. Marked weight loss with little overt manifestation of tumor growth, occult hepatosplenomegaly, or an infiltrating tumor of the muscle, brain, or almost any tissue may be the presenting sign. A leukemic phase of the illness occurs much more rarely than in lymphosarcoma.

For the most part pathogenetic mechanisms in non-Hodgkin's lymphomas resemble those in Hodgkin's. Although chronologic patterns of progression may be capricious, spread usually occurs from the lymphatic system to the liver, spleen, and other tissues. Death may be caused by the tumor itself or it may come as a result of infectious complications which follow in the footsteps of the damage done to the immunologic system. Autoimmune phenomena, such as hemolytic anemia or thrombocytopenia, occur in a minority of patients before, concomitant with, or following the first overt sign of lymphoma. About 5 per cent of sera from non-Hodgkin's lymphoma have an IgM or IgG M-component, a finding which is rare in Hodgkin's. Other abnormalities of immunoglobulin production, such as Bence Jones proteinuria or hypogammaglobulinemia, are observed in some patients with non-Hodgkin's lymphoma but not as a rule in Hodgkin's. The several principles of staging and therapy outlined in the management of Hodgkin's lymphoma would hypothetically appear also to represent sound approaches to the patient with non-Hodgkin's types.

M-Component Disorders. An "M-component" is the secretory product of a single monoclonal line of immunoglobulin-producing immunocytes. The abnormal protein is recognized as a narrow homogeneous band or "spike" in the electrophoretic pattern of serum or concentrated urine. It is the product of a cellular clone which has undergone an unusual degree of proliferation, often of a neoplastic character. The absolute production rate of the M-component can be used as a measure of the mass of the abnormal cell line, assuming that each cell produces a fixed quantity of immunoglobulin per unit time. The production rate thus can be estimated from measurement of its concentration and a knowledge of its turnover rate. An imbalance in the production rates of the subunits which combine to make up the immunoglobulin molecule causes overproduction of one of the subunits, usually L chains, which spill out readily into the urine because of their low molecular weight. The L chains, called "Bence Jones protein" in the premolecular era, are either κ or λ in type, but not both, a further demonstration of the monoclonal character of the cell of origin. Excesses of H chains in the serum and urine are a much more seldom observed event.

The presence of these abnormal proteins is sometimes uncovered by sheer diligence on the part of physicians, but increasingly they are discovered accidentally because of the frequency with which serum electrophoresis is used as a routine test. The heat test for Bence Jones protein in the urine is unreliable and should be replaced by electrophoresis of sufficiently concentrated urine. Paper dip techniques in common use for the routine detection of albuminuria are not sensitive to the presence in the urine of other proteins, such as L chains. L chains may be detected in the serum, but since they are so rapidly excreted by the kidney, their concentration is very low unless there is renal insufficiency. The concentration of the serum M-component varies from the range of 1 gram per 100 ml. to more than 10 grams per 100 ml. The daily urinary excretion of L chains may vary from less than 1 gram per day to 15 to 20 grams per day. Immunoelectrophoretic techniques are now in common use to classify the M-components of the serum and urine. Quantitation of immunoglobulins will frequently show depressed serum concentrations of the uninvolved types. The ability to produce specific antibody is often impaired. Recurrent bacterial pneumonia and other infectious complications then appear.

M-components in the serum sometimes confer strange properties upon it which may be of pathophysiologic significance. Reversible precipitation or gelation in the cold (i.e., the M-component is a "cryoglobulin") may cause circulatory embarrassment in exposed body parts. Red cells readily aggregate into "rouleaux," and the erythrocyte sedimentation rate is often rapid, but significant hemolysis usually does not occur. Bleeding may stem from antagonistic effects on plasma coagulation factors, fibrin polymerization, and platelet function. The M-component, especially if it is an IgM type, may increase plasma viscosity by 8- to 10-fold. The "hyperviscosity syndrome" is then prone to develop, with visual disturbances and retinal venous congestion with a sausage-like periodicity of the vein walls ("boxcar effect"), mental confusion, stupor, and even coma. Since the patients are usually aged, prompt recognition is not always achieved. Symptoms are quickly ameliorated by plasmapheresis. The excretion in the urine of large amounts of L chains is significantly related to the development of renal insufficiency, presumably through deposition of L chains as amyloid, as described by Glenner and coworkers. There may be a direct toxic effect of this small protein on the renal endothelial and tubular epithelial cells (see Mogielnicki et al. reference). Hypercalcemia and hyperuricemia also contribute to the multifactorial renal disease which complicates plasma cell myeloma.

Plasma cell myeloma is a malignant proliferation of plasma cells, usually in the bone marrow, sometimes forming solitary or multiple tumors, but almost always going on to widespread dissemination as diffuse "myelomatosis." Destructive bone disease is the major pathologic consequence. Localized osteolytic punched-out lesions affecting the skull, ribs, pelvis, or proximal portions of the long bones, as well as diffuse osteoporosis of the whole skeletal system are common. Extramedullary myelomas may rarely form almost anywhere. Lymphatic involvement is not a feature of the disease, and hepatosplenomegaly is generally not detected. Localized bone pain and pathologic fractures are the most fearsome consequences. Symptomatic hypercalcemia, apparently related to bone dissolution, is common and may require emergency treatment. A mild normocytic and normochromic anemia is common, and about one third of patients have pancytopenia related to replacement of the marrow by the neoplastic plasma cells. Morphologic confirmation of the diagnosis is always necessary, either by biopsy of a plasma cell tumor or by random aspiration of bone marrow. If sheets containing more than 50 per cent plasma cells replace the normal marrow cellular elements, the morphologic picture is diagnostic, but if the plasma cells are fewer, great care must be exercised in morphologic interpretation. Reactive plasmacytosis may increase the marrow plasma cells to 25 or 30 per cent of the total, although usually a reactive plasmacytosis is not in excess of 10 to 15 per cent. "Benign monoclonal gammopathy" and primary amyloidosis must also be distinguished from plasma cell myeloma. Increasing degrees of plasma cell immaturity along with frequent polyploid forms favor the latter diagnosis.

Three fourths of plasma cell myeloma patients have either an IgG or an IgA M-component in the serum, IgG occurring twice as commonly as IgA. Almost all the remaining one fourth who lack such a serum component will have an M-component in the urine, often with decreased serum immunoglobulin concentrations. In all, about one half to two thirds have demonstrable L chains in the urine. Rare cases of IgD and IgE myeloma have been reported, the latter in association with plasma cell leukemia. A few plasma cells are commonly seen in the peripheral blood in myeloma, but overt plasma cell leukemia is a rare and rapidly fatal variant.

Primary macroglobulinemia of Waldenström typically affects older people in their eighth decade. The clinical picture often overlaps that of chronic lymphatic leukemia and lymphosarcoma, in which about 5 per cent of patients have an M-component, usually IgM. The typical presentation of primary macroglobulinemia is one of a dense infiltration of the bone marrow with small mature lymphoid cells, many of which have plasmacytoid features. A number of typical plasma cells may also be seen. There is no leukemic infiltration of the blood; generalized lymphadenopathy and splenomegaly are present but are not marked. The diagnosis is confirmed by demonstrating the presence in the serum of an IgM M-component in excess of 2 grams per 100 ml. L chains may be found in the urine. Anemia is common and may be severe. Pancytopenia is not uncommon. Osteolytic bone lesions are exceptionally rare.

Finding an M-component in the serum or urine alone cannot be considered diagnostic of either of the above immunoproliferative conditions without the assistance of supporting information. The term "benign monoclonal gammopathy" has been applied to those patients with an M-component in the serum, usually less than 2 grams per 100 ml., without decreases in the other serum immunoglobulins, significant abnormalities in blood counts, bone disease, or more than a minority of mostly mature plasma cells in the marrow (see Abramson and Shattil, Michaux and Heremans references). In some instances the M-component spontaneously disappears, suggesting that it may have been evoked as a physiologic but monoclonal response to some undetermined but highly specific antigen. The question of antibody activity of M-components has been recently reviewed by Potter. About 15 per cent of these patients are discovered to have an associated carcinoma. A low concentration of monoclonal IgM occurs with cold agglutinin hemolytic anemia. Amyloidosis is thought to bear some relationship to an underlying process of plasma cell proliferation either of a secondary reactive nature, as in chronic infections, Hodgkin's lymphoma, or rheumatoid arthritis, or of a primary nature (see Cohen reference). M-components and marrow plasmacytosis are thus common findings in primary amyloidosis, the diagnosis of which is most readily confirmed by biopsy of the gum or rectal mucosa. In the absence of these associated conditions, patients with "benign monoclonal gammopathy" commonly remain stable and asymptomatic for many years and require no treatment, but in some instances the condition exists as the asymptomatic preclinical stage of plasma cell myeloma.

Heavy chain diseases are rare, having been first described by Franklin, who observed γ type H chains in the serum and urine of a patient with a lymphoma-like illness. A peculiar variant of H chain disease is the α type, which presents as a lymphoma of the small intestine in association with the signs and symptoms of sprue (see Bonomo et al. reference). The relationship is particularly intriguing because of the known abundance of IgA-secreting plasma cells in the normal gastrointestinal tract.

Therapy of the symptomatic M-component disorders is often successful and may arrest progression of the disease for years (see Alexanian et al. reference). The chemotherapeutic agents of greatest utility have been alkylating agents (melphalan, cyclophosphamide, and chlorambucil) and adrenal glucocorticoids. Palliative radiation therapy is helpful for local bone pain and for such dread complications as spinal cord compression, for which surgical decompression may also be necessary.

THROMBOCYTES

STRUCTURE

In 1906, Wright first proposed that the megakaryocyte, a well-known but mysterious bone marrow giant cell, produced blood platelets. Numerous subsequent morphologic and kinetic studies have supported this proposal and shown that this cell plays a key role in hemostasis. The average megakaryocyte measures about 5000 cu. microns in volume (Fig. 22-6) but cells almost twice that size and with diameters of more than 100 microns are often seen. The megakaryocytes descend from megakaryoblasts, which morphologically are quite similar to other blast cells. The megakaryoblasts first become recognizable as distinct entities when their diameter reaches 20 to 30 microns and their nucleus, because of polyploidy, becomes denser than those of other blast cells. The nucleus divides synchronously without cleavage and forms a lobulated mass containing 2, 4, 8, or even 16 times the normal diploid content of DNA. The basophilic cytoplasm increases proportionally in volume, but visible cytoplasmic maturation does not commence until DNA synthesis and nuclear endoduplication have ceased. When the cell has reached its final ploidy, usually 8 times normal, specific cytoplasmic organelles appear and the cytoplasm takes on a pale blue granular appearance. At this stage the cytoplasm becomes burrowed out by tubular channels forming demarcation membranes and facilitating the final peeling-off of platelets. After the lobulated megakaryocytic nucleus has become depleted of cytoplasm it is rapidly disposed of by macrophages.

As is true for the red blood cells, the newly formed platelets are larger than more mature forms, and careful sizing of blood platelets on a peripheral blood smear may provide information about the rate of platelet production. The mature platelets measure about 2 to 3 microns in diameter and are pale blue with a granular core. On electron microscopy (Fig. 22-111), the core is found to consist of glycogen granules, mitochondria, vacuoles, and various dense particles. The glycogen and mitochondria provide energy essential for viability and function. The vacuoles appear to be part of a spongelike system of in-

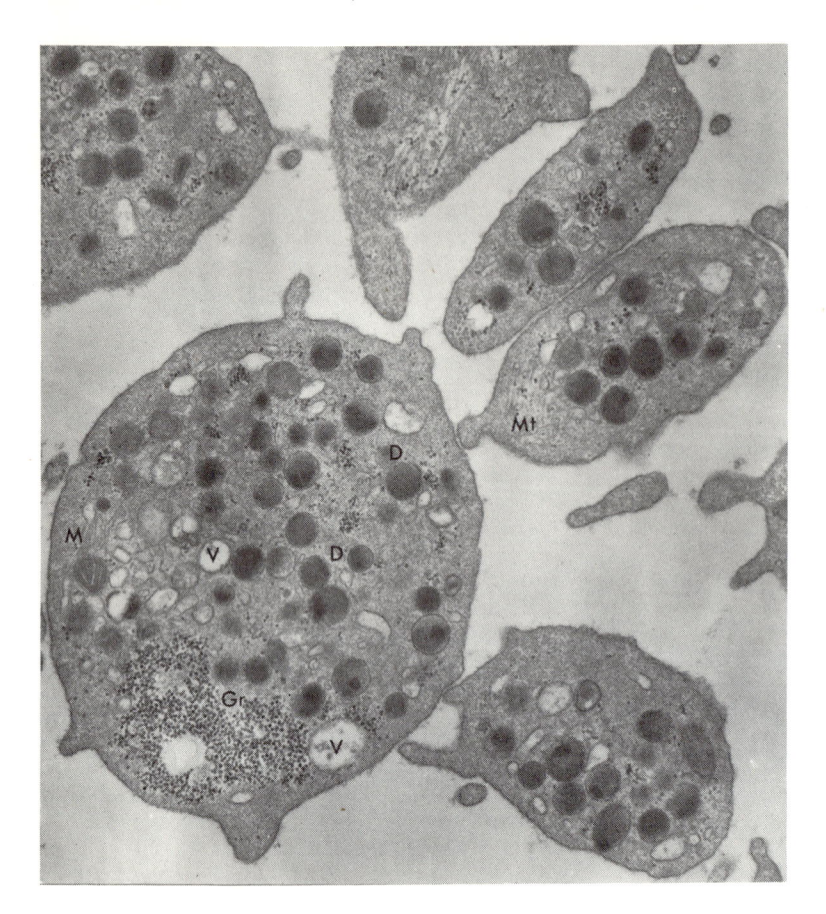

Figure 22-111 Electron microscopic picture of normal platelets showing dense particles (D), vacuoles (V), mitochondria (M), micro-tubules (mt), and glycogen granules (Gr). (Courtesy of Dr. D. Zucker-Franklin.).

teriorized phospholipid-containing surface membrane, facilitating the absorption of and interaction with various coagulation factors. Some of the dense particles are enzyme-containing lysosomes, whereas others contain ADP and serotonin and are released during early aggregation. The platelets also contain a network of microfilaments which are organized into microtubules under the platelet membrane. These structures contain contractible proteins and may be responsible for the change in shape which takes place during aggregation and subsequent clot retraction.

FUNCTION

Platelets constitute our first and foremost line of defense against accidental blood loss. They accumulate almost instantaneously at the site of a vascular injury and attempt first to provide a temporary seal by plugging the vascular leak and then to promote the formation of a permanent seal by releasing an essential coagulation factor. The aggregation of nonsticky, circulating platelets into a firm platelet plug is a remarkable feat which involves the interaction of platelets with collagen fibers and ADP. Observations recently summarized by Zucker have shown that the addition of small amounts of ADP to platelet-rich suspensions in vitro causes a change in the suspension stability, with smooth, disc-shaped granulated platelets being transformed reversibly into an aggregate of spiny, sticky degranulated spheres (Fig. 22–112). Large amounts of ADP will result in an irreversible aggregation of platelets, whereas intermediate amounts cause a characteristic biphasic response with aggregation, disaggregation, and renewed aggregation (Fig. 22–113). The second wave of aggregation is believed to be induced by endogenous ADP from granules extruded during the first wave of aggregation. The addition of collagen to a platelet-rich suspension causes degranulation but only one wave of aggregation corresponding in time to the second ADP wave and believed to be caused by the release of endogenous ADP from platelets. These observations of in-vitro activity provide the framework for our current concept of the mechanism responsible for the formation of a hemostatic platelet plug.

The initiating event in hemostasis is vascular injury with exposure of otherwise concealed collagen fibers to circulating blood. Within a few

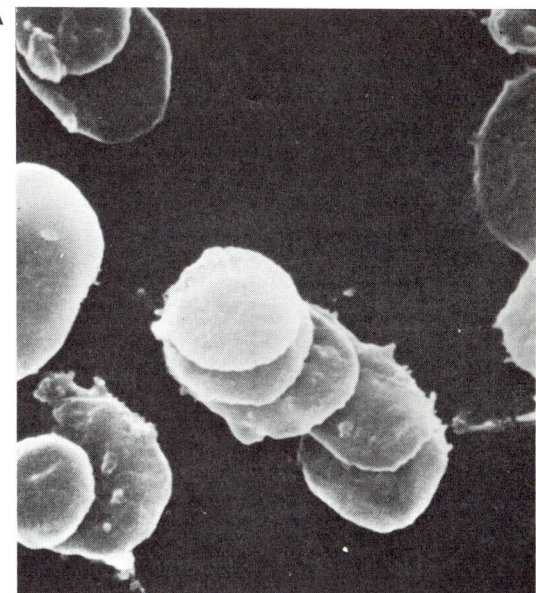

Figure 22-112 Pictures made by the scanning electron microscope of free disc-shaped platelets (A) and aggregates of spiny transformed platelets (B). (From Hovig, T.: Series Hematologica, 3:47, 1970.)

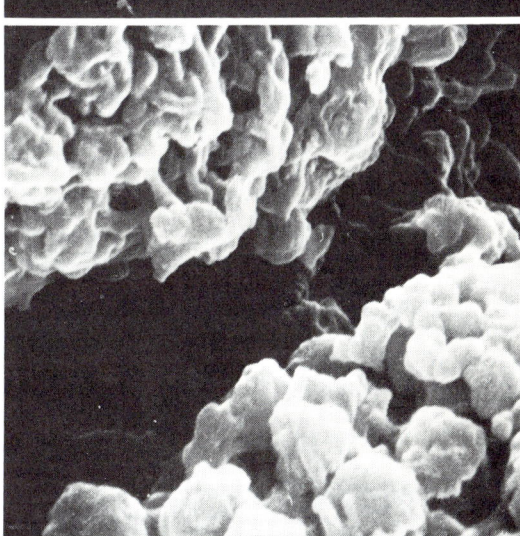

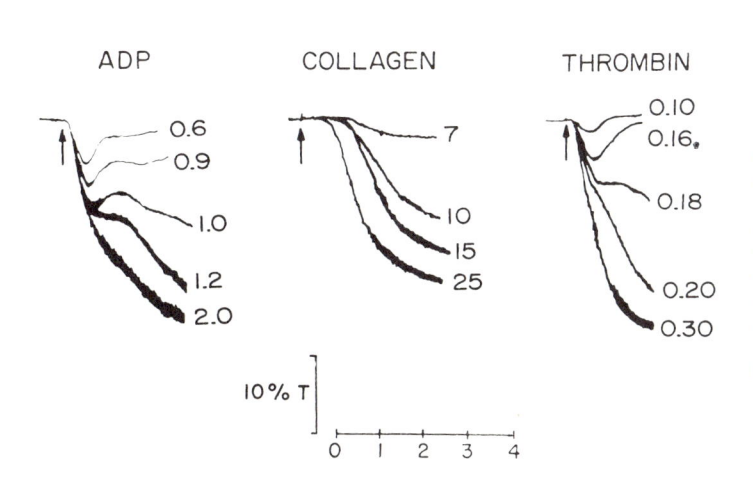

Figure 22-113 Aggregation of human platelets in citrated platelet-rich plasma at 37°C. ADP, collagen suspension, or thrombin was added (arrow) to give the fluid concentrations shown (μ moles/liter, μ liter/ml., or μ/ml., respectively). Photometric recordings indicate the increase in light transmission as the platelets aggregate over a period of about 3 minutes. (Courtesy of Dr. D. C. B. Mills.)

seconds platelets passing by will adhere to the raw collagen fibers, become degranulated, and release ADP, which in turn causes adhesion and aggregation of new platelets, further ADP release, and further platelet adhesion and aggregation. In this fashion a chain reaction is established, with the formation of a firm platelet aggregate covering the vascular break. In addition to ADP, the transformed platelets will release a phospholipoprotein, so-called platelet factor 3, which augments thrombin formation and results in the coating of the platelet plug with resilient fibrin and the formation of a white thrombus. Thrombin also causes platelet aggregation and ADP release and contributes to both the platelet and the fibrin phases in the formation of a hemostatic seal. A certain amount of intravascular coagulation and red thrombus formation takes place before the flow of blood has diluted and dissipated ADP, thrombin, and other procoagulants. Final clot retraction and consolidation are caused by thrombosthenin, a contractile platelet protein. Similar to other contractile proteins, it acts as an ATPase and requires ATP as an energy source. Degranulation during the early phase of platelet adhesion and aggregation will also result in the release of serotonin and lysosomal enzymes which in part are responsible for the inflammatory reaction that may occur around a newly formed thrombus.

In addition to sealing vascular breaks, platelets appear to play an almost continuous role in maintaining normal vascular integrity. Patients with thrombocytopenia have a decreased capillary resistance, and petechiae appear following the slightest extrinsic trauma or intrinsic change in blood pressure. It seems probable that these petechiae are caused by superficial endothelial desquamations which under normal conditions are sealed immediately by platelets but in patients with thrombocytopenia remain open and permit the escape of a small amount of blood.

KINETICS

Until recently, kinetic studies of megakaryocytes and thrombocytes have appeared quite forbidding because of difficulties in quantitating the rate of production of platelets, the size of the circulating platelet mass, and the life span of individual platelets. However, careful planimetric measurements of megakaryocytes in bone marrow sections, the introduction of phase contrast microscopic measurements, automatic particle counting, and the use of random and cohort labeling with various isotopes have provided valuable and reproducible kinetic data. These data indicate that platelet production, like red cell production, is controlled by a feedback system which regulates the transformation of a committed but undifferentiated stem cell to a differentiated blast cell.

As previously emphasized, our current concept of the bone marrow stem cell pool is that it is made up of a multipotential compartment and several unipotential compartments, one of them committed to the megakaryocytic cell line. The interrelationship between these compartments is not clear, but it appears that the multipotential stem cells are predominantly dormant (G_0) and are called into supportive action only if the committed stem cell compartments become depleted. Because increased erythropoiesis after blood loss or hemolysis is often associated with increased thrombopoiesis and under certain conditions with decreased granulocytopoiesis, questions have been raised but not answered about specific cooperation or competition among the committed stem cell compartments. In response to demands for platelets, the stem cells committed to megakaryocytes undergo blast transformation and differentiate to megakaryoblasts. During the next 2 to 3 days and before visible cytoplasmic maturation, the nucleus divides 2 to 4 times, resulting in the formation of a large blast cell with a multilobulated nucleus. After the endomitotic division has ceased, the cytoplasm matures, granulated material segregates, and platelets are finally peeled off 2 to 3 days later. It has been estimated that the normal human bone marrow contains about 6×10^6 megakaryocytes per kg. body weight and that each megakaryocyte produces about 2000 to 7000 platelets. Since the average megakaryocytic volume is about 5000 cu. microns, the total megakaryocytic mass is about 3×10^{10} cu. microns per kg. body weight, about 15 times less than the total mass of nucleated red cell precursors ($5 \times 10^9 \times 90$ cu. microns). Since the mean volume of the platelets is also about 15 times smaller than that of the erythrocytes, it is not surprising that the daily production of platelets, about 2.5×10^9 per kg. body weight, is close to that of erythrocytes, about 3.0×10^9 per kg. body weight.

After the release from the bone marrow, the platelets will circulate for about 8 to 10 days before they are removed and destroyed by the reticuloendothelial tissue, primarily in liver and spleen. During their circulating life span, the platelets are distributed between the spleen and the bloodstream. Aster has pointed out that, at any one time, about one third of the circulating platelets are present in the spleen, probably in a slow transit through the tortuous splenic cords rather than in the form of trapped and starved cells. A transit time of merely 8 minutes would explain such a segregation of the total platelet mass between spleen and blood. It has been proposed that the youngest platelets are sequestered preferentially by the spleen but this may be due to a slower transit time of cells of larger size. Certainly, the sequestration of platelets in the spleen does not appear to last long enough to produce cellular injury, and splenic contraction induced by epinephrine will expel perfectly normal platelets into the circulation. The physiologic significance, if any, of the splenic pooling of platelets is not known, but its existence does explain that the platelet count almost invariably is higher in splenectomized than in normal individuals. In patients with splenomegaly, a significant proportion of the circulating platelets is slowly meandering through the large spleen, and although total platelet mass may be normal, the platelet count can be quite low. This splenomegalic thrombocytopenia is rarely as severe as thrombocytopenia caused by hypersplenic destruction of platelets. However, hemostasis depends on the number of circulating platelets, and if a large spleen cannot mobilize its content of platelets in time, the effect is the same as if the platelets had been permanently destroyed.

Since platelets are consumed during their function as hemostatic agents, it could have been anticipated that their destruction would be random rather than age dependent. In other words, survival curves should be exponential rather than linear with time. Somewhat surprisingly, however, most studies of platelet life span utilizing random labels such as chromium-51 or cohort labels such as phosphorous-32 have indicated an age-dependent linear life span (Fig. 22–114). Furthermore, studies by Abrahamsen of individuals receiving anticoagulants have failed to show a change in the slope of the survival curve or a prolongation of the platelet life span. This would tend to rule out the existence of major continuous intravascular coagulation with random platelet utilization. However, the spread of the survival curve is wide enough to conceal the presence of some minor random utilization in addition to the major age-dependent destruction.

Under physiologic conditions, the platelet count and especially the platelet mass is kept constant, indicating the existence of a feedback system adjusting platelet production to platelet destruction. This feedback has a built-in delay that causes a considerable rebound thrombocytosis after induced thrombocytopenia and rebound thrombocytopenia after induced thrombocytosis (Fig. 22–115). The magnitude of this delay in humans can be estimated from careful measurements of the platelet count in patients who have undergone splenectomy. In such patients the platelet count tends to oscillate, with a period twice as long as the time it takes from the initiation of a signal for increased platelet production until the produced platelets have finished their life span. This oscillating pattern is occasionally very pronounced (Fig. 22–93), making it easy to discern a period which in most cases is quite uniformly about 28 days. Since the life span of platelets is about 10 days, the delay from the triggering effect of a stimulus until the platelet is released from the bone marrow must be around 4 days, which is about the time it takes for the megakaryoblast to mature into a megakaryocyte and release platelets. Either the stimulus could cause the megakaryoblast to undergo additional

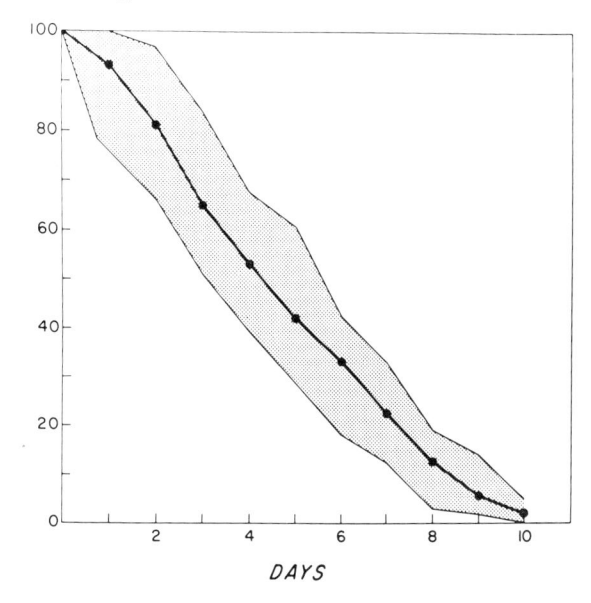

Figure 22–114 Survival of ^{51}Cr-labeled human platelets. Shaded area from 30 normal subjects. (From Aster, R. H.: J. Clin. Invest., 45:645, 1966.)

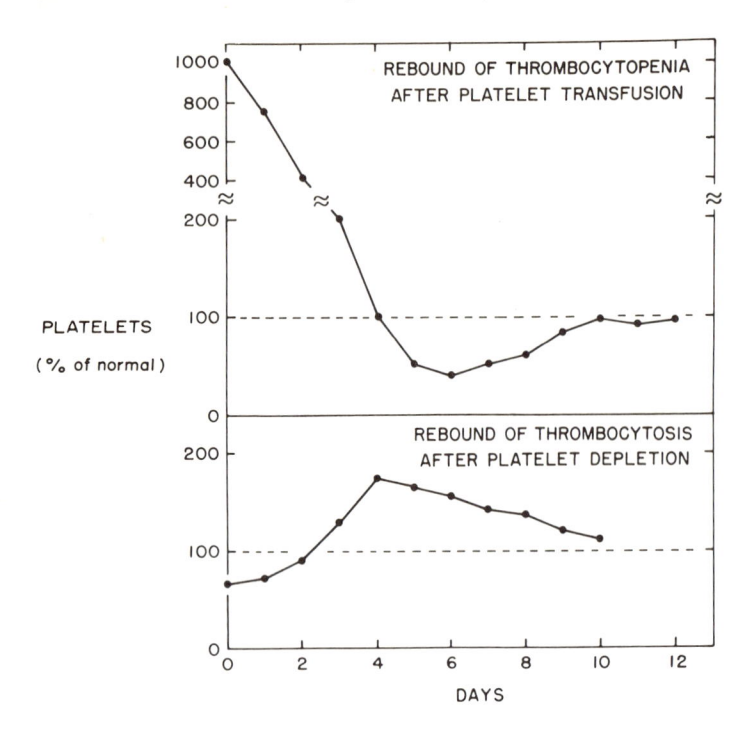

Figure 22-115 Rebound thrombocytopenia after platelet transfusion and rebound thrombocytosis after platelet depletion in normal rats. (Adapted from Odell, T. T., Jr., et al.: Acta Haemat., 38:34, 1967, and Odell, T. T., Jr., et al.: Acta Haemat., 27:171, 1962.)

endomitotic divisions, increase its volume, and produce more platelets, or it could act on committed stem cells and cause the production of an increased number of megakaryoblasts. Since the megakaryocytes of patients with thrombocytopenia due to increased platelet destruction are both larger and more numerous than normal, Harker concluded that the stimulus does both. It has also been suggested that the stimulus shortens maturation time, a suggestion more difficult to accept because the introduction of additional endomitotic divisions should lengthen the total maturation time, unless of course the generation time is cut way down.

Numerous investigators have suggested that the responsible stimulus is transmitted by a specific humoral factor, a so-called thrombopoietin, but it is just recently that Evatt and Levin, and Harker and Finch have provided the first convincing experimental data in support of this suggestion. Utilizing selenium-75 methionine to label megakaryocytic cytoplasm, Levin and co-workers showed that injection into normal animals of serum from donors with thrombocytopenia will cause a greater isotope incorporation into new platelets than injection of serum from normal donors. The difference becomes more pronounced if endogenous thrombopoiesis of the recipient is suppressed by platelet transfusions (Fig. 22-116). Although the technique is similar to the technique which has been used successfully in the study of erythropoietin, the logistic problems of maintaining a preparatory thrombocytosis are so large that very little additional information about thrombopoietin has been obtained.

Since platelets are needed for the maintenance of vascular integrity, it would seem likely that impaired hemostasis causes the release of a thrombopoietin. However, as shown by the age-dependent life span of platelets, most platelets do not get involved in hemostatic activities. Furthermore, hemostatic function remains normal until the platelet count is reduced far below the level at which a compensatory increase in platelet production is initiated. Finally, the patients with congestive splenomegaly in whom up to 80 per cent of the total platelet mass is in the spleen fail to show a compensatory increase in platelet production despite low circulating platelet count and impaired hemostatic function. These observations suggest that it is the platelet mass rather than the platelet count which triggers the release of thrombopoietin. On the other hand, it is very difficult to envision a sensor which can perceive the size of the platelet mass, distributed as it is between the spleen and the circulating blood. It seems possible that rather than being the number or mass, it is the surface area which is involved in sensing and adjusting the concentration of thrombopoietin. The platelet surface is well known to act as a sponge and absorb a variety of plasma factors. Actually, deGabriele and Penington have shown that thrombopoietic activity of plasma could be removed by

Figure 22-116 Effect of plasma upon incorporation of selenomethionine-75 (^{75}SeM) into the platelets of rabbits previously transfused with platelet concentrates. The plasma, in volume from 20 ml. to 150 ml., was administered in three divided doses and ^{75}SeM was given 6 hours after the last infusion (solid lines). The broken line is the mean ^{75}SeM utilization in six platelet transfused control rabbits. (From Shreiner, D. P., and Levin, J.: J. Clin. Invest., 49:1709, 1970.)

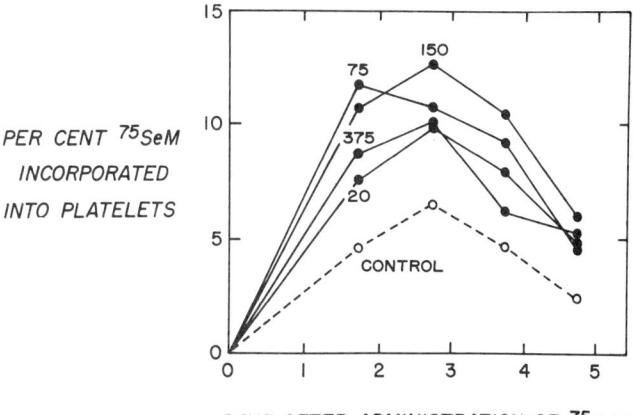

preincubation with normal platelets. Consequently, platelet function, mass, and surface have had to be incorporated into the hypothetical model of the feedback circuit controlling platelet production and depicted in Figure 22-117.

PATHOPHYSIOLOGY

Classification and General Considerations

The thrombocytic disorders are usually classified according to number and function of platelets into "quantitative abnormalities" and "qualitative abnormalities" (Table 22-16).

In general, patients with platelets in inadequate numbers or with inadequate functional competence will have petechiae, hemorrhages, prolonged bleeding time, and impaired clot retraction. Since platelets are primarily responsible for hemostasis in small superficial vessels, petechiae are the hallmark of platelet deficiency disorders. Local pressure from tissue tension will tend to diminish blood loss from deep vessels, and the presence of many petechiae and hemorrhages on the skin or visible mucous membrane does not necessarily mean that similar bleedings are present throughout the body. Actually, deep bleedings into tissues or joint spaces are much more characteristic of a deficiency in coagulation proteins than of a deficiency in platelets. The

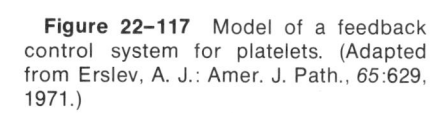

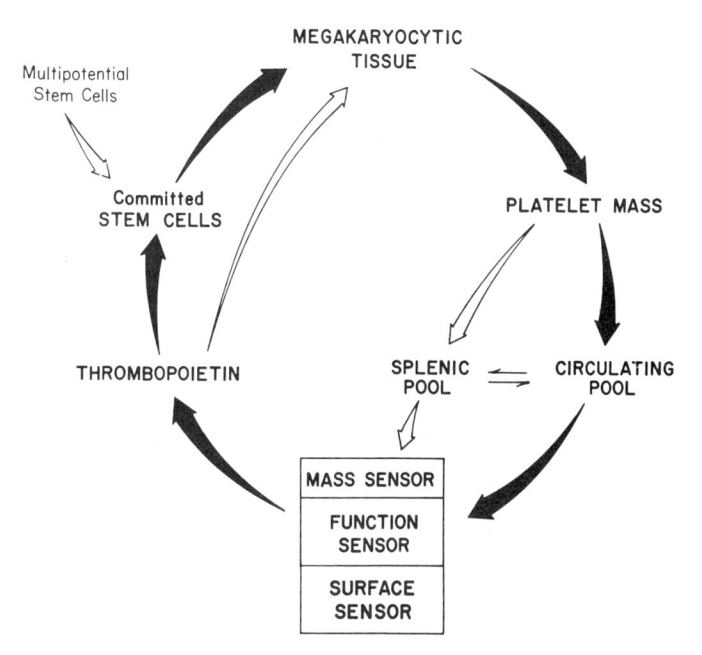

Figure 22-117 Model of a feedback control system for platelets. (Adapted from Erslev, A. J.: Amer. J. Path., 65:629, 1971.)

TABLE 22–16 CLASSIFICATION OF THROMBOCYTIC DISORDERS

I. *Quantitative Abnormalities*
    Thrombocytopenia
        Decreased production
            Congenital
            Acquired
                Megakaryocytic disorders
                Bone marrow replacement
        Increased destruction
            Immune
            Consumptive
        Uneven distribution
            Hypersplenism
    Thrombocytosis
        Reactive
        Myeloproliferative disorders
II. *Qualitative Abnormalities*
    Congenital
    Acquired

---

minimal number of platelets needed for normal hemostasis is usually considered to be about 50,000 per cu. mm. However, spontaneous hemorrhages are rare until the platelet count is reduced to less than 20,000 per cu. mm. Observations by Karpatkin and others indicate that the hemostatic competence of young, large platelets is greater than that of old platelets, explaining that hemorrhagic problems tend to be less at a given platelet level for individuals with thrombocytopenia due to peripheral destruction than for those with thrombocytopenia due to decreased production.

Elevated platelet counts are usually tolerated well but may cause either thrombosis or bleeding. The thrombotic tendency is probably related to an excessive response to minor vascular injury, but the reason for the bleeding tendency in face of an increased number of functional platelets is still unknown.

Quantitative Abnormalities

Thrombocytopenia. *Decreased platelet production* occurs in a bewildering collection of congenital and acquired disorders. In some the pathogenesis has been unraveled but in most the responsible dysfunction of the megakaryocytes awaits identification.

Of special interest among the many descriptions of individual cases is a report by Shulman and coworkers about a child with severe congenital thrombocytopenia who was found to respond to infusions of normal plasma with brief increases in platelet count and who for many years has been kept alive and functioning on regularly spaced plasma infusions. The responsible plasma factor was named thrombopoietin and was found to cause maturation of existing megakaryocytes. Since only one case with a deficiency of this factor has been described, the general physiologic significance of the factor is unknown, but it probably is different from the thrombopoietin believed to control platelet production.

Acquired abnormalities of megakaryocytes causing moderately severe thrombocytopenia are usually found in patients with megaloblastic anemia due to folic acid or B_{12} deficiency, and specific treatment causes a prompt return of platelet count to normal. Patients with chronic alcoholism also may have maturation problems of both nucleated red cells and megakaryocytes, but the cause is difficult to pinpoint, since such patients usually suffer from a multitude of nutritional deficiencies and hepatic abnormalities. Recent metabolic studies by Post and Des Forges have demonstrated that one cause may be alcohol which apparently impairs megakaryocytic function per se. Although iron deficiency has been associated with thrombocytopenia, thrombocytosis is observed far more commonly. If decreased platelet production is found in iron-deficient patients, it is usually assumed that complicating deficiencies of folic acid or B_{12} are responsible.

Viral infections and exposures to certain drugs are often associated with megakaryocytic dysfunction and thrombocytopenia. During pregnancy, such infections and exposures may lead to neonatal thrombocytopenia, usually of short duration. However, if the bone marrow insult occurs during the first trimester, a specific syndrome characterized by amegakaryocytic thrombocytopenia, malfunction of the heart, and absence of the radius may occur. Since the megakaryocytes, heart, and radius all appear at about the sixth to eighth week of gestation, an infectious or toxic insult at that time may explain the development of this seemingly unrelated triad. In both children and adults, viral infections frequently cause thrombocytopenia. For example, inoculation with live measles vaccine will, as Oski and Naiman have shown, regularly cause a temporary decrease in platelet production. As a general principle, a self-limited viral infection should always be suspected as the etiology in every patient with unexplained thrombocytopenia. Despite this frequent association, drugs are actually the most common cause of defective platelet production. The many myelosuppressive agents used in the treatment of neoplastic and autoimmune disorders make up the majority of thrombocytopenic agents. The anticipated response to such drugs is a general bone marrow suppression, but certain drugs such as cytosine arabinoside have a reputation for causing an almost selective suppression of platelet production. More capricious and still unexplained is the megakaryocytic suppression which may follow the use of thiazide diuretics. However, taken in general, drug-induced megakaryocytic injury is a far less common cause for drug-related thrombocytopenias than drug-induced, immunologic destruction of circulating platelets.

Immunologic destruction of platelets can cause thrombocytopenia at any age. In the newborn the pathogenetic mechanism is similar to that causing erythroblastosis fetalis. During pregnancy and at time of delivery, platelets from the fetus pass into the circulatory system of the mother, and if they contain antigens different from hers, they will evoke an antibody response. The subsequent transfer of the antibody across the placenta results in platelet destruction and thrombocytopenia. Such isoimmune thrombocytopenia does not depend on ABO or Rh incompatibility but on incompatibility in the HL-A tissue antigen system. Since tests for antigens and antibodies in this system are time-consuming and difficult, the diagnosis is usually made by exclusion. First, thrombocytopenia due to infections has to be ruled out immediately. Maternal viremia can cause changes in the fetal production and destruction of platelets, and bacteremia in the newborn may be associated with disseminated intravascular coagulation and thrombocytopenia. Second, thrombocytopenia due to transfer of the antibody characterizing idiopathic thrombocytopenic purpura has to be excluded by obtaining a platelet count and a thorough history from the mothers.

In children and adults, the cause for immunologic rejection and destruction of platelets is usually idiopathic, but the possibility that it is drug related should always be considered. Quinidine and Sedormid are the most widely recognized offenders, and their mechanism of action is slowly being unraveled. When attached to a protein these drugs act as haptens, causing the production of antibodies in sensitized individuals. It was first assumed that the hapten attached itself to a platelet protein and that this hapten-platelet complex elicited and responded to antibody. However, recent data suggest that the hapten is bound to a plasma protein carrier and that it is this complex which elicits and combines with antibody. The subsequent binding of the antigen-antibody complex to platelet membrane is due to a chance affinity between the complex and the membrane, and the platelet is actually an "innocent bystander" in the immunologic reaction (Fig. 22–118). Unfortunately for the platelets the coating with antigen-antibody complexes causes agglutination, complement-fixation, and destruction. A great number of drugs have been implicated in immunologic platelet destruction but only in a few instances have in-vivo and in-vitro testing convincingly shown a drug to be causa-

Figure 22–118 Possible mechanism for drug-induced and other immunologic thrombocytopenias. *Left,* the platelets are directly involved by initially being coated by antigen. *Right,* the platelets act as "innocent bystanders." (From Shulman, N. R.: Ann. Intern. Med., 60:506, 1964.)

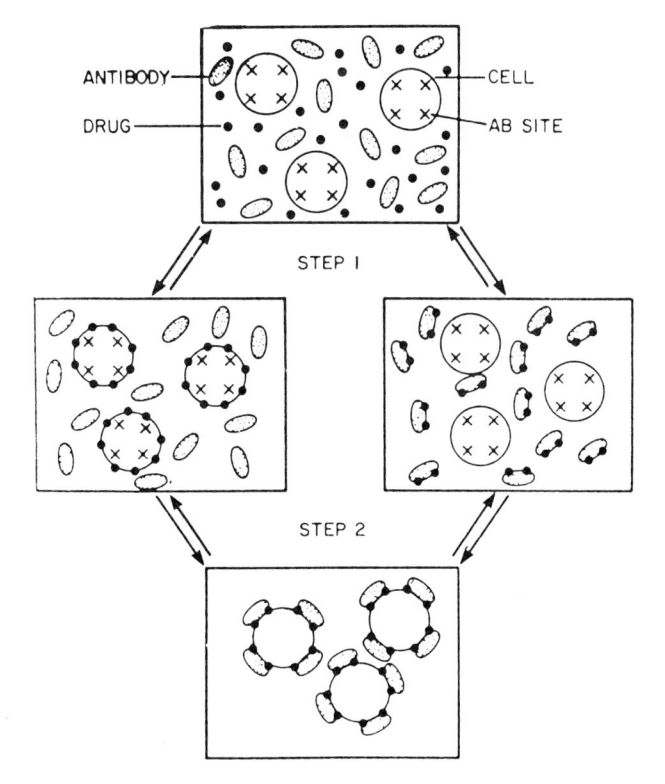

tive. In addition to Sedormid and quinidine, quinine, stibophen, digitoxin, methyldopa, sulfonamides, and gold have been so identified. The association of aspirin or birth control pills with thrombocytopenia has been of interest, but the possibility of a mere coincidence rather than a cause-effect relationship has not been ruled out. Recently, it has been suggested that the thiazide diuretics which cause megakaryocytic hypoplasia may do so through an immunologic process of rejection, similar to the immunologic rejection of nucleated red cells observed in patients with pure red cell aplasia. In order to establish a diagnosis of drug-induced thrombocytopenia several in-vitro tests have been developed. These are based on finding impaired platelet function after the addition of the drug to the patient's plasma. Inhibition of normal clot retraction is the easiest test, but it probably is less sensitive than tests depending on agglutination, lysis, complement fixation, or release of platelet factor 3.

Idiopathic thrombocytopenic purpura (ITP) is a disorder characterized by increased platelet destruction in an otherwise healthy individual. In childhood, ITP is usually acute and time-limited, and many studies have related it immunologically to a preceding viral infection. In adults, ITP is usually chronic and, although also believed to be immunologically determined, its etiology is still truly idiopathic.

Acute thrombocytopenia may follow well-established viral infections such as rubella, rubeola, or chicken pox, but in most cases the preceding illness consists merely of a mild respiratory or gastrointestinal upset, so frequently experienced in childhood that it is often overlooked. The thrombocytopenia is usually first noticed after the "viral symptoms" have subsided, suggesting that the platelet injury is caused by antibodies rather than by the virus itself. It has been proposed that platelet antibodies are elicited by platelet membranes antigenically altered by the attachment of viral particles. However, similar to the mechanism believed to operate in drug-induced thrombocytopenia, the platelets may merely be "innocent bystanders" with a fatal affinity for viral antigen-antibody complexes. In either case, the antibody production and action would depend on the presence of a circulating viral antigen, and the disease would be of limited duration. Complete recovery can be expected if the patient is carried through the dangerous thrombocytopenic period by the judicious use of careful observation, protection against trauma, platelet transfusions, and corticosteroids. Splenectomy, although undoubtedly effective, need rarely be contemplated in the acute time-limited ITP of childhood.

The chronic variety of ITP is a disease of adults, although children who fail to recover from acute ITP must be included. Like acute ITP, it is believed to be immunologically induced, but if a foreign antigen is involved, this antigen must be an almost permanent component of the body, since the disease despite remissions is rarely cured.

The immunologic nature of this disorder was first suspected when Harrington and coworkers found that plasma or its gamma globulin fraction from patients with chronic ITP caused thrombocytopenia when infused into normal subjects. Supportive evidence for the existence of an autoimmune mechanism was provided by the fact that infants of mothers with chronic ITP often have transient thrombocytopenia at birth and that in-vitro immunologic tests indicate the presence of an antiplatelet antibody in plasma from a large number of patients with chronic ITP. So far the antibody has reacted with all platelets, regardless of antigenic composition, and it appears that it is directed against a common platelet component rather than a specific HL-A antigen. The agent responsible for the production of autoantibodies is unknown, but the lifelong presence of certain viral antigens in tissue cells makes a viral etiology an attractive hypothesis.

The severity of chronic ITP and its response to splenectomy seems to be dependent on the amount of antibody coating the platelets. Heavy coating will cause agglutination with easy recognition, sequestration, and destruction by all reticuloendothelial tissues in the body, and splenectomy by removing merely a fraction of these tissues will be of only moderate therapeutic benefit. Light coating, however, will not cause significant agglutination of circulating platelets, and only the spleen with its slow percolation of blood through vessels densely lined with reticuloendothelial cells will recognize and sequester coated platelets. In this condition, splenectomy will be of definite benefit, and the life span and function of lightly coated platelets will be almost normal after surgery. In a few cases the titer of antiplatelet antibodies has decreased after splenectomy, suggesting that the spleen preferentially produces these antibodies and that splenectomy not only removes a filter but also eliminates a major site of antiplatelet antibody production.

One of the most controversial findings in chronic ITP has been the presence of megakaryocytes of unusual morphologic appearance. Not only are they increased in number, as would be expected as a compensation for increased destruction of mature platelets, but they are also immature, are devoid of intracytoplasmic demarcations, and show no evidence of active platelet production (Fig. 22–119). It has been suggested that the antibody to circulating platelets also reacts with megakaryocytes and prevents platelet formation. However, platelet turnover studies show an increased rate of platelet production, and it seems more likely that accelerated thrombo-

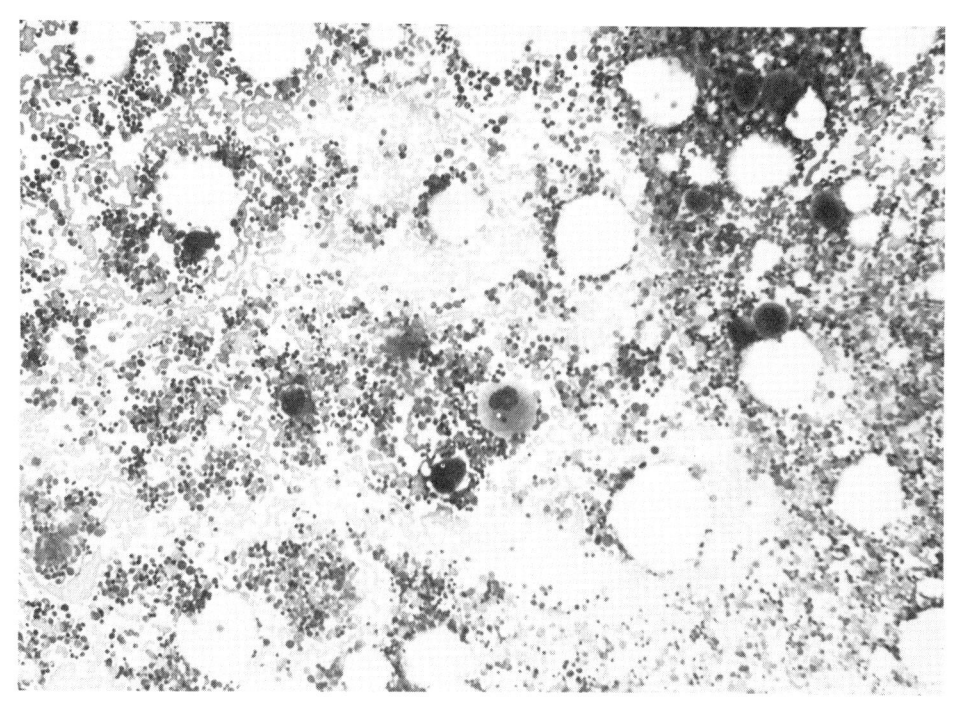

Figure 22-119 Megakaryocytic hyperplasia in patient with chronic ITP.

poietic activity causes an early release of platelets from still immature cells and a shift to the left in the megakaryocytic series. The presence of unusually large platelets in the blood of patients with chronic ITP also suggests a hurried production with the release of unfinished pieces of megakaryocytic cytoplasm.

The clinical manifestations of chronic ITP are determined entirely by the number of available platelets, and the treatment is directed toward maintaining the number at an asymptomatic level. As expected, platelet transfusions are of very brief effect, since transfused platelets are destroyed as fast as endogenous platelets. Adrenocortical steroids are usually quite effective in increasing the platelet count in patients with chronic ITP. They may act by suppressing phagocytic activity, but the exact reason for their beneficial effect has still not been established (see Claman reference). In patients who do not respond to steroids with an increase in platelet count, the bleeding manifestations are nevertheless reduced, as if the steroids in some way enhance capillary stability. In the treatment of chronic ITP, steroids are usually administered for a few months in the hope that the disease will remit spontaneously. If the thrombocytopenia recurs immediately after discontinuation of the drug or if the patient is only partly responsive, splenectomy is the treatment of choice. Splenectomy will result in a sustained improvement in 70 to 90 per cent of patients. In almost all, the operation will be followed by a brief thrombocytosis which reaches its peak at about the tenth day and then slowly decreases over the next few months (Fig. 22-120). This sequence corresponds well to the fact that in the absence of the spleen the platelets produced by the increased number of megakaryocytes live a normal 10-day life span, and it suggests that it must take some time to adjust the number of megakaryocytes in the bone marrow to the actual need for platelets in the circulation. Postsplenectomy thrombocytosis is of concern in patients in whom postoperative complications force them to rest immobile in bed, and in such patients the use of preventive anticoagulants may be indicated. It is assumed that platelets of patients who do not derive lasting benefit from splenectomy are so heavily coated with antibody that they are removed by all reticuloendothelial organs, not merely the spleen. In such patients, immunosuppression has been attempted using drugs developed for the treatment of neoplastic disorders. In some patients gratifying remissions have been obtained, but the decision to use these potentially leukemogenic agents certainly has to be made with great reluctance and only if other methods of treatment fail.

Nonimmunologic destruction of circulating platelets in bacterial or viral infections is often difficult to separate from immunologic destruction since these infections may be associated with

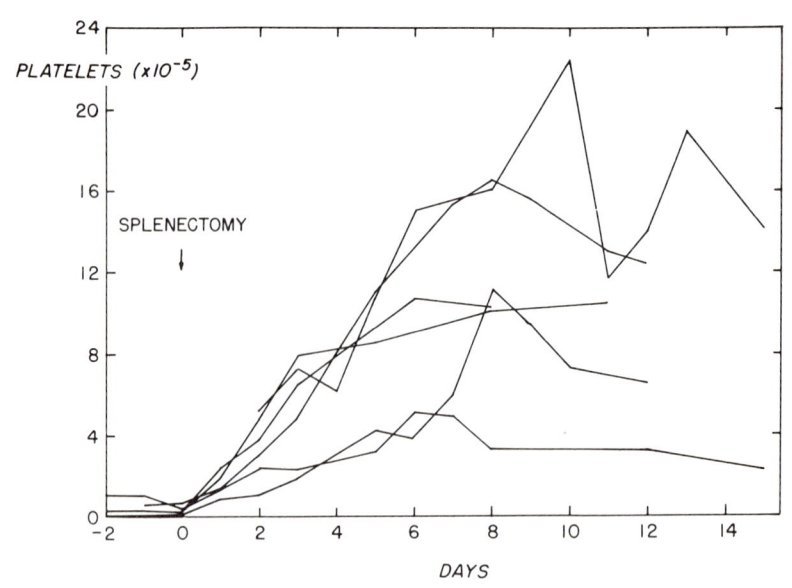

Figure 22–120 Thrombocytosis following splenectomy in patients with ITP.

both. However, nonimmunologic destruction usually occurs at the height of the infectious illness and is accompanied by decreased levels of several coagulation proteins such as fibrinogen and Factors V and VIII. The pathogenesis is believed to be increased platelet consumption due to disseminated intravascular coagulation (see Deykin reference). The thrombocytopenia characterizing "thrombotic thrombocytopenic purpura" or the "hemolytic uremic syndrome" is probably also caused by excessive intravascular coagulation. The fibrin deposits in the microvasculature are probably responsible for the specific manifestations of these syndromes by causing red cell destruction and embolization of cerebral and renal vessels. Despite the presence of purpura and increased bleeding tendency, heparin is the treatment of choice whenever laboratory studies indicate an increased rate of consumption of platelets and coagulation proteins.

Thrombocytopenia is observed regularly in patients with splenomegaly, and in the past many explanations were given for the development of this hypersplenic thrombocytopenia. The most obvious explanation for the thrombocytopenia would appear to be increased platelet destruction by the large spleen, but this explanation was made untenable some years ago when Cohen, Gardner, and Barnett found that the platelet life span in patients with hypersplenic thrombocytopenia was normal. The alternate explanation, that platelet production was decreased owing to the effect of megakaryocytic inhibitors released by the large spleen, was also found to be untenable because platelet turnover studies did not suggest a decreased rate of platelet production. Recent studies by Aster of platelet kinetics have provided a third and much more likely explanation.

As described earlier, the spleen, because of its tortuous vascular channels, always contains a considerable number of platelets in slow transit. In patients with splenomegaly, the transit time becomes longer, and instead of containing about 30 per cent of all circulating platelets, a large spleen may contain up to 80 per cent of the platelets. Since platelet production appears to be aimed at maintaining a constant total platelet mass, the uneven distribution of platelets between spleen and circulating blood is not being compensated for by an increased rate of platelet production, and the hypersplenic patient will stay thrombocytopenic. This explanation is supported by the observation that the infusion of platelets to patients with hypersplenic thrombocytopenia results in lower peripheral recovery than normal (Fig. 22–121) and that large numbers of viable platelets can be mobilized from an intact spleen by giving epinephrine and from an excised spleen by flushing its vascular system with saline. Supporting evidence is also provided by the fact that hypersplenic thrombocytopenia is not always proportional to the size of the spleen but is more closely related to its vascularity. For example, congestive splenomegaly secondary to liver cirrhosis is usually associated with lower platelet counts than "meaty" splenomegaly secondary to lymphomas or lipidosis. The potential

Figure 22-121 Recovery of transfused platelets in the circulating blood of asplenic patients, normal patients, and patients with congestive splenomegaly. (Gardner, F.: Clin. Haemat., 1:307, 1972.)

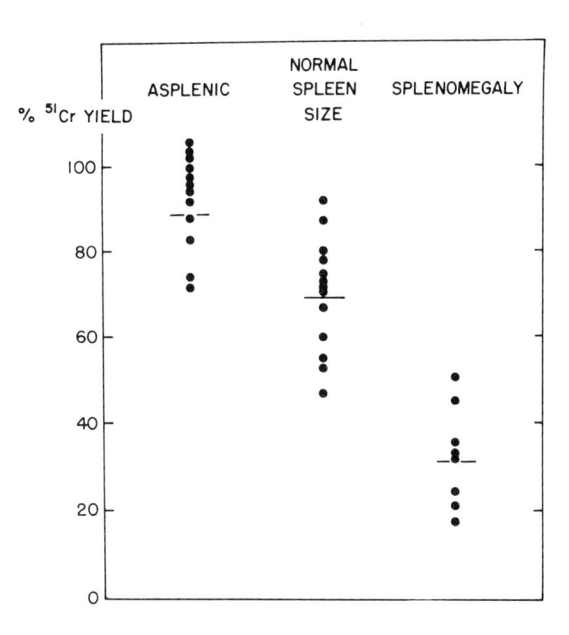

availability of splenic platelets and the distributional limits to the number of platelet which can be present in the spleen make this thrombocytopenia rather mild and rarely in need of treatment per se.

Thrombocytosis. Thrombocytosis occurs as an obscure reactive response to a number of illnesses and as a manifestation of the myeloproliferative syndrome. A high platelet count is a useful diagnostic clue in patients with anemia, since iron deficiency regularly causes an increase in platelet production, and counts in excess of one million per cu. mm. may be found in children with nutritional iron deficiency anemia. Other conditions in which a high platelet count may be of diagnostic help are Hodgkin's disease, disseminated malignant diseases, and chronic inflammatory disorders. (See Schloesser et al., Levin and Conley, and Marchasin et al. references). Pronounced thrombocytosis with levels of several millions per cu. mm. is usually seen only after splenectomy or in myeloproliferative disorders, such as polycythemia vera, myelosclerosis, chronic myelogenous leukemia, or essential thrombocytosis. The clinical manifestations of very high platelet counts consist of a capricious combination of thrombotic episodes and increased bleeding tendency. The thromboses are probably caused by aggregation and platelet factor 3 release by the expanded platelet mass, but the bleeding tendency is more difficult to explain. Cardamone and coworkers have found a platelet dysfunction in some cases, but in most cases the only abnormality found has been an increase in the number of circulating platelets.

Qualitative Abnormalities

Qualitative abnormalities of platelet function have been found in a confusing collection of rare hereditary disorders and more commonly in uremia or after ingestion of aspirin. The congenital disorder most often reported has been named Glanzmann's thrombasthenia and is characterized by a prolonged bleeding time, impaired clot retraction, and absent ADP-induced aggregation. The number and morphology of platelets and megakaryocytes are normal, but the patients suffer from a mild, lifelong increased bleeding tendency. Impaired platelet glycolysis with decreased ATP production and decreased reductive capacity have been found in some cases (see Karpatkin and Weiss reference), whereas in others the adsorption of fibrinogen to platelets appears to be defective. The so-called thrombopathies are congenital platelet disorders with even less of a common metabolic denominator than the thrombasthenias. The platelets may be defective in platelet factor 3 activity, in ADP release, in adhesive capacity, and so on, but so far the cases are collectors' items and have failed to provide unifying clues.

Of the acquired disorders of platelet function, the clinically most important is the disorder found associated with chronic renal failure. Purpura and increased bleeding tendency are important manifestations of uremia and occur regularly despite normal platelet counts. Platelets from affected individuals have been found to be lacking in platelet factor 3 release. However, of probably greater significance is the finding that these platelets fail to aggregate normally in response to ADP. Intensive dialysis rectifies this response and also normalizes the bleeding time, and it seems most likely that a retention product of small molecular size is responsible for the platelet defect. Horowitz has proposed that this chemical is guanidinosuccinic acid, a metabolite of urea, but definite proof is still lacking. The effect of aspirin on in-vitro platelet function is quite remarkable. The ingestion of only one to two aspirin tablets will cause a week-long impairment in the release of platelet ADP in response to collagen or other aggregating agents. Recent studies by Smith and Willis suggest that this impaired ADP release may be caused by irreversible aspirin-induced inhibitors of the synthesis of platelet prostaglandin E-2. Although aspirin clinically has been associated with an increased bleeding tendency, it must be conceded that bleeding problems are rare among the millions who daily consume aspirin preparations and that the striking in-vitro changes cause in-vivo hemorrhages only rarely.

HEMOSTASIS: PLASMA COAGULATION FACTORS

NORMAL STRUCTURE AND FUNCTION

The circulatory system is self sealing, thanks to the clotting ability of the blood and the contractility of the vascular wall. Leakages ranging from pinpoint hemorrhages to life-threatening exsanguination may occur when the coagulation mechanism breaks down. On the other hand, the pathologic formation of clots within the intact circulatory system is equally serious. The cause and nature of clot formation within the circulatory system vary with the site. The "white thrombus," consisting of platelets enmeshed in a fibrin meshwork, forms in rapid-flow arterial systems at points where the continuity of the endothelial lining is interrupted. The "red thrombus" has a white head with growth downstream of a red tail and is found in the venous system as a result of stasis of blood flow. Clots in large vessels are likely to undergo fibrous organization and recanalization, whereas those formed in the microvasculature are dissolved by virtue of the presence in the vascular wall of potent activators of the fibrinolytic system.

Although platelets are the "prime movers" in the formation of the white thrombus, the substance and strength of the clot, whether white or red, lie in the physical nature of the fibrin polymer which is formed as the end-product of a complex and controlled series of sequential reactions of the plasma coagulation factors. The no-

TABLE 22-17 PLASMA COAGULATION FACTORS AND THEIR SYNONYMS

Factor I	Fibrinogen
Factor II	Prothrombin
Factor III	Tissue thromboplastin
Factor IV	Calcium
Factor V	Proaccelerin
Factor VII	Proconvertin; SPCA
Factor VIII	Antihemophilic globulin (AHG)
Factor IX	Plasma thromboplastin component (PTC), Christmas factor
Factor X	Stuart-Prower factor
Factor XI	Plasma thromboplastin antecedent (PTA)
Factor XII	Hageman factor
Factor XIII	Fibrin stabilizing factor

menclature of the plasma coagulation factors has undergone revision over the years. Current and past usage is summarized in Table 22–17. Factors V and VII through XIII are in fact most commonly designated by their numbers today, while Factors I and II are generally called fibrinogen and prothrombin, respectively. There is no Factor VI. Factor III is tissue thromboplastin and should not be confused with platelet factor 3.

The cascade (or "waterfall") concept of clotting, as proposed by Davie and Ratnoff and by MacFarlane, has marvelously enhanced our ability to comprehend this complex series of reactions. Succinctly stated, this hypothesis conceives of coagulation factors existing in an inactive (or procoagulant) and an activated state. The activated form of one factor specifically activates the next one in the sequential series, with a progressive amplification of the effect culminating in the formation of the fibrin clot. But coagulation, like other biological systems, does not consider consistency a virtue, and the cascade hypothesis may well not apply to all the plasma factors, as will be subsequently discussed.

Fibrinogen, the raw material for the production of the clot, is a major constituent of the plasma, with a normal concentration of 200 to 400 mg. per 100 ml. The other plasma factors, present in much lower concentration, stand poised as a loaded gun with trigger cocked, aimed at fibrinogen. Most of the body pool of fibrinogen circulates in the plasma with a catabolic rate having a half-life of four days. The plasma concentration readily increases secondary to a large number of stimuli, including pregnancy, acute or chronic inflammatory states, and injury or surgical operation. The increase is entirely accounted for by increased synthesis, which takes place in the liver.

Among the plasma clotting factors, the structure of fibrinogen is best understood. Its molecular weight of about 340,000 is equally divided between two identical subunits with their like ends bound centrally together, giving the molecule a symmetrical mirror-image structure (Fig. 22–122). Each of the subunits consists of an alpha, a beta, and a gamma polypeptide chain, the N-terminal ends of which are found at the ends of the symmetrical molecule. The C-terminals occupy the center. Disulfide bonds connect the polypeptide chains together, thus forming an "N-terminal disulfide knot" at either end of the molecule. The appearance of thrombin on the scene causes polymerization with the formation of a long fibrin strand. Thrombin acts enzymatically on fibrinogen at arginyl-glycyl bonds by splitting off small pieces from the ends of the alpha and beta chains amounting to about 3 per cent of the total molecular weight. The pieces split off are called fibrinopeptides A and B, respectively. Their cleavage from the parent molecule leaves behind "fibrin monomer," which then rapidly undergoes intermolecular association to form hydrogen-bonded polymers. The clot is finally strengthened by the action of Factor XIIIa ("a" is used to designate the activated form of the procoagulant) (see Schwartz et al. reference). This causes strong side-to-side linkage between adjacent fibrin threads through crosslinking peptide bonds which join alpha to gamma polypeptide chains in an intermolecular association. Such "stabilization" renders the clot insoluble in 5 M urea.

Certain snake venoms resemble thrombin in their action on fibrinogen. Pit viper venom hydrolyzes only the alpha polypeptide chains, releasing fibrinopeptide A. The parent molecule, like fibrin monomer, polymerizes into a clot. However, the clot is weak and is readily dissolved through the action of plasmin.

In contrast to the limited fibrinogen degradation which sets off its polymerization into a firm clot, the degradative process of clot dissolution by plasmin involves a much more aggressive attack upon the molecule at multiple points in its structure. Plasmin (or "fibrinolysin") is an enzyme which resembles trypsin in its breadth of action as an endopeptidase which splits lysine and arginine bonds. Like trypsin, it attacks a variety of proteins, including plasma proteins. It is active at neutral pH; trypsin has a more alkaline pH optimum. The circulating plasma proteins are not physiologically exposed to its broadly destructive propensity, since it circulates as an inactive precursor, plasminogen, which is activated locally at the site of clot deposition. Plasmin attacks fibrinogen with the same fervor that characterizes its assault upon fibrin. The degradation products of the two cannot be distinguished and therefore are referred to as fibrinogen-fibrin degradation products, or "split products."

In the first stage of fibrinogen degradation, the molecular weight of the molecule is reduced from 340,000 to 270,000 by the release of low molecular weight fragments from the ends of the polypeptide chains in the region of the N-terminal disulfide knot. The macromolecular structure which remains, called the "X" fragment, resembles fibrin monomer, since it retains the property of engaging in clot formation and thus is not found in serum. However, it clots slowly and its presence weakens the clot structure. The X fragment retains the three "nodular" regions which make up the fibrinogen molecule, the two at either end designated "D" and that at the center "E". The second stage of degradation involves a further reduction of the molecular weight by the separation of a D–E linkage, yielding a smaller D piece of MW 90,000 and a larger DE (or "Y") segment of MW 155,000. Since each of these fragments retains some portions of the N-terminal disulfide knot, they retain the capacity of poly-

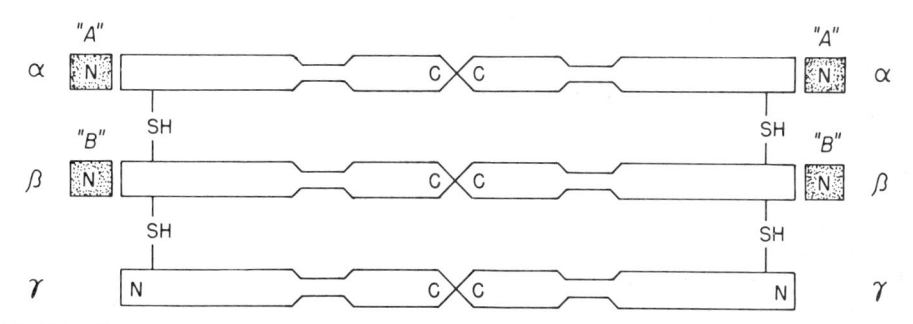

Figure 22–122 The structure of fibrinogen. The N-terminal amino acids (N) of the paired α, β, and γ chains are at opposite ends of the molecule. The subunits are held together by disulfide bonds. The C-terminal amino acids (C) are represented in the center of the molecule. The cleavage from the main molecule of fibrinopeptides "A" and "B" by thrombin is represented. (Modified from Blombäck, B.: Brit. J. Haemat., 17:145, 1969.)

merizing with fibrin monomer or with X fragment, but the strand length is limited to short complexes which do not go on to completion of the clot ("paracoagulation"). Thus, these fragments, by interfering with fibrin strand formation, are potent anticoagulants demonstrable as complexes in serum. In the third and final stage, the DE piece is further reduced from MW 155,000 to a D piece of MW 90,000 and an E piece of MW 30,000 to 50,000. The latter, coming from the center of the fibrinogen molecule, is relatively impotent with regard to its activity on clot formation (Fig. 22–123).

The terms "intrinsic" and "extrinsic" refer to clotting inside and outside the vascular system, respectively. The intrinsic system is relatively slow and the extrinsic somewhat faster, thanks to the action of tissue thromboplastin. In either case the final common pathway is the conversion of prothrombin to thrombin, the active enzyme which acts upon fibrinogen as its substrate.

The sequential reaction of clotting factors which brings about this conversion involves aspects of the cascade hypothesis as well as the concept of complex formation on phospholipid micelles (Fig. 22–124). The first phase of the intrinsic system is the surface activation of Factors XII and XI. The baring of collagen in vivo has as its in-vitro counterpart exposure to glass, bentonite, or kaolin surfaces. The conversion of Factor XII to XIIa seems to require prior complex formation with Factor XI, which in turn is changed to XIa. Factor XIa then triggers coagulation by activating IX to IXa, a potent procoagulant. A complex is then formed of Factors IXa and VIII with platelet phospholipid. The formation of this "Factor VIII complex" is accelerated by the presence of small quantities of thrombin. This complex then converts Factor X to Xa, which by itself has "prothrombinase" activity. The rate of reaction, however, is markedly accelerated by the presence of Factor V and platelet phospholipid.

The extrinsic system short circuits the first two phases of the intrinsic system by directly activating Factor X through the formation of a complex between Factor VII and tissue thromboplastin, which is composed of phospholipid and protein. Tissue thromboplastin is found in many tissues, but brain, lung, and placenta are particularly rich sources.

Calcium is required for most of the coagulation reactions, a point of considerable laboratory importance. Citrate, which complexes calcium, is the most commonly used anticoagulant for sample collection for coagulation testing. However, it is virtually impossible for hypocalcemia to be of sufficient magnitude in vivo to cause abnormal bleeding. Whether activated forms of Factors V, VII, and VIII exist or whether their activity is mediated solely through complex formation with phospholipid remains uncertain. The thrombin formed as the end-product of this accelerating series of reactions, in addition to forming fibrin monomer and activating Factor XIII, also engages in "positive feedback" by increasing platelet aggregation and promoting Factor VIII complex formation. Modulating influences on the negative side come from enzyme antagonists in the plasma, such as antithrombins and alpha-2-macroglobulin. The activated forms of the coagulation factors are cleared from the circulation rapidly, which is also of considerable importance in keeping the process of clot formation under physiologic control.

Most of the tests of the clotting mechanism depend on the appearance of a fibrin clot in the test tube. The simplest of these is the whole blood clotting time, which is a crude measure of the intrinsic system. A much more convenient, accurate, and reproducible method of measuring the clotting time in the laboratory rather than at the bedside is to collect citrated plasma and subsequently to measure the plasma clotting time after restitution of the calcium concentration. The normal "recalcification time" is about 1.5 to 4.0 minutes, compared to 5 to 15 minutes for the whole blood clotting time. The addition of various reagents to recalcified plasma gives considerable information about the coagulation mechanism. The addition of a substitute for platelet phospholipid (a "partial thromboplastin") shortens the time to about 1.0 to 1.5 minutes in the "partial thromboplastin time," which reflects the status of the intrinsic system. The activation of Factors XII and XI by surface-active materials, such as bentonite or kaolin, shortens the time to about 0.5 minute and gives a more reproducible test ("activated partial thromboplastin time"). If tissue (i.e., complete) thromboplastin is added, the plasma clotting time is about 13 seconds, and the corresponding test, somewhat erroneously called the "prothrombin time," is a measure of the extrinsic system. The addition of Russell's viper venom ("Stypven time") activates Factor X directly and thus eliminates Factor VII as a variable in the assessment of the extrinsic system. The addition of thrombin ("thrombin time") is a direct measure of the ability to form a fibrin clot in the test plasma and normally produces a clot so rapidly (about 6 seconds) that dilution of the thrombin is necessary in order to lengthen the time and thus to obtain more accurate and meaningful results. It is obvious that all tests which depend on the appearance of a fibrin clot require an adequate concentration of fibrinogen in the test plasma as well as the absence of substances which would prevent the development of a clot, such as high concentrations of plasmin or of fibrinogen-fibrin degradation products.

Most of the coagulation factors are made in the

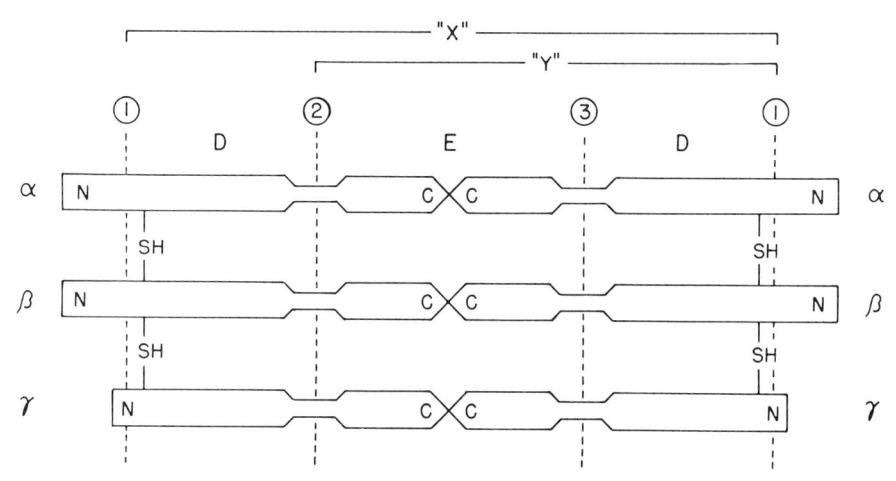

Figure 22-123 The degradation of fibrinogen by plasmin. 1, 2, and 3 represent the stages of degradation discussed in the text. (Modified from Marder, V. J.: Scand. J. Haemat., Suppl. *13*:21, 1971.)

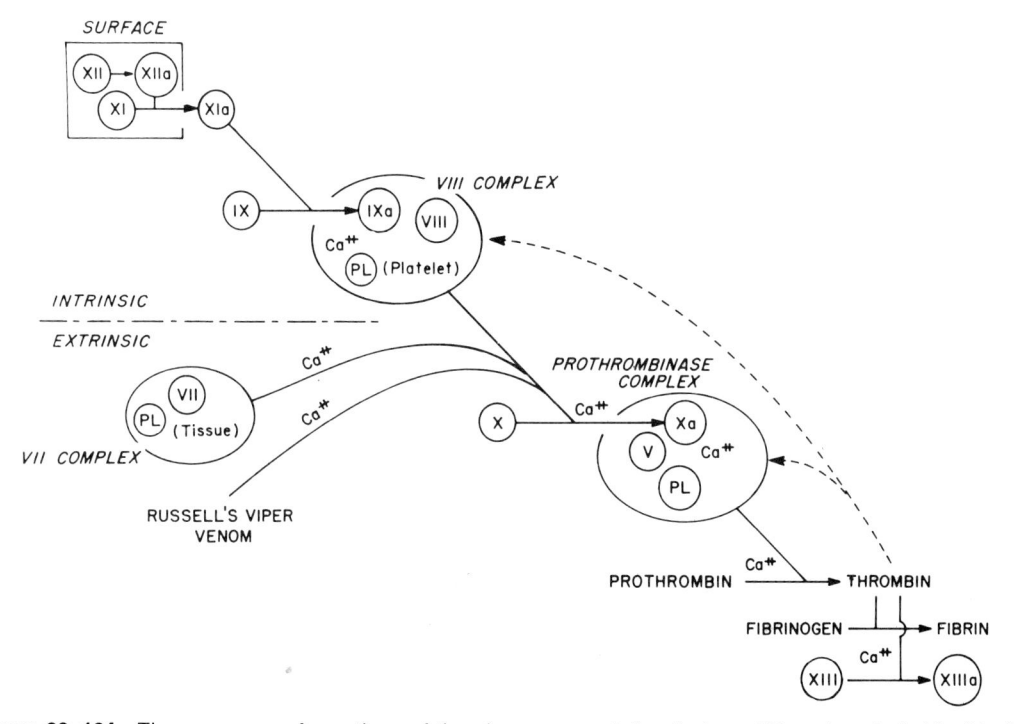

Figure 22-124 The sequence of reactions of the plasma coagulation factors. (*PL* = phospholipid). (Modified from Williams, W. J.: *In* Williams et al. (Eds.): Hematology. New York, McGraw-Hill Book Co., 1971, p. 1086.)

liver, but the site of synthesis of Factor VIII remains something of a mystery. Along with fibrinogen, its concentration in the plasma increases readily in response to pregnancy, surgery, or inflammatory states. There is a splenic pool of Factor VIII which can be mobilized along with the splenic pool of platelets by epinephrine, which causes not only a prompt increase in platelet count but also a rise in plasma Factor VIII concentration. The synthesis of Factors II, VII, IX, and X is dependent upon an adequate supply of vitamin K, as reviewed by Suttie. Treatment of plasma with certain adsorbents selectively removes the "vitamin K-dependent factors," a convenient tool for the preparation not only of concentrates of these factors for therapeutic purposes but also of test plasma deficient in these factors for use in laboratory diagnosis. Not all the plasma coagulation factors are consumed during the process of clotting. Serum differs from plasma in that it lacks fibrinogen, prothrombin, and Factors V and VIII. Factors V and VIII are also noteworthy for their instability. They rapidly lose activity in stored plasma. The biological half-lives of most of the clotting factors are relatively short, Factor VII having the shortest and fibrinogen and Factor XIII the longest values (Table 22-18).

Fibrinogen spends an uneasy existence in the plasma, circulating between the forces of clot promotion, represented by thrombin, and those of clot dissolution, represented by plasmin (see Spaet reference). The process of fibrinolysis is designed by nature to be a local phenomenon at the site of clot formation only and not in the general circulation.

Plasminogen is present in the plasma at a concentration of 10 to 20 mg. per 100 ml. Potent and specific plasminogen activators are present in many tissues and body fluids. As an example, the plasminogen activator of the urinary tract keeps this system free of clots and the potential disaster they could cause by obstructing the flow of urine. Especially large quantities of plasminogen activators are found in white cell lysosomes, from which they are released with difficulty, and also in the endothelial cells which line the vascular walls, from which release easily occurs. The development of a fibrin clot causes a rapid release of plasminogen activator into the clot, where it converts plasminogen to plasmin (Fig. 22-125). The activation is accomplished by the simple splitting of a single peptide bond between a valine and an arginine residue without reduction in molecular weight. Plasmin thus appears mostly at the site of the clot, with relatively little spilling over into the general circulation. Plasmin is unstable and its activity soon disappears. Circulating plasmin inhibitors also contribute to the systemic protection of fibrinogen and other plasma proteins. Since the ratio of surface endothelium to cross-sectional area is greatest in the microcirculation, this is the site within the circulatory system with the greatest potential for plasminogen activation and complete clot dissolution.

A variety of influences other than fibrin deposition also bring about the release of plasminogen activators from the endothelium. These include exercise, acute stress of almost any kind, and pharmacologic and other kinds of vasoreactive stimuli. The increase in plasma fibrinolytic activity, however, is transient and mild, since the plasminogen activators are rapidly cleared from the plasma by the liver with a half-life of only 13 minutes. The impairment of this clearing mechanism will lead to somewhat less transient and less mild degrees of systemic fibrinolysis, a situation which occasionally arises in liver disease (see Fletcher et al. reference).

ABNORMAL STRUCTURE AND FUNCTION

The hereditary abnormalities of the coagulation factors, reviewed by Prentice and Ratnoff, are readily classified because they are definable in terms of a single inherited abnormality in either the amount or the structure of a single protein. Acquired defects are often more difficult to categorize in that they frequently affect many different aspects of the coagulation sequence as well as multiple coagulation factors (Table 22-19).

The general effects are those of bleeding and/or clotting. The clinical nature of the bleeding gives clues about its underlying cause. Intra-articular hemorrhage is highly characteristic of hemophilia and is only rarely seen in other disorders, while petechiae are strongly suggestive of thrombocytopenia. Ecchymoses and purpura are very nonspecific; deep hemorrhage into muscles or retroperitoneally is more a feature of hemophilia or of adverse effects of anticoagulants. Intracranial hemorrhage, regardless of the underlying hemostatic defect, is probably the most dread complication. Bleeding from the umbilical stump

TABLE 22-18 BIOLOGIC HALF-LIVES OF PLASMA COAGULATION FACTORS

Factor VII	1.5 to 5 hours
Factor VIII	9 to 18 hours
Factor V	15 to 20 hours
Factor IX	20 to 24 hours
Factor X	1 to 2 days
Factor XI	1.7 to 3.5 days
Factor II	2.8 to 4.4 days
Factor XII	2 days
Factor I	3.2 to 4.5 days
Factor XIII	4.5 to 7 days

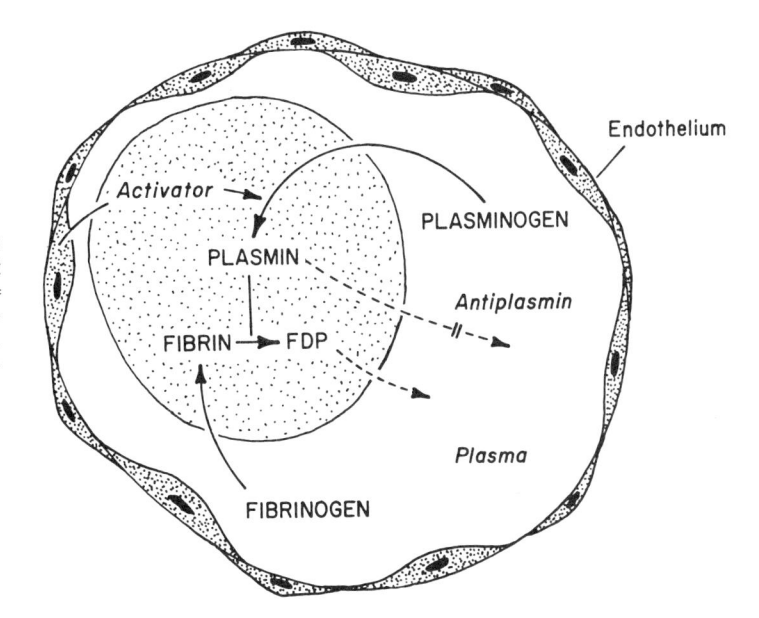

Figure 22-125 The local activation of plasminogen at the site of fibrin clot within a small blood vessel. (*FDP* = fibrin degradation products.) (Modified from Sherry, S.: *In* Williams et al. (Eds.): Hematology. New York, McGraw-Hill Book Co., 1972, p. 1111.)

TABLE 22-19 CLASSIFICATION OF DISORDERS OF PLASMA COAGULATION AND VASCULAR FACTORS

I. *Disorders of Fibrinogen and Related Factors*
    Hereditary
        Afibrinogenemia
        Dysfibrinogenemia
        Factor XIII deficiency
    Acquired
        Disseminated intravascular coagulation
        Primary fibrinolysis
        Liver disease
II. *Disorders of the Intrinsic and Extrinsic Systems*
    Hereditary
        Hemophilia A
        Hemophilia B
        Deficiencies of surface active Factor XII or XI
        Other deficiencies: Factor VII, X, V, or II
        von Willebrand's disease
    Acquired
        Vitamin K deficiency
        Liver disease
        Hemorrhagic diseases of the newborn
        Exogenous anticoagulants
        Endogenous anticoagulants (antibodies to Factor VIII and other Factors)
III. *Vascular Disorders*
    Hereditary
        Hereditary hemorrhagic telangiectasia
        Ehlers-Danlos syndrome and other connective tissue disorders
    Acquired
        Superficial purpura
        Scurvy
        Cushing's syndrome
        Amyloidosis
        Allergic purpura

or after circumcision may be the first sign of a hereditary disorder. Later in life, the onset of the menses, dental extraction, and surgical procedures are natural tests of hemostasis. Delayed hemorrhage several days after the completion of a procedure raises the index of suspicion that a coagulation disorder exists.

Disorders of Fibrinogen and Related Factors

A low level of circulating fibrinogen may be secondary to decreased production, as in liver disease, to a rare inherited deficiency, or more frequently to an increase in the rate of its degradation. The excess in fibrinogen consumption above its production rate is most often due to a process of intravascular coagulation. Rarely it is caused by the presence of a high level of circulating plasmin.

Several different terms have been used to describe the process of extensive intravascular clotting, none of them entirely satisfactory. "Consumption coagulopathy" placed emphasis on the depletion of the plasma coagulation factors, but not all the factors are consumed, and the "panel" of depressed factor levels is neither uniform nor predictable. "Disseminated intravascular coagulation" placed major emphasis on the pathogenetic importance of the deposition of large quantities of fibrin throughout the microcirculation but does not fit those situations in which the fibrin deposition is extensive and yet mostly or entirely localized to the vascular beds of certain tissues.

If not fatal, the process may be acute and self-limited, subacute, or chronic, depending on the underlying cause, as reviewed by Bachman and by Deykin. It may be set off by a pathologic activation of the extrinsic or the intrinsic clotting systems; in many circumstances the triggering mechanism is not known. The activation of the extrinsic system is caused by the entry into the circulation of large amounts of tissue thromboplastin. Examples of such extrinsic syndromes are the hypofibrinogenemic states associated with pregnancy: abruptio placentae, amniotic fluid embolism, toxemia, and retained dead fetus. Since fibrinogen concentration normally increases in pregnancy, the finding of a plasma concentration within the normal range may be indicative of significant consumption if found late in pregnancy in association with one of the aforementioned complications. Widespread carcinoma may incite intravascular clotting, also presumably on account of the tumor content of tissue thromboplastin which finds its way into the circulation. The intrinsic system may be activated by bacterial septicemia and certain rickettsial and viral infections (Rocky Mountain spotted fever, epidemic hemorrhagic fever) which lay bare the vascular endothelium and expose collagen (see Yoshikawa et al. reference). Antigen-antibody complexes trigger intrinsic clotting by an unknown mechanism in massive transfusion reactions (although the thromboplastic properties of red cell membrane may play some role) and in anaphylactic reactions. It has been suggested that an immunologic mechanism underlies purpura fulminans, a serious and often fatal disorder of children which characteristically follows shortly after recovery from a minor viral infection. Properly timed injections of endotoxin given to animals have been experimentally used to produce the so-called generalized Shwartzman reaction, a disseminated intravascular coagulation syndrome, but in this model the precise initiating event also remains obscure. The classification of intravascular coagulation syndromes is given in Table 22-20.

Local factors may prepare the vascular bed of a certain organ or tissue for selective fibrin deposition. In pregnancy the kidney is particularly vulnerable, and the syndrome which may ensue is bilateral renal cortical necrosis with oliguric renal failure. In cavernous hemangiomas, a large vascular bed with a high ratio of endothelial surface area to vascular cross-sectional area accommodates a large volume of blood with static flow. This may be sufficient to set up a chronic process of extensive but localized fibrin deposition, the endothelium contributing high plasminogen activating activity and thus releasing fibrin degradation products into the circulation.

The reticuloendothelial system is responsible for rapidly clearing activated coagulation factors as well as fibrinogen-fibrin degradation products

TABLE 22-20 CLASSIFICATION OF DISSEMINATED INTRAVASCULAR COAGULATION SYNDROMES

I. Pregnancy
    Abruptio placentae
    Amniotic fluid embolism
    Toxemia
    Retained dead fetus
    Septic abortion with septicemia
    Hydatidiform mole
II. Malignant Disease
    Metastatic carcinoma
    Acute leukemia (promyelocytic)
III. Infectious Disease
    Bacterial septicemia (meningococcal, other gram negative and gram positive)
    Rickettsial (Rocky Mountain spotted fever)
    Viral (epidemic hemorrhagic fever)
    Parasitic (malaria)
IV. Pediatric Syndromes
    Neonatal (respiratory distress syndrome, retained dead twin fetus, septicemia, rubella, abruptio placentae)
    Purpura fulminans
    Hemolytic uremic syndrome
V. Antigen-Antibody Complexes
    Anaphylactic reaction
    Massive transfusion reaction
VI. Miscellaneous
    Postoperative (open heart and other thoracic surgery, prostatic surgery)
    Massive trauma (including burns)
    Heat stroke
    Drowning
    Snake bite
    Giant hemangioma

and their complexes from the circulation. Any impairment of this process will prolong and aggravate the severity of the coagulopathy. Clinical states of shock, whatever the underlying primary cause, cause poor perfusion of reticuloendothelial clearing mechanisms and thus seriously increase the magnitude of the syndrome. Reticuloendothelial blockade with substances such as Thorotrast markedly contributes to the severity of intravascular coagulation syndromes experimentally in animals. A similar blockade may be of pathogenetic significance in septicemia or in massive hemolysis.

The resultant defects in the hemostatic mechanism are those of depletion of coagulation factors along with interference with the polymerization of fibrin monomer by the presence of fibrin degradation products. The paradox thus arises that hypercoagulability leads to hemorrhage. The process of consumption resembles that of the in-vitro conversion of plasma to serum. The most consistent changes are decreases in the platelet count and in the fibrinogen level, while Factors

II, V, and VIII are also commonly depressed. Serial observations which demonstrate decreases in several of these during the onset or increases following recovery from a suspected clinical episode of intravascular coagulation provide inferential support for the diagnosis. Plasminogen activation, a process which is especially brisk in the small vessels, releases fibrin degradation products in the general circulation. These form complexes with fibrin monomer and with each other and may cause serious interference with clot formation.

The ischemic consequences to local tissues of the blockage of the microcirculation are fortunately usually self-limited, owing to the local fibrinolytic efficiency, which rapidly removes the fibrin deposits. However, renal failure is one of the most dire of the ischemic effects. Cutaneous patches of gangrene and acrocyanosis are more externally visible effects seen in purpura fulminans and sometimes in septicemia. Erythrocyte fragmentation, occurring as red cells are forced through the obstructing fibrin meshwork, causes the morphologic appearance of microangiopathic hemolytic anemia on the peripheral blood film. The picture may be accompanied by clinical signs of hemolysis. Intravascular coagulation causing oliguric renal failure and erythrocyte fragmentation is therefore one of the "hemolytic uremic" syndromes.

The diagnosis is aided by laboratory tests which, in the most severe circumstances, show widespread derangements of the coagulation system due to either the presence of fibrin degradation products or low levels of plasma coagulation factors or both (see Merskey et al. reference). The test tube clot will be small and easily broken up. Thus, a prolonged prothrombin and partial thromboplastin time may also be accompanied by a prolonged thrombin time. Tests which detect paracoagulation (protamine sulfate, ethanol gelation, staphylococcal clumping, cryofibrinogen) may be positive. Serial measurements of the concentrations of coagulation factors may also be useful, especially of platelets, fibrinogen, and Factor VIII. Laboratory confirmation may be difficult to obtain in mild cases.

Treatment varies with the individual circumstances. In acute syndromes, the prompt and vigorous treatment of the primary underlying cause and the correction of shock are the most important measures. Heparin is sometimes used in order to arrest the deposition of fibrin, not without fear of increasing the bleeding tendency. Repletion of coagulation factors is rarely required, barring immediate needs such as those imposed by emergency surgery. Replacement therapy is best combined with heparin in order to avoid the unwanted possibility that more fibrin deposition will further worsen the situation. By the same reasoning, inhibitors of fibrinolysis such as epsilon aminocaproic acid are contraindicated, since they will delay the physiologic resolution of the fibrin clots within the vasculature.

Primary fibrinolysis is an acute severe bleeding state which resembles intravascular clotting but must be distinguished from it because the treatments differ. The high levels of circulating plasmin which set up this state are sometimes secondary to metastatic carcinoma of the prostate, thoracic surgery, injury to the genitourinary tract with extravasation of urokinase-containing urine into tissues, or cirrhosis or shock with impaired ability to clear plasminogen activators from the circulation. Plasmin attacks circulating fibrinogen and causes a decrease in its concentration along with the appearance of fibrinogen degradation products in the circulation. These unfortunately cannot be distinguished from the fibrin degradation products of disseminated intravascular coagulation. Other coagulation factor levels may also be depressed. However, in contrast to intravascular coagulation syndromes, the test-tube clot which initially forms completely dissolves within one or two hours, the platelet count is normal, the red cell morphology does not show fragmentation, and the bleeding improves with the therapeutic use of fibrinolytic inhibitors.

Inherited disorders of fibrinogen are rare (see Jackson et al. reference). Afibrinogenemia is a quantitative deficiency secondary to a profound lack of synthesis, while dysfibrinogenemia refers to a variation in the structure of the molecule. Only trace quantities of fibrinogen are detectable in hereditary afibrinogenemia, an autosomal recessive condition which is of clinical significance only in the homozygous form. Whole blood or recalcified plasma clotting times are indefinitely long and are not corrected with the addition of thrombin. Successful arrest of hemorrhage is achieved by replacement therapy sufficient to raise the fibrinogen level above 60 mg. per 100 ml. Hereditary dysfibrinogenemia is a mild or even asymptomatic disorder. Several different types have been described, presumably differing in the specific amino acid substitution in the molecule (see Beck et al. reference). The detailed abnormalities involved and the molecular mechanisms with respect to the altered function of the molecule remain for the most part to be worked out. Clot formation, however, is prolonged, and clot structure, though weak, is insoluble in 5 M urea. Plasma coagulation tests therefore may be broadly deranged. Fibrinogen concentration measured by immunochemical or physical methods is normal, but methods which depend on "clottable fibrinogen" give low values. The condition is autosomal, and affected heterozygotes therefore have normal fibrinogen along with the variant molecule.

Hereditary deficiency of Factor XIII is properly included among disorders of fibrinogen, since

Factor XIII also affects clot structure. Deficiency is detectable in the laboratory by virtue of the fibrin clot solubility in 5 M urea. The defect, also autosomal recessive, is clinically severe and, as in hereditary afibrinogenemia, may first come to attention because of bleeding at the site of the sloughed umbilical cord (see Duckert and Beck reference). Wound healing is impaired presumably because fibroblastic organization of the clot is not normal. Affected homozygotes have less than 1 per cent of the normal concentration and respond particularly well to replacement therapy because Factor XIII has a relatively long half-life and only small quantities are required. Acquired failure of Factor XIII synthesis occurs in liver disease.

Intrinsic and Extrinsic System Disorders

Hemophilia A and hemophilia B are hereditary deficiencies of Factor VIII and Factor IX, respectively. The two disorders are clinically indistinguishable except by laboratory test. Both are sex-linked and thus transmitted by asymptomatic carrier females to half their sons. Female homozygotes, offspring of affected fathers and carrier mothers, are exceedingly rare. Hemophilia A occurs with a frequency of 1 per 10,000, 5 to 10 times the frequency of hemophilia B. Severe hemophilia is characterized by repeated hemarthroses and ultimately by chronic arthritis and joint destruction. Ankles, knees, and elbows are most susceptible. The normal ineffectiveness of the extrinsic clotting system in the articular structures may explain the particular susceptibility of this tissue to hemorrhage in the face of severe deficiencies of the intrinsic system. Patients with hemophilia of moderate severity may have only occasional joint hemorrhages, whereas mild cases usually have normal joints. Deep hematomas may dissect along fascial planes and cause nerve compression or compromise the vascular supply of an extremity. Even with intensive treatment the surgical risk is great, and intracranial hemorrhage often provoked by minor head trauma may be untreatable and have a fatal outcome.

Decades of investigation have still not resolved controversy about the pathogenesis of hemophilia A. Until recently the defect clearly appeared to be one of lack of Factor VIII. However, the successful production in the rabbit of a specific antiserum against human Factor VIII has permitted the demonstration that almost all patients with hemophilia A have antiserum neutralizing activity equal to that of normal plasma. Because of this immunochemical evidence that Factor VIII antigens circulate in the plasma of hemophilia A patients, the disorder is now viewed by Zimmerman and others as a qualitative defect of a structurally abnormal and functionally inept protein which is produced in normal amounts. Similar immunochemical studies using naturally occurring human Factor VIII antibodies rather than rabbit antiserum have given evidence that there are two types of hemophilia A, one constituting about 10 per cent of the total which possess antibody neutralizing activity, the remaining 90 per cent having no such activity (see Feinstein et al. and Hoyer and Breckenridge references). The pathogenetic significance of this observation and its possible relationship to genetic polymorphism are still not clear. Similar immunochemical approaches suggest that analogous pathogenetic mechanisms may also apply to hemophilia B.

The accurate diagnosis and classification as to degree of severity of hemophilia A and B ultimately rest upon the direct measurement of the levels of Factor VIII and Factor IX activity (Fig. 22–126). The treatment of major hemorrhagic episodes or the preparation of patients for surgery also requires the ability to measure the specific factor level to ensure that it remains in excess of 30 per cent at all times. The partial thromboplastin time is sensitive to levels below 20 per cent and thus is almost always prolonged in untreated patients of any degree of severity. The prothrombin time and the bleeding time are normal. Female carriers cannot be identified with certainty because their functional levels, 25 to 75 per cent for hemophilia A heterozygotes and 9 to 90 per cent for hemophilia B heterozygotes, overlap considerably with the range of normal, 50 to 150 per cent. Positive identification may eventually become possible by virtue of the discrepancy that heterozygotes show between the functional level and the immunochemical concentration of Factor VIII or IX in comparison with the corresponding value in normals.

Replacement therapy with plasma or plasma derivatives is effective in both hemophilia A and hemophilia B (Fig. 22–127). Treatment must be specific, however, an axiom which has become of crucial importance since plasma fractionation procedures have come into common use. Cryoprecipitate and other Factor VIII-rich preparations lack Factor IX activity, whereas fractions containing Factor IX and the other vitamin K-dependent factors lack Factor VIII (see Hoag et al. reference). Factor IX is relatively stable and is present in stored plasma or serum, both of which are poor sources of Factor VIII. The longer biological half-life of Factor IX (about 24 hours as compared to 12 for Factor VIII) is also of importance in that less frequent infusions of Factor IX are required to maintain its functional activity at the desired level.

Von Willebrand's disease is also a hereditary disorder of Factor VIII but, in contrast to hemophilia A, it is inherited as an autosomal dominant

Figure 22-126 The method of measurement of plasma Factor VIII and IX levels based on a modification of the partial thromboplastin time made dependent upon the concentration of the specific factor by using dilutions of test plasma mixed with deficient plasma. A standard curve using normal plasma is shown. (Redrawn from Gaston, L. W.: Hosp. Pract., August, 1969, p. 76.)

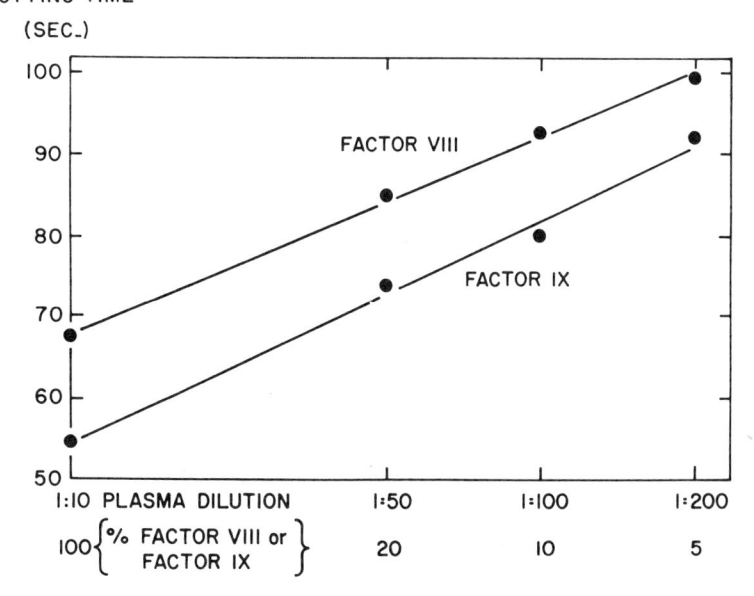

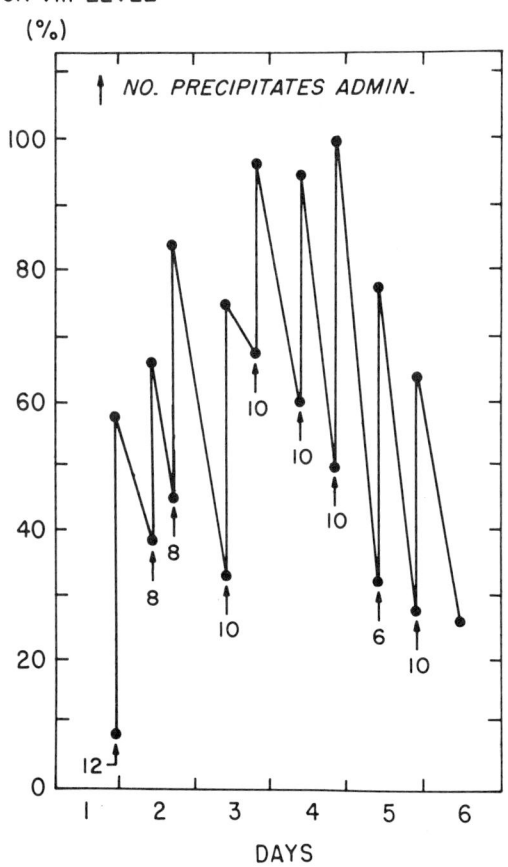

Figure 22-127 Plasma Factor VIII levels measured during treatment of a patient with hemophilia A by repeated infusions of cryoprecipitate. (Redrawn from Pool, J. G., and Shannon, A. E.: New Eng. J. Med., 273:1443, 1968.)

and in addition has an associated defect of platelet adhesion to injured blood vessels, causing a prolonged bleeding time (see Weiss reference). Platelet adhesion to glass beads is also impaired, but other platelet functions, such as the aggregation reactions and ADP release, are typically normal. Epistaxis, menorrhagia, and gastrointestinal hemorrhage are common, but joint hemorrhage is rare. The Factor VIII level is reduced below 50 per cent to as low as 1 to 5 per cent. The partial thromboplastin time is not adequate to detect those cases with less severely depressed levels. Factor VIII levels fluctuate in individual cases, in contrast to their constancy in hemophilia A. Pregnancy stimulates an increased Factor VIII level, as in normal women, and thus may ameliorate hemorrhagic manifestations. Immunochemical evidence indicates that Factor VIII in von Willebrand's disease, in contrast to that in hemophilia A, is qualitatively normal but is produced in short supply (see Zimmerman et al. reference).

One of the most intriguing differences between the two disorders lies in their response to plasma infusions. The increase in Factor VIII level in hemophilia A is entirely acccounted for by the amount of infused material; the maximum occurs immediately after infusion and the declining level thereafter follows the known biological half-life of Factor VIII, about 12 hours. Plasma infusions given to patients with von Willebrand's disease actually stimulate the production of Factor VIII; levels reaching a peak at 4 to 24 hours are higher than those which could be explained on the basis of the amount of infused material. The subsequent decline to original pretreatment levels occurs slowly over several days (Fig. 22-128). Donor plasma taken from patients with hemophilia A indeed has more potent Factor VIII-stimulating activity than normal plasma. Thus, Factor VIII production is in some manner controlled by loci on two different chromosomes, one X and one autosomal. Possibly the latter locus controls the synthetic rate of an X-linked structural locus. An alternate hypothesis states that the autosomal locus, deficient in von Willebrand's disease, produces a Factor VIII precursor or component present in normal plasma and in greater than normal quantities in hemophilia A plasma. In addition to the Factor VIII-stimulating activity of normal and hemophilia A plasma, there is a second activity distinct from the first—the "bleeding time factor." Thus, these plasmas correct the abnormal bleeding time after infusion, but the duration of action is shorter than that of the Factor VIII-stimulating activity. Furthermore, the latter activity is rather stable in stored plasma, whereas the "bleeding time factor" is labile. Curiously, platelet transfusion does not correct the bleeding time defect as it does in hereditary or acquired defects of platelet aggregation, further evidence that the poor platelet adherence in von Willebrand's disease is related to a plasma deficiency.

Acquired defects in Factor VIII, other than those found in the intravascular coagulation syn-

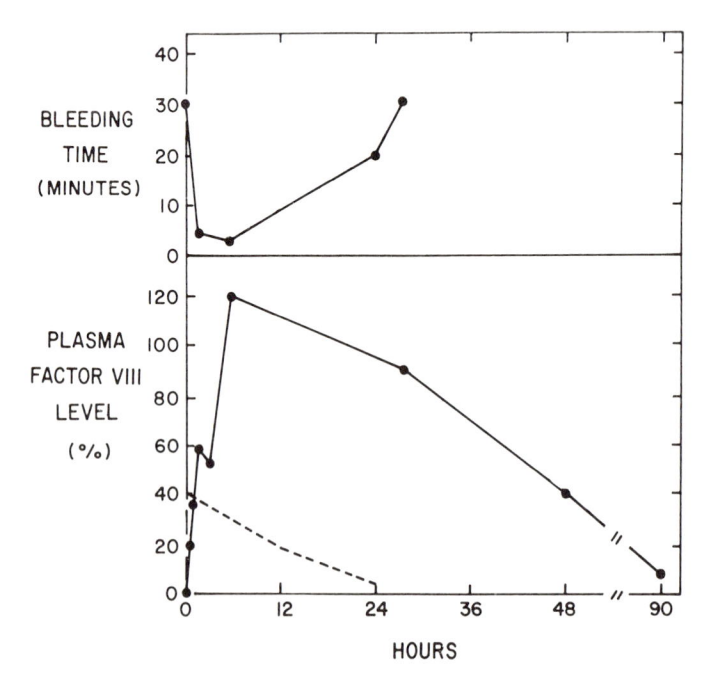

Figure 22-128 Response of Factor VIII level and of bleeding time in a patient with von Willebrand's disease given at time zero a single infusion of a fraction prepared from normal plasma. The interrupted line represents the response in Factor VIII level to be expected in a patient with hemophilia A. (Modified from Williams, W. J.: *In* Williams et al. (Eds.): Hematology. New York, McGraw-Hill Book Co., 1972, p. 1340.)

dromes, result from the pathologic production of autoantibodies directed against Factor VIII (see Robboy et al. reference). Somewhat paradoxically, about 20 per cent of patients with hemophilia A develop antibodies against Factor VIII after repeated replacement therapy, as reported by Strauss. These greatly complicate successful therapy when they are present in high titer. Fortunately, the titer falls with time, and if the intervals between hemorrhagic episodes are sufficiently spaced, intensive replacement therapy may successfully arrest the bleeding before the anamnestic response to the infused Factor VIII raises the antibody titer to levels which would preclude successful treatment. Acquired antibodies to Factor VIII are also seen in association with such autoimmune disorders as lupus erythematosus, rheumatoid arthritis, ulcerative colitis, and regional enteritis. A third variant occurs days to weeks postpartum. A fourth type is found without obvious relationship to other coexisting factors, especially in older people. The antibody behaves as a natural circulating anticoagulant and its addition to normal plasma will delay its clotting time (see Shapiro reference). Specific confirmation is made by measuring the neutralization of the Factor VIII activity of normal plasma by plasma containing the natural antibody. Therapy may be difficult if spontaneous disappearance does not alleviate the problem. Immunosuppressive therapy has been successfully used in a few instances. Autoantibodies to other plasma coagulation factors have also been discovered, but the great majority have been directed against Factor VIII.

Hereditary deficiencies of the remaining plasma coagulation factors are uncommon. Of the surface-active factors, Factor XII deficiency is usually not associated with any bleeding abnormality, and the hemorrhagic diathesis of Factor XI deficiency is mild. Deficiency of Factor VII, X, V, or II will produce a prolonged prothrombin time as well as partial thromboplastin time. All are associated with mild to moderate bleeding manifestations.

Inadequate supplies of vitamin K, normally synthesized by intestinal bacteria, cause depletion of the vitamin K-dependent factors: II, VII, IX, and X. Absorptive impairment secondary to gastrointestinal disease or to obstruction of the biliary tract causes clotting factor depletion which is correctable by parenterally administered vitamin K. The coumarin and indandione derivatives antagonize the hepatic synthesis of the vitamin K-dependent factors by mechanisms which are still not known. Thus, they are active in vivo as orally administered anticoagulants, but they are inactive in vitro. The Factor VII level is the first to fall after hepatic synthesis stops because of its short biological half-life. Factors II, IX, and X reach their nadir at about 5 to 10 days after anticoagulant therapy is begun. Vitamin K, occasionally required to arrest hemorrhage in patients treated with anticoagulant, will significantly increase the levels of the dependent factors within 6 hours. If more rapid correction is necessary, replacement therapy with plasma or with concentrates of the vitamin K-dependent factors can be given. Vitamin K therapy is ineffective if the low factor levels are the result of severe liver disease, which in addition to the vitamin K-dependent factors is associated with failure of synthesis of other factors, such as Factor V, fibrinogen, and Factor XIII.

The normal newborn infant has lower concentrations of the vitamin K-dependent factors than the adult, partially because of the immaturity of the fetal liver and partially because of low vitamin K stores (see Sutherland et al. reference). Prematurity exaggerates the phenomenon. Breast milk is a poor source of vitamin K, but cow's milk contains significant quantities. A hemorrhagic disease occurring two to three days after birth owing to low levels of the vitamin K-dependent factors has been associated with a sufficiently high mortality rate that prophylactic administration of a small quantity of vitamin K is considered warranted, even though only a partial correction of the coagulation abnormalities is achieved. The syndrome must be distinguished from other neonatal hemorrhagic syndromes, such as the thrombocytopenias, disseminated intravascular coagulation disorders, and hemophilia (see Hathaway et al. reference). The coumarin drugs cross the placental barrier and therefore are not given to pregnant women.

Hemorrhagic complications following heparin therapy are relatively infrequent, considering how extensively this drug is used. Heparin acts most impressively on the intrinsic clotting system, and its major effect is thus on the partial thromboplastin time (see Wessler and Gaston reference). It also prolongs the prothrombin time slightly, probably by virtue of antithrombin activity as well as inhibition of Factor Xa. The duration of action of heparin is limited to 4 to 6 hours and thus the use of protamine, which neutralizes heparin, is rarely necessary in the management of hemorrhagic complications. Hemorrhagic complications may also occur following therapy with plasminogen activators, such as streptokinase or urokinase, but these agents are also rapidly removed if reticuloendothelial clearing mechanisms are functioning normally.

HEMOSTASIS: VASCULAR FACTORS

The vascular wall stands closely juxtaposed to the normal process of hemostasis. Platelets adhere at cut surfaces and aggregate where collagen is bared. Serotonin is released by platelets, causing vasoconstriction which may assist the task of vessel plugging. Collagen also activates the intrinsic coagulation system. The vascular endothelium then finally initiates the process of clot lysis by releasing plasminogen activator. However, intrinsic defects of the vascular wall itself may be of pathogenetic importance in the etiology of hemorrhage. The supporting structures around the vessels may lose elasticity and turgor, an important factor in the superficial purpura commonly seen in the inelastic skin of normally aging individuals. This syndrome, somewhat injudiciously named "senile purpura," is clinically benign and is not associated with clinical bleeding, its most serious consequence being cosmetic. Hereditary disorders of connective tissues, such as Ehlers-Danlos syndrome, also decrease the compliance of perivascular tissues, sometimes sufficiently to cause significant hemorrhage. Scurvy, sometimes seen in combination with alcoholic liver disease and other nutritional deficiencies, affects the integrity of connective tissue of the vascular wall. Perifollicular hemorrhages resembling petechiae suggest vitamin C lack. Excessive amounts of adrenal glucocorticoids weaken the structure of the vascular wall. Purpura and ecchymoses of Cushing's syndrome are explained on this basis. Amyloid deposition within vascular walls is another example of an acquired intrinsic disorder of the vessel wall. The abnormality in hereditary hemorrhagic telangiectasis, an autosomal dominant condition, is still not understood in terms of primary etiology but leads to localized dilatations of small vessels which appear as tiny punctate vascular spots which blanch on pressure. These nonpulsatile spots are found commonly on the lips and mucous membranes of the mouth and nose as well as on the fingertips. However, internal involvement commonly occurs in the gastrointestinal tract as well as in other organs, including the lungs and the central nervous system. The telangiectasias usually do not develop until the fifth or sixth decade of life, when the weakened vascular wall finally becomes apparent. Epistaxis and gastrointestinal hemorrhage are the most common symptoms.

Damage to the vascular wall as a consequence of various infections has already been mentioned. Immunologic vascular damage leads to the syndrome of allergic purpura, which resembles thrombocytopenic purpura in the sense that a petechial eruption forms with predilection for the dependent portions of the body. The eruption appears more violaceous and more confluent than thrombocytopenic purpura, and also has a tendency to involve the buttocks and flexor surfaces of the legs. When the purpuric signs are combined in a triad together with gastrointestinal hemorrhage and arthritis, the term "Henoch-Schönlein purpura" is appropriate. The condition may affect the pediatric age group, in which a postinfectious cause appears to be most common, or adults, in which case drug reactions may be more likely trigger mechanisms (see Cream et al. reference). In either group, nephritis is the most serious complication (see Meadow et al. reference).

The diagnosis of the primary vascular purpuric syndromes rests primarily on clinical recognition. Laboratory confirmation is at present unsatisfactory. The bleeding time and the tourniquet test (in which the appearance of petechiae is observed after inflation of a blood pressure cuff to the level sufficient to occlude venous return but not arterial filling) are primarily tests of adequacy of platelet numbers and function, and although abnormalities may be detected in the primary vascular disorders, the information is not of great assistance in establishing their presence. The fact that almost 10 per cent of normal people have a positive tourniquet test also diminishes the diagnostic value of this procedure.

REFERENCES

Bone Marrow

Baikie, A. G., Court Brown, W. M., Buckton, K. E., Harnden, D. G., Jacobs, P. A., and Tough, I. M.: A possible specific chromosome abnormality in human chronic myeloid leukaemia. Nature (London), *188*:1165, 1960.

Boggs, D. R., and Chervenick, P. A.: Hemopoietic stem cells. *In* Greenwalt, T. J., and Jamieson, G. A. (Eds.): Formation and Destruction of Blood Cells. Philadelphia, J. B. Lippincott Co., 1970, p. 240.

Craddock, C. G., Longmire, R., and McMillan, R.: Lymphocytes and the immune response. New Eng. J. Med., *285*:324, 1972.

Erslev, A. J.: Feedback circuits in the control of stem cell differentiation. Amer. J. Path., *65*:629, 1971.

Finch, C. A.: Pathophysiologic aspects of sickle cell anemia. Amer. J. Med., *53*:1, 1972.

Fliedner, T. M., Calvo, W., Haas, R., Fortega, J., and Bohne, F.: Morphologic and cytokinetic aspects of bone marrow stroma. *In* Stohlman, F., Jr. (Ed.): Hemopoietic Cellular Proliferation. New York, Grune and Stratton, 1970, p. 67.

Gregersen, M. I., and Rawson, R. A.: Blood volume. Physiol. Rev., *39*:307, 1959.

Hudson, G.: Bone marrow volume in the human foetus and newborn. Brit. J. Haemat., *11*:446, 1965.

Huggins, L., and Blockson, B. H.: Changes in outlying bone marrow accompanying a local increase of temperature within physiologic limits. J. Exp. Med., *64*:253, 1956.

Killmann, S. A., Cronkite, E. P., Fliedner, T. M., and Bond, V. P.: Mitotic indices of human bone marrow cells. III. Duration of some phases of erythrocyte and granulocytic proliferation computed from mitotic indices. Blood, *24*:267, 1964.

Knospe, W. H., Blom, J., and Crosby, W. H.: Regeneration of locally irradiated bone marrow. II. Indication of regeneration in permanently aplastic medullary cavities. Blood, *31*:400, 1968.

Kretchmar, A. L.: Erythropoietin: Hypothesis of action tested by analog computer. Science, 152:367, 1966.
Till, J. E., and McCulloch, E. A.: A direct measurement of the radiation sensitivity of normal mouse bone marrow cells. Radiat. Res., 14:213, 1961.
Trentin, J. J.: Determination of bone marrow stem cell differentiation by stromal hemopoietic inductive microenvironment (HIM). Amer. J. Path., 65:621, 1971.
Weiss, L.: The histology of the bone marrow. In Gordon, A. S. (Ed.): Regulation of Hematopoiesis. New York, Appleton-Century-Crofts, 1970, p. 79.
Wu, A. M., Till, J. E., Siminovitch, L., and McCulloch, E. A.: A cytological study of the capacity for differentiation of normal hemopoietic colony-forming cells. J. Cell. Physiol., 69:177, 1967.

Erythrocytes

Abramson, N., LoBuglio, A. F., Jandl, J. H., and Cotran, R. S.: The interaction between human monocytes and red cells. Binding characteristics. J. Exp. Med., 132:1191, 1970.
Alving, A. S., Johnson, C. F., Tarlov, A. R., Brewer, G. J., Kellermeyer, R. W., and Carson, P. E.: Mitigation of the haemolytic effect of primaquine and enhancement of its action against exoerythrocytic forms of the Chesson strain of plasmodium vivax by intermittent regimens of drug administration. Bull. WHO, 22:621, 1960.
Arderman, S., Chanarin, I., and Doyle, J. C.: Studies on secretion of gastric intrinsic factor in man. Brit. Med. J., 2:600, 1964.
Balcerzak, S. P., Westerman, M. P., Lee, R. E., and Doyle, A. P.: Idiopathic hemochromatosis. Amer. J. Med., 40:857, 1966.
Baugh, C. M., Krumdieck, C. L., Baker, H. J., and Butterworth, C. E., Jr.: Studies on the absorption and metabolism of folic acid. J. Clin. Invest., 50:2009, 1971.
Beck, W. S.: Vitamin B_{12} deficiency. In Williams, W. J., et al. (Eds.): Hematology. New York, McGraw-Hill Book Co., 1972, p. 256.
Bellingham, A. J., and Huehns, E. R.: Compensation in hemolytic anemias caused by abnormal hemoglobin. Nature, 218:924, 1968.
Bert, P.: La pression barométrique. Paris, Masson, 1878.
Bertles, J. F., and Milner, P. F.: Irreversibly sickled erythrocytes: A consequence of the heterogeneous distribution of hemoglobin types in sickle cell anemia. J. Clin. Invest., 47:1731, 1968.
Bessis, M.: Life Cycle of the Erythrocyte. Sandoz Monographs, 1966.
Beutler, E.: The effect of methemoglobin formation in sickle cell disease. J. Clin. Invest., 40:1856, 1961.
Beutler, E., Yeh, M., and Fairbanks, V. F.: The normal human female as a mosaic of X-chromosome activity: Studies using the gene for G-6-PD deficiency as a marker. Proc. Nat. Acad. Sci., 48:9, 1962.
Bookchin, R. M., and Nagel, R. L.: Ligand induced conformational dependence of hemoglobin in sickling interactions. J. Molec. Biol., 60:273, 1971.
Bookchin, R. M., Nagel, R. L., and Ranney, H. M.: The effect of beta 73 Asn on the interactions of sickling hemoglobins. Biochim. Biophys. Acta, 221:373, 1970.
Bothwell, T. H., and Finch, C. A.: Iron Metabolism. Boston, Little, Brown and Co., 1962.
Brain, M. C.: Microangiopathic hemolytic anemia. Ann. Rev. Med., 21:133, 1970.
Brewer, G. J., and Eaton, J. W.: Erythrocyte metabolism: Interaction with oxygen transport. Science, 171:1205, 1971.
Bull, B. S., and Kuhn, I. N.: The production of schistocytes by fibrin strands (a scanning electron microscopic study). Blood, 35:104, 1970.
Bunn, H. F.: Erythrocyte destruction and hemoglobin catabolism. Seminars Hemat., 9:3, 1972.
Bunn, H. F., and Jandl, J. H.: The renal handling of hemoglobin. II. Catabolism. J. Exp. Med., 129:925, 1969.
Castle, W. B.: Current concepts of pernicious anemia. Amer. J. Med., 48:541, 1970.

Chanarin, I.: The Megaloblastic Anemias. Philadelphia, F. A. Davis Co., 1969.
Charache, S., Conley, C. L., Waugh, D. E., Ugoretz, R. J., and Spurrell, J. R.: Pathogenesis of hemolytic anemia in homozygous hemoglobin C disease. J. Clin. Invest., 46:1795, 1967.
Chodos, R. B., Wells, R., Jr., and Chaffee, W. R.: A study of ferrokinetics and red cell survival in congestive heart failure. Amer. J. Med., 36:553, 1964.
Clarke, C. A.: The prevention of Rh isoimmunization. Hosp. Pract., January, 1973, p. 77.
Condon, P. I., and Serjeant, G. R.: Ocular findings in homozygous sickle cell anemia in Jamaica. Amer. J. Ophthal., 73:533, 1972.
Conrad, M. E., and Crosby, W. H.: Intestinal mucosal mechanisms controlling iron absorption. Blood, 22:406, 1963.
Cooper, R. A.: Lipids of human red cell membrane: normal composition and variability in disease. Seminars Hemat., 7:296, 1970.
Cooper, R. A., and Jandl, J. H.: Bile salts and cholesterol in the pathogenesis of target cells in obstructive jaundice. J. Clin. Invest., 47:809, 1968.
Cooper, R. A., and Jandl, J. H.: The selective and conjoint loss of red cell lipids. J. Clin. Invest., 48:906, 1969.
Corcino, J. J., Waxman, S., and Herbert, V.: Absorption and malabsorption of vitamin B_{12}. Amer. J. Med., 48:562, 1970.
Crichton, R. R.: Ferritin: Structure, synthesis and function. New Eng. J. Med., 284:1413, 1971.
Croff, J. D., Jr., Swisher, S. N., Jr., Gilliland, B. C., Bakemeier, R. F., Leddy, J. P., and Weed, R. I.: Coombs test positivity induced by drugs: Mechanisms of immunologic reactions and red cell destruction. Ann. Intern. Med., 68:176, 1968.
Cronkite, E. P., and Bond, V. P.: Radiation Injury in Man. Springfield, Illinois, Charles C Thomas, 1960.
Dacie, J. V., and Mollin, D. L.: Siderocytes, sideroblasts and sideroblastic anemia. Acta Med. Scand., Supple. 445, p. 237, 1966.
Dacie, J. V., and Worlledge, S. M.: Autoimmune hemolytic anemias. Prog. Hemat., 6:82, 1969.
Davidson, R. J. L.: March or exertional hemoglobinuria. Seminars Hemat., 6:150, 1969.
deFuria, F. G., Miller, D. R., Cerami, A., et al.: The effects of cyanate in vitro on red blood cell metabolism and function in sickle cell anemia. J. Clin. Invest., 51:566, 1972.
Diggs, L. W.: Sickle cell crises. Amer. J. Clin. Path., 44:1, 1965.
Donohue, D. M., Reiff, R. H., Hanson, M. L., Betson, Y., and Finch, C. A.: Quantitative measurements of the erythrocytic and granulocytic cells of the marrow and blood. J. Clin. Invest., 37:1571, 1958.
Erslev, A. J.: Humoral regulation of red cell production. Blood, 8:349, 1953.
Erslev, A. J.: The role of erythropoietin in the control of red cell production. Medicine, 43:661, 1964.
Erslev, A. J.: Anemia of chronic renal disease. Arch. Intern. Med., 126:774, 1970.
Erslev, A. J.: The search for erythropoietin (Editorial). New Eng. J. Med., 284:849, 1971.
Filmanowicz, E., and Gurney, C. W.: Studies on erythropoiesis. XVI. Response to a single dose of erythropoietin in polycythemic mouse. J. Lab. Clin. Med., 57:65, 1961.
Finch, C. A.: Iron metabolism. Nutrition Today, Summer, 1969, p. 2.
Finch, C. A., Deubelbeiss, K., Cook, J. D., et al.: Ferrokinetics in man. Medicine, 49:17, 1970.
Finch, C. A., and Lenfant, C.: Oxygen transport in man. New Eng. J. Med., 286:407, 1972.
Gabuzda, T. G.: Hemoglobin H and the red cell. Blood, 27:568, 1966.
Gabuzda, T. G., Nathan, D. G., and Gardner, J. H.: The turnover of hemoglobins A, F and A_2 in the peripheral blood of three patients with thalassemia. J. Clin. Invest., 42:1678, 1963.
Gallo, R. C., Fraimow, W., Cathcart, R. T., and Erslev, A. J.: Erythropoietic response in chronic pulmonary disease. Arch. Intern. Med., 113:559, 1964.
Gardner, F. H., Nathan, D. G., Piomelli, S., and Cummins, F. J.:

The erythrocythaemic effects of androgen. Brit. J. Haemat., 14:611, 1968.

Gardner, F. H., and Pringle, J. C., Jr.: Androgens and erythropoiesis. II. Treatment of myeloid metaplasia. New Eng. J. Med., 264:103, 1961.

Gartner, L. M., and Arias, I. M.: Formation, transport, metabolism, and excretion of bilirubin. New Eng. J. Med., 280:1339, 1969.

Giblett, E. R.: Genetic Markers in Human Blood. Oxford, Blackwell Scientific Publications Ltd., 1969, p. 349.

Gilette, P., Manning, J. M., and Cerami, A.: Increased survival of sickle cell erythrocytes after treatment in vitro with sodium cyanate. Proc. Nat. Acad. Sci., 68:2791, 1971.

Goldberg, A.: Lead poisoning and heme biosynthesis. Brit. J. Haemat., 23:521, 1972.

Gordon, A. S., Cooper, G. W., and Zanzani, E. D.: The kidney and erythropoiesis. Seminars Hemat., 4:337, 1967.

Götze, O., and Müller-Eberhard, H. J.: Paroxysmal nocturnal hemoglobinuria. Hemolysis initiated by the C3 activator system. New Eng. J. Med., 286:180, 1972.

Granick, S., and Levere, R.: Controls of hemoglobin synthesis. Plenary Session Papers. XIIth Internat. Soc. Hemat. Congress, 1968, p. 274.

Gräsbeck, R.: Intrinsic factor and the transcobalamins with reflections on the general function and evolution of soluble transport proteins. Scand. J. Clin. Lab. Invest., 19:(Suppl. 95), 1967.

Gräsbeck, R.: Intrinsic factor and other vitamin B_{12} transport proteins. Progr. Hemat., 6:233, 1969.

Hall, C. A.: Transport of vitamin B_{12} in man. Brit. J. Haemat., 16:429, 1969.

Harris, J. W.: Notes and comments on pyridoxine responsive anemia and the role of erythrocyte mitochondria in iron metabolism. Medicine, 43:803, 1964.

Harris, J. W., and Kellermeyer, R. W.: The Red Cell. Cambridge, Harvard University Press, 1970.

Hartmann, R. C., and Jenkins, D. E., Jr.: Paroxysmal nocturnal hemoglobinuria: Current concepts of certain pathophysiologic features. Blood, 25:850, 1965.

Haurani, F. I., Burke, W., and Martinez, E. J.: Defective reutilization of iron in the anemia of inflammation. J. Lab. Clin. Med., 65:560, 1965.

Haurani, F. I., Sherwood, W., and Goldstein, F.: Intestinal malabsorption of vitamin B_{12} in pernicious anemia. Metabolism, 13:1342, 1964.

Herbert, V.: Experimental nutritional folate deficiency in man. Trans. Amer. Assoc. Physicians, 75:307, 1962.

Hillman, R. S., and Finch, C. A.: Erythropoiesis: normal and abnormal. Seminars Hemat., 4:327, 1967.

Hines, J. D., Hoffbrand, A. V., and Mollin, D. L.: The hematologic complications following partial gastrectomy. Amer. J. Med., 43:555, 1967.

Horowitz, H. J., Stein, J. M., Cohen, B. D., and White, J. M.: Further studies on the platelet-inhibitory effect of guanidinosuccinic acid and its role in uremic bleeding. Amer. J. Med., 49:336, 1970.

Huehns, E. R., and Shooter, E. M.: Review article: Human haemoglobins. J. Med. Genet., 2:48, 1965.

Hurtado, A.: Acclimatization to high altitudes. In Weihe, W. H. (Ed.): Physiological Effects of High Altitude. New York, Pergamon Press, 1964, p. 1.

Itano, H. A.: The human hemoglobins; their properties and genetic control. Advances Protein Chem., 12:216, 1957.

Jacob, H. S.: Mechanisms of Heinz body formation and attachment to the red membrane. Seminars Hemat., 7:341, 1970.

Jacobs, A.: Iron balance and its disorders. Proc. Roy. Soc. Med., 63:1215, 1970.

Jacobson, L. O., Goldwasser, E., Fried, W., and Plzak, L.: Role of the kidney in erythropoiesis. Nature (London), 179:633, 1957.

Jaffé, E. R., and Hsieh, H. S.: DPNH-dependent methemoglobin reductase deficiency and hereditary methemoglobinemia. Seminars Hemat., 8:417, 1971.

Jenkins, D. E., Jr., Hartmann, R. C., and Kerns, A. L.: Serum-red cell interactions at low ionic strength: erythrocyte complement coating and hemolysis of paroxysmal nocturnal hemoglobinuria cells. J. Clin. Invest., 36:753, 1967.

Jensen, W. N., and Lessin, L. S.: Membrane alterations associated with hemoglobinopathies. Seminars Hemat., 7:409, 1970.

Katz, J. H.: The delivery of iron to the immature red cell. A critical review. Scand. J. Haemat., Suppl. 6, 1965, p. 15.

Kirschbaum, J. D., Matsno, T., Sato, K., Ishimarn, M., Tsucchmoto, T., and Ishimarn, T.: A study of aplastic anemia in an autopsy series with special reference to atomic bomb survivors in Hiroshima and Nagasaki. Blood, 38:17, 1971.

Knospe, W. H., Blom, J., and Crosby, W. H.: Regeneration of locally irradiated bone marrow. II. Induction of regeneration in permanently aplastic medullary cavities. Blood, 31:400, 1968.

Krantz, S. B., and Kuo, V.: Studies on red cell aplasia. II. Report of a second patient with an antibody to erythroblast nuclei and a remission after immunosuppressive therapy. Blood, 34:1, 1969.

Kushner, J. P., Lee, G. R., Wintrobe, M. M., and Cartwright, G. E.: Idiopathic refractory sideroblastic anemia. Clinical and laboratory investigation of 17 patients and review of the literature. Medicine, 50:139, 1971.

Landaw, S. A., Callahan, E. W., Jr., and Schmid, R.: Catabolism of heme in vivo: comparison of the simultaneous production of bilirubin and carbon monoxide. J. Clin. Invest., 49:914, 1970.

Lehmann, H.: Different types of alpha thalassemia and significance of hemoglobin Bart's in neonates. Lancet, 2:73, 1970.

Lessin, L. S., and Bessis, M.: Morphology of the erythron. In Williams, W. J., et al. (Eds.): Hematology. New York, McGraw-Hill Book Co., 1972, p. 62.

Lessin, L. S., Jensen, W. N., and Klug, P.: Ultrastructure of the normal and hemoglobinopathic red blood cell membrane. Arch. Intern. Med., 129:306, 1972.

Lewis, S. M., and Dacie, J. V.: The aplastic anemia: Paroxysmal nocturnal hemoglobinuria syndrome. Brit. J. Haemat., 13:236, 1967.

Lie-Injo Luan Eng: Pathological findings in hydrops fetalis due to alpha thalassemia. A review of 32 cases. Trans. Roy. Soc. Trop. Med. Hyg., 62:874, 1968.

Marks, P. A., and Rifkind, R. A.: Protein synthesis in erythropoiesis. Science, 175:955, 1972.

Marsh, G. W., and Lewis, S. M.: Cardiac hemolytic anemia. Seminars Hemat., 6:133, 1969.

Martland, H. S.: The occurrence of malignancy in radioactive persons. Amer. J. Cancer, 15:2435, 1931.

Maugh, T. H.: Vitamin B_{12}: After 25 years, the first synthesis. Science, 179:266, 1973.

McIntyre, P.: Radioactive tracers in hematologic disease. Hosp. Pract., March, 1972, p. 99.

Mengel, C. E., Kann, H. E., Jr., and Meriwether, W. D.: Studies of paroxysmal nocturnal hemoglobinuria erythrocytes: increased lysis and lipid peroxide formation by hydrogen peroxide. J. Clin. Invest., 46:1715, 1967.

Metcalfe, J., Dhindsa, D. S., Edwards, M. J., and Mordjinis, A.: Decreased oxygen affinity of blood for oxygen in patients with low-output heart failure. Circ. Res., 25:47, 1969.

Miller, M. E.: Thymic dysplasia ("Swiss agammaglobulinemia"). I. Graft vs. host reaction following bone marrow transfusion. J. Pediat., 70:730, 1967.

Milner, P. F., Clegg, J. B., and Weatherall, D. J.: Hemoglobin H disease due to a unique hemoglobin variant with an elongated alpha-chain. Lancet, 1:729, 1971.

Modan, B., and Lilienfeld, A. M.: Polycythemia vera and leukemia—the role of radiation treatment. A study of 1,222 patients. Medicine, 44:305, 1965.

Mollin, D. L., Waters, A. H., and Harriss, E.: Clinical aspects of the metabolic inter-relationships between folic acid and vitamin B_{12}. Vitamin B_{12} and intrinsic factor, 2. In Heinrich, H. C. (Ed.): Europaisches Symposion, Hamburg. Stuttgart, Enke, 1961, p. 737.

Morley, A., and Stohlman, F., Jr.: Erythropoiesis in the dog: the periodic nature of the steady state. Science, 165:1025, 1969.

Motulsky, A. G.: Hemolysis in glucose-6-phosphate dehydrogenase deficiency. Fed. Proc., 31:1286, 1972.

Muirhead, H., Cox, J. M., Mazzarella, L., and Perutz, M. F.: Structure and function of haemoglobin III. A three-dimensional Fourier synthesis of human deoxyhaemoglobin at 5.5 A resolution. J. Molec. Biol., 13:646, 1965.

Muldowney, F. P., Crooks, J., and Wayne, E. F.: The total red cell mass in thyrotoxicosis and myxoedema. Clin. Sci., 16:309, 1957.
Murayama, M.: Molecular mechanism of red cell "sickling." Science, 153:145, 1966.
Murray, J. F., Gold, P., and Johnson, B. L., Jr.: The circulatory effects of hematocrit variations in normovolemic and hypervolemic dogs. J. Clin. Invest., 42:1150, 1963.
Nathan, D. G.: Thalassemia. New Eng. J. Med., 286:586, 1972.
Nathan, D. G., and Shohet, S. B.: Erythrocyte ion transport defects and hemolytic anemia: "Hydrocytosis" and "Desiccytosis." Seminars Hemat., 7:381, 1970.
Owren, P. A.: Congenital hemolytic jaundice: The pathogenesis of the "hemolytic crisis." Blood, 3:231, 1948.
Pape, L., Multani, J. S., Stitt, C., and Saltman, P.: In vitro reconstitution of ferritin. Biochemistry, 7:606, 1968.
Perutz, M. F.: Stero chemistry of cooperative effects in haemoglobin. Nature, 228:726, 1970.
Pillow, R. P., Epstein, R. B., Buckner, C. D., Giblett,, E. R., and Thomas, E. D.: Treatment of bone marrow failure by isogeneic marrow infusion. New Eng. J. Med., 275:94, 1966.
Pollycove, M.: Iron metabolism and kinetics. Seminars Hemat., 3:235, 1966.
Ratto, O., Brescoe, W. A., Morton, J. W., and Comroe, J. H., Jr.: Anoxemia secondary to polycythemia and polycythemia secondary to anoxemia. Amer. J. Med., 19:958, 1955.
Reissmann, K. R.: Studies on the mechanism of erythropoietic stimulation in parabiotic rats during hypoxia. Blood, 5:372, 1950.
Robinson, S. H.: Formation of bilirubin from erythroid and nonerythroid sources. Seminars Hemat., 9:43, 1972.
Rosenberg, L. E., Lilljeqvist, A-C., and Hsia, Y. E.: Methylmalonic aciduria: metabolic block localization and vitamin B_{12} dependency. Science, 162:805, 1968.
Rosse, W. F.: Effects of immune reactions on the red cell membrane. Seminars Hemat., 7:323, 1970.
Rosse, W. F.: Quantitative immunology of immune hemolytic anemia. II. The relationship of un-bound antibody to hemolysis and the effect of treatment. J. Clin. Invest., 50:734, 1971.
Rosse, W. F., Dourmashkin, R., and Humphrey, J. H.: Immune lysis of normal and paroxysmal nocturnal hemoglobinuria (PNH) red blood cells. II. The membrane defects caused by complement lysis. J. Exp. Med., 123:969, 1966.
Schmid, R.: Cutaneous porphyria in Turkey. New Eng. J. Med., 263:397, 1960.
Schroeder, W. A., Huisman, T. H. J., Shelton, R., Shelton, R. B., Kleihauer, E. F., Dozy, A. M., and Robberson, B.: Evidence for multiple structural genes for the α-chain of human fetal hemoglobin. Proc. Nat. Acad. Sci., 60:537, 1968.
Shahidi, N. T., and Diamond, L. K.: Testosterone-induced remission in aplastic anemia of both acquired and congenital types. New Eng. J. Med., 264:953, 1961.
Shohet, S. B.: Hemolysis and changes in erythrocyte membrane lipids. New Eng. J. Med., 286:577, 1972.
Silber, R., and Moldow, C. F.: The biochemistry of B_{12} mediated reactions in man. Amer. J. Med., 48:549, 1970.
Skalak, R., and Brånemark, P. I.: Deformation of red blood cells in capillaries. Science, 164:717, 1969.
Spaet, T. H., Bauer, S., and Melamed, S.: Hemorrhagic thrombocytopenia. A blood coagulation disorder. Arch. Intern. Med., 98:377, 1956.
Stamatoyannopoulos, G., Bellingham, A. J., Lenfant, C., and Finch, C. A.: Abnormal hemoglobins with high and low oxygen affinity. Ann. Rev. Med., 22:221, 1971.
Stewart, W. B., Yuile, C. L., Claiborne, H. A., Snowman, R. T., and Whipple, G. H.: Radio iron absorption in anemic dogs. Fluctuations in the mucosal block and evidence for a gradient of absorption in the gastrointestinal tract. J. Exp. Med., 92:375, 1950.
Streiff, R. R.: Folate deficiency and oral contraceptives. J.A.M.A., 214:105, 1970.
Sullivan, L. W.: Vitamin B_{12} metabolism and megaloblastic anemia. Seminars Hemat. 7:6, 1970.
Tabulation of reports compiled by the Panel on Hematology of the Registry on Adverse Reactions. Council on Drugs. American Medical Association, May, 1965, and June, 1967.
Taddeini, L., and Watson, C. J.: The clinical porphyrias. Seminars Hemat., 5:335, 1968.
Thomas, E. D., et al.: Aplastic anemia treated by bone marrow transplantation. Lancet, 1:284, 1972.
Thorling, E. B.: Paraneoplastic erythrocytosis and inappropriate erythropoietin production: A Review. Scand. J. Haemat., Supple. 17, 1972.
Thorling, E. B., and Erslev, A. J.: The "tissue" tension of oxygen and its relation to hematocrit and erythropoietin. Blood, 32:332, 1968.
Valentine, W. N.: Hereditary hemolytic anemias associated with specific erythrocyte enzymopathies. Calif. Med., 108:280, 1968.
Vincent, P. C., and de Gruchy, G. C.: Complications and treatment of acquired aplastic anemia. Brit. J. Haemat., 13:977, 1967.
Ward, H. P., Kurnick, J. E., and Pisarczyk, M. J.: Serum level of erythropoietin in anemias associated with chronic infection, malignancy and primary hematopoietic disease. J. Clin. Invest., 50:332, 1971.
Waxman, S., Metz, J., and Herbert, V.: Defective DNA synthesis in human megaloblastic bone marrow: Effects of homocysteine and methionine. J. Clin. Invest., 48:284, 1969.
Weatherall, D. J., and Clegg, J. B.: The Thalassemia Syndromes. London, Blackwell Scientific Publications Ltd., 1972.
Weed, R. I., LaCelle, P. L., and Merrill, E. W.: Metabolic dependence of red cell deformability. J. Clin. Invest., 48:795, 1969.
Weed, R. I., and Reed, C. F.: Membrane alterations leading to red cell destruction. Amer. J. Med., 41:681, 1966.
Weintraub, L. R., Weinstein, M. B., Huser, H. J., and Rafal, S.: Absorption of hemoglobin iron: Role of heme-splitting substance in intestinal mucosa. J. Clin. Invest., 47:531, 1968.
Wiley, J. S.: Red cell survival studies in hereditary spherocytosis. J. Clin. Invest., 49:666, 1970.
Yataganas, X., and Fessas, P.: The pattern of hemoglobin precipitation in thalassemia and its significance. Ann. N.Y. Acad. Sci., 165:270, 1969.
Yunis, A. A., Smith, U. S., and Restrepo, A.: Reversible bone marrow suppression from chloramphenicol. A consequence of mitochondrial injury. Arch. Intern. Med., 125:272, 1970.

PHAGOCYTES

Baehner, R. L., and Nathan, D. G.: Quantitative nitroblue tetrazolium test in chronic granulomatous disease. New Eng. J. Med., 278:971, 1968.
Bizzozero, O. J., Johnson, K. G., and Ciocco, A.: Radiation-related leukemia in Hiroshima and Nagasaki, 1946–1964. New Eng. J. Med., 274:1095, 1966.
Blume, R. S., Bennett, J. M., Yankee, R. A., and Wolff, S. M.: Defective granulocyte regulation in the Chediak-Higashi syndrome. New Eng. J. Med., 279:1009, 1968.
Boggs, D. R.: The kinetics of neutrophilic leukocytes in health and disease. Seminars Hemat., 4:359, 1967.
Cline, M. J.: Monocytes and macrophages – differentiation and function. In Greenwalt, T. J., and Jamieson, G. A. (Eds.): Formation and Destruction of Blood Cells. Philadelphia, J. B. Lippincott Co., 1970, p. 222.
Cline, M. J.: Biochemistry and function of monocytes and macrophages. In Williams, W. J., et al. (Eds.): Hematology. New York, McGraw-Hill Book Co., 1972, p. 741.
Craddock, C. G., Perry, S., Lawrence, J. S., Buxbaum, L., and Pieper, G.: Production and distribution of granulocytes and the control of granulocyte release. In Wolstenholme, G. E. W., and O'Connor, M. (Eds.): Ciba Foundation Symposium on Haemopoiesis. London, Churchill, 1960, p. 237.
Dameshek, W.: Some speculations on the myeloproliferative syndromes. Blood, 6:392, 1951.
Fialkow, P. J., Thomas, E. D., Bryant, J. J., and Neiman, P. E.: Leukaemic transformation of engrafted human marrow cells in vivo. Lancet, 1:251, 1971.
Gross, L.: Viral etiology of leukemia and lymphomas. Blood, 25:377, 1965.
Holmes, B., Quie, P. G., Windhorst, D. B., and Good, R. A.:

Fatal granulomatous disease of childhood: An inborn abnormality of phagocytic function. Lancet, 1:1225, 1966.
Karnofsky, M. L., Noseworthy, J., Simmons, S., and Glass, E. A.: Metabolic patterns that control the functions of leukocytes. *In* Greenwalt, T. J., and Jamieson, G. A. (Eds.): Formation and Destruction of Blood Cells. Philadelphia, J. B. Lippincott Co., 1970, p. 207.
Kennedy, B. J.: Cyclic leukocyte oscillations in chronic myelogenous leukemia during hydroxyurea therapy. Blood, 35:751, 1970.
Killmann, S. A.: Acute leukemia: the kinetics of leukemic blast cells in man. An analytical review. Series Haemat., 1(3):38, 1968.
March, H. C.: Leukemia in radiologists, ten years later. Amer. J. Med. Sci., 242:137, 1961.
Miller, M. E., Oski, F. A., and Harris, M. B.: Lazy leucocyte syndrome. Lancet, 1:665, 1971.
Nowell, P. C., and Hungerford, D. A.: A minute chromosome in human chronic granulocytic leukemia. Science, 132:1497, 1960.
O'Riordan, M. L., Robinson, J. A., Buckton, K. E., and Evans, H. J.: Distinguishing between the chromosome involved in Down's syndrome (trisomy 21) and chronic myeloid leukemia (Ph[1]) by fluorescence. Nature, 230:167, 1971.
Pisciotta, A. V.: Studies on agranulocytosis X. A biochemical defect in chlorpromazine-sensitive marrow cells. J. Lab. Clin. Med., 78:435, 1971.
Richard, K. A., Morley, A., Howard, D., and Stohlman, F., Jr.: The in vitro colony-forming cell and the response to neutropenia. Blood, 37:6, 1971.
Skipper, H. E.: Cellular kinetics associated with "curability" of experimental leukemia. *In* Dameshek, W., and Dutcher, R. M. (Eds.): Perspectives in Leukemia. New York, Grune and Stratton, 1968, p. 187.
Spiers, A. S. D.: Chemotherapy of acute leukaemia. Clin. Haemat., 1:127, 1972.
Ward, P. A.: Insubstantial leukotaxis. J. Lab. Clin. Med., 79:873, 1972.
Ward, P. A., Cochrane, C. G., and Müller-Eberhard, H. G.: Further studies of the chemotactic factor of complement and its formation in vivo. Immunology, 11:141, 1966.
Warner, H. R., and Athens, J. W.: An analysis of granulocyte kinetics in blood and bone marrow, in leukopoiesis in health and disease. Ann. N.Y. Acad. Sci., 113:523, 1964.
White, J. G.: The Chediak-Higashi syndrome: A possible lysosomal disease. Blood, 28:143, 1966.
Zucker-Franklin, D., Elsbach, P., and Simon, E. J.: The effect of the morphine analog levorphanol on phagocytosing leukocytes. Lab. Invest., 25:415, 1971.
Zuelzer, W. W., and Cox, D. E.: Genetic aspects of leukemia. Seminars Hemat., 6:228, 1969.

Immunocytes

Abdou, N. I., and Abdou, N. L.: Bone marrow: The bursa equivalent in man? Science, 175:446, 1972.
Abramson, N., and Shattil, J. J.: M-components. J.A.M.A., 223:156, 1973.
Alexanian, R., Bonnet, J., Gehan, E., Haut, A., Hewlett, J., Lane, M., Monto, R., and Wilson, H.: Combination chemotherapy for multiple myeloma. Cancer, 30:382, 1972.
Bonomo, L., Dammacco, F., Marano, R., and Bonomo, G. M.: Abdominal lymphoma and alpha chain disease. Amer. J. Med., 52:73, 1972.
Claman, H. N.: Corticosteroids and lymphoid cells. New Eng. J. Med., 287:388, 1972.
Cohen, A. S.: Amyloidosis. New Eng. J. Med., 277:512, 574, 628; 1967.
Cole, P.: Epidemiology of Hodgkin's disease. J.A.M.A., 222:1636, 1972.
Craddock, C. G., Longmire, R., and McMillan, R.: Lymphocytes and the immune response. New Eng. J. Med., 285:324 and 378, 1971.
David, J. R.: Lymphocytic factors in cellular hypersensitivity. Hosp. Pract., March, 1971, p. 79.
DaVita, V. T., Jr., and Canellos, G. P.: Treatment of lymphoma. Seminars Hemat., 9:193, 1972.

Fahey, J. L.: Function of lymphocytes and plasma cells—immunoglobulin synthesis. *In* Williams, W. J., et al. (Eds.): Hematology. New York, McGraw-Hill Book Co., 1972, p. 791.
Franklin, E. C., Lowenstein, J., Bigelow, B., and Meltzer, M.: Heavy chain disease. A new disorder of serum γ-globulins: report of the first case. Amer. J. Med., 37:332, 1964.
Glenner, G. G., Ein, D., Eanes, E. D., Bladen, H. A., Terry, W., and Page, D. L.: Creation of "amyloid" fibrils from Bence Jones proteins in vitro. Science, 174:712, 1971.
Holland, J. F., and Glidewell, O.: Oncologists reply: survival expectancy in acute lymphocytic leukemia. New Eng. J. Med., 287:769, 1972.
Jones, S. E., Rosenberg, S. A., Kaplan, H. S., Kadin, M. E., and Dorfman, R. F.: Non-Hodgkin's lymphomas. II. Single agent chemotherapy. Cancer, 30:31, 1972.
Keller, A. R., Kaplan, H. S., Lukes, R. J., and Rappaport, H.: Correlation of histopathology with other prognostic indicators in Hodgkin's disease. Cancer, 22:487, 1968.
Lampkin, B. C., McWilliams, N. B., and Mauer, A. M.: Cell kinetics and chemotherapy in acute leukemia. Seminars Hemat., 9:211, 1972.
Levine, A. S., Graw, R. G., Jr., and Young, R. C.: Management of infections in patients with leukemia and lymphoma. Current concepts and experimental approaches. Seminars Hemat., 9:141, 1972.
Mathé, G.: Immunotherapy in the treatment of acute lymphoid leukemia. Hosp. Pract., December, 1971, p. 43.
Mauer, A. M., Saunders, E. F., and Lampkin, B. C.: Possible significance of nonproliferating leukemic cells. National Cancer Institute Monograph No. 30, Human Tumor Cell Kinetics, p. 63.
Michaux, J. L., and Heremans, J. F.: Thirty cases of monoclonal immunoglobulin disorders other than myeloma or macroglobulinemia. Amer. J. Med., 46:562, 1969.
Mogielnicki, R. P., Waldman, T. A., and Strober, W.: Renal handling of low molecular weight proteins. I. L-chain metabolism in experimental renal disease. J. Clin. Invest., 50:901, 1971.
Pinkel, D.: Five year followup of "Total Therapy" of childhood lymphocytic leukemia. J.A.M.A., 216:648, 1971.
Potter, M.: Myeloma proteins (M-components) with antibody-like activity. New Eng. J. Med., 284:831, 1971.
Prosnitz, L. R., Hellman, S., vonEssen, C. F., and Kligerman, M. M.: The clinical course of Hodgkin's disease and other malignant lymphomas treated with radical radiation therapy. Amer. J. Roentgen., 105:618, 1969.
Rappaport, H.: Tumors of the hematopoietic system. Armed Forces Institute of Pathology, Washington, D.C., 1966, pp. 91–206.
Rubin, P.: Updated Hodgkin's disease. A. Introduction. B. Curability of localized disease. C. Advanced disease and special problems. J.A.M.A., 222:1292, 1972; and 223:49 and 164, 1973.
Saunders, E. F., Lampkin, B. C., and Mauer, A. M.: Variation of proliferative activity in leukemic cell populations of patients with acute leukemia. J. Clin. Invest., 46:1356, 1967.
Saunders, E. F., and Mauer, A. M.: Reentry of nondividing leukemic cells into a proliferative phase in acute childhood leukemia. J. Clin. Invest., 48:1299, 1969.
Smith, R. T., and Bausher, J. A.: Epstein-Barr virus infection in relation to infectious mononucleosis and Burkitt's lymphoma. Ann. Rev. Med., 23:39, 1972.
Tomasi, T. B.: Secretory immunoglobulins. New Eng. J. Med., 287:500, 1972.
Wilson, J. D., and Nossal, G. J. V.: Identification of human T and B lymphocytes in normal peripheral blood and in chronic lymphatic leukemia. Lancet, 2:788, 1971.
Wood, T. A., and Frenkel, E. P.: The atypical lymphocyte. Amer. J. Med., 42:923, 1967.
Young, R. C., Corder, M. P., Haynes, H. A., and DeVita, V. T.: Delayed hypersensitivity in Hodgkin's disease. Amer. J. Med., 52:63, 1972.

Thrombocytes

Abrahamsen, A. F.: Platelet survival studies in man—with special reference to thrombosis and atherosclerosis. Scand. J. Haemat., Suppl. 3, 1968, p. 7.

Aster, R. H.: Pooling of platelets in the spleen: Role in the pathogenesis of "hypersplenic" thrombocytopenia. J. Clin. Invest., 45:645, 1966.

Cardamone, J. M., Edson, J. R., McArthur, J. R., and Jacob, H. S.: Abnormalities of platelet function in the myeloproliferative disorders. J.A.M.A., 221:270, 1972.

Claman, H. N.: Corticosteroids and lymphoid cells. New Eng. J. Med., 287:388, 1972.

Cohen, P., Gardner, F. H., and Barnett, G. O.: Reclassification of the thrombocytopenias by the ^{51}-Cr-labeling method for measuring platelet lifespan. New Eng. J. Med., 264:1294, 1961.

de Gabriele, G., and Penington, D. G.: Regulation of platelet production: "thrombopoietin." Brit. J. Haemat., 13:210, 1967.

Deykin, D.: The clinical challenge of disseminated intravascular coagulation. New Eng. J. Med., 283:636, 1970.

Erslev, A. J.: Feedback circuits in the control of stem cell differentiation. Amer. J. Path., 65:629, 1971.

Evatt, B. L., and Levin, J.: Measurements of thrombopoiesis in rabbits using ^{75}selenomethionine. J. Clin. Invest., 48:1615, 1969.

Gardner, F. H.: Platelet kinetics and lifespan. Clin. Haemat., 1:307, 1972.

Harker, L. A., and Finch, C. A.: Thrombokinetics in man. J. Clin. Invest., 48:963, 1969.

Harrington, W. J., Minnich, V., Hollingsworth, J. W., and Moore, C. V.: Demonstration of a thrombocytopenic factor in the blood of patients with thrombocytopenic purpura. J. Lab. Clin. Med., 38:1, 1951.

Horowitz, H. J.: Uremic toxins and platelet function. Arch. Intern. Med., 126:823, 1970.

Hovig, T.: Influence of various compounds on blood platelets and platelet aggregation. A scanning electron microscopic study. Series Hemat., 3:47, 1970.

Karpatkin, S.: Heterogeneity of human platelets. II. J. Clin. Invest., 48:1083, 1969.

Karpatkin, S., and Weiss, H. J.: Deficiency of glutathione peroxidase associated with high levels of reduced glutathione in Glanzmann's thrombasthenia. New Eng. J. Med., 287:1062, 1972.

Levin, J., and Conley, C. L.: Thrombocytosis associated with malignant disease. Arch. Intern. Med. (Chicago), 114:497, 1964.

Marchasin, S., Wallerstein, R. D., and Aggeler, P. M.: Variation of the platelet count in disease. Calif. Med., 101:95, 1964.

Odell, T. T., Jr., Jackson, C. W., and Reiter, R. S.: Depression of the megakaryocyte platelet system in rats by transfusion of platelets. Acta Haemat., 38:34, 1967.

Odell, T. T., Jr., McDonald, T. P., and Asano, M.: Response of rat megakaryocytes to bleeding. Acta Haemat., 27:171, 1962.

Oski, F. A., and Naiman, J. L.: Effect of live measles vaccine on the platelet count. New Eng. J. Med., 275:352, 1966.

Post, R. M., and Des Forges, J. F.: Thrombocytopenia and alcoholism. Ann. Intern. Med., 68:1230, 1968.

Schloesser, L. L., Kipp, M. A., and Wenzel, F. J.: Thrombocytosis in iron-deficiency anemia. J. Lab. Clin. Med., 66:107, 1965.

Shreiner, D. P., and Levin, J.: Detection of thrombopoietic activity in plasma by stimulation of suppressed thrombopoiesis. J. Clin. Invest., 49:1709, 1970.

Shulman, I., Pierce, M., Lukens, A., and Currimbhoy, Z.: Studies on thrombopoiesis. I. A factor in normal human plasma required for platelet production; chronic thrombocytopenia due to its deficiency. Blood, 16:943, 1960.

Shulman, N. R.: A mechanism of cell destruction in individuals sensitized to foreign antigens and its implications in autoimmunity. Ann. Intern. Med., 60:506, 1964.

Smith, J. B., and Willis, A. L.: Aspirin selectivity inhibits prostaglandin production in human platelets. Nature, 231:235, 1971.

Wright, J. H.: The histogenesis of the blood platelets. J. Morph., 21:263, 1910.

Zucker, M. B.: Platelet function. *In* Williams, W. J., et al. (Eds.): Hematology. New York, McGraw-Hill Book Co., 1972, p. 1014.

HEMOSTASIS: PLASMA COAGULATION FACTORS

Bachman, F.: The paradoxes of disseminated intravascular coagulation. Hosp. Pract., September, 1971, p. 113.

Beck, E. A., Shainoff, J. R., Vogel, A., and Jackson, D. P.: Functional evaluation of an inherited abnormal fibrinogen: fibrinogen "Baltimore." J. Clin. Invest., 50:1874, 1971.

Blombäck, B.: The N-terminal disulphide knot of human fibrinogen. Brit. J. Haemat., 17:145, 1969.

Cream, J. J., Gumpel, J. M., and Peachey, R. D.: Schönlein-Henoch purpura in the adult. A study of 77 adults with anaphylactoid or Schönlein-Henoch purpura. Quart. J. Med., 39:461, 1970.

Davie, E. W., and Ratnoff, O. D.: Waterfall sequence for intrinsic blood clotting. Science, 145:1310, 1964.

Deykin, D.: The clinical challenge of disseminated intravascular coagulation. New Eng. J. Med., 283:636, 1970.

Duckert, F., and Beck, E. A.: Clinical disorders due to the deficiency of factor XIII (fibrin stabilizing factor, fibrinase). Seminars Hemat., 5:83, 1968.

Feinstein, D., Chouy, M. N. Y., Kasper, C. K., and Rappaport, S. I.: Hemophilia A: Polymorphism detectable by a factor VIII antibody. Science, 163:1071, 1969.

Fletcher, A. P., Ziederman, O., Moore, D., Alkjaersig, N., and Sherry, S.: Abnormal plasminogen-plasmin system activity ("fibrinolysis") in patients with hepatic cirrhosis. Its causes and consequences. J. Clin. Invest., 43:681, 1964.

Gaston, L. W.: When to hospitalize for hypocoagulability. Hosp. Pract., August, 1969, p. 76.

Hathaway, W. E., Mull, M. M., and Pechet, G. S.: Disseminated intravascular coagulation in the newborn. Pediatrics, 43:233, 1969.

Hoag, M. S., Johnson, F. F., Robinson, J. A., and Aggeler, P. M.: Treatment of hemophilia B with a new clotting factor concentrate. New Eng. J. Med., 280:581, 1969.

Hoyer, L. W., and Breckenridge, R. T.: Immunologic studies of antihemophilic factor (AHF, factor VIII): Cross reacting material in a genetic variant of hemophilia A. Blood, 32:962, 1968.

Jackson, D. P., Beck, E. A., and Charache, P.: Congenital disorders of fibrinogen. Fed. Proc., 24:816, 1965.

MacFarlane, R. G.: An enzyme cascade in the blood clotting mechanism and its function as a biochemical amplifier. Nature, 202:498, 1964.

Marder, V. J.: Identification and purification of fibrinogen degradation products produced by plasmin: considerations on the structure of fibrinogen. Scand. J. Haemat. (Supple.), 13:21, 1971.

Meadow, S. R., Glasgow, E. F., White, R. H. R., Moncrieff, M. W., Cameron, J. S., and Ogg, C. S.: Schönlein-Henoch nephritis. Quart. J. Med., 41:241, 1972.

Merskey, C., Johnson, A. J., Kleiner, G. J., and Wohl, H.: The defibrination syndrome: clinical features and laboratory diagnosis. Brit. J. Haemat., 13:528, 1967.

Pool, J. G., and Shannon, A. E.: Production of high-potency concentrates of antihemophilic globulin in a closed bag system. New Eng. J. Med., 273:1443, 1965.

Prentice, C. R. M., and Ratnoff, O. D.: Genetic disorders of blood coagulation. Seminars Hemat., 4:93, 1967.

Robboy, S. J., Lewis, E. J., Schur, P. H., and Colman, R. W.: Circulating anticoagulants to factor VIII. Amer. J. Med., 497:42, 1970.

Schwartz, M. L., Pizzo, S. V., Hill, R. L., and McKee, P. A.: The effect of fibrin stabilizing factor on the subunit structure of human fibrin. J. Clin. Invest., 50:1506, 1971.

Shapiro, S. S.: The immunologic character of acquired inhibitors of antihemophilic globulin (factor VIII) and the kinetics of their interaction with factor VIII. J. Clin. Invest., 46:147, 1967.

Sherry, S.: Mechanisms of fibrinolysis. *In* Williams, W. J., et al.

(Eds.): Hematology. New York, McGraw-Hill Book Co., 1972, p. 1111.

Spaet, T. H.: Hemostatic homeostasis. Blood, 28:112, 1966.

Strauss, H. S.: Acquired circulating anticoagulants in hemophilia A. New Eng. J. Med., 281:866, 1969.

Sutherland, J. M., Glueck, H. I., and Gleser, G.: Hemorrhagic disease of the newborn. Amer. J. Dis. Child., 113:524, 1967.

Suttie, J. W.: Control of clotting factor biosynthesis by vitamin K. Fed. Proc., 28:1696, 1969.

Weiss, H. J.: von Willebrand's disease—diagnostic criteria. Blood, 32:668, 1968.

Wessler, S., and Gaston, L. W.: Pharmacologic and clinical aspects of heparin therapy. Anesthesiology, 27:475, 1966.

Williams, W. J.: Sequence of coagulation reactions. In Williams, W. J., et al. (Eds.): Hematology. New York, McGraw-Hill Book Co., 1972, p. 1085.

Yoshikawa, T., Tanaka, K. R., and Guze, L. B.: Infection and disseminated intravascular coagulation. Medicine, 50:237, 1971.

Zimmerman, T. S., Ratnoff, O. D., and Littell, A. S.: Detection of carriers of classic hemophilia using an immunologic assay for antihemophilic factor (factor VIII). J. Clin. Invest., 50:255, 1971.

Zimmerman, T. S., Ratnoff, O. D., and Powell, A. E.: Immunologic differentiation of classic hemophilia (factor VIII deficiency) and von Willebrand's disease. J. Clin. Invest., 50:244, 1971.

CHAPTER 23

THE SPLEEN AND RETICULO-ENDOTHELIAL SYSTEM*

SPENCER O. RAAB

INTRODUCTION

Existence of a reticuloendothelial system (RES) has, for the most part, been a rather nebulous concept. One reason for this confusion is that the cellular components of the RES are so widely scattered, so diverse in their structural elements, and so pleomorphic that there exists a confusion of terms and concepts concerning their morphology and function. These cells include macrophages lining the sinuses of various organs, microglia, reticulum cells of lymphatic tissue, tissue macrophages (histiocytes), and the specialized cells such as Kupffer cells in the liver, spleen, and bone marrow. Another reason is that only recently has a body of knowledge been obtained which is based on solid experimental data to explain the functions of this wide variety of cells. The development of the German dye industry gave the first impetus to understanding this system. Ehrlich and his associate, Goldmann, performed the first injection of these dyes into animals and made a rather extensive study of the resultant vitally stained tissues. Although they did not attach a specific name to the system, it was evident that the endothelium of organs such as the liver, lymph nodes, and spleen was richly endowed with phagocytic powers and ingested these dyes. Later, Aschoff (1924) suggested the name reticuloendothelial system. He was not unduly worried by the morphologic diversity because the cells had in common the property of phagocytosis. In an effort to provide a unifying definition of the RES, Aschoff divided the system into four structures:

1. Splenic phagocytes and blood histiocytes.
2. Reticulum cells of the pulp cords of the spleen, cortical nodules, and pulp cords of lymph nodes and other lymphatic tissues.
3. Histiocytes of connective tissue. (These are now regarded as tissue macrophages.)
4. Reticuloendothelium of lymph sinuses, splenic sinuses, capillaries of the liver, bone marrow, adrenal cortex, and anterior lobe of the pituitary.

Although this type of classification is useful in understanding the morphology of the RES, it has little use in defining function.

Recently, the main thrust of research has been toward the study of specific reticuloendothelial cells rather than the system as a whole in an effort to understand how they function. This approach has been quite successful. Table 23-1 lists the types of cells commonly found in the reticuloendothelial system and the commonly proposed functions and origins for each of these cells. Clearly, the reticuloendothelial system does not fit into any one discipline, and a study of it requires a background knowledge of many fields.

At the present time, the functions of the RES may thus be listed as follows:

1. Immune responses—antibody formation, cell-borne and humorally mediated responses.
2. Phagocytosis of bacteria (implies killing which is not always accomplished) and phagocytosis of various particles.

---

*Based on the Chapter "The Spleen and Reticuloendothelial System" by James H. Jandl, which appeared in the previous edition of this book.

TABLE 23-1 DISTRIBUTION AND FUNCTION OF CELLS OF THE RES

Cell Type	Subtypes	Principal Distribution	Mobility	Principal Functions
Reticuloendothelial cells (RE cells)	Reticulum cells Endothelial cells	Spleen, lymphatics, liver, bone marrow	Remain in tissue of origin, except for histiocytes, small numbers of which circulate	RES structure, filtration of particles, phagocytosis, stem cell compartment
Immunocytes a. Lymphocytes	Small lymphocytes Large lymphocytes	Spleen, lymphatics, thymus, blood	Circulate readily through blood and lymphatics	Immunologic responsiveness*, stem cell compartment, "T" cell (cell borne), "B" cell (humoral)
b. Plasma cells	——	Spleen, lymphatics, bone marrow	Circulate to a minor extent in blood	Antibody formation
Monocytes	——	Blood (probably formed in bone marrow)	Circulate readily in blood	Phagocytosis
Tissue macrophages	——	Alimentary tract, bone marrow, intestinal tract	Originate in bone marrow; migrate to tissues but do not recirculate to any major extent	Phagocytosis, filtration of particles
Specialized tissue macrophages	——	Lung, central nervous system, Kupffer cells (liver)	Originate in bone marrow; migrate to tissues but do not recirculate to any major extent	Phagocytosis, filtration of particles

*"T" designates thymus-derived lymphocytes. "B" designates "bursa-equivalent" or bone marrow-derived lymphocytes.

3. Blood cell formation.
4. Filtration of blood and extravascular fluids and removal of senile cells, damaged cells, or cells coated with antibodies.
5. Hematopoiesis and replenishment of a stem cell compartment.

Table 23-2 lists the four major organs of this system, their cellular classification, and the principal functions they perform in the human organism.

It is obvious that there is a considerable amount of duplication of function in these geographically separate but closely related organs. All of them, for example, filter the blood and/or extravascular fluid, but each of the major structures appears to have a specialized function in this regard. The RE cells of the spleen remove inclusions from the erythrocytes, while the Kupffer cells of the liver have a somewhat different function. Consequently, it is helpful to classify the RES in this manner, since treatment of some diseases is based on these special functions. The bone marrow also has a special "role" within this system, but the spleen and liver may act as "understudies" in some instances.

This chapter concerns the various functions of the reticuloendothelial system from the standpoint of both the organ involved and the single type of cell line involved. Some of these functions will be covered in greater detail elsewhere, and the reader will be referred to the appropriate chapters. The spleen, second only to the bone marrow, is the focus of attention. It will receive the first consideration in this chapter. The most important function of the bone marrow, that of blood cell formation, is reviewed in Chapter 22 and will not be discussed here.

THE SPLEEN

Historical Perspectives

The spleen has a long, distinguished history as the object of scientific scrutiny. For example, Galen regarded the spleen as an organ "full of

TABLE 23-2 PRINCIPAL FUNCTIONS OF THE RES ORGANS IN MAN

Organ	Cellular Composition	Estimate Blood Flow	Principal RES Functions
Lymph nodes	RE cells Lymphocytes Plasma cells	Small (probably <1% of cardiac output)	Filtration of extravascular fluids, antibody formation
Spleen	RE cells Lymphocytes Plasma cells	Approximately 3 to 5% of cardiac output	Filtration of blood, antibody formation
Liver	RE cells Hepatocytes	20 to 25% of cardiac output	Filtration of blood
Bone marrow	RE cells Blood cell precursors Fat cells	Approximately 5% of cardiac output	Filtration of blood, blood cell formation*

*In certain pathologic states all organs of the RES may contribute to blood cell formation.

mystery" and believed it to be the source of "black bile" or melancholy. This belief is, of course, an extension of the theory of Hippocratic medicine concerning the doctrine of the four humors. Almost simultaneously, another society viewed the spleen in a mystical fashion. In the great Chinese medical classic, *The Canon of Medicine* (Nei Ching), the spleen was regarded as the seat of thought. The liver according to the *Canon* was the seat of anger, the heart of happiness, the lung of sorrow, and the kidney of fear. In this same treatise, it was thought that the liver formed tears and the spleen formed saliva. Obviously, the anatomic and physiologic precepts of the *Canon* are based upon neither observation nor experiments. Be that as it may, over the centuries two facts emerged about the spleen: first, the spleen is not essential to life; second, enlargement of the spleen is usually, but not always, accompanied by poor health. Splenomegaly, in most instances, is a result of underlying disease such as leukemia, lymphoma, or infection. Therefore, it is not, in itself, a cause of ill health but rather an accessory finding. However, in some cases, an enlarged spleen and even a normal-sized spleen may play a major role in the pathophysiology of disease, such as in hereditary spherocytosis. Understanding the mechanism involved in these instances requires a detailed knowledge of the anatomy and histology of this organ.

THE STRUCTURE OF THE NORMAL SPLEEN

Traditionally, the spleen is said to consist of a capsule and trabeculae enclosing a pulp (Fig. 23-1). The pulp itself is divided into three zones: the white pulp, a marginal zone, and the red pulp.

The capsule and trabeculae in the human spleen consist of dense white fibrous tissue and carry the major afferent and efferent blood and lymphatic vessels and nerves. Although this structure contains a small amount of elastic tissue, it is not thought to be contractile in the usual meaning of the word. In contradistinction, the dog spleen possesses a muscular capsule which is capable of contraction. Therefore, the dog spleen has the unusual capacity to become engorged with blood during sleep or anesthesia and, in some cases, an increase in weight to several times greater than normal has been reported. Although the human spleen may become engorged, it appears to be incapable of contraction and of spilling stored contents into the bloodstream as occurs in the dog. This is an important concept to remember when considering the splenic red cell pool in health and disease.

The white pulp consists for the most part of lymphoid tissue. It thus appears "white" or lighter colored as compared to the other areas of the organ. Two major components are present in the white pulp: the periarterial lymphatic sheath and the secondary lymphoid follicles. Periarterial lymphatic sheaths consist of cylinders of white pulp coaxially surrounding the major arterial vessels which enter the pulp of the spleen from the trabeculae. The secondary lymphatic follicles are nodular thickenings of white pulp occurring here and there within the periarterial lymphatic sheaths. They occur especially at the bifurcations of the arterial vessels. The secondary follicle consists of a central germinal center of large cells and a surrounding mantle zone of small lymphocytes. Interlaced through these two major components of the white pulp is a fine reticular meshwork which acts as a scaffolding to support the blood vessels containing the so-called free cells,

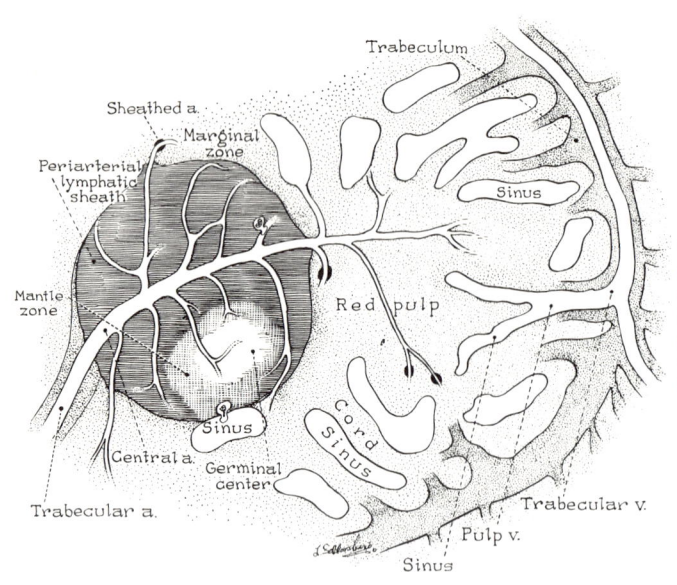

Figure 23–1 Diagrammatic representation of splenic circulation. (From Weed, R., and Weiss, L.: Trans. Assoc. Amer. Physicians, 79:426, 1966. Reprinted from Greep: Histology. New York, McGraw-Hill Book Co., Blakiston Division, 1966, p. 397. Copyright 1966. Used with permission of McGraw-Hill Book Company.)

that is, the lymphocytes and other related cells. This meshwork, which is stained with special silver stain, is referred to as a fibrillar reticulum, or the term "reticulum" is sometimes used alone. This substance is probably produced by the reticular cells that closely follow the reticular fibers. This reticular cell meshwork is sometimes termed cellular reticulum. While they may be phagocytic to a slight degree, they do not appear to differentiate the lymphocytes or other cell types. The primary functions of these reticular cells appear to be supporting the free cells and producing extracellular reticulum. The free cells of the white pulp consist of lymphocytes, monocytes, macrophages, plasma cells, and occasional granulocytes.

The marginal zone is a poorly defined junction of tissue which surrounds the white pulp and lies between the white and red pulp. It is significant because it receives many arterial terminations. Consequently, many cells and particles trapped in the spleen end up in the marginal zone, and pathologic processes such as argyria and amyloidosis are noticed first in this particular zone. Like other areas of the pulp, the marginal zone also consists of three different elements: the reticular meshwork, the blood vessels, and free cells. In hemolytic anemia, damaged erythrocytes are concentrated in the marginal zone and are phagocytized, creating a relative increase in the number of erythrocytes and macrophages in this area.

The red pulp contains arterial vessels, sinuses, and cords. The cords are reticular tissues similar in structure to the reticular tissue of the marginal zone. The cords receive almost all the arterial vessels reaching the red pulp. Within the interstices of this fibrillar reticulum substance there is a variety of cells, again including lymphocytes, macrophages, and plasma cells. When the spleen is sectioned, the cords appear as bands of tissue separating sinuses, but in fact they are a continuous extensive tissue, honeycombed with sinuses. Sinuses are elongated, broad efferent vessels consisting of an endothelium or lining cell and a basement membrane. The lining cells are reticular cells that are cytologically similar to those forming the meshwork in the white pulp, marginal zone, and cord. But instead of having the branch form of reticular cells in these places, the reticular cells of sinuses are elongated tapering rods lining the sinus walls, their axes parallel to the long axis of the vessel. These reticular cells lie side by side, and although their lateral surfaces touch, they are not held together by any modification of cell membrane. Consequently, free cells may pass between adjacent lining cells, pressing them apart. The lining cells lie upon a basement membrane which is remarkable in that it is pierced by large regular fenestrations with the result that the substance of the basement membrane is reduced to a system of fine strands. Thus, the basement membrane, which controls passage of materials across the cell wall, would appear to allow for the ready passage of cells but retains sufficient structure to support the vessel.

Thus, a groundwork has been laid for discussion of the blood flow through the spleen. The splenic artery penetrates the spleen capsule at the hilar notch in the medial aspect of the organ. Beyond this point, the artery branches within the trabeculae in company with veins and with an efferent system of lymphatics. These branches are named trabecular arteries, and they enter the periarterial lymphatic sheaths as the central artery. As the artery passes through the white pulp, a number of small vessels permeate this area. Other vessels, as mentioned earlier, escape the white pulp and empty into the marginal zone. The bulk of the blood flow, however, passes through arterial vessels into the red pulp. These arterial vessels entering the red pulp may terminate in two different ways. A few communicate directly with the sinuses and thus flow directly into the pulp veins and into the trabecular veins and the splenic veins. Under normal conditions, this represents a rather small amount of the total blood flow. Virtually all arterial blood from arteries terminating in red pulp empties into the cords. Accordingly, the blood cells then pass between the lining cells and also through the basement membrane into the pulp veins, which in turn flow into the trabecular veins. This type of flow has been called "open circulation," since the blood leaves its closed system of endothelium-lined vessels and invades the pulp spaces before entering the openings in the walls of the venous sinusoids.

It is obvious that the phagocytic function of the spleen would be extremely efficient under these conditions, since the red blood cells can move only slowly among the interstices of the pulp and therefore come in contact with many reticuloendothelial cells.

Although this "open circulation" theory, which denotes rather slow passage of cells through the red pulp, is attractive, much of the experimental data supports a second type of blood flow in which the blood passes quite rapidly through the pulp tissue into the splenic veins. This type of circulation is thought to occur through anatomically closed circuits, i.e., the indirect anastomoses between the pulp arteries and the sinuses.

The normal circulation of erythrocytes through the spleen is of the rapid transit type. This rapid transit probably involves both methods mentioned above. In a normal spleen, erythrocyte transit may proceed equally rapidly through the "open circulation," even though the erythrocytes must pass through the rather narrow spaces between the RE cells.

However, when the spleen is enlarged and diseased because of an accumulation of cells in the splenic cords, the relatively short journey between arterial termination and the sinus lumen becomes longer and much more difficult. These changes undoubtedly lead to pooling of blood in the cord and a subsequent slow passage through the spleen. This leads to "conditioning" of the cells, which in turn causes their premature death. The phenomenon will be discussed later in this chapter. It is obvious that the structure of the spleen and the mechanism of blood flow through the spleen play key roles in the removal of "damaged" red cells from the circulation.

RELATIONSHIP OF THE SPLEEN AND THE ERYTHROCYTES

Sequestration Without Destruction of Erythrocytes

Under physiologic conditions, very little blood is sequestered in the normal spleen. The total blood content of the spleen, despite its rich vascularity, is only about 50 ml., which represents about 1 per cent of the total blood volume. Most of this blood appears to exchange rapidly with peripheral blood and is therefore judged to be in complete equilibrium. The blood flow to the normal human spleen is believed to be about 3 or 4 per cent of the cardiac output, or approximately 150 ml. per minute.

Jandl has performed direct studies of normal spleen blood mixture in man by injecting ^{51}Cr-labeled autologous red cells into a peripheral vein and monitoring radioactivity over the spleen. Such studies have shown that the time for complete mixing of peripheral blood with splenic blood is as short as 20 seconds and no more than 2 minutes (Fig. 23–2). Although it is quite conceivable that in these results there is the concealed factor of a minor compartment in which the ex-

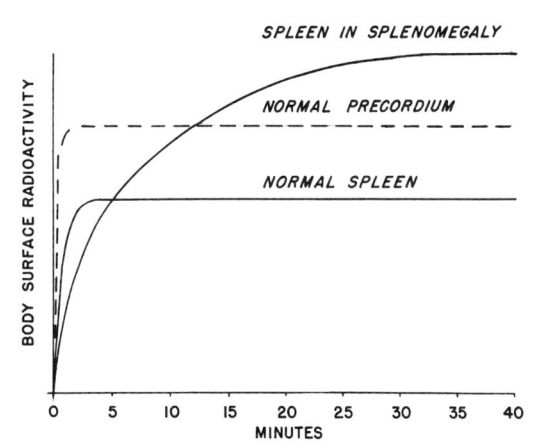

Figure 23–2 Rates of mixing of red cells in normal and enlarged spleens. Following the intravenous injection of normal Cr^{51}-labeled red cells, mixing of labeled and unlabeled cells can be monitored with a directional scintillation counter. As indicated by the interrupted line, radioactivity over the normal precordium reaches a plateau indicating complete mixing within less than a minute, and that over the normal spleen is very slightly slower. However, mixing of circulating and intrasplenic blood often is not completed for 30 or 40 minutes in patients with splenomegaly and may require longer than an hour.

change rate is slower, it is clear that the transit time for most of the blood flowing through the spleen is only slightly slower than in other organs.

The hemodynamics are altered, however, in patients having splenomegaly for any variety of reasons. In such patients, the total number of labeled red cells entering the splenic pool is increased. Moreover, the period required for the systemic pool of labeled cells to equilibrate with the splenic pool may be remarkably prolonged, frequently 30 or 40 minutes (Fig. 23-2). In some patients, over an hour is necessary for complete equilibration to take place. Harris et al. have shown that normal mixing of blood in the spleen follows a single exponential function of time. Many patients with splenomegaly and delayed mixing showed two component curves.

These studies provide strong kinetic evidence for two vascular compartments: one conducts blood rapidly with a transit time of less than two minutes and appears to be the predominant normal pathway; the second exchanges much more slowly and in splenomegaly may be much larger. Splenomegaly tends to detain red cells, and in those patients with large spleens, an appreciable "extravascular" red cell pool appears to exist. The anatomic counterparts of these two kinetic vascular compartments are not clear. It is reasonable to suppose, however, that the larger and patent sinuses supply the rapid flow in the normally predominant compartment, and that under certain conditions the second (cordal) compartment is entered or opened up. It is possible, of course, that the direct endothelium lined connection with the sinuses has a limited capacity to expand, and when this capacity is exceeded the excess blood is shunted into the splenic cords.

The splenic cords may, on the other hand, have an almost infinite capacity to expand as increasing blood is fed into this very loosely bound group of reticulum and free cells. The more blood fed into this pool, however, the longer it would take any one individual cell to reach the sinuses and the veins draining the pulp substance.

Another factor that may play a role in slowing blood flow through the spleen is the ability of this organ to induce hemoconcentration. Barcroft and others demonstrated that the dog spleen had a marked ability to concentrate red cells in the splenic pulp while skimming off plasma in the white pulp and marginal area of the spleen.

Normal human spleens do not show such a striking change in hemoconcentration, but Rothchild et al. have demonstrated that in individuals with large spleens there is a significant increase in the total body hematocrit as compared to the peripheral hematocrit, indicating existence of a hemoconcentrated splenic pool. Subsequent calculations by others have revealed that the red cell pool in splenomegaly is highly variable, depending presumably on whether enlargement represents vascular or nonvascular tissue; in some patients with splenomegaly, however, studies with ^{51}Cr-labeled red cells indicate that as much as 20 to 25 per cent of the total splenic red cell mass may be in the splenic pool.

Up until now, we have been discussing the sequestration of normal cells into normal-sized or enlarged spleens. Altered red cells may be handled in a somewhat different fashion than normal cells by a normal spleen. In some instances, they may be sequestered for several hours and then released back into the circulation to survive fairly normally thereafter (Fig. 23-3). In other words, altered red cells are not invariably lysed in the spleen following sequestration. It has been known for many years that following splenectomy, red cells containing certain kinds of inclusion bodies appeared in the circulation that had not been recognized prior to the removal of the spleen. Two examples are cells with Howell-Jolly bodies and cells with iron granules. Crosby showed in a series of elegant experiments that transfused red cells containing iron granules (siderocytes) lost these granules in normal spleens without the cells themselves being destroyed (Fig. 23-4). He called this phenomenon the "pitting function" of the spleen. Other investigators demonstrated that the spleen normally sequestered immature red cells, including many reticulocytes, and that many of these apparently ripened there, and then proceeded into the circulation. The finding that immature red cells possess a protein coating (largely as attached transferrin) and behave like antibody-coated cells in vitro suggests a common mechanism for their splenic sequestration. Keene demonstrated that the bone marrow and spleen are the two RES organs most avid in trapping nucleated red cells. Thus, in a sense, the spleen acts in the role of inspector in the assembly line. The spleen scrutinizes the circulating red cells and removes from circulation those which do not, so to speak, meet specifications. This has been called a "culling" effect, and it is probably performed by the phagocytes, the fixed and wandering group of cells in the red pulp of the spleen. These fixed phagocytes are the littoral cells that line the sinusoids, and their increase in size and number in certain hemolytic diseases would indicate their role in destruction of abnormal red blood cells.

Although the spleen performs this function in an extremely efficient manner, its ability is not limitless. Splenectomy in normal subjects results in only a few cells with Howell-Jolly bodies or siderocytes appearing in the circulation. Probably only relatively few such cells are released from the bone marrow. On the other hand, splenectomy in patients who exhibit a severe degree of

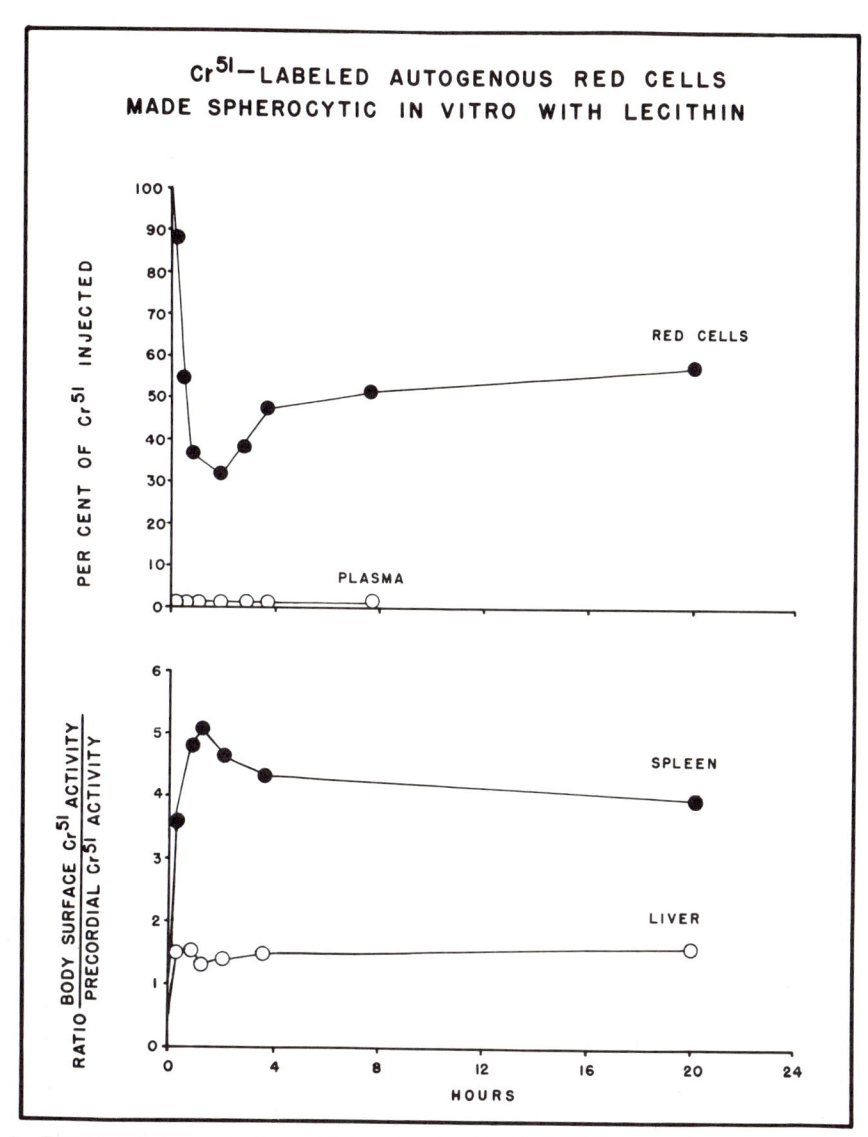

Figure 23-3 Temporary sequestration of injured red cells. Cells that had been injured by lecithin, which makes red cells spheroidal in shape, were at first taken up by the spleen of this normal individual. After about an hour many of the trapped cells were released from the spleen (lower portion) into the circulation (upper portion), which releasing continued for several hours thereafter. Presumably in this instance splenic sequestration exerted a beneficial or at least a temporizing influence, for the survival of the labeled cells thereafter was normal. (Reproduced with the kind permission of the publishers, from Jandl, J. H., and Tomlinson, A. S.: J. Clin. Invest., 37:1202, 1958.)

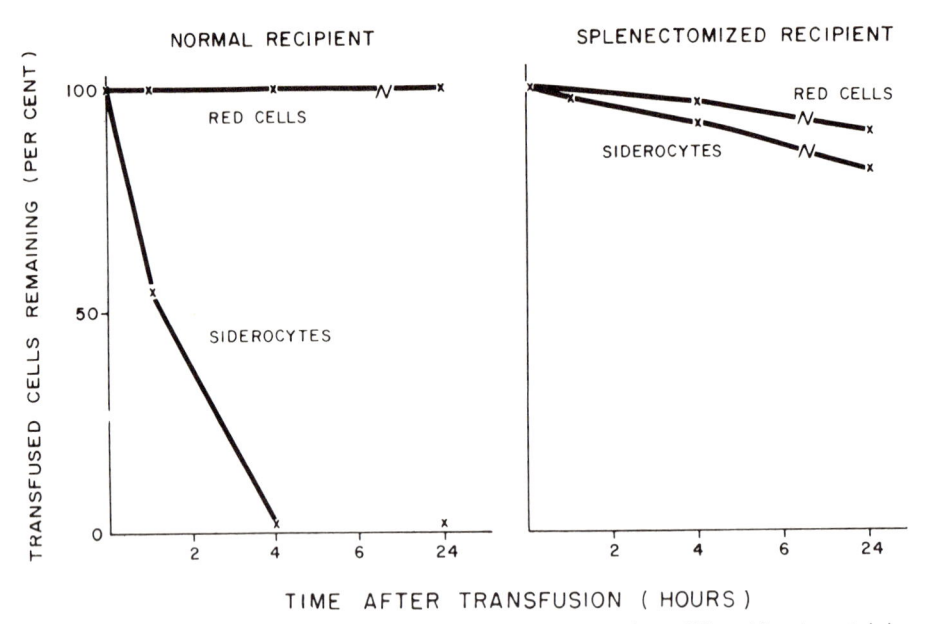

Figure 23-4 Removal of red cell inclusion granules by the normal spleen. When blood containing numerous siderocytes (red cells possessing inclusion granules of iron) was transfused to a normal recipient, as depicted on the left, these red cells survived normally but the inclusions were removed. When the same blood was transfused to a splenectomized recipient (right), these iron granules persisted. This attribute of the spleen was termed by Crosby the "pitting function." (Reproduced with the kind permission of the author and publisher, from Crosby, W. H.: Blood, *14*:399, 1959.)

abnormal red cell production results in the appearance of numerous bizarre forms in the circulation. Some forms may be present even before splenectomy, which may indicate that the capacity of the spleen was exceeded. Such forms occur in thalassemia major, myelofibrosis, and carcinomatosis.

An example of a condition in which the splenic sequestration of red cells serves a useful purpose is latent endemic bartonellosis. In this disorder, seen in rats or dogs, apparently healthy animals develop severe, often fatal hemolytic disease after splenectomy. This bacilliform organism clings to red cell surfaces and causes their destruction. Evidently, the intact spleen efficiently removes minimally "infected" red cells from the blood, destroys the organisms, and thereby suppresses the disease. Removal of the spleen allows the Bartonella organisms to remain and survive in the circulation, to proliferate, and within a few days to hemolyze the red cells.

In Table 23-3 are listed the changes that occur in the red cells, leukocytes, and platelets following splenectomy or in those rare individuals who are born without a spleen. There is a great variety in a number of these changes that occur in any one particular individual following a splenectomy. In some normal individuals, a splenectomy (for a ruptured spleen) may result in the appearance of only a few Howell-Jolly bodies and an occasional target cell; no nucleated red cells will be seen. In other individuals, a large number of these cells will appear in the circulation.

TABLE 23-3 HEMATOLOGIC FINDINGS AFTER SPLENECTOMY OR IN CONGENITAL SPLENIC AGENESIS (ASPLENISM)

A. Red cells
  1. No change in numbers or life span
  2. Flattening of cell, increase in surface, target cells
  3. Usually slight increase in reticulocytes
  4. Inclusion bodies: siderocytes, Howell-Jolly bodies, basophilic stippling, Heinz bodies
  5. Occasional nucleated red cells
B. Leukocytes
  1. Leukocytosis, moderate at first; later usually slight or moderate
  2. Occasional immature forms
  3. Frequently a delayed increase in lymphocytes, monocytes and eosinophils
C. Platelets
  1. Thrombocytosis; may be striking at first, later usually slight
  2. No change in life span
  3. Occasionally atypical and giant forms

Sequestration with Destruction of Erythrocytes

It has been evident for many years that clearance from the blood of senescent or injured red cells is, under all circumstances except the unusual case of acute intravascular hemolysis, a function of the reticuloendothelial system and its mononuclear macrophages. The most important organ of the reticuloendothelial system in this regard is the spleen. Emerson, Shen, and Castle provided evidence that the spleen detained red cells in hereditary spherocytosis and subjected them to what they called "erythrostasis."

Dacie and Young also demonstrated that the spleen can indeed selectively retain red cells in this disease. It was apparent, therefore, that a spleen that permits normal red cells to pass through unmolested can trap and destroy an abnormal cell.

Knowledge in this field was further enhanced by the use of a gamma-emitting isotope, ^{51}Cr, as a red cell label. Using this label, Jacob and Jandl found that certain kinds of abnormalities of red cells would cause the cells to be sequestered very selectively in the spleen. There was little or no sequestration elsewhere in the RES. Examples of alterations predisposing to splenic sequestration are cell-coating with "incomplete" antibodies, spherocytosis induced by exposure of cells to mild heat or lecithin, and certain chemical abnormalities such as inhibition of membrane sulfhydryl groups with N-ethylmaleimide (Fig. 23-5). These investigators showed that a normal individual's red cells moderately injured in these ways are cleared from the circulation at slow or moderate rates, the half-survival time being not less than about 20 minutes. In individuals with large spleens, on the other hand, sequestration by the spleen may be faster, with a half-survival time as short as 8 to 10 minutes. In splenectomized individuals, red cells similarly altered are cleared much less rapidly, half-survival time being 5 to 10 or more hours (Fig. 23-5).

Recently, a number of investigators, Weed in particular, have added greatly to our knowledge of the mechanisms by which destruction of red cells occurs within the spleen in the RE system. Weed and coworkers suggested that red cell fragmentation, defined as loss from the cell of a piece of membrane which may or may not contain hemoglobin, may be an important aspect of the loss

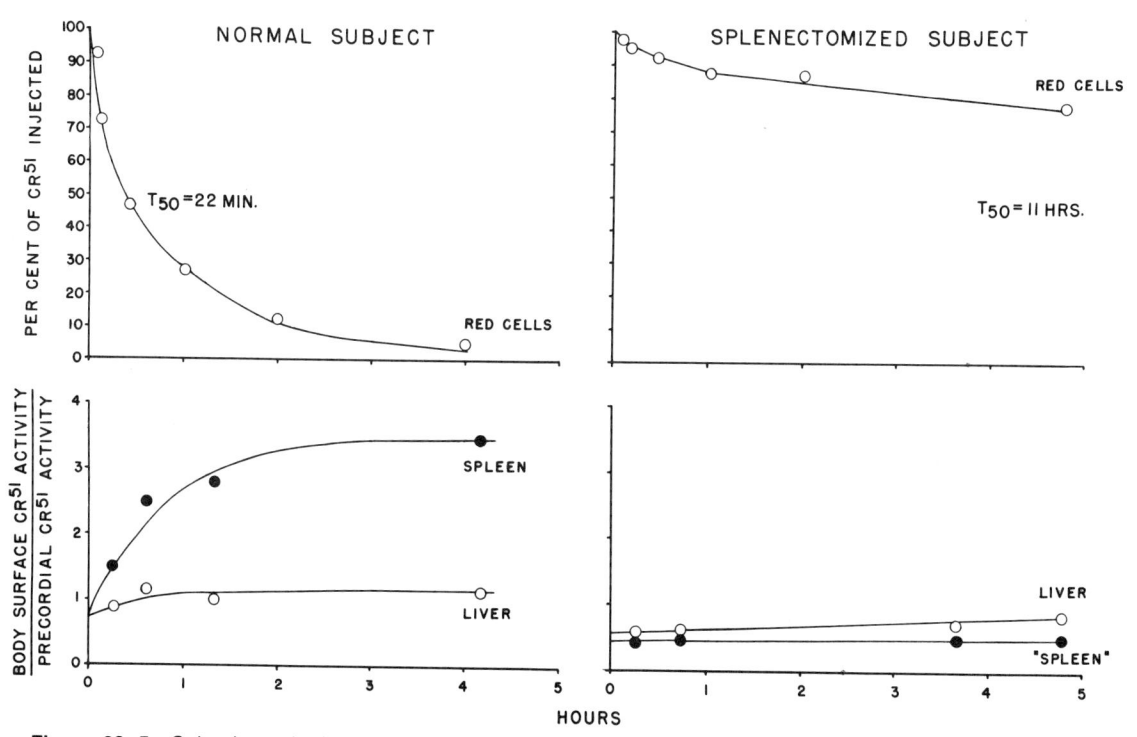

Figure 23-5 Selective splenic sequestration of mildly injured red cells. The special facility of the spleen for trapping and destroying red cells is revealed here by injecting autogenous red cells that had been exposed to low concentrations of the sulfhydryl-blocking agent, NEM. As shown on the left, such cells are cleared readily by the spleen at a rate probably limited by its blood flow. In a splenectomized individual, however, clearance is markedly impaired. (Reproduced with the permission of the publishers, from Jacob, H. S., and Jandl, J. H.: J. Clin. Invest., 41:1514, 1962.)

TABLE 23-4 MECHANISMS OF HEMOLYSIS

1. Injury
   Changes in permeability, colloid osmotic lysis, or direct hemoglobin loss
2. Sequestration of damaged cells
3. Phagocytosis of damaged cells
4. Loss of membrane content
   a. Fragmentation
   b. Phagocytosis of fragmented cells

Modified from Weed, R., and Weiss, L.: Trans. Assoc. Amer. Physician, 79:426, 1966.

of integrity of the cell and its consequent removal from the circulation. The role of the spleen in this fragmentation phenomenon was suggested by prior observations of Weiss, who called attention to the hazards imposed on red cells by passage through the normal circulation of the spleen. Table 23-4 lists the processes in sequential order that occur with in-vivo hemolysis. In this discussion, injury denotes any mechanism that may effect a change in the red cell membrane. These lesions include normal aging, intracorpuscular biochemical defects, or an extracorpuscular agent. Sequestration represents the selective filtration of injured cells from the general circulation and their concentrations within the vascular spaces of the RES.

Weed and coworkers have shown that a wide variety of injuries to the cell result in a rigid cell membrane. A prime example is the spherocyte, which has been shown by these investigators to have less deformability when the cell is made to pass through a fine capillary tube. If the spherocytosis is due to a hereditary disease, it is an example of an intracorpuscular defect. If it is acquired, it is an example of injury due to an extracorpuscular agent. Hemoglobin C disease is another example. In this disease, the precipitation of the abnormal hemoglobin in the cell membrane causes the membrane to become more rigid and therefore less likely to pass through an opening in the basement membrane of the cord into the sinuses. The precipitation of antibody on the cell membrane will also cause rigidity and is yet another example of an extracorpuscular agent.

These cells, which have a more rigid membrane as compared with normal cells, must squeeze through a narrow space imposed by an endothelium of terminal arteries and then pass through the narrow confines of the splenic cords, which are lined by many phagocytic cells. If they survive this passage, the erythrocytes must then squeeze through openings in the basement membrane separating the cord from the sinuses and then back into general circulation. The dimensions of the lumen connecting cords and sinus are about 0.5 micron in diameter under normal circumstances. This requires considerable deformability of erythrocytes for passage. Normal red cells, for the most part, have this ability. Injured cells, on the other hand, do not have this ability to deform infinitely. They become "hung up" as they try to pass through the very small openings in the splenic cords and thus become readily available for the phagocytic cells to engulf part of the membrane. This membrane loss causes the cells to become even more spherocytic and rigid, and on the next passage through the splenic circulation ultimate lysis of the cell may occur. It is probable that most cells require two or more passages through the spleen before this occurs. Figure 23-6 summarizes this sequence of events. Figure 23-7 is an electron micrograph illustrating the fragmentation of a red cell containing a Heinz body as it passes from the cord into the sinus. One can readily see that a "vicious cycle" occurs in this process. Initial fragmentation produces a more rigid membrane, and this in turn causes a decreased deformability of the cell, thus setting the stage for more loss of membrane by phagocytosis on the next passage through the spleen. Thus, lysis of the cell ultimately occurs. The common mechanism of red cell destruction in hemolytic anemias appears to be an alteration of the deformability of the cell membrane.

RELATIONSHIP OF THE SPLEEN AND THE PLATELETS

Sequestration Without Premature Destruction

Platelet concentration in the circulation can be thought of as an equilibrium between the production of platelets in the bone marrow and the destruction of platelets somewhere in the periphery of the body. In the past, increased destruction was believed to be the only mechanism responsible for low platelet counts in those individuals who had normal or increased numbers of megakaryocytes in the bone marrow. However, it is apparent that another mechanism, that is, sequestration of platelets, could also cause a decrease in the concentration in the blood if the process were so marked as to exceed the capacity of the bone marrow to "keep up."

The spleen has long been known to act as a sequestrating organ. Using platelets labeled with ^{51}Cr, Aster demonstrated that the spleen contains an exchangeable pool for platelets that varies roughly in magnitude in proportion to the spleen size. These cells can be discharged into the circulation by epinephrine infusion. Furthermore, Aster's studies indicated that normally about one third of the total platelet mass is contained in the spleen. In splenomegaly, the spleen platelet pool may be greatly enlarged and may contain up to

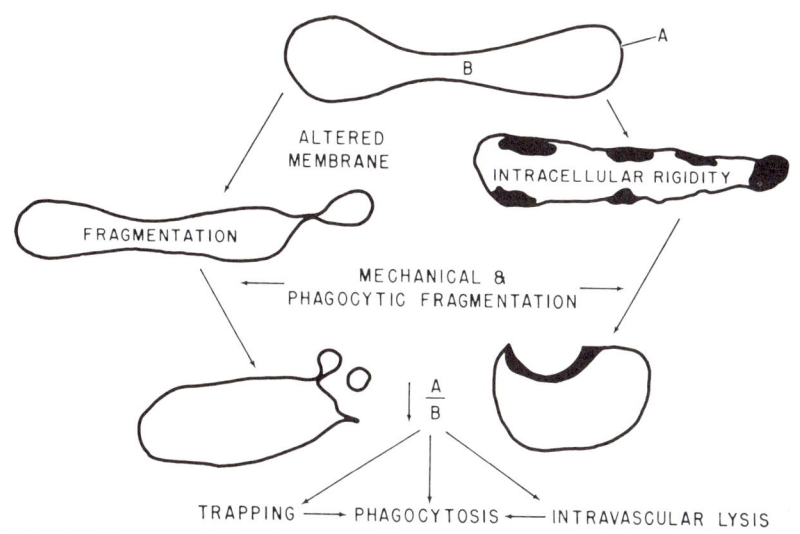

Figure 23-6 Splenic effects on rigid erythrocytes. (From Weed, R., and Weiss, L.: Trans. Assoc. Amer. Physicians, 79:426, 1966.)

90 per cent of the total platelet mass. Thus, both the normal and the abnormal spleen have a marked capacity for sequestrating platelets under a variety of conditions. These platelets are merely sequestrated and are not destroyed. This concept has been shown to be true by Aster and a large number of other investigators using ^{51}Cr-labeled cells. In these studies the platelets were labeled in vitro with ^{51}Cr and then infused into the donor. After equilibrium was established, usually in 1 to 2 hours (by which time the radioactivity had fallen to approximately two thirds the initial value), epinephrine was given to the subjects. Within a few minutes, the platelet count had increased significantly but the amount of label per unit number of platelets remained ex-

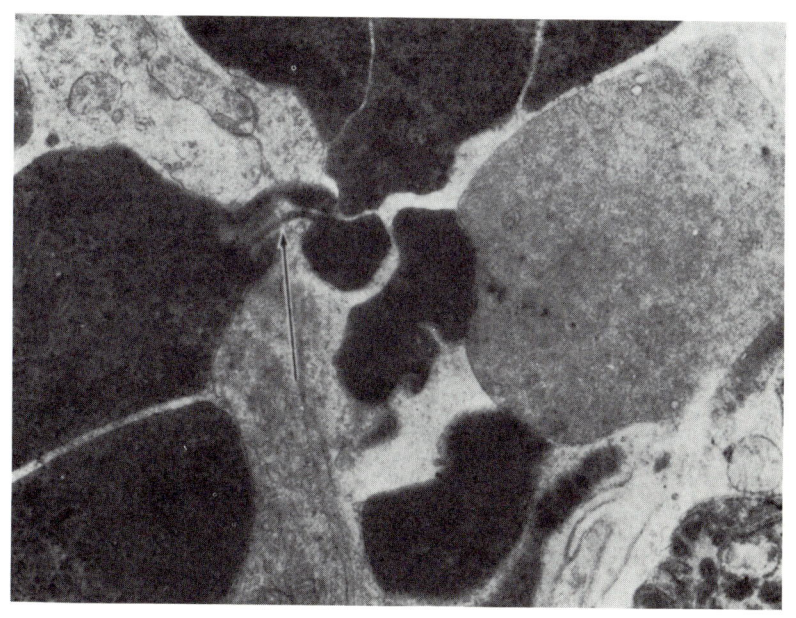

Figure 23-7 Electron micrograph of Heinz body containing fragment breaking off from red cell upon passage from cord into sinus. Arrow indicates fragment breaking off from cell. (From Weed, R., and Weiss, L.: Trans. Assoc. Amer. Physicians, 79:426, 1966.)

actly the same when compared to the number of platelets in the circulation at the time equilibrium was established. Therefore, we can conclude that (1) the increased platelet count was not due to new unlabeled cells released from the bone marrow or from other pools and (2) that this recovery of cells represented the same cells that were initially labeled and infused. In addition, the survival time of the labeled platelets was found to be normal, which would not be the case if these cells were destroyed at an accelerated rate in the spleen.

This same mechanism was demonstrated to be present in a patient with a large spleen by Harker (Fig. 23-8). In this patient, splenomegaly was associated with a marked thrombocytopenia. Notice, however, that the platelet survival time was normal and that the bone marrow megakaryocyte mass was increased. The recovery of labeled platelets injected was quite low at the start of the study, indicating a marked increase in splenic pooling immediately after the infusion.

The removal of a normal spleen is another situation in which there is sequestration without destruction of platelets. When such a spleen is removed, the platelet increase is quite marked immediately following splenectomy and it is greater and more prolonged than after other surgical procedures. This suggests that the increase is not due to the surgical procedure alone. After removal of a large spleen in disorders *not* related to platelets or megakaryocytes such as in hereditary spherocytosis, the platelet count may soar into the millions. This suggests that a big spleen stimulates a chronic increase in platelet production by sequestrating large numbers of platelets.

Sequestration with Increased Destruction of Platelets

The spleen may play a major role in destroying platelets in certain disease states. The most common and best studied entity in this category is chronic idiopathic thrombocytopenic purpura (ITP). Many studies have shown that the platelets have a decreased survival time in these individuals. Furthermore, following splenectomy, at least 66 to 75 per cent of these patients experience a complete clinical recovery and, in addition, the platelet survival time as measured by ^{51}Cr returns to normal. This sequence of events suggests that the spleen is acting as the end organ or agent to filter out and destroy the platelets in these subjects (Fig. 23-9). The platelet numbers rise fairly rapidly after splenectomy, usually within the first 24 to 48 hours, although a peak is not reached until five to seven days have passed. Not all patients respond in this fashion, and in a few individuals, thrombocytopenia may persist for years. It should be remembered that these observations are based on an abnormal state, such as that of patients with ITP.

Studies using normal autologous platelets labeled with ^{51}Cr in normal subjects revealed the liver to be the principal normal source of platelet removal. Therefore, some other factor must be present in order to explain the picture of increased destruction of platelets in the spleen. This factor is the existence of a humoral antiplatelet antibody. Over 20 years ago, Harrington reported the existence of such a factor in approximately 65 per cent of patients with ITP. This factor was capable of lowering the platelet count precipitously when injected into normal volun-

D.S.

Count 55,000

Survival 9.0

Production
 E   2.2
 T   2.1

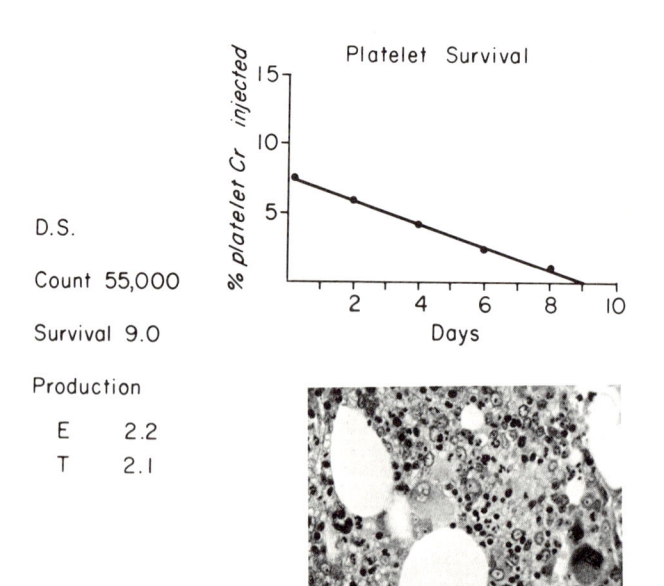

Figure 23-8 Massive splenomegaly due to chronic active hepatitis and a platelet count of 55,000 per μl. in a 15-year-old girl. Platelet survival was normal with a marked *increase in splenic pooling*. Platelet turnover (effective production) and megakaryocyte mass (total production) were comparably increased. (From Harker, L. A.: *In* Brinkhous, K. M., et al. (Eds.): Platelet (Monograph). Baltimore, Williams and Wilkins Co., 1971.)

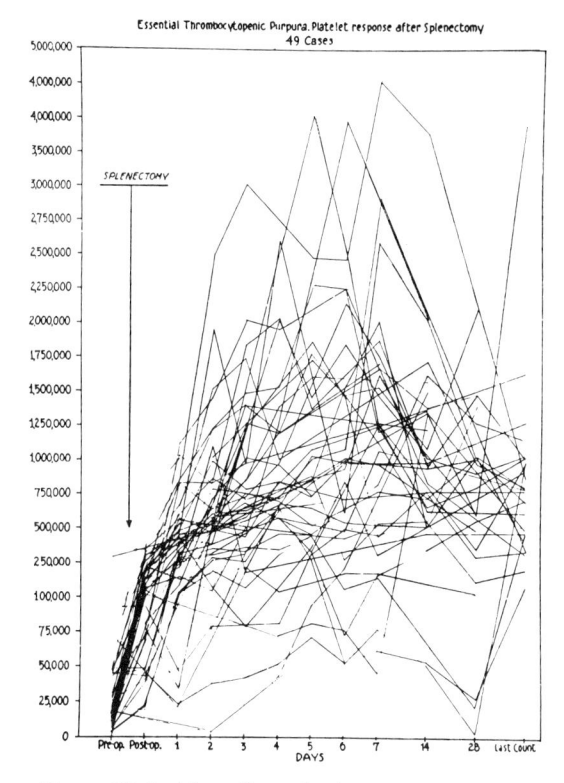

Figure 23-9 The effect of splenectomy on peripheral blood platelet levels in 49 consecutive cases of thrombocytopenic purpura. An immediate rise in platelet levels occurred in all but five patients at the operating table on the day of surgery. In most patients platelets rose steadily thereafter to reach a peak level within a week. (Reproduced with the kind permission of the author and publisher, from Doan, C. A.: Bull. New York Acad. Med., 25:625, 1949.)

teers. In-vitro demonstration had been difficult, however, until recently, when Karpatkin and coworkers, using a more sensitive and refined test, demonstrated an antibody to be present in two thirds of patients with ITP, whether the platelet count was normal or low, and in 96 per cent of the same patients who demonstrated thrombocytopenia (Table 23-5). These investigators employed a platelet factor 3 "immuno-injury" technique (PF-3) and demonstrated that the antiplatelet antibody was an immunoglobulin of the IgG variety. The antibody was also found to be present in patients with other so-called autoimmune diseases associated with thrombocytopenia, such as systemic lupus erythematosus (SLE), autoimmune hemolytic anemia, and rheumatoid arthritis. It was not found in patients with drug-induced thrombocytopenia, hypersplenism, prosthetic heart valve disease, disseminated intravascular coagulation, and thrombotic thrombocytopenic purpura. Of great interest was the finding that the antibody was also present in patients with SLE and normal platelet counts. The platelet survival time was decreased in these subjects. The authors postulated the presence of a "compensatory thrombolytic state," and suggested that the existence of such a state can be readily determined by examination of a blood smear, which in these individuals shows an increased number of large platelets (megathrombocytes). These large platelets are actually young platelets. The concept is analogous to the one of a compensated hemolytic state in which anemia is not present but the number of reticulocytes (larger than normal RBCs) is increased.

Equally or perhaps more fascinating was the finding by Karpatkin et al. that the level of an-

TABLE 23-5 CLINICAL DISORDERS IN WHICH ANTIPLATELET ANTIBODY CAN GENERALLY BE DETECTED*

Clinical Diagnosis	Total No.	No. Detectable	% Positive	Average Positive Titer†	% of Patients with Thrombocytopenia‡
ITP	80	52	65	1:26	96
SLE	50	39	78	1:29	14
Rheumatoid arthritis	5	4	80	1:25	20
Lymphoma	9	6	65	1:21	100
Autoimmune hemolytic anemia	5	3	60	1:16	100
Hepatitis	4	2	50	1:12	75
Blood transfusions§	5	4	80	1:17	40

*Globulin fractions of serum assayed for antiplatelet activity by the PF-3 test for platelet injury.
†Arithmetic average of positive titers. Negative titers not included in average.
‡One or more platelet counts below 150,000/cu. mm.
§Multiple blood or platelet transfusions.

From Karpatkin, S., et al.: Amer. J. Med., 52:776, 1972.

tibody decreased significantly in 7 of 8 patients with ITP following splenectomy. In addition, the antiplatelet antibody could be eluted from the spleen in 10 of 12 patients with ITP. These data suggest that the spleen either contains or synthesizes antiplatelet antibody. The possibility of the spleen being an organ of antibody synthesis is not unreasonable. Antiplatelet antibody synthesis by the spleen in patients with ITP could help to explain the paradoxical positive response after splenectomy of some patients with predominantly hepatic sequestration of platelets as well as a positive response of some patients who do not respond to steroid therapy. An alternative explanation is that the rise in platelet count after splenectomy results in the increased absorption of circulating antiplatelet antibody.

In summary, the mechanisms involved in thrombocytopenia and autoimmune states may be outlined as follows:

1. An antiplatelet antibody (IgG) is present in the circulation. This antibody attaches to the platelet membrane.

2. The splenic macrophage system recognizes these coated cells as either a "damaged cell" or possibly as a "foreign" substance and the cells are destroyed in the splenic cords and sinuses. Although the spleen is the major site for platelet sequestration and death, other organs may be involved, e.g., the liver.

3. The spleen may be a major source for the production of the antibody in some patients as well as the end organ that removes the damaged cells in patients with ITP.

4. Evidence suggests the presence of a "compensated thrombolytic state" in patients with normal platelet counts, the presence of antiplatelet antibodies, and a shortened survival time. In these patients, the bone marrow is able to increase production sufficiently to maintain a normal equilibrium.

RELATIONSHIP OF THE SPLEEN AND THE GRANULOCYTES

Early investigators believed that the spleen was a large reservoir for granulocytes. Their beliefs were based on their observation that in dogs the circulating granulocyte count dramatically increased and sometimes doubled following injection of epinephrine. Since the dog spleen had been shown to possess contractural ability, the same characteristic was attributed to the human spleen. Discrepancies in this theory first appeared when it was shown that the same response to epinephrine was obtained in patients who had had a splenectomy for a number of diverse conditions including trauma, ITP, thalassemia, and autoimmune hemolytic anemias. In addition, anatomic studies revealed that the human spleen has very little contractural ability.

Later, Athens and coworkers developed a method utilizing DFP-32 as a cell label for measuring the total number of cells in the circulation (total blood granulocyte pool [TBGP]). They found that this pool of cells consisted of two pools of equal size in complete equilibrium with each other; the circulating granulocyte pool (CGP), which is a product of the blood volume and the absolute venous granulocyte count, and the marginal granulocyte pool (MGP). This latter pool consists of cells that transiently adhere to the walls of the capillaries throughout the body. They can readily be brought back into the circulation with epinephrine or exercise, hence, the rapid increase in the number of circulating granulocytes following epinephrine injection. The splenic vasculature apparently is only a very small part of this marginal pool. This was shown to be the case by Raab et al. when they measured the TBGP, CGP, and MGP in normal dogs before and after splenectomy. There was no significant difference in any of these measurements.

The marginal granulocyte pool has been measured in patients with varying degrees of leukocytosis ranging up to 500,000 per cu. mm. In most of these patients, the MGP and the CGP were found to be of equal size.

The role of the spleen in leukopenia has not been clearly defined. Some, but not all, patients with splenomegaly and leukopenia exhibit an increased rate of disappearance of the granulocytes from the circulation when they are measured with a radioactive label. However, it has not been possible to prove the role of the spleen in this regard. It is likely that the spleen plays only a minor role, if any, in this abnormal granulocyte kinetic pattern.

SPLENOMEGALY

The spleen, in association with the other organs of the RES, has a notorious capacity for enlargement. Consequently, it has gained an undeserved reputation as a sinister organ. However, this capacity for enlargement is probably relatively no greater, and in many instances less, than the enlargement we see in the ordinary lymph node under the same circumstances. The discovery of splenomegaly seems to be a much more dramatic finding to the average physician as compared to the finding of scattered lymphadenopathy. Perhaps that is one reason for the greater interest in this organ. Another reason is that the finding of splenomegaly represents the presence of a more specific group of disease processes, whereas lymphadenopathy is a rather nonspecific phenomenon. The degree of enlargement that is necessary before the spleen can be palpated has always been a common question that eager students pose. Precise measurements are lacking, but the generally accepted belief is that the spleen is usually enlarged two to four times its normal size before it can be palpated. It is obvious, of course, that a great many environmental factors may hinder estimation of splenic size. Obesity, guarding of the abdominal wall, presence of other masses (an enlarged uterus, for example), and, perhaps most important of all, the skill of the examiner are possibilities that must be taken into consideration.

Tables listing all the possible causes of splenomegaly are so inclusive as to be virtually useless clinically. It is perhaps more helpful to distinguish certain magnitudes of splenomegaly. The more common causes of splenomegaly (as seen in temperate regions) are listed in Table 23–6 in terms of the degree of enlargement. Obviously, there is a great deal of overlap within a particular disease state. For example, patients with chronic granulocytic leukemia may present with spleens that are barely palpable, and other patients may have spleens that extend to the iliac crest. Some of this variability may be due to the stage of the disease when it is first seen by the physician. In addition, true variability from one patient to another is undoubtedly operating in many disease processes. In certain geographic regions, the list of common causes of marked splenomegaly would include kala-azar, chronic malaria, and echinococcosis.

In a very large number of patients with slight splenomegaly, the underlying cause of the enlargement is never ascertained. Furthermore, the splenic enlargement resulting from transient illnesses may regress quite slowly thereafter, persisting often for weeks, frequently for months, and occasionally for years after recovery is complete. Therefore, a palpable spleen does not always imply the presence of any active disease. McIntyre and Ebaugh, as a part of a routine physical examination, were able to palpate the spleen in 3 per cent of college freshmen. Three years later, 30 per cent of these students still had palpable spleens and had had no discernible disease.

Further perusal of Table 23–6 would tend to show that the greatest magnitude of splenomegaly is seen in those instances in which an infiltrative process is present. In addition to the examples of chronic granulocytic leukemia and myelofibrosis, Gaucher's disease, Niemann-Pick disease, and diffuse amyloidosis can result in spleens weighing over 2000 grams.

Although most of the factors governing splenic size are not well understood, some clinical observations and experimental data support the hypothesis that the major stimulus appears to be the "workload" that is presented to this organ. The chronic hemolytic anemias are an excellent demonstration of this regulatory phenomenon. These diseases have in common the following microscopic changes in the splenic structure:

1. Varying degrees of hyperemia and dilatation of the sinuses and red pulp.
2. Hyperplasia of the reticuloendothelial cells.
3. Increase in reticulum fibers in the red pulp, particularly above the sinus sites.
4. Increase in number, diameter, and height of the littoral cells lining the sinuses.

Thus, the cells most closely concerned with fragmentation of the red cell and phagocytosis of particles of the red cell membrane are greatly increased in these individuals.

Jacob et al. confirmed these clinical observations in a series of experiments using spleen autotransplants in rats. They show that the regeneration of these spleens was associated with acquisition of sequestering function as determined by injecting labeled red cells. When a particular workload was imposed by creating a hemolytic process, splenic transplant growth and sequestering function were markedly stimulated.

The rate of synthesis of DNA using ^{3}HTDR as the radioautograph label was performed in both the spleen and the livers of rats. The authors demonstrated that the spleen had a very high DNA turnover rate when phagocytosis took place in this organ. The same authors, using heat-

TABLE 23–6 COMMON CAUSES OF SPLENOMEGALY

	Magnitude of Splenomegaly		
Category	Cm. Below Left Costal Margin	Spleen: Weight, gm.	*Causative Diseases*
Normal	0	100 to 200	None
Slight	0 to 4	200 to 500	Infections (tuberculosis, SBE, hepatitis), hypersensitivity reactions, connective tissue disorders
Moderate	4 to 8	500 to 2000	Cirrhosis, hemolytic anemia, infectious mononucleosis, leukemia and lymphoma, polycythemia vera
Marked	>8	>2000	Chronic granulocytic leukemia, myelofibrosis

treated red blood cells, revealed that this increased rate of synthesis of DNA occurred mainly in the marginal zone and in the red pulp. This increased production of DNA represents hyperplasia in these areas. This hyperplastic reaction subsides over a period of several days, but if the stimulus is sustained, the hyperplasia is cumulative and gross splenomegaly ensues. Presumably this chain of events accounts for the hyperplastic splenomegaly observed in patients with intracorpuscular defects of the red cells as in hereditary spherocytosis or in thalassemia.

Thus, increasing the function and demands of the spleen stimulates its growth; presumably the lymph nodes have a similar response. Therefore, it should not be inferred that patients with functional splenic hyperplasia will all improve following splenectomy. If the spleen is the primary reticuloendothelial organ responsible for removing abnormal cells, such as in hereditary spherocytosis, and elliptocytosis, then recovery may be expected. However, when other areas of reticuloendothelial tissue in addition to the spleen perform this culling action, for example, in congenital nonspherocytic anemia, the hemoglobinopathies, and some cases of acquired hemolytic anemia, no improvement or perhaps only partial improvement will follow splenectomy. Sickle cell anemia is perhaps a case in point. In these patients, a so-called "auto-splenectomy" is the rule after the patient reaches adolescence and adult life. Autopsy findings in these individuals reveal the spleen to be very fibrotic and remarkably small, and in some instances it has been difficult even to recognize the existence of this organ. Howell-Jolly bodies, siderosis, and Pappenheimer bodies are present in the circulating red cells, supporting the diagnosis of a hyposplenic state. However, the hemolytic process in red cell destruction goes on at an undiminished rate in the other organs of the RES. These clinical and laboratory findings suggest that whereas the culling action of the spleen is taken over by the remainder of the RES, the "pitting" function is for the most part unique for the spleen and is not a part of the function of the lymph nodes, bone marrow, or liver.

ACCESSORY SPLEENS

Accessory spleens have been observed in from 20 to 30 per cent of all post-mortem examinations. The numbers vary from single spherical nodules to multiple nodules found most commonly near the tail of the pancreas in the gastrosplenic ligamentum and in the mesentery of the small and large intestines. They are histologically and functionally similar to the main organ. Splenosis is a term used when, following traumatic rupture or surgery of the spleen, fragments are liberated into the peritoneal cavity and into the retroperitoneal space. These seedlings will grow and occasionally have been implicated in intestinal obstruction that necessitates later surgery.

Occasionally patients who have responded well to splenectomy for disorders such as idiopathic thrombocytopenic purpura or hemolytic anemia have had relapses attributable to the presence of accessory spleens. In many of these individuals, exploration would undoubtedly reveal aberrant spleen tissue or so-called accessory spleen, since they can occur, as noted above, in a significant number of normal patients at autopsy. The role of these spleens in causing relapse is not clear. It is unlikely that a relapse of hemolytic anemia would occur unless this accessory spleen were at least of a size approaching that of a normal organ. Such a hemolytic relapse has been documented by McKinsey et al. in a splenectomized patient with hereditary spherocytosis; at surgery a splenunculus was found to weigh 217 grams. Stobie reported a similar case.

Patients with idiopathic thrombocytopenic purpura present a more complicated picture. Although an accessory spleen has not been demonstrated to be the major offender responsible for the removal of damaged platelets in most patients, it may produce an antiplatelet antibody, as discussed previously. It is conceivable that a very small accessory spleen could produce sufficient antibody to coat the platelets which would then be destroyed in other reticuloendothelial organs. Although this hypothesis has yet to be tested, it would appear to be an attractive alternative to the belief that an extremely small spleen is capable of removing enough platelets to cause thrombocytopenia.

RUPTURE OF THE SPLEEN

There have never been reports of spontaneous rupture of a normal spleen. Consequently, rupture should be considered to occur in only two circumstances—in patients who have some underlying disease and in trauma. Smith and Custer reported 45 cases of spontaneous rupture of the spleen from the records of the Armed Forces Institute of Pathology. The following distribution was documented:

Underlying Disease	Number of Cases
Recurrent malaria	22
Infectious mononucleosis	7
Congestive splenomegaly	5
Leukemia	3
Torsion	3
Cause unknown	5

Other authors have reported that the most common single cause of spontaneous rupture of the spleen is malaria, followed by infectious mononucleosis. In the temperate zones, the latter disease is by far the most likely cause of spontaneous splenic rupture. Other conditions predisposing to rupture of the spleen are amyloidosis, typhoid fever, tularemia, and the myeloproliferative diseases. The mechanism of rupture is basically a weakening of the capsule and trabeculae through either infarction or actual infiltration of these structures.

Infectious mononucleosis is a special culprit, It causes cellular infiltration around the intratrabecular vessels which separate them from the connective tissue sheath (Fig. 23-10). The loosening of the supporting structure, particularly evident in the second or third week of illness, markedly increases the fragility of the vessels and sets the stage for traumatic hematomas and rupture.

Trauma to the spleen, usually due to a severe blow or crushing injury, is a major cause of delayed death. The incidence of ruptured spleen in automobile accidents in which injury occurs is high. Two kinds of injury may be seen. When the splenic capsule is actually torn, internal bleeding may be massive, and death may ensue promptly. More often, the tear is subscapular, that is, initially there is no defect in the splenic capsule. Following the injury, blood may seep into the splenic substance and a large growing hematoma may develop. Extravasation gradually occurs throughout the spleen and expands the capsule, causing extreme tenderness and splenomegaly. Eventual rupture of the capsule and shock may then occur. The laboratory values may mirror those of a gradual blood loss, as in gastrointestinal hemorrhage. In many cases, the trauma may be so slight that the patient has forgotten the incident unless closely questioned. Prompt surgical intervention is mandatory in most cases.

HYPERSPLENISM

For years the term hypersplenism aroused heated controversy among the world's outstanding hematologists. It elicited numerous definitions and almost as many theories regarding the mechanisms by which the spleen was responsible for anemia, leukopenia, thrombocytopenia, or any of a combination of these manifestations. Chauffard originally used the term to describe the role of the spleen in hereditary spherocytosis. Later, Dameshek, Doan, and others revived the term to encompass a spectrum of disorders in which splenomegaly was associated with depression of one, two, or three formed elements of the blood. Dameshek and coworkers attributed the syndrome to an influence of the spleen on bone marrow function, notably to the release of some humoral substance which affected the maturation and delivery of immature blood cells. This theory was probably the cause of most of the controversy in the use of this term, since numerous experimental attempts to demonstrate a splenic humoral effect in bone marrow activity were unsuccessful or were difficult to interpret. It may well be that such a regulatory influence exists, but proof is still lacking.

In the past, hypersplenism has been classified as either primary or secondary. Accordingly, hereditary spherocytosis and idiopathic thrombocytopenic purpura are classified as "primary" hypersplenism. The term secondary hypersplenism was used when an underlying disease could be recognized. We now know that in patients with hereditary spherocytosis and in other congenital hemolytic anemias splenomegaly is probably secondary to the hemolytic anemia. Therefore, these diseases are no longer regarded by most hematologists as true examples of hyper-

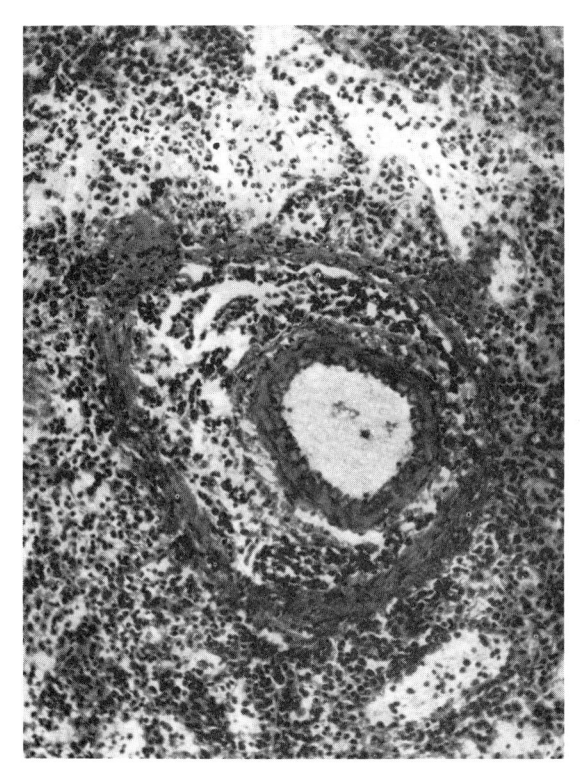

Figure 23-10 Characteristic lesion of the intratrabecular vessels of the spleen in infectious mononucleosis. The separation of the vessels from their supporting connective tissue sheaths by the lymphocytic infiltrate and edema creates vascular friability and predisposes to splenic hematoma or rupture. Similar changes may occur in leukemia. Other disorders such as malaria or congestive splenomegaly appear to predispose to rupture by causing simple vascular engorgement. (Reproduced with the kind permission of the authors and publisher, from Jambon, M., and Bertrand, L.: Sang, *31*:235, 1960.)

splenism. In the overwhelming majority of cases, therefore, the term is reserved for those individuals in whom splenomegaly is the initial occurrence and hematologic manifestations are manifested at a later date. Another disease is almost always present.

Confusion often exists as to the criteria necessary for the diagnosis of hypersplenism in any particular instance. The following are the accepted principal features of hypersplenism as outlined in its usual sense: (1) splenomegaly; (2) one or more of the following—anemia, leukopenia, thrombocytopenia, or any combination; (3) hyperplasia of the bone marrow; and (4) correction of the cytopenia(s) by splenectomy.

Unfortunately, if all four criteria were strictly required, the diagnosis of hypersplenism could be made only in retrospect. Obviously, it is of little help to the clinician to include the correction of the cytopenia by splenectomy, since the decision of whether or not to operate must be based on the first three factors alone.

Mechanism of Hemolysis in Hypersplenism

The evidence that a large spleen can sequester and destroy red cells at an increased rate is unequivocal. Jandl and coworkers have investigated the mechanism of anemia in congestive splenomegaly and a variety of splenomegalic states. They have found the red cell survival to be diminished and the splenic uptake of labeled cells to be increased (Fig. 23–11).

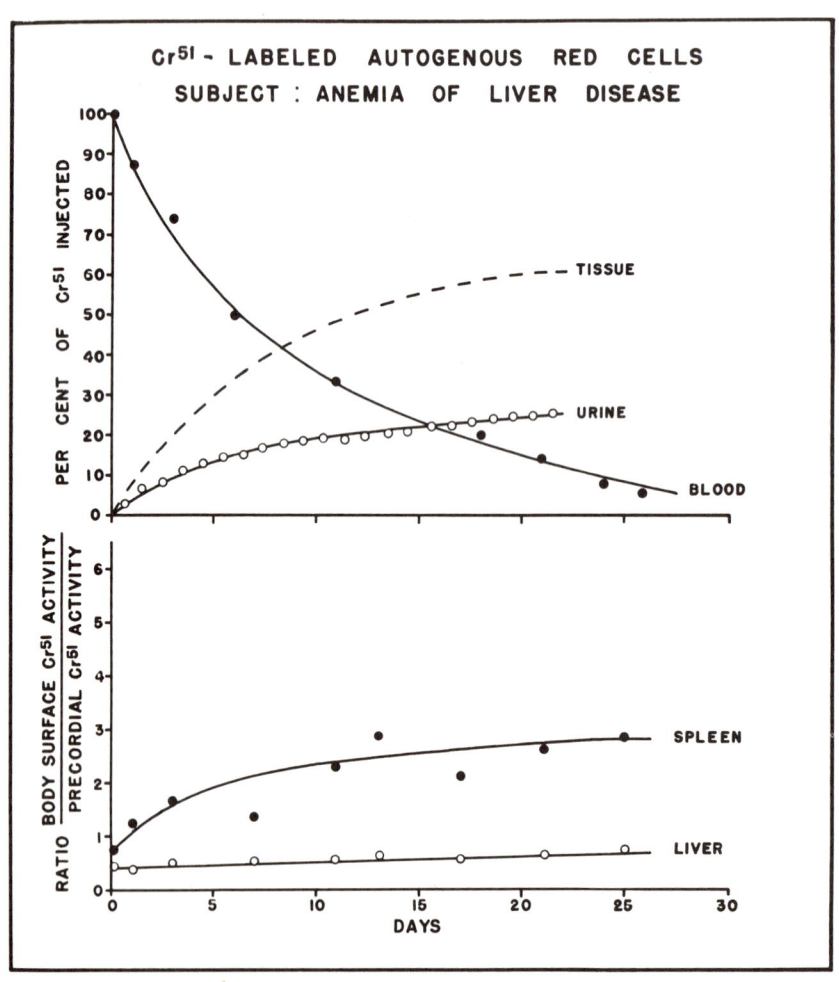

Figure 23–11 Hemolytic anemia and splenic sequestration of red cells in congestive splenomegaly. A common cause of hypersplenism with increased red cell destruction in the spleen is congestive splenomegaly secondary to cirrhosis of the liver. (Reproduced with the kind permission of the publisher, from Jandl, J. H., Greenberg, M. S., Yonemoto, R. H., and Castle, W. B.: J. Clin. Invest., *35*:842, 1956.)

Of all the combinations of cytopenias that are described in hypersplenism, the mechanism of increased destruction of the red cell is perhaps based on the most firm theoretical and experimental grounds. The hazards that beset normal cells in passage through the normal spleen have been described earlier in this chapter. These dangers include mechanical hazards, metabolic and rheologic hazards, hazards of stasis, and immunologic hazards. It is assumed that in the large spleen these dangers are increased to the extent that normal red cells suffer an early death. For example, if a red cell should spend one hour in the red pulp during each passage through the spleen as compared to the usual 20 to 40 seconds, it is reasonable that stasis, with its concomitant changes in the metabolic environment of the cell, may eventually create too much stress for even a normal healthy red cell.

At present, suggestions as to what metabolic stresses are actually applied to a red cell wedged within a cord or sinus and how long the stress can be withstood are conjectural. Almost certainly glucose deprivation, lactate accumulation, and a fall in pH take place. If one judges from studies in vivo, viability is lost within a few hours of erythrostasis when the cells are packed together. Undoubtedly, this injury is much more rapid when red cells are packed in close proximity to cells having high metabolic requirements, as would be the case in splenic red pulp. The ability of cells to withstand this repetitious splenic conditioning will be a function of the time spent in the spleen as opposed to the metabolic capacity to recuperate while circulating elsewhere. When the red cell is essentially normal, the process of conditioning will cause destruction of only a relatively limited number of cells, which is usually the case in hypersplenism. In general, hemolytic anemia and hypersplenism are mild or moderate, not necessitating splenectomy. On the other hand, when hypersplenism develops in patients with impaired marrow function or with preexisting intrinsic defects of the red cell, as may be the case in thalassemia and myelofibrosis, severe anemia may result.

Mechanism of Leukopenia and Thrombocytopenia in Hypersplenism

It is difficult to engender enthusiasm for implication of the above mechanisms as a cause of the leukopenia and/or thrombocytopenia observed in the syndrome we commonly call hypersplenism. Granulocytes have an almost infinite capacity to deform and consequently to pass through the vessel walls. The role of the granulocytes is to police the body perimeters, and this work takes place, for the most part, outside the vascular system. The blood serves merely as a conduit for these cells to proceed to the areas where they are most needed. Investigations of Athens et al. demonstrate that in normal individuals, half the cells have disappeared from the circulation in less than 7 hours, with a range of 4 to 9 hours. This fast disappearance time of granulocytes has been studied in a large number of individuals with large spleens, and no consistent abnormality was noted in the majority of instances unless an extremely high white count was also present.

Felty's syndrome has been used as a prime example of leukopenia and hypersplenism. It is of interest, however, that in this disease, an abundance of serologic changes is frequently found. Studies with latex and bentonite particles show that the rheumatoid factor is almost always positive in high titers. Antinuclear antibodies of IgG, IgA, and IgM are similarly detected, usually in a shaggy pattern that suggests an antibody reaction to the deoxynucleoprotein complex of the nucleus. These titers are not consistently decreased following splenectomy. Initial descriptions of a leukocyte-specific antinuclear factor, that is, one not absorbed by thyroid, and other tissue nuclei in 8 patients with Felty's syndrome have raised the possibility that immune mechanisms may be operative in causing the leukopenia. We know that selective decreases of red blood cells and platelets may be associated with specific antibodies directed toward these respective cells. The finding of leukocyte-specific antinuclear factor suggests a similar mechanism in which antibody-engaged leukocytes are sequestered and perhaps destroyed in the spleen. Additional documentation is necessary. Furthermore, the natural history of leukopenia in chronic rheumatoid disease has not been defined. One is not able to predict whether or not persons with asymptomatic leukopenia in conjunction with rheumatoid arthritis will progress to hypersplenism and recurrent infections. It may well be that in the future the defect causing leukopenia in patients with hypersplenism may be shown to exist in the cell itself rather than in the spleen.

The same reasoning may apply to the platelets in patients with large spleens. Although a great deal of knowledge has been gained about the size of the platelet pool in the sequestration of normal platelets in the spleen, little is known about the factors which actually cause lysis under these conditions. The consistent finding of an antiplatelet antibody in patients with idiopathic thrombocytopenic purpura by Karpatkin and coworkers suggests a mechanism for the reinvestigation of patients with a previous diagnosis of hypersplenism. It is conceivable that in some of these patients the spleen may have antibodies directed toward the platelets and that the large spleen happened to be a coexistent factor in those patients with immunologic disease. It should be noted that appearance of marrow megakaryocytes seen in hypersplenism is quite similar to that found in ITP. The megakaryocytes are increased in number and have smooth margins and less grainy cytoplasm. Evidence at the present time would indicate that these changes are not due to any hormone released by the spleen acting on the marrow but are secondary to increased destruction of platelets in the periphery. Therefore, it appears that this type of megakaryocyte reflects cellular immaturity and rapid platelet utilization and does not necessarily imply suppressed production.

In summary, the thrombocytopenia present in at least some patients with large spleens, i.e., hypersplenism, would appear to represent a disordered distribution of platelets rather than excessive splenic cell destruction. In these patients, splenic pooling, alluded to earlier, is presumed to be exaggerated. It has been demonstrated by Aster and by Harker that in patients with splenomegaly, the equilibrium for the normal surviving platelets between systemic and splenic intravascular compartments markedly favors the splenic pool. The resultant decrease in the circulating platelet level stimulates thrombopoiesis as shown by parallel increases in the megakaryocyte mass and the platelet turnover rate. A normal platelet count results if thrombopoiesis compensates sufficiently, but thrombocytopenia results if the splenic pooling exceeds the compensatory capacity of the existent marrow. If a compromised marrow is present, the thrombocytopenia may be much more severe. While this mechanism may be operating in the majority of patients with splenomegaly and thrombocytopenia, increased platelet destruction has been demonstrated in others. As noted above, an immune mechanism may be present. If thrombocytopenia is severe, large prematurely released platelets appear in the circulation. This finding may be a clue in the differentiation between these two mechanisms.

Indications For Splenectomy in Hypersplenism

Splenectomy is employed more widely today than it was in the past, when the only generally accepted indication for operation was trauma to the organ or its massive enlargement. This is due, for the most part, to better understanding of splenic disorders, to better supportive therapy with antibiotics, platelets, and in some cases white cell transfusions, and to the radical reduction in operative risks. But despite advances, the procedure may be underutilized in two controversial areas: hypersplenism associated with progressive incurable disease, and hypersplenism of any sort in the elderly patient. Therefore, the indications for splenectomy in various diseases with large spleens will be discussed in further detail.

"Primary" Hypersplenism

HEREDITARY SPHEROCYTOSIS. Splenectomy is permanently curative in almost every case of hereditary spherocytosis; the only exceptions are patients in whom substantial residuum of splenic tissue remains after operation. The general rule in this disease is that splenectomy should be performed as soon as the diagnosis has been made, with few exceptions. Splenectomy in children under 5 years of age has been reported to be accompanied by the severe complications of bacterial infection, meningitis, and pneumococcal sepsis. Therefore, it might be wise, if possible, to wait until the child is at least 5 years of age. Another exception would be during pregnancy in any trimester. The risk of inducing abortion is probably greater than the danger of waiting until after the pregnancy has terminated.

IDIOPATHIC THROMBOCYTOPENIC PURPURA. Splenectomy is usually reserved for those patients who fail to maintain a response to corticosteroids. Some patients may have a complete response to steroid therapy and then suffer a relapse after the drug is stopped. In those cases, it is recommended that another trial of steroids be initiated; if the patient fails to respond to the second trial, or fails to maintain a response, splenectomy should be performed.

SPLENIC NEUTROPENIA. Results in this disease are somewhat more equivocal than in those discussed above. However, if the patient has severe neutropenia with numerous attacks of severe infections, splenectomy in some cases has been quite helpful.

"Secondary" Hypersplenism

CONGESTIVE SPLENOMEGALY. When cirrhosis of the liver is associated with splenomegaly and hematologic evidence of hypersplenism, the clinical considerations relating to splenectomy are considerably more complex. Although many patients with this syndrome have some degree of hypersplenism, in only a small minority does it ever pose a clinical problem. If hypersplenism is present one must then consider whether or not portal hypertension poses the most serious threat to the patient. With large esophageal varices and a history of bleeding, decompression of portal hypertension is the principal measure and is probably best accomplished by construction of a portacaval shunt. If, on the other hand, the hypertension produces only moderate manifestations while the hypersplenism is severe or progressive, and particularly if there is bleeding that can be attributed to thrombocytopenia, splenectomy is indicated. The correction of portal hypertension alone will seldom abolish either splenomegaly or hypersplenism. In more than two thirds of cases, cytopenia persists following portal decompression without splenectomy. On the other hand, removal of a large spleen with its blood supply reduces to a considerable extent the blood coming into the portal system. This may result in a reduction of the portal pressure.

NON-HODGKIN'S LYMPHOMA. Occasionally a patient with lymphosarcoma will exhibit a classic picture of hypersplenism. The decision to perform splenectomy should come early in the course of management. The belief that treatment with chemotherapy will reduce the size of the spleen and thus reduce the extent of the hypersplenism has not, in most cases, been successful. Rather, the bone marrow response to the increased cell destruction is further depressed, and more severe anemia, leukopenia, and thrombocytopenia may develop. Consequently, splenectomy should be performed as soon as discernible evidence appears, that is, before the extensive use of chemotherapy or irradiation.

HODGKIN'S DISEASE. The same criteria as those described above for lymphoma apply here. However, the widespread use of laparotomy and splenectomy for staging may make this a moot question in the future.

MYELOFIBROSIS. Splenectomy in these individuals should be reserved for the rare patient in whom numerous blood transfusions or numerous platelet transfusions are necessary to keep the patient out of danger. This is a relative judgment and would depend upon the patient's age, rapidity of progression of the disease, and the existence of any contraindications, such as advanced cardiac, pulmonary, or renal disease.

Splenectomy is contraindicated in the following conditions: acute leukemia, erythroleukemia (DiGuglielmo syndrome), benign self-limiting infections, neoplastic proliferation, poor prognosis for long-term survival, and advanced cardiac, pulmonary, or renal disease. The role of splenectomy in thrombotic thrombocytopenic purpura is equivocal at the present time.

THE RETICULOENDOTHELIAL SYSTEM

The kinds of cells found in the reticuloendothelial system and their distribution are outlined in the introduction to this chapter. Although no one function can be classified as more important than another, it is obvious that a major concern of the RES is the "policing" of both the extravascular and the intravascular fluids. This vital role serves to preserve the normal fluidity of the blood and to rid it of toxic or infectious particles. Among the particulate matter with which the system may deal are bacteria, microemboli, fibrin and other coagulation products, antigen-antibody complexes, and certain lipids. The overall process by which this is accomplished by the RE system is often referred to as phagocytosis.

Metchnikoff introduced the term "phagocyte" or "eating cell" in a paper published in the Zoological Institute at the University of Odessa in 1884. During a visit to a friend's house, he noticed that some of the water fleas in an aquarium had lost their transparency and were opaque and cloudy. This was due to an infection of the colony by a microorganism and he was able to observe phagocytosis by large mesenchymal cells. Thus, Metchnikoff's contribution was the realization that the ability of phagocytes to take up microorganisms was a component of the body's defense system against invading parasites. His experiments were so clear and convincing that the concept of phagocytes as scavenger cells has been dominant until the present time. However, the collection of knowledge, for the most part, was only a scattering of empirical observations until recently. Within the past ten years, there has been considerable progress in understanding of the origin and function of the tissue macrophages and of the blood monocytes. Consequently, the processes by which bacteria are engulfed and eventually killed have been slowly unraveled. Presumably, these processes are common properties of all the monocytes and of the tissue macrophages scattered throughout the body, whether they reside in the lung, alimentary tract, liver, or spleen. The special role of the spleen in the sequestration and removal of cellular elements from the blood has already been discussed. Therefore, we shall now direct our attention to analogous mechanisms of phagocytosis occurring in the other organs of the RES.

ORIGIN AND KINETICS OF MONOCYTES AND TISSUE MACROPHAGES

The superb investigations by Cohn and Hirsch and coworkers in this country and by Van Furth in the Netherlands have led to far better understanding of the origin and kinetics of these cells. Reports of early studies based on morphologic criteria and functional information obtained from cell markers such as vital dyes or carbon particles appeared shortly after Metchnikoff's theories were published. Over the years, two opinions about the origin of these cells emerged: one, that mononuclear phagocytes were derived from lymphocytes; the other, that they originated from a separate cell line. According to these early concepts, the source of peripheral blood monocytes was attributed to histiocytes of the reticuloendothelial system or to bone marrow cells. One of the drawbacks of these earlier studies was that the cell markers applied were not sufficiently specific and stable to permit reliable identification of the phagocytic cells.

The application of tritiated thymidine, which is incorporated into nuclear DNA by the cells preparing for division and which remains in such cells as a fairly stable label, has made it possible to draw more definite conclusions concerning the origin and kinetics of mononuclear phagocytes. These authors have shown that the life history of these phagocytic cells is as follows: the stem cells in this line are located in the bone marrow; the young forms (monocytes) produced by this group of progenitor cells then enter the blood, and a short time later immigrate into the tissues; the tissue forms then undergo further maturation, which varies, depending upon the particular tissue environment, and become macrophages. These tissue macrophages have a long life span and apparently in some instances can be stimulated to undergo cell division. A schematic representation of this cycle is shown in Figure 23-12.

In mice, after a single injection of tritiated thymidine, labeled monocytes arrive in the circulating blood within 2 hours. This rapid arrival of labeled monocytes in the circulation means that newly formed monocytes leave the bone marrow almost immediately after they are labeled and implies that the pool of mature monocytes in the bone marrow is rather small.

Van Furth has estimated that labeled monocytes disappear exponentially from the circulation with a half-disappearance time of 22 hours. This is calculated under normal steady-state conditions. Using this half-time value, he then estimates that the average transit time of monocytes has been calculated to be 32 hours for mice. It is not clear why these cells remain in the circulation for such a prolonged period of time before they enter the extravascular or tissue pool. A certain degree of recirculation of these cells could explain the phenomenon. After arrival at the tissues, the mononuclear phagocytes undergo varying degrees of stimulation and become avidly phagocytic. They are now called macrophages. The ratio of tissue macrophages to circulating monocytes has been estimated to be 400:1 in man. The electron microscopic changes that occur as a mouse peripheral blood monocyte is transformed into a mouse peritoneal macrophage are shown in Figures 23-13, and 23-14 as determined by Fedorko and Hirsch. It is apparent that the monocyte is a large cell with prominent nucleoli, a well-developed Golgi apparatus, and abundant cytoplasmic ribosomal aggregates. Macrophages, on the other hand, show increased cytoplasmic vesicles and granules. Ribosomal aggregates are absent or markedly decreased in number, and there is an increase in the rough endoplasmic reticulum.

The turnover time of tissue macrophages, that is, the time required for replacement of the total population of cells, has been studied in a number of tissues using tritiated thymidine as a pulse label. The turnover time in mouse peritoneal macrophages has been estimated to be between 20 and 40 days; the Kupffer cells in the liver have been estimated to turn over about once in 60 days; alveolar macrophages of the lung have been estimated to have a turnover time of approximately 50 days.

The ultimate fate of the tissue macrophage is not known at the present time. Under certain conditions, in vivo or in vitro, macrophages can be stimulated to undergo mitosis. In this case, they would function as any fixed cellular tissue in the body, and calculation of their life span would be difficult if one uses present-day techniques. However, most observations are in agreement with the finding that under usual circumstances multiplication of these cells does not occur within the tissues. Furthermore, the observations of Hirsch and coworkers and Van Furth would indicate that the total life span of tissue macrophages is more likely a matter of months rather than days. Another problem in calculating the life span of tissue macrophages is the question of whether these cells recirculate through the bloodstream or migrate to other sites of the body. The

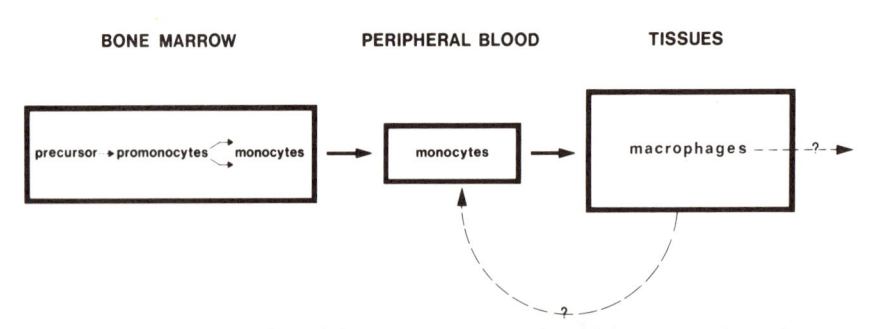

Figure 23-12 Schematic representation of three compartments in which mononuclear phagocytes reside. In bone marrow compartment, promonocytes proliferate and give rise to monocytes. In peripheral blood compartment, monocytes are transported from bone marrow to tissues. In tissue compartment, mononuclear phagocytes become avidly phagocytic macrophages. Possible elimination of mononuclear phagocytes from body and possible recirculation of tissue macrophages are also indicated. (From Van Furth, R.: Seminars Hemat., 7:125, 1970. Used by permission of Grune and Stratton, Inc.)

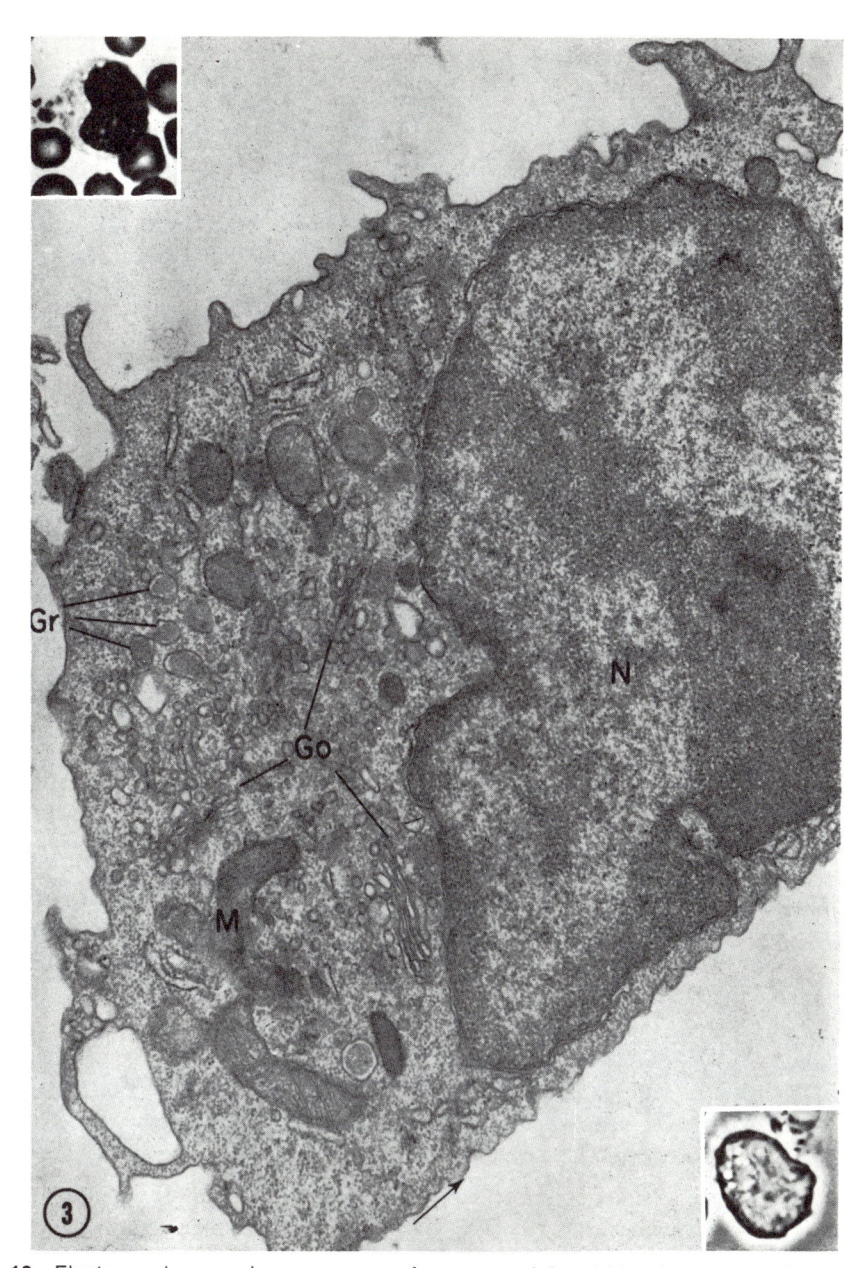

Figure 23–13 Electron microscopic appearance of mouse peripheral blood monocyte after settling on glass two hours. Cell margin at lower right (arrow) has been attached to glass, and free cell margin shows many microprojections. Nucleus (N) is elongate and shows indentations. Peripheral cytoplasm contains a few short strips of endoplasmic reticulum and rare ribosomal aggregates. Moderately prominent Golgi apparatus (Go) surrounded by a few mitochondria (M) and cytoplasmic granules (Gr) (×24,000).
 Insert lower right, Phase microscopic appearance of peripheral blood monocyte. Reniform-shaped nucleus occupies right half of cell. In nuclear hof area there are a few phase dense granules and lucent vacuoles (×1000).
 Insert upper left, Mouse marrow monocyte on blood smear, stained with Wright–Giemsa. Deeply stained reniform nucleus occupies right part of cell. Nuclear cytoplasmic ratio is greater than one. Cytoplasm is granular in appearance and contains rare vacuoles (×1000). (From Fedorko, M., and Hirsch, H.: Seminars Hemat., 7:109, 1970. Used by permission of Grune and Stratton, Inc.)

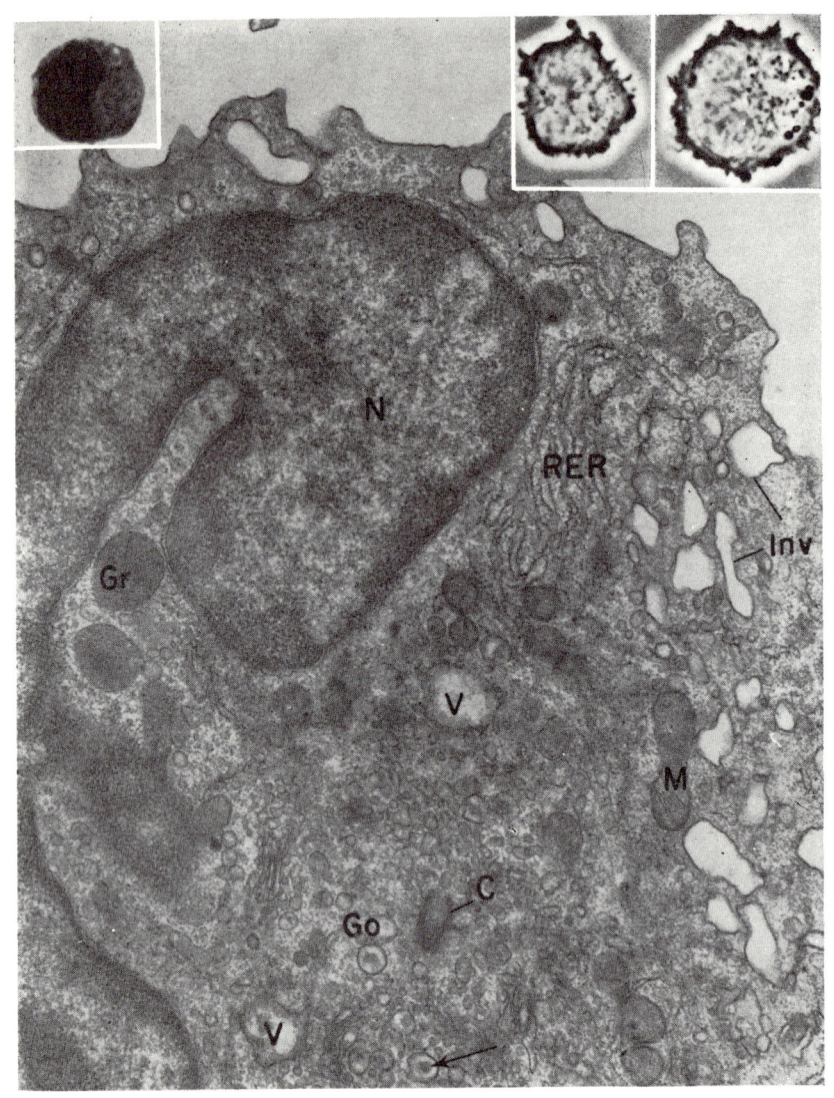

Figure 23-14 Electron microscopic appearance of mouse peritoneal macrophage. Cell membrane is ruffled and shows small microprojections, as well as deeper invaginations (*Inv*), which appear as peripheral clear cytoplasmic vacuoles in thin sections. Nucleus (*N*) is long and narrow. Focal stacks of rough endoplasmic reticulum (*RER*) are present; ribosomal aggregates are not seen. Golgi complex (*Go*) is extensive, characteristically multicentric, and surrounds centrioles (*C*). At periphery of Golgi complex are seen vacuoles (*V*), probably of pinocytic origin, granules (*Gr*), mitochondria (*M*), and vesicles with dense cores (arrow) (×19,200).

Inserts upper right, Phase microscopic appearance of two mouse peritoneal macrophages demonstrates range of size and structural variations in cell population. On left is an example of small cell with moderate numbers of cytoplasmic organelles; that on the right is larger and has more phase dense organelles. In both cells microprojections and ruffling of cell membrane are marked. Nuclei of both cells are reniform in shape and cell organelles are gathered in and about nuclear hof (×1000).

Insert upper left, Appearance of mouse peritoneal macrophage on Wright-Giemsa-stained smear. Nuclear cytoplasmic ratio is approximately equal to or less than one. Nucleus is densely stained and reniform in shape. Cytoplasm shows several vacuoles and some suggestion of granularity (×1000). (From Fedorko and Hirsch; Seminars Hemat., 7:109, 1970. Used by permission of Grune and Stratton, Inc.)

data are confusing on this matter and apparently depend on the type of label that is used. It is conceivable that the so-called free macrophages of the peritoneal cavity and of the spleen can be mobilized and enter the circulation moving into other organs, but the fixed tissue macrophages may not be mobile under any of their normal or pathologic conditions (inflammation or antigen stimulation).

Inflammation, either acute or chronic, has been shown to increase the migration of monocytes to the site of the lesion. For example, when a sterile inflammation is induced in the mouse peritoneal cavity, the number of peritoneal macrophages increases two- to threefold during the first three days. Since the labeling index of these cells using tritiated thymidine is no higher than in normal animals, this increase in the number of macrophages is apparently not due to any augmented mitotic activity of these cells.

Similar results have been seen in the skin using either a skin window technique or subcutaneous insertion of cover slips into the skin of the animal to be tested. Again, labeling studies have shown that these cells are truly monocytes originating from the bone marrow and not from any mitotic activity within the skin itself.

The data are not clear as to the origin of the increase in Kupffer cells in the liver of experimental animals. The type of inflammatory agent may play a decisive role in this regard, since the liver macrophages were found to be mainly of lymphocytic origin during the proliferative phase of a graft-versus-host reaction. This is in contrast to the findings in normal animals as well as those obtained with animals in which the accumulation of Kupffer cells had been induced by partial hepatectomy. These latter results clearly demonstrated the monocytic origin of the Kupffer cells. In addition, animals infected with *Listeria monocytogenes* showed that a labeling index of Kupffer cells 30 minutes after a tritiated thymidine pulse rises as much as 18 per cent, indicating considerable proliferation of the mononuclear phagocytes during the development of the state of cellular immunity. The origin of the phagocytic cells of the nervous system, the microglia cell, is still not known with certainty, but it is thought that it is probably monocytic in origin. Labeling studies in animals with experiment-induced allergic encephalomyelitis revealed that the mononuclear cell in these lesions was of hematogenous origin.

Endocytosis

The next step in the policing of the body perimeters by the macrophages of the RES is the process by which the cell engulfs the bacterium or particle under question. This entire process has been called endocytosis and is defined as the action by which the cell ingests part of the external environment, enclosing it within the invaginations or evaginations of its nuclear membrane. No description of the role of the macrophage would be complete without a description of this endocytotic activity, since its function is the one upon which the success of almost all mechanisms of acquired antimicrobial immunity depends. The term encompasses pinocytosis and phagocytosis. Pinocytosis refers to the ingestion of phase translucent fluid droplets (or colloid) at the surface of the undulating hyaline cytoplasm of macrophages. Phagocytosis refers to the ingestion of particles visible with a light microscope. Micropinocytosis refers to uptake of extracellular material too small to be seen with a light microscope but visible with an electron microscope.

Phagocytosis. The act of phagocytosis cannot begin until a particle makes contact with and adheres to the plasma membrane of a phagocytic cell. The phagocytic mechanism is triggered, therefore, by an interaction between components of the cell surface and the particle. The importance of surface requirements for phagocytosis was realized many years ago when it was shown that some bacteria had to be "coated" by certain factors in serum before they were ingested by phagocytic cells. The responsible serum components are called *opsonins*, and their importance is now well established. The best source of opsonins is specific immune serum, and there is no doubt that the active molecules are specific antibodies. More recently, opsonins have been identified with certain classes of specific immunoglobulins. Studies in vivo have shown IgM to be more efficient in promoting phagocytosis by macrophages than IgG. In vitro studies, on the other hand, have shown that under complement-free conditions IgG shows a higher opsonic efficiency than IgM.

The mechanisms which enable the cell to respond phagocytically to opsonized surfaces is not known. There is no evidence that the cell is capable of recognizing and reacting with specific combining sites of antibodies. Therefore, it apparently recognizes a peculiar molecular configuration common to all antigen antibody complexes.

In some instances, it has been demonstrated that phagocytic cells are able to ingest some particles in the apparent absence of serum factors. However, even if some particles are ingested in the absence of opsonins, there is little doubt that most particles are ingested better in their presence.

The function of opsonins is not simply to insure the establishment of a force of adhesion between particle and cell surface. Something more than adhesion is required. Rabinovitch has demonstrated that aldehyde-treated red cells bind firmly to macrophages in balanced salt solutions but are not phagocytized unless opsonins are also available. This indicates that special molecules in the cell surface must participate in the adhesion before the mechanism of phagocytosis is triggered. Thus, phagocytic cells appear to be endowed with receptors which are capable of reacting with antigen-antibody complexes. North has postulated that the special ability of phagocytic cells to recognize and respond phagocytically to surfaces containing antigen-antibody molecules may one day form the basis of functional definition of these cells.

Pinocytosis. Pinocytosis by macrophages has been studied in vitro and in vivo. The intensity of pinocytotic activity in vitro has been shown to be influenced by the presence of certain types of molecules in the incubation media. Cohn and Parks, for example, have demonstrated that the rate of pinocytosis by mouse macrophages is significantly increased in the presence of certain anionic proteins, carbohydrates, and amino acids. In contrast, they demonstrated that neutral and cationic molecules had little or no effect. The same authors have also shown that the induction of pinocytosis may also be dependent, in some cases, on immunologic factors. In this experiment, they showed that pinocytosis in mouse macrophages could be triggered by the presence in heat-inactivated newborn calf serum of antibody molecules directed against components of the macrophage plasma membrane.

The postulated differences between pinocytosis and phagocytosis are shown in Figure 23–15. According to North, the most obvious difference between pinocytosis and phagocytosis is seen in the mechanical events which lead to formation of the surface vesicle. In phagocytosis, the size and shape of the newly formed vesicles are determined by the size and shape of the particle. After contact, the cell progressively increases its area of contact with a particle, and when the area of contact is maximal, the particle is completely closed in the vacuole. In contrast, the size and shape of a pinocytotic vesicle cannot be molded on its contents, which are fluid and lacking in rigidity. There have been studies of phagocytosis using a diverse number of particles in association with macrophages. One common property seems to be that each particle is capable, in itself, of inducing a separate act of phagocytosis. In other words, each phagocytic vacuole contains a single particle. This mechanism has not been found to operate when the same cells are allowed to ingest colloidal gold when the particle diameter is of the order of 0.03 micron. In this instance, each newly formed endocytic vacuole contains a large number of gold particles. Apparently, a single gold particle on a plasma membrane is not a sufficient stimulus to induce the formation of a surface vacuole. This finding would suggest that a morphologic distinction between phagocytosis and pinocytosis is that a particle is phagocytosed when it is large enough to induce the formation of a vacuole, whereas a particle can only be pinocy-

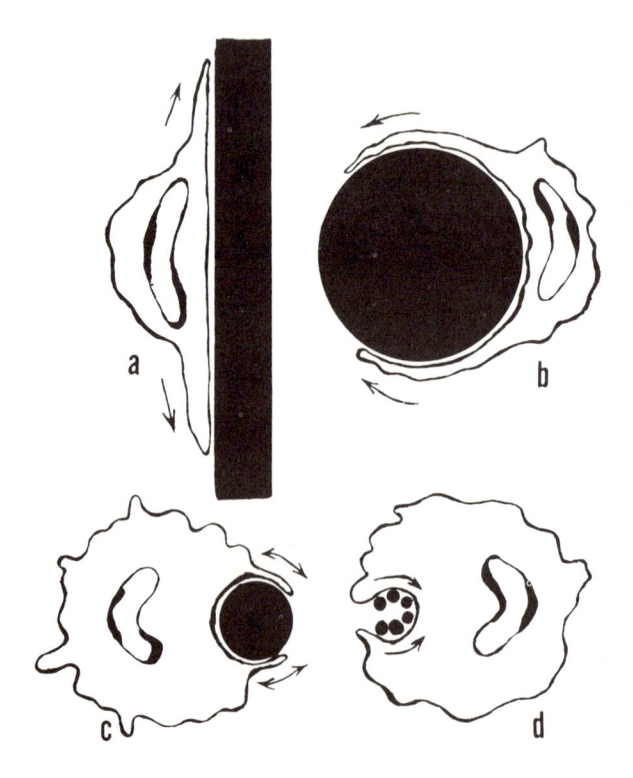

Figure 23–15 Diagrammatic representation of different ways mechanism of endocytosis can express itself. Indentation of cell surface to enclose small particles (c,d), outward extensions of peripheral cytoplasm to enclose much larger particles (b), and attempt by macrophage to increase area of contact with planar surface (a) are all interpreted as being due to mechanical activity of endocytotic mechanism. Pinocytosis (d) is distinguished from phagocytosis (a,b,c) on grounds that pinocytotic vesicle encloses more than one particle. (From North, R. J.: Seminars Hemat., 7:168, 1970. Used by permission of Grune and Stratton, Inc.)

tosed if it is too small by itself to trigger vacuole formation. Thus, the macrophage is induced to form a pinocytotic vacuole only after a given number of small particles accumulate on a given area of the cell surface.

Another difference between phagocytosis and pinocytosis is the finding that polymorphonuclear leukocytes, although well equipped for phagocytosis, do not form pinocytotic vesicles of the type observed in macrophages.

Intracellular Digestion

Effective policing of the body perimeters implies not only the phagocytosis of bacteria but the efficient killing of the ingested bacteria within a reasonable period of time. Cohn investigated the fate of bacteria ingested by rabbit peritoneal macrophages and found that intracellular inactivation was followed by extensive degradation of bacterial lipids, nucleic acids, and proteins. The rate of degradation was somewhat variable, depending upon the nature of the particle ingested. When experiments were performed using ^{32}P-labeled *E. coli,* 80 per cent of the labeled RNA and DNA and 50 per cent of the labeled lipid were recovered within two hours as acid-soluble labeled products. The principal breakdown products were nucleotides and ^{32}P$_i$. The same kinds of experiments were performed with ^{14}C-labeled bacteria. Again, two hours after phagocytosis more than 45 per cent of the ^{14}C was recovered in the acid-soluble fraction. The labeled products of digestion were identified as peptides and amino acids.

In 1957, a condition was first described which demonstrated the extreme importance of the ability of the neutrophil or macrophage to kill bacteria. This condition, named chronic granulomatous disease of childhood (CGD), is manifested by severe widespread and repeated bacterial infections with *Staphylococcus aureus* and also with a number of gram-negative organisms, beginning in the first year of life and progressing relentlessly unto death at an early age. Purulent granuloma frequently involving the neck or inguinal areas is one of the hallmarks of this disease. The neutrophils and macrophages from patients with CGD were shown to have an impaired ability to kill those bacteria generally found in the lesions, that is, *S. aureus* and the other low-grade gram-negative pathogens. Other bacteria, that is, streptococci, lactobacilli, and pneumococci were readily killed. Further experiments revealed that the phagocytic function of the neutrophils and macrophages in these patients was unimpaired. Rather, the ingested bacteria of the *S. aureus* and other types were able to exist and multiply within the cell.

The enzymic basis for the defect in CGD is controversial. Klebanoff demonstrated that the neutrophils in this disease demonstrated a deficiency in H_2O_2 production, which in turn is associated with the decreased microbicidal activity. The mechanism by which the decreased H_2O_2 is responsible for the decreased degradation and killing of bacteria is not known. It is interesting that bacteria that supply their own H_2O_2 are killed in a normal fashion by cells from patients with CGD. This is the explanation offered for normal intracellular destruction of streptococci, lactobacilli, and pneumococci in this disease. In contrast, *S. aureus* does not produce enough H_2O_2 to trigger the metabolic activity necessary for intracellular killing, and thus the organism escapes its just fate.

Metabolic Requirements

The phagocytic process is associated with a burst of metabolic activity. Oxygen consumption is considerably increased. Respiration in the absence of exogenous substrate is due, in part at least, to glycogen breakdown, since glycogen levels fall during phagocytosis. Glucose consumption and lactic acid production are also increased, particularly under anaerobic conditions. The respiratory burst is associated with H_2O_2 formation and with the reduction of nitro blue tetrazolium (NBT) to blue Formazan. Lipid turnover is increased by phagocytosis, but the process has no effect on protein synthesis. RNA turnover, however, is increased, but the metabolic burst is independent of RNA synthesis. Thus, there is unequivocal evidence that the processes of phagocytosis and intracellular destruction of bacteria require metabolic energy. In addition, it has been demonstrated that pinocytosis in mouse peritoneal macrophages can be significantly depressed by the presence of inhibitors which block either anaerobic glycolysis or oxidative phosphorylation.

IMMUNITY

For many years, the study of immunology was, in essence, a study of the reticuloendothelial system. However, within the last two decades the tremendous expansion of knowledge in this area has been astounding. In fact, the field has grown from a stepchild of the reticuloendothelial system to a full-grown, independent discipline. Therefore, detailed discussions of immunology will be found in Chapters 4, 5, and 22. These chapters approach the subject of immunity mainly from the standpoint of the origin, kinetics, and functions of the immunocyte, which includes the large and small lymphocytes and the plasma cell.

Recent studies have demonstrated that monocytes and phagocytes of the reticuloendothelial system also play an important role in host susceptibility to and defense against viral pathogens.

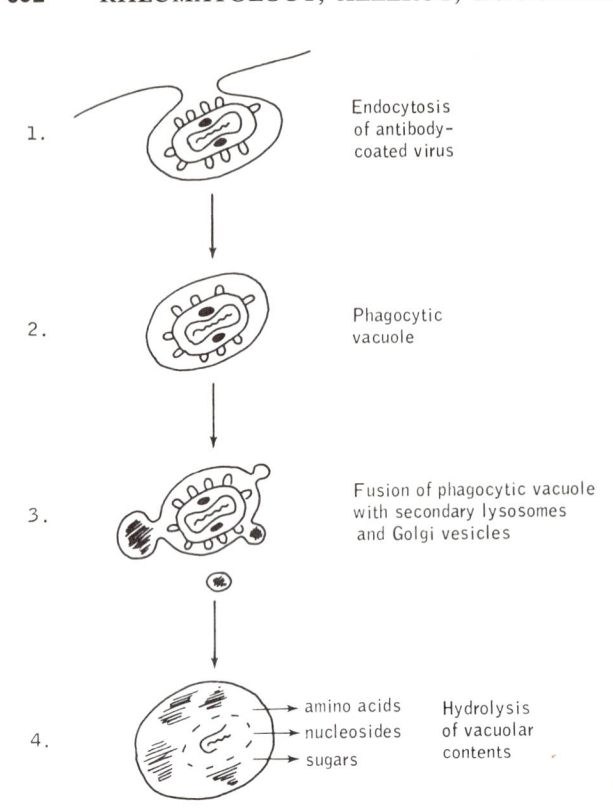

Figure 23–16 Cellular pathway through which antibody-neutralized vaccinia virus is degraded. (From Silverstein, S.: Seminars Hemat., 7:185, 1970. Used by permission of Grune and Stratton, Inc.)

1. Endocytosis of antibody-coated virus
2. Phagocytic vacuole
3. Fusion of phagocytic vacuole with secondary lysosomes and Golgi vesicles
4. Hydrolysis of vacuolar contents → amino acids, nucleosides, sugars

Macrophages remove antibody-neutralized virus from the circulation and degrade the antibody-virus complexes to low molecular weight metabolites. In some circumstances, viruses enter the macrophage cytoplasm but are unable to replicate within a cell type and thus are eliminated as a potential source of continued infection. When viral replication in macrophages does occur, other mechanisms of host defenses are summoned to combat the progress of the infection. Under these circumstances, however, the first line of defense, i.e., the macrophage, has been breached. The relationship between viruses and macrophages has been demonstrated by the use of mouse hepatitis virus. The steps by which an antibody-coated virus is degraded by the macrophage are shown in Figure 23–16. Although not all viruses are handled in this fashion, it is apparent that at least in some virus infestation in animals, and presumably in man, the macrophage may play a vital role in viral immunity.

PATHOLOGIC DISORDERS OF THE RES

Aplasia and hypoplasia of the large and small lymphocytes and of the plasma cells are discussed in Chapter 5. These abnormalities constitute a fascinating but somewhat frightening group of diseases. They are extremely important, since recognition of complete or partial deficiencies of a single cell line has led to important discoveries in the understanding of the entire immune system.

The malignant diseases of the RES are discussed in Chapter 22. These entities have also contributed greatly to the understanding of the physiology and biochemistry of this system. For example, important clues concerning the structure and function of various types of globulins were first obtained in patients with multiple myeloma and Waldenström's macroglobulinemia.

The malignant diseases of the RES constitute a rather heterogenous group, insofar as the variety of pathologic morphology within any one group of diseases is concerned. For example, Hodgkin's disease has been subclassified into four types, depending on the presence of lymphocytes, the depletion of lymphocytes, the presence of histiocytes (previously classified as reticulum cells), and the structure of the involved nodes (see Chapter 22). A similar classification of non-Hodgkin's lymphoma is another case in point. In spite of this refinement in classification, numerous patients are still found to have variants of this disease; histiocytic medullary reticuloendotheliosis and leukemic reticuloendotheliosis represent disease entities which cannot be placed in any one specific morphologic category. It is apparent that much more information concerning the spectrum of pathologic responses of each cell line of the RES to a wide variety of insults is necessary before we can meaningfully understand the malignant perturbations of this system.

LIPIDOSES

In this group of genetically determined diseases, Gaucher's disease and Neimann-Pick disease are well known examples. They illustrate the unique role of the phagocytic cells in the RES. For many years, the cells found in Gaucher's disease were thought to be special, unique for that particular entity. A specific enzymatic defect has now been described, glucocerebrosidase, which is an enzyme necessary to cleave glucocerebroside. This abnormality, present at birth, leads to a pathologic increase of the substrate, which is then ingested by the macrophages. Thus, a Gaucher's cell represents merely a macrophage filled with glucocerebroside. The granulocytes are apparently major contributors of this material to the body pool. It is theoretically possible to have a disease in which the granulocyte mass and turnover rate are so increased that the glucocerebrosidase activity is saturated, giving rise to Gaucher's cells in otherwise normal individuals. This has indeed proved to be the case; Gaucher's cells have been found to be present in the bone marrow of some patients with chronic granulocytic leukemia.

REFERENCES

General and Historical

Ashoff, L.: Das reticulo-endothelial System. Ergeb. Inn. Med. Kinderheilk., 26:1, 1924.

Chauffard, A., and Troisier, J.: Des Rapports de certaines anémies splénomégaliques avec l'ictère hémolytique congénital. Bull. Mém. Soc. Med. Hop. Paris, 27:293, 1909.

Metchnikoff, E.: Lectures on a comparative pathology of information. Translated by Starling, F. A., and Starling, E. H., London, Kegan, Paul, Trench and Trubes, 1901.

Stuart, E. A.: The Reticulo-endothelial System. Edinburgh, E. & S. Livingstone, 1970, 255 pp.

Spleen; Structure and Normal Function

Barcroft, J., and Florey, H. W.: Some factors involved in the concentration of blood by the spleen. J. Physiol., 66:231, 1928.

Blaustein, A. U. (Ed.): The Spleen. New York, McGraw-Hill Book Co., 1963.

Crosby, W. H.: Normal functions of the spleen relative to red blood cells: A review. Blood, 14:399, 1959.

Harris, I. M., McAlister, J., and Prankard, T. A. J.: Splenomegaly and the circulating red cell. Brit. J. Haemat., 4:97, 1958.

Jacob, H. S., MacDonald, R. A., and Jandl, J. H.: The regulation of spleen growth and sequestering function. J. Clin. Invest., 42:1476, 1963.

Jacob, H. S., and Jandl, J. H.: Effects of sulfhydryl inhibition on red blood cells. II. Studies in vivo. J. Clin. Invest. 41:1514, 1962.

Jandl, J. H., Files, N. M., Barnett, S. B., and MacDonald, R. A.: Proliferative response of the spleen and liver to hemolysis. J. Exp. Med., 122:299, 1965.

Keene, W. R., and Jandl, J. H.: The sites of hemoglobin catabolism. Blood, 26:705, 1965.

Knisely, M. H.: Spleen studies. I. Microscopic observations of the circulatory system of living unstimulated mammalian spleen. Anat. Rec., 65:23, 1936.

Wennberg, E., and Weiss, L.: The structure of the spleen and hemolysis. Ann. Rev. Med., 20:29, 1969.

Weiss, L.: The structure of the normal spleen. Seminars Hemat., 2:205, 1965.

Disorders of the Spleen, Hypersplenism and Splenic Sequestration, Rupture and Splenosis

Aster, R. H.: Pooling of platelets in the spleen: Role in the pathogenesis of "hypersplenic" thrombocytopenia. J. Clin. Invest., 45:645, 1966.

Athens, J. W., Raab, S. O., Haab, O. P., Mauer, A. M., Ashenbrucker, H. E., Cartwright, G. E., and Wintrobe, M. M.: Leukokinetic Studies III. The distribution of granulocytes in the blood of normal subjects. J. Clin. Invest., 40:159, 1961.

Athens, J. W., Raab, S. O., Haab, O. P., Mauer, A. M., Ashenbrucker, H. E., Cartwright, G. E., and Wintrobe, M. M.: Leukokinetic Studies IV. The total blood, circulating and marginal granulocyte pools and the granulocyte turnover rate in normal subjects. J. Clin. Invest., 40:189, 1961.

Bishop, C. R., Rothstein, G., Ashenbrucker, H. E., and Athens, J. W.: Leukokinetic Studies XIV. Blood neutrophil kinetics in chronic steady state neutropenia. J. Clin. Invest., 50:1678, 1971.

Cartwright, G. E., Athens, J. W., Haab, O. P., Raab, S. O., Boggs, D. R., and Wintrobe, M. M.: Blood granulocyte kinetics in conditions associated with granulocytosis. Ann. N. Y. Acad. Sci., 113:963, 1964.

Crosby, W. H.: Hypersplenism. Ann. Rev. Med., 13:127, 1962.

Emerson, C. P., Shen, S. C., Ham, T. H., Fleming, E. M., and Castle, W. B.: Studies on the destruction of red blood cells. IX. Quantitative methods for determining the osmotic and mechanical fragility of red cells in the peripheral blood and spleen pulp; the mechanism of increased hemolysis in hereditary spherocytosis as related to the functions of the spleen. Arch. Intern. Med., 97:1, 1956.

Faber, V., and Elling, P.: Leukocyte-specific anti-nuclear factors in patients with Felty's syndrome, rheumatoid arthritis and systemic lupus erythematosus and other diseases. Acta Med. Scand., 179:257, 1966.

Giblett, E. R., Motulsky, A. G., Casserd, F., Houghton, B., and Finch, C. A.: Studies on the pathogenesis of splenic anemia. Blood, 11:1118, 1956.

Harker, L. A.: Thrombokinetics in the platelets. Brinkhous, K. M., et al. (Eds.): Platelet. Baltimore, Williams & Wilkins Co., 1971, p. 13.

Harrington, W. J., Minnick, V., Hollingsworth, J. W., and Moore, C. V.: Demonstration of a thrombocytopenic factor in the blood of patients with thrombocytopenic purpura. J. Lab. Clin. Med., 38:1, 1951.

Jandl, J. H., Jones, A. R., and Castle, W. B.: The destruction of red cells by antibodies in man. I. Observations on the sequestration and lysis of red cells altered by immune mechanisms. J. Clin. Invest., 36:1428, 1957.

Jensen, W. N., and Lessen, L. J.: Membrane alteration associated with hemaglobinopathies. Seminars Hemat. 7:409, 1970.

Karpatkin, S., Strick, N., Karpatkin, M., and Sisskind, G.: Cumulative experience in the detection of anti-platelet antibody in 234 patients with idiopathic purpura, systemic lupus erythematosus and other clinical disorders. Amer. J. Med., 52:776, 1972.

LaCelle, P. L.: Alteration of membrane deformity in hemolytic anemia. Seminars Hemat., 7:355, 1970.

Louie, J., and Pearson, C.: Felty's syndrome. Seminars Hemat., 8:216, 1971.

McIntyre, O. R., and Ebaugh, F. G., Jr.: Palpable spleens in college freshmen. Ann. Intern. Med., 66:301, 1967.

Raab, S. O., Athens, J. W., Haab, O. P., Boggs, D. R., Ashenbrucker, H. E., Cartwright, G. E., and Wintrobe, M. M.: Granulocytic kinetics in normal dogs. Amer. J. Physiol., 200:83, 1964.

Rifkind, R. A.: Destruction of injured red cells in vivo. Amer. J. Med., 41:7011, 1966.

Smith, E. B., and Custer, R. P.: Infectious mononucleosis. Blood, 1:317, 1946.

Weed, R. I., and Reed, C. F.: Membrane alteration leading to red cell destruction. Amer. J. Med., *41*:681, 1966.

Weed, R. I., and Weiss, L.: The relationship of red cell fragmentation occurring within cell to cell destruction. Trans. Assoc. Amer. Physicians, *79*:426, 1966.

The RES

Berendes, H., Bridges, R. A., and Good, R. A.: The fatal granulomatosis of childhood. Minn. Med., *40*:309, 1957.

Cohn, Z. A.: The fate of bacteria within phagocytic cells. I. Degradation of isotopically labelled bacteria by polymorphonuclear leukocytes and macrophages. J. Exp. Med., *117*:27, 1963.

Cohn, Z. A.: The structure and function of monocytes and macrophages. Adv. Immun., *9*:163, 1968.

Dales, S., and Kajioka, R.: The cycle of multiplication of vaccinia virus in Earl's strain L-cells. I. Uptake and penetration. Virology, *24*:278, 1964.

Fedorko, M. E., and Hirsch, J.: Structure of Monocytes and Macrophages. Seminars Hemat., *7*:109, 1970.

Klebanoff, S. J.: Intraleukocytic microbiocidal defects. Ann. Rev. Med., *22*:39, 1971.

Mims, C. A.: Aspects of the pathogenesis of virus disease. Bact. Rev., *28*:30, 1964.

North, R. J.: Endocytosis. Seminars Hemat., *7*:161, 1970.

Rabinovitch, M.: The role of antibody in the ingestion of aldehyde-treated erythrocytes attached to macrophages. J. Immun., *99*:233, 1967.

Silverstein, S., and Dales, S.: The penetration of reovirus RNA and initiation of its genetic function in L-strain fibroblasts. J. Cell Biol., *36*:197, 1968.

Van Furth, R. (ed.): Mononuclear Phagocytes. Oxford, Blackwell Scientific Publications, 1970.

Van Furth, R.: Origin and kinetics of monocytes and macrophages. Seminars Hemat., *7*:125, 1970.

Van Furth, R., and Cohn, Z. A.: The origin and kinetics of mononuclear macrophages. J. Exp. Med., *128*:415, 1968.

Volkman, A., and Gowans, J. L.: The origin of macrophages from bone marrow in the rat. Brit. J. Exp. Path., *46*:62, 1965.

SECTION IV

GASTROENTEROLOGY, ENDOCRINOLOGY, AND METABOLISM

CHAPTER 24   THE ESOPHAGUS

DAVID B. SKINNER

INTRODUCTION

The primary function of the esophagus is the transportation of ingested material from the pharynx to the stomach. A second function is the prevention of involuntary regurgitation of stomach contents. Abnormalities of the esophagus can be considered in relation to the four major components contributing to normal esophageal function. These components are the cricopharyngeal sphincter at the upper end, the muscular layers of the esophagus, the mucosal lining of the esophagus, and the sphincter mechanism at the cardia. The esophagus plays no important role in the digestion or absorption of food, although the initial breakdown of starches by salivary gland secretions may occur during the transportation of food through the length of the esophagus.

STRUCTURE

The cricopharyngeal sphincter consists of skeletal muscle fibers which are arranged obliquely in its upper portion and blend into those of the inferior pharyngeal constrictor muscle. In the lower portion of the sphincter the fibers are arranged transversely and are continuous with the muscle layers of the esophagus. The muscle bundles composing the sphincter arise from the back and sides of the cricoid cartilage anteriorly and insert into a fibrous raphe in the posterior midline. In the resting state the sphincter is contracted, maintaining a mean pressure of approximately 30 mm. Hg. During swallowing, relaxation occurs. When studied by intraluminal pressure recordings, the sphincter ranges from 3 to 5 cm. in length, but appears somewhat shorter in radiographic examinations. It is located at the level of the sixth cervical vertebra.

Esophageal muscle fibers are of the striated or skeletal type in the upper one third of the esophagus and are of smooth muscle in the lower esophagus. The transition between skeletal and smooth muscle is indistinct and somewhat variable in location. Esophageal muscle is arranged in two layers, the outer layer running longitudinally, and the inner layer positioned transversely or obliquely around the lumen. There is no serosal layer on the surface of the esophagus, and the outer longitudinal muscle fibers blend into the overlying fibrous tissue of the pleura and pericardium and the fibrofatty tissue of the mediastinum.

The mucosa of the esophagus is squamous epithelium continuous with that of the pharynx at the upper end. At the distal esophagus there is a sharp transition to simple columnar epithelium which may be visible during esophagoscopy as the ora serrata or "Z" line. Scattered unevenly throughout the esophageal submucosa are intrinsic glands. These produce mucus which reaches the lumen through small excretory ducts and provides lubrication for the passage of ingested material. Simple tubular glands similar to those at the cardia of the stomach may be located at the upper and lower ends of the esophagus and are confined to the lamina propria mucosae. In some individuals there may be islands of gastric columnar epithelium replacing squamous epithelium. These are more commonly encountered in the distal esophagus. Occasionally, acid-secreting or oxyntic cells are encountered in these patches of columnar epithelium. The esophageal mucosa is separated from the muscle layers by a submucosal layer which permits considerable movement of the mucosa in relation to the muscle.

In man, a lower esophageal sphincter cannot be identified by anatomic dissection. However, functionally, the distal esophagus behaves as a sphincter, in that the resting luminal pressure at the gastroesophageal junction is greater than in the esophagus above or the stomach below. This contracted segment relaxes in response to a swallow. The characteristics of this sphincter are described by manometric studies. Normally the sphincter straddles the gastroesophageal mucosal junction and ranges in length from 2 to 4 cm. Resting pressure is generally 8 or more mm. Hg greater than gastric pressure. The reversal of pressure deflections caused by respiration occurs near the center of this high pressure zone. Below the pressure reversal point, inspiration causes an increase in pressure similar to that in the abdomen, whereas proximal to this level inspiration causes a decrease in pressure similar to the intrathoracic pattern. When manometric studies and cineradiography are performed simultaneously, the lower portion of the distal esophageal sphincter corresponds to the submerged or closed segment within the diaphragmatic hiatus while the upper portion of the sphincter corresponds to the distal half of the phrenic ampulla radiographically.

The esophagogastric junction is located at the level of the tenth thoracic vertebra within the esophageal hiatus of the diaphragm. The hiatus is a muscular tunnel, 2 to 3 cm. long, through which pass the esophagus, vagus nerves, and extensions of endo-abdominal fascia. The endo-abdominal fascia and endothoracic fascia join together to form the phreno-esophageal membrane. This sheet of fibrous and elastic tissue extends from the muscular margins of the hiatus to the esophagus circumferentially and blends into the esophageal muscle slightly above the upper margins of the hiatus and above the mucosal junction.

Disease of the esophagus may be classified and understood by considering its effect upon the two primary functions of the esophagus—transportation of ingested material and the prevention of reflux—and the four above-mentioned major components which contribute to normal function: the cricopharyngeal sphincter, the muscle layers, the mucosal lining, and the lower esophageal sphincter. Since dysphagia or difficulty in swallowing is almost a universal complaint in patients with any disease interfering with esophageal function, this symptom must be regarded as nonspecific. However, dysphagia must be regarded as a strong indication for complete diagnostic evaluation of esophageal structure and function. Only in this way will a precise diagnosis of the individual pathologic condition be made at a time when therapy can be instituted to restore esophageal function to normal.

TRANSPORTATION OF INGESTED MATERIAL

Normal Swallowing

When food or liquid is swallowed, the bolus is transmitted from the pharynx to the stomach by the coordinated action of all four esophageal components. Instantaneously, with the onset of swallowing, the cricopharyngeal sphincter relaxes and luminal pressure level falls to that in the body of the esophagus. This sphincter relaxation lasts for a short time, often one second or less, and is followed by a contraction of the sphincter which may produce a luminal pressure of up to 80 mm. Hg.

The arrangement of circular and longitudinal esophageal muscle fibers allows both constriction of the lumen and shortening of the esophagus which are essential for effective peristalsis. A primary peristaltic wave triggered by a swallow is characterized by a progressive contraction which moves down the body of the esophagus at the rate of 2 to 4 cm. per second and generates intraluminal pressures which generally range between 30 and 60 mm. Hg above resting pressure. Preceding the peristaltic contraction, relaxation occurs. The arrangement of mucosal folds, their loose adherence to the muscle, and the marked ability of the relaxed muscle to stretch permit distention of the esophagus to several centimeters without disruption. A single swallow generates a peristaltic contraction which progresses completely down the full length of the esophagus. However, if a second swallow is performed immediately, the initial peristaltic wave is interrupted and a second wave begins in the upper esophagus and progresses downward. In older persons the proportion of swallows followed by a primary progressive peristaltic contraction is diminished when compared to that of younger individuals.

Other types of esophageal contractions are observed. Secondary peristalsis is a progressive peristaltic wave that occurs without initiation by a swallow. These may be triggered by a bolus in the esophagus or by regurgitation of gastric contents or may occur spontaneously. Tertiary or segmental contractions are nonperistaltic and may follow a swallow in an older patient with disordered esophageal function, may result from stimulation by an oversized bolus, or may be initiated by irritants such as regurgitated acid in the lumen. High-amplitude tertiary contractions are considered spastic and may persist for prolonged periods.

In response to a swallow, the lower esophageal sphincter segment relaxes promptly, permitting intraluminal pressure to drop to gastric level. This relaxation lasts until the peristaltic wave reaches the lower esophagus. As the peristaltic wave reaches the upper portion of the sphincter, it participates in the contraction with a marked increase in pressure, whereas the lower portion of the sphincter simply regains its resting tone of approximately 8 mm. Hg above intragastric pressure. The concentric contraction of the distal esophagus is useful in differentiating between esophagus and stomach radiographically, since the latter does not contract concentrically. The termination of the peristaltic contraction can be employed to locate the muscular junction between esophagus and stomach.

The entire action of the esophagus in response to a swallow is coordinated by vagal or parasympathetic nerve fibers which provide the major innervation of the esophagus. Both central and local neural pathways appear to be involved in the peristaltic contraction. Anticholinergic drugs or vagotomy causes a decrease in the strength of the peristaltic contraction and diminishes the resting pressure in the lower esophageal sphincter. Sympathetic innervation has been demonstrated anatomically, but the function of these nerve fibers is not completely understood.

Disorders of the Cricopharyngeal Sphincter

Failure to Relax. The importance of precise neuromuscular coordination of swallowing is perhaps most critical at the level of the cricopharyngeal sphincter. Since this sphincter normally remains in the tonic or contracted state, it must relax to permit a swallowed bolus to enter the esophagus. As previously noted, the time of relaxation is short and must precede and overlap the time of pharyngeal contraction. Relaxation is controlled by branches from the vagus nerves. A number of neurologic disorders may interfere with this coordinated function and cause faulty timing or failure of sphincter relaxation, which in turn prevents passage of the bolus into the esophagus and favors the likelihood of aspiration of swallowed material through the larynx into the tracheobronchial tree. Failure of the sphincter to open may cause symptoms of obstruction in the throat, with periodic choking or frequent cough accompanying swallowing. In some patients the symptoms are not very dramatic and the disorder may lead to chronic pulmonary damage from aspiration of small quantities without the patient being aware of difficulty in swallowing. Underlying diseases which may interfere with neuromuscular coordination include minor or major vascular occlusions in the brain stem, peripheral neuropathies involving the vagus nerve, and skeletal abnormalities such as cervical osteoarthritis.

Spasm. A second source of failure of the cricopharyngeal sphincter to relax is spasm of this muscle. Radiographic studies have demonstrated that patients with disorders lower in the esophagus such as severe gastroesophageal reflux may have regurgitation or retention of material in the upper esophagus. This in turn irritates the sphincter and causes spasm. In addition to aspiration during swallowing, such patients may be aware of a chronic irritation in the throat and may develop a fear of swallowing which has been previously categorized as "globus hystericus." Some patients with neurologic or muscular dysfunction of the cricopharyngeal sphincter will develop secondary laryngeal changes, causing symptoms of hoarseness and chronic pharyngitis. Inflammatory polyps of the vocal cords and trachea may be found.

Cricopharyngeal (Zenker's) Diverticulum. Zenker's diverticulum is the most common type encountered in the esophagus. It is a false or acquired diverticulum characterized by pouching of the mucosal or submucosal layers through a defect in the muscular wall. The defect is located just proximal to the cricopharyngeal sphincter in the posterior wall of the inferior pharynx. Recent studies suggest that the pouch is secondary to dysfunction of the cricopharyngeal sphincter. When a bolus is forced into the lower pharynx against a closed sphincter, high pressures build up just above the sphincter. There is a weak place posteriorly in the musculature of the inferior pharynx where the oblique muscle fibers of the inferior constrictor blend into the transverse fibers of the sphincter. At this point a blowout of mucosa or diverticulum may develop.

In patients with a fully developed cricopharyngeal diverticulum it is common to elicit a history of swallowing difficulty dating back several years prior to awareness of the pouch. Initially the symptoms are cervical dysphagia and occasional bouts of aspiration or choking. As the pouch enlarges, solid particles and fluid become trapped and later regurgitate into the pharynx. When the patient lies down or stoops forward he may notice undigested food eaten hours earlier now regurgitating back into the mouth. The swallowing of large solid particles such as pills, capsules, or pieces of meat may be particularly difficult, as these routinely lodge in the pouch. A patient with a fully developed pouch finds that he must eat slowly and carefully to avoid aspiration. Friends and family frequently notice gurgling noises when the patient eats or swallows.

Complications of this disorder include chronic or acute aspiration, the risk of a large solid bolus lodging in the larynx that may cause asphyxiation, an increased risk of perforation from foreign bodies, and the development of ulcerations in the pouch from retained irritating particles. Carcinomas have developed within such pouches. There is a particular risk of perforation during endoscopic or intubation procedures for patients with this disorder.

Disorders of Esophageal Muscle

Esophageal muscular disorders may interfere with transmission of a swallowed bolus in several ways.

Other Esophageal Diverticula. Pulsion diverticula may occur at levels in the esophagus other than the cricopharyngeal region. The next most common site is the lower esophagus. These epiphrenic diverticula also consist of mucosal protrusions through the muscular layer and normally develop just proximal to the lower esophageal sphincter or just proximal to a segment of spastic esophageal muscle. The mechanism for development of such a diverticulum appears similar to that for the cricopharyngeal diverticulum. Although aspiration and laryngeal irritation do not occur, other symptoms from retention of swallowed material are similar.

When studied manometrically, the esophagus distal to the pulsion diverticulum characteristically demonstrates spastic or tertiary contractions, or failure to relax as the peristaltic wave progresses down the esophagus. When viewed radiographically, the usual finding is a segment of tonic or contracted muscle just beyond the opening of the pouch. Dysphagia frequently accompanies pulsion diverticulum. This has been attributed to the large size of the pouch hanging in a dependent position and compressing the adjacent lower esophagus. However, dysphagia may accompany a small diverticulum, in which case such a mechanical explanation cannot be invoked, and it is now thought that the dysphagia represents a primary disorder in the esophageal muscle rather than a secondary effect of the diverticulum.

More rare are true diverticula which may occur at any level and in which the body of the esophagus appears to be normal above and below the opening of the pouch. The wall of the true diverticulum consists of both mucosal and muscular layers. Distinction is sometimes made between those diverticula which appear rounded and have a narrow orifice similar to that of pulsion diverticula and are considered of congenital origin, and those with broad openings, generally in the midesophagus, which are commonly called traction diverticula. This latter term derives from the theory that the esophagus is pulled out of its normal course by contractions of adhesions to adjacent inflammatory lymph nodes or chronic mediastinal infection; however, clear evidence of this is frequently not demonstrable. Normally these diverticula cause no or few symptoms unless they reach a large size.

Systemic Sclerosis. Systemic sclerosis or scleroderma is a generalized disease involving smooth muscle and connective tissues throughout the body. Esophageal involvement is the most common alimentary tract manifestation and may precede other clinical evidence of the disease. The esophageal changes consist of atrophy of the smooth muscle in the lower two thirds of the organ distal to the segment of skeletal muscle. The smooth muscle is gradually replaced by fibrosis. The muscle atrophy causes a failure of the peristaltic wave to progress into the lower esophagus and causes weakness or obliteration of the lower esophageal sphincter mechanism. This in turn permits increased gastroesophageal reflux which may lead to secondary esophagitis. The fibrosis of the muscle may lead to a stricture of the distal esophagus, or stricture may develop owing to the severity of the esophagitis accompanying gastroesophageal reflux. The effects of reflux in such patients may be particularly severe because of the inability of the esophagus to respond by secondary peristalsis and empty itself of regurgitated gastric contents. Either aperistalsis or stricture may cause the symptom of dysphagia.

The absence of peristalsis when observed manometrically or by radiographic techniques and systemic manifestations of the disease differentiate this disorder from abnormal gastroesophageal reflux due to an incompetent lower esophageal sphincter in an otherwise healthy patient. The common radiographic finding is failure of ingested barium to pass the level of the carina when the patient is in a supine position. When the patient sits upright, the barium falls under the influence of gravity. When a stricture develops in such patients the esophageal disease may become the most prominent feature of systemic sclerosis and lead to progressive weight loss and starvation. Because of the atrophic esophageal wall and frequent secondary esophagitis, attempts to treat this disorder by dilatation may be difficult and the risks of esophageal perforation are high.

Esophageal Spasm. When esophageal spasm is encountered, it is generally secondary to another esophageal disorder. The majority of patients who demonstrate spasm will be found to have either abnormal gastroesophageal reflux which appears to trigger spasm, particularly in the lower esophagus, or a partial obstruction such as a ring, web, hypertensive lower esophageal sphincter, or tumor. Occasionally, patients are encountered in whom none of these disorders can be identified, and spasm on a primary neurogenic or functional basis must be diagnosed. Whenever this diagnosis is made, a careful search for an underlying cause should be undertaken.

Characteristically, spasm is localized or segmental in distribution, with the most prominent spastic contractions occurring repeatedly at the same level. Complete or partial obstruction to the passage of ingested food may result from spasm. A prominent feature of this disorder is severe substernal pain which may be suggestive of the symptoms accompanying ischemic heart disease. Since the spasm may be reduced by the use of nitrites, response to nitroglycerin is not a useful way to differentiate between this disease and coronary heart disease. The diagnosis of esophageal spasm is made by the characteristic x-ray appearance of a corkscrew esophagus or multiple constrictive rings which do not dilate during fluoroscopic observation. Another useful diagnostic technique is manometry, which shows failure of progressive peristalsis and the presence of high-pressure contractions occurring spontaneously or in response to a swallow and located at the same level in the esophagus on repeated studies.

Leiomyoma. Benign tumors of smooth muscle in the esophagus are occasionally encountered. Normally, these are incidental findings in the course of barium swallow radiography, but occasionally these tumors may reach sufficient size to interfere with the passage of an ingested food bolus and cause dysphagia. They are not normally fixed to the esophageal mucosa and cannot be diagnosed endoscopically. When a leiomyoma is suspected from radiographic findings, a biopsy should not be attempted through the esophagoscope because of the dangers of introducing infection and causing inflammatory adhesion of the tumor to the mucosa, which interferes with later surgical removal.

Disorders of Mucosa

Neoplasm. Benign neoplasms of the esophageal mucosa are infrequent and generally of little clinical importance. Occasionally, squamous polyps or papillomas may be encountered. Adenomas arising in the esophageal glands are rare. The most common esophageal neoplasm is carcinoma. This most frequently causes the symptom of dysphagia and occurs with sufficient frequency that any patient complaining of persistent dysphagia should be thoroughly investigated for the possibility of this disease.

Carcinoma of the esophagus is a virulent neoplasm causing approximately five deaths per hundred thousand population in the United States each year. The disease is more frequent in males than in females, and in nonwhite than in white Americans. It occurs more commonly in the sixth, seventh, and eighth decades of life. Carcinoma may develop in association with conditions contributing to esophageal retention or irritation such as excessive use of alcohol or tobacco, and among patients having achalasia or lye strictures. Patients with the Plummer-Vinson syndrome (see below) are susceptible to squamous cell carcinoma of the cervical esophagus and hypopharynx.

Carcinoma may present a variety of appearances, including ulceration, fungating tumor, or diffuse scirrhous strictures. The most common site of origin appears to be in the middle third of the esophagus. Microscopically, squamous cell carcinoma is by far the most common type. Adenocarcinoma truly arising in the esophagus separated from the stomach is rare. Adenocarcinoma at the cardia is more common and probably arises from gastric mucosa. Carcinomatous change in esophageal mucosa may be multifocal. The disease spreads by direct extension, lymphatic invasion, and blood-borne metastases. The rich lymphatic network of the esophageal submucosa permits early and extensive spread of the tumor up and down the length of the esophagus. It is not uncommon to encounter malignant cells 5 cm. or more from the visible margins of a tumor. Direct invasion of adjacent structures such as the trachea or aorta is common and a frequent cause of life-threatening complications. One reason for the poor prognosis of these tumors is the advanced state which they reach before causing symptoms. Because of the ability of smooth muscle to stretch, involvement of the esophageal lumen must be nearly circumferential before dysphagia and obstruction develop.

Although the patient may recall a sensation of substernal fullness or poorly localized chest pain, the usual presenting complaint is dysphagia or difficulty in swallowing. The level of the obstruction may be quite accurately localized by the patient's symptoms. Rapid weight loss and emaciation accompany the dysphagia. As the obstruction becomes more complete, regurgitation of swallowed food, vomiting, or choking and aspiration are noted. Hoarseness may develop from recurrent nerve involvement by the primary tumor or lymph node metastases. Horner's syndrome, hematemesis, or melena may occur. When the tumor invades the trachea or bronchus, cough, hemoptysis, or dyspnea result. Complications of the tumor may be heralded by the presence of lymph nodes in the neck, bone pain from metastases, hemorrhage from invasion of mediastinal vessels, fever from perforation or abscess, and severe cough from tracheobronchial involvement. Tracheo-esophageal fistula may develop in advanced cases and be the terminal event.

Because the obvious symptoms from carcinoma of the esophagus represent complications of the disease at an advanced stage, it is especially important that the diagnosis be made whenever possible at any earlier stage, when treatment is more favorable and symptoms are less apparent. Any patient complaining of symptoms which might arise from the esophagus should undergo radiographic examination and have specimens of esophageal washings submitted for cytologic examination. In addition to the standard barium swallow observed fluoroscopically and recorded on permanent x-ray films, it is often helpful to examine the esophagus by cineradiographic techniques, so that the course of the barium may be examined repeatedly if questionable regions in the esophagus are observed. Just as the pathologic presentation of esophageal carcinoma is variable, the radiographic manifestations may take many forms such as a fungating mass, ulceration, stricture, or polypoid tumor. In some patients the radiographic appearances may be more suggestive of benign disease.

Cytologic examination of cells obtained from esophageal washings offers a high diagnostic yield in patients with this disease. In addition to the patients whose symptoms or x-ray findings suggest a possible neoplasm, those having a high risk of the disease such as individuals with long-standing lye stricture, achalasia, or the Plummer-Vinson syndrome are good candidates for repeated cytologic examinations at six-month or yearly intervals.

To confirm or establish the diagnosis of carcinoma in patients whose symptoms or x-ray findings are suggestive, esophagoscopy is an essential diagnostic procedure. A biopsy will provide confirmatory evidence of the diagnosis and indicate the cell type. Because of the tendency for esophageal neoplasms to spread up and down the mucosa, biopsies are generally taken above the level of the tumor to ascertain whether submucosal spread has occurred. This has great importance in planning treatment for the disease. In patients whose neoplasm is located in the middle third of the esophagus, bronchoscopy should also be performed to detect evidence of tracheal or left main bronchial invasion or vocal cord paralysis.

Web or Ring. Benign rings or webs of the esophageal mucosa may cause symptoms by obstructing the passage of solid food through the lumen. Although these mucosal constrictions may occur at any level in the esophagus, there are two specific clinical forms in which this lesion is more frequently encountered.

The Plummer-Vinson syndrome, when fully developed, includes a hypochromic microcytic anemia, spoon-shaped fingernails, atrophy of the tongue and of the pharyngeal and esophageal mucosa, fissures at the corners of the mouth, and dysphagia. This syndrome occurs more frequently in fair-complexioned females of Northern European descent. The dysphagia may result from a hypopharyngeal or upper esophageal mucosal web. These patients have a higher than normal incidence of carcinoma of the upper esophagus and must be carefully observed for a change in symptoms suggesting the development of a neoplasm. Such patients are candidates for periodic cytologic examination of esophageal washings.

Schatzki and Gary (1953) and Ingelfinger and Kramer (1953) independently described the condition of lower esophageal ring causing dysphagia. This clinical syndrome often occurs in older male patients and is manifested by sudden severe dysphagia after ingestion of a large bolus of solid food. The sensation of food sticking under the lower sternum and severe pain are prominent symptoms. As the food digests or is gradually propelled through the narrow segment, the symptoms subside and may not recur for prolonged periods until a large bolus is once again ingested. The symptoms of severe pain which may accompany this disorder are due to spasm of the esophageal muscle above the ring as the esophagus contracts upon the impacted bolus. In this regard the symptoms of pain come from a mechanism similar to that which causes pain lower in the intestinal tract, namely, vigorous contraction of gut muscle above an obstructing point.

Pathologically, the "Schatzki" ring is often found to have esophageal squamous mucosa on the superior surface and columnar mucosa on the inferior surface. A thin layer of fibrous tissue is seen in the submucosa between the two layers of mucosa. Deeper layers of the esophagus are normal. Occasional cases have been described in which the ring is located completely within the zone of esophageal squamous epithelium.

The effect of the ring is to limit esophageal distention. Thus, when the esophagus is empty, no ring is visible. It is only when the lumen of the esophagus is distended beyond the diameter of the ring that it becomes noticeable. For this reason the ring may be missed in radiographic examinations unless the lower esophagus is studied in the dilated condition. The diameter of the ring has a strong correlation with the presence of symptoms. Patients whose rings measure less than 13 mm. in diameter almost always have symptoms of dysphagia, whereas those whose rings are larger than 13 mm. may be asymptomatic. Rings of large diameter are frequent findings in routine barium swallow examinations but those which progress to a narrow aperture and cause symptoms are uncommon. Because the ring represents a zone of restricted distensibility rather than a constant weblike defect in the esophagus, it may be easily missed by esophagoscopy. The diagnosis is generally made only on radiographic study.

Stricture. Stricture or abnormal narrowing with contraction of the esophagus may occur from a variety of causes. Malignant neoplasms may present as a stricture. The ingestion of corrosive substances such as lye may cause destruction of the esophageal wall, with stricture formation. The most common type of benign esophageal stricture is caused by reflux esophagitis. The diagnosis of a stricture is made by x-ray examination demonstrating a persistent narrowing or contraction of the esophagus. However, the specific type of stricture can generally not be diagnosed solely by x-ray but is determined by the clinical history and esophagoscopic findings.

Strictures secondary to gastroesophageal reflux are thought to occur through the following mechanisms: An incompetent lower esophageal sphincter permits free reflux of upper gastrointestinal secretions, including acid, pepsin, bile, and pancreatic secretions, into the lower esophagus. Prolonged contact of these substances with the esophageal mucosa causes penetration and breakdown of the mucosa, superficial ulceration, and submucosal inflammation. The damage is repaired by deposition of inflammatory tissue followed by collagen deposition and fibrosis, just as injured tissue heals elsewhere in the body. If the reflux decreases, the mucosa may be restored by migration and regeneration of columnar epithelial cells rather than the squamous epithelium which normally lines the lower esophagus. Continuous or repeated insults to the mucosa lead to increasing amounts of tissue destruction and fibrosis. Initially this occurs in the superficial layers, but as the condition becomes more severe the muscle fibers are damaged and replaced by fibrous tissue as well. As the collagen matures, it contracts, causing rigidity, narrowing, and shortening of the esophageal wall until a tight stricture develops. As the lumen is gradually occluded by the contracting fibrous tissue, the amount of reflux diminishes, and the mucosa and esophagus above the level of the stricture are spared from further insult and appear normal. The development of a stricture through these steps has been documented sequentially in individual patients and has been seen in various stages in numerous patients, providing evidence for this theory of stricture development.

At the time when a stricture is apparent by x-ray, the fibrosis may still be limited to the submucosal layers, or the x-ray finding of a stricture may represent far advanced disease, with total breakdown and replacement of the esophageal wall by fibrosis and granulation tissue. Thus, the clinical and radiographic diagnosis of esophageal stricture may represent pathologic conditions of varying degrees of severity. This must be taken into account when therapy is planned and the results of treatment are assessed.

The physiologic effects of reflux esophagitis and stricture are initially those of disordered peristalsis. Partial esophageal narrowing as well as esophageal reflux can disrupt or alter progression of the peristaltic wave and cause synchronous or tertiary contractions. Inability of the esophagus to empty permits prolonged contact of refluxed material with the mucosa and aggravates the esophagitis. It is only when the stricture becomes far advanced that the bolus of food is mechanically obstructed by the narrowing. By this time, the patient's intake of solid food is markedly restricted. As the stricture tightens, the reflux may be less, so that the symptoms of heartburn and regurgitation are diminished. Dysphagia may be the only complaint. This leads to a paradox in which the most severe stages of esophagitis may be associated with few symptoms of reflux, although this is thought to be the underlying cause of the inflammation and stricture. In patients whose esophagus is relatively insensitive to reflux, dysphagia may be the earliest complaint leading the patient to the physician.

In addition to symptoms of reflux, dysphagia, and inanition, the patient with a stricture is likely to have pulmonary complaints of nocturnal cough or choking or coughing when eating, and may develop pulmonary infection secondary to aspiration. Other complications of a stricture include hemorrhage, normally from ulceration in areas of ectopic columnar mucosa, or perforation of the esophagus, again usually due to ulceration in areas of ectopic gastric epithelium.

Between the two common types of benign esophageal strictures—those due to reflux esophagitis and those secondary to ingestion of caustic materials—important differences exist. The stricture secondary to reflux is almost always rather short and localized to the region just above columnar epithelium, whether this be at the gastroesophageal junction or high in the esophagus in patients whose esophagus is lined with columnar or gastric epithelium. Thus, the patient with a short stricture in the midesophagus caused by reflux will probably have columnar epithelium below the stricture. On the other hand, a patient whose stricture is due to ingestion of lye or other corrosives will often have long segments of esophagus damaged by the chemicals and replaced with fibrous tissue. Damage may be particularly severe at the levels of the esophagus where there is a shelf or transient holdup of the bolus, such as the cricopharyngeal region, the level of the aortic arch, and just above the lower esophageal sphincter.

A second distinction between the reflux and corrosive strictures is that the cause of the reflux stricture persists, so that the condition continues to worsen rather than improve with time. Methods of therapy which do not prevent the underlying reflux may fail to provide relief from further stricture development. On the other hand, the stricture secondary to ingestion of corrosives is caused by a single injury. Taking this into account, one may employ methods of therapy which differ from those used in treatment of a reflux stricture.

Malignant strictures of the esophagus are considered in a preceding section and will not be discussed further here. The secondary effects and complications of the malignant stricture may be similar to those of the benign stricture.

Disorders at the Cardia Interfering With Transportation of Ingested Material

Achalasia. Achalasia is an uncommon disease of unknown etiology in which the lower esophageal sphincter fails to relax in response to a swallow, and there is an absence of peristalsis in the body of the esophagus. Pathologic findings on visual or radiographic examination include a normally contracted distal esophageal segment of approximately 2 to 4 cm. in length composed of normal muscle. The body of the esophagus is generally dilated and may distend to a very large size sufficient to contain several quarts of fluid. Generally, the muscle of the esophageal wall in its midportion is thickened, but in far advanced cases it may become atrophic and fibrotic. Microscopically, the distinctive feature of achalasia is the absence or decrease in number of the ganglion cells in Auerbach's plexus. Fibrosis of the plexus may be noted. These changes are found throughout the esophagus but are more conspicuous in the lower portion. The inner circular muscle layer may be hypertrophied or sclerotic, and scarring of the muscle cells may be noticed microscopically. Although several reports have suggested that there may be abnormalities of the vagus nerves or the central nervous system in patients with achalasia, these findings have not been thoroughly substantiated or generally accepted.

While the etiology of achalasia is unknown, a similar type of mega-esophagus with similar pathologic changes in the muscle and Auerbach's plexus may be seen in Chagas' disease. This disease occurs in South America and is caused by *Trypanosoma cruzi*. Evidence suggests that the organism secretes a neurotoxin which affects the ganglion cells. Although this disease is clinically similar to achalasia, the organism has not been found in the vast majority of patients suffering from typical achalasia in North America or Europe.

The physiologic disorder of achalasia may best be studied by esophageal manometry. The characteristics of the lower esophageal sphincter segment in the resting state are the same as in normal individuals. However, in the body of the esophagus the resting intraluminal pressures are generally high and may exceed the pressures of the gastric fundus. The manometric abnormalities of achalasia are most striking when the response to a swallow is studied. The lower esophageal sphincter fails to relax following a swallow, and contraction may occur prematurely in the upper portion of the sphincter, so that the sphincter is effectively closed when the peristaltic wave would normally reach the lower esophagus. In addition to the failure of the sphincter to relax, passage of the bolus is further impeded by the absence of peristalsis in the body of the esophagus. Following the swallow, a simultaneous contraction generally occurs throughout the length of the esophagus with no progression of the pressure waves. In far advanced cases in which the muscle has become sclerotic, atrophic, and fibrotic, no contraction at all may be observed.

A further physiologic abnormality in the patient with achalasia is the response to methacholine. In the normal subject, injection of this drug generally causes no change in pressure in the body of the esophagus. In a patient with achalasia, subcutaneous injection of 5 to 10 mg. of methacholine chloride may cause an increase in resting esophageal pressure of 20 cm. of water or more. This may be associated with severe substernal pain, similar to that in patients with esophageal spasm. The methacholine response may be abolished by administration of atropine sulfate.

The symptoms caused by these specific pathologic and physiologic changes are often sufficiently distinctive to separate this disease from other esophageal disorders. Initially, the patient will notice intermittent obstruction to swallowing which is generally localized to the lower substernal region. The obstruction is generally less when a meal is taken slowly and the food is warm. The obstruction may be intermittent and may be more severe when the patient is tense or nervous. As the symptoms become more pronounced, the patient becomes aware of regurgitation whenever he stoops forward. Unlike gastroesophageal reflux, the regurgitated material is not acid or sour, and undigested food can often be identified. Pain is generally not associated with the regurgitation. The pain which occurs with achalasia, if any, is usually of the spastic type, rather than heartburn. It may be quite severe, is located substernally, and persists for a long time.

When esophageal retention becomes marked, pulmonary symptoms secondary to aspiration become prominent. The patient may awaken to find ingested food material regurgitated onto the pillow. Secondary pulmonary complications including lung abscess may occur. Nutrition may be impaired and the patient suffers weight loss and vitamin deficiency. Although bleeding is quite uncommon in these cases, a retention esophagitis may develop and cause chronic anemia from blood loss. In addition to these complications from obstructed swallowing, patients with achalasia are thought to have a higher than normal incidence of carcinoma in the midportion of the esophagus.

Hypertensive Lower Esophageal Sphincter. A rare variation of the spastic esophageal motor disorders may be increased tone in the lower esophageal sphincter, causing dysphagia and severe pain. Generally, retention of ingested food in the esophagus is not prominent in these patients; this finding differentiates it from achalasia, as does the finding of increased sphincter pressure during manometric studies. In other respects, this syndrome is similar to that of esophageal spasm described above. Whether the hypertensive sphincter syndrome occurs as a secondary manifestation of a gastroesophageal reflux remains uncertain.

Other Diseases Affecting Transportation of Ingested Material

A variety of diseases which involve the esophagus may have a secondary effect of blocking transportation of ingested material. Extrinsic conditions such as neoplasm metastatic to the mediastinum or esophageal wall may interfere with swallowing in a manner similar to that of primary carcinoma of the esophagus. An enlarging thoracic aortic aneurysm may compress the esophagus and cause secondary dysphagia. Primary bronchogenic carcinoma adjacent to the esophagus may involve the esophageal wall and block ingestion of food. Lodgment of a foreign body in the esophagus generally interrupts swallowing, owing to both its physical presence and the edema and inflammation which it causes in the wall of the esophagus.

Esophageal atresia with tracheo-esophageal fistula is a fairly common abnormality of the newborn which obviously interferes with transportation of ingested food. Following surgical correction of the atresia and fistula, function of the esophagus will generally return to normal unless a stricture develops at the anastomosis. Acquired tracheo-esophageal fistulas may occur from malignant disease in the mediastinum or rarely from inflammatory diseases such as tuberculosis or histoplasmosis. Such fistulas permit transportation of food material from the esophagus directly into the lungs, with resulting severe cough and pulmonary infection.

Rupture of the esophagus may occur spontaneously, from penetrating wounds or external trauma, from foreign bodies, or during the course of esophageal intubation. This catastrophic event occurs most commonly during esophagoscopy or gastroscopy. When perforation accompanies endoscopy, the common sites are just distal to the cricopharyngeal sphincter and in the lower esophagus. Spontaneous rupture of the esophagus is almost always caused by vomiting and occurs most frequently along the left lateral aspect of the lower esophagus. During vomiting, the antrum of the stomach contracts and the upper stomach and esophagus relax, permitting increased intra-abdominal pressure to force the gastric contents cephalad. The distal esophagus may increase dramatically in diameter fivefold or more. The left lower esophageal wall is the weakest point of the organ and can be ruptured by pressures of 5 lbs. per square inch or less, providing the setting for spontaneous rupture during vomiting.

Following esophageal rupture, the patient experiences a sudden severe substernal or epigastric pain. If the rupture occurs when the patient is anesthetized or sedated for endoscopy, this initial symptom may be absent. Following rupture, mediastinal dissection of air or pneumothorax develops. This is manifested by crepitus felt in the neck or a mediastinal crunching sound heard on auscultation over the back. If the rupture does not penetrate the pleura, an effusion secondary to the mediastinitis develops in the pleura within the course of several hours. Free perforation into the pleura causes a hydropneumothorax and empyema. A tension pneumothorax may occur. The patient rapidly becomes gravely ill, with signs of shock. This illness may be mistaken for perforated duodenal or gastric ulcer, acute pancreatitis, acute myocardial infarction, or dissecting aortic aneurysm. The diagnosis can be resolved by abdominal and thoracic x-rays, serum amylase levels, electrocardiogram, and x-ray visualization of the esophagus by a swallow of radiopaque water-soluble substance.

PREVENTION OF GASTROESOPHAGEAL REFLUX

The second major function of the esophagus is the prevention of involuntary regurgitation of stomach contents. The responsibility for this function is vested in the esophagogastric junction or cardia.

Mechanisms for Competency of the Cardia

In normal individuals the mechanism which permits unimpeded passage of swallowed material into the stomach while preventing regurgitation of gastric contents back through the esophageal orifice is remarkably effective. Withdrawal of a pH electrode across the cardia often reveals a 5 unit change in pH over a distance of approximately 0.5 cm. This represents a 100,000-fold difference in hydrogen ion concentration across this short distance. In spite of a great deal of investigation as to the structure and function of the esophagogastric junction, precise understanding of the mechanism which prevents reflux remains incomplete.

A variety of factors have been suggested as contributing to competency of the cardia. The strength or resting pressure of the lower esophageal sphincter has a statistical correlation with the control of reflux. Yet, in individual patients a high pressure in the sphincter may be present, and free reflux occurs. Conversely, a low sphincter pressure may be found in a patient without reflux. Since no anatomic sphincter can be demonstrated in humans, the source of the pressures recorded in the distal esophagus remains uncertain. The high-pressure zone probably represents a summation of intrinsic pressure generated from the lower esophageal muscle, extrinsic pressure resulting from the diaphragmatic hiatus, and positive abdominal pressure exerted against the endo-abdominal fascia, which inserts at or above the level of the sphincter. An active role of the distal esophageal muscle in generating the measured sphincter pressure and in the prevention of reflux is suggested by the observation that pressures in the lower esophageal sphincter rise markedly when the hormone gastrin is administered. The ability of the sphincter to adapt its tension to changes in abdominal pressure further suggests an intrinsic role of the lower esophageal muscle in preventing reflux. Most investigators now accept the lower esophageal muscle as being at least partially responsible for competency of the cardia.

The esophageal hiatus of the diaphragm may play a role in the normal control of reflux, but it is not essential. Some patients with a hiatal hernia have a competent cardia, whereas others in whom a hiatal hernia cannot be demonstrated may have an incompetent cardia.

The location of a portion of the lower esophageal sphincter within the positive pressure abdominal environment appears to be important in the prevention of reflux. The pressure gradient across the diaphragm is usually 10 mm. Hg or more and increases during inspiration. The compressing effect of abdominal pressure during all phases of respiration supplements the intrinsic pressure generated by the lower esophageal muscle segment. Intra-abdominal pressure may remain effective even in patients with hiatal hernia if the extension of endo-abdominal fascia through the hiatus inserts into the esophagus above the sphincter. Thus, compression by the right crus of the diaphragm or muscular contraction of the diaphragm does not appear important, but an intra-abdominal location of the distal esophageal segment probably does contribute to competency of the cardia.

Other suggested factors for which there is less evidence of effectiveness include an acute esophagogastric angle of entry and the plugging of the esophageal orifice by redundant gastric folds. Further investigations are necessary to determine precisely how competency of the cardia is achieved in the normal human being.

Hiatal Hernia. Hiatal hernia is one of the most common disorders of the alimentary tract. Its significance varies greatly, depending upon type, size, and associated complications. It is essential to understand that gastroesophageal reflux and hiatal hernia, which often appear together, are separate entities, each of which may occur without the other. For this reason, it is important to differentiate the symptoms, diagnosis, and complications for each of the two conditions.

Hiatal hernia is defined as stomach passing into the thorax through the esophageal hiatus of the diaphragm. There are two basic types of hiatal hernia which can be differentiated by the anatomic and physiologic abnormalities of each. Combinations of the two types constitute a third group of hiatal hernias, and the presence of other organs in addition to the stomach passing through the esophageal hiatus make up a fourth category of hiatal hernia.

In Type I, the axial or sliding hiatal hernia, the esophagogastric junction is displaced through the diaphragm as the leading point of the hernia. In Type II, the parahiatal or rolling hernia, the esophagogastric junction remains fixed at the level of the hiatus, but a portion of the gastric fundus advances above the cardia into a hernia sac. It is the Type I hiatal hernia which may be accompanied by gastroesophageal reflux and its distinctive symptoms and complications. Type II hiatal hernia is rarely associated with abnormal reflux. The combined Type III hiatal hernia, in which the esophagogastric junction is herniated through the diaphragm, but a portion of the gastric fundus is more cephalad than the cardia, may be associated with the symptoms and complications of both Type I and II hernias.

The diagnosis of a hiatal hernia is established primarily by radiographic study and is confirmed by surgical dissection. Diagnostic methods such as manometry, mucosal potential difference measurements, and pH recordings are more useful in diagnosing gastroesophageal reflux and its complications than in establishing the presence of a hiatal hernia.

Generally, the common small Type I hiatal hernia is asymptomatic and causes no complications unless abnormal gastroesophageal reflux is present. The symptoms and complications often attributed to this hernia are really those of reflux and will be described in the next section.

The Type II hiatal hernia may be asymptomatic, even though quite large, or may cause symptoms related to the abnormal position of the stomach in the hernia sac. These symptoms are most commonly mild discomfort or fullness in the epigastrium or chest after eating. This may be relieved by belching or vomiting. Dysphagia may occur because of extrinsic compression of the esophagus by the adjacent large hernia pouch. This type of hernia is associated with a substantial incidence of serious mechanical complications involving the gastric pouch. Complications include hemorrhage from ulcers or gastritis in the supradiaphragmatic stomach, gastric obstruction, or volvulus, which may lead to strangulation and gastric infarction. Very large Type II hernias are commonly combined with displacement of the cardia proximally and may be associated with reflux and its complications. Large hernias introduce a risk of intrathoracic gastric dilatation with respiratory embarrassment. When the sac is sizable, other organs such as colon, small intestine, or spleen may herniate and provide a further source of complications.

Gastroesophageal Reflux. Regurgitation of gastric contents through the esophagogastric junction probably occurs at times in everyone. Manometric study has shown that newborn infants lack a lower esophageal sphincter and they frequently regurgitate. During the first year of life, competency of the cardia is acquired and regurgitation ceases. Although occasional reflux may occur as a normal event in older patients, frequent reflux into an esophagus sensitive to the irritating gastrointestinal secretions may cause symptoms and complications. When this occurs, the clinical condition of abnormal gastroesophageal reflux results. This rarely develops in the interval between infancy and late teen age. Thereafter the incidence of abnormal reflux rises, and the problem is most common in patients over 40 years of age. There seems to be an increased tendency for reflux to occur in obese individuals.

Although abnormal reflux commonly is associated with Type I or sliding hiatal hernia, a causal relationship between these two conditions is not established. Individuals without a hiatal hernia demonstrated radiographically or at surgery may experience reflux through an incompetent cardia, and, as mentioned in the preceding section, patients having a hiatal hernia do not necessarily experience abnormal reflux.

In the typical patient with gastroesophageal reflux, manometric studies often demonstrate a decreased resting pressure in the lower esophageal sphincter. Generally, the sphincter segment will be of normal length unless a large hiatal hernia is present which distorts the pressure recordings. Relaxation to swallowing is normal. As described above, however, there is not a precise one-to-one relationship between sphincter pressure and competency of the cardia, so that the manometric studies alone are not acceptable as diagnostic evidence of abnormal reflux.

Radiography is the most useful technique for detecting a hiatal hernia, but it is less successful in demonstrating reflux. The diagnosis of abnormal reflux can be made by the radiologist, if he sees reflux at a time other than when the patient swallows. If reflux is suspected as the cause of the patient's complaint but cannot be demonstrated radiographically, the use of pH recordings is a more sensitive and reliable method for making the diagnosis. In patients with severe reflux there may be a disorder of esophageal motor function manifested by an increased proportion of simultaneous contractions rather than progressive peristalsis. A bolus of acid placed in the esophagus in such subjects may not be cleared normally.

The typical symptoms caused by gastroesophageal reflux are pain and regurgitation aggravated by postural positions such as stooping or lying down. Discomfort is usually felt beneath the sternum and in the subxiphoid region, with occasional radiation to one side. The pain may radiate to the shoulders, neck, arms, ears, or between the scapulae, but it nearly always includes the substernal region. The nature of the pain is a burning sensation and is frequently called heartburn by the patient. Regurgitation may be noted as a sour or bilious taste in the mouth or as the "repeating" of food. Effortless vomiting after meals may occur in severe cases. Aggravation of the symptoms by bending over or lying flat permits the diagnosis of reflux clinically. If the patient's complaints are not related to posture, heartburn or regurgitation may be the result of other causes and cannot be attributed to abnormal reflux on the basis of symptoms alone.

Other symptoms which may be caused by reflux include vague epigastric or substernal discomfort, a foreign sensation, fullness or tightness in the neck, hoarseness, change in voice, chronic pharyngitis from reflux through the cricopharyngeal sphincter, or symptoms which mimic those of angina pectoris. When atypical symptoms are noted, the diagnosis cannot be made on clinical grounds and must depend upon objective evidence of reflux and exclusion of other causes. Recordings of pH in the esophagus to document reflux may be especially helpful. In patients with atypical symptoms, the perfusion of acid and saline alternately into the esophagus may be useful in determining whether the symptoms are of esophageal origin. Reproduction of the patient's spontaneous symptoms by infusion of acid and not with saline represents a positive acid perfusion test.

The complications of gastroesophageal reflux include esophagitis, stricture, bleeding, ulceration, spasm, and aspiration of regurgitated material into the lungs. Esophagitis is the most common complication of reflux. Since the severity of the patient's symptoms correlate poorly with esophagitis, this diagnosis can be made with certainty only by esophagoscopy. Patients who present with advanced esophagitis and stricture may have minimal or no symptoms of reflux prior to the onset of obstruction, whereas some who complain most bitterly of heartburn and regurgitation are found on esophagoscopy and biopsy to have no or minimal esophagitis. The reason for such variability in sensitivity of the esophagus to reflux is not completely understood. One symptom which does suggest the presence of esophagitis and mediastinal inflammation is soreness between the scapulae following ingestion of hot or alcoholic liquids. When dysphagia develops, esophagitis is more likely to be present. However, reflux alone may trigger esophageal muscle spasm, causing dysphagia in the absence of esophagitis, and therefore this symptom is not diagnostic.

Because of the lack of specific symptoms for

reflux esophagitis, esophagoscopy is essential in diagnosing this condition. The esophagoscopic findings may be categorized based upon severity. These include no visible esophagitis and Grade I esophagitis, when the mucosa is reddened but not ulcerated. In such cases, biopsy may show only thinning of the mucosa and perhaps dilatation of epithelial vessels without other change. Grade 2 esophagitis is recorded when superficial erosions and ulcerations are noted. When the wall of the esophagus becomes somewhat stiffened and fibrotic in addition to being ulcerated, Grade 3 esophagitis is present. When the fibrosis and contraction has caused a stricture, Grade 4 esophagitis is observed. Stricture is discussed in detail in a preceding section. Ulceration of the esophageal mucosa commonly takes the form of circumferential destruction of the squamous epithelium just above the columnar epithelial border. Localized penetrating ulcers into the wall of the esophagus, particularly in islands of ectopic gastric mucosa, may occur and cause rapid hemorrhage. Bleeding may also be severe in milder forms of esophagitis when diffuse oozing of blood from the mucosal surface is encountered.

Another common complication of an incompetent cardia is aspiration. Mild degrees manifested by nocturnal cough and occasional hoarseness are frequently noted in the histories of patients who prove to have reflux. When aspiration becomes more severe, pulmonary complications such as recurring pneumonitis or lung abscess may occur.

REFERENCES

Allen, T. H., and Clagett, O. T.: Changing concepts in the surgical treatment of pulsion diverticula of the lower esophagus. J. Thorac. Cardiovasc. Surg., 50:455, 1962.

Belsey, R.: The pulmonary complications of oesophageal disease. Brit. J. Dis. Chest, 54:342, 1960.

Belsey, R.: Functional disease of the esophagus. J. Thorac. Cardiovasc. Surg., 52:164, 1966.

Bennett, J. R., and Hendrix, T. R.: Diffuse esophageal spasm: A disorder with more than one cause. Gastroenterology, 59:273, 1970.

Bernstein, L. M., Fruin, R. C., and Pacini, R.: Differentiation of esophageal pain from angina pectoris: Role of the esophageal acid perfusion test. Medicine (Balt), 41:143, 1962.

Bombeck, C. T., Dillard, D. H., and Nyhus, L. M.: Muscular anatomy of the gastroesophageal junction and role of phrenoesophageal ligament. Autopsy study of sphincter mechanism. Ann. Surg., 164:643, 1966.

Botha, G. S. M.: The Gastro-oesophageal Junction. Boston, Little, Brown and Co., 1962.

Castell, D. O., and Harris, L. D.: Hormonal control of gastroesophageal sphincter strength. New Eng. J. Med., 282:866, 1970.

Cauthorne, R. T., VanHoutte, J. J., Donner, M. W., and Hendrix, T. R.: Study of patients with lower esophageal ring by simultaneous cineradiography and manometry. Gastroenterology, 49:632, 1965.

Cohen, B. R., and Wolfe, B. S.: Roentgen localization of the physiologically determined esophageal hiatus. Gastroenterology, 43:43, 1962.

Cohen, S., and Harris, L. D.: The adaptive response of the lower esophageal sphincter. Clin. Res., 17:300, 1969.

Cohen, S., and Harris, L. D.: Does hiatus hernia affect competence of the gastroesophageal sphincter? New Eng. J. Med., 282:866, 1970.

Delahunty, J. E., Alonso, W. A., Margulies, S. I., and Knudson, D. H.: Relationship of reflux esophagitis to pharyngeal pouch (Zenker's diverticulum) formation. Laryngoscope, 81:570, 1971.

Ellis, F. H., Jr., and Olsen, A. M.: Achalasia of the Esophagus. Philadelphia, W. B. Saunders Co., 1969.

Foster, J. H., Jolly, P. C., Sawyers, J. L., and Daniel, R. A.: Esophageal perforation: Diagnosis and treatment. Ann. Surg., 161:701, 1965.

Fyke, F. E., Jr., Code, C. F., and Schlegel, J. G.: The gastroesophageal sphincter in healthy human beings. Gastroenterologia (Basel), 86:135, 1956.

Gephart, T., and Graham, R.: The cellular detection of carcinoma of the esophagus. Surg. Gynec. Obstet., 108:75, 1959.

Gryboski, J. D., Thayer, W. R., Jr., and Spiro, H. M.: Esophageal motility in infants and children. Pediatrics, 31:382, 1963.

Harris, L. D., and Pope, C. E., II: "Squeeze" vs. resistance: An evaluation of the mechanism of sphincter competence. J. Clin. Invest., 43:2272, 1964.

Hayward, J.: The lower end of the oesophagus. Thorax, 16:36, 1961.

Hiebert, C. A., and Belsey, R.: Incompetency of the gastric cardia without radiologic evidence of hiatal hernia. J. Thorac. Cardiovasc. Surg., 42:352, 1961.

Holder, T. M., and Ashcraft, K. W.: Esophageal atresia and tracheoesophageal fistula. Curr. Probl. Surg., August, 1966.

Hunt, P. S., Connell, A. M., and Smiley, T. B.: The cricopharyngeal sphincter in gastric reflux. Gut, 11:308, 1970.

Ingelfinger, F. J.: Esophageal motility. Physiol. Rev., 38:533, 1958.

Ingelfinger, F. J., and Kramer, P.: Dysphagia produced by contractile ring in lower esophagus. Gastroenterology, 23:419, 1953.

Ismail-Beigi, F., Horton, P. F., and Pope, C. E., II: Histological consequences of gastroesophageal reflux in man. Gastroenterology, 58:163, 1970.

Just-Viera, J. O., Morris, J. D., and Haight, C.: Achalasia and esophageal carcinoma. Ann. Thorac. Surg., 3:526, 1967.

Katz, D., and Hoffman, F. (Eds.): The Esophagogastric Junction. Amsterdam, Excerpta Medica, 1971.

Mackler, S. A.: Spontaneous rupture of the esophagus, an experimental and clinical study. Surg. Gynec. Obstet., 95:345, 1952.

Mossberg, S. M.: The columnar lined esophagus (Barrett syndrome): An acquired condition? Gastroenterology, 50:671, 1966.

Olsen, A. M., and Schlegel, J. F.: Motility disturbances caused by esophagitis. J. Thorac. Cardiovasc. Surg., 50:607, 1965.

Schatzki, R.: The lower esophageal ring: Long-term followup of symptomatic and asymptomatic rings. Amer. J. Roentgen., 90:805, 1963.

Schatzki, R., and Gary, J. E.: Dysphagia due to diaphragm-like localized narrowing in lower esophagus ("lower esophageal ring"). Amer. J. Roentgen., 70:911, 1953.

Skinner, D. B., Belsey, R. H. R., Hendrix, T. R., and Zuidema, G. D. (Eds.): Gastroesophageal Reflux and Hiatal Hernia. Boston, Little, Brown and Co., 1972.

Sutherland, H. D.: Cricopharyngeal achalasia. J. Thorac. Cardiovasc. Surg., 43:114, 1962.

Terracol, J., and Sweet, R. H.: Diseases of the Esophagus. Philadelphia, W. B. Saunders Co., 1958, p. 247.

Wilkins, E. W., Jr., and Skinner, D. B.: Recent progress in surgery of the esophagus: I. Pathophysiology and gastroesophageal reflux. II. Clinical entities. J. Surg. Res., 8:41, 90; 1968.

Wynder, E. L., and Fryer, J. H.: Etiologic considerations of Plummer-Vinson (Paterson-Kelly) syndrome. Ann. Intern. Med., 49:1106, November, 1958.

CHAPTER 25 THE STOMACH

JOSEPH B. KIRSNER

ANATOMIC VARIATIONS

The form and position of the stomach vary in different persons and in the same person at various times, depending upon the degree of filling, the size and position of the adjacent organs, the condition of the anterior abdominal musculature, and the physical habitus. In the relatively short, obese person with a tense abdominal wall the stomach often lies high in the left upper abdomen and is steer-horn in shape, whereas in the tall, thin person the greater curvature may extend to the brim of the true pelvis and the stomach is in the shape of the letter J. Such variations in the position of the stomach are of no clinical significance; they do not produce symptoms. The important consideration is not the location but rather the structure and physiologic activity of the stomach.

CONGENITAL ANOMALIES

Congenital absence of the stomach has been reported but, of course, is extremely rare.

Hypertrophic Stenosis of the Pylorus

Obstructive narrowing of the pylorus by hypertrophy of the pyloric muscle is most common in infants 2 or 3 weeks old, although it may be observed at any time between the ages of 10 days and 3 or 4 months. Males are involved more often than females. Occasionally, more than one member of a family is affected. The available data have been interpreted as indicating that the liability to pyloric stenosis is polygenic and modified by sex in such a way that girls require much more genetic liability before they develop the clinical condition. Because of the concentration of autosomal genetic factors in an affected female, her offspring will receive a greater number of these genes than do the offspring of an affected male. The condition generally is attributed to congenital hypertrophy, with or without spasm. The pylorus is represented by an oval mass of muscular tissue approximating 3.0 cm. in length and 1.5 cm. in diameter, with hypertrophy, especially of the circular layer of the muscularis propria, and fibrotic thickening of the submucosa. Microscopically, the muscular layer may be edematous and infiltrated with leukocytes. Symptoms begin usually during the second to fourth weeks after birth and consist of projectile vomiting after a feeding, constipation or obstipation, rapid loss of weight, and undernutrition. Dehydration and alkalosis develop as a consequence of the loss of fluid and electrolytes in the gastric content.

Hypertrophy of the pylorus occurs in adults with and without stenosis, and with and without symptoms. The congenital origin of the hypertrophy is less certain, although some instances may represent persistence of pyloric hypertrophy from infancy into adulthood. The condition may be associated with acquired gastric disease, such as peptic ulcer, and may be the result of work-hypertrophy of the muscle or of chronic inflammation. The chief symptoms are nausea, vomiting, and epigastric discomfort aggravated by the ingestion of food. Pain may or may not be present; if present, it usually is caused by the associated lesion. Hematemesis may occur from an associated hemorrhagic gastritis or mucosal erosions.

Diverticula

Diverticula of the stomach are rare, being seen once in every 2000 roentgen studies of the upper digestive tract. True diverticula contain all the coats of the normal stomach and are either congenital or secondary to pulsion and traction. False diverticula lack the muscular coats and are attributed to weakening of the gastric wall. Any region of the stomach may be involved, but diverticula occur most frequently (75 per cent) near the cardia, close to the esophageal junction on the posterior wall, suggesting a congenital weakness in the muscular wall at this site. Approximately 15 per cent occur in the prepyloric area of the stomach. Duodenal diverticula are much more common. Almost all diverticula of the duodenal bulb are "pseudo-diverticula," produced by the scarring associated with duodenal ulcer. Gastric and duodenal diverticula do not cause distress, except unusually in the presence of inflammation or ulceration, or unless they are huge in size and are so situated as to fill readily with food and gastrointestinal contents but empty poorly, resulting in stagnation associated with bacterial infection and inflammation.

Gastric Torsion and Volvulus

The stomach may rotate about its long axis so that the greater curvature turns upward or at a 90-degree angle to this axis, when the pylorus turns forward to the left and the cardia passes backward. Torsion is present when the degree of rotation is less than 180 degrees and obstruction is not complete. Some degree of rotation of the stomach is a common radiologic finding and probably of little clinical significance. Volvulus is an extension of torsion in which the degree of rotation is more than 180 degrees, so that obstruction occurs at each end of the twisted segment. Volvulus may develop as an exacerbation of torsion; or it may occur in a previously normally situated stomach. Diaphragmatic anomalies, including large paraesophageal hernias, contribute to the development of volvulus. The onset of gastric volvulus is sudden and acutely painful. The exciting cause may be a large meal, a minor injury, or a sudden movement. Pain is severe and continuous and is experienced chiefly in the epigastric and left subcostal regions. It then radiates through to the back or remains retrosternal in site. There may be repeated attempts at vomiting but only with the emission of small amounts of mucoid material. These symptoms are accompanied by the rapid development of severe epigastric distention. Perhaps the most important clinical observation is inability to pass a Levin tube to relieve the gastric distention. The triad of acute distention, futile retching, and inability to pass a tube are pathognomonic of gastric volvulus.

SENSORY DISTURBANCES

Appetite and Hunger

The sensations of appetite and hunger are closely related. Appetite is a pleasant sensation conditioned by previous agreeable experiences with the smell, taste, and appearance of food. Hunger is an unpleasant sensation of abdominal emptiness, epigastric discomfort, or pangs of dull pain, produced by the intermittent contractions of the empty stomach and/or intestine. The distinction between hunger and appetite is not always sharp, and accentuation of the appetite often is interpreted as a part of the total complex of hunger. The following sensory components may be enumerated:

1. Pleasant olfactory and gustatory sensations with their associated pleasant memories of the taste and smell of food are the classic features of appetite.
2. Painful hunger pangs result from contractions of the empty stomach and intestines.
3. An indefinite, unpleasant, generalized, steady and continuous sensation is interpreted as hunger and is vaguely referred to the abdomen.
4. Accessory phenomena such as lassitude, weakness, drowsiness, faintness, irritability, restlessness, and headache may occur concomitantly.

As summarized by Janowitz, "At the physiologic level of regulation of intake, deficits of the body's stores of calorically significant nutrients activate feeding reflexes which are facilitated by areas in the lateral hypothalamus and are inhibited by the ventromedial hypothalamus. These deficits concomitantly give rise to hunger sensations which may be cues for food intake. These hypothalamic centers are sensitive to local temperature changes and appear to be influenced also by the body stores of water. Day-to-day regulation of the amount of food consumed is regulated in part by oropharyngeal receptors; and the size of an individual meal is controlled by gastric and upper intestinal receptors responding to distention, probably mediated by the vagus nerve. The hypothalamic areas also are believed to be influenced by the metabolic consequences of food absorbed and assimilated. The specific dynamic action of food, the utilizable blood glucose, the concentration of other metabolites in the blood, the level of protein in the diet and depot fat, all have been proposed as cues to the central nervous system, but none has been firmly established as governing short- or long-term control."

Excessive appetite and hunger occur in various conditions, as in convalescence from an acute infectious disease, but the mechanism is unexplained. A similar situation obtains in thyrotoxicosis, in which the requirement of food is maintained at a high level because of the excessive metabolism. In diabetes mellitus the glucose in the blood is not available to the tissues; hunger and polyphagia result. Excessive appetite also may be observed in the emotionally disturbed individual. In peptic ulcer the distress may be interpreted as hunger, because the patient fails to differentiate it from a hunger pang or because it occurs when the stomach is thought to be empty and is relieved by eating.

Loss of appetite is a variable but common symptom in many diseases. It is an early and prominent feature of hepatitis and of gastric or pancreatic neoplasm. Loss of appetite often is nervous in origin, a manifestation of an emotional disturbance, usually depression. As such it is the outstanding symptom of *anorexia nervosa*, a psychoneurotic state observed chiefly in adolescent girls, infrequently in males. The age of onset usually is within a year or two of the advent of puberty, but it does occur during the "teens" and occasionally in early adult life. The problem is regarded as a "self-inflicted" starvation disorder, pivoting around the maturational changes of puberty and their psychosocial implications for the patient. The clinical features include cachexia, amenorrhea, constipation, and hypothermia. Laboratory findings include hypoproteinemia and anemia. The mortality rate is considerable, ranging from 5 to 15 per cent. The diagnosis is established principally in terms of differentiation from panhypopituitarism. Death occurs from inanition or suicide, especially when the disorder is of 10 years' duration or longer. According to Bruch, primary anorexia nervosa is characterized by "body-image disturbances of delusional proportions, with a distortion in the accuracy of perception or recognition of bodily states, regression of ego, and a pervading sense of ineffectiveness, conceived as the outcome of a transactional pattern between mother and child which is deficient in confirmation of child-initiated behavior."

Vomiting

Vomiting is defined as the forceful expulsion of gastric and intestinal contents through the mouth. Immediately preceding vomiting are tachypnea, copious salivation, dilatation of the pupils, sweating, pallor, and rapid heartbeat, all signs of general autonomic stimulation. Vomiting begins with deep inspiration. The glottis is closed and the nasopharynx is shut off partly or completely. Inspiration is converted to an expiratory effort, with simultaneous contraction of the abdominal muscles. Because the glottis is closed, the increase in intrathoracic and intra-abdominal pressure is transmitted to the stomach and esophagus. The body of the stomach and the muscle of the esophagus relax. At the same time a strong annular contraction, at approximately the angulus of the stomach, nearly divides the body from the antrum. While the body of the stomach remains flaccid, peristaltic waves sweep aborally over the antrum. The positive intrathoracic and intra-abdominal pressures force expulsion of the gastric contents through the mouth. The esophagus then is emptied partly by the elevated intrathoracic pressure and partly by peristaltic waves stimulated by vomitus in the esophagus and mouth. Finally, the voluntary muscles relax and respiration resumes.

The vomiting center is located in the dorsolateral border of the lateral reticular formation, just ventral to the tractus solitarius and its nucleus, near the sensory nucleus of the vagus. It may be excited directly by mechanical stimuli such as increased intracranial pressure, by chemical stimuli in the form of such drugs as digitalis or emetine, by afferent impulses produced by distention of the stomach and duodenum, or by impulses from any region of the body. Vomiting is associated with such metabolic problems as renal failure, hyperparathyroidism and alkalosis, and clinical situations such as migraine and labyrinthine disorders. Vomiting also may be produced in susceptible persons by impulses from the higher cerebral centers, as when unpleasant subjects are discussed or when offensive odors are encountered. Nervous vomiting is a manifestation of a psychiatric difficulty; the characteristic feature is the continued, effortless vomiting of food, usually immediately after eating, without loss of weight. The symptom presumably reflects physiologically a state of reverse peristalsis in the intestine and in the stomach, initiated by stimuli from the central nervous system. The afferent impulses reach the center along many routes, the chief ones being the vagal and sympathetic nerves from the stomach and other abdominal viscera. The efferent fibers are contained chiefly in the phrenic, vagus, and sympathetic nerves.

Nausea

Nausea denotes an unpleasant sensation, ordinarily referred to the back of the throat, the epigastrium, or both, and often culminating in vomiting. It may be accompanied by vasomotor manifestations or autonomic stimulation, such as salivation, sweating, vertigo, and tachycardia. The clinical significance of nausea is identified with that of vomiting. It may be produced by gastric or pancreatic disease, by pyloric or intestinal obstruction, by reverse peristalsis of functional origin, by various biochemical abnormalities associated with metabolic disorders, or by intense pain from any source.

Belching

Belching is the eructation of swallowed air. Normally a small amount of air is swallowed in the process of eating; larger amounts are swallowed with the rapid eating of food, the chewing of gum, or excessive smoking. Most of the swallowed air does not reach the stomach, but is regurgitated immediately from the lower esophagus as a part of the act of belching. Some of the gas passes into the stomach and accumulates in the gastric air bubble until it is eliminated in a more or less spontaneous belch. The chronic belcher then renews the cycle of swallowing more air, most of which he regurgitates with each belch, but some of which passes into the stomach, until once more a spontaneous belch occurs. In time, the act becomes almost involuntary. Belching is not related specifically to disease of the gallbladder, stomach, or any other organ. It is primarily a functional event, often induced by a sensation of abdominal fullness or discomfort which the patient attempts to relieve by the gastroesophageal expulsion of air.

MOTOR DISTURBANCES

Gastric tone and peristalsis are subject to wide physiologic variations. The factors normally influencing gastric emptying include the pressure gradient between the antrum and duodenum, the opening of the pylorus, the consistency and size of the bolus, the osmolarity and temperature of the chyme, and the pH and volume of the gastric contents. Added bulk in the diet, pleasant sensory stimuli, and emotional reactions such as anxiety, resentment, or hostility increase the motor activity of the stomach, whereas the presence of fat in the food, unpleasant sensory stimuli, fear, and sadness depress it. Tone and peristalsis are not dependent upon secretion; there is, however, some relation between the motor and secretory functions. Vagal stimulation increases and vagal section decreases both. After vagotomy gastric tonus is reduced, the peristaltic waves are shallow, and gastric emptying is delayed. With the passage of time, there is more or less recovery, attributable perhaps to control regained by the intrinsic neurogenic mechanism. Gastric peristalsis may be decreased in patients with diabetes mellitus, resembling the situation after vagotomy. Symptoms may be absent or include gradual loss of weight, vague abdominal discomfort, nausea or vomiting, and unexplained difficulty in controlling the diabetes. According to some observers, gastric motility may be increased in patients with uncomplicated duodenal ulcer and reduced in gastric ulcer. The decreased activity allegedly contributes to stimulation of the antrum and to the increased production of gastrin. Hyperperistalsis and hypertonicity of the stomach, observed in nervous persons, are not the basis for symptoms.

Spasm of the entire stomach or of a portion of the stomach has been described in lesions of the central nervous system, and also in the presence of cholelithiasis or pancreatic disease. The relationship of such spasm to abdominal pain is questionable. Localized muscular spasm occurs not infrequently with gastric lesions, as in hourglass contracture with a benign ulcer, the contracture disappearing when the ulcer heals. Contraction of the stomach along the greater curvature also has been observed in emotionally disturbed patients who ruminate. The incisura-type indentation presumably is spastic in nature but it is not accompanied by pain. Painless spasm of the pylorus, as evidenced by rather persistent closure, occurs with intrapyloric peptic ulcer, with gastric and duodenal lesions adjacent to the pylorus and occasionally with gastric ulcers located proximal to the pylorus, on the lesser curvature.

GASTRIC SECRETION

Physiologic Considerations

The secretion of hydrochloric acid physiologically is a composite of three interrelated phases: neurogenic (vagal), gastric (gastrin), and, to a lesser extent, intestinal. The neurogenic phase is initiated by stimuli such as the sight, smell, or taste of food acting upon receptors in the cerebral cortex and subsequent stimulation of the vagal nucleus. The process presumably is mediated chemically by acetylcholine acting upon the parietal cells, in conjunction with gastrin from the antrum, probably sensitizing the parietal cells to the action of histamine. Similar effects are noted with the chief cells. Stimulation of the vagus nerve elicits a copious secretion of gastric juice, rich in acid and pepsin. Truncal division of the vagi is followed by a pronounced reduction in the volume and acidity of the gastric secretion in patients with duodenal ulcer, but the production of hydrochloric acid is not eliminated completely and is demonstrable with sufficient stimulation of the secretory mechanism. Stimulation of the splanchnic nerves evokes an alkaline secretion, chiefly from the pyloric glands, rich in mucus and poor in peptic activity. Emotional disturbances exert an important influence upon the secretory and motor functions of the stomach. Prolonged anxiety, hostility, and resentment cause engorgement of the gastric mucosa and increased secretion, whereas depression and fear induce pallor of the mucosa and a reduction in acid output; these changes are related to the rate of blood flow through the gastric vasculature.

The gastric phase of secretion is mediated by the hormone gastrin, produced by the antrum in response to distention by food and fluid, by vagal stimulation with release of acetylcholine, and probably by exposure of the mucosa of the antrum to the products of protein digestion. Gastrin has been identified as two nearly identical peptides (gastrins I and II), each much more potent than histamine in stimulating acid secretion when given in low concentrations, but inhibiting acid secretion when administered in high concentrations. The gastrin molecule is composed of 17 linearly arranged L-amino acids (Fig. 25–1). Gastrin II differs from gastrin I in the presence of an esterified SO₃H attached to tyrosine in position 12. Both terminals are blocked, the N-terminal with pyroglutamyl and the C-terminal with an amide. Human gastrin is identical with hog gastrin except that in man leucine is substituted for methionine in the number 5 position. The C-terminal four amino acids of the gastrin molecule (Try-Met-Asp-Phe-NH₂) possess the full physiologic range of actions of the parent molecule. This material, with 4 butyloxycarbonyl-beta-alanine attached to the N-terminus, now is available commercially as the gastrin-like pentapeptide pentagastrin. It is noteworthy that pancreozymin-cholecystokinin, which shares many physiologic actions with gastrin, possesses five terminal amino acids in common with gastrin.

Gastrin exerts a wide spectrum of motor and secretory actions involving multiple target organs. These include strong stimulation of acid gastric secretion (apparently acting directly on the parietal cells), weak to moderate stimulation of gastric pepsin, increased gastric intrinsic factor, stimulation of gastric motility, weak to moderate stimulation of pancreatic secretion (water, bicarbonate) but strong stimulation of pancreatic enzymes, and weak stimulation of biliary flow. Utilizing fluoresceinated antibodies to human gastrin I, gastrin has been localized within mucosal cells of the antrum of man and of the hog. The immunofluorescence is restricted to numerous conspicuous cytoplasmic granules in differentiated interspersed mucosal cells present along the course of pyloric antral glands. The gastrin-producing cell in the antrum has not been identified conclusively, but interest has focused upon the D (delta) cell (the third type of cell in the pancreas, the other cells designated as alpha and beta). The size, shape, distribution, and presence of cytoplasmic granules suggest that the cells are similar to members of the argentaffin or argyrophil classes of cells. Electron microscopy reveals characteristic granules 150 to 250 millimicrons in size, intermediate in electron density between the granules of the alpha and beta cells. Histochemically similar "G" cells also have been noted in the antral pyloric area of the stomach. The staining properties of granules stored in G cells suggest the presence of an acid protein with many side-chain carboxyl groups, in accord with the chemical properties of gastrin. The identity or possible interrelationship of the D and G cells and their role in the production of gastrin remains to be determined. The release of gastrin from the cells may involve emiocytosis, recognized as the releasing mechanism for a variety of hormones from cytoplasmic granules. The mechanism of emiocytosis involves the migration of hormone-containing granules, each encased in a membranous sac, to the surface of the cell. The enclosing sac fuses with the plasma membrane of the cell surface, rupturing with extrusion of the contents of the granule into the intracellular space where it undergoes rapid dissolution, the hormone thereby becoming available for circulation.

Radioimmunoassay techniques indicate normal fasting plasma gastrin levels from 0 to 200 picograms per ml., apparently rising with increasing age. After feeding or gastric alkalinization, the gastrin concentrations increase more than 200 per cent over basal levels. In general, gastrin levels in patients with gastric ulcer and duodenal ulcer apparently do not differ significantly from normal. According to McGuigan, "There is considerable variability among serum gastrin levels in patients with gastric ulcer disease. Some patients with a gastric ulcer have levels which are definitely higher than those with duodenal ulcer and those assigned as controls. It

CAERULEIN

└Glu · Gln · | Asp · Tyr (SO₃H) | · Thr · | Gly · Try · Met · Asp · Phe-NH₂ |

C-TERMINAL OCTAPEPTIDE OF
CHOLECYSTOKININ-PANCREOZYMIN

| Asp · Tyr (SO₃H) | · Met · | Gly · Try · Met · Asp · Phe-NH₂ |

HUMAN GASTRIN II

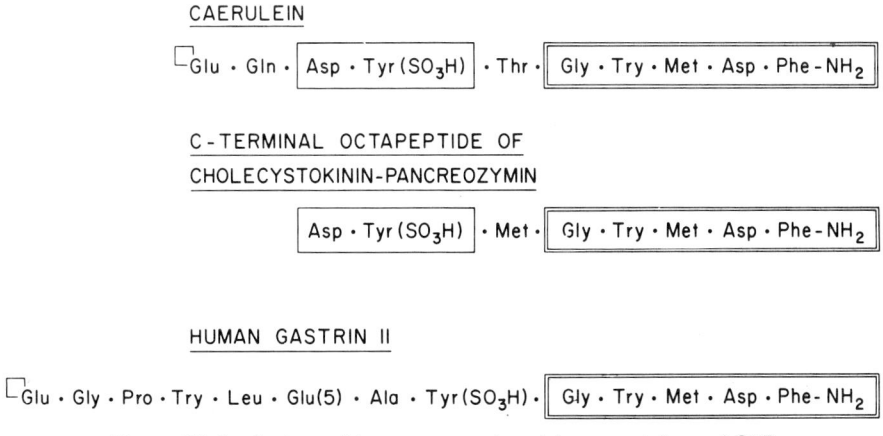

└Glu · Gly · Pro · Try · Leu · Glu(5) · Ala · Tyr(SO₃H) · | Gly · Try · Met · Asp · Phe- NH₂ |

Figure 25–1 Amino acid sequences of gastrin, caerulein, and CKP.

appears that serum gastrin levels in patients with gastric ulcer disease may, when compared with appropriate controls, be higher than those of the controls. The increase in serum gastrin levels among some patients with gastric ulcer disease may reflect decreased rates of acid secretion and thereby decreased inhibition of gastrin release." Gastrin values are greatly increased in patients with the Zollinger-Ellison syndrome, ranging from 700 to 62,000 pg. per ml., and this disorder now is diagnosed regularly by gastrin radioimmunoassay. Elevated gastrin values are noted also in patients with pernicious anemia; the levels average 1079 pg., with a range from 300 to 9000 pg. per ml. These levels overlap with those for the Zollinger-Ellison syndrome but the clinical conditions differ greatly. The gastrin content of the antral mucosa is greatly increased above normal, and the G cells in the antrum are much more numerous in patients with pernicious anemia and elevated serum gastrin levels. The high levels of serum gastrin in patients with the Zollinger-Ellison syndrome reflect the activity not of the antral gastrin cells but of the hyperfunctioning polypeptide-secreting tumor cells. The increased concentrations of gastrin in pernicious anemia have been attributed to the extensive gastric atrophy and to the lack of acid secretion; the levels apparently can be lowered by the administration of hydrochloric acid. Increased serum gastrin levels also are demonstrable in atrophic gastritis associated with antibodies to parietal cells and with adequate absorption of B_{12}, but not in simple atrophic gastritis without parietal cell antibodies. Hypergastrinemia thus may be characteristic only of gastritis associated with autoimmune reactions to gastric antigens and of pernicious anemia. Simple atrophic gastritis appears to be a different disease and the nonelevated serum gastrin levels may reflect involvement of the antral mucosa, whereas in "autoimmune gastritis" the antral mucosa is spared. Elevated serum gastrin levels also have been recorded in patients with pheochromocytoma. The diminished output of acid after atropine results from withdrawal of the acetylcholine potentiation of gastrin. The calcium-induced secretion of gastric acid apparently is caused by calcium-induced hypergastrinemia. Vagal synergism with the increased levels of serum gastrin is required for the stimulation of acid secretion.

The intestinal phase of gastric secretion is initiated by the entrance of partly acidified or neutralized food into the small intestine, initiating a humoral mechanism, with the release of gastrin, a hormone resembling gastrin, or a secretory stimulant produced by the digestion of food. An interesting clinical observation is the gastric hypersecretion observed occasionally after partial resection of the small bowel, especially after removal of the more proximal segments of small intestine.

Histamine elicits from the parietal cells a large amount of hydrochloric acid and relatively small quantities of pepsin and mucus. Histalog, the analogue of histamine (3-beta aminoethyl pyrazole), stimulates gastric secretion similarly, but with fewer side-effects; it also is effective when administered orally. The gastric hypersecretion after portacaval anastomosis involves the effect of a secretory stimulant, possibly histamine, produced in the alimentary canal and not inactivated within the liver, as a consequence of the shunt. The physiologic activity of the gastric chief and parietal cells appears to depend also upon adequate circulating quantities of pituitary, adrenal, thyroid, and parathyroid hormones. In their insufficiency or absence, gastric secretory activity is greatly diminished. The growth of the gastric mucosa probably depends upon growth hormone from the pituitary gland and a normal pituitary gland is essential to the structural integrity of the gastric mucosa and to the normal secretory function. The adrenal glucocorticoids are the only steroids capable of influencing gastric acid and peptic activity, and adrenal corticotropic hormone is the only one capable of stimulating gastric secretion. This effect is not observed with deoxycorticosterone acetate, testicular and adrenal androgens, progesterone, and potent estrogenic preparations.

The target of the various secretory stimuli is the parietal cell, with varying numbers of cells responding at a given time, depending upon the physiologic state of the stomach and upon the strength of the stimuli, principally nervous (vagal) and chemical (gastrin). The absolute number of acid-secreting parietal cells estimated from measurements of the maximum acid output approximates 2.2×10^9 parietal cells in a thin man. The number appears to be less in some population groups (e.g., India). In health, the maximal acid output can be related to the lean body mass or, more conveniently, to the total body mass.

Gastric secretion may be inhibited under various circumstances, such as emotional disturbances, presumably via inhibitory fibers in the vagus and splanchnic nerves. Gastric secretion also is influenced by at least two autoregulatory mechanisms: local inhibition of gastrin release by exposure of the antral mucosa to a pH of 1.5 or lower; and release of an inhibitory hormone, possibly enterogastrone, produced in the upper small intestine in the presence of bile salts and pancreatic lipase, or very possibly the release of pancreatic secretin, produced by the action of acid content in the upper small intestine. The inhibition of gastric acid caused by fat in contact with the duodenum and upper small intestine appears to be equally effective against both endogenous and exogenous gastrin; suggesting that the humoral agent released by fat acts predominantly or solely by inactivating circulating gastrin rather than by preventing the release of gastrin. Other postulated gastric secretory inhibiting mechanisms include an inhibitory substance from the pancreas, and an intraduodenal "brake." A depressant of gastric secretion, gastrone, has been identified in human gastric juice, mostly in anacid gastric specimens. Its physiologic significance and possible relationship to other inhibitory materials are not yet known. Various drugs and biological substances are known to depress gastric secretion, including central nervous system depressants (chlorpromazine), inhibitors of histidine decarboxylase, estrogens and prostaglandins, and long-chain, oxygenated, unsaturated fatty acids.

The principal components of gastric secretion are hydrochloric acid; various mucosubstances (acid aminopolysaccharides, fucomucins, sialomucins); proteolytic enzymes including at least three pepsins; rennin, cathepsins, gastric intrinsic factor, water-soluble blood group substances and other biologically active materials, nonproteolytic enzymes; gastric intrinsic factor; the anions—chloride, phosphate, and sulfate; and the cations—sodium, potassium, calcium, and magnesium. The alkaline component of gastric secretion is a mixture of various constituents, including mucus from the surface mucous cells, cytoplasm of desquamated cells, and a transudate of interstitial fluid. Pepsinogen is secreted by the chief cells and is converted to pepsin in the gastric lumen. Thus far, seven human pepsinogen fractions have been identified, five of which are group I pepsinogens and two of which are group II pepsinogens. The relative proportions of the different pepsinogens in human gastric mucosa and of the pepsins in human gastric juice apparently vary from person to person. Vagally mediated influences are the major stimuli to the sustained secretion of pepsin. The output of pepsin also may be increased by gastrin and by large quantities of histamine. A very small proportion of pepsinogen is secreted into the plasma and thence into the urine; and its measurement has been utilized in an attempt to indirectly assess the level of gastric secretion. The protein content of gastric juice originates in several sources: (a) the protein moiety of mucoproteins; (b) cell desquamation; (c) enzymes; (d) exudates from inflamed and ulcerated areas; and (e) the secretion and/or transudation of protein. Electrophoretic studies of the gastric mucous substances, as well as of other high molecular components of gastric content, provide additional quantitative parameters of gastric secretion. The known sources of the various gastric secretory products are listed in Figure 25-2.

The volume of gastric juice secreted daily under fasting conditions in the average normal adult ranges from 1000 to 1500 ml., with an acid concentration of approximately 40 mEq. per L. Although the normal stomach may secrete gastric juice as acidic as that in peptic ulcer, significant quantitative differences are observed. In duodenal ulcer, the 24-hour volume often exceeds 2000 ml., with an average acid concentration of approximately 100 mEq. per L.; the output of hydrochloric acid may exceed normal by 3 to 20 times. The volume of secretion in patients with gastric ulcer usually is normal but the concentration of acid is lower. The output of acid is smallest in patients with gastric carcinoma, the decreased

CELLS	PRODUCTS
Fundic Glands	
Parietal cells	HCl
	Water
	Blood group substances, (alcohol-soluble)
	Intrinsic factor
Chief (peptic cells)	Pepsinogen and other proteolytic proenzymes
	Electrolytes (chlorides, bicarbonates, phosphates)
Mucous neck cells	Mucosubstances
Surface epithelium and crypts	Mucosubstances
	Blood group substances (water-soluble)
	Electrolytes (chlorides, bicarbonates, phosphates)
	Gastrone (?)

Figure 25-2 Sources of gastric secretory products. (After McGuigan, 1970.)

secretory activity often preceding the development of cancer.

Under theoretically optimal conditions, hydrochloric acid is secreted by the parietal cells as a relatively pure solution, with an initial acid concentration of 160 to 170 mEq. per L, a pH of slightly less than 1.0, and isosmotic or slightly hyperosmotic in relation to the blood. The factors affecting the concentration of hydrochloric acid include (a) the rate of parietal cell secretion; (b) the rate of nonparietal buffering and diluting secretion; (c) the amount of buffering, neutralizing, and diluting secretion; (d) extragastric secretion (saliva, bile, duodenal content, pancreatic secretion); and (e) the buffering and diluting effect of food. The lower acid values observed clinically are the result of (1) neutralization by buffer substances such as protein, phosphate, and bicarbonate present in food, saliva, gastric and regurgitated intestinal secretion; (2) dilution by these fluids; and (3) rediffusion of hydrogen ions into the blood or tissues.

Hollander postulated that hydrochloric acid is formed by the hydrolysis of the neutral chlorides (chiefly sodium chloride) of the cytoplasm, the residual alkali being neutralized immediately by intracellular buffers. The wall of the intracellular canaliculus presumably functions as a membrane permeable to water and to hydrogen and chloride ions. The application of any secretory stimulus to the parietal cell initiates a process, driving water from the cell in two directions. The fluid passing forward into the intracellular canaliculus carries hydrogen and chloride ions with it, thus effecting a membrane hydrolysis of the neutral chloride, with simultaneous separation of the hydrochloric acid so formed. At the same time, the "alkalinized" buffers of the cytoplasm are transported across the cell wall proper back into the tissue fluids and into the general circulation, obviating pronounced or prolonged elevation of the intracellular pH. Davies regards the fundamental reaction as that expressed in the formula $H_2O \to H + OH^-$. The hydrogen ions are thought to be elaborated by means of energy available from the metabolism of glucose. The hydrogen ions are secreted, and the OH^- ions are finally neutralized by the carbon dioxide and passed into the blood. This process is regarded as comparable with the theory of membrane hydrolysis. The chemical sequence may be as follows:

$$NaCl + H_2O \to NaOH + HCl$$
$$NaOH + H_2CO_3 \to NaHCO_3 + H_2O$$
$$H_2O + CO_2 \to H_2CO_3$$
$$NaCl + CO_2 + H_2O \to NaHCO_3 + HCl$$

The secretion of hydrochloric acid requires large amounts of energy, derived presumably via ATP During active secretion, blood flow through the stomach is greatly increased.

Disturbances in Gastric Secretion

Pathologic alterations in gastric secretion occur more often in the direction of diminution in total volume, acid concentration, or both. These variations do not correspond exactly with anatomic changes in the mucosa, although true anacidity occurs most frequently in association with atrophy of the stomach. Normal persons with apparently normal mucosae exhibit a wide variety of secretory responses, ranging from achlorhydria, with a pH value of approximately 8.0, to a highly acid juice, with a pH of 1.0. These differing secretory rates are not correlated with specific symptoms or disease, except that chronic peptic ulcer does not occur in the continued absence of acid gastric juice. The complete absence of all gastric juice (achylia gastrica) is rare, for some secretion containing enzymes in small amounts is almost always present. The term "achlorhydria" or "anacidity," therefore, may be preferable. Anacidity may be defined as a decrease in the pH of the gastric content less than one unit or a pH above 6.0 following maximal stimulation of the gastric secretory mechanism with histamine, histalog, or pentagastrin. The hydrogen ion concentration of anacid specimens obtained after histamine stimulation varies in different diseases, although not consistently. The pH of the gastric secretion in pernicious anemia ranges usually between 7.0 and 8.0; the pH in atrophy of the gastric mucosa unaccompanied by other disease is similar, although more variable; values between 3.5 and 7.0 may be observed in gastric carcinoma. Anacidity is not a normal variant, since it is associated with an almost total loss of functioning parietal cells, as in severe gastric atrophy. The gastric content in "true" gastric atrophy is characterized by progressive secretory failure involving initially hydrochloric acid, then pepsin, and, finally, intrinsic factor. Maximal histamine tests indicate that anacidity is rare in patients with gastric carcinoma and with gastric polyps. Patients with true anacidity who do not have pernicious anemia require careful observation for the later development of pernicious anemia or gastric carcinoma. In gastric carcinoma, the stomach content is characterized by reduced acid secretion and by elevation of certain enzyme constituents, including beta glucuronidase, lactic dehydrogenase, glutamic oxaloacetic transaminase and phosphohexose isomerase. Whether or not these alterations precede as a reflection of a vulnerable mucosa or accompany the neoplasm remains unclear. Histologic studies indicate that the number of parietal cells in the fundus of the stomach is relatively high in patients with duodenal ulcer and decreases progressively in benign gastric ulcer and in gastric cancer, especially in patients without acid; parietal cells are virtually absent in pernicious anemia. Human gastric content also contains a secretory inhibiting substance, present in larger amounts in patients with pernicious anemia and extensive gastric atrophy.

Hypersecretion of hydrochloric acid refers to an excessive quantity of acid rather than to an increased concentration. The clinical conditions associated with gastric hypersecretion are duodenal ulcer, stomal ulceration, the Zollinger-Ellison syndrome, and retained, excluded antrum after gastric surgery. An excessive output of hydrochloric acid is observed in approximately 50 per cent of patients with duodenal ulcer. The hypersecretion is demonstrable continuously, between meals, during the night, and after the ulcer has healed. The Zollinger-Ellison syndrome is characterized by extremely high basal outputs of hydrochloric acid, usually with less than a 50 per cent rise following stimulation with maximal doses of histamine, Histalog, or pentagastrin.

The cause of the gastric hypersecretion in duodenal ulcer is not established completely. Anatomically, it is correlated with an increased number of parietal cells, possibly a genetically determined trait or perhaps the result of chronic stimulation by neurogenic and humoral influences. The total number of parietal cells has been estimated as 0.65 billion for gastric ulcer, 0.82 billion for the average normal stomach, and 1.72 billion for duodenal ulcer. Physiologically, the continuous hypersecretion of gastric juice in duodenal ulcer is chiefly of neurogenic origin and decreases significantly after vagotomy. Other mechanisms contributing to the acid hypersecretion of duodenal ulcer include excessive humoral stimulation (gastrin) and, possibly, impairment in the homeostatic mechanisms regulating gastric secretion.

MECHANISM OF PAIN

The normal gastric mucosa is insensitive to touch, cutting, pinching, tearing, and exposure to solutions of varying hydrogen ion concentration. Heat and cold are experienced as such. Vigorous pressure on the gastric wall elicits a steady, dull, gnawing pain, experienced approximately in the region of the stimulus. This pain, like that produced by distention or by powerful contractions, arises from stretching of the muscular and peritoneal layers of the stomach. Its mechanism involves a local rise in smooth muscle tension produced by spasm, obstruction, or rapid distention, and subsequent contraction or stretching of the nerve terminals lying between the circular muscle fibers. The intensity of the distress is proportional to the state of contraction of the stomach at the time and to the rapidity of the stimulus. The entire reflex involved in the transmission of such impulses may be via the afferent visceral fibers accompanying the sympathetic pathways; the cerebrospinal nerves need not participate. The threshold for pain in the stomach and, therefore, for the development of symptoms is influenced by the condition of the gastric mucosa. Vascular engorgement and acute inflammation diminish the threshold for pain, and in their presence stimuli such as hydrochloric acid or gastric contractions not causing discomfort when the mucosa is normal elicit painful sensations. Vascular ischemia causes pain presumably by altering the motor activity of the stomach. By virtue of its location, the stomach is in proximity to numerous other organs with differing nerve supplies; their involvement contributes additional components to the symptomatology of gastric disease.

The pain of peptic ulcer is caused primarily by the hydrochloric acid in the gastric content. The acid evokes a chemical inflammation and thereby lowers the pain threshold of the nerve endings present in large numbers in the base and in the margins of the ulcer. The pain is a true visceral sensation, arising directly at the site of the lesion. It is not dependent upon hyperperistalsis, gross spasm of the musculature, pylorospasm, or distention of the antrum. However, the acid may activate not only the pain mechanism but also motor activity; under these circumstances, ulcer pain originating in a sensitive ulcer may be increased by motility or muscle spasm. The importance of acid in the development of ulcer pain is further indicated by the occurrence of the distress only when the gastric content is acid. The concentration of hydrochloric acid at the time of distress is not necessarily excessive, nor does it exceed that present in the same stomach without pain when the ulcer is healed or in the healing phase. The threshold of acidity necessary to evoke pain varies from one patient to another and in the same patient from time to time. The presence of pain is dependent, therefore, upon the presence of both an inflamed lesion lowering the pain threshold and an adequate stimulus, acid gastric juice. The pain is relieved by emesis or aspiration of the stomach, which removes the acid, or by the ingestion of food or alkali, which neutralizes hydrochloric acid. When the pain mechanism is sensitive, pain may be induced by the introduction of hydrochloric acid in physiologic concentrations (0.1 N) or by acid gastric juice; it is alleviated by withdrawal or neutralization of the acid. The pain induced by the hydrochloric acid is not prevented by prior parenteral or oral administration of anticholinergic compounds. Pain sensitivity disappears quickly, presumably as the acute inflammatory process in the ulcer subsides. The absence of pain in some instances and the occurrence of hemorrhage or perforation without antecedent pain are difficult to explain, except on the vague basis of an individually high pain threshold, protection of the ulcer crater from the hydrochloric acid by blood during the course of hemorrhage, and the very rapid formation of an acute perforating ulcer, encompassing development and penetration into a blood vessel within hours.

Location of Pain

Ulcer pain is located almost always in the epigastrium and usually is limited to an area several centimeters in diameter. The pain of gastric ulcer is likely to be experienced in the left epigastrium or just below the xiphoid process and, with ulcers in the upper portion of the stomach, occasionally in the anterior or left lateral portion of the chest. Such shifts of pain occur usually with progressive deepening of the ulcer. So long as gastric ulcers remain shallow and do not actively penetrate or perforate, the distress usually is indistinguishable from that of duodenal ulcer. In duodenal ulcer, the pain is located in the right epigastrium and slightly above the umbilicus. In jejunal ulcer, it is located usually in the left midabdomen and also in the left lower abdominal quadrant. The pain may be referred laterally to the left chest in the area supplied by the sixth and seventh thoracic nerves or may extend through to the back at the level of the eighth to tenth dorsal vertebrae. This latter radiation is more common in duodenal ulcer located on the posterior wall.

Sudden, severe abdominal pain frequently indicates an acute perforation. Perforation of an ulcer on the posterior wall of the duodenum causes pain in the location characteristic of pancreatic pain, i.e., in the region between the twelfth thoracic and second lumbar vertebrae. The pain is characteristic in its occurrence at night, aggravation by the supine position, partial relief by sitting or by lying with the trunk flexed, or by pressure over the midabdomen while the patient leans forward over folded arms or a pillow. Perforation of an ulcer on the anterior wall of the duodenum may cause pain in the right lower abdominal quadrant, where the lesion may be confused with acute appendicitis, or it may produce pain in the right groin or testis, simulating right ureteral pain. Its distribution also depends partly on the course taken by the escaping gastric contents. Gravitation of the contents to the right paracolic gutter produces pain in the right lower abdominal quadrant. Pain in front, behind, or on top of the shoulder and at the base of the neck denotes involvement of the diaphragm and the phrenic innervation. When an ulcer on the lesser curvature of the stomach perforates into the lesser omental tissues, undersurface of the liver, anterior aspect of the pancreas, or the diaphragmatic crura, there may be an upward and left shift of pain into the anterior part of the thorax and left hypochondrium, and a referred or somatic pain often is present in the interscapular region usually at the level of the sixth thoracic vertebra. If pain is transmitted to the left shoulder cap, the lesion usually is located high in the stomach.

Pain in Gastric Carcinoma

The pain originating in gastric carcinoma may be of several types. In the presence of hydrochloric acid, the pain often is indistinguishable from that produced by benign peptic ulcer, because the mechanism is the same: acid irritation. An ulcerating carcinoma perforating the greater curvature may simulate a benign ulcer and also may cause pain in the left shoulder cap, pancreatic pain, and pain in the left lower abdominal quadrant, secondary to involvement of the left transverse mesocolon, perisplenitis, and parietal involvement of peritoneum in the eleventh or twelfth thoracic segment. In the absence of acid and peptic activity, gastric cancer is painless until the tumor progresses beyond the confines of the stomach and involves somatic tissue. The pain then becomes constant, is unrelated to the nature of the gastric content, and is relieved only by opiates. This pain is attributable to malignant infiltration of both the somatic and splanchnic nerves. Benign gastric tumors, e.g., polyps, leiomyomas, do not produce pain unless they obstruct the pylorus or the cardioesophageal orifice.

Transmission of Pain

At least three distinct mechanisms may be involved in pain originating within the abdomen: true visceral pain, with impulses transmitted over afferent visceral fibers accompanying the sympathetic trunks; referred pain, with impulses carried over both afferent visceral and cerebrospinal nerve fibers; and the peritoneocutaneous reflex of Morley, with impulses transmitted only via cerebrospinal nerves. True visceral pain alone may be present, or all three mechanisms may participate, as in the perforation of peptic ulcer with peritonitis.

Pain impulses arising in the stomach and duodenum are conducted along sensory fibers in the splanchnic branches of the sympathetic nerves. The splanchnic nerves enter first the celiac ganglion, travel via the greater splanchnic nerves to the spinal cord, probably to the corresponding posterior roots of the eighth through thirteenth thoracic spinal nerves, and thence to the higher centers by way of the spinal thalamic tract. The parasympathetic supply of the stomach and duodenum arises in the dorsal vagal nucleus in the floor of the fourth ventricle, and the afferent fibers end in the same nucleus, which is a mixture of visceral efferent and afferent cells. The fibers are conveyed to and from the abdomen through the vagus nerves, esophageal plexus, and vagal trunks. The reproduction of ulcer pain after complete section of the vagi, by introducing hydrochloric acid into the stomach of a patient with a sensitive ulcer, demonstrates that pain impulses travel via the splanchnics. The skin area to which visceral pain is referred is determined by the segment of the spinal cord receiving the visceral afferent (sympathetic) fibers. Ulcer distress arising from lesions not penetrating to the serosa has a cutaneous reference, indicating that visceral nerves are capable of mediating pain referred to somatic segments.

CHRONIC NONSPECIFIC GASTRITIS

Gastric mucosa is normal histologically when the parietal and chief cells of the gastric glands display a regular arrangement and normal nuclei; there are no abnormalities in the surface epithelium or in the foveolae; the glands are normal in outline and are disposed regularly throughout the mucosal surface; the lamina propria is complete at both its surface and deep layers, with capillaries, collagenous fibers, and cellular elements; the lumina of the foveolae are empty; and the muscularis mucosae forms a lamina at the bottom of the glands, with fibers extending all along the lamina propria. An absolutely normal mucosa is found only during infancy or the first decade of life. Subsequently there is a progressive interstitial infiltration with lymphocytes, plasma cells, and eosinophils and metaplasia of the glandular epithelium in virtually every adult stomach. Such changes, although not normal and probably reflecting local inflammatory and possibly immunologic influences, are not accompanied by clinical symptoms or identifiable clinical consequences and hence are regarded as within the range of "normal." When these changes are accompanied by hemorrhages in the superficial layers of the mucosa, erosion of the papillae, and cellular infiltration of the submucosa, muscularis, and serosa, the diagnosis of gastritis may be regarded as established.

Clinically, chronic gastritis is classified on the basis of gastroscopic observation into three types. (1) In *superficial gastritis* the mucosa is reddened, edematous, and covered with adherent mucus; mucosal hemorrhages and small erosions are frequent. The histologic findings include flattening and irregularity of the epithelium, distortion and dilatation of the glands, penetration of the glandular epithelium by polymorphonuclear cells, and lymphocytic infiltration of the deep layers of the lamina propria. (2) *Atrophic gastritis* is characterized by a thinned, gray or greenish-gray hemorrhagic mucosa; the folds are diminished in number and size, so that the mucosa presents an unusually smooth surface. The histologic features are thinning of the gastric wall, distortion and disappearance of the glandular structure, inflammatory cells, decreased numbers of parietal and chief cells, so-called intestinal metaplasia of the glandular epithelium, the presence of Paneth cells and Russell bodies, and proliferation of fibrous tissue. In early chronic atrophic gastritis, patches of altered surface epithelium present morphologic and histochemical features of a regenerating mucosa, suggesting prior injury to the neck and crypt areas of the normal gastric surface epithelium. Gastric atrophy is characterized by the almost complete disappearance of the gastric glands. Parietal cells and chief cells are scarce. Inflammatory infiltration is minimal. Intestinal metaplasia is pronounced. The normal cells of the gastric epithelium are replaced by cells identical with those of the normal small intestine. The surface epithelium of the normal stomach is columnar, but in intestinal metaplasia it has a prominent brush border and may contain goblet cells and Paneth cells. Histochemically, this mucosa is identical to that of the small intestine and functionally it acquires the absorptive capacity of the small intestine. (3) In *hypertrophic gastritis* the mucosa is dull, spongy, or nodular in appearance; the rugae are irregular, thickened, or nodular; hemorrhages and superficial erosions are frequent. This category is reserved for the unequivocal evidence of enlarged, inflamed gastric rugae. The mucosa is thickened, measuring 2 to 7 mm. or more in width, in contrast to the normal width of 0.7 mm. The rugae may be so nodular and fixed as to resemble the convolutions of the brain. The glands are increased, and parietal and chief cells are greatly multiplied in number. Inflammatory changes may be present, together with cysts and small collections of lymphocytes. The mucosal changes associated with the Zollinger-Ellison syndrome are identical to those of hypertrophic glandular gastritis.

Giant hypertrophy of the mucosal folds of the gastric mucosa (Menetrier's disease) is a disorder of unknown etiology, characterized by conspicuous increases in the height and thickness of the gastric folds, especially along the greater curvature of the stomach. The hypertrophy is limited to the mucosa; the submucosa and the muscle layers of the stomach remaining normal. The disorder is restricted to the body and fundus of the stomach and usually stops abruptly at the margin of the antrum. Microscopically, there is striking hyperplasia of the gastric glands of varying size and shape, the crypts are tortuous and cystic, and, in sections, their profile resembles a corkscrew cut sagittally. The gastric glands may retain the normal chief and parietal cells, or there may be metaplasia, replacing the normal cells with cuboidal or flattened epithelium interspersed with mucin-secreting goblet cells. Often the gastric glands are increased in length and in many areas penetrate the muscularis mucosae. The portion of the gland below the muscularis mucosae retains its continuity with the dilated portion above. Considerable inflammation may be present in the lamina propria. The gastric mucosa is abnormally permeable, and the pronounced exudation of serum proteins into the gastric content and their subsequent digestion may lead to hypoproteinemia. The clinical manifestations in addition to the edema associated with the protein loss include vague, nonspecific gastrointestinal complaints. Gastric bleeding may be the sole manifestation. While gastric secretion may be normal, low, or even increased, most patients have achlorhydria either as a result of the gastritis, the inflammatory cells blocking the gastric glands, or as a consequence of later replacement of acid-secreting cells by an atrophic mucosa.

The etiology and pathogenesis of chronic gastritis are not known. Dietary indiscretions, alcohol, tobacco, coffee, infections, and nutritional deficiencies have been implicated, but the evidence is inconclusive. The process may develop as a consequence of long-continued "irritation" from almost any source, ranging from foods, alkaline reflux, drugs, or as the outcome of genetic and immunologic mechanisms. The stomach is subjected constantly to a variety of influences, physiologic, psychogenic, physical, chemical, and bacterial, the individual significance of which is difficult to evaluate. All types of chronic gastritis are observed in association with peptic ulcer, but atrophy is more frequent in gastric than in duodenal ulcer, whereas a hyperplastic mucosa is more common in duodenal ulcer than in gastric ulcer. Atrophy of the gastric mucosa is invariably present in pernicious anemia and gastric polyposis and not infrequently in patients with sprue, pellagra, and iron-deficiency anemia. The condition is characterized by progressive failure of gastric secretory function involving initially hydrochloric acid, then pepsin, and finally intrinsic factor. Although atrophy may be observed in young people, it is more common in the older age groups. In one study, chronic atrophic gastritis was associated with blue eyes, low social class, heavy cigarette smoking, heavy consumption of alcohol, drinking hot tea, and possibly aspirin-taking. An isolated granulomatous gastritis also has been observed, distinct from regional enteritis or sarcoidosis. The condition often presents clinically as pyloric obstruction with radiologic features of antral narrowing, simulating neoplasm.

A possible immune mechanism in the development of gastric atrophy has been suggested on the basis of interesting observations in patients with pernicious anemia: resemblance of the gastric mucosal lesion in pernicious anemia to that of the thyroid in autoimmune thyroiditis; the frequent clinical interrelations of pernicious anemia with autoimmune disease of the thyroid (thyroiditis, myxedema, Hashimoto's disease); the high incidence of circulating thyroid antibodies in patients with pernicious anemia and, conversely, the high incidence of gastric antibodies in serum from patients with these thyroid diseases; the familial tendencies in both disorders; the frequent presence of circulating antibodies reacting specifically with parietal cell cytoplasmic antigen and/or gastric intrinsic factor in patients with pernicious anemia; and the presence of the same parietal cell antibody in serum from patients with atrophic gastritis without pernicious anemia, presumably candidates for the later development of pernicious anemia. Treatment with corticosteroids may permit regeneration of gastric mucosal glands with recovery of acid and intrinsic factor secretion and normal absorption of vitamin B_{12}. Those who respond tend to have the highest titers of circulating parietal cell antibodies. There is no correlation in this regard with the presence of antibodies to intrinsic factor. Patients with extensive intestinal metaplasia of the gastric mucosa are least likely to benefit from steroid therapy.

Parietal cell antibodies are circulating antibodies of the IgG variety with an affinity for the cytoplasm of parietal cells. They are demonstrable in 80 to 90 per cent of patients with pernicious anemia and in 60 per cent of patients with other forms of gastritis without hematologic abnormality. Parietal cell antibodies also are more common in older patients. However, their presence is not necessarily correlated with the severity of the gastritis. Parietal cell antibodies are absent in patients with extensive or severe gastritis associated with partial gastric resection, gastric carcinoma, or iron deficiency. The presence of parietal cell antibodies suggests that such patients have a genetically determined ability to form antibodies, but there is no evidence in such patients that the gastritis is the result of these antibodies or that the antibodies predispose to the severity and the chronicity of the gastritis. Antibody-containing mononuclear inflammatory cells in the gastric mucosa of patients with pernicious anemia have been shown to contain antibodies to parietal cells and antibodies of the blocking type to intrinsic factor. Parietal cell antibodies are found commonly in patients with impaired absorption of vitamin B_{12}. Interestingly, gastric antibodies are not found in patients with postgastrectomy gastritis. The concentration of immunoglobulins, especially IgA, is increased in conjunction with the increased number of immunoglobulin-producing plasma cells.

Intrinsic factor antibodies are more complex. They are found in only about 50 to 60 per cent of patients with pernicious anemia (see p. 557). Antibodies to intrinsic factor almost never are detected in patients with chronic gastritis alone. In some patients with pernicious anemia, intrinsic factor antibodies are found only in the gastric content or the intestinal secretion. Such antibodies interfere with the absorption of vitamin B_{12} by preventing its complexing with IF ("blocking antibody") or with the B_{12}-IF complex to prevent absorption ("precipitating antibody").

Antibodies to intrinsic factor are associated almost invariably with poor absorption on vitamin B_{12}. Evidence of a pernicious anemia-like disorder was found in 4 of 10 patients with clinically significant primary immunoglobulin deficiency. Histologic evidence of atrophic gastritis was found in 4. In a fifth patient secretion of gastric acid and intrinsic factor was greatly reduced. Additional findings were absence of plasma cells in gastric mucosal infiltrates and absence of demonstrable circulating parietal cell, intrinsic factor, or thyroid antibodies. These observations suggest that detectable specific serum antibodies are not essential for the development of atrophic gastritis.

The consequences of chronic nonspecific gastritis are not known. Minor surface alterations, such as erosions, hemorrhages, and hyperemia, usually heal completely. Severe and complete atrophy of the stomach generally tends to continue unchanged. In elderly patients, especially among women, minimal deficiency of vitamin B_{12} may develop; but it does not progress to pernicious anemia. The associated clinical manifestations include weakness, loss of memory, mental depression, paresthesias, and abdominal discomfort with flatulence, which respond to treatment with B_{12}. Deficiencies of iron and other vitamins also may be associated with atrophy of the gastric mucosa.

The evaluation of symptoms in patients with chronic gastritis often is difficult. Experimentally, acute inflammation and sustained hyperemia of the gastric mucosa lower the threshold for pain. Chronic inflammation, therefore, may be expected a priori to facilitate the occurrence of gastric symptoms. Clinically, however, chronic gastritis is noted gastroscopically in the absence of abdominal distress. In patients with chronic gastritis, the symptoms are varied and vague; their incidence, type, or severity cannot be correlated with the character and degree of the gastritis. The most frequent complaints enumerated by patients found to have gastritis are loss of appetite, fullness, belching, vague epigastric pain, nausea, and vomiting. These also are the symptoms of functional gastrointestinal distress. On the other hand, erosive and ulcerative gastritis may cause symptoms identical with those of peptic ulcer.

Acute erosive gastritis is a transient inflammation involving the mucosa of the stomach, characterized by small round or linear submucosal hemorrhages and shallow erosions, usually 2 to 3 mm. in diameter, involving only part of the glandular layer and never extending to the muscularis mucosae. The inflammation may involve all or part of the gastric mucosa or remain limited to the surfaces of gastric rugae. The development of erosions has been ascribed to necrosis of the neck cells. In general, cell degeneration begins with vacuolization of the cytoplasm, swelling of the mitochondria and enlargement of the tubules of the endoplasmic reticulum. The lamina propria is infiltrated to a variable degree with polymorphonuclear leukocytes, lymphocytes, and occasional eosinophils. Another concept emphasizes capillary and venous congestion as the characteristic lesion of acute gastritis, with localized areas of mucosal hemorrhage confined to the lamina propria. Further development of this process leads to degeneration and desquamation of epithelial cells as a consequence of anoxia. The hemorrhagic lesion often involves the entire thickness of the lamina propria, stopping abruptly at the muscularis mucosae. More advanced lesions occasionally may include necrosis of portions of the muscularis mucosae and hemorrhage into the submucosa. A "typical" fully developed lesion often includes a defined area of hemorrhagic infarction, characterized by linear zones of necrosis extending from the muscularis mucosae to the mucosal surface. Occasionally, thrombi are present in small capillaries adjacent to the zones of hemorrhagic infarction.

Acute hemorrhagic and erosive gastritis is one of the more common (25 per cent) and important causes of severe hemorrhage from the upper gastrointestinal tract. The inciting causes are multiple, including "stress" associated with serious illness, burns, head injury, other trauma, infections, surgical operations, psychogenic disorders, and other circumstances associated with poor vascular perfusion through the stomach via submucosal arteriovenous shunting, increasing the susceptibility of the mucosa to injury, the excessive intake of alcohol, and the ingestion of various medications, among which aspirin represents a prototype. The mechanism of the gastric mucosal injury has been clarified initially by Davenport, who describes the gastric mucosal barrier as a lipid and protein layer permeable to fat-soluble compounds but not to water-soluble materials. A potentially destructive drug must penetrate the surface mucosa before damage occurs. Aspirin apparently is harmless when it is merely in contact with the mucosa but it becomes toxic when it penetrates the mucosa. The physicochemical constants determine the difference. At pH 2, aspirin is more than 95 per cent in the unionized fat-soluble form so that it can diffuse readily across the mucosa. In this circumstance, the aspirin breaks the tight junctions between cells, enhancing the back-diffusion of hydrogen ions. However, at pH 7, it is completely ionized and water-soluble and therefore poorly suited for absorption by the stomach. When aspirin is given in the presence of hydrochloric acid, it causes bleeding and the chemical reflections of gastric irritation—pronounced losses of Na, K, and H ions and chloride into the gastric content. When aspirin is given in a neutral solution, there are no damaging effects.

Gastric mucosal permeability to the back-diffusion of hydrogen ions is increased also by alcohol, fatty acids, bile salts, and other lipid-soluble substances. In addition to salicylates, the potentially injurious drugs include steroids, indomethacin, reserpine, insulin, tolbutamide, antibiotics, anticoagulants, digitalis preparations, nitrofurazone, xanthine derivatives, potassium chloride, and thiazides. According to Silen, increased mucosal permeability may be a critical factor in the pathogenesis of gastritis, stress ulcerations, and gastric ulcer.

According to Davenport, H^+ diffuses slowly through the normal mucosal barrier and rapidly through the broken barrier. H^+ releases histamine within the mucosa, and histamine stimulates H^+ secretion. Histamine also dilates mucosal capillaries and increases their permeability. These effects on capillaries, facilitated by the decreased colloid osmotic pressure difference across the capillary wall, cause filtration of plasma into interstitial spaces, producing edema and increased interstitial pressure. Interstitial fluid containing electrolytes, proteins, and glucose is filtered across the mucosa and, as modified by the filtration process, it enters the gastric lumen. H^+ also breaks some mucosal capillaries, and this effect is intensified when mucosal capillary hydrostatic pressure is induced by concurrent cholinergic stimulation. H^+ stimulates intramucosal plexuses, and gastric motility is enhanced through a cholinergic reflex. The action of H^+ on intramucosal plexuses also may contribute to stimulation of acid secretion. A contributory factor may involve concomitant injury to mast cells by the back-diffusion of hydrogen ions, causing the rapid release of other vasoactive amines, including, in addition to histamine, serotonin, 5-hydroxytryptamine, heparin, kinins, and other products of cellular injury. Experimental studies indicate that the injurious effect of aspirin on the gastric mucosa is mediated also by lowering the protective mucous barrier. Mucin secretion is greatly reduced, the outputs of fucomucin and sulfomucin being lowered much more than that of sialomucin.

Acute erosive gastritis often develops suddenly in previously healthy gastric mucosa and usually heals within a few days. Acute erosive gastritis may produce no symptoms or nonspecific symptoms such as postprandial discomfort, especially after a large meal. The most common clinical manifestation is almost completely unheralded and unexpected gastrointestinal bleeding. Treatment includes the restoration of blood volume, low temperature gastric lavage, and gastric aspiration. Uncontrolled bleeding requires surgical intervention, the procedures including partial gastric resection with and without truncal vagotomy and the combination of vagotomy and pyloroplasty.

PEPTIC ULCER

Pathogenesis

Pure acid gastric juice is capable of destroying and digesting all living tissues, including the stomach. Under normal circumstances, the gastric mucosa is protected, partially at least, by compactly arranged epithelial cells with very tight junctional relationships and by a thick layer of tenacious adherent mucus. Protection also is afforded by the regenerative capacity of the mucosal cells; the alkaline, pancreatic, and intestinal secretions; and an adequate blood supply. There are other protective factors, but their nature is not known. Under certain conditions the resistance of the stomach to digestion fails. The mechanism of this failure is not clear. In duodenal ulcer there is an excessive secretion of acid, neurogenic and probably humoral in origin, and abnormal in that it continues when the stomach is empty and in the absence of the usual stimuli for gastric secretion. The gastric secretory mechanism probably also is more responsive than usual to secretory stimuli. Presumably, the hydrogen ion concentration and the proteolytic activity of the gastric juice exceed in destructive effect the defensive capacity of the mucosa.

Experimentally, peptic ulcer may be produced by various operations interfering with the normal neutralization of the acid by the intestinal content, by the administration of acid, or by the continuous stimulation of highly acid gastric secretion. The occurrence of jejunal ulcer following experimental diversion of bile and pancreatic juice by a duodenal-jejunal conduit (as in the McCann modification of the Mann-Williamson operation) is attributable to hypersecretion of acid gastric juice because of loss of the "duodenal brake" upon gastric secretion; canceling the neutralization of the acid gastric content by the alkaline duodenal secretions. The role of emotional stress in the pathogenesis of peptic ulcer remains clinically impressive but the mechanism whereby nervous tension influences tissue resistance is not known. Emotional pressure presumably increases gastric secretion via the vagal nerves, with the probable participation of the gastrin mechanism. Presumably, the excitatory effects of brain stimulation are mediated by the vagus nerve. An increase in neural activity in the vagus nerve increases gastric motility and secretion, but the vagus nerve also mediates inhibitory influences on the physiologic activities of the stomach. Increase in stomach size and in parietal cell mass may account for the excessive gastric secretion in patients with duodenal ulcer, but other pathogenetic factors also must be involved. The most important type of tension is the long-continued inability to deal with psychogenic problems and internal conflicts, resulting from the frustrations of susceptible individuals. The association of peptic ulcer with sustained heavy cigarette smoking has been attributed, in part at least, to the inhibition of pancreatic and biliary buffering secretions and to the consequently less effective neutralization of hydrochloric acid.

Tissue resistance presumably depends upon multiple factors, including the integrity of the gastric and duodenal mucosal cells, the abundant vascular supply, the rapid, continuous regeneration of the epithelium, the mucus barrier, and the permeability of the gastroduodenal mucous membrane, among other considerations. The gastric mucosal barrier includes (a) the overlying layer of viscous mucus; (b) underlying tall columnar cells; (c) low cuboidal and columnar cells lining the crypts of the gastric glands; (d) the membrane that forms the surface of the cells; and (e) the band of fission linking each cell to its neighbor in a tight junction.

The factor of decreased tissue resistance is implicated in both duodenal and gastric ulcer but appears to be especially important in patients with gastric ulcer, in whom the output of hydrochloric acid may be normal or less than normal. According to Bralow, the mucosa is unable to maintain "cellular homeostasis" after mucosal injury. Nevertheless, complete neutralization of the acid or its prolonged inhibition invariably results in healing of the ulcer. The lower incidence and lesser severity of duodenal ulcer and its complications in women, and the apparently beneficial influence of pregnancy in women with peptic ulcer suggest a sex-linked influence, but the nature of this factor, if indeed present, is not known.

Regardless of the initial causes, the subsequent development and extension of the lesion, its chronicity, and its failure to heal are attributable to the destructive action of acid gastric juice upon a susceptible mucosa. Tissue necrosis and digestion result eventually in the typical peptic ulcer. The ulcerogenic effects of drugs such as the salicylates, adrenal corticosteroids, indomethacin, and phenylbutazone seem attributable to direct irritation and inflammation of the mucosa, and perhaps also to a depletion of gastric mucus, whereas the ulcerogenic effect of reserpine seems to be related more completely to its potent stimulation of gastric secretion.

Most peptic ulcers occur along the lesser curvature of the stomach and in the first 3 or 4 cm. of the duodenum, the "duodenal bulb." Acute and chronic ulcers differ chiefly in the amount of granulation tissue and fibroplasia. The incidence of peptic ulcer is difficult to establish but generally is assumed to approximate 15 per cent. It is more common in patients with rheumatoid arthritis, obstructive bronchopulmonary disease, and possibly in patients with cirrhosis of the liver treated by portacaval shunt. The mechanisms involved are not known entirely. Duodenal ulcer appears to be more frequent in individuals with blood group O, especially those not secreting A, B, and H blood group factors in saliva and gastric juice. The significance of this relationship is not apparent, but it suggests perhaps that duodenal ulcer represents the outcome of an interplay between environmental and hereditary factors. The output of hydrochloric acid is significantly higher in patients of blood group O than in those of groups A, B, and AB, and especially in those nonsecretor individuals of blood group O. Apparently, individuals of blood group O are approximately 35 per cent more liable to duodenal ulcer than individuals of groups A, B, and AB. Nonsecretors are about 50 per cent more liable. People who are both group O and nonsecretor (the most susceptible group) are about 2.5 times more liable than the individuals who are at least sick, the secretors of groups A and B. The association with group O has been found to apply particularly to those people whose ulcers have bled or perforated, indicating that group O may influence the severity of peptic ulcer. Constitutional factors are suggested by the occurrence of ulcers occasionally in families and in twins living separately. The incidence of peptic ulcer increases significantly among relatives of ulcer patients, especially among male relatives of male propositi.

Gastric ulcers are one tenth as common as duodenal ulcers. They occur together with duodenal ulcer in approximately 20 per cent of patients, although in some geographic areas the incidence may be higher. The age range is higher and more women are affected by gastric than by duodenal ulcer. Gastric ulcer may be single or multiple, large or small, acute or chronic. The diameter varies from several millimeters to several centimeters, and the depth from 10 to 20 mm. or more. They occur anywhere in the stomach but especially on the lesser curvature proximal to the angulus, and in the area distal to the border zone formed by the junction of fundic and pyloric gland tissue.

Gastric ulcer resembles duodenal ulcer in its chronicity, recurrences, complications, and tendency to healing, especially when the acid gastric content is neutralized or abolished. Gastric ulcer differs from duodenal ulcer in its lower output of hydrochloric acid and the intermittency of the secretion, and in its increased frequency among women, older age groups, and the poorly nourished and impoverished social classes. An increased frequency of gastric ulcer has been noted in young women in Australia and is attributed to the increased ingestion of salicylates. Gastric ulcer is attributed by Dragstedt to the "hypersecretion" of gastric juice of humoral or gastrin origin induced by stasis of food in the stomach in contact with the gastric antrum. This stasis may result from pyloroduodenal stenosis from an accompanying duodenal ulcer or from decreased gastric tonus and motility. Another major pathogenetic concept of gastric ulcer involves diminished tissue resistance, abetted by exogenous irritants including drugs (e.g., aspirin), reflux of bile, excess use of cigarettes and alcohol, and the ingestion of irritants such as hot tea and hot rice. The role of bile reflux appears supported by the following observations: (1) gastritis is an invariable accompaniment of gastric ulcer; (2) regurgitation of intestinal contents is common in gastric ulcer; (3) exposure of the normal gastric mucosa to intestinal content causes gastritis; and (4) gastritis increases the susceptibility of the gastric mucosa to ulcer formation. An increased reflux of intestinal content containing bile has been reported in patients with gastric ulcer and has been implicated both in the production of a gastritis favoring the development of gastric ulcer and/or the gastric ulcer itself. Experimentally, drainage of bile into the stomach of the dog causes morphologic changes similar to gastritis in man. Also, bile acids increase the transmural flux of sodium and hydrogen ions, disrupting the physiologic mucosal barrier in a manner similar to that induced by salicylates. The reflux of duodenal content also exposes the gastric mucosa to lysolecithin, fatty acids, and pancreatic enzymes, all of which could be injurious to the gastric mucosa. Other observers maintain that the bile reflux in gastric ulcer is a secondary phenomenon, possibly a consequence of the release of gastrin. In the experimental studies of Dragstedt and his colleagues, the formation of ulcers at the efferent stoma where there is contact with the acid gastric content and not in the esophagus or stomach where there is contact with bile and pancreatic juice suggests that the latter are relatively impotent as ulcerogenic agents.

Endocrine Relationships

There is no etiologic relationship between the ordinary peptic ulcer and primary endocrine disorders. However, certain endocrine (humoral) abnormalities may be associated with refractory peptic ulcer and gastric hypersecretion. The *Zollinger-Ellison syndrome* is characterized by single or multiple nonbeta islet cell adenomas of the pancreas; by enormous outputs of hydrochloric acid and pepsin; by single or multiple ulcers in the esophagus, second, third, and fourth portions of the duodenum, and in the jejunum and ileum, in addition to the stomach and duodenal bulb; and by refractoriness to medical or surgical treatment, short of total gastric resection. The parietal cell mass is sixfold larger than normal and threefold larger than in patients with the usual duodenal ulcer. Gastric rugae and mucosal folds in the small intestine often are enlarged. The Zollinger-Ellison syndrome is relatively uncommon but it is not rare. The disorder is more common in men, the ratio being 6 males to 4 females. It occurs in all age groups but especially during the third to fifth decades.

Ulcer pain is present in approximately 95 per cent of patients. Symptoms exceed 1 year in duration in more than 80 per cent and range from 5 to 10 years in duration in 30 per cent. Atypically located and multiple peptic ulcers (esophagus, distal duodenum and jejunum) strongly suggest the disorder. However, three fourths of the ulcers in the Zollinger-Ellison syndrome are not located atypically and they are not multiple. While case reports often describe the severe, occasionally dramatic complications of atypically located peptic ulceration, the symptoms often are indistinguishable from those of ordinary peptic ulcer, until operation removes the anatomic integrity of the stomach and duodenum and disrupts normal homeostatic mechanisms controlling acid gastric secretion. The course then usually, although not invariably, is more complicated, with severe ulcer pain, bleeding, and perforation, the entire sequence occasionally developing very rapidly after ulcer surgery.

Diarrhea occurs in approximately one third of patients and may or may not be associated with peptic ulcer, including a profuse watery diarrhea without steatorrhea, resulting in hypokalemia and dehydration. The secretion of hydrochloric acid is low or absent (see p. 744). Hypokalemic nephropathy may be an initial manifestation of the Zollinger-Ellison syndrome. Steatorrhea is not uncommon and is attributable to multiple factors: acid inactivation of pancreatic lipase; precipitation of bile salts, with defective micelle formation; direct injury to the intestinal mucosa by the excessive hydrochloric acid; and acid injury to the vitamin B_{12}-intrinsic factor complex.

Occasionally there is no adenoma in the pancreas but an increased number of islet cells and a higher proportion of nonbeta to beta cells. Approximately 60 per cent of the tumors are malignant. The adenomas have a low grade of malignancy but, like carcinoids, they may metastasize to the liver. They occur anywhere in the pancreas but especially in the body and tail. Aberrant adenomas may be found in the hilus of the spleen, in the gastric wall, and along the liver curvature of the second position of the duodenum.

The most characteristic laboratory finding is the enormous "basal" secretion of hydrochloric acid, exceeding 200 ml. or 20 mEq. hydrochloric acid per hour, with a comparatively small increment (less than 60 per cent) following the injection of histamine, Histalog, or pentagastrin. The volume of the 12-hour nocturnal gastric secretion averages 2000 ml., with recorded volumes exceeding 5 and 10 liters. However, low gastric acidity has been observed in approximately 5 per cent of patients.

The gastric hypersecretion is humoral in origin, gastrin having been extracted from the pancreatic adenoma and from metastases in the liver, duodenum, or lymph nodes, and also identified immunochemically with the amino acid constituents of human gastrin types I and II. The carboxyl-terminal tetrapeptide amide, Try-Met-Asp-Phe-NH_2, is the active center of gastrin, producing the full spectrum of actions of the entire gastrin molecule but, on a molar basis, about one fifth as active. Antibodies to gastrin have been produced by immunization with the C-terminal tetrapeptide amide of gastrin conjugated to carrier protein macromolecules. These antibodies react equivalently on a molar basis with the C-terminal tetrapeptide amide, with the gastrin-like pentapeptide amide, and with a variety of intact gastrin molecules.

Utilizing radio-immunoassays for gastrin, fasting serum from patients with the Zollinger-Ellison syndrome contains gastrin levels tenfold or higher than normal. Normal fasting levels of gastrin range from 10 to 300 pg. per ml., with a mean of 100 pg. Similar levels apparently are found in "ordinary" peptic ulcer. In both normal persons and in patients with peptic ulcer, gastrin levels increase with age. The range in patients with the Zollinger-Ellison syndrome is 800 to 165,000 pg. Serum levels of gastrin in 3 patients with histologically verified Zollinger-Ellison syndrome were 3550, 7880, and 21,000 pg., respectively. Since some Zollinger-Ellison tumors apparently secrete gastrin intermittently, repeated analyses may be required for diagnosis. Serum gastrin levels also appear to relate directly to the plasma calcium concentration, decreasing with hypocalcemia after parathyroidectomy and increasing with infusions of calcium but not of parathormone. The humoral abnormality in the Zollinger-Ellison syndrome is not limited to the overproduction of gastrin. Blood and urine levels of various biologically active amines also may be elevated.

The Zollinger-Ellison ulcer and its complications are not controlled by the usual antacid and antisecretory therapy; by gastric irradiation; or by surgery, including vagotomy with pyloroplasty, gastroenterostomy, or antrum resection. The treatment of choice at present is complete removal of the stomach. Active immunization with the gastrin tetrapeptide may induce resistance in rats to the acid-secretory effects of exogenous gastrin. This technique and the possible development of specific gastrin antagonists eventually may provide an effective medical approach to the gastrin-mediated hypersecretion of hydrochloric acid in patients with the Zollinger-Ellison syndrome.

Polyendocrine adenomatosis (Wermer's syndrome) is a familial disorder characterized by the concomitant presence of multiple tumors or hyperplasia of several endocrine glands. The parathyroid glands are most frequently involved, followed by the pancreatic islets and pituitary, adrenals, and thyroid glands. Bronchial and intestinal carcinoid tumors, pheochromocytomas, and lipomas are included in the syndrome. The adenomas may or may not be hormonally active in one or more glands and in any combination. Peptic ulcer is present in more than 50 per cent of cases; the sexes are affected equally; and the disease has been described in all age groups after the first decade, with the peak occurrence in the third and fourth decades. Multiple endocrine adenomatosis appears to have a genetic basis attributable to the action of an autosomal dominant gene of high penetrance. Approximately one half the ulcers are multiple and in atypical locations. The most common presenting feature of the syndrome is peptic ulcer and its complications. The symptoms of hypoglycemia are next in frequency. Acromegaly, pituitary dwarfism, hypogonadism, Cushing's syndrome, hyperaldosteronism, and hyperthyroidism may occur alone or in any combination. Complications of perforation, obstruction, and hemorrhage are common. Diarrhea and steatorrhea occur in 10 per cent of patients in association with ulcer. Although gastrin has been extracted from the pancreatic adenomas, all attempts to isolate gastrin or a gastric secretagogue from adenomas of other endocrine glands have failed. The peptic ulcer associated with polyendocrine adenomatosis seems identical in all respects to that of the Zollinger-Ellison syndrome. On the basis of present information, therefore, it perhaps is justifiable to regard the Zollinger-Ellison syndrome as the "gastrin-secreting, pancreatic islet-cell tumor component" of polyendocrine adenomatosis.

Treatment of each endocrine abnormality follows the usual measures; management of the ulcer in polyendocrine adenomatosis is the same as for the Zollinger-Ellison syndrome. In a recent survey of five families with multiple endocrine adenomatosis, all families had members with parathyroid and pancreatic islet-cell tumors, and some families also had pituitary tumors, lipomas, and bronchial carcinoids. In the total sample of 38 patients, the most common abnormality was hypercalcemia and the next most common was pancreatic tumors. The most useful screening methods were the clinical history and measurement of the serum calcium. Multiple endocrine adenomatosis appears to have a genetic basis attributable to the action of a mutated gene which is dominant, carried in an autosome, and is of high penetrance. Duodenal ulcer may be more common in patients with parathyroid adenomas and hyperparathyroidism, especially among men. Acute ulcers may develop during adrenocortical insufficiency but they heal rapidly when adrenal function is restored. Peptic ulcers are not more frequent in patients with adrenocortical hyperfunction.

Peptic ulcer is a penetrating process, beginning in the mucosa, gradually extending through the muscularis mucosae into the muscularis propria, in some cases perforating through the wall, and in others eroding into blood vessels. Regenerative activity is present almost always and may at any time lead to healing of the ulcer, especially if it is protected from gastric juice. Healing of peptic ulcer occurs from below upward with the growth of granulation tissue and young fibroblasts. In small superficial lesions, healing is complete. In large, chronic ulcers, healing is slower; new glands are not formed and tissue is replaced by fibrous and elastic tissue.

Clinically, chronic peptic ulcer occurs only in those parts of the digestive tract exposed to the action of acid gastric juice: the lower part of the esophagus, the stomach, the upper part of the duodenum, or the small bowel adjacent to a patent gastroenterostomy or a Meckel's diverticulum containing ectopic gastric glands. It occurs only in patients whose gastric glands are able to secrete acid. It does not develop in patients with complete achlorhydria. Prolonged emotional turmoil tends to produce vascular engorgement, increased secretory and motor activity of the stomach, and heightened susceptibility of the mucosa to injury. Frequently, a chronological parallelism exists between the onset, recurrence, and course of peptic ulcer and emotional disturbances. The development of gastric ulcer in patients with stenosing duodenal ulcers and delayed gastric emptying has been attributed to stimulation of the gastric antrum and the consequent overproduction of gastrin.

Thus, peptic ulcer may be described as the product of a pathologic physiologic condition in which the mucosa fails to withstand the destructive action of acid-pepsin gastric juice and is unable to repair adequately the mucosal injury. Tissue susceptibility as well as acid and pepsin and "ulcerogenic" influences all play significant pathogenetic roles. The local factors responsible probably include a diminution of cellular resistance, possibly a loss of protective intracellular substances, increased mucosal permeability, decreased cellular protection from an insufficient production and possibly biological changes in the nature of the gastric mucus, excessive secretion of hydrochloric acid, or a combination of these.

Symptoms

The outstanding symptom of peptic ulcer is pain, characterized by its chronicity, periodicity, and relation to the ingestion of food. The average duration at the time the patient is first seen by the physician is 6 or 7 years. In occasional cases the symptoms have been present for only a few days or weeks; in others, they have continued for 40 or 50 years. The periodicity of the distress is striking, the symptoms lasting a few days, weeks, or months, with periods of remission of similar duration. The explanation for this intermittent pattern remains unknown. Periodicity of ulcer distress is observed under all circumstances: environmental, social, and climatic. Exacerbations of peptic ulcer occur at all times of the year, but in some patients they may be confined to the spring and fall seasons of the year. In some patients the tendency is for the periods of distress to become more frequent and of longer duration, whereas the remissions are less frequent and shorter. On the other hand, progression is not inevitable; in many individuals recurrences become less frequent, and eventually the ulcer may heal completely.

The pain is usually a gnawing or aching sensation, sometimes described as burning, boring, heartburn or pressure in the upper abdomen, cramplike, or, indeed, as hunger. It differs from the intermittent pangs of true hunger in that ulcer distress is almost always steady and continuous for 15 minutes to an hour or more unless relieved, whereas the hunger pang lasts for only a minute or so. The rhythm of pain in peptic ulcer is related to the digestive cycle; it is the same for both gastric and duodenal ulcer. Pain attributable to peptic ulcer usually is absent before breakfast, appears 1 to 4 hours after breakfast, and lasts 30 minutes or more, perhaps until relief is obtained at the noon meal. The distress recurs 1 to 4 hours later and usually is more severe than in the forenoon. The afternoon pain likewise may

TABLE 25–1 COMPARATIVE OUTPUTS OF HYDROCHLORIC ACID

	Basal (mEq./hr.)	Maximal Histamine (mEq./hr.)	Nocturnal (mEq./12 hr.)
Normal	2	20	18
Gastric ulcer	4	20	8
Duodenal ulcer	8	35	60
Zollinger-Ellison syndrome	30	45	120

disappear spontaneously, but more often food or alkali is required to obtain relief. In the evening, the pain may recur 1 to 4 hours after eating; it may be less severe than in the afternoon. The patient may be awakened with pain, usually between midnight and 3:00 in the morning. Rarely does nocturnal pain appear unless pain has been present in the evening, and rarely indeed does pain attributable to ulcer develop later in the night, unless it has been present earlier. The presence of nocturnal pain often is interpreted as evidence of pyloric obstruction or high-grade stenosis, but it occurs also in nonobstructive, acutely inflamed lesions.

The site of peptic ulcer cannot be predicted accurately by the topographical location of the pain. Ulcer pain usually is localized in the epigastrium, to the left of the midline and in the left upper quadrant in gastric ulcer, and halfway between the xiphoid and umbilicus to the right of the midline or immediately above the umbilicus in duodenal ulcer. In postbulbar ulcer, the pain may be in the right upper quadrant, penetrating to the right side of the back. The pain of esophageal ulcer is in the substernal or subxiphoid area. The pain of jejunal ulcer often is in the left midabdomen and in the left lower quadrant. Pain in the back at the level of the eighth to tenth thoracic vertebrae may occur in the presence or absence of a penetrating ulcer. With penetration of an ulcer into the pancreas or other adjacent structures, ulcer pain becomes more persistent and more severe. In young children with peptic ulcer the distress may lack the usual rhythmicity and periodicity, the pain is vague, and vomiting is common. In older children, the symptoms resemble those of adults. Nausea, vomiting, anorexia, and weight loss, as in older patients with gastric ulcer, initially may suggest the presence of malignant disease.

Nausea is not a common symptom. Vomiting may result from severe pain, but usually indicates pyloric obstruction. Painless vomiting may occur with nonobstructive ulcer, presumably owing to a reflex disturbance of the intrinsic neuromuscular coordination. The appetite and weight usually are well preserved, but severe loss of weight may result from continued vomiting or the patient's fear of eating. The frequent ingestion of food to relieve pain, on the other hand, may produce a gain of weight. Constipation and flatulence reflect an associated irritable colon. Diarrhea may result from various causes: the excessive use of laxative antacids; gastric hypersecretion, the acid inactivating intestinal and pancreatic enzymes and thus interfering with normal digestive processes; and a gastrojejunocolic fistula, short-circuiting the gastrointestinal content.

Bleeding occurs in the life history of at least 25 per cent of patients with peptic ulcer; the ulcers associated with bleeding vary in size and duration with all gradations from superficial erosions to huge penetrating lesions. They may be located in the esophagus, stomach, duodenum, or jejunal stoma after a gastroenterostomy. The ulcers usually are on the posterior wall. The anterior surfaces of the stomach and duodenum do not contain major vessels, and the vascular channels are smaller than on the posterior wall. The associated symptoms are determined by the rapidity and severity of the blood loss. The manifestations of severe hemorrhage include sudden weakness, faintness, perspiration, dizziness, headache, palpitation, chilliness, abdominal cramps, thirst, dyspnea, syncope, and collapse as a consequence of the pronounced decrease in blood volume and diminished cardiac output. These symptoms respond promptly to the transfusion of whole blood and other supportive measures. Ulcer pain is absent or infrequent.

In the absence of a definite diagnosis of peptic ulcer, upper gastrointestinal bleeding requires differentiation from a variety of other conditions associated with bleeding. These include erosive gastritis, esophageal varices, carcinoma of the stomach, vascular abnormalities, and the Mallory-Weiss syndrome. The latter condition is characterized by longitudinal lacerations in the cardioesophageal region varying from 3 to 20 mm. in length and from 2 to 3 mm. in width. They occur during the retching and straining associated with intense vomiting. The mucosal tears are attributed to unequal distensibility of the mucosa and musculature and severe pressure in the cardioesophageal area.

Pyloric or duodenal obstruction results from spasm, edema, and inflammation in an active pyloric or duodenal ulcer, from cicatricial stenosis, or from a combination of these changes. The obstruction in the majority of patients is temporary and disappears during medical treatment, as the inflammation and edema subside. Permanent narrowing may result from frequent recurrences of ulcer. Each episode results in the proliferation of connective tissue, followed eventually by cicatricial contraction. The end result is a firmly contracted scar narrowing the lumen. The most significant symptoms of obstruction are the vomiting of retained food and gastric content, loss of weight, and weakness. Obstruction in gastric ulcer may result from inflammation and narrowing of the gastric antrum and from shortening of the lesser curvature of the stomach, with upward retraction of the antrum and distortion of the pylorus.

The loss of large quantities of chloride ion and a smaller but significant amount of sodium as well as of potassium and fluid in the vomitus produces alkalosis, characterized by an increase in the carbon dioxide content and pH and a decrease in the concentration of chloride and sodium ions in the plasma. The consequent diminution in blood volume, reduction in the flow of blood through the kidneys, and tissue dehydration lead to a temporary impairment of renal function. The symptoms of the electrolyte imbalance (alkalosis) include loss of appetite, distaste for food, increased nausea, weakness, lassitude, headache, nervous irritability, and occasionally coma. Tetany is rare, since the carbon dioxide tension of the blood usually is maintained above the critical level, but muscular twitchings and hyperirritability of the reflexes may be present. These manifestations disappear rapidly with correction of the biochemical disturbance by the intravenous administration of appropriate amounts of chloride, sodium, and water.

Perforation

Approximately 1 to 2 per cent of all ulcers perforate, and perforations recur in 1 to 2 per cent of these cases. Pyloroduodenal perforations exceed gastric perforations in a proportion of 20:1 for men and 5:1 for women. The incidence in males exceeds that in females in a ratio of 50:1. The ulcers usually are on the anterior wall of the stomach or duodenum, unsupported by contiguous structures. Ulcers on the posterior wall tend to penetrate rather than perforate, and their further extension is limited by adjacent solid organs. Perforations occur more often after eating and during the latter part of the afternoon or evening. Ulcers perforate at all times of the year but probably less often during the summer and more frequently during the winter. The symptoms begin with sudden, extremely severe pain in the upper abdomen, extending rapidly throughout the abdomen as a consequence of the escape of the irritating gastric and intestinal contents and the development of a chemical peritonitis. The pain may be referred to one or both shoulders because of irritation of the diaphragm, innervated by the phrenic nerves. The sudden severe pain is replaced within 6 to 12 hours by a dull discomfort and may disappear within 24 hours. The subsequent development of a bacterial peritonitis produces fever, tachycardia, increasing abdominal distention, and toxemia. Death occurs within 5 to 7 days if surgical and medical management proves inadequate.

Jejunal ulcer is a complication of the surgical treatment of peptic ulcer developing under circumstances of ineffective control of gastric secretion and exposure of the vulnerable jejunal mucosa to the acid-pepsin gastric content. Jejunal ulcers are most frequent in the efferent loop, approximately 1 cm. beyond the anastomosis. Jejunal ulcer also may develop in the absence of surgery in patients with the Zollinger-Ellison syndrome. Incidence in males predominates 10:1. The pain of jejunal ulcer may be in the left lower quadrant or in the lower abdomen. It often is more severe than previously and less responsive to treatment. In perforated jejunal ulcer the pain may extend to the left groin, testes, the left flank, and the back. The characteristic relationship to the intake of food may disappear, and nocturnal distress is frequent. Nausea and vomiting may signify an associated malfunction or obstruction of the stoma. Loss of weight is common but is not pronounced when a jejunocolic fistula develops.

Other Complications

A gastrojejunocolic fistula may develop from penetration of an ulcer at the anastomosis between the stomach and jejunum into the adjacent transverse colon. The principal symptoms are the pain of peptic ulceration and diarrhea of varying intensity. The diarrhea and the bypass of small intestine result in rapid and severe loss of weight, electrolytes, and water. Regurgitation of colonic contents into the stomach produces fecal vomiting. The associated malnutrition often is pronounced. Rarely, duodenal ulcer may cause an obstructive jaundice as a consequence of ulceration into the common bile duct, inflammatory obstruction of the duct, penetration into the head of the pancreas causing pancreatitis, or penetration into the gastrohepatic ligament, obstructing the common bile duct proximally.

Various surgical procedures are available for the management of peptic ulcer unresponsive to medical treatment and for the complications of peptic ulcer. These procedures include gastroenterostomy, partial gastric resection, truncal "selective" vagotomy with pyloroplasty or with antral resection, and so-called superselective vagotomy. The most important postsurgical problems, gastrointestinal and metabolic, follow gastric resection. These include the mechanical difficulties of reduced gastric capacity, stomal dysfunction, jejunogastric intussusception, diarrhea, uncovering of a latent malabsorption (gluten enteropathy), chronic obstruction of the afferent loop, recurrent ulcer formation, and the dumping syndrome. The nutritional and metabolic problems after gastric resection occur later, sometimes many years later, as in the disordered calcium metabolism with demineralization of bone, associated with deficiency of vitamin D, resulting from the combination of diminished oral intake and impaired absorption. The late difficulties include deficiencies of vitamin B_{12} intrinsic factor and folic acid, decreased absorption of iron and iron-deficiency anemia, intestinal leakage of albumin, increased susceptibility to infections including pulmonary tuberculosis, and, in emotionally vulnerable patients, addiction to alcohol or drugs or psychotic episodes. Late gastrointestinal problems may include the development of gastric carcinoma involving the gastric stump, bezoar formation, and milk intolerance. The evidence for an increased incidence of cholelithiasis after gastric resection is inconclusive.

The dumping syndrome is caused by accelerated gastric emptying following gastric surgery, especially partial gastric resection but also after gastroenterostomy, pyloroplasty, and vagotomy, with the entrance of large amounts of gastric content into the proximal jejunum. The hyperosmolar intestinal content initiates the movement of extracellular fluid from the plasma to the lumen to achieve isotonicity, decreasing the circulating blood volume and inducing compensatory vasoconstriction. The distention of the jejunum and the presence of a hypertonic solution also activate a humoral mechanism which stimulates the production and release of serotonin from the argentaffin cell mass in the proximal jejunum. The serotonin presumably acts upon target organs, including the circulatory system. Bradykinin has been implicated in the early vasomotor symptoms and serotonin in the delayed response. The early manifestations, within 5 to 30 minutes after eating, include such vasomotor phenomena as warmth, sweating, weakness, palpitation, vertigo, or desire to lie down, and such digestive complaints as abdominal discomfort, nausea, and explosive diarrhea. The late manifestations relate to the rapid entrance of glucose into the blood, producing hyperglycemia before sufficient insulin has been mobilized to facilitate its metabolism. The hyperglycemia elicits an overproduction of insulin causing hypoglycemia two to three hours after a meal. Recent studies suggest that postgastrectomy hypoglycemia is caused by an inducible gastrointestinal insulin-secretory factor, possibly related to glucagon, potentiating glucose-mediated insulin release. Dumping may be precipitated by any food, but especially by foods rich in glucose and disaccharides when fluids are taken simultaneously, and by nervous tension. Dumping is more frequent after surgery for duodenal ulcer in women and among emotionally labile patients.

BENIGN GASTRIC TUMORS

Gastric neoplasms may be classified pathologically as of mesenchymal, epithelial, or endothelial origin. Their clinical differentiation, however, is difficult. The mesenchymal tumors include myoma, fibromyoma, leiomyoma, leiomyoblastoma, hemangioma, angioma, lipoma, osteoma, osteochondroma, and the malignant sarcomas. The epithelial tumors include polyps, papillomas, and adenomas. Endothelial tumors include hemangioma, lymphadenoma, and endothelioma. Gastric teratomas arise from the visceral wall, the embryonic splanchnopleure, and are composed of tissues representing all three embryonic germ layers. They apparently occur exclusively among males. Tumors originating in the neural tissue, such as neurofibroma, neuroepithelioma, and neurilemoma, also may occur. The pathogenesis of most benign gastric tumors is as obscure as that of carcinoma of the stomach.

Adenomatous polyps may be smooth and lobulated or the epithelium may be thrown into frond-like processes, the villous adenoma. The proliferating epithelial tubules are packed closely together, and the epithelium shows a diminution in the number of goblet cells, crowding of the nuclei with much hyperchromatism, and an increased number of mitotic figures, all features of a neoplastic process. All stages in the development of a malignant disease from "carcinoma in situ" to invasive cancer may be seen. Polyps may be single or multiple; they vary in size from a few millimeters to 7 cm. in diameter. Some polyps are sessile; others are pedunculated. The histologic appearance of most polyps is that of glandular proliferation, without hyperchromatism or excessive mitoses.

Leiomyomas constitute perhaps 2 per cent of all gastric tumors. They originate from the smooth muscle of the gastric wall and may remain for some time as an intramural structure. As the tumor enlarges, it may grow either into the gastric mucosa toward the lumen or outward toward the serosa, sometimes growing in both directions to assume an hourglass appearance. About one third present as an ulcerated intragastric polypoid tumor and one fourth as a polypoid lesion covered by intact mucosa. The risk of evolution to leiomyosarcoma is small. Because of their tendency to remain silent, leiomyomas may grow to a very large size. They may outgrow their blood supply, leading to central necrosis and large antral cavities in the tumor connected by fistulous tracts to the gastric lumen. The most common symptom is hemorrhage, either acute or chronic. Abdominal discomfort, partially suggestive of peptic ulcer, may be present. Leiomyomas situated close to the pylorus induce symptoms of obstruction.

A variety of benign inflammatory disorders may simulate malignant disorders. These include inflammatory fibroid polyps, inflammatory pseudotumors, and lymphomatous lesions, "pseudolymphomas." The most important distinguishing feature is follicular formation with true germinal centers. The predominant cell type is the mature lymphocyte. A mixed inflammatory infiltrate and reactive changes are additional features. Two histologic types of pseudolymphoma are described. The monomorphic type is composed of lymphocytes, lymphoblasts, or histiocytes. The polymorphic form is composed of a mixed inflammatory infiltrate with an abundance of plasmocytes.

There is no clinical syndrome characteristic of

benign tumor of the stomach. Symptoms are determined by the size and position of the lesion and by its tendency to ulcerate, bleed, or become malignant. Tumors located away from the orifices of the stomach are symptomless until complicated by ulceration or hemorrhage. Large tumors indicate their presence by the mechanical effects of pressure, causing sensations of fullness and distention and such variable symptoms as distress after meals, heartburn, and nausea. Tumors, sessile or pedunculated, situated near the pylorus may produce an intermittent pyloric obstruction, with episodes of pain, nausea, and vomiting; complete pyloric obstruction may develop. Pain, as a rule, is mild or absent; it is evident usually when prolapses or intussusception of the tumor through the pylorus occurs or when the tumor is sufficiently large to be caught and pulled by gastric peristalsis. Hemorrhage and anemia are the important clinical manifestations. Bleeding occurs more readily in adenomas, leiomyomas, and hemangiomas, and more often in large tumors than in small growths. The hemorrhage is attributed usually to torsion of the pedicle, with vascular congestion, ulceration of the overlying mucosa, and sloughing of the polypoid tumor.

CARCINOMA OF THE STOMACH

The cause of gastric carcinoma remains obscure, but it is not congenital; it does not develop from embryonal rests; it is not directly inherited (although a predisposition to it may be inherited); it is neither infectious nor contagious, although a viral etiology has become an intriguing possibility. Its "spontaneous" occurrence among animals is extremely rare except possibly in the Australian mastomys. The use of alcohol, tobacco, coffee, and condiments apparently is of no etiologic significance. The possible relationship between gastric carcinoma and various chemical carcinogenic substances, especially their ingestion in foods, e.g., hot rice, fish, cabbage, and superheated fats, continues to be intriguing. The role of ethnic-related factors is suggested by the observation in Sumatra of the high incidence of gastric carcinoma among the Chinese and its rarity among the Javanese. The high incidence of cancer of the stomach among both Japanese men and women is noteworthy and unexplained; the average age of appearance of gastric cancer in Japan is at least a decade earlier than in the white population of the United States. In Israel, gastric carcinoma appears to be more common among Jews of northern European ancestry than among Jews of Mediterranean or Asian origin. The incidence of gastric cancer also is higher in people of lower socioeconomic status, but again the biological significance of this relationship is not evident at present. The pronounced variations in incidence of gastric cancer in different countries (decreasing in the United States, Canada, and England, and remaining high in Finland, Iceland, Chile, and Japan), the higher incidence in higher latitudes, and the inverse correlation with economic status suggest environmental, principally dietary, influences (hot liquids and foods, seasonings, smoked fish). The increased ingestion of wheat cereals containing "antioxidants" alleged to be anticarcinogenic has been implicated in the declining incidence of gastric cancer in the United States and in other countries where the consumption of cereals is high. The importance of mucus and the mucous cells as a barrier to the diffusion of carcinogens and of bile and gastric juice as vehicles for carcinogenic agents remains unclear. Trauma appears to be significant only in relation to the sequelae of corrosion of the mucosa, as in acid or alkali poisoning. Although a sequence of ulceration and inflammation, regenerative hyperplasia, and unregulated cell growth is appealing theoretically, there is no conclusive evidence that benign gastric ulcer undergoes neoplasia. There may be a relationship between polyps of the stomach and gastric carcinoma, though direct evidence also is lacking.

The relationship of atrophic gastritis to carcinoma is obscure. Some degree of atrophy is observed in almost all cancer-bearing stomachs. Extensive atrophy of the gastric mucosa is invariably present in pernicious anemia and gastric polyposis, diseases in which the incidence of gastric carcinoma is distinctly higher than among similar age groups of the general population. In pernicious anemia the severe gastric atrophy affects the mucosa of the body of the stomach. Yet, when cancer develops it may be in either the body or the antrum; suggesting that some factor other than the gastritis may be responsible for predisposing to the development of the tumor. The transitional changes from chronic atrophic gastritis with small areas of hyperplasia to papilloma and to carcinoma have been demonstrated. On the other hand, atrophic gastritis occurs in association with gastric disease other than carcinoma and in the absence of any other apparent disorder. Perhaps the associated intestinal metaplasia of the gastric epithelium is more significant than the atrophy as a vulnerable substrate for gastric neoplasia. Possibly the gastritis is associated with a high cell turnover, creating an unstable cellular situation and increasing the vulnerability to neoplasia. An increased incidence of blood group A among patients with gastric cancer has been observed throughout the world and presumably represents a significant, albeit weak, genetic link. The very occasional strong family histories of gastric carcinoma and its occurrence among identical twins support the implication of a genetic influence in some instances.

The possible role of achlorhydria in the development of gastric carcinoma is closely related to that of atrophic gastritis. Complete anacidity is present in only a very small proportion of patients with carcinoma; in many the output of hydrochloric acid is reduced; but in some instances the acidity is high. The cause of the decreased gastric secretion has not been established. If achlorhydria were responsible, it might be expected that patients with gastric carcinoma without pernicious anemia, whatever the site of the tumor, would have a uniform secretory pattern. But there is no correlation between the extent and the site of the tumor and the suppression of acid and intrinsic factor secretions. Neither the atrophy nor the anacidity appears to be of direct etiologic significance; rather, they represent detectable abnormalities produced by some as yet undefined defect in the cells of the gastric mucosa. The apparently increased incidence of gastric carcinoma in the residual stomach after operations (especially gastrojejunostomy) for peptic ulcer, especially among males with blood group A, represents still another clinical situation reflecting an increased tissue vulnerability to neoplasia.

Gastric carcinoma thus may be regarded as an acquired disease, developing in an abnormal gastric mucosa and probably arising on the basis of cellular reaction to continued injury, presumably from unknown chemical carcinogens. The frequency of gastric carcinoma in the United States has decreased during the past 25 years. The incidence of carcinoma of the pancreas and cancer of the colon and of the lung, on the other hand, has increased substantially.

Carcinoma may involve any part of the stomach but develops most frequently from the mucus-secreting cells of the antrum and pylorus, especially along the lesser curvature, an area probably more exposed to carcinogenic influences. The majority of gastric tumors are adenocarcinomas, originating in the mucus-secreting cells of the mucosa. The tumor does not necessarily begin with a single cell, but many cells throughout an area of variable size may undergo neoplasia, as in multiple polyposis and frank multicentric carcinoma. Gastric carcinoma, like other neoplasms, varies enormously in its rate of growth, from the "acute" rapidly metastasizing tumors to "subacute" and "chronic" neoplasms. Nothing is known of the factors accelerating its progress in some instances and retarding it in others, nor of the conditions inhibiting growth in some directions and favoring it in others. Some tumors project into the lumen with little penetration into the wall, others extend directly through the gastric wall, and still others spread chiefly along the wall, primarily along the mucosa, the so-called superficial spreading carcinoma. This neoplasm extends no deeper than the muscularis mucosae. Surgical removal offers an excellent prognosis for long-term survival. Spread occurs by direct extension through the stomach, involving adjacent organs. Lymphatic spread involves the regional nodes along the lesser curvature, in the greater omentum, the hilum of the spleen, the subpyloric and suprapancreatic nodes.

The resistance of the body to cancer is not well understood, but it exists, as indicated in part by the sharp circumscription of some tumors, with atrophy and pyknosis of cancer cells at the margins of the lesion and the proliferation of fibrous tissues. Other histologic features associated with a favorable prognosis include the presence of an inflammatory reaction around the tumor, cellular differentiation, and, of course, the absence of lymph node metastases. Some lesions are associated with early ulceration; in others it is a late manifestation, and in some ulceration never occurs. The immunologic aspects of gastric (and other) carcinoma are only now attracting attention. An antigen related to blood group A has been demonstrated occasionally in the tumor cells.

Symptoms

There are no symptoms pathognomonic of early gastric carcinoma. The onset of the disease usually is so insidious and its course so latent that it is seldom suspected by the patient or the physician until it is advanced. An interval of 6 to 12 months usually elapses between the initial manifestations and establishment of the diagnosis. The development and nature of the symptoms depend chiefly upon the location of the growth, the presence of hydrochloric acid, the size and extent of the carcinoma, and its tendency to ulcerate, bleed, or metastasize. A tumor at the cardiac end of the stomach, sufficiently large to narrow the lumen of the esophagus, causes the progressive difficulty in swallowing characteristic of esophageal neoplasm. Severe vomiting often is the first indication of neoplasm, obstructing the pylorus. On the other hand, a carcinoma on the lesser or greater curvature of the stomach, or the body, may not cause symptoms until ulceration, bleeding, secondary infection, or metastases develop.

Symptoms include some type of indigestion, such as vague upper abdominal discomfort, a sense of fullness, ulcer-like distress but without the usual relief after the taking of food or antacid, or continuous epigastric pain. Anorexia is common, although in many instances the appetite initially may be unimpaired. The patient experiences a sense of fullness after eating less than the customary amount of food. The cause of the anorexia is not known. Loss of appetite in later stages is attributed generally to a diminution of gastric tone and peristalsis secondary to neoplastic infiltration, but this explanation is not entirely satisfactory. The decreased desire for food reduces the total caloric intake and results in progressive loss of weight. The inadequate diet and the loss of nutrient substances by vomiting or diarrhea may lead to protein and vitamin deficiencies; in patients with pyloric obstruction, the malnutrition may become extreme.

Pain may occur early or late in the disease, or occasionally not at all. It seldom is severe until the carcinoma has ulcerated or invaded the wall of the stomach. The distress may be only a vague sensation of dullness or burning in the epigastrium. When hydrochloric acid is present, the pain often is indistinguishable from that of benign peptic ulcer. In general the pain tends to appear earlier and to be more severe in patients with acid gastric secretion than in those with anacidity, presumably because of peptic ulceration. In many cases, however, the distress of carcinoma differs from that of peptic ulcer in that it is aggravated by the ingestion of food and relieved only partially or not at all by alkali or emesis. With progression and extension of the carcinoma to involve the celiac plexus and the spinal nerves, the pain may become severe and constant and may be relieved only by opiates.

Nausea and vomiting may occur relatively early in the disease, regardless of the location of the lesion, but these symptoms are much more frequent when the tumor obstructs the pylorus. The vomitus may or may not contain food, bile, or blood, but the so-called coffee-ground emesis is common. Dysphagia and substernal distress are characteristic of a tumor involving the cardiac orifice of the stomach and the lower end of the esophagus. Ulceration of a comparatively small tumor located in a "silent" area, with penetration into the wall of a blood vessel, may cause hematemesis or melena before other symptoms appear. Anemia is frequent, usually hypochromic and microcytic in type, and is caused by the occult loss of blood. However, the hematologic picture may be that of a true pernicious anemia, owing probably to coexistence of the two diseases. The anemia very occasionally results from carcinomatous infiltration of the bone marrow and displacement of the hematopoietic cells into the liver and spleen. Weakness, increasing fatigue, and lack of energy are related usually to the loss of weight and anemia, but they may precede these latter manifestations. Diarrhea is not uncommon, and in patients with diffusely infiltrating linitis plastica of the stomach it may be ascribed to rapid gastric emptying, in addition to increased bacterial invasion of the upper gastrointestinal tract as a consequence of the diminished acid secretion. An elevation of body temperature may originate in an associated pyogenic gastritis. Infrequently, the "initial" manifestations are those of metastatic lesions such as carcinomatosis of the peritoneum, massive enlargement of the liver, or severe backache caused by extension of the neoplasm into the celiac plexus or the spine. Severe progressive dyspnea results from diffuse pulmonary lymphatic spread of gastric carcinoma.

REFERENCES

Ballard, H. S., Frame, B., and Hartsock, R. J.: Familial multiple endocrine adenoma-peptic ulcer complex. Medicine, 43:481, 1964.

Bastiaans, J., and Weiner, H. (Eds.): Duodenal Ulcer, Vol. 6. Advances in Psychosomatic Medicine. Basel, S. Karger, 1971.

Berson, S. A., and Yalow, R. S.: Nature of immunoreactive gastrin extracted from tissues of gastrointestinal tract. Gastroenterology, 60:215, 1970.

Bralow, S. P.: Current concepts of peptic ulceration. Amer. J. Dig. Dis., 14:655, 1969.

Bruch, H.: Anorexia nervosa. Int. Psychiat. Clin., 7:3, 1970.

Byrnes, D. J., and Lazarus, L.: Serum gastrin and gastric acidity. Austr. New Zeal. Med. J., 1:26, 1971.

Creutzfeldt, W., Arnold, R., Creutzfeldt, C., Feurle, G., and Ketterer, H.: Gastrin and G-cells in the antral mucosa of patients with pernicious anemia, acromegaly and hyperparathyroidism and in a Zollinger-Ellison tumour of the pancreas. Europ. J. Clin. Invest., 1:461, 1971.

Davenport, H. W.: Back diffusion of acid through the gastric mucosa and its physiological consequences. In Glass, G. B. J. (Ed.): Progress in Gastroenterology. New York, Grune and Stratton, 1970, p. 42.

Davenport, H. W.: Salicylate damage to the gastric mucosal barrier. New Eng. J. Med., 276:1307, 1970.

Davenport, H. W.: Physiology of the Digestive Tract. 3rd ed. Chicago, Year Book Medical Publishers, 1971.

Davies, R. E., Longmuir, N. W., and Crane, E. E.: Elaboration of hydrochloric acid by gastric mucosa. Nature, 159:468, 1947.

Dragstedt, L. R.: On the cause of gastric and duodenal ulcers. J. Roy. Coll. Surg. Edinb., 16:251, 1971.

Dragstedt, L. R., Woodward, E. R., Seito, T., Isaza, J., Rodriguez, J. R., and Samijan, R.: The question of bile regurgitation as a cause of gastric ulcer. Ann. Surg., 174:548, 1971.

Edwards, F. C., and Coghill, N. F.: Aetiological factors in chronic atrophic gastritis. Brit. Med. J., 2:1409, 1966.

Ellison, E. H., and Wilson, S. D.: The Zollinger-Ellison syndrome: Reappraisal and evaluation of 260 registered cases. Ann. Surg., 160:512, 1964.

Gregory, R. A., and Tracy, H. J.: The constitution and properties of the two gastrins from hog antral mucosa. I. The isolation of two gastrins from hog antral mucosa. II. The properties of two gastrins isolated from hog antral mucosa. Gut, 5:103, 107; 1964.

Grossman, M. I., Kirsner, J. B., Gillespie, I. E., and Ford, H.: Basal and histalog-stimulated gastric secretion in control subjects and in patients with peptic ulcer or gastric cancer. Gastroenterology, 45:14, 1963.

Hollander, F.: The chemistry and mechanics of hydrochloric acid formation in the stomach. Gastroenterology, 1:403, 1943.

Holmes, K. D.: Mallory-Weiss syndrome. Review of 20 cases and literature review. Ann. Surg., 164:810, 1966.

Ivey, K. J.: Gastric mucosal barrier. Gastroenterology, 61:247, 1971.

Jaffe, B. M.: The measurement of serum gastrin. J. Surg. Res., 10:193, 1970.

Janowitz, H. D.: Hunger and appetite – physiologic regulation of food intake. Amer. J. Med., 25:327, 1958.

Kirsner, J. B.: Peptic Ulcer. *In* Beeson, P. B., and McDermott, W. (Eds.): Cecil-Loeb Textbook of Medicine. 13th ed. Philadelphia, W. B. Saunders Co., 1971, p. 1259.

Kirsner, J. B., Clayman, C. B., and Palmer, W. L.: The problem of gastric ulcer. Arch. Intern. Med., *104*:995, 1959.

Kirsner, J. B., Levin, E., and Palmer, W. L.: Observations on the excessive nocturnal gastric secretion in patients with duodenal ulcer. Gastroenterology, *11*:598, 1948.

Kirsner, J. B., Nutter, P. B., and Palmer, W. L.: Studies on anacidity: The hydrogen-ion concentration of the gastric secretion, the gastroscopic appearance of the gastric mucosa and the presence of a gastric secretory depressant in patients with anacidity. J. Clin. Invest., *14*:619, 1940.

Kirsner, J. B., and Palmer, W. L.: Symposium on Peptic Ulcer. Multiple authors. Amer. J. Med., *29*:5, 1960.

Lipkin, M.: In "defence" of the gastric mucosa. Gut, *12*:599, 1971.

Littman, A.: The Veterans Administration cooperative study on gastric ulcer. Gastroenterology, *61 (part 2)*:567, 1971.

McConnell, R. B.: Genetics and gastroenterology – progress report. Gut, *12*:592, 1971.

McGuigan, J. E.: On antibodies to gastrin: concerning their production, behavioural characteristics and uses. Gut, *11*:363, 1970.

McGuigan, J. E.: Personal communication, 1971.

McGuigan, J. E., and Greider, M. H.: Correlative immunochemical and light microscopic studies of the gastrin cell of the antral mucosa. Gastroenterology, *60*:223, 1970.

Menguy, R.: Pathophysiology of peptic ulcer. Amer. J. Surg., *120*:282, 1970.

Naik, S. R., Bajaj, S. C., Goyal, R. K., Gupta, D. N., and Chuttani, H. K.: Parietal cell mass in healthy human stomachs. Gastroenterology, *61*:682, 1971.

Palmer, W. L.: The "acid test" in gastric and duodenal ulcer. J.A.M.A., *89*:1778, 1927.

Palmer, W. L.: Causality in peptic ulcer. Arch. Intern. Med., *106*:786, 1960.

Prolla, J. C., Kobayashi, S., and Kirsner, J. B.: Gastric cancer. Arch. Intern. Med., *124*:238, 1969.

Samloff, I. M.: Pepsinogens, pepsins and pepain inhibitors. Gastroenterology, *60*:586, 1970.

Schrager, J.: The chemical composition and function of gastrointestinal mucus. Gut, *11*:450, 1970.

Silen, W.: Personal communication, 1972.

Smith, B. M., Skillman, J. J., Edwards, B. G., and Silen, W.: Permeability of the human gastric mucosa. New Eng. J. Med., *285*:716, 1971.

Snyder, N., III, Scurry, M. T., and Deiss, W. P., Jr.: Five families with multiple endocrine adenomatosis. Ann. Intern. Med., *76*:53, 1972.

Taylor, K. B.: Gastritis. New Eng. J. Med., *280*:818, 1970.

Trudeau, W. L., and McGuigan, J. E.: Serum gastrin levels in patients with peptic ulcer disease. Gastroenterology, *59*:6, 1970.

Twomey, J. J., Jordan, P. H., Jr., Laughter, A. H., Meuwissen, H. J., and Good, R. A.: The gastric disorder in immunoglobulin-deficient patients. Ann. Intern. Med., *72*:499, 1970.

Wermer, P.: Endocrine adenomatosis and peptic ulcer in a large kindred. Amer. J. Med., *35*:205, 1963.

Yalow, R. S., and Berson, S. A.: Further studies on the nature of immunoreactive gastrin in human plasma. Gastroenterology, *60*:203, 1970.

Yalow, R. S., and Berson, S. A.: Radioimmunoassay of gastrin. Gastroenterology, *58*:1, 1970.

Zollinger, R. M., and Ellison, E. H.: Primary peptic ulceration of the jejunum associated with islet cell tumors of the pancreas. Ann. Surg., *142*:709, 1955.

CHAPTER 26 THE SMALL INTESTINE

DAVID W. WATSON
WILLIAM A. SODEMAN, Jr.

The small intestine is a complex tube whose structure is well designed to subserve such seemingly diverse but related functions as the aboral transport of luminal contents, the secretion of enzymes and hormones, the digestion and absorption of ingested materials, and the mounting of an immune response. These functions are modified by neurohumoral influences and are materially aided by contributions from the pancreas and hepatobiliary system. The primary function of the small bowel, however, is digestion and absorption. All other activities either regulate or facilitate this process.

The pathophysiologist seeks to explain the signs or symptoms of intestinal disease in terms of an alteration in this structure and these functions. Implicit in such an undertaking is an understanding of normal structure and function and the manner in which they are modified by those processes which we call disease. In the small intestine, as elsewhere, structure and function are intimately though not always obviously related, and the greater our knowledge of how this relationship operates to ensure the gut's contribution to health the easier it will be to predict the consequences of changes induced by disease.

Although our understanding of small intestinal pathophysiology has increased, many unanswered questions remain. This discussion is based upon information that is firmly established for the human small intestine and does not present concepts based solely upon presumably parallel animal models, however applicable they may appear. Sufficient species differences in small bowel structure and function exist so as to make such carte blanche applications hazardous.

We will present an outline of normal structure from the gross to the electron microscopic level and discuss normal function and abnormal structure-function relationships as they apply to motor function, digestion and absorption, secretion, and immune responses. Circulatory disturbances have wide-ranging effects involving several of the aforementioned functions and will be discussed separately.

NORMAL STRUCTURE

By means of postmortem measurements the length of the small intestine has been estimated to be 6.5 to 7.0 meters. In life, however, tubes 3 meters long may pass into the cecum. Its caliber diminishes slightly from duodenum to terminal ileum, in part accounting for the fact that foreign bodies such as gallstones more frequently obstruct the lower ileum. The division of the small bowel into duodenum (20 to 30 cm.), jejunum (2.5 meters) and ileum (3.5 meters) is imprecise and based upon rather slight modifications of structure and relatively more important differences in function. Certain of the latter, such as the absorption of monosaccharides, amino acids, and β-monoglycerides, occur mainly in the jejunum. Other portions of the small intestine, however, can to a large extent compensate for loss of this segment. On the other hand, the physiologic absorption of vitamin B_{12} and the active transport of bile salts are exclusive functions of the terminal ileum.

The wall of the small bowel is composed of four basic layers: the mucosa, submucosa, muscularis externa, and serosa. The mucosa is composed of an epithelial cell layer with its filamentous basement membrane, a lamina propria containing blood vessels, lymphatics, smooth muscle cells, nerve fibers, plasma cells, lymphocytes, fibroblasts, eosinophils, macrophages, reticular cells, mast cells, collagen, and reticular fibrils and is separated from the submucosa by the muscularis mucosa. The submucosa contains larger blood vessels, lymphatics, more connective tissue, nerves and ganglia, and more lymphoid elements. The muscularis externa is divided into an inner circular layer and an outer longitudinal layer of smooth muscle, with the myenteric plexus interspersed between the two. In the past the longitudinal muscle has been described as a long, drawn-out spiral and the circular layer as a tight spiral. More recent studies indicate that fibers in both layers deviate from a strictly longitudinal or circular orientation at random, both right and left, so that the net direction in the two layers is axial and circumferential.

The small intestine is distinguished by three and possibly four structural features which together enormously increase its luminal surface area. The valvulae conniventes are circumferential folds of mucosa and submucosa absent from the duodenal bulb but prominent in the duodenum and jejunum, and disappearing in the mid-ileum. They are responsible for the feathery appearance of the small bowel on barium studies and constitute the transverse folds seen in plane x-rays of air-filled intestine. The villi are projections of mucosa, readily discernible with a hand lens, which are usually fingerlike or leaflike but under some conditions appear as ridges or convolutions. Figure 26-1 is an illustration of villi as viewed with the scanning electron microscope. The individual cells of the villi and to a lesser extent the crypts possess filamentous microvilli, which in turn are coated with a finely filamentous material or "fuzz."

The mucosal crypts lie between the villi and extend basally to the muscularis mucosa. This relationship is depicted in Figure 26-2. In normal Americans and Europeans the villi constitute two thirds to three fifths of the mucosal thickness and the crypts two fifths to one third. As many as 20 crypts surround each villus but a functional ratio of 3:1 seems likely.

The surfaces of the villi and the linings of the crypts are covered by a continuous single layer of five different types of columnar cells: goblet cells, Paneth cells, enterochromaffin cells, undifferentiated crypt cells, and the differentiated villous epithelial cells (enterocytes or absorptive cells).

The majority of cells in the crypts are undifferentiated cells which have a high mitotic index. They have numerous ribosomes and polysomes but little endoplasmic reticulum, scant microvilli, and undeveloped terminal webs. Although they contain what appear to be secretory granules no secretory function has been established and their main purpose is to serve as a source of

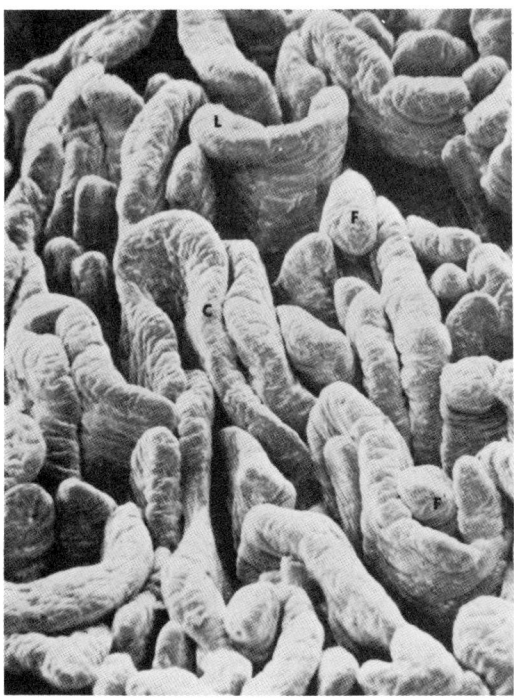

Figure 26-1 *A*, Human jejunal biopsy. Scanning electron micrograph (SEM) showing a leaf-shaped villus, *L;* finger-shaped villi, *F;* and a convolution, *C*. Surface creases can be distinguished (× 110). *B*, Human jejunal biopsy. SEM of part of the surface of a single villus. The mouths of two goblet cells are prominent and the hexagonal cell outlines are clearly seen (× 2300). (Toner, P. G., and Carr, K. E.: J. Path., *97*:611, 1969.)

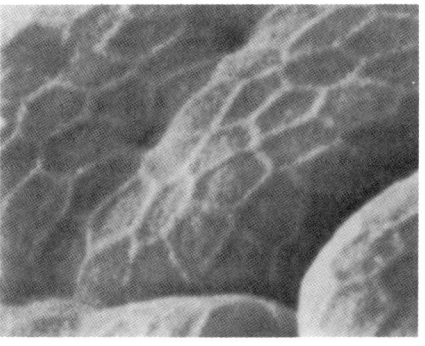

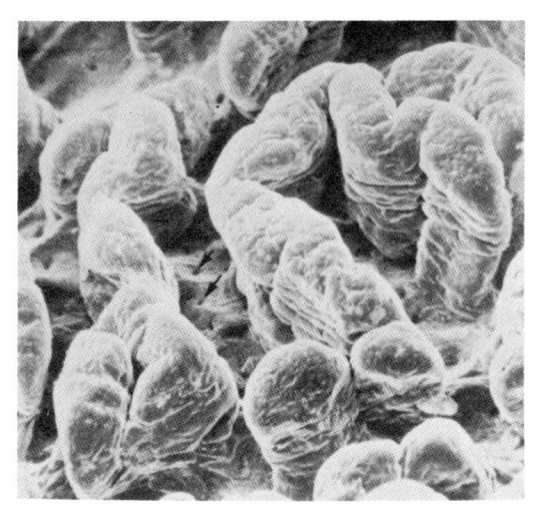

Figure 26-2 Human duodenal biopsy. SEM showing various shapes of villi. The mouths of intestinal crypts opening into the circumvillar basin are arrowed (× 210). (Toner, P. G., and Carr, K. E.: J. Path., 97:611, 1969.)

the differentiated epithelial cell types. Newly formed cells migrate up the crypts and as they reach the junction of the crypt and villus they undergo morphologic, biochemical, and functional maturation to become villous absorptive cells, goblet cells, or Paneth cells. The origin of the enterochromaffin cells is less certain. During this migration-maturation process the differentiating cells develop larger and more numerous microvilli, a well-demarcated terminal web, more numerous mitochrondria and rough endoplasmic reticulum, and there is a decrease in free ribosomes and polysomes, loss of secretory granules, and the formation of large apical dense bodies which represent lysosomal derivatives. As these cells differentiate into villous absorptive cells they acquire enzymes, receptors, and carriers essential for the final phases of digestion and the processes of absorption. Cells migrating up the villus continually push the older, more differentiated cells toward the villous tip, from which they are eventually extruded into the lumen. This renewal process is accomplished in a period of 3 to 7 days.

The absorptive cells are the most numerous and functionally most important cells on the villous surface. They are simple columnar cells in which the luminal surface is specialized to form a striated or brush border. This brush border is composed of microvilli ranging in length from 0.75 to 1.50 micron and in width from 0.10 to 0.20 micron. They number 3000 to 6500 per cell and are closely and regularly spaced with an intervillous distance of 0.01 to 0.05 micron. They are enclosed by an extension of the same trilaminar-appearing plasma membrane that surrounds the remainder of the cell. The microvillous core contains a central zone of 10 to 50 closely packed parallel filaments or tubules extending from the microvillous tip to the terminal web, which is the area just basal to the microvilli. It contains no organelles but only nonparallel tubular filaments similar to those in the microvilli and a few structures termed apical vesicles, thought to represent lysosomes. These tubular filaments are smaller and quite distinct from the cytoplasmic microtubules which lie roughly parallel to the long axis of the absorptive cell in the supranuclear cytoplasm. The microvillous plasma membrane is coated with a strongly adherent, filamentous "fuzz" termed the glycocalyx. It is composed of a sulfated, weakly acidic mucopolysaccharide which appears to be continuously synthesized by the Golgi apparatus of the epithelial cell, transported to the microvillous surface, and eventually shed into the lumen. The glycocalyx is most prominent on the absorptive cells, especially at the villous tips. Figure 26-3 illustrates the fine structural relationships of these cells.

The microvillous plasma membrane and its glycocalyx constitute a digestive-absorptive unit. Several enzymes have been localized to this structure, including alkaline phosphatase, the disaccharidases, aminopeptidases, dipeptidases, adenosine triphosphatase, thiamine triphosphatase, and folic acid conjugase. The active transport of glucose, galactose, and amino acids as well as the uptake of the vitamin B_{12}-intrinsic factor complex is mediated by receptors and carriers localized to this region.

The epithelial cells covering the villi and lining the crypts are joined at their lateral margins by a junctional complex composed of three parts. Just basal to the origin of the microvilli the outer leaflets of the lateral plasma membranes fuse to form the tight junction (zonula occludens). Just basal to this lies the intermediate junction (zonula adherens) and beneath it the desmosome (macula adherens), so named because the cytoplasm underlying the plasma membrane at this point is condensed. These latter two structures represent only close approximations of the plasma membranes, not fusion. The epithelial cells with their junctional complexes form a tight unbroken membrane lining the luminal surface of the small intestine.

This epithelial membrane is a complex dynamic "organ" regulating the flux of materials between the lumen and the lamina propria. Its integrity depends upon the continual replication, maturation, and metabolism of its cells. Interruption of any of these vital processes will lead to a failure of this organ, which will usually be expressed as a malabsorption syndrome.

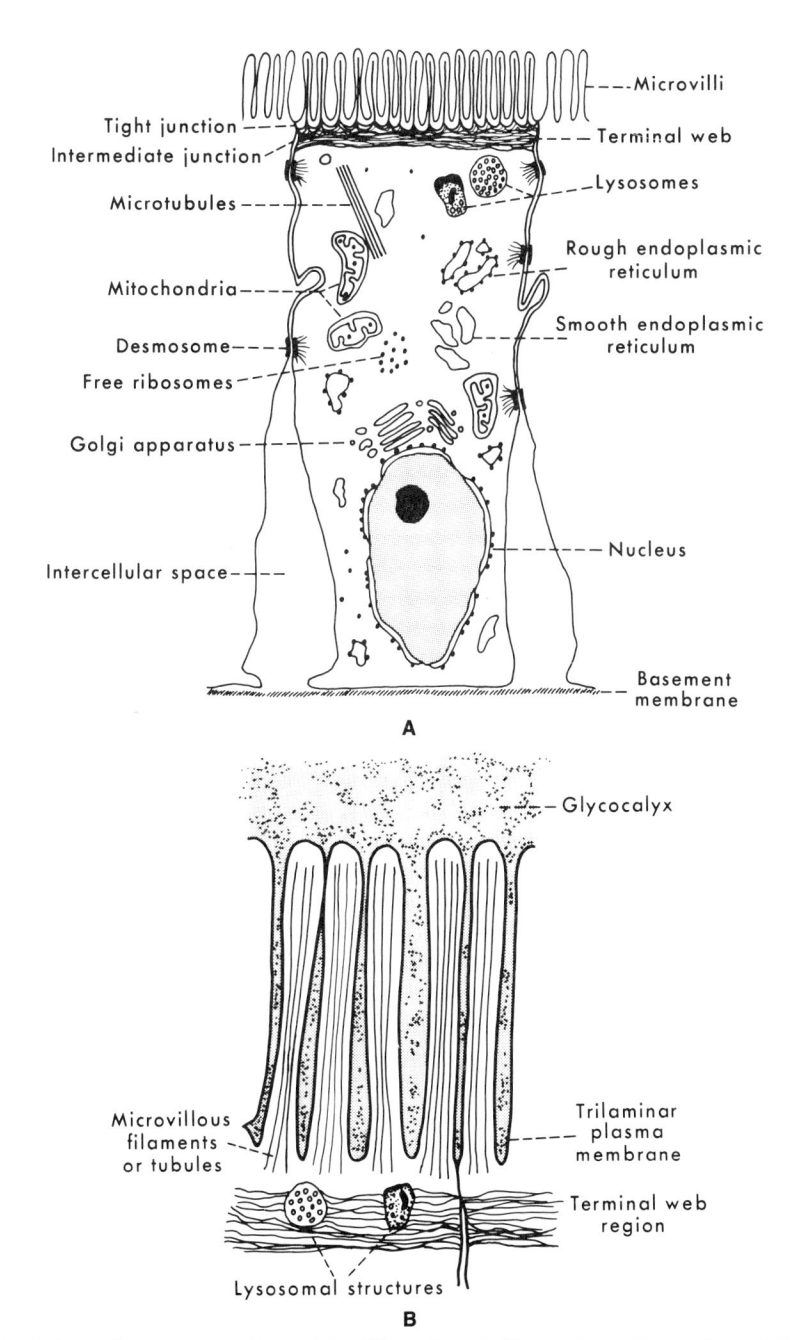

Figure 26–3 Schematic representation of A, differentiated villous absorptive cell, and B, the glycocalyx-microvillus structure.

MOTOR FUNCTION

Normal Motor Function

The overall concept of small intestinal motor activity becomes more meaningful when it is not viewed as the primary function of the small bowel but rather as complementary to the organ's major activity. To facilitate the digestive-absorptive process, small intestinal movements must do two things: mix ingested materials with pancreatic and hepatobiliary secretions and propel luminal contents from one end to the other at a rate suitable for both optimal absorption and the continuing entry of gastric contents. Normally this rate is approximately 1 cm. per minute, and as a result the residue from the previous meal leaves the ileum at about the same time the next meal enters the stomach. An understanding of how these two activities are accomplished requires a consideration of the electrical and contractile events taking place in the small intestine.

Intestinal smooth muscle exhibits spontaneous contractions, can be stimulated by stretch, and will conduct impulses independently of nerves. Its resting membrane potential is unstable and varies irregularly with basal tension and the general level of contractile activity, but it also fluctuates in two consistent patterns. The first is a rhythmically occurring, omnipresent fluctuation arising in the longitudinal muscle and identified as either the slow wave, the basic electrical rhythm (BER), or the pacesetter potential. As visualized by Code et al., if at any one instant the electrical activity of the small bowel could be stopped or frozen in place, each slow wave or pacesetter potential would be fixed in the wall and would extend over a distance which may be termed its cycle length or wavelength for that particular segment. The bowel beneath each cycle would then represent a physiologic motor unit, with the slow wave prescribing its dimensions and controlling the nature of motor activity occurring within it at any one instant. These pacesetter potentials evoke no muscular contractions themselves but instead govern the rate at which the second type of electrical activity may take place. These are termed spike potentials and are responsible for the contractions of the circular muscle. Spike potentials can only occur during the periods of maximal depolarization of the pacesetter potentials. This relationship between pacesetter potentials, spike potentials, and circular muscle contraction is presented in Figure 26-4.

The pacesetter potential passes caudally as a sheath or ring whose front constitutes a rapid depolarization reaching all circumferential points simultaneously. An intact intrinsic nerve plexus is required for this to occur. Its frequency is rather constant with time but displays a declining gradient over the small bowel from 11.8 cycles per minute in the duodenum and first 10 cm. of the jejunum to 9.0 cycles per minute in the ileum. This decline may be stepwise through a sequence of frequency plateaus, each representing the distance traversed by the pacesetter potentials originating in that segment, but there is no agreement on this point. Since pacesetter potentials of a given frequency pass over relatively long segments and exhibit this declining frequency, they serve to integrate the activity of the whole organ.

The conduction of either pacesetter or spike potentials is made possible by tight side-to-side or end-to-end junctions between the individual muscle cells. These nexuses represent a partial fusion of the outer leaflets of the trilaminar plasma membranes and provide low resistance electrical shunts between cells.

The pacesetter potential therefore sets the frequency but not the magnitude of circular muscle contraction. An alteration in frequency of the pacesetter potential may be brought about in several ways. Duodenal compression or transection causes a decrease in frequency distal to the injury. A decrease in frequency is also seen with hypothermia, hypothyroidism, hypoglycemia, malabsorption syndromes, substances interfering with active membrane transport, and damage to the intrinsic nerve plexuses. Serotonin, Pituitrin, and Pitressin also cause a decrease in frequency, the latter two by reducing blood supply to the

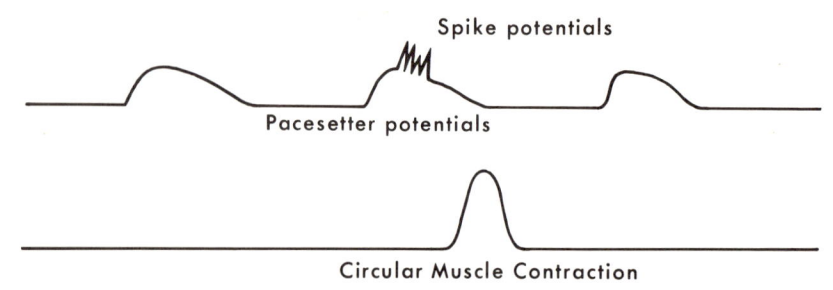

Figure 26-4 Digrammatic presentation of the relationship between pacesetter potentials, spike potentials, and circular muscle contraction.

longitudinal muscle. An increase in frequency occurs with pyrexia, hyperthyroidism, adrenergic stimulation, and morphine administration. Pacesetter potentials are relatively insensitive to drugs, and cholinergics, anticholinergics, and topical anesthetics are mostly without effect. Extrinsic nerve stimulation, the ingestion of food, and changes in electrolyte concentrations also have little or no effect on the frequency of pacesetter potentials.

Spike potentials are the electrical counterparts of circular muscle contraction and therefore are associated with luminal pressure changes. They are not propagated and their sequential occurrence in successive segments (peristalsis?) is due rather to propagation of the pacesetter potentials to which they are coupled. Not every pacesetter potential need evoke a spike potential but the frequency of spike potentials can never exceed the frequency of pacesetter potentials. The latter are conducted from their origin in the longitudinal muscle to the circular muscle probably via the nexuses.

The electrical response, if any, of the circular muscle to a given pacesetter potential is governed by an interplay of influences provided by the activity of the intrinsic nerve plexuses acting as part of local or central reflexes and various circulating or locally produced hormones. The amplitude of circular muscle contraction is proportional to the number, duration, and amplitude of the spike potentials. The factors which influence the generation of spike potentials are somewhat different from those that alter the frequency of pacesetter potentials. Spike potentials are initiated by rapid radial stretch or distention of the bowel wall, vagal stimulation, and ingestion of food. In contrast to pacesetter potentials, spike potentials are relatively sensitive to the effects of drugs, hormones, and other pharmacologically active substances. They are initiated by cholinergic drugs, hydrochloric acid, serotonin, and morphine and are eliminated by anticholinergics, ganglionic blocking agents, barbiturates, and sympathomimetics. Mechanical obstruction at first results in an increase in spike potentials proximal to the obstruction and a decrease distally. Anoxia causes an initial stimulation but eventually results in their disappearance.

Although coordinated intestinal motor activity may occur in the absence of extrinsic autonomic innervation this system is important in modifying motor activity in relationship to other physiologic responses within the body. Unfortunately, its structure and function are still not well understood. The vagi contain motor preganglionic parasympathetic fibers making synaptic connections with secondary parasympathetic motor neurons in the subserosal, myenteric, and submucosal plexuses. Postganglionic sympathetics also traverse the vagi but their termination is unclear. Motor fibers in the splanchnic nerves are preganglionic sympathetic fibers terminating in the abdominal sympathetic ganglia and postganglionic sympathetic fibers arising in the paravertebral ganglia. Postganglionic sympathetic fibers are then distributed to the gut with branches of the associated arteries. Their sites of termination are not known, although some catecholamine-containing fibers form meshes around cholinergic ganglion cells and others enter the muscle layers. Sensory nerves travel in both systems, with vagal fibers originating in the unipolar cells of the nodose ganglion. The nerve cells lying within the gut are postganglionic parasympathetic or internuncial neurons and perhaps cells with sensory function, although no specialized neural structures have been identified as sensory. The enteric plexuses appear to be interconnected but the anatomic relationship between fibers originating in them and secretory and smooth muscle cells is unknown.

The influence of extrinsic nerve stimulation on spike potentials is imperfectly understood, and for the present only the following generalization can be made. In the absence of significant small intestinal activity both parasympathetic and sympathetic stimulation initiate spike potentials, whereas an actively contracting bowel tends to be inhibited. The small intestine contains both alpha- and beta-adrenergic receptors. Alpha receptors have an affinity for epinephrine and act to eliminate spike potentials. Beta receptors bind isoproterenol and, in the duodenum at least, their stimulation tends to elicit spike potentials, but the remainder of the intact human small intestine has not been adequately studied. Alpha receptors predominate in the small bowel, and the net effect of either alpha or beta stimulation is an inhibition of small intestinal smooth muscle activity. How this is mediated in the case of beta receptors is not clear.

Apart from serving as a source of pacesetter potentials, the contribution of the longitudinal muscle layer to small intestinal motor function is not well understood. No electrical events corresponding to its contraction have been recorded. Current views suggest that it serves largely to regulate the overall "tone" of the bowel wall and the caliber of its lumen, its contraction producing a net increase in luminal diameter and thereby a decrease in pressure.

Little is known about the electrochemical events involved in the contractile process. It appears that the release of calcium ions from a site of storage triggers contraction. The term smooth is not strictly apt, however, since faint striations are in fact present as uniform small filaments of actin. Myosin has also been identified in "smooth" muscle but its location is unknown.

The interaction of these electrical and contractile events under the direction of various local and systemic neurohumoral influences results in intestinal *motility*. This is an ambiguous term at best, however, and may refer to movements of the bowel wall, smooth muscle contraction, luminal pressure changes, or propulsion of luminal contents. Since circular muscle contraction and the rate of flow of luminal contents may have an inverse relationship, the term becomes self-contradictory. The ambiguity is further compounded by adding the prefixes hyper and hypo. From the standpoint of small intestinal function, only two types of motor activity are important—mixing and propulsion, which correspond grossly to Type I and Type III waves, as seen in motility records.

Mixing is accomplished predominantly by Type I waves occurring either as isolated stationary "standing ring" contractions of circular muscle involving a 1 to 2 cm. segment of bowel or as a series of such contractions, referred to as rhythmic segmentation. This latter type of motor pattern is diagrammatically represented in Figure 26–5. Segmenting activity decreases in frequency from the duodenum to the ileum, and although it is the predominant type of activity recordable, it is present only 2 per cent of the time in the resting small intestine. Segmenting contractions are more frequent after a meal or following morphine administration and have the effect of slowing transmit. In patients with rapid transit, segmenting activity is decreased.

Flow through the alimentary canal can be thought of as analogous to flow through the vascular system, albeit more complex and less well understood. Both systems possess pacemakers, pressure receptors, and osmoreceptors, and flow is enhanced as viscosity decreases. The rate at which intestinal contents move through the small intestine is dependent upon a pressure gradient generated by the bowel wall and the peripheral resistance of the gut. The resistance varies with the diameter of the lumen and the contractility or tone of the intestinal wall. The prime regulator of transit, however, is peripheral resistance. Precisely how this resistance is varied and in what manner contractile activity is ordered to bring about the required pressure differential for transit to occur is still a matter of debate. Peristalsis, a moving ring contraction, is controversial. It must occur infrequently and over short distances, if at all, since normally it takes several hours for contents to traverse the small bowel. There is no quantitative information about the frequency, velocity, or range of movement of peristalsis in the human small intestine. The so-called "peristaltic rush" connotes a vigorous ring contraction progressing rapidly from the duodenum to the ileum. Its existence is debated and if it does occur it is probably always pathologic. Some aboral movement of contents will occur with isolated or rhythmic segmenting contractions. As Texter has pointed out, the aboral transport of luminal contents is more closely related to the pressure gradient between proximal and distal segments than to the activity of any single type of contraction. With the probable exception of waves that progress over a considerable distance (peristalsis) and of rhythmic sequences, pressure waves contribute more to the increase of peripheral resistance than to the promotion of propulsion. Since there is a progressive decrease in the level of activity in sequentially more distal segments of the small intestine, the resulting gradient probably constitutes the most important mechanism for transit. It is therefore the total motor pattern of the entire small bowel that underlies transit rather than any one or another specific kind of contractile activity. A generalized increase in activity will just as effec-

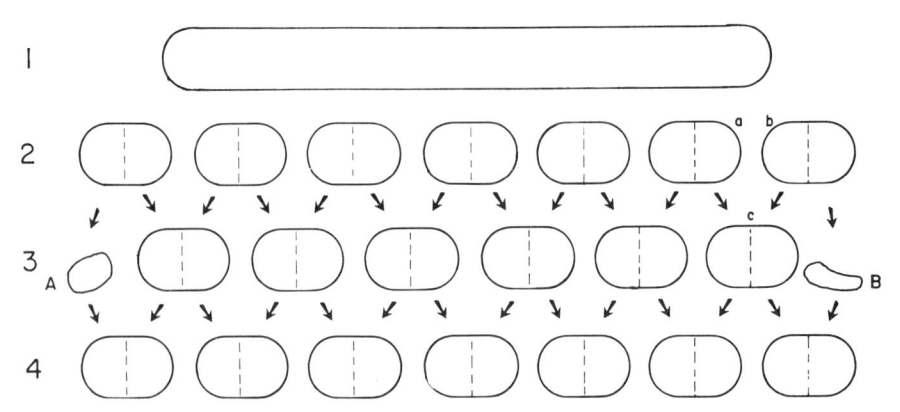

Figure 26–5 Diagram representing process of rhythmic segmentation. Rows 1, 2, 3, and 4 indicate sequence of appearances in loop. Dotted lines mark regions of division. Arrows show relation of particles to segments they subsequently form. (Hightower, N. C., Jr.: *In* Code, C. F. (Ed.): Handbook of Physiology. Vol. IV. Washington, D.C., American Physiological Society, 1968.)

tively retard transit as complete atony, since in neither case will a pressure gradient be produced.

Abnormal Motor Function

Without a satisfactory knowledge of normal motor function an understanding of pathologic processes must also be incomplete. Furthermore, the definition of abnormal motor function depends upon one's point of view. To the physiologist it is an alteration of smooth muscle contractility; the radiologist finds it reflected in some abnormality of the distribution and movement of barium; those interested in "motility" patterns will be impressed by unusual fluctuations in intraluminal pressures, while the physician at the proverbial bedside wonders about the origin of abdominal pain, constipation, and diarrhea. Unfortunately it is not possible to describe any consistent or reproducible relationship between these different kinds of measurements, and in many instances signs and symptoms of altered function remain largely unexplained.

On the clinical level, disturbed motor function will be manifest primarily as abdominal pain or some alteration in transit perceived as constipation or diarrhea. The only known stimulus for pain production in the small bowel is an increase in intramural tension. Distention therefore will only produce pain when accompanied by significant tone in the intestinal wall or marked contraction involving a relatively broad segment. The intensity of pain is proportional to the rapidity with which the tension develops and its magnitude. Any stimulus capable of eliciting such increases in tension may produce pain. Most commonly they arise as a result of luminal obstruction, vascular insufficiency, ulceration, increased levels of certain pharmacologically active substances or the administration of drugs such as parasympathomimetics or codeine. Whether ulceration and ischemia produce pain by causing secondary intramural tension changes or by some other mechanism is not clear. Like other visceral forms of pain, that arising in the small intestine is not sharply localized. The sensory innervation of the small intestine derives largely from the tenth thoracic spinal segment, and small bowel pain is perceived in the corresponding somatic dermatome. Since pain originating in midline-derived structures tends to be referred to the midline, small bowel pain is characteristically periumbilical, with some spillover into the adjacent supra- and infra-umbilical areas. The increased intramural tension, regardless of cause, tends to wax and wane episodically and therefore the pain is usually described as cramping or colicky. In the presence of a pain-causing lesion, the superimposition of factors contributing to increased motor activity will lead to intensification; for example, the pain of intestinal obstruction or mesenteric vascular insufficiency is more prominent after eating. This classic description is often modified, however, by individual variations in pain threshold, prior abdominal surgical procedures, and the presence of concurrent disease. Although bilateral vagotomy has no effect on pain perception, it appears that bilateral abdominal sympathectomy, like midthoracic cord lesions, may reduce or abolish it.

Diarrhea and constipation as expressions of altered motor function cannot be as readily interpreted in terms of small intestinal disease or transit times. They are described by events occurring or not occurring at the anal opening, and interposed between this point of awareness and the small bowel are the colon and rectum. Transit times through the small bowel vary within a wide range under presumably normal conditions and only extremes will be manifest as an alteration in bowel habit. Complete obstruction of the small bowel will eventually lead to constipation. Partial obstruction may do so as well, but not infrequently the process causing the partial obstruction leads to more rapid emptying of the small bowel and colon distal to the obstruction, causing diarrhea.

The small intestine may initiate diarrhea in two ways: by exposing the colon to intestinal contents at a rate-volume relationship which exceeds its absorptive capacity or by allowing the entry into the colon of substances stimulating rapid emptying as may occur in the malabsorption syndromes. Small intestinal causes of diarrhea which are the result of abnormalities involving secretion (for example, cholera) or malabsorption (for example, nontropical sprue) will be discussed in relationship to the pathophysiology of those disorders.

Lesions which do reflect primarily, although not exclusively, abnormal motor function include obstruction, ileus, and humoral influences provided by the products of certain tumors and endocrine disorders.

Obstruction and Ileus. The term obstruction should be reserved for partial or complete occlusion of the intestinal lumen, regardless of cause. Simple obstruction implies luminal occlusion only, whereas a strangulating obstruction involves both luminal occlusion and interference with blood supply. Closed loop obstruction implies a segment of intestine with its lumen occluded at both ends. Ileus, on the other hand, refers to an adynamic state of the intestine occurring either segmentally or throughout its entire length.

Small intestinal obstruction may follow external compression from tumors or abscesses, torsion or volvulus usually in relationship to a fibrous adhesion, intussusception, intramural fibrosis as in Crohn's disease, intramural hemorrhage or edema, intraluminal tumors, or foreign bodies such as gallstones. The manifestations of an obstruction depend upon its site, degree, duration, rapidity of development, and whether or not it is a simple, closed loop or strangulating obstruction.

When the obstruction is in the duodenum or proximal jejunum, distention is slight and there is early vomiting of large amounts of bile-stained fluid. With lesions of the lower jejunum and ileum, distention is often marked by the time vomiting of fecal-appearing material occurs. Periumbilical, cramping pain is the most prominent symptom. With complete obstruction, constipation is usual, but with partial obstruction, diarrhea or constipation may be present. Bowel sounds are more frequent and often of higher pitch in partial obstructions and early in complete obstruction, with increases in intensity often coinciding with crescendos of pain. Abdominal examination in the patient with early simple obstruction usually discloses only distention, occasional visible contractile activity, and the auscultatory findings mentioned. Percussion may reveal increased resonance but this will depend upon the relative amounts of fluid and gas within the bowel lumen. Signs of peritonitis appear rapidly with strangulating obstructions, somewhat later in untreated closed loop obstructions, and relatively late in untreated simple obstructions. Although rigidity of the abdominal wall signifies peritonitis, rebound tenderness may be elicited with a distended, inflamed bowel in the abscence of actual peritoneal inflammation.

Acute obstructions are usually the result of torsion or volvulus, intussusception, or herniation. Chronic obstructions are more often due to inflammatory strictures or tumors. The more slowly the obstruction develops, the more indolent and less pronounced the symptoms will be. In acute, high-grade obstruction as distention progresses, even in a localized segment, the initial intestinal hyperactivity is replaced by generalized ileus. This is due to the activation of alpha- and beta-adrenergic receptors by a sympathoadrenal discharge, with inhibition of contractile activity which can be reversed by propranolol and phenoxybenzamine in the experimental situation.

Chronic partial obstruction leads to generalized protein-calorie malnutrition, but acute obstruction causes marked abnormalities of fluid and electrolyte balance.

In contrast to obstruction, ileus represents inadequate or absent propulsive motor activity occurring segmentally or throughout the entire small intestine. It occurs with such regularity following abdominal operations that postoperative ileus has been referred to as physiologic ileus even though at times it may represent a mortal complication. More severe and protracted ileus results from bacterial and chemical peritonitis or sudden and usually painful distention of other hollow structures such as the bile ducts, ureters, and urinary bladder. It may also be a sequel to complete or near complete luminal occlusion, intestinal ischemia, or hypokalemia. Ileus under these circumstances has been termed paralytic as opposed to physiologic but the difference is in degree rather than kind. All true ileus can properly be described as adynamic. Reference has occasionally been made to something called dynamic ileus, supposedly representing functional obstruction due to intestinal spasm. This is a contradiction in terms and it is doubtful that such a condition exists, at least within the small intestine.

In the case of postoperative ileus the stomach may remain atonic for several days but the small intestine usually exhibits activity within a few hours. If the ileus persists, the bowel becomes progressively distended with gas and fluid. The gas is largely swallowed air but colonic bacteria may contribute significant amounts, especially if the small bowel has become colonized.

The most prominent findings in the patient with ileus are those related to the postoperative abdomen or the underlying disease process, usually peritonitis. There is abdominal distention, and bowel sounds are minimal or absent. Signs of dehydration and evidence of ineffective circulating plasma volume may also be present.

It has been known for some time that the gut is not intrinsically paralyzed but is capable of contraction when properly stimulated. Neely and Catchpole have redrawn attention to this fact and have proposed that ileus is due to inhibition of contractile activity by sympathetic overactivity brought about by increased levels of circulating adrenal catecholamines and/or sympathetic nerve stimulation. As previously pointed out, this reaction is mediated by alpha-adrenergic stimulation. The experimental observation that postoperative or paralytic ileus can be prevented by abdominal sympathectomy or splanchnic anesthesia has strengthened this view.

Such a mechanism readily suggests a rational approach to management, first utilizing drugs to block the sympathetic overactivity, followed by parasympathetic stimulation of the "liberated" intestine. Guanethidine and bethanechol, guanethidine and prostigmine, or phentolamine and prostigmine have been utilized with good results. Since guanethidine blocks the release of norepinephrine rather than causing alpha blockade, phentolamine, an alpha blocker, may be required if there are already increased circulating levels of epinephrine and norepinephrine. Since alpha receptors predominate in the small intestine, beta blockers appear not to be required. Patients selected for this therapy must fulfill certain criteria. Hypovolemia must be corrected first to prevent hypotension from sympathetic blockade; electrolyte imbalance, especially hypokalemia, must be managed and intestinal obstruction carefully excluded. Nasogastric suction remains a useful adjunct to minimize distention. Long tubes of the Miller-Abbott type have been employed but it is often difficult to obtain passage through an adynamic gut.

Radiologic examinations utilizing plane films of the abdomen may be of help in substantiating the presence of obstruction or ileus and occasionally in differentiating the two. Dilated air-filled loops of bowel with air-fluid levels are characteristic of both. In ileus the air-filled bowel may not be as dilated as in obstruction but many exceptions will be found. Perhaps most helpful is the distribution pattern of intestinal gas. With ileus, gas is characteristically found throughout the small and large bowel, although not necessarily in a continuous column, whereas in obstruction, gas is usually not evident distal to the occlusion. A localized ileus may mimic obstruction, however. It must be remembered that as the fluid-gas ratio increases, little of note may be seen radiologically.

The consequences of obstruction or ileus are reflected in marked alterations of fluid and electrolyte distribution. The severity of fluid loss and the extent of acid-base derangement depend not only upon the area and amount of bowel involved but also upon the duration of the process. In high obstruction there is external loss through vomiting of large amounts of gastric, pancreatic, biliary, and duodenal secretions, with a lesser amount remaining sequestered within the gastrointestinal lumen. As much as 5 liters may be lost within a 24-hour period. Most commonly a metabolic acidosis develops, since the amount of bicarbonate lost usually exceeds the loss of hydrogen ion. With lower obstructions or generalized ileus, as much as 40 per cent of the circulating blood volume may accumulate within the gut without evidence of external fluid loss. As the bowel distends, there is increasing fluid and electrolyte accumulation within its lumen, representing a shift from the extracellular compartment. This loss is nearly isosmotic with plasma with regard to the concentrations of major ions. It represents both a decrease in insorption and an increase in exsorption. Elevations of intraluminal pressure up to 20 cm. of water increase insorption, but above this level insorption falls off while exsorption continues to increase. The mechanism underlying this effect is unknown. Initially, the serum sodium concentration remains relatively normal but gradually hyponatremia develops as sodium loss exceeds that of water. The reason for this is not clear. Both clinical and experimental observations indicate that hypotonic dehydration leads to more profound circulatory abnormalities than isotonic dehydration. The resulting decrease in plasma volume is at first compensated for by generalized vasoconstriction, so that blood pressure and pulse rate remain normal for a time. When these homeostatic mechanisms are interfered with by general anesthesia, precipitous drops in blood pressure may occur, underscoring the need for preoperative fluid replacement in all patients. Depending upon the stage of the process and the rapidity of its development, various degrees of dehydration and circulatory collapse will be observed. Because of starvation, dehydration, ketosis, loss of alkaline secretions, and declining renal function, a metabolic acidosis develops. If ischemia is present, as in a strangulating obstruction, a profound and often fatal lactic acidosis may occur. Losses of potassium are high and the resulting hypokalemia may contribute to atonicity and distention. The fully developed clinical picture is one of an acutely ill patient exhibiting signs of dehydration, abdominal distention, tachycardia, hypotension, diaphoresis, hemoconcentration, normal or low serum concentrations of sodium and potassium, normal or elevated BUN and serum creatinine, and metabolic acidosis.

Strangulating obstructions develop the same pattern of fluid and electrolyte abnormalities but because of the associated intestinal ischemia also exhibit signs of tissue necrosis. Closed loop obstructions also commonly result in ischemia of the bowel wall as do simple obstructions if they remain untreated for a sufficient length of time. As pointed out by Bynum and Jacobson, however, it is doubtful that increased intraluminal pressure per se can cause ischemic necrosis of the intestine. Decreased flow, mainly involving the mucosa, occurs at pressures above 30 mm. Hg but marked anoxia is prevented by the phenomena of autoregulation and autoregulatory escape (see section on mesenteric vascular disease). Additional factors such as decreases in plasma volume and reflex vasoconstriction are probably of material importance. In simple and closed loop obstructions, venous outflow is usually impeded first, whereas in strangulating obstructions, both arterial and venous occlusion occur early. The result is tissue anoxia, increased capillary permeability, and intramural and mucosal hemorrhage. Intramural edema and marked losses of protein develop and the integrity of the epithelial membrane is disrupted, resulting in bacterial invasion with peritonitis and bacteremia. Progressive ischemia, gangrene, and peritonitis rapidly ensue. This stage is accompanied by high fever and leukocytosis in addition to the previously discussed fluid and electrolyte disturbances. With tissue necrosis and compromised renal function, hypokalemia may be replaced by hyperkalemia. Materials produced by tissue necrosis, hemorrhage, and infection accumulate in the peritoneal cavity and their absorption is a major factor in the profound cardiovascular collapse which too often characterizes the terminal phase of this condition.

Management of patients with intestinal obstruction or ileus requires early recognition of the problem, prompt differentiation of various forms of obstruction and ileus, replacement of fluid and electrolyte losses, correction of acidosis, nasogastric suction to minimize distention, and prompt surgical correction of the obstructing lesion. Therapy with adrenergic blocking agents and parasympathomimetics may be important adjuncts to the successful management of the patient with simple ileus.

Motor Dysfunction Due to Humoral Mechanisms. The electrical and contractile processes which underlie normal intestinal motor function are integrated and modified by various humoral substances, the concentrations of which under certain circumstances may be markedly altered. Hyperthyroidism, hypoparathyroidism, adrenal insufficiency, carcinoid tumors, medullary carcinomas of the thyroid, gastrin-producing tumors of the pancreas (Zollinger-Ellison syndrome), certain nongastrin-producing pancreatic tumors (Verner-Morrison syndrome), and neural crest tumors may be associated with crampy abdominal discomfort and diarrhea, while hypothyroidism and hyperparathyroidism are often characterized by constipation. Carcinoid tumors and medullary carcinomas of the thyroid may be taken as examples of this type of abnormality. It is to be emphasized, however, that most of the above conditions affect small bowel secretion as well as motor activity, so that the clinical expression observed is a net effect of the two processes.

Carcinoids may appear in any entodermally derived tissue or teratomas. In the small intestine they arise from enterochromaffin cells (Kulchitsky cells, argentaffin cells). They are the most common neoplasms of the small intestine, the appendix being the overall most frequent site of origin (53 per cent) followed closely by the jejunum and ileum (28 per cent). The remainder arise in other portions of the gastrointestinal tract, biliary tree, pancreas, ovary, and bronchi. They are generally small, 95 per cent being less than 2 cm. in diameter. Most appear cytologically benign and the only reliable criteria of malignancy are invasion and metastasis. The majority are asymptomatic, being discovered in the course of investigating and treating other conditions such as appendicitis.

Clinical manifestations may be due to ulceration or obstruction or to the carcinoid syndrome. This syndrome occurs most commonly with tumors of the jejunum or ileum which have metastasized to the liver. The pharmacologically active principles of these tumors are inactivated by hepatic enzyme systems and therefore no systemic symptoms will be produced unless tumor tissue can release its products into the systemic circulation. Systemic manifestations include characteristic attacks of flushing involving the head, neck, and upper trunk, at times precipitated by eating, alcohol, emotion, or pressure on the tumor; abdominal cramping pain and diarrhea; bronchoconstriction; right-sided heart failure; and pellagra-like skin lesions and ascites. Usually only a few of these features are present intermittently in any one patient.

The tumors are known to contain serotonin, 5-hydroxytryptophan, kallikreins, histamine, and ACTH. Increased serotonin levels are probably responsible for the increased intestinal motor activity and diarrhea as well as the endocardial fibrosis leading to pulmonary and tricuspid valve deformity. The metabolic pathway of serotonin is presented in Figure 26–6. Serotonin lowers the excitation threshold of intestinal smooth muscle, resulting in increased responsiveness to otherwise inadequate stimuli. In keeping with this mechanism is the sometimes beneficial effect of serotonin antagonists such as methysergide or cyproheptadine and the deleterious response to monoamine oxidase inhibitors. Improvement may also occur with p-chlorophenylalanine, which inhibits the hydroxylation of tryptophan and is the rate-limiting step in serotonin synthesis, or, with methyldopa, a decarboxylase inhibitor. Serotonin is known to produce fibroblastic proliferation and its administration to experimental animals has resulted in endocardial lesions similar to those encountered in patients. Serotonin is metabolized primarily in the liver and lungs to 5-hydroxyindoleacetic acid, and increased urinary excretion of the latter is presumptive evidence for the

TRYPTOPHAN
↓ tryptophan 5-hydroxylase
5-HYDROXYTRYPTOPHAN
↓ aromatic L-amino acid decarboxylase
5-HYDROXYTRYPTAMINE (SEROTONIN)
↓ monoamine oxidase
5-HYDROXYINDOLE ACETALDEHYDE
↓ aldehyde dehydrogenase
5-HYDROXYINDOLE ACETIC ACID

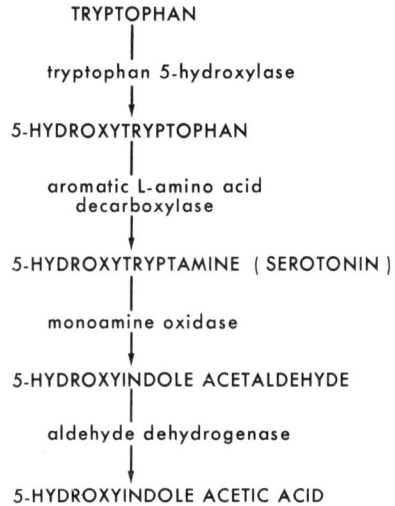

Figure 26–6 Outline of tryptophan metabolism.

presence of a functioning carcinoid. Slight increases in urinary 5-hydroxyindoleacetic acid, however, may be found after the ingestion of foods high in serotonin such as bananas, tomatoes, avocados, red plums, walnuts, and eggplant. Cough syrups containing glyceryl guaiacolate may cause false positive reactions for 5-hydroxyindoleacetic acid, and patients with nontropical sprue may exhibit slight elevations. The pellagra-like syndrome seen in some patients results from the diversion of large amounts of tryptophan to serotonin synthesis.

The substances responsible for the attacks of flushing and bronchoconstriction are less certain. Serotonin appears to be a less likely cause than histamine or bradykinin. Increases in circulating bradykinin levels are brought about by the mechanism outlined in Figure 26–7. Since epinephrine may provoke flushing as well as release kallikreins from tumor tissue, alpha-adrenergic blocking agents may ameliorate flushing by blocking their release.

Efforts to treat the various components of the syndrome are worthwhile even if only partially successful, since the average duration of life from the onset of symptoms to death is 8 years, with a 21 per cent 5-year survival for patients with liver metastases.

The most recent substances to be incriminated in disturbances of intestinal motor activity are the prostaglandins. They are derivatives of prostanoic acid and occur in four forms, designated E, F, A, and B, which differ in the structure of the attached 5-membered carbon ring. Although no clear role for prostaglandins in normal gut motor physiology has been demonstrated, types E and F do affect intestinal smooth muscle function. Prostaglandins $F_{1\alpha}$ and $F_{2\alpha}$ generally cause contraction of both longitudinal and circular muscle, and prostaglandins E_1 and E_2 produce contraction of longitudinal muscle and inhibition of circular muscle. The intravenous infusion of E_1 in man causes abdominal cramps and $F_{2\alpha}$ results in diarrhea. The F series act via a direct effect on circular muscle, while the E compounds affect longitudinal muscle directly as well as stimulate cholinergic nerve fibers within the small intestine. The resulting net effect is smooth muscle contraction. Some medullary carcinomas of the thyroid and neural crest tumors contain large amounts of prostaglandins E_1 and $F_{2\alpha}$ and patients often exhibit increased blood levels of these substances and have diarrhea. Since the prostaglandins probably also augment intestinal secretion via cyclic AMP, this may further contribute to the diarrhea in such patients.

Such conditions, such as scleroderma, appear to interfere with normal intestinal motor responses by structurally altering smooth muscle. Others, like diabetes mellitus, may affect function by way of lesions involving the autonomic nerve supply

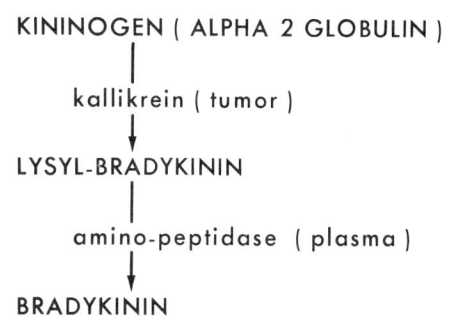

KININOGEN (ALPHA 2 GLOBULIN)
↓ kallikrein (tumor)
LYSYL-BRADYKININ
↓ amino-peptidase (plasma)
BRADYKININ

Figure 26–7 Outline of bradykinin formation.

(autonomic neuropathy, diabetic enteropathy). There is no general agreement, however, on the underlying pathophysiologic mechanisms involved.

DIGESTIVE-ABSORPTIVE FUNCTION

Advances in our knowledge of normal digestive and absorptive mechanisms have enabled the physician to understand better the pathophysiology of the different malabsorption syndromes. The terms digestion and absorption merely emphasize different phases of a single continuing process initiated by events taking place within the small intestinal lumen and completed by the specialized functions of the villous absorptive cell, the plasma membrane of which maintains differences in composition and electrical charge between the luminal and intracellular environment by influencing the rates at which molecules enter the cell. The differences between the function of this membrane at the cell's apical and basal surfaces result in a net movement of molecules through the cell which we call absorption.

Substances traverse this membrane by processes having different kinetics and energy requirements. These transport mechanisms include passive diffusion, nonionic diffusion, carrier-mediated transport, facilitated transport, and exchange diffusion. The term active or "uphill" transport is best used in a general sense to refer to a process requiring energy and coupled directly to cellular metabolism. Net movement is usually but not invariably against a concentration gradient and electrochemical potential difference. In this sense, only carrier-mediated processes constitute true active transport. Passive diffusion is movement due solely to the kinetic energy and electrical charge of molecules and the electrical field in which they exist. Free fatty acids and beta-monoglycerides are examples of substances absorbed by this mechanism. Nonionic diffusion suggests the association between an anion and cation on one side of a membrane with the complex then crossing the membrane and dissociating on the opposite side to the original anion and cation. The net effect is the transfer of ionized compounds. In contrast to passive diffusion, nonionic diffusion accounts for the movement of a charged species independent of the electrical potential difference. Such processes are highly dependent on the H^+ concentration, however. This type of transport characterizes the absorption of unconjugated bile salts and many drugs. Carrier-mediated transport is coupled to cell metabolism and exhibits substrate specificity, saturation kinetics, competitive inhibition, and counter transport. The transported substance binds reversibly to a carrier on one side of the membrane and is released on the opposite side. Solutes such as hexoses, amino acids, and pyrimidines are absorbed by this mechanism. Facilitated transport refers to a process that also exhibits substrate specificity, saturation kinetics, competitive inhibition, and counter transport and results in net movement of substrate but is not directly coupled to cell metabolism and cannot produce net transport against an electrochemical potential difference. Fructose absorption is in part accomplished in this way. Exchange diffusion implies the obligatory exchange of a molecule on one side of a membrane for a molecule of the same species on the opposite side. It is not directly coupled to cell metabolism and cannot produce net transport but may result in substantial fluxes across membranes. Sodium transport under certain conditions may constitute an example of exchange diffusion.

Normal Digestion and Absorption

The digestion of dietary lipids, carbohydrates, and proteins is initiated in the lumen of the duodenum and proximal jejunum and completed at the glycocalyx and microvillous plasma membrane of the jejunal absorptive cells. Normally, the resulting fatty acids, beta-monoglycerides, monosaccharides, and amino acids as well as water- and fat-soluble vitamins (with the exception of vitamin B_{12}) are absorbed predominantly in the jejunum. The ileum is capable of transporting these substances but absorption is usually complete before this portion of the intestine is reached. Ileal absorption may become quantitatively important when the jejunum is abnormal or no longer present. Figure 26–8 outlines the basic steps involved in the digestion and absorption of fat, carbohydrates, and protein.

Fat Absorption. The average American and Northern European diet contains 60 to 100 grams of fat, the majority of which is in the form of neutral fat or triglyceride. Most is hydrolyzed in the proximal small intestine by pancreatic lipase which preferentially splits the ester bonds in the α and α' positions, forming free long-chain fatty acids and beta-monoglycerides. Pancreatic lipase has a pH optimum between 6 and 7 and is inactivated by higher H^+ concentrations. Cephalic stimulation via the vagus causes the release of cholecystokinin-pancreozymin from the duodenal and jejunal mucosa which in turn increases the secretion of lipase and other enzymes from the pancreas. Fatty acids and especially essential amino acids further augment this hormonal re-

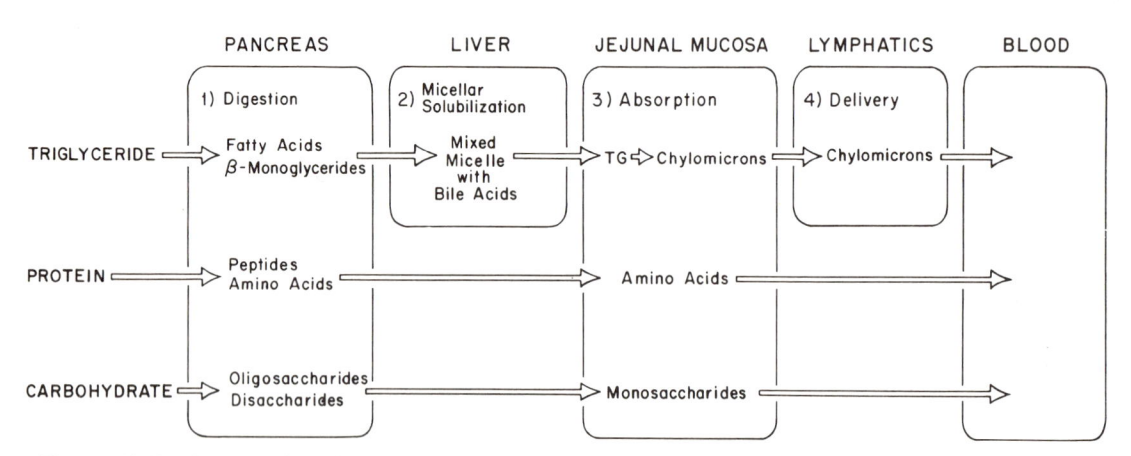

Figure 26–8 A comparison between the four major steps of fat digestion and absorption and the corresponding processes involved in the assimilation of protein and carbohydrates. This diagram emphasizes that the processes of micellar solubilization and delivery of chylomicrons through the intestinal lymphatics are not involved in the absorption of these latter two nutrients. Thus, diseases that cause dysfunction at the level of step 2 or 4 result in the malabsorption only of fat, i.e., isolated steatorrhea, whereas diseases that exert their effect at the level of step 1 or 3 may produce significant malabsorption of fat, protein, and carbohydrate. (Wilson, F. A., and Dietschy, J. M.: Gastroenterology, *61*:911, 1971.)

sponse, which also causes contraction of the gallbladder, increasing the delivery of bile salts and other biliary constituents to the intestinal lumen. Lipolysis does not directly alter dietary lipid solubility but the resulting fatty acids and beta-monoglycerides differ from triglycerides in being amphipaths. The bile salts are detergent-like molecules which when present in a concentration greater than 1 to 2 millimoles per liter (the critical micellar concentration) aggregate into macromolecular complexes known as micelles. The fatty acids and beta-monoglycerides, being amphipaths, will dissolve into the micelle structure of the bile salts to form mixed micelles and so achieve aqueous solubilization. Micelle formation also indirectly increases the rate of lipid hydrolysis by removing the end products of the reaction. An important characteristic of the bile salts participating in this process is their conjugation with either taurine or glycine. Normally there are no unconjugated bile salts in bile. Unconjugated bile salts are weaker detergents and less efficient contributors to micellar solubilization.

When the mixed micelle reaches the epithelial cell membrane the fatty acids and beta-monoglycerides enter the cell by passive diffusion. There is then rapid re-esterification to triglyceride, which becomes associated with protein, cholesterol, cholesterol esters, and phospholipid to form a specific class of lipoproteins called chylomicrons. The chylomicrons are then released from the basal portion of the epithelial cell, cross the interstitial space and enter the lacteal. The important steps involved in the digestion and absorption of fat are outlined in Figure 26–9.

The lacteal has a blind distal end at the villous tip and proximally anastomoses with the submucosal lymphatics. The manner in which chylomicrons gain entry into the lacteal is still debatable. Electron microscopy has demonstrated no pores in the lacteal wall, but pinocytotic vesicles appear to occupy approximately 15 per cent of the endothelial cell cytoplasm, suggesting to some that this is a major pathway of chylomicron uptake. Others, however, maintain that these macromolecular aggregates enter the lacteal through gaps at the endothelial cell junctions.

The flow of lymph through the lacteal appears to be dependent upon the "pumping" action of the villus, which occurs independently of intestinal motor activity. The smooth muscle fibers of the villus are responsible for this movement and may be under the control of a hormone, villikinin, found only in small intestinal mucosa and released in response to mechanical and chemical stimuli.

Some deconjugation of bile salt molecules occurs normally in the intestinal lumen and the unconjugated bile salts are absorbed largely by nonionic diffusion throughout the small bowel. Conjugated bile salts are taken up by an active transport mechanism in the terminal ileum. Approximately 96 per cent of the bile salt pool is reabsorbed during each cycle of the enterohepatic circulation, and each day the pool is cycled 6 to 10 times. This results in a normal 24-hour loss of only 500 mg. of bile salts in the feces. This loss is exactly compensated for by hepatic synthesis and to an extent increased losses can be balanced by increased production. Active ileal absorption is crucial, however, to maintaining the integrity of the total bile salt pool and normal micellar solubilization.

In contrast to dietary fat, the medium-chain triglycerides now widely used as dietary supplements in certain gastrointestinal disorders are composed of fatty acids of 6 to 12 carbon atoms and are handled by the gut in a somewhat different manner. They are hydrolyzed largely by pancreatic lipase, which is more active against triglycerides composed of short-chain fatty acids. Effective hydrolysis appears to occur in the presence or absence of bile salts and the hydrolytic products are mainly free fatty acids with little monoglyceride. They are not incorporated into chylomicrons but are transported by the portal venous system. Micelle formation is probably not obligatory for their effective absorption, since bile diversion has little effect on their uptake by the epithelial cells. Furthermore, a small but significant amount of medium-chain triglycerides is absorbed intact. In some patients with defective lipolysis and/or fat absorption they may constitute important forms of diet therapy because they are more efficiently handled by the gut.

Carbohydrate Absorption. Western diets contain approximately 350 grams of carbohydrate, with an average composition of 60 per cent starch, 30 per cent sucrose, and 10 per cent lactose. The conversion of these substances to monosaccharides is a necessary process for normal absorption. Salivary and to a greater extent pancreatic α-amylase attacks the interior 1,4 α-linkages of amylose (starch), producing maltose and maltotriose. Amylopectin, a branched-chain carbohydrate having similar 1,4 α-linkages but in addition 1,6 α-linkages at the branching points, yields maltose, maltotriose, and branched saccharides called α-dextrins containing an average of eight glucose molecules. Isomaltose, the disaccharide with 1,6 α-linkages, is not a physiologic substrate in the small intestine. Since amylase has little or no activity for the outer 1,4 α-linkages in these molecules, no glucose is formed in the intestinal lumen under physiologic conditions. Although the intestinal mucosa is the site of some intrinsic and adsorbed amylase activity, most hydrolysis takes place within the lumen. The resulting maltose, maltotriose, and α-dextrins as well as ingested lactose and sucrose are then presented to the brush

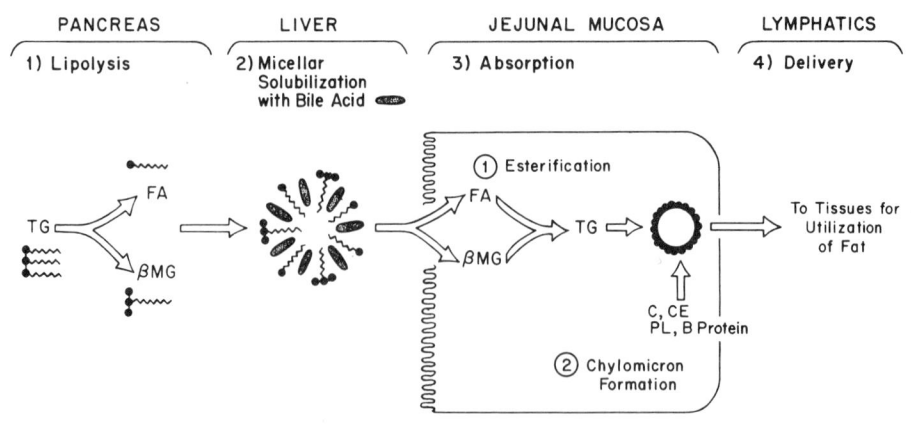

Figure 26-9 Diagrammatic representation of the major steps in the digestion and absorption of dietary fat. These include (*1*) the lipolysis of dietary triglyceride (TG) by pancreatic enzymes; (*2*) micellar solubilization of the resulting long-chain fatty acids (FA) and beta-monoglycerides (βMG) by bile acids secreted into the intestinal lumen by the liver; (*3*) absorption of the fatty acids and beta-monoglyceride into the mucosal cell, with subsequent re-esterification and formation of chylomicrons; and finally (*4*) movement of the chylomicrons from the mucosal cell into the intestinal lymphatic system. During the process of chylomicron formation small amounts of cholesterol (C), cholesterol ester (CE), and phospholipid (PL) as well as triglyceride are incorporated into this specific lipoprotein class. (Wilson, F. A., and Dietschy, J. M.: Gastroenterology, *61*:911, 1971.)

border, where they are converted to their component monosaccharides by enzymes (maltase, sucrase, lactase, and α-dextrinase) located in the glycocalyx-plasma membrane structure. From a pathophysiologic point of view, lactase is the most important of these enzymes. Lactase activity has been demonstrated to reside in three different beta galactosidases: enzyme I, a neutral lactase with a pH optimum of 5.5 to 6.0, located in the brush border and active against lactose and synthetic beta galactosides; enzyme II, an acid beta galactosidase with a pH optimum of 4.5, located in the cellular lysosomal fraction and active against lactose and synthetic beta galactosides; and enzyme III, a cytoplasmic neutral hetero beta galactosidase, having a pH optimum of 5.5 to 6.0 and hydrolyzing only synthetic beta galactosides. Enzyme I is responsible for most normal intestinal lactase activity.

Some monosaccharides diffuse back into the lumen but most of the glucose, galactose, and fructose is absorbed. Existing data are compatible with the hypothesis that glucose and galactose are transported from the intestinal lumen across the brush border into the epithelial cell by a shared carrier-mediated process and that the rate and direction of movement depend upon the distribution ratio of Na^+ and possibly K^+ across this membrane. Sodium is therefore required for absorption and this asymmetrical distribution of cations depends directly on energy production. Fructose, however, appears to be absorbed to a large extent by facilitated transport, since it does not accumulate against its own concentration gradient, but the mechanism is saturable and its absorption is more rapid than pentoses but slower than that of glucose or galactose. The events involved in the digestion and absorption of carbohydrates are schematically summarized in Figure 26-10.

An important concept, not yet fully developed, involves the dietary regulation of small intestinal enzyme activity. Rosensweig has studied the adaptive responses of disaccharidase and glycolytic enzymes (common to all cells) in man following dietary manipulation. Sucrose or fructose feeding increases the activities of sucrase and maltase but not lactase, whereas glucose and galactose also enhance glycolytic enzyme activity, but the increase is less than that observed after feeding isocaloric amounts of noncarbohydrate calories. In the case of disaccharidases, the adaptive response occurs within a 2- to 5-day period (the time required for intestinal cell renewal), suggesting an action on the undifferentiated crypt cells. In the experimental animal, lactase activity adapts in a period of 8 to 10 weeks, but short-term experiments in man have failed to show lactase adaptation.

The full implication of this phenomenon is not yet apparent but it is obvious that dietary habits must be taken into consideration when abnormalities of epithelial enzyme activity are present.

Protein Absorption. The usual dietary intake of 70 to 90 grams of protein presents the digestive-absorptive mechanism with a more complex task than that presented by fat or carbohydrate. A much larger group of enzymes is required to reduce native proteins to their amino acid components. This process is initiated in the gastrointestinal lumen by pepsin, which is dispensable for adequate protein assimilation, and the numerous pancreatic proteases including trypsinogen, chymotrypsinogen, procarboxypeptidase A, procarboxypeptidase B, leucine aminopeptidase, proelastase, and nucleases. They are released largely in response to vagal influences and the action of cholecystokinin-pancreozymin. These mechanisms are described more fully in the chapter dealing with the pancreas and in the portion of this section discussing the endocrine function of the small intestine. The inactive trypsinogen is converted to active trypsin by enterokinase, and the trypsin then acts to complete the conversion of the various proenzymes to their active forms. Trypsin and chymotrypsin are endopeptidases which split the peptide bonds within the protein molecule, while the carboxypeptidases are exopeptidases acting only on the terminal peptide bonds. These various enzymes differ in both topographical activity and amino acid specificity, and because of their restricted sites of action, protein digestion occurs only by virtue of their sequential activity.

A large proportion of the pancreatic proteases are adsorbed onto the epithelial cell surface, and whether their activity is exerted mainly within the lumen or in the region of the microvilli is uncertain. In either case, peptides that are 3 to 6 amino acid residues long are released and presented to the brush border and intracellular enzyme systems, where three groups of peptidases complete the process of amino acid liberation. The amino-oligopeptidases have been partially localized to the brush border and hydrolyze the longer peptides probably to amino acids, dipeptides, and tripeptides. The amino-tripeptidases, also partially localized to the brush border, split the N-terminal residues from tripeptides. Lastly, there are several dipeptidases including glycyl-glycine peptidase, leucyl-glycine peptidase, glycyl-leucine peptidase and imino and imido peptidases hydrolyzing proline-containing peptides, the precise localization of which is not known.

From studies comparing normal and cystinuric patients it is clear that both free amino acids and dipeptides can enter the epithelial cell and significant dipeptidase activity probably takes place within the cytoplasm. Only certain amino acids are in fact readily released within the lumen in free form. Appreciable amounts of the basic amino acids (arginine and lysine) and neutral amino acids (valine, phenylalanine, tyrosine, methionine, and leucine) are released and transported by the epithelial cell membrane. In contrast, glycine, the imino acids (proline and hydroxyproline), the hydroxyl-substituted amino acids (serine and threonine), and the dicarboxylic amino acids (aspartic and glutamic) remain about 90 per cent peptide-linked until their disappearance from the lumen, and they presumably enter the cell as constituents of small pep-

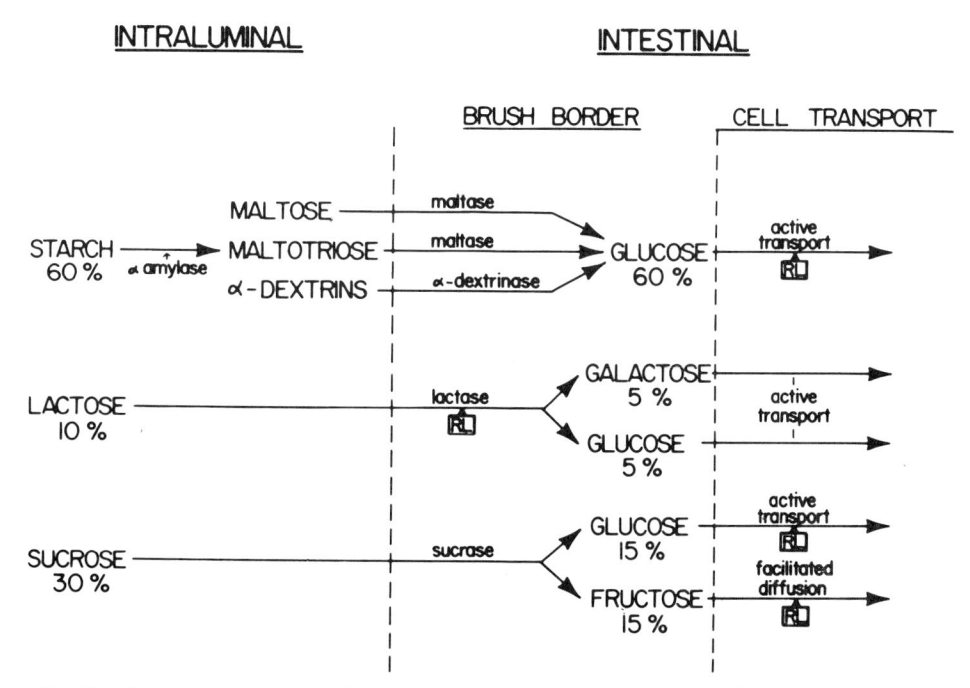

Figure 26-10 Schematic representation of the events involved in the digestion and absorption of carbohydrates. RL is the rate-limiting step in the particular reaction. (Gray, G. M.: Gastroenterology, *58*:96, 1970.)

tides. It is clear that glycine is more rapidly and efficiently absorbed as the di- and tripeptide than as the free amino acid. The physiologic importance of oligopeptide absorption, however, remains unclear. Most peptides are hydrolyzed by several electrophoretically distinct enzymes and, conversely, each enzyme hydrolyzes several different peptides. The specificity and localization of the many intestinal peptidases are still uncertain and their role in protein digestion is obviously more complex than the brush border disaccharidase system.

The manner in which peptides cross the plasma membrane is unknown. It has been proposed that amino acids are transported via a carrier-mediated process that, like hexose absorption, is stimulated by Na^+. Amino acid influx is not tightly coupled to Na^+ influx, however, and in the absence of Na^+ amino acid transport still exhibits saturation kinetics and competitive inhibition. Sodium does not affect the maximum velocity of amino acid influx but does increase the apparent affinity of the carrier system. Hereditary defects of amino acid transport have provided evidence for several different transport systems, each having different affinities for different groups of amino acids. These are presented in Table 26-1.

Somewhat analogous to carbohydrate digestion, it is apparent that the absorption rates of essential amino acids at least can be influenced by dietary, caloric, or protein deprivation in man. Adibi and Allen subjected patients to a 14-day period of either protein or protein-calorie deprivation and found a decreased rate of jejunal amino acid transport with a corresponding increase in fecal nitrogen, which could not be correlated with any light or electron microscopic changes. This sort of observation again emphasizes the potential modifications in intestinal absorptive function that may follow dietary manipulation.

Folic Acid and Vitamin B_{12} Absorption. Folic acid is 2-amino,4-hydroxypteridine joined to a p-aminobenzoic acid residue and linked to one molecule of L-glutamic acid. Naturally occurring folates contain additional L-glutamic acid molecules linked by the unusual γ-peptide bond, with pteroylheptaglutamic acid being the principal species in most plant and animal tissues. This conjugated form is converted in the small intestine to the free monoglutamate by γ-glutamyl carboxypeptidase ("conjugase"), an enzyme associated with the mucosal cell but of which the precise site of action is unknown. Absorption of pteroylmonoglutamic acid occurs largely in the proximal small intestine but its transport mechanism has not been defined. Within the intestinal cell the monoglutamate is converted by dihydrofolate reductase and a methylating mechanism to reduced methyl folate (largely 5-methyltetrahydrofolate) prior to entry into the portal circulation. Tetrahydrofolic acid functions as a cofactor in various important enzyme systems.

Vitamin B_{12} in food is bound to protein by peptide bonds which are hydrolyzed by cooking, acidification, and proteolytic enzymes. In the presence of the free vitamin, intrinsic factor produced by the gastric parietal cells dimerizes and one mole of the dimer binds two moles of the vitamin. In addition to being essential for its active ileal absorption, intrinsic factor probably serves to protect vitamin B_{12} from digestion and to a limited extent from bacterial utilization. The free vitamin can be absorbed by passive diffusion throughout the small intestine but only 1 per

TABLE 26-1 INTESTINAL AMINO ACID TRANSPORT MECHANISMS

Type	Amino Acids Transported	Type of Transport	Rate
Neutral (monoamino-monocarboxylic)	Aromatic (tyrosine, tryptophan, phenylalanine) Aliphatic (glycine,* alanine, serine, threonine, valine, leucine, isoleucine) Methionine, histidine, glutamine, asparagine, cysteine	Active, Na^+-dependent	Very rapid
Dibasic (diamino)	Lysine, arginine, ornithine, cystine	Active, partially Na^+-dependent	Rapid (10% of neutral)
Dicarboxylic (acidic)	Glutamic acid, aspartic acid	Carrier-mediated, ?active, partially Na^+-dependent	Rapid
Imino acids and glycine	Proline, hydroxyproline, glycine*	Active, ?Na^+-dependent	Slow

*Shares both the neutral and imino mechanism with low affinity for the neutral.
From Gray, G. M., and Cooper, H. L.: Gastroenterology, *61*:535, 1971.

cent is handled in this way. The absorption of physiologic amounts (>2 micrograms) is intrinsic factor-mediated and takes place only in the terminal ileum where 60 to 80 per cent is absorbed. The B_{12}-intrinsic factor complex attaches to receptors located in the glycocalyx-plasma membrane complex of the terminal ileal absorptive cells. This attachment requires the presence of Ca^{++} and/or Mg^{++} amd a pH above 5.6. The vitamin B_{12} is released from intrinsic factor in or on the ileal absorptive cell and is transported to the portal blood bound to a carrier, transcobalamin. Vitamin B_{12} has an enterohepatic circulation with two thirds to three fourths of biliary B_{12} reabsorbed in the ileum, provided that intrinsic factor is adequate. The fate of intrinsic factor is not clear but it does not appear to be absorbed (see Chapter 27).

The absorption of other water-soluble vitamins has been little studied and the manner in which ascorbic acid, riboflavin, and other members of the B group are handled by the small intestine is largely unknown. Absorption of the fat-soluble vitamins A, D, E, and K in general parallels that of lipid absorption. Vitamin A deserves special comment here, since its absorption has been utilized as a form of lipid tolerance test. It is ingested largely in an esterified form which requires hydrolysis by pancreatic and brush border enzymes prior to micellar solubilization. After entering the epithelial cell it is re-esterified with long-chain fatty acids and transported via the lymph in association with the chylomicrons. It has recently been appreciated, however, that significant absorption occurs by way of the portal vein. Consequently, vitamin A transport is a more general index of absorption and is not strictly equatable with lipid tolerance. The absorption of the other fat-soluble vitamins as well as iron and calcium is discussed in those sections dealing with their overall metabolism and pathophysiology.

The digestive-absorptive process therefore involves not only the handling of a wide range of ingested materials but numerous enzymes and hormones, each requiring its own optimal environment, as well as highly specialized cellular structure-function relationships. Although such physiologic complexity quite naturally predisposes to pathophysiologic diversity, it is in most instances possible to understand the different malabsorption syndromes in terms of one or more alterations in this overall process.

Abnormalities of Digestion and Absorption

Many disease processes directly or indirectly alter gastrointestinal physiology in such a manner that normal absorptive mechanisms are compromised and maldigestion or malabsorption of one or more dietary constituents occurs. There may be malabsorption of fat alone or of protein and carbohydrate as well. A defect may be so severe and widespread that it precludes the normal absorption of any ingested nutrient, or so circumscribed that only single substances are affected. Furthermore, some disorders cause malabsorption by more than one pathophysiologic mechanism.

A large number of tests have been utilized in the differential diagnosis of malabsorption syndromes. However, many are of little value despite their continued use. The physician who has a sound understanding of the normal mechanisms of digestion and absorption as well as the tests useful in their investigation will be able to arrive at a correct diagnosis in the vast majority of cases by correlating clinical information with the following diagnostic procedures: the quantitative determination of stool fat, the quantitative determination of stool nitrogen, the xylose absorption test, the lactose tolerance test, the vitamin B_{12} absorption test, and peroral intestinal biopsy. Hemoglobin concentrations and red cell morphology as well as serum levels of albumin, cholesterol, carotene, prothrombin activity, iron, calcium, phosphorus, and alkaline phosphatase are *nutritional indices* and not tests of absorption. Abnormalities may reflect not only malabsorption but inadequate intake and increased utilization or loss by other routes.

The quantitative chemical determination of fecal fat is the most reliable measure of steatorrhea. The amount of fat appearing in the stool of normal individuals is usually less than 7 per cent of the dietary intake. With the usual intake of 60 to 100 grams, this will result in the excretion of less than 6 grams per 24 hours. Even with intakes as high as 200 grams, only 8.7 plus or minus 0.7 grams will appear in the stool. With zero fat intake, approximately 3 grams will still be present, presumably from sloughed epithelial cells and bacterial lipids. In the patient with compromised digestive or absorptive capacity the amount of fat excreted in the stool is more directly related to the amount ingested. The van de Kamer method is most commonly employed for quantitating fecal fat, but this procedure must be modified for the patient receiving medium-chain triglycerides, since medium-chain fatty acids will otherwise be underestimated.

The normal fecal nitrogen excretion is in the range of 2.0 to 2.5 grams in persons with intakes between 80 and 100 grams. Desquamation of epithelial cells, secretory proteins, and leakage of plasma proteins contributes to the intraluminal nitrogen pool and, provided that significant protein-losing enteropathy is not present, fecal nitrogen determinations are a useful measure of protein malabsorption.

Xylose, a 5-carbon monosaccharide, is absorbed primarily by passive means in the proximal small intestine. The amount excreted in the urine during the first five hours following an oral dose of 25 grams should be greater than 4.5 grams. Artifactually low values may be due to vomiting, delayed gastric emptying, dehydration, impaired renal function, or the presence of massive ascites. The mean normal excretory rate also decreases with advancing age and probably is reflective of declining renal function. Values less than 2.5 to 3.0 grams are encountered in disease states in which there is significant loss of the functional integrity of the jejunum or massive bacterial overgrowth in the proximal small intestine, resulting in bacterial utilization. The administration of antibiotics may correct abnormal values due to the latter condition.

Vitamin B_{12} absorption is usually assessed by some variation of the standard Schilling test. Excretion of greater than 5 to 8 per cent in 24 hours of the orally administered radiolabeled B_{12} is generally regarded as normal. Provided that the patient has or has been given adequate amounts of intrinsic factor, excretory rates below 1 to 3 per cent per 24 hours are found in two situations: (1) in the presence of massive bacterial overgrowth or infestation with certain tapeworms involving the proximal small intestine, in which there is binding of both free B_{12} and the B_{12}-intrinsic factor complex by the microorganisms; and (2) disease states or surgical procedures that lead to significant loss of the functional integrity of the terminal ileum. The administration of appropriate antibiotics will often correct the Schilling test in the former but not the latter situation.

Peroral intestinal biopsy has considerably facilitated the diagnosis of certain malabsorption syndromes. Knowledge of normal histology at various levels of the intestine as well as variations encountered in different populations is a definite requisite for making comparisons with diseased tissues. In at least five specific disorders the histologic findings are sufficiently unique to be diagnostic: nontropical sprue, Whipple's disease, a beta-lipoproteinemia, amyloidosis, and mast cell disease. In radiation enteritis, lymphangiectasia, tropical sprue, nongranulomatous ulcerative jejunitis, scleroderma, eosinophilic gastroenteritis, dermatitis herpetiformis, hypogammaglobulinemia, and some parasitic infestations the changes are usually compatible with but not diagnostic of the particular disorder. In most other conditions leading to maldigestion and malabsorption small intestinal histology is normal, at least to light microscopy.

The signs and symptoms exhibited by the patient with a malabsorption syndrome will quite naturally vary with the disease responsible. The manifestations of the malabsorption itself will depend upon the nature and amount of the substances involved and the duration of the process. Weight loss, muscle wasting, anemia, tetany, edema, bleeding tendencies, osteomalacia, osteoporosis, fatigue, abdominal distention, multiple vitamin deficiencies, steatorrhea, and even diarrhea are commonly observed in various combinations. Classically, with steatorrhea the stools are described as voluminous or bulky, foul smelling, greasy, frothy, pale yellow, and floating. Unfortunately, not all such descriptions by the patient will be associated with an increase in fecal fat, and significant steatorrhea may exist in the absence of any of these characteristics. True diarrhea may be produced by disorders causing a decrease in transit time, the malabsorption of water and electrolytes, or the cathartic action of hydroxylated fatty acids. Hypocalcemia and hypophosphatemia result in part from the formation of insoluble calcium soaps with unabsorbed fatty acids, vitamin D deficiency, and loss of calcium-binding protein normally located in the glycocalyx.

Radiologic examination of the small intestine with a barium meal may be helpful in disclosing a "malabsorption pattern" but is rarely capable of providing an etiologic diagnosis. The characteristic features are illustrated in Figure 26-11 and include localized dilatations, segmentation of the barium column, loss of mucosal detail (moulage), flocculation of the barium due to the presence of increased amounts of water and mucus in the intestinal lumen, and often thickening of the valvulae conniventes.

The presence of a malabsorption syndrome therefore must be suspected under a variety of clinical circumstances. An understanding of the pathophysiologic mechanisms that may be responsible is essential to the proper interpretation of clinical signs and symptoms as well as abnormalities reported by the clinical laboratory. A classification of malabsorption syndromes based upon the type of defect responsible is presented in Table 26-2. The normal digestive-absorptive process may be disrupted by abnormalities occurring within the intestinal lumen, at the level of the mucosa (involving the absorptive cells or the lamina propria) or the intestinal lymphatics.

Intraluminal Abnormalities. The intraluminal phase of the digestive-absorptive process is concerned with the digestion of fats, carbohydrates, and proteins, and the micellar solubilization of free fatty acids and beta-monoglycerides. Maldigestion will result from any disorder interfering with *effective* pancreatic enzyme activity. This may be due to abnormalities of pancreatic exocrine function secondary to chronic pancreatitis, carcinoma of the pancreas, mucoviscidosis, or pancreatic resection, which reduce the absolute amount of enzyme available, or to acid hypersecretion and gastric resection, which result in ineffective activity of otherwise adequate amounts of enzyme.

Several factors appear to play a role in the

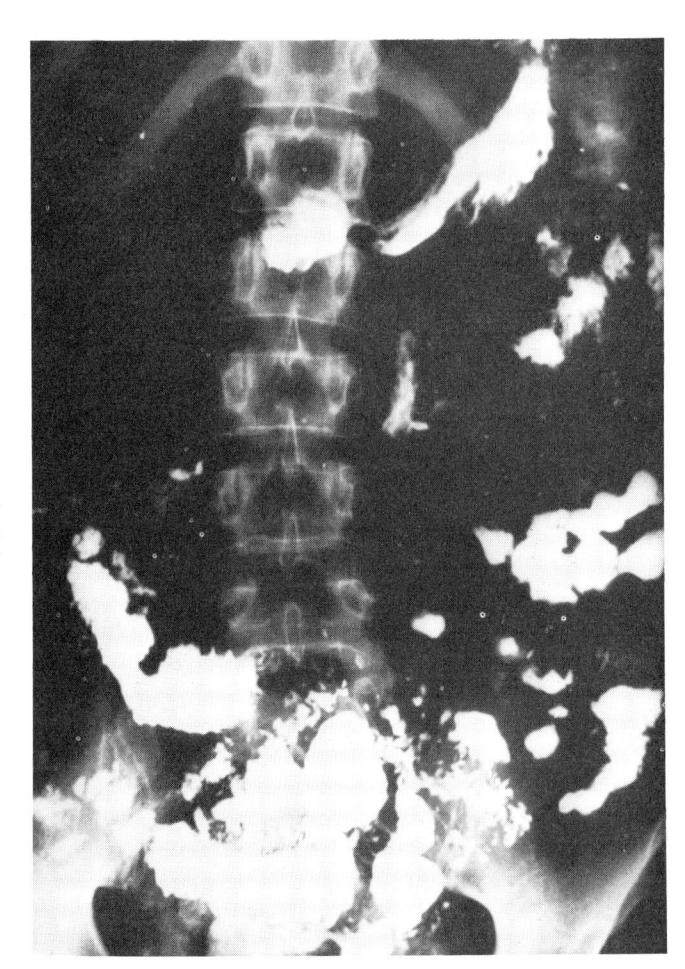

Figure 26-11 Barium meal demonstrating a typical malabsorption pattern, consisting of segmentation, localized dilatation, and moulage formation.

malabsorption associated with the acid hypersecretion of the Zollinger-Ellison syndrome. The low intraluminal pH denatures or inactivates pancreatic enzymes, especially lipase, and conjugated bile salts may be precipitated from solution. It is also possible that the absorptive capacity of the mucosal cells may be impaired by acid injury. Pancreatic exocrine insufficiency results in severe steatorrhea and nitrogen loss, but xylose absorption, vitamin B_{12} absorption, and jejunal histology are normal. Patients with the Zollinger-Ellison syndrome exhibit moderate increases in fecal fat and slight impairment of xylose absorption. B_{12} absorption and jejunal histologic findings are normal. No values for fecal nitrogen have been reported.

Following gastric resection particularly with a Billroth II-type anastomosis, malabsorption may involve interference with absorptive processes at several steps. Duodenal bypass leads to a poor secretory response of the pancreas and inadequate mixing of food with bile salts and pancreatic enzymes. Rapid intestinal transit may occur, with a reduction of contact time between the intestinal contents and the mucosal absorptive cells. The reasons for the abnormal transit time are essentially unknown. An additional factor in certain patients is massive bacterial overgrowth in the afferent loop giving rise to an intestinal stasis syndrome (see below). Steatorrhea is generally mild, and nitrogen excretion and xylose absorption are usually normal, although the latter may be reduced in the presence of a stasis syndrome. Jejunal biopsy is usually normal but occasionally reveals mild villous atrophy of doubtful functional significance. Vitamin B_{12} absorption may be reduced for three possible reasons: (1) inadequate intrinsic factor secretion by the gastric remnant; (2) rapid passage of B_{12} through the gastric remnant, preventing the formation of the B_{12}-intrinsic factor complex; or (3) the presence of an afferent loop stasis syndrome. Correction of an abnormal Schilling test with exogenous intrinsic factor or antibiotics will help in determining the precise cause. Although many inconsistencies are encountered, malabsorption

TABLE 26–2 A PATHOPHYSIOLOGIC CLASSIFICATION OF DISORDERS ASSOCIATED WITH MALABSORPTION

Abnormalities of intraluminal events
    Inadequate digestion
        Pancreatic insufficiency
        Acid hypersecretion
        Gastric resection
    Altered bile salt metabolism
        Intraluminal binding of bile salts
        Hepatobiliary disease
        Ileal resection or disease
        Bacterial overgrowth
Abnormalities of mucosal transport
    Generalized defects
        Nontropical sprue (celiac disease, gluten enteropathy)
        Tropical sprue
        Crohn's disease
        Intestinal resection or bypass
        Nongranulomatous ulcerative jejunitis
        Radiation enteritis
        Whipple's disease
        Drug-induced malabsorption
        Hypothyroidism
        Addison's disease
        Hyperthyroidism
        Hypoparathyroidism
        Parasitic disease
        Mast cell disease
        Dermatitis herpetiformis
        Intestinal ischemia
        Intestinal lymphoma
        Protein malnutrition
        Amyloidosis
    Selective defects
        A-β-lipoproteinemia
        Disaccharidase deficiency
        Monosaccharide malabsorption
        Amino acid malabsorption
        Vitamin B_{12} malabsorption
Abnormalities of lymphatic transport
    Primary intestinal lymphangiectasia
    Whipple's disease
    Crohn's disease
    Radiation enteritis
    Intestinal lymphoma
    Constrictive pericarditis
    Congestive heart failure
Unclassified abnormalities
    Carcinoid syndrome
    Dysgammaglobulinemias
    Diabetic gastroenteropathy
    Scleroderma

---

achieve adequate micellar solubilization may result from one or more of several different mechanisms. The intraluminal binding of bile salts occurs with the administration of cholestyramine, a nonabsorbable anion exchange resin used in the management of intractable pruritis due to increased tissue levels of bile salts. In general, steatorrhea is present only in patients receiving in excess of 12 grams per day and fecal fat losses are relatively mild. Portal-systemic shunts that lower the extraction of bile salts from portal venous blood, hepatocellular disease that reduces bile acid synthesis, and intra- or extrahepatic cholestasis with or without jaundice which limits biliary excretion all may contribute to a micellar defect. The result is an isolated, mild steatorrhea. The reason why the steatorrhea is not more severe is that the two most important steps in fat absorption remain intact: lipolysis and epithelial cell uptake. Furthermore, the ileum, which does not normally participate significantly in fat absorption, in part compensates for decreased jejunal uptake. In patients with an external biliary fistula, for example, fat absorption is little impaired on a low fat intake and as much as 75 per cent of an intake of 120 grams may be absorbed. With increasing intake, however, there is increasing steatorrhea.

Blind loop or intestinal stasis syndromes may be due to a variety of anatomic or motor disturbances of the intestine including afferent loops following gastric resection, enteroenterostomy or internal fistulas with bypass of a segment of small bowel, multiple strictures, jejunal diverticulosis, scleroderma, diabetic enteropathy, and gastrocolic fistula. The common denominator is stasis and bacterial colonization of the small intestine with a more fecal type of flora. Bacterial counts in luminal fluid from the duodenum, jejunum, and proximal ileum normally are low, in the range of less than 10^4 per ml., and consist primarily of streptococci, aerobic lactobacilli, and diphtheroids as well as fungi. The distal ileum represents a transitional zone, with bacterial counts between 10^5 and 10^8 per ml. In two thirds of cases there are appreciable numbers of gram-negative organisms, largely aerobic coliforms with very few anerobic bacteria such as bacteroides. The two most important factors controlling the "relative sterility" of the proximal small intestine are gastric acid secretion and the cleansing action of propulsive motor activity. It is also probably important that bacterial generation times are much longer in the intestinal lumen than under in-vitro conditions. Interference with either may permit the establishment of a colonic type of flora containing large numbers of bacteroides, coliforms, and clostridia. This bacterial overgrowth has several important metabolic effects. First, and most importantly, there is deconjugation and dehydroxylation of bile salts

tends to occur with a decreasing order of severity subsequent to the following surgical procedures: total gastrectomy with esophagojejunostomy, subtotal gastrectomy with gastrojejunostomy, subtotal gastrectomy with gastroduodenostomy, and vagotomy and pyloroplasty.

Altered bile salt metabolism with failure to

resulting in decreased micelle formation. Second, the bacteria are capable of binding the B_{12}-intrinsic factor complex, preventing its absorption, and of metabolizing xylose. The characteristic findings in patients with an intestinal stasis syndrome therefore include mild steatorrhea and abnormal B_{12} absorption. Fecal nitrogen values and jejunal histologic findings are usually normal, while xylose absorption may be normal or decreased. The abnormal values for fecal fat and the diminished B_{12} and xylose absorption most often return to normal after several days of antibiotic therapy, especially with lincomycin.

Bacterial stasis syndromes may result in some additional effects unrelated to malabsorption: (1) increased serum folate levels due to bacterial synthesis and release of folic acid; (2) increased urinary indican excretion from the conversion of tryptophan to indole which is hydroxylated and sulfated in the liver to indoxysulfate or indican; and (3) increased ammonia production by the deamination of dietary protein to form urea, with subsequent conversion to ammonia by intestinal ureases.

Abnormalities of Mucosal Transport. Most disorders affecting the small intestinal mucosa result in widespread defects characterized by malabsorption of most normally transported materials. Any process causing structural or functional abnormalities of the glycocalyx-plasma membrane digestive-absorptive unit, the remainder of the epithelial cell proper, or the surrounding lamina propria may produce a generalized malabsorption syndrome. Most, if not all, tests of absorption will be abnormal and the fecal losses of fat and nitrogen are often severe. On the other hand, highly specific defects may occur with only single substances exhibiting abnormal transport.

Nontropical sprue (celiac disease, gluten enteropathy) provides a good example of generalized primary intestinal malabsorption. Jejunal biopsies of patients with untreated celiac disease almost always show total or near total villus atrophy. In order for this to be apparent it is important that the sections be properly oriented so that they are cut perpendicular to the luminal surface. The total mucosal thickness is relatively normal and as a result the crypts appear elongated. The surface epithelial cells exhibit several abnormalities: (1) their vertical height is decreased and they assume a more cuboidal shape, (2) the simple columnar orientation is replaced by a stratified configuration, (3) cytoplasmic degenerative changes are apparent, (4) the brush border structure is attenuated or even inapparent, (5) there is a relative decrease in goblet cells, and (6) there is infiltration of the epithelial cell layer by lymphocytes. The crypt cells generally appear normal by both light and electron microscopy but there is a relative increase in the number of Paneth and enterochromaffin cells, and the undifferentiated cells at the bases of the crypts exhibit increased mitoses. In fact, Trier and Browning, using tissue cultures of intestinal epithelium from untreated patients, found an increased proliferation and migration of crypt cells similar to the recovery phase of sublethal ionizing radiation. The cells also reverted to a more normal appearance after only 24 hours in a gluten-free medium. The lamina propria contains increased numbers of plasma cells and eosinophils and the interstitial spaces appear to be filled with a lightly staining amorphous material. Morphologic changes are most marked in the duodenum and jejunum and tend to be less prominent in the ileum.

Although the cereal protein gluten (wheat, rye, barley, and oats) is firmly established as the offending agent, the mechanism of its noxious effect remains unknown. Gluten is the starch-free portion of the cereal grain and the toxic factor is contained in its 70 per cent alcohol-soluble fraction (gliadin). This consists of a complex mixture of several electrophoretically and chromatographically separable proteins of varying molecular weight. Clinical challenge with peptic-tryptic digests suggests that the toxic factor is a polypeptide of molecular weight less than 1000. Efforts to demonstrate abnormal peptidase activity in treated patients, however, have failed. Antibodies to gluten fractions are present in the serum and intestinal secretions of untreated and to a lesser extent of treated patients, but their significance is debated. No antibodies in the diseased tissue itself react with gluten fractions and no complement-fixing immune complexes have been demonstrated. Interestingly enough, however, the celiac jejunal epithelial cells uniquely bind gluten fractions in vitro. Whatever the reason, the basic problem appears to be an inadequately compensated, shortened life span of the villous absorptive cells.

The net result is a decrease in intestinal surface area, a loss of enzymes and carriers, and compromised absorptive cell function. The main physiologic defect is a failure of transport by the epithelial cell. The result is malabsorption of most dietary constituents, including fat, carbohydrate, protein, vitamins, iron, and calcium. The fecal losses of fat and nitrogen tend to be relatively severe and the absorption of xylose is markedly impaired. Jejunal histology in the untreated case is essentially diagnostic. Vitamin B_{12} absorption may be normal or low, depending upon the severity of the ileal abnormality. The anemia which develops is most commonly due to iron deficiency, but macrocytic anemias due to foic acid and less often to B_{12} deficiency are also frequent. With the loss of brush border enzymes, disaccharidase deficiencies occur, of which lactose intolerance is clinically the most prominent. Water and electrolyte transport is also affected, and perfusion of the jejunum with isotonic electrolyte solutions results in a net secretion of water, sodium, and potassium instead of absorption.

Improvement of absorption coincides with the removal of gluten-containing cereals and cereal products from the diet. Cytologic abnormalities begin to disappear within a matter of days, whereas villous architecture reverts toward normal over a period of weeks and months. It is doubtful, however, whether villi ever achieve a totally normal appearance.

Other clinical entities which are characterized by abnormal villous architecture and distorted morphology of intestinal absorptive cells include tropical sprue, dermatitis herpetiformis, and nongranulomatous ulcerative jejunitis. The absorptive defect therefore is qualitatively similar to that of celiac disease.

In contrast, the morphologic changes in Whipple's disease are most striking in the lamina propria, where the normal cellular elements are replaced by macrophages containing periodic acid-Schiff positive glycoprotein within their cytoplasm. In addition, rod-shaped structures can be seen in the lamina propria that under the electron microscope have the features of bacteria. The villous absorptive cells and mucosal surface area, however, are relatively well preserved. Nonetheless, in-vitro studies of tissue biopsy specimens have demonstrated impaired amino acid transport and fatty acid esterification. There is also morphologic evidence suggesting an impaired delivery of triglyceride to the lymphatics. Precisely how the observed structural abnormalities are translated into functional defects is not clear. Characteristically, patients with Whipple's disease exhibit severe malabsorption of fat and protein but very little alteration of xylose or B_{12} absorption.

The malabsorption associated with intestinal resection can be divided into three essentially distinct syndromes: massive resection or bypass, removal of the jejunum, and ileectomy. It is patently obvious why the first of these results in severe malabsorption of fat and protein as well as of xylose and vitamin B_{12}. On the other hand, removal of the jejunum causes only a mild defect in fat absorption, presumably because the ileum can almost totally compensate for its loss. This may simply represent the expression of functions not normally called upon in the presence of an intact jejunum. In a number of experimental animals, however, there has been an actual increase in villus height and mucosal thickness of the ileum following jejunal resection. Conversely, loss of the ileum leads to a more severe malabsorption of fat and B_{12}. This is because disruption of the enterohepatic circulation of bile salts results in ineffective micellar solubilization. Ordinarily this would produce only a modest steatorrhea, because the ileum would partially compensate for the resulting reduced jejunal absorption. When the ileum is missing or diseased, however, this cannot occur. Furthermore, the coexisting B_{12} deficiency itself appears to affect the maturation of villous absorptive cells, thereby contributing to the absorptive defect. Loss of the ileum is also frequently associated with watery diarrhea which is thought to be due to the cathartic action of the large amount of unabsorbed bile salts entering the colon.

A number of drugs have been implicated in the production of mucosal transport defects primarily involving fat. Cholestyramine has been discussed in relation to its effect on micelle formation. Colchicine produces a diffuse alteration of absorptive function manifested by slightly increased fecal losses of fat and nitrogen and decreased xylose absorption. It probably exerts this effect by disturbing epithelial cell function and inhibiting cell renewal. A variety of cathartic agents may also cause slight steatorrhea, hypokalemia, and protein-losing enteropathy, but no satisfactory explanation of their effect has been put forward. Neomycin, the most widely studied of the drugs producing malabsorption, has been shown to produce morphologic changes in intestinal villi, to inhibit the intraluminal hydrolysis of triglycerides, and to precipitate bile salts. Neomycin is a polybasic aminoglucoside and it has been suggested that an interaction between its cationic amino groups and the anionic fatty acids and bile acids leads to precipitation of the whole micellar complex. Triparanol produces an intestinal lesion indistinguishable from celiac disease and results in mild fat and nitrogen losses. High doses of para-aminosalicylic acid have also induced a reversible defect in fat and xylose absorption.

The remainder of the mucosal transport defects listed in Table 26-2 lead to malabsorption by even less well understood mechanisms. Some disorders such as amyloidosis, radiation enteritis, parasitic infestation, and mast cell disease are associated with morphologic abnormalities while the various endocrinopathies appear to represent mucosal cell dysfunction induced by metabolic influences.

In contrast to these generalized absorptive defects, a few conditions represent defective transport of a single substance. Except for a-beta-lipoproteinemia they are not characterized by any morphologic abnormalities, and only lactase deficiency and pernicious anemia occur with any frequency.

A-beta-lipoproteinemia is a rare disorder involving a partial or total absence of plasma beta-lipoprotein. It is probably inherited as an autosomal recessive, and total deficiency is associated with lipid malabsorption, acanthocytosis, peripheral neuropathy, and retinal lesions. The defect in lipid absorption and the absence of beta-lipoproteins appear to be due to an inability of the epithelial cell to synthesize the protein moiety of chylomicrons. Jejunal biopsies reveal a normal villous architecture, but in the fasting state numerous cytoplasmic fat droplets are found in the absorptive cells. Mild steatorrhea is the only abnormality observed.

Isolated vitamin B_{12} deficiency is most commonly due to inadequate intrinsic factor activity in association with pernicious anemia, chronic atrophic gastritis, and subtotal or total gastrectomy. As discussed previously, gastrectomy may or may not be associated with the malabsorption of other substances. Resection or disease of the ileum is seldom if ever characterized by defective B_{12} transport alone. A condition referred to as selective B_{12} malabsorption (Imerslund's syndrome) has been described, however, which may represent absence of ileal B_{12}-intrinsic factor receptors. Those affected are most often children of North African non-Ashkenazic origin who have renal abnormalities with proteinuria, normal intrinsic factor activity, and no intrinsic factor antibodies.

Abnormalities of hexose transport may also involve a single substance. Congenital glucose-galactose malabsorption presents in infancy as intractable diarrhea until these monosaccharides or their disaccharide precursors are excluded from the diet. In some, there is an associated glycosuria, suggesting a coexisting renal tubular transport defect. It seems likely that the specific carrier involved in glucose-galactose transport is lacking or defective, since sodium flux and other sodium-dependent processes such as amino acid absorption are normal.

Spontaneously occurring defects of amino acid transport have contributed important information to our understanding of the different types of carrier systems involved in normal amino acid transport. They have also emphasized the great similarity between intestinal and renal tubular transport systems. Cystinuria, an inherited disorder of basic amino acid transport, is perhaps the best studied of such defects. These patients have defective renal and intestinal transport systems for cystine, arginine, ornithine, and lysine. Three forms have been described, depending upon the type of intestinal transport defect: Type I, in which there is absent intestinal transport of both cystine and the dibasic amino acids; Type II, in which only dibasic amino acids are improperly absorbed; and Type III, in which there is abnormal transport only by the renal tubule. Patients with Hartnup's disease have defective renal tubular transport systems for neutral amino acids but only tryptophan malabsorption has thus far been demonstrated in the small intestine. This accounts for the increased urine indican characteristic of such patients. Joseph's syndrome (prolinuria, iminoglycinuria) involves the urinary loss of proline and glycine with a variable defect present in the intestine; some individuals demonstrate transport defects for both amino acids, some for proline alone, and others have no intestinal transport defect. Patients with Lowe's syndrome (oculocerebrorenal syndrome) have a renal tubular defect involving neutral and dibasic amino acids but apparently only dibasic amino acids are handled abnormally by the intestine.

Isolated deficiencies of the various disaccharidases have also been described, lactase deficiency being the most frequent and best understood. Its prevalence remains disputed, but it may appear as a congenital or presumably acquired abnormality affecting Negroes, Orientals, and Cypriot Greeks somewhat more frequently than Caucasians. Its more frequent occurrence in patients with ulcerative colitis, Crohn's disease (uninvolved intestine), and even viral hepatitis has been alleged by some and denied by others. A previously asymptomatic lactase deficiency may become manifest when combined with other gastrointestinal disease, however, because of (1) an increased lactose load contained in an ulcer diet, (2) an increased rate of gastric emptying following gastric resection, or (3) the concurrent development of functional or inflammatory intestinal disease. Several criteria have been proposed for a diagnosis of lactase deficiency: (1) diarrhea, cramping abdominal pain, and flatulence upon ingesting lactose; (2) absent or diminished lactase activity in mucosal biopsy specimens; (3) a flat lactose tolerance curve after the oral administration of 50 grams of lactose, with normal tolerance curves for glucose and galactose; (4) a fall in the stool pH after ingestion of lactose due to the conversion of the unabsorbed lactose to lactic acid by the colonic bacteria; and (5) disappearance of symptoms upon the removal of lactose from the diet. The severity of the defect varies widely, and since there is a gradient of lactase activity in the small bowel with peak levels in the jejunum and proximal ileum, it is not possible to measure total intestinal lactase activity using biopsy specimens and this information therefore may be misleading. Spuriously flat lactose tolerance curves may occur in the presence of delayed gastric emptying or a rapid rise and fall of the blood glucose during the first 30 minutes of the test. Direct instillation of lactose into the duodenum will resolve the first problem and the measurement of capillary rather than venous blood glucose will obviate the latter.

Abnormalities of Lymphatic Transport. Any condition interfering with the normal flow of lymph from the lacteal through the abdominal lymphatic systems to the thoracic duct and thence to the general circulation may result in increased losses of lymph constituents, namely, plasma proteins, chylomicron fat, and small lymphocytes.

From a pathophysiologic point of view, such conditions are not, strictly speaking, absorptive defects as much as they are disorders of lymph flow. However, fat does tend to accumulate in the villous absorptive cells, in the intercellular spaces between absorptive cells, in the extracellular space of the lamina propria, and in the endothelial cells of the lacteals; from the standpoint of lipid absorption, these conditions can be considered as exit blocks.

Disorders of lymphatic transport may be congenital, as in the case of primary intestinal lymphangiectasia, or acquired secondary to structural abnormalities occurring as part of other primary intestinal disease or to an increase in lymphatic pressure due to increases in central venous pressure. Because of the associated loss of plasma proteins, lymphatic abnormalities also represent one type of protein-losing gastroenteropathy. Pure lymphatic abnormalities result in mild steatorrhea, modest elevations of fecal nitrogen, hypoalbuminemia, hypogammaglobulinemia, and, not infrequently, lymphocytopenia. Circulating immunoglobulins may therefore be low and cellular immune responses impaired. Clinical manifestations related to the lymphatic abnormality may include diarrhea, edema, and sometimes repeated infections and cutaneous anergy, including the ability to accept homografts. The edema in patients with primary intestinal lymphangiectasia may be asymmetrical since there is often an asymmetrical hypoplasia of peripheral lymphatics as well. Small intestinal x-ray examination shows thickening of the mucosal folds and sometimes suggestive features of a mild malabsorption pattern. Lymphangiography will demonstrate the structural lymphatic defect and occasionally puddling of the dye in the intestinal lumen. Mucosal biopsy reveals the dilated mucosal lymphatics but cannot provide an etiologic diagnosis. Ideally, therapy should be directed toward relief of the responsible lymphatic obstruction; however, this may be possible in only a few situations, such as constrictive pericarditis or congestive heart failure. In the other conditions, especially primary intestinal lymphangiectasia, a reduction in lymph flow and pressure can be achieved by reducing the dietary intake of long-chain triglycerides and replacing them with medium-chain triglycerides which are absorbed by the portal vein.

Protein-Losing Gastroenteropathies. Although not strictly disorders of absorption it is convenient to discuss other aspects of the protein-losing gastroenteropathies at this point, since they do represent states of increased intestinal nitrogen loss. A classification of the major protein-losing states is presented in Table 26–3. Over 40 disorders have been associated with abnormal protein loss, many representing only single case reports, and the reader is referred to the review by Waldmann for a more complete listing of these conditions. Generally, protein-losing states fall into one of the following categories: (1) benign or malignant tumors largely of the stomach or colon; (2) any condition associated with gastrointestinal inflammation with loss of epithelial cell integrity; (3) primary or secondary structural abnormalities of lymphatic channels from the lacteal to the termination of the thoracic duct; and (4) a sustained and significant increase in central venous pressure, which is then transmitted to the thoracic duct. Fecal nitrogen is often mildly elevated but is not diagnostically helpful because of the digestion and absorption of variable amounts of the protein lost and the inability to distinguish between increased loss and malabsorption. Therefore, techniques using radiolabeled macromolecules are utilized in an attempt to document and quantitate gastrointestinal protein loss.

An ideal substance should fulfill the following requirements: (1) the labeled substance should have a normal metabolic behavior, (2) there should be no excretion of the label into the gastrointestinal tract unless it is bound to protein, and (3) there should be no absorption of the label from the gastrointestinal tract after its catabolism. None of the readily available substances completely fulfills these requirements.

Using intravenously administered ^{131}I-labeled albumin, one may determine the plasma volume, the total albumin pool, the rate of albumin degradation, and, in the steady state, the rate of albumin synthesis. Patients with protein loss, regardless of the mechanism involved, have reduced circulating and total body pools of albumin, a normal or slightly increased rate of albumin synthesis, and a markedly shortened al-

TABLE 26–3 CLASSIFICATION OF PROTEIN-LOSING GASTROENTEROPATHIES

Loss of epithelial integrity
    Menetrier's giant hypertrophic gastritis
    Gastric carcinoma
    Carcinoma of the colon
    Nontropical sprue
    Crohn's disease
    Gastrointestinal lymphoma
    Acute gastroenteritis
    Ulcerative colitis
    Gastrointestinal polyposis syndromes
Lymphatic hypertension
    Primary intestinal lymphangiectasia
    Retroperitoneal tumors
    Retroperitoneal fibrosis
    Constrictive pericarditis
    Congestive heart failure
    Whipple's disease
    Crohn's disease
    Gastrointestinal lymphomas

bumin survival. Data obtained from serum and urinary radioactivity curves, however, indicate only that hypercatabolism or increased loss is the cause of the hypoproteinemia but do not necessarily implicate the gastrointestinal tract. The fecal output of ^{131}I cannot be used as an estimate of protein loss, since most of the label entering the intestinal tract is removed, reabsorbed, and excreted in the urine. Also there is active secretion of ^{131}I into the gastrointestinal tract regardless of where in the body it is removed. Amberlite IRA-400, an ion exhange resin, has been utilized in an effort to trap the ^{131}I in the lumen but with only partial success. The half-life of ^{131}I-albumin is 14 to 22 days.

^{131}I-labeled polyvinylpyrrolidone is a synthetic polymer with an average molecular weight of 40,000 that is unaffected by digestive enzymes and is poorly absorbed. Normal subjects excrete 0 to 1.5 per cent of an intravenous dose, while patients with protein loss excrete 2.9 to 32.5 per cent. Variable but significant amounts of the label are removed and absorbed; nevertheless, it can be of great value as a screening test.

^{51}Cr-labeled albumin is perhaps the most useful of the readily available substances, since the label is neither significantly absorbed from nor secreted into the gastrointestinal tract. Normals excrete 0.1 to 0.7 per cent of an intravenous dose, while patients with protein loss excrete 2 to 40 per cent of the radioactive substance. A disadvantage is its short apparent half-life of 3 to 10 days due to the elution of the label from the protein. For this reason, ^{51}Cr-albumin cannot be used to determine pool sizes or rates of protein synthesis and catabolism.

A more complete analysis of protein metabolism can be achieved by the simultaneous use of ^{51}Cr-albumin and ^{125}I-albumin. The size of the albumin pool and rates of albumin catabolism and synthesis can be determined from the ^{125}I data and the magnitude of gastrointestinal protein loss estimated by the ^{51}Cr-albumin.

SECRETORY FUNCTION

There is as yet very little clear understanding of the importance of secretion in the normal physiology of the small intestine. Both water and electrolytes as well as certain hormones and enzymes appear to be secreted by the intestinal mucosa but the older concept of a succus entericus has not proved useful or accurate. By virtue of its apparent link to cyclic AMP, the secretory process is subject to complex and varied forms of regulation. Potentially, therefore, many agents may alter the secretory rates of various substances through effects on adenyl cyclase or phosphodiesterase activity. Although our knowledge in this area is limited, certain observations related to the secretion of water, electrolytes, hormones, and enzymes do have clinical application.

Water and Electrolyte Secretion

The usual concentrations of electrolytes in small intestinal fluid vary somewhat between the jejunum and the ileum. Sodium and potassium concentrations are similar in the two areas, the former being approximately 140 mEq. per liter and the latter 7 mEq. per liter. Jejunal chloride concentrations, however, are higher than in the ileum (129 mEq. per liter as compared to 81 mEq. per liter), while the reverse is true for bicarbonate (17 mEq. per liter versus 63 mEq. per liter). The manner in which water and electrolyte fluxes are regulated to maintain these differing concentrations under normal circumstances is virtually unknown. Somewhat paradoxically, more information is available about their fluxes in certain disease states. The most notable of these is cholera, and studies in cholera patients have provided some insight into the handling of water and electrolytes by the small intestine.

The diarrhea of cholera, almost entirely of small bowel origin, offers an impressive demonstration of the secretory capacity of this organ. In the adult with acute cholera the secretory capacity amounts to 1 to 2 liters per hour. The fluid is approximately isosmotic with plasma and is nearly protein-free. The predominant cation is sodium and the predominant anions are chloride and bicarbonate, the latter two exhibiting the same relationships in the jejunum and ileum as under normal circumstances. The *Vibrio cholerae* does not invade the intestinal wall and as a result there is no disruption of the epithelium or significant inflammation. Consistent with the absence of epithelial cell damage is the fact that glucose absorption and glucose-coupled sodium transport remain normal. Once this was realized, the oral administration of glucose to stimulate fluid absorption became an important adjunct to therapy. The epithelium of the small intestine can be triggered to secrete chloride actively by both cholera exotoxin and cyclic AMP. Furthermore, the exotoxin results in an increase in the cyclic AMP concentration in the intestinal mucosa. Despite its gradual development, secretion is difficult to reverse once the toxin has come into contact with the epithelium. There are two possible driving forces for the massive intestinal secretion encountered in cholera: active transport by the epithelium and a hydrostatic pressure difference from the interstitial tissue to the lumen. On the basis of present evidence it is highly probable that the fluid loss results from an active secretory process. The massive diarrhea characteristic of acute cholera ensues because the absorptive capacity of the colon is readily overwhelmed by the large quantity of water and electrolytes presented to it.

The products of several other bacteria also elicit small intestinal fluid secretion, including *E. coli*, *Shigella*, and *Clostridium perfringens*. The massive diarrhea occasionally occurring in association with several hormone-secreting tumors such as malignant carcinoids, medullary carcinomas of the thyroid, and some nonbeta cell tumors of the pancreatic islets may also in part be due to an enhancement of cyclic AMP activity. This possibility rests upon the concept of a two-messenger system of hormone action. The first messenger is a hormone stimulating adenyl cyclase activity within the target cell. This results in the formation of increased amounts of cyclic AMP (the second messenger) from ATP. In view of the large number of agents that increase cyclic AMP concentrations in this way, it is likely that this secretory mechanism plays an important part not only in cholera but in other disorders associated with diarrhea.

The Secretion of Hormones and Enzymes

The small intestine is known to secrete three hormones (secretin, cholecystokinin-pancreozymin, and glucagon) and is suspected of producing another (enterogastrone). Although most small bowel enzymes are fixed in that they function at sites in the glycocalyx-plasma membrane structure or epithelial cell cytoplasm, one enzyme is released into the lumen in physiologic concentrations (enterokinase).

Secretin is released from the duodenum and probably the proximal jejunum in response to H^+ the magnitude of response being proportional to the amount rather than to the concentration of the H^+. It shares a 14 amino acid sequence with glucagon, but no fragment with superior biological activity has been identified. Cholecystokinin-pancreozymin is secreted from the duodenum and jejunum following vagal stimulation but especially in response to free fatty acids and essential amino acids in the intestinal lumen. It contains the same C-terminal pentapeptide as gastrin but most of its activity is contained in the C-terminal heptapeptide. Also, a glucagon-like immunoreactive substance distinct from pancreatic glucagon is released from the duodenum in response to intraluminal glucose. The activities of these three hormones are summarized in Table 26-4. Their function in coordinating the various phases of the digestive-absorptive process is related to their effects on gastric emptying, gastroduodenal motor responses, and the secretion of acid, bile, and pancreatic juice.

The specific cells responsible for the synthesis and release of these three hormones have not been identified and no primary disorders of their secretion have been reported. In diffuse mucosal lesions of the small intestine such as nontropical sprue, however, the activities of secretin and cholecystokinin-pancreozymin may be reduced. These patients often exhibit delayed emptying of the gallbladder; decreased luminal concentrations of pancreatic lipase, bile acids, and micellar lipid; and decreased intestinal motor activity. Furthermore, the secretion of bicarbonate by the pancreas is impaired following duodenal acidification.

The glucagon-like immunoreactive material released in response to an oral glucose load may be important to the development of reactive hypoglycemia. The insulin response to oral glucose is greater and more prolonged than the response to intravenous glucose, and in the presence of reactive hypoglycemia there is a rise in the blood glucagon-like immunoreactive material but not in pancreatic glucagon. This substance is then thought to stimulate insulin release, resulting in the hypoglycemia. Oral glucose loading also stimulates the release of secretin and cholecystokinin-pancreozymin and they may play some role in this sequence of events, since they too are capable of insulin release.

The existence of enterogastrone continues to remain uncertain. Substances from various tis-

TABLE 26-4 PHYSIOLOGIC EFFECTS OF INTESTINAL HORMONES

	Cholecystokinin-Pancreozymin (CCK–PZ)	Secretin	Glucagon
Gallbladder contraction	S	0	?
Stomach			
H^+	Sw	I	Iw
Pepsin	Sw	S	0
Motility	S	I	I
Exocrine pancreas			
HCO_3^-	Sw	S	I
Enzymes	S	Sw	I
Endocrine pancreas			
Insulin	S	S	S
Glucagon	S	0	—
Intestine			
Brunner's glands	S	S	S
Motility	S	I	I
Hepatic bile			
HCO_3^-	Sw	Sw	Sw

S — Stimulates
Sw — Stimulates weakly
I — Inhibits
Iw — Inhibits weakly
0 — No effect

Modified from Go, V.L.W., and Summerskill, W.H.J.: Amer. J. Clin. Nutr., 24:160, 1971.

sues collectively referred to as "gastrones" inhibit gastric acid secretion. The duodenal instillation of acid, fat, or hypertonic solutions results in an inhibition of acid secretion. Some maintain that the release of secretin and cholecystokinin-pancreozymin provides an adequate explanation for this effect. Others point out that fat in the duodenum blocks histamine-stimulated acid secretion, whereas secretin and cholecystokinin-pancreozymin do not. An extract of duodenal mucosa has been shown to diminish the acid response to histamine, and it is probable that an enterogastrone does exist.

As previously discussed, enterokinase is concerned with the conversion of pancreatic proenzymes to their active forms. The enzyme is located in the proximal duodenum in relationship to the microvilli, but its mechanism of release into the duodenal lumen has not been established. Bile salts appear to constitute one effective stimulus and in their presence enterokinase activity is increased. Recently, several cases of enterokinase deficiency have been recognized in infants presenting with diarrhea from birth, showing failure to thrive, and exhibiting a good clinical response to pancreatic extracts.

IMMUNOLOGIC FUNCTION

Normal Structure and Function

Unlike most other organs such as the heart or kidney, the gastrointestinal tract is replete with immunologically competent tissue. It is capable not only of experiencing but also of mounting an immune response. In this respect it maintains functional identity with other peripheral lymphoid tissues such as the lymph nodes and spleen. Little is known, however, regarding either the qualitative or quantitative contributions of the gut to the body's immune responses. Of further importance is the realization that all the currently recognized, so-called central lymphoid tissues which determine the immunological capabilities of the whole organism are lymphoepithelial derivatives of the gut. The small intestine, therefore, assumes a position of considerable importance to the immunologist as well as to those who seek an understanding of its more classic functions. Any attempt to relate abnormalities of the small bowel to concurrently observed immunologic changes must proceed from an awareness of the potential of the small intestine as both a central and peripheral lymphoid organ as well as an immunologic target.

The lymphoid elements of the small bowel are arranged in different ways, but the functional implications of these structural variations are unknown. The Peyer's patches lie in the lamina propria and submucosa and consist of lymphoid follicles containing germinal centers. The lymphocytes in the follicular cortex appear to represent a separate population when compared to similar areas of spleen and lymph nodes. Small lymphocytes from thoracic duct lymph preferentially "home" to the Peyer's patches as well as lymph nodes and spleen. These structures are well developed by the fifth month of fetal life, increase in size and number until the age of 10 or 12, and gradually atrophy thereafter. Although Peyer's patch cells are capable of antibody synthesis and probably of both primary and secondary immune responses, the importance of this function in relation to their location is unclear. The lamina propria also contains a second population of lymphoid cells differing in certain respects from the Peyer's patches. Its lymphocytes and plasma cells also contain various immunoglobulins but they are not arranged in any structured fashion. Large lymphocytes from the thoracic duct lymph preferentially seed the lamina propria as do lymphoblasts formed in lymph nodes following antigenic stimulation. It is not known, however, whether primary or secondary immune responses occur in situ within this nonaggregated lymphoid tissue of the lamina propria. The third type of lymphoid elements found in the small intestine are the theliolymphocytes. They lie within and between the mucosal epithelial cells but their source, nature, function, and fate are unknown.

The lymphoid tissues of the Peyer's patches and lamina propria are sparse and appear undeveloped prior to birth and in the germ-free state. With the development of an intestinal flora, lymphocytes and plasma cells become more numerous and germinal centers develop.

It is apparent that all three of these lymphoid "structures" maintain a lymphoepithelial relationship which is similar to that of the thymus and the avian bursa of Fabricius. The former is responsible for the development of the cellular immune system and the latter, in avian species at least, regulates the development of the humoral immune system. This has led to considerable speculation concerning which, if any, of the small intestinal lymphoid elements constitute a human bursal equivalent.

Most immunoglobulin-containing cells in the small intestine are mature plasma cells, although some immunoglobulins are found within immature plasma cells and lymphocytes. It is well established that IgA is the predominant immunoglobulin in the lymphoid cells and secretions of the small intestine. IgM, IgG, and IgD are also present in that order; recently, IgE has been identified in the small intestine but its relative amount has yet to be established. The IgA found in the small intestine and its secretions differs from 7S serum IgA in that it is an 11S globulin with a molecular weight of 390,000. This secretory IgA appears to represent a dimer of the 7S serum IgA coupled to a nonimmunoglobulin glycoprotein, referred to as secretory piece or T (transport) component. This secretory component has been identified as a product of the epithelial cells and is associated with the mucus-containing area of intestinal goblet cells. Its precise function is not known, although it no doubt confers some biological advantage on IgA in the external secretions. There are two subclasses of IgA — IgA_1 and IgA_2. IgA_2 appears to predominate in the intestinal secretions and differs from IgA_1 in that it contains no disulfide bonds linking the light and heavy chains, and contains a genetic marker, Am_2 within its heavy chain structure.

The human infant is born totally lacking IgA in serum and external secretions, and secretory IgA appears sooner and reaches adult levels more quickly than serum IgA. The small intestine therefore has been regarded as a potentially important source not only of secretory but also of serum IgA. Secretory IgA has been demonstrated to possess antiviral and antibacterial activity as well as the properties of isohemagglutinins. Although the precise role played by secretory IgA in the external secretions remains unsettled, it probably constitutes an important defense against certain microorganisms and perhaps other potentially harmful substances.

Abnormal Structure and Function

Chronic diarrhea and malabsorption are common in immunodeficiency syndromes presenting later in life. Gastrointestinal symptoms, however, are characteristically absent in congenital sex-linked agammaglobulinemias. Two distinctive histologic patterns have been described in the small intestine of patients with immunodeficiency syndromes and gastrointestinal symptoms: The first, nodular lymphoid hyperplasia of the small intestine, has been so named because of the multiple small lymphoid nodules present within the mucosa. These nodules contain hyperplastic germinal centers but plasma cells are sparse throughout the intestine and the epithelial and villous architecture remain well preserved. The second pattern has been referred to as hypogammaglobulinemic "sprue" because there is villus atrophy and the mucosa often presents a flat appearance. These patients differ, however, from those with gluten-sensitive enteropathy not only in the presence of the immunodeficiency but also in failing to respond in the majority of instances to a gluten-free diet. Plasma cells are also nearly completely absent in the small intestine of patients with this type of pattern.

In their initial report, Hermans and his associates described five characteristic features of patients with nodular lymphoid hyperplasia: (1) dysgammaglobulinemia, consisting of the virtual absence of IgA and IgM, with a moderate reduction in IgG; (2) susceptibility to sinopulmonary infections; (3) diarrhea; (4) *Giardia lamblia* in the stools; and (5) nodular lymphoid hyperplasia of the small intestine. Additional cases have been described with idiopathic acquired hypogammaglobulinemia, and two subjects have been reported with a selective absence of IgA. In those patients studied, cellular immune mechanisms appear to be intact. Mild steatorrhea is often present and in many instances both the diarrhea and steatorrhea respond favorably to treatment of the Giardia infestation. The radiographic findings in nodular lymphoid hyperplasia are characteristic, demonstrating innumerable small filling defects measuring only a few millimeters in diameter which are uniform in size and smooth in contour. Segmental involvement of the small intestine and colon may be present or the entire small bowel may be involved, and a mild malabsorption pattern is at times superimposed.

In so-called hypogammaglobulinemic sprue, steatorrhea is often more marked. These patients also frequently harbor *Giardia lamblia* in the small intestinal secretions, and in many instances the associated diarrhea and steatorrhea are improved after treatment of the giardiasis. These patients generally exhibit an acquired type of hypogammaglobulinemia, although again selective IgA deficiency has been encountered.

The relationship between the immunodeficiency and the structural and functional abnormalities present in the small intestine is unknown. It should be noted that selective IgA deficiency is not uncommon in the general population, occurring in approximately 1 of every 700 individuals. Many of these patients are without any intestinal symptoms and many patients with acquired hypogammaglobulinemia fail to demonstrate structural abnormalities or symptoms related to the small intestine. At the present time, therefore, these various structural and functional changes cannot be understood in pathophysiologic terms.

VASCULAR DISORDERS OF THE SMALL INTESTINE

Normal Physiology

The splanchnic circulation receives 28 per cent of the cardiac output and contains 20 per cent of the total blood volume, with 65 per cent distributed to the mucosa. After eating, there is a 30 per cent increase in splanchnic flow which correlates with the processes of secretion and absorption. This effect is probably in part mediated by the release of gastrin, secretin, and cholecystokinin-pancreozymin, all of which act to increase superior mesenteric artery flow.

Intestinal blood flow is regulated primarily by the sympathetic nervous system via alpha receptor activity. Stimulation can virtually interrupt flow, especially to the mucosa, while the elimination of normal constrictor activity results in a 20 to 40 per cent increase. When all factors capable of augmenting blood flow are operative, the maximal possible increase is in the range of 500 per cent. A decrease in splanchnic flow may result from a number of influences, including exercise, standing, intraluminal pressures above 30 mm. Hg, and increased sympathetic neurohumoral activity. Although muscle contraction leads to a decrease in flow, the net effect of intestinal motor activity is to increase flow probably as a result of increased cholinergic activity and the release of various metabolites.

Intestinal blood flow also exhibits autoregulation and autoregulatory escape. Autoregulation involves the coordination of physiologic mechanisms to maintain blood flow in the face of a decrease in arterial pressure, while autoregulatory escape is the intrinsic ability of the intestinal vasculature to "escape" from persistent vasoconstrictor activity imposed by alpha-adrenergic stimulation. It therefore represents a protective mechanism within the intestinal circulation to counter ischemia during prolonged sympathetic activity.

An additional concept important to an understanding of intestinal ischemia is that of countercurrent exchange (Fig. 26–12). The effect of such an arrangement is that arterial substances (for example, oxygen) entering at the base of the villus will progressively decrease in concentration toward the villous tip, whereas absorbed materials entering at the villous tip will leave the villus more slowly. Countercurrent exchange operates at low perfusion rates and aggravates mucosal ischemia.

Intestinal Ischemia and Infarction

A compromise in the arterial supply of the small intestine may result in either chronic intestinal ischemia or infarction. Approximately 60 per cent of infarctions result from nonocclusive disease, while 30 per cent are due to either thrombosis or embolism, the former probably being more frequent. The remaining 10 per cent follow venous occlusion.

Chronic intestinal ischemia is best understood as a series of recurring attacks of acute ischemia which do not result in infarction. Although any disease process which results in a decrease in arterial flow may be responsible, the vast majority of cases are a result of atherosclerotic narrowing of the celiac axis and superior or inferior mesenteric arteries. The constriction is asymmetrical and most evident in the first centimeter of the involved vessel. The most prominent manifestation is cramping, periumbilical pain (intestinal angina) which characteristically occurs 10 to 15 minutes after eating and lasts 2 to 3 hours. Larger meals produce more pain and there is a tendency for it to become worse with the passage of time. As noted previously, ischemia causes increased contractility of smooth muscle and the mechanism responsible for pain production is probably smooth muscle spasm. Patients tend to restrict their food intake in an effort to avoid these episodes of pain, and as a result weight loss may be marked. Not uncommonly, mild diarrhea with or without a slight increase in stool fat and nitrogen occurs, probably as a result of impaired

Figure 26–12 The functional implications of the mucosal countercurrent exchanger schematically illustrated. *A*, Absorbed materials are delayed in their egress from the villus, and *B*, arterial O_2 achieves a progressively lower concentration at the villous tip.

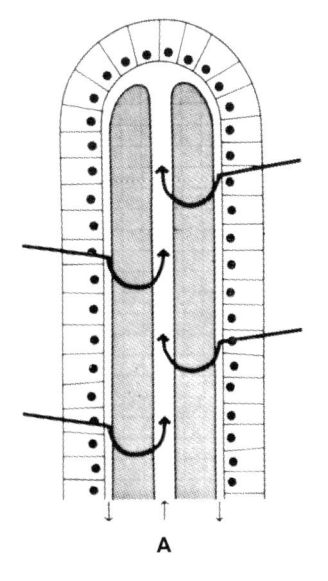

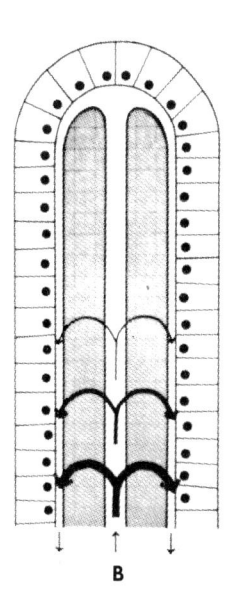

epithelial cell function and an increase in propulsive motor activity.

It must be recognized, however, that symptom production cannot always be correlated with anatomic abnormalities demonstrated by arteriography. Even occlusion of all three major arterial branches of the abdominal aorta has been encountered in the absence of apparent symptoms. Granting such inconsistencies, the general view is that a patient with characteristic abdominal pain and weight loss not explained by a primary disorder of the gut, pancreas, or hepatobiliary system and who has significant (> 50 per cent of the lumen) narrowing in two of the three mesenteric arteries should be regarded as having a clinical disturbance of the mesenteric arterial circulation. If a gradient of >35 mm. Hg is present at the time of operation, this assumption is strengthened. Surgical correction will result in relief of pain in 90 per cent of such patients and reversal of the malabsorption in 75 per cent. Protection from future fatal infarction, however, is less well established.

Main stem occlusion of the superior mesenteric artery is characterized by two phases: initially there is mucosal ischemia, necrosis, and hemorrhage, with associated intestinal muscle spasm; this is followed by paralysis of smooth muscle, intestinal dilatation, and necrosis of the entire bowel wall, with peritonitis and major fluid and blood loss into the gut. Significant inflammatory changes are characteristically absent, with hemorrhage and edema being the predominant features. Patients at first complain of colicky periumbilical pain which gradually becomes continuous, severe, and poorly localized. Initially there is a disproportionate lack of physical findings followed by signs of sympathetic overactivity, peritonitis, and cardiovascular collapse. Occlusion by an embolus may occur at different levels. In the presence of significant atheromatous disease, the main stem of the superior mesenteric artery may be involved (18 per cent) but 55 per cent of emboli lodge at the origin of the middle colic artery.

Nonocclusive infarction results from an interplay of several factors. The common denominator is a decrease in splanchnic flow resulting in a reduced perfusion pressure. This may be due to a reduced cardiac output or a decrease in the fraction entering the mesenteric circulation. A further decrease in flow, especially to the mucosa, is brought about by the activation of alpha-adrenergic receptors and the renin-angiotensin mechanism. The gut is therefore placed in an impossible situation. Autoregulatory escape will not maintain flow, and continued sympathetic activity reduces flow especially to the mucosa. An increase in blood viscosity and the collapse of small vessels at low perfusion pressure no doubt provide aggravating factors. Furthermore, many patients are taking digitalis, which has a mesenteric constrictor effect, and this may be a contributing influence. The result is mucosal necrosis and hemorrhage and, if the process is severe enough, transmural infarction.

Venous occlusion affects the superior mesenteric vein 20 times more frequently than it affects the inferior mesenteric vein, but it is doubtful that occlusion of the latter leads to symptoms. Venous occlusion is associated with the gradual onset of vague abdominal discomfort, anorexia, and a change in bowel habits associated with slight abdominal tenderness and diminished bowel sounds. Intramural edema is marked and the sequence of events described previously takes place, albeit more slowly. Most often it represents a complication of hypercoagulable states, polycythemia, carcinomas, portal hypertension, sepsis, or surgical injury.

REFERENCES

Adibi, S. A., and Allen, E. R.: Impaired jejunal absorption rates of essential amino acids induced by either dietary caloric or protein deprivation in man. Gastroenterology, 59:404, 1970.

Asp, N. G., and Dahlqvist, A.: Multiplicity of intestinal beta-galactosidases. Contribution of each enzyme to the toal lactase activity in normal and lactose intolerant patients. Acta Paediat. Scand., 60:364, 1971.

Asp, N. G., Dahlqvist, A., and Koldovsky, O.: Small intestinal beta-galactosidase activity. Gastroenterology, 58:591, 1970.

Balcerzak, S. P., Lane, W. C., and Bullard, J. W.: Surface structure of intestinal epithelium. Gastroenterology, 58:49, 1970.

Bass, P.: In vivo electrical activity of the small bowel. In Code, C. F. (Ed.): Handbook of Physiology. Vol. IV. Washington, D.C., American Physiological Society, 1968, p. 2051.

Bayless, T. M., Swanson, V. L., and Wheby, M. S.: Jejunal histology and clinical status in tropical sprue and other chronic diarrheal disorders. Amer. J. Clin. Nutr., 24:112, 1971.

Bennett, A., and Fleshler, B.: Prostaglandins and the gastrointestinal tract. Gastroenterology, 59:790, 1970.

Bentley, D. W., Nichols, R. L., Condon, R. E., et al.: The microflora of the human ileum and intra-abdominal colon: Results of direct needle aspiration at surgery and evaluation of the technique. J. Lab. Clin. Med., 79:421, 1972.

Binder, H. J.: A comparison of intestinal and renal transport systems. Amer. J. Clin. Nutr., 23:330, 1970.

Braddock, L. E., Fleisher, D. R., and Barbero, G. J.: A physical chemical study of the van de Kamer method for fecal fat analysis. Gastroenterology, 55:165, 1968.

Brandborg, L. L.: Structure and function of the small intestine in some parasite diseases. Amer. J. Clin. Nutr., 24:124, 1971.

Brooks, F. P.: Absorption. In Control of Gastrointestinal Function. London, The Macmillan Co., 1970.

Bynum, T. E., and Jacobson, E. D.: Blood flow and gastrointestinal disease. Digestion, 4:109, 1971.

Bynum, T. E., and Jacobson, E. D.: Blood flow and gastrointestinal function. Gastroenterology, 60:325, 1971.

Christensen, J.: The control of gastrointestinal movements: some old and new views. New Eng. J. Med., 285:85, 1971.

Code, C. F., Szurszewski, J. H., and Kelly, K. A.: A concept of motor control by the pacesetter potential in the stomach and small bowel. Amer. J. Dig. Dis., 16:601, 1971.

Corcino, J. J., Waxman, S., and Herbert, V.: Absorption and malabsorption of vitamin B_{12}. Amer. J. Med., 48:562, 1970.

Cornes, J. S.: Number, size and distribution of Peyer's patches in the human small intestine. I. The development of Peyer's patches. Gut, 6:225, 1965.

Daniel, E. E., Robinson, K., Duchon, G., et al.: The possible role of close contacts (nexuses) in the propagation of control electrical activity in the stomach and small intestine. Amer. J. Dig. Dis., 16:611, 1971.

Demling, L.: The motility of the gastrointestinal tract. Digestion, 2:362, 1969.

Dixon, J. A., Harman, C. G., Nichols, R. L., et al.: Intestinal motility following luminal and vascular occlusion of the small intestine. Gastroenterology, 58:673, 1970.

Dobbins, W. O., III: Morphologic and functional correlates of intestinal brush borders. Amer. J. Med. Sci., 258:150, 1969.

Dobbins, W. O., III: Intestinal mucosal lacteal in transport of macromolecules and chylomicrons. Amer. J. Clin. Nutr., 24:77, 1971.

Donaldson, R. M., Jr.: Small bowel bacterial overgrowth. Advances Intern. Med., 16:191, 1970.

Dowling, R. H.: The enterohepatic circulation. Gastroenterology, 62:122, 1972.

Editorial: Ileus: Paralytic or sympathetic? Lancet, 1:329, 1971.

Editorial: "Enterogastrone(s)." Lancet, 1:1224, 1971.

Eggermont, E., Molla, A. M., Rutgeerts, L., et al.: The source of human enterokinase. Lancet, 2:369, 1971.

Elsas, L. J., Hillman, R. E., Patterson, J. H., et al.: Renal and intestinal hexose transport in familial glucose-galactose malabsorption. J. Clin. Invest., 49:576, 1970.

Farrar, J. T., and Zfass, A. M.: Small intestinal motility. Gastroenterology, 52:1019, 1967.

Fasel, J., Hadjikhani, H., and Felber, J. P.: The insulin secretory effect of the human duodenal mucosa. Gastroenterology, 59:109, 1970.

Fichtelius, K. E.: The gut epithelium—a first level lymphoid organ? Exp. Cell Res., 49:87, 1968.

Field, M.: Intestinal secretion: Effect of cyclic AMP and its role in cholera. New Eng. J. Med., 284:1137, 1971.

French, A. B.: Protein-losing gastroenteropathies. Amer. J. Dig. Dis., 16:661, 1971.

Freter, R.: Locally produced and serum derived antibodies in "local immunity." New Eng. J. Med., 285:1375, 1971.

Go, V. L. W., and Summerskill, W. H. J.: Digestion, maldigestion, and the gastrointestinal hormones. Amer. J. Clin. Nutr., 24:160, 1971.

Gorbach, S. L.: Intestinal microflora. Gastroenterology, 60:1110, 1971.

Gray, G. M.: Carbohydrate digestion and absorption. Gastroenterology, 58:96, 1970.

Gray, G. M., and Cooper, H. L.: Protein digestion and absorption. Gastroenterology, 61:535, 1971.

Greenberger, N. J.: The intestinal brush border as a digestive and absorptive surface. Amer. J. Med. Sci., 258:144, 1969.

Hall, J. G., and Smith, M. E.: Homing of lymph-borne immunoblasts to the gut. Nature, 226:262, 1970.

Harrison, L. A., and Jacobson, E. D.: Gastrointestinal hormones. J. Okla. Med. Assoc., 63:157, 1970.

Hellier, M. D., Perrett, D., and Holdsworth, C. D.: Dipeptide absorption in cystinuria. Brit. Med. J., 4:782, 1970.

Hellier, M. D., Perrett, D., Holdsworth, C. D., et al.: Absorption of dipeptides in normal and cystinuric subjects. Gut, 12:496, 1971.

Hendrix, T. R., and Bayless, T. M.: Digestion: Intestinal secretion. Ann. Rev. Physiol., 32:139, 1970.

Henry, C., Faulk, W. P., Kuhn, L., et al.: Peyer's patches: Immunologic studies. J. Exp. Med., 131:1200, 1970.

Hermans, P. E., Huizenga, K. A., Hoffman, H. N., et al.: Dysgammaglobulinemia associated with nodular lymphoid hyperplasia of the small intestine. Amer. J. Med., 40:78, 1966.

Hightower, N. C., Jr.: Motor action of the small bowel. In Code, C. F. (Ed.): Handbook of Physiology. Vol. IV. Washington, D.C., American Physiological Society, 1968, p. 2001.

Holt, P. R.: Medium chain triglycerides: Their absorption, metabolism and clinical applications. In Glass, G. B. J. (Ed.): Progress in Gastroenterology. New York, Grune and Stratton, 1968, p. 277.

Hughes, W. S., Cerda, J. J., Holtzapple, P., et al.: Primary hypogammaglobulinemia and malabsorption. Ann. Intern. Med., 74:903, 1971.

Jacobson, E. D., Brobmann, G. F., and Brecher, G. A.: Intestinal motor activity and blood flow. Gastroenterology, 58:575, 1970.

Jeffries, G. Y. H., Weser, E., and Sleisenger, M. H.: Malabsorption. Gastroenterology, 56:777, 1969.

Jordan, P. H., Jr., Boulafendis, D., and Guinn, G. A.: Factors other than major vascular occlusion that contribute to intestinal infarction. Ann. Surg., 171:189, 1970.

Kraft, S. C., and Kirsner, J. B.: Immunological apparatus of the gut and inflammatory bowel disease. Gastroenterology, 60:922, 1971.

Kriebel, G. W., Jr., Kraft, S. C., and Rothberg, R. M.: Locally produced antibody in human gastrointestinal secretions. J. Immun., 103:1268, 1969.

Lenz, H., Blomer, A., and Dux, A.: Analysis of the propulsive movements of the small intestine. Cineradiographic and experimental studies. Amer. J. Dig. Dis., 16:1107, 1971.

Lundgren, O.: Countercurrent exchange in the small intestine. Amer. Heart. J., 79:285, 1970.

Marsh, M. N., and Swift, J. A.: A study of the small intestinal mucosa using the scanning electron microscope. Gut, 10:940, 1969.

Neely, J., and Catchpole, B.: Ileus: The restoration of alimentary tract motility by pharmacologic means. Brit. J. Surg., 58:21, 1971.

Nordstrom, C., and Dahlqvist, A.: Intestinal enterokinase. Lancet, 1:1185, 1971.

Pearse, A. G. E., Coulling, I., Weavers, B., et al.: The endocrine polypeptide cells of the human stomach, duodenum, and jejunum. Gut, 11:649, 1970.

Peters, T. J.: Intestinal peptidases. Gut, 11:720, 1970.

Pettersson, T., and Wegelius, O.: Biopsy diagnosis of amyloidosis in rheumatoid arthritis. Malabsorption caused by intestinal amyloid deposits. Gastroenterology, 62:22, 1972.

Porter, H. P., Saunders, D. R., Tytgat, G., et al.: Fat absorption in bile fistula man. A morphological and biochemical study. Gastroenterology, 60:1008, 1971.

Rosenberg, I. H., and Godwin, H. A.: The digestion and absorption of dietary folate. Gastroenterology, 60:445, 1971.

Rosenweig, N. S., Herman, R. H., and Stifel, F. B.: Dietary regulation of small intestinal enzyme activity in man. Amer. J. Clin. Nutr., 24:65, 1971.

Rubin, W.: Celiac disease. Amer. J. Clin. Nutr., 24:91, 1971.

Rubin, W.: The epithelial "membrane" of the small intestine. Amer. J. Clin. Nutr., 24:45, 1971.

Sadikali, F.: Dipeptidase deficiency and malabsorption of glycylglycine in disease states. Gut, 12:276, 1971.

Savilahti, E., Visakorpi, J. K., and Pelkonen, P.: Morphological and immunohistochemical findings in small intestinal biopsy in children with IgA deficiency. Acta Paediat. Scand., 60:363, 1971.

Schiff, E. R., and Dietschy, J. M.: Steatorrhea associated with disordered bile acid metabolism. Amer. J. Dig. Dis., 14:432, 1969.

Scratcherd, T., and Case, R. M.: The role of cyclic adenosine-3′,5′-monophosphate (AMP) in gastrointestinal secretion. Gut, 10:957, 1969.

Sessions, J. T., Jr., de Andrade, S. R. V., and Kokas, E.: Intestinal villi: Form and motility in relation to function. In Glass, G. B. J. (Ed.): Progress in Gastroenterology. New York, Grune and Stratton, 1968, p. 248.

Shanbour, L. L., and Jacobson, E. D.: Autoregulatory escape in the gut. Gastroenterology, 60:145, 1971.

Shih, V. E., Bixby, E. M., Alpers, C. S., et al.: Studies of intestinal transport defect in Hartnup disease. Gastroenterology, 61:445, 1971.

Storer, E. H.: The pharmacologic and biochemical nature of carcinoid tumors. Curr. Probl. Surg., November, 1970, p. 41.

Tarlow, M. J., Hadorn, B., Arthurton, M. W., et al.: Intestinal enterokinase deficiency. A newly recognized disorder of protein digestion. Arch. Dis. Child., 45:651, 1970.

Texter, E. C., Jr.: Pressure and transit in the small intestine. The concept of propulsion and peripheral resistance in the alimentary canal. Amer. J. Dig. Dis., 13:443, 1968.

Thompson, G. R., Barrowman, J., Guterrez, L., et al.: Action of neomycin on the intraluminal phase of lipid absorption. J. Clin. Invest., 50:319, 1971.

Tidball, C. S.: The nature of the intestinal epithelial barrier. Amer. J. Dig. Dis., 16:745, 1971.

Tomasi, T. B., Jr., Tan, E. M., Solomon, A., et al.: Characteristics of an immune system common to certain external secretions. J. Exp. Med., 121:101, 1965.

Toner, P. G., and Carr, K. E.: The use of scanning electron microscopy in the study of the intestinal villi. J. Path., 97:611, 1969.

Toner, P. G., Carr, K. E., Ferguson, A., et al.: Scanning and transmission electron microscopic studies of human intestinal mucosa. Gut, 11:471, 1970.

Toner, P. G., and Ferguson, A.: Intraepithelial cells in the human intestinal mucosa. J. Ultrastruct. Res., 34:329, 1971.

Trier, J. S., and Browning, T. H.: Epithelial-cell renewal in cultured duodenal biopsies in celiac sprue. New Eng. J. Med., 283:1245, 1970.

Trier, J. S., Phelps, P. C., Eidelman, S., et al.: Whipple's disease: Light and electron microscope correlation of jejunal mucosal histology with antibiotic treatment and clinical status. Gastroenterology, 48:684, 1965.

van de Kamer, J. H., ten Bokkel, H., and Weyers, H. A.: Rapid method for determination of fat in feces. J. Biol. Chem., 177:347, 1949.

Waldmann, T. A.: Protein-losing enteropathy. Gastroenterology, 50:422, 1966.

Watson, D. W.: Immune responses and the gut. Gastroenterology, 56:944, 1969.

Weser, E.: Intestinal adaptation to small bowel resection. Amer. J. Clin. Nutr., 24:133, 1971.

Weser, E., and Sleisenger, M. H.: Pathophysiology of sprue syndromes. Advances Intern. Med., 15:253, 1969.

Williams, L. F., Jr.: Vascular insufficiency of the bowels. D. M., August, 1970.

Williams, L. F., Jr.: Vascular insufficiency of the intestines. Gastroenterology, 61:757, 1971.

Wilson, F. A., and Dietschy, J. M.: Differential diagnostic approach to clinical problems of malabsorption. Gastroenterology, 61:911, 1971.

Wilson, H.: Carcinoid syndrome. Curr. Probl. Surg., November, 1970, p. 36.

Wilson, H., Cheek, R. C., Sherman, R. T., et al.: Carcinoid tumors. Curr. Probl. Surg., November, 1970, p. 4.

CHAPTER 27

THE LARGE INTESTINE

WILLIAM A. SODEMAN, Jr.
DAVID W. WATSON

INTRODUCTION

The colon, including the rectum, forms the multifunctional termination of the gastrointestinal tract. Its anatomy is substantially differentiated from the relatively simple muscular tube of the small intestine. The colon is approximately 150 cm. long. It is highly variable in diameter, though as a general rule the cecum is the widest part and the angulation at the rectosigmoid juncture forms its narrowest constriction. The cecum, ascending colon, and proximal one half of the transverse colon are derived from the midgut and share innervation and vascular supply with the small intestine. The distal colon is a hindgut derivative and utilizes the inferior mesenteric artery and sacral parasympathetic innervation. There is substantial anastomosis between the two vascular beds and considerable overlap of innervation, so that these embryonic divisions are indistinct. In adult life, the left and right colon perform distinctly different tasks, though there is no evidence that this is a reflection of embryonic origin.

The wall of the colon has the same four layers as the small intestine: mucosa, submucosa, muscularis externa, and serosa. The mucous membrane is not thrown into villous extensions. Scanning electron microscopy (Fig. 27–1) shows a flat epithelial surface broken into polygonal units by a cleft. Openings of the numerous goblet cells are apparent, and the center of each polygonal unit is perforated by a crypt of Lieberkühn that is lined with goblet cells and penetrates down to the muscularis mucosa. On conventional microscopic examination the surface epithelial cells that are presumably engaged in absorption present a striated border similar to that of small intestinal cells. Under the electron microscope the striated border resolves into microvilli complete with a fuzzy coat. There are scattered argentaffine cells. Cell renewal is initiated in the crypts, and cells migrate upward to the surface where they are extruded at the midpoint between crypts. The cell renewal time, based on cultured biopsy specimens of the rectum, averages 90 hours. Crypts disappear in the anal canal and the mucosa is replaced by stratified squamous cell epithelium. The lamina propria is represented by a thin layer of connective tissue that extends between the crypts. The submucosa resembles that of the small intestine and it contains nerves, plexuses, larger blood vessels, and scattered lymphoid follicles.

The muscular wall of the colon consists of two layers: an inner circular and outer longitudinal layer. Muscle fibers of the inner circular layer deviate from a strict circular orientation; however, because of close attachment to the taeniae it has, thus far, been impossible to identify a helical orientation. The longitudinal layer is gathered into three strips or bundles, the taeniae coli. The taeniae are spaced approximately equally around the circumference of the bowel. One taenia follows the mesenteric attachment. A thin layer of longitudinal muscle bridges the gap between the taeniae. The colon wall presents the appearance of being drawn into multiple loose sacculations, the haustra. Haustrations are most apparent in the transverse colon and may be absent from the descending colon and sigmoid. The haustral folding is a dynamic process that is a result of circular muscle contraction, not puckering by taenial shortening. Each individual apparently has some

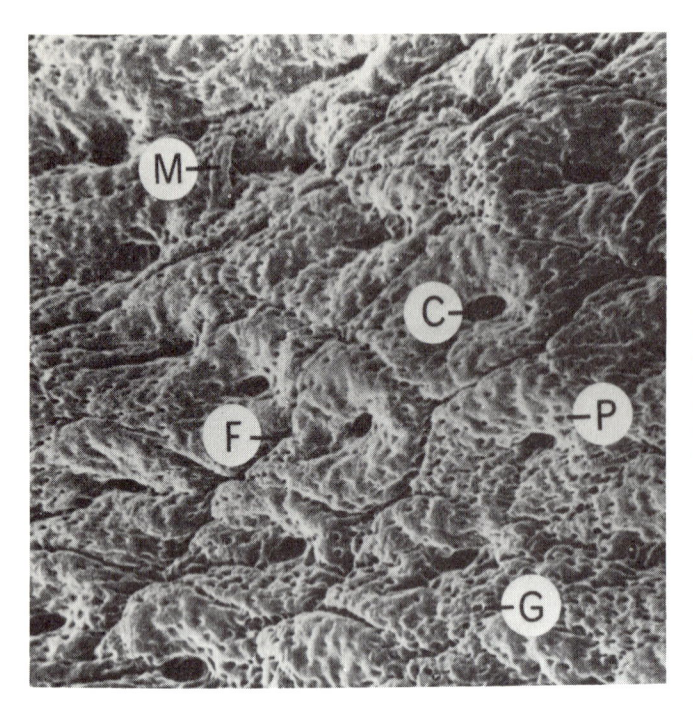

Figure 27-1 Scanning electron micrography of normal rectal mucosa. Each polygonal unit is surrounded by a furrow (F) with the crypt lumen (C) opening centrally. Filled (P) and empty (G) goblet cells and a mucus thread (M) can be identified (× 240). (Kavin, H., et al. Gastroenterology, 59:426, 1970.)

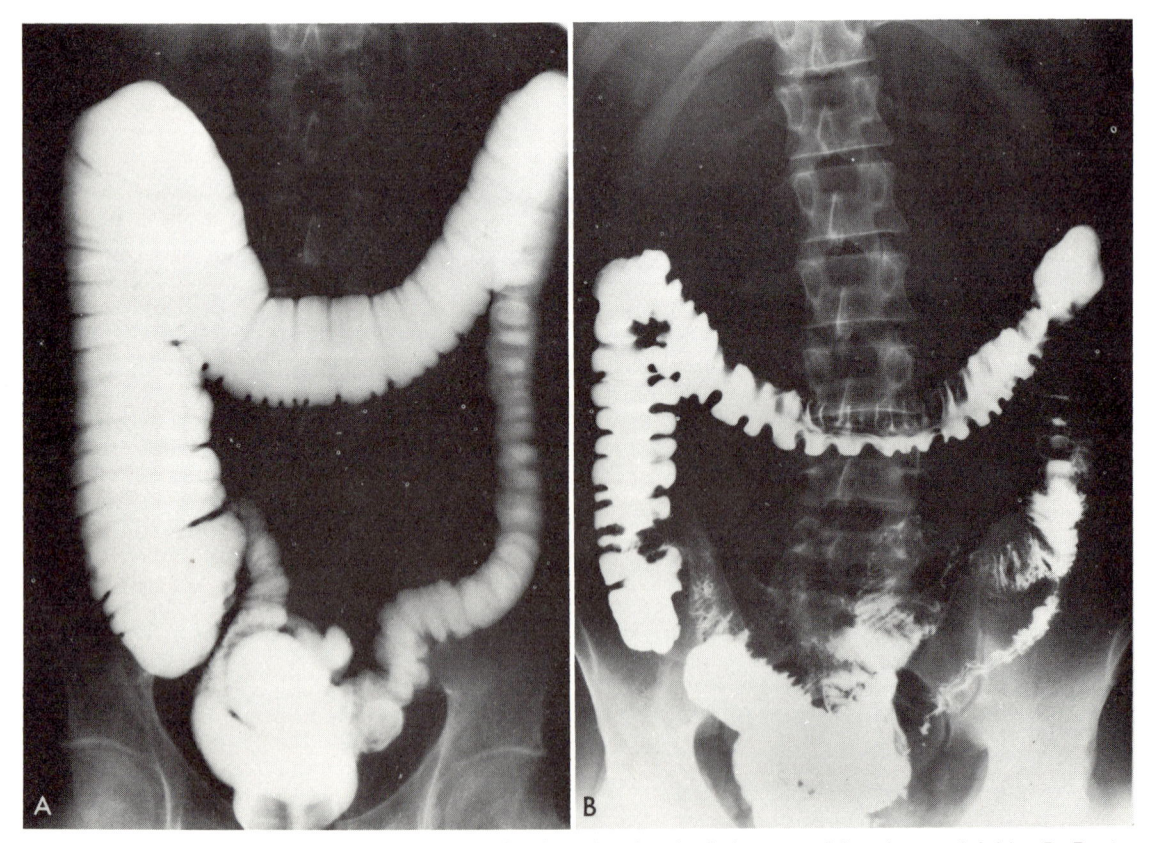

Figure 27-2 A, Normal barium enema examination showing both inter- and intrahaustral folds. B, Postevacuation film of the same patient showing the position of interhaustral folds.

points of regular haustral folding that are marked histologically by a concentration of muscular tissue and bridging by the serosa; however, intrahaustral folding can occur, so that the x-ray appearance of haustration may seem to vary from time to time (Fig. 27-2).

The mesenteric attachments permit substantial mobility of the colon. Only the descending colon and rectum are relatively fixed structures. The colon is supplied with external sympathetic and parasympathetic innervation and an extensive ganglionic plexus that permits intrinsic reflex innervation. Classic teaching holds that sympathetic innervation is inhibitory and parasympathetic innervation is stimulatory toward colonic musculature. Although there is extensive support from animal experimentation, it is difficult to apply to man. Neurogenic tumors that secrete epinephrine have been noted to result in intractable diarrhea in children. Truncal vagotomy may result in diarrhea. While it is reasonable to accept the concept of parasympathetic stimulation and sympathetic inhibition, it must be remembered that the final expression of any sort of stimulation in terms of motility will depend upon the state of the intrinsic innervation and that paradoxical responses may occur. From the anatomic standpoint, parasympathetic fibers to the right colon are carried in the vagus and those that arrive at the left colon come from the second through fourth sacral segments by way of the pelvic nerves. Sympathetic innervation is derived from cord segments thoracic 11 through lumbar 2 and arrives from the mesenteric ganglia in mesenteric and hypogastric nerves.

Integration of motility is the responsibility of the myenteric and submucosal plexuses. When they are absent, as in megacolon, contractions may continue in the aganglionic segment, but integrated motility is absent. As in the small intestine, the colon contains α and β receptors, with β receptors predominating; however, their function remains poorly elucidated. Central innervation may modify the ganglia activity but it cannot substitute for it. There also is substantial evidence for some degree of humoral control of intestinal activity. Although this is poorly understood at the present time, it clearly implies further difficulty in assigning roles to the various components of intestinal innervation.

The normal function of the colon encompasses controlled transit, absorption, and, to a limited degree, secretion. These culminate in defecation, a mechanism for elimination of metabolic wastes and dietary residue. It is customary to speak in relatively laudatory terms of the colon's ability to desiccate and evacuate fecal contents, but it seems to us that the task, relative to the magnitude of small intestinal function, is unimpressive. The degree of mixing of intestinal content in the colon makes transit time only a relative approximation. Material ingested as a bolus will become dispersed over a substantial length of bowel and aliquots may appear over several days. When glass beads are ingested, a different color at each of the three meals, their appearance in the stool, including their distribution in the fecal pellet, is completely mixed and it is impossible to tell which color was ingested first.

NORMAL MOTOR FUNCTION

Electrical Activity

All evidence suggests that the membrane electrical properties of colonic smooth muscle, including the rectum and anal sphincter, resemble those of the remainder of the gastrointestinal tract. Innervation, both extrinsic and intrinsic, plus circulating humoral substances must combine to provide integrated function in the colon. The pacesetter potential or basic electric rhythm (BER) in the small intestine seemingly acts as a governor initiating and integrating its function. The decreasing aboral gradient of the rhythm of slow wave depolarization integrates the pattern of flow of small intestinal content, resulting in transit down the intestine. Net flow down the colon is slower than in the small intestine and is modified by a degree of voluntary control. A simple gradient of BER has not been established in the colon. There have been few studies in man, largely because of technical difficulties. Slow waves have been recorded throughout the colon, in the rectum and anal sphincter in man. No BER has been identified in the ascending colon. The slow waves are irregular in occurrence. A BER of 9 to 16 cycles per minute has been identified in the transverse and descending colon. No gradient has been identified. Results in the sigmoid have been variable. A rhythm ranging from 8.4 to 10.6 cycles per minute has been recorded; however, such rhythmic activity has been present for only brief intervals in one study, averaging 5 per cent of the total observation time. BER in the rectum has been recorded as 3 to 6 cycles per minute. Spike waves have also been recorded, frequently appearing in bursts. In the small intestine, spikes appear related to circular muscle contraction and can result in intraluminal pressure changes. No such relationship has been identified in the colon. The internal anal sphincter claims a BER with the highest frequency thus far identified in the intestinal tract, averaging 17 cycles per minute. This has been correlated with high resting tone suggesting active closure of the sphincter. Sphincter relaxation correlates with inhibition of the BER. Curiously, the internal anal sphincter represents the only identification of BER in circular muscle thus far. Our sketchy knowledge of BER in the colon provides us little insight concerning integration of colonic motor activity.

Motility Mechanisms

Bayless and Starling initiated manometric studies of colonic motility in 1899. Cannon performed contrast studies of the colon in cats in 1902. Holzknecht described mass movement in man in 1909. To the present, no completely satisfactory description of motility mechanisms in the colon has been forthcoming. A number of technical problems remain. Access to proximal colon has been difficult and the lumen size plus the character of its contents make motility recording either by a balloon or by open-tip manometry difficult. Radiologic study utilizing contrast material has been hampered by the overall slowness of colonic mechanisms. Transit is regularly measured in days, yet motility events may be of short duration, with long quiet intervals. It is difficult to identify a decisive moment. The definitive combined radiologic and manometric studies have been burdened with both sets of technical difficulties and too few such studies have been performed.

It is important for the interpretation of available information concerning colonic motility to identify the strengths and weaknesses of the methods utilized in its study. The classic approach to motility study utilizes liquid-filled open-tipped tubes or liquid-filled balloon-tipped tubes which are connected to strain gauge manometers. Balloon-tipped tubes not only introduce the artifactual stimulus of the balloon itself, but they seem to vary in their response, depending on the proximity of the balloon to the wall of the colon. Open-tipped tubes, even if perfused, face artifactual hazards from the semisolid colonic contents. Finally, in the saccular colon it is clear that pressure changes do not always reflect contraction of muscle immediately adjacent to the sensor tip. A capsule containing a miniature radiomanometer has been devised but its localization has been difficult. A series of wave patterns of the classic types I, II, III, and IV have been described but they have been difficult to translate into motility events. From the standpoint of manometry, colonic activity is best separated into segmentation or kneading by alternate formation and relaxation of haustral-like folds, and transportation, which implies peristaltic-like movement over longer segments of bowel. From the clinical standpoint, manometry's most significant contribution has been the identification of the negative relationship between colonic activity and motility. Segmenting activity produces in the colon a state of high resistance to flow. Normal, that is, slow or controlled, transit is associated with a substantial degree of manometric activity, much of which is segmenting. Peristalsis and mass transit, which can sweep colonic contents over distances of 10 to 100 cm., are found only in the absence of segmenting activity. Colons are manometrically quiet except presumably at the instant when the wave of mass movement passes down the bowel. For this reason drugs, particularly anticholinergics that quiet the bowel and reduce segmenting activity, are likely to worsen simple diarrhea. Drugs that increase tone and thus trigger spike activity will retard stools of simple diarrhea.

Radiologic assessment of motility likewise has it strengths and weaknesses. Roentgenograms of hollow viscera all produce negative shadows that depend upon the use of contrast material. Both the physical and chemical qualities of the contrast can modify motility. Most contrast media will form a diffuse nonparticulate shadow and one must be satisfied with several assumptions to interpret changes in size, shape, and density of the opacified masses in terms of motility. Changes in density may as easily be the result of dilution by nonopacified material as of the loss of material by transit. Finally, colonic movements are slow and ill-suited to cine recording. The static films are poor records of dynamic events. Recently, several groups of investigators, most notably Ritchie and coworkers, have utilized time-lapse roentgenography to identify motility mechanisms. They administered a suspension of barium orally and on the following day performed a time-lapse x-ray study, taking films at intervals of one a minute for a period of 1 to 3 hours. Both control observations and a variety of stimuli have been utilized.

Ritchie's analysis has demonstrated two separate classes of activity (Table 27–1). The first is produced by haustral systole. It may involve one or several haustra. It may or may not result in transit and transit may be in either direction. The second is progressive contraction of the bowel, a ringlike wave of activity that is propulsive and may go in either direction. These are not the exact equivalents of manometric segmentation and transit. These two broad classes of activity have been further subdivided on the basis of their apparent mechanical effect. The simplest activity is haustral shuttling. This consists of successive formation of a constriction at the midpoint of the haustra, with relaxation of the immediately preceding and following folds. Colonic content in effect shuttles back and forth from haustra to haustra, with mixing but without a net aboral or adoral transit. Ritchie's observations were based on studies of 190 individuals. This sort of activity was observed in 38 per cent of individuals at rest but in only 13 per cent after a meal. As an extension of this simple activity there is haustral propulsion and retropulsion. This is simple, successive, sequential contraction of single haustra that does result in movement in one or the other direction. This occurred in 36 per

TABLE 27-1 COLONIC MOTILITY, TYPES OF CONTRACTIONS

Type of Movement	At Rest (%)	Postprandial (%)	Distance Traveled	Rate
Haustral shuttling	38	13	0	0
Haustral propulsion	36	57	5 to 10 cm.	2.5 cm./min.
Haustral retropulsion	30	52	5 to 20 cm.	2.5 cm./min.
Multihaustral propulsion				
Systolic	9	17	Variable	5 cm./min.
Serial				2.5 cm./min.
Peristaltic ripples	Not Reported	Not Reported	5 to 10 cm.	0.1 to 2.0 cm./min.
Peristalsis	6	8	18 to 20 cm.	1 to 2 cm./min.
Mass propulsion	Rare	12	30 cm.+	5 to 35 cm./min.

Frequency of Occurrence

Data taken from Ritchie, J. A.: Gut, 9:442, 1968.

cent of the individuals as aboral movement and in 30 per cent as adoral movement at rest. After a meal, aboral movement occurred in 57 per cent of individuals and adoral movement in 52 per cent. Some individuals experienced movement in both directions during the period of observation. The distances covered ranged from 5 to 20 cm. at a rate of 2 to 2.5 cm. per minute. A more complex variety of movement was termed multihaustral propulsion. This could be systolic or serial. Systolic movement occurred when three or more haustra merged. Transit occurred by the addition of single haustra to the head of the mass, with formation of empty haustra at the tail. Multihaustral propulsion was termed serial when three haustra would join. The contents merged and then subsequently one empty haustra re-formed, with the net transfer of its contents to the remaining two.

Activity involving either of these mechanisms was observed in 9 per cent of these individuals at rest and 17 per cent postprandially. Transit could be in either direction and at rates up to 5 cm. per minute. Systolic activity appeared best suited to moving fluid contents either alone or around more solid contents without displacement of the solid stool.

Progressive contractions appeared to occur with several degrees of magnitude. Peristaltic ripples are ring contractions that are progressive and that do move contents over 5 to 10 cm. lengths. They move at a rate that is usually less than 1 cm. a minute. At their maximum they merge with peristalsis proper, which is a propagated ring contraction carried over a distance of 18 to 20 cm. It is preceded by relaxation and often followed by tonic contraction of the bowel. Some sort of peristalsis was noted to occur in 6 per cent of colons at rest and 8 per cent postprandially. Contractions of this sort have been noted to move both aborally and adorally. Finally, there is mass propulsion, which is thought to be peristaltic movement of the colon contents of a magnitude that may empty up to one half the length of the large bowel. This sort of activity was observed in only a few of the nearly 190 individuals studied. Mass propulsion seemed rare in the resting state and in most cases was observed postprandially. Mass propulsion has been noted to move aborally only and at a rate of progression which is rapid, in the range of 5 to 35 cm. per minute. Progressive waves depend on relaxation of interhaustral folds. If the relaxation fails, progressive waves are aborted. Progressive waves move the entire intestinal content, solid or liquid.

There are two other components in motility, the significance of which is not clearly defined. The first is colonic shortening by taenial contraction. This does occur in combination with many of the activities mentioned above, but its role in transit is not clear. Secondly, there are the postural or gravity effects. In an organ in which the lumen is partially open, such as the colon, and which is filled with gaseous, fluid, and semisolid contents, gravity and postural changes have observable effects, but these have been difficult to define and their significance remains unclear. They are important, however, in pathologic states. Those individuals suffering from diarrhea may achieve some control over their bowel action by simple bed rest. The constipation which plagues many patients upon admission to the hospital with enforced bed rest probably has its origin in the same mechanism.

Transit

Contractile mechanisms not only are complex but also have segmental or regional expression. It is rare to observe a completely inactive colon.

It is similarly rare to observe a normal colon that is active throughout its entire length. There are nearly always inactive portions. In general, the right colon is responsible for the largest absorption of water and solute. Haustral shuttling and systolic propulsion yield the maximum mucosal contact necessary to make this process efficient.

The left colon is faced with semisolid colonic contents, which it stores and evacuates. This is carried out most economically in terms of effort by serial propulsion and peristalsis. While this is generally true if viewed as a net response, all varieties of activity have been observed throughout the colon. Again the clearest documentation of the spectrum of segmental activity has come from the work of Ritchie (Table 27-2). He noted marked changes in activity postprandially, with haustral activity most notable in the right colon. Other investigators have suggested that the activity of the distal colon, as measured by the motility index, is similarly enhanced by eating. A similar increase in motility index has been produced by the administration of gastrin and this would support the suggestion that at least some of the integration of colonic activity may rest upon hormonal basis.

In Western man with normal bowel habits, colonic activity is punctuated three times a day by a change in activity that follows eating. Activity as a general rule is enhanced in the postprandial state but transit down the colon as a whole remains unchanged. Retropulsion apparently balances increased propulsion. Following the ingestion of a meal there is an increase in ileal activity, with resultant slow filling of the cecum and ascending colon. The ileal influx is shuttled and propelled by systolic haustral contractions. Fluid contents may flow around masses of solid material, which accounts for mixing and the apparent length of transit time. Peristaltic movements may occur. Gradually, as the prandial stimulus subsides, areas of inactive bowel re-emerge. Retropulsive movements occur in the right colon under the stimulus of a meal but are uncommon at rest. At rest the net propulsion amounts to about 1 cm. per hour. In this fashion the fluid contents of the right colon are rocked back and forth over the absorptive epithelium with each fresh surge of ileal influx. The contents are desiccated and as the left colon is approached the character of the colonic activity changes. At 18 to 24 hours, some portion of the ileal influx will have entered the rectum, but because of mixing, the colon clearance times for the entire bolus will be much longer. Retropulsion increases as the sigmoid region is approached. Gradually the sigmoid fills and periodically material passes on into the rectum. This distention initiates a defecatory urge. Response to this is governed, as will be discussed, by a number of physiologic and environmental variables. Defecation may result in simply local rectal emptying or it may lead to mass propulsion emptying the entire distal colon.

Variations of this normal sequence result not only from changes in the stimulus in the muscle, as by inflammation or distention, but also from changes in the character of the colonic content. This explains why a response to a barium enema bears so little relationship to normal function. The propulsion of gas through the colon and its passage reflect its relatively unaltered state during its passage down the large intestine.

Defecation

The rectum constitutes the distal 15 cm. of the large intestine. The rectosigmoid junction is indistinct, but the caudal level is well marked by the junction of mucous membrane with the anal canal's transitional epithelium. The rectum below its junction with the sigmoid enlarges to form the rectal ampulla. Above the peritoneal reflection, the rectum is bound to the pelvis by a fibrous sheath and below the support is provided by the muscles of the pelvic diaphragm. The musculature of the rectum is formed by a continuation of the colonic muscular coats. The outer longitudinal layer spreads from the taeniae of the

TABLE 27-2 COLONIC MOTILITY, DISTRIBUTION OF ACTIVITY

	Proportion of Section Remaining Inactive		Proportion of Colon Showing (Nonpropulsive Segmentation)	
	At Rest (%)	Postprandial (%)	At Rest (%)	Postprandial (%)
Cecum and ascending colon	42	16	38	45
Transverse colon	8	5	44	20
Descending colon	25	19	31	18
Pelvic colon	34	26	22	28
Rectum	60	59	20	22
Whole colon (mean)	32	21	35	25

Data taken from Ritchie, J. A.: Gut, *9*:502, 1968.

sigmoid to form a continuous even coat. The superficial fibers insert into the perineal body and merge with the levator. The deep fibers insert into the perianal skin. The circular muscle differentiates into the internal sphincter surrounding the anal canal. The anus forms the terminal 2 to 4 cm. of the intestinal tract. The pectinate line marks the boundary between the anal canal and the rectum. The anus is lined with stratified squamous epithelium.

The external sphincter is made up of striated muscle which lies outside the internal sphincter and extends down below it to encircle the terminal portion of the anal canal. This muscle arises in the central perineum and inserts into the coccyx. The integrated function of the colon, rectum, and sphincters depends upon both sensory and motor innervation. Sensory endings are provided with both somatic and autonomic pathways. Sensory pathways for the anal canal and the perianal skin ascend through the somatic nerves to segments S2, S3, and S4. Proprioceptive spindles are present in the striated muscles of the external sphincter. Autonomic sensory innervation for the rectum passes to the same segments, though along parasympathetic pathways. A wide variety of sensory endings are present in both the rectum and anal canal. Motor fibers to the striated external sphincter arrive through the pudendal nerve and the coccygeal plexus, and originate in segments S2 to S5. Parasympathetic motor nerves to the internal sphincter descend from L5 and S1 to S3 through the pelvic nerves. These stimuli are inhibitory. Sympathetic fibers arrive via the hypogastric nerve and are excitatory motor stimuli. Sympathetic innervation of the rectum is drawn from L2 to L4 and parasympathetic fibers arrive from S2 to S4.

A variety of mechanisms combine to maintain fecal continence. None is as important as the variety of reflex responses that are capable of operating without central control. A degree of basal tone is the feature of both rectum and sphincter. Flow of feces into the rectum gives rise to immediate increase in pressure, which at a critical volume stimulates rectal contraction and produces an urge to defecate. If this is denied, the rectum will relax and accommodate the feces, as evidenced by a fall in pressure. When defecation is denied, some feces may be returned to the sigmoid or higher. Both sphincters are in a continuous state of contraction. BER identified in the internal sphincter is inhibited by sphincter relaxation. Of the two, the internal sphincter seems to contribute the largest share of the squeeze closing the anal canal. Distention of the rectum results in relaxation of the internal sphincter. This relaxation is short-lived, but it will allow rectal contents to descend into the anal canal far enough to permit their identification by sensory receptors. Voluntary contraction of the external sphincter can maintain continence during the short interval of internal sphincter relaxation. There is a prompt (but poorly understood) increase in external sphincter squeeze which defends continence against increases in intra-abdominal pressure from straining and other activity. Micturition results in reflex relaxation of the external sphincter.

With such a wide variety of reflex controls, anorectal function is susceptible to many sorts of neurologic lesions. These may be grouped into three broad categories: (1) Loss of central innervation with intact sensation. This results in defecatory urge, which, while it cannot be denied, does remain under some local voluntary control. (2) Loss of both sensory and motor control above the sacral outflow results in a reflex colon. (3) Loss of the sacral cord or peripheral nerves results in an absence of reflex control.

Defecation is initiated in a continent man when the central nervous system accepts the information that the left colon and rectum are primed for defecation and when the environment is deemed acceptable for this activity. Intra-abdominal pressure increases, the sphincters relax, the pelvic floor tenses, and the colon contracts. Evacuation of the distal rectum may be coupled with mass peristalsis which can empty the colon as high as the splenic flexure, but as often as not it seems to be related to multihaustral movement that empties only the distal end of the colon. Edwards and Beck obtained pre- and postdefecation films of individuals with radiopacified feces. They noted that small quantities of feces moved in and out of the rectum regularly and that a "call to stool" is initiated only when a critical volume to which the individual person is habituated is reached. This differs from the established teaching that the rectum remains empty until immediately prior to defecation but it confirms the regular clinical observation of feces palpable at the rectal examination. Some individuals empty the rectum only partially but others empty it completely. A number of factors remain to be defined to understand completely the controls of normal defecation.

NORMAL ABSORPTION AND SECRETION

In addition to transportation and elimination of dietary and metabolic waste, the colon is charged with the task of defending fluid and electrolyte homeostasis in the gastrointestinal tract. Fine regulation of electrolyte and fluid balance belongs to the renal and respiratory systems, yet the flux of liquid and electrolytes across the gastrointestinal mucosa is of such a magnitude that highly developed gastrointestinal regulation is essential.

Water and Electrolytes

Under ordinary circumstances the gastrointestinal tract is presented with a volume of 8 to 9 liters of combined secretion and ingested fluid daily. Absorption by the small intestine will reduce this to a volume of 500 to 600 ml. This daily volume will pass the ileocecal valve carrying an electrolyte load of 40 to 70 mEq. of sodium, 3 to 6 mEq. of potassium, 20 to 40 mEq. of choloride, and 30 to 35 mEq. of bicarbonate. Passage through the colon will reduce the volume to 100 ml. of water. Electrolyte concentrations, based on fecal dialysis studies by Wrong and colleagues, will average sodium 30 mEq. per liter, potassium 75 mEq. per liter, chloride 15 mEq. per liter, and bicarbonate 30 mEq. per liter. Approximately 50 per cent of the anion in fecal water will be made up of organic anion which results from bacterial action on carbohydrates. The resultant stool will be hyperosmolar (376 mOsm.).

The absorptive work is not uniformly distributed down the colon and there is evidence of regional specialization. The largest fluid volume and electrolyte absorption occurs in the right colon. The rectum is apparently impermeable to electrolytes and water. These values for absorption and secretion represent the net result and underlying this net result there may be a substantial effort in terms of flux of electrolytes in both directions across the mucosa (Table 27-3).

In terms of mechanisms, the absorption of water seems to be passive following the osmotic gradient produced by the absorption of sodium. The absorption of sodium is an active process. Absorption may be accomplished against a significant concentration gradient. Absorption has been noted from colonic luminal concentrations as low as 25 mM. sodium. Sodium is absorbed along an electrical gradient of 30 to 40 mv., mucosa negative.

Potassium can be secreted into the colon. Several mechanisms may be involved in the entry of potassium into the lumen. Mucus secreted by goblet cells in the colon may contain extraordinary quantities of potassium. Concentrations of up to 140 mEq. per liter have been noted. The potassium is not bound and may be reabsorbed, so that the contribution of mucus to potassium secretion will vary with the rapidity of transit and the total quantity of mucus secreted. The majority of potassium passing into the colon does go passively down an electronegative gradient. When luminal potassium concentrations rise above 15 mEq. per liter, the flux of potassium changes to absorption rather than excretion. There is no apparent interaction between the transfer of sodium and potassium.

The colon is sensitive to aldosterone and other mineralocorticoids. The effect, increased sodium absorption and potassium secretion, resembles the steroid action on the kidney.

Chloride has a net absorption which exceeds that of sodium. Chloride transport itself is not active and it seems to be absorbed as a paired ion with sodium. The absorption of chloride and the secretion of bicarbonate are coupled. In the absence of chloride, bicarbonate will be absorbed as a paired ion with sodium. When chloride is present, bicarbonate will be secreted apparently in exchange for chloride. Some secreted bicarbonate will combine with organic acids produced by bacteria in the feces. The absorptive capacity of the colon is limited. Calculations based on extrapolations of perfusion results are indicated in Table 27-3, along with the magnitude of the flux and the usual daily load.

Nutrients and Metabolic Products

The large intestine also has a meager digestive and synthetic role which only rarely may achieve clinical significance but should be remembered. Ordinarily, ingested cellulose passes through the intestinal tract largely unaltered. Bacterial digestion does break down some but this contribution is minimal. In constipated individuals with markedly prolonged transit times, colonic digestion of cellulose and absorption can become a significant factor in the diet. This circumstance is one that Davenport terms the "greedy colon." In addition to cellulose digestion, colonic bacteria can synthesize a number of vitamins, most notably folic acid but including riboflavin, biotin, vi-

TABLE 27-3 COLONIC ABSORPTION AND SECRETION FROM THE COLON

	Average/24 Hours	Maximum Capacity/24 Hours Flux Absorbed	Secreted	Net
Water	400 ml.+	10,800 ml.	7800 ml.	3000 ml.+
Na+	66 mEq.+	878	418	460+
K+	3 mEq.−	26	58	32−

Data taken from Shields, R., and Miles, J. B.: Postgrad. Med. J., *41*:435, 1965.

tamin K and nicotinic acid. Failure to produce these compounds can occasionally result in a clinical deficiency. An enterohepatic circulation involving the colon has been identified for several compounds. A urea-ammonia cycle is apparently limited to the colon. The colon also participates, though to a much more limited degree, in the enterohepatic circulation of bile acids. Urea is synthesized by the liver and enters the systemic circulation. The small intestinal mucosa is permeable to urea which may diffuse into the lumen, but quantitatively the amount involved is small, less than 500 mg. of the 7 grams normally degraded by the gut daily. The colonic mucosa is relatively impermeable to the diffusion of urea in either direction. Circulating blood urea is hydrolyzed in the colonic epithelial wall by bacterial ureases that either penetrate or are closely applied to the mucosa. Most of the ammonia that is produced is absorbed by the circulation. The alkaline pH in the lumen favors the dissociation of any ammonium that may diffuse into it. Free ammonia readily penetrates the mucosa and the nitrogen is returned to the liver for resynthesis of urea or use in protein synthesis. This colonic conservation of nitrogen may achieve clinical importance in the face of protein malnutrition. The apparent involvement of blood urea rather than luminal urea helps to explain the success of immunization against urease and systemic urease inhibitors such as acetohydroxamic acid in treatment of hepatic encephalopathy.

Synthesis of bile acids by the liver is limited. The bile acid pool which varies from 1.2 to 6.0 grams is conserved by cycling through the enterohepatic circulation. In the course of 6 to 10 cycles a day, a small amount escapes the small intestinal absorption mechanism. The daily fecal excretion amounts to an average of 500 mg. of bile acid. Chenodeoxycholic acid escaping into the colon is dehydroxylated by bacteria to form lithocholic acid, which is nonabsorbable and is excreted. It accounts for 300 mg. of the 500 mg. of bile acid lost daily. Cholic acid is dehydroxylated to desoxycholic acid and about half of this will be reabsorbed by the colon. Since 200 mg. is lost in the feces, there must be addition to the bile acid pool of approximately 200 mg. of this secondary bile acid daily from the colon.

Drugs

A wide variety of drugs are regularly administered by enema or suppositories. Salicylates, sedatives, antiemetics, opiates, bronchodilators, tranquilizers, and selected antibiotics all have significant absorption and systemic effect. A number of agents administered for local action, such as corticosteroids, may have significant systemic absorption which will limit their use. Neomycin is also in this category.

A seemingly endless number of drugs have been administered rectally without success. Chloramphenicol, tetracycline, and sulfonamides are erratically absorbed by the rectal mucosa, though they may be well absorbed by the oral route. There are no identified carrier mechanisms in the colonic mucosa. Absorption depends on several factors. Small molecules may diffuse through the pores in the colonic epithelium. They could be carried in by water during its passive absorption. Rectal absorption of water and electrolytes is markedly restricted if it occurs at all, and hence the absorption of a drug by diffusion will depend on the level to which the preparation is carried in the colon. Its retention time will also be a critical factor that determines absorption. This may well account for the erratic absorption of many of the antibiotic compounds. As a general rule, compounds which remain in a lipid-soluble state at colonic pH are better absorbed. They presumably dissolve through the lipid-containing cell membrane. Some drugs such as neomycin are as well absorbed rectally as they are orally and the absorption appears completely unaffected by retention time or other identifiable factors. The mechanism of their absorption remains to be defined. An additional avenue for absorption may be available for those agents which are used topically in the treatment of inflammatory bowel disease. The ulcer bed and denuded mucosa expose deeper, perhaps barrier-free areas which may permit absorption.

Gas

The gastrointestinal tract contains an average of 100 ml. of gas. This may be subject to wide variation with changes in diet. While gas may be distributed down the entire length of the intestinal tract, a substantial percentage of it accumulates in the colon. Gas passed by rectum is made up of swallowed air, gas diffusing across the mucosa from the circulation, and gas produced by bacteria in the small intestine and colon. Its final composition will obviously reflect the activity of these various sources. In addition to oxygen, nitrogen, and carbon dioxide, methane and hydrogen may be major components of flatus. A number of gaseous components are present in trace amounts. Swallowed air contains small quantities of the rare gases and a number of volatile metabolic products may be present. These can include ammonia, hydrogen sulfide, skatole, indole, and fatty acids. Ordinarily, these represent less than 1 per cent of flatus.

Hydrogen is produced by bacteria, and in the absence of bacterial overgrowth of the small intestine it is derived primarily from the colon. There is no other source for production of gaseous hydrogen in the human body. Methane is similarly produced by bacterial fermentation in the intestine. Bacteria utilize only substrate found within the lumen, and production of gas is related to the dietary availability of suitable substrate. Carbon dioxide may be swallowed but more significant amounts are produced in the intestinal tract as a consequence of neutralization of acid by bicarbonate. Free carbon dioxide is in equilibrium with bicarbonate and with circulating carbon dioxide. It can diffuse across the mucosa. A similar equilibrium exists for nitrogen and oxygen. In the colon, bacterial utilization of oxygen may result in extremely low or negligible concentrations of oxygen. In this fashion, an anaerobic environment may be maintained within the colon.

Passage of gas through the colon may be far more rapid than liquid or semisolid feces. Resistance to flow by haustration is substantially less effective for gases than it is for liquids. Also, colonic activity is usually sufficient to prevent layering of fluid and solid fecal contents into separate phases but it is insufficient to prevent the separation of a gaseous phase. This makes possible the differential motility of gas in the colon.

DISORDERS OF MOTOR AND ABSORPTIVE FUNCTIONS

DIARRHEA WITH NORMAL-APPEARING COLON

Diarrhea may be a result of a wide variety of stimuli. The final common path resulting in frequent stools lies with an increase in the volume load, a decrease in the absorptive capacity, or in rapid transit. On occasion, stimulation of colonic secretion may be a factor. The number of pathophysiologic mechanisms that may lead through one or several of these pathways is huge and a comprehensive discussion is beyond the limits of this chapter. In this and subsequent sections, examples utilizing each of the pathways will be presented and it should be remembered that these are illustrative and not a complete portrayal. It is rare to find only a single mechanism operative, and even in an apparently pure disorder, there may be secondary involvement of several mechanisms ultimately producing the diarrhea. This feature has important therapeutic implications. Without this concept clearly in mind, the use of some agents in the treatment of diarrhea (and their success) may seem paradoxical. This is particularly true with regard to the use of hydroscopic, bulk-producing materials in the treatment of diverticulosis and irritable bowel syndrome.

The primary causes of most diarrheal disease without structural abnormality remain either hidden, i.e., idiopathic, or beyond any reasonable hope of control, i.e., viral gastroenteritis, and one relies on a number of nonspecific agents to obtain symptomatic relief. There are a few circumstances in which the primary pathologic condition is identifiable and susceptible to modification. Diarrhea associated with hyperthyroidism presumably represents an extension of the general hypermetabolic state. Control of excess circulating thyroid hormone, medically or surgically, offers primary control of diarrhea. Similarly, epinephrine-producing neurogenic tumors offer an identifiable mechanism. In addition, the case for an excitatory role for sympathetic innervation is strengthened by the clinical observation of the result of these tumors. Although resection of the tumor may not always be feasible, the use of epinephrine-blocking agents offers a therapeutic avenue. Diarrhea may be associated with certain medullary tumors of the thyroid. This is thought to be related to release of a prostaglandin. The identity of the diarrheogenic hormone found in some nonbeta islet cell tumors of the pancreas is not clear. It may well be a secretory agent similar to the prostaglandin released by medullary tumors of the thyroid. The syndrome of watery diarrhea and hypokalemia has occurred in individuals with the Zollinger-Ellison syndrome, but it does also appear in a pure form unrelated to gastric hypersecretion. Primary mechanisms of this sort deserve specific therapy. However, in absolute numbers they form a relatively insignificant proportion of the diarrheal diseases. One identifiable primary mechanism that does seem to form a significant portion of diarrheal diseases is related to lactose malabsorption. Many individuals on a constitutional or acquired basis will have a decline in lactase activity in the small intestine following weaning. The final level of lactase activity seems to vary from individual to individual. When the small intestinal mucosa is stressed with a lactose load beyond its metabolic capacity, the unsplit disaccharide will be carried down the small intestine and discharged into the colon. In the colon, lactose can serve as a substrate and it will be fermented by a variety of bacteria. The fermentation process produces lactic acid and gas. The combination of volume and the acid stimulus produces intestinal hyperactivity that may be manifested by audible intestinal sounds, cramping abdominal pain, and occasionally diarrhea. Small intestinal lactase does appear to be an inducible enzyme in some animals. However, it remains to be demonstrated that the enzyme level is inducible in man. The only effective therapy at this time is the elimination of lactose from the diet to produce a reduction to levels that an individual may tolerate.

Simple Diarrhea—"Precolonic Cholera"

Volume overload of the colon resulting in frequent stools probably represents the commonest of gastrointestinal afflictions. The colonic overload in simple diarrhea is a product of disturbed small intestinal function. Cholera is a classic example. Exposure of small intestinal mucosa to cholera toxin results in activation of the adenyl cyclase system regulating sodium secretion. Massive flux of sodium and fluid into the bowel lumen is the result. This secretion exceeds the reabsorptive capacity of the small intestine and the colon. The colon simply fills to capacity and watery diarrhea ensues. The radiologist can ordinarily fill a colon at the time of barium enema with 1500 ml. of barium suspension. Patients with full-blown cholera ordinarily produce watery stools at the rate of 500 ml. per hour. Cholera as a clinical entity is exotic. The diarrhea of travelers, enteropathogenic *E. coli* infection, viral gastroenteritis, Clostridium and staphylococcal toxin-containing food, and the use of saline cathartics represent more practical clinical extensions of the concept of simple volume overload of the colon. Although the colon is capable of absorbing up to 3000 ml. of fluid daily (Table 27-3), this represents a relatively meager absorption capacity of 125 ml. per hour or slightly more than 2 ml. a minute. It is not difficult for a volume load to exceed these limits in a short period of time. One effect of the volume load is a change in the composition of the stool. As the volume increases so does the sodium concentration and the potassium content of the stool decreases. Gradually, at a volume of approximately 3000 ml. of stool a day, the composition approaches that of normal plasma. Clearly, there must also be some alteration in intestinal motility; however, this is less impressive in simple diarrhea than in the irritable colon syndrome and inflammatory bowel disease. Perhaps the absence of the motility components is more apparent than real, since, as will be discussed, the motility alterations associated with diarrhea produce a quiet colon.

Irritable Colon Syndrome

A great deal of human emotion is expressed by conscious voluntary activity such as a smile, clearing of the throat, or a nod of the head. Often, the translation of the emotional content into activity, such as applause, will vary from culture to culture. There is a similar body of reflex emotional expression, such as blushing or weeping, over which voluntary control has never been remarkably effective. Some reflex emotional responses cross the rather indistinct boundary that separates physiologic from pathologic response. It is not uncommon to identify individuals who respond to stress with urticaria, asthma, or emesis. When the emotional expression alters intestinal motility and absorption, producing pain and/or diarrhea, often alternating with constipation, the condition is described as the irritable colon syndrome.

The stringent limits that we as individuals set to identify as our normal bowel habits are more often culturally than physiologically inspired. Much, but not all, of what is diagnosed as irritable bowel syndrome is hardly disease. If public defecation at the roadside were considered a poetic expression rather than vulgar display, individuals with an irritable bowel would be the laureates of the land.

Two other factors seem to have a strong impact on the expression of irritable colon. One is an ill-understood constitutional or familial factor, about which little more can be said than that it exists. The other is related to irritants. These may be infections, respiratory as well as gastrointestinal, or, more commonly, food irritants. Food as an irritant seems as often as not to represent an idiosyncratic response of an individual rather than rational expression of a toxic food. The kind of food which precipitates symptoms varies widely from individual to individual. This brings the full circle back to emotional factors.

There is, to be sure, an element of emotional overlay that will accompany any of the colonic afflictions discussed in this chapter. Also, there is great individual variation in terms of colonic response to emotional stress. The various appellations applied to the irritable colon syndrome, i.e., spastic gut, psychophysiologic gastrointestinal reaction, functional bowel syndrome, and mucous colitis, indicate that in many people it represents an emotional disturbance alone. When irritable colon syndrome is seemingly not an extension of organic disease, that is, when it is truly idiopathic, it poses a challenge to physicians to continue symptomatic control. It is true that irritable colon syndrome must once have included those individuals with lactose intolerance, amebiasis, and a wide variety of other identifiable colonic diseases and there probably remain some primary mechanisms yet to be identified and extracted. However, this does not make it a wastebasket diagnosis. Clearly, an exaggerated response to stress can, alone and unaided, be responsible for both the spastic and diarrheal varieties of irritable colon syndrome.

From the standpoint of pathologic physiology, irritable colon syndrome may be separated into two varieties—spastic and diarrheal. The spastic variety presents clinically with an alteration in bowel habits and abdominal pain. Diarrhea may alternate with constipation. The cramping abdominal pain seems to be the key clinical feature in determining the pathophysiology. These individuals experience a stimulation of haustral contractions. Vigorous segmental contractions produce closed chambers containing trapped fluid and gas. Further contractions result in increased tension in the colonic wall and cramping abdominal pain. Increased segmentation yields a high resistance state within the colon and there will be little effective transit. As the increased segmentation subsides, haustral transit may occur and peristaltic activity may be stimulated; thus, the cramping abdominal pain may terminate in a diarrheal rush. The diarrheal variety is relatively more simple in clinical appearance. Patients do not have cramping abdominal discomfort, though there may be ample audible intestinal activity. The call to stool may be precipitated and result in passage of a liquid stool. A sequence of response with a number of watery stools in progressively smaller volume, beginning in the morning and terminating in the forenoon, with the patient remaining relatively symptom-free for the remainder of the day, is not uncommon.

With this variety the mechanism seems to be related to a quiet colon. Manometrically, there is an absence of the phasic contractions that are usually identified with segmentation. In this case, small changes in pressure may result in substantial flow down the low resistance colon. Absence of haustral propulsion sets the stage for peristalsis and mass movement. The response to food in the sigmoid colon may be a normal increase in phasic contraction, but this quickly fades at the termination of the meal and the colon returns to its basic hypotonic state.

Either variety of irritable colon syndrome may be associated with increased mucus secretion. Occasionally, this may present as spectacular ropy strands of mucus passed in the stool without apparent associated feces. More often, small amounts of mucus will collect in the rectum, just above the sphincter. The quantity will be too small to act as a stimulus, but the patient quickly learns that the passage of flatus may prove embarrassing. This additional anxiety and the necessity to retreat to the toilet to pass flatus further compound the irritable colon syndrome.

Each mechanism implies specific therapy. In the spastic variety, anticholinergics, which have been noted manometrically to inhibit phasic activity, may give a measure of control over the cramping abdominal pain. To do this the dose must be carried to a critical level. The inhibition of phasic activity carried to completion may exacerbate the diarrheal component as the colon is reduced to a low resistance state. It takes great patience to direct anticholinergic therapy in this situation. Irritable bowel of the diarrheal variety obviously responds poorly to anticholingercics alone. The addition of opiates, which enhance tone and may stimulate phasic activity, and the use of hydroscopic bulk agents, which act to increase resistance to fluid flow, constitute a better and more effective regimen. In either case, the thoughtful selection of sedatives and tranquilizers may support the regimen.

Bile Acid Diarrhea

Bile acid diarrhea illustrates a third general response to the development of diarrhea in a normal-appearing colon. Suitable concentrations of conjugated and unconjugated dehydroxy bile acids in the colon stimulate secretion of sodium and water. This produces diarrhea by a volume overload that has its primary genesis within the colon itself.

Disorders of the enterohepatic circulation of bile acids may lead to diarrhea by a number of mechanisms. When the bile acid circulation is broken and the pool size falls, the concentration of bile entering the duodenum may be insufficient to permit complete fat absorption. Steatorrhea, often with diarrhea, may result. In small intestinal stasis syndrome, bacterial deconjugation of bile acids may lead to similarly insufficient levels of bile acid for the formation of micelles and fat absorption. The diarrhea under these circumstances is a result of hepatic and small intestinal failure. When the enterohepatic circulation is broken because of ileal dysfunction and failure of active ileal absorption of bile acids, larger than normal quantities of bile acids may pass into the colon. Experimentally, perfusion of the human colon with deconjugated dehydroxy bile acids in a concentration of 3 to 5 mM. produces a marked secretion of sodium and water. Equimolar mixtures of conjugated bile acids cause similar secretion of sodium and water plus additional secretion of potassium and bicarbonate. The magnitude of secretion is sufficient to explain diarrhea associated with an enterohepatic circulation broken at the ileal level. Successful therapy of bile acid diarrhea has been described using cholestyramine, a resin which binds bile acid. Successful application of cholestyramine requires a careful selection, for though it reduces bile acid effects, it increases steatorrhea. There is a relatively limited zone in which the net result is an effective reduction of diarrhea.

DIARRHEA WITH STRUCTURAL CHANGES IN THE COLON – INFLAMMATORY BOWEL DISEASE

Specific Inflammatory Disease

Inflammatory disease of the wall of the colon results in diarrhea by one or a combination of several mechanisms. Mucosal erosion and ulceration destroy the epithelial barrier and leave a raw exuding surface. When the stool content is primarily exudate, blood, and necrotic epithelium, the clinical diagnosis of dysentery is appropriate, and widespread colonic disease may be suspected. Shigella, amebae, and Staphylococcus that produce pseudomembranous enterocolitis are perhaps the commonest specific agents producing dysenteric symptoms. Pathologic changes are not limited to the mucosal inflammation. Inflammatory cell infiltration and ulceration may extend into the submucosa and the muscularis. Rarely, septic perforation will occur. The extension of inflammatory disease to deeper levels, with resultant infiltration and edema, changes the physical characteristics of the wall, particularly the stiffness, and, because of irritation of nerve plexuses, may alter motility mechanisms. In the presence of active inflammation it is common to see absence of haustration, with resultant low resistance to flow down the colonic lumen. As inflammation subsides and healing occurs, several varieties of derangement are possible, depending on the pattern of fibrosis that evolves. If the fibrotic reaction is diffuse, the pattern of absent haustration may solidify. This is best exemplified in the hosepipe appearance of the colon in burnt-out chronic ulcerative colitis and is a less frequent but not unheard of sequela of specific infectious colitis. Changes of this sort require rather massive involvement of the colon or prolonged repetitive bouts of inflammation. When fibrosis is localized, a partial or complete stricture may result. Complete obstruction in the large intestine, whether by stricture or volvulus or whatever mechanism, results in changes similar to those described in the small intestine. In individuals with a competent ileocecal valve, the added complication of closed loop obstruction with toxic dilatation can occur. When stricture produces only partial obstruction, the distention may result in an irritable focus with a distal increase in transit, producing diarrhea.

Several agents which produce inflammatory bowel changes do not ordinarily present with widespread colonic disease. Amebic, tuberculous, and fungal infections typically present with a regional involvement. The usual involvement is cecal and is thought to be related to stasis in the cecal segment. For most organisms this location represents the first point of slowing of the intestinal stream, affording an opportunity for prolonged contact by multiple organisms that is necessary for penetration of the epithelial barrier. It is also possible that the relative fluidity and concentration of nutrients plus the favorable redox potential in the cecum play an important role in the establishment of infection in this area. Regional infection is also common in the rectosigmoid, the other point of relative stasis of the fecal stream. In addition to an ulcerative inflammatory response, a proliferative granulomatous response to most of these agents may occur. These infectious pseudotumors can disorder motility and result in diarrhea. Several of the parasites, particularly schistosomes, produce colonic lesions by embolization or deposition of ova in the intestinal wall. With the development of delayed immune sensitivity, a granulomatous reaction surrounds these lesions, which may ulcerate through the mucosa or may produce proliferative granulomatous polyps. In all these cases, specific and effective chemotherapy can halt progression of these lesions. However, their resolution may lead to significant structural changes and to the production of additional symptoms.

Diverticular Disease of the Colon

Diverticula in the colon represent outpouchings or herniations of mucosa and submucosa between fasciculi of the circular muscle of the colonic wall. True diverticula contain all coats of the colon wall, similar to Meckel's diverticulum in the small intestine. These do occur, but they are exceedingly rare. The usual diverticula form in response to two sets of circumstances. In the colon there are, in effect, two kinds of diverticular disease. These two varieties are simple diverticulosis and spastic diverticulosis. Both may eventuate in inflammatory bowel disease; however, in both the inflammation is a late phenomenon complicating the end stage of the disease. In the absence of inflammation, simple diverticula are silent and usually unassociated with any symptoms. Some workers have felt that they are the sequelae of the diarrheal variety of irritable bowel syndrome. The diverticula of spastic diverticulosis are not asymptomatic. Here the disease is felt to be an extension of the spastic variety of irritable bowel syndrome. Thus, pain and alteration of bowel habits will precede the development of diverticula. Simple diverticula are outpouchings through weakened portions of an otherwise normal circular muscle. They increase in frequency with age and after age 40, 5 per cent or more of the population of the United States will have demonstrable diverticula. Constitutional and environmental factors are thought to be major factors in their occurrence. Diverticula are rare among African and Asian populations. Simple diverticula represent herniations at points of anatomic weakness, often at points of penetration of the musculature by arteries. While single scattered diverticula are common, occasional individuals may present with massed simple diverticula. With massed diverticula, each herniation is thought to be the result of increased pressure pushing the mucosa through the muscular defect. The result is an apparent shortening of the colon, because the total area of the mucosa remaining to line the lumen is inadequate. This apparent shortening is unassociated with inflammation and is a simple mechanical phenomenon. Simple diverticula may become inflamed, just as any outpouching of the gut may in a fashion similar to the appendix develop intraluminal inflammation. This sort of inflammation seems to be a rare occurrence. However, rupture of inflamed simple diverticula with peritonitis, abscess, and fistula have been reported. Inspissated contents may produce ulceration of the diverticulum neck. Because of the close association of many simple diverticula with small arteries, the ulceration can lead to spectacular lower gastrointestinal bleeding. Right-sided diverticula may bleed for this reason as readily as those on the left. Selective angiography currently is apparently the most reliable method of identifying the bleeding diverticula. Bleeding diverticula are notoriously inapparent at surgery and may require multiple colotomies for their identification. Selective infusion of epinephrine or vasopressin through arterial catheters offers some hope for medical therapy of massive bleeding from this source. It certainly represents a step up over blind resection of portions of the colon in the therapeutic armamentarium for bleeding diverticula.

Spastic diverticulosis, which is limited in distribution to the sigmoid and distal descending colon, is an entirely different entity in terms of its pathologic physiology. The circular muscle in the distal colon is organized into fasciculi or rings. There are fibers that bridge from one ring to another ring, but the general structural orientation remains and is visible in a longitudinal cross section of the bowel. In certain individuals with a spastic variety of irritable colon syndrome, these rings of sigmoid musculature begin to undergo remarkable muscular hypertrophy with a crowding together of the muscle fibers. This hypertrophy may be eccentric and usually will involve only a portion of the circumference of the ring. The portion of the colonic wall running between the mesenteric taenia and the two antimesenteric taeniae is involved. The remaining one third of the circumference of the wall lying between the two antimesenteric taeniae is relatively spared. The muscular hypertrophy permits the formation of multiple closed chambers from the lumen of the sigmoid, and within these chambers there may be significant increase in intraluminal pressure as a result of contraction of the hypertrophied circular muscle (Fig. 27-3). This increase in tension results in cramping abdominal pain. The muscular thickening and crowding of the circular muscle yields a characteristic pattern on radiographic examination, often termed a sawtooth deformity (Fig. 27-4). The wall thickening may also present as a palpable mass. All these features—the pain, the mass, and the radiologic abnormality—may present in the absence of inflammation and have been reported in the absence of diverticula. Diverticula form in a fashion similar to simple diverticula as herniations of mucosa blown out through weakened areas between the hypertrophied fasciculi of the circular muscle. On occasion the increased pressure generated in the closed chamber will cause a perforation of the tip of the diverticulum. This can give rise to the formation of pericolitis, abscess, peritonitis, and fistula formation. This then repre-

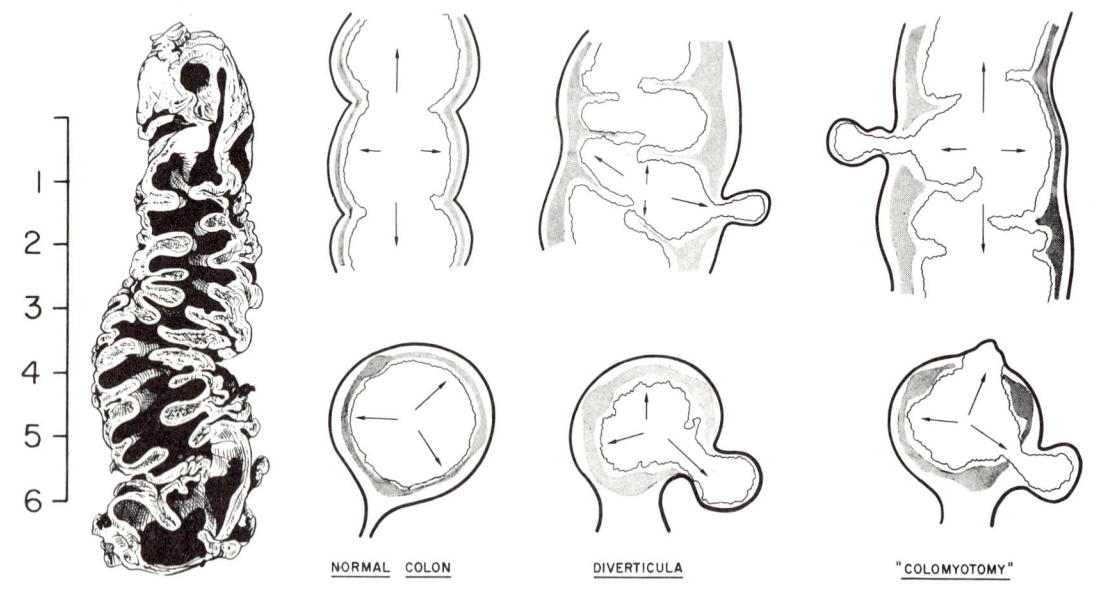

Figure 27–3 Figure on left is a drawing of a gross specimen of sigmoid colon which is involved in sigmoid diverticulitis. The hypertrophied rings of circular muscle which give rise to the saw-tooth deformity on x-ray are clearly apparent. The remainder of the illustration indicates the mechanism of formation of diverticula and their relief by colomyotomy. (See also Figure 27–4.) (Ranson, J. H. C., et al.: Amer. J. Surg., *123*:185, 1972.)

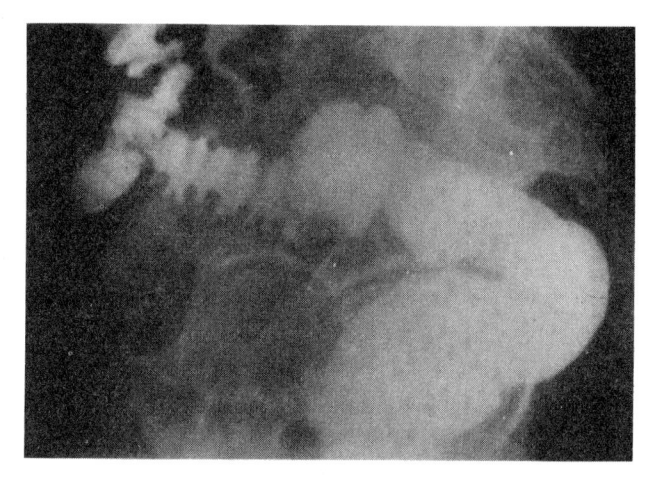

Figure 27-4 Photograph of a gross specimen of sigmoid colon (*bottom*) and a preoperative barium enema of this colon (*top*) showing the abrupt change from normal sigmoid to that involved with hypertrophy of the circular muscle. The saw-tooth or serrated deformity is easily visible on x-ray. (Arfwidsson, S.: Acta Chir. Scand., Supplement *342*:40, 1964.)

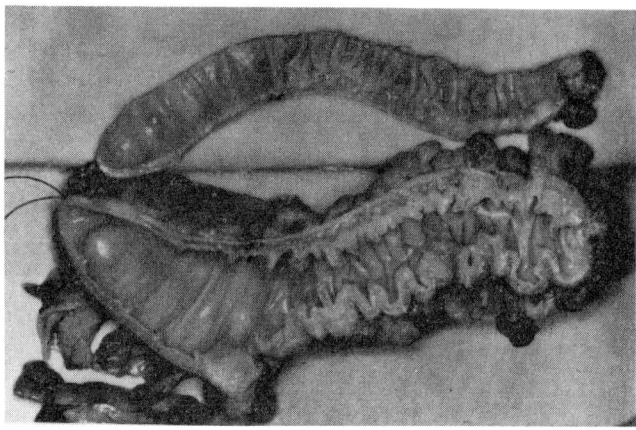

sents true diverticulitis and will also give rise to a palpable mass and pain. It may be distinguished from the noninflammatory "diverticulitis" by the presence of fever, leukocytosis, and the finding of extravasated barium at the time of enema. Treatment will vary with the stage of the disease. When perforation and pericolitis occur, the patient must be treated as any perforated viscus is treated. Recurrent diverticulitis may be a management problem. Connell treats recurrent pericolitis with intermittent courses of nonabsorbable sulfa for periods of 4 to 5 days each month. In the absence of inflammation, two courses are currently open. Long sigmoid myotomy dividing the hypertrophied rings of muscle but without penetrating the mucosa has been reported to give symptomatic relief (Fig. 27-3). Recently, the use of high-residue diets based largely on bran content has been reported to yield relief of symptoms that is maintained indefinitely. Critical evaluation and controlled trials of bran have not been performed. If the relationship between spastic irritable bowel and spastic diverticulitis is verified, earlier and more aggressive therapy of the former may be preventative.

Idiopathic Chronic Inflammatory Bowel Disease

On the basis of certain clinical and histopathologic features, two distinct forms of chronic inflammatory bowel disease are currently recognized. The utility of this separation derives from differences in histologic appearances and clinical events which reflect different patterns of morbidity and mortality. The terms ulcerative colitis and Crohn's disease have been most frequently applied to these disorders, but in the colon the latter has also been frequently referred to as granulomatous colitis, transmural colitis, or ileocolitis when disease is present in both small and large bowel. The differential features of the two conditions are summarized in Table 27-4. This separation into two seemingly distinct conditions, however, should not obscure their obvious

TABLE 27-4 PATHOLOGIC FEATURES OF CROHN'S DISEASE AND ULCERATIVE COLITIS

	Crohn's Disease	Ulcerative Colitis
Gross Features		
Anal and perianal lesions	Major and common	Minor and uncommon
Bowel wall	Thickened	Normal to slight increase
Strictures	Common	Uncommon
Fistulas	Common	Rare
Pseudopolyps	Rare	Common
Ulcers	"Fissure"	Punctate to troughlike
Distribution	More proximal	More distal
Continuity	Often "skip" areas	Always contiguous
Toxic megacolon	Uncommon	More common
Carcinoma	Rare	Increased
Microscopic Features		
Primary impact	Submucosa	Mucosa
Type of reaction	Productive	Exudative
Lymphoreticular hyperplasia	Marked and transmural	Minimal and superficial
Granulomas	40 to 80%	Occasionally
Crypt abscesses	Occasionally	Usual
Vascular ectasia and edema	Marked	Related to acute inflammation
Epithelial regeneration	Rare	Common

Watson, D. W.: Calif. Med., *117*:25, 1972.

interrelationship, which is expressed most fully in the colon, in which the distinction between ulcerative and granulomatous colitis at times may not be possible. If the morbid anatomy characteristic of each form is kept in mind, the clinical differences between the two are more readily appreciated. In classic Crohn's disease the submucosal edema and fibrosis and the deep fissure ulcers often lead to partial intestinal obstruction and fistulae, whereas the mucosal ulceration characteristic of ulcerative colitis more commonly results in hemorrhage and perforation. In the colon, however, chronic inflammatory bowel disease often presents a mixed histologic appearance, with a corresponding overlapping of clinical manifestations.

Ulcerative Colitis

Although occurring most frequently in Great Britain, North America, New Zealand, and Australia, ulcerative colitis has a worldwide distribution, as evidenced by reports from Costa Rica, Africa, and India. The peak incidence occurs in the second and third decades with a smaller peak after age 60. A genetic predisposition appears likely for the following reasons: (1) the higher incidence in Jews and the relative rarity among Blacks; (2) a familial occurrence ranging between 5 and 12 per cent which is interdependent with Crohn's disease; (3) an association with ankylosing spondylitis, which itself has genetic determinants; and (4) the presence of anticolon antibodies in healthy relatives.

Efforts to determine cause have emphasized infectious, psychogenic, and immunologic factors. An infectious origin appears highly unlikely and the potential influence of psychogenic factors probably has been overemphasized. It has been widely held that patients with ulcerative colitis exhibit a characteristic personality type, but the few controlled studies available fail to demonstrate a relationship between ulcerative colitis and various psychological parameters. Some type of immune reaction involving small lymphocytes and bacterial or colonic antigens appears most likely, but present evidence is inconclusive.

Although primarily a disorder of the colon, it is clear that ulcerative colitis is often a systemic disease exhibiting a wide range of extracolonic manifestations. These are listed in Table 27-5.

The colon's contribution to the clinical picture is in the form of some combination of diarrhea, hematochezia, and cramping lower abdominal pain. The intensity of these symptoms varies widely between patients and from time to time in the same patient. Onset may be gradual or fulminant and the course chronic and continuous or remittent and relapsing. Asymptomatic intervals vary from a few weeks to many years, but eventual relapse is the rule, the rate varying between 27 and 50 per cent per year. Fever and leukocytosis may occur with acute attacks and anemia is common. The latter is most often due to blood loss but other causes include malabsorption of iron, autoimmune hemolytic anemia, microangiopathic hemolytic anemia, G-6-PD deficiency, and Heinz body anemia related to Azulfidine therapy.

Diagnosis depends upon observing characteristic features of the disease by proctosigmoidos-

TABLE 27-5 EXTRACOLONIC MANIFESTATIONS OF ULCERATIVE COLITIS

Skin lesions
    Erythema nodosum
    Erythema multiforme
    Pyoderma gangrenosum
    Nonspecific pustular dermatosis
Mucous membrane lesions
    Aphthous stomatitis
    Ulcerative esophagitis
Eye lesions
    Episcleritis
    Uveitis
    Iritis
    Conjunctivitis
    Marginal corneal ulceration
Bone and joint lesions
    Arthralgias
    Sacroiliitis
    Arthritis of ulcerative colitis
    Ankylosing spondylitis
    Rheumatoid arthritis
Hepatobiliary lesions
    Active chronic hepatitis
    Pericholangitis
    Unclassified inflammatory changes
    Cirrhosis (postnecrotic and biliary)
    Carcinoma of extrahepatic bile ducts
    Primary sclerosing cholangitis
Pericarditis
Renal calculi

copy or barium enema. Since both gross and microscopic features are nonspecific, it is also important to exclude bacterial and parasitic infections, especially in patients with acute disease of recent onset. Classically the mucosa appears hyperemic, edematous, granular, and friable, often with fine ulcerations and active bleeding. Involvement is always continuous over the length involved. Rectal biopsy may reveal characteristic but nonspecific changes and will always be abnormal in the presence of active disease or demonstrable disease elsewhere in the colon. A histologically normal rectum in the presence of more proximal disease is highly unlikely in ulcerative colitis and favors a diagnosis of Crohn's disease. The radiologic appearance of ulcerative colitis is well known and only a few comments are appropriate here. In more acute phases there will be rather broad-based mucosal ulcerations, edema of the mucosa, and often loss of haustrations. More chronic involvement is manifested by loss of mucosal detail, loss of haustrations, shortening, widening of the retrorectal space, pseudopolyps, and occasionally rectovaginal or rectovesical fistulae. The terminal ileum may be involved with a superficial "backwash" ileitis in about 10 per cent of cases. Involvement begins distally and proceeds proximally always in a continuous fashion without skip areas. There is little or no fibrosis even with long-standing disease, and the majority of radiologic findings, including shortening and loss of haustrations, are potentially reversible.

Complications include severe hemorrhage, perforation, toxic megacolon, malnutrition, carcinoma of the colon, and, in children, failure of sexual development and growth retardation. Three high-risk factors have been identified with respect to the development of carcinoma of the colon: (1) onset in childhood, (2) total or near total colonic involvement, and (3) duration of disease longer than 10 years. Obstruction and fistulization are seldom encountered in patients with ulcerative colitis.

All nonsurgical treatment is empirical and symptomatic. Emphasis has been placed upon the administration of Azulfidine (salicylazosulfapyridine), measures to control diarrhea, and the use of systemic or topical steroids. The aforementioned complications are obvious indications for colectomy, but the most frequent reason for surgical intervention in patients with ulcerative colitis continues to be intractability and failure of medical management. Although some continue to employ subtotal colectomy, there is a growing emphasis upon one-stage total proctocolectomy and permanent ileostomy.

The outcome of the disease is most dependent on the age of the patient, the extent of the involvement, and the severity of the current attack. Mortality is highest in those above the age of 60, those with total involvement and the severest attacks. The single most important factor governing prognosis is the severity of a given attack. The reported mortality for severe attacks varies between 11 and 26 per cent and that for mild or moderate attacks is less than 1 per cent. The late outcome or long-term mortality remains inadequately defined, since most studies are based upon projected values involving relatively small numbers of patients.

Crohn's Disease

Crohn's disease most frequently is confined to the small intestine with 90 per cent of cases involving the terminal ileum. The colon may be the only site of involvement in some 10 to 17 per cent of patients or may be involved as part of an enterocolitis in 17 to 40 per cent. It has an ethnic and age distribution similar to ulcerative colitis except for the lack of a secondary peak in the older age group. Reliable data concerning its incidence and prevalence in the general population and its geographic distribution are not available, however, owing to the uncertain frequency of granulomatous colitis, since a firm diagnosis of the latter often requires surgical material. Again a genetic predisposition seems probable, but hypotheses concerning etiology are even less well formulated than in the case of ulcerative colitis. Similar to the latter, these patients frequently possess anticolon antibodies and circulating lymphocytes which are cytotoxic for allogenic colon epithelial cells. A major difference from ulcerative colitis is the presence of anergy in a significant proportion of patients. This anergy and the granulomatous nature of the disorder have prompted a comparison with sarcoidosis, and although both exhibit a response to Kveim antigen, there is little else to suggest an etiologic relationship. Furthermore, from a clinical standpoint, they appear to be quite different disorders.

The proclivity to transmural involvement with edema and fibrosis often results in chronic partial intestinal obstruction. The mucosa may become secondarily involved but to a much less extent, so that hemorrhagic ulceration is not as frequently encountered as in patients with ulcerative colitis. Similarly, the thickened bowel wall rarely is the site of a free perforation. Instead, the deep cleft-like fissure ulcers, characteristic of this disease, lead to fistulization and abscess formation. The relative sparing of the mucosal layer probably also accounts for the infrequent development of carcinoma in these patients.

Sigmoidoscopic examination presents a variable appearance. Fully one half of patients with large bowel involvement and all the patients with disease limited to the small bowel will have a normal rectum, both grossly and histologically. In the known presence of more proximal inflammatory disease this in itself strongly favors a diagnosis of Crohn's disease as compared to ulcerative colitis. A small proportion of patients have rectal involvement that will not be microscopically distinguishable from ulcerative colitis. The remainder exhibit features suggesting the presence of Crohn's disease. These include skip areas; large ulcerations and various anal and perianal lesions including indolent, undermined anal fissures, sometimes extending to involve the perineum and even to the inguinal regions; enterocutaneous fistulae; solitary ulcers; and edematous anal tags. These anal lesions at times are the initial manifestation of disease, and biopsy of an ulcer, fissure, or fistulous tract may demonstrate granulomas and greatly assist in diagnosis. The point of demarcation between normal and abnormal bowel is relatively sharp in contrast to ulcerative colitis. Opinions differ regarding the usefulness of rectal biopsy in establishing a diagnosis, since the major thrust of the disease is in the submucosa and therefore a biopsy, to be helpful, must be deep enough to include a substantial portion of this area. This is often safe only on the rectal valves or the margin of an ulcer, and if characteristic changes are observed, including marked submucosal fibrosis and inflammation with granulomas, a diagnosis of Crohn's disease may be possible.

Radiologically, the presence of certain features strongly suggests a diagnosis of Crohn's disease as opposed to ulcerative colitis. These include skip areas, asymmetrical involvement of the bowel wall, fissure ulcers, enteric or enterocutaneous fistulae, disease limited to the more proximal portions of the colon, and the presence of clear-cut abnormalities within the small intestine. Many cases, however, will be indistinguishable from ulcerative colitis on radiologic grounds and many of these will exhibit overlapping histologic features. The spectrum of extraintestinal manifestations seen in patients with ulcerative colitis is also encountered in patients with Crohn's disease, although they are seen somewhat less frequently. Nonsurgical therapy in Crohn's disease follows the same general pattern of that utilized in patients with ulcerative colitis except that corticosteroids have a much less profound effect on patients with Crohn's disease, and the evidence presented by Cooke and Fielding suggests that mortality and complications are actually increased in patients with Crohn's disease receiving long-term steroid therapy. The surgical management of Crohn's disease is less satisfactory than in the case of ulcerative colitis. This is due to the frequent necessity for resection of physiologically important amounts or areas of bowel and the relatively high recurrence rate. Recurrence rates vary from 30 to 65 per cent, depending upon the distribution of disease at the time of surgery. Recurrence is least frequent with disease limited to small bowel, especially terminal ileum, is somewhat more frequent with colon involvement, and is most likely in the presence of ileocolitis. Some 30 per cent of patients will require more than one operation, with the risk of recurrence rising somewhat with each successive procedure.

The prognosis of Crohn's disease has been difficult to define, since it often depends on confirmation of the diagnosis by surgical means and the length of observation. It has generally been considered to be a chronic disease of high morbidity and low mortality, with physicians often trying to recall when they had last witnessed an autopsy on a patient with the disorder. The overall mortality is probably in the range of 15 per cent. In a study by Prior et al. of 295 patients followed for 1 to 38 years there were 53 deaths, more than twice the number expected for either sex. There was also a tendency for mortality to be higher in those with onset before age 40 and when corticosteroids had been employed.

It is obvious from the foregoing discussion that in many, probably most, instances ulcerative colitis and Crohn's disease appear to be distinct and separable entities, clinically, radiologically, and histopathologically. It is also true that they share many familial, ethnic, and immunologic similarities and as many as 20 per cent of cases of large bowel disease cannot be fitted into one of the two available types. Whether we are dealing with distinct entities having overlapping manifestations or a spectrum of a single disease remains unclear. In either case, differences exist which have prognostic and therapeutic relevance. Although the clinical course and complications encountered in the classic forms of the two extremes of chronic inflammatory bowel disease are readily understood in terms of histopathologic events characteristic of each, the latter cannot at present be understood in etiologic or pathogenetic terms.

CONSTIPATION

There is remarkably wide variation in human bowel habits. Diarrhea is present when stool frequency increases to the point at which formed stools are no longer produced. The end point for constipation is less easy to define. Davenport reports human tolerance for fecaliths of up to 100 lbs. and intervals between defecation as long as one year. Under normal circumstances failure to defecate regularly at intervals of at least 7 days probably requires prompt investigation. Many individuals may be appropriately diagnosed as constipated, with smaller changes in bowel habit. Except for the emotional turmoil, the only pathologic changes that may regularly be associated with constipation are the development of hemorrhoids, anal fissure, and the consequences of straining at stool.

Constipation may occur by several mechanisms. Congenital failure of the formation of intramural ganglia will result in a constricted colonic segment. Failure of integrated contraction causes a functional obstruction, with the back-up of feces and the presentation of megacolon. Excision of the offending segment results in return of transit and a resumption of bowel function. The pathophysiology of simple constipation is substantially less clear. Two varieties are recognized. In spastic or colic constipation, individuals demonstrate a motility abnormality of the sigmoid and descending colon. In the resting state there is a substantial increase in segmentation and nonpropulsive activity and there is delay of transfer of feces into the rectum. Rectal examination reveals a relatively empty rectum containing at best a few small lumps of hard feces. The underlying cause of the motility abnormality remains unclear. There has been a demonstration of the failure of normal physiologic mechanisms such as the effect of eating to stimulate a change of activity in the sigmoid colon. Stool softeners and a thoughtful use of contact laxatives orally or in suppository form and the use of bulk agents may effect a return to normal bowel habits.

Sensory constipation is an extension of the normal social inhibition of bowel action necessary to control defecation. When the rectum is distended to a critical volume, the urge to defecate is initiated. If it is denied, the rectum will relax and distend to accommodate the feces. The addition of larger quantities of feces will be required to reactivate the reflex. When voluntary denial is frequent, the rectum may become desensitized and a failure of call to stool by rectal distention results. On examination, these individuals will be found to have a rectum full of soft feces. This resembles the circumstances that result from cord transection with sensory failure. Therapy is more difficult with sensory constipation and requires re-education of the patient to achieve normal bowel habits.

Local pain and fear of its recurrence can inhibit defecation. Careful evaluation for rectal inflammatory lesions is an essential part of the therapy of constipation.

DISORDERS OF SECRETORY FUNCTION

Normal function of the colon includes net absorption of sodium and chloride and absorption of water. Potassium and bicarbonate may be absorbed or secreted. Because there is a substantial flux of sodium and potassium into and out of the lumen, it often is difficult to identify a disorder that is the result of enhanced secretion. The net secretion of sodium and water when the colon is exposed to conjugated bile acids may as well be the result of decreased active sodium absorption as an increase in secretion. There are two disorders in which abnormal electrolyte secretion seems to be a primary defect—chloridorrhea and the hypokalemia associated with villous adenoma of the rectum. In addition, the colon shares with the small intestine a role in the immune system. The colon may mount its own immune response, secreting coproantibodies into the lumen.

Chloridorrhea

Chloridorrhea occurs in both a congenital and an acquired form. Normal handling of chloride in the colon results in passive absorption as paired ion with sodium. In the absence of chloride in the lumen, bicarbonate is absorbed. When chloride is present in the lumen, the chloride absorption seems to be coupled with an exchange for bicarbonate. The acquired form of chloridorrhea occurs in individuals who suffer from both diarrhea, due to some primary colonic disease, and severe hypokalemia. It is thought that the potassium deficiency affects the permeability of the mucosa, and the chloride-bicarbonate exchange is interrupted.

Increased delivery of chloride into the gut is postulated. While the chloride secretion may be reabsorbed in individuals with normal colons, in individuals with some primary colonic disease absorptive failure due to mucosal abnormality or increased transit results in chloridorrhea. In congenital chloridorrhea, a similar mechanism exists. The primary colonic lesion is the congenital inability to absorb chloride adequately through the colonic mucosa. The excess fecal chloride acts as an osmotic cathartic. With development of hypokalemia, additional chloride loss by secretion results. Fecal chloride concentrations regularly exceed the sum of fecal sodium and potassium concentrations. Correction of potassium defect by supplementation and by limiting dietary chloride results in a significant improvement in diarrhea and electrolyte balance. Similar therapy should prove effective in acquired chloridorrhea.

Villous Adenoma

Villous adenomas are benign tumors of the colon. They may occur throughout the colon, though they are most common in the rectosigmoid. Their gross and microscopic appearance is that of multiple frondlike extensions. The folds are lined with numerous goblet cells and may produce truly astounding quantities of mucus secretion. Villous adenomas are distinguished clinically by a well-established potential for malignant transformation and for the production of mucus diarrhea which may on occasion lead to severe hypokalemia. Although the frequency of carcinomatous change has been reported to be as high as 50 per cent, the biological activity of this tumor is low and successful secondary resections are reported. Mucus secretion is a result of the large number of goblet cells contained in the tumor. The occasional villous adenoma that is found in the colon higher than the rectosigmoid does not result in diarrhea, since reabsorption of electrolytes secreted in the mucus may occur. As was indicated earlier, there is little or no reabsorption from the rectum and therefore tumors in the rectal segment are the prime offenders. Colonic mucus generally contains concentrations of sodium which are isotonic with plasma, 140 mEq. per liter. Concentrations of potassium are very much higher than serum concentrations. Concentrations as high as 140 mEq. per liter have been reported. However, the potassium concentration in mucous diarrhea usually remains only 3 to 10 times the serum level. The resultant loss of potassium will involve not only electrolyte changes but can precipitate kaliopenic nephropathy, digitalis toxicity, muscle weakness, and fatigue. Losses of a magnitude sufficient to cause death have been reported. The proper treatment is surgical removal of the tumor.

TUMORS OF THE COLON

The colon may play host to a full range of neoplasms, both benign and malignant. By far the most common benign tumor is the adenomatous polyp and the most common malignant tumor is adenocarcinoma. Villous adenomas have been presented under disorders of secretion. The benign adenoma, whether sessile or pedunculated, rarely produces significant symptoms. Occasionally, a benign tumor will bleed significantly or a low-lying polypoid adenoma will cause enough rectal irritation to produce diarrhea, but for the most part they are silent lesions. Extensive discussion of polyps would be unrewarding were it not for the controversy over whether benign adenomatous polyps are inclined to develop into adenocarcinoma. The simple adenomatous polyp is a neoplasm. Studies by Lane and coworkers of small polyps reveal distinct changes in glands with absence of papillary infolding and increase in cellularity. Mitotic figures may be found well above their normal zone of occurrence in the crypts and there are distinct changes in nuclei and distribution of cell types. In addition there are changes in the pattern of secretion and the basement membrane. Hyperplastic polyps frequently occur in the colon, but the above features serve to distinguish adenomatous polyps from them. The question of whether they are prone to undergo malignant transformation is controversial. There are two views: One suggests that adenomatous polyps have no greater potential for becoming carcinomatous than any of the remaining colonic epithelium. The latter do admit that the cytologic appearance of cellular atypia may develop in polyps but state that regardless of cytologic appearance their biological behavior remains that of a benign tumor. They further admit the presence of polypoid carcinomas. These are felt to represent cancers from the time of their origin and not malignant degeneration in a polyp. Generally, all cancers are felt to be larger than 1.5 cm. in diameter. Thus risk of operation has been felt to be greater than the risk that a polypoid lesion less than 1.5 cm. in diameter is a carcinoma. Long pedicles tend to favor slow-growing tumors of longer duration (Fig. 27–5). Both groups agree that villous adenomas can undergo malignant degeneration. The other group, believing in malignant potential of an adenomatous polyp, has yet to demonstrate unequivocally that a metastasizing carcinoma has developed from a benign adenomatous polyp in any individual. The group favoring no malignant potential appears to have the balance in their favor; however, a barium enema never permits one to make a cytologic differentiation between villous adenoma, polypoid carcinoma, and adenomatous polyp. The resolution of the problem at this time lies with the endoscopist. Flexible fi-

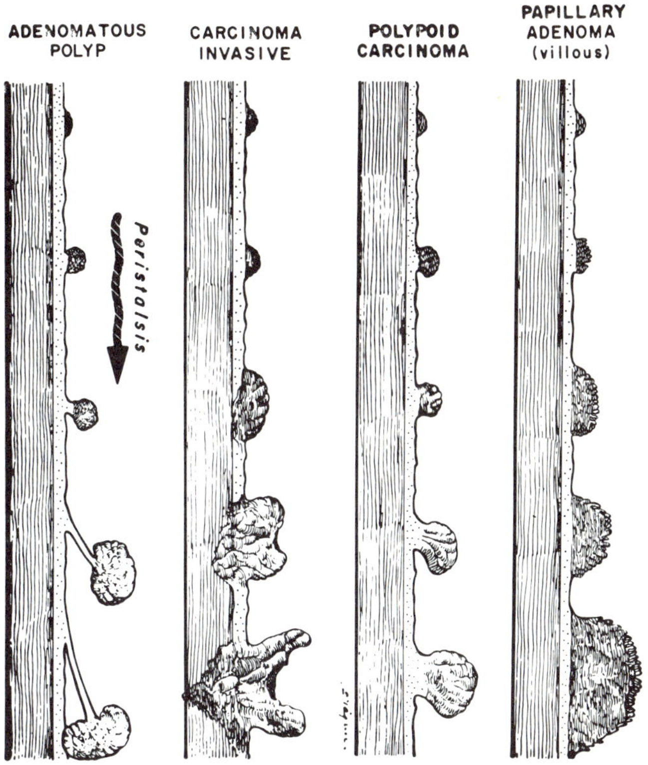

Figure 27-5 Castleman's conception of pedicle formation. With papillary adenomas, the broad base prevents prolapse, so that pedicles are rare. Polypoid cancer may develop with a short pedicle. Invasive cancer rapidly fixes mucosa to muscularis, so that pedicle formation becomes impossible. Simple adenomas, by proliferation at the tip, develop large heads, so that the underlying mucosa is soon pulled into a pedicle by peristalsis. (From Welch, C. E.: Polypoid Lesions of the Gastrointestinal Tract. Philadelphia, W. B. Saunders Co., 1964.)

beroptic colonoscopes are available in lengths suitable to permit examination of the entire colon from the cecum to the anus. As experience broadens, it appears technically feasible to reach the cecum in greater than 90 per cent of cases. Snares with electrocoagulation and forceps are available to permit biopsy at any depth. The safety of the procedure, the effect of sampling error, and the economic feasibility of extensive use of these endoscopes remain to be evaluated, but at the present time colonoscopy represents the most reasonable approach to the diagnosis and therapy of small polypoid lesions. If one accepts the suggestion that adenomatous polyps remain benign, even fragmentary biopsy will provide the necessary differentiation of the polypoid lesions. There will of course always be individuals for whom colonoscopy, for medical, technical, or emotional reasons, cannot be performed. A like group for similar reasons will not be operable. With regard to carcinoma proper, several additional points bearing on the pathologic physiology of their presentation should be mentioned. Carcinomatous lesions remain silent until they encroach on the lumen, bleed, or present with metastasis. The fluid contents in the right colon make obstruction a late occurrence. Right-sided lesions characteristically come to attention because of blood loss from the ulcerated and friable tumor surface or because of distant metastasis. The semisolid contents of the left colon, particularly the rectum and sigmoid, permit obstruction with smaller, earlier tumors. The critical feature of colonic cancer and practically any cancer is not its size or location as much as its biological activity. Cancers of low biological activity may remain resectable after long intervals and after reaching large size. Tumors of high biological activity will metastasize before any hope of identification is present. There is no practical measure of biological activity that may be used clinically at this time. Some hope exists for the use of quantitative determination of fetal intestinal tract proteins and other endogenous substances produced by cancer. Apparently gastrointestinal tumors, particularly colonic cancer plus a number of nongastrointestinal tumors, undergo regression to an embryonic cellular activity at the time of malignant transformation. Gold and coworkers have described a radioimmunoassay for carcinoembryonic antigen (CEA), one of these fetal intestinal tract proteins. The full range of the specificity and sensitivity of testing for this protein is yet to be identified. LoGerfo and coworkers have utilized a similar assay for a tumor associated antigen (TAA) which may be different from CEA. It is similarly incompletely evaluated. CEA and TAA testing remain the current hope for any increase in sensitivity for the diagnosis and management of colon carcinoma.

COLONIC MICROFLORA

The colon is best known for the lush growth of bacteria that inhabits the lumen. The difference in numbers of microorganisms in samples aspirated from the distal ileum in the cecum may be in the order of 4 to 6 $\log_{10}$. The bacterial flora of the large intestine does not represent an uncontrolled growth of a mass of organisms, for there appear to be a variety of mechanisms for qualitative and quantitative control of the flora. Normal flora performs several "functions." The digestion of cellulose and the production of a variety of vitamins have been discussed. Balanced normal flora may inhibit the overgrowth of pathogenic organisms, particularly staphylococci. The risk of staphylococcal overgrowth with enterocolitis is always present when normal flora is rendered unstable by antibiotic therapy. There also is an apparent necessity for specific bacterial flora to be present for full clinical expression of ameba infection. Normal flora may contribute to local and systemic pathologic changes in a number of other ways. Fermentation of lactose produces symptoms in lactase deficiency, and bacterial metabolism of bile acids may alter the enterohepatic circulation. The urea-ammonia cycle is also dependent upon bacterial action and may achieve significance in protein malnutrition and hepatic encephalopathy. Specific infections such as Shigella have been discussed. The colon may also harbor a range of other pathogenic organisms, particularly *Vibrio cholerae* and Salmonella, contributing to the carrier state. The full significance in terms of the pathologic physiology of colonic disease of alterations of controls over bacterial flora remains to be identified.

REFERENCES

Allen, F. D.: Essentials of Human Embryology. 2nd ed. New York, Oxford University Press, 1969.
Bentley, D. W., Nichols, R. L., Condon, R. E., and Gorbach, S. L.: The microflora of the human ileum and intraabdominal colon: Results of direct needle aspiration at surgery and evaluation of the technique. J. Lab. Clin. Med., 79:421, 1972.
Bleiberg, H., Mainguet, P., Galand, P., Chretien, J., and Dupont-Mairesse, N.: Cell Renewal in the Human Rectum. In vitro autoradiographic study on active ulcerative colitis. Gastroenterology, 58:851, 1970.
Bloom, A. A., LoPresti, P., and Farrar, J. T.: Motility of the intact human colon. Gastroenterology, 54:232, 1968.
Breen, K. J., Bryant, R. C., Levinson, J. D., and Schenker, S.: Neomycin absorption in man. Studies of oral and enema administration and effect of intestinal ulceration. Ann. Intern. Med., 76:211, 1972.
Casarella, W. J., Kanter, I. E., and Seaman, W. B.: Right-sided colonic diverticula as a cause of acute rectal hemorrhage. New Eng. J. Med., 286:450, 1972.
Castleman, B., and Krickstein, H. I.: Do adenomatous polyps of the colon become malignant? New Eng. J. Med., 267:469, 1962.
Castleman, B., and Krickstein, H. I.: Current approach to the polyp-cancer controversy. Gastroenterology, 51:108, 1966.
Chaudhary, N. A., and Truelove, S. C.: The irritable colon syndrome. A study of the clinical features, predisposing causes, and prognosis in 130 cases. Quart. J. Med., 31:307, 1962.
Christensen, J.: The controls of gastrointestinal movements: Some old and new views. New Eng. J. Med., 285:85, 1971.
Connell, A. M.: The motility of the pelvic colon. Part II. Paradoxical motility in diarrhoea and constipation. Gut, 3:342, 1962.
Connell, A. M.: Motor action of the large bowel. *In* Code, C. F. (Ed.): Handbook of Physiology. Vol. IV. Washington, D.C., American Physiological Society, 1968.
Cooke, W. T., and Fielding, J. F.: Corticosteroid or corticotrophin therapy in Crohn's disease (regional enteritis). Gut, 11:921, 1970.
Couturier, D., Roze, C., Couturier-Turpin, M. H., and Debray, C.: Electromyography of the colon in situ. An experimental study in man and in the rabbit. Gastroenterology, 56:317, 1969.

Crane, C. W.: Observations on the sodium and potassium content of mucus from the large intestine. Gut, 6:439, 1965.
Davenport, H. W.: Physiology of the Digestive Tract. 3rd ed. Chicago, Year Book Medical Publishers, Inc., 1971.
deDombal, F. T.: Ulcerative colitis. Epidemiology and aetiology, course and prognosis. Brit. Med. J., 1:649, 1971.
Derjanecz, J. J., and Clark, C. W.: Papillary adenomas of the colon and rectum: Clinical and pathological behavior. A plea for more conservative treatment. Canad. J. Surg., 7:389, 1964.
Devroede, G. J., and Phillips, S. F.: Conservation of sodium, chloride and water by the human colon. Gastroenterology, 56:101, 1969.
Devroede, G. J., and Phillips, S. F.: Failure of the human rectum to absorb electrolytes and water. Gut, 11:438, 1970.
Dowling, R. H.: The enterohepatic circulation. Gastroenterology, 62:122, 1972.
Edwards, D. A. W., and Beck, E. R.: Fecal flow, mixing and consistency. Amer. J. Dig. Dis., 16:706, 1971.
Edwards, D. A. W., and Beck, E. R.: Movement of radiopacified feces during defecation. Amer. J. Dig. Dis., 16:709, 1971.
Elsen, J., and Arey, L. B.: On spirality in the intestinal wall. Amer. J. Anat., 118:11, 1966.
Evanson, J. M., and Stanbury, S. W.: Congenital chloridorrhoea or so-called congenital alkalosis with diarrhoea. Gut, 6:29, 1965.
Feldman, F., Cantor, D., Soll, S., and Bachrach, W.: Psychiatric study of a consecutive series of 34 patients with ulcerative colitis. Brit. Med. J., 3:14, 1967.
Field, M.: Intestinal secretion: Effect of cyclic AMP and its role in cholera. New Eng. J. Med., 284:1137, 1971.
Fleischner, F. G.: Diverticular disease of the colon; new observations and revised concepts. Gastroenterology, 60:316, 1971.
Fordtran, J. S., and Ingelfinger, F. J.: Absorption of water, electrolytes and sugars from the human gut. *In* Code, C. F. (Ed.): Handbook of Physiology. Vol. III. Washington, D.C., American Physiological Society, 1968.
Goligher, J. C., deDombal, F. T., Watts, J. M., and Watkinson, G.: Ulcerative Colitis. Baltimore, Williams and Wilkins Co., 1968.
Gorbach, S. L.: Intestinal microflora. Gastroenterology, 60:1110, 1971.
Hellmans, J., Vantrappen, G., Valembois, P., Janssens, J., and

Vandenbroucke, J.: Electrical activity of striated and smooth muscle of the esophagus. Amer. J. Dig. Dis., 13:320, 1968.

Hofmann, A. F.: The syndrome of ileal disease and the broken enterohepatic circulation: Cholerheic enteropathy. Gastroenterology, 52:752, 1967.

Hofmann, A. F., and Poley, J. R.: Cholestyramine treatment of diarrhea associated with ileal resection. New Eng. J. Med., 281:397, 1969.

Holzknecht, G.: Die normale Peristaltick der Kolon. Muench Med. Wschr., 56:2401, 1909.

Lane, N., Kaplan, H., and Pascal, R. R.: Minute adenomatous and hyperplastic polyps of the colon: Divergent patterns of epithelial growth with specific associated mesenchymal changes. Contrasting roles in the pathogenesis of carcinoma. Gastroenterology, 60:537, 1971.

Levitan, R., and Ingelfinger, F. J.: Effect of d-aldosterone on salt and water absorption from the intact human colon. J. Clin. Invest., 44:801, 1965.

Levitt, M. D., and Bond, J. H., Jr.: Volume, composition, and source of intestinal gas. Gastroenterology, 59:921, 1970.

LoGerfo, P., Herter, F., and Hansen, H. J.: Tumor associated antigen in patients with carcinoma of the colon. Amer. J. Surg., 123:127, 1972.

Matsumoto, K. K., Peter, J. B., Schultze, R. G., Hakim, A. A., and Franck, P. T.: Watery diarrhea and hypokalemia associated with pancreatic islet cell adenoma. Gastroenterology, 50:231, 1966.

Mekhjian, H. S., Phillips, S. F., and Hofmann, A. F.: Colonic secretion of water and electrolytes induced by bile acids: Perfusion studies in man. J. Clin. Invest., 50:1569, 1971.

Mendeloff, A. I., Monk, M., Siegel, C. I., and Lilienfeld, A.: Illness experience and life stresses in patients with irritable colon and with ulcerative colitis. New Eng. J. Med., 282:14, 1970.

Morson, B. C.: The muscle abnormality in diverticular disease of the sigmoid colon. Brit. J. Radiol., 36:385, 1963.

Morson, B. C.: Current concepts of colitis. Trans. Med. Soc. London, 86:159, 1970.

Painter, N. S., Almeida, A. Z., and Colebourne, K. W.: Unprocessed bran in treatment of diverticular disease of the colon. Brit. Med. J., 2:137, 1972.

Phillips, R. A.: Cholera in the perspective of 1966. Ann. Intern. Med., 65:922, 1966.

Phillips, S. F.: Absorption and secretion by the colon. Gastroenterology, 56:966, 1969.

Phillips, S. F., and Edwards, D. A. W.: Some aspects of anal continence and defecation. Gut, 6:396, 1965.

Prior, P., Waterhouse, J. A., Fielding, J. F., and Cooke, W. T.: Mortality in Crohn's disease. Lancet, 1(3):1135, 1970.

Provenzale, L., and Pisano, M.: Methods for recording electrical activity of the human colon in vivo. Amer. J. Dig. Dis., 16:712, 1971.

Reilly, M.: Sigmoid myotomy – interim report. Proc. Roy. Soc. Med., 62:715, 1969.

Ritchie, J. A.: Colonic motor activity and bowel function. Part I. Normal movement of contents. Gut, 9:442, 1968.

Ritchie, J. A.: Colonic motor activity and bowel function. Part II. Distribution and incidence of motor activity at rest and after food and carbachol. Gut, 9:502, 1968.

Ritchie, J. A.: Movement of segmental constrictions in the human colon. Gut, 12:350, 1971.

Ritchie, J. A., Truelove, S. C., Ardran, G. M., and Tuckey, M. S.: Propulsion and retropulsion of normal colonic contents. Amer. J. Dig. Dis., 16:697, 1971.

Rosch, J., Gray, R. K., Grollman, J. H., Jr., Ross, G., Sterkel, R. J., and Weiner, M.: Selective arterial drug infusions in the treatment of acute gastrointestinal bleeding. A preliminary report. Gastroenterology, 59:341, 1970.

Samuel, P., Saypol, G. M., Meilman, E., Mosbach, E. H., and Chafizadeh, M.: Absorption of bile acids from the large bowel in man. J. Clin. Invest., 47:2070, 1968.

Schanker, L. S.: Absorption of drugs from the rat colon. J. Pharmacol. Exp. Ther., 126:283, 1959.

Schultz, S. G., and Curran, P. F.: Intestinal absorption of sodium chloride and water. In Code, C. F. (Ed.): Handbook of Physiology. Vol. IV. Washington, D.C., American Physiological Society, 1968.

Shields, R., and Miles, J. B.: Absorption and secretion in the large intestine. Postgrad. Med., 41:435, 1965.

Shorter, R. G., Huizenga, K. A., Spencer, R. J., Aas, J., and Guy, S. K.: Cytophilic antibody and the cytotoxicity of lymphocytes for colonic cells in vitro. Amer. J. Dig. Dis., 16:673, 1971.

Solomon, S. S., Moran, J. M., and Nabseth, D. C.: Villous adenoma of rectosigmoid accompanied by electrolyte depletion. J.A.M.A., 194:5, 1965.

Thompson, D. M. P., Murphy, J., Freedman, S. O., and Gold, P.: The radioimmuno assay of circulating carcinoembryonic antigen of the human digestive system. Proc. Nat. Acad. Sci., 64:161, 1969.

Torsoli, A., Ramorino, M. L., and Crucioli, V.: The relationships between anatomy and motor activity of the colon. Amer. J. Dig. Dis., 13:462, 1968.

Ustach, T. J., Tobon, F., Hambrecht, T., Bass, D. D., and Schuster, M. M.: Electrophysiological aspects of human sphincter function. J. Clin. Invest., 49:41, 1970.

Waller, S. L., and Misiewicza, J. J.: Colonic motility in constipation or diarrhoea. Scand. J. Gastroent., 7:93, 1972.

Watson, D. W.: The problem of chronic inflammatory bowel disease. Calif. Med., 117:25, 1972.

Williams, I.: Changing emphasis in diverticular disease of the colon. Brit. J. Radiol., 36:393, 1963.

Wolpert, E., Phillips, S. F., and Summerskill, W. H. J.: Transport of urea and ammonia production in the human colon. Lancet, 4:1387, 1971.

Wrong, O., Metcalfe-Gibson, A., Morrison, R. B. I., Ng, S. T., and Howard, A. V.: In vivo dialysis of faeces as a method of stool analysis. I. Technique and results in normal subjects. Clin. Sci., 28:357, 1965.

Zamcheck, N., Moore, T. L., Dhar, P., and Kupchik, H.: Immunologic diagnosis and prognosis of human digestive-tract cancer: Carcinoembryonic antigens. New Eng. J. Med., 286:83, 1972.

Zetzel, L.: Granulomatous (ileo) colitis. New Eng. J. Med., 288:600, 1970.

CHAPTER 28

NORMAL AND PATHOLOGIC PHYSIOLOGY OF THE LIVER*

F. L. IBER

On physical examination the liver is well protected by the ribs. Secretion is difficult to sample, and examination of the stool, urine, and changes in the blood must be relied upon for information about the liver. Liver biopsy reveals infiltrations and cell changes; scintiscans reveal overall shape; and visualization of the blood vessels and bile ducts within the liver is possible by radiologic techniques.

ANATOMIC CONSIDERATIONS AND TECHNIQUES FOR GAINING INFORMATION (TABLE 28–1)

Liver Size and Shape

There is marked variation in liver shape but very little variation in liver weight (2 per cent of body). Palpation primarily provides information about the inferior descent of the anterior edge of the liver; it is not surprising that the location of the palpable edge correlates poorly with liver mass. Percussion reveals the span and the anterior projection of the liver. Scintiscanning, or isotope imagery, is the best technique to outline the liver in two or more dimensions and not only accurately estimates liver mass but reveals large collections of a nonliver mass (such as cancer) within the liver substance.

---

*Recognition is given to Mr. Barry O'Neil for the artwork done in preparation of this chapter.

Scans

Rose bengal, an anionic dye, can be readily labeled with radioiodine. This dye, when administered intravenously, is taken up by the liver cells, as is bilirubin, and is actively excreted into the biliary passages. Ten to 45 minutes after intravenous administration, the dye is uniformly distributed throughout the hepatic parenchymal cells. A scintillation camera will show a homogeneous distribution of radioactivity. Thirty to 90 minutes after administration, dye is in the biliary passages and in the intestinal tract. Approximately two hours after administration no radioactivity remains in the liver. Radioactive rose bengal is now utilized to show patency of the

TABLE 28–1 APPRAISAL OF LIVER STATUS

Gross Anatomic Measures

1. Scans
   a. Liver cell uptake – rose bengal ^{131}I
   b. Reticuloendothelial uptake; gold, iodine, technetium colloids
2. Hepatic artery angiograms*
3. Portal venography
   a. Splenic†
   b. Umbilical*
   c. Venous phase of arteriography*
4. Peritoneoscopy*

*Skilled or trained person needed.
†Increased risk.

TABLE 28-2 USES OF SCANS*

1. Size, shape, and volume of liver.
2. Presence of nonliver nodules within image.
3. Identification of chest or abdominal mass as liver.
4. Showing impaired or irregular vascularity of liver.
5. Patency of common bile duct—serial rose bengal.
6. Enlargement of hilar bile ducts—rose bengal and colloid.
7. Size, shape, and volume of spleen.

*Colloid, unless specified.

biliary passages by serial scanning but is not used for liver scanning because anionic dye uptake is impaired in liver disease and the scans are poor. Colloidal substances (gold-198 on phosphate colloid, technetium or iodine on either sulfur colloid or denatured albumin) of the correct molecular size or range are preferentially taken up by the reticuloendothelial cells of the liver and spleen. These cells remain active in the presence of major hepatic cellular disease and therefore the scans are adequate. These scanning agents are widely utilized for determining the size, shape, and homogeneity of the liver. Table 28-2 indicates the utilization of scanning.

The surfaces of the liver reflect sound. Ultrasound devices may be employed to indicate the projection of the liver, but as yet these are not widely used in clinical medicine.

Arteriograms

The splenic or hepatic artery may be directly cannulated by percutaneous introduction of catheters. In the early phase, arteriograms will outline the arterial vessels of the liver or spleen and, in the late phase, the portal or hepatic veins. By employing this technique, the patency and anatomic course of all groups of blood vessels may be determined. Nodularity, erosion, new blood vessel formation, tumor blush, and collateral circulation may also be indicated. Portovenograms are made either by injecting radiopaque dye into the spleen (the dye is subsequently picked up and returned via the splenic and portal veins) or by cannulating the vestigial umbilical vein or a branch of the mesenteric vein. Direct techniques more clearly demonstrate collaterals of the portal vein.

Peritoneoscopy

The peritoneal cavity is distended with air, and a lighted telescope is inserted to inspect the surfaces of the anterior organs. The liver, a portion of the gallbladder, some of the mesenteric circulation, and portions of the intestine are nearly always seen. A great expanse of peritoneal surface may also be observed. Nodular lesions of the liver are usually seen and biopsy specimens may be taken if indicated.

Histology

Approximately two thirds of the liver consists of hepatocytes arranged in highly ordered plates. Each 8- to 12-surfaced cell has surface contact with blood vessels called sinusoids, but one or two surfaces remain in close contact with an adjacent cell and contain a minute bile duct or bile canaliculus (Fig. 28-1). The sinusoids are lined with en-

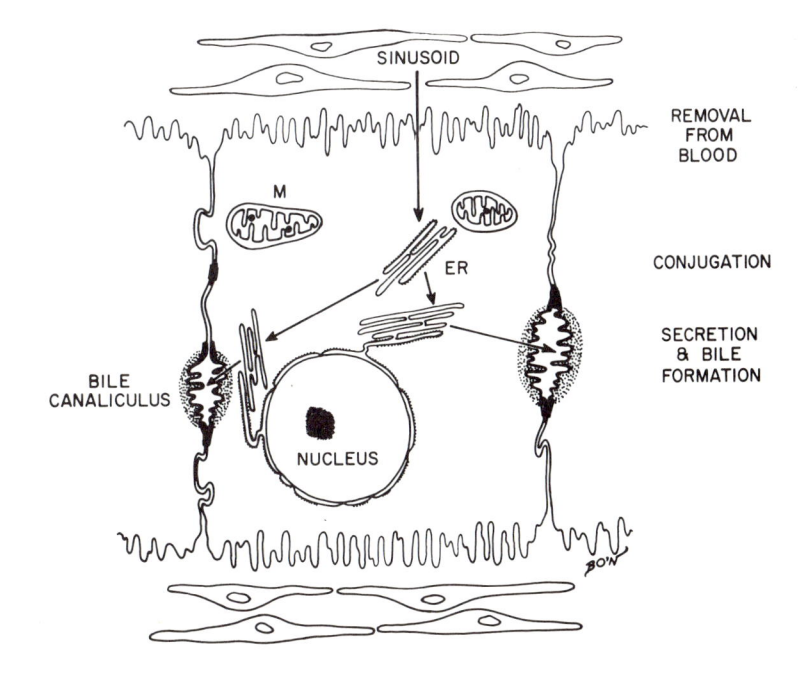

Figure 28-1 Schematic model of liver cell indicating the smooth and rough endoplasmic reticulum (*ER*), the mitochondria (*M*), and other structures.

dothelial cells and large reticuloendothelial cells called Kupffer cells. Proper polygonal cell function is highly dependent upon a rich intimate blood supply and adequate bile capillary drainage. The wall of the sinusoid is probably the most permeable capillary in the body, as indicated by the crossing of large proteins synthesized by the liver. The reticuloendothelial system of the liver, one of the most active in the body, offers optimal opportunity for phagocytosis, owing to the slow flow of blood through the sinusoids.

Pathologic processes may directly affect the liver polygonal cells or the Kupffer cells. They may alter the blood supply or the biliary drainage. The invasion of inflammatory cells may produce major pathologic changes. The liver is normally undergoing constant repair and it is estimated that liver cell renewal occurs each 50 to 75 days. A newly formed liver cell is less enzymatically mature than an older one and many liver functions cannot be efficiently performed.

Regeneration

The mammalian liver possesses a remarkable capacity both to regenerate its polygonal cells when portions are damaged and to cease regeneration when the proper mass is present. (Regeneration occurs in areas receiving portal blood.) Any form of dietary deficiency, particularly folic acid B_{12} and protein, will restrict regeneration, but no known material will stimulate it. Animal perfusion studies clearly indicate that a humoral factor stimulates hepatic mitosis, but the nature of this substance is unknown. Regeneration is much more striking in the young than in the old. There is no evidence that regeneration is impaired in liver disease, and most data support an increased destructive activity.

In all forms of hepatic damage, the bile ducts and large blood vessels seem to emerge more intact than the other hepatic elements. Mesenchymal elements (connective tissue) grow predominantly following certain types of liver damage (alcoholic, as an example). New blood vessel formation is far more prominent in tumor nodules than in regenerative liver nodules.

CLINICALLY IMPORTANT BIOCHEMISTRY OF THE LIVER

Rather than offering a complete survey of biochemistry, this section will discuss some arbitrary principles useful to later discussions. If one looks at the emergence of the liver by means of comparative physiology, it is apparent that processing of food, conversion of food from one form to another, food storage, and formation of an important digestive fluid are activities common to nearly all species. Removal of noxious substances, both those in the environment and those produced metabolically, is another major function. Finally, most species use the liver to make substances used elsewhere in the body.

The Great Toxin Remover—Ammonia and Purine Metabolism

Three substances are produced in quantity each day in the human body, and all seem to be toxic, since they are excreted. These are ammonia, porphyrins, and purines. The body has developed complex mechanisms that involve the liver and the kidney working in conjunction to remove these substances, without producing harm and with a great deal of energy expenditure. Thus, ammonia is converted to urea, porphyrins are converted to bilirubin, and purines are converted to uric acid. The liver has a major role in the removal of all these substances from the body. Many other molecules are modified and removed by the liver. Ammonia and purine metabolism will be briefly considered in this section.

Ammonia arises metabolically from the breakdown of amino acids when they are used for energy production and as a by-product of renal production of ammonia to conserve base. Additional ammonia arises from the intestinal tract. The intestinal production is usually the most important. Intestinal ammonia is predominantly the result of action of intestinal bacteria on dietary nitrogen-containing food and of metabolically produced urea. The portal blood contains from 4 to 50 times the ammonia content of other blood of the body, yet the liver so successfully removes it that hepatic venous blood is the lowest in content of any in the body. The liver contains the enzyme machinery that condenses ammonia with bicarbonate in the presence of carbamyl phosphate synthetase as the first step in the formation of urea. Despite the predominant role of the liver in urea formation, impairment of ammonia uptake is more prominent in liver disease than is overall urea synthesis. Clinical data suggest that urea formation is almost never significantly impaired in any stage of liver disease, but that ammonia removal is often a problem. Increased peripheral blood ammonia is frequently found in liver disease. It arises most notably from the shunting of portal blood directly to the systemic circulation. Increased production of ammonia is also due to the increased small intestinal flora in liver disease and to the diminished uptake of ammonia by damaged liver cells.

Purines are progressively oxidized to uric acid in primates and the final enzyme in this oxidation, xanthine oxidase, is contained solely in the liver. As far as can be determined, there seem to be no clinical consequences of mild impairment of this system in liver cell disease.

Bilirubin Metabolism (Fig. 28-1)

The liver plays a varied and intimate role in bilirubin metabolism. The prominent and unique yellow color of the patient with liver disease (jaundice) invites attention to those factors basic to an understanding of liver physiology.

All bilirubin in the body results from the breakdown of cyclic tetrapyrroles, functioning as electron transport pigments. Hemoglobin is the most significant of these pigments in the production of bilirubin, but myoglobin, P-450, and various cytochromes all contribute cyclic tetrapyrroles which are catabolized and eliminated via the bilirubin pathway.

The liver plays no apparent role in the destruction of erythrocytes, and although its reticuloendothelial cells will occasionally ingest a damaged erythrocyte, there is evidence that the red cell is not broken down. On the other hand, lysed red cells and hemoglobin bound or not bound to haptoglobin are taken up by specialized Kupffer cells and converted successively to biliverdin and free bilirubin. For each molecule of cyclic tetrapyrrole converted to bilirubin, a molecule of CO is released and eventually eliminated through the lungs. A precise measure of the rate of formation of CO is an exact measure of bilirubin formation.

The majority of free bilirubin is formed in the reticuloendothelial system of the body outside the liver. The iron and globin are stripped from the hemoglobin before the ring is opened. Free bilirubin is formed and is released into the bloodstream. Free bilirubin, although containing several polar groups, is highly insoluble in water or body fluids; this is due to a tight intramolecular arrangement that renders the active groups unavailable. Free bilirubin is tightly bound to serum albumin to be soluble in blood; the binding constant is about the same as that between albumin and free fatty acids. Because of this nearly total association with albumin, the volume of distribution is identical to that of albumin. Free bilirubin is lipid soluble and over several days is extracted into body fat. This extraction and subsequent tissue staining is responsible for jaundice; bilirubin confined to the blood is not apparent to an external observer regardless of the level.

Functions of the Liver. Three separate functions of the liver are commonly distinguished: (a) uptake of albumin-bound free bilirubin by the liver cell, (b) combination of free bilirubin with glucuronide into conjugated bilirubin, and (c) active secretion of conjugated bilirubin into the bile. Each of these operations illustrates important liver physiologic characteristics, and abnormalities of each occur that result in a disease (Fig. 28-1).

UPTAKE. The liver contains a protein of about 30,000 m.w. that binds bilirubin in the liver cell and seems responsible for the transfer of albumin-bound bilirubin into the liver cell. This process occurs at the cell surface, the albumin does not enter the liver cell, and no energy is required in this transfer. It seems to maintain an equilibrium in which bilirubin moves from the tightly bound state on albumin to an equally tight or slightly tighter binding on this intrahepatic transport and storage protein, called Y protein; movement continues from blood to liver because the Y protein in the liver cell is constantly being freed of its bilirubin load.

Normal albumin is saturated with 2 moles of free bilirubin per mole of albumin; thus, each gram of albumin can convey about 8 mg. of free bilirubin, a state seldom reached in disease. Many molecules share the same binding sites on albumin as bilirubin and if present in sufficient concentration may lessen bilirubin binding. Synthetic vitamin K and certain salicylates are examples. The rate of transfer of free bilirubin into the liver cell is dependent upon (a) the concentration of bilirubin in the blood, (b) the concentration of albumin in the blood, (c) the blood flow to the liver, (d) the concentration of Y protein in the liver cell, and (e) the concentration of bilirubin on the Y protein in the liver cell. Two- or threefold increases in this transport may be achieved over a period of time, probably by increasing (e) and (d), but abrupt lesser increases or chronic increases exceeding this range can be accomplished only by increasing the level of bilirubin in the blood. At levels of bilirubin of 6 or 7 mg. per 100 ml. any achievable amount of free bilirubin may be transported. If serum free bilirubin level is above this, the transport machinery is defective.

The Y protein has a short half-life, and its rate of restoration is impaired by protein starvation. Thus, any form of free hyperbilirubinemia is exaggerated by a 24-hour fast or in chronically starved patients in whom this form of jaundice may be apparent. The same transport system is utilized by a number of albumin-bound organic acids. Sulfobromophthalein, bile salts, acids, and many acidic drugs removed by the liver initially enter the liver cell bound to Y protein.

CONJUGATION. Conjugation occurs inside the liver cell. This process combines two proprionic acid side chains on the bilirubin molecule with glucuronide molecules. In this fashion the tight intramolecular arrangement of bilirubin is destroyed and a water soluble molecule called conjugated bilirubin is produced. Conjugation occurs on the smooth endoplasmic reticulum (ER) and requires activated glucuronic acid to combine with bilirubin through the intervention of an enzyme called glucuronyl transferase. There is evidence that portions of the ER adjacent to the bile canaliculus are principally responsible for this enzyme activity.

Conjugation enzymes mature late in the development of the fetus and are not fully developed until the tenth month after conception. Thus, premature infants have impaired conjugation, and varying degrees of impairment may be commonly found in underweight newborns. This is emphasized by the abrupt destruction of erythrocytes that occurs at the time of birth (hemoglobin decreases from about 19 to 14 gm. per 100 ml.) and its concomitant pigment load. Under this circumstance, free bilirubin accumulates in the blood in large amounts. When the level exceeds 20 mg. per 100 ml., the possibility of entry into central nervous tissues and subsequent brain damage is quite high. Birth brain anoxia due to birth injury makes this possibility a likelihood. Such brain damage resulting from free bilirubin is called kernicterus after the yellow staining of basal ganglia of the brain. The abnormal hemolysis produced by maternal anti-Rh positive serum reaching the Rh positive fetus most often produces such damage. If the hazard arises *after* birth, the level of bilirubin may be monitored; if above 20 mg. per 100 ml., it may be lowered by removing about one fifth of the patient's blood and replacing it with normal blood. This exchange transfusion is highly effective in lowering the circulating free bilirubin. A series of circumstances combine to make bilirubin brain damage feasible in childhood but nearly impossible later in life. These are

(a) Physiologic or abnormal breakdown of red cells in large amounts.

(b) Conjugation impairment due to prematurity.

(c) Failure of immature blood-brain barrier to exclude bilirubin.

(d) Anoxic birth injury.

Conjugation of bilirubin is impaired by several experimental drugs, by a steroid occasionally occurring in maternal milk, and by certain plant toxins. Two inborn errors of metabolism are associated with impairment of bilirubin conjugation. The first of these, Crigler-Najjar syndrome, is present at birth, is associated with a high degree of brain damage (two thirds of cases), and is unresponsive to any known treatment. The second, the Arias type of Crigler-Najjar, appears shortly after birth, does not result in brain damage, and is apparently controlled by inducing microsomal enzymes with phenobarbital, lowering the bilirubin to normal. The diagnostic features of both forms are very high free bilirubin (more than 10 mg. per 100 ml.), presence early in and throughout life, and absence of any apparent bilirubin conjugation in liver biopsy specimens. The bile in Crigler-Najjar syndrome contains no conjugated bilirubin; some is present in the A types. Table 28-2 indicates circumstances in which free bilirubin accumulates in the serum. In acquired disease, conjugated impairment almost never accounts for jaundice.

SECRETION. Conjugated bilirubin is produced in proximity to the bile canaliculus and is rapidly secreted into the bile. Under normal conditions it does not escape from the hepatic cell. However, if there is necrosis of liver cells, conjugated bilirubin in the bile ducts may reach the space of Disse. Accumulation of conjugated bilirubin in the liver cells for any reason may also lead to conjugated bilirubin in the blood and in the urine. Conjugated bilirubin passes freely into all the fluids of the body; it is partially bound to albumin, so that its distribution is influenced by the protein content. Conjugated bilirubin stains most protein-containing subcutaneous fluids and is readily observed in the sclerae of the eye and in the loose connective tissue beneath the tongue. It enters urine, spinal fluid, ascites, and most edema fluid. The most clinically useful difference between free and conjugated bilirubin is the regular appearance of conjugated bilirubin in the urine, whereas free bilirubin cannot reach the urine. If no bilirubin is excreted at all, the daily production rate (250 mg. per day) will raise the serum bilirubin 4 to 6 mg. per 100 ml. per day. Conjugated bilirubin is the only form in the bile.

Urobilinogen. Intestinal bacteria reduce conjugated bilirubin progressively to compounds called stercobilin or urobilinogen. These products, which number approximately 20 different substances, account for the color of stool. If intestinal bacterial reduction occurs normally, no bilirubin is found in the stool. Several of these products undergo extensive enterohepatic circulation. The sum of all known tetrapyrrole products does not equal the amount of bilirubin excreted; other small metabolic products occur. The determination of urobilinogen in the urine and the stool are useful assessments of overall pigment metabolism.

Normally, about 70 mg. of urobilinogen is absorbed via the portal vein and excreted almost entirely via the liver. Less than 5 per cent of this absorbed urobilinogen reaches the urine. Urobilinogen is a weak acid and as such is more concentrated in alkaline urine than an acid one. Normally, fresh urine with a pH of 5.5 or more contains urobilinogen, reflecting that conjugated bilirubin is reaching the gut and normal bacterial reduction and intestinal absorption of the urobilinogen are occurring. The total absence of urobilinogen in fresh urine of pH 5.5 or higher indicates that this cycle is broken. Most commonly, total obstruction of the biliary passages is present; less commonly, bacterial reduction (such as after extensive antibiotic use) is interrupted. Marked increase in urine urobilinogen suggests an increased production of urobilinogen, inefficient hepatic cell removal (such as in liver cell disease), or abnormal vascular communications between the portal and systemic circulation, bypassing the liver.

Tests of Bilirubin Metabolism. *Total bilirubin* in blood and urine may be accurately measured. However, partition into free and conjugated may be only crudely approximated by the "direct reacting" and "indirect reacting" bilirubin. Pure free bilirubin will almost always be less than 20 per cent direct reacting. Conjugated bilirubin, on the other hand, may be as much as 50 per cent indirect reacting. In clinical situations, if less than 25 per cent of the bilirubin is direct reacting, it may be presumed that *all* the bilirubin is free. If 50 per cent or more of the bilirubin is direct reacting, it should be assumed that all is conjugated. Determination of bilirubin in a fresh urine sample is the most precise method of determining whether bilirubin is entirely in the free form or not; in such cases the Ictotest or Harrison spot test will show it to be absent from the urine.

Aside from the serum and urine bilirubin, assessment of bilirubin metabolism either is available in only a limited number of highly specialized laboratories or is indirect. Table 28-3 indicates the problems and the direct and indirect tests commonly used in diagnosis. These tests and their utility in certain clinical examples are discussed below.

SULFOBROMOPHTHALEIN (BSP) AND INDOCYANINE GREEN (ICG) TESTS. These materials behave similarly in assessing liver metabolism. Both are intravenously administered anionic dyes. Both travel tightly adherent to albumin, both are taken up by the Y protein of the liver (in direct competition with bilirubin), and BSP but not ICG is conjugated by an enzyme on the endoplasmic reticulum with glutathione. Conjugated BSP and ICG are then secreted by the anion pump into the bile. In clinical use, a fixed dose of the dye is administered intravenously (5 mg. per kg. BSP–0.5 mg. per kg. ICG) and a blood sample is taken 45 minutes later for BSP (20 minutes for ICG) to determine how much dye has persisted in the blood. If more than 6 per cent is found, liver cell uptake

TABLE 28-3 TESTS OF BILIRUBIN METABOLISM

I. Increased Production	
A. Direct and specific	
1. CO production	1 mol. CO for each mol. bilirubin, any source
2. Fecal urobilinogen	Only about 2/3 total measured
3. ^{51}Cr RBC survival	Adult RBC only
B. Indirect but useful	
1. Serum haptoglobin	Only detects hemoglobin release
2. Reticulocyte levels	Marrow reaction
C. Indirect and rarely helpful	
1. Coombs' test	
2. Osmotic fragility	Only 1 or 2 specific diseases detected with these
3. Hemoglobin electrophoresis	
II. Impaired Conjugation	
A. Assay of glucuronyl transferase activity in liver biopsy	Require special laboratory procedures
B. Comparison of glucuronide excretion of other agents	
III. Impaired Excretion of Conjugated Bilirubin Associated with Extensive Malfunction of Liver Cells	
A. BSP maximal excretory rate	
B. I.V. cholangiography	Useful if bilirubin less than 3
C. Serial rose bengal scans	
D. Urobilinogen in the urine	
E. Tests of protein, or injury of cells	See Table 28-6
IV. Impaired Excretion of Conjugated Bilirubin with Preservation of Other Liver Cell Function (Cholestasis)	
A. Tests of anion pump (also abnormal if severe and prolonged impaired biliary flow)	
1. Appearance of conjugated BSP in venous blood after 90 minutes	
2. BSP maximal excretory rate	
3. Accumulation of bile salts in serum	
4. Lipoprotein of cholestasis	
B. Intermediate bile ductule disease	
1. Antimitochondria antibody	
2. Liver biopsy	
C. Patent large biliary passages	
1. I.V. cholangiography	
2. Transhepatic cholangiography	
3. Operative cholangiography	
4. Rose bengal scans, serial	

is considered defective. Any form of jaundice competes with the removal of both dyes, but in the nonjaundiced patient the removal from blood is mainly a measurement of the uptake and storage of the liver cell. On a research basis, both tests may be modified to measure maximal storage and maximal transport by the anion pump. Less damage is required to produce BSP or ICG retention than bilirubin retention.

URINE UROBILINOGEN. A fresh urine sample should be used and the pH determined; only if the pH is 5.5 or higher should urobilinogen be measured. The serial dilution which contains detectable material should be ascertained. The important questions are (a) is there some urobilinogen present and (b) is it present in a dilution of 1 to 50 or greater. Absence of urobilinogen indicates either (a) absence of conjugated bilirubin reaching the intestine or (b) absent bacterial conversion to urobilinogen usually due to antibiotics but occasionally due to colectomy or rapid diarrhea preventing sufficient numbers of the correct bacteria. An excess of urobilinogen indicates one of the following: increased production of bilirubin, an impaired removal of urobilinogen from portal blood due to damaged liver cells, or increased shunting of portal blood into the systemic circulation.

Classification of Jaundice. The problems of jaundice in the first year of life and much later are sufficiently different that the approach is usually kept separate. Table 28-4 indicates the major classification and cause of jaundice in the first year of life.

Some jaundice in the first days of life is normal as a function of transfer from the anoxic intrauterine existence to the open world. About one third of the hemoglobin is destroyed, and this sudden pigment load is sufficient to produce jaundice. If the child weighs under 3000 grams (an index of fetal maturity), bilirubin conjugation is probably impaired and will enhance greatly the level of indirect reacting bilirubin. Several acquired blockages of normal glucuronyl transferase have been reported; one of the most interesting is due to an abnormal steroid in mothers' milk absorbed by nursing babies. An occasional congenital defect is failure of bile ducts to develop. This may be a defect in just small segments in the large bile ducts, which is amenable to surgical repair, or total absence of intralobular ducts.

Jaundice in the older child and adult may be approached in a similar way. It is useful to divide the problems into those which have predominantly unconjugated or free bilirubin in the serum in contrast to those which have predominantly direct reacting pigment. Table 28-5 indicates a useful classification along these lines. Two predominant forms of unconjugated hyperbilirubinemia occur—those due to increased production and those due to inborn errors of metabolism. Unless some of the specialized tests indicated in Table 28-3 are applied, it may prove very difficult to specifically assign a case to one or the other.

Patients with predominantly direct reacting pigment are most conveniently divided into those with multifunctional liver cell impairment and those with cholestasis, which is predominantly failure of excretion of bilirubin and bile salts. This distinction, though it includes some overlapping diseases, is the way in which one must approach clinical problems.

Protein Synthesis — A Function of the Rough Endoplasmic Reticulum

Granular or rough endoplasmic reticulum receives RNA from the nucleus (see p. 72) and is the site at which the extensive protein synthesis of the hepatocyte occurs. Table 28-6 indicates the wide variety of proteins that are made almost exclusively by the liver and many are subsequently released into the blood. To support this extensive synthetic factory there is a rich array of systems in the liver cell which store amino acids, convert an amino acid present in excess to one present to a lesser degree, and are sources of energy. Because of these many complex interrelated functions, protein synthesis will be completely normal only when there are adequate numbers of completely normal liver cells, few or no inhibitors of protein synthesis affecting this complex function, and an adequate supply of dietary protein to assure availability of those amino acids that cannot be adequately synthesized within the body.

The blood level of a given protein is a function of both its rate of synthesis and its rate of removal. Some proteins persist a very short time in the

TABLE 28-4 CLASSIFICATION OF JAUNDICE IN FIRST YEAR OF LIFE

I. Predominantly Indirect Reacting
  A. Increased breakdown of red cells
    1. Physiologic
    2. Hemolysis, Rh and other
  B. Conjugation defects
    1. Prematurity
    2. Lack of glucuronyl transferase, permanent Crigler-Najjar
    3. Lack of glucuronyl transferase, inducible, Arias type
    4. Inactivation of glucuronyl transferase, abnormal breast milk steroid
II. Predominantly Direct Reacting
  A. Hepatic cell defect
    1. Giant cell hepatitis
  B. Cholestasis
    1. Giant cell hepatitis
    2. Biliary atresia

TABLE 28-5 CLASSIFICATION OF JAUNDICE IN OLDER CHILDREN AND ADULTS

I. Predominantly Indirect Reacting Bilirubin
   A. Increased production of bilirubin
      1. Chronic—Hemoglobin or red cell membrane abnormality
      2. Acute—Red cell damage, drug, thermal, or immunologic
   B. Impaired transfer albumin to Y-protein
      1. Familial unconjugated hyperbilirubinemia—Gilbert's
      2. Nonfamilial cases
      3. Acquired cases
   C. Conjugation defects (rare)
      1. Toxins
      2. Crigler-Najjar
      3. Arias type
II. Predominantly Direct Reacting Bilirubin
   A. Associated with multifunctional impairment of the liver
      1. All forms of hepatitis
      2. Infiltrative liver disease
         a. Tumor
         b. Amyloid, lipid
   B. Cholestasis
      1. Anion pump injury—hepatitis
      2. Bile capillary injury—drugs
      3. Obstruction to large hepatic and common bile ducts

blood after release. Factors operative in disease may hasten the removal of the protein from blood (such as loss of albumin into the intestinal tract or the urine, or depletion of serum fibrinogen due to accelerated coagulation).

Under normal circumstances, serum proteins synthesized in the liver vary widely in removal rates. Thus, albumin persists in the serum with a half-time of approximately 30 days; fibrinogen with a half-time of approximately 4 days, and prothrombin with a half-time of approximately 12 hours. This means that total cessation of hepatic manufacture and release would result in a fall of prothrombin to 5 per cent, of fibrinogen to 60 per cent, and of albumin to 92 per cent of initial level in two days. The small change in albumin might well be overlooked. Use of the persistence time of these several proteins is helpful in dating the onset of severe liver cell failure.

The wide variety of proteins made by the liver and present in the serum is of less use in diagnosing than in comprehending the many changes present in long-standing liver cell disease.

Albumin. A lowering of the serum albumin level (often to less than one half normal) is common in cirrhosis and is clinically apparent in fluid retention of edema and ascites. Many physiologic substances and drugs are tightly bound to albumin and are altered in their effective blood levels and in their hepatic and renal transport by this lowering.

Coagulation Abnormalities. These are common in acute and long-standing liver disease. The four liver-made proteins requiring vitamin K as a cofactor for synthesis (II, VII, IX, X) and measured as the one-stage prothrombin time are the most frequently abnormal. Substantial hemorrhage may be a complication of liver disease. Absorptive defects of vitamin K, increased activation of intravascular clotting with subsequent consumption of coagulation factors, and platelet defects due to persistence of products of fibrinolysis are additional commonplace problems of coagulation that require detailed evaluation.

The many transport protein abnormalities in liver disease suggest the wide groups of functions that may be abnormal in liver disease. Thus, iron transport is often abnormal in hepatic disease; haptoglobin (used to assess the amount of free hemoglobin being formed to diagnose hemolysis) may be misleading. Lipoproteins and lipid transport may be quite abnormal. The liver produces specific binding proteins for most nonpeptide hormones and in liver disease the level produced may be less than normal. Many tissue effects of hormones depend upon the amount of free or nonprotein-bound hormone.

Alcohol, many antibiotics, a few cancer chemotherapy drugs, and some toxins impair protein synthesis as their means of action. Nearly all affect lipoprotein synthesis by hepatic cells and result in an accumulation of fat within the liver cell.

Function of the Smooth Endoplasmic Reticulum

Large numbers of enzymes are bound to the smooth endoplasmic reticulum. The orderly arrangement seems essential because sequential chemical reactions that oxidize or reduce complex organic molecules are accomplished. The substrates are usually of limited solubility and are

TABLE 28-6 PROTEINS MADE PREDOMINANTLY BY THE LIVER

1. Albumin
2. Coagulation Proteins
   a. Fibrinogen (Factor I)
   b. Prothrombin (Factor II)
   c. Factors III, V, VIII, IX, X, and XI
3. Transport Proteins
   a. Haptoglobin
   b. Transferrin
   c. Ceruloplasmin
   d. Hormone transport proteins
   e. Y protein
   f. Alpha-lipoprotein
   g. Beta-lipoprotein
4. Reaction to Injury
   a. Alpha-globulin
   b. Beta-globulin

often combined by these enzymes with highly polar molecules (such as sulfate, glucuronide, glutathione, glycine, acetate) to permit subsequent excretion by liver or renal tubular cells. Figure 28-2 indicates that portions of the chain are used for many different reactions requiring an electron transport system to molecular oxygen.

A few normal substances are metabolized using these membrane-bound enzymes. Most steroids are reduced by this system. Fatty acids are oxidized by this system. The system is also important for many trace materials and particularly important in drug metabolism. Many drugs are fairly insoluble in water and resist excretion. The liver is a major organ responsible for biotransformation—the chemical modification of a drug that usually alters its biological activity and renders it more susceptible to excretion by both the kidney and the liver. Oxidation reactions such as N- and O-dealkylization, aromatic ring and side chain hydroxylation, N-oxidation, N-hydroxylation, and deamination of primary and secondary amines are common. Reduction of nitro groups, reductive cleavage of azo groups, and reduction of ring double bonds may occur. Conjugation of phenols, alcohols, carboxylic acids, and amines with glucuronides, sulfates, acetates, or glycine is a common mode of rendering molecules more polar for excretion. Specific enzymes for each reaction are usually necessary to activate the drug or to carry out portions of the chemistry. However, certain of the enzymes in the endoplasmic reticulum are used in common by many systems. NADPH and cytochrome P-450 are common requirements for most of these. Figure 28-2 indicates a common relationship between these.

Lipid solubility seems an important determinant of which drugs utilize the endoplasmic reticulum enzymes. The rates of reaction vary markedly and, similarly, the effect of liver disease on these drug removal reactions varies. Steroid inactivation is usually slow in almost any form of liver cell disease, and sex hormone, adrenal cortical hormone, and aldosterone may persist in liver cell disease. Bilirubin conjugation is usually not altered in liver cell disease, bile salt conjugation is often impaired, and the normal threefold increase of glycine conjugations over taurine is reduced.

Antibiotics, hypnotics, and hypoglycemic agents all show unusual persistence in the presence of liver disease. One can best generalize by stating that any drug using the hepatic endoplasmic reticulum should be used with caution and its blood level or biological effects observed.

An important and unique aspect of the endoplasmic reticulum is its near total hypertrophy (with all the contained enzymes) after treatment with certain agents that saturate one or more of its enzymes. Phenobarbital is the best known drug causing generalized hypertrophy of the enzymes in the endoplasmic reticulum. Drug removal rates are accelerated for nearly all agents using enzyme on the ER. For this reason, many patients with hepatic disease may have increased rather than impaired endoplasmic reticulum enzymes. This may be from drugs they have received in the course of treatment or it may be from alcoholism. The Arias type of impairment of liver conjugation of bilirubin, an inborn error of metabolism, is effectively treated with phenobarbital—the increased enzyme removes the excess bilirubin.

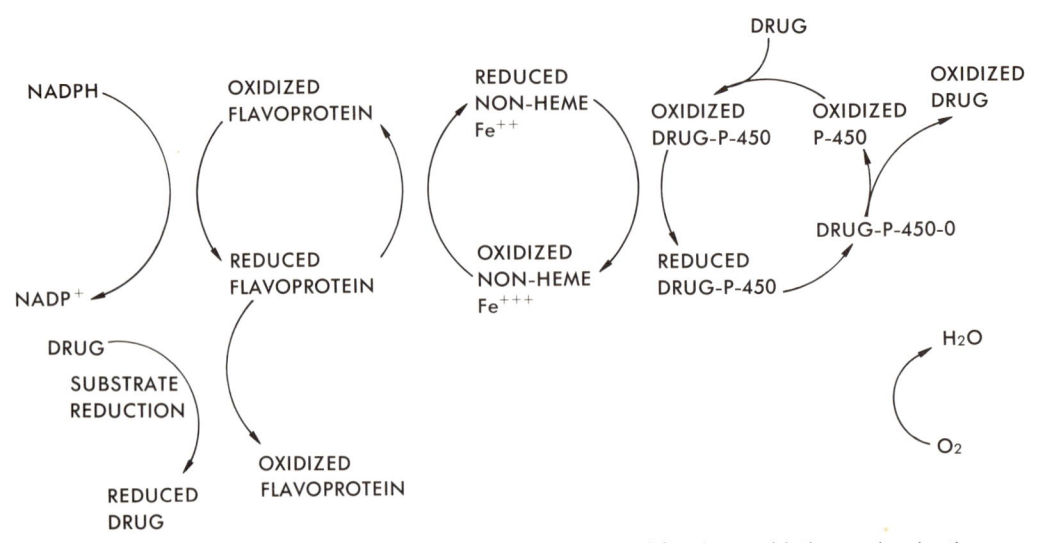

Figure 28-2 Endoplasmic reticulum electron transport used for drug oxidation and reduction.

Carbohydrate Metabolism

The liver has an active role in glucose and carbohydrate metabolism (see pp. 847 and 900). The liver stores glucose as glycogen in the absorptive period, preventing the blood glucose from reaching a diabetic level. Even in a well-nourished person the glycogen supply is adequate to maintain the blood glucose for only a few hours. The liver constantly converts lactic acid and amino acids into glucose to maintain adequate glucose in the blood. In severe liver cell failure, symptomatic hypoglycemia may be a major problem. This occurs after prolonged fasting. In the alcoholic patient, conversion of protein and fat to glucose may be impaired.

Insulin is normally released into the portal vein and reaches the liver in much higher concentration than it is in the peripheral blood. Portal hypertension and portal shunts to the systemic circulation may account for abnormal levels and effects of both insulin and glucose. Thus, hyperglycemia and hypoglycemia may accompany liver disease.

Acute damage to large numbers of liver cells may result in substantial amounts of lactic, pyruvic, citric, and alphaketoglutaric acids in the serum; these may replace other anions and result in both acidosis and a 10 to 30 mEq. per liter increase in the undetermined anion (the numerical difference between the sum of the sodium and potassium and the sum of the bicarbonate and chloride).

BILE FORMATION, BILE FLOW, AND CHOLESTASIS

Bile contains water and electrolytes in amounts approximately the same as those in plasma, but in addition contains four major organic components (bile salts, lecithin, cholesterol, bilirubin) and many others. Bile is initially formed in the bile canaliculus at the juncture of two hepatocytes as a result of active secretion of anions by the liver cell. Water diffuses passively to maintain isotonicity. The thick epithelium of intermediate-sized bile ducts may add or remove water and/or electrolytes. The gallbladder markedly concentrates hepatic bile by the removal of water and electrolytes (see p. 819). Remarkably, the contents of the biliary tree remain nearly isotonic throughout all these alterations, largely owing to the propensity of the organic molecules to form loose molecular complexes (called micelles). These micelles principally serve to keep the more insoluble components (cholesterol) in solution. Many substances are secreted by the liver into bile for excretion; almost any organic acid may be so excreted. The normal composition of the major components of bile are indicated in Table 28-7.

Mechanism of Bile Formation

The wall of the bile canaliculus, with the likely participation of adjacent endoplasmic reticulum and possibly components of the Golgi apparatus, is capable of actively secreting a variety of materials into the lumen. The most active transport system excretes a number of organic anions; bile salts are by far the most important single material secreted by this system. This is commonly called the anion pump. Table 28-8 indicates the variety of substances actively transported into bile, at the level of the liver cell. The wall of the bile canaliculus seems freely permeable to water and uncharged molecules up to a molecular weight of about 900, but charged molecules seem retarded in their passage. As a result of the active secretion of bile salt and other molecules, water moves to preserve isotonicity and bile flow begins. Bile volume is highly dependent upon total bile salt secretion; normal flow is 450 to 700 ml. per 24 hr. The epithelium of intermediate bile ducts is capable of both absorbing and secreting into bile; water, electrolytes, and possibly glucose seem to be the principal substances transported.

TABLE 28-7 COMPOSITION OF HUMAN HEPATIC BILE

Component	mg. per 100 ml.	% Total Solids	mEq./L.
Bile salts	140–2230	8–53	3–45*
Lecithin	140–810	9–21	2–8*
Cholesterol	97–320	3–11	2–6*
Bilirubin	12–70	0.4–2.0	less than 1
Urobilinogen	5–45	0.2–1.5	less than 1
Sodium			146–165
Potassium			2.7–4.9
Chloride			88–115
Bicarbonate			27–55

*Variability due to micelle formation.
After Thureborn, E.: Acta Chir. Scand. (Suppl.) *303*:1, 1962.

TABLE 28-8 REPRESENTATIVE COMPOUNDS ACTIVELY EXCRETED BY HEPATIC CELLS

Organic Acids
    Naturally occurring:
        bile salts*
        bilirubin
        urobilinogen*
        lecithin**
    Therapeutic agents:
        sulfonamides**
        penicillin**
        ampicillin*
        chlorthiazide**
        streptomycin*
        tetracycline*
    Used Diagnostically:
        sulfobromophthalein**
        indocyanine green
        iopanoic acid**
        iodipamide
Bases
    procaine amide ethobromide
Neutral
    adrenal and sex sterols
    cholesterol*
    digitalis glycosides**

*Highly active enterohepatic circulation.
**Mildly active enterohepatic circulation.

Similar to the pancreas, these epithelial cells are responsive to the hormone secretin; a voluminous secretion elevated in bicarbonate results.

Enterohepatic Circulation

Many of the organic molecules contained in the bile are reabsorbed by the intestine into the portal venous blood and are transported to the liver, where they are re-excreted. Intestinal reabsorption may be highly efficient (95 per cent for bile salts), of intermediate efficiency (30 to 50 per cent for urobilinogen), or very slight (bilirubin). The process of liver bile excretion, gut absorption, and liver re-excretion is called enterohepatic circulation. The hepatic extraction of the reabsorbed material may be so efficient that little reaches the peripheral venous blood. This recycling of substances through the biliary tree is employed to treat biliary tract infections. An antibiotic which is recycled through the biliary tract many times is chosen. Occasionally, iopanoic acid (radiopaque dye) when given orally and recirculated enterohepatically will deposit in gallstones and they become visible with a rim of dye on x-ray after a week or so. Enterohepatic circulation assumes substantial importance when interrupted. In intestinal disease, bile salt conservation is impossible and depletion occurs. When inefficient liver cell extraction occurs, products normally removed by the liver appear in the urine, as, for example, urobilinogen. If portal blood is shunted to the periphery, higher peripheral blood levels may occur. Cholestyramine, an insoluble resin taken orally, binds certain materials undergoing enterohepatic circulation (bile salts, digitalis glycosides) in the intestine and thus depletes the body of them.

Bile Salts and Bile Salt Metabolism

Bile salts are synthesized exclusively by the liver from cholesterol. Cholic acid and chenodeoxycholic acid are the two bile salts made by the liver of man. Adult man forms about 200 to 300 mg. of cholic acid per day and a similar amount of chenodeoxycholic. Under stimulation cholic acid synthesis can increase seven- to tenfold and chenodeoxycholic acid synthesis two- or threefold. Bile salts are conjugated in the acid group with either glycine or taurine, with two to three times as much in the glycine form.

Conjugation of bile salts is important for both hepatic excretion and distal ileal reabsorption. If intestinal bacteria deconjugate large quantities of bile salts in the intestine, they are lost via the stool, because reabsorption becomes inefficient.

The normal human possesses about 4 grams of bile salt and this is utilized two to ten times daily, depending upon the amount of fat in the diet and the efficiency of the enterohepatic circulation. About 0.5 gram is lost from the body each day and about 0.5 gram is newly formed each day. Intestinal bacteria are active in reducing bile acids and producing new compounds that are not manufactured de novo by man but function nonetheless as important bile salts undergoing all the same reactions. Deoxycholic acid is the most important of these; small amounts of lithocholic acid are also found (see Fig. 28-3). It is apparent that an intact enterohepatic circulation of bile acids is essential for homeostasis of bile salt metabolism and fat absorption.

Bile salts are clearly responsible for two abnormalities in man. The increased accumulation in the bloodstream for any reason is associated with pruritus. The itching seems to result from concentration of bile salt in the sweat glands. If increased amounts of bile salts reach the colon, they may interfere with absorption of water and electrolyte and produce watery diarrhea (see p. 778). This condition, common after ileal resection of less than 100 cm. and occasionally occurring in primary ileal disease, is controlled by administering an ion exchange resin, cholestyramine, which is capable of binding bile salts.

Alteration of Bile Salts in Disease. Any process interfering with either the delivery of bile salts into the bile ducts or the flow of bile through the bile ducts will obviously result in diminished bile salts in the intestine, and fat malabsorption is produced. Accumulation of bile in the bloodstream produces pruritus, and accumulation of bile salts in the liver cell may possibly produce injury. The entire group of such processes is discussed below under cholestasis.

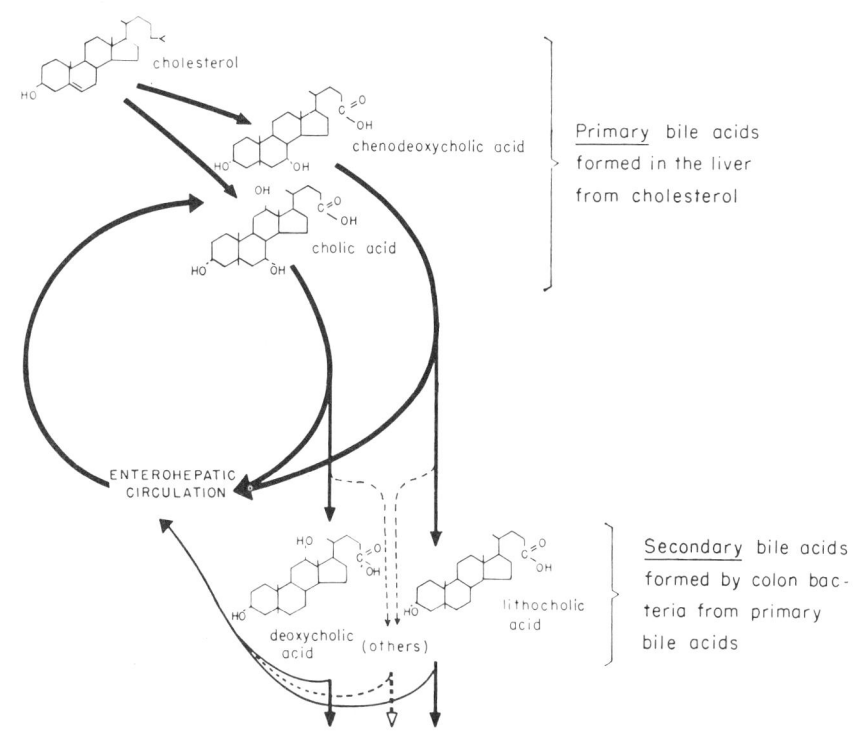

Figure 28-3 Formation of primary and secondary bile acids from cholesterol. (Reproduced from Carey, J.: In Schiff, L. (Ed.): Diseases of the Liver. 3rd ed., Philadelphia, J. B. Lippincott Co., 1969.)

Since the liver manufactures bile acids and salts, abnormalities due to liver cell disease might be anticipated. The most prominent abnormality seems to be a decrease in cholic acid and a relative increase in deoxycholic acid and chenodeoxycholic acid. The reasons for this shift are obscure, but it has been observed in a wide variety of different forms of hepatocellular disease.

Although conjugation of bile acids is mildly impaired in disease, it seems less important than the increased production of dihydroxy acids.

Cholestasis

Clinically, bilirubin and bile salts are the two most prominent components of bile. Whenever there is evidence that adequate amounts of *both* of these substances have failed to reach the intestinal tract and have accumulated in the blood, the condition is designated cholestasis. This concept is useful, since there are marked similarities in patients with jaundice from the extreme of disease of the anion pump to mechanical obstruction at the level of the ampulla of Vater (Fig. 28-4).

Cholestasis is ordinarily diagnosed with evidence from three different sources (Table 28-9). Lack of bilirubin and bile salts in the stool produces steatorrhea, vitamin K deficiency and its prolongation of the prothrombin time, light stools, and lack of urobilinogen in the urine. Accumulation of bilirubin and bile salts in the blood produces pruritus and jaundice. If the cholestasis is severe and prolonged for months, the blood cholesterol and phospholipid levels will rise markedly. The cholesterol may deposit in the skin as xanthomas. The high cholesterol is caused by increased rate of hepatic and intestinal manufacture. Bile salts reaching the gut normally repress hepatic and intestinal synthesis of cholesterol. Finally, in cholestasis some evidence of stimulation or injury to the hepatic and biliary epithelial cells is present. This is demonstrated most prominently by marked elevation of the enzyme, alkaline phosphatase; and by a marked induction of hepatic production. The result of bile salt injury of liver cell membranes is a modest elevation of serum transaminase. Injury and mild inflammation are also apparent on liver biopsy. This takes the form of distorted bile canaliculi, bile lakes (lysed cells due to bile accumulation), and occasional inflammatory cells.

In practice, cholestasis is diagnosed when there is jaundice, elevation of the serum alkaline phosphatase, and little or no evidence of major hepatocellular damage. If the stools are light (owing to both increased fat content and reduced pigment) and there is no urine urobilinogen, the syndrome is even more firmly established.

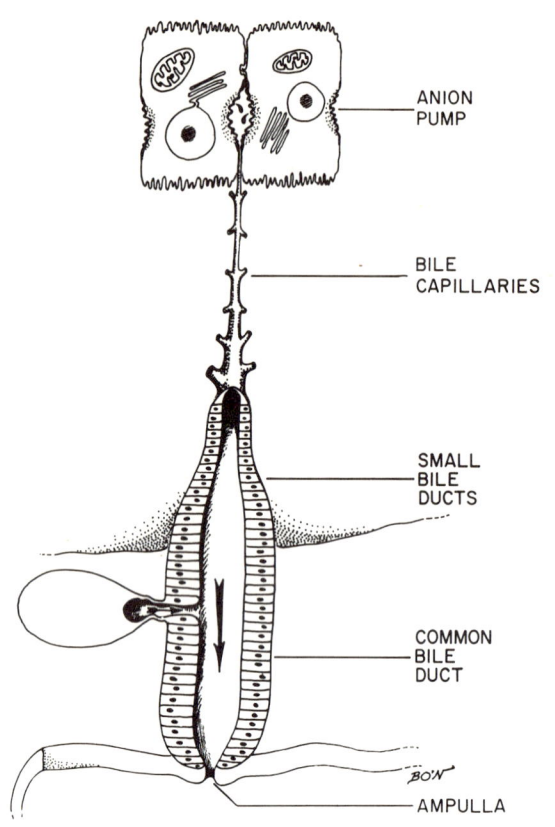

Figure 28–4 Various levels of abnormality producing cholestasis. Changes within the liver cells and the smallest bile capillaries produce similar clinical presentations. Bile ducts 1 mm. in diameter and larger are capable of secretion and absorption and dilate markedly with distal obstruction. Blockage of the drainage at any level produces cholestasis.

The practical problem of cholestasis is to determine at what level from the liver cell to the ampulla the block has occurred (Fig. 28–4). Studies of bile salt and bilirubin metabolism are usually not helpful in this determination. From the level of the bifurcation of the hepatic ducts distally, surgical removal or bypass of the lesion producing cholestasis is indicated; at higher levels, surgical intervention is not practical and often exaggerates the underlying condition.

Two little-known factors about the common causes of cholestasis often permit one to suspect correctly the proper cause: (1) bile ducts larger than 1 mm. in diameter are capable of tremendous dilatation with the secretory pressure of the liver and (2) cholestasis at the level of the anion pump or the bile capillaries rarely is complete for more than a few days. Each factor is useful in several ways. If cholestasis is caused by a surgical lesion, dilatation of the many ducts and moderate to marked enlargement of the liver must be present. If a patient with cholestasis has a normal-sized liver, a surgical lesion is very unlikely. The most common cause of surgical cholestasis is a gallstone impacted in the common bile duct. This most often lodges in the narrowest and least distensible portion of the common bile duct, which is the portion of the duct traversing the wall of the duodenum (Fig. 28–5). Dilatation proximal to such an obstruction will usually produce a 2- to 4-cm. turgid tube passing beneath the duodenal bulb (Fig. 28–6). A standard barium meal will usually reveal this garden-hose-like mass, producing a silhouette as it passes posteriorly. Such a mass clearly indicates a distended common bile duct. Occasionally the ducts in the hilum are sufficiently enlarged to produce a defect on colloid scan of the liver; this defect may disappear on rose bengal scan. Sometimes the turgid distended gallbladder is clearly and diagnostically palpable, indicating this problem. Visualization of the ducts by direct or radiologic means (direct laparotomy or peritoneoscopy, transhepatic or direct cholangiography) should indicate substantial dilatation beyond the normal 8 to 10 mm. in diameter.

The lack of complete obstruction in medical cholestasis is best appreciated by serial observations over several days. If small amounts of pigment appear in the stools or urobilinogen in the urine, incomplete obstruction is present. An anion excreted by the liver into the bile—radioactive rose bengal—may be used both for scans and for demonstrating the patency of the common bile duct. A trace of rose bengal given intravenously is completely taken up by the normal liver in 30 to 60 minutes and completely excreted into the

TABLE 28–9 FINDINGS SOMETIMES PRESENT IN CHOLESTASIS

Clinical	Laboratory
Due to Accumulation in Blood	
Jaundice	Elevated bilirubin
Itching	Elevated bile salts
Due to Lack in Intestine	
Bulky, loose stools	Increased stool fat and weight
Ecchymoses	Prolonged prothrombin time
White or light stools	No bile pigment, no urobilinogen
	Decreased urine urobilinogen
Xanthoma	Elevated serum cholesterol (after prolonged cholestasis)
Injurious Effects on Liver	
Mild hepatomegaly	Elevated serum alkaline phosphatase
	Elevated SGOT, SGPT
	Liver biopsy changes

NORMAL AND PATHOLOGIC PHYSIOLOGY OF THE LIVER

Figure 28–5 Anatomic course of the common bile duct. Note the course posterior to the duodenum and passage through the substance of the head of the pancreas. The common bile duct traverses the wall of the duodenum obliquely for a portion. This is the least dilatable portion of the duct and the site of most mobile obstructions. The gallbladder usually presses on the duodenal bulb. The close anatomic proximity of the pylorus, duodenum, gallbladder, pancreas, and common bile duct emphasizes the possibility of similarity of symptoms.

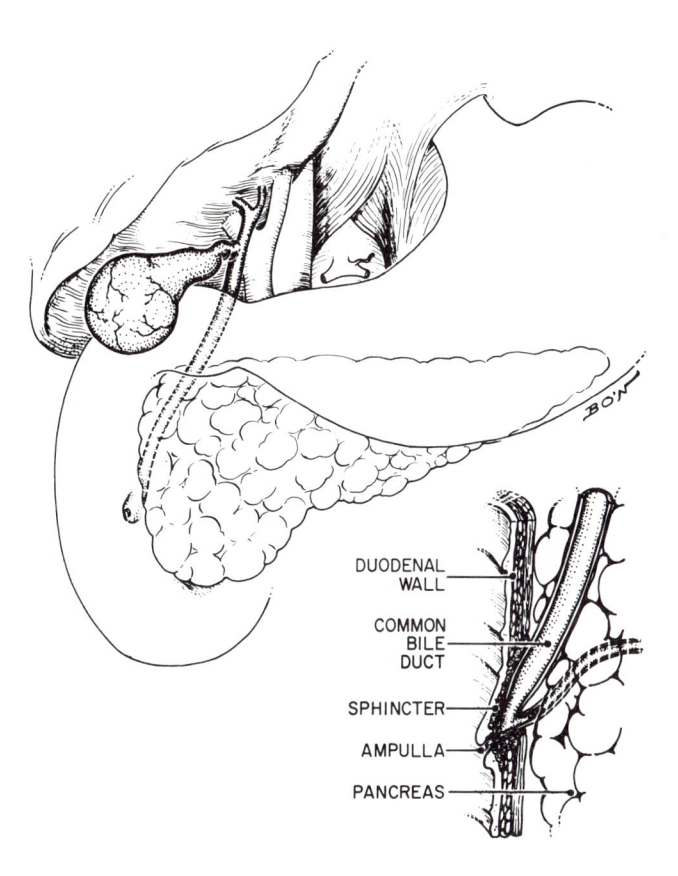

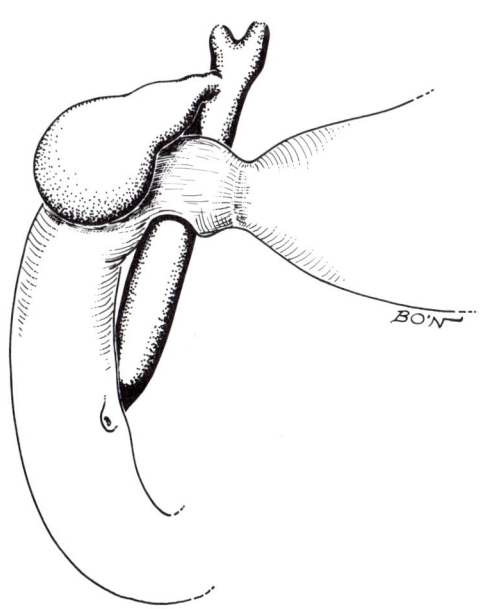

Figure 28–6 Detail of a common duct obstructed in the wall of the duodenum in the area of the ampulla. Note the marked dilatation of the common duct compared to Figure 28–5 and the filling defect produced in the duodenal area by the turgid dilated duct.

bile within 2 hours. In cholestasis, the uptake by the liver is normal but the subsequent excretion is retarded. However, in surgical cholestasis the obstruction is usually complete, so that scans done 1 hour and 24 hours after a single dose of radioactive rose bengal are essentially identical; in contrast, in the less complete intrahepatic cholestasis the scan at 24 hours is decreased in intensity usually by 50 per cent or more and often all the dye has passed into the gut.

In difficult cases it may be necessary to conduct an exploratory laparotomy to determine the correct diagnosis. If the diagnosis is not immediately apparent upon entering the peritoneal cavity, a radiologic demonstration of the ducts by injection of radiocontrast media via the gallbladder is necessary. If this does not indicate the cause, a liver biopsy should be taken and the abdomen closed. Occasionally, liver biopsy or transhepatic cholangiography is undertaken to clarify cases that are not explored. The liver biopsy is done to confirm hepatocellular or bile capillary causes; it is risky and less often of value in surgical problems. In transhepatic cholangiography a needle is passed blindly into the liver parenchyma toward the hilum. A bile duct is located either by aspirating to find bile or by injecting radiocontrast medium under fluoroscopy. Bile is then evacuated and replaced by radiocontrast media to obtain x-ray pictures of the bile ducts. This is most likely to demonstrate only abnormal bile ducts and is used when surgical problems are most likely.

The safer demonstration of the bile ducts by introduction of radiocontrast dye via duodenoscopy is now widely available.

HEPATIC BLOOD FLOW AND PORTAL HYPERTENSION

Blood Flow Through the Liver

All portal venous blood and all hepatic arterial blood combine into a single capillary bed that drains from the liver via the hepatic veins. The total blood flow in the liver is the same as the hepatic venous blood flow or the sum of the hepatic arterial and portal venous flow. About 20 per cent (or 1 to 2 liters per min.) of the resting cardiac output reaches the liver, one third via the hepatic artery and two thirds via the portal vein. The portal venous flow varies markedly during the day because the arterial flow to the stomach and intestines varies. Stimulation of gastric or pancreatic secretion enhances both arterial flow and venous drainage. Similarly, food in the intestine stimulates motility and blood flow. Inflammation of these organs or of the spleen also increases blood flow.

The hepatic artery seems more responsive to the needs of the liver. Hepatic anoxia lowers intrahepatic resistance and increases arterial flow. Hepatic inflammation also increases hepatic arterial flow. The hepatic, splenic, and superior mesenteric arteries are similarly responsive to many regulatory agents. Bradykinin, low doses of epinephrine and some prostaglandins are arterial vasodilators, whereas serotonin, pitressin, high doses of epinephrine, noradrenaline, and other prostaglandins diminish arterial flow.

Both the portal and hepatic arterial supply come together in the sinusoids. These are highly permeable capillaries which surround three to six surfaces of each liver cell. The blood comes into sufficient contact with the reticuloendothelial cells (Kupffer cells) and liver cells to assure that more than 99 per cent of substances taken up by either cell will be removed in a single passage through the liver. In the resting state, blood actively flows in only about one fifth of the sinusoids. The remaining four fifths are temporarily static but the actual flow into the sinusoids can change from moment to moment. A higher proportion of the total number of sinusoids is conducting blood when the total liver blood flow increases. The liver resistance changes with flow, so that a doubling of portal venous flow is associated with only a slight rise of pressure in the portal vein.

Liver blood flow may be measured in man by three methods (Table 28–10). The dyes sulfobromophthalein (BSP) and indocyanine green (ICG) are almost entirely removed by the liver. If either is infused at a constant rate for 30 to 45 minutes,

TABLE 28–10 METHODS TO MEASURE PORTAL PRESSURE AND LIVER BLOOD FLOW AND TO ASSESS LIVER COLLATERAL FLOW

---

1. Liver Blood Flow
   a. Sulfobromophthalein or indocyanine green constant infusion with samples from hepatic venous catheter.*
   b. Radioactive colloid injection intravenously and determine the rate of removal from peripheral blood.
   c. Infuse substance into hepatic artery and sample at hepatic vein. Calculate dilution.*
2. Portal Pressure Measurement
   a. Catheterize the occluded umbilical vein.*
   b. Splenic pulp manometry.*
   c. Wedged hepatic venous pressure.*
3. Collateral Veins
   a. All methods in part 2.
   b. Venography phase of splenic and superior mesenteric artery injection.*
   c. Esophageal varices:
     (1) Esophagoscopy
     (2) Barium swallow

---

*Skilled operator required.

the blood level rises and increases until the liver removal rate can keep up with the rate of infusion. At this time, simultaneous samples of mixed hepatic venous blood and peripheral arterial blood are obtained by appropriately placed catheters. The arterial level of dye represents that entering both the hepatic artery and the portal vein, and the hepatic venous level represents the concentration after some dye removal from the liver. The difference represents the amount of dye removed from each ml. of blood perfusing the liver. Since the rate of infusion and the rate of hepatic removal are the same, the infusion rate for the dye may be utilized to determine the liver blood flow.

The reticuloendothelial system of the liver specifically removes particles within a narrow range of size; the RE system of other organs will not remove such particles. If a trace dose of such particles is injected intravenously, the removal rate is a function of how much of the cardiac output is actually reaching the liver. Isotopic techniques have been so defined that an estimate of liver flow may be made from external counting.

A precise third method of determining liver flow, particularly applicable when shunts are present and liver cell function is diminished, is available by constant infusion of labeled albumin into the hepatic artery and constant sampling via the hepatic vein through appropriately positioned catheters. The dilution of the infused albumin reveals the total hepatic blood flow.

In practice, liver blood flow is of limited value in either diagnosis or understanding hepatic disorders. All forms of stable chronic liver disease seem to alter blood flow when need for oxygen is present. Any form of splenic disease and most forms of pancreatic, small intestinal, gastric, and colonic inflammatory disease are associated with enhanced portal blood flow. Inflammatory liver diseases increase liver flow but diseases associated with loss of total numbers of available liver cells are associated with diminished flow.

Portal Pressure

The pressure measured in the portal vein, or its feeding veins, fluctuates not only with each respiration but also with intra-abdominal pressure and modestly increases following each meal. Knowledge of the pressure at only one point in time may be misleading or unrepresentative; one desires to know whether the pressure is persistently above normal levels.

The pressure may be persistently elevated because of an obstruction in the portal vein or in any of the branches (up to the level of the right auricle). In the presence of a totally normal liver increased liver blood flow usually will not result in an elevated pressure. Minor abnormalities of the liver, however, along with an increased portal blood flow, may be responsible for some forms of portal hypertension.

Measurement of portal pressure is complex and requires a highly skilled physician and complex apparatus (Table 28-10). One accurate procedure is to dissect out the occluded umbilical vein in the umbilicus under local anesthetic and pass a catheter into the portal vein for direct measurement. Less directly, a needle may be passed into the pulp of the spleen and the pressure in the splenic sinusoids will indicate a close approximation of the portal pressure. Still more indirect, but of somewhat unique value, is the pressure recorded when a straight catheter is passed retrograde into a hepatic vein until it occludes the lumen. The pressure in the occluded vein will rise until blood is forced through available collateral channels proximal to this blockage; these are at the level of hepatic sinusoids. If such a recorded pressure is normal, this indicates that the resistance to flow from sinusoids is normal. In some diseases the pressure recorded in this manner is much elevated, indicating an increased resistance to the escape of blood from the sinusoids. This pressure, called the wedged hepatic venous pressure, is a measurement of postsinusoid resistance. Table 28-10 lists the available methods of measuring portal pressure.

The detailed evaluation of portal pressure requires the measurement of pressure in the portal vein or one of its branches. If it is elevated, the site of increased resistance must be determined. Wedged hepatic venous pressure may be measured to determine whether the elevation arises between that point and the heart or on the portal vein side of the sinusoid. Peripheral venous pressure may sometimes indicate a cardiac or peripheral localization of the resistance producing portal hypertension. Table 28-11 indicates some forms of portal pressure elevation and the anatomic localization of the increased resistance. Figure 28-7 emphasizes these anatomic locations.

Consequences of Portal Hypertension. There are many abnormalities that result from portal hypertension regardless of the basic cause. The severity and duration of portal hypertension seem more important determinants than the exact level of obstruction. The level of obstruction is of greatest importance in the mode of treatment and prognosis. The sequelae of portal hypertension are conveniently divided into three groups—splanchnic sequestration of blood, high pressure and development of collaterals, and congestion. These are listed for convenience in Table 28-12 and detailed below.

It is apparent that the portal pressure rises in order to permit blood to leave the splanchnic bed (all blood vessels which normally drain into the portal system). If for any reason there is an increased entry of blood into the portal system

TABLE 28-11 CAUSES OF PORTAL PRESSURE ELEVATION AND ANATOMIC LOCATION

Disease	Frequency	Anatomic Level of Block	Comment
Extrahepatic portal vein occlusion	Infrequent	Portal vein	
Schistosomiasis	Common	Tiny portal veins	Endemic areas
Cancer nodules			
Extramedullary hematopoiesis			
Fat, lipid, amyloid accumulation	Common	Sinusoids	
Hypertrophy of endoplasmic reticulum			
As above plus increased portal blood flow due to splenomegaly or inflammation	Rare	Sinusoids	
Cirrhosis	Common	Postsinusoid	
Budd-Chiari syndrome			
Veno-occlusive disease	Rare	Hepatic veins	
Inferior vena cava			
Constrictive pericarditis			
Heart failure	Common	Right auricle	

(such as following a meal or any temporary boost in the cardiac output), this blood cannot promptly return to the heart. It must pool in the splanchnic bed to raise the pressure slightly and then the return flow to the heart will increase. This increase in portal volume and pressure occurs concomitantly with a diminution in the blood volume available to the remainder of the body. As a result, the renal mechanisms to increase blood volume become operative and a portion of the sodium retention is a direct result of this maldistribution of the blood volume. Because of this, every patient with portal hypertension develops an increased blood volume compared to normal. The increase is entirely sequestered behind the obstructed portal circulation. No matter how

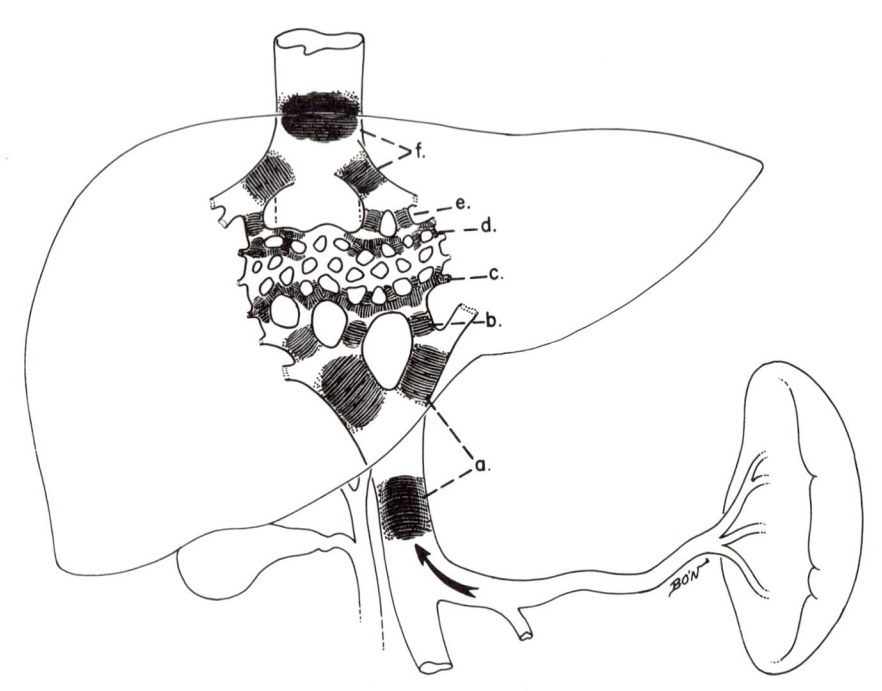

Figure 28-7 Schematic representation of the levels of obstruction of the portal vein producing portal hypertension. (*a*) Blockage of the extrahepatic or large intrahepatic branches of the portal vein. (*b*) Blockage of the tiny portal veins, such as is found in noncirrhotic portal hypertension of India. (*c*) Blockage immediately presinusoidal, as produced by embolism and granuloma with schistosomiasis. (*d*) Postsinusoidal block common in alcoholic cirrhosis. (*e*) Block as in veno-occlusive disease. (*f*) Hepatic vein, subhepatic vein, and inferior vena cava blockage.

TABLE 28–12 SEQUELAE OF PORTAL HYPERTENSION

1. Splanchnic Sequestration
   a. Increases portal pressure after meal.
   b. Diminishes nonsplanchnic blood volume.
   c. Enhances renal retention of sodium.
   d. Increases overall plasma volume.
   e. Impairs vascular homeostasis in bleeding.
2. High Portal Pressure
   a. Promotes development of collaterals—esophageal varices common.
   b. Promotes hemorrhage from varices.
   c. Promotes flow of blood through collaterals—shunting of portal blood promotes liver coma.
3. Congestion of Viscera
   a. Splenomegaly—hypersplenism.
   b. Impaired intestinal and stomach function.
   c. Thrombosis of spleen and mesenteric veins.
   d. Enhanced liver and mesenteric lymph formation—ascites.

large the volume, each time more blood enters the splanchnic circulation there is a temporary maladjustment. Should hemorrhage occur, this portion of the blood volume is only slowly available to the heart because of the high resistance before entering the systemic circulation.

The elevated pressure, over weeks or months, promotes formation of collaterals to permit blood to return to the heart through other channels. Rarely, if ever, do these collateral channels restore the pressure to normal. Collaterals prevent pressure from reaching levels that would rupture vessels but are constantly associated with marked elevation as compared to normal. Wherever the inferior vena cava and portal vessels have a common distribution, significant anastomoses may occur. The more important clinical areas are (a) directly from the portal vein along the stomach, up the esophagus, and anastomosing with the intercostal veins; (b) the area of the spleen between the diaphragm and the posterior abdominal wall; (c) along the umbilical vein or the mesentery through adhesions with the anterior abdominal wall; (d) posterior from branches in the area of the pancreas to the lumbar veins; and (e) around the rectum in the area of the hemorrhoidal vessels. These various collateral channels may be seen by various techniques. Sometimes they are visually prominent (abdominal, periumbilical, hemorrhoidal areas) or loud bruits (over the umbilicus) are detectable. They often produce large protrusions into the esophagus (opacified by a barium sulfate swallow) or similarly into the stomach. They are sometimes seen in the esophagus (esophagoscopy) or in the peritoneum (peritoneoscopy) and may also be demonstrated radiographically by the injection of a radiocontrast medium into the portal vein or its branches. The same techniques may be used to measure portal pressure directly, or large quantities of radiopaque media may be injected into the splanchnic arteries and thus opacify the portal veins and its branches (see Table 28–10).

Finally, the presence of collateral channels may sometimes be suspected when divergence of large amounts of materials normally limited to the portal circulation appear in the systemic circulation. Extremely high levels of glucose (postprandially), extremely high levels of ammonia, and extremely high levels of urinary urobilinogen may be produced by large quantities of portal blood bypassing the liver and directly reaching the systemic circulation. The role of ammonia in liver coma is discussed in a later section.

Enlarged submucosal veins of the esophagus, known as esophageal varices, serve as collateral vessels between the portal venous system and the inferior and superior venae cavae. These vessels are tortuous and distended up to 8 mm. in diameter. The submucosa of the esophagus has little or no supportive-connective tissue. Esophageal varices are produced when portal pressure of more than 20 mm. Hg above right heart pressure persists for months. At pressures above 35 mm., they tend to rupture and bleed profusely. Bleeding almost always occurs in the vicinity of the transition from intra-abdominal pressure to intrathoracic and is mainly caused by a temporary elevation in portal pressure. Surface irritation in the esophagus occasionally plays a role. Once bleeding begins, it is kept active by the sustained pressure, and the consequences of such hemorrhage are serious in that at least one sixth of such episodes produce death. Significant bleeding from other collateral beds in portal hypertension is infrequent. The surgical construction of a large low-resistance communication between the portal bed and the vena cava (portacaval shunt) will eliminate portal hypertension. Shunting, if adequate, is effective in removing the hazard of variceal bleeding and may facilitate disappearance of varices.

Techniques for demonstrating collateral vessels and particularly esophageal varices are indicated in Table 28–10. Congestion of viscera is prominent in portal hypertension and occurs more frequently when the inflow to the splanchnic bed increases. In a few months' time this leads to prominent splenomegaly. Over many months, it is rare for a patient with portal hypertension not to have an enlarged spleen, usually apparent on palpation but invariably demonstrated by scanning. Infarction, a common occurrence in portal hypertension, may develop owing to an enlarged, congested spleen and the slow turnover of blood. The congested sinusoids of the spleen and the prolonged contact of the active RE cells of the spleen with the formed elements of the blood (platelets, erythrocytes, leukocytes) may injure and destroy some or all three of these. The loss of any of these formed elements due to enlarged spleen is sometimes called hypersplenism. This is most apparent in the lowering of the peripheral counts. Platelets are often lowered from a normal of 250,000 to half that level or less; leukocytes are lowered to less than 4,000, mostly owing to loss of polymorphonuclear leukocytes. Lowering of the red blood cells is less frequent. Despite the frequent occurrence of these lowered levels, this is rarely of clinical consequence in producing bleeding (due to platelet lack), increased infection (due to leukocyte lack), or symptoms of anemia. The lowering is reversed invariably by splenectomy and often is removed by a portacaval shunt to correct the congestion.

Congestion of the mesenteric vessels may lead to mesenteric infarction. Small thromboses of the mesenteric veins seem frequent in portal hypertension. They produce altered motility of the small intestine and occasionally damage the wall, producing peritonitis and septicemia, but they are difficult to recognize unless they are major. Whenever there are abrupt changes in congestion, intestinal function and motility may be temporarily impaired and edema of the gut and impaired absorption may result. This congestion is one of the factors contributing to ascites, which is discussed in a later section.

Lymph Flow. The hepatic sinusoid is possibly the most permeable capillary in the body; it is estimated that normally 0.3 per cent of the blood flow through the liver passes through the walls of the sinusoid and appears as liver lymph (compared to approximately 0.01 per cent for muscle). This lymph mainly follows the bile channels in lymphatic vessels, exits from the liver in the porta hepatis, and joins the cisterna chyli along with the mesenteric and large leg lymphatics. Any process which increases sinusoidal pressure (such as cirrhosis) may markedly increase liver lymph formation. In patients with cirrhosis this increased lymph may exude from the surface of the liver and flow into the peritoneal cavity as ascites. This happens only when the rate of production exceeds the ability of the lymphatics to convey it back into the circulation. Protein elevation in lymph content reflects protein production by the liver (above 3.0 mg. per 100 ml.). Any interruption of hepatic lymphatics, such as may occur in biliary tract surgery or during surgery on the portal veins, may lead to large lymph fistulas into the peritoneal cavity.

In a similar fashion, any form of portal hypertension will increase the forces forming intestinal lymph in all parts of the bowel. If the increase is only slight, the lymphatics can convey it at about the same rate that it is formed. If the formation is acute or extremely rapid, it will produce edema of the cells of the bowel and may cross into the peritoneum and appear as ascites. Intestinal lymph is lower in protein content but may contain large amounts of lipid (chyle), particularly after fatty meals. Chylous ascites may result in patients with portal hypertension, though it is more frequent in patients with blockage of the lymphatics from obstruction. It has been observed that in all forms of portal hypertension the flow of lymph in the thoracic duct is markedly increased from 3 to 60 times the normal level.

Portacaval Shunts. A surgical collateral between the portal vein and the inferior vena cava may be constructed to lower portal pressure. Figure 28–8 indicates the forms that are frequently used. If properly constructed, all the pressure, congestion, and adverse effects disappear (Table 28–12), but the amount of portal blood shunted to the systemic circulation increases markedly.

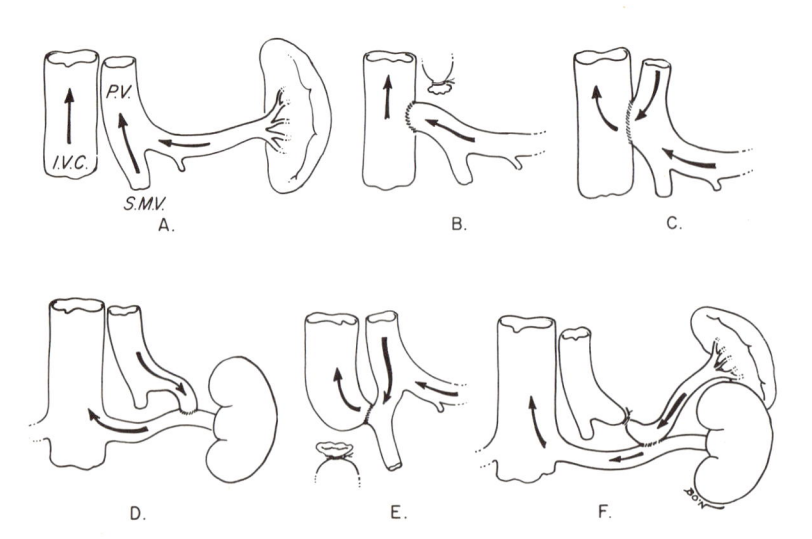

Figure 28–8 Types of portal systemic shunts constructed surgically. *A*, Normal. I.V.C., inferior vena cava; P.V., portal vein; S.M.V., superior mesenteric vein. *B*, End-to-side portacaval shunt—the portal vein is transected and the intestinal side anastomosed to I.V.C. *C*, Side-to-side portacaval shunt. *D*, Splenorenal shunt—usually the spleen is resected. *E*, Mesocaval shunt. The I.V.C. is transected and the proximal portion anastomosed to the S.M.V. Reverse splenorenal shunt, used to preserve S.M.V. blood flow to liver, but decompress varices by permitting splenic venous flow and the variceal collaterals to drain through the renal circulation.

Shunts are most widely used to prevent subsequent hemorrhage from esophageal varices in patients in whom this has occurred at least once. Shunts produce some additional morbidity largely from the increased shunting of blood to the systemic circulation (liver encephalopathy), and this has led to a modification of procedures. These modified procedures have the advantage of preventing bleeding without producing such a total shunt of intestinal blood.

LIVER FUNCTION TESTS

A wide variety of tests assess aspects of the liver. Those tests listed in Tables 28-1, 28-3, 28-6, and 28-10 are liver function tests. Usually one restricts the term "liver function test" to those blood and urine tests indicated in Table 28-13. The meaning and method of performance of each of these will now be discussed. Of the several thousand known biochemical functions of the liver only a few are abnormal during the early stages of liver disease. Some tests have been abandoned because they are abnormal too frequently, others because the patient must be close to death before an abnormality appears.

Liver Biopsy

A special needle is inserted into the liver and a core of tissue 1 to 2 mm. in diameter is removed for histologic or other examination. Continued hemorrhage accounts for some mortality (1 per 10,000) during this procedure. The cellular injury and nature of inflammatory response are revealed in all diffuse processes. If there is diffuse cancer, metabolic storage disease, or infection, it will be seen. Focal conditions such as tumor metastases or diseases affecting only some of the hepatic lobules (such as congenital fibrosis or biliary cirrhosis) are often missed completely. A biopsy examination is the most definite of the commonly employed procedures and is used in almost every patient with liver disease in whom the diagnosis is unknown or the prognosis uncertain. Even in liver clinics 10 to 20 per cent of biopsies performed reveal a major unsuspected diagnosis.

Tests of Cellular Necrosis

Intact hepatocytes contain a number of substances in the cystosol in concentrations much higher than in the circulating blood. These substances may be released into the serum following damage to the cell wall. Persistence of each abnormal substance is determined by a balance between its rate of release and its duration of survival in the bloodstream. Serum glutamic pyruvic transaminase is the most specific and widely used measure of hepatocellular necrosis. In a person in good nutritional state, with good stores of intracellular enzyme, damage to as little as 1 per cent of the liver cells will raise the serum level. Serum glutamic oxaloacetic acid transaminase acts similarly but is less specific for all forms of striate muscle containing this material. Serum iron and vitamin B_{12} behave similarly but remain elevated longer than the transaminase.

In severe necrosis, amino acids are released from the liver cells and appear in high concentration in the blood; the more insoluble ones (tyrosine and cysteine) appear in the urine as crystals.

The cephalin-cholesterol flocculation test, now rapidly disappearing because of the delay of 48 hours for its final reading, is a sensitive test for liver necrosis. Suspensions of cephalin and cholesterol are stabilized by normal serum but sera containing minute quantities of protein released from necrotic liver cells will produce flocculation. A positive test indicates acute liver necrosis. High gammaglobulin levels also produce flocculation. Thymol turbidity, Takata-Ara flocculation, colloidal gold flocculation, and Weltmann tests are all similar to the cephalin-cholesterol flocculation test.

The liver biopsy may reveal damaged cells with pyknotic nuclei or feathery degeneration, but more commonly it reveals inflammatory cells surrounding the place where the cell was or distorted

TABLE 28-13 TESTS OF LIVER CELL DAMAGE

A. Cell Necrosis
 1. SGOT
 2. SGPT
 3. Cephalin cholesterol flocculation
 4. Bilirubinuria
 5. Biopsy[r*]
 6. Serum Fe
 7. Serum B_{12}
 8. Amino acidemia and aciduria
 9. Increased undetermined anion
B. Too Few Functioning Liver Cells
 1. Bilirubin
 2. Sulfobromophthalein, indocyanine green
 3. Albumin
 4. Prothrombin
 5. Fibrinogen
 6. Urine urobilinogen
C. Inflammation
 1. α, γ immunoglobulin
D. Specific Etiology
 1. Hepatitis-associated antigen
 2. Antimitochondrial antibody
 3. Amebae, hydatid complement fixation
 4. Eaton Barr agent antibody
E. Intrahepatic or Extrahepatic Shunts
 1. Ammonia

*r Increased risk.

liver cords due to loss of many cells or rapid regeneration, indicating their replacement. Very active necrosis may leave cellular debris in the form of eosinophilic or hyaline bodies (Mallory body, Councilman body).

Tests of Insufficient Functioning Liver Cells

It is apparent from partial hepatic ablation studies in animals and in man needing major liver surgery that most of these liver tests are normal until about half the liver is gone. At this level the BSP test (sulfobromophthalein test) or the indocyanine green test becomes abnormal. Alterations of liver blood flow alter this transport only if the normal flow is reduced by more than 50 per cent.

When 60 per cent or more of the liver cells are not functioning, jaundice occurs. If the pigment load is enhanced for any reason (hemolysis or transfusion), lesser amounts of liver damage are needed. The principal cause of jaundice is impairment at the level of the anion pump. Conjugation is usually adequate.

The liver makes many proteins that are released into the bloodstream and can serve as liver function tests; albumin and prothrombin are the most useful. If the liver ceased to function totally, the albumin level on the third day would be reduced only about 10 per cent but the prothrombin level would be about 5 per cent of normal. Prothrombin (half-time 12 hours) and fibrinogen (half-time 4 days) reflect acute liver damage more readily than does albumin, with its 30-day half-life. Prothrombin requires adequate amounts of vitamin K as a cofactor in its hepatic synthesis; vitamin K malabsorption is common in cholestasis. Any patient with a prolonged prothrombin time should have the level checked again 12 hours after administration of 5 mg. of parenteral vitamin K. A marked change in the circulating level is seen if the cause is malabsorption.

Tests of Inflammation

The globulin level is the most widely used test of inflammatory response and antibody formation. This is prominently elevated in any form of liver disease infiltrated with round cells. This is usually gamma globulin on electrophoresis.

Tests of Specific Etiology

Hepatitis-Associated Antigen. A portion of the long-incubation hepatitis virus may be detected with sensitive antisera. This is called the hepatitis-associated antigen, sometimes called Australia antigen, and seems diagnostically specific. It appears in the serum of 90 per cent or more of all patients weeks or months before the onset of active disease. At the time of hepatocellular manifestations it is present in about 60 per cent of such patients and persists for about 15 additional days and then disappears. It persists in the serum of about 20 per cent of the patients with chronic hepatitis and is present in 60 per cent or more of patients who have received transfusions transmitting viral hepatitis. Antibody to HAA indicates postinfection and is less clearly associated with existing disease.

Antimitochondrial Antibody. Antibody to mitochrondria of a variety of species (rat or guinea pig liver mitochrondria are commonly used) seems a feature of primary biliary cirrhosis. This test is of great value if the techniques are sensitive and the limit of normal is set sufficiently high to exclude many common inflammatory diseases. There is no clear understanding of its meaning.

Fetoglobulin, Placental Alkaline Phosphatase, and Carcinoembryonic Antigen. These three substances, produced by carcinoma in the adult, seem a part of the development of embryonic cells but are lost by normal adult tissues. Fetoglobulin found in an adult nearly always indicates liver carcinoma; placental alkaline phosphatase in a person without a placenta indicates a carcinoma of entodermal origin; colon and pancreatic carcinomas seem responsible for production of the carcinoembryonic antigen. Sensitive complement fixation tests for etiologic agents are useful in detecting amebiasis, hydatid disease, and certain fungus disorders.

APPROACH TO THE PROBLEM OF CLINICAL LIVER DISEASE

Liver disease may start predominantly as a focal process; such processes use the rich blood supply of the liver but interfere little with the hepatocyte function. In contrast, liver disease may indicate diffuse involvement of the hepatocytes. These two types of initial disease are quite distinct in typical cases but may completely overlap as they advance. There is some value in having a clear understanding of each.

Focal Liver Disease and Its Typical Syndromes

Two prototypes of focal liver disease must be considered. One is a single abscess or metastasis within the liver that progressively grows but, even when massive, interferes but slightly with overall liver function. The other consists of myriad small foci (such as miliary tuberculosis or extramedullary hematopoiesis) which similarly may grow without affecting liver function.

Systemic symptoms are a function of the basic

pathologic condition invading the liver but are important to keep in mind. Abscesses, specific infectious agents (amebae, hydatid, tuberculosis), and cancer with necrosis may produce impressive systemic signs of fever and weight loss; however, these signs may not reveal themselves in the history, physical examination, or laboratory screening to indicate that the liver is the host to the problem. This is particularly true in the diseases mentioned and in some cases of lymphoma.

Modest hepatomegaly is most readily detected by scanning. Uniform distribution of an increased mass of 20 per cent throughout the liver would result in an average increase in each dimension of 1 cm. and this amount cannot be detected upon ordinary physical examination. If the increase is not uniformly distributed or produces symptoms (fullness in the abdomen, pulling on the side), hepatomegaly might well be found. Tight clothing in women often brings about the finding of abdominal masses, and hepatomegaly is also found in this way. If the enlargement is rapid or if the underlying process is one that may hemorrhage into itself, pain may result.

Painful sensations in the liver seem to arise from end organs lying in the liver capsule and along the fibrous tissue following the portal veins and its branches. These sensations pass from the liver via the sympathetic nerves, through the celiac plexus, and on to the seventh through twelfth paravertebral ganglia. These nerve endings seem particularly sensitive to distention but are not affected by penetration, heat, or cold. Acute distention of the capsule, as produced by vascular or bile congestion or rapid infiltration of inflammation, produces exquisite pain and tenderness. Pain and tenderness will disappear after a few days of steady distention. Other innervated portions include the hepatic veins and bile ducts, which produce the sensation of pain when they are acutely distended or in spasm. The parietal peritoneum overlies much of the liver capsule and is particularly sensitive after inflammation or occurrence of fibrin deposits. Thus, focal processes may alter the capsule, vessels, or overlying peritoneum and produce pain and tenderness.

Slow-growing, usually benign tumors or infiltrations of the liver may remain indefinitely silent. Moderate infiltrations of fat, amyloid, Gaucher's lipid, or hamartomas may remain silent during life.

Generalized Liver Disease and Its Typical Syndromes (Table 28-14)

Jaundice. In liver cell disease, jaundice is due to either damage to the anion pump or cholestasis. Both produce jaundice that is more than half direct-reacting. If there is no increased production of bile pigments, the degree of jaundice is a general reflection of the severity of the disease, and the level of jaundice may increase as its course progresses. Stable jaundice of liver cell origin is usually an indication of increased destruction of liver cells exceeding their replacement rate. If there is no evidence of liver cell destruction, cholestasis is usually prominent, owing to the huge regenerative capacity of the liver.

Acute Liver Cell Failure. Destruction of about 90 per cent or more of liver cells within a few weeks or less results in a rapid, devastating, often fatal syndrome in which jaundice and confusion are nearly always present but often mild, and in which metabolic changes, hemorrhage, and cardiovascular collapse may be so prominent as to produce death. Many of the common manifestations of liver disease, such as jaundice, require time to occur while material accumulates in the blood; and the course, until death due to liver failure, may be so rapid that these manifestations do not occur prominently.

The totally failing liver is unable to clear amino acids or the citric acid cycle intermediates from the blood (lactate, pyruvate, alpha-ketoglutarate), and these materials are acidic. Prominent acidosis and a marked increase in the undetermined anion may be observed. The undetermined anion is the numerical difference between the sum of the sodium and potassium minus the sum of the chloride and bicarbonate. It is usually less than 16 mEq. per L. but may be as high as 60 mEq. per L. in acute liver failure.

The liver manufactures nearly all coagulation proteins and many of these are diminished in any form of liver disease. The one-stage prothrombin time measures a complex relationship of Factors I (fibrinogen), II (prothrombin), V, VII, and X, all of which are manufactured by the liver. Activated coagulation with further removal of clotting factors by consumption may occur in acute inflammatory liver disease, and this may result in prominent oozing into all tissues.

In animals it has been noted that when liver tissue is removed and permitted to autolyze under sterile conditions and is then reinjected, peripheral vasodilatation and increased cardiac output result. It is likely that the sudden release of destroyed liver tissue is responsible for many

TABLE 28-14 SYNDROMES OF GENERALIZED LIVER DISEASE

---

1. Jaundice, including cholestasis
2. Acute liver failure
3. Fluid retention
4. Portal hypertension
5. Confusion, including hepatic encephalopathy and hypoglycemia
6. Systemic wasting

---

cardiovascular changes. In addition, acute liver failure may have manifestations in all the other areas.

Fluid Retention. Any form of liver cell disease is associated with prominent fluid retention mediated via sodium retention by the kidney. Any experimental design leading to congestion within the liver results in profound sodium retention. It is possible that a portion of this is due to sequestration of an important proportion of the plasma volume behind the liver, but other factors may also be important. Sodium retention is mediated by the renin-angiotensin-aldosterone mechanisms, but after a few days a fundamental alteration in blood distribution occurs within the kidney and is probably hormonally mediated (third factor). The common pathway of sodium retention by the kidney is clearly understood. Most patients with liver cell failure have 6 to 30 lb. of increased extracellular fluid and will secrete increasing amounts of sodium and water as the liver disease improves.

This increased extracellular fluid will distribute itself in a variety of places. It will be manifest as edema or ascites, dependent upon local factors. If there is mostly erect posture or venous stasis of the legs, the fluid will be most visible in the legs. If there is portal hypertension, the venous pressure in either the hepatic or mesenteric bed must exceed that in the legs, and ascites results. Fluid retention usually corrects itself when the disease improves. If this is unlikely or complications are feared, it is appropriate to stimulate sodium excretion by the kidney.

The important relationship between plasma volume and portal pressure was discussed earlier. An ambulatory patient with fluid is often put to bed, the result being redistribution of leg fluid, increased portal pressure, and finally hemorrhage. Patients exhibiting increased fluid stores should be gently controlled before bed rest is enforced.

Portal hypertension has been discussed in an earlier section, including its major complications—hypersplenism and esophageal varices with hemorrhage—and its indirect complications—ascites and increased collateral circulation.

Confusion, Including Hepatic Encephalopathy and Hypoglycemia. Hypoglycemia occurs so frequently that it should be the first problem suspected when a patient with liver disease becomes confused. Hypoglycemia usually arises from impaired gluconeogenesis in (a) severe liver cell damage; (b) congestive heart failure; and (c) alcoholics, particularly after a prolonged fast.

Liver encephalopathy is an altered metabolic state of the central nervous system. It is brought about by the direct shunting of some material from the intestinal tract bypassing the liver to the brain. This material seems to be present in proteins in the intestinal tract and may be ammonia. Once encephalopathy is present, a variety of noxious materials seem to affect the central nervous system adversely in a similar manner. The signs and symptoms of liver encephalopathy are aggravated by ammonia, hypokalemia, anoxia, sedative drugs, and central nervous system depressants (such as morphine).

The shunting of intestinal blood through or around the liver cells seems more important in the production of liver coma than does the presence of damaged liver cells. This syndrome is known to occur in the presence of a normal liver cell mass.

In its mildest form there is a slight disturbance of thought processes and a disturbance of the diurnal sleep-awake rhythm, so that the patient is awake at night and dozes all day. At the next stage there is mental-motor dissociation, which shows far more impairment than is revealed by any routine neurologic testing. Thus, if the patient is asked to copy a simple line drawing or to write his name, it cannot be done, even though the patient tries. Still later, the "flapping tremor" or asterixis becomes apparent. This tremor is elicited by asking the patient to hold the arms and hands extended maximally against gravity and encouraging him to hold them perfectly still. Periodically, the sustained stimulus to hold them against gravity will be relaxed owing to a temporary block in the signal, and despite the will of the patient the hand will drop; the patient, in trying to comply, will quickly jerk the limb back into position, and a flapping effect is produced. Subsequently, stages are progressive loss of memory and then unconsciousness. Finally, deep coma may intervene and death occurs. The level of consciousness has been raised by treatments aimed at interrupting the supply of ammonia reaching the brain. This is achieved by discontinuing oral intake of all protein- and nitrogen-containing materials. The G.I. tract is purged to remove blood and other foodstuffs and to lessen the stasis that promotes accumulation of ammonia-forming bacteria. Nonabsorbed antibiotics, particularly neomycin, are highly effective in inhibiting the function of intestinal flora.

An alternative hypothesis on the cause of liver coma (and also the hepatorenal syndrome) is the false transmitter hypothesis. Biological amines, related structurally to noradrenaline, may accumulate in liver disease and make the usual neurotransmitter substance noradrenaline less effective owing to the accumulation of these false transmitters at the synapse. Such a problem could be overcome by providing the nerve cells with more precursor for noradrenaline synthesis such as dopa or dopamine. Animal and human data consistent with this hypothesis exist, but there is not yet sufficient proof to warrant widespread application in treatment.

REPRESENTATIVE HEPATIC DISEASES

Vascular Impairment

An example of vascular impairment is congestive heart failure due to myocardial disease. The liver has two vascular supplies and either is sufficient to maintain a fully functioning liver. However, when the venous drainage is blocked from the liver owing to either intrahepatic or extrahepatic disorders, it produces a profound derangement of liver function which is largely due to damage from anoxia. Initially, there is vascular stasis throughout the liver without death of liver cells, but all metabolic function of the liver is inefficient. The liver becomes enlarged owing to vascular congestion and may become very tender. Fluid retention, a result of sodium retention, usually is present. After several weeks, liver cells die with prominent transaminase elevation. Lack of liver cells is apparent from marked BSP retention, jaundice, hypoalbuminemia, and low prothrombin time. In order for blood to continue to flow through the liver, portal hypertension, splenomegaly, and in extreme cases even portal collateral circulation must develop.

Hepatitis

Viral hepatitis, alcoholic hepatitis, and allergic or idiosyncratic hepatitis (from drugs or other environmental agents) are the principal forms of hepatitis. Coincidental with the injury to liver cells are systemic symptoms such as fever, nausea and vomiting, and malaise. The exact cause of these symptoms is unclear. The liver soon becomes enlarged from edema of injury which is caused by the infiltration of inflammatory and regenerative cells (they are larger than the destroyed cells). Tenderness may be prominent at this stage. Jaundice, a cumulative phenomenon, becomes most marked usually after healing has started. Transaminase elevation is most prominent during the maximal injury phase.

Self-limited hepatitis from the preceding causes is usually not associated with either hyperglobulinemia or hypoalbuminemia. The majority of all forms of hepatitis completely heal and at a subsequent time the liver is completely normal. In cases of viral hepatitis among previously healthy young people, 85 per cent recover completely within 3 months and in total 95 per cent recover completely. In cases of alcoholic hepatitis, about 50 per cent later develop cirrhosis; in cases of viral hepatitis, about 3 per cent have cirrhosis and about 2 per cent have a chronically active (destructive) form of the disease that may persist for years or until death.

There are hepatotoxic substances in nature and medicine but the latter have usually been eliminated with the advent of safer agents. A hepatotoxic substance is an agent that, if given in a sufficient amount, will cause liver damage; the toxic pattern is readily reproduced in animals but not in all species. Idiosyncratic or allergic hepatitis is the most common and troublesome form of liver disease. It develops only in a small number of people, is not dose related, and cannot be predicted from animal testing. Nearly every drug and many environmental chemicals have produced this form of hepatitis. Some drugs, such as phenothiazine tranquilizers, isonicotinic acid hydrazide, and Fluothane, are very frequent causes.

Cirrhosis

The term cirrhosis as used in medicine has two definitions; occasionally they are synonymous, but very often they are quite different. The most precise description is a pathologic entity which has three features: (1) Present or deduced major hepatic necrosis sufficient to destroy total lobules in at least two thirds of the liver. This may occur in a single wave or many small waves of necrosis. (2) Major scarring as a result of this necrosis which becomes a permanent type of connective tissue. (3) Formation of new liver through the process of regeneration. As a result, the architecture of the liver is completely destroyed and is largely formed of scars and regenerative nodules. To the clinician the term cirrhosis refers to any form of long-standing liver disease in which the features of portal hypertension are prominent. Although these conditions are usually presumed to be synonymous, only with some element of proof is this actually the case.

The cirrhotic liver (in pathologically confirmed cases) is strikingly different from the normal or precirrhotic liver in the following ways:

— The necrosis usually continues and may be the most prominent feature.

— The new liver cells have a very inefficient relationship to the blood supply. They are usually very deficient and much less subject to increase with need. There is little to no portal blood supply, and if the perfusion pressure is not maintained high, the blood supply, already marginal, will drop precipitously and may produce additional ischemic damage. A regenerative nodule grows concentrically like a berry, and the blood supply and drainage come in from the outside like fingers surrounding a ball. The growth of a nodule is dependent upon its success in developing a blood supply. Soon competition develops for space, and the growing nodule presses against the contracting scars. This pressure is detrimental to the veins. The nodule, if successful, becomes totally arterially dependent. Because the venous drainage is under high pressure, there is increased lymph flow from the sinusoids. This interferes with efficient cellular exchange and thus causes postsinusoidal resistance or outflow obstruction which is found in cirrhosis.

— Regeneration is rarely complete — there is always liver cell deficiency.

— Major shunts of portal blood exist in vascularized scars, portal collaterals, and plexuses surrounding bile ducts.

— Sequestration of additional portions of the plasma volume behind the liver due to portal hypertension impairs vascular homeostasis.

Despite the fact that on the average there is 20 per cent increase in total blood volume, the blood volume available to perfuse the kidneys, heart, and brain is less than normal. These features explain many of the problems that patients with cirrhosis have in common, but in varying degrees. These features are (a) Liver destruction (activity) and liver cell insufficiency. (b) Usually inefficient metabolism of food — mild malabsorption (reflecting bile salt insufficiency), frequent glycosuria, and weight loss despite adequate calorie intake. (c) Portal hypertension, esophageal varices, and enlarged spleen with hypersplenism are frequently present. The collateral circulation is responsible for elevated urinary urobilinogen, extremely high postprandial blood sugar, and often hyperammonemia. (d) Poor tolerance of hemorrhage or electrolyte depletion resulting from impaired vascular homeostasis. The frequent postural hypotension and impaired renal function may be features of this problem. (e) Prominent ascites.

Patients with cirrhosis show a propensity for the complications of gastrointestinal hemorrhage (usually from esophageal varices), liver encephalopathy, liver cell failure, and renal insufficiency. It is likely that the poor vascular homeostasis and possibly a small hemorrhage are the principal precipitants of the additional liver cell failure and renal insufficiency.

In the cirrhotic liver there is an increased tendency for a primary tumor called a hepatoma to form. This tumor often produces a primitive protein made in the fetus (fetoglobulin), which enters into the blood. This is found in about 50 per cent of the patients with hepatoma and seems to occur in no other tumor.

Cirrhosis may result from many different causes of liver damage. Viral hepatitis, alcoholic liver damage, biliary cirrhosis, and hemochromatosis are the principal forms. In approximately one third of all cases a cause cannot be assigned. Prognosis is far more dependent upon continuation of destructive activity and upon the maximal functioning liver cell mass that can be attained from the specific complication. Except for hepatoma and renal insufficiency, highly effective treatments exist for the other complications, including portal hypertension, hypersplenism, bleeding esophageal varices, liver coma, and ascites.

EFFECT OF LIVER DISEASE ON OTHER ORGANS

Cardiovascular Effects

Acute hepatic necrosis may release vasodilating substances into the blood. Wide pulse pressure, warm palms, and high cardiac output may be manifestations of this. An inflamed liver may have such a high blood flow that it creates cardiac overload by acting as an arterial venous shunt. Most forms of active liver disease cause a 20 to 50 per cent increase in cardiac output.

Plasma volume is usually increased by one third in chronic liver disease; this increased volume is entirely sequestered in the obstructed splanchnic circulation. It has no influence on cardiovascular function except that the return of blood to the systemic circulation is retarded and occasionally leads to hypovolemia and postural hypertension. Regulation of plasma volume following hemorrhage is limited.

Lowered arterial Po_2 commonly accompanies liver disease, particularly when associated with ascites. Many patients regain normal Po_2 by breathing high concentrations of oxygen. This suggests ventilatory perfusion abnormalities brought about by the large liver or the prominent ascites. Rarely, an unresponsive lowering of the Po_2 after oxygen inhalation is found and is caused by anatomic shunts within the substance of the lung. This is most prone to occur after 3 to 7 years of cirrhosis, and clubbing of the fingers is often seen at this stage.

Many hepatic alterations of pH are possible. Liver disease is often associated with nausea, vomiting, or diarrhea, and large depletions of potassium may occur. Depletion may be accompanied by an intracellular acidosis and an extracellular alkalosis. Impairment of renal acidification is often present in chronic hepatic disease and further accentuates potassium depletion. In any form of hepatocellular damage, acidic products of metabolism, amino acids, and carbohydrate intermediates may be released into the blood and produce acidosis. This is most commonly seen as a persistent lowering of the serum bicarbonate.

In liver encephalopathy, hyperventilation due to an altered central threshold is common and alkalosis results.

Renal Changes

Renal blood flow and glomerular filtration are well preserved in most cases of mild and moderately severe liver disease. Chronic sodium retention by the kidney in association with liver disease initially involves the aldosterone mechanism, but when severe or prolonged it involves a different system. A far higher proportion of the glomerular filtrate is reabsorbed by the proximal loop of Henle (as high as 98 per cent), thus limiting the amount of sodium that reaches the distal convoluted tubule. A hormone called "third factor" is postulated to be the cause. Severe limitation of sodium on the distal convoluted tubule impairs excretion of free water and impairs responsiveness to diuretics acting on the distal convoluted tubule (spironolactones, thiazides).

In cirrhosis, a higher than normal portion of renal blood flow goes to the medulla. This high flow cleanses the high concentration of medullary solutes, so that in the water-deprived person with cirrhosis there is only about a twofold increase in medullary osmolality compared to the three- or fourfold increase in the normal subject. This makes urine concentration more difficult for the patient with cirrhosis.

It may be concluded that the person with chronic hepatic disease excretes sodium poorly and is unable either to excrete large volumes of free water or to concentrate the urine as markedly as the normal person in order to conserve water.

Renal tubule acidosis is commonly observed in the presence of liver disease. This condition is simply an expression of the kidney's production of an inappropriately alkaline urine, even in the presence of a large acid load and systemic acidosis. This reflects the limited ability of the cirrhotic kidney to make and excrete hydrogen ion. To compensate for this defect, there are increased losses of potassium into the urine and increased formation of ammonia. Thus, if hydrogen ions cannot be excreted, an acid load is excreted which is largely neutralized with sodium, potassium, or ammonium. Since sodium cannot be easily secreted, potassium is the predominant ion and losses of 150 mEq. per day have been observed. Ammonia for the urine is manufactured in the renal tubular cells from glutamate. Increased ammonia due to an acid pH and rapid flow is diffused into both urine and blood. In these patients approximately twice as much ammonia is delivered into the renal venous blood as into the urine, further increasing the load to be removed by the liver.

The hepatorenal syndrome is progressive oliguria and azotemia occurring without apparent cause in patients with liver disease. There is an abrupt increase in glomerular filtration resistance, with the maintenance of normal renal histology and overall blood flow. There is shunting of blood from the glomeruli, the cause of which is unknown but is probably a hormone.

Studies of arteriography and of the washout curves of radioactive krypton indicate that glomerular flow to such kidneys is markedly reduced but that tubular and medullary flow is preserved. If the urine is carefully examined, its sediment is normal but the urine sodium content is extremely low (less than 5 mEq. per L.). If the kidney from such a patient who has died is transplanted into a normal recipient, it functions normally, indicating that it was the original environment that caused the malfunction.

Since there are oliguria and azotemia, the principal differential diagnosis is shock kidney or necrosis of the tubular epithelium. In the hepatorenal syndrome the amount of urinary sodium is less than 5 mEq. per L. and the ratio of urine to blood creatinine or urea is greater than 1:3 and usually greater than 1:15. In contrast, in the disease with renal tubular damage the urinary sodium is rarely less than 30 mEq. per L. and the ratio of urine to plasma creatinine or urea is 1:3 or less, indicating that there is little tubular function.

Endocrine Changes

The liver is not considered an endocrine organ, yet it plays a significant role in hormone metabolism, because most nonpeptides are biotransformed by the liver into an inactive form. Most nonpeptide hormones are bound to a carrier protein in the plasma that limits the level of free hormone; the liver usually manufactures these carriers. These two functions may lead to increases in the circulating level of the free hormone which may persist longer than normal. If the production of the hormone is under careful feedback regulation (that is, the rate of release of hormone is also controlled by the tissue level of the hormone), this will have no effect. However, if this regulatory mechanism is insensitive, the hormone levels may be altered in liver disease.

Peptide hormones may be inactivated by the liver. Careful study of blood hormone levels in patients with liver cell disease often reveals many abnormalities.

Coagulation Difficulties

The release of coagulation protein was discussed earlier. The liver seems to be the principal organ responsible for the removal of activated coagulation factors from the plasma and for the removal of fibrinogen degradation released by the action of fibrinolysin or fibrin. The persistence of activated coagulation factors in the blood may account for consumptive coagulopathy. All aspects of coagulation may be affected; even platelet levels may be reduced owing to hypersplenism or consumptive coagulation. Additionally, platelets may be less active in contraction, owing to release of serotonin. Although the final pattern of abnormality in liver disease is not settled, it is apparent that many possible coagulation difficulties exist in the presence of liver disease.

REFERENCES

GENERAL

Popper, H., and Schaffner, F. (Eds.): Progress in Liver Diseases. New York, Grune and Stratton, Vol 1, 1961; Vol. 2, 1965; and Vol. 3, 1970. In-depth monographs on a single topic.

Schiff, L. (Ed.): Diseases of the Liver. 3rd edit. Philadelphia, J. B. Lippincott and Co., 1969. A multiauthored, extremely accurate collection of monographs for details on all areas of liver disease.

Sherlock, S.: Diseases of the Liver and Biliary System. 4th ed. Oxford, Blackwell Scientific Publications, 1969. A text that makes clinical problems clear and accurate. Clear pictures and concise prose often make it the best source for further reading.

ANATOMY AND TESTING

Baum, S.: Hepatic Angiography. In Popper, H., and Schaffner, F. (Eds.): Progress in Liver Diseases. Vol. 3. New York, Grune and Stratton, 1970, p. 444.

Castell, D. O., O'Brien, K. D., Muench, H., and Chalmers, T. C.: Estimation of liver size by percussion in normal individuals. Ann. Intern. Med., 70:1183, 1969.

Eyler, W. R., Schuman, B. M., Du Sault, L. A., and Hinson, R. A.: Rose Bengal I^{131} liver scan. J.A.M.A. Vol. 194 (No. 9):990, November, 1965.

McAfee, J. G., Ause, R. G., and Wager, H. N.: Diagnostic value of scintillation scanning of the liver. Arch. Intern. Med., 116:25, 1965.

Wagner, H. N., Jr., McAfee, J. G., and Mozley, J. M.: Diagnosis of liver disease by radioisotope scanning. Arch. Intern. Med., 107:324, 1961.

BIOCHEMISTRY

Arias, I. M., Gartner, L. M., Cohen, M., Ben-Ezzer, J., and Levi, A. J.: Chronic nonhemolytic unconjugated hyperbilirubinemia with glycuronyl transferase deficiency. Evidence for genetic heterogeneity. Trans. Assoc. Amer. Physicians, 81:66, 1968.

Arias, I. M., and London, I. M.: Bilirubin glucuronide formation in vitro. Demonstration of a defect in Gilbert's disease. Science, 126:563, 1957.

Bloomer, J. R., Berk, P. D., Howe, R. B., and Berlin, N. I.: Interpretation of plasma bilirubin levels based on studies with radioactive bilirubin. J.A.M.A., 218:216, 1971.

Bourke, E., Milne, M. D., and Stokes, G. S.: Mechanism of renal excretion of urobilinogen. Brit. Med. J., 2:1510, 1965.

Collins, J. R., and Crofford, O. B.: Glucose intolerance and insulin resistance in patients with liver disease. Arch. Intern. Med., 124:142, 1969.

Combes, B., and Schenker, S.: Laboratory tests. In Schiff, L. (Ed.): Diseases of the Liver. 3rd ed. Philadelphia, J. B. Lippincott and Co., 1969, p. 165.

Fingl, E., and Woodbury, D. M.: In Goodman, L. S., and Gilman, A. (Eds.): The Pharmacological Basis of Therapeutics. New York, The Macmillan Co., 1970.

Gray, C. H., and Nicholson, D. C.: Recent developments in our knowledge of the urobilins. Medicine, 46:83, 1967.

Hecker, R., and Sherlock, S.: Electrolyte and circulatory changes in terminal liver failure. Lancet, 2:1121, 1956.

Levi, A. J., Gatmaitan, Z., and Arias, I. M.: Deficiency of hepatic organic anion binding protein as a possible cause of nonhemologic unconjugated hyperbilirubinemia in the newborn. Lancet, 2:139, 1969.

Levi, A. J., Gatmaitan, Z., and Arias, I. M.: Two hepatic cytoplasmic protein fractions Y and Z and their possible role in hepatic uptake of bilirubin, sulphobromophthalein and other anions. J. Clin. Invest., 48:2156, 1969.

McFadzean, A. J., and Yeung, R. T. T.: Further observations on hypoglycemia in hepatocellular carcinoma. Amer. J. Med., 47:220, 1969.

Odell, G. B., Ryan, W. B., and Richmond, M. D.: Exchange transfusion. Pediat. Clin. N. Amer., 9:605, 1962.

Powell, L. W., Hemingway, E., Billing, B. H., and Sherlock, S.: Idiopathic unconjugated hyperbilirubinemia (Gilbert's syndrome). New Eng. J. Med., 277:1108, 1967.

Remmer, H.: Detoxification of drugs in the liver. In Popper, H., and Schaffner, F. (Eds.): Progress in Liver Diseases. Vol. 2. New York, Grune and Stratton, 1965, p. 116.

Schoenfield, L. J.: Sulfobromophthalein transport and metabolism. Gastroenterology, 48:530, 1965.

Summerskill, W. H. J.: Ammonia metabolism in the gastrointestinal tract. In Glass, G. B. J. (Ed.): Progress in Gastroenterology. Vol. 2. New York, Grune and Stratton, 1970.

BILE FORMATION, BILE FLOW, AND CHOLESTASIS

Carey, J. B., Jr.: Bile salts and hepatobiliary disease. In Schiff, L. (Ed.): Diseases of the Liver. 3rd ed. Philadelphia, J. B. Lippincott and Co., 1969.

Danzinger, R. G., Hofmann, A. F., Schoenfield, L. J., and Thistle, J. L.: Dissolution of cholesterol gallstones by chenodesoxycholic acid. New Eng. J. Med., 286:1, 1972.

Gorbach, S. L.: Intestinal microflora. Gastroenterology, 60:1110, 1971.

Havel, R. J.: The abnormal lipoprotein of cholestasis. New Eng. J. Med., 285:578, 1971.

Javitt, N. B.: Symposium on bile salt. Amer. J. Med., 51:565, 1971.

Kaplan, M. M., and Righalli, A.: Induction of rat liver alkaline phosphatase. Mechanism of serum elevation in duct obstruction. J. Clin. Invest., 49:508, 1970.

Seidel, D.: The abnormal lipoprotein of cholestasis. New Eng. J. Med., 285:1538, 1971.

Strack, P. R., Newman, H. K., Lerner, A. G., Green, S. H., Meng, C., Del Guercio, L. R. M., and State, D.: Integrated procedure for rapid diagnosis of hepatobiliary disorders. New Eng. J. Med., 285:1225, 1971.

Thureborn, E.: Human hepatic bile. Composition changes due to altered enterohepatic circulation. Acta Chir. Scand. (Suppl.) 303:1, 1962.

HEPATIC BLOOD FLOW, PORTAL HYPERTENSION

Chiandussi, L.: Umbilical-portal catheterization in diagnosis of liver disease. In Popper, H., and Schaffner, F. (Eds.): Progress in Liver Diseases. Vol. 3. New York, Grune and Stratton, 1970, p. 466.

Dumont, A. E., and Mulholland, J. H.: Hepatic lymph in cirrhosis. In Popper, H., and Schaffner, F. (Eds.): Progress in Liver Diseases. Vol. 2. New York, Grune and Stratton, 1965, p. 427.

Kimber, C., Deller, D. J., Ibbotson, R. N., and Lander, H.: The mechanism of anemia in chronic liver disease. Quart. J. Med. (new series), 34:33, 1965.

Liebowitz, H. R.: Pathogenesis of ascites in cirrhosis of the liver. N. Y. State J. Med., I. 69:1895; II. 69:2012; July, 1969.

Reynolds, T. B.: Portal hypertension. In Schiff, L. (Ed.): Diseases of the Liver. 3rd ed. Philadelphia, J. B. Lippincott and Co., 1969, p. 268.

Reynolds, T. B., and Redeker, A. G.: Hepatic hemodynamic and portal hypertension. In Popper, H., and Schaffner, F. (Eds.): Progress in Liver Diseases. Vol. 2. New York, Grune and Stratton, 1965, p. 457.

LIVER FUNCTION TESTS

Discombe, G.: Flocculation tests. Lancet, 1:1005, 1959.

Feizi, T.: Immunoglobulins in chronic liver disease. Gut, 9:193, 1968.

Moore, T. L., Kupchik, H. Z., Marcon, N., and Zamcheck, N.: Carcino-embryonic antigen assay in cancer of the colon and pancreas and other digestive tract disorders. Amer. J. Dig. Dis., 16:1, 1971.

Paronetto, F.: Immunologic aspects of liver diseases. In Popper, H., and Schaffner, F. (Eds.): Progress in Liver Diseases. Vol. 3. New York, Grune and Stratton, 1970, p. 299.

Rachmilewitz, N., Stein, Y., Aronovitch, J., and Grossowicz, N.: The clinical significance of serum cyanocobalamine in liver disease. Arch. Intern. Med., 102:1118, 1958.

Ratnoff, O. D.: Disordered hemostasis in hepatic disease. In Schiff, L. (Ed.): Diseases of the Liver. 3rd ed. Philadelphia, J. B. Lippincott and Co., 1969, p. 147.

Schiff, L., and Gall, W. E. A.: Needle biopsy of the liver. *In* Schiff, L. (Ed.): Diseases of the Liver. 3rd ed. Philadelphia, J. B. Lippincott and Co., 1969, p. 209.

Smith, J. B., and O'Neill, R. T.: Alphafetoprotein occurrence in germinal cell and liver malignancies. Amer. J. Med., *41*: 767, 1971.

Stolbach, L., Krant, M. J., and Fishman, W.: Ectopic production of an alkaline phosphatase isoenzyme in patients with cancer. New Eng. J. Med., *281*:757, October, 1969.

Wright, R., McCollum, R. W., and Klatskin, G.: Australia antigen in acute and chronic liver disease. Lancet, *2*:117, 1969.

Zieve, L., Hill, E., Hanson, M., Falcone, A. B., and Watson, C. J.: Normal and abnormal variations and clinical significance of the one minute and total serum bilirubin determinations. J. Lab. Clin. Med., *38*:446, 1951.

CLINICAL LIVER DISEASE

Davidson, C. S., and Gabuzda, G. J.: Hepatic coma. *In* Schiff, L. (Ed.): Diseases of the Liver. 3rd ed. Philadelphia, J. B. Lippincott and Co., 1969, p. 378.

Losowsky, M. D., Jones, D. P., Lieber, C. S., and Davidson, C. S.: Local factors in ascites formation during sodium retention in cirrhosis. New Eng. J. Med., *268*:651, 1963.

Rake, M. O., Pannell, G., Flute, P. T., and Williams, R.: Intravascular coagulation in acute hepatic necrosis. Lancet, *1*:533, 1970.

Shear, L., Cheng, S., and Gabuzda, G. J.: Compartmentalization of ascites and edema in patients with hepatic cirrhosis. New Eng. J. Med., *282*:1391, 1970.

EFFECT OF LIVER DISEASE ON OTHER ORGANS

Abelmann, W. H., Kramer, G. E., Verstraete, J. M., Gravallese, M. A., Jr., and McNeely, W. F.: Cirrhosis of the liver and decreased arterial oxygen saturation. Arch. Intern. Med., *108*:34, 1961.

Baldus, W. P., Summerskill, W. H. J., Hunt, J. C., and Maher, F. T.: Renal circulation in cirrhosis. Observations based on catheterization of the renal vein. J. Clin. Invest., *43*:1090, 1964.

Maddrey, W. C., Sen Gupta, K. P., Basu Mallick, K. C., Iber, F. L., and Basu, A. K.: Extrahepatic obstruction of the portal venous system. Surg. Gynec. Obstet., *127*:989, 1968.

Murray, J. F., Dawson, A. M., and Sherlock, S.: Circulatory changes in chronic liver disease. Amer. J. Med., *24*:358, 1958.

Shear, L., Bonkowsky, H. L., and Gabuzda, G. J.: Renal tubular acidosis in cirrhosis. A determinant of susceptibility to recurrent hepatic precoma. New Eng. J. Med., *280*:1, 1969.

Shorr, E.: *In* Liver Injury. Transactions of the Sixth Conference. Edited by F. W. H. Offbauer. Sponsored by Josiah Macy, Jr., Foundation, 1947, p. 33.

Summerskill, W. H. J.: Hepatic failure and the kidney. Gastroenterology, *51*:94, 1966.

Summerskill, W. H. J.: Ascites: The kidney in liver disease. *In* Schiff, L. (Ed.): Diseases of the Liver. 3rd ed. Philadelphia, J. B. Lippincott and Co., 1969.

Walls, W. D., and Losowsky, M. S.: The hemostatic effect of liver disease. Gastroenterology, *60*:108, 1971.

CHAPTER 29 PATHOPHYSIOLOGY OF GALLBLADDER DISEASE

FRANZ GOLDSTEIN

Since antiquity the gallbladder has been the subject of superstitious misconceptions based on erroneous ideas about its function. The ancient Greeks, believing the gallbladder to be the source of bile, one of the main body "humors," thought that human behavior was dependent on the type of bile secreted. To this day our language, if not our thinking, reflects these antiquated ideas when we use such terms as melancholy (referring to black bile), choleric, or bilious to describe human moods. The disease cholera remains misnamed to this date. Of greater importance, however, are other currently held misconceptions shared by large segments of the medical profession with the lay public regarding the function of this small pear-shaped organ. Its true contributions to health and normal bodily functions are minimal but its potential for disease production is great, exceeded only by the frequency with which it is mistakenly blamed for causing troubles originating elsewhere.

ASPECTS OF STRUCTURE

The gallbladder is a distensible hollow organ with an average capacity of about 50 cc. The thin wall of the normal gallbladder consists of mucosa, muscularis, and serosa but has no submucosa, and the mucosa contains no glands. The delicately woven mucosal folds and villi normally project into the muscular layer as crypts. In diseased gallbladders these mucosal invaginations may become larger and more deeply penetrating, imitating on histologic cross sections actual gland formation. These pseudoglandular sacculations are known as Rokitansky-Aschoff sinuses and signify either chronic inflammation or degenerative gallbladder disease (cholecystosis), depending on one's viewpoint.

The cystic duct connects the gallbladder with the juncture of the common hepatic and common bile ducts. It is tortuous and its mucous membrane is thrown into folds, forming the spiral valves of Heister. A true sphincter is probably not present and the direction of bile flow to and from the gallbladder is determined primarily by pressure differences between the gallbladder and bile ducts. The tortuosity of the cystic duct presents an obstacle to the passage of solid objects such as stones.

GALLBLADDER FUNCTION

The gallbladder is not essential to life and some mammalian species (e.g., rat, horse) have no gallbladder. Extirpation of the gallbladder in man does not interfere with good health and usually causes mild and temporary physiologic disturbances, if any.

The *functions* of the gallbladder are (1) storage and concentration of micellar bile complexes, (2) discharge of stored bile into the duodenum during periods of digestion, and (3) stabilization of bile pressure within the biliary system. Normally, the liver secretes about 800 to 1000 ml. of bile per day. Instead of entering the duodenum directly, part of the bile is diverted through the cystic duct into the gallbladder whenever the lower end of the common bile duct is closed by contraction of the sphincter of Oddi and whenever the pressure in the common duct exceeds the pressure in the gallbladder. The sphincter is closed most of the time and thus normally prevents entry of intestinal contents into the biliary tract. Relaxation of the sphincter occurs normally in response to the ingestion of fat-containing food and is synchronized with gallbladder contractions. The secretory pressure of bile normally varies between 15 and 25 cm. of water. The sphincter of Oddi offers resistance to bile flow at pressures of the same order of magnitude. When the gallbladder is filled and a pressure of 25 cm. is reached in the common duct, sphincter resistance is overcome and bile trickles into the duodenum. Bile ceases to enter the extrahepatic bile ducts from the liver when, owing to obstruction, intraductal pressure rises above about 35 cm. of water. After prolonged bile duct obstruction, all bile pigment proximal to the obstruction is absorbed and the bile ducts become filled with white fluid and mucus ("white bile") produced by the lining cells of the ducts.

The gallbladder concentrates bile 5 to 10 times through the absorption of water. The main solids of bile—conjugated bile acids, cholesterol, lecithin and conjugated bilirubin—are concentrated to a comparable extent, whereas the ordinary electrolytes are partially absorbed with water to maintain osmotic equilibrium with plasma (Table 29–1). Even though bile is isosmotic with plasma, the total cation concentration of bile may greatly exceed that of plasma and may reach 350 mM. per L. This phenomenon is related to the presence of large molecular aggregates known as micelles. Bile micelles, consisting chiefly of bile salts, cholesterol, and lecithin, contain on their surface many negative charges which bind cations, especially sodium and calcium. The bound cations exert no osmotic pressure. Bile acids, upon entering the duodenum, play an important role in fat digestion. Bile acids aid the solubilization of lipids by means of micelle formation, and they appear to activate pancreatic lipase. Both actions are necessary for normal fat digestion (i.e., hydrolysis) and subsequent absorption. It has been debated whether the gallbladder is able to secrete cholesterol. Evidence in favor of cholesterol secretion derives mostly from the presence of cholesterol underneath the mucosa of the gallbladder, at times in large quantities (cholesterolosis of the gallbladder or "strawberry gallbladder"). However, this does not constitute proof of secretion and may reflect absorption and deposition of cholesterol underneath the mucosa. There is evidence of minimal absorption of the organic constituents of bile through the normal gallbladder mucosa, whereas an inflamed gallbladder mucosa becomes more permeable to a variety of bile solids, including bile salts, and other substances such as gallbladder dyes.

The volume and concentration of liver bile is affected by certain agents. Substances that increase the volume flow of bile are called hydrocholeretics, whereas those that increase the concentration of bile solids are called choleretics. Naturally occurring bile salts are the most potent agents, with both hydrocholeretic and choleretic activities. Unconjugated, oxidized bile acid derivatives are also potent hydrocholeretics; their ability to produce copious flow of dilute bile has been thought to have therapeutic value, but their safety has recently been called into question, especially their potential to cause gallstone formation.

Substances which stimulate gallbladder contraction are called cholagogues; they include fats, proteins and peptones, hydrochloric and other acids, magnesium sulfate, and especially the hormone cholecystokinin (CCK), which likely is the common pathway for all stimuli initiating gallbladder contraction. CCK is a single-chain polypeptide with 33 amino acid units. Its C-terminal octapeptide is structurally almost identical with that of gastrin, with which it shares many physiologic actions, and is more active than CCK itself in respect to its action both on the gallbladder and on enzyme secretion of the pancreas. This and other pieces of evidence strongly suggest that a single peptide, of identical structure, exerts two major hormonal actions, those of CCK and of pancreozymin (PZ). CCK is released from duodenal and upper jejunal mucosa in response to fat ingestion and appears to be the most important physiologic agent producing gallbladder contraction. In response to cholecystokinin, the sphincter of Oddi relaxes simultaneously with the evacuation of the gallbladder. Caroli and his associates have claimed the existence of an anticholecystokinin and have expressed the hypothesis that the relative amounts of the two hormones control the tone and contraction of the gallbladder, bile

TABLE 29–1 APPROXIMATE COMPOSITION OF NORMAL GALLBLADDER BILE*

Sodium	210	mEq./L.
Potassium	13	"
Calcium	23	"
Chloride	25	"
Bicarbonate	10	"
Bile salts	300	mM./L.
Bilirubin	300	mg./100 ml.
Cholesterol	500	"
Lecithin	3000	"
Protein	30	"
Osmolality	280	mOsm./L.

*After Bouchier, I. A. D., and Freston, J. W.: Lancet, 1:340, 1968.

ducts, and sphincter of Oddi. Autonomic nervous stimuli and autonomic drugs also affect gallbladder motor activity at least by mediating the release of cholecystokinin and possibly also by more direct action. Although some investigators believe that gallbladder evacuation is a purely passive process brought about by reduction in both sphincter tone and intraductal pressure, there is good evidence for the presence of active gallbladder contractions. This is illustrated clinically by the occasional dissociation between the action of the gallbladder and that of the sphincter of Oddi in which forceful bladder contraction occurs in the absence of sphincter relaxation (biliary dyskinesia).

Tests of Gallbladder Function

Among the numerous substances excreted in bile and concentrated in the gallbladder are certain organic iodinated radiopaque compounds called dyes. The recognition of this fact led Graham and Cole to the development of oral cholecystography. At a suitable interval after the ingestion of a dye such as iodopanoic acid, x-ray films of the gallbladder area are taken which permit visualization of the gallbladder shadow, demonstrate radiolucent stones as filling defects, and document evacuation of the gallbladder after the administration of a cholagogue (a fat meal or intravenous CCK). Nonvisualization of the gallbladder indicates a nonfunctioning and, usually, diseased gallbladder, provided that the following conditions can be excluded: (1) failure of the patient to have ingested the dye, (2) vomiting of dye, (3) pyloroduodenal obstruction, (4) poor excretory liver function as evidenced by jaundice or marked Bromsulphalein retention, (5) unsuspected cholecystectomy, (6) intrahepatic gallbladder obscured by the liver shadow, and (7) congenital absence of the gallbladder. Diarrhea may follow the intake of some gallbladder dyes but does not usually interfere with their absorption. In rare instances the gallbladder does not concentrate dye because it is filled with thick mucus after prolonged periods of inactivity resulting from a fat-free diet. Following the ingestion of fatty foods for several days, a normal cholecystogram may be obtained. Apparent lack of filling may also be produced by irritability of the gallbladder in some cases of cholecystosis.

Stones in the common duct and gallbladder of mildly jaundiced patients can occasionally be demonstrated by the 4-day oral administration of dye (calculography), and tiny accretions of bile solids, clinically spoken of as sand or gravel, can be detected by a recent modification of the dye method called sabulography. When the oral administration of dyes is not feasible, or when higher concentrations of dye are required for optimal outlining of the biliary tree, especially after cholecystectomy, intravenous cholangiography is often used. However, none of the above procedures is applicable in the presence of jaundice. Jaundice is evidence of impaired excretory liver function with respect to bilirubin. Gallbladder dyes are excreted by the liver by mechanisms similar to bilirubin excretion. Hence, in the presence of jaundice the liver generally does not excrete sufficient dye to produce x-ray contrast in the biliary tree, and no conclusions regarding gallbladder function can be drawn from oral cholecystography or I.V. cholangiography in jaundiced patients. In such patients one can resort to transhepatic percutaneous cholangiography, in which dye is injected via needle or catheter inserted directly into the liver, aiming for dilated bile radicles such as are present in extrahepatic obstructive jaundice. In patients with parenchymal jaundice the method is not indicated. In patients who undergo operations for biliary tract disease, operative cholangiography is performed in selected patients with suspected stones or other lesions of the common duct, the dye being injected through a catheter or a T-tube inserted into the common bile duct (operative or T-tube cholangiography). This procedure is often repeated within 10 days or later, before removing the T-tube from the common duct, to ascertain the patency of the duct.

An older test which retains limited usefulness is biliary drainage (Lyon-Meltzer test). The recovery of calcium bilirubinate and cholesterol crystals from bile obtained by duodenal intubation may clinch the diagnosis of cholelithiasis in patients with a poorly functioning or nonfunctioning gallbladder. Duodenal drainage also permits the recovery of parasites (e.g., *Giardia lamblia*) and pathogenic bacteria (e.g., *E. typhosa*) residing in the duodenum or gallbladder. More recently, bile obtained by drainage has been subjected to physicochemical analysis to determine the state of cholesterol saturation in relation to potential stone formation.

The above tests have done much to place the diagnosis of gallbladder disease on a sound objective basis but have not totally eliminated the misconceptions about gallbladder disease created around the turn of the century.

GALLSTONE FORMATION

Cholelithiasis (the presence of gallstones) constitutes the pivotal problem in gallbladder disease. Gallstones not only may give rise to symptoms but may lead to cholecystitis and its various complications and, rarely, to the development of carcinoma of the gallbladder. The importance of gallstones is related to their frequency. Once thought to be confined largely to females who were fat, fertile, and forty or older, gallstones are now recognized to exist in both sexes, admittedly with a female predominance, in fat as well as lean people and with an age incidence that rises from childhood on. Recent estimates place the number of people with gallstones in the United States at 12 million women and 4 million men, leading to about 5000 to 8000 deaths and a direct economic loss of 1 billion dollars annually.

Traditionally, gallstones have been classified into three types: cholesterol, pigment, and mixed stones. Such a classification lacks scientific precision but aids the clinician in preliminary identification of stone type. Recent analyses of large numbers of stones by modern methods employing microradiography, microdiffraction, infrared spectrophotometry, and gas chromatography have revealed the mixed composition of almost all stones containing cholesterol monohydrate, calcium carbonate, calcium bilirubinate, and also bile salts, proteins, mucopolysaccharides, fatty acids, and small quantities of several minerals. Nevertheless, cholesterol is the major component in about 90 per cent of stones recovered from the American population, and in virtually all stones found in American Indians. Despite the admixture of other matter, such stones are best referred to as cholesterol stones. In other populations, e.g., Japanese, calcium bilirubinate stones predominate but cholesterol stones are also increasing in frequency. The highest prevalence of gallstones among various population groups studied is found among Southwestern American Indians, among whom close to 50 per cent of a sampled population revealed the presence of cholesterol stones. Less pronounced differences in stone prevalence can be found among various other ethnic groups within the United States, with Negroes having the lowest prevalence, and Italians and Jews apparently having higher than average frequency of stones. To what extent these differences are attributable to genetic, dietary, or other patterns, remains unclear.

Obesity probably predisposes to stone formation, but total caloric intake, rather than fat or cholesterol intake alone, appears to be more important. Ileal disease or resection is another condition clearly predisposing to stone formation. In the course of their enterohepatic circulation, bile salts are reabsorbed from the ileum and re-excreted by the liver into the bile ducts and ultimately the intestine, several cycles being completed in the course of a large meal (see p. 747). The total bile acid pool, normally 2 to 3 grams, may be severely reduced as the result of an impaired enterohepatic circulation and loss of bile acids into the colon with ultimate fecal excretion. Increased hepatic synthesis of bile acids can only partially compensate for such losses. Pigment stones are far more common in patients with hemolytic disorders because of increased bilirubin formation secondary to increased hemoglobin breakdown. Infection appears to be an important etiologic factor in calcium bilirubinate stones, especially in Japan and other oriental countries where such stones are frequent. Presumably, *E. coli* and other bacteria with beta-glucuronidase activity enter the biliary system and cause hydrolysis of bilirubin glucuronide, the formed free bilirubin readily precipitating in the aqueous bile medium. The role of infection in initial cholesterol stone formation is probably minor. Infection superimposed upon cholelithiasis, by favoring bile salt absorption, raising the pH, and providing desquamated epithelial nuclei, may possibly favor stone growth and the development of mixed stones.

Important progress has been made in recent years in the understanding of cholesterol stone formation. Cholesterol is almost totally insoluble in aqueous solutions, yet gallbladder bile contains an average of about 500 mg. of cholesterol per 100 ml. in water-clear solution. This is made possible by the process of micelle formation, aided by the physicochemical properties of bile salts and lecithin. The two main primary bile salts of human bile secreted by the liver are cholic and chenodeoxycholic acid, conjugated to glycine or taurine (Fig. 29-1). Normal human bile also contains small and usually insignificant amounts of deoxycholate, formed by bacterial dehydroxylation of cholate in the gut, absorbed, and recirculated. The two chief bile salts, in their conjugated forms, are crucial in micelle formation because of their abundance and their amphiphilic or detergent-like properties. Amphiphilic molecules contain both water-soluble, or polar, and lipid-soluble, or nonpolar, portions in their molecules. In aqueous solution, bile salts, like household detergents, arrange themselves in spherical or other geometric shapes, with their polar portions facing the outside and the nonpolar lipid-soluble portions oriented toward the center. These molecular aggregates, or micelles, are able to solubilize water-insoluble lipids in their centers. Micelles in bile are composed chiefly of bile salts, lecithin, and cholesterol. Lecithin, first discovered to be a major ingredient of human bile by Isaksson in 1951, while water-insoluble itself, has an important function in the formation of mixed bile micelles and greatly increases their cholesterol solubilizing ability. Admirand and Small have plotted the concentrations of cholesterol, bile salt, and lecithin on triangular coordinates and have been able to define the relative concentrations of these three major bile components within which cholesterol is held in micellar solution (Fig. 29-2). "Abnormal" bile resulting from an increase in cholesterol concentration relative to the amounts of the other two components can thus be clearly identified as supersaturated or lithogenic, i.e., leading to cholesterol precipitation and stone formation.

Figure 29-1 Chemical structure of cholesterol, of human primary bile acids and normally present secondary deoxycholic acid, and of normal bile acid conjugates with glycine and taurine.

With an understanding of the basic physicochemical phenomena controlling cholesterol solubility in bile, as outlined in much abbreviated form above, has come progress in unraveling the pathogenesis of stone formation. It has become clear that the liver secretes bile in the form of micellar complexes containing cholesterol in solution and that in patients with stones, or those seemingly predisposed to form stones, the liver secretes abnormal bile supersaturated with cholesterol. This appears to be the first stage in cholesterol stone formation and has led to the concept that cholelithiasis may be considered to be a liver disease. Just what leads to the formation of such supersaturated bile remains unclear. The work of Vlahcevic and associates has suggested a reduced bile acid pool in patients with gallstones as a major

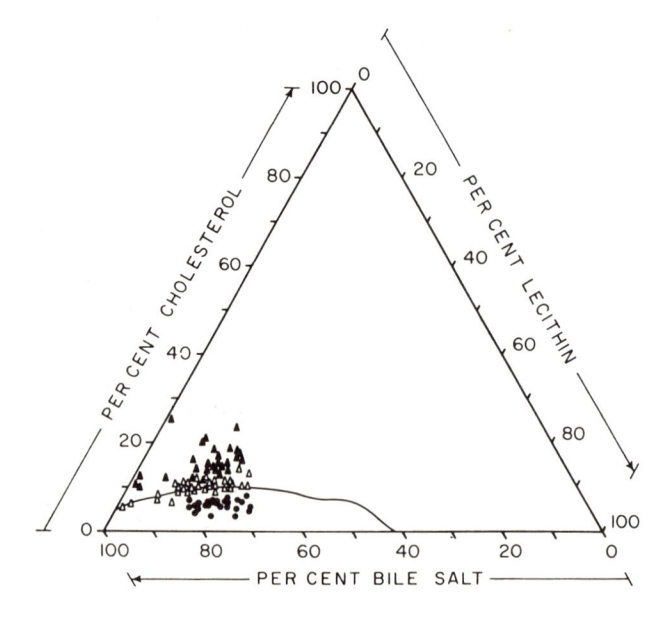

Figure 29-2 Diagram plotting relative concentrations of cholesterol, lecithin, and bile salts on triangular coordinates, with zone of micellar solubility shown by line in left lower portion of triangle. Black circles within zone of solubility reflect measurements of bile from patients without gallstones. Open triangles reflect bile samples from patients with cholesterol or mixed stones in which no microcrystals were present. Black triangles reflect bile from gallstone patients with microcrystals in bile. (After Admirand, W. H., and Small, D. M.: J. Clin. Invest., 47:1043, 1968.)

abnormality. This would tend to explain the propensity for stone formation in patients with diseased or absent ileums, the site of bile salt reabsorption. Other investigators have suggested altered ratios of dihydroxy to trihydroxy (i.e., chenodeoxy to cholic) acids. Although hepatic bile is frequently supersaturated with cholesterol, precipitation of cholesterol and stone formation rarely occur outside the gallbladder, emphasizing the role played by the latter organ in cholelithiasis. Thus, cholecystectomy is rarely followed by stone formation in the major bile ducts, even though there is no reason to expect any change in liver bile composition following the removal of the gallbladder.

Among suspected causes of precipitation of cholesterol from supersaturated bile in the gallbladder are bacteria, reflux of intestinal contents from the duodenum, abnormal bile pigments or abnormal bile salts secreted by the liver, abnormal mucoproteins, and foreign bodies. Any of these may form the nidus or lead to the formation of the nidus around which stones form. Stone formation may occur very suddenly, given the proper conditions. Small stones have been observed to grow in size, leading to the recognition of a third or growth phase of stone formation, a process which may be reversible and on which much hope for eventual treatment is based. Dissolution of gallstones after feeding of chenodeoxycholate for prolonged periods of time has recently been reported.

Clinical Significance of Gallstones

As long as stones remain confined to the gallbladder, they tend to cause little, if any, trouble. Occasionally, stones may disappear spontaneously, owing to passage or dissolution, but such instances are quite rare. All too often stones are forced into the biliary ducts, presumably by contractions of the gallbladder, initiating a series of potentially dangerous as well as unpleasant events. The lodgement of stones in, or passage through, the cystic and common duct usually is accompanied by a pain syndrome known as "biliary colic." This pain is not actually colicky, if colic is to denote a crampy intermittent pain. The pain produced by stone passage, resulting in spasm of the ducts and forceful contraction of the gallbladder with or without dilatation, is an example of visceral pain transmitted by sympathetic nerve fibers. Like most visceral abdominal pain, it is referred to the midline, usually the midepigastrium, and is quite severe. It often radiates diffusely along both costal margins, but mostly the right, and through to the back. The pain usually builds up in crescendo fashion and then remains constant for hours. It may subside either spontaneously, presumably when the stone drops back into the gallbladder or passes into the duodenum, or following the injection of antispasmodics or opiates. The pain is frequently accompanied by nausea and vomiting, probably by reflex vagal stimulation.

If the stone remains impacted in the cystic duct, partial or complete obstruction and distention of the gallbladder (hydrops) may lead to the development of acute cholecystitis. Attacks of biliary colic tend to occur at unpredictable intervals ("episodic pain"), in contrast to the "rhythmic" and "periodic" recurrence of peptic ulcer pain. Most attacks follow heavy meals, usually by several hours, and are probably related to events in the digestion of fats and forceful gallbladder contractions. Single large stones are less commonly set in motion by gallbladder contractions, and hence less commonly give rise to colic. Larger stones, by exerting constant pressure, may erode the wall of the gallbladder and perforate into the peritoneal cavity or they may produce fistulous communications into surrounding structures such as the common bile duct, duodenum, more distal small intestine, and colon. As such fistulas may divert most bile from the proximal small bowel, steatorrhea may be induced as not enough bile is present in the proximal small bowel for lipid solubilization. Large stones entering the intestine may cause partial or complete intestinal obstruction.

Despite the presence of stones in it, the gallbladder may continue to function, as evidenced by the results of cholecystographic examination and biliary drainage. The presence of gallstones per se has no demonstrable effects on fat digestion or absorption unless stones enter and block the common duct, thus preventing bile from entering the duodenum. When this happens, other clinical manifestations usually appear, especially jaundice and intermittent fever and chills (Charcot's fever).

It is difficult to understand the alleged causation of chronic "dyspeptic symptoms," "flatulent indigestion," gaseousness, and indigestion after ingestion of fatty food by the mere presence of stones in the gallbladder. Recent objective analyses of symptoms by Price in England and by Koch and Donaldson in the United States have shown that indigestion and dyspeptic symptoms occur with equal frequency in patients with and without gallstones. Interestingly, around the turn of the century, leading medical authorities considered most gallstones to be asymptomatic and held biliary tract pain to be the only symptom reliably attributable to gallstones, as we are gradually coming to believe again. Moynihan, a highly influential British surgeon, was the chief champion of a causal relationship between gallstones and indigestion. His belief was based on the finding of gallstones and the absence of gastric lesions on autopsies of patients with histories of indigestion, and the illogical conclusion that the stones had to have caused the deceased patients' indigestion, since their stomachs were normal.

When digestive symptoms are encountered in patients with gallstones, it is likely that they either are caused by organic disease of other gastrointestinal structures or are "functional" in origin, associated with the irritable bowel syndrome, aerophagia, or the prolonged abstinence from fatty foods. The latter may in itself lead to intolerance of fats, manifested by an exaggerated delay in gastric emptying and nausea following the unaccustomed ingestion of fat. Even a *nonfunctioning diseased gallbladder,* with or without stones, offers no satisfactory explanation for indigestion and flatulence. The removal of a *nonfunctioning* gallbladder does not produce any change in the transport and character of bile and could hardly be expected to affect digestive function. Cholecystectomy, cannot, therefore, be expected to ameliorate dyspeptic symptoms and should not be recommended for that purpose. Digestive symptoms are not usually encountered following the removal of the gallbladder for painful calculous cholecystitis in patients without digestive symptoms preoperatively.

INFLAMMATION OF THE GALLBLADDER

Cholecystitis, or inflammation of the gallbladder, occurs in association with stones in about 90 per cent of cases. It is assumed that intermittent or chronic blockage by stones of the gallbladder outflow tract, i.e., gallbladder neck or cystic duct, is related to the causation of cholecystitis. Other causes of cystic duct or infundibular obstruction account for a small percentage of cases of cholecystitis. The initial inflammation is chemical or ischemic in nature, and bacterial cultures during the early stage of inflammation are usually sterile. After prolonged distention of the organ, resulting in stasis of gallbladder contents and impairment of its blood supply, bacterial invasion is likely to occur. While *E. coli* is the most common bacterial organism involved, most enteric organisms may be encountered.

In about half of all patients with acute cholecystitis the initial symptom is midepigastric pain of visceral origin, the biliary colic described earlier. Unless specific inquiry is made, the early pain may not be mentioned by the patient who may be too preoccupied with the later right upper quadrant pain caused by local inflammation of the gallbladder and parietal peritoneal irritation transmitted by spinal nerve fibers. The pain of cholecystitis is frequently referred to the right scapula or the interscapular area. While physical examination of patients with biliary colic and visceral pain alone usually reveals no abnormalities, examination of patients with acute cholecystitis will elicit signs of local inflammation, such as tenderness and muscle guarding approximately over the area of the gallbladder. When the gallbladder is distended, it can often be palpated and, when tender, the presence of hydrops is suggested. Systemic evidence of inflammation in the form of fever and leukocytosis can also be expected. Slight hyperbilirubinemia, rarely exceeding 2.0 mg. per 100 ml., may be encountered in the absence of choledocholithiasis and is explained by edema of the cystic duct and its encroachment on the lumen of the common duct. The acute inflammation may subside or progress to empyema, gangrene, and rupture of the gallbladder, with resulting peritonitis or abscess formation. In other instances chronic cholecystitis may ensue. The diagnosis of the latter should not be accepted without cholecystographic proof of impaired gallbladder function; in many instances stones can be demonstrated, as well, in a shrunken, contracted gallbladder. Impaired gallbladder function, with or without crystals, may be demonstrable by bile drainage. Patients with chronic cholecystitis may be totally asymptomatic or may experience repeated attacks of symptoms as described for acute cholecystitis; others may complain of mild right upper quadrant pain and tenderness, especially after fatty meals.

In about 80 per cent of cases jaundice due to common duct stones is associated with chronic cholecystitis and hence with a nondistensible and sometimes contracted gallbladder. In contrast, jaundice due to carcinomatous obstruction of the common duct is usually accompanied by a dilated gallbladder (Courvoisier's law), unless previous unrelated cholecystitis prevents distention of the diseased organ.

Occasionally, obstruction of the cystic duct and low-grade chronic cholecystitis leads to the absorption of all bile pigment. The material filling the gallbladder in such patients, mostly mucus and calcium salts secreted by the mucosa of the gallbladder, is white and pasty and contains much calcium carbonate, hence the term "milk of calcium" bile. The high calcium content is responsible for the radiopacity of the affected gallbladder on scout films of the abdomen.

LESS COMMON GALLBLADDER DISEASES

Jutras and his associates have in recent years described under the term of "hyperplastic cholecystoses" a condition, or group of conditions, of alleged degenerative gallbladder disease. Included are previously recognized forms of gallbladder disease such as cholesterolosis, adenomyomatosis, and Rokitansky-Aschoff sinuses. Jutras postulates that in the degenerative cholecystoses hyperplasia of mucosal, muscular, and neural elements takes place and leads to a "hyperfunctional state" which in turn may produce severe and prolonged postprandial pain, intermittent colics, and indigestion. The diagnosis heretofore has been based mostly on radiologic criteria. Further work will be required to show whether the described condition constitutes a pathologic entity or a conglomeration of unrelated conditions, some possibly of inflammatory or congenital origin.

The clinical significance of the hyperplastic cholecystoses is also not clearly defined at this time. It appears that a "hyperfunctional state" of the gallbladder exists, characterized clinically by postprandial pain after fatty meals, with the radiologic counterpart of excessive gallbladder contraction after fat or CCK stimulation. In other instances impaired gallbladder evacuation can be demonstrated, possibly due to partial obstruction of the gallbladder outflow tract caused by the hyperplastic mucosa, diffuse adenomyomatosis, or cholesterol polyps. In such cases one could interpret the muscular hypertrophy as a form of work hypertrophy resulting from chronic hypercontraction of the gallbladder against resistance.

The pain observed in some patients with hyperplastic cholecystosis, diagnosed on the basis of Jutras' radiographic criteria, is identical to the pain of patients with motility disturbances of both functional and organic origin. So-called functional biliary dyskinesia was first clearly defined by Westphal in 1922 and is believed to represent a loss of synchronization of gallbladder contraction with sphincter of Oddi relaxation. The net result is the inability of the gallbladder to effectively empty itself because of sphincter spasm and painful hypercontractions of the gallbladder against resistance occurring after fatty meals. Westphal postulated autonomic nervous dysfunction as the cause of biliary dyskinesia. The rarity of the condition has made some clinicians dubious of its existence. The diagnosis should be made only if rigid criteria can be met, specifically the demonstration of impaired gallbladder evacuation in the course of CCK cholecystography, with prominent filling of the common bile and hepatic ducts and failure of dye to enter the duodenum. Preferably, sublingual nitroglycerin and/or anticholinergics should relieve the spasm and, when combined with CCK cholecystography, should lead to dye entering the duodenum and to gallbladder emptying. The term dyskinesia is often used incorrectly in connection with unrelated flatulence and indigestion before or after cholecystectomy. When sphincter spasm cannot be relieved with nitroglycerin and anticholinergics, sphincter stenosis is likely to be found and requires surgical correction in the form of sphincterotomy or sphincteroplasty with cholecystectomy.

Identical postprandial biliary pain can also be produced by partial mechanical obstruction of the cystic duct due to bands, adhesions, or cystic duct stenosis. The term cystic duct syndrome has been given to this syndrome and its diagnosis requires CCK cholecystography for reliable confirmation. As in functional dyskinesia and sphincter stenosis, CCK injection reproduces the patient's spontaneous postprandial pain as the gallbladder is induced to contract against resistance, but in contrast to the other two syndromes, the common duct fills minimally, if at all, and a block is evident at the level of the cystic duct. This interesting condition is far more common than is generally believed but is gradually gaining wider recognition. It appears that an overlap exists between chronic acalculous cholecystitis, the hyperplastic cholecystoses of Jutras, and the cystic duct syndrome, and further studies will undoubtedly be required to clarify the true relationships.

Carcinoma of the gallbladder is a relatively rare malignant condition, found in about 0.35 per cent of autopsies in this country and not necessarily related to the cause of death. Most, but not all, cases follow calculous cholecystitis, with chronic inflammation and "irritation" believed to be predisposing factors. Since this cancer is relatively rare and encountered mostly in older age groups (peak incidence in seventh decade) and since cholelithiasis is so very common, cholecystectomy in all calculous individuals for the prevention of carcinoma is not generally recommended. The number of lives lost from the resulting operative mortality would likely exceed the number of lives saved by the prevention of carcinoma occurrence, and the disparity would be even greater if the loss of years of life rather than crude mortality figures alone were compared.

REFERENCES

Admirand, W. H., and Small, D. M.: The physicochemical basis of cholesterol gallstone formation in man. J. Clin. Invest., 47:1043, 1968.

Berry, H., and Flower, R. J.: The assay of endogenous cholecystokinin and factors influencing its release in the dog and cat. Gastroenterology, 60:409, 1971.

Bouchier, I. A. D.: Gallstone formation. Lancet, 1:711, 1971.

Bouchier, I. A. D., and Freston, J. W.: The aetiology of gallstones. Lancet, 1:340, 1968.

Camishion, R. C., and Goldstein, F.: Partial, noncalculous cystic duct obstruction (cystic duct syndrome). Surg. Clin. N. Amer., 47:1107, 1967.

Caroli, J., Plessier, J., and Plessier, B.: Endogenous cholecystokinin and its inhibitor: method of assessment in humans; its role in normal and pathologic physiology. Amer. J. Dig. Dis., 6:646, 1961.

Cohen, S., Kaplan, M., Gottlieb, L., and Patterson, J.: Liver disease and gallstones in regional enteritis. Gastroenterology, 60:237, 1971.

Cozzolino, H. J., Goldstein, F., Greening, R. R., and Wirts, C. W.: The cystic duct syndrome. J.A.M.A., 185:920, 1963.

Danziger, R. G., Hofmann, A. F., Schoenfield, L. J., and Thistle, J. L.: Dissolution of cholesterol gallstones by chenodeoxycholic acid. New Eng. J. Med., 286:1, 1972.

Editorial: Classification of human gallstones. Lancet, 1:1416, 1968.

Editorial: Gallstones: a new liver disease. New Eng. J. Med., 283:96, 1970.

Fotopoulos, J. P., and Crampton, A. R.: Adenomyomatosis of the gallbladder. Med. Clin. N. Amer., 48:9, 1964.

Hofmann, A. F.: Clinical implications of physicochemical studies on bile salts. Gastroenterology, 48:484, 1965.

Isaksson, B.: On the dissolving power of lecithin and bile salts for cholesterol in human bile. Acta Soc. Med. Upsal., 59:296, 1954.

Jorpes, J. E.: The isolation and chemistry of secretin and cholecystokinin. Gastroenterology, 55:157, 1968.

Juniper, K., Jr.: Physicochemical characteristics of bile and their relation to gallstone formation. Amer. J. Med., 39:98, 1965.

Jutras, J. A.: Hyperplastic cholecystoses. Amer. J. Roentgen., 83:795, 1960.

Kaye, M. D., and Kern, F.: Clinical relationships of gallstones. Lancet, 1:1228, 1971.

Koch, J. P., and Donaldson, R. M., Jr.: A survey of food intolerance in hospitalized patients. New Eng. J. Med., 271:657, 1964.

McMaster, P. D., and Elman, R.: On the expulsion of bile by the gallbladder and a reciprocal relationship with the sphincter of Oddi. J. Exper. Med., 44:173, 1926.

Moynihan, B.: Gall stones. Brit. Med. J., 1:8, 1913.

Nakayama, F., and van der Linden, W.: Bile composition: Sweden versus Japan. Its possible significance in the difference in gallstone incidence. Amer. J. Surg., 122:8, 1971.

Price, W. H.: Gallbladder dyspepsia. Brit. Med. J., 2:138, 1963.

Salzman, E., Spurck, R. P., and Watkins, D. H.: X-ray diagnosis of bile duct calculi. Gastroenterology, 37:587, 1959.

Sampliner, R. E., Bennett, P. H., Comess, L. J., Rose, F. A., and Burch, T. A.: Gallbladder disease in Pima Indians. New Eng. J. Med., 283:1358, 1970.

Sarles, H. H., Planche, J., Lafont, H., and Gerolami, A.: Diet, cholesterol gallstones and composition of bile. Amer. J. Dig. Dis., 15:251, 1970.

Small, D. M.: Gallstones. Current Concepts. New Eng. J. Med., 279:588, 1968.

Small, D. M.: Gallstones 1971. Viewpoints on Dig. Dis., 3:3, 1971.

Small, D. M., and Rapo, S.: Source of abnormal bile in patients with cholesterol gallstones. New Eng. J. Med., 283:53, 1970.

Swell, L., Bell, C. C., Jr., and Vlahcevic, Z. R.: Relationship of bile acid pool size to biliary lipid excretion and the formation of lithogenic bile in man. Gastroenterology, 61:716, 1971.

Thistle, J. L., and Schoenfield, L. J.: Induced alterations in composition of bile of persons having cholelithiasis. Gastroenterology, 61:488, 1971.

Thistle, J. L., and Schoenfield, L. S.: Lithogenic bile among young Indian women. Lithogenic potential decreased with chenodeoxycholic acid. New Eng. J. Med., 284:177, 1971.

Valberg, L. S., Jabbari, M., Kerr, J. W., Ramchand, S., and Prentice, R. S. A.: Biliary pain in young women in the absence of gallstones. Gastroenterology, 60:1020, 1971.

Verschure, J. C. M., and Mijnlieff, P. F.: The dominating macromolecular complex of human gallbladder bile. Clin. Chim. Acta, 1:154, 1956.

Vlahcevic, Z. R., Bell, C. C., Jr., and Swell, L.: Significance of the liver in the production of lithogenic bile in man. Gastroenterology, 59:62, 1970.

Wheeler, H. O.: Flow and ionic composition of bile. Arch. Intern. Med., 108:156, 1961.

Wheeler, H. O.: Concentrating function of the gallbladder. Amer. J. Med., 51:588, 1971.

CHAPTER 30 # PATHOPHYSIOLOGY OF THE PANCREAS

FRANZ GOLDSTEIN

ASPECTS OF NORMAL ANATOMY AND PHYSIOLOGY

The pancreas is a large intra-abdominal digestive gland, located retroperitoneally, its head surrounded by the bend of duodenum and its body extending transversely and slightly upward along the posterior wall of the stomach and toward the vicinity of the hilum of the spleen where its tail is located. The human pancreas weighs about 85 to 100 grams. Functionally, it is divided into two major parts: an endocrine portion confined to the islets of Langerhans, and an exocrine portion consisting of glandular acini, intercalated and larger collecting ducts eventually leading to the duodenum by way of the two major ducts of Wirsung and Santorini. Life without the pancreas is possible but barely so and only with complex replacement therapy of both endocrine and exocrine secretions. The endocrine portion, elaborating insulin and glucagon under normal conditions and occasionally other humoral agents such as gastrin from islet tumors, is discussed elsewhere.

The exocrine pancreas is further subdivided according to function. Pancreatic fluid is secreted primarily by cells lining the intercalated and smaller collecting ducts, whereas the acinar cells are the site of enzyme production. From 800 to 3000 cc. of pancreatic juice is secreted daily in man. While isosmotic with plasma, pancreatic juice may contain bicarbonate in concentrations up to 150 mEq. per L., with chloride concentrations dropping in inverse proportion. Other ions tend to be closely related to their corresponding plasma concentrations. The high bicarbonate concentration renders pancreatic juice the most alkaline secretion in the body and constitutes the major buffering system to neutralize gastric hydrochloric acid. In normal individuals, bicarbonate concentration rises with increasing rate of secretion, but this relationship is disturbed in pancreatitis. Fluid and bicarbonate secretion are stimulated chiefly by the hormone secretin, released from duodenal and proximal jejunal mucosa upon contact with acid, peptones, fatty and amino acids, and even water but apparently not with carbohydrates. With the exception of acid the same stimuli, particularly fats, trigger the release from upper intestinal mucosa of cholecystokinin-pancreozymin, the major hormonal stimulant of pancreatic enzyme secretion. Nervous stimuli, mediated through both vagal and local reflexes, appear to integrate further pancreatic function. Recent investigations have shown that nicotine inhibits pancreatic fluid and electrolyte, but not enzyme, secretion, both by direct action on the pancreas and by decreasing the endogenous release of secretin from duodenal mucosa.

The acinar cells constitute a sack of enzymes, accounting for the fact that 20 per cent of the dry weight of pancreas is enzyme protein. The pancreas has 13 times the protein-producing capacity of the liver and reticuloendothelial system combined despite its disproportionately smaller weight. The rate of enzyme production is high; studies with labeled amino acids have shown that enzyme molecules can be synthesized in 1 to 3 minutes. The main known "exportable" pancreatic enzymes are trypsinogen and chymotrypsinogens A and B, procarboxypeptidases A and B, phospholipase A, several ribonucleases, elastase, possibly collagenase, and, of course, amylase and lipase. All these enzymes are proteins and many details of their structure are known. They are synthesized in ribosomes, concentrated, and packaged into zymogen granules in the vacuoles of the Golgi area. Phospholipids play an important role in the transport of zymogen granules into the cavities of the endoplasmic reticulum and across the plasma membrane into the intercalated ducts. Most of the enzymes are produced and stored in their precursor forms. For additional protection against premature activation, several protease inhibitors are known to be present within acinar cells. In addition, the cells produce lysosomal hydrolases which have an as yet undefined role in the pathogenesis of pancreatic inflammation. Another important enzyme heavily concentrated in the pancreas is kallikrein, present in lower concentrations in many other body tissues. This enzyme, secreted in inactive form, is activated by Factor XII (Hageman); its active form cleaves one of the widely available plasma alpha-globulin kininogens at a lysyl-arginine bond to produce an active kinin. Pancreatic kallikrein is known to produce lysyl-bradykinin, a peptide variation of 10 amino acids. All kinins, in nanogram quantities, have profound effects on small blood vessels and can induce by themselves the cardinal features of inflammation, i.e., vasodilation, capillary permeability, leukotaxis, and pain. The role of kallikrein in pancreatitis has only recently been widely appreciated.

Pancreatic enzymes hydrolyze complex foodstuffs (e.g., starches, triglycerides, proteins) into smaller components including disaccharides and peptides, which either can be absorbed as such or are further broken down by intestinal brush border disaccharidases and peptidases before being absorbed. Pancreatic exocrine secretions appear to have effects also on iron and vitamin B_{12} absorption, but these effects are less clear and not fully explained as yet. Impaired absorption of B_{12} is encountered in a significant number of patients with exocrine pancreatic insufficiency.

PANCREATITIS

Pancreatitis or inflammation of the pancreas is the most common, most complex, and most interesting disease of the pancreas. Despite great advances made in research into the mechanisms of pancreatitis, its pathogenesis remains incompletely understood. It is important to differentiate between the etiologic factors, many but not all of which are known; the chemical nature and pathology of the disease, which are reasonably well understood; the pathogenesis of pancreatitis, which remains least well understood; and the complex clinical manifestations of pancreatitis and their mechanisms.

Two major causes account for approximately 50 to 90 per cent of cases of pancreatitis in this country: alcoholism and gallstones. Approximately 5 to 50 per cent of cases are caused by a wide variety of other known causes, including infection due to mumps and coxsackie viruses, trauma, a variety of metabolic disturbances such as hyperlipemia and hypercalcemia, various drugs acting either through direct toxicity or through hypersensitivity, and probably immunologic and vascular factors. Table 30–1 lists many of the known etiologic agents in pancreatitis. Most larger groups of patients with pancreatitis include a substantial number of cases for which the cause cannot be identified and these are therefore termed "idiopathic."

The chemical and pathologic events constituting pancreatitis reflect the effects of activated enzymes released inside the pancreas and their destructive, autolytic effects on the pancreatic tissue itself as well as on contiguous and remote structures. Amylase does not cause appreciable damage even when it leaves the cells. Lipase causes fat necrosis, denoting the formation of calcium soaps from the interaction of calcium with fatty acids liberated by the action of lipase on triglycerides. Whitish deposits of fat necrosis can be found at operation or autopsy in patients with severe pancreatitis but this alteration itself does not have any serious consequences unless it is very extensive and thus leads to severe hypocalcemia. The most severe damage is done by the release of proteolytic enzymes, but recent evidence suggests a major role also for phospholipase A.

Trypsin, sometimes referred to as the queen of pancreatic enzymes, has long been held to be the major villain in the production of pancreatic necrosis. Stored, inactive trypsinogen is activated through contact with duodenal enterokinase by splitting off a portion of its polypeptide chain. Once formed, trypsin itself further activates trypsinogen as well as other proteolytic enzyme precursors. The penetration of these activated proteases into the pancreatic tissue appears to be responsible for much of the observed edema, necrosis, nuclear pyknosis, and karyolysis. Entire acini may necrose, with hemorrhage and thrombosis supervening, indicating simultaneous damage to the vascular wall which likely is produced by elastase and collagenase.

Recently, the role of phospholipase A has been intensely investigated, especially by Creutzfeldt and Schmidt. This enzyme acts on phospholipids with resultant release of lysolecithin and related compounds which have strong cytotoxic effects. The cytotoxicity of phospholipid derivatives is in part caused by their incorporation in membrane structures which consist mainly of lecithin and cephalin. Since bile contains large amounts of lecithin, bile reflux into the pancreas may serve

TABLE 30-1 CAUSATIVE FACTORS IN PANCREATITIS

Factor or Agent	Presumed Mechanism(s) of Action
Gallstones	a, b, c
Ethyl alcohol	b, c, d
Methyl alcohol	d
Ethionine	d
L-Asparaginase	d
Obstruction of afferent loop of enterostomy	b, c, g
Ascaris lumbricoides and other parasites	a, g
Carcinoma of pancreas	a, g, b
Duodenal diverticulum	a, g, b
Surgical damage to sphincter of Oddi	b
Polyp of pancreatic duct	g
Polyp of common duct	a, b, g
Regional enteritis of duodenum	b, g
Annular pancreas	b, g
Trauma to pancreas	h
Trauma away from pancreas	i, f
Hyperparathyroidism	g, j, ?
Hypercalcemia	g, j, ?
Hyperlipidemia	g
Hemochromatosis	d
Hereditary pancreatitis	g, ?
Malnutrition	d, ?
Protein malnutrition	d, ?
Diabetic ketoacidosis	d, ?
Thiazides and sulfa drugs	d, e
Immunosuppressant drugs	d, e
Isoniazid	d, e
Adrenal corticosteroids	i, ?
ACTH	i, ?
Excessively heavy meal	c, b
Radiation injury	d, f
Vascular insufficiency	f
Postpartum state	e, b, ?, i
Postoperative state	i, ?
Multiple myeloma (see Hypercalcemia)	
Scorpion bite	d
Renal transplantation (see immunosuppressants)	
Extracorporeal circulation	f, i, ?
Mumps infection	d
Bacterial infection	d
Coxsackie and other viral infections	d
Polyarteritis, collagen disease	f, e
Carbon tetrachloride toxicity	d
Electric shock	f, ?
Idiopathic	?

Key:
(a) Blockage of common channel
(b) Duodenal reflux
(c) Obstruction-hypersecretion
(d) Direct toxicity
(e) Hypersensitivity
(f) Vascular
(g) Blockage of pancreatic duct(s)
(h) Spillage of enzymes
(i) "Stress"
(j) Inappropriate activation of enzymes
(?) Unknown

as a substrate for lysolecithin formation. Upon injecting purified phospholipase A into the pancreas in the presence of small amounts of bile, severe necrosis of pancreatic and surrounding tissue rapidly occurs. The type of coagulation necrosis induced experimentally by injecting phospholipase A into the pancreas closely resembles acute human pancreatitis.

Enzymes liberated from damaged pancreatic cells readily spread beyond the confines of the gland and find their way into the nearby lesser peritoneal sac and other surrounding structures and by way of the bloodstream may reach remote sites. Thus, lipase not only produces fat necrosis in the pancreas itself but may induce similar changes over a wide area of contiguous structures and rarely in the bone marrow or skin. Damage to muscles from the spreading of trypsin has also been noted. In some patients pancreatic damage is relatively mild and confined to edema and mild necrosis ("edematous pancreatitis"), while in other patients a cascading of events takes place with progressive spreading of the inflammatory process leading to total or near total destruction of the pancreas and severe systemic manifestations with a high mortality. This form of the disease is referred to as necrotizing or hemorrhagic pancreatitis.

In chronic pancreatitis the gland may become markedly fibrotic or atrophic, fibrosis replacing many acini. Microscopic alterations of the duct system, often filled with gelatinous material, include dilatation, hyperplasia, and squamous metaplasia. Calcium deposition may be heavy, and the islands of Langerhans may show varying degrees of degeneration or destruction.

Pathogenesis

The actual pathogenesis, or the sequence of events leading to the human disease of pancreatitis, is not completely understood. When Opie found a large gallstone lodged in the common channel formed by the common bile duct and main pancreatic duct of Wirsung in a patient who had died of pancreatitis, he thought he had solved the problem. The *common channel theory*, as basically formulated by Opie's observations, held that pancreatitis was produced by bile reflux leading to the activation of pancreatic enzymes, with a stone embedded in the common channel leading to bile reflux. Experimentally, bile reflux produces significant pancreatitis at high pressures but not at more physiologic pressures. Generally, secretory pressure in the pancreatic duct is higher than in the common bile duct and reflux of bile into the pancreatic duct would not likely occur even if a common channel were present and blocked. Many patients with pancreatitis have no common channel, the respective ducts entering the duodenum separately. It is now estimated that gallstones blocking the common channel may at most account for approximately 6 per cent of cases of acute pancreatitis, as indicated by anatomic dissections and by surgical and autopsy findings of stones embedded in a common channel.

The *obstruction-hypersecretion theory,* which until recently was most widely accepted, holds that pancreatitis results from active pancreatic secretion in the presence of ductal obstruction of any cause, leading to breaks in cell membranes and leakage of activated enzymes back into the gland. Many flaws in this theory have been detected. Ligation of the pancreatic duct in the dog with simultaneous secretin stimulation produces merely transient edema. Ligation of major pancreatic ducts in various species produces atrophy rather than pancreatitis. Organic obstruction of the pancreatic ducts is absent in the majority of patients with acute or chronic pancreatitis. Secretin tests performed in patients with chronic and even acute pancreatitis have failed to show reduced flow of pancreatic juice in most patients. Pancreatic ductal obstruction is present in a small number of patients with severe chronic pancreatitis, but this appears to be a secondary phenomenon, the result rather than the cause of the original inflammatory process.

In recent years, McCutcheon has revived interest in reflux of duodenal contents into the pancreatic duct, independent of gallstones blocking the common channel, and has thus created the *duodenal reflux theory* of pancreatitis. Such reflux would carry both duodenal juice, with its enterokinase, and bile. Two components of bile have been found to be extremely toxic to the pancreas when reflux was induced experimentally; they are lysolecithin, derived from lecithin, which has been mentioned previously, and unconjugated bile salts produced by the action of certain bacteria on bile acid conjugates. Normally, bile does not contain unconjugated bile salts. Reflux of duodenal contents into the pancreatic duct is normally prevented by a number of mechanisms: the oblique course of the duct, which bends and narrows as it passes through the layers of duodenal muscle; the constricting effect of the intestinal muscle; the sphincter of Oddi; and the transverse mucosal folds or valvules that block the entrance to the pancreatic duct. Thus, distention of the duodenum for a short time in healthy males does not cause reflux into the pancreatic duct. Various operative procedures leading to reflux through interference with normal anatomic and pressure relationships are known to lead to pancreatitis. According to McCutcheon, a variety of factors in individual patients may lead to reflux of duodenal contents into the pancreatic duct: increased intraduodenal pressure and a normal papilla of Vater; normal intraduodenal pressure and a relaxed sphincter of Oddi; or relatively low intraduodenal pressure and a damaged papilla of Vater. It remains unexplained why reflux may and does occur at times without inducing pancreatitis and what it is that leads to pancreatitis in other instances of reflux. Numerous toxic substances, derivatives of heme pigments, bacterial metabolites, increased pressure, and so on have been suggested in explanation, but in individual patients the actual sequence of events and causative factors frequently remain unexplained.

Alcoholic Pancreatitis

Since ethyl alcohol is a definite etiologic factor in a large percentage of patients with pancreatitis, the most common etiologic factor in some parts of the world, various hypotheses have been advanced to explain its effects. Alcohol stimulates pancreatic secretion primarily by way of stimulating gastric acid secretion, which in turn is a potent stimulant of secretin release. Alcohol may also stimulate the release of gastrin and further add to the acid-secretin mechanism. Alcohol has been claimed to induce pancreatic ductal obstruction but the evidence is less clear. Presumably, alcohol may induce duodenitis, edema, and spasm at the sphincter of Oddi, with resultant partial obstruction to the outflow of pancreatic juice. McCutcheon suggests that alcohol predisposes to reflux of duodenal contents by producing edema of the papillary region or atony of the sphincter. The evidence for any of the preceding sequences is not entirely convincing.

Alcohol appears also to have direct toxic effects on the pancreas. Subnormal responses of volume, bicarbonate concentration, and amylase output were found in about half the patients drinking more than 1 quart of whiskey per day for a prolonged period of time. Mezey and coworkers demonstrated that these abnormalities in pancreatic function returned to normal in about three weeks with adequate diet while the subjects continued to drink alcohol. These observations illustrate a complex interaction between alcohol and malnutrition. In the rat, prolonged alcohol ingestion produces deposition of fat, injury to the mitochondria, and occasional focal death of pancreatic cells, changes similar to those induced by alcohol in liver cells. Perhaps the rapidly metabolizing cells of the pancreas show a particular susceptibility to the effects of ethanol. Since ethyl alcohol produces direct toxic actions on other actively metabolizing tissues, it is likely that its actions on the pancreas have a similar basis, perhaps by interfering with nucleic acid metabolism. Perhaps there is a similarity to the mechanism of pancreatitis induced by ethionine, a metabolic antagonist of methionine, an amino acid avidly taken up by pancreatic acinar cells for incorporation in enzyme synthesis. Similarly, the administration of L-asparaginase, a chemotherapeutic agent interfering with amino acid synthesis, frequently induces pancreatitis.

Recent electron microscopic investigations of Darle et al. demonstrate that chronic ingestion of alcohol indeed has a direct toxic effect on the acinar cell. Whether this finding is related to plugs found in the ductules and acini in chronic human pancreatitis by Sarles et al. is unknown. Methyl alcohol, when ingested accidentally or otherwise, has a tendency to cause damage to the pancreas; severe pancreatitis is a consistent feature in patients dying of methanol toxicity.

Pathogenetic Considerations in Other Etiologic Forms of Pancreatitis

The great variety of other known infectious, metabolic, and mechanical causes of pancreatitis makes it unlikely that a single pathogenetic chain of events could ever be successfully forged. Presumably, a direct toxic effect on the pancreas is exerted by viral agents known to cause pancreatitis. The role of vascular insufficiency in the pathogenesis of pancreatitis has been known for over 20 years, thanks to the experiments of Popper and Necheles, who demonstrated that under proper experimental conditions impaired blood supply to the pancreas could convert a mild edematous to a severe hemorrhagic pancreatitis. It is likely that pancreatitis in older people with a compromised mesenteric circulation may be correspondingly more severe, given a relatively mild stimulus.

The association of pancreatitis with parathyroid adenoma and hyperparathyroidism and its relationship to pancreatic calcinosis is particularly intriguing. Between 6.5 and 10 per cent of patients with hyperparathyroidism develop pancreatitis. The postulated mechanisms have included obstruction of pancreatic ducts by calcium stones, inappropriate activation of trypsin by calcium in pancreatic cells, and secondary vasculitis within the pancreas. Banks has recently reviewed the evidence critically and found it to be inconclusive. About 25 to 45 per cent of patients with pancreatitis associated with hyperparathyroidism develop parenchymal calcinosis or ductal stones. Such stones are also seen in patients with alcohol pancreatitis and hereditary pancreatitis but rarely with pancreatitis associated with biliary tract disease. Calcinosis with severe pancreatitis has been reported in a high percentage of patients studied in India with other aspects reflecting severe acinar damage combined with ductal obstruction.

Hereditary pancreatitis, which appears to be transmitted as an autosomal dominant trait, is also associated with pancreatic calcifications in 40 to 50 per cent of cases. In the hereditary form of pancreatitis there has also been noted an association with amino aciduria, but this has not been confirmed in recent cases. While the prognosis in most of the hereditary cases is better than average, in some patients fatal complications have developed. The mechanism of pancreatitis in this form of disease is entirely unknown. Patients with familial hyperlipidemia may manifest recurrent pancreatitis, also without an established mechanism. Idiopathic familial hyperlipemia with hypertriglyceridemia occasionally antedates attacks of pancreatitis, whereas alcoholic pancreatitis not infrequently is followed by hyperlipemia with predominantly type IV lipoprotein electrophoretic patterns (see p. 852).

Postoperative pancreatitis may be explained by direct trauma to the pancreas resulting in enzyme leakage but occasionally operations are performed far away from the pancreas, with pancreatitis following for unexplained reasons. Stress and the release of corticotropin have been invoked, supported by the observation that the administration of corticotropin and adrenal corticosteroids may produce pancreatitis in animals and man. Pancreatitis may develop in association with pregnancy, especially in the immediate postpartum period. This form of pancreatitis carries a high mortality. Because of the known alterations in immune responses manifested by women during the parturition period, immunologic mechanisms are suspected to play a role in this form of pancreatitis. Allergy and hypersensitivity to a variety of drugs have been known to cause pancreatitis, and several agents have induced a necrotizing hypersensitivity angiitis in the pancreas as well as in other organs. In Trinidad, the most common cause of pancreatitis is the sting of a scorpion, presumably with direct toxicity to the pancreas from the released poison.

While most of the above remarks referred chiefly to acute pancreatitis, they are also applicable with minor qualifications to the chronic variety. In this country by far the largest percentage of patients suffering from chronic pancreatitis are alcoholics, not necessarily out-and-out drinkers. Some patients develop chronic pancreatitis with socially acceptable, noninebriating alcohol intake, presumably owing to a higher than average susceptibility possibly caused by a less than average ability to detoxify or otherwise metabolically to handle ethanol. Alcoholic pancreatitis and alcoholic hepatitis and cirrhosis do not necessarily coexist and in fact rarely do. Gallbladder disease is a rare cause of chronic pancreatitis, because most such patients are cured surgically after one or two attacks unless they succumb to their acute disease. The various metabolic causes account for a fair proportion of chronic pancreatitis, and a proportionately higher percentage of cases than in acute disease remain unexplained. Malnutrition and its extreme forms of kwashiorkor and marasmus are major causes of chronic pancreatitis and of pancreatic atrophy in some developing countries. The high rate of protein turnover in the pancreas appears to make this organ especially vulnerable to the effects of protein deprivation.

Just as the exact pathogenesis of pancreatitis is incompletely understood, so is the exact relationship of acute to chronic pancreatitis. Most observers believe that the same factors causing acute pancreatitis can also cause chronic disease and that the two forms of the disease are closely related etiologically and pathogenetically. According to the Marseilles classification adopted by a group of experts in 1963, one can distinguish between (1) acute and acute relapsing pancreatitis and (2) chronic and chronic relapsing pancreatitis. In the acute forms of the disease, restitution of the pancreatic gland to normal occurs between bouts of acute inflammation, while in the chronic forms there is irreversible and often progressive damage to the pancreas. This classification recognizes the importance of the pancreas' potential ability to regenerate even after severe acute attacks of inflammation.

Mechanisms of the Clinical Manifestations in Pancreatitis

Pain, while occasionally absent, is the most consistent manifestation in *acute pancreatitis* and often the most distressing symptom of chronic pancreatitis. The pain is generally severe and not well localized. In patients with gallstone pancreatitis the initial pain is frequently midepigastric, resembling the visceral pain of biliary colic, complete with its radiation to the back. Unlike the pain of uncomplicated biliary colic, the pain of pancreatitis tends to persist longer and tends to involve the left side and back more prominently. Patients are restless and, unlike victims of a perforated viscus, often shift around in a futile effort to find a comfortable position. Several mechanisms have been suggested to explain the various components of pancreatic pain. Initial ductal obstruction in gallstone pancreatitis undoubtedly elicits the severe visceral pain that so closely resembles biliary colic. Edema and distention of the gland are likely to cause pain by stimulation of nerve endings in the pancreatic capsule. Exudation of fluid into the lesser peritoneal sac produces local peritonitis which may well be a major cause for the frequent and prolonged back pain. Recent emphasis on kinin release has focused on another cause of the severe pain of pancreatitis. Kinins produce pain by causing arteriolar constriction, increased capillary permeability, smooth muscle spasm, and possibly direct excitation of nerve endings. Pain in pancreatitis may also be accentuated by diffuse or localized ileus, a frequent feature of severe acute pancreatitis. The pain of acute pancreatitis is difficult to control, especially since large doses of narcotics should be avoided because they can induce spasm of the sphincter of Oddi and thereby aggravate both the pancreatitis and the resultant pain. Nausea and vomiting may accompany the pain, presumably owing to reflex action resulting from any severe pain, as well as from abdominal distention and ileus.

Systemic manifestations of the inflammatory reaction, such as fever and leukocytosis, are common with severe pancreatitis. *Tenderness* is not as distinct in pancreatitis as it is in some other forms of intra-abdominal inflammatory disease, probably because of the retroperitoneal location of the pancreas and its distance from the anterior abdominal wall. When associated with cholecystitis, localized tenderness over the gallbladder may be expected. The tenderness of pancreatitis more often is of moderate severity and diffuse, more pronounced with deep palpation, and not associated with rigidity of the abdominal wall, such as is encountered in the presence of a perforated viscus and free anterior peritonitis. *Bowel sounds* may be depressed or absent in the presence of diffuse ileus, but hyperactive gurgling-type bowel sounds are occasionally present in patients with localized ileus. These sounds then emanate from the relatively normal bowel proximal to the area of localized ileus, which behaves like a segment of mechanically obstructed intestine. *Jaundice* is usually seen in gallstone pancreatitis due to obstruction by stones of both the pancreatic and the common bile ducts. In alcoholic pancreatitis, jaundice is less commonly encountered and is then usually caused by edema of the head of the pancreas encroaching upon the common bile duct, thus blocking the free flow of bile. This occurs both in acute pancreatitis, in which it is usually of relatively short duration, and in chronic disease when progressive fibrosis of the region of the pancreatic head constricts the common duct and may lead to a chronic, fluctuating, usually low-grade obstructive jaundice.

Hypovolemic shock is the most dreaded manifestation of acute pancreatitis. Several mechanisms are known to contribute to it: the loss of appreciable quantities of protein-rich exudate and blood into the area surrounding the pancreas, including the lesser peritoneal cavity, results in a contracted blood volume; the release of kinins produces vasodilation and capillary permeability; necrotic pancreatic tissue may become infected by bacteria normally circulating in blood in small numbers, producing localized abscesses and leading to gram-negative bacteremia, with release of endotoxins and their disastrous effects on blood pressure; the severe necrosis of pancreatic tissue may erode into the stomach or duodenum and lead to massive hemorrhage, a rare but ominous complication of pancreatitis. Rarely, acute pancreatitis is ushered in by severe diabetes and *diabetic ketoacidosis* that can lead to coma and shock. Measures designed to counteract the shock of pancreatitis include replacement of blood, plasma, and other colloid substances; maintenance of fluid and electrolyte balance; antibiotic coverage against gram-negative bacteria; and other supportive measures including insulin and vasoconstrictor substances. In extreme situations steroids should be tried, but their potentially harmful effects and their known ability to induce pancreatitis must be weighed before deciding on their use.

Severe acute pancreatitis may lead to *hypocalcemia*, presumably because of the large amounts of calcium deposited in areas of fat necrosis, and possibly also because of release of corticotropin and adrenal corticosteroids with their hypocalcemic effects. Hypocalcemia in acute pancreatitis indicates massive necrosis and constitutes a poor prognostic sign proportional to the depth of the hypocalcemia. It rarely proceeds to tetany, however, which is more common in severe chronic alcoholic pancreatitis. In that situation calcium losses may be prolonged, leading to depletion of body calcium stores and to osteomalacia. Secondary hyperparathyroidism may ensue. The calcium losses in chronic pancreatitis are caused chiefly by fecal excretion of calcium bound to unabsorbed fatty acids in the form of soaps as well as by frequent avitaminosis D and resultant impairment of calcium absorption.

Ascites may accompany acute and sometimes chronic pancreatitis, occasionally associated with pleural effusions on the left or right sides or both. Presumably, fluid from the injured pancreas leaks into the peritoneal and hence into the pleural cavities by way of lymphatic channels crossing the diaphragm. This fluid is characterized by very high amylase activities, considerably higher than simultaneously measured serum amylase activity. In nonpancreatic fluid effusions, amylase values closely approximate normal serum amylase levels. When bloody fluid of pancreatic origin leaks from the retroperitoneal spaces into subcutaneous tissue, it may produce a reddish ecchymotic discoloration around the umbilicus known as Cullen's sign, or it may extend into the groin and flank areas, producing the Grey-Turner sign.

Distant fat necrosis rarely occurs in pancreatitis but may produce bone lesions as well as subcutaneous nodules resembling the lesions of erythema nodosum and of Weber-Christian disease. Arthritis may accompany the manifestations of subcutaneous fat necrosis.

Acute pancreatitis may mimic myocardial infarction with its severe pain involving the epigastric region, its shock, and even its *electrocardiographic changes*. The latter, if present in pancreatitis, usually are nonspecific and involve the ST-T complex, resulting from hypotension, shock, or electrolyte imbalance, and are often indicative of *coronary insufficiency*. Occasionally, a myocardial infarction, especially of the subendocardial type, may be induced by acute pancreatitis in an older person with an already compromised coronary circulation. Acute *renal failure* also occurs in severe acute pancreatitis, presumably also secondary to hypotension and reduced renal blood flow or secondary to general "toxicity."

Abnormalities in *blood coagulation* have long been observed in both acute and chronic pancreatitis as well as in pancreatic neoplasm. Trypsin-like proteolytic activity has been found in the blood of patients with acute pancreatitis, attributed to release of proteolytic enzymes from necrotic pancreatic tissue. Increased proteolytic activity has been described in association with defibrination, accelerated use of fibrinogen, and other coagulation factors in patients with acute pancreatitis. Thromboembolic complications have been noted in various pancreatic disorders, including pancreatitis, attributed both to altered clotting factors and to mechanical pressure of an enlarged gland on the retroperitoneal venous trunks. Low molecular weight dextran has been used in recent years in an effort to help control the vascular and thrombotic factors in pancreatitis. This substance with its antithrombotic action is believed to prevent both stasis and the formation of hemagglutination thrombi in the pancreatic microcirculation. Its use in dogs with experimentally produced hemorrhagic pancreatitis has markedly reduced mortality and morbidity. In human pancreatitis, low molecular weight dextran has not been used extensively enough to judge its effect.

The protean manifestations of acute pancreatitis are rounded out by manifestations of *acute psychosis,* including transient hallucinations, delusions, agitation, and disorientation. In patients with alcoholic pancreatitis these manifestations may be difficult to separate from those of acute alcoholic encephalopathy. The cause of these mental aberrations is not at all clear. Psychiatric disturbances have long been noted in patients with pancreatic carcinoma and chronic pancreatitis and remain equally poorly understood.

Most of the manifestations of *chronic pancreatitis,* including pain, have already been discussed, and except for their chronicity or recurrence they do not differ from those of acute pancreatitis. However, with repeated bouts of chronic relapsing pancreatitis or in other forms of progressive pancreatic disease, a state of pancreatic insufficiency may eventually be reached. Because of its considerable functional reserve, the pancreas may continue to deliver sufficient enzymes and hormones to meet the body's requirements until 80 to 90 per cent of its glandular acini and insulin-producing islets are destroyed.

Exocrine pancreatic insufficiency is manifested chiefly by fatty stools, steatorrhea, azotorrhea, and eventual weight loss. The stool in pancreatic insufficiency typically looks oily on the surface and remains formed or semiformed, in contrast to the amorphous, more liquid stool in sprue. Microscopically, the stool contains stainable fat globules and striated meat fibers indicative of impaired digestion and absorption of fats and meat proteins, respectively.

Endocrine pancreatic insufficiency leads to a form of diabetes mellitus. Recent immunoassay measurements of insulin suggest that patients with pancreatic diabetes have decreased serum levels of insulin in the fasting state and a diminished response to various insulin stimuli, such as the infusion of glucose, intravenous tolbutamide, glucagon, or secretin. Because alpha-cell function is also disturbed in patients with advanced pancreatic insufficiency, glucagon secretion is diminished, resulting in impaired homeostasis and a relatively brittle form of diabetes, even though the insulin requirements tend to be lower than in many patients with idiopathic diabetes mellitus. The manifestations of chronic pancreatic insufficiency due to chronic pancreatitis can nevertheless be controlled reasonably well by the judicious use of insulin and by supplements of pancreatic extract containing high concentrations of pancreatic enzymes. These must be administered just before or with meals to be available when food reaches the small intestine. In patients with preserved gastric acid secretion, pancreatic enzymes must be given together with bicarbonate or other antacids to protect the administered enzyme from the destructive effects of gastric hydrochloric acid. Pancreatic enzymes not only are inactive in an acid pH but can be irreversibly destroyed by acid. In patients with pancreatic insufficiency, both enzyme and bicarbonate secretion are severely impaired, the latter normally constituting a major buffering system against gastric acid.

Diagnostic Aspects in Pancreatitis

Because pancreatitis can present with such a variety of clinical manifestations, it often presents diagnostic difficulties. Until the use of serum amylase measurements became widespread after World War II, the diagnosis of acute pancreatitis was rarely made, and then mostly at operation or autopsy. With greater awareness of the clinical spectrum of pancreatitis and a better understanding of its pathogenetic mechanisms, the present-day clinician more often correctly suspects the presence of acute or chronic pancreatitis and has available the laboratory means of confirming, or excluding, his diagnostic impressions.

The major requirements for confirming the diagnosis of acute pancreatitis are increases in serum amylase and lipase activities. These usually begin shortly after the onset of the disease, often when the patient is first seen with abdominal pain. Amylase values tend to occur and disappear slightly earlier than lipase values, but the differences in these time relationships are not as great as some older texts would have one believe. In most instances serum amylase and lipase activities remain elevated for several days and occasionally they remain high for weeks. When prolonged beyond 10 days, serum enzyme elevations suggest the presence of pancreatic cysts or abscesses. The height of the elevation in serum enzymes, especially amylase, does not necessarily bear a direct relationship to the severity of the inflammatory process, but prolonged high enzyme activities tend to suggest a more severe process. On the other hand, when severe necrosis of the pancreas has occurred, not enough enzyme may remain to be released and to produce high serum levels. Very high enzyme levels are often encountered in stone pancreatitis, because of the suddenness of onset and the intactness of the previously uninjured pancreas.

In chronic relapsing alcoholic pancreatitis, severe disease may be accompanied by only moderate enzyme elevations. Renal function and renal clearance rates affect serum enzyme activities, since the enzymes are excreted through the kidneys after entering the bloodstream. Thus, misleadingly high amylase levels are occasionally found in the serum of patients with renal failure.

In recent years another important aspect of serum amylase measurements has been elucidated. Normal amylase has a molecular weight of about 50,000, is not bound to any serum proteins, and is easily cleared by renal glomerular filtration. In some patients with persistent serum amylase elevations, macromolecular complexes of amylase bound to several globulins of 7S, 11S, and even 19S classes, unable to be cleared through the kidneys, have been found. This condition, termed macroamylasemia, is characterized by persistently high serum amylase activities, low or absent amylase activities in urine, and absence of clinical manifestations of pancreatitis. It is unrelated to pancreatitis and has to be differentiated from it. In acute pancreatitis, high urinary amylase activities are consistently encountered, unless renal function is severely impaired. Urinary amylase measurements are preferred by some in the diagnosis of acute pancreatitis, but they are subject to wide fluctuations in normal persons, thus limiting their practical usefulness. Serum measurements of other pancreatic enzymes have not proved to be of diagnostic value. Serum calcium measurements have already been mentioned as signifying the presence of severe necrotizing pancreatitis in the appropriate clinical setting. Other serum enzyme elevations occur in pancreatitis, including SGOT, LDH, and alkaline phosphatase, but they have no specific diagnostic value and reflect associated phenomena pertaining chiefly to impairment of liver function or hepatic ductal obstruction.

Serum amylase elevations occur in conditions other than pancreatitis, including mumps with or without pancreatic involvement, perforated duodenal ulcer, intestinal obstruction, and ruptured tubal pregnancy. Elevations greater than three times the upper limit of normal serum amylase activities occur rarely in these conditions. Lipase values are of greater specificity, but lipase measurements are more time-consuming to perform, not always available on an emergency basis, and subject to more laboratory error.

Blood glucose levels or glucose tolerance tests may be abnormal in acute pancreatitis but only in very severe situations, and they obviously are not specific indicators of pancreatitis but merely reflect possible effects of pancreatitis on glucose metabolism.

The confirmation of the diagnosis of chronic pancreatitis is also heavily dependent on laboratory findings. While serum enzyme activities may be elevated in chronic relapsing pancreatitis, they are normal, and hence of little value, in the majority of patients with chronic pancreatitis. Low serum amylase levels are not a diagnostic finding in chronic pancreatic disease, possibly because the normal serum amylase activity is at least in part derived from sources other than the pancreas. Since chronic pancreatitis by definition leads to destruction of pancreatic tissue and hence to impaired pancreatic function, measurements of pancreatic function are important in this diagnosis. Several modifications of tests depending upon analysis of duodenal contents after stimulating the pancreas either with a test meal, or with secretin alone, or combined with pancreozymin are available for this purpose. The simplest and most widely used of these is the secretin test in which volume and bicarbonate concentration of pancreatic juice after secretin stimulation are measured. Varying degrees of impairment in pancreatic function may be encountered in chronic pancreatic disease of all types. Pancreatic insufficiency is indicated by marked impairment in pancreatic function as measured by the various parameters of the secretin test as well as by impaired digestion and absorption of food, clinically marked by frequent diarrhea and steatorrhea and most readily quantitated by fecal fat measurements. Measurements of pancreatic enzymes in duodenal aspirates after pancreozymin stimulation appear to raise the sensitivity of the secretin test, but perhaps not enough to justify the increased complexity and expense of the added measurements for routine clinical purposes. On the other hand, Lundh, in Sweden, has advocated measurements of duodenal trypsin concentrations alone after a test meal as a reasonably simple and reliable method of assessing pancreatic function. Not enough experience has been accumulated to make meaningful comparisons of this technique with the more standard secretin test. Stool measurements of pancreatic enzymes have also been tried but have been of limited value in the diagnosis of chronic pancreatitis, largely because of great variability in the results among normal individuals. The total or near total absence of trypsin or chymotrypsin in the stool has been found more helpful in the diagnosis of cystic fibrosis, in which complete cessation of pancreatic secretion is not uncommon.

A variety of radiologic abnormalities can also be useful in the diagnosis of pancreatitis. In acute pancreatitis one may encounter various radiologic signs of local or general adynamic ileus, including so-called cutoff signs. Intravenous cholangiography may reveal abnormal deflections of the distal common duct by edematous or fibrotic pancreatic tissue. Edema of the head of the pancreas may cause characteristic impressions on adjacent portions of the duodenal loop as seen on upper gastrointestinal contrast studies. In chronic pancreatitis, localized or diffuse calcifications in the pancreas may be encountered. Pancreatic scanning using radioactive selenium-tagged methionine has been used for about a decade, but the method has not proved sensitive or accurate enough to gain wide acceptance. A normal scan usually indicates a normal pancreas, but abnormal scans cannot be used as proof of pancreatic disease, since many false positive scans are obtained. Angiographic visualization of the pancreas has been used primarily in the diagnosis of pancreatic neoplasm, in which its enormous value is being increasingly appreciated.

Reference has already been made to associated diabetes mellitus, impaired glucose tolerance, and insulin reserve in patients with advanced chronic pancreatitis. These are generally insensitive measures of pancreatic function and lack specificity but may be useful adjuncts in the overall diagnostic profile of patients with pancreatitis.

Therapeutic Considerations in Pancreatitis

No specific pharmacologic treatment of pancreatitis exists and that which is available is based on an understanding of the pathogenetic mechanisms in pancreatitis and efforts to counteract them. In acute pancreatitis, nasogastric suction is instituted to minimize pancreatic stimulation by way of the food-acid-secretin-pancreozymin chain of events. When eating is resumed, antacids should be given between multiple small "bland" meals. Anticholinergics are also used to minimize pancreatic secretion, but their usefulness is limited and they should not be given in the presence of ileus, which they can aggravate. Other measures have been referred to already in the discussion on pathogenesis. When such complications as pancreatic cysts and abscesses are strongly suspected or verified, surgical drainage is indicated. In chronic pancreatic insufficiency enzyme supplements, bicarbonate, and vitamins are helpful in reducing the impact of exocrine insufficiency, while insulin may be needed to control the endocrine defect.

When pain persists in chronic pancreatitis, its control can be extremely difficult. Many patients thus affected are chronic alcoholics, and every effort must be made to remove the cause of the disease, i.e., induce the patient to stop drinking.

When pancreatic ductal obstruction can be documented, e.g., by a low volume of secretion and a rise in serum levels of pancreatic enzymes after secretin stimulation, or by pancreatography recently made possible through endoscopes, surgical drainage of the distal pancreas or longitudinal pancreaticojejunostomy (Puestow operation) may prove helpful. Stones or other mechanical obstacles to the free flow of pancreatic juice should be surgically removed. However, caution must be exercised in the interpretation of cholecystograms taken early in the course of acute pancreatitis. For reasons not entirely explained, the gallbladder often does not fill on oral cholecystography during the first week or two after a bout of pancreatitis due to any cause, even in the absence of cholecystitis with or without stones. Thus, a nonfilling gallbladder should be confirmed after a suitable time interval by repeat cholecystography or cholangiography before performing cholecystectomy. Efforts to counteract enzyme activity by means of available antitrypsin or antikallikrein preparations have not stood the test of clinical trial.

CARCINOMA OF THE PANCREAS

This lesion has been increasing in frequency during the past 40 years, as documented by the American Cancer Society and other agencies gathering cancer statistics in the United States. The reasons for this increase are not apparent, but one must wonder as to what, if any, environmental and dietary factors may be responsible. At the present time deaths from pancreatic cancer in the United States exceed deaths from gastric cancer, once near or at the top of the list of all fatal carcinomas, but declining in frequency for similar unknown reasons concurrently with the increase in pancreatic cancer.

Pancreatic carcinoma, the most common type of pancreatic neoplasm, is an ominous disease. Unless the lesion arises in the main duct or ampullary region, representing in effect an ampullary lesion and giving rise to early jaundice, symptoms usually do not arise until the tumor has spread to adjacent lymph nodes and more distal structures by both lymphatic and blood routes. The pancreas is surrounded by many lymphatic and venous channels draining into numerous medium-sized and larger vessels in all directions, making localization of tumor spread difficult. For these and other reasons, cures of pancreatic carcinomas are rare. The "earliest" symptoms of pancreatic carcinoma may be anorexia, vague but distressingly persistent epigastric and back pain, early satiety, weight loss, abdominal distention caused by ascites, jaundice, and occasionally fatty stools. The pain tends to get more severe as time progresses, tends to persist day and night, prevents patients from sleeping, and is often partially relieved by leaning forward or assuming the fetal position. This posture is thought to relieve pressure on nerve structures adherent to the pancreas. It is a frequent clue to the correct diagnosis.

Presumably because of the intensity and duration of the pain, and possibly due to unknown biochemical factors, patients with pancreatic carcinoma have often developed psychiatric disturbances, including psychotic manifestations. Before this association was recognized, and possibly even now, such patients have not infrequently been referred to mental hospitals for shock treatment while the primary cause of pain and associated symptoms was overlooked. Physical examination of patients with pancreatic neoplasm may detect large tumor masses, ascites, jaundice, an enlarged liver, or arterial bruits from compression of various arteries by tumor tissue. Unfortunately, all the above symptoms and signs herald far advanced tumor growth. Intensive efforts have been under way to develop more sensitive methods of detecting pancreatic carcinoma in earlier, curable stages. The secretin test combined with cytologic examination of duodenal aspirates, pancreatic photoscanning, and various radiographic examinations has long been employed. Recent progress in selective mesenteric, celiac, and smaller vessel angiography has raised hope modestly of finding operable, resectable lesions. Exciting progress has also been made in detection of gastrointestinal, including pancreatic, cancer by means of immunologic methods such as immunoassays of carcinoembryonic antigen (CEA). A high index of suspicion, early application of the most sensitive available diagnostic techniques, early laparotomy with transduodenal pancreatic needle biopsy, and cytologic examination of suspicious areas might possibly lead to earlier curative resections. Chemotherapy of pancreatic neoplasm has also been disappointing up to the present, even for purely palliative purposes.

Other tumors of the pancreas such as cystadenocarcinomas or islet cell adenomas and carcinomas are less common. Functioning islet cell adenomas and carcinomas and the rare carcinoid tumors of the pancreas are of great interest physiologically and biochemically and are discussed in detail elsewhere (see pp. 744 and 903).

CYSTIC FIBROSIS

Cystic fibrosis is the most common and most important among the hereditary and congenital disorders affecting the pancreas. It is a familial disease chiefly of infants and children, transmitted as an autosomal recessive trait predominantly among Caucasians, and is estimated to occur in approximately 1 to 2000 live births. Cystic fibrosis is a disorder of exocrine glands and affects the pancreas, lungs, paranasal sinuses, liver, gallbladder, intestinal glands, and salivary glands. The underlying molecular or metabolic cause of cystic fibrosis has not been elucidated. However, two defects stand out—abnormal electrolyte transport and physicochemical abnormalities of glycoprotein-rich secretions such as mucus. Many of the clinical symptoms and morphologic changes in affected organs are produced by obstruction of small ducts by the excessively viscid mucoid secretions.

The pancreas is the main target organ of cystic fibrosis in the gastrointestinal tract and second in importance only to chronic obstructive pulmonary disease, the latter usually determining the course and life expectancy of affected individuals. Approximately 80 per cent of patients with cystic fibrosis have practically total loss of pancreatic enzyme activity. Pancreatic dysfunction may be evidenced shortly after birth or it may occur later and be progressive in severity. Some patients maintain relatively normal secretion of pancreatic enzymes following stimulation with pancreozymin while manifesting impaired secretion of water and bicarbonate in response to secretin stimulation. It has been suggested that the deficiency in pancreatic fluid secretion leads to concentrated enzyme secretion as a cause for the destructive changes in the pancreas, with rupture of obstructed ductules and destruction of acini. Diabetes mellitus is rare in cystic fibrosis but occurs in relatively older patients, i.e., late adolescents, with severe cystic fibrosis.

Pancreatic insufficiency in patients with cystic fibrosis is similar to pancreatic insufficiency of other causes, but because it affects children, it frequently leads to stunted physical growth unless adequate pancreatic replacement therapy is instituted early. Patients tend to have a good appetite, yet may manifest diarrhea, steatorrhea and azotorrhea, abdominal distention, poor muscle tone, and vitamin deficiencies. The latter have been seen less frequently in recent years because of the widespread use of water-miscible vitamins in infant formulas and supplements. In inadequately treated patients, deficiencies of various fat-soluble vitamins, demineralization of bones, secondary hyperparathyroidism, and osteomalacia may occur.

The diagnosis of cystic fibrosis in children has been facilitated by the sweat test, demonstrating markedly elevated sweat electrolyte concentrations in affected patients. Since the advent of the sweat test, measurements of pancreatic enzymes in duodenal aspirates have been used less often for diagnosis in children. Stool assays for trypsin and chymotrypsin activity are helpful in the diagnosis of cystic fibrosis because so many patients with this disease have total absence of pancreatic enzyme secretion and hence have no pancreatic enzyme activity in stools. However, the presence of enzyme in stool does not exclude the diagnosis of cystic fibrosis.

Replacement of pancreatic enzymes, water-miscible multivitamin preparations, and adequate diet are reasonably effective ways to correct the pancreatic exocrine deficiency. These measures are often less effective than they are in patients with pancreatic insufficiency of other causes, presumably because a concomitant defect of intestinal mucosa is often present, related to dysfunction of intestinal glands. Intestinal dysfunction and production of abnormally viscid mucus may lead to meconium ileus at birth in from 5 to 10 per cent of infants born with cystic fibrosis. A meconium ileus equivalent having similar causes has been described in older infants and children and even adults. In the past, meconium ileus has always necessitated surgical relief but recently some success has been had with the use of enemas containing pancreatic enzymes, mucolytic substances, or Gastrografin, a water-soluble x-ray contrast medium.

Whether cystic fibrosis can first manifest itself in adult life remains debatable. Some case reports making such claims have appeared in the literature, basing the diagnosis on concomitant pancreatic insufficiency and chronic pulmonary disease as well as abnormal sweat tests. However, the sweat test in adults does not offer clear-cut differentiation between normal and abnormal individuals, and the association of pulmonary and pancreatic disease may be coincidental in any given patient.

REFERENCES

Achord, J. L., and Gerle, R. D.: Bone lesions in pancreatitis. Amer. J. Dig. Dis., 11:453, 1966.

Albrink, M. J., and Klatskin, G.: Lactescence of serum following episodes of acute alcoholism and its probable relationship to acute pancreatitis. Amer. J. Med., 23:26, 1957.

Ammann, R. W., Tagwercher, E., Kashiwagi, H., and Rosenmund, H.: Diagnostic value of fecal chymotrypsin and trypsin assessment for detection of pancreatic disease. Amer. J. Dig. Dis., 13:123, 1968.

Anderson, M. F., Davison, S. H. H., Dick, A. P., et al.: Plasma insulin in pancreatic disease. Gut, 11:524, 1970.

Bagdade, J. D.: Diabetic lipaemia complicating acute pancreatitis. Lancet, 2:1041, 1969.

Banks, P. A.: Acute pancreatitis. Gastroenterology, 61:382, 1971.

Berk, J. E., Kizu, H., Wilding, P., and Searcy, R. L.: Macroamylasemia. New Eng. J. Med., 277:941, 1967.

Bock, O. A. A., Bank, S., Marks, I. N., et al.: Effect of propantheline bromide upon exocrine pancreatic secretion. Gastroenterology, 55:199, 1968.

Boijsen, E., and Tylen, U.: Angiography in diagnosis. Clin. Gastroent., 1:85, 1972.

Brooks, F. P.: Testing pancreatic function. New Eng. J. Med., 286:300, 1972.
Burch, G. E., Tsui, C. Y., Harb, J. M., and Colcolough, H. L.: Pathologic findings in the pancreas of mice infected with coxsackievirus B4. Arch. Intern. Med., 128:40, 1971.
Burton, P., Evans, D. G., Harper, A. A., et al.: A test of pancreatic function in man based on the analysis of duodenal contents after administration of secretin and pancreozymin. Gut, 1:111, 1960.
Carone, F. A., and Liebow, A. A.: Acute pancreatic lesions in patients treated with ACTH and adrenal corticoids. New Eng. J. Med., 257:690, 1957.
Chey, W. Y., Shay, H., and Nielsen, O. F.: Diagnosis of diseases of the pancreas and biliary tract. J.A.M.A., 198:167, 1966.
Choi, H. J., Goldstein, F., Wirts, C. W., and Menduke, H.: Normal duodenal trypsin values in response to secretin-pancreozymin stimulation with preliminary data in patients with pancreatic disease. Gatroenterology, 53:397, 1967.
Colman, R. W., Mason, J. W., and Sherry, S.: The kallikreinogen-kallikrein enzyme system in human plasma. Assay of components and observations in disease states. Ann. Intern. Med., 71:763, 1969.
Creutzfeldt, W., and Schmidt, H.: Aetiology and pathogenesis of pancreatitis (current concepts). Scand. J. Gastroent., 5(Suppl. 6):47, 1970.
Darle, N., Ekholm, R., and Edlund, Y.: Ultrastructure of the rat exocrine pancreas after long-term intake of ethanol. Gastroenterology, 58:62, 1970.
Davidson, P., Costanza, D., Swieconek, J. A., and Harris, J. B.: Hereditary pancreatitis. A kindred without gross aminoaciduria. Ann. Intern. Med., 68:88, 1968.
di Sant'Agnese, P. A., and Talamo, R. C.: Pathogenesis and physiopathology of cystic fibrosis of the pancreas. New Eng. J. Med., 277:1287, 1967.
Dreiling, D. A.: Investigation of pancreatic function. In Beck, I. T., and Sinclair, D. G. (Eds.): The Exocrine Pancreas. London, Churchill Ltd., pp. 154–163.
Eaton, S. B., Fleischli, D. J., Pollard, J. J., et al.: Comparison of current radiologic approaches to the diagnosis of pancreatic disease. New Eng. J. Med., 279:389, 1968.
Editorial: Vascular factors in acute pancreatitis. Lancet, 2:830, 1969.
Gambill, E. A.: Pancreatitis associated with pancreatic carcinoma: A study of 26 cases. Mayo Clin. Proc., 46:174, 1971.
Geokas, M. C., van Lancker, J. L., Kadell, B. M., and Machleder, H. I.: Acute pancreatitis (U.C.L.A. Conference). Ann. Intern. Med., 76:105, 1972.
Goldberg, D. M., and Wormsley, K. G.: The interrelationships of pancreatic enzymes in human duodenal aspirate. Gut, 11:859, 1970.
Goldstein, F., Wirts, C. W., Cozzolino, H. J., and Menduke, H.: Secretin tests of pancreatic and biliary tract disease. Arch. Intern. Med., 114:124, 1964.
Greipp, P. R., Brown, J. A., and Gralnick, H. R.: Defibrination in acute pancreatitis. Arch. Intern. Med., 76:73, 1972.
Hadorn, B.: Diseases of the pancreas in children. Clin. Gastroent., 1:125, 1972.
Iber, F. L.: Alcohol and the gastrointestinal tract. Gastroenterology, 61:120, 1971.
Janowitz, H. D.: Pancreatic secretion. Physiology for physicians. 2:1, 1964.
Jorpes, J. E.: The isolation and chemistry of secretin and cholecystokinin. Gastroenterology, 55:157, 1968.
Kalser, M. H., Leite, C. A., and Warren, W. D.: Fat assimilation after massive distal pancreatectomy. New Eng. J. Med., 279:570, 1968.
Kellermeyer, R. W., and Graham, R. C., Jr.: Kinins—possible physiologic and pathologic roles in man. New Eng. J. Med., 279:754, 1968.
Konturek, S. J., Dale, J., Jacobson, E. D., and Johnson, L. R.: Mechanisms of nicotine induced inhibition of pancrcatic secretion of bicarbonate in the dog. Gastroenterology, 62:425, 1972.
Kopel, F. B.: Gastrointestinal manifestations of cystic fibrosis. Gastroenterology, 62:483, 1972.
Legge, D. A., Hoffman, H. N., and Carlson, H. C.: Pancreatitis as a complication of regional enteritis of the duodenum. Gastroenterology, 61:834, 1971.

Levitt, M. D., Rapoport, M., and Cooperbrand, S. R.: The renal clearance of amylase in renal insufficiency, acute pancreatitis, and macroamylasemia. Ann. Intern. Med., 71:919, 1969.
Lundh, G.: Pancreatic exocrine function in neoplastic and inflammatory disease: a simple and reliable new test. Gastroenterology, 42:275, 1962.
McCutcheon, A. D.: A fresh approach to the pathogenesis of pancreatitis. Gut, 9:296, 1968.
Menguy, R. B., Hallenback, G. A., Bollman, J. L., and Grindlay, J. H.: Intraductal pressures and sphincteric resistance in canine pancreatic and biliary ducts after various stimuli. Surg. Gynec. Obstet., 106:306, 1958.
Mezey, E., Jow, E., Slavin, R. E., and Tobon, F.: Pancreatic function and intestinal absorption in chronic alcoholism. Gastroenterology, 59:657, 1970.
Mixter, C. G., Jr., Keynes, W. M., and Cope, O.: Further experience with pancreatitis as a diagnostic clue to hyperparathyroidism. New Eng. J. Med., 266:265, 1962.
Moreland, J. J., and Johnson, L. R.: Effect of vagotomy on pancreatic secretion stimulated by endogenous and exogenous secretin. Gastroenterology, 60:425, 1971.
Mullin, G. T., Caperton, E. M., Jr., Crespin, S. R., and Williams, R. C., Jr.: Arthritis and skin lesions resembling erythema nodosum in pancreatic disease. Ann. Intern. Med., 68:75, 1968.
Nothman, M. M., and Callow, A. D.: Investigations on the origin of amylase in serum and urine. Gastroenterology, 60:82, 1971.
Nusbaum, M., Baum, S., Kuroda, K., and Blakemore, W. S.: Selective mesenteric arteriography in the diagnosis of pancreatic lesions. Amer. J. Gastroent., 48:421, 1967.
Pirola, R. C., and Davis, A. E.: The sphincter of Oddi and pancreatitis. Amer. J. Dig. Dis., 15:583, 1970.
Popper, H. L., Necheles, H., and Russell, K. C.: Transition of pancreatic edema into pancreatic necrosis. Surg. Gynec. Obstet., 87:79, 1948.
Rogers, J. B., Howard, J. M., and Pairent, F. W.: Serum insulin levels in patients with chronic pancreatitis. Amer. J. Surg., 119:171, 1970.
Sarles, H., and Gerolami-Santandrea, A.: Chronic pancreatitis. Clin. Gastroent., 1:195, 1972.
Sarles, H., Lebreuil, G., Tasso, F., et al.: A comparison of alcoholic pancreatitis in rat and man. Gut, 12:377, 1971.
Schrier, R. W., and Bulger, R. J.: Steroid-induced pancreatitis. J.A.M.A., 194:176, 1965.
Schuster, M. M., and Iber, F. L.: Psychosis with pancreatitis. Arch. Intern. Med., 116:228, 1965.
Schwachman, H., and Holsclaw, D. S.: Complications of cystic fibrosis (Editorial). New Eng. J. Med., 281:500, 1969.
Shamma'a, M. H., and Rubeiz, G. A.: Acute pancreatitis with electrocardiographic findings of myocardial infarction. Amer. J. Med., 32:827, 1962.
Strum, W. B., and Spiro, H. M.: Chronic pancreatitis. Ann. Intern. Med., 74:264, 1971.
Toffler, A. H., and Spiro, H. M.: Shock or coma as the predominant manifestation of painless acute pancreatitis. Ann. Intern. Med., 57:655, 1962.
Toskes, P. P., Hansell, J., Cerda, J., and Deren, J. J.: Vitamin B_{12} malabsorption in chronic pancreatic insufficiency. New Eng. J. Med., 284:627, 1971.
Veeger, W., Abels, J., Hellemans, N., and Nieweg, H. O.: Effect of sodium bicarbonate and pancreatin on the absorption of vitamin B_{12} and fat in pancreatic insufficiency. New Eng. J. Med., 267:1341, 1962.
Weinstein, B. R., Korn, R. J., and Zimmerman, H. J.: Obstructive jaundice as a complication of pancreatitis. Ann. Intern. Med., 58:245, 1963.
White, T. T., Morgan, A., and Hopton, D.: Postoperative pancreatitis. Amer. J. Surg., 120:132, 1970.
Williams, L. F., and Byrne, J. J.: The role of bacteria in hemorrhagic pancreatitis. Surgery, 64:967, 1968.
Woods, J. E., Anderson, C. F., Frohnert, P. P., and Petrie, C. R.: Pancreatitis in renal allografted patients. Mayo Clin. Proc., 47:193, 1972.
Zamcheck, N., Moore, T. L., Dhar, P., and Kupchik, H.: Immunologic diagnosis and prognosis of human digestive-tract cancer: carcinoembryonic antigens. New Eng. J. Med., 286:83, 1972.

CHAPTER 31

NUTRITIONAL FACTORS IN DISEASE

GEORGE A. BRAY

The nutritional factors in human physiology include all the necessary as well as all the usable environmental elements taken in through the mouth. Carbohydrates, proteins, and lipids are the elements ingested in quantity, but the vitamins and minerals, although small in quantity, are of equal importance in maintenance of normal health. In this chapter, the effects of abnormal amounts of these elements upon human disease will be examined. Certain aspects of biochemistry and physiology will be reviewed as they relate to the mechanisms by which deviations from normal nutrition produce their pathologic consequences.

OBESITY

Obesity is appropriately defined in terms of body fatness. In its extreme forms, obesity can be recognized at a glance. The round-jowled, puffing, often red-faced individual weighing in excess of 300 pounds is a familiar sight. However, quantitative assessment of the degree of obesity in these individuals and in lesser degrees of obesity is difficult for the physician. Neither the usual recording of body weight nor the criteria based upon weight in relation to height are sufficiently accurate in many instances. For example, above average muscle development or an unusually large skeleton could be mistaken for obesity. It is fair to say, however, that when weight exceeds the norm by more than 30 per cent in any but the most athletic male, there is almost certainly obesity, i.e., an above-normal percentage of fat.

Measurement of body weight on a scale does not distinguish between mass occurring as excess fat, as bone, as muscle, or as water, and this lack of distinction can have significant clinical implications. Obese patients often fail to lose weight and may even gain weight when put on a diet. This is usually attributed to "cheating" by the patient when it may, in fact, be the result of the wrong measurement. This can happen even when caloric intake is severely restricted, and careful measurements show that food intake is less than that required to maintain weight. This paradox is explained in terms of the oxidation of fatty acids (Fig. 31-1). This equation shows that when 256 grams of palmitic acid are completely oxidized, 288 grams of water are produced. When gaseous exchange of O_2 and CO_2 is completed, the body is left with a net gain in weight of 32 grams of water for every mole of palmitic acid which is oxidized. Until this excess water is excreted, a patient may gain weight when fatty-acids are the principal

$$\text{Chemical Structure:} \quad CH_3 - (CH_2)_{14} - COOH + 23\ O_2 \rightarrow 16\ CO_2 + 16\ H_2O$$
$$\text{(palmitic acid)}$$

Molecular Weights: 256   736   704   288

Figure 31-1 Oxidation or complete combustion of palmitic acid to CO_2 and water. During this oxidation, a compound weighing 256 g./mole is burned. Since the CO_2 and O_2 will equilibrate with the environment, 288 g. of water remain after the combustion of only 256 g. of fatty acid. This explains how the oxidation of fat can lead to the temporary accumulation of weight in individual patients.

metabolic fuel. Such a phenomenon has been observed frequently and has been known to persist for more than 30 days, even when patients have been hospitalized under strictly controlled conditions. Measuring body weight on a scale would be misleading under these circumstances, since the scale could not assess changes in the various components of the body weight. For this reason, more sophisticated techniques are necessary to understand the nature of the weight in obesity and its relation to the normal composition of the human body.

Analysis of Human Body Components

Several techniques have been used to assess the components of the human body (Table 31-1). The most direct method is analysis of individual cadavers for lipid, water, protein, and ash components. Technical difficulty in such analyses and the rarity of opportunities to obtain cadavers for this purpose have led to publication of only seven complete studies. The data from five of these analyses of total body composition are shown in Figure 31-2. Water represented just under two thirds of the total body weight. Fat and protein were at least 15 per cent of body weight. Since direct analyses cannot be performed on the living subject, three alternative methods have been used. Measurement of density of the human being is the first of these. This can be accomplished by weighing the subject in and out of water, a principle that Archimedes discovered centuries ago. It allows an assessment of the fraction of body weight which is fat and that which is nonfat. Measurement of body density has been widely applied, since it is simple and highly accurate.

The second approach to measurement of body composition in vivo is the use of isotope dilution. When a known quantity of isotope is injected into the bloodstream and its concentration is measured after allowing for equilibration with the body stores of that compound, the ratio of radioactivity in plasma to the quantity injected will give a measure of the apparent volume of distribution for the substance. Radioactively labeled water

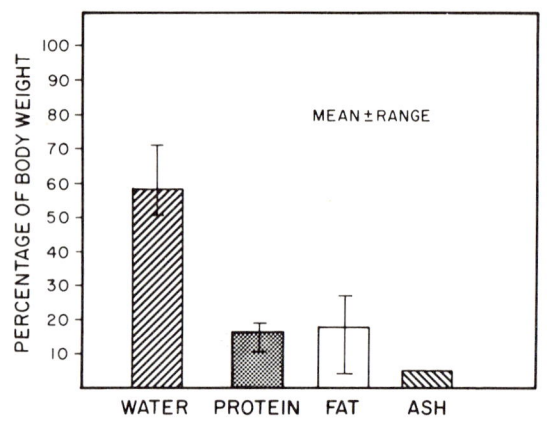

Figure 31-2 Analysis of body composition in five cadavers. The heights of individual bars are the mean for five patients, and the vertical lines represent the range. Body components are plotted as per cent of total body weight. (Adapted from Widdowson, E. M.: In Brozek, J. (Ed.): Human Body Composition: Approaches and Application. New York, Pergamon Press, 1965.)

(^3H_2O), potassium (^{42}K or ^{40}K), and sodium (^{22}Na or ^{24}Na) have been among the most widely used substances for obtaining measurements of body composition by this technique. The data from the measurements obtained by isotopic dilution are similar to those obtained using body density and direct analysis. However, measurements by isotopic dilution provide additional information, since they allow for an estimate of intra- and extracellular fluid.

Studies on humans during gain and loss of weight have provided important insights into the nature of the components which are accumulated or lost. In normal volunteers gaining 10 to 20 kg. over a period of six months, nearly two thirds of the increase in weight is fat; the remainder is extracellular fluid and cellular components. Direct measurements of the size of fat cells from such individuals have shown that the size of the fat cells has increased with weight gain. Conversely, when obese patients in a hospital lose weight, the largest fraction of the loss is fat and only small amounts of protein and fluid are lost. These data therefore illustrate the complexity of body composition and the difficulties in assigning a diagnosis of obesity based on body weight alone.

Measuring the thickness of skin folds is another approach to assessing the amount of body fat. Some have suggested that the thickness of the folds on the dorsal side of the triceps muscle midway between the olecranon process and the acromioclavicular joint should be less than 1 inch in normal subjects. Unfortunately, comparative studies failed to show that this method is more reliable than the scale. So, at present, the scale,

TABLE 31-1 TECHNIQUES FOR MEASURING "FATNESS"

A. Direct carcass analysis
B. Indirect methods
  1. Densitometric
  2. Dilutional
    a. Radioactive (^3H_2O, ^{40}K)
    b. Chemical (cyclopropane)
  3. Anthropometric
    a. Height and weight
    b. Skin folds

despite all its limitations, is the best tool available for patients and most physicians to use in determining the degree of excess weight. When this overweight is sufficiently great, i.e., 30 per cent or more above values in standard tables for height and weight (Table 31–2), one can assume that the patient is obese.

Imbalance Between Caloric Intake and Expenditure

There is little argument at present that obesity results from an excess intake of food in relation to body needs. The basis for this proposition resides in the work published in 1783 by Lavoisier and Laplace using the guinea pig. This early work was given a theoretical basis in the physical chemistry of the 19th century as the "law of the conservation of energy." That it applied to other than the guinea pig was readily shown. In classic experiments, Rubner showed that the amount of heat produced by a dog in the absence of food equals the heat from combustion of the fat and protein which were burned during starvation minus the heat of combustion in the urine. Atwater and Benedict made similar observations in man and concluded that "for practical purposes we are, therefore, warranted in assuming that the law of conservation of energy obtains in general in the living organism as indeed there is every a priori reason to believe that it must." A demonstration that this law applied to the obese subject was delayed until the 20th century. It has been amply demonstrated that obese subjects, like their lean counterparts and all other known living systems, obey the law of conservation of energy.

Measurements of the energy contained in food are expressed in calories. A calorie measures the quantity of heat required to raise the temperature of 1 gram of water by 1° between 15 and 16° C. As noted above, the quantity of heat obtained by the combustion of a foodstuff outside the body is equal to the quantity of heat obtained by combustion of the same foodstuff to the same end product. In the cases of carbohydrate and lipid, the end products are carbon dioxide and water and the heat produced during their combustion in vitro is directly related to the heat produced in vivo. Since protein is incompletely oxidized in the living organism, a correction is required. The end products of protein catabolism are carbon dioxide, water, and urea. The urea excreted in the urine represents a significant number of calories. Thus, to obtain an accurate assessment of total caloric utilization, the quantity of urea must be known.

Measurement of O_2 consumption and CO_2 production with a correction for urinary nitrogen allows an indirect quantitation of energy expenditure. This technique of indirect calorimetry (measurement of oxygen consumption and carbon dioxide production) has been widely used in assessing the caloric needs of the human organism. Figure 31–3 is a presentation of the energy expenditure for a reference man and a reference woman as estimated by the National Research Council in 1968. The male, aged 22 and weighing 70 kilos, required 2800 calories; the female, aged 22 and weighing 58 kilos, required 2000 calories. The total requirements for the reference subjects in 1968 are about 10 per cent lower than in 1963. Yet, even these current estimates are probably too high. The increased use of the automobile and decreased amount of physical activity have accounted for a steady reduction in total caloric requirements of men and women. Since these are "reference" figures, they must be modified before being applied to a given individual. Factors such as age, the degree of activity, pregnancy, and the presence of certain diseases all serve to modify energy requirements. There are convincing data that the caloric needs decline with age at approximately 5 per cent per decade. Since activity also declines, the actual caloric need declines even more rapidly. Pregnancy, as well as several hormones, can increase the body's oxygen consumption. Thyroid hormone was the first hormone shown to have a calorigenic action. In conditions of thyroid hormone excess, total energy requirements are increased, and in the absence of this hormone, total caloric requirements drop sharply. Other hormones which have a ca-

TABLE 31–2 DESIRABLE WEIGHT IN RELATION TO HEIGHT*

Height	Men Average	Men Range	Women Average	Women Range
4′ 10″			102	92–119
4′ 11″			104	94–122
5′ 0″			107	96–125
5′ 1″			110	99–128
5′ 2″	123	112–141	113	102–131
5′ 3″	127	115–144	116	105–134
5′ 4″	130	118–148	120	108–138
5′ 5″	133	121–152	123	111–142
5′ 6″	136	124–156	128	114–146
5′ 7″	140	128–161	132	118–150
5′ 8″	145	132–166	136	122–154
5′ 9″	149	136–170	140	126–158
5′ 10″	153	140–174	144	130–163
5′ 11″	158	144–179	148	134–168
6′ 0″	162	148–184	152	138–173
6′ 1″	166	152–189		
6′ 2″	171	156–194		
6′ 3″	176	160–199		
6′ 4″	181	164–204		

*Adapted from data courtesy of the Metropolitan Life Insurance Company.

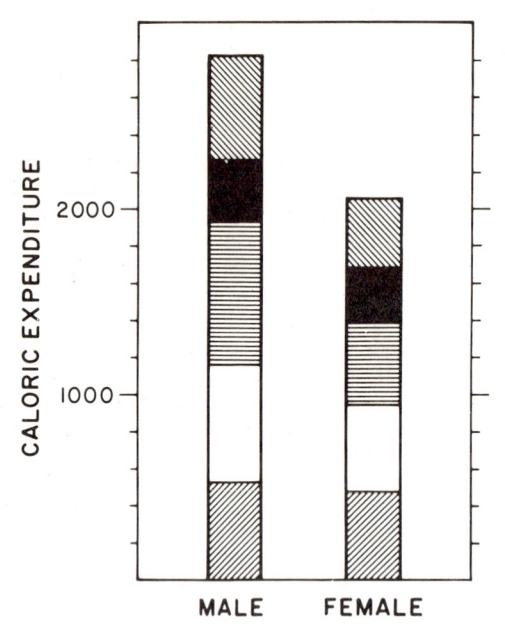

Figure 31-3 Estimated average energy expenditure of men and women. The lower hatched bars represent the energy expended during sleeping and reclining (1.0 to 1.1 kcal./min.). The unshaded open portion represents the average energy expended during sitting (1.1 to 1.5 kcal./min.). The horizontally shaded section represents the energy expenditure during standing (1.5 to 2.5 kcal./min.). The solid segment represents the energy expended during walking (2.5 to 3 kcal./min.). The top portion of each bar represents other activities (3 to 4.5 kcal./min.). The lower value within each preceding set of parentheses represents the average value for females and the upper value the average for males. (Adapted from Recommended Dietary Allowances.)

lorigenic action include the catecholamines (epinephrine and norepinephrine), human growth hormone, and the androgenic steroids.

Regulation of Food Intake

As noted earlier, obesity represents an imbalance between caloric intake and caloric expenditure. It now appears that the regulation of food intake, as well as the utilization of calories, is defective in the obese individual. This net effect appears as an increase in the efficiency for food utilization. Efficiency may be defined in a number of ways. We will consider efficiency from the point of view of food storage. The more weight gained for a given food intake, the greater the efficiency. Thus, a more efficient animal or human being will store a greater fraction of total calories ingested. That is, for every 1000 calories ingested, the efficient animal might store 20 per cent, while the inefficient animal would store only 10 per cent. This means that for the same caloric intake, it is possible for one animal to become considerably heavier and more obese than another. Such considerations have obvious commercial significance and it has been observed that animals which are bred for obesity will store a larger fraction of their calories in their carcass than lean animals. Differences in efficiency have also been noted in laboratory animals in which obesity is inherited as a recessive trait. In these obese animals, more fat will accumulate per gram of food ingested than in lean littermates. Although few measurements are available, the current data would suggest that this form of efficiency results from inactivity of the fat animal. Thus, for any given food intake, fewer calories are used for activity than in the lean animal. We must conclude that the efficiency of the fat animal may be substantially greater than for lean animals.

Control of food intake involves several factors. These include components of the central nervous system, metabolic factors, and the external environment.

Central Nervous System. The classic experiment of Hetherington and Ranson demonstrated that injury to a portion of the hypothalamus near the midline in the so-called ventromedial nucleus would consistently induce increased food intake and obesity in laboratory animals. This syndrome in experimental animals is analogous to the development of obesity noted by Fröhlich in his classic case report in 1903. Hypothalamic obesity resulting from injury to the ventromedial nucleus is accompanied by a number of alterations. The animals are consistently and uniformly hyperphagic and prefer a diet with a high fat content rather than a high carbohydrate or a high protein diet. They will avoid eating food which tastes bad or which has an unpalatable consistency. They show increased levels of insulin and enlargement of the pancreatic islets of Langerhans. Finally, these animals, though initially hyperactive following introduction of these lesions, become hypoactive, although they can easily be aroused to rage. Injury to this region of the brain is followed by a period of rapid weight gain (dynamic phase) and then by a plateau weight (static phase), at which they will again regulate their food intake and body weight. Lateral to this ventromedial nucleus is a second hypothalamic area, destruction of which leads to total, but temporary, aphagia. If animals are tube-fed following this initial injury, they will eventually begin eating again but will maintain weight at a lower level than normal. Animals with this lateral hypothalamic lesion will no longer eat in response to insulin-induced hypoglycemia but will eat in response to cold or to other metabolic stimuli. Thus, there appear to be two hypothalamic centers involved in the regulation of food intake: a ventromedial system, which is involved in controlling signals for satiety, and a lateral system, which is involved in regulating the drive for food intake. Recent studies have demonstrated that these hypothalamic centers are probably under adrenergic control. Injection of small quantities of norepinephrine into these regions will lead to feeding behavior in the fed animals, while the injection of isoproterenol will lead to inhibition of food intake. In current terminology, the regulation of food intake may be described as an alpha-adrenergic feeding center and a beta-adrenergic satiety center. These new findings have extended our understanding of the physiologic control of food intake to the cellular level.

Metabolic Factors. Metabolic factors are a second group of regulatory mechanisms for food intake. In most animals, the body fat is a fairly constant fraction of total body weight. Although there is a tendency for the human being to gain weight with increasing age, the number of calories which are stored in fat in relation to the total numbers of calories eaten is very small. This is illustrated in Figure 31-4. No more than 0.34 per cent of calories need be stored to gain 1 pound per year. The nature of the mechanism involved in providing information about the quantity of metabolic energy is unknown. Several theories have been put forward, but they are as yet too limited to provide a sufficient explanation. That the body does regulate its food intake based on metabolic stores is, however, clearly shown by two kinds of experiments. In the first, the available food is diluted with various indigestible substances such as cellulose. In normal animals, the total amount of nutritional value is maintained constant, although the quantities of diluted food that are ingested varies. A similar result has been obtained by giving part of the food by stomach tube. As the quantity of food provided through a tube is increased, the amount ingested orally is decreased. Thus, there are mechanisms by which the feeding centers discern the metabolic needs of the organism and respond by food-seeking behavior.

The External Environment. The external environment provides a third category of factors which regulate food intake. As noted above, animals with injury to the hypothalamus become finicky in what they will eat. A similar observation has been made in obese human subjects. When exposed to ice cream adulterated with small amounts of quinine, the obese patient will eat less than the lean one, though he eats much more normal ice cream. Similarly, other factors in the external environment also influence food intake. The experiments of Shachter and his colleagues have shown that the obese individual eats more when food is readily available. It appears from these and other experiments that the obese subject is more responsive to external cues than he is to metabolic cues. In contrast, the lean subject eats largely in response to metabolic needs, with external cues from taste, smell, and sight playing a much smaller role.

Caloric Storage and Utilization

Triglycerides represent the primary form of energy storage in most mammalian species (Table 31-3). Whether the excess caloric intake occurs as protein, fat, or carbohydrate seems to be of little importance. The storage form is primarily triglyceride. This has obvious advantages. A gram of triglyceride contains 9 calories. The adipocyte has about 7 to 7.5 calories per gram, with the aqueous components making up the difference. The caloric value of a gram of lean body mass, in contrast, is in the range of 1.5 calories, since approximately two thirds of this weight is fluid. Storage of carbohydrate as glycogen, though of importance as an immediate source of glucose, has the disadvantage of requiring a substantial addition of water and therefore a substantial addition of total weight relative to caloric storage. The rapid storage and subsequent utilization of large stores of triglyceride are of prime importance in two situations—the migratory bird and the hibernating mammal. Prior to the flight across the Gulf of Mexico, birds will eat enormous quantities of food and store it as fat which can be released and burned during long-distance flight. A similar mechanism is involved in energy storage for the hibernating animal.

Three mechanisms are available for the storage of excess calories as triglycerides. The triglyceride can be stored by an increase in the size of the existing fat cells. It is also possible for

$$2{,}800 \text{ cal/d} \times 365 \text{ days/year} \times 20 \text{ yrs.} = 20.5 \times 10^6 \text{ cal}$$

$$\text{Gained 20 lbs.} \times 3{,}500 \text{ cal/lb.} = 70 \times 10^3 \text{ cal}$$

$$\text{or } 0.34\% \text{ of ingested calories stored}$$

Figure 31-4 Caloric intake and expenditure to accumulate 20 pounds. This figure assumes the average caloric intake of the standard male to be 2,800 kcal./day and calculates the total number of calories expended during a period of 20 years. If 20 pounds are gained and if each pound is assumed to have 3,500 calories, only 70,000 calories, or less than 0.34 per cent of the total calories, are stored. This shows the high efficiency of the human body for regulating energy intake and expenditure over prolonged periods of time.

TABLE 31-3 METABOLIC FUELS IN MAN*

Fuel Supply	Normal Man (70 kg.)		Obese Man (140 kg.)	
Fat	15.00 kg.	141,000 kcal.	80.000 kg.	752,000 kcal.
Protein	6.00 kg.	24,000	8.000 kg.	32,000
Glycogen				
Muscle	0.12 kg.	480	0.160 kg.	640
Liver	0.07 kg.	280	0.700 kg.	280
Glucose	0.02 kg.	80	0.025 kg.	100
		165,840 kcal.		785,020 kcal.

*Adapted from Cahill, G. F., and Owen, O. E.: *In* Rowland, C. V., Jr.: Anorexia and Obesity. Boston, Little, Brown and Co., 1970.

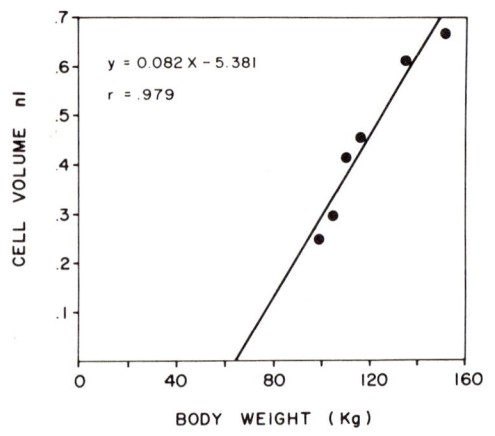

Figure 31-5 Effect of weight loss on the size of fat cells. The individual dots represent the cell volume of fat cells from one patient during a period of caloric restriction. During hospitalization, this woman lost 100 kg. and had a reduction in the size of fat cells of more than 50 per cent. Calculation of the total number of fat cells showed no change during weight loss. Thus, the loss of 100 kg. in weight had occurred entirely by a decrease in size of individual cells (Bray, G. A.: Ann. Intern. Med., 73:565, 1970.)

the number of fat cells to increase, with little or no change in the size of individual cells. Finally, it is possible for both the size and number of adipocytes to increase. The adipocyte is a highly differentiated cell which arises from a mesenchymal precursor. During the process of growth and development, a number of these precursor cells differentiate into fat cells. The mature fat cell does not divide and does not dedifferentiate into fat-free cells. Thus, once developed, the fat cell appears to remain throughout the life of the organism. In detailed studies of obesity, it has been clearly established that almost all obesity is accompanied by an increased size of fat cells. This form of adaptation to glyceride storage is probably the principal mechanism when obesity develops in adult life. In the forms of obesity which develop in early years of life, however, an increase in the total number of fat cells appears to be a major mechanism for adapting to the increased demands for triglyceride storage. Thus, individuals with gross obesity having its genesis in the early years of life accumulate an increased mass of fat cells which do not subsequently dedifferentiate, although significant amounts of weight may disappear. This has been demonstrated on a number of occasions and one such example is shown in Figure 31-5. In this individual, the size of adipocytes from the abdominal wall were measured on six occasions during a loss of 50 kg. Calculations showed no change in the total number of fat cells during this period, although the size of individual adipocytes had decreased by two thirds. By the time the patient was discharged, the fat cells had returned to the size found in normal individuals, yet body weight was still substantially above normal. This, without doubt, reflects the increased total mass of the adipose organ.

A series of biochemical reactions are involved in the formation of fatty acids and their conjugation with α-glycerophosphate (sn-glycerol-3-phosphate) to form triglycerides. Lipogenesis, i.e., the formation of fatty acids, appears to be controlled by nutritional state, by the presence of hormones, and by the size of the adipocyte. There is now substantial evidence in studies of human fat that incorporation of radioactivity into long-chain fatty acids can occur and that this process is dependent upon the nutritional state of the individual from whom the fat is obtained. Rapid formation of fatty acids is observed in adipose tissue taken from overfed patients. With caloric restriction, the rate of lipogenesis is severely depressed. Of the hormonal factors, insulin is of primary importance in controlling the rate of lipogenesis both in vivo and in vitro. The size of the adipose cell is also a determining factor in the rate of lipogenesis. With large fat cells, the rate of fatty acid synthesis is reduced. However, overfeeding for a short period of time will increase lipogenesis in large fat cells to a striking degree. The frequency with which food is ingested is a final factor which seems to be of importance in controlling lipogenesis. In experimental animals and in man, the ingestion of food in one or two large meals produces significant changes in the metabolic and biochemical function. When an individual eats a few large meals, he tends to have an impaired ability to metabolize glucose, to have a higher level of plasma cholesterol, to be more obese, and to show a greater rate of fatty acid formation in adipose tissue than is observed in individuals eating more frequent meals, but of smaller size.

The triglyceride stores in adipose tissue generally serve the body's needs during the intermeal periods. Thus, storage of carbohydrate and fatty acids in adipose tissue represents a transitory storage form for many fatty acids which are released following food ingestion. Following food ingestion, there is an increase in the output of insulin which is stimulated both by ingestion of glucose and by the presence of amino acids and, in turn, there is stimulation by gastrointestinal factors which facilitate the release of insulin. As the nutrients absorbed from the gastrointestinal tract enter the blood, the concentration of insulin is rising and this augments the storage of glucose in the liver as glycogen and of fatty acids and glucose in adipose tissue as triglycerides. As the concentration of glucose returns toward normal, there is a concomitant decline in the concentration of insulin and a return of the concentration of fatty acids toward their initial levels. This transition from the fed to the fasting state is facilitated by a reduction in insulin and may also be facilitated by the rise in growth hormone which is frequently observed 4 to 5 hours after ingesting a meal. The release of fatty acids from adipose tissue is essential to provide for the metabolic needs of peripheral tissues during the intermeal period. Studies from several laboratories originally suggested that obese patients had an impaired ability to release and utilize fatty acids. The evidence supporting this hypothesis came from two observations. First, it was observed that with fasting there was a very small rise in the concentration of free fatty acids. Second, it was observed that the injection of hormones which tend to increase free fatty acids and to enhance lipolysis in adipose tissue had less effect in obese patients than in normal subjects. This conclusion has not been supported by testing with more sophisticated techniques. Measurement of the turnover and metabolism of fatty acids has shown that obese patients release and metabolize fatty acids more rapidly than lean subjects. Supporting evidence has also come from studies of adipose tissue in vitro which have shown that the breakdown of triglycerides with the formation of free fatty acids and glycerol in vitro occurs at a higher rate with large adipose cells of the kind obtained from obese subjects, as compared with adipocytes from normal-weight subjects. Present evidence would thus suggest that the utilization of adipocyte triglycerides is normal or supernormal in obese individuals.

Endocrine Consequences of Obesity

The consequences of obesity can be divided into several groups, but we will consider only those of hormonal or metabolic origin. The most frequent endocrine change is hyperinsulinemia. Figure 31–6 shows that the level of insulin in the fasting state has a highly significant, positive correlation with the degree of obesity. The more obese an individual, the higher his fasting insulin. Similarly, the release of insulin in response to such stimuli as glucose, leucine, and tolbutamide is greater in obese individuals than in lean subjects. Thus, not only are their basal levels of insulin elevated, but output of insulin in response to several stimuli is increased. Moreover, when glucose utilization and insulin are related, the obese individual requires more insulin to stimulate the utilization of glucose than normal. This implies that obese people are resistant to insulin. Studies by Salans and his collaborators have suggested that the adipocyte may be one site for this resistance. Other studies have shown, however, that muscle membrane is also resistant to insulin. With a technique for perfusing the human forearm, it is possible to examine the response of muscle and adipose tissue simultaneously. The muscle of the obese individual behaves as does the muscle of a normal individual after hyperin-

Figure 31–6 Relation of immunoreactive insulin to body weight. Fasting levels of immunoreactive insulin have been plotted against the per cent of ideal body weight. Thus, body weight is a primary factor in determining the fasting serum insulin. (Reproduced with permission from Bagdade, J. D., et al.: J. Clin. Invest., 46:1549, 1967.)

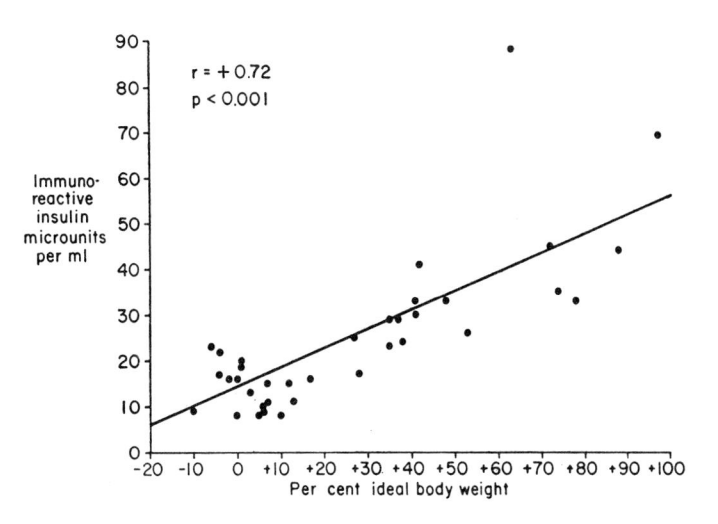

sulinemia is induced. Thus, the obese individual has an induced resistance to insulin in muscle and adipose tissue and probably liver. The physiologic and biochemical basis for this insulin resistance, however, remains to be established.

A second consistent alteration in obesity is an impaired output of growth hormone. Basal concentrations of growth hormone are normal or slightly reduced. Most striking is the impaired response to stimuli which usually increase growth hormone. The concentration of this hormone can usually be increased 4 to 5 hours after the administration of glucose orally by the induction of hypoglycemia with insulin and by the administration of arginine by the intravenous route. In the obese individual, the output of growth hormone is impaired to all these stimuli.

The third consistent alteration in endocrine function of obese subjects is the increased production rate of adrenocortical steroids. Although the concentrations of plasma cortisol remain normal, the production rate of cortisol by the adrenal gland and the excretion of its metabolites in the urine are increased in obesity.

These three endocrine adaptations are ones that would be expected from an internal milieu which favored the synthesis of fatty acid and deposition of triglycerides. It might be supposed that these endocrine alterations were causally related to obesity. However, it is possible that they are the consequence of overeating rather than a cause of corpulence. To gain insight into this question, Sims and his collaborators induced a weight gain of 30 to 40 pounds in a group of normal volunteers and studied their endocrine and metabolic responses. In all cases, the pattern of endocrine adaptation was similar to that observed in the patients with spontaneous obesity. That is, normal volunteers who gained weight by overeating demonstrated hyperinsulinemia, a reduced output of growth hormone in response to arginine, and increased production of cortisol by the adrenal gland. They also demonstrated insulin resistance of the muscle in the forearm similar to that observed in patients with spontaneous obesity. It would thus seem that the endocrine alterations in obesity are probably a consequence rather than a cause of the disease.

PROTEIN AND/OR CALORIE DEFICIENCY

Several clinical syndromes result from the deficiency of proteins and/or calories. These conditions can occur when there is an insufficient supply of food, as in times of war or famine, or when the quality of the available food is inadequate for human needs. The presence of severe disease of the gastrointestinal tract which prevents absorption of essential nutrients, toxemia associated with acute or chronic diseases, or the use of fasting as a treatment of obesity also impairs intake. Our knowledge of the consequences of starvation increased rapidly during the first and second World Wars and more recently with the introduction of fasting as a treatment for obesity. Several clinical and pathologic features of the syndromes with caloric or protein deprivation are presented in Table 31–4. Three of these—starvation or subnutrition, anorexia nervosa, and marasmus in children—represent deficiencies of both protein and calories and may more appropriately be named protein-calorie malnutrition, although there are some features unique to each. Kwashiorkor develops when protein is the element which is deficient in the diet.

Starvation

Death is the ultimate consequence of total starvation and is frequently observed during periods of acute famine or in concentration camps during international conflagrations. The duration of survival following restriction of intake depends upon the severity of the deprivation and upon the adaptive mechanisms of the body. The presence of concurrent diseases accelerates deterioration. In classic studies on animals, Howe showed that dogs could be trained to starve. After 45 days during an early fast, his champion dog was near death. After a period of recovery with refeeding, the same animal was able to "learn" to starve for more than 117 consecutive days. In each case the nutritional needs during this period were supplied by the stores in the body. The distribution of calories in the fat source, protein, and carbohydrate in a normal and an obese individual is shown in Table 31–3. Carbohydrates stored in the form of glycogen in liver and muscle, or as circulating glucose, represent only a small fraction of total body calories. The mechanisms by which the body adapts to the deficiency of carbohydrate intake are examined in detail below. Although the maintenance of glucose is essential for survival, it is clear that the triglycerides in adipose tissue are the principal source of calories. These represent nearly 80 per cent of the total caloric stores of the normal individual and well over 95 per cent in an obese subject. With a caloric requirement of 2000 calories daily, a normal man would be expected to survive between 30 and 60 days. In contrast, the obese subject exemplified in Table 31–3 could survive for nearly a year. Indeed, obese individuals have been starved for therapeutic purposes in excess of 250 days without apparent ill effects.

The supply of glucose is clearly limited, yet it is an obligatory substrate for the brain under normal circumstances and is the primary fuel used by red cells, leukocytes, the renal medulla, and peripheral nerves. If glycogen were supplying

TABLE 31-4 A COMPARISON OF SOME FORMS OF MALNUTRITION

	Starvation	Anorexia Nervosa	Kwashiorkor	Marasmus
Primary deficiency	Calories	Calories	Protein	Calories
Age	Any age	10 to 30	At weaning	Children
Sex	Either	90% Female	Both	Both
Growth retardation	—	—	Slight	Significant
Body water	Decreased	Decreased	Increased	Decreased
Subcutaneous fat	Decreased	Decreased	May be normal	Decreased
Skin and hair lesions	—	—	Increased	Absent
Edema	Late	Late	Present	None
Diarrhea	Late	None	Present	Marked
Weight loss	Marked	Marked	Mild or absent	Marked
Serum albumin	Normal	Normal	Decreased	Normal
Hemoglobin	Normal	Normal	Decreased	Normal
Mg	Decreased	Decreased		Decreased
Liver	Normal	Normal	Enlarged and fatty	Normal
Pancreatic enzyme			Decreased	Normal

total caloric needs, the available supply would provide the body for only 10 hours. In the absence of carbohydrate intake, therefore, protein or fat must provide for most of the caloric needs. In addition, glucose must be formed from one of these substances. There is no evidence that fatty acids or acetate can be converted to carbohydrate and, therefore, essentially all the new glucose formed during starvation comes from alanine, lactate, or pyruvate. This process of gluconeogenesis occurs primarily in the liver, with the kidney participating to a small extent. The oxidation of fatty acids activates the conversion of amino acids to glucose. In the short-term fast, lasting several hours to 2 to 3 days, the needs of the body for glucose are supplied from protein and Cori cycle intermediates (lactate) and are stimulated by the release of free fatty acids from the adipose tissue. Evidence from studies of Cahill and his collaborators suggest that insulin is the principal hormone concerned with regulating the initial process of adaptation to fasting. This is most clearly seen by comparing the period of food ingestion with the intermeal period. Following the ingestion of food, insulin is released from the pancreas and serves to increase the uptake of glucose into muscle and adipose tissue and to enhance the conversion of glucose to glycogen in the liver. Insulin similarly diminishes the release of free fatty acids from adipose tissue by inhibiting lipolysis and simultaneously accelerating the conversion of glucose into long-chain fatty acids within the adipocytes. Thus, the outpouring of insulin following the ingestion of foods containing carbohydrate or amino acids accelerates the storage of fuels for the coming period without food. With fasting, the concentration of insulin declines and the entry of glucose into tissues falls. Triglycerides are hydrolyzed and the fatty acids are released into the circulation to be metabolized in liver and peripheral tissues. The low levels of insulin similarly reduce the conversion of carbohydrate to glycogen in muscle. Thus, in a short-term fast, reduction in the concentration of insulin increases the release of free fatty acids from adipose tissue and of amino acids from muscle. In this way the substrates for gluconeogenesis and energy metabolism in peripheral tissues are supplied. This is shown schematically in Figure 31-7.

As fasting is continued, the excretion of nitrogen falls, indicating that mobilization of amino acids has diminished. In time, the supply of carbon precursors for the formation of glucose from amino acids falls below the metabolic requirements of the brain, red cells, and renal medulla. Two possibilities exist to permit survival. One is that the glucose-requiring tissue can adapt to utilize other substrates; the other is that glucose could be formed from long-chain fatty acids. There is, at present, no evidence for the latter possibility. There is, however, evidence to indicate that with prolonged fasting the brain can adapt to utilize ketone bodies to provide a significant fraction of the total caloric needs. Thus, after a prolonged period of fasting, 5 to 6 weeks, a number of adaptations have occurred in fuel consumption by the organisms. The brain which was previously consuming 140 grams of glucose has decreased its consumption to 80 grams, the remainder being derived by oxidation of ketone bodies. Release of ketogenic amino acids is significantly reduced. With prolonged fasting, gluconeogenesis from the liver is decreased and the kidney becomes a more significant source of new glucose (Fig. 31-7). Indeed, during prolonged fasting the kidney provides as much or more glucose than the liver primarily because of the renal ammonia production. With fasting there is also a reduction in total caloric requirements which can represent 15 to 20 per cent, thus reduc-

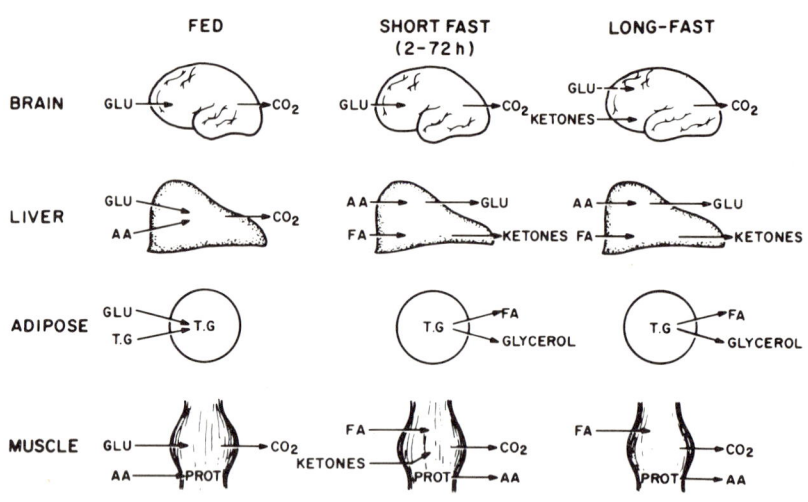

Figure 31–7 Effect of fasting on substrate utilization. Effects of substrate utilization by brain, liver, adipose tissue, and muscle in the fed state after short fast of 2 to 72 hours and following a prolonged fast. In the fed state and during a short fast, glucose is the principal substrate for the brain. With prolonged fasting, however, the brain adapts to the use of ketones for a significant fraction of its total energy requirements. With fasting, the liver adapts from burning glucose and amino acids to converting amino acids to glucose and converting free fatty acids to ketones which are then used in the peripheral tissues. In the fed state, adipose tissue stores fatty acids as triglyceride, and in the short- and long-term fast it releases these triglycerides as their fatty acid and glycerol moieties. Muscle during the fed state utilizes glucose and amino acids, but with fasting uses free fatty acids or ketones. (Adapted from Cahill, G. F., Jr., and Owen, O. E.: *In* Rowland, C. V., Jr. (Ed.): Anorexia and Obesity. Boston, Little, Brown and Co., 1970.)

ing the total requirements for calories in the form of fatty acids. The mechanism underlying these long-term adaptations to fasting is unknown. The decreased concentration of insulin appears to provide the principal signal for the early responses to fasting. Insulin, however, remains low during prolonged fasting and does not seem to be a signal for the adaptive processes observed primarily in the brain and liver. Human growth hormone and glucocorticoids have also been explored as possible agents in the adaptation of fasting but do not appear to provide the needed hormonal signal. Glucagon has not as yet been completely evaluated. Recent studies have suggested that small doses of this hormone will produce a marked decrease in the concentration of amino acids without changes in insulin or glucose. The final answer to the role of glucagon in the adaptation to prolonged fasting will await the result of further research. The major differences between the fed state and short- or long-term fasts is shown in Figure 31–7.

In addition to the endocrine and metabolic changes already described, fasting produces a number of other alterations that warrant brief comment. A thorough discussion of this subject, however, is beyond the purpose of this chapter. The decrease in circulating levels of insulin and glucose has already been noted. Changes in the concentration of growth hormone are variable, but it is frequently increased. The excretion of 17-hydroxycorticosteroids and 17-keto steroids is decreased. Concentrations of gonadotropins and testosterone show no change with fasting. Plasma levels of amino acids undergo a variety of changes. Alanine, which is an important precursor for gluconeogenesis, falls to one third of its normal level. Valine, leucine, and isoleucine initially increase in concentration but subsequently decline. Glycine, on the other hand, rises significantly with continued fasting. In addition to these changes in amino acids, there are significant losses of sodium, potassium, and magnesium from the body. The changes in magnesium are particularly interesting, since plasma magnesium remains normal, yet magnesium depletion can amount to 20 per cent. A mild ketoacidosis is uniformly found along with hyperuricemia. The increased concentrations of uric acid probably result from an increase in concentrations of keto acids, primarily β-hydroxybutyrate. This has been supported by the fact that the excretion of uric acid is reduced by the infusion of lactate or β-hydroxybutyrate. Riboflavin is decreased most rapidly but there is also a delayed fall in pantothenic acid, pyridoxine, and thiamin.

Several significant consequences can occur during fasting. Postural hypotension and collapse have been observed. Gouty arthritis and precipitation of uric acid stones have been reported and can be prevented by treatment with the appropriate drugs. The most serious consequence, however, is death. It has been reported in several patients undergoing therapeutic starvation and indicates that such treatment should only be undertaken with careful medical supervision.

Anorexia Nervosa

Anorexia nervosa represents a second form of protein-calorie deficiency with loss of tissue. Although this is a clinically defined entity, it represents a physiologic pattern of change similar to that observed with caloric restriction or total starvation. This disease affects primarily females in the age range of 10 to 30 years. Not infrequently, these individuals have been modestly overweight and suddenly go into a catabolic phase. Patients with anorexia nervosa show little concern about their relatively cachectic state. Weight loss is marked and subcutaneous fat is often nearly absent. Adipocytes can be expected to be very small indeed. Breast development remains little changed and there is no loss of axillary or pubic hair and no development of skin lesions. The concentration of adrenocortical hormones in the plasma remains normal, but it is reduced in the urine. Reproductive function is deficient in these individuals as it is in individuals with marasmus and frequently during total starvation. Plasma growth hormone is elevated.

Marasmus and Kwashiorkor

The findings in the various forms of starvation are to be contrasted with those observed when protein deficiency is the principal defect. This illness, known as kwashiorkor, is seen in its relatively pure form occasionally but is more frequently observed with various degrees of simultaneous caloric deficiency. In its relatively pure form, kwashiorkor begins at the time of weaning when the infant is deprived of protein intake but supplied with an adequate number of calories. Growth retardation is slight in comparison with the significant growth retardation observed with caloric restriction. Subcutaneous fat may be normal in the individual with kwashiorkor but is uniformly reduced in patients with marasmus or caloric deficiency. This is readily explained in terms of the alterations in the ingested fuel mixture. When protein is deficient but calories are adequate, these calories must be either carbohydrate or fat. The ingestion of carbohydrate as noted above stimulates the release of insulin and serves as a stimulus for the production and storage of triglyceride and glycogen. It is thus not surprising that body fat stores are relatively well preserved.

A second consequence is that body weight loss is mild or absent in contrast to starvation, in which marked weight loss occurs. Edema, however, is a common feature in kwashiorkor and can be attributed largely to the striking reduction in serum albumin. Since the intake of protein is reduced, the supply of amino acids to the liver from the gastrointestinal tract is inadequate. In the presence of normal carbohydrate intake, the release of amino acids from muscle sources is reduced, and consequently the supply from this source is also lower than normal. Thus, protein supplies to the liver are insufficient for the synthesis of normal amounts of serum albumin. With the reduction in serum albumin to levels of 1 to 2 grams per 100 ml. blood (20 to 30 per cent of normal), the oncotic pressure in plasma is reduced. Plasma osmotic pressure becomes insufficient to counterbalance the hydrostatic and osmotic forces in the extracellular fluid, and there is a tendency for fluid to accumulate in the extravascular compartment. This has been confirmed by the measurements of increased quantities of total body water and of extracellular fluid in patients with kwashiorkor. The deficiency in protein is also accompanied by an enlarged, fatty liver which is usually not seen when both calories and protein are deficient. The appearance of skin and hair lesions in kwashiorkor may be a reflection of vitamin deficiencies which are often observed when protein is deficient. Diarrhea, a late event in starvation, is less common in the patients with kwashiorkor. It is thus possible to distinguish between the various forms of protein-calorie malnutrition on clinical grounds and using laboratory measurements. Particularly prominent in the patient with protein depletion but adequate caloric intake are the marked reduction in albumin, the enlarged fatty liver, and nearly normal amounts of subcutaneous fat. With starvation, however, adipose stores are mobilized to provide energy for body stores and to spare protein and carbohydrate.

LIPIDS

Interest in the role of lipids in human disease has been continually reinforced by the observations that cardiovascular disease, particularly acute myocardial infarctions, occurs with significantly higher frequency in individuals with high serum cholesterol. The major lipid components of blood are listed in Table 31–5. Cholesterol is a 25-carbon molecule with four rings and is a normal constituent of animal and plant fats. Triglycerides are esters of fatty acids and glycerol. Phospholipids are a class of diglycerides with a phosphate ester on the third hydroxyl of glycerol. Fats or lipids account for approximately 40 per cent of the calories available for consumption in the retail market of the United States. Over the past 20 years there has been a gradual decrease

TABLE 31–5 LIPID COMPONENTS OF BLOOD

Serum Lipids	Concentration
Total cholesterol mg./100 ml.	230 ± 35*
Phospholipids mg./100 ml.	220 ±
Triglycerides mg./100 ml.	105 ± 25
Free fatty acids µEq./L.	400 to 800

*Mean ± S.D.

in the sources of animal fat from 75 to 66 per cent, while the fraction of fats available from vegetable sources has increased from 25 to 34 per cent. This transition has been accelerated by observations that the quality of fats in the diet, as well as their total quantity, may play a role in the development of human cardiovascular disease. A relationship between changes in serum cholesterol and the intake of fats and cholesterol has been derived by Keys from the data of many investigators (see formula below). This reduction in saturated fats would have a more significant effect on cholesterol than increasing unsaturated fats. The effect of dietary cholesterol is small, since it appears as the square root of its concentration.

Fat Ingestion and Metabolism

The ingestion of fats is followed by their cleavage into smaller moieties prior to absorption. Considerable interest has been focused on the mechanism for hydrolysis, absorption, and transport of dietary lipids. Triglycerides are cleaved by a pancreatic lipase into monoglycerides or glycerol and fatty acids. In the presence of bile acids, water-soluble micelles composed of fatty acids and monoglycerides are formed. These micellar aggregates are then absorbed into the mucosal cells of the ileum. The bile acids are recycled into the portal circulation, taken up by the liver, and secreted into the bile again. The fate of the fatty acids depends upon their chain length. For fatty acids with less than 12 carbon atoms, the triglycerides formed in the intestinal epithelium are released into the portal circulation and transported directly to the liver. With the long-chain fatty acids of more than 12 carbon atoms, however, transport is more complex. These fatty acids, after conversion to triglycerides, are surrounded by a protein coat to form chylomicrons. Although chylomicrons consist predominantly of triglycerides, they also contain small amounts of cholesterol and phospholipid. These aggregates are secreted into the lacteals of the intestinal villi and enter the general circulation through the thoracic duct. In high concentration they give the serum a creamy appearance. Chylomicrons are removed from circulation after hydrolysis of the triglyceride by lipoprotein lipase which is present in many tissues. This enzyme is increased by insulin and glucose and is activated by heparin. The fatty acids and glycerol thus formed enter adipose or muscle cells for metabolism or storage.

In addition to the chylomicrons formed in the gastrointestinal tract, pre-beta-lipoproteins can also be assembled in the liver and secreted into the circulation. The fatty acids in these lipoproteins can be synthesized from glucose in the liver or from fatty acids taken up from the blood. The fate of the lipoproteins is similar to that of the chylomicrons, i.e., the triglycerides are hydrolyzed by lipoprotein lipase. The cholesterol and phospholipid remaining after cleavage of the triglycerides are partly transferred to higher density lipoproteins, with the remainder becoming β-lipoproteins. There are thus two sources of the large triglyceride-rich lipoproteins: (1) chylomicrons formed from dietary lipid and (2) hepatic lipoproteins formed from fatty acids synthesized in the liver or taken up from the circulation.

Our understanding of lipid metabolism was greatly expanded by the introduction of techniques for separating the various serum lipoproteins by electrophoresis. By using this technique along with measurements of triglyceride and cholesterol and in some instances using flotation methods in the ultracentrifuge, it is possible to distinguish chylomicrons from alpha-, beta-, and pre-beta-lipoproteins. A typical electrophoretic pattern of normal serum is shown in Figure 31–8. When analyzed quantitatively, the components of these various lipoproteins differ. The cholesterol content is highest in the alpha-lipoprotein and lowest in chylomicrons and pre-beta-lipoproteins, with the beta-lipoprotein being intermediate. In contrast, the triglyceride concentration is highest in chylomicrons and lowest in the alpha-lipoproteins.

Defects in Fat Metabolism and Their Determination by Electrophoretic Techniques

At least two proteins make up the envelope for the circulating lipoproteins. These are an A pro-

$$\Delta \text{Cholesterol} = 1.2 [2(\Delta S) - \Delta U] + 1.5 \Delta \left(\sqrt{\text{Chol} \frac{\text{mg.}}{1000 \text{ cal.}}} \right)$$

ΔS = Glycerides of saturated fatty acids (C_{12} to C_{16}) as a percentage of total calories.

ΔU = Glycerides of polyunsaturated fatty acids in the diet as a percentage of total calories.

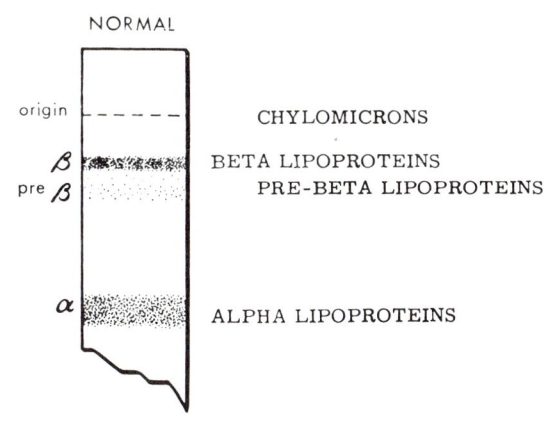

Figure 31-8 Electrophoretic pattern for lipoproteins. This schematic diagram shows the pattern obtained during electrophoresis of normal serum. The sample applied at the origin undergoes electrophoresis in an albumin buffer. Chylomicrons, if present, remain at the origin. The first band contains β-lipoproteins and the faint band running just in front of the β-lipoproteins contains the pre-β-lipoproteins. The high density α-lipoproteins migrate farthest on paper electrophoresis.

tein associated in highest concentration with the alpha-lipoproteins and a B protein associated in highest concentration with the beta-lipoproteins. Deficiency of the B protein has been described in more than 30 individuals and presents a characteristic clinical picture. As might be expected, the concentrations of chylomicrons and beta-lipoproteins are very low, since the protein which provides the principal coating is absent. Indeed, some patients have no detectable beta-lipoproteins. Serum cholesterol is also strikingly reduced. These patients also demonstrate neurologic abnormalities and an irregularity of the red blood cells called acanthocytosis. Persons lacking the B protein manifest their disease in infancy as a failure to grow and the appearance of fat in the stools. The basic pathophysiology is failure to form the protein coat by which triglycerides of long-chain fatty acids can be transported. Since triglycerides formed from short- and medium-chain fatty acids do not require a protein coat for transport, they have proved useful in treating patients with a beta-lipoproteinemia.

A second defect in transport of lipoproteins is observed with absence of the A protein. This disease was originally found on Tangier Island in Chesapeake Bay and has since been called Tangier disease. The defect is an absence of A protein associated with a reduction in the concentration of cholesterol and phospholipid in the plasma, but triglyceride shows only mild changes. The most striking abnormality in individuals with this disease is the large orange-colored tonsils which result from the deposition of cholesterol esters in this tissue. Similar esters are also deposited in the reticuloendothelial cells of liver and spleen. In the absence of alpha-lipoprotein, lipid is carried primarily by the beta-lipoproteins which appear to be normal by immunoelectrophoresis.

Absence of lipoprotein lipase from peripheral tissues produces a third defect in lipid metabolism and is inherited as an autosomal recessive trait. This enzyme is essential for the hydrolysis of triglycerides carried on chylomicrons and pre-beta-lipoproteins prior to their entry and storage in adipose cells and other peripheral tissues. Absence of this enzyme would lead to an accumulation of these lipoproteins in the serum. On visual examination the serum from such patients is creamy. The marked elevation in serum triglycerides and chylomicrons results from the dietary intake of triglyceride. If fat is excluded from the diet, the chylomicrons disappear and lipid levels return almost to normal. Thus, exclusion of fat from the diet represents the principal mode of treatment for individuals with this disease. The symptom complex observed is also susceptible to treatment by dietary restriction of fat and therefore probably results from the high levels of chylomicrons. These symptoms include abdominal pain, a creamy color to the retinal vessels, and the appearance of reddish-yellow lipid-containing plaques in the skin.

By using the technique illustrated in Figure 31-8, the lipoprotein patterns can be segregated into six groups, as illustrated in Table 31-6, which is adapted from the currently recommended international classification.

Type I results from deficiency of lipoprotein lipase and was described above. As would be expected with a deficiency of this enzyme, the pattern on electrophoresis shows a marked increase in concentration of chylomicrons.

The second type of pattern observed with this technique is a marked increase in the beta-lipoprotein fraction without elevation of triglycerides (IIa) or when this moiety is also elevated (IIb). This protein carries a significant fraction of the total cholesterol and is accompanied by significant elevations in concentration of plasma cholesterol. The familial form is inherited as an autosomal dominant and Types IIa and IIb appear in the same families. The specific biochemical defect has not yet been elucidated. This disease is often associated with accumulations of lipid (xanthomas) in tendons. Early cardiovascular death has often been associated with this syndrome. Recent evidence indicates that high levels of cholesterol can be detected in up to 0.5% of newborns, making it an easily detectable and optimistically treatable affliction.

The third abnormality in the electrophoretic pattern (Type III) is known by its description as

TABLE 31-6 CLASSIFICATION OF HYPERLIPOPROTEINEMIA

Type	Chylo-microns	LDL β	VLDL pre-β	Floating β	Appearance of Standing Plasma	Cholesterol	Tri-glyceride	Chol./TG
I	+				Creamy	↑	↑↑	<0.2
IIa		+			Clear	↑↑	N	>15.0
IIb		+	+		Clear or faintly turbid	↑	↑	Variable
III				+	Turbid	↑	↑	Frequently >1.0
IV			+		Clear or turbid	N or ↑	↑	Variable
V	+		+		Creamy	↑	↑↑	>0.15; <0.06

Key:
+ = Present
↑ = Increased
↑↑ = Greatly Increased
N = Normal

broad beta disease. This is observed when the beta band is increased in width and streaks over into the pre-beta region but without a separate band. This a rare disease and must be distinguished from IIb by showing that the lipoprotein floats at a density of 1.006. The familial form of this disease is inherited as an autosomal recessive and is manifested mainly in adult life. The increased amounts of triglyceride and cholesterol often result in lipid deposition in the skin. Such individuals are also plagued by coronary artery disease at an early age. Glucose metabolism is often abnormal in patients with this disease.

The fourth type of electrophoretic abnormality (Type IV) shows a striking increase in the concentration of pre-beta-lipoproteins and is among the two most common types. This disease is inducible by a high-carbohydrate diet and is often termed endogenous or "carbohydrate-inducible" hyperlipoproteinemia. This abnormality and that of Type II are frequently seen as complications of other diseases including diabetes, hypothyroidism, and the nephrotic syndrome. The serum from patients is usually cloudy. Glucose tolerance is often abnormal and these patients are frequently obese.

The final syndrome (Type V) is manifested by an elevation in both chylomicrons and pre-beta-lipoproteins. The activity of lipoprotein lipase is frequently low in patients with Type V disease and may account for their increased level of chylomicrons. As with Type I, patients suffering from Type V abnormalities frequently have abdominal pain and usually show abnormal metabolism of glucose. Progestational and anabolic steroids have been found to enhance the activity of lipoprotein lipase and to lower levels of triglyceride.

To summarize, the absorption, digestion, transport, and storage of the lipid components of the diet represent a complex and well-integrated system. Lipoproteins represent the principal form for transporting lipids in plasma. The introduction of electrophoretic techniques for separating the lipoproteins in plasma has provided significant new insights into the pathogenesis of a number of disease states. The two principal lipoproteins, alpha- and beta-lipoproteins, are associated primarily with A and B proteins in their coats. Disease syndromes have been described which result from the deficiency of one or the other of these proteins. Elevated chylomicrons result from a deficiency of lipoprotein lipase, the enzyme which hydrolyzes circulating triglycerides, so that they can be absorbed and stored in adipose tissue. Four other types of abnormality in lipoprotein patterns have also been described which can occur as genetically transmitted forms or in association with other diseases.

VITAMINS

Vitamins may be defined as small chemical molecules which are essential for maintenance of normal metabolic processes but which cannot be synthesized within the body. These substances must therefore be provided in adequate amounts from dietary sources. Over the past 70 years, a number of vitamins have been elucidated and their clinical correlates put into focus. A listing of these vitamins is presented in Table 31-7. They can be divided into two groups: the water-soluble vitamins, comprising the B-complex vitamins and vitamin C, and the fat-soluble vitamins, A, D, E, and K. The precise metabolic role of some vitamins has been clearly described, but the role of others is less well understood. The B-complex vitamins as a group are involved in the metabolism of carbohydrate as cofactors either for the

TABLE 31-7 RECOMMENDED DAILY ALLOWANCES FOR VITAMINS

Vitamins	Recommended Daily Allowances
Water-Soluble Vitamins	
Thiamin (B$_1$)	0.2 to 1.5 mg.
Riboflavin (B$_2$)	0.4 to 1.7 mg.
Pyridoxine (B$_6$)	0.2 to 2.0 mg.
Niacin	5.0 to 20.0 mg.
Pantothenic acid	—
Folacin (folic acid)	0.05 to 0.4 mg.
Cyanocobalamin (B$_{12}$)	1.0 to 5.0 µg.
Biotin	—
Ascorbic acid (C)	35 to 55 mg.
Fat-Soluble Vitamins	
Vitamin A	5000 I.U.
Vitamin D	400 I.U.
Vitamin E	5 to 25
Vitamin K	—

transfer of hydrogen or for decarboxylation or transamination. Pyridoxine is involved in transfer of amino groups and biotin in the fixation of CO_2 during fatty acid synthesis and gluconeogenesis. Folic acid and vitamin B_{12} are involved in nucleic acid synthesis. The precise role for vitamin C is unclear. Vitamin A has several functions but its role in the visual cycle has been most clearly defined. Vitamin D has an essential role in bone metabolism, but the function of vitamin C in bone metabolism is still unclear. Vitamin K will be dealt with in more detail in the section on hematology.

Defining the requirements for these nutritional factors has occupied considerable research effort. Since most of them are intimately involved in intermediary metabolism, their requirements in general vary with the overall rate of metabolism. It would thus be expected that diseases which altered metabolism would alter the rates at which the vitamins are metabolized and thus increase or decrease their requirements. Hyperthyroidism which increases oxygen consumption, enhances the need for thiamine and riboflavin. When thyroid function is decreased, the requirements for these vitamins fall. The definition of requirements for many vitamins must, therefore, be stated in terms of total caloric requirements. In general, however, the minimum daily requirements are high enough to allow a reasonable margin of safety for individual variation.

Water-Soluble Vitamins

Thiamin (Vitamin B$_1$). Thiamin was among the first of the B-complex vitamins to be chemically identified and serves as an important cofactor in the decarboxylation of pyruvic and α-ketoglutaric acids. Deficiency of this vitamin is manifested by defective metabolism of carbohydrates. One of the cardinal biochemical alterations accompanying the clinical states of thiamin deficiency is an increase in circulating levels of pyruvic acid. The inability to utilize pyruvate in thiamin deficiency is accompanied by the development of two clinical syndromes, one involving the peripheral nervous system and the other the cardiovascular system. Peripheral involvement of the nervous system, known as peripheral neuritis, is manifested as increased pain, a loss of sensation, or an aching or burning sensation. Significant alterations in the central nervous system also occur and are most commonly observed in patients ingesting large quantities of alcohol. The cardiovascular manifestations are primarily those of inadequate energy supply to the myocardium and the periphery with an increase in cardiac output. Arterioles are dilated, leading to an increased flow of blood between the arterial and venous circulation. As a result of the high cardiac output and defective carbohydrate metabolism, heart failure occurs associated with shortness of breath, increased heart rate, subjective feelings of palpitation, and objective findings of irregular rhythms. The heart is usually enlarged and, as might be expected in a heart which is unable to pump blood at a sufficient rate, there is an increase in venous pressure. These neurologic and cardiovascular symptoms are most prominent in severe deficiencies, but careful studies of hospitalized patients have revealed significantly reduced levels of thiamin in approximately one third of such patients. Since the requirements for thiamin are related to the metabolic rate, both deficient food intake and hypermetabolism can produce symptoms of disease. Patients with prolonged alcoholic intake or people eating hypocaloric diets can suffer from mild symptoms of thiamin deficiency, while individuals with hypermetabolism (usually hyperthyroidism) will suffer from similar symptoms even though thiamin intake may be adequate normally.

Riboflavin (Vitamin B$_2$). Although riboflavin was chemically identified for the first time in 1879, its role in the production of disease was not appreciated for some years thereafter. Normal subjects on a riboflavin-deficient diet developed characteristic lesions within three months. Among the pathologic changes were vascularization of the cornea and cheilosis. Riboflavin and its two active nucleotides, flavin mononucleotide (FMN) and flavinadeninedinucleotide (FAD), are the hydrogen-accepting cofactors for several enzymes including xanthine oxidase, succinic dehydrogenase, triphosphopyridine nucleotide, and mitochondrial glycerophosphate oxidase. Like thiamin, the requirements for riboflavin depend on overall metabolic activity and have been defined as 0.25 to 0.30 mg. per 1000 kcal. of food oxidized. Thyroid hormones play a major role in the control of flavoproteins. Hyperthyroidism clearly produces an increased metabolic rate and alters the metabolism of riboflavin. This latter effect is manifested as an increase in the enzymes which convert riboflavin to its active form, flavin mononucleotide. Hypothyroidism, on the other hand, produces a decrease in hepatic flavin-containing enzymes which are similar to those produced by riboflavin deficiency. The metabolic rate is reduced in riboflavin-deficient animals as it is in hypothyroidism. Similarly, α-glycerophosphate dehydrogenase, a mitochondrial enzyme, is decreased in hypothyroidism and in riboflavin deficiency. These observations suggest that certain clinical features of hypothyroidism may be attributable to the inability to metabolize riboflavin in a normal manner.

Niacin (Nicotinamide). Deficiency of niacin produces pellagra, or black tongue. This illness is characterized by symptoms referable to the skin, gastrointestinal tract, and central nervous system. In experimentally induced deficiency in man, the earliest manifestations are a red eruption on the skin resembling sunburn which first appears on the back of the hand. Other areas which are exposed to light are subsequently involved. The lesions, which are symmetrical, may darken, shed skin, and eventually scar. Sores on the mucocutaneous membranes, a swelling of the tongue, nausea, and vomiting are present in a significant number of individuals. Symptoms referable to the central nervous system include headache, insomnia, depression, dizziness, and difficulty with memory. The presence of a nutritional factor which could cure these symptoms was demonstrated in the classic work of Goldberger and his colleagues, and this substance was subsequently found to be nicotinamide or niacin. This vitamin is a critical part of two cofactors, NAD and NADP, which are involved in the transfer of hydrogen in most biological oxidations. Although the role of NAD and NADP in biological oxidations and biochemical synthesis are well known, the mechanism by which the symptoms observed with deficiency of niacin relate to the levels of these cofactors remains unclear. One thing is clear, however—the administration of nicotinic acid to patients suffering from pellagra produces dramatic alterations within 24 hours.

Pyridoxine (Vitamin B$_6$). After the identification of thiamin, riboflavin, and niacin, it became clear that other water-soluble nutritional factors were also necessary for normal metabolic function. In the period between 1930 and 1935 several groups of workers described an additional factor, vitamin B$_6$, subsequently called pyridoxine. This compound is activated by conversion to pyridoxal phosphate and is involved in a number of metabolic reactions with amino acids including decarboxylation and transamination. Pyridoxine deprivation can produce symptoms in man and other species. These include changes in the skin, central nervous system, and production of red blood cells. In man, the skin lesions consist of seborrheic changes around the eyes, nose, and mouth and of swelling and redness of the tongue. With prolonged deficiency, convulsive activity in the central nervous system has been demonstrated. The anemia which accompanies pyridoxine deficiency is microcytic and hypochromic in type. All these symptoms can be promptly relieved by the administration of small doses of pyridoxine. The recommended dose of pyridoxine is related to protein intake, since its principal role is in the metabolism of amino acids. The range is between 1.25 and 2.00 mg. with protein intakes of 100 grams or less. With high protein intake, more pyridoxine may be needed.

In addition to the symptoms of deficiency which are cured by low doses of pyridoxine, there are a group of clinical states in which symptoms can be cured by much higher doses of this vitamin. These include some forms of convulsions, particularly in children; vitamin B$_6$-dependent anemia; xanthinuric aciduria; cystothionuria; and homocystinuria. The doses of vitamin B$_6$ required for control or amelioration of these conditions are in the range of 200 to 600 mg. daily as compared to a range of 1.5 to 2.0 mg. per day for normal maintenance. The convulsive activity in the brain would appear to be related to altered levels of gamma-amino butyric acid (GABA). This amino acid is produced by decarboxylation of glutamate, a process involving transamination and requiring pyridoxal phosphate. A reduction in the level of GABA increases the tendency for convulsive activity and probably accounts for the convulsions observed in such patients. The physiologic basis for the effect of pyridoxine in the other conditions is unknown at present.

Pantothenic Acid and Biotin. These two water-soluble agents are important cofactors in the metabolism of fats. Pantothenic acid was first identified in 1933 and was clearly associated with a nutritional deficiency disease in fowl by Wooley and his collaborators in 1939. Pantothenic acid is an essential component of coenzyme A which is of prime importance in both synthesis and degradation of fatty acids. The presence of biotin was demonstrated from studies showing the production of a disease by feeding egg white. It is now known that raw egg white contains avidin, a glycoprotein of high molecular weight which irreversibly binds biotin. The structure of biotin was established in 1942, and it is an important enzyme in the fixation of CO_2 during synthesis of fatty acids and during gluconeogenesis. Although specific syndromes can be produced in man by feeding synthetic diets deficient in pantothenic acid or biotin, these are almost unknown under natural conditions because of the wide availability of these two substances in foods.

Folic Acid and Vitamin B$_{12}$ (Cobamide). These two vitamins are essential for the maintenance of normal hematopoiesis. Because of their integral relationship with the blood, discussion of vitamin B$_{12}$ and folic acid is included in Chapter 22.

Vitamin C. Vitamin C or ascorbic acid, the last water-soluble vitamin, is essential for the prevention of scurvy. The existence of a nutritional factor which would prevent scurvy was recognized in 1753 by Lind, who demonstrated that oranges, lemons, and limes could prevent and cure scurvy among sailors, hence the nickname "limey" for British sailors. The chemical identification of this antiscurvy or antiscorbutic factor was not made for nearly 200 years. Progress was greatly aided by the demonstration that guinea pigs could be made scorbutic, i.e., develop scurvy. With this bioassay, several groups of workers demonstrated the essential nature of ascorbic acid. It was a hexuronic acid present in high concentrations in the adrenal gland, as well as in citrus fruits and cabbages.

The physiologic and biological functions for ascorbic acid are far less clearly defined than for the other water-soluble vitamins. Most of the other vitamins function as cofactors for a specific enzymatic step in a chain of biochemical reactions. No such enzymatic step has been defined which requires ascorbic acid as a cofactor. The vitamin rather appears to function in its reduced form, dehydroascorbic acid, in oxidation-reduction reactions. Its role in the metabolism of tyrosine has been studied in some detail. The first step in metabolism is the transamination of tyrosine to p-hydroxyphenylpyruvic acid. The next step is conversion to homogentisic acid by parahydroxyphenylpyruvic acid oxidase, an enzyme which is inhibited by its substrate unless ascorbic acid is present. This effect occurs when the quantities of tyrosine are large. The functional role of the high concentrations of ascorbic acid found in the adrenal gland and in the ovary are unclear at present.

When vitamin C deficiency is produced, two groups of symptoms occur: those involving growth of bones and those involving blood vessels. During periods of rapid growth, a separation of the periosteum from the cortex occurs and subperiosteal hemorrhages may result. When growth is less rapid, the lesions in the epiphyseal-diaphyseal junction may lead to disunion and/or fragmentation. Changes in the capillary walls are also prominent, and hemorrhages into the space around hair follicles are common. All these symptoms are rapidly reversed by the administration of ascorbic acid, which is required in the range of 50 to 75 mg. per day. It is of interest that only man, certain primates, and the guinea pig have a requirement for vitamin C; other mammals are able to synthesize the vitamin by a series of reactions involving the glucuronic acid pathway. The correlation between the clinical symptoms and the biochemical reactions is unclear. Definition of this area again awaits further understanding of the biochemical mechanisms by which ascorbic acid acts at the cellular level.

Fat-Soluble Vitamins

The vitamins A, D, E, and K differ from the group discussed previously because they are soluble in fat. Toxicity from overdosage has been reported for vitamins A and D because body fat serves as a storage depot. Toxicity is not observed with the water-soluble vitamins because any excess is excreted in the urine.

Vitamin A. The discovery of vitamin A stemmed from studies on the skin lesions and xerophthalmia in rats fed artificial diets containing lard. The chemical factor which prevented this deficiency was identified in 1929 as beta-carotene, and its structure was proved in 1931. Subsequent work on the physiologic role of beta-carotene and other carotenoid pigments has taken two lines: (1) studies on its effect on vision and (2) studies on growth and development. The actions in the visual cycle have been clearly elucidated by work from several laboratories. Deficiency of vitamin A impairs adaptation of the retina to the dark. It also impedes growth. The mechanism for the stimulation of growth by vitamin A has not yet been clearly established. Retinoic acid, an oxidation product of retinal, is a potent promoter of growth in the vitamin A-deficient animal, yet it is ineffective in restoring visual function. It may thus be that the components of vitamin A which are essential for growth may not be those which are involved in maintenance of the visual response to dark. The nature of this growth-promoting component of vitamin A awaits further investigation.

Induction of vitamin A deficiency requires prolonged periods of a deficient intake due to the fat solubility of this vitamin. The clinical symptoms which eventually appear involve desiccation and ulceration of the cornea and conjunctiva in the eye, increased frequency of respiratory infection, and keratinization and drying of the skin, with an occasional papular eruption. Kidney stones and alterations in the pancreatic ducts are frequently found. These symptoms of vitamin A deficiency are most commonly seen in patients suffering from impaired intestinal fat absorption. Thus, pancreatic disease, disease of the biliary tract, sprue, and ulcerative colitis are the primary causes of vitamin A deficiency; only rarely does dietary deficiency alone produce symptoms.

Overzealous treatment with preparations containing vitamin A can, however, induce symptoms of toxicity. These symptoms, which usually take six months or more to develop, require doses in excess of 50,000 units of vitamin A per day and consist of irritability, loss of appetite, and itching of the skin. Fatigue, myalgia, changes in body hair, and enlargement of the liver and spleen have also been observed. Withdrawal of the vitamin leads to rapid regression of most of the symptoms. The one exception is the bony hyperostoses which develop on the extremities and in the occipital region of the skull.

Vitamin D, Calcium, Magnesium, and Their Control. *Vitamin D* is a fat-soluble sterol which can prevent rickets. Much of the early work on this disease was prompted by the significant numbers of afflicted children in urban areas of the temperate zones. By 1920 it had been established that the disease was the result of a dietary deficiency and a lack of sunlight. Irradiation of dietary rations and the skin were effective in preventing the disease. Demonstration of an antirachitic factor in various fish oils was followed by intensive chemical studies leading to the identification and elucidation of the structure of vitamin D_2 by 1937. The next major advance in the physiology of vitamin D was the synthesis of radioactively labeled vitamin D_2 of high specific activity. With radioactive vitamin D_2, it was shown that orally administered vitamin D_2 is converted to an active metabolite now known to be 25-hydroxycholecalciferol. This metabolite is active in vitro, whereas the native vitamins D_2 and D_3 require conversion. In the presence of parathyroid hormone renal tissue converts 25-hydroxylcholecalciferol to 1,25-dihydroxycholecalciferol, which acts even more rapidly than its precursor. The dihydroxy derivative may thus be the "active" form of vitamin D.

Vitamin D has two principal actions. The first is to increase the absorption of calcium from the intestine and the second is to facilitate the reabsorption of calcium from bone in the presence of parathyroid hormone. The effects of vitamin D on the absorption of calcium from the gastrointestinal tract are dependent upon the formation of a transport protein in the gastrointestinal mucosa. When isolated intestine is perfused with solutions of vitamin D, it takes four hours or more to increase calcium absorption. The active metabolite 1,25-dihydroxycholecalciferol produces an increase in calcium transport in less than one and one-half hours. This effect is blocked by actinomycin D, an inhibitor of nucleic acid synthesis, suggesting that the synthesis of new protein is involved. Parathyroid hormone also plays a role in calcium absorption from the gut. In the hypoparathyroid animal, normal intake of vitamin D does not produce a normal rate of calcium absorption, although increased intake of vitamin D can restore calcium absorption to normal. Injections of parathyroid hormone lead to normal calcium absorption in the presence of normal intake of vitamin D. Similarly, in vitamin D-deficient animals, absorption of calcium is deficient, although there is excess secretion of parathyroid hormone. In the mechanisms of calcium absorption from the gut, vitamin D would appear to have the primary role, with parathyroid hormones making a secondary or minor contribution.

The actions of vitamin D on bone have been less extensively studied, but an essential interaction with parathyroid hormone is again evident. In tissue cultures of bone, the addition of 25-hydroxycholecalciferol will stimulate bone reabsorption in a manner similar to that observed with parathyroid hormone. Moreover, this metabolite of vitamin D acts synergistically with parathyroid hormone. Although recent evidence suggests that parathyroid hormone acts on the kidney and bone to increase the production of cyclic-AMP, vitamin D does not influence this system. Thus, the synergism of parathyroid hormone and vitamin D on the reabsorption of bone appears to occur at different sites. Raisz has suggested that "the synergism could be explained if parathyroid hormone controlled entry of calcium into the nucleus and thus controlled the nuclear events of transcription and cellular transformation."

The maintenance of normal levels of circulating *calcium* is of prime importance for neuromuscular transmission and for cellular transport. The control mechanisms involved in maintaining the normal levels of serum calcium are determined not only by vitamin D but by parathyroid hormone, phosphorus, magnesium, and calcitonin. It is beyond the scope of this chapter to review these interactions in detail, but certain effects of pathologic derangements are worthy of note. Osteomalacia and rickets are the consequences of vitamin D deficiency which result from lack of sunlight, from deficiency of this vitamin in the diet, from resistance at the cellular level, or from malabsorption in the gastrointestinal tract. Pathologic consequences also occur with increased amounts of vitamin D. When parathyroid hormone is present, the ingestion of markedly increased amounts of vitamin D can induce a pathologic state similar to that observed with an excess excretion of parathyroid hormone. The state of vitamin D intoxication increases the concentrations of serum calcium and reduces the level of circulating phosphate. Calcium absorption from the gastrointestinal tract is increased, and bony abnormalities can be induced by increased absorption of calcium from bones. The consequences of hypercalcemia on the electrocardiogram and on neuromuscular conduction can be observed. Finally, persistent hypercalcemia can produce renal failure by damaging the kidney.

In the metabolism of *magnesium*, increased concentrations of parathyroid hormone can increase magnesium excretion and induce a state of magnesium deficiency. Such a change would tend to reduce the effects of parathyroid hormone. Magnesium deficiency can also be induced by dietary means and by alcoholism, and such a state is usually associated with hypocalcemia. The pathologic mechanism by which magnesium deficiency leads to hypocalcemia is unclear, although it has been attributed to resistance of the skeleton to the action of parathyroid hormone. One would expect that with hypomagnesemia the output of parathyroid hormone would be increased, as observed under in vitro and in vivo conditions, yet serum calcium is usually below normal. Support for diminished effectiveness of parathyroid hormone with magnesium depletion has been shown in studies with bone cultures and in measurements of cyclic-AMP excretion in the urine. By use of the technique of bone culture, it was shown that the effect of parathyroid hormone on calcium mobilization was reduced when the concentration of magnesium was low. Similarly, magnesium-deficient patients failed to excrete normal amounts of cyclic-AMP after the administration of parathyroid hormone. Since the action of parathyroid hormone on bone and kidney appears to involve cyclic-AMP, this may be the essential biochemical defect in this interaction. It is known from other studies on this membrane-bound enzyme complex that magnesium is essential for the conversion of ATP to $3',5'$-AMP (cyclic-AMP). Thus, in magnesium deficiency the impaired response of parathyroid hormone might be due to the slowed rate of conversion of ATP to cyclic-AMP in the absence of this divalent cation.

Vitamin E. The place of vitamin E, or alpha-tocopherol, in human nutrition is still unsettled. It was originally discovered as an essential factor for the maintenance of pregnancy in rats. Because this is a fat-soluble vitamin, depletion of the body stores occurs very slowly. Prolonged feeding of diets deficient in vitamin E to adults failed to produce clear-cut evidence of a deficiency state. However, in infants with protein-calorie malnutrition, vitamin E could reverse the hemolytic anemia which was often present. A similar hemolytic anemia occurs in monkeys fed a diet free of alpha-tocopherol, suggesting that this vitamin may play a role in hematopoiesis.

Vitamin K. Vitamin K is a fat-soluble vitamin which is essential for hepatic synthesis of clotting factors II, VII, IX, and X (see Chapter 22). Because it is a fat-soluble quinone, it is often deficient in states of malabsorption. Indeed, this is one of the observations which led to its discovery. Although the quinone structure was rapidly elucidated, it is still not known how the vitamin acts to enhance the synthesis of clotting factors. Of pathophysiologic importance is that this vitamin is competitively antagonized by such drugs as aspirin. Thus, bleeding disorders from deficiency of vitamin K can occur with hepatic disease or malabsorption or by use of drugs which are competitive antagonists.

Pathophysiologic Mechanisms of Disease States Resulting from Vitamin Deficiencies

A number of pathogenetic mechanisms can lead to deficiencies of one or another vitamin and thus to the production of clinical or subclinical syndromes resulting from a lack of vitamins. *Deficient dietary intake* is the first such mechanism. This can result from selective absence of one or more vitamins or its precursor in the diet, or to a generalized deficiency of all vitamins as observed in malnutrition or during total stravation. In other diseases such as alcoholism, dietary intake is frequently reduced but loss of vitamins is also accelerated.

Absence of vitamin D in the diet or inadequate exposure to sunlight is associated with rickets. The failure to calcify bony matrix which characterizes this disease is now rare in this country because vitamin D is added to most milk supplies and because most infants receive supplements of vitamins. However, rickets is still seen occasionally when vitamin D is insufficient or when the response is impaired by genetic defects. Although relatively rare, it must be pointed out that cases of rickets due to vitamin deficiency are still seen even in the major metropolitan centers of the United States.

Severe generalized malnutrition and *therapeutic starvation* are also mechanisms for producing vitamin deficiency. Over the past decade, the use of starvation as therapy for human obesity has become widespread. During starvation there is a marked reduction in the circulating concentration of many vitamins. Thiamin, niacin, biotin, pantothenic acid, folate, riboflavin, and pyridoxine are among the vitamins which are lost. The decline in pyridoxine is progressive with the duration of starvation and reaches very low levels by 5 to 6 months. With starvation, riboflavin also drops progressively but rises promptly when food is returned to the diet. Thiamin is also reduced. In one particular patient with hypotension, vomiting, and weakness occurring after three weeks of fasting, the symptoms disappeared following the intravenous administration of thiamin. Other vitamin supplements had no effect.

Total absence of food, however, is not the only mechanism for nutritional reduction in vitamin levels. Surveys of hospitalized patients, particularly children, have shown that numbers ranging up to 45 per cent had lowered serum concentrations of one or more vitamins. This reduction varied with the ethnic origin of the patients. For example, Puerto Rican children showed lower circulating levels of thiamin, niacin, vitamin B_{12}, and folate than children from other ethnic groups in New York City. In contrast, Chinese children showed many instances of higher levels than other groups. Protein intake was of primary importance in determining the levels of many vitamins. When less than 38 grams of protein was ingested daily, there were marked reductions in the levels of biotin, thiamin, and ascorbic acid. Supplements with oral vitamins did not raise the serum levels to normal until protein intake was increased. Thus, protein deficiency per se influences the circulating levels of vitamins in a manner which is as yet poorly understood.

Alcoholism is a third pathologic state associated with reduced serum levels of some vitamins. These individuals frequently have a deficiency of folic acid and they are often deficient in thiamin. The deficiency in folic acid probably accounts for the frequent association of hematologic abnormalities and megaloblastic anemia. However, folic acid deficiency may also impair the ability of the liver to regenerate, since it is necessary for synthesis of DNA and for cell replication. The deficiency of thiamin in alcoholics is associated with a characteristic group of symptoms which include a wobbling gait, inability to move the eye muscles appropriately, and confusion. This symptom complex can be rapidly reversed by the intravenous administration of thiamin.

Malabsorption is another pathologic mechanism that induces vitamin deficiency. A number of disease states are associated with ineffective absorption of one or more vitamins and/or minerals from the gastrointestinal tract. Thus, food intake may be normal, but body supplies of essential elements may be deficient. This is more often seen when the pathologic alteration leads to increased loss of fat in the stools. As might be expected with increased fat excretion, the amount of fat-soluble vitamins A, D, and K is most frequently affected.

Similarly, calcium, which complexes with fatty acids formed during hydrolysis of triglyceride, is also lost with fatty acids. Thus, deficiencies of vitamin D and calcium can lead to impaired formation of bone, with decreased circulating levels of calcium. This complex of symptoms in adults is known clinically as osteomalacia and is analogous to rickets in children. It is characterized by a loss of mineral from the skeleton with ensuing deformities of the weight-bearing bones. Pseudo-fractures may be detected on x-rays as symmetrical lines at bony areas of reabsorption where nutrient arteries penetrate the bone. There is relative impairment of normal bone reabsorption and histologically defective mineralization of the newly formed bony matrix. The hypocalcemia which is usually present is relatively unresponsive to the injection of parathyroid hormone. Urinary excretion of calcium and increased secretion of phosphate from the kidney are observed. As a result of the lowered levels of circulating calcium, parathyroid hormone is secreted from the parathyroid gland in increased amounts but appears to be relatively less active than normal in improving calcium reabsorption from bone.

In addition to osteomalacia which results from loss of vitamin D and calcium, malabsorption also produces a loss of vitamin A. As noted earlier, vitamin A affects visual function and growth. Impaired adaptation of the retina to the dark is the principal effect of vitamin A deficiency. The chemical process of dark adaptation requires the synthesis of rhodopsin, a combination of a protein opsin and a prosynthetic group, 11-cis-retinal, which is derived from vitamin A. After exposure to light, this pigment undergoes a number of changes which lead to initiation of the nerve impulse. When vitamin A is deficient, the essential prosthetic group 11-cis-retinal is reduced and the production of rhodopsin, the photosensitive pigment, is impaired. Thus, malabsorption of fat can impair both bone formation and visual adaptation to darkness.

The third effect of malabsorption is the loss of vitamin K. This is an essential vitamin for the synthesis of prothrombin. In its absence, prothrombin levels are reduced and coagulation of blood is impaired, with a tendency to hemorrhage. In contrast to the other two fat-soluble vitamins, water-soluble forms of vitamin K can be administered and overcome this defect in formation of prothrombin.

Specific forms of malabsorption can also influence vitamin absorption. Pernicious anemia is a case in point in which vitamin B_{12} is not absorbed because intrinsic factor is lacking from the gastrointestinal mucosa. Injections of vitamin B_{12} will bypass this abnormality.

Although vitamin ingestion and absorption are normal, the *administration of antimetabolites or drugs* which compete directly or indirectly with vitamins for their active sites on enzymes may lead to symptoms of vitamin deficiency. Antimetabolites of folic acid are among the best known examples of this type of induced vitamin deficiency. Megaloblastic anemia responsive to folate therapy can be produced by two classes of drugs. The first class includes the anticonvulsants such as diphenylhydantoin (Dilantin) or phenobarbital. Both these drugs induce folate deficiency presumably by interfering with its reduction to dihydrofolic acid or by interfering with its role in the formation of DNA. A second group of antifolic acid metabolites includes those used in the treatment of certain cancers. These drugs interfere directly with folic acid metabolism. Aspirin is an example of the second group of drugs which will inhibit the effects of a vitamin. Salicylates compete with vitamin K and thus lower the production of prothrombin. Hypoprothrombinemia is frequently observed in patients treated with high doses of aspirin, and this effect can be overcome by administering supplements of vitamin K. Isoniazid (INH) is the final example of a drug which inhibits vitamin metabolism. This drug is widely used for the treatment of tuberculosis and has been observed to increase the excretion of pyridoxine (vitamin B_6). With high doses of isoniazid, a peripheral neuropathy, convulsions, and anemia have been observed. All three of these untoward effects resulting from the administration of isoniazid can be prevented or treated by supplements of pyridoxine.

Increased vitamin utilization in the presence of a normal dietary intake is another mechanism by which the effects of vitamin deficiency can be produced. This can occur in hypermetabolic states, such as those due to prolonged fever or other causes. There are three such common clinical states. The first is increased levels of thyroid hormone (hyperthyroidism or administration of exogenous thyroid hormone), the second is pregnancy, and the third is childhood. In hyperthyroidism, the metabolic rate is significantly increased. As noted earlier, the requirement for thiamin, riboflavin, niacin, and possibly the other water-soluble B-complex vitamins is a function of the total caloric expenditure. As caloric expenditure rises in hyperthyroidism, the daily requirements for each of these vitamins increases. To avoid induction of nutritional deficiency, it is often wise to treat patients with hyperthyroidism with supplements of B vitamins during the period of time when their disease is being controlled. A second physiologic state of hypermetabolism is observed during pregnancy and a third in the growing child. Caloric requirements per kilogram body weight are increased in children, and vitamin requirements for this age group are similarly higher than for adults. Many illnesses in children are accompanied by vitamin deficiencies as shown by low circulating levels of vitamins. Vitamin requirements are also increased in pregnancy. During gestation, a second body is formed and the increased metabolism required by this procedure demands more vitamins. It is customary to give vitamin supplements during this period to prevent depletion of maternal supplies, with potential pathologic consequences for the developing infant.

TRACE ELEMENTS

Improvements in analytical methods within the past decade have expanded our understanding of the role of trace elements in human nutrition and disease. In this section some of these elements and their role in the production of disease will be examined. The ability to induce pathologic changes by selective removal of one element from the diet provides one of the best examples of the correlation between pathologic and physiologic alterations. We will illustrate, when possible, the biochemical basis of these changes. However, it is clear that in many instances such a fundamental understanding is not yet possible because our knowledge of the role of many of these trace elements is as yet incomplete. A summary of the data concerning body content, plasma concentration, functional role, and deficiency appears in Table 31-8. Calcium, magnesium, iron, and zinc are quantitatively the largest, present in gram quantities. Copper, chromium, manganese, iodine, and fluoride, on the other hand, are found in only milligram quantities.

Zinc

The content of zinc is approximately 1.4 to 2.3 grams in a 70 kg. man, with 20 per cent of this amount in the skin. Circulating concentrations can be readily measured and average 121 μg. per 100 ml. in serum and somewhat more than ten times this concentration in red blood cells. Although intake is between 10 and 15 mg. per day, absorption is usually low, representing less than 10 per cent, and is decreased by certain binding

TABLE 31-8 TRACE ELEMENTS

Element	Body Content	Concentration Whole Blood	Plasma or Serum	Average Intake	Absorption
Calcium	1000 g.	9–10.5 mg./100 ml.	9–10.5 mg./100 ml.	0.2–1.5 g./d.	0.1–0.5 g.
Magnesium	25 g.	3.0 mEq./liter	1.8–2.5 mEq./liter	400 mg./d.	100 mg.
Iron	5 g.	43 mg./100 ml.*	70–180 μg./100 ml.	12–15 mg./d.	0.6–1.5 mg.
Zinc	2	800 μg./100 ml.	120 μg./100 ml.†	10–15 mg./d.	1 mg.
Copper	100–150 mg.	98 μg./100 ml.	109 μg./100 ml.	2.5–5 mg./d.	0.6–1.6 mg.
Iodine	10–20 mg.	—	4–8 μg./100 ml.	50–1000 μg./d.	50–1000 μg.
Manganese	12–20 mg.	9.8 μg./100 ml.	1.4 μg./100 ml.	2–8 mg./d.	
Molybdenum	10–20 mg.	1.4 μg./100 ml.	1.4 μg./100 ml.	100 μg./d.	90 μg.
Chromium	6 mg.	15 μg./100 ml.	1–6 μg./100 ml.	50 μg./d.	0.5 μg.
Cobalt	1 mg.	53	4.3 μg./100 ml.	300 μg./d.	30–60 μg./d.

*As iron in hemoglobin (0.34% × 12.7 g./100 ml.).
†Serum 16% higher than plasma (lysis of platelets releases zinc).

agents, particularly phytates, which are present in various cereals. Zinc is a factor in a number of enzymes including alkaline phosphatase, found in liver and bone; carbonic anhydrase; carboxypeptidase from the pancreas; as well as lactate, malate, and alcoholic dehydrogenase. Zinc is also of importance in the beta cells of the pancreas and may be involved in the crystallization of insulin in the granules within these cells. This element also has an important role in the synthesis of DNA and protein, as shown by the reduced incorporation of radioactivity from thymidine into nuclear DNA in zinc deficiency. This impairment can be overcome by injecting zinc a short time before giving thymidine. The effects of zinc on the activity of ribonuclease offer one explanation for these effects on nucleic acid synthesis. Zinc is an inhibitor of this enzyme in the deficient state and the activity of ribonuclease might be enhanced.

Experimental zinc deficiency has been produced in several experimental animals and has been documented with reasonable certainty in human beings. Zinc deficiency in man is characterized by dwarfism and hypogonadism. Most cases have come from villages in Egypt and Iran where the ingestion of clay and diets high in cereal might impair the absorption of zinc. The subjects in question are usually males and show a marked delay in onset of sexual development. Pubic hairs are sparse or absent, and the testes are small. Facial hair is sparse and hepatosplenomegaly is frequent. Administration of zinc accelerated growth of these boys and led to an enhanced rate of sexual development. On this basis, it appears that zinc might be a causative factor of human disease.

The mechanism by which zinc impairs growth is unclear. It is known to be an essential part of the enzyme alkaline phosphatase, which is found in bone but the role of which in bone growth and development is still unsettled. The zinc deficiency is also accompanied by slow rates of growth in experimental animals, an effect which is independent of growth hormone. Although reproductive function is impaired in zinc-deficient dwarfs, the mechanism has not been established. Pituitary function, as indicated by thyroid status, is normal, and adrenal function is only slightly impaired. From the failure to develop sexually, one presumes that the output of gonadotropins is deficient.

Zinc deficiency also impairs the healing of wounds. Over 20 per cent of the total zinc stores are located in skin. Zinc supplements were shown to accelerate the rate of wound healing in groups of apparently normal men. Detailed studies of this phenomenon, however, showed that the effects of zinc were only detectable in those individuals with mild degrees of zinc deficiency. Little or no effect was present in individuals with normal levels of this element. A mild zinc deficiency thus occurs in a significant number of people. Among the groups in which the levels of zinc are reduced are cirrhotics who show enhanced urinary zinc levels and patients with the nephrotic syndrome.

Copper

Although copper has been known for centuries, its importance in nutrition has only been appreciated since 1930. At that time, an anemia in rats due to copper deficiency was clearly demonstrated. Since that time, it has been possible to show that patients with protein-calorie malnutrition have copper deficiency. The body stores approximately 80 mg. of copper. The largest fraction of this is in the liver and significant abnormalities in liver and brain occur in Wilson's disease, in which the transport protein for copper is markedly reduced. In this disease, the copper content of the liver and of brain is increased, with the development of neurologic symptoms and hepatic failure. Copper is part of several enzymes including cytochrome oxidase, tyrosinase, and uricase. Deficiency of copper produces three changes. The first is a hypochromic, microcytic anemia. Although copper is not known to be an important element in the production of the enzymes involved in hemoglobin synthesis, it appears to play a critical role in the overall process for utilization of iron. Copper-deficient infants recovering from protein-calorie malnutrition develop an anemia which is cured by administration of copper. These infants also have brittle bones. Leukopenia is the second principal manifestation of copper deficiency. Induction of this state in adults is difficult because of the ubiquity of copper. However, in severe malnutrition in which initial replacement is with milk for sustained periods, a deficiency in copper can be observed.

Chromium

Interest in the element chromium has been stimulated by the work of Mertz and his collaborators, who demonstrated that chromium deficiency in experimental animals was accompanied by abnormalities in the metabolism of glucose. This diabetes-like syndrome would be reversed by the administration of chromium. The body only contains 6 mg. of chromium. It is transported in blood by a specific protein known as siderophilin. Most, if not all, chromium is present with a valence of +3. This element appears to be an integral part of membranes and is contained in the enzyme phosphoglucomutase. The induction of experimental chromium deficiency impairs glucose tolerance in rats, in addition to lowering the sensitivity to the effects of insulin in vitro. The suggestion that chromium acts at the cell membrane is supported by the observation that the addition of certain chromium-containing compounds restores the response to insulin in vitro. These observations in experimental animals may be relevant to diabetes in man. It has been established that the concentration of chromium declines with age, paralleling reduced metabolism of glucose. There is suggestive evidence that in some individuals with impaired glucose tolerance, supplements of chromium can restore their metabolism of glucose toward normal. The possibility thus exists, and presents a fascinating challenge to medical science, that chromium deficiency may play a significant role in certain types of human diabetes.

Fluoride Metabolism

Fluoride is widely distributed in nature and is present in small concentrations in most supplies of soil and water. Whether this element is essential for nutrition, however, has not yet been established. Animals fed diets with very low levels of fluoride show little difference in growth rate and metabolic characteristics from animals fed diets supplemented with this element. The principal interest in fluoride has come from its inhibition of dental decay and the toxic state of fluorosis, i.e., the disease of excess fluoride intake. The initial studies demonstrating that fluoride had an effect on dental caries were conducted in the 1930s. The results of one such experiment are shown in Table 31-9. It is clear from this table that in a 5-year period there was a significant reduction in the number of carious teeth in children receiving fluoride supplements but no significant change in the control groups. This effect of fluoride was most striking in the younger children and decreased as the age of the children increased. These data and many other controlled experiments clearly demonstrate that fluoride supplement at a level of 1 part per million (ppm.) in drinking water is capable of reducing dental caries. The mechanism by which this occurs, however, is unclear. Fluoride is found in its highest concentrations in bone and teeth and appears to be involved in the formation of bone matrix. An intake of water of 1 to 2 liters per day with a fluoride concentration of 1 ppm. will provide an intake of 1 to 2 mg. of fluoride. This appears to be optimal for reducing dental caries. At higher levels, fluoride poisoning or fluorosis occurs. This is primarily observed in animals but can be seen in man following industrial accidents. The symptoms develop after the compensatory mechanisms for disposition of fluoride have been exhausted. When the intake of fluoride increases sharply, the urinary excretion also rises until the maximum is achieved. Bone uptake also increases but has a finite capacity. When the capacities of the kidney and bone have been saturated, the extra fluoride is stored in tissue and induces the symptoms of fluorosis, which consist of a loss of appetite and a loss of body weight. Symptoms referable to the gastrointestinal and neuromuscular systems also occur, as do pulmonary congestion and respiratory and cardiac failure. It must be noted, however, that such levels of fluoride are hardly ever reached in man.

One of the principal sources of fluoride in the human diet is tea. This plant absorbs large quantities of fluoride from the soil and is in this sense unique. For most other foods, concentrations of 1 to 2 ppm. of fluoride are maximal. Fluoride concentrations in tea, however, can be up to 100 ppm. or 100 times that usually seen in almost all other sources of food.

Iodine

The importance of iodine in human metabolism has been known for over 50 years. This element which was discovered in the early part of the 19th century was studied extensively by Chatin, who correlated the prevalence of goiter with availability of iodine supplies in the soil, food, and water. His work in the middle of the 19th century strongly suggested that the regions with a high incidence of thyroid enlargement (goiter) were those regions with low iodine in food and water. His analytical methods were relatively crude by present standards and his work went largely unnoticed. Revival of interest in iodine came from the observations by Baumann that the thyroid gland contained iodine. Within a short time, the presence of thyroxine was demonstrated by Kendall, and in 1927 the structure and synthesis of this hormone were reported by Harington. At the same time, studies by Marine and his collaborators demonstrated the efficacy of iodine supplements as a treatment for thyroid enlargement. In a series of studies carried out in the school system of Akron, Ohio, in 1916 to 1920, these investigators showed that supplements of

TABLE 31-9 EFFECT OF FLUORIDE ON DENTAL CARIES IN CHILDREN*

Age in Years	Control Areas 1956	Control Areas 1961	Areas with Fluoride Added in 1956 — 1956	Areas with Fluoride Added in 1956 — 1961	Per cent Reduction with Fluoride
3	3.53	3.32	3.80	1.29	66%
4	5.18	4.83	5.39	2.31	57%
5	5.66	5.39	5.81	2.91	50%
6	6.32	6.22	6.49	4.81	26%
7	7.08	6.89	7.06	6.05	14%

*Fluoride added to drinking water of one area in 1956 at 1 part per million. Adapted from British Ministry of Health: Roy. Soc. Health J., 82:173, 1962.

iodine significantly reduced the incidence of goiter among school children. From their work and the observations of many since that time, the essential nature of iodine intake for prevention of goiter and the need to supplement iodine intake in regions with low iodine content in the food and water has become clear. The principal supplementary sources of iodine in diet have come by the addition of iodide to salt in the form of iodized salt and more recently by the use of iodates in bread.

The iodide ingested in the diet is absorbed and circulates at a concentration of 0.06 to 0.80 μg. per ml. of serum. This iodide has two principal exit routes from the serum: (1) into the thyroid gland and (2) into the urine by filtration at the glomerulus. The fraction of iodide concentrated by the thyroid gland and converted to hormone is related to the total quantity of iodine already present in the thyroid. In areas of iodine deficiency, i.e., when intake is less than 75 μg. per day on the average, the iodine stores in the thyroid become deficient, since the daily requirements for hormone synthesis are approximately 80 μg. Thus, as deficiency develops, compensatory mechanisms increase the fraction of circulating iodine which is trapped by the thyroid gland and decrease the fraction which is excreted in the urine. Conversely, when iodine intake is high, the thyroid stores become saturated and further uptake of iodine is inhibited, and the relative fraction concentrated by the gland falls as the fraction appearing in the urine increases. This reciprocal relationship between uptake of iodine by the thyroid gland and its excretion in the urine has been used by Oddie, Fisher, and their collaborators to evaluate levels of iodine intake in various parts of the United States. Regional differences in dietary intake are clearly apparent (Fig. 31–9). It is the regions with low iodine intake where the incidence of endemic goiter is highest.

Severe iodine deficiency occurs in several regions of the world. One of the earliest studies of the pathophysiologic consequences of iodine deficiency was carried out by Stanbury and his collaborators in the Mendoza region of Argentina. More recent studies have been conducted in the Congo, in New Guinea, and in portions of South America and the Middle East. The more severe the lack of iodine, the greater the frequency of enlarged thyroid glands. However, even in the most severely deficient areas, enlargement of the thyroid gland does not occur in all persons. This observation suggests significant variability between individuals in their ability to compensate for severe iodine deficiency. Several mechanisms are involved in this compensation. The first of these is an increase in the fraction of ingested iodine which is trapped by the thyroid gland. In many areas, iodine uptake is frequently above 70 per cent and may reach 100 per cent of an administered dose. The iodide which is trapped by the thyroid is attached to tyrosine to form mono- and diiodotyrosine which are in turn coupled to form thyroxine and tri-iodothyronine. As iodine becomes scarce, the percentage of monoiodotyrosine is increased in the thyroid gland relative to di-iodotyrosine. Similarly, the proportion of 3,5,3'-tri-iodothyronine increases relative to

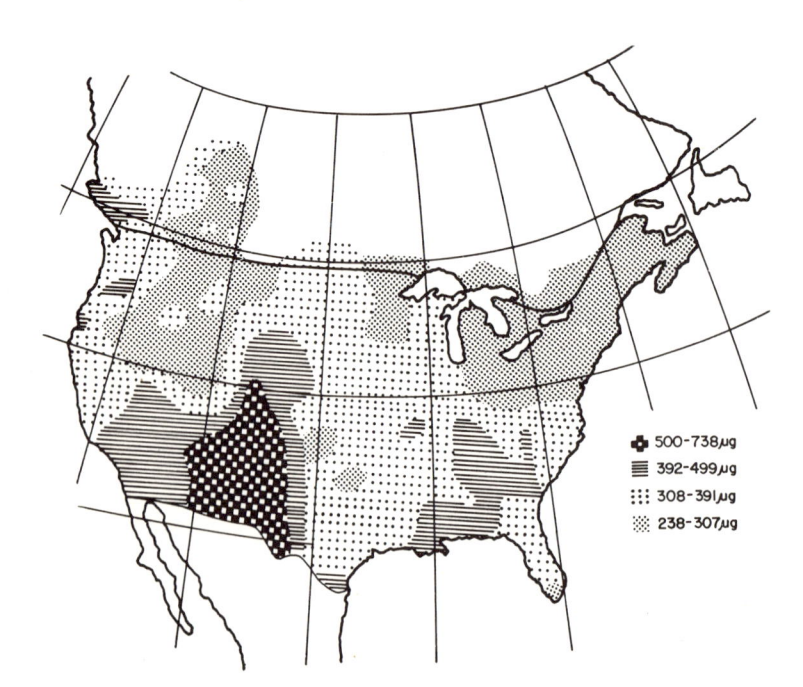

Figure 31–9 Iodine intake in the United States. These data on iodine intake in the United States were calculated from data on the regional uptake of radioactive iodine. The areas of highest iodine intake are in the southwest United States and the lowest regions are in the Midwest, along the east coast and in some sections of the upper Rocky Mountains. (Reproduced with permission from Oddie, T. H., et al.: J. Clin. Endocr., *30*:659, 1970.)

thyroxine. Thus, the quantities of monoiodotyrosine and tri-iodothyronine are increased and the concentrations of di-iodotyrosine and thyroxine are reduced in areas of iodine deficiency. Because the iodine stores are low, the turnover rate of thyroid iodine increases. Thus, tri-iodothyronine becomes a larger fraction of the circulating thyroactive hormone in iodine deficiency than when iodine stores are adequate. Finally, the thyroid gland itself enlarges in an attempt to compensate for the low iodine intake. Two underlying mechanisms are thus involved in the adaptation to iodine deficiency. The first are the intrathyroidal mechanisms of autoregulation. By this term one means that the responsiveness of the thyroid to the thyroid-stimulating hormone from the pituitary gland is increased in iodine deficiency. Thus, the uptake of iodide, the conversion to hormone, the release of hormone, and enlargement of the thyroid gland are all increased in an iodine-deficient thyroid. The second mechanism for regulating thyroidal iodine stores is the increase in the concentrations of thyroid-stimulating hormone (TSH). This mechanism is presumably activated by a reduction in the concentration of circulating thyroxine and tri-iodothyronine detected by the hypothalamic receptors which control the output of thyrotropin-releasing hormone from the pituitary.

The enlarged thyroid which occurs in iodine-deficient areas can be reduced in size in many individuals given iodine supplementation. This has been shown repeatedly by giving iodine supplements to deficient groups. Thus, iodine is an essential element for human nutrition and in its absence compensatory processes occur which lead to thyroid enlargement. Failure of the compensatory mechanism to provide a reasonable circulating level of thyroid hormone is accompanied by hypothyroidism and failure to grow normally. Areas of severe iodine deficiency show an increase in the number of such goiterous cretins suffering from deficiency of thyroid hormones.

In some regions of the world, iodine supplies occur in excess. In these regions, thyroid glands tend to be smaller than normal, but in some individuals, thyroid enlargement occurs. This consequence of high intake of iodine has been termed iodide myxedema. The mechanism for this effect appears to be suppression of thyroid function by high iodide intake resulting in a drop in circulating thyroid hormone and compensatory increase in the output of thyrotropin by the pituitary. This, in turn, stimulates the thyroid gland to enlarge. A comparable effect of high iodide intake was observed in animals by Wolff and Chaikoff, and the mechanism of this effect is currently under intensive investigation.

REFERENCES

OBESITY

Anand, B. K.: Nervous regulation of food intake. Physiol. Rev., *41*:677, 1961.

Bagdade, J. D., Bierman, E. L., and Porte, D., Jr.: The significance of basal insulin levels in the evaluation of the insulin response to glucose in diabetic and nondiabetic subjects. J. Clin. Invest., *46*:1549, 1967.

Bray, G. A.: Measurement of subcutaneous fat cells from obese patients. Ann. Intern. Med., *73*:565, 1970.

Bray, G. A.: Lipogenesis in human adipose tissue: Some effects of nibbling and gorging. J. Clin. Invest., *51*:537, 1972.

Bray, G. A., Schwartz, M., Rozin, R. R., and Lister, J.: Some relationships between oxygen consumption and body composition of obese patients. Metabolism, *19*:418, 1970.

Bray, G. A., and York, D. A.: Genetically transmitted obesity in rodents. Physiol. Rev., *51*:598, 1971.

Bray, G. A., Raben, M. S., Londono, J., and Gallagher, T. F., Jr.: Effects of triiodothyronine, growth hormone and anabolic steroids on nitrogen excretion and oxygen consumption of obese patients. J. Clin. Endocr., *33*:293, 1971.

Bruch, H.: The Fröhlich syndrome. Amer. J. Dis. Child., *58*:1282, 1939.

Fabry, P., Hejda, S., Cerny, K., Osancova, K., and Pechar, J.: Effect of meal frequency in school children. Changes in the weight-height proportion and skinfold thickness. Amer. J. Clin. Nutr., *18*:358, 1966.

Gordon, E. A.: Metabolic aspects of obesity. In Levine, R., and Luft, R., (Eds.) Advances in Metabolic Disorders. Vol. 4. New York, Academic Press, 1970, p. 229.

Hetherington, A. W., and Ranson, S. W.: Hypothalamic lesions and adiposity in the rat. Anat. Rec., *78*:149, 1940.

Hirsch, J., and Knittle, J. L.: Cellularity of obese and nonobese human adipose tissue. Fed. Proc., *29*:1516, 1970.

Hoebel, B. G.: Feeding: Neural control of intake. Ann. Rev. Physiol., *33*:533, 1971.

Hollenberg, C. H., Vost, A., and Patten, R. L.: Regulation of adipose mass: Control of fat cell development and lipid content. Recent Progr. Hormone Res., *26*:463, 1970.

Keys, A., and Grande, F.: Body weight, body composition and calorie status. In Wohl, M. G., and Goodhart, R. S. (Eds.): Modern Nutrition in Health and Disease. 4th Ed. Philadelphia, Lea and Febiger, 1968, pp. 3–30.

Lusk, G.: The Elements of the Science of Nutrition. Philadelphia, W. B. Saunders Co., 1928.

Mayer, J., and Thomas, D. W.: Regulation of food intake and obesity. Science, *156*:328, 1967.

Moore, R. D., Olesen, K. H., McMurrey, J. D., Parker, H. V., Ball, M. B., and Boyden, C. M.: The Body Cell Mass and Its Supporting Environment. Philadelphia, W. B. Saunders Co., 1963.

Rabinowitz, D.: Some endocrine and metabolic aspects of obesity. Ann. Rev. Med., *21*:241, 1970.

Recommended Dietary Allowances. 7th Ed. Washington, D.C., National Academy of Sciences, 1968.

Salans, L. B., and Dougherty, J. W.: The effect of insulin upon glucose metabolism by adipose cells of different size. Influence of cell lipid and protein content, age, and nutritional state. J. Clin. Invest., *50*:1399, 1971.

Salans, L. B., Horton, E. S., and Sims, E. A. H.: Experimental obesity in man: Cellular character of the adipose tissue. J. Clin. Invest., *50*:1005, 1971.

Schachter, S.: Obesity and eating. Internal and external cues differentially affect the eating behavior of obese and normal subjects. Science, *161*:751, 1968.

Sims, E. A. H., Goldman, R. F., Gluck, C. M., Horton, E. S., Kelleher, P. C., and Rowe, D. W.: Experimental obesity in man. Trans. Assoc. Amer. Physicians, *81*:153, 1968.

Sims, E. A. H., Horton, E. S., and Salans, L. B.: Inducible metabolic abnormalities during development of obesity. Ann. Rev. Med., *2*:235, 1971.

Widdowson, E. M.: Chemical analysis of the body. *In* Brozek, J. (Ed.): Human Body Composition: Approaches and Applications. New York, Pergamon Press, 1965, pp. 31–55.

PROTEIN AND/OR CALORIE DEFICIENCY

Cahill, G. F., Jr., Herrera, M. G., Morgan, A. P., Soeldner, J. S., Steinke, J., Levy, P. L., Reichard, G. A., Jr., and Kipnis, D. M.: Hormone-fuel interrelationships during fasting. J. Clin. Invest., 45:1751, 1966.

Cahill, G. F., Jr., and Owen, O. E.: Body fuels and starvation. *In* Rowland, C. V., Jr. (Ed.): Anorexia and Obesity. Boston, Little, Brown and Co., 1970, pp. 25–36.

Crisp, A. H.: Anorexia Nervosa – "Feeding Disorder," "Nervous Malnutrition," or "Weight Phobia"? World Rev. Nutr. Diet., 12:452, 1970.

McCance, R. A., and Widdowson, E. M.: Calorie deficiencies and protein deficiencies. Boston, Little, Brown and Co., 1968.

Own, O. E., Morgan, A. P., Kemp, H. G., Sullivan, J. M., Herrera, M. G., and Cahill, G. F., Jr.: Brain metabolism during fasting. J. Clin. Invest., 46:1589, 1967.

Young, V. R., and Scrimshaw, N. S.: The physiology of starvation. Sci. Amer., 225:14, 1971.

LIPIDS

Beaumont, J. L., Carlson, L. A., Cooper, C. R., Fejfar, Z., Fredrickson, D. S., and Strassen, T.: Classification of hyperlipidemias and hyperlipoproteinemias. WHO Bull., 43:891, 1970.

Fredrickson, D. S., Levy, R. I., and Lees, R. S.: Fat transport in lipoproteins. An integrated approach to mechanisms and disorders. New Eng. J. Med., 276:32, 94, 148, 215, 273; 1967.

Glueck, C. J.: Effects of oxandrolone on plasma triglycerides and postheparin lipolytic activity in patients with types III, IV, and V familial hyperlipoproteinemia. Metabolism, 20:691, 1971.

Glueck, C. J., Heckman, F., Schoenfeld, M., Steiner, P., and Pearce, W.: Neonatal familial type II hyperlipoproteinemia: Cord blood cholesterol in 1800 births. Metabolism, 20:597, 1971.

VITAMINS

Baker, H., and Frank, O.: Vitamin status in metabolic upsets. World Rev. Nutr. Diet., 9:124, 1968.

Braun, I. G.: Vitamin A: Excess, deficiency, requirement, metabolism, and misuse. Pediat. Clin. N. Amer., 9:935, 1962.

Darby, W. J.: Tocopherol-responsive anemias in man. Vitamins Hormones, 26:685, 1968.

DeLuca, H. F.: Recent advances in the metabolism and function of vitamin D. Fed. Proc., 28:1678, 1969.

Frimpter, G. W., Andelman, R. J., and George, W. F.: Vitamin B_6-dependency syndromes. Amer. J. Clin. Nutr., 22:794, 1969.

Hodges, R. E., Hood, J., Canham, J. E., Sauberlich, H. E., and Baker, E. M.: Clinical manifestations of ascorbic acid deficiency in man. Amer. J. Clin. Nutr., 24:432, 1971.

Kleeman, C. R., Massry, S. G., and Coburn, J. W.: The clinical physiology of calcium homeostasis, parathyroid hormone, and calcitonin. Calif. Med., 114:16, March, 1971.

Raisz, I. G.: Physiologic and pharmacologic regulation of bone resorption. New Eng. J. Med., 282:909, 1970.

Rivlin, R. S.: Riboflavin metabolism. New Eng. J. Med., 283:463, 1970.

Stewart, C. P., and Guthrie, D.: Lind's Treatise on Scurvy. Edinburgh, The Edinburgh University Press, 1953.

Terris, M.: Goldberger on Pellagra. Baton Rouge, Louisiana State University Press, 1964.

TRACE ELEMENTS

British Ministry of Health: Report on the five year fluoridation studies in the United Kingdom, July 3, 1962. Roy. Soc. Health J., 82:173, 1962.

Mertz, W.: Chromium occurrence and function in biological systems. Physiol. Rev., 49:163, 1969.

Oddie, T. H., Fisher, D. A., McConahey, W. M., and Thompson, C. S.: Iodine intake in the United States: A reassessment. J. Clin. Endocr., 30:659, 1970.

Sandstead, H. H., Prasad, A. S., Schulert, A. R., Farid, Z., Miale, A., Bassilly, S., and Darby, W. J.: Human zinc deficiency, Endocrine manifestations and response to treatment. Amer. J. Clin. Nutr., 29:422, 1967.

Underwood, E. J.: Trace Elements in Human and Animal Nutrition. 3rd Ed. New York, Academic Press, 1971.

CHAPTER 32   ENDOCRINOLOGY

THOMAS W. BURNS

INTRODUCTION

The endocrine system is composed of glands which secrete one or more hormones directly into the bloodstream. The ductless glands of the endocrine system are in contrast to the exocrine glands, the secretions of which pass into the lumen of the gastrointestinal tract or onto the skin. Over 100 years ago Claude Bernard introduced a fundamental concept of biology—homeostasis of the internal milieu. Survival of mammalian species has required mechanisms to maintain the constancy of the internal environment despite wide fluctuations in the physical environment and in the availability of essential nutrients. The endocrine system provides many of these mechanisms.

If a principal function of the endocrine system is the preservation of homeostasis, its method of accomplishing this is communication. Increasingly it appears that the nervous system and the endocrine system form a complementary "wire" and "wireless" communications network regulating a broad array of metabolic processes. Neural signals from higher centers impinge on the hypothalamus, thereby modulating the synthesis and secretion of neurohumoral substances which either regulate the release of anterior pituitary hormones or pass directly to the posterior pituitary. Once these hormones are released into the circulation, they in turn stimulate the secretion of hormones by specific target glands or act directly on other tissues of the body. At the distal end of the communications circuit, these hormones powerfully affect intracellular events. At the proximal end, many of these hormones, including those secreted by the thyroid, gonads, parathyroids, and pancreas, are essential for the proper development and function of the central nervous system. While in no instance has the precise mechanism of action of the hormone on a tissue been elucidated, recent work suggests that hormone action commences with the interaction of the hormone with a specific receptor protein in either the cellular membrane or cytosol. The hormone-receptor protein complex then activates the first of a series of enzymatic steps leading to the overt expression of the hormone's biological activity. Thus, the central nervous system, the endocrine system, and the intracellular enzymatic systems form an interlocking triad of regulation, each element capable of directing and responding to appropriate signals which allow the transfer of information from the integrated center of the organism to its smallest operating unit.

BASIC PHYSIOLOGIC NOTIONS

ELEMENTS OF THE ENDOCRINE SYSTEM

The endocrine system comprises the hypothalamus, the anterior and posterior pituitary, the thyroid, the parathyroids, the pancreas, the adrenal cortex, the adrenal medulla, and the gonads (ovaries and testes). The endocrine function of the human pineal gland has not been established and will not be considered. The placenta elaborates several hormones, but there are few data implicating the endocrine placenta in human disease and it will not be commented upon further. The secretory activity of the adrenal cortex, the thyroid, and the gonads is subservient to the tropic hormones of the anterior pituitary. The secretion of parathyroid hormone is regulated by the level of plasma ionized calcium, and that of insulin principally by the serum glucose concentration. The secretion of epinephrine by the adrenal medulla is controlled by the sympathetic nervous system.

HORMONES: DEFINITION AND BASIC CHARACTERIZATION

The term "hormone" was first used by Starling and Bayliss in 1906 to describe secretin and gastrin. They defined hormones as chemical substances released into the circulation by one group of cells and affecting one or more different groups of cells. A more useful definition, proposed by Huxley in 1935, emphasizes the biological function of hormones rather than their means of transport. According to Huxley, hormones are molecules whose essential purpose is the transfer of information from one set of cells to another to meet the needs of the total organism.

At the present time it is possible to distinguish two groups of hormones. Those in the first group clearly subserve the transfer of information role of Huxley's definition. Examples include epinephrine, parathyroid hormone, insulin, and most of the hormones of the anterior pituitary. In general, the response of the body to these hormones is rapid and proportionate to the quantity of hormone present. The response promptly ceases when the concentration of hormone falls below a critical level. These hormones appear to act through the adenylate cyclase-cyclic AMP system to be described later. The second group of hormones is exemplified by the steroids, thyroxine, and growth hormone. The response of cells to these hormones is slow and may persist after the plasma concentration of the hormone has fallen below a physiologically effective level. Their primary function appears to be growth and maintenance. Since, in their absence, cells may not be able to respond to the first group of hormones, hormones of the second group have been termed permissive. Their mechanism of action appears to involve modification of protein synthesis. Thus far, there has been no demonstration that they activate the cyclic AMP system.

FEEDBACK CONTROL IN THE REGULATION OF HORMONE SECRETORY ACTIVITY

The concept of negative and positive feedback control is basic to a clear understanding of the normal and pathologic physiology of the endocrine system. The interrelations between the anterior pituitary and the thyroid exemplify the principles involved. The secretory rate of thyroid hormone is increased by plasma thyroid-stimulating hormone (TSH) which is secreted by the anterior pituitary. [*Note:* Throughout this chapter, thyroid hormone is intended to include thyroxine (T_4) and triiodothyronine (T_3)]. As the level of thyroid hormone in the plasma increases, it reaches a concentration called the "set point," which causes the cessation of TSH secretion and hence of the secretion of thyroid hormone itself. The plasma concentration of thyroid hormone then falls and when it declines below the set point, TSH secretion resumes. An analogy may be drawn between this process and the control of room temperature by the interaction of a thermostat and a furnace. The thermostat setting, for example 70°, is similar to the set point. Heat from the furnace will be delivered until the room temperature exceeds 70°. At that point, the thermostat signals the furnace to shut off and delivery of heat ceases. When the temperature falls below the set point, the thermostat is activated and signals the furnace to turn on. In this analogy, the furnace represents the thyroid gland, heat represents plasma thyroid hormone, the thermostat represents the anterior pituitary, and the electrical signal between the thermostat and the furnace is analogous to TSH.

The control of parathyroid hormone secretion is based on a simpler negative feedback. The principal stimulus to its secretion is a fall in plasma calcium concentration below a set point of approximately 10 mg. per 100 ml. The increase in plasma parathyroid hormone, by its action on kidney, bone, and gut, increases serum calcium until the set point is reached. The relationship between insulin secretion by the pancreas and the plasma concentration of glucose exemplifies a positive feedback system. When glucose concentration exceeds a level of about 120 mg. per 100 ml., insulin secretion increases and diverts glucose into the liver and peripheral tissues, thus reducing the blood glucose. The advantages of these feedback systems, which have many counterparts in the servomechanisms in industry, are obvious. They permit maintenance of closely controlled concentrations of hormones, metabolites, and nutrients in the plasma, and thus preserve the homeostasis of the internal milieu. As will be repeatedly emphasized, the diagnosis of an endocrine disease frequently is based on the interpretation of laboratory data in light of the feedback concept.

CHEMICAL NATURE, ELABORATION, SECRETION, AND TRANSPORT OF HORMONES

If hormones are classified on the basis of chemical structure, four broad categories emerge:
1. Small peptides
2. Large polypeptides
3. Steroids
4. Derivatives of amino acids

The structures of some neurohumoral substances elaborated by the hypothalamus are only now being elucidated. They appear to be small peptides with only a few amino acid residues. Vasopressin, also formed in hypothalamic nuclei, has 8 amino acids. The hormones of the anterior pituitary are large polypeptides, as are insulin, glucagon, and parathyroid hormone. The steroid hormones include secretions of the adrenal cortex, the ovaries, and the testes. Both thyroxine and epinephrine are amino acid derivatives.

Much information is accruing regarding the molecular events involved in the biosynthesis, storage, and release of hormones, especially thyroid hormone, insulin, and the steroid hormones. The fabrication of a hormone requires a number of enzymatic steps, and many diseases are now recognized which are due to a deficiency of a biosynthetic enzyme. This leads either to the absence of hormone production by the involved gland or to the synthesis of a defective hormone. It should be recalled that many hormones have the secondary function of interacting with either the hypothalamus or the pituitary to assist in the regulation of their own secretion. The structural requirements for both the primary and secondary functions of a hormone are thought to be the same. The consequences of a target endocrine gland secreting a biologically inactive hormone are predictable from the negative feedback concept. An affected individual will display not only the effects of hormonal deficiency but also enlargement of the affected gland, because of an increase in the specific circulating tropic hormone. Examples of this phenomenon involving deficiencies in the biosynthesis of thyroid hormone will be discussed later.

After their release into the circulation, many hormones quickly combine with a carrier protein. In general, the structure of the carrier protein is highly specific for its client hormone. Since only the free hormone is metabolically active, the binding of hormone to a specific protein provides another means of regulating its activity. The concentrations of carrier proteins are influenced by various factors including sex hormones, drugs, and certain diseases. Instances of genetically induced deficiency, and also excess, of the thyroid-binding protein (thyroid-binding globulin or TBG) have been observed. As discussed below, carrier proteins have become of great value in the laboratory for the measurement of the specific hormones they bind.

MECHANISM OF ACTION OF HORMONES

It is gratifying to students of biology when a unifying concept becomes established as fact. Such was the case when the nucleotide adenosinetriphosphate (ATP) was identified as the final donor of energy in almost all biological reactions. A similar event may be imminent concerning the mechanism of hormone action, since most, if not all, appear to act through one of two pathways.

Adenylate Cyclase–Cyclic AMP System

Largely through the patient and creative investigations of Sutherland and coworkers 10 years ago, the nucleotide cyclic AMP was recognized as a key mediator of the action of epinephrine on liver glycogen. Since then, research on the role of cyclic AMP has proliferated at a fantastic rate. Hormone tissue interactions in which cyclic AMP has been implicated are summarized in Table 32-1. Not only has cyclic AMP been found in cells of all animal species studied, but recently Pastan demonstrated its necessity for the induction of certain enzymes in the bacterium *E. coli*. Cyclic AMP has also been identified as the attractant substance that signals individual cells of the social ameba, the slime mold, to aggregate. Thus, the significance of cyclic AMP in biology rivals that of ATP.

The manner in which cyclic AMP mediates hormonal action appears constant for all hormones and animal species thus far studied. The hormone circulating in plasma interacts with a receptor in the plasma membrane of the cell. The receptor may be an integral part of the enzyme adenylate cyclase or may merely be linked to it. In any event, the hormone-receptor interaction leads to activation of adenylate cyclase. This enzyme catalyzes the formation of cyclic AMP from ATP. Cyclic AMP then triggers the response that is recognized as the hormone's biological action. In this scheme, the hormone is frequently designated as the "first messenger" and cyclic AMP as the "second messenger." Besides being increased by adenylate cyclase, the intracellular level of cyclic AMP is regulated by the activity of a potent, specific esterase, phosphodiesterase. This enzyme is inhibited by xanthine derivatives such as theophylline and caffeine. These agents cause an increase in cyclic AMP and tend to mimic hor-

TABLE 32-1 HORMONES WHICH UTILIZE CYCLIC AMP AS A SECOND MESSENGER

Hormone	Tissue
Catecholamines	Various tissues
Glucagon	Liver, pancreatic islets, adipose tissue
ACTH	Adrenal cortex and adipose tissue
LH or ICSH	Ovarian and testicular tissue
Vasopressin	Various epithelial tissues
Parathyroid hormone	Kidney and bone, gut
TRH	Anterior pituitary
TSH	Thyroid tissue
MSH	Frog skin
Prostaglandins	Various tissues
Histamine	Brain
Serotonin	Fasciola hepatica

From Robison, G. A., Butcher, R. W., and Sutherland, E. W.: Cyclic AMP. New York, Academic Press, 1971.

mone action in in-vitro systems. Additional details are now known regarding the mechanism by which cyclic AMP initiates the cellular response to a hormone. The nucleotide reacts with a specific protein-receptor, which then interacts with a cyclic AMP-dependent protein kinase. This enzyme in turn activates another enzyme or enzymes, presumably by phosphorylation, and this secondary enzyme (or enzymes) catalyzes the final step leading to the hormone's action and is thought to be inhibited or destroyed by a phosphatase. This schema is depicted in Figure 32–1.

Sutherland and his coworkers have suggested four criteria which ideally should be met if cyclic AMP is to be considered the "second messenger" for a given hormone. These are (1) The hormone should be capable of stimulating adenylate cyclase in broken cell preparations from appropriate tissue. (2) A physiologic concentration of hormone should be able to increase the cyclic AMP concentration of intact cells. This increase in cyclic AMP should precede the physiologic response. (3) Phosphodiesterase inhibitors such as theophylline should potentiate the response to the hormone. (4) The activity of the hormone should be mimicked by cyclic AMP or its more soluble dibutyryl derivative.

A question that often arises when one views Table 32–1 is how can the same compound, cyclic AMP, mediate the highly specific responses of such a diverse array of hormones? There are at least two sites at which specificity could be endowed. Presumably all cells of the body (exclusive of those in the central nervous system) are equally exposed to a hormone circulating in the plasma. However, only the cells of responsive tissue have receptor sites that "recognize" the hormone. The receptor site has a conformational structure complementary to that of the hormone, permitting the latter to bind to the former with high affinity. Additional specificity is imparted by the nature of the substance(s) available to serve as substrates for the cyclic AMP protein kinase catalytic unit. In adipose tissue, the substance is a lipase; in liver, it is a phosphorylase. Specificity could also result if cyclic AMP were compartmentalized within the cell, but this has not been demonstrated thus far.

Interaction of Hormones with Cytoplasmic Receptor Protein and Nuclear Acceptors

At present it appears that the steroid hormones (testosterone, estradiol, progesterone, aldosterone, and cortisol) all exert their metabolic effects in a similar fashion (Fig. 32–2). Each appears to combine with a specific receptor protein located in the cytoplasm; the steroid-receptor

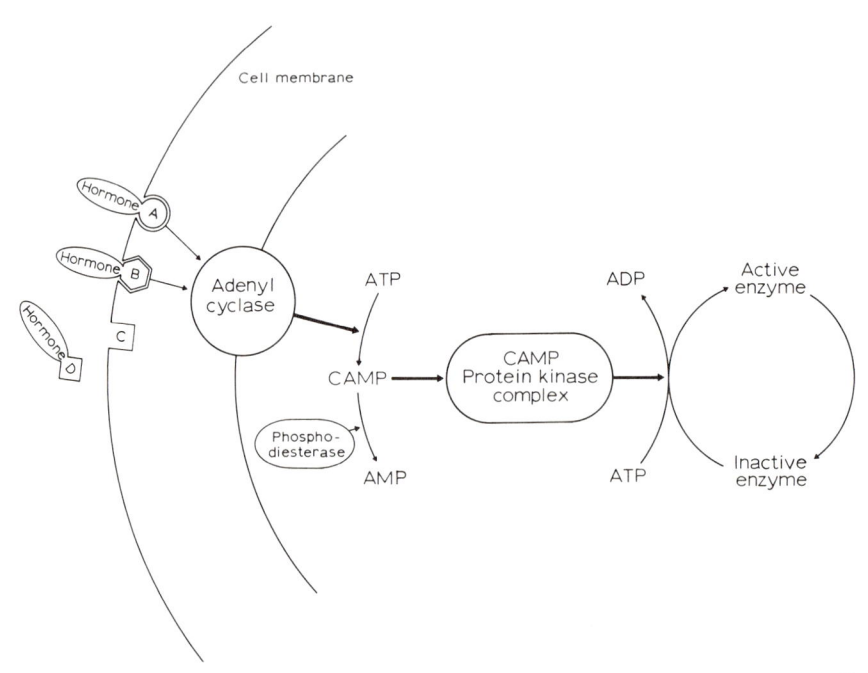

Figure 32–1 Cyclic AMP-mediated hormone action. Circulating hormones ("first messengers") interact with specific receptor sites on the plasma membrane of responsive cells, causing stimulation of adenylate cyclase. Adenylate cyclase catalyzes the conversion of ATP to cyclic AMP (CAMP). The nucleotide activates a protein kinase which, in turn, causes the activation of the enzyme(s) responsible for the expression of the hormone. Free cyclic AMP is quickly destroyed by a specific phosphodiesterase (see text).

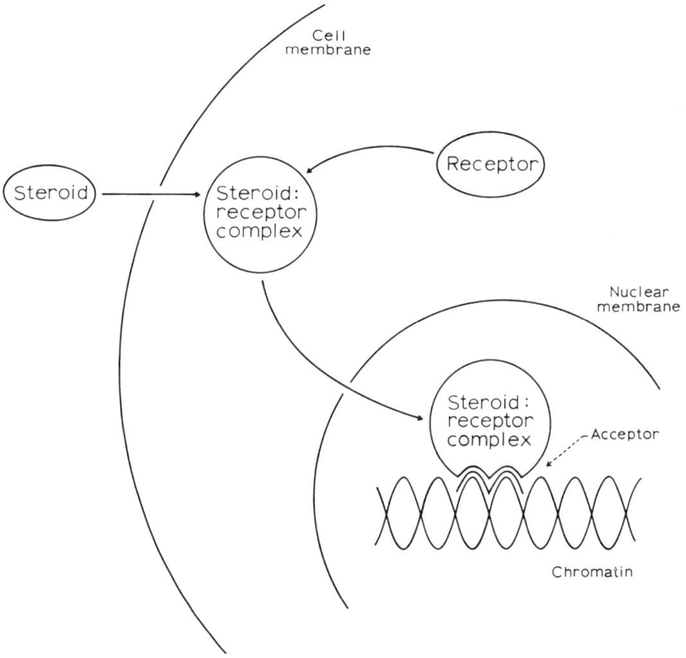

Figure 32-2 Mechanism of action of steroid hormones. Steroid hormones penetrate the cell membrane and combine with highly specific receptor molecules in the cytosol. The steroid-receptor complex then enters the nucleus and binds to an acceptor. The aggregate stimulates the production of messenger RNA which stimulates the synthesis of the protein substances that are responsible for the hormone's action (see text).

complex is translocated to the nucleus, where it combines with specific acceptors located on chromatin. The steroid-receptor-acceptor complex causes the nuclear genetic material to produce messenger RNA, which in turn signals the fabrication of the enzyme which is more directly responsible for the biological expression of the hormone's activity. Specificity results from the conformational structure of the receptor protein and the nuclear acceptor sites.

Other Modes of Hormone Action

Although the mechanisms just described account for the action of a large number of hormones, they do not appear to apply to thyroid hormone or, possibly, insulin. In spite of intense investigation, the manner in which these two hormones modify the metabolic activity of virtually every cell in the body remains obscure.

MANIFESTATIONS OF ENDOCRINE DISORDERS

The majority of endocrine diseases are secondary to either an excess or a deficiency of one or more hormones. Commonly, the clinical description of an endocrine disorder has antedated by many years an appreciation of the gland and hormone involved. Progress in relating clinical syndromes to deficient or excessive hormone was relatively slow until techniques were derived for the measurement of hormones and their metabolites in blood and urine. The protean modes of presentation of endocrine disease are best appreciated by considering the specific examples in the following sections. However, it is important to appreciate the close symbiosis that exists between bedside medicine and laboratory physiology in the field of endocrinology. Perhaps in no other field of medicine has clinical observation been more important in shaping the direction of physiologic experimentation, and similarly there is no area in which the physician is more dependent on an understanding of physiologic principles in diagnosing and treating his patient.

Generally, the clinical manifestations of hormone excess and deficiency are extremely slow in evolving. With few exceptions, even the abrupt loss of a given hormone causes no immediate distress. Thus, when one recognizes clear-cut evidence of excessive or deficient endocrine function, one can usually conclude that the patient's condition began many months or even years earlier. Before he becomes critically ill, the patient passes through a prolonged period of increasing disability. Unfortunately, the early symptoms of the underlying disease are often vague and not very convincing to either patient or physician. Early diagnosis is further handicapped by the not infrequent occurrence of predominantly psychiatric symptoms, which distract the physician from a realization of the organic basis of the patient's illness.

LABORATORY PROCEDURES

Although the presence of an endocrine problem is frequently suggested by symptoms, signs, or an abnormal finding among screening laboratory procedures, establishing the diagnosis usually requires one or more relatively sophisticated laboratory procedures. Increasingly, the latter include direct measurement of the hormone under suspicion. Capability in this area has been greatly enhanced by the development of two new approaches to hormone analysis: radioimmunoassay and competitive protein-binding assay. These methods have in common the use of a reagent protein that is highly specific for the substance to be measured. In the radioimmunoassay, the reagent protein is an antibody generated by a laboratory animal in response to injections of the foreign, human hormone to be measured. In the competitive protein-binding procedure, the reagent protein is usually the binding protein that normally transports in plasma the hormone to be measured.

Radioimmunoassay was first applied to the measurement of insulin in human serum by Yalow and Berson. At the present time, satisfactory procedures for most of the pituitary tropic hormones, glucagon, and parathyroid hormone have been developed, but most are not yet generally available. One requires not only a potent antiserum but also a small supply of pure hormone to serve both as a standard and as a radioactively labeled tracer. To perform an assay, small aliquots of antiserum and labeled hormone are mixed. The latter is in excess, so that there is both labeled hormone bound to the antiserum and free (unbound) labeled hormone. Known quantities of highly purified, *nonlabeled* hormone are now added to one series of flasks. Aliquots of unknown serum are added to the remaining flasks. All flasks are incubated, during which time a certain amount of bound, labeled hormone is displaced from antibody by free, nonlabeled standard or nonlabeled hormone in test plasma. The more nonlabeled hormone present, the greater the quantity of labeled hormone displaced from antibody and the greater the reduction in the so-called bound to free (B/F) ratio (of labeled hormone). To determine this ratio, it is necessary to separate bound hormone from free hormone. A number of satisfactory methods (physical, chemical, and immunologic) have been developed for this purpose. Following the separation, the radioactivity of either (or both) fraction(s) of each flask is counted, and its B/F ratio calculated. A standard curve is prepared by plotting B/F against the quantity of pure, unlabeled hormone in each set of standards; from this curve, the quantity of hormone in the unknown samples can be calculated using the B/F ratio.

The competitive protein-binding procedure was introduced recently by Murphy and Pattee to measure serum thyroxine. Methods available prior to this technique were acceptable in all respects except for their failure to discriminate between thyroid hormone and iodinated organic compounds which frequently contaminate a patient's serum as a result of radiographic procedures. Murphy and Pattee overcame this difficulty by utilizing a highly specific reagent that combined readily with thyroxine but not with other organic iodinated moieties. The reagent is thyroid-binding globulin or TBG. In performing the test, TBG is saturated with thyroxine labeled with radioactive isotopic iodine. This reagent is added to one series of flasks containing known quantities of nonlabeled thyroxine and to a second series containing alcohol extracts of serum samples containing unknown quantities of thyroxine. All flasks are incubated during which time a portion of the bound, labeled thyroxine is displaced from the TBG by unlabeled thyroxine. The greater the quantity of unlabeled thyroxine present, the greater the amount of thyroxine displaced and the greater the reduction in the B/F ratio. The bound fractions of thyroxine are separated from the free by column chromatography, and the radioactivity of one of the fractions is counted. A standard curve is prepared, and the amount of thyroxine in unknown samples is read off the curve. This same approach has been used to determine serum levels of numerous hormones, including testosterone, progesterone, and cortisol.

In summary, the advantages of radioimmunoassay and competitive protein-binding assays are these:

1. *Sensitivity.* The ability to measure the nanogram and picogram quantities of hormone that normally are present in the plasma.

2. *Simplicity.* Once the assay has been established, hundreds of samples per week can be processed.

3. *Specificity.* Because of the high binding affinity for the reagent protein, be it antibody or transport protein, great specificity is inherent in these methods.

One potential disadvantage of these assays is that they measure the immunologically active portion of the hormone rather than the biologically active portion.

HYPOTHALAMUS

PHYSIOLOGY

One of the most exciting advances in endocrinology in the past decade has been the discovery that the secretory activity of the anterior pituitary is subservient to hormones elaborated by the hypothalamus of the central nervous system. The notion that nervous tissue could elaborate hormones was not new. For some time it has been appreciated that the hormones of the posterior pituitary, vasopressin and oxytocin, were elaborated by nuclei of the hypothalamus and then transmitted down neurons to the posterior pituitary. Comparable neural connections between the hypothalamus and the anterior pituitary have not been found. However, it is now established that there are vascular connections between the hypothalamus and the anterior pituitary. The median eminence of the hypothalamus contains a capillary network that drains into the hypophyseal portal veins. The latter enter the anterior pituitary and subdivide into a second network. Thus, substances produced by cells of the median eminence and adjacent areas in the hypothalamus have ready access to the cells of the anterior pituitary via the hypophyseal portal system. In 1969, two groups working independently succeeded in establishing the identity of one such factor, thyrotropin-releasing hormone (TRH). TRH is a tripeptide, pyroglutamyl-histidyl-proline amide, that has now been synthesized in large quantities and is being evaluated for its diagnostic usefulness in man. Although they have not yet been identified structurally, it is evident that specific releasing factors stimulate the secretion of human ACTH, LH, FSH, and growth hormone. The secretion of two other anterior pituitary hormones, melanocyte-stimulating hormone (MSH) and prolactin, appears to be chronically suppressed by hypothalamic inhibiting factors.

If one assumes that anterior pituitary secretion is regulated by humoral substances from the hypothalamus, the question arises as to what in turn regulates the release of the latter? It has long been known that the hypothalamus is a major relay station of the central nervous system. Presumably neural signals from many parts of the brain could activate the cells of the median eminence, either directly or via a neurohumoral substance such as dopamine. Another question that arises is how the hypothalamic factors interact with the target gland hormones which have been known, or thought, to inhibit anterior pituitary secretion in a negative feedback fashion. The mode of interaction may be unique for each pituitary hormone. For example, thyroid hormone appears to oppose TRH at the level of the TSH-producing cells of the anterior pituitary. Cortisol, on the other hand, may act by inhibiting the production and/or release of corticotropin-releasing factor (CRF) at the level of the median eminence.

From the foregoing, it is clear that the central nervous system has a profound influence on the endocrine glands, the interface being the hypothalamus. Although less well documented, the converse may also be true, that is, the endocrine system may have profound influences on the central nervous system. For example, it has been shown that if newborn male rats are castrated and not treated with male hormones for only four or five days, they will subsequently fail to exhibit normal male mating behavior as adult animals even though they are given androgen replacement therapy. This observation suggests an intriguing, though unproved, explanation for some instances of human homosexual activity. Impaired testicular function during a critical perinatal period conceivably could prevent the induction of the normal male behavior pattern in the central nervous system. Consistent with such a hypothesis is the fact that the testes of the newborn male are normally adult-like histologically; later in infancy, the testes regress to the prepubertal pattern and remain so until adolescence. Perhaps in man, as in the rat, male hormone is required in the neonatal period to induce modification in the central nervous system necessary for the development of male behavior in later life. It has long been held that testicular function in adult homosexuals is normal. However, recent studies of large numbers of males with varying degrees of homosexuality revealed an inverse relationship between serum testosterone concentration and homosexual behavior. Subjects who were overtly homosexual had distinctly lower testosterone values.

NEUROENDOCRINE DISORDERS

In light of the new knowledge regarding the dominant role of the hypothalamus in regulating pituitary function, it seems likely that some diseases previously attributed to malfunction of the pituitary may actually be due to disordered function of the hypothalamus. For example, Cushing's syndrome results from prolonged excessive secretion of cortisol by the adrenal cortex. In a large number of cases, the abnormal secretion of cortisol is associated with adrenal hyperplasia secondary to abnormal, excessive secretion of ACTH. It may well be that the latter is also a secondary phenomenon, i.e., that the anterior pituitary is being subjected to an excessive stimulation by CRF. With this possibility in mind, one might consider adrenal hyperplasia a disease of the hypothalamus or of even higher loci in the central nervous system. However, this reasoning will remain speculation until the cause of the excessive secretion of ACTH is elucidated. For the present, it would seem prudent to consider Cushing's syndrome in the section on the adrenal cortex. Comparable reasoning applies to several other endocrine disorders that in the future may well be established as hypothalamic in origin.

ANTERIOR PITUITARY

PHYSIOLOGY

The pituitary is a small gland, weighing approximately 0.6 grams and measuring about 1 cm. in diameter. The anterior lobe, derived from endodermal tissue embryologically, makes up about 75 per cent of the gland by weight. It is contained in a bony socket, the sella turcica ("Turkish saddle"), situated at the base of the brain above the sphenoid sinus. The anterior pituitary elaborates a number of peptide hormones of which six have clearly defined functions in man. Adrenocorticotropic hormone (ACTH, corticotropin) stimulates the biosynthesis and release of cortisol by the adrenal cortex. Thyroid-stimulating hormone (thyrotropin, TSH) stimulates the uptake of iodine and the release of thyroid hormone by the thyroid. Follicle-stimulating hormone (FSH) stimulates the development of the Graafian follicle and secretion of estrogen in the ovary and spermatogenesis in the testes. Luteinizing hormone (LH) prompts ovulation and the luteinization of the mature follicle in the ovary. In the male, this hormone is also called the interstitial cell-stimulating hormone (ICSH). ICSH or LH stimulates the production and release of testosterone by the Leydig cells of the testes. Prolactin (lactogenic hormone, LTH) stimulates the secretion of milk by the breast of the postpartum female. Growth hormone (GH, somatotropin) promotes growth of all tissues in the immature subject. Its primary physiologic function in the adult is not clear. Melanocyte-stimulating hormone (MSH) promotes pigmentation in many species but its role in human physiology has not been established.

On the basis of their staining characteristics, the cells of the anterior pituitary have classically been characterized as chromophobic (without granules), eosinophilic, and basophilic. With more sophisticated techniques, cells previously believed to be chromophobes have been found to contain small basophilic or eosinophilic granules; these cells have been labeled amphophils. In the traditional view, chromophobe cells were believed to be either precursor or supportive cells without secretory activity; eosinophilic cells were considered responsible for the secretion of growth hormone, lactogenic hormone, and prolactin; and basophilic cells for the secretion of ACTH, TSH, and MSH. Such a schema is undoubtedly greatly oversimplified. For example, some tumors producing excessive quantities of ACTH or of growth hormone have consisted of chromophobe cells. It should be remembered, however, that stained granules represent stored hormone. Conceivably, tumor cells could release hormone as rapidly as it is formed and thus be agranular when stained. Using the electron microscope, attempts have been made to relate the hormone secreted to granule size. Basophilic cells with granules of about 50 mμ in size are thought to elaborate TSH, while those with larger granules (200 mμ or more) are believed to produce gonadotropins. Much work remains to be done in this area before hormone-cell type relationships of the anterior pituitary are clearly established.

Control of Anterior Pituitary Secretion

The fact that anterior pituitary hormone secretion is under dual control has already been stated. These control mechanisms are (1) negative feedback, in which the target gland hormone, acting at the level of the pituitary or hypothalamus, inhibits secretion of its tropic hormone; and (2) control by hypothalamic hormones arising from neuronal cells in or near the median eminence and secreted into the hypophyseal portal circulation.

These mechanisms are so important from both conceptual and pragmatic points of view that their repeated emphasis is warranted. The interaction among the three hormonal elements controlling thyroid hormone secretion is the most firmly established and can serve to illustrate the principles involved.

The evidence suggests that the normal pituitary can secrete TSH at a low level *independent* of influences from high centers. Presumably, TRH tonically maintains the secretory rate of TSH at a basal rate that constitutes the set point. The rate of TRH release is thought to be determined by neural signals, but the source of such signals and their relationship to physiologic phenomena such as temperature regulation is poorly understood. The evidence for a diurnal variation in circulating TSH is conflicting; if such a variation occurs, it is small in magnitude.

TRH stimulates both the synthesis and the release of TSH; these two actions can be dissociated. The latter is very prompt; in man, an increase in plasma TSH is detectable within minutes of an intravenous infusion of TRH. This release process appears to be mediated by the adenylate cyclase-cyclic AMP system.

Thyroid hormone blocks the releasing action of TRH on the pituitary *if* the thyroid hormone is administered some time before TRH is given. If the two hormones are administered simultaneously, or thyroid hormone just a few minutes before TRH, no block occurs. There is evidence that thyroid hormone stimulates the synthesis of a protein within the pituitary that inhibits TRH action. Whether thyroid hormone also acts on the hypothalamus or higher in the central nervous system to inhibit the formation or secretion of TRH is not known. These interrelations are illustrated in Figure 32–3.

The very marked biological activity of TRH

Figure 32-3 Pathways of iodine metabolism and the relationships among the hypothalamus, pituitary, and thyroid. Ingested iodine is assimilated as iodide ion which is selectively taken up or "trapped" by the thyroid. Normally, the gradient between intrathyroidal and plasma iodide is about 25 to 1. Once in the thyroid, iodide is rapidly oxidized and combined with tyrosyl residues in a series of steps, collectively termed "organification," which take place in thyroglobulin molecules. Thyroglobulin is stored as colloid in the lumina of follicles. Iodine from the thyroid hormone precursors (diiodotyrosine [DIT] and monoiodotyrosine [MIT]) is recycled. Thyroid hormone (T_4 and T_3) is released from thyroglobulins by enzymatic cleavage. Both thyroid hormone release (X_1) and iodide "trapping" (X_2) are TSH dependent. Nearly all circulating T_4 and most T_3 is bound to proteins such as thyroid-binding globulin (TBG). Thyroid hormone interferes with the action of TRH on the TSH-synthesizing cells of the anterior pituitary. Whether thyroid hormone has a direct action on the hypothalamus is not known (see text).

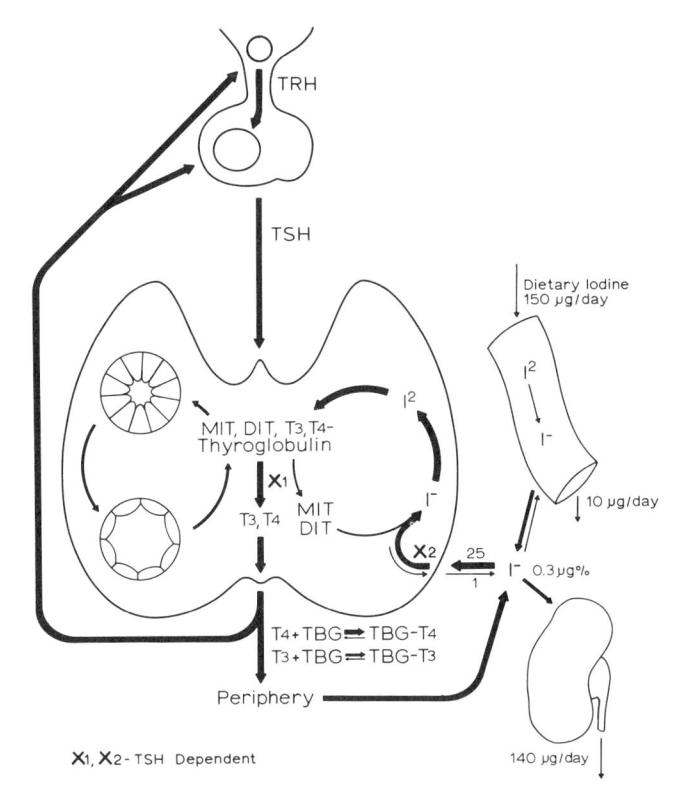

illustrates the phenomenon of amplification, in which a relatively minute amount of hormone acting as a primary signal stimulates the secretion of a much larger amount of a second hormone. It has been estimated that this amplification factor is about 100,000 in the case of the TRH-TSH interaction, i.e., 10 ng. of TRH will cause the secretion of 1 mg. of its tropic hormone.

Data tabulated by Catt which depict pituitary hormone size, storage, secretion rate, and other parameters are contained in Table 32-2.

CLINICAL ENTITIES

Pituitary Tumors

The pathophysiology of pituitary tumors involves two basic considerations: (1) the effects of a space-occupying mass in the strategic area above and lateral to the sella turcica and (2) the effects of excess or deficiency of one or more pituitary hormones.

From the standpoint of the first consideration, all pituitary tumors are similar in that presenting symptoms may be headache and visual impairment. The latter manifestation usually results from pressure of the tumor on the decussating fibers of the optic chiasma. The characteristic pattern of visual field loss involves the upper outer quadrant followed by the lower outer quadrant. The resulting defect, bitemporal hemianopsia, is often apparent when the visual fields are assessed by gross confrontation at the patient's bedside.

From the standpoint of the second consideration, pituitary tumors may be divided into four groups: (1) chromophobe adenomas, nonsecretory; (2) craniopharyngiomas; (3) eosinophilic tumors; (4) the tumors of Nelson's syndrome. Tumors in the first two groups do not elaborate hormones but frequently cause manifestations owing to a deficiency of one or more hormones. Similarly, hormonal deficiencies may arise in any of the four groups above because of (a) the effects of the pressure of the tumor on normal cells, (b) the consequences of treatment, or (c) rarely from apoplexy or hemorrhage into the tumor. The consequences of deficiencies of anterior pituitary hormones are discussed below, as are the consequences of excessive growth hormone produced by an eosinophilic tumor.

Because of the underlying mechanisms it illustrates, the fourth group of tumors requires additional comment. Nelson et al. have reported intense pigmentation in patients who were previously subjected to bilateral adrenalectomy for Cushing's disease. Each patient was found to have a chromophobe adenoma of the pituitary and a very high level of plasma ACTH. Clinical

TABLE 32-2 SIZE, PITUITARY CONTENT, SECRETORY RATE, PLASMA LEVEL, CLEARANCE RATE, AND ESTIMATED ACTIVITY OF THE ANTERIOR PITUITARY HORMONES

Hormone	Molecular Weight	Pituitary Content (µg.)	Secretory Rate (µg./day)	Plasma Level (ng./ml.)	Clearance Rate (L./day)	Estimated Specific Activity of Pure Hormone (units/mg.)
ACTH	4,500	300	10	0.03	300	200
HGH	21,500	8,500	500	1.0–5.0	280	2
TSH	26,000	300	110	1.0–2.0	61	30
LH	30,000	80	30	0.5–1.5	36	14,000
FSH	41,000	35	15	0.5–1.0	19	14,000

From Catt, K. J.: Lancet, *1*:830, 1970.

experience since Nelson's original report indicates that as many as 20 per cent of all patients undergoing adrenalectomy for adrenal hyperplasia due to Cushing's disease will develop this complication. The chromophobe tumor in these patients is more aggressive than the typical variety. Complications due to pressure on the surrounding structures are frequent, as is pituitary apoplexy. According to one hypothesis, the syndrome is best explained by assuming that the initial pathologic event is excessive secretion of CRF that is inadequately suppressed by the resultant abnormally high levels of plasma cortisol. Over a period of many months, the latter leads to Cushing's disease, which can be treated by removal of the hyperplastic adrenal glands and replacing their secretions with an exogenous glucocorticoid in physiologic amounts. The manifestations of Cushing's disease regress over a period of time. Unfortunately, the diminished, now normal levels of plasma cortisol permit a further increase in CRF secretion. The long-term excessive stimulation of the ACTH-producing cells of the anterior pituitary by CRF leads to tumor formation and to extremely high levels of plasma ACTH. It is the latter event that leads to pigmentation which may be so intense that a previously white person may be mistaken for a black. It has been established that ACTH has pigmenting capability, which is very likely a result of the similarity of its N-terminal amino acid sequence to that of melanocyte-stimulating hormone. Thus, despite receiving appropriate therapy for Cushing's disease, these unfortunate patients trade the severe disabilities of Cushing's disease for the crippling ones of a pervasive pituitary tumor.

Acromegaly and Gigantism

Acromegaly (excessive size of the distal parts of the body) results from sustained, excessive secretion of growth hormone in the adult. The source of the growth hormone is an eosinophilic, or less often a chromophobic, tumor of the anterior pituitary. When such a tumor develops in childhood or adolescence before closure of the epiphyses, growth in height is greatly accelerated with resulting gigantism. In this circumstance, the disease process usually continues into adult life, so that the typical patient with gigantism also has the striking features of acromegaly. Massive enlargement of the hands, feet, and skull, particularly the mandible, occurs. The broadened nose together with the large head has suggested the term "leonine facies" to describe some acromegalic patients. Acromegaly is an outstanding example of an endocrine disorder that was being recognized decades before the hormone involved was discovered. The classic features of acromegaly were first described in 1886 by Pierre Marie. The metabolic effects of long-standing growth hormone excess are often surprisingly mild. Impairment of glucose tolerance is commonly seen, and frank diabetes mellitus occurs in perhaps 15 per cent of cases.

The normal hypothalamic-pituitary-target tissue interrelations of human growth hormone (HGH) are poorly understood. It is known that there is a hypothalamic HGH-releasing factor that stimulates the growth hormone-producing cells of the anterior pituitary. Perhaps some of the tumors in acromegalics arise from chronic overstimulation of the pituitary by this HGH-releasing factor—a mechanism comparable to that postulated for the ACTH-secreting tumor of Nelson's syndrome. The occurrence in some acromegalic individuals of tumors which are chromophobic or of mixed histology suggests an unusually low storage and rapid discharge of growth hormone. As discussed below, a number of stimuli capable of increasing plasma growth hormone have been identified, but relatively few inhibitors are known. One of these, hyperglycemia, is of practical value in the diagnosis of acromegaly. When a glucose load is administered to normal subjects, the ensuing hyperglycemia is associated with a decline in HGH to undetectable or normal levels. The basal HGH level of the acromegalic individual not only is typically elevated but can not be suppressed to within normal limits by hyperglycemia.

Pituitary Infantilism

The outstanding manifestation of pituitary deficiency which develops prior to puberty is failure to grow. This is true whether the deficiency is restricted to HGH alone or includes deficiencies of other tropic hormones. The term pituitary infantilism implies dwarfism and immaturity of the secondary sexual characteristics. The latter finding, of course, can only be appreciated clinically in the post-adolescent patient. The most common cause of pituitary infantilism is the craniopharyngioma; frequently, however, no organic lesion can be demonstrated. In pituitary infantilism, impaired secretion of tropic hormones other than HGH can almost always be demonstrated. There are uncommon forms of pituitary *dwarfism* studied extensively by McKusick and Merimee and collaborators in which only HGH secretion or peripheral responsiveness to HGH is deficient (see Table 32-3).

Before discussing these, we should consider briefly what is known about the mechanism of action of growth hormone. In terms of promoting growth, the hormone acts in the intact, immature animal to stimulate cartilage formation. One can study this process in vitro by incubating cartilage from immature rats with labeled sulfate and measuring the incorporation of the label, as chondroitin sulfate, into cartilage. When one adds growth hormone itself to such a system, no increase in sulfate incorporation occurs. Similarly, serum from an animal that has undergone hypophysectomy has little activity. However, serum from such an animal *treated with growth hormone* is very active. These findings led Daughaday (1971) to speculate that growth hormone does not affect growth directly; rather it interacts with receptors that in turn generate a "sulfation factor" which actually stimulates cartilaginous growth. Relevant to this hypothesis are findings from patients with a rare form of dwarfism first described in oriental Jews in Israel by Laron. These individuals resemble pituitary dwarfs in their physical characteristics. However, there are abundant levels of growth hormone in their sera as determined by radioimmunoassay. Like true pituitary dwarfs they have very low levels of sulfation factor in the sera. Unlike pituitary dwarfs, however, the administration of therapeutic amounts of growth hormone fails to induce an increase in sulfation factor and promotes relatively little increase in stature. One explanation for these findings is that these patients have a defect in the proposed sulfation factor generation system that cannot be overcome by the administration of even large amounts of growth hormone. Alternatively, their pituitary glands could be elaborating an abnormal growth hormone which lacks biological activity but is antigenically normal and thus measurable by radioimmunoassay. It is conceivable that such a molecule could interfere with exogenous growth hormone by competitive inhibition. In attempting to explain the possible value of the sulfation factor mechanism, Daughaday has pointed out that growth hormone is secreted in bursts throughout the day in response to a host of metabolic and neurogenic stimuli. This irregular and intermittent pattern of secretion would seem inappropriate for the gradual progressive processes involved in orderly cell growth. The interaction of growth hormone with a system generating the actual growth substance, e.g., sulfation factor, would provide an attractive mechanism to explain the normal regulation of skeletal growth.

Sexual Ateliotic Dwarfism

As mentioned, Merimee and coworkers have described a variety of familial dwarfism due to a selective inability of the pituitary to secrete growth hormone; in these patients, all other anterior pituitary hormones are secreted normally. These authors applied the term sexual ateliotic (*ateliosis* = imperfect development) dwarfism to this disorder to denote normal sexual development in an individual with short stature. Theoretically, many mechanisms involving growth hormone synthesis, secretion, and tissue interaction might occur which would interfere with normal growth. Some of these are as follows:

— An absence or reduction in the hypothalamic growth hormone-releasing factor.
— An absence or abnormality of the growth hormone-producing cells of the anterior pituitary.
— Deficiency of the enzyme(s) required for the release of stored growth hormone.
— Production of a biologically abnormal growth hormone molecule, that is, one without metabolic activity but antigenically intact and thus measurable by immunoassay.
— Production of an abnormal growth hormone molecule with partial biological activity which may or may not be measurable by immunoassay.
— A circulating antagonist(s) to growth hormone in the bloodstream.
— Increased destruction of normally secreted growth hormone.
— A defect in the sulfation factor generation system.
— End-organ resistance to growth hormone or the growth principle (sulfation factor).

TABLE 32-3 SOME FEATURES OF SEXUAL ATELIOTIC DWARFISM

Type	Basal HGH	GH Response to I.V. INS/ARG	Response to HGH	Response to Insulin	Insulin Response to I.V. GLU/ARG	Mode of Inheritance	Nature of Defect
I	0	0	+	Sensitive	Decrease	Autosomal Recessive	Inability to produce HGH
II	0	0	+	Normal	Increase	Autosomal Dominant	Inability to produce HGH
III	High (Non-suppressible)	0 or +	0	Sensitive	Decrease	?(Yemenite Jews)	"Warped HGH" plus end-organ resistance
IV	Normal	Normal	0	Sensitive	Decrease	Pygmy	End-organ resistance

Modified from Merimee, T. J., et al.: Lancet, *1*:963, 1969.
HGH = Human growth hormone
INS = Insulin
ARG = Arginine
GLU = Glucose

Obviously a number of these proposed mechanisms could overlap, and most, it should be emphasized, are hypothetical. Similarly, the classification proposed by Merimee et al. (1969) and contained in Table 32-3 should be regarded as tentative. Patients with Types I and II dwarfism have undetectable levels of plasma growth hormone which remain low during hypoglycemia or arginine infusion. They differ, however, in their mode of inheritance and in their responsiveness to insulin. Type I dwarfism is inherited as an autosomal recessive, while Type II is transmitted as an autosomal dominant trait. Patients with Type I dwarfism are highly sensitive to administered insulin, while those with Type II are resistant to it. Type III dwarfism is characterized by a high plasma level of HGH, as determined by radioimmunoassay, which may or may not be suppressed by hyperglycemia. In Type IV dwarfism, exemplified by the Pygmies of central Africa, growth hormone appears to be secreted normally. The administration of HGH, however, fails to elicit the expected changes in plasma free fatty acids and blood urea nitrogen. This could be due either to peripheral tissue unresponsiveness to normal growth hormone or to the secretion of a biologically defective but antigenically intact growth hormone molecule which saturates peripheral receptors.

To evaluate the ability of the anterior pituitary to secrete growth hormone, two stimuli are commonly used. The first is hypoglycemia induced by the intravenous administration of 0.1 to 0.2 units of regular insulin per kg. of body weight to a fasting patient. The second is the infusion of 30 grams of the amino acid arginine monohydrochloride. In these tests, blood samples are obtained every 15 to 30 minutes over a 1- to 2-hour period for growth hormone and blood sugar determinations. Most normal individuals respond to these stimuli with a maximum plasma GH or 20 ng. per ml. or more.

It should be emphasized that most of the current information concerning growth hormone was obtained in the last ten years following the development of a highly sensitive radioimmunoassay and the availability of purified growth hormone suitable for administration to man. Unfortunately, growth hormone is highly species specific. Preparations from domestic animals do not elicit metabolic effects in man. Since human growth hormone is necessarily prepared from pituitary glands obtained at autopsy, the supply available is obviously limited. Perhaps a metabolically active preparation can be synthesized after the precise identification of the amino sequence(s) which governs the hormone's biological expression.

Panhypopituitarism (Postpubertal)

The term panhypopituitarism signifies a deficiency of all anterior pituitary hormones. The most common cause in the adult is an expanding, nonsecretory chromophobe adenoma. It may also occur as a sequela of hemorrhagic shock at the time of delivery. For reasons which are not entirely clear, the pituitary of the pregnant female at term is highly vulnerable to hypotension. When excessive blood loss occurs during delivery, a definite risk of pituitary necrosis is present. The resulting panhypopituitarism bears the eponym Sheehan's syndrome. Less common causes of adult hypopituitarism include craniopharyngioma and long-standing pituitary tumors associated with acromegaly.

The peripheral manifestations of panhypopituitarism in the adult are largely the consequence of deficiencies of four hormones: the gonadotropins (LH and FSH), ACTH, and TSH. Characteristically, evidence of target gland deficits appear in that order, i.e., gonadal, adrenal cortical, and thyroidal. Thus, loss of libido in the male and amenorrhea in the female are early symptoms. Loss of thyroid function causes dry skin, cold intolerance, somnolence, bradycardia, and constipation. Decrease in adrenal cortical function causes symptoms of hypovolemia and hypoglycemia and, in the female, loss of axillary and pubic hair. Typically, the patient with panhypopituitarism has pale skin and premature, fine wrinkles about the eyes and mouth. The loss of pigment has been attributed to ACTH deficiency.

As is so often the case in endocrinology, the definitive diagnosis of panhypopituitarism requires the judicious selection of certain laboratory procedures. The traditional approach has been the demonstration of hypofunction of the adrenal cortex and thyroid, which may be reversed by the administration of ACTH and TSH, respectively. The advent of radioimmunoassays for several anterior pituitary hormones has permitted a more direct approach to the diagnosis. The use of arginine infusion or induced hypoglycemia to provoke growth hormone secretion has already been mentioned, as has the use of TRH to stimulate TSH release. In panhypopituitarism, the responses of HGH and TSH to these stimuli would be severely impaired or absent.

Much less common than panhypopituitarism are instances of isolated deficiency of a single pituitary hormone, so-called monotropic hypopituitarism. Monotropic growth hormone deficiencies (sexual ateliotic dwarfism) have already been described. Deficiency of both pituitary gonadotropins is a relatively common cause of hypogonadism in the male and may also afflict females. It is usually familial and may be associated with a decrease or absence in the sense of smell, hyposmia or anosmia (Kallman's syndrome). Selective deficiencies of LH, TSH, ACTH, and prolactin have also been well documented.

POSTERIOR PITUITARY

PHYSIOLOGY

The principal secretion of the posterior pituitary, the octapeptide vasopressin (antidiuretic hormone, ADH), has the major physiologic role of regulating water metabolism. Unlike anterior pituitary hormones, this hormone is actually produced in the hypothalamus by the supraoptic and paraventricular nuclei. It is transported down the axons of the hypothalamic-hypophyseal tracts to the posterior pituitary, where it is stored until secreted. It has been established, however, that the storage of ADH in the posterior pituitary is not essential for its normal function. Normal water metabolism can persist after complete destruction of the posterior pituitary if the hypothalamus and proximal pituitary stalk are not damaged.

The primary stimulus to ADH secretion is an increase in plasma osmolality or tonicity. Normally, it is closely maintained at 280 mOsm. per liter. When extracellular water is lost, plasma osmolality increases, causing the activation of osmoreceptors which signal the release of ADH. The precise location of the osmoreceptors and the manner in which they stimulate the release of ADH are not known. Increased plasma osmolality also stimulates the thirst center, which is anatomically adjacent to, or connected with, the supraoptic nuclei.

The action of ADH to conserve water is exerted primarily on the cells of renal collecting ducts. At this site, ADH exerts its unique ability of changing permeability of the epithelial cell membranes to enhance the egress of water from the tubules to the hypertonic fluid of the peritubular or interstitial space. This action of ADH is probably mediated by the adenylate cyclase-cyclic AMP system. The consequent shift of water reduces urine volume and increases its concentration. Thus, an increased serum osmolality tends to correct itself by reducing water loss and increasing water intake as depicted in the accompanying diagram.

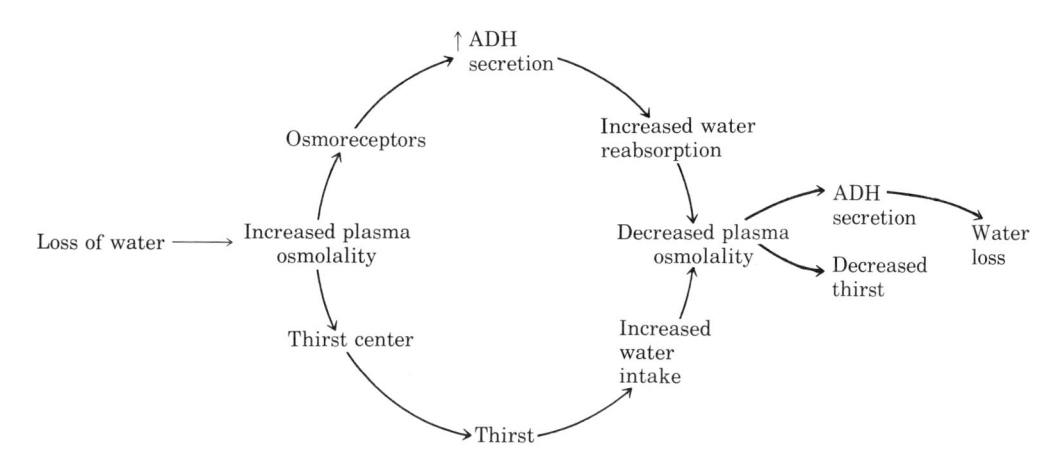

The integrated activity of ADH and thirst is highly effective in maintaining the osmolality of the body fluids within very narrow limits. These interrelations provide an ideal example of the precision with which the endocrine system normally functions to maintain the constancy of the internal milieu. Although plasma osmolality is the most important regulator of ADH secretion, other factors also influence it. For example, an abrupt decrease in plasma volume due to acute blood loss stimulates ADH secretion. Neural signals triggered by painful stimuli may also prompt ADH release, as do certain drugs such as nicotine. The posterior pituitary also secretes oxytocin. Although large doses of this substance will induce contractions of the gravid uterus, its physiologic importance in man has not yet been established.

CLINICAL ENTITIES

Diabetes Insipidus

Diabetes insipidus is the clinical condition that results from an impaired or absent capacity to secrete ADH. The term "diabetes" signifies copious amounts of urine; "insipidus" implies dehydration. The causes of diabetes insipidus are numerous. In one large series, one third of the cases were due to tumor, one third were of unknown cause, and one third were of a variety of causes including trauma, inflammation, and granuloma (Thomas). The principal manifestation of diabetes insipidus is the excretion of large volumes of urine—5 to 15 liters or more daily—of low specific gravity (1.007 or less). To compensate for this prodigious water loss, the patient must drink large volumes of fluid. These two symptoms are particularly troublesome during the sleeping hours. Frequent urination and the need to satisfy thirst substantially encroach on the patient's rest, and loss of sleep is frequently his presenting complaint. For reasons that are not clear, the onset of symptoms is typically dramatically abrupt. The patient often recalls the precise day or hour when polyuria and thirst began. Another peculiar feature of the disease is the patient's marked preference for chilled fluids. He will go to considerable trouble to relieve his thirst with ice water.

A number of other disorders associated with the passage of large volumes of urine may simulate diabetes insipidus. An abbreviated differential diagnosis of polyuria is summarized in the accompanying chart in the next column.

The presence of diabetes mellitus, chronic renal failure, or disturbances in calcium and potassium metabolism is easily established. Patients with psychogenic thirst should theoretically respond to water deprivation in a normal manner, that is, by decreasing urine volume and increasing urine concentration. Thus, after water is withheld from the patient who is an obsessive water drinker, the specific gravity of his urine should rise above 1.012 within a few hours and reach 1.020 or more after 12 hours. Unfortunately, the results of this procedure may be obscured by the patient's ability to obtain water surreptitiously and, conversely, by the ability of some patients with diabetes insipidus to concentrate urine to a specific gravity of 1.012 or 1.014. Lastly, water deprivation in a patient with unequivocal, total diabetes insipidus is potentially dangerous.

Differential Diagnosis of Polyuria	Mechanism
1. Diabetes insipidus	Decreased ADH secretion
2. Diabetes mellitus	Osmotic diuresis
3. Renal disease	
a. Nephrogenic diabetes insipidus	End-organ resistance to ADH
b. Hypercalcemia	Impaired concentrating ability
c. Hypokalemia	Impaired concentrating ability
d. Psychogenic thirst	Obsessive water drinking

A second method of diagnosing diabetes insipidus involves the use of hypertonic saline and vasopressin. After the patient is well hydrated, with a urine flow rate of at least 5 ml. per min., a 3 per cent sodium chloride solution is infused for 45 minutes. If no antidiuresis occurs within the next 30 minutes, aqueous vasopressin (ADH) is given, and urine collection is continued for another 30 minutes. If both kidney function and neurohypophyseal function are normal, the hypertonic saline infusion should cause a prompt fall in urinary flow and an increase in urinary specific gravity and osmolality. If ADH secretion is impaired, the saline infusion will be ineffective, but there will be a prompt decline in urine volume in response to vasopressin. If the defect is caused by an inability of the renal tubules to respond to ADH (i.e., nephrogenic diabetes insipidus), neither hypertonic saline nor Pitressin infusion will influence the rate of urine flow.

Inappropriate Secretion of Antidiuretic Hormone

This syndrome was first described by Schwartz in 1957 in patients with cancer of the lung. It has subsequently been noted as a complication of various underlying conditions, including head trauma, myxedema, tuberculosis, and meningitis, to name a few. In all instances, the manifestations are those which would be expected from the inappropriate release of ADH into the circulation. (In some instances, e.g., cancer of the lung, presumably the tumor does indeed elaborate and release autonomously an ADH-like peptide. In contrast to the anterior pituitary, no example of a hormone-producing tumor of the posterior pituitary or hypothalamus has been described.) There is retention of water and consequently dilution of body fluids. The increase in plasma volume leads to an increase in glomerular filtration and a decrease in aldosterone secretion, both factors that increase loss of sodium into the urine. Thus, the concentration of serum sodium is decreased by at least two mechanisms: (1) dilution by inappropriate water retention and (2) excessive urinary sodium excretion. When evaluating a patient for this syndrome, one should carefully rule out conditions that would *appropriately* lead to an increase in ADH secretion or to sodium wasting.

THYROID

PHYSIOLOGY

Essential to understanding thyroid disorders is an appreciation of normal iodine metabolism and the normal interrelations between the thyroid and the pituitary-hypothalamic unit (see Figure 32–3).

Iodine Metabolism

A daily absorption of approximately 100 to 200 μg. of dietary iodine is required to ensure adequate thyroid hormone synthesis. With the exception of that contained in organic compounds, ingested iodine is reduced to ionic iodide (I^-) before being assimilated into the bloodstream. During the first hour after absorption, iodide is distributed in a space representing approximately 35 per cent of body weight, or about 25 liters in a 70 kg. man. The concentration of circulating iodide has been estimated at less than 0.1 μg. per 100 ml. of plasma.

Uptake (Trapping). Normally, the thyroid has an iodide clearance rate between 10 and 35 ml. of plasma per minute. This uptake by the thyroid is an active, energy-requiring process, sometimes referred to as the "iodide pump." It is stimulated by TSH and is blocked by a number of anions such as thiocyanate and perchlorate. Normally, a concentration gradient of 1 to 25 exists between plasma and thyroidal I^-. This gradient may be increased 10-fold or more in toxic goiter. Iodide ion constitutes approximately 10 per cent of the total intrathyroidal iodine which normally amounts to 5000 to 7000 μg. The iodide pool may be increased when organification is impaired by drug action, inflammation, or genetically determined enzyme defects. Careful studies indicate that there are in fact two independent iodide pools within the thyroid gland. The first, normally about 10 μg., is composed of newly trapped iodide. Its uptake can be blocked by perchlorate or thiocyanate. The second pool, estimated at about 490 μg., consists of iodide released by enzymatic dehalogenation of monoiodotyrosine (MIT) and diiodotyrosine (DIT). This pool, apparently part of an internal recycling process which conserves iodide, is not directly affected by agents that block trapping. One can view the action of perchlorate or thiocyanate in "discharging" iodide as one of inhibition of inward transport of iodide while outward diffusion is unaffected.

Oxidation and Organification. After being trapped, iodide ions are rapidly transported into the luminal space of follicles and are either incorporated into an organic molecule or diffuse out of the follicles unchanged. Oxidation of iodide to molecular iodine (I_2) occurs prior to its displacement of hydrogen at the C_3 position of tyrosine. These reactions which lead to the formation of MIT and DIT occur rapidly, and their exact sequence has not been established. The oxidation step is probably catalyzed by a peroxidase. MIT is then iodinated at the C_5 position to form DIT. Probably the tyrosyl residues are attached to thyroglobulin or to other iodoproteins during these reactions. The oxidation-organification steps can be blocked by thiourea drugs such as propylthiouracil and are stimulated by TSH. The formation of the iodothyronines, thyroxine (T_4), and triiodothyronine (T_3), probably results from the condensation of iodotyrosines, either two DIT molecules or one DIT and one MIT molecule, with the extrusion of one side chain. DIT and MIT molecules that are not utilized in the formation of T_4 and T_3 undergo catalytic deiodination by a dehalogenase. The regenerated iodide (the second iodide pool) is subsequently reutilized in hormone synthesis in the thyroid (see earlier discussion). T_4 and T_3 are not susceptible to deiodination.

Storage and Release. Most of the iodinated compounds of the thyroid are in combination with thyroglobulin, a 650,000 M.W. protein, which is the principal iodoprotein in thyroidal colloid. Analysis of the globulin-bound iodinated compounds reveals the following relative amounts: MIT, 17 to 28 per cent; DIT, 25 to 42 per cent; T_3, 5 to 8 per cent; and T_4, 35 per cent. These stored compounds alone are sufficient to maintain normal hormonal activity in an adult for several months. The large size of thyroglobulin precludes its escape from the intraluminal colloid under normal circumstances. The secretion of the thyroid hormone (T_3 and T_4) requires that it first be cleared from thyroglobulin by proteolytic enzymes. T_3 and T_4, being freely diffusible, then readily enter the circulation. This process is stimulated by TSH and may be inhibited by large amounts of iodine. While the principal secretion of the thyroid is thyroxine (90 per cent or more), there is a small but significant amount of T_3 in the venous effluent of the thyroid. It is estimated that approximately 80 to 90 µg. of thyroxine is secreted per day.

Transport of Thyroid Hormones. Once released, free thyroxine and triiodothyronine quickly bind with one of several carrier proteins. The protein with the strongest affinity for T_4 and T_3 is thyroxine-binding globulin (TBG), an interalpha (α_1–α_2) glycoprotein. The normal concentration of TBG is about 1 mg. per 100 ml. of serum, a quantity sufficient to bind 10 to 26 µg. of T_4. A second protein, thyroxine-binding prealbumin (TBPA), also effectively binds thyroxine. Lastly, serum albumin binds T_4 but with less affinity than either TBG or TBPA. The equilibrium between TBG and bound and free T_4 is reversible, as illustrated by the equation

$$TBG \cdot T_4 \rightleftarrows TBG + T_4$$

The concentration of free T_4 is normally about 1.0 to 2.0 ng. per 100 ml. (les than 1.0×10^{-10} Molar), representing about 0.05 per cent of total T_4. The binding affinity of T_3 for the protein carriers is substantially less than that of T_4. However, since it is the free hormone that penetrates cells to regulate metabolism, the metabolic contribution of T_3 is in fact important. Despite an absolute concentration, which is small compared to that of total T_4, the amount of free T_3 approaches that of free T_4 because of the weaker affinity of T_3 for its carrier proteins. Moreover, recent evidence indicates that T_4 can be converted to T_3 in peripheral tissues (Ingbar et al., 1970); how important this transformation is in normal man remains to be seen.

There are numerous drugs that affect either the binding capacity or the amount of circulating thyroid-binding proteins. For example, diphenylhydantoin competes with T_4 for TBG binding sites, and salicylates displace T_4 from TBPA. Estrogenic compounds increase the amount of carrier protein. Familial deficiencies and excesses of TBG have been well documented. However, the concentration of *free* thyroxine is normal in these patients, hence they are euthyroid.

It is estimated that the total extrathyroidal content of thyroxine-iodine in the normal adult is about 500 µg. Assuming a normal plasma volume and a T_4 concentration of 5 µg. per 100 ml. of plasma, only 150 µg. can be accounted for in the bloodstream. The large amount of remaining thyroxine-iodine is presumed to be bound to tissue protein. According to recent studies the liver is the major storage organ, containing up to 30 per cent of total body thyroxine-iodine. Normally the fractional turnover of thyroxine-iodine is about 10 per cent per day, reflecting a biological half-life of 6.7 days. The fractional turnover rate is increased in hyperthyroidism and decreased in hypothyroidism. These findings are consistent with the observation that the fractional turnover rate may be regulated by the plasma concentration of *free* thyroxine. An alternate hypothesis proposes that the content of exchangeable cellular T_4 is the factor which determines turnover rate.

Cell Entry, Intracellular Metabolism, and Fate of Thyroxine. *Free* thyroxine and triiodothyronine appear to cross most cellular membranes; however, thyroxine is not present in cerebral spinal fluid and it crosses the human placenta slowly and in small amounts. Factors which control the entry of thyroxine into cells are poorly understood. The presence within the cell membrane of one or more proteins with a high binding affinity for T_4 is one possibility. Once in the cell, the manner in which thyroxine or an active derivative acts to increase cellular metabolism is yet another enigma. A once widely held hypothesis implicates the stimulation of uncoupling of oxidative phosphorylation. In contradiction to this possibility is the failure of other uncoupling agents such as 2,4-dinitrophenol to mimic the full spectrum of physiologic actions of T_4. Currently, studies are being conducted to test the hypothesis that changes in mitochondrial membrane function and alterations in nuclear RNA, RNA polymerase, and protein synthesis represent the initial manifestations of T_4 action within the cell. Three principal pathways for disposal of T_4 have been described: (1) conjugation of the phenolic portion of the molecule with formation of the glucuronide or sulfate; (2) degradation of the alanine side chain, and (3) deiodination.

Excretion of Iodide. Nearly all the iodide circulating through the kidneys is filtered by the glomeruli. However, much of the filtered iodide is reabsorbed, so that the renal iodide clearance rate is about 40 ml. per minute. In man, iodide reabsorption appears to be a passive, unregulated process. As indicated in Figure 32–3, urinary loss of iodine normally nearly balances iodine ingestion, with only small quantities of iodine being excreted in the feces.

The Hypothalamic-Pituitary-Thyroid Axis

The interactions between the hypothalamus, the anterior pituitary, and the thyroid have been described earlier in this chapter.

TESTS OF THYROID FUNCTION

To discuss the pathophysiology of thyroid disease in a meaningful fashion, it is helpful to refer to certain tests that are used in assessing thyroid function. Most of the tests that are currently available fit into one of three categories: (1) those that measure the concentration of thyroid hormone in the plasma, (2) those that depend on thyroidal iodine kinetics, and (3) those that reflect the impact of thyroid hormone on body metabolism.

The first group can be exemplified by the serum protein-bound iodine concentration (PBI). The major shortcoming of the PBI has been the elevated values caused by exogenous iodinated substances, such as contrast media used in radiography, which do not reflect circulating thyroid hormone. This disadvantage has been obviated by the development of a protein (TBG) binding assay for T_4 which is not affected by organic iodides (see earlier discussion). The second group of tests is illustrated by the 24-hour uptake of radioactive iodine by the thyroid gland. In this procedure, a small (approximately 10 microcuries) amount of radioactive iodine (^{131}RAI) is administered orally and radioactivity over the thyroid gland is determined 24 hours later. As already mentioned, both the normal uptake of iodine and the discharge of thyroid hormone require TSH and a functioning thyroid gland. The last category is exemplified by the basal metabolic rate (BMR). In this procedure, the patient's rate of oxygen consumption is measured and compared to normal values based on the patient's age, size, and sex.

The value of these procedures in assessing thyroid function is best conveyed by citing examples of their application.

Example	PBI	RAI	BMR
1. Hyperthyroidism	Increased	Increased	Increased
2. Hypothyroidism secondary to thyroid atrophy	Decreased	Decreased	Decreased
3. Goitrous cretinism	Decreased	Increased	Decreased
4. Normal subject on 2 to 3 grains thyroid extract	Normal	Decreased	Normal

The results in examples 1 and 2 are straightforward and require no comment. In the third example, goitrous cretinism due to either a severe dietary deficiency of iodine or an abnormality in the biosynthesis of thyroid hormone, the patient is unable to secrete an adequate amount of thyroid hormone. As a result, the level of circulating hormone is low and the patient is hypothyroid. The low concentration of hormone stimulates an increase in TSH release from the pituitary which, in turn, causes an increase in iodine uptake and, over a period of time, thyroid enlargement or goiter. In the fourth example, a patient with normal thyroid function has been placed on a therapeutic dose of thyroid extract. Because of the negative feedback relation between the thyroid and anterior pituitary, this exogenous thyroid is not additive; rather it suppresses TSH release as reflected by a low to absent uptake of radioactive iodine, and endogenous thyroid hormone secretion virtually ceases. The normal metabolic rate (BMR) and PBI merely reflect the euthyroid condition caused by the ingestion of physiologic quantities of thyroid extract.

CLINICAL ENTITIES

Primary Adult Hypothyroidism (Myxedema)

The cause of adult hypothyroidism is usually unknown. The pathologic findings are quite nonspecific, the thyroid being atrophic and largely replaced by fibrous tissue. In some cases, the presence of high titers of serum antithyroglobulin antibodies suggests that at least in these instances the disease resulted from autoimmune thyroiditis. Not infrequently, hypothyroidism follows the treatment of Graves' disease with either radioactive iodine or surgery. The onset of the clinical disease in the idiopathic variety is extremely gradual. Thus, one can be reasonably confident that the manifestation of florid myxedema is the result of a condition that has been slowly developing for many years. Since all cells of the body are affected by the deficiency of thyroid hormone, the physician may encounter manifestations of the disease which arise from any major organ. As one might expect, these manifestations are often the opposite of those seen in hyperthyroidism (Table 32–4). The term "myxedema" refers to the infiltration of the dermis by a mucinous substance containing a mucopolysaccharide. The hypothyroid patient may be hypothermic, and his skin is usually dry and cold. He is comfortable during the hot days of summer and distressed by cool weather. His slow mentation and poor memory are often erroneously attributed to aging. The generalized decline in metabolic activity is reflected in the cardiovascular system by bradycardia and in the gastrointestinal tract by constipation.

The biochemical consequences are formidable. Although cholesterol synthesis is decreased, its disposal rate is slowed to an even greater extent, resulting in a high level of cholesterol in the plasma. It is likely that chronic hypercholesterolemia is responsible at least in part for the increase in coronary artery disease encountered in patients with hypothyroidism. These patients are also extremely sensitive to most drugs and anesthetic agents, presumably because of marked slowing of the metabolic pathways involved in drug disposal.

TABLE 32-4 CONTRASTING FEATURES OF HYPERTHYROIDISM AND HYPOTHYROIDISM

	Hyperthyroidism	Hypothyroidism
Appetite	Increased	Decreased or no change
Weight	Decreased	No change
Cold tolerance	Increased	Decreased
Perspiration	Excessive	Absent
Menses	Amenorrhea	Menorrhagia
Skin	Satin smooth	Coarse, dry
Pulse	Rapid	Slow
Mentation	Rapid	Sluggish
Reflexes	Brisk	Slow

Cretinism and Juvenile Hypothyroidism

Since both the skeletal and nervous systems are profoundly dependent on thyroid hormone for normal development, it is predictable that the manifestations of thyroid hormone deficiency in childhood are increasingly severe with an earlier age of onset. Hypothyroidism in the infant may result from congenital absence of the thyroid (athyreotic cretinism) or from an abnormal biosynthesis of thyroid hormone. In the latter circumstance, there is compensatory goiter formation. Occasionally, thyroid function is normal during infancy, but then fails for unknown reasons during childhood or adolescence. As with the infant, a marked retardation in skeletal and mental development is observed. The importance of making an early diagnosis of hypothyroidism at any age cannot be overly stressed. An intriguing exception to the overall impairment in growth and development has been described in juvenile hypothyroidism. This is the occurrence of sexual precocity, manifested by menstruation and breast development in the female and penile and testicular enlargement in the male. A popular hypothesis invoked to explain this manifestation is that normally in children there is an "overlap" in the suppressive effect of thyroid hormone on the anterior pituitary and hypothalamus, i.e., thyroid hormone suppresses not only TSH but also pituitary gonadotropin release. Thus, when there is a deficiency of circulating thyroid hormone, not only TSH but also the gonadotropins are secreted in increased quantities, the latter leading to the premature development of secondary sexual characteristics.

Toxic Diffuse Goiter (Graves' Disease)

The most common cause of thyrotoxicosis or hyperthyroidism (the terms are used interchangeably) is Graves' disease, a syndrome in which there is diffuse enlargement of the thyroid gland associated with excessive secretion of thyroid hormone, no longer responsive to normal controls. Exophthalmos is a common but not invariable feature of the syndrome. However, the eye signs may appear before thyrotoxicosis is evident, or not until after the thyrotoxicosis has been treated and the patient is euthyroid. The enlargement of the gland is highly variable. It may be so slight that no goiter is evident. Thus, the three major components of the syndrome—diffuse thyroid enlargement, thyrotoxicosis, and exophthalmos—need not be present concurrently.

Although its cause is unknown, Graves' disease is characterized by certain features which may be clues to the underlying cause. It is a common disease, second only to nontoxic sporadic goiter as the most frequent disorder of the thyroid gland. As in most thyroid diseases, women are afflicted much more commonly than men; among patients with Graves' disease, the ratio of women to men is approximately 9:1. A family history of thyroid disease is commonly present; close relatives have a high incidence of nontoxic goiter, thyroiditis, or Graves' disease itself. It is a common clinical observation that symptoms of the disease often begin shortly after a major psychological or physical disturbance. Until recently, it was believed that the diffuse enlargement and increased function of the thyroid might be due to an excessive secretion by the pituitary of TSH. If this were so, Graves' disease would be analogous to Cushing's disease, in which an excessive secretion of ACTH leads to adrenal hyperplasia and elevations in plasma corticoids. With the availability of a highly sensitive radioimmunoassay for TSH, it is now apparent that the serum concentrations of TSH in patients with Graves' disease are decreased or undetectable; thus, the anterior pituitary and hypothalamus are eliminated as the primary pathogenic sites.

The diffuse hyperplasia of the gland in Graves' disease does suggest that it is being stimulated by some extrathyroidal substance. About 17 years ago, Adams and Purves (1956) reported that sera from patients with Graves' disease contained a factor with TSH-like activity. This substance was capable of discharging thyroid hormone from the glands of experimental animals. Unlike the response to TSH which was evident within one hour, the serum factor did not cause detectable changes until four to six hours after administration. Because of this characteristic it was labeled "long-acting thyroid stimulator," or LATS. Subsequent investigations have disclosed that LATS is a 7S gamma globulin antibody which is capable of interacting with thyroid cells. It has the capability to stimulate protein synthesis and glucose metabolism of thyroid tissue and to effect the release of thyroid hormone. Serious doubts remain, however, about the etiologic role of LATS in Graves' disease. One such doubt is based on the inability to detect LATS, using current techniques, in the sera of many patients with Graves' disease.

Other common causes of hyperthyroidism include multinodular toxic goiter and toxic adenoma. In these disorders, autonomously functioning thyroid tissue secretes excessive amounts of thyroid hormone. If one administers radioactive iodine to a patient with toxic adenoma and then scans over the neck, radioactivity is found only over the adenoma. This occurs because the excessive thyroid hormone secreted by the adenoma has suppressed TSH secretion and hence iodine trapping by the normal tissue surrounding the adenoma (Fig. 32-4).

Since all cells of the body are influenced by thyroid hormone, it is not surprising that, as in hypothyroidism, manifestations of thyroid hormone excess may involve all systems of the body. The clinical picture of florid thyrotoxicosis is a memorable one. Typically, the patient is thin, hyperkinetic, and impatient with the relatively slow pace of those around him. Palpitation, increased cold tolerance, and diarrhea are common symptoms. On physical examination, characteristic eye signs and goiter are usually present. The skin is satiny smooth and warm; the pulse rate is elevated and the pulse pressure widened. The latter results from mild systolic hypertension and a decrease in diastolic pressure due in part to dilatation of peripheral vessels. There is often evidence of muscle wasting, particularly of the temporalis, shoulder girdle, and quadriceps. The deep tendon reflexes are very brisk. Infrequently, the manifestations of hyperthyroidism are markedly exaggerated. In this condition, termed "thyroid storm," the patient becomes agitated, delirious, and febrile and has a sustained tachycardia. Such an occurrence is a true medical emergency which often terminates fatally despite prompt and appropriate therapy.

The description of thyrotoxicosis as presented in the foregoing paragraphs is applicable to patients of middle age or younger. When patients over 60 develop the disease, the clinical picture is often not so clear-cut. Frequently a second disease such as congestive heart failure obscures the underlying thyrotoxicosis. The older person may not respond to excessive thyroid with the marked increase in energy and physical activity that is characteristic of the younger patient. The terms "masked hyperthyroidism" and "apathetic hyperthyroidism" are thus frequently appropriate for the disease as it presents in the older patient.

Usually, the laboratory tests discussed above (PBI, radioactive iodine, and BMR) confirm the presence of hyperthyroidism suspected on clinical grounds. There are circumstances in which additional laboratory data are helpful in establishing the diagnosis. Two such situations will be described because they illustrate facets of the pathophysiology underlying thyrotoxicosis.

The first circumstance is exemplified by a young woman with weight loss, nervousness, palpitations, and a small goiter. Laboratory examinations reveal a PBI of 8 μg. per 100 ml. (normal, 3.4 to 8.0); a radioactive iodine uptake of 20 per cent in 24 hours (normal, 8 to 15); and a BMR of +20 (normal, −10 to +15). The question then is whether the patient's thyroid function is within the normal range, albeit near the upper limit, or if it is definitely but minimally elevated. To answer this question, the physician can make use of the thyroid suppression test in which the radioactive iodine uptake is repeated after administering physiologic amounts of thyroid hormone for 10 days, e.g., 75 μg. of triiodothyronine daily. If the patient is normal, the second radioactive iodine uptake should be significantly reduced compared to the first; if the patient has early hyperthyroidism, the RAI uptake will be virtually unchanged, since the gland is no longer being normally regulated by TSH.

The second circumstance concerns the finding of a normal PBI in a patient who by clinical appearance is clearly thyrotoxic and in whom radioactive iodine uptake and BMR are both abnormally high. When the sera of such patients have been analyzed for triiodothyronine as well as thyroxine, abnormally high concentrations of the former thyroid hormone have been found coexis-

Normal "Cold" nodule Toxic adenoma

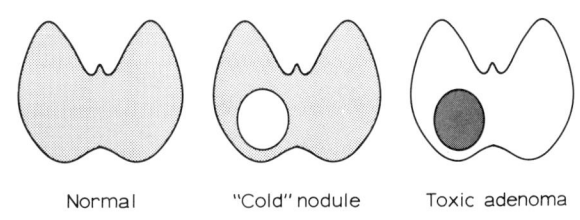

Figure 32–4 Thyroid scans. The *normal thyroid gland* picks up radioactive iodine (RAI) uniformly, resulting in a homogeneous distribution of radioactivity as shown. *"Cold" nodule.* Lesions such as cysts or tumors that occupy space but lack normal biological activity appear as deficits on scan. *Toxic adenomas ("Hot" nodule).* Occasionally adenomas develop which produce thyroid hormone autonomously; when the production of thyroid hormone from this source exceeds physiologic quantities, the patient becomes mildly toxic, TSH production is curtailed, and uptake of iodide by the surrounding normal thyroid virtually ceases.

tent with normal levels of thyroxine. Since plasma normally contains only about 0.3 µg. per 100 ml. of triiodothyronine, a fivefold increase in this hormone would cause little increase in the PBI. In hyperthyroidism usually both triiodothyronine and thyroxine are increased. In this variant, which has been termed "T_3 toxicosis," only triiodothyronine is elevated or it is disproportionately high.

ADRENAL CORTEX

PHYSIOLOGY

The classic description by Addison in 1849 of the disease which ensues following the destruction of the adrenal cortex first attracted attention to the critical importance of this gland in the maintenance of life. Much later, cortisol and aldosterone, the principal secretions of the adrenal cortex, were identified as steroid molecules of basically similar structure. It is of interest that the other endocrine glands of mesodermal origin, the testes and ovaries, also elaborate steroidal hormones which have a structure and mode of action similar to those of the adrenal cortex.

Regulation of Cortisol Secretion

The negative feedback control of cortisol secretion has already been alluded to (see earlier discussion). Normally, a rising level of plasma free cortisol inhibits the release of CRF from hypothalamic sites into the hypophyseal portal circulation, thereby causing a decrease in ACTH release by the anterior pituitary. This fall in plasma ACTH leads to a decline in cortisol secretion by the adrenal glands and, hence, a corresponding reduction in its plasma concentration; thus, the negative feedback loop is completed. This mechanism is modulated by several additional factors. There is evidence that elevations of ACTH in the plasma perfusing the median eminence of the hypothalamus suppress CRF release, creating a "short loop" negative feedback control. Since the plasma concentration of cortisol required to inhibit CRF release (the so-called "set point") varies diurnally, presumably on the basis of neural signals reaching the CRF-synthesizing neurons, ACTH and, in turn, cortisol are secreted in a cyclic fashion. Thus, the peak level of cortisol in the plasma normally occurs between 6 and 8 A.M. By 5 P.M. the concentration has decreased by about 50 per cent, and the fall continues until the nadir is reached around midnight, following which plasma cortisol increases. This normal circadian rhythm is lost in Cushing's syndrome. Other neural signals such as those triggered by various forms of "stress" can also override the normal feedback control and transiently increase cortisol secretion. CRF, which can cause ACTH release within minutes, is thought to be a small peptide similar to TRH, but its structure has not been positively established. ACTH is a 39 amino acid peptide with all biological activity, including MSH-like activity, residing in the first 24 amino acids. This sequence has been synthesized and is available commercially. The amino acids from 25 to 39 vary from one species to another and account for the molecule's immunologic specificity.

ACTH is thought to exert its action through the adenylate cyclase-cyclic AMP system. The interaction of ACTH with the adenylate cyclase of adrenal cortical cell membranes leads to an increase in intracellular cyclic AMP which then promotes the synthesis of a protein capable of catalyzing the conversion of cholesterol to 20 alpha hydroxycholesterol. The latter compound in turn is converted to pregnenolone, the precursor of all steroidal hormones of the adrenal cortex.

Regulation of Aldosterone Secretion

The principal regulator of aldosterone secretion is the renin-angiotensin system. Renin is produced in the kidney by specialized cells of the juxtaglomerular apparatus. Although the complete details regarding its synthesis and release are not yet clear, it is known that a decrease in plasma volume causes an increase in renin release and, conversely, an increase in plasma volume inhibits its release. Once in the plasma, renin is converted to angiotensin I through interaction with a protein substrate which cleaves off a decapeptide fragment. In the lung, angiotensin I is converted to angiotensin II, the compound which stimulates aldosterone secretion. Aldosterone, by prompting sodium retention, causes plasma volume expansion which then shuts off renin release, and the feedback loop is completed.

Aldosterone release is also influenced by potassium. An increase in plasma potassium promptly increases aldosterone secretion. Conversely, depletion of body potassium inhibits aldosterone release. ACTH administration also increases aldosterone secretion but this effect is transient; aldosterone production declines to normal within 48 hours despite continued ACTH administration.

Biological Actions

In man, cortisol and aldosterone are the principal representatives of glucocorticoids and mineralocorticoids, the two main classes of adrenal cortical steroids. The biological activities of these steroids can be inferred from the descriptions of the classic clinical entities in which they are either deficient or in excess. An important action of cortisol is to promote the conversion of protein into glucose by induction of enzymes of gluconeogenesis. In its role in regulating glucose homeostasis, cortisol frequently acts in opposition to insulin. The primary functions of aldosterone are interlinked: regulation of extracellular fluid volume and potassium metabolism. Unlike cortisol, which affects all cells of the body, the action of aldosterone appears limited to the kidney and the sweat and salivary glands. In the kidney, aldosterone acts on the distal tubule to promote the absorption of sodium ions in exchange for potassium and hydrogen ions. In excess, aldosterone initially stimulates sodium reabsorption by the proximal renal tubules, but after a short time "escape" from this effect occurs. Escape from the action of aldosterone on the distal tubule does not occur. Thus, in chronic aldosterone excess (primary aldosteronism) there is expansion of the extracellular fluid volume and profound potassium depletion, but no edema. In the female the androgenic steroids constitute a third functional group of steroids elaborated by the adrenal cortex. The androgenic steroids have anabolic effects and are thought to be required for the development of libido and the capacity to achieve orgasm. At least part of their effect on female sexuality depends on their tropic action on the clitoris. The mechanism of action of all steroid hormones probably involves interaction with specific protein receptors in the cytosol and nucleus, leading to modification of a portion of the genome, transcription of messenger RNA, and protein synthesis.

Biosynthesis, Transport, and Metabolism of the Adrenal Steroids

Cholesterol is the basic precursor of steroid biosynthesis. It is initially converted to its 20-α hydroxyl derivative in a reaction stimulated by ACTH via the adenylate cyclase-cyclic AMP system. There is then cleavage of the terminal, 6-carbon side chain of cholesterol, resulting in pregnenolone. Pregnenolone is transformed to progesterone by the action of a 3-β-hydroxysteroid dehydrogenase and an isomerase. Thereafter, a series of hydroxylations occur, each catalyzed by a specific hydroxylase and requiring TPNH to form successively compounds with a hydroxyl group at C_{17}, C_{21}, and finally C_{11}. As discussed below, inborn errors of metabolism exist in which these enzymes are deficient.

In the mineralocorticoid pathway, progesterone is hydroxylated at the C_{21} position to form 11-desoxycorticosterone. There is then hydroxylation at the 11 position to form corticosterone, followed by hydroxylation at the 18 position to form 18-hydroxycorticosterone. Oxidation of this C_{18} hydroxyl group yields a final product, aldosterone. Another principal pathway involves the formation of dehydroepiandrosterone, a major metabolite of the adrenal cortex. This compound is formed by dehydroxylation of pregnenolone and cleavage of the C_{20}, C_{21} side chain to form the C_{19} steroid. Dehydroepiandrosterone is converted to androstenedione by a 3-β-hydroxysteroid-dehydrogenase and an isomerase. The latter steroid is the immediate precursor of testosterone. In females, testosterone is derived from the peripheral conversion of circulating androstenedione rather than from secretion by the adrenal gland.

Following its secretion, cortisol is transported and bound to an alpha-2-globulin called transcortin or cortisol-binding globulin (CBG). It is estimated that approximately 45 per cent of circulating cortisol is thus bound and only 5 per cent is in the biologically active, free form; the remainder conjugated with glucuronide is not included in the usual procedures used to measure plasma cortisol. Aldosterone circulates loosely bound to albumin. Both hormones are metabolized in the liver by the reduction of ring A to tetrahydro derivatives which are conjugated with glucuronide. These water-soluble biologically inactive derivatives are excreted in the kidneys. The biological half-life of cortisol, normally about two hours, is prolonged in liver disease and decreased in thyrotoxicosis; the half-life of aldosterone is 30 minutes. Adrenal steroid secretory rates and concentrations in body fluids are listed in Table 32-5.

TABLE 32-5 SECRETORY RATES AND CONCENTRATIONS IN BODY FLUIDS OF THE ADRENAL CORTICAL HORMONES

	Plasma Level (μg./100 ml.) Total	Plasma Level (μg./100 ml.) Free	Secretion Rate (mg./day)	Urinary Metabolites (mg./day)
Cortisol	15	1	15–30	4–8
Aldosterone	0.003–0.015	0.003	0.050–0.250	0.025–0.035
Dehydroepiandrosterone	65	65	15–30	4–8

Modified from Catt, K. J.: *Lancet*, 1:1279, 1970.

CLINICAL ENTITIES

Addison's Disease

As mentioned above, the clinical features of chronic adrenal insufficiency were first described by Addison over a hundred years ago. The underlying pathologic process may be tuberculosis or other granulomatous disease such as histoplasmosis; metastatic carcinoma; or, most commonly, simple atrophy. Although the cause of the latter is unknown, there is reason to believe that it may be the consequence of an autoimmune reaction. Typically, the clinical manifestations of primary adrenal insufficiency are extremely insidious; rare exceptions are the acute adrenal insufficiency of meningococcemia (the Waterhouse-Friderichsen syndrome) and that due to heparin overdosage.

The manifestations, regardless of cause, are attributable to deficiencies of cortisol and aldosterone and, in the female, androgenic steroids. Cortisol deficiency results in loss of appetite, weight loss, severe weakness, gastrointestinal disturbances, and emotional lability. Because of impaired gluconeogenesis, patients may become hypoglycemic after an overnight fast. The persistently low or absent plasma concentrations of cortisol lead to hypersecretion of ACTH and MSH, resulting in a characteristic increased pigmentation of the skin and mucous membranes. Aldosterone deficiency results in unregulated loss of body sodium and retention of potassium, with consequent reduction in plasma volume and hyperkalemia. The hypovolemia leads to prerenal azotemia, orthostatic hypotension, and ultimately shock. Because of its deleterious effect on cardiac rhythm, hyperkalemia is potentially a lethal complication of Addison's disease. Although the course of Addison's disease is typically prolonged, it may abruptly worsen if the patient is severely stressed by trauma or infection. Under these conditions, acute adrenal crisis may develop, manifested by vomiting, shock, high fever, and coma.

The laboratory findings in Addison's disease include a reduction in serum sodium, elevation in serum potassium, a reduced fasting blood glucose, and mild azotemia. These findings are of course not diagnostic of Addison's disease. To establish the diagnosis, it is necessary to demonstrate the inability of the adrenal glands to respond normally to ACTH stimulation. This may be done by analyzing the response of 17-hydroxycorticoids in 24-hour urine samples to the administration of ACTH over a 3- to 5-day period. In Addison's disease the control excretion of 17-hydroxycorticoids is typically less than 2 mg. per day and does not increase by more than 2 to 3 mg. during ACTH administration. In contrast, when adrenal insufficiency is secondary to hypopituitarism, the control values of urinary 17-hydroxycorticoids may be very low but will progressively increase with each day of stimulation to values which equal or exceed 8 to 10 mg. per day.

One particularly common form of secondary adrenal insufficiency deserves special comment. Large doses of cortisone and related glucocorticoids are often used in the chronic treatment of a variety of diseases such as asthma and rheumatoid arthritis. When such treatment is extended beyond four or five weeks, a semipermanent suppression of CRF and ACTH secretion ensues. If the steroid is then abruptly discontinued, the hypothalamic-pituitary axis is unable to respond normally to the reduction in circulating cortisol. The result is a mild degree of hypoadrenocorticism, which can become particularly significant if the patient is subjected to stress. This potential problem is minimized by gradually tapering the dose of steroid before discontinuing it entirely.

Cushing's Syndrome

Cushing's syndrome is the clinical condition that results from chronic exposure to excessive circulating levels of glucocorticoids. Four etiologic subsets of the disorder have been identified. First, the primary lesion may be either an adenoma or a carcinoma within the adrenal cortex which elaborates cortisol autonomously. Alternatively, the disease may be due to disordered hypothalamic-pituitary function, with a persistent overproduction of CRF and in turn ACTH, resulting in hyperplasia and hyperfunction of both adrenal glands. Characteristic of this disorder is a loss of the diurnal or circadian rhythm of ACTH secretion and a relative inability of cortisol to suppress ACTH secretion. The pituitary itself may be normal morphologically, or it may contain small basophilic tumors, as did the pituitary glands of the patients originally described by Cushing. This variety of Cushing's syndrome is often called "Cushing's disease." Thirdly, the adrenal cortex may be stimulated excessively by ACTH or an ACTH-like peptide elaborated by a nonpituitary tumor. This variety of Cushing's syndrome has been called the "ectopic ACTH syndrome." Carcinoma of the lung is perhaps the most frequent neoplasm responsible. Fourthly, and the most common form of Cushing's syndrome, is that resulting from chronic therapy with pharmacologic doses of glucocorticoids for an illness such as rheumatoid arthritis, asthma, or ulcerative colitis.

The clinical manifestations of Cushing's syndrome are explicable on the basis of known effects of cortisol. Principal actions of cortisol include the promotion of protein catabolism and the diversion of amino acids into gluconeogenesis. When these physiologic processes are exaggerated by chronic cortisol excess, marked loss of protein occurs. The clinical consequences are

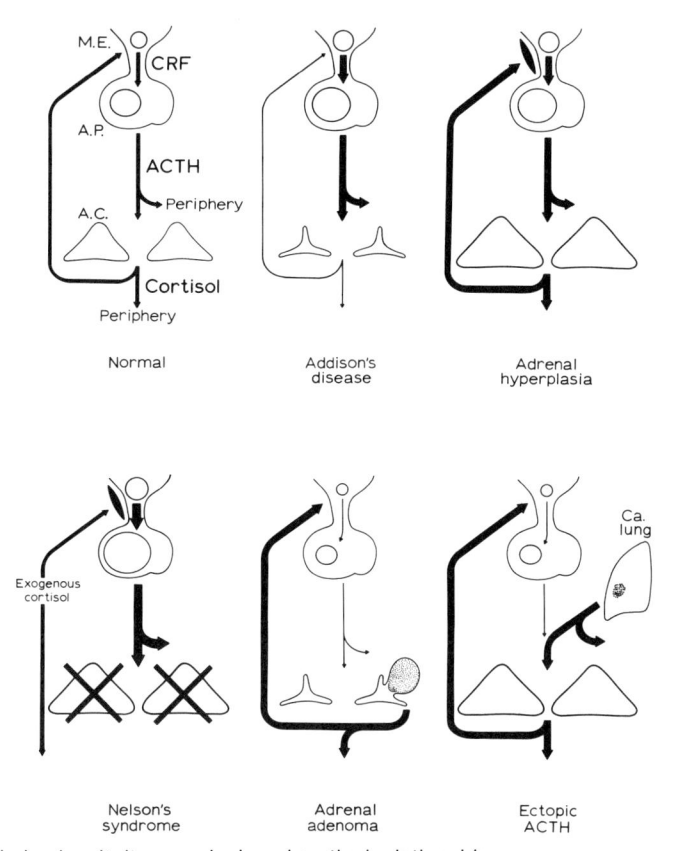

Figure 32-5 Hypothalamic, pituitary, and adrenal cortical relationships.

Normal: CRF elaborated by the median eminence (*M.E.*) stimulates the secretion of ACTH by the anterior pituitary (*A.P.*). ACTH triggers the synthesis and release of cortisol, the principal glucocorticoid of the adrenal cortex (*A.C.*); a rising level of cortisol inhibits CRF release, completing the negative feedback loop.

Addison's disease: In primary disease of the adrenal cortex, the level of plasma cortisol falls drastically and CRF release proceeds without inhibition, causing a marked increase in secretion of ACTH. High levels of the latter hormone promote the pigmentary changes characteristic of Addison's disease.

Adrenal hyperplasia: The primary lesion is probably at the level of the hypothalamus or higher. Production of CRF is excessive, leading to increased ACTH and cortisol secretion. The latter causes the peripheral manifestations of the disorder (Cushing's disease). Cells of the M.E. are resistant to the high levels of circulating cortisol.

Nelson's syndrome: When Cushing's disease is treated by bilateral adrenalectomy, the physiologic quantity of cortisol used to treat the patient is a relatively weak brake on CRF production. The latter increases substantially, causing intense stimulation of the ACTH-producing cells of the A.P., eventually leading to tumor formation and extreme pigmentation, which are characteristic features of the syndrome.

Adrenal adenoma: An adenoma or carcinoma of the adrenal may produce cortisol autonomously. When the rate of production exceeds physiologic quantities, Cushing's syndrome results; CRF release is inhibited by the high level of circulating cortisol, with resultant diminished ACTH secretion and atrophy of the normal adrenal tissue.

Ectopic ACTH: In this syndrome, an ACTH-like peptide is elaborated by a tumor such as carcinoma of the lung. The adrenals are stimulated; circulating cortisol increases inhibiting CRF production.

muscle wasting, thinning of the skin, easy bruisability, abdominal striae, and osteoporosis. Cortisol, in addition to promoting glucose formation in the liver, also antagonizes the action of insulin in transporting glucose into cells. Predictably, diabetes mellitus is a common complication of Cushing's syndrome. In a number of ways, cortisol alters the normal response to infection and injury. Antibody formation is suppressed, and the accumulation and migration of polymorphonuclear cells at inflammatory sites are inhibited. Some manifestations of the disease are much less well understood, for example, the characteristic redistribution of adipose tissue causing moon facies, buffalo hump, supraclavicular fat pads, and truncal obesity. Also obscure is the basis of the mental aberrations commonly seen in Cushing's syndrome.

Because cortisol has some mineralocorticoid activity, a few patients with Cushing's syndrome

TABLE 32-6 TYPICAL LABORATORY FINDINGS IN CUSHING'S SYNDROME DUE TO HYPERPLASIA, ADENOMA, CARCINOMA, AND ECTOPIC ACTH PRODUCTION

	Normal	Adrenal Pathologic Condition			
		Hyperplasia	Adenoma	Carcinoma	Ectopic ACTH
Plasma:					
Cortisol (μg./100 ml., A.M./P.M.)	17/8	30/25	35/35	50/50	35/35
ACTH (pg./ml.)	< 150	50 to 500	< 50	< 10	500 to 1000
Urine: 17 OHC (mg./24 hr.)					
Basal	2 to 10	15	30	50	30
After ACTH stimulation	2 to 5× ↑	3 to 5× ↑	↑/↔	↔	2× ↔
Dexamethasone suppression (2 mg./day)	< 3	> 4	30	50	30
Dexamethasone suppression (8 mg./day)	< 3	< 3	30	50	30

↑ = increase
↔ = no change

Modified from Williams, G. H., and Lauler, D. P.: Laboratory evaluation of adrenocortical function. *In* Harvey, J. C. (Ed.): Practice of Medicine. Vol. II, Hagerstown, Maryland, W. F. Prior Co., 1966.

have elevations in blood pressure and hypokalemia, findings typical of primary aldosteronism.

Although clinical findings may strongly suggest the diagnosis of Cushing's syndrome, laboratory confirmation is essential. One such approach entails the estimation of the 17-OHC content of 24-hour urine samples collected in the basal state and then during the sequential administration of intravenous ACTH and oral dexamethasone, 2 mg. daily for 3 days, followed by 8 mg. per day for 3 days. The results of these procedures should establish the presence of Cushing's syndrome and, moreover, provide information regarding its cause. Illustrative data are summarized in Table 32-6 and shown graphically in Figure 32-5. It should be noted that the basal urinary excretion of 17-OHC in Cushing's syndrome due to hyperplasia may be normal (15 per cent of cases) or only slightly elevated. The hyperplastic glands ordinarily respond very briskly to ACTH stimulation.

Congenital Adrenal Hyperplasia (CAH)

The term congenital adrenal hyperplasia embraces an interesting spectrum of disorders characterized by progressive virilization which results from an inherited deficiency of a specific enzyme involved in the biosynthesis of the adrenal steroids. Although manifestations of the condition are usually present at birth, they are often unrecognized or misinterpreted. Clinically, three forms can be distinguished: (1) Virilization alone, (2) virilization plus salt wasting, and (3) virilization plus hypertension. The virilization may be pronounced. The external genitalia of the female infant with this disorder may be sufficiently masculine to lead to an erroneous conclusion regarding the patient's sex. Thus, CAH is a common cause of female pseudohermaphroditism. In the salt-losing form of CAH, the infant fails to thrive, vomits, becomes dehydrated, and often expires if untreated. Laboratory examination reveals the electrolyte pattern of severe adrenal insufficiency—decreased serum sodium and increased serum potassium concentrations.

Deficiency of C_{21} Hydroxylase. Deficiency of C_{21} hydroxylase is by far the most common cause of CAH. Its absence results in an increase in 17-hydroxyprogesterone and other precursors of androgens, including androstenedione and testosterone. The excessive quantities of the latter hormones cause virilization. When the enzymatic deficiency is mild, as it is in about 50 per cent of the cases, cortisol production is maintained at normal or near normal rates by a compensatory increase in the pituitary secretion of ACTH, which is prompted by the initially low levels of circulating cortisol. As expected, however, the increased stimulation of the adrenal cortex causes hyperplastic changes and an increase in the production of androgenic substances. When the enzymatic defect is more severe, this compensatory mechanism is inadequate to maintain a normal secretion of cortisol, and adrenocortical insufficiency ensues. The steps in the pathogenesis of CAH may be summarized as follows:

1. The primary lesion is a deficiency of an enzyme required for the formation of cortisol.
2. Deficiency of cortisol leads to a compensatory increase in ACTH secretion.
3. The increase in ACTH secretion causes adrenal hyperplasia and an increase in total

adrenal steroid production, including virilizing steroids.

While the salt-losing variety of CAH is clinically quite distinct from the "virilizing only" form, there is no firm evidence of qualitative differences in the underlying defect in steroidogenesis. It is possible that in salt-losing CAH, relatively large quantities of steroids capable of competitively inhibiting aldosterone are produced. Such substances, probably derived from progesterone, would be similar to the synthetic steroid spirolactone, which is widely used by clinicians as a diuretic.

All newborn infants with ambiguous secondary sexual characteristics should be examined for the presence of Barr bodies. The female infant with CAH and malelike external genitalia will have a positive chromatin pattern (i.e., Barr bodies will be present indicating a female genotype) on examination of a buccal mucosa smear. Once suspected, the diagnosis can be substantiated by the determination of pregnenetriol levels in the urine. Pregnenetriol, the principal excretory product of 17-hydroxyprogesterone, is greatly increased when C_{21} hydroxylation is blocked.

Once the diagnosis is established, the management of CAH is both straightforward and gratifying. A glucocorticoid such as cortisone acetate is given orally in physiologic doses. This exogenous replacement supplies the need of the peripheral tissues for cortisol; salt wasting, if present, is corrected. At the same time, ACTH secretion is suppressed, adrenal hyperplasia regresses, and the excessive production of androgens ceases.

Other Defects in Adrenal Steroidogenesis. In addition to 21-hydroxylase deficiency, CAH may arise from lack of 11-β-hydroxylase, 17-hydroxylase, or 3-β-hydroxysteroid dehydrogenase. The latter two conditions are extremely rare. Deficiency of 11-hydroxylase constitutes about 10 per cent of the cases of CAH. In this form of the disease, hypertension is a prominent clinical feature. Impairment of hydroxylation of C_{11} leads to the accumulation of both 11-desoxycortisol and, by loss of the C_{17} hydroxyl group, desoxycorticosterone. Whereas 11-desoxycortisol is biologically inert, excessive serum levels of desoxycorticosterone cause hypertension by a mechanism which has not been fully elucidated. Confirmation of a clinical diagnosis of 11-hydroxylase deficiency requires the demonstration of excessive quantities of tetrahydrodesoxycortisol (the excretory product of 11-desoxycortisol) in the urine. It is of interest that the pharmacologic agent, metyrapone, used to test for pituitary ACTH reserve, acts by inhibiting 11-hydroxylase, thus transiently simulating the inborn error of metabolism under discussion. CAH due to 11-β-hydroxylase deficiency also responds to physiologic doses of glucocorticoid.

Primary Aldosteronism (Conn's Syndrome)

Primary aldosteronism is the clinical condition caused by excessive, unregulated secretion by the adrenal cortex of the potent, salt-retaining steroid, aldosterone. The underlying pathologic lesion is almost always a small adenoma. The history of both the clinical entity and the hormone is brief but instructive. By 1950 the research of many investigators had indicated that certain known actions of the adrenal cortex could not be attributed to cortisol alone. Greep and Deane were among those who postulated that there was an unidentified substance responsible for the powerful effect exerted by the adrenal cortex on mineral metabolism. In search of this missing "mineralocorticoid," Tait and coworkers isolated a factor they termed "electrocortin." This substance was soon characterized chemically and named aldosterone because of an aldehyde group on C_{18}. In 1955 the first case of primary aldosteronism was reported by Conn, who stated: "When in April, 1954, I was confronted with a patient who exhibited a most fascinating disturbance in electrolyte metabolism similar to a few cases which had been reported as potassium-losing nephritis, it could not have been presented to anyone more conscious of the possibility of aldosteronism in man than I was at that moment." Dr. Conn modestly goes on to say, "It actually required little imagination."

Chronic excessive secretion of aldosterone leads to hypertension and hypokalemia, the two characteristic findings in primary aldosteronism. Although the hypertension is usually mild or moderate in severity, it may result in manifestations of sustained hypertension such as left ventricular hypertrophy and narrowing of the retinal arterioles. The hypokalemia may cause intestinal atony and characteristic electrocardiographic alterations. Muscle weakness may be so severe that an ascending neuritis such as that found in the Guillain-Barré syndrome is suggested. The electrolyte disturbance also leads to other symptoms such as polyuria, muscle cramps, and paresthesias. On laboratory examination, the serum potassium is typically below 3.6 m Eq. per L., serum sodium is normal or slightly elevated, bicarbonate is increased, and choloride is decreased (hypokalemic, hypochloremic alkalosis).

Although the occurrence of hypokalemia in a hypertensive patient should suggest the diagnosis, confirmation requires the demonstration of both increased aldosterone secretion and low plasma renin activity. Urinary aldosterone should exceed 20 μg. per day in a patient with primary aldosteronism who is receiving ample dietary sodium, e.g., greater than 120 mEq. per day. In addition, the plasma renin activity should be low and remain suppressed despite a low-sodium diet and several hours of ambulation. Patients with malignant hypertension, or hypertension due to chronic renal disease or renal artery stenosis, will also excrete large amounts of aldosterone, but in contrast the plasma renin activity will be elevated. The most common form of hypertension is termed "essential," since no specific etiologic factor can currently be identified. Although these patients have normal urinary aldosterone levels, approximately one third will display suppressed plasma renin values for reasons which are not yet clear. A scheme recommended by Conn and coworkers (1969) for the evaluation of primary aldosteronism is given below.

Procedures
1. Two weeks: Unrestricted diet, no diuretics
2. Day 1: 120 mEq. Na diet.
   Day 2: 120 mEq. Na diet.
   Day 3: 120 mEq. Na diet; collect 24-hour urine for aldosterone; take fasting blood for plasma renin activity (PRA) after 2-hour ambulation.
3. Day 4: 10 mEq. Na diet.
   Day 5: 10 mEq. Na diet.
   Day 6: 10 mEq. Na diet; collect 24-hour urine for aldosterone; take fasting blood for plasma renin activity (PRA) after 2-hour ambulation.

Results
Aldosterone Excretion (μg./24 hr.)
	(120 mEq. Na diet)	(10 mEq. Na diet)
Normals	10.7 ± .6	39.5 ± 3.9
Patients	21 to 72	16 to 75
(n = 13)		

Plasma Renin Activity (ng./100 ml.)
	(120 mEq. Na diet)	(10 mEq. Na diet)
Normals	370 ± 36	1181 ± 117
Patients	0 to 372	0 to 446
(n = 13)		

The treatment of primary aldosteronism consists of surgical extirpation of the adenoma. Preoperative localization of the tumor may be made by the use of isotopically labeled cholesterol which is concentrated by the involved adrenal. The prognosis is variable; if the process has been going on for many years, the cardiovascular complications of long-standing hypertension are usually irreversible and the hypertension itself tends to be fixed.

PARATHYROIDS

PHYSIOLOGY

The parathyroid glands are minute, with a total mass of only 200 mg.; they are of endodermal origin, being derived from the pharyngeal pouches. In the adult, they are usually located either in close proximity to or within the thyroid gland. They secrete parathyroid hormone, a polypeptide with a molecular weight of approximately 8500, which has the principal and perhaps only function of maintaining calcium homeostasis. The narrow range within which the serum calcium concentration normally varies attests to the high priority of calcium homeostasis in vertebrate evolution. Calcium plays an important role in such vital processes as neuromuscular excitability, muscular contraction, membrane permeability, and coagulation of blood. Furthermore, it is required for the activation of many critical enzymes and provides the major structural support for the organism. In the skeleton, and to a much lesser extent in the plasma, calcium is chemically linked to phosphate. Like calcium, phosphate has great importance outside the skeleton. Phosphorylated compounds (e.g., ATP) are the currency of energy in cellular metabolism. Although parathyroid hormone has a dominant effect on plasma phosphate, there is no evidence that plasma phosphate has any direct effect on parathyroid hormone secretion. Apparently, the release of parathyroid hormone in man is determined by only one factor—the level of ionized calcium perfusing parathyroid tissue. Two other substances—vitamin D and calcitonin—are also of major importance in calcium homeostasis and bone metabolism. The latter is a hypocalcemic hormone first described by Copp and coworkers in 1962.

Gastrointestinal Tract

The gastrointestinal tract is a critical site in the regulation of calcium metabolism. Intestinal absorption of calcium occurs either from the duodenum by active transport or at any point along the entire small bowel by simple diffusion. The latter movement of calcium across the intestinal mucosa is bidirectional; hence, fecal calcium consists of calcium excreted into the gut, as well as nonabsorbed dietary calcium. Although vitamin D has effects on other tissues, its primary action is to promote calcium absorption from the gastrointestinal tract by stimulation of its active transport. Parathyroid hormone also enhances calcium absorption but to a lesser extent. The absorption of intestinal phosphate is probably linked to that of calcium. The optimum ratio of intestinal calcium to phosphate for calcium absorption is 2 to 1. Absorption of calcium is impaired by diseases of the small bowel such as sprue and celiac disease and by hepatic disease such as biliary cirrhosis. It is also influenced by the acidity of the intestinal content and by dietary factors such as acetic acid, phytic acid, and oxalates.

Calcium absorbed from the gastrointestinal tract enters the extracellular pool of calcium, estimated at about 950 mg. in the adult. Extracellular calcium is in dynamic equilibrium with calcium in the intracellular component of soft tissue (about 11,000 mg.), and with the so-called exchangeable calcium pool of the skeleton. The latter pool is estimated to turn over 40 to 50 times each day. The precise quantity and even the location of this exchangeable pool of bone calcium are not known. Some believe that it is contained within partially calcified bone, and others contend that it is calcium released from bone undergoing active resorption.

Bone

In the adult in calcium balance, approximately 300 mg. of calcium per day is resorbed from bone and the same amount deposited each day. This turnover largely reflects the continuous process of bone remodeling. While a number of factors influence bone remodeling, such as age, bone disease, deficiency of calcium or phosphate, and hormones other than parathyroid hormone and calcitonin, the principal controlling factors are (1) parathyroid hormone and calcitonin and (2) the effects of mechanical stress on the skeleton. The actions of parathyroid hormone and calcitonin on bone resorption subserve calcium homeostasis. Thus, when a conflict arises between maintenance of a normal serum calcium and skeletal integrity, bone is sacrificed to provide the needed calcium. Mechanical stress, the second factor, causes a remodeling of bone to meet changing requirements for structural strength. Within physiologic limits, it appears that parathyroid hormone (and perhaps calcitonin) is the principal determinant of the magnitude of remodeling, while mechanical stresses are the principal determinants of the locations where remodeling occurs.

The mechanism of action of parathyroid hormone on bone at the cellular level has not been determined. One line of evidence suggests that parathyroid hormone stimulates both the osteolytic activity of osteocytes, causing an early rise in plasma calcium, and also the differentiation of mesenchymal cells into osteoclasts, the cells responsible for bone resorption.

The Kidneys

The normal kidney is extraordinarily efficient in its conservation of calcium. Despite filtration by the glomeruli of an estimated 10,000 mg. of calcium daily, no more than 300 mg. of this is normally excreted in the urine. Tubular reabsorption of calcium is enhanced by parathyroid hormone, but this effect is usually overshadowed by hypercalcemia caused by the action of parathyroid hormone on bone. Vitamin D has a weak calciuric effect. Calcitonin reduces calcium excretion, but this may in part reflect its hypocalcemic action. The kidney's efficiency in conserving calcium is not matched by an equal ability to excrete it when the need arises. Even with continued severe hypercalcemia, the 24-hour urinary excretion of calcium will rarely exceed 500 mg. This limitation is detrimental if calcium is being absorbed from the gut or mobilized from bone in an excessive and unregulated fashion as occurs, for example, in vitamin D intoxication or metastatic bone disease. Calcium virtually disappears from the urine when the serum calcium falls below 7 mg. per 100 ml. A major renal action of parathyroid hormone is to inhibit the tubular reabsorption of phosphate. In the absence of parathyroid hormone, about 90 per cent or more of filtered phosphate is reabsorbed, whereas in hyperparathyroidism this value usually is less than 70 per cent. Parathyroid hormone may also stimulate the secretion of phosphate by the tubules as well as decrease its reabsorption. The major actions of parathyroid hormone are summarized in Table 32-7. The mechanism of action of parathyroid hormone on the renal tubules involves the adenylate cyclase-cyclic AMP system. Following the injection of parathyroid hormone, the urinary excretion of cyclic AMP is markedly increased.

CLINICAL ENTITIES

Metabolic Bone Disease

The concept of metabolic bone disease was introduced over 30 years ago by Albright. The term applies to those disorders of bone in which—at the molecular level—all parts of the skeleton are involved. The qualification "at the molecular level" is important, since clinically, radiographically, and even histologically the disease may appear to be limited to only one or several sites. As might be predicted from its generalized nature, the identified causes of metabolic bone disease are usually hormonal or nutritional. Features of the three "classic" examples of metabolic bone disease—osteitis fibrosa cystica, osteoporosis, and

TABLE 32–7 SITES OF ACTION OF PARATHYROID HORMONE AND RELATIVE IMPORTANCE OF EACH ACTION IN MAINTAINING CALCIUM HOMEOSTASIS

Site	Action	Degree of Influence
Renal tubule	↑ PO$_4$ Excretion	++++
	↑ Ca^{++} Reabsorption	+
Bone	↑ Bone Resorption	++++
Gut	↑ Ca^{++} Absorption	+

TABLE 32-8 COMPARISON OF THE MAJOR METABOLIC BONE DISEASES

	Osteitis Fibrosa Cystica	Osteoporosis	Osteomalacia
Etiology	Excessive PTH	Varied but usually unknown	Vitamin D deficiency; malabsorption; etc.
Serum			
Calcium	Increased	Normal	Decreased or normal
Phosphate	Normal or decreased	Normal	Decreased
Alkaline phosphatase	Normal or increased	Normal	Increased
Pathophysiology	Increased bone resorption	Decreased bone mass (resorp. > accret.)	Decreased mineralization
Histopathology	Cysts; fibrosis; "Brown" tumor	Normal histology	Increased osteoid tissue
Radiology	Subperiosteal resorption; cysts	Rarefaction of axial skeleton; "codfish" vertebrae compression fractures	Rarefaction of appendicular skeleton; pseudofractures (Looser's zones)

osteomalacia—are given in Table 32-8. Other forms of bone disease may be widely disseminated, as for example in metastatic cancer, but between metastatic sites the bone will be normal, and thus the process can not be considered under the above classification.

Hypoparathyroidism

By far the leading cause of parathyroid hormone deficiency is inadvertent removal or damage to the parathyroids during thyroid surgery. Permanent hypoparathyroidism is a serious complication of thyroidectomy, occurring with a frequency of about 1 per cent. Idiopathic hypoparathyroidism, a rare disorder, is noteworthy in several respects. It is often familial and may be associated with generalized moniliasis and deficiencies of other endocrine glands. The sera of some patients with idiopathic hypoparathyroidism have high titers of antibody to human parathyroid tissue, suggesting an autoimmune cause.

The manifestations of hypoparathyroidism are directly attributable to impaired calcium homeostasis due to parathyroid hormone deficiency. Both total and ionized serum calcium are low, and serum phosphate is high. Hypocalcemia causes an increase in neuromuscular irritability. When the total serum calcium falls below 7 to 8 mg. per 100 ml., the patient develops symptoms such as numbness, tingling, formication, and muscle cramping. With a further depression in serum calcium, the physical manifestations of hypocalcemia, termed tetany, ensue. These include carpopedal spasm, laryngeal spasm and stridor, muscle twitching, and generalized convulsions. The latter occasionally lead to the erroneous diagnosis of epilepsy. This tragic mistake can be avoided by routinely determining the serum calcium in all patients undergoing their initial evaluation for a seizure disorder. The altered myocardial contractility due to hypocalcemia is reflected in the electrocardiogram by prolongation of the Q-T interval. Such a finding on a routine electrocardiogram should always arouse suspicion of occult hypocalcemia. Factors that alter the protein binding of calcium in the serum can either enhance or diminish the symptoms of hypocalcemia. For example, alkalosis will increase the quantity of calcium bound to protein with a corresponding reduction in ionized calcium; thus, hyperventilation commonly precipitates tetany in the presence of a normal total serum calcium. Conversely, acidemia increases the dissociation of bound calcium, and thus may prevent tetany even when the total calcium is 5 or 6 mg. per 100 ml.

Chronic hypocalcemia results in cataract formation and calcification within the central nervous system. The basal ganglia and cerebellum appear to be especially vulnerable. It has been thought that such calcification is the result of supersaturation of body fluids with calcium phosphate. Although the calcium × phosphate product may indeed be elevated in hypoparathyroidism, this fails to explain the peculiar distribution of calcification in hypoparathyroidism, which differs strikingly from that found in other diseases with a high calcium × phosphate product.

Pseudohypoparathyroidism

In 1942, Albright and his colleagues introduced the term pseudohypoparathyroidism to describe a 28-year-old female with a seizure disorder, short stature, and the serum calcium and phosphate findings of hypoparathyroidism. However, large quantities of administered parathyroid hormone corrected neither the serum chemical abnormalities nor the hypophosphaturia, suggesting that the basic problem was an inability to respond to parathyroid hormone rather than a deficiency of the hormone. Subsequently, similar patients have been reported and have manifested, in addition to hypocalcemia and an elevated serum phosphate, short stature and a short neck, a rounded face, short metacarpal and metatarsal bones, extraosseous calcification, and mental retardation. The syndrome is inherited as an autosomal dominant trait with partial penetrance. Patients with the characteristic physiognomy but without serum chemistry abnormalities have been identified and labeled with the rather awkward term "pseudopseudohypoparathyroidism." Since pseudopseudohypoparathyroidism and pseudohypoparathyroidism have occurred in the same kindred and also in the same patient at different times, the former condition is regarded as a less severe genetic expression (or "forme fruste") of the latter.

Considerable evidence now supports Albright's thesis that pseudohypoparathyroidism is a disorder involving end-organ unresponsiveness to parathyroid hormone rather than a deficiency of the hormone. Hyperplastic parathyroid glands have been demonstrated in these patients at surgery, and their sera have been shown to contain abnormally high levels of immunoassayable parathyroid hormone. As mentioned above, the action of parathyroid hormone on the renal tubular cells is mediated by the adenylate cyclase-cyclic AMP system. When parathyroid hormone is administered to normal subjects or patients with hypoparathyroidism or pseudopseudohypoparathyroidism, the urinary content of cyclic AMP is greatly increased; contrariwise, no increase in cyclic AMP occurs in patients with pseudohypoparathyroidism. Thus, unresponsiveness of the renal tubular cells to parathyroid hormone is clearly implicated in the pathogenesis of the hypocalcemia and hyperphosphatemia of pseudohypoparathyroidism. This observation also tends to localize the biochemical defect in the kidneys to either the interaction of parathyroid hormone with adenylate cyclase or of adenylate cyclase with cyclic AMP. An additional question of importance in pseudohypoparathyroidism concerns the responsiveness of the other parathyroid hormone-sensitive tissues, especially bone. Since occasional patients with pseudohypoparathyroidism have developed osteitis fibrosa cystica, it would appear that bone is at least partially responsive to parathyroid hormone in some patients with this disorder. As is so often true in endocrinology, studies undertaken to clarify the nature of a relatively obscure disorder, pseudohypoparathyroidism, have yielded information of basic importance to an understanding of hormone action.

Primary Hyperparathyroidism

Primary hyperparathyroidism refers to the disorder in which parathyroid hormone is secreted autonomously and excessively by one or more of the parathyroid glands. It is to be distinguished from secondary hyperparathyroidism which occurs in response to chronic renal disease, malabsorption, and other disorders characterized by long-standing hypocalcemia. The underlying pathologic disorder in primary hyperparathyroidism is either one or more adenomas (90 per cent of cases), hyperplasia of all four glands (10 per cent), or carcinoma (less than 1 per cent). Infrequently, when hyperparathyroidism is familial, there is a high incidence of neoplasms involving other endocrine glands, especially the pituitary and the pancreas, or the thyroid and adrenal medulla. These pluriglandular syndromes are termed multiple endocrine adenomatosis (MEA). Certain neoplasms arising in other organs, especially the lung, liver, and genitourinary tract, occasionally elaborate a peptide with parathyroid hormone activity. The resulting biochemical disturbance which may closely mimic primary hyperparathyroidism is often referred to as "pseudohyperparathyroidism."

The major manifestations of primary hyperparathyroidism are due to (1) the physiologic effects of hypercalcemia, (2) the effects of chronic hypercalcemia on the kidney, and (3) the effects of chronic excessive parathyroid hormone on bone. Hypercalcemia per se impairs the concentrating ability of the kidney and polyuria is an early symptom of hyperparathyroidism. Precipitation of fine crystals of calcium salts in the renal tubules (nephrocalcinosis) impairs both glomerular and tubular function. Renal stone formation occurs in up to 60 per cent of patients with hyperparathyroidism. A vicious cycle may ensue in which renal calculi predispose to infection, and alkalinization of the urine by infecting organisms in turn leads to further stone formation. If uninterrupted, this sequence of events may progress to uremia and death. Clearly, any patient who has or has had a renal stone should be investigated for hyperparathyroidism.

For reasons that are not yet clear, bone involvement in hyperparathyroidism sufficient to cause symptoms or to be detected by x-ray is becoming increasingly uncommon. An unproved hypothesis attempting to explain this trend has implicated the protective effect provided by the high calcium content of the typical American diet.

The high incidence of peptic ulcer disease which has been observed in patients with primary hyperparathyroidism may be a consequence of hypercalcemia. It has been shown experimentally that increasing the level of serum calcium stimulates an increase in circulating gastrin and an increased rate of secretion of hydrochloric acid by the stomach. Hypertension is also a frequent finding in hyperparathyroidism; although it is usually a benign complication which disappears after correction of the primary disorder, it often persists following surgery in those patients with nephrocalcinosis.

Renal Osteodystrophy

Although it has long been appreciated that chronic hypocalcemia can lead to hyperplasia of the parathyroids, the full implications of this phenomenon as it applies to chronic renal disease are just beginning to emerge. The term "renal osteodystrophy" embraces a syndrome in uremic patients that includes profound disturbances in divalent ion metabolism; metabolic bone disease including osteomalacia, osteitis fibrosa cystica, and osteosclerosis; and hyperplasia of the parathyroids and soft tissue calcification. In the past, the brief life span of a patient with severe renal failure probably precluded the development of advanced metabolic bone disease. With the advent of chronic dialysis and renal transplantation, the patient with uremia may survive for extended periods but frequently develops severe renal osteodystrophy. It is estimated that 25 per cent of uremic patients treated with conventional therapy and 80 per cent of those in chronic dialysis programs have this form of bone disease.

Although many questions remain unanswered, a working hypothesis (see Figure 32–6) which explains the development of renal osteodystrophy has been provided by Stanbury, Dent, and others. Probably, the earliest contributing event in renal failure is the development of resistance to vitamin D. Careful studies by Friis have shown that in mild renal failure, serum phosphate concentration is initially decreased and phosphate clearance increased. Before the serum phosphate increased as renal failure progressed, the serum calcium was noted to fall. These findings can be explained by a resistance to vitamin D, which leads to a decreased absorption of calcium from the gut. (The mechanism underlying the develop-

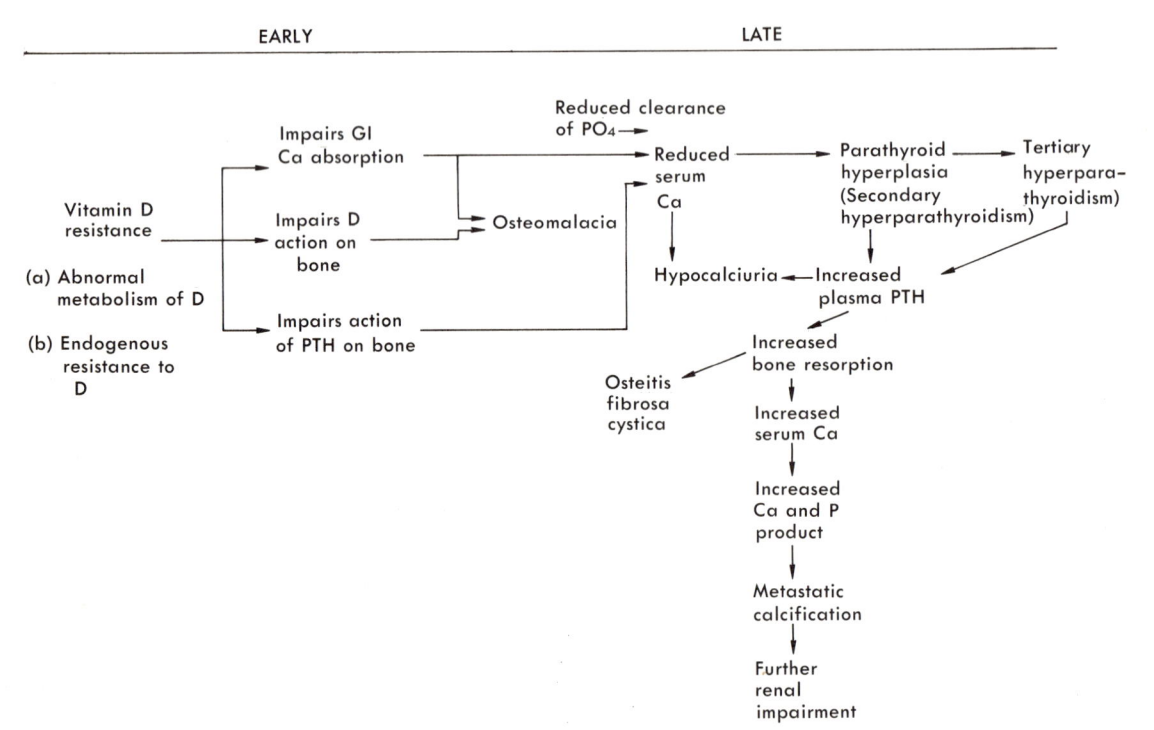

Figure 32–6 The effect of progressive renal failure on calcium and phosphate metabolism and bone. Although osteomalacia and osteitis fibrosa cystica are seen in advanced renal failure, the pathogenesis of these bone disorders remains speculative. The sequence of events depicted in the figure undoubtedly will be modified as new information becomes available (see text).

TABLE 32-9 BIOCHEMICAL FINDINGS IN PATIENTS WITH EARLY AND LATE RENAL OSTEODYSTROPHY

	Plasma Calcium* (mg./100 ml.)	Plasma Phosphate* (mg./100 ml.)	Product Ca × P	BUN* (mg./100 ml.)
Early (Azotemic osteomalacia)	7.6	6.0	46	78
Late (Osteitis fibrosa cystica)	10.1	8.8	87	131

*Normal range: calcium 8.5 to 10; phosphate, 3.0 to 4.5; BUN, 10 to 22.
From Stanbury, S. W., and Lumb, G. A.: Parathyroid function in chronic renal failure. Quart. J. Med., 35:1, 1966.

ment of vitamin D resistance may be related to the role the kidney normally plays in vitamin D metabolism. Deluca and his colleagues demonstrated that the conversion of vitamin D_3 to the metabolite active in the intestine—1,25-dihydroxycholecalciferol—takes place in the kidney.) To maintain serum calcium, an increase in parathyroid hormone secretion is required, and this is reflected in an increased phosphaturia and a decrease in serum phosphate. Maintenance of calcium homeostasis at this early stage might be entirely due to the action of parathyroid hormone in increasing the reabsorption of calcium from the renal tubule. Later, however, the reduced absorption of calcium from the gut, secondary to vitamin D resistance, causes a decrease in the miscible pool of calcium, with resultant demineralization of bone. Thus, osteomalacia evolves as renal failure advances. Eventually, the diseased kidney becomes unresponsive to parathyroid hormone, the level of serum phosphate rises, and serum calcium falls.

The inverse relationship between serum calcium and phosphate emphasized by Albright many years ago appears to be valid today, and one cause of hypocalcemia in renal failure is the hyperphosphatemia directly resulting from the renal disease. Stimulated by chronic hypocalcemia, the parathyroids become markedly hyperactive. In fact, the serum levels of parathyroid hormone are higher in chronic renal failure than in primary hyperparathyroidism. Eventually, the level of parathyroid hormone becomes sufficient to overcome vitamin D resistance at the level of bone, and a marked increase in bone resorption results. This is reflected radiographically in the development of osteitis fibrosa cystica and biochemically by an increase in the serum calcium. The increase in the calcium × phosphate product in body fluids may result in precipitation of calcium phosphate in the soft tissues. Such deposits in the kidney further reduce renal function.

The clinical manifestations of disordered calcium and bone metabolism in chronic renal disease are usually late findings. Typically, bone pain occurs in the patient with advanced renal failure, particularly when his life has been prolonged by repeated hemodialysis. In such patients, bone pain may be the chief complaint, since manifestations of uremia have been minimized by dialysis. Pathologic fractures may result from severe osteitis fibrosa cystica, and symptomatic, soft tissue calcification may also occur. Distressing itching of the skin is another late manifestation of renal failure. The basis of this intractable pruritus is not clear, but it disappears promptly following parathyroidectomy. Typical biochemical findings in early and late renal osteodystrophy are given in Table 32-9.

Osteoporosis

Osteoporosis is by far the most frequently encountered form of metabolic bone disease. It occurs most commonly in postmenopausal Caucasian females and in males over 60 years of age. The Negro race is infrequently affected. The basic abnormality is loss of bone substance which is seen radiographically as demineralization. The principal symptom is low back pain. Serum calcium, phosphate, and alkaline phosphatase are normal, as is the histologic and biochemical examination of biopsy samples of the bone itself.

The cause of primary or idiopathic osteoporosis is not known. As discussed earlier, maintenance of normal skeletal integrity requires a balance between bone formation and bone resorption. In osteoporosis, the latter exceeds the former. Whether resorption is pathologically increased or formation abnormally decreased, or both, is not clear. In recent years sophisticated methodology has been applied to the problem. Calcium kinetics, using ^{45}Ca, have been determined in patients with osteoporosis; in addition, their bones have been analyzed by microradiography and morphometric techniques using tetracycline labeling. Unfortunately, these different approaches have not yielded consistent results, and the cause (or causes) of primary osteoporosis remains unknown. However, studies have eliminated a number of factors once suspected as being causally important in osteoporosis. For example, it is now clear that calcium deficiency, a known cause of osteoporosis under experimental conditions, is infrequently present. Deficiencies of estrogenic and androgenic hormones have long been considered to play important roles in the development of this disease. This view is supported by the high incidence of osteoporosis in postmenopausal women, young women with ovarian agenesis, and older men. However, long-term treatment with estrogens has not caused a detectable increase in bone mass in women with postmenopausal osteoporosis. At the present time, it appears likely that primary osteoporosis may be the result of several coexistent factors.

A number of specific conditions are recognized that lead to osteoporosis. These include Cushing's syndrome, prolonged treatment with glucocorticoids, immobilization, thyrotoxicosis, and pregnancy. In hyperparathyroidism, there may be osteoporosis coexistent with the more specific lesions of subperiosteal bone resorption and cyst formation.

Low back pain is the most frequent symptom of osteoporosis. Typically, it is insidious in onset. Occasionally the onset is acute or there is an acute exacerbation of pain superimposed on the chronic discomfort. These latter events are associated with compression fracture of a vertebral body. Not infrequently, advanced osteoporosis is discovered in x-rays taken for an unrelated condition in a patient who is free of back pain. Progressive shortening of stature due to collapsed vertebrae may occur with little or no pain.

The diagnosis depends on finding characteristic changes in the x-ray films of the skeleton, particularly the spine. The end plates of the vertebrae are less rarefied than the bodies, causing an increased contrast between the two. The end plates may be depressed centrally, leading to the so-called "codfish" appearance of the spine. With further advance in the disease, the nucleus pulposus herniates through the end plate, producing an irregular area of increased density in the central portion of the vertebral body, a finding known as the "Schmorl node." When compression fracture occurs, typically the anterior portion of the body gives way, producing a "wedgelike" deformity of the vertebral body. Cortical bone is less affected than cancellous bone in osteoporosis. One can grossly assess the long bones by comparing the combined thickness of the bone's cortices with its total thickness. Normally, the former accounts for approximately 45 per cent of the latter.

ADRENAL MEDULLA

PHYSIOLOGY

The primary function of the adrenal medulla is to secrete catecholamines. These are substances with diverse effects on intermediary metabolism, contractility of cardiac and smooth muscle, and neurotransmission. To accomplish these effects, the catecholamines reach target cells by two different routes: (a) epinephrine is secreted by the adrenal medulla into the circulation to perfuse peripheral tissues and (b) norepinephrine is released by nerve endings of the sympathetic nervous system to act on neighboring cells. Strictly speaking, only case (a) fulfills the criteria for a hormone; however, from an operational point of view, it is helpful to discuss metabolic responses to catecholamines regardless of their origin. The following discussion will consider the biosynthesis, metabolic actions, and degradation of the catecholamines.

Biosynthesis

The primary precursor in the biosynthesis of the catecholamines is phenylalanine. Successive hydroxylations, decarboxylation, and methylation yield norepinephrine and epinephrine as follows:

phenylalanine → tyrosine → diphenylalanine (Dopa) → dopamine → norepinephrine → epinephrine

Epinephrine is the principal circulating catecholamine elaborated by the adrenal medullary cells, but they also secrete small quantities of norepinephrine. Norepinephrine is the principal neurotransmitter of the sympathetic nervous system and probably of the central nervous system as well.

Mechanism of Action

The concept of alpha- and beta-adrenergic receptors is basic to an understanding of the mechanism of action of epinephrine and norepinephrine. As mentioned in the introduction to this chapter, the response to a hormone begins when it combines with a specific receptor in either the cell membrane or the cytosol. No example of this phenomenon has been studied more thoroughly than the interaction of catecholamines with their receptor sites.

The characterization of adrenergic receptors as alpha and beta originated with pharmacologic studies designed to measure the relative potencies of epinephrine, norepinephrine, and synthetic catecholamines such as isoproterenol on selected responses, including myocardial and smooth muscle contractility. Isoproterenol possessed the greatest potential for stimulating the myocardium, and norepinephrine the least; contrariwise, norepinephrine was the most effective vasoconstrictor, and isoproterenol the least effective. It was postulated that the stimulatory effect of these agents on myocardial contractility was mediated by alpha sites. The significance of this hypothesis was strengthened following the discovery of phentolamine, an agent that blocks alpha-site activity, and propranolol, a beta-site blocker. Extensive studies with these and similar drugs demonstrated that epinephrine and norepinephrine are agonists for both alpha and beta sites, while isoproterenol is essentially a beta agonist. The effect of epinephrine on adipose tissue and pancreatic islet cells, two tissues of fundamental metabolic importance, will illustrate the concept of adrenergic receptor sites.

Epinephrine has long been known to stimulate lipolysis via the adenylate cyclase-cyclic AMP system. Recent studies with isolated human fat cells which were incubated with epinephrine alone, or epinephrine with phentolamine or propranolol, indicate that both alpha- and beta-adrenergic sites are present on the adipocyte and that they mediate divergent effects on lipolysis. Epinephrine alone stimulates lipolysis and causes an increase in cyclic AMP, effects that are greatly enhanced if phentolamine is also present. Contrariwise, the addition of propranolol to epinephrine causes a sharp fall in both intracellular cyclic AMP and lipolysis. Thus, stimulation of beta sites increases the lipolytic response, while the activation of alpha sites has the opposite effect. The beta effect predominates, since epinephrine alone causes an increase in lipolysis.

Similar in-vitro studies have been performed with isolated pancreatic islets of the rat. Epinephrine alone sharply decreases insulin release by the islets, and a further reduction occurs when the cells are exposed to both epinephrine and propranolol. Conversely, the addition of phentolamine to epinephrine causes a marked increase in insulin release. Thus, islet cells appear to have both alpha and beta sites which mediate divergent effects on insulin release. In contrast to adipose tissue, the alpha effect predominates, since epinephrine alone decreases insulin release.

The major actions of the catecholamines include:
- Inotropic and chronotropic actions on the myocardium
- Blood vessel constriction and dilatation
- Bronchodilatation and constriction
- Contraction and relaxation of smooth muscle of gut and uterus
- Neurotransmission in the central nervous system
- Metabolic effects including those on lipolysis, insulin secretion, and hepatic glycogenolysis

The major metabolic effects of epinephrine result from its action on four major tissues: adipose tissue, pancreas, liver, and muscle. Catecholamine interactions with the first two have already been mentioned. In the liver, epinephrine stimulates adenylate cyclase, and the resultant increase in cyclic AMP promotes glycogenolysis and an increase in gluconeogenesis. It has not been firmly established that adrenergic receptor sites are involved in the initiation of these effects. In muscle, epinephrine stimulates glycogenolysis by beta-site activation. Unlike liver, muscle does not have a phosphatase capable of dephosphorylating glucose-6-phosphate. Hence, the products of glycogenolysis are either CO_2 and water or, in the presence of hypoxemia, lactate.

The principal metabolic effects of epinephrine in the intact organism are hyperglycemia and an increase in free fatty acids in the plasma. Hyperglycemia results from the release of glucose by the liver, the suppression of insulin release, and the stimulation of muscle glycogenolysis resulting in a release of lactic acid into the circulation. The latter serves as substrate for gluconeogenesis by the liver. Lipolysis is increased by direct stimulation of adipose tissue by epinephrine and also by the decline in plasma insulin. Thus, the responses of these four tissues to epinephrine are complementary in that each promotes an increase in the available supply of circulating free fatty acids and glucose. The increased levels of these two metabolic fuels ensure that the nervous system and muscle will have ample substrate during physiologic stress. The catecholamines have thus been characterized as the hormones of "flight or fight," since they are discharged most conspicuously at times of great threat to the animal's survival. Similarly, the cardiovascular and smooth muscle responses to catecholamines assist the organism in meeting such a threat successfully. It is likely that the changes that occur during stress are but exaggerations of responses that take place continuously as the sympathetic nervous system and adrenal medulla act to modulate the flow of nutrients to and from the liver, adipose tissue, and muscle.

Degradation of the Catecholamines

The two principal pathways for the biochemical disposal of epinephrine and norepinephrine involve methylation and oxidation:

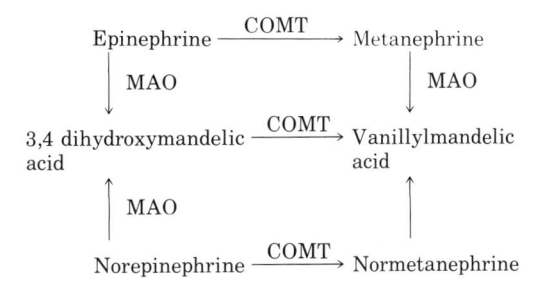

$$\begin{array}{ccc}
\text{Epinephrine} & \xrightarrow{\text{COMT}} & \text{Metanephrine} \\
\downarrow \text{MAO} & & \downarrow \text{MAO} \\
\text{3,4 dihydroxymandelic acid} & \xrightarrow{\text{COMT}} & \text{Vanillylmandelic acid} \\
\uparrow \text{MAO} & & \uparrow \\
\text{Norepinephrine} & \xrightarrow{\text{COMT}} & \text{Normetanephrine}
\end{array}$$

COMT (catechol-O-methyltransferase) is widely distributed throughout the body and acts rapidly to inactivate circulating catecholamines. MAO (monoamine oxidase) catalyzes the oxidative deamination of the catecholamines; it is located within nerve endings and acts to prevent excessive storage of norepinephrine.

CLINICAL ENTITIES

Loss of adrenal medullary function appears to cause little or no disability. Thus, patients who have undergone bilateral adrenalectomy respond satisfactorily to treatment with only adrenal cortical hormones. Such a procedure, of course, leaves the sympathetic nervous system intact. However, its function has been reduced both surgically and pharmacologically in the treatment of hypertension. Although patients who undergo such treatment are subject to orthostatic hypotension, impaired metabolism among such patients has not been reported.

Pheochromocytoma

Pheochromocytomas (from the Greek, meaning "darkly staining cells") are tumors arising from chromaffin cells that secrete excessive amounts of epinephrine or both epinephrine and norepinephrine. Although usually located in the adrenal medulla, they may develop anywhere in the body where rests of chromaffin cells are found. The preeminent manifestation of pheochromocytoma is hypertension. In a series of 507 cases reviewed by Hermann and Mornex, 26 per cent of patients had paroxysmal hypertension, 61 per cent showed sustained hypertension, and 4 per cent were found to be hypertensive during pregnancy. In 9 per cent of cases, hypertension was not present. Among all patients with hypertension, however, pheochromocytoma is exceedingly rare, probably less than 0.1 per cent. Nevertheless, in most cases pheochromocytomas are benign and accessible to the surgeon and are an important cause of curable hypertension.

Most of the manifestations of pheochromocytoma can be anticipated from the known actions of epinephrine and norepinephrine. Often, they occur in paroxysmal fashion, as in the patient who has had normal or moderately elevated blood pressure but who suddenly becomes severely hypertensive, blanches, and complains of headache, chest pain, and palpitation. The metabolic effects of excessive circulating catecholamines, hyperglycemia and an increase in free fatty acids, can usually be demonstrated. In most patients, however, the presentation of pheochromocytoma is less dramatic, consisting of sustained hypertension and nonspecific symptoms such as weakness, tremor, palpitation, and anxiety. In either event, a firm diagnosis can be established only by appropriate laboratory testing.

In the past, reliance was placed on pharmacologic tests. For example, the prompt attenuation of severe hypertension by the administration of the alpha blocker phentolamine was highly suggestive of pheochromocytoma. The usefulness of phentolamine has now shifted from the sphere of diagnosis to that of therapy. Diagnosis is currently dependent on the demonstration of abnormally high concentrations of epinephrine, norepinephrine, or their metabolites in the urine. The upper limits of normal for the daily excretion of these substances in the adult are as follows:

epinephrine, 20 μg.
norepinephrine, 80 μg.
metanephrines, 1.3 mg.
vanillylmandelic acid (VMA), 6.5 mg.

However, to be meaningful, these tests must be performed by a competent laboratory on specimens which are not contaminated with interfering drugs or dietary constituents. If the patient has paroxysmal hypertension, urine must be collected during such an episode and the amount of catecholamine present expressed per gram of urinary creatinine.

PANCREAS

PHYSIOLOGY

The principal function of the endocrine pancreas is the secretion of insulin, a hormone necessary for the orderly intracellular storage and retrieval of dietary nutrients such as glucose, amino acids, and triglyceride. It is not difficult to perceive the survival value of insulin. With food supply erratic, the animal capable of storing nutrient fuel during times of plenty had a great advantage over the species that could not. Furthermore, since muscle and adipose tissue require insulin for glucose transport while nervous tissue does not, the insulin regulatory mechanism is necessary for the adequate development and function of the central nervous system, which is dependent on glucose for survival. Without insulin, glucose would flow into muscle and adipose tissue cells in an unregulated fashion resulting in recurrent hypoglycemia.

Biosynthesis and Release of Insulin

Insulin is elaborated by the beta cells of the islets of Langerhans. These cells of endodermal origin occur in clusters throughout the pancreas. It has been estimated that the human pancreas contains about 1.5 million islets with a total weight of about 1 gram. Approximately 75 per cent of the cells of human islets are beta cells. The remainder are either alpha cells, which elaborate glucagon, or delta cells, which secrete gastrin. The average adult pancreas contains approximately 200 units of insulin (equivalent to 8 mg.); the average daily secretion of insulin is estimated at between 35 and 50 units. Insulin has a molecular weight of 6000 and is composed of two chains; the A chain has 21 amino acids, the B chain has 30. Recently, Steiner and coworkers demonstrated that insulin is derived from a larger molecule, termed proinsulin. Proinsulin contains a connecting peptide, the C chain, composed of 33 amino acids which join the N terminus of chain A to the carboxyl terminus of the B chain. Proinsulin is not biologically active and normally little of it is secreted; the C peptide is cleaved off by trypsin-like enzymes as part of the biosynthetic process. The full significance of proinsulin in both health and disease is currently under active investigation.

Although numerous physiologic events may alter insulin secretion, the most important regulatory factor is the concentration of glucose in the plasma perfusing the pancreas. When blood glucose levels exceed approximately 100 mg. per 100 ml., insulin release is stimulated; as glucose falls, so does the rate of insulin secretion. However, even during prolonged fasting when the plasma level of glucose remains low, a continuing basal secretion of insulin can be demonstrated. Certain amino acids such as leucine and arginine, given in pharmacologic amounts, can also stimulate insulin release, as can the intestinal hormones gastrin, secretin, pancreozymin, and glucagon-like peptide. Release of these intestinal hormones during digestion appears to intensify the pancreatic insulin response to glucose and amino acids. Insulin secretion is also influenced by catecholamines interacting with islet cell adrenergic receptor sites. Stimulation of alpha-adrenergic sites decreases insulin secretion, whereas stimulation of beta sites increases it. Epinephrine interacts with both sites, but apparently the alpha effect is dominant, since epinephrine causes a sharp decrease in insulin release.

Depending on the method of analysis, the fasting level of insulin ranges from 10 to 20 μU. per ml. and increases to 50 to 150 μU. per ml. following a meal or a glucose load. Its biological half-life is less than 10 minutes, being rapidly cleared from the circulation by the liver and kidneys. It should be appreciated, however, that the peak effect of intravenously administered insulin occurs between 30 and 60 minutes after infusion.

Action of Insulin

The primary mechanism by which insulin exerts its metabolic effects is not known despite a vast international effort aimed at answering this question. A great deal is known about *what* insulin does, but relatively little is known regarding *how* it does it.

The action of insulin on three metabolically important tissues—adipose tissue, muscle, and liver—is summarized below. These actions are illustrated more graphically in subsequent paragraphs in which the consequences of insulin deficiency are discussed.

Adipose Tissue. Insulin stimulates the transport of glucose into the fat cell or adipocyte and probably the initial phosphorylation of glucose to glucose-6-phosphate. The ensuing metabolism of glucose-6-phosphate to acetyl-CoA affects fat metabolism in several ways:

1. Metabolism of glucose via the hexose monophosphate shunt generates TPNH, the coenzyme required for fatty acid synthesis.
2. Metabolism of glucose via the Embden-Meyerhof pathway generates α-glycerol phosphate which is necessary for the esterification of fatty acids to form triglyceride. Unphosphorylated glycerol is not reactive. Since adipose tissue does not contain a glycerol kinase, glycerol derived from hydrolysis of triglyceride cannot be used in re-esterification.
3. The metabolism of glucose provides two carbon fragments for fatty acid synthesis.

Unrelated to its effect on glucose metabolism, insulin has two additional effects on fat metabolism:

1. Regulation of the disposal of triglyceride in the peripheral tissues.
2. Regulation of lipolysis.

Circulating triglyceride does not enter the fat cell as such; it is hydrolyzed by a lipoprotein lipase present between the basement membrane of the capillary and the plasma membrane of the adipocyte. This enzyme, necessary for the clearing of exogenous and endogenous triglyceride particles from the plasma, is insulin dependent. The regulation of fat mobilization or lipolysis is incompletely understood. Lipolysis is stimulated by norepinephrine released by sympathetic nerve endings, which acts via the adenylate cyclase-cyclic AMP system to activate the hormone-sensitive lipase which hydrolyzes triglyceride. Lipolysis is also stimulated by a fall in plasma insulin concentration and is inhibited by an increased concentration of insulin. The mechanism of action of insulin in altering lipolysis is not clear. It is tempting to suggest that it acts by inhibiting adenylate cyclase, but this has not been established.

In summary, insulin affects adipose tissue metabolism by promoting transport of glucose into the cell, stimulating fatty acid synthesis, inhibiting lipolysis, and inducing the enzyme necessary for the disposal of plasma triglyceride.

Muscle. Insulin is necessary for the transport of glucose into muscle cells in the resting state. Once in the cell, glucose is oxidized either completely to CO_2 or, if oxygen is limited, to lactic acid. Lactic acid then diffuses into the circulation, from which it is extracted by the liver and used as a substrate for glucose formation. The movement of carbon from the liver to muscle in the form of glucose and its return as lactic acid is known as the Cori cycle. It should be emphasized that muscle metabolizes ketones and fatty acids in preference to glucose, and that fat is the principal fuel of muscle. In the process, both fatty acids and ketones are oxidized to CO_2 and water.

Muscle serves as the major reservoir of amino acids for the body. Insulin stimulates the transport of amino acids into muscle cells and their conversion into protein. Cortisol opposes this action. During fasting, the cortisol influence predominates, and glycogenic amino acids are released from muscle and circulate to the liver, where they serve as a substrate for gluconeogenesis.

Liver. Insulin is not necessary for the transport of glucose into the liver, since hepatic cells are freely permeable to it. However, insulin powerfully influences glucose metabolism within the cell. Insulin promotes the formation of glycogen and stimulates the disposal of glucose via glycolytic pathways. It suppresses those enzymes necessary for gluconeogenesis and glycogenolysis. Thus, insulin antagonizes the hepatic effects of cortisol, epinephrine, and glucagon. The overall effect of insulin is to increase glucose utilization by the liver. During fasting, plasma insulin concentration falls, the influence of the gluconeogenic hormone cortisol predominates, and the liver releases the glucose required for metabolism by the central nervous system.

During fasting, or with insulin deficiency, the release of fatty acids from adipose tissue is greatly increased. The liver disposes of fatty acids through several pathways. Some are completely oxidized to CO_2 and water. The majority are oxidized to two carbon fragments, which are directed into new glyceride synthesis or into ketogenesis. The basic ketone body, acetoacetic acid, is formed by the condensation of two acetyl-CoA moieties. Beta-hydroxybutyric acid and acetone are metabolites of acetoacetic acid. The survival advantage of ketogenesis is not clear. Ketones are readily used as metabolic fuel by muscle, but so are fatty acids. Two important differences between the liver, on one hand, and muscle and adipose tissue, on the other, deserve emphasis. Insulin is not required for glucose transport into the liver, and hepatic cells have a phosphatase capable of cleaving glucose-6-phosphate to produce free glucose, which readily diffuses into the plasma.

CLINICAL ENTITIES

Diabetes Mellitus

A relative or absolute deficiency of insulin results in the disease, diabetes mellitus. (The term diabetes, from the Greek, meaning "a siphon," denotes excessive urine formation; mellitus is derived from the Greek word mel, meaning honey). Diabetes mellitus is by far the most important disorder of the endocrine system, afflicting several million people in the United States alone. The term covers a wide spectrum of disability from the elderly asymptomatic individual with mild glucose intolerance to the youthful patient dependent on exogenous insulin. The pathophysiology of the disease is more clearly illustrated by the insulin-dependent diabetic and, unless otherwise specified, it is this variety of the illness that will be referred to in the following discussion. The manifestations of diabetes mellitus are divisible into two groups: (1) the acute diabetic syndrome characterized by hyperglycemia, ketoacidosis, and, if untreated, death; and (2) the chronic diabetic syndrome characterized by diffuse microangiopathy involving vital tissues and organs such as the kidney, retina, and nervous system.

At the present time, controversy exists as to whether insulin lack causes these vascular changes or whether they occur independently. One school of thought, for example, contends that thickening of the capillary basement membrane is responsible for both the acute manifestations and the chronic complications of diabetes mellitus. It is generally agreed that diabetes mellitus is a heritable disease. If this is so, one can formulate the conflicting views regarding its pathogenesis as follows:

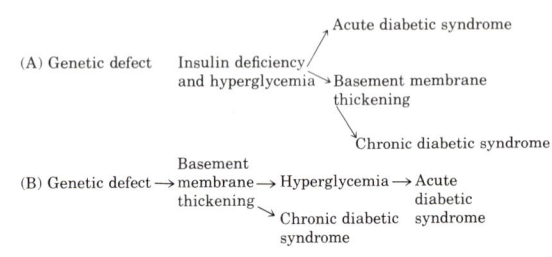

(A) Genetic defect → Insulin deficiency and hyperglycemia → Acute diabetic syndrome / Basement membrane thickening → Chronic diabetic syndrome

(B) Genetic defect → Basement membrane thickening → Hyperglycemia → Acute diabetic syndrome / Chronic diabetic syndrome

The question is of more than academic interest, because if hypothesis A is correct, intensive effort to minimize hyperglycemia would be justified to prevent late vascular complications, whereas if B is correct, the argument for rigid control of the blood glucose concentration would be considerably weakened.

If indeed diabetes mellitus arises from one or more genetically determined defects, one can consider that the disease begins at conception. From that point on, one can divide its natural history as illustrated in Figure 32-7.

The manifestations of diabetes mellitus are predictable from the known actions of insulin discussed earlier. Insulin deficiency results in hyperglycemia, the central biochemical feature of the disease. It is due to impaired transport of glucose into muscle and adipose tissue and to the

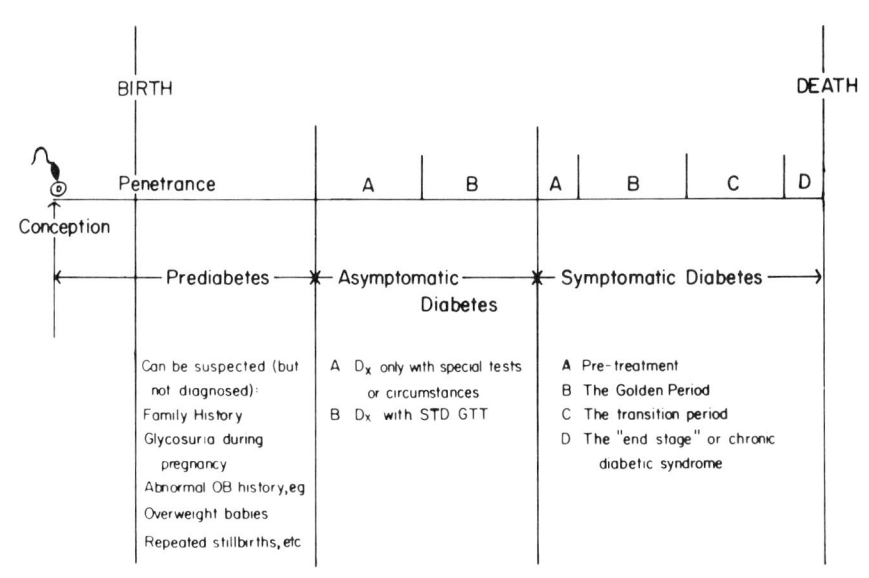

Figure 32-7 Natural history and sequelae of diabetes mellitus. Progression from one stage of the disease to another is unpredictable. Many individuals remain at the "prediabetic" or asymptomatic stage throughout life. The course of patients with symptomatic diabetes is also variable; with proper management they may remain free of significant complications throughout life. Whether or not attempts at very rigid control of the blood glucose level improves prognosis remains a controversial question (see text).

release of glucose by the liver. Above a blood level of about 160 mg. per 100 ml., the renal tubules are unable to absorb all the glucose filtered by the glomeruli. The renal excretion of glucose requires concomitant excretion of water and thus produces an osmotic diuresis. Loss of water causes an increase in the serum osmolality, which stimulates the thirst center in the hypothalamus. The three "polys" of diabetes mellitus (polyuria, polydipsia, and polyphagia) are thus explicable by the body's loss of large quantities of glucose and water with a compensatory increase in hunger and thirst.

Ketoacidosis. As a more severe insulin deficiency ensues, hyperglycemia and glycosuria intensify, and ketonemia develops owing to a marked increase in lipolysis and in serum fatty acids. Both acetoacetic acid and beta-hydroxybutyric acid dissociate to yield hydrogen ions, depressing the plasma pH. At a pH level of 7.2, the respiratory center is stimulated and the patient's breathing becomes deep and rapid (Kussmaul respirations). This hyperventilation is a defensive effort to prevent a further decline in plasma pH. It will be recalled from the Henderson-Hasselbalch equation that pH is determined by the ratio of plasma bicarbonate to carbonic acid $\frac{HCO_3^-}{H_2CO_3}$, which normally is about 20 to 1. With loss of bicarbonate (utilized to buffer hydrogen ions derived from ketone bodies), this ratio decreases, as does the pH. The increased loss of CO_2 from the lungs reduces plasma carbonic acid and tends to restore the ratio to normal. A further decline in the pH is associated with increasing depression of cerebral function, eventually culminating in coma and death. The major components in the pathogenesis of ketoacidosis are depicted schematically in Figure 32-8. At several points the consequences of ketonemia and hyperglycemia act synergistically with one another to accelerate the course of events. For example, the cations sodium and potassium are lost into the urine secondary to the osmotic diuresis and in association with the acidic ions acetoacetate and beta-hydroxybutyrate. Hyperosmolality, dehydration, hypotension, and acidosis abet one another in causing deterioration of cerebral function.

Insulin deficiency prompts protein catabolism which results in the release of nitrogen and potassium into the circulation. Late in the course of ketoacidosis, when dehydration and hypovolemia have occurred, renal perfusion falters, with a consequent increase in plasma sodium and potassium concentrations in spite of the total body deficiency of these substances. It is not uncommon to see hyperkalemia, followed by hypokalemia during the initial hours of therapy for diabetic ketoacidosis. With the administration of insulin, potassium re-enters cells along with glucose. Fluid therapy causes expansion of plasma volume and a return of normal renal function. In the past, patients often did well initially only to

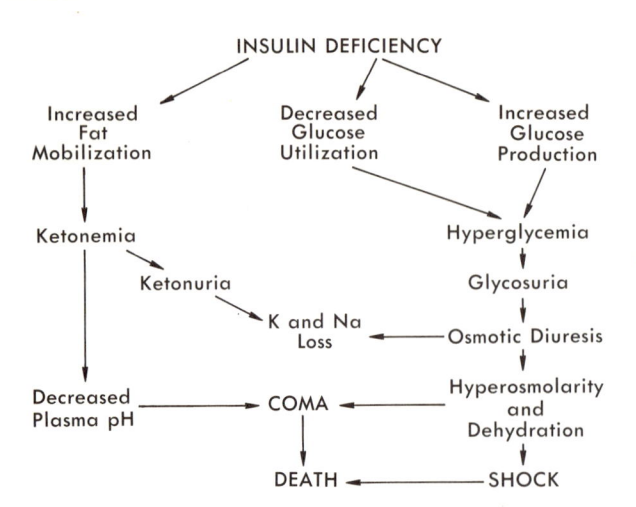

Figure 32-8 The pathogenesis of diabetic ketoacidosis (see text).

develop profound muscle weakness and cardiac dysfunction without apparent cause. With the advent of frequent monitoring of plasma electrolytes, hypokalemia was soon identified as the cause of these complications. They are now readily prevented by the judicious administration of potassium.

Although initially ketonemia is the only cause of acidosis, the subsequent occurrence of hypotension and tissue hypoxia leads to lactate accumulation and a further lowering of the plasma pH. Lactate accumulation sufficient to produce acidosis can also occur in nondiabetic patients severely ill from a variety of causes in which tissue hypoxia is found.

Hyperosmolar Nonketotic Coma. In recent years a variant of hyperglycemic diabetic coma has been recognized. In this syndrome, descriptively named hyperosmolar nonketotic coma, hyperglycemia is usually extreme, between 900 mg. and 3000 mg. per 100 ml., while ketonemia is mild or undetectable, and acidosis is absent. It usually affects patients with mild diabetes not requiring insulin. Characteristically, the diabetic state worsens insidiously, often from the stress of unrelated illness or trauma. Initially the increasing fluid loss due to glycosuria can be balanced by an increase in the patient's fluid intake. Ultimately, however, this intake becomes insufficient, and progressive dehydration develops. The large loss of water in the urine continues but is no longer matched by a commensurate oral intake of water. Because the loss of water exceeds that of glucose, the serum rapidly becomes hyperosmolar. Associated with this rise in serum osmolality, and probably because of it, the patient becomes increasingly obtunded and unable to respond to his thirst. Thus, a vicious cycle ensues which rapidly leads to coma and, if not treated, to death.

The puzzling feature of the syndrome is that the affected diabetic patients are severely hyperglycemic but not acidotic. Available evidence suggests that this apparent paradox may be due to the relative potency of insulin in promoting glucose transport, on one hand, and inhibiting fat mobilization, on the other. Thus, patients with hyperosmolar nonketotic coma seem to have sufficient circulating insulin to retard the massive release of fatty acids that occurs in ketoacidosis but not enough insulin to stimulate the entry of glucose into peripheral tissues. This view is supported by data such as those reported by Gerich et al. and summarized in Table 32-10.

Hyperlipidemia. Although ketoacidosis and hyperosmolar nonketotic coma are the most dramatic life-threatening manifestations of acute insulin deficiency, others deserve mention. Infrequently, the uncontrolled diabetic will present with evidence of hyperlipidemia as the major manifestation of his disease. On physical examination there may be a widespread skin eruption of recent origin. These lesions, which are yellow-orange in color, papular, and about 2 to 4 mm. in diameter, are eruptive xanthomas. On funduscopic examination, the color of the venules is startling; instead of being deep red, they are white, gray, or light pink. This finding, lipemia retinalis, is directly related to the character of the patient's blood, which is pink or rose when aspirated by venipuncture. After clotting, the appearance of the supernatant serum is indistinguishable from cream. Chemical analysis reveals a marked increase in triglycerides to several thousand mg. per 100 ml. Analysis by paper electrophoresis or ultracentrifugation reveals that the increased triglyceride consists mostly of dietary chylomicrons, although endogenous triglycerides are usually present as well. This impaired

TABLE 32–10 HORMONAL AND METABOLIC DIFFERENCES BETWEEN DIABETIC KETOACIDOSIS AND HYPEROSMOLAR NONKETOTIC COMA

	Hyperosmolar Nonketotic Coma (9 Patients)	Diabetic Ketoacidosis (6 Patients)
Blood Sugar (mg./100 ml.)	1058	798
CO_2 (mEq./L.)	22	9.6
Osmolarity (mOsm./L.)	368	327
Free Fatty Acids (mEq./L.)	880	2053
Immunoreactive Insulin (μU./ml.)	0 to 15	0 to 15
Growth Hormone (ng./ml.)	2	12
Cortisol (μg./100 ml.)	21	40

Data adapted from Gerich, J. E., Martin, M. M., and Recant, L.: Diabetes, *19*:354, 1970.

TABLE 32–11 PRINCIPAL CAUSES OF HYPOGLYCEMIA

Underlying Condition	Mechanism
I. FASTING	
A. Addison's disease, panhypopituitarism	Impaired gluconeogenesis
B. Liver disease	Impaired gluconeogenesis, glycogen storage
C. Fasting + Alcohol	Impaired gluconeogenesis, depleted glycogen
D. Mesothelial tumors	Unknown
E. Insulin-dependent diabetes	Excessive insulin, iatrogenic
F. Islet cell adenoma	Excessive, unregulated insulin release
II. FED (Reactive)	
G. Postgastrectomy	Tachyalimentation of glucose
H. Functional	Tachyalimentation of glucose
I. Early ("chemical") diabetes	Abnormal "glucostat" ($\uparrow$ insulin secretion)

disposal of triglyceride results from relative inactivity of the insulin-dependent lipoprotein lipase, described earlier. Treatment with insulin promptly increases the activity of this enzyme; the plasma triglyceride level falls to normal in a short time, and the skin and retinal changes disappear. It is curious that hyperlipidemia occurs uncommonly in untreated diabetics. Other factors in addition to insulin must be important in influencing the activity of the lipoprotein lipase of the peripheral tissues.

Hypoglycemia

The common causes of hypoglycemia are listed in Table 32–11. The time of day at which hypoglycemia occurs provides a clue to the underlying cause. Since hepatic production of glucose sustains the blood level during periods of fast, impaired glycogen storage and gluconeogenesis will lead to fasting hypoglycemia, which typically occurs in the early morning after 8 or 9 hours of fasting. This pattern also is seen with hypoglycemia due to insulin-secreting islet cell adenomas; hypoglycemia, minimized during the waking hours by constant eating, becomes apparent during the hours of sleep.

In contrast to these "fasting" hypoglycemias are those that are reactive, that is, triggered by the assimilation of glucose following a meal. Normally, the secretion of insulin is approximately commensurate with the degree of hyperglycemia. However, following gastrectomy and, occasionally in the absence of surgery, glucose is very rapidly assimilated into the circulation. The resulting excessive hyperglycemia stimulates a brisk release of insulin which causes hypoglycemia as assimilation from the gastrointestinal tract wanes. The situation in the prediabetic is somewhat different. In this case, glucose is assimilated at a normal rate, but the insulin secretory response is delayed, as if the sensing mechanism or "glucostat" were not functioning; when the response does occur it is excessive, causing hypoglycemia 3 to 5 hours after a meal.

The most frequent cause of clinically significant hypoglycemia is insulin self-administration by the diabetic patient. This may be the result of an improper insulin regimen or, as very often happens, dietary omission or excessive physical activity. Overnight hypoglycemia secondary to insulin overdose is frequently not recognized because the patient is asleep and therefore unaware of the early subjective symptoms of mild hypoglycemia. Furthermore, hypoglycemia occurring at 2 A.M., for example, stimulates increases in the hormones that counter hypoglycemia—epinephrine, cortisol, and possibly growth hormone. These hormones cause the blood glucose to rise at an accelerated rate when the level of plasma insulin falls, and consequently the patient finds glucose in his urine prior to breakfast. This overshoot or rebound in glucose concentration that follows hypoglycemia, first emphasized by Somogyi, has great clinical significance; it is often misinterpreted as evidence of insufficient insulin rather than too much insulin. Thus, the dosage of insulin is increased, the overnight hypoglycemia is more marked, and the rebound in blood glucose greater. The latter finding, of course, tends to perpetuate the mistake.

Regardless of its underlying cause, the manifestations of hypoglycemia tend to evolve in a characteristic pattern. With mild hypoglycemia, the patient experiences hunger, tremor, perspiration, weakness, blurred vision, and impaired mentation. Mental confusion is often followed by bizarre behavior. The patient may become bellicose and resistant to help. Neuromuscular function becomes impaired. Staggering gait and irrational hostile behavior are frequently misinterpreted as drunkenness. Finally, the patient becomes comatose. If the hypoglycemia is profound, epileptoid seizures occur; if severe hypoglycemia remains untreated, permanent brain damage or death results. The sequence of events just described is typical, but the exact pattern varies among patients and even in the same patient from one episode to another. For example, on one occasion the patient may wander about in a confused state for 2 to 3 hours at approximately the same level of function; another time, he might pass from an alert and rational state to coma in a half hour or less.

The correct diagnosis of coma in the diabetic patient is critical, since the two commonest causes—too much or too little insulin—require diametrically opposite therapy. The major features that distinguished the two disorders, listed in Table 32-12, are explicable in terms of the pathophysiologic consequences of insulin deficiency and excess described previously.

TESTES

PHYSIOLOGY

The dual role of the testes in procreation and maintenance of male attributes has been appreciated from antiquity. Throughout history, castration has been practiced in many societies, usually with the goal of rendering the victim devoid of both the desire and capability of sexual activity. Thus, in contrast to pituitary, thyroid, or adrenal deficiencies which occurred as the result of various diseases, one form of male gonadal deficiency, eunuchism, was deliberately induced. If the history of the involvement of the testes in reproduction is an old one, it is far from complete. In the following paragraphs, the current status of our knowledge of testicular physiology will be briefly reviewed.

In 1949, Barr and Bertram described a darkly staining chromatin material located at or very near the inner side of the nuclear membrane of neural tissue from female cats. This clump was conspicuously absent in tissue from males. In the ensuing years, comparable findings were obtained with human tissues. Properly stained material obtained from the buccal mucosa of the female was found to contain nuclear sex chromatin in 50 to 60 per cent of cells examined. Cells derived from males contained nuclear sex chromatin, presumably artefactual, in 1 to 2 per cent

TABLE 32-12 DIFFERENTIAL DIAGNOSIS OF COMA DUE TO DIABETIC KETOACIDOSIS AND HYPOGLYCEMIA

	Acidosis	*Hypoglycemia*
Onset	Hour to days	Minutes
Background events	Intercurrent disease, omission of insulin	Exercise, omission of meal
Symptoms	Thirst, polyuria, headaches, nausea, vomiting, abdominal pain	Hunger, headache, perspiration, *confusion*, stupor
Physical findings	Kussmaul respirations, dehydration, flushed face, fast pulse: *appears ill*	Normal pulse, respirations: appears well
Typical laboratory findings		
Urine		
Glucose	5%	0 to 5%
Ketones	Strongly positive	0 to positive
Serum		
Glucose	400 mg./100 ml. or more	Less than 40 mg./100 ml.
Ketones	Positive, 1:8	Negative
HCO_3	Less than 10 mEq./L.	26 mEq./L.
Response to 50% glucose, I.V.	None	Dramatic

of cells counted. Davidson and Smith (1954), studying smears of human blood cells, found several clumps of chromatin lying beyond the main mass of nuclear material of the polymorphonuclear leukocytes of females but not of males. The ovoid clump was attached to the nucleus by a fine strand, producing a characteristic "drumstick" form. It is now generally accepted that the female nuclear sex chromatin of buccal mucosal cells (the "Barr" body) and the "drumstick" of the polymorphonuclear leukocyte represent the same phenomenon, presumably an (inactivated) X sex chromosome or gonosome.

Normal Human Sex Determination

Using the technique of tissue culture coupled with mitotic arrest, Tjio and Levan in 1956 were able to correct a long-standing misconception about the actual number of human chromosomes in somatic cells. Their work, which was soon amply confirmed, indicated that each somatic cell (i.e., all cells other than germ cells) normally contains 46 chromosomes, 22 pairs of autosomes and two sex chromosomes. This number is double (or diploid) the basic complement (termed the haploid number) contained in mature germ cells. In the normal female, the sex chromosomes are both X; in the normal male, there is one X and one Y chromosome. When the cell divides in the process of mitosis, these 23 pairs are replicated, producing two sets of 23 pairs. The germ cell or gamete, however, must contain the basic complement or haploid number of chromosomes to match an equal haploid number of the gamete of the opposite sex at time of fertilization (see Chapter 3). This reduction in the number of chromosomes occurs during the first maturation division. In the testes, the primary spermatocyte with 44 autosomes, plus X and Y sex chromosomes, divides to form two secondary spermatocytes, each containing 22 autosomes and either a Y or an X chromosome. This process of reduction division is termed meiosis. The comparable reduction division in the ovary occurs when a primary oocyte divides to produce a daughter cell, the secondary oocyte, containing 22 autosomes plus one X sex chromosome and a functionless polar body. In meiosis, homologous chromosomes line up in pairs. Before the cell actually divides, members of each pair separate and each complement moves away, one from the other, migrating toward the new central locus of the cell to be. This separation and migration of equal complements of chromosomes is termed disjunction. Disjunction thus is the basic process responsible for the haploid number of chromosomes of the mature gamete, be it spermatozoon or ovum. The ovum contains 22 autosomes plus one X chromosome; the spermatozoon contains 22 autosomes and either an X or a Y chromosome. At the time of conception, the union of ovum with spermatozoon produces a fertilized ovum with the diploid number of chromosomes, i.e., 44 autosomes (22 pairs) with either two X chromosomes or one X and one Y chromosome. A male develops in the latter instance (44 + XY), and a female in the former (44 + XX). Thus, the sex of the fetus is determined by the chromosomal constitution of the spermatozoon; if it carries an X sex chromosome, a female results (44 + XX); if it contains a Y chromosome, the issue is male (44 + XY). The role of the female at this point is notably passive.

Embryogenesis of the Gonads and Genitalia

The embryogenesis of reproductive structures involves the following four sets of primordia: the gonads, the genital ducts, and the urogenital sinus and groove. These give rise, respectively, to the mature gonad, the internal genitalia, and the external genitalia. Regardless of the genetic sex, there are both male and female anlagen in the primordial gonad and genital ducts. The urogenital groove and sinus on the other hand are bipotential. The gonads of the male become differentiated by the seventh week and those of the female by the tenth week. In the former instance, a substance elaborated by the testes causes development of the male genital duct (the mesonephros, or wolffian duct) and regression of the female one (müllerian duct). In the absence of the testes, the müllerian duct develops, and the other structures regress. Similarly, the bipotential urogenital sinus and groove respond to the presence of the testes by differentiating into the male external genitalia, and in the absence of testes, into female genitalia. The inductor substance of the testes responsible for the development of the mesonephros appears to act locally, since the ipsilateral testis must be present for both development of the mesonephros and regression of the müllerian duct. It is probably not an androgen, since administration of androgen to an experimental animal whose gonads have been removed results in the development of the mesonephros but no evidence of müllerian duct regression. This substance may be the factor which, through its effect on the central nervous system, is responsible for the development of male behavior during adolescence (see earlier discussion). The secretory activity of the testes in utero is probably stimulated by the high levels of placental chorionic gonadotropin. Not surprisingly, the fetal testis resembles the adult gonad histologically.

Postnatal Testicular Function

Following delivery, the testes become quiescent but probably not completely inactive. Recent careful studies indicate that there are measurable levels of both gonadotropins and androgens beginning in early childhood. The mechanisms that initiate pubescence are poorly understood. Presumably, the primary signal arises from the hypothalamus or higher sites in the central nervous system. In any event, at an average age of about 13 years LH plasma levels increase (FSH increases occur at an earlier age) and the testes enlarge, mainly owing to an increase in the volume of the seminiferous tubules. Leydig cell function is stimulated by LH, resulting in a marked increase in plasma testosterone. The latter is responsible for the development of male secondary sexual characteristics, including changes in external genitalia, body hair, voice, musculature, libido, and potentia. Eventually, this surge of androgens causes closure of the epiphyses of the long bones and growth ceases, but only after a pubescent growth spurt of 6 or more inches.

The Adult Testis; Biosynthesis, Transport, and Action of Testosterone

The adult testis is approximately 4.5 cm. by 2.5 cm. and weighs between 15 and 20 grams. It comprises two major elements: (a) Leydig or interstitial cells, which make up approximately 10 per cent of testicular volume, and (b) the seminiferous tubules, lined with the spermatogonia and Sertoli cells, composing about 75 per cent of the volume of the testes. Each day the Leydig cells elaborate approximately 7 mg. of testosterone and 2 mg. of its immediate precursor, androstenedione, and the seminiferous tubules release about 150,000,000 spermatozoa.

The biosynthesis of testosterone follows the same basic pathway as that of the adrenal cortical steroids. Either acetate or cholesterol can serve as the basic precursor; pregnenolone and 17-alpha-hydroxyprogesterone are important intermediaries. Once secreted, 95 per cent of testosterone circulates in the plasma bound to a specific beta globulin. The normal range of testosterone in young adults is 440 to 1000 ng. per 100 ml. of plasma. There is a progressive decline in plasma testosterone after middle age. In females, the normal range is from 34 to 100 ng. per 100 ml. In the peripheral tissues, testosterone is converted to dihydrotestosterone, the compound which is currently thought to be the active metabolite mediating androgenic function. The proposed mechanism of action of the sex steroids including testosterone has already been alluded to.

Regulation of Testicular Function

The evidence for a negative feedback relationship between the Leydig cells and the hypothalamic-pituitary axis is quite convincing (Fig. 32-9). In 1968, Masao et al. reported on the effects of a partially purified FSH-releasing factor prepared from beef hypothalami. Kastin et al. have now identified the hypothalamic substance capable of initiating LH release from the anterior pituitary; this factor has been termed the LH-releasing hormone (LRH). LH acts on the testes to increase the conversion rate of cholesterol to pregnenolone, the rate-limiting step in the formation of testosterone. Cyclic AMP appears to function as an intermediary or second messenger in this reaction. Above a critical concentration (the set point), plasma testosterone interferes with the release of LH. It is not clear whether this is accomplished by inhibition of LRH secretion or by a direct inhibitory effect of testosterone on the anterior pituitary. In either event, the decline in plasma LH results in a decrease in testosterone secretion, completing the negative feedback loop.

The relationship between the anterior pituitary and the seminiferous tubules is not so obvious. It appears certain that FSH is required for spermatogenesis. In the absence of FSH, the germinal epithelium desquamates and the seminiferous tubules become fibrotic. Contrariwise, in those circumstances in which there is primary injury to the germinal epithelium, there is an increase in FSH secretion (Paulsen, 1968). This occurs even when Leydig cell function (and hence testosterone production) remains normal, as, for example, in primary seminiferous tubular failure. Such observations certainly suggest that a substance capable of retarding FSH secretion is elaborated by the germinal epithelium. Indeed, a number of investigators have labeled this hypothetical material "inhibin." Unfortunately, attempts to prepare an extract from testicular tissue capable of suppressing FSH release have been unsuccessful.

CLINICAL ENTITIES

Klinefelter's Syndrome (Seminiferous Tubule Dysgenesis)

Klinefelter's syndrome is probably the most common cause of male infertility and hypogonadism. Although reports of this entity had been published earlier, Klinefelter, Reifenstein, and Albright in 1942 emphasized the features of the syndrome in a paper significantly entitled "A Syndrome Characterized by Gynecomastia, Aspermatogenesis without A-Leydigism and Increased Excretion of Follicle-Stimulating Hormone." This report described nine patients with small testes, gynecomastia, and increased FSH titers. The stature of the patients varied from normal to slightly eunuchoid, but all had good muscular development and masculine secondary sexual characteristics. The histologic alterations in the testes consisted of hyalinization of the

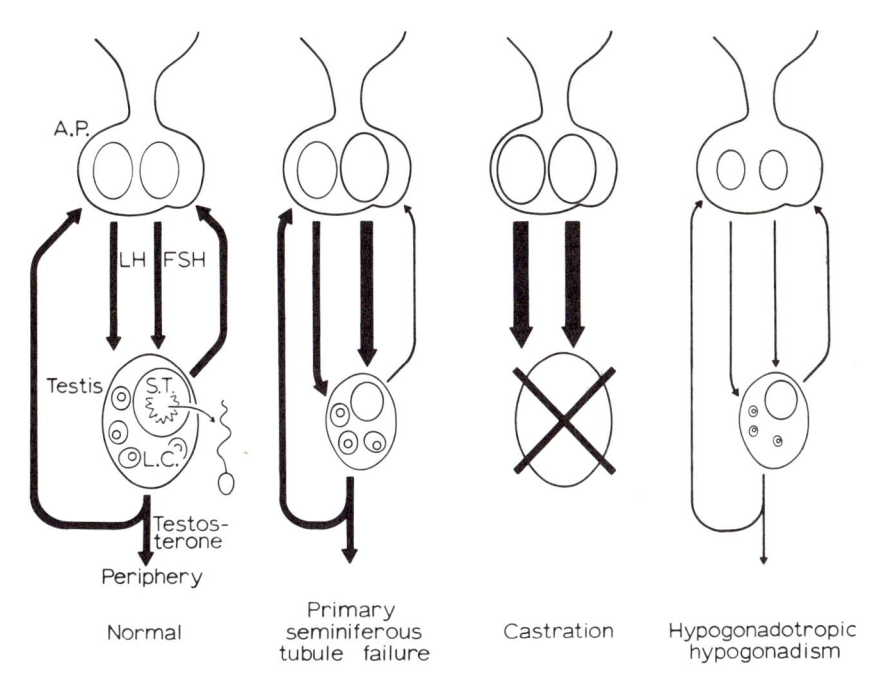

Figure 32-9 Anterior pituitary-testicular relationships.
Normal: The anterior pituitary (*A.P.*) secretes LH, which stimulates the Leydig cells (*L.C.*) to secrete testosterone. Rising levels of testosterone inhibit further LH secretion, completing the negative feedback loop. The anterior pituitary also secretes FSH, which stimulates the seminiferous tubules (*S.T.*) and spermatogenesis. The release of a humoral substance by cells of the seminiferous tubules (right hand arrow) is suspected but not established.
Primary seminiferous tubule failure: For unknown causes the seminiferous tubules undergo atrophy, and spermatogenesis ceases; urinary excretion of FSH is high. Leydig cell function remains intact.
Castration: When both Leydig cell and seminiferous tubular elements of the testes are lost, gonadotropin secretion is markedly increased.
Hypogonadotropic hypogonadism: Isolated loss of gonadotropin secretin by the pituitary in the pubescent male results in both sterility and underdeveloped male secondary sexual characteristics.

seminiferous tubules with loss of Sertoli cells and spermatogonia elements, while interstitial cells appeared normal. Subsequent experience with large numbers of patients has made it clear that impaired Leydig cell function, reflected by subnormal levels of circulating testosterone and underdeveloped secondary sexual characteristics, is a common feature of the syndrome.

The realization of the etiologic role of chromosomal abnormalities in the manifestations of Klinefelter's syndrome represents one of the most exciting events in the history of endocrinology. Plunkett and Barr reported chromatin-positive cells in patients with Klinefelter's syndrome. The disparity between the chromatin sex pattern ("female") and the physiognomy of the patients (male) was clarified when the chromosomal constitution of patients with classic Klinefelter's syndrome was identified as 44 + XXY. Thus, it now appears certain that the pathogenesis of Klinefelter's syndrome begins with an abnormal meiotic phase in one of the parents. The most common abnormality consists of failure of the sex chromosomes of the dividing cell to move away from one another and is termed nondisjunction. In the male parent, the gamete that results from nondisjunction has a chromosomal constitution of either 22 + XY or 22 + O; in the female, it is 22 + XX or 22 + O. The possible chromosomal constitutions of fertilized ova resulting from union of an abnormal with a normal gamete are summarized here.

	Father	*Mother*	*Offspring*
I. Nondisjunction in the father:	(a) 22 + O	22 + X	44 + XO
	(b) 22 + XY	22 + X	44 + XXY
II. Nondisjunction in the mother:	(c) 22 + X	22 + XX	44 + XXX
	(d) 22 + X	22 + O	44 + XO
	(e) 22 + Y	22 + XX	44 + XXY
	(f) 22 + Y	22 + O	44 + YO

Thus, Klinefelter's syndrome can arise from abnormal meiosis either in the father, as in (b) above, or in the mother, as in (e) above.

Although classic Klinefelter's syndrome is usually associated with a karyotype of 44 + XXY, a number of variants of the syndrome have been reported. For example, if there is mosaicism (or more than one stem line), of the sex chromosomes (e.g., XXY/XY), there may be few clinical abnormalities. On the other hand, when there is more than one abnormality of chromosomal division, as rarely occurs, there may be more than one supernumerary X chromosome, such as 44 + XXXY and 44 + XXXXY. In general, these patients have more profound disturbances of gonadal function. The spectrum of Klinefelter's syndrome from both the clinical and chromosomal standpoints has been reviewed by Paulsen et al. in 1968.

The "Fertile Eunuch" Syndrome

Patients have been reported with eunuchoid habitus but normal fertility and normal or near normal height. Histologic examination of testicular biopsy specimens has revealed normal seminiferous tubules but greatly reduced numbers of Leydig cells. The presumed pathogenesis of this uncommon condition—an isolated deficiency of pituitary LH, with normal FSH secretion—has recently been confirmed by radioimmunoassay determinations of plasma gonadotropins.

Hypogonadotropic Hypogonadism

As already stated, the gonadotropins, FSH and LH, are required to maintain normal testicular function in the male. When these hormones are deficient or absent, as frequently occurs in patients with pituitary tumors, both the germinal and Leydig cell elements of the testes become atrophic; spermatogenesis ceases, and the level of circulating testosterone falls dramatically. The consequences of the latter event emerge slowly; the patient's libido falters, and there is loss of muscle mass and eventually loss of facial and body hair. For a time, the testicular changes are reversible, as demonstrated by their response to the administration of replacement therapy such as human chorionic gonadotropin (HCG). However, after a period estimated at one to five years, the testes become unresponsive to hormonal stimulation.

If the gonadotropins are deficient at the time of pubescence, the changes characteristic of that period do not take place. The external genitalia remain infantile; body form, hair distribution, and voice remain feminine; and the epiphyses of the long bones remain open, permitting an increase in eventual height. The eunuchoid habitus which often occurs in this situation is characterized by excessive stature and span. Normally, the length of the lower segment of the body (measured from the top of the symphysis pubis to the floor) is about equal to that of the upper segment (measured from the top of the symphysis to the crown); in the eunuchoid patient, the lower segment length significantly exceeds the upper one.

An interesting familial variety of prepubertal hypogonadotropin deficiency has been described in which the affected patients have a greatly impaired or absent sense of smell (hyposmia or anosmia). Since the original report by Kallman et al., numerous case reports have appeared. In one careful study of seven patients, the urinary FSH and LH titers were very low but detectable. This finding suggests that the signal that normally triggers the pubertal increase in gonadotropins fails to occur in Kallman's syndrome. The significance of impaired sense of smell is obscure. Since olfaction is critical to the reproductive behavior of mammalian species, it is conceivable that both olfaction and the regulation of gonadotropin secretion could be influenced by a common site in the central nervous system.

The Syndrome of Feminizing Testes

This is a rare familial disorder in which the patient possesses male gonads but manifests a normal female physiognomy. The testes, usually located intra-abdominally or along the inguinal canals, are unremarkable histologically. The external genitalia are those of the female, and the internal genitalia are usually deficient. The pathophysiology of this puzzling disorder may involve an abnormality in the metabolism of testosterone. Recent reports indicate that in tissues especially responsive to androgens, such as the skin of the scrotum, testosterone is converted to dihydrotestosterone. It is believed that the latter substance is the active metabolite of testosterone, comparable to 1,25-dihydroxycholecalciferol in vitamin D metabolism (see earlier discussion). Wilson and Walker in 1969 studied the ability of tissue from patients with the feminizing testes syndrome to convert testosterone to dihydrotestosterone. Skin samples from the labia majora of three patients were relatively inadequate in promoting this critical conversion. Thus, this syndrome may be an inborn error of metabolism in which the enzymes(s) necessary to convert testosterone to its active metabolite is deficient.

OVARIES

PHYSIOLOGY

Menstrual Cycle: Follicle Development, Ovulation, Corpus Luteum Formation, Menstruation, and Pregnancy

The human ovaries are nodular bodies the morphology and function of which are dynamically interwoven. Each weighs about 4 grams and measures 4 cm. long by 2 cm. wide. The adult ovary is estimated to contain 400,000 primordial follicles: oocytes encased in an avascular envelope of granulosa cells. At the onset of each menstrual cycle, several follicles migrate from the periphery of the ovary toward its center; concomitantly, there is proliferation of both the granulosa cells to form a multilayer band and the cells of the theca, which develops as an outer vascular mantle. As these processes progress, indentation of each follicle occurs, producing a cavity or antrum. Although these early events apparently do not require gonadotropins, FSH is required for the subsequent development of the mature graafian follicle. Of the several follicles that have undergone the changes just described, only one continues to develop; the remaining follicles regress into atretic forms. Under FSH stimulation, the chosen follicle accumulates fluid in its antrum, the cells of the granulosa and theca proliferate, and the whole mass migrates to the periphery. The ripened follicle comes to lie just beneath the outer covering of the ovary, creating a detectable bulge in its surface. As the follicle matures, the theca differentiates into the vascular theca interna and a theca externa, made up of stroma-like cells. The theca interna is composed of large glandular cells which under FSH stimulation elaborate estrogen. Their secretory activity accelerates throughout the preovulatory stage, reaching a peak just before ovulation. There is evidence that the rising level of estrogen (estradiol) triggers the release of LH — a positive feedback phenomenon — and that the high concentration of plasma LH acts on the theca cells to effect the release of the ovum from the ripened follicle. Following the extrusion of the ovum, the graafian follicle is transformed into the corpus luteum under the continued influence of LH. This complex process of luteinization includes cellular hypertrophy of both the granulosa and theca interna and their development into tissues which are capable of steroid hormone synthesis. If pregnancy does not occur, the corpus luteum continues to secrete progesterone and estrogen for two weeks, and as this function ceases, the levels of plasma estrogen and progesterone fall abruptly and menstruation occurs. The morphologic and functional changes that the ovary undergoes during the menstrual cycle have been lucidly described in a review by Franchi. During the preovulatory or follicular phase of the cycle, proliferation of the endometrium occurs under the stimulation of estrogen. During the postovulatory or luteal phase of the cycle, both progesterone and estrogen act to slow down endometrial growth and to so alter its structure that it is prepared for the nidation of a fertilized ovum. Glandular elements become engorged with secretions and there is a substantial increase in vascularization. These uterine phases, corresponding to the follicular and luteal periods of ovarian function, are termed proliferative and secretory, respectively.

There is evidence that the ovum is susceptible to fertilization for only a brief time following its release. When spermatozoa are present, fertilization usually occurs within six hours of ovulation in the distal third of the fallopian tube. The fertilized ovum then slowly migrates to the uterine cavity and becomes implanted in the secretory endometrium about eight days after conception. Almost immediately, the implanted blastocyst or trophoblast begins to secrete chorionic gonadotropin which stimulates the continued secretion of progesterone and estrogen by the corpus luteum. The latter hormones cause a continuing buildup of the endometrium, forming the decidua. Very early in pregnancy, the ovaries are the principal source of the necessary sex steroids; later, the fetal placental unit assumes this responsibility, and pregnancy proceeds without further assistance from the ovaries. It should be noted that the function of the corpus luteum becomes nearly autonomous following ovulation, secreting estrogen and progesterone with but little stimulation from pituitary gonadotropins. Thus, the pituitary is not necessary for the maintenance of pregnancy, and only a very low level of circulating gonadotropins is required for corpus luteum function. This conclusion was recently substantiated by a report describing the induction of ovulation by the administration of human menopausal and chorionic gonadotropins in a woman who had undergone hypophysectomy (Corral et al.). The patient conceived, and the pregnancy proceeded uneventfully to a normal spontaneous delivery at term. Plasma levels of estrogen, pregnanediol (a metabolite of progesterone), and chorionic gonadotropin were normal throughout the pregnancy.

Hypothalamic-Pituitary-Ovarian Interactions

Current evidence, albeit incomplete, indicates that the secretion of FSH and LH by the anterior pituitary is subservient to regulation by hypothalamic releasing factors, as mentioned earlier in this chapter. These, in turn, are influenced by plasma levels of estrogen, progesterone, and, undoubtedly, neural signals from higher centers. An understanding of the interactions among hypothalamic, pituitary, and ovarian factors in regulating the complex sequence of events of the menstrual cycle is gradually emerging. FSH stimulates follicle growth during the first (follicular) phase of the cycle; ovulation has been attributed to a rapid increase in plasma LH. Actually, both FSH and LH increase sharply just before ovulation. Most investigators believe that the surge in LH is stimulated by the rapidly rising concentration of estrogen. Others believe that 17-hydroxyprogesterone, possibly in conjunction with estradiol, may be involved (Odell et al.). The latter investigators treated postmenopausal women for 22 days with a potent estrogen; FSH and LH levels fell progressively. On the twelfth day, a single intramuscular injection of progesterone was given, and 24 hours later the levels of both FSH and LH increased sharply. Despite continued administration of oral progesterone, FSH and LH promptly declined. Although FSH appears to be the principal factor which stimulates estrogen formation by the follicle, it is probable that both FSH and LH are necessary for optimal estrogen synthesis and release. Little if any progesterone is secreted by the developing follicle, a finding inconsistent with the thesis that progesterone stimulates the preovulatory surge of LH. It is generally agreed that following ovulation, the corpus luteum secretes the sex steroids with relatively little stimulation from the pituitary for about 14 days. The abrupt fall in plasma estrogen and progesterone at the end of this time is responsible not only for initiating menstruation but, in all likelihood, for the re-institution of FSH secretion. Thus, the first day of menstruation signifies both the end and the beginning of the cycle.

Biosynthesis, Transport, Mechanism of Action, and Disposal of Estrogen and Progesterone

The formation of both estrogens and progesterone follows the basic pathway already described for cortisol synthesis. In this sequence, cholesterol is converted to pregnenolone, the intermediate common to all the steroid hormones. Conversion of pregnenolone to progesterone requires two enzymes: an isomerase to shift the double bond in ring B to ring A, and a dehydrogenase to oxidize the hydroxy- at the 3 position to a keto- structure. Cleavage of the $C_{20, 21}$ side chain yields an androgen, androstenedione, the major precursor of estrogen. Removal of C_{19} and aromatization of ring A yields estrone. Estrone and 17-beta-estradiol, the most potent estrogen, are interconvertible.

The ovarian hormones circulate bound to carrier proteins. The plasma levels of estrone and estradiol in normal females range from 10 to 100 ng. per 100 ml. of plasma, depending on the time of the cycle. Plasma progesterone concentrations average about 140 ng. per 100 ml. during the follicular phase and about 1000 ng. per 100 ml. during the luteal phase. These steroid hormones are inactivated primarily in the liver by conversion to water-soluble glucuronide and sulfate derivatives. Pregnanediol is the chief excretory metabolite of progesterone, and its content in a 24-hour urine collection provides a reasonable index of progesterone activity.

The principal functions of the ovarian hormones are to interact with both the hypothalamic-pituitary unit and the uterus to orchestrate the tightly integrated sequence of follicular development, ovulation, corpus luteum formation, and either menstruation or pregnancy. Beyond their direct effects on reproduction, the ovarian hormones, especially estrogen, are necessary for the development and maintenance of secondary sexual characteristics in the female. Estrogens also appear to promote epiphyseal closure and thus the termination of longitudinal growth, a role comparable to that of testosterone in the male. Estrogen deficiency in the adult female can be associated with osteoporosis.

CLINICAL ENTITIES

Gonadal Aplasia (Turner's Syndrome)

In 1938, Turner described seven females with distinctive phenotypic abnormalities, including sexual infantilism, short stature, webbed neck, and an increased carrying angle of the upper extremities. Surgical explorations revealed gonadal tissue consisting only of a primitive streak in the broad ligaments. On histologic examination, this tissue was sufficiently undifferentiated that it could not definitely be identified as ovarian. Because of the scanty amount and primitive nature of the gonadal tissue, the term "gonadal aplasia" was introduced and is currently the accepted, noneponymic designation of the syndrome.

Although uncommon, the syndrome has been a focal point for the elucidation of sex determination. The determination of nuclear chromatin revealed that the majority of patients with Turner's syndrome have negative patterns (Polani et al.). This finding, coupled with the high incidence of color blindness (Polani et al.), led to the hypothesis that a deficient X chromosome was a basic factor in the pathogenesis of the syndrome. When it became possible to characterize the chromosomal constitution of individuals, the validity of the hypothesis was borne out. Patients with gonadal aplasia and a negative nuclear chromatin pattern were found to have a karyotype of 44 + XO. Without the protection of a normal X chromosome, these individuals are subject to color blindness with the same frequency as males. The 44 + XO karyotype can be explained on the basis of nondisjunction occurring during gametogenesis in either parent. It is of academic interest that the site of abnormal meiosis can be determined in some instances by the pattern of red-green color blindness in the patient and her family. For instance, if both the patient and her father were color blind, one would suspect that nondisjunction occurred in oogenesis, depriving the patient of a maternal X chromosome.

The principal clinical features of Turner's syndrome are (1) primary amenorrhea, underdevelopment of secondary sexual characteristics, and infantile female internal genitalia; (2) short stature, usually less than 5 feet; (3) increased carrying angle of the arms (cubitus valgus); (4) webbed neck (pterygium colli); (5) shield chest;

(6) mental deficiency; (7) coarctation of the aorta; (8) hypertension of unknown cause; and (9) skeletal defects. Of these, the first two are most consistently seen. As with Klinefelter's syndrome, a spectrum of variants has been reported. Some of these result from mosaicism, in which some clonal lines have the deficiency of a sex chromosome (XO) while others are normal. Partial forms of the syndrome may also be due to deletion of a portion of an X chromosome, the karyotype being expressed as Xx. If the deletion is of the short arm of the X chromosome, the patient has short stature and the somatic features of the syndrome but may experience normal sexual development. If the deletion is of the long arm, the patient manifests sexual infantilism but is of normal stature and has few if any of the somatic anomalies.

The disorder does not seem to be familial. Only a few instances have been reported in which more than one member of a family has been affected. Neither does maternal age seem to be a causal factor; in a series of 27 cases, the mean maternal age was 24 years, the same as in a control group. Although theoretically one might expect Turner's syndrome to occur with the same frequency as Klinefelter's syndrome, this is not the case. The determination of nuclear sex chromatin patterns in 1800 consecutive newborn females failed to demonstrate a single instance of the negative pattern. In contrast, comparable studies suggest an incidence of the positive pattern in about 1 of 500 newborn males.

The occurrence of short stature in an individual with severe gonadal deficiency is at first glance inconsistent with the observation that castration in the prepubescent youth leads to a tall eunuchoid individual. The latter event is presumably related to delayed closure of epiphyses of long bones due to the absence of the gonadal hormones. If the basic abnormality in Turner's syndrome was limited to gonadal aplasia, i.e., equivalent to castration in infancy or youth, one would not expect short stature. Actually, Turner's is a multiple system disease, and short stature is but one of several defects that are associated with, but not caused by, gonadal aplasia.

The typical patient with Turner's syndrome seeks medical advice during early adolescent years because of a delay in menarche and in the development of secondary sexual characteristics. The differential diagnosis of the triad of short stature, sexual infantilism, and primary amenorrhea involves Turner's syndrome and hypopi-

TABLE 32-13 DIFFERENTIAL DIAGNOSIS—PITUITARY INFANTILISM AND GONADAL APLASIA (TURNER'S SYNDROME)
In the Adolescent or Young Adult Female

	Turner's Syndrome	**Pituitary Infantilism**
Stature	Usually < 5 feet	< 5 feet
Bone age	Delayed-Normal*	Marked delay
Secondary sexual characteristics		
Breasts, vagina, uterus, tubes	Infantile	Infantile
Sexual hair	Delayed	Absent
Axillary hair	Delayed	Absent
Urinary findings		
Gonadotropins	High titer, usually	0 titer
17-OHC (mg./24-hr.)	1 to 2	0.5 or less
17-KS (mg./24 hr.)	1 to 3	1.0 or less
Mental status	Normal or defective	Normal
Nuclear chromatin pattern	Negative	Positive
Chromosomal constitution	44 + XO, XX/XO, or XX	44 + XX
Hypertension	Frequent (even in absence of coarctation)	Absent
Other findings	Webbed neck, cubitus valgus, coarctation of aorta, skeletal defects	Headaches, visual field defects

*Because of delay in epiphyseal closures, bone age appears retarded in the adolescent. By early adulthood (e.g., 25 years) bone age is normal, adult.

tuitarism. Often, additional clinical findings point to the correct diagnosis with near certainty. A webbed neck, coarctation of the aorta, or other stigmata of Turner's syndrome in a patient with this triad would be virtually diagnostic. On the other hand, findings such as bitemporal hemianopsia would implicate a primary disease of the pituitary. When such features are absent or equivocal, the diagnosis can be established by appropriate laboratory studies. Examination of buccal mucosal scrapings reveals a negative chromatin pattern in 80 per cent of cases of Turner's syndrome. Karyotypes prepared from leukocytes reveal a modal chromosomal constitution of 44 + XO in the majority of cases. Determination of urinary 24-hour gonadotropins usually provides a clear separation between the two entities, the amount being very low or absent in hypopituitarism and higher than normal in Turner's syndrome. The latter finding reflects the absence of feedback inhibition of the anterior pituitary by sex steroids. Another test of pituitary function, determination of growth hormone secretory capacity, is nearly always abnormal in pituitary infantilism. The clinical and laboratory findings in these two conditions are contrasted in Table 32–13.

In the past, physicians have occasionally erred in considering patients with Turner's syndrome as being "genetically male." This attitude probably arises from equating a *negative* chromatin pattern with genetic maleness. When the karyotype is 44 + XO, as in Turner's syndrome, such an interpretation is illogical. Without deliberate investigation, one has no way of knowing the nature of the missing chromosome. Maleness is determined by the presence of a Y chromosome, not the presence of a single X. Thus, the physician has scientific reasons, as well as those dictated by tact, to use great caution in discussing the genetic basis of Turner's syndrome with the patient and *her* family.

REFERENCES

General

Bondy, P. K. (Ed.): Duncan's Diseases of Metabolism. 6th ed. Philadelphia, W. B. Saunders Co., 1969.
Catt, K. J.: An ABC of Endocrinology. Boston, Little, Brown and Co., 1971.
Stanbury, J. B., Wyngaarden, J. B., and Fredrickson, D. S. (Eds.): The Metabolic Basis of Inherited Disease. New York, McGraw-Hill Book Co., 1966.
Williams, R. H. (Ed.): Textbook of Endocrinology. 4th ed. Philadelphia, W. B. Saunders Co., 1968.

Introduction

Huxley, J. S.: Chemical regulation and the hormone concept. Biol. Rev., *10*:427, 1935.
Liddle, G. W., et al.: Clinical and laboratory studies of ectopic humoral syndromes. Recent Progr. Hormone Res., *25*:283, 1969.
Murphy, B. E.: Protein binding and the assay of non-antigenic hormones. Recent Progr. Hormone Res., *25*:563, 1969.
Odell, W. D., and Moyer, D. L.: Hormone measurement. In Physiology of Reproduction. St. Louis, The C. V. Mosby Co., 1971, pp. 1–13.
O'Malley, B. W.: Mechanisms of action of steroid hormones. New Eng. J. Med., *284*:370, 1971.
O'Malley, B. W.: Unified hypothesis for early biochemical sequence of events in steroid hormone action. Metabolism, *20*:981, 1971.
Pastan, I., and Perlman, R. L.: Regulation of gene transcription in *Escherichia coli* by cyclic AMP. In Greengard, P., Paoletti, R., and Robison, G. A.: Advances in Cyclic Nucleotide Research. Vol. 1. New York, Raven Press, 1972.
Robison, G. A., Butcher, R. W., and Sutherland, E. W.: Cyclic AMP. New York, Academic Press, 1971.

Hypothalamus

Anderson, M. S., et al.: Synthetic thyrotropin-releasing hormone. New Eng. J. Med., *285*:1279, 1971.
Bauer, H. G.: Endocrine and other clinical manifestations of hypothalamic disease. J. Clin. Endocr., *14*:13, 1954.
Fleischer, N., et al.: Synthetic thyrotropin-releasing factor as a test of pituitary thyrotropin reserve. J. Clin. Endocrinol. Metab., *34*:617, 1972.
Frohman, L. A.: Clinical neuropharmacology of hypothalamic releasing factors. New Eng. J. Med., *286*:1391, 1972.
Hall, R., et al.: The thyrotrophin-releasing hormone test in diseases of the pituitary and hypothalamus. Lancet, *1*:759, 1972.
Heuser, G. (Moderator): Trends in clinical neuro-endocrinology. Clinical Case Conference, Ann. Intern. Med., *73*:783, 1970.
Kastin, A. J., et al. Release of LH and FSH after administration of synthetic LH-releasing hormone. J. Clin. Endocrinol. Metab., *34*:753, 1972.
McCann, S. M., and Porter, J. C.: Hypothalamic pituitary stimulating and inhibiting hormones. Physiol. Rev., *49*:240, 1969.
Pittman, J. A., Jr., Haigler, E. D., Jr., Hershman, J. M., and Pittman, C. S.: Hypothalamic hypothyroidism. New Eng. J. Med., *285*:844, 1971.
Reichlin, S.: Function of the hypothalamus (Editorial). Amer. J. Med., *43*:477, 1967.

Anterior Pituitary

Bardin, C. W., et al.: Studies of the pituitary-Leydig cell axis in young men with hypogonadotropic hypogonadism and hyposmia: Comparison with normal men, prepubertal boys, and hypopituitary patients. J. Clin. Invest., *48*:2046, 1969.
Daughaday, W. H.: Sulfation factor regulation of skeletal growth: A stable mechanism dependent on intermittent growth hormone secretion (Editorial). Amer. J. Med., *50*:277, 1971.
Gill, G. N.: Mechanism of ACTH action. Metabolism, *21*:571, 1972.
Goodman, H. G., Grumbach, M. M., and Kaplan, S. L.: Growth and growth hormone. II. A comparison of isolated growth-hormone deficiency and multiple pituitary-hormone deficiencies in 35 patients with idiopathic hypopituitary dwarfism. New Eng. J. Med., *278*:57, 1968.
Laron, Z., Pertzelan, A., and Mannheimer, S.: Genetic pituitary dwarfism with high serum concentration of growth hormone: A new inborn error of metabolism? Isr. J. Med. Sci., *2*:152, 1966.
McKusick, V. A., and Rimoin, D. L.: General Tom Thumb and other midgets. Sci. Amer., *217*:102, July, 1967.
Merimee, T. J., Hall, J. D., Rimoin, D. L., and McKusick, V. A.: A metabolic and hormonal basis for classifying ateliotic dwarfs. Lancet, *1*:963, 1969.
Merimee, T. J., et al.: Glucose and lipid homeostasis in the absence of human growth hormones. J. Clin. Invest., *50*:574, 1971.
Murdoch, R.: Sheehan's syndrome—Survey of 57 cases since 1950. Lancet, *1*:1327, June, 1962.
Purnell, D. C., Randall, R. V., and Rynearson, E. H.: Postpartum pituitary insufficiency (Sheehan's syndrome): Review of 18 cases. Mayo Clin. Proc., *39*:321, 1964.

Rimoin, D. L., Merimee, T. J., Rabinowitz, D., Cavalli-Sforza, L. L., and McKusick, V. A.: Peripheral subresponsiveness to human growth hormone in the African pygmies. New Eng. J. Med., 281:1383, 1969.

Sheehan, H. L., and Summers, V. K.: The syndrome of hypopituitarism. Quart. J. Med., 18:319, 1949.

POSTERIOR PITUITARY

Barlow, E. D., and de Wardener, H. E.: Compulsive water drinking. Quart. J. Med., 28:235, 1959.

Coggins, C. H., and Leaf, A.: Diabetes insipidus. Amer. J. Med., 42:807, 1967.

Lauson, H. D.: Metabolism of antidiuretic hormones. Amer. J. Med., 42:713, 1967.

Martin, F. I. R.: Familial diabetes insipidus. Quart. J. Med., 28:573, 1959.

Sachs, H.: Biosynthesis and release of vasopressin. Amer. J. Med., 42:687, 1967.

Sachs, H., et al.: Biosynthesis and release of vasopressin and neurophysine. Recent Progr. Hormone Res., 25:447, 1969.

Schwartz, I. L., and Schwartz, W. B.: Symposium on antidiuretic hormones: Dedication to Vincent du Vigneaud. Amer. J. Med., 42:651, 1967.

Thomas, W. C.: Diabetes insipidus (Teaching Clinic). J. Clin. Endocr., 17:565, 1957.

Wakim, K. G.: Reassessment of the source, mode and locus of action of antidiuretic hormone. Amer. J. Med., 42:394, 1967.

THYROID

Adams, D. D., and Purves, H. D.: Abnormal responses in the assay of thyrotrophin. Proc. Otago Med. Sch., 34:11, 1956.

Braverman, L. E., Ingbar, S. H., and Sterling, K.: Conversion of thyroxine (T_4) to triiodothyronine (T_3) in athyreotic human subjects. J. Clin. Invest., 49:855, 1970.

Burke, G.: The triiodothyronine suppression test. Amer. J. Med., 42:600, 1967.

Fore, W., and Wynn, J.: The thyrotropin stimulation test. Amer. J. Med., 40:90, 1966.

Hershman, J. M., and Pittman, J. A., Jr.: Control of thyrotrophin secretion in man. New Eng. J. Med., 285:997, 1971.

Ivy, H. K., Wahner, H. W., and Gorman, C. A.: "Triiodothyronine (T_3) toxicosis." Its role in Graves' disease. Arch. Intern. Med., 128:529, 1971.

Leon-Sotomayor, L., and Bowers, C. Y.: Myxedema Coma. Springfield, Illinois, Charles C Thomas, Publ., 1964.

Means, J. H., DeGroot, L. H., and Stanbury, J. B.: The Thyroid and Its Diseases. 3rd ed. New York, McGraw-Hill Book Co., 1963.

Mitsuma, T., Nihei, N., Gershengom, M. C., and Hollander, C. S.: Serum triiodothyronine: Measurements in human serum by radioimmunoassay with corroboration by gas-liquid chromatography. J. Clin. Invest., 50:2679, 1971.

Selenkow, H. A., and Hoffman, F. (Eds.): Symposium on the diagnosis and treatment of common thyroid diseases. San Francisco, 1970. Amsterdam, Excerpta Med., 1971.

Sterling, K.: The significance of circulating triiodothyronine. Recent Progr. Hormone Res., 26:249, 1970.

Werner, S. C. and Ingbar, S. H. (Eds.) The Thyroid. 3rd ed. New York, Harper and Row, 1971.

ADRENAL CORTEX

Bongiovanni, A. M., and Root, A. W.: The adrenogenital syndrome. New Eng. J. Med., 268:1283, 1342, 1391; 1963.

Conn, J. W.: Primary aldosteronism, a new clinical syndrome. J. Lab. Clin. Med., 45:6, 1955.

Eisenstein, A. B.: Addison's disease: Etiology and relationship to other endocrine disorders. Med. Clin. N. Amer., 52:327, 1968.

Frawley, T. F.: Adrenal cortical insufficiency. In Eisenstein, A. B. (Ed.): The Adrenal Cortex. Boston, Little, Brown and Co., 1967, p. 439.

Liddle, G. W.: Cushing's syndrome. In Eisenstein, A. B. (Ed.): The Adrenal Cortex. Boston, Little, Brown and Co., 1967, p. 523.

Melby, J. C.: Assessment of adrenocortical function. New Eng. J. Med., 285:735, 1971.

Nelson, D. H., Meakin, J. W., and Thorn, G. W.: ACTH-producing pituitary tumors following adrenalectomy for Cushing's syndrome. Ann. Intern. Med., 52:560, 1960.

Nichols, T., Nugent, C. A., and Tyler, F. H.: Steroid laboratory tests in the diagnosis of Cushing's syndrome. Amer. J. Med., 45:116, 1968.

Ross, E. J., Marshall-Jones, P., and Friedman, M.: Cushing's syndrome: Diagnostic criteria. Quart. J. Med., 35:149, 1966.

Siegal, A. M., Kreisbert, R. A., Hershman, J. M., and Owen, W. C.: Recurrent Cushing's disease following total adrenalectomy. Arch. Intern. Med., 129:642, 1972.

Smilo, R. P., and Forsham, P. H.: Diagnostic approach to hypofunction and hyperfunction of the adrenal cortex. Postgrad. Med., 46:146, November, 1969.

Thorn, G. W.: The adrenal cortex. I. Historical aspects. II. Clinical considerations. Johns Hopkins Med. J., 123:49, 1968.

Weiss, E. R., Rayyis, S. S., Nelson, D. H., and Bethune, J. E.: Evaluation of stimulation and suppression tests in the etiological diagnosis of Cushing's syndrome. Ann. Intern. Med., 71:941, 1969.

PARATHYROIDS

Albright, F., Burnett, C. H., Smith, P. H., and Parson, W.: Pseudohypoparathyroidism, an example of the "Seabright-Bantam syndrome." Report of three cases. Endocrinology, 30:922, 1942.

Albright, F., and Reifenstein, E. C., Jr.: The Parathyroid Glands and Metabolic Bone Disease. Baltimore, Williams and Wilkins, 1948.

Bollet, A. J.: Osteoporosis, or the osteoporosities? (Editorial). Amer. J. Med. Sci., 256:271, 1968.

Condon, O. O., et al.: Osteoporosis (Editorial). Lancet, 1:180, 1970.

Copp, D. H.: Endocrine regulation of calcium metabolism. Ann. Rev. Physiol., 32:61, 1970.

Copp, D. H., et al.: Evidence for calcitonin – A new hormone from the parathyroid that lowers blood calcium. Endocrinology, 70:638, 1962.

Goldsmith, R. S.: Hyperparathyroidism. New Eng. J. Med., 281:367, 1969.

Greenberg, S. R., Karabell, S., and Saade, G. A.: Pseudohypoparathyroidism, a disease of the second messenger (3'5'-cyclic AMP). Arch. Intern. Med., 129:633, 1972.

Haines, S.: Symposium on hyperparathyroidism. Amer. J. Med., 50:557, 1971.

Harris, W. H., and Heaney, R. P.: Skeletal renewal and metabolic bone disease. New Eng. J. Med., 280:193, 1969.

Hermans, P. E., Gorman, C. A., Martin, W. J., and Kelly, P. J.: Pseudopseudohypoparathyroidism (Albright's hereditary osteodystrophy): A family study. Mayo Clin. Proc., 39:81, 1964.

Hirsch, P. F., and Munson, P. L.: Thyrocalcitonin. Physiol. Rev., 49:548, 1969.

Kleeman, C. R., Massry, S. G., Coburn, J. W., and Popostzer, M. M.: The problem and unanswered questions: Renal osteodystrophy, soft tissue calcification and disturbed divalent ion metabolism in chronic renal failure. Arch. Intern. Med., 124:262, 1969.

Krane, S. M.: Selected features of the clinical course of hypoparathyroidism. J.A.M.A., 178:472, 1961.

Lafferty, F. W.: Pseudohyperparathyroidism. Medicine, 45:247, 1966.

Lee, J. B., Tashyian, A. H., Streato, J. A., and Frantz, A. G.: Familial pseudohypoparathyroidism. New Eng. J. Med., 279:1179, 1968.

Pyrah, L. N., Hodgkinson, A., and Anderson, C. K.: Primary hyperparathyroidism. Brit. J. Surg., 53:245, 1966.

Raisz, L. G.: The diagnosis of hyperparathyroidism (or what to do until the immunoassay comes). New Eng. J. Med., 285:1106, 1971.

Rasmussen, H.: Ionic and hormonal control of calcium homeostasis. Amer. J. Med., 50:567, 1971.

Redding, T. W., Schally, A. V., Arimura, A., and Matsuo, H.: Stimulation of release and synthesis of luteinizing hormone (LH) and follicle stimulating hormone (FSH) in tissue cultures of rat pituitaries in response to natural and synthetic LH and FSH releasing hormone. Endocrinology, 90:764, 1972.

Stanbury, S. W., and Lumb, G. A.: Parathyroid function in chronic renal failure. Quart. J. Med., 35:1, 1966.

Stanbury, S. W., Lumb, G. A., and Mawer, E. B.: Osteodys-

trophy developing spontaneously in the course of chronic renal failure. Arch. Intern. Med., *124*:274, 1969.
Wessler, S., and Avioli, L. V.: The parathyroid adenoma. J.A.M.A., *205*:105, 1968.

ADRENAL MEDULLA

Hermann, H., and Mornex, R.: Human Tumors Secreting Catecholamines. New York, The Macmillan Co., 1964.
Page, L. B., and Copeland, R. B.: Pheochromocytoma. Disease-A-Month, *1*:1, 1968.
Sjoerdsma, A. (Moderator): Pheochromocytoma: Current concepts of diagnosis and treatment. Clinical Staff Conference at National Institutes of Health, Ann. Intern. Med., *65*:1302, 1966.

PANCREAS

Arieff, A. I. and Carroll, H. J.: Nonketotic hyperosmolar coma with hyperglycemia: Clinical features, pathophysiology, renal function, acid-base balance, plasma-cerebrospinal fluid equilibria and the effects of therapy in 37 cases. Medicine, *51*:73, 1972.
Arky, R. A., and Knopp, R. H.: Evaluation of islet-cell function in man. New Eng. J. Med., *285*:1130, 1971.
Bressler, R.: Investigative issues in diabetes mellitus. Arch. Intern. Med., *123*:219, 1969.
Cahill, G. F.: The physiology of insulin in man. Diabetes, *20*:785, 1971.
Clinicopathological Conference: Diabetes mellitus with hyperosmotic coma. Amer. J. Med., *52*:115, 1972.
Ellenberg, M., and Rifkin, H. (Eds.): Diabetes Mellitus: Theory and Practice. New York, McGraw-Hill Book Co., 1970.
Fajans, S. S., and Sussman, K. E. (Eds.): Diabetes Mellitus: Diagnosis and Treatment. Volume III. New York, American Diabetes Association, 1971.
Flatt, J. P.: On the maximal possible rate of ketogenesis. Diabetes, *21*:50, 1972.
Gerich, J. E., Martin, M. M., and Recant, L.: Clinical and metabolic characteristics of hyperosmolar nonketotic coma. Diabetes, *20*:228, 1971.
Gorman, C. K.: Hypoglycemia. Med. Clin. N. Amer., *49*:947, 1965.
Levin, M. E.: Endocrine syndromes associated with pancreatic islet cell tumors. Med. Clin. N. Amer., *52*:295, 1968.
Siperstein, M. D., Unger, R. H., and Madison, L. L.: Studies of muscle capillary basement membranes in normal subjects, diabetic, and pre-diabetic patients. J. Clin. Invest., *47*:1973, 1968.
Somogyi, M.: Exacerbation of diabetes by excess insulin action. Amer. J. Med., *26*:169, 1959.
Steiner, D. F., et al.: Proinsulin and the biosynthesis of insulin. Recent Progr. Hormone Res., *25*:207, 1969.
Unger, R. H.: Glucagon physiology and pathophysiology. New Eng. J. Med., *285*:443, 1971.
Williams, R. H., and Ensinck, J. W.: Current studies regarding diabetes. Arch. Intern. Med., *128*:820, 1971.
Yalow, R. S., and Berson, S. A.: Dynamics of insulin secretion in hypoglycemia. Diabetes, *14*:341, 1965.

TESTES

Barr, M. L., and Bertram, E. G.: A morphological distinction between neurones of the male and female, and the behavior of the nucleolar satellite during accelerated nucleoprotein synthesis. Nature, *163*:676, 1949.
Davidson, W. M., and Smith, D. R.: A morphological sex difference in the polymorphonuclear neutrophil leukocytes. Brit. Med. J., *2*:6, 1954.
Federman, D. D.: Disorders of sexual development. New Eng. J. Med., *277*:351, 1967.
Hecht, F., Wyandt, H. E., and Erbe, R. W.: Revolutionary Cytogenetics (Editorial). New Eng. J. Med., *285*:1482, 1971.
Kallman, F. J., Schoenfeld, W. A. and Barrera, S. E.: The genetic aspects of primary eunuchoidism. Amer. J. Ment. Defic., *48*:203, 1944.
Kastin, A. J., et al.: Stimulation of LH release in men and women by LH-releasing hormone purified from porcine hypothalami. J. Clin. Endocr., *29*:1046, 1969.
Keats, T. E., and Burns, T. W.: The radiographic manifestations of gonadal dysgenesis. Radiol. Clin. N. Amer., *2*:297, 1964.
Klinefelter, H. F., Jr., Reifenstein, E. C., Jr., and Albright, F.: Syndrome characterized by gynecomastia aspermatogenesis without A-Leydigism, and increased excretion of follicle stimulating hormone. J. Clin. Endocr., *2*:615, 1942.
Masao, I., et al.: Clinical effects with partially purified beef hypothalamic FSH-releasing factor. Amer. J. Obstet. Gynec., *100*:867, 1968.
Paulsen, C. A.: Disorders of spermatogenesis in man. *In* Astwood, E. B., and Cassidy, C. E. (Eds.): Clinical Endocrinology. Vol. II. New York, Grune and Stratton, 1968.
Paulsen, C. A., et al.: Klinefelter's syndrome and its variants: A hormonal and chromosomal study. Recent Progr. Hormone Res., *24*:321, 1968.
Plunkett, E. R., and Barr, M. L.: Cytologic tests of sex in congenital testicular hypoplasia. J. Clin. Endocrinol. Metab., *16*:829, 1956.
Plunkett, E. R., and Barr, M. L.: Testicular dysgenesis affecting the seminiferous tubules principally, with chromatin-positive nuclei. Lancet, *2*:853, 1956.
Tjio, J. H., and Levan, A.: The chromosome number of man. Hereditas, *42*:1, 1956.
Wilson, J. D., and Walker, J. D.: Conversion of testosterone to 5 alpha-androstan-17 beta-ol-3-one (dihydrotestosterone) by skin slices of man. J. Clin. Invest., *48*:371, 1969.

OVARIES

Corral, J., Calderon, J., and Goldzieher, J. W.: Induction of ovulation and term pregnancy in a hypophysectomized woman. Obstet. Gynec., *39*:397, 1972.
Franchi, L. L.: The ovary. *In* Philipp, E. E., Barnes, J., and Newton, M. (Eds.): Scientific Foundations of Obstetrics and Gynaecology. Philadelphia, F. A. Davis Co., 1970.
Gemzell, C. A.: Ovulation. *In* Philipp, E. E., Barnes, J., and Newton, M. (Eds.): Scientific Foundations of Obstetrics and Gynaecology. Philadelphia, F. A. Davis Co., 1970.
Israel, S. L.: Menstruation. *In* Philipp, E. E., Barnes, J., and Newton, M. (Eds.): Scientific Foundations of Obstetrics and Gynaecology. Philadelphia, F. A. Davis Co., 1970.
Lipsett, M. B., Cargille, C. M., and Ross, G. T.: Methodologic advances and clinical studies. National Institutes of Health Conference on Reproductive Endocrinology, Ann. Intern. Med., *72*:933, 1970.
Means, A. R., and O'Malley, B. W.: Mechanism of estrogen action: Early transcriptional and translational events. Metabolism, *21*:357, 1972.
Odell, W. D., and Swerdloff, R. S.: Progestogen-induced luteinizing and follicle-stimulating hormone surge in postmenopausal women: Simulated ovulatory peak. Proc. Natl. Acad. Sci., *61*:529, 1968.
Penny, R., et al.: Correlation of serum follicular stimulating hormone (FSH) and luteinizing hormone (LH) as measured by radioimmunoassay in disorders of sexual development. J. Clin. Invest., *49*:1847, 1970.
Penny, R., Foley, T. P., Jr., and Blizzard, R. M.: Serum follicular-stimulating hormone and luteinizing hormone as measured by radioimmunoassay correlated with sexual development in hypopituitary subjects. J. Clin. Invest., *51*:74, 1972.
Polani, P. E., Hunter, W. F., and Lennox, B.: Chromosomal sex in Turner's syndrome with coarctation of the aorta. Lancet, *267*:120, 1954.
Polani, P. E., Lessof, M. H., and Bishop, P. M. F.: Color blindness in "ovarian agenesis" (gonadal dysplasia). Lancet, *271*:118, 1956.
Prunty, F. T. G.: Hirsutism, virilism and apparent virilism and their gonadal relationship. J. Endocr., *38*:85, 1967.
Richardson, G. S.: Ovarian physiology. New Eng. J. Med., *274*:1008, 1966.
Ross, G. T., et al.: Pituitary and gonadal hormones in women during spontaneous and induced ovulatory cycles. Rec. Progr. Horm. Res., *26*:1, 1970.
Turner, H. H.: A syndrome of infantilism, congenital webbed neck and cubitus valgus. Endocrinology, *23*:566, 1938.

SECTION V

TOXIC PHYSICAL AND CHEMICAL AGENTS

CHAPTER 33

EFFECTS OF PHYSICAL AGENTS

CHARLES E. BILLINGS[*]

INTRODUCTION

There exist within man's physical environment a great number of stressors or stimuli, nearly all of which in some dose over some time period are capable of causing dysfunction, disease, or death. These agents, however, are unique in that nearly all are essential to life and in that too little, as well as too much, of many of them may be injurious. It is the intent of this chapter to outline the tolerance envelope for each of these agents and to indicate what physiologic alterations occur when man encounters unusual environments.

We may consider the physical environment as being made up of three parts, each necessary to life. One is the *gaseous* environment: the atmospheric envelope which surrounds our planet, exerting a pressure upon every living thing on its surface and containing the oxygen, carbon dioxide, and nitrogen without which life, either animal or plant, could not have come to be.

Another facet of the environment is what we may call the *electromagnetic* environment: the sum of the electromagnetic waves and energetic particles which constantly bathe the earth. The infrared radiation upon which we depend for warmth, the light which allows us to visualize our surroundings and which triggers the photosynthetic reactions upon which we depend for food, the ultraviolet rays which produce vitamin D within our skin—all are necessary to life, yet each in insufficient or excessive amounts is harmful.

We may call the third part of our surroundings the *kinetic* environment—the accelerative forces which act upon us. Although many of the accelerations which we encounter are a consequence of our technology, gravity subjects us all to a constant acceleration toward the earth's center of mass. With our present dependence upon machines for transportation, we must consider other linear and radial accelerations as well, and also the effects of rapid deceleration or impact. Vibration and noise are other products of our technology which evoke physiopathologic responses.

Life has been characterized as "the struggle of an organism to remain distinct from its environment." The attribute of biological systems which allows them to carry on this struggle is adaptability—the ability to respond *actively* to imposed stresses. The sum of these responses is what we know as the physiology of man; it is this which allows him, for a time, to withstand the universe's inexorable march toward greater entropy. Man cannot avoid his physical environment as he can toxic chemicals or microorganisms; indeed, he depends upon his environment for the oxygen, food, and energy necessary for survival. He must therefore learn to cope with naturally occurring alterations in the physical environment. It is the mechanisms of this coping behavior which we shall examine here.

THE GASEOUS ENVIRONMENT

Under this heading, we must consider man's tolerance envelope for barometric pressure, his ability to withstand changes in pressure, and his tolerance limits for each of the gases found in his environment: oxygen, carbon dioxide, nitrogen, and the noble gases, argon, neon, helium, krypton, and xenon. In general, we shall examine the

---

[*]The author wishes to thank Dr. Paul Webb and Dr. Ebtissam Hamdi, who read the manuscript and offered helpful criticisms.

lower end of the tolerance spectrum first, then attempt to define optimal levels for productive existence, and finally define the upper limits of tolerance as a time-dependent phenomenon.

First a word about units of measurement: Although the Système Internationale (S.I.) has been recommended for universal adoption, its unit of pressure being the Newton per square meter, nearly all texts on physiology still define pressures in millimeters of mercury. In order not to burden the reader unduly, we shall use mm. Hg as our primary unit here, though we shall sometimes include in parentheses the equivalent in $N/m.^2$ or in the more commonly used equivalent, millibars (mb.). One additional pressure unit will also be used in discussing life at high pressures—atmospheres absolute (ATA). Since several systems of pressure measurement are in common use in Western countries, Figure 33–1 is provided as a convenient reference. It is a nomogram which shows the quantitative relationships among the various systems. It also shows barometric pressure as a function of pressure, altitude above mean sea level in meters and feet, and depth in sea water. (See formula below.)

Barometric Pressure

Normal Range. While 760 mm. Hg (1.013×10^5 $N/m.^2$, 29.92 in. Hg) is the "standard" pressure exerted by the weight of the atmosphere upon the surface of the earth at mean sea level, the actual barometric pressure at any point on the earth's surface at a given time fluctuates with weather phenomena, with elevation, and with the acceleration due to gravity, which varies with latitude. Fluctuations caused by weather are generally in the range 745 to 785 mm. Hg (980 to 1045 mb.), though pressures at the center of severe thunderstorms or hurricanes may be as low as 956 and occasional readings as high as 1062 mb. are reported. Pressures through the range of terrestrial elevations are shown in Figure 33–1.

Tolerance Limits for Low Barometric Pressure. The lowest barometric pressure at which a sea-level equivalent alveolar gas composition can be maintained if 100 per cent oxygen is breathed is about 187 mm. Hg ($P_{A_{O_2}} = 100$, $P_{A_{CO_2}} = 40$, $P_{H_2O} = 47$). This pressure is encountered at an altitude of 34,000 feet. At pressures below this, alveolar and therefore arterial oxygen tension decreases. A modest degree of hyperventilation occurs when the carotid sinus chemoreceptors sense a drop in arterial oxygen tension. The limit for continued consciousness occurs at an alveolar P_{O_2} of about 30 mm. Hg, thus, at barometric pressures below about 100 mm. Hg ($P_{O_2} = 30$, $P_{CO_2} = 25$, $P_{H_2O} = 47$), human function ceases.

The ultimate limit for human tolerance of low barometric pressure is roughly 47 mm. Hg (63,000 feet), the vapor pressure of water at body temperature. Sudden exposure to lower pressures causes rapid evolution of water vapor bubbles within the blood and tissues, the condition known as *ebullism*. Central venous pressure rises as bubbles form in the more distensible venous reservoir and soon meets or exceeds mean arterial pressure. Circulation then ceases. Ventricular fibrillation may ensue within 90 seconds, though animals (dogs, primates) have sometimes recovered after exposure at 2 mm. Hg absolute for as long as 180 seconds.

Humans breathing 100 per cent oxygen have survived and functioned for long periods of time at barometric pressures in the range 187 to 285 mm. Hg (250 to 380 mb.) The pressure suits used in lunar exploratory missions provide a total pressure of 187 mm. Hg, 3.5 psi, and the Apollo spacecraft are pressurized at 285 mm. Hg, 5.5 psi. There have been problems at these pressures (see Inert Gases) but they do not appear to have been caused by pressure as such.

For men breathing air, tolerance limits for low barometric pressures are related to hypoxia and will be discussed under that heading.

Effects of Pressure Fluctuations on Earth. A number of investigators have inferred from epidemiologic studies that psychological depression and suicide rates are more common during periods of weather which involve very low barometric pressures. Conclusive evidence is lacking. Patients with various forms of arthropathy commonly state that they can predict weather changes by observing changes in the pain and stiffness of their diseased joints. We are not

---

1 atmosphere absolute (ATA)
    = 1.013×10^5 Newtons per square meter ($N/m.^2$)
    = 1013.6 millibars (mb.)
    = 760.0 millimeters of mercury (mm. Hg)
    = 29.92 inches of mercury (in. Hg)
    = 14.70 pounds per square inch (psi)
    = 33.0 feet of sea water
    = 34.2 feet of fresh water

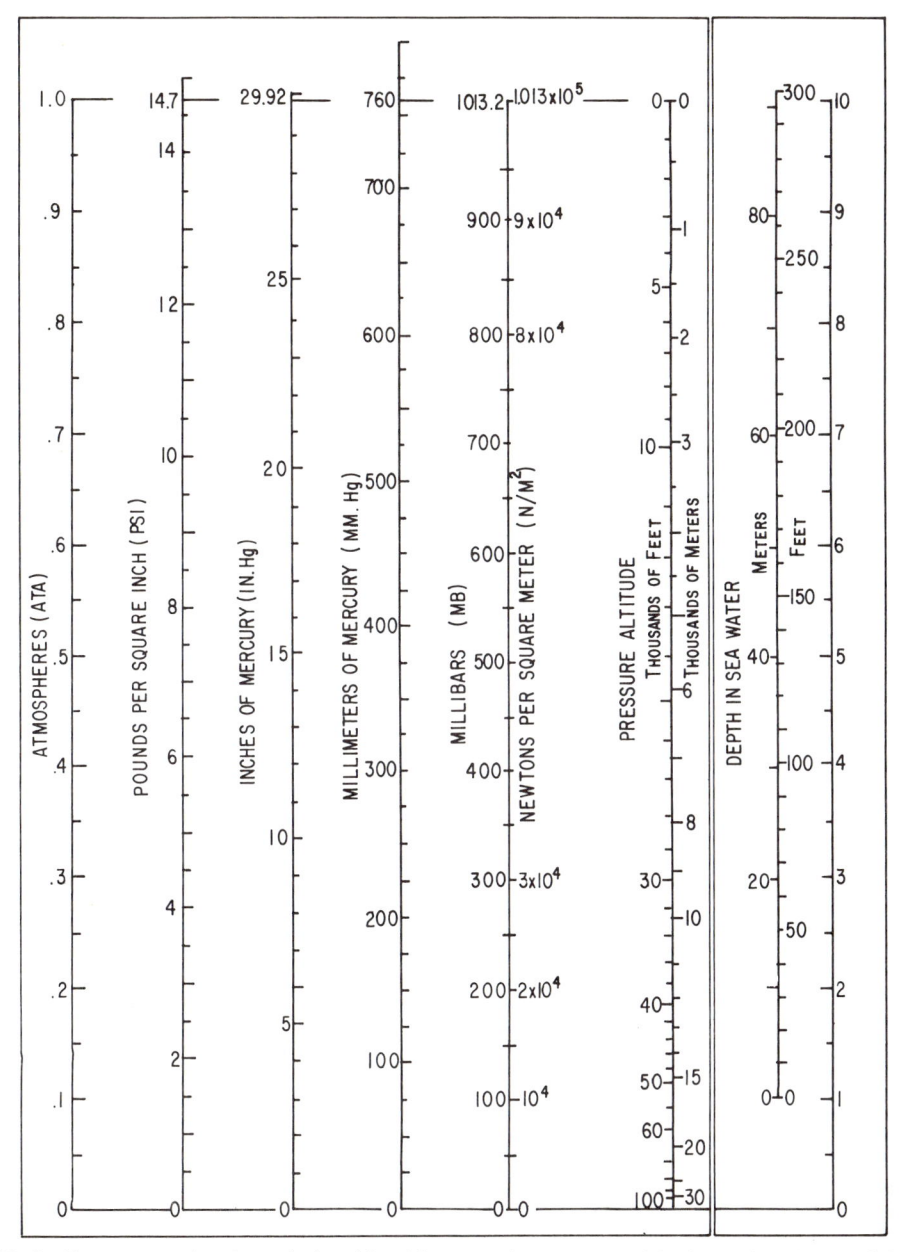

Figure 33-1 Nomogram showing relationship of barometric pressure, altitude or elevation, and depth in sea water. Several equivalent systems of pressure measurement are shown.

aware of controlled studies of this phenomenon, but neither are we inclined to reject it out of hand.

Effects of High Barometric Pressure. We do not know what the ultimate tolerance limit for high pressures will be. Leaving aside the effects of high partial pressures of the various gases in man's breathing medium and the effects of relatively rapid changes in pressure, we know that normal men can live and work at pressures of 31 ATA (equivalent to 1000 feet depth in sea water) for a week: briefer exposures to 45 ATA have been successfully tolerated, and studies at higher pressures are in the offing. Fenn has suggested that the limits will occur at the point at which oxidative biochemical reactions, many of which involve increases in molecular volume, are inhibited by hydrostatic pressures. It seems more likely that limits will be imposed by impairment of distribution and mixing of inspired with alveolar air, and by limitations in the ability to perform the work involved in breathing extremely dense gas mixtures, though Lambertson has recently demonstrated that fit young men can perform moderate work while breathing gas the density of which approximates that which will be encountered at 150 ATA (5000 feet depth in sea water).

Effects of Rapid Changes in Barometric Pressure. Under this heading, we must consider the effects of both increases and decreases in total pressure as they act on gases within the various gas-containing cavities of the body (middle ear, paranasal sinuses, lungs, gut) and on gases dissolved in body fluids according to Henry's law. Dissolved gases can only evolve as bubbles when the total pressure on them is decreased, whereas trapped gas in body cavities will attempt to obey Boyle's law as the pressure on the body changes in either direction.

Increasing Barometric Pressures. Any increase in barometric pressure will cause a decrease in the volume of a given quantity of gas. If the gas is in free communication with a gaseous environment, more gas will flow into a rigid cavity of a given size. If such gas is not available from the environment (as in underwater swimming or breath-hold diving), a relative negative pressure will occur within the cavity.

The human middle ear is a cavity of relatively fixed volume which is ventilated only through the eustachian tube. The mucosal lining of the eustachian tube is so constructed that air within the middle ear can leave the cavity passively. Re-entry of air, however, is impeded and in most people requires voluntary action (yawning, swallowing) to contract the pharyngeal muscles and open the tubal orifices. Attempts to ventilate the middle ear during a descent from altitude or a dive in shallow water may be impeded by swelling of the nasopharyngeal mucosa or lymphoid hypertrophy (as found in upper respiratory infections, allergic rhinitis, and so on).

If a substantial negative pressure differential is allowed to build up within the ear, voluntary attempts to reopen the eustachian tubes may become difficult or impossible. The Valsalva maneuver may help by forcing air into the ear. If the relative vacuum persists, however, fluid is drawn into the middle ear; it may be serous or hemorrhagic in character. Rarely, the tympanic membrane may rupture. Treatment of this condition, known as aerotitis or barotitis, is physiologic: air is introduced into the middle ear by myringotomy or eustachian tube catheterization to neutralize the pressure differential across the eardrum.

If the paranasal sinus ostia are occluded by mucosal swelling, a similar condition may arise in these cavities. This condition is called aero- or barosinusitis. Unlike the middle ear, however, sinus pain may occur during either ascent or descent. The pain may be intense and incapacitating. It is caused by either a positive or negative differential pressure in the sinus cavities.

The lungs, unlike the middle ears and sinuses, are contained in a cavity of variable volume. The thoracic cavity is thus free to contract, within limits, even when air is not available from the environment (e.g., breath-hold diving). Limits are imposed on the contraction in volume, however; once the residual volume of the lungs is reached, further increases in barometric pressure cause a relative negative pressure to occur within the thorax (thoracic squeeze). This is compensated for in part by an increase in the volume of blood in the lesser circulation and the intrathoracic portion of the venous reservoir, but at high negative pressures, pulmonary parenchymal injury results. The world's record for a breath-hold dive is 231 feet, 760 to 6080 mm. Hg.

If gas is available outside the body, very rapid increases in pressure are tolerated. Some people appear able to ventilate their eustachian tubes continuously; such subjects can tolerate pressure increases on the order of 60 mm. Hg per sec. (1 psi per sec.) without difficulty. Entry of air into the lungs is not a limiting factor in these circumstances.

Blast waves in free air, however, may be a problem, since very high overpressures with very short rise times may occur. In these circumstances, air does not have time to enter the lungs and very considerable differential pressures may occur across the chest wall, followed by marked underpressures in the environment during the rarefaction wave which follows the initial overpressure. These events occur so rapidly that the lung-chest system does not have time to adapt; it acts as a rigid system in which shear forces may cause tearing of delicate structures.

Decreasing Barometric Pressures. Relatively rapid decreases in barometric pressure occur during an ascent from depth to the surface in water, during decompression of a caisson, and during ascent to altitude in aircraft. The effects of such decreases in pressure are expansion of trapped gas and, when a substantial decrease in pressure is involved, evolution of gases from solution in the blood and body fluids.

Because of the peculiar structure of the eustachian tube, ear discomfort is almost never a problem when barometric pressure decreases. Barosinusitis or barodontalgia, however, may occur owing to expansion of trapped gas. The latter disorder is due to pockets of gas in improperly filled or infected teeth.

Under normal circumstances, the gastrointestinal tract contains relatively small amounts of gas. As this gas expands, stretch receptors in the wall of the gut are stimulated and peristalsis becomes more active. Relief from cramps is obtained by belching or passing flatus. During an extremely rapid decompression, however, massive expansion may occur before a muscular response is possible; the result may be vagovagal syncope. Rapid decompressions can occur in the event of a window, door seal, or wall failure in pressurized jet aircraft.

The foregoing comments suggest that the physician should be careful about allowing patients with hypomotile gut disorders to fly at high altitudes in unpressurized aircraft. Modern passenger aircraft are pressurized to keep cabin altitude at or below 8000 feet (564 mm. Hg). Even at this moderate pressure, however, relative gas volume (saturated) is 38 per cent over sea-level values. In unpressurized light aircraft, altitudes of 12,000 feet (P_B 483 mm. Hg) are common.

The human lung-airway system at resting expiratory level has a time constant in the neighborhood of 0.05 to 0.10 seconds. During rapid decompression of an aircraft, if the time constant of the cabin (a function of its volume and the orifice through which air is escaping) is appreciably longer than that of the lungs and airway, no substantial overpressure will occur within the chest. If the reverse is true, however, overpressures will occur within the lungs. If the magnitude of the pressure drop is great enough, the lungs can become distended; a further buildup of differential pressure within the lungs can cause parenchymal tears and possibly air embolism. Such rapid decompressions are very rare in civil aircraft but can occur in military jets which have small cabin volumes and large canopies.

It should be noted that during ascent from deep water to the surface, pressure decreases at the rate of 1 ATA per 33 feet. If a diver inspires from a breathing apparatus at depth, then attempts breath-holding during an ascent, he is in grave danger of lung rupture. It is necessary to expire actively throughout this maneuver and to limit the ascent rate. Naval divers are warned to "follow their bubbles" during such ascents, which gives them an ascent rate of about 60 feet per minute. This same precaution is necessary during emergency escape from submarines, which is accomplished through pressurized air locks.

Decompression Sickness. When the total pressure on a fluid containing dissolved gas is sharply decreased, the gases emerge from solution as bubbles (the phenomenon of effervescence observed when a bottle of soda or beer is uncapped). In the body, inert gas as well as oxygen and carbon dioxide are dissolved, both in water and in fat. The amount of inert gas in solution is a function of the alveolar partial pressure of the gas and its solubility coefficients in water and in oil.

Once bubbles of gas form in the tissues or the blood, they obey Boyle's law. If the pressure on the body is reduced further, they expand; if the pressure is increased, they contract, but they do not disappear until the pressure is increased considerably above the pressure at which they were formed.

During any ascent to high altitude or from depth, the amount of inert gas in solution in blood and various tissues is the limiting factor, since decompression at too rapid a rate will favor formation of bubbles. The rate at which inert gas is eliminated from any tissue is a function of the perfusion of that tissue and the partial pressure of inert gas in the perfusing blood. Since different tissues contain different proportions of lipid and water and have different rates of perfusion, some (such as depot fat) give up inert gas very slowly, whereas diffusion proceeds rapidly in muscle and liver.

The symptoms which occur when man is decompressed too rapidly are known collectively as *decompression sickness*. While it is not certain that all the manifestations of decompression sickness are due to evolved gas, this is the most consistent explanation which has been offered to date. Regardless of the cause, however, the symptoms of decompression sickness are consistent. They fall into five distinct categories.

The most common and least ominous form of this disorder is called the bends, after the grotesque postures effected in an effort to minimize the often excruciating joint and periarticular pain which characterizes the syndrome. Bends may come on suddenly or insidiously. Pain in or around a joint is the first symptom. It often afflicts a joint in use, or one which has previously been injured. The pain may remain localized, may migrate, or may affect several joints sequentially. A relatively small increase in barometric pressure may produce complete relief. If decompression continues, however, the pain may become incapacitating, or other forms of decompression sickness may supervene.

Localized paresthesias, itching, and rashes may also occur, presumably owing to bubbles in the skin or subcutaneous tissues. They are not dangerous. Much more ominous is a painless mottling of the skin which resembles patchy cyanosis. Its precise etiology is uncertain, but it is often seen in combination with or preceding the onset of the more severe forms of decompression sickness listed below.

A more serious form of decompression sickness is the symptom complex known as the chokes. This form is characterized by tachypnea, burning substernal pain, which worsens on deep inspiration, and dry cough. It is believed that these symptoms, together with pulmonary hypertension, are caused by showers of bubbles arising in the venous circulation, which lodge in pulmonary arterioles and capillaries. The chokes are a grave development, for they often precede the most serious forms of decompression sickness.

Central nervous system decompression sickness may occur in isolation or in combination with other forms of the disease. The symptoms may mimic virtually any acute discrete or disseminated CNS lesion. Hemianopsia, hemiparesis, aphasia, confusion, delirium, and other equally frightening symptoms and signs may be observed. These are thought to be caused by gas bubbles which either block or evoke severe spasm in cerebral arterioles. Despite the serious nature of this syndrome, dramatic relief is usually produced by immediate recompression to a pressure well above that at which the symptoms appeared. With effective treatment, permanent sequelae are rare though not unknown.

Syncope may be the first or a secondary symptom of decompression sickness. Particularly when recompression is prompt, the patient will usually return to consciousness rapidly. After some time, however, such a patient may quite suddenly begin to show signs of shock, which can progress rapidly to severe levels, with anuria, refractory peripheral vascular collapse, coma, and death.

The treatment of decompression sickness is relatively simple if, and only if, adequate facilities are at hand. Recompression is the specific treatment for this disorder. In the case of decompression sickness occurring at high altitude, and persisting after return to sea level, overcompression in hyperbaric chambers has been remarkably successful. Although such treatment does not make gas bubbles dissolve immediately, it does make them smaller and probably promotes more rapid dissolution. Details as to the compression treatment of this disorder may be found in the U.S. Navy Diving Manual, the basic source document for anyone involved in situations in which decompression sickness can occur.

A late finding in caisson workers and divers who are repeatedly exposed to compression and marginally adequate decompressions is aseptic bone necrosis, which often occurs in the heads of the long bones but may be seen elsewhere as well. This disorder may be serious and disabling. Once present, it does not differ appreciably from aseptic necrosis caused by other agents. It is probably due to compromise of the circulation to these areas.

Oxygen

The oxygen concentration in the lower atmosphere (below 50,000 feet) is remarkably constant at about 20.9 per cent. Since barometric pressure changes geometrically with altitude (Fig. 33–1), the partial pressure of oxygen in air changes in the same manner. The reader will recall that humidification of air in the upper airways causes a decrease in the partial pressure of oxygen in the inspirate; another more marked drop in oxygen pressure or tension occurs in the alveoli due to continuous extraction of oxygen from and addition of carbon dioxide to the alveolar air. A further drop is seen when pulmonary venous blood is examined (the alveolar-arterial gradient); there is another slight decrease in arterial oxygen tension due to admixture of venous with arterial blood. The relatively long diffusion pathway for oxygen in the tissues means that the oxygen tension at the mitochondria is usually remarkably low. This entire pathway must be considered when we deal with alterations in oxygen partial pressures in the environment or in the human.

Absence of Oxygen; Anoxia. True tissue anoxia probably occurs only when circulation ceases. With the exceptions of oxygen dissolved in tissue fluids and oxygen bound to myoglobin and hemoglobin, the body has no storage capacity for this vital substance. When circulation to the brain ceases completely, as in ventricular fibrillation or rapid decompressions to near-vacuum conditions, consciousness is lost within 5 to 10 seconds; in animals, anoxic brain damage is seen after 90 to 180 seconds. It is interesting that even after such extreme exposures, if consciousness is regained at all, signs of cerebral dysfunction may be transitory and apparently complete recovery usually follows. This may also be true following accidental electrocution.

Decreases in Oxygen; Hypoxia. As noted earlier, man's ultimate tolerance for hypoxia of a duration longer than a few minutes is governed by his ability to maintain a state of consciousness. Consciousness is usually lost within 10 to 15 seconds after alveolar oxygen tension drops below 30 mm. Hg. The arterial oxygen tension under these circumstances is generally below 20 mm. Hg. The retina and brain have the highest oxygen uptakes per unit mass of any tissues in the body, and thus are the tissues most rapidly and severely affected by hypoxia.

In persons breathing air, time of useful consciousness varies from hours at a barometric pressure of 350 to 380 mm. Hg to about 10 to 20 seconds at a barometric pressure of 120 to 140 mm. Hg.

At pressures greater than 380 mm. Hg, indefinite survival on air is possible, though not without severe dysfunction. Impaired mentation and coordination are common during acute exposures to hypoxia of this degree. The symptoms of moderate hypoxia include dyspnea, difficulty in concentrating, and altered judgment and mood; euphoria or depression may be noted. The symptoms may be similar to those of intoxication with ethanol and are due to impaired cerebral oxygenation, magnified by hypocapnia, which causes a degree of cerebral ischemia.

If exposure to alveolar oxygen tensions below about 50 mm. Hg is prolonged for more than 6 to 12 hours, as in mountain climbing, symptoms of acute altitude sickness begin to appear. These symptoms include malaise, headaches (which may be severe), nausea, anorexia, and insomnia. They are made worse by strenuous physical activity or exposure to cold. Breathlessness and dyspnea may be extreme. The incidence of this syndrome reaches its height between 24 to 48 hours and usually subsides thereafter.

The cause of the disorder is not known, though it occurs during a period of multiple physiologic changes. In response to hyperventilation and hypocapnia, fixed base is excreted in the urine. Plasma and extracellular water decrease; the intracellular fluid space increases. A generalized stress response is observed. Roy and others have observed that diuresis usually occurs on the second or third day at altitude, and that symptoms usually decline in severity at this time.

Nearly all persons going to high altitudes experience symptoms of acute altitude sickness. The severity of the symptoms may be lessened by taking acetazolamide for 24 hours prior to ascent.

A few people, instead of feeling better after an initial period of discomfort at altitude, may continue to have difficulty. If hypoxic exposure is continued, some will develop one or more symptoms of a more serious disorder known as chronic altitude sickness. The most ominous forms of this condition involve either cerebral edema or acute pulmonary edema or both. These are life-threatening if hypoxic exposure is not terminated.

Again, the ultimate cause is not known. Hultgren has performed cardiac catheterization studies at altitude on persons susceptible to high altitude pulmonary edema and has found grossly elevated pulmonary arterial pressures; wedge pressures were normal. Some persons can endure repeated hypoxic exposures without showing these signs; others appear inordinately susceptible. The young are more affected; physical activity by susceptible persons hastens the onset of symptoms.

As exposure to hypoxia is prolonged past 3 to 5 days, hematologic changes begin to be evident. The hemoglobin, red cell count, and hematocrit all rise. The latter reaches values of 60 per cent or so after a month of exposure. Concomitant with these changes, heart rates at rest and during work decline; work tolerance increases, though not to sea-level values. Appetite improves and fluid intake increases.

The changes noted here, and others beyond the scope of this review, gradually revert toward sea-level values following cessation of exposure to hypoxia. Normal sea-level values are reached within 2 to 3 weeks after return from altitude.

Exposure to hypoxia in the range of barometric pressures 640 to 520 mm. Hg (5,000 to 10,000 feet) normally evokes only mild to moderate exertional dyspnea, mild fatigue for a few days, and subtle psychomotor defects, though scotopic visual thresholds are moderately to markedly elevated.

Oxygen Tensions at Sea Level; Normoxia. It can be shown that the oxygen tension of arterial blood at sea level (95 to 105 mm. Hg) is still low enough to cause a mild tonic ventilatory stimulus in the carotid chemoreceptors. Nonetheless, persons with normal oxygen transport systems appear to have no other symptoms of hypoxia at rest at barometric pressures in the neighborhood of 760 mm. Hg. During severe physical exercise, the administration of high concentrations of oxygen produces substantial reductions in minute ventilation and increases endurance and work capacity.

Increases in Oxygen; Hyperoxia. Since the arterial blood is virtually fully saturated with oxygen at an alveolar partial pressure of 100 mm. Hg, an increase in alveolar oxygen tension above its normal sea-level value of 100 to 110 mm. Hg results in an increase only in the quantity of oxygen dissolved in plasma, normally about 0.3 ml. per 100 ml. at an oxygen tension of 100 mm. Hg. It is possible to attain alveolar oxygen tensions as high as 670 mm. Hg by breathing 100 per cent oxygen at sea level for several hours. The gain in oxygen content of whole blood is only about 2 ml. per 100 ml., however, in a normal person. If arterial desaturation is present owing to an increased A:a gradient, of course, the use of increased concentrations of oxygen can have much more substantial results. It should be emphasized, however, that the prolonged use of oxygen in persons who do not have either a ventilation or diffusion defect is not physiologic and may be harmful.

Oxygen at pressures above 200 to 250 mm. Hg is toxic to man. The toxicity is a time-dependent phenomenon. The most important manifestations of this toxicity at oxygen pressures up to 1 ATA are pulmonary—inflammatory changes, and later pulmonary edema. It also appears that high oxygen tensions interfere with surfactant formation or excretion, with the result that small areas of atelectasis are observed. One should note that all these pulmonary changes interfere with oxygenation of the blood, which is the reason oxygen is being administered. Such administration, therefore, is a two-edged sword. There is considerable evidence that intermittent administration of oxygen delays or prevents the appearance of pulmonary oxygen toxicity; this should be kept in mind when the gas is to be used for long periods of time.

At pressures of 2 to 3 ATA, oxygen begins to cause central nervous system dysfunction. Tremors, anxiety, and grand mal convulsions are seen. Again, the effects are time- and pressure-dependent, an increase in either causing more severe signs. Oxygen at these pressures is used in the initial treatment of carbon monoxide poisoning, in treatment of gas gangrene and clostridial sepsis, and to enhance the radiosensitivity of certain tumors. It has been useful in cardiac surgery, though hyperbaric oxygen causes coronary and cerebral vasoconstriction; one study has shown as much as a 40 per cent decrease in cerebral oxygen uptake. Again, oxygen administration is clearly a two-edged sword.

Nitrogen

There is no evidence that the human organism is able to "fix" or incorporate molecular nitrogen into chemical compounds. In the absence of such evidence, we are unable to state with finality that gaseous nitrogen is an essential substance. It is necessary, in any discussion of this gas, to distinguish between its role as a unique element and its role as a diluent gas for oxygen, in which latter role any physiologically inert gas will serve as well.

The Role of Nitrogen. As we have said, there is no clear evidence that gaseous nitrogen is essential to human survival, though Allen has shown that chick embryos fail to develop in environments free of the gas. Adult males have functioned effectively for up to 2 weeks in atmospheres virtually devoid of nitrogen in Gemini and some Apollo space flights.

There is absolutely no evidence that nitrogen at sea-level pressures of roughly 600 mm. Hg is toxic. At substantially higher pressures, however, gaseous nitrogen begins to exert a narcotic effect. This effect limits the depth to which divers can descend breathing air. Nitrogen narcosis is pronounced at total pressures of 10 ATA (P_{N_2} of 6000 mm. Hg), equivalent to a depth of about 270 feet of sea water.

This effect is not unique; we shall see that virtually all physiologically inert gases are narcotic at some pressure. The narcotic effect of nitrogen is enhanced by physical activity; it appears to be lessened by repeated exposure to narcotic pressures.

The Role of Inert Gases. While nitrogen as such has not been shown to be essential, it has been shown that the absence of inert diluent gases has specific and predictable effects. Pure oxygen is absorbed rapidly in the lung, and even at pressures below toxic levels, patchy atelectasis has been demonstrated in subjects breathing 100 per cent oxygen. A similar phenomenon occurs in the middle ear if that cavity, after depressurization, is ventilated with pure oxygen. The gas is absorbed slowly, and the resulting pressure decrease within the ear causes symptoms of barotitis.

Inert diluent gases are necessary at sea level and higher barometric pressures, if only to prevent oxygen pressures from reaching toxic levels. At considerable depth, other inert gases must be substituted for nitrogen to avoid nitrogen narcosis. The most commonly used substitute is helium; neon is also used under special circumstances, though it is extremely expensive.

Helium

Effects of High Pressures of Helium. Helium is not an essential element and is normally present in air in only minute amounts. Helium-oxygen mixtures may be substituted for the usual nitrogen-oxygen mixture at sea level with predictable effects but without causing harm even over extended periods of exposure.

Helium is much less dense than nitrogen, though its viscosity is slightly higher than that of nitrogen. The work of breathing at rest at sea level is largely expended in producing laminar air flow and is a function of the viscosity of the gas mixture. Turbulent air flow, however, is a function of density; when the proportion of turbulent air flow is increased, either during intense work or in the presence of significant airway narrowing (as in bronchial asthma), the use of helium-oxygen mixtures appreciably reduces the work of breathing.

Also, helium has a very high thermal conductivity. Comfort temperatures in a helium-oxygen environment are several degrees higher than in air, as a result. The convective heat loss in helium environments is a serious problem in deep diving, particularly when hard work is being performed; respiratory heat loss under these circumstances may exceed the capacity of the diver to produce heat.

Only minimal narcotic effects of helium are seen even at the highest barometric pressures to which man has thus far been exposed. The narcotic potency of all the noble gases is proportional to molecular weight, however; there is no reason to believe that helium will not be narcotic at some pressure, as yet undefined.

The relative insolubility of helium in body fluids, its low density, and its low narcotic potential have made it the diluent of choice in diving. Its disadvantages are its high thermal conductivity and its effects on speech; in the latter, the fundamental frequency is shifted upward and the harmonic structure is sharply modified by altered gas density. At high helium pressure, human speech may become virtually unintelligible.

Other Inert Gases

Neon has been used in diving and in experimental sojourns at moderate depths. It is less narcotic than nitrogen and more dense than helium, so that speech is less altered; heat loss is sharply reduced compared to helium. Its major disadvantages are its expense and its narcotic action at pressures above 10 ATA, though research in this range is inadequate.

Argon is more soluble in fat than nitrogen. Its

use in diving therefore prolongs decompression time. *Krypton* and *xenon* are both potent narcotics at pressures near atmospheric. For these reasons, these gases have not been used in diving, or as other than tracer gases at sea level.

THE ELECTROMAGNETIC ENVIRONMENT

Figure 33-2 is a schematic representation of the electromagnetic environment. It serves to remind us of the reciprocal relation of frequency and wavelength, of the increasing energy of radiation as frequency increases, and of a few of the important effects of electromagnetic waves: molecular excitation at low frequencies, molecular interactions at higher frequencies, and molecular ionization and disruption at the highest frequencies.

In this section, we shall also consider briefly the effects of electric currents which may pass through the body, and we shall mention certain questions which have been raised about the effects of continuous and alternating magnetic fields on the human organism.

The reader will recall that electromagnetic waves are propagated at the speed of light. Since the speed of light varies in different materials, these waves, upon encountering matter, may be reflected, refracted, transmitted, or absorbed. When matter is truly transparent to waves, they transfer none of their energy to that matter. Only if matter is opaque or translucent to waves can energy transfer take place. The student interested in pursuing this area in more detail should review briefly the thermodynamics of heat transfer.

Magnetism

Almost since the discovery of the lodestone, man has speculated about the possible effects of magnetic fields upon physiological function. Much medical quackery has been based on the supposed beneficial effects of magnetic fields. More recently, with the advent of manned space flight, there has been genuine concern about the possible detrimental effects of prolonged existence in environments virtually free of such fields. Beischer and others have devoted several years to animal and human studies.

Exposure to high-intensity magnetic fields causes the appearance of visual phosphenes, though whether these are due to the magnetic or to an induced electrical field in the retina is uncertain. Growth disturbances have been observed in very high, nonuniform magnetic fields. Behavioral effects have also been reported. In theory, very high field strengths can cause migration of cell substances, though it should be noted that fields of several thousand gauss are not strong enough to overshadow the normal thermal movement of such molecules.

Electricity

Electricity is so much a part of our lives, and is so easily kept under our control, that we tend to overlook its considerable dangers. Nearly everyone in a technological society has been "bitten" by an electric current at some time; the overwhelming majority of such incidents cause nothing more than momentary annoyance. Yet electrical deaths are daily occurrences, and the difference between mere annoyance and a fatal outcome may be nothing more than fortuitous: a matter of whether one's hands are dry, whether shoes are being worn, and the like.

In medicine, where biomedical sensors and monitors are increasingly useful, the hazards of inadvertent electrocution are compounded, since these devices are attached to the body in ways which minimize resistance to the passage of stray currents.

When the body is exposed to an electrical current, the electrical characteristics of the exposed part will determine how much current enters the body. Within the body, the conductivity of tissues between the entrance and exit points will determine the path taken by the current and the proportion of the total energy dissipated within the body as heat. Wide variations in individual responses are the rule.

In general, the threshold of perception for current entering the hand is about 5 milliamperes (mA) for direct current, and less than 1 mA for 60 Hz alternating current. Little more than these amounts is generally reported as painful by some investigators; others report the range of 3 to 10 mA as the pain threshold.

With direct current, involuntary muscular contractions sufficient to prevent the exposed person from removing his hand from a source of current are produced by less than 60 mA in men, 40 mA in women. With alternating currents, corresponding values are 9 and 6 mA.

The most serious hazard in accidental contacts with electricity is ventricular fibrillation, since currents passing from a hand to any other extremity must traverse the chest. The heart is absolutely refractory to the induction of ventricular fibrillation except during a short period during the repolarization phase of the ventricles; thus, the timing of brief shocks is important.

Speaking generally, a 60 Hz alternating current of 100 mA crossing the chest for 1 second or more will often induce fibrillation. About 5 times this current, delivered during the sensitive phase of the cardiac cycle, is required with direct current. Much smaller currents are sufficient when they are delivered directly to the heart.

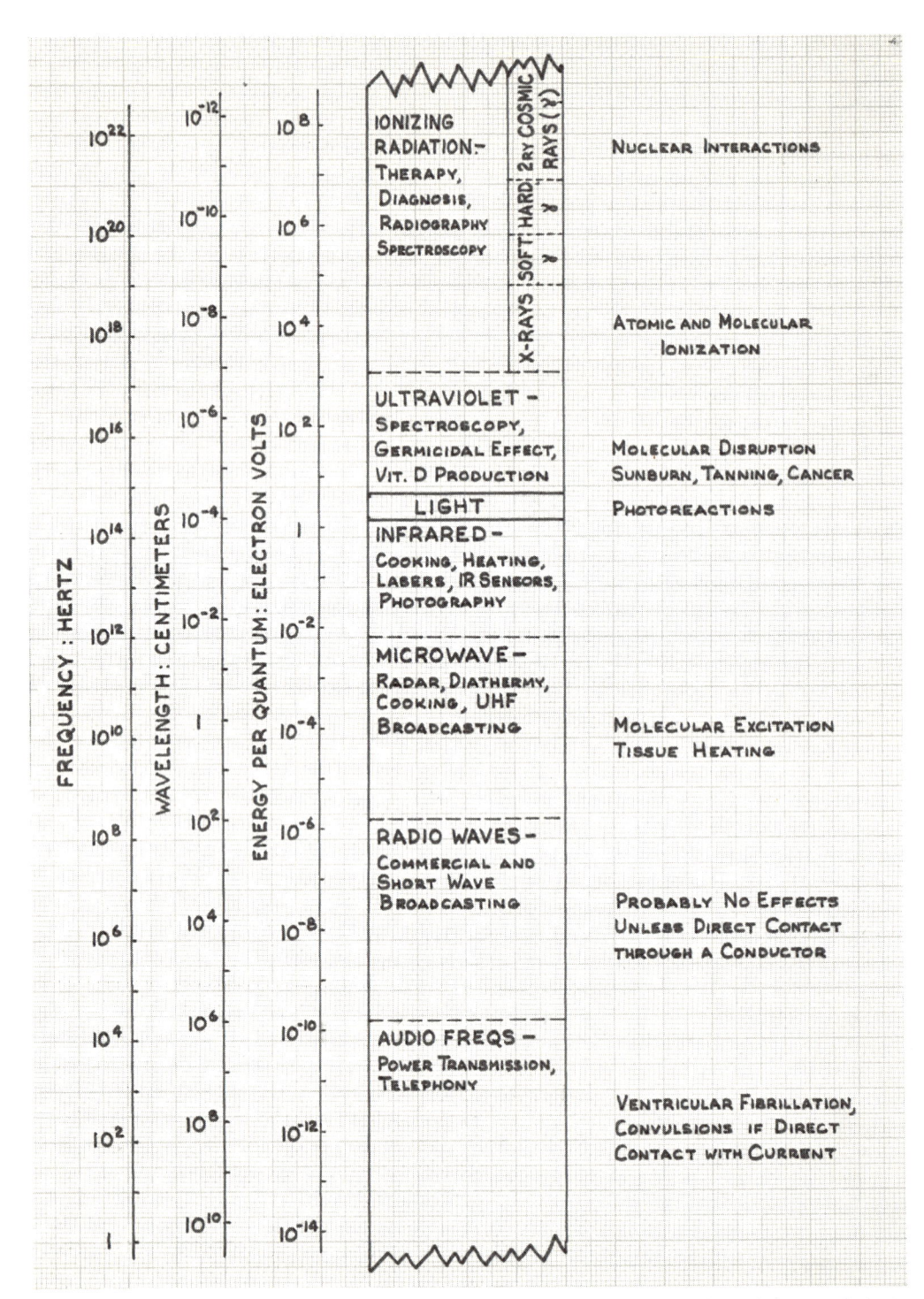

Figure 33-2 This chart shows the relationship between frequency, wavelength, and energy of electromagnetic waves, together with the commonly used division of the spectrum and comments on biological effects.

Electrical currents are used in electroconvulsive therapy of neurotic and psychotic depressive reactions. Currents of several hundred mA (60 Hz AC) passed transversely across the cerebrum produce momentary respiratory arrest and tonic, then clonic, convulsions, unconsciousness, and amnesia. Much smaller currents passed longitudinally through the brain stem produce severe physiologic respiratory arrest, often without other dysfunction or injury. It may be for this reason that recovery from accidental electrocution may occur after even protracted assisted ventilation. More severe shocks, as in legal electrocution, cause gross disruption of brain tissues and hemorrhage.

Electrical defibrillation of the heart can be lifesaving in cases of "spontaneous" ventricular fibrillation. It is generally agreed that direct currents are safer than alternating currents for this purpose. Most defibrillators make use of a condenser discharge at controlled levels. The energy delivered to the chest wall can be varied from 25 to several hundred watt-seconds (joules).

When an electric current is delivered to a tissue the resistance of which is high, a considerable proportion of the energy appears as heat. The resistance of the skin is usually much higher than that of the interior of the body; this is the reason for the often serious electrical burns at entrance and exit points, even when the current through the body has not caused permanent injury. Use is made of this in electrocautery, which is also used to coagulate small blood vessels during surgery. Controlled electrical coagulation of portions of the central nervous system has also been used, both experimentally and therapeutically.

It should be noted that both the rate at which heat energy is generated in a tissue and the rate at which it can be dissipated by conduction or by convective transfer in blood are equally important in determining whether irreversible denaturation of tissue proteins will occur. Poorly vascularized tissues in the body, such as the lens of the eye, are particularly susceptible to injury by electricity or other radiation which can cause rapid energy transfer. Lenticular cataracts have been produced by electrical currents as well as by infrared and microwave radiation.

Electromagnetic Waves; Radio Frequencies

The human body is essentially transparent to low-frequency electromagnetic waves. Waves of frequencies above 200 megahertz (MHz), however, are absorbed to an increasing degree by biological tissues. The energy thus absorbed appears as heat (molecular excitation). Such waves are encountered in ultra-high-frequency radio and television broadcasting, in which they are usually propagated omnidirectionally, and in Radar (*r*adio *d*etection *a*nd *r*anging), in which they are usually focused into a narrow beam by a parabolic antenna and reflector. Transmission may be continuous (CW) in broadcasting or pulsed (PW) in most radar applications. Microwave diathermy units, operating at about 2500 MHz, and microwave ovens, at similar frequencies, are usually CW devices, though some recent studies have suggested that PW devices may be more effective in diathermy.

A detailed description of this exceedingly broad band of radiation is beyond the scope of this review. Certain general principles can be stated, however. As frequency increases, penetration of these waves decreases in water or biological tissues; the radiation is absorbed, therefore, by a smaller cone of tissue and the local heating increases. For example, 1 joule transferred through 1 cm.^{2} of skin and absorbed in a depth of 1 cm. would yield the heat equivalent of 1 joule per cm.^{3}, whereas the same energy transfer at a higher frequency, absorbed in the top 1 mm. of skin, would yield the heat equivalent of 10 joules per cm.^{3}.

Since the body has temperature receptors only at its surface, it has no way of sensing the presence of low-frequency microwave energy, which passes into the body core. High-intensity fields at high frequencies, however, may be sensed as warmth or a burning sensation.

Microwave radiation is reflected by metals and to a lesser extent by earth. Metal screens can be used to protect persons working in microwave fields.

Some investigators in this area have reported effects of microwave radiation other than thermogenic effects. The most consistent findings have been in the hematopoietic system, though these reports are disputed by others. Interference with nerve conduction has also been reported.

There is little question that microwave radiation in large doses can cause cataracts. Reports of such lesions in industry have been rare, however, as have authentic reports of systemic injury caused by microwave radiation in general. Nonetheless, the introduction of microwave heating and cooking equipment into homes, with the attendant possibilities for misuse, warrant a degree of caution on the part of physicians. Microwave transmitters may also interfere with the function of cardiac pacemakers.

Infrared or Thermal Radiation

It is not possible to set a clear boundary between microwave and thermal, or infrared, radiation. As we have seen, tissue heating is produced by electromagnetic waves of much lower than infrared frequencies. Most authors place the boundary in the neighborhood of 10^6 MHz, or a wavelength of 3×10^7 Ångström units (A.U.).

Since thermal radiation is effectively absorbed

by the body, and since metabolism results in endogenous heat production, we must consider in some detail the physiopathology evoked by both excessive and insufficient heat.

It will be recalled that the human must maintain rather precise internal temperature control in the face of widely varying environmental temperatures and levels of heat production. Thermal inputs to the body come by radiation, convection, or conduction from the environment, and from metabolic heat production. Man can lose heat to his environment by radiation, convection, conduction, and evaporation of water or sweat. His range of tolerance for heat is remarkably narrow: if we consider him purely as a container of heat, his total heat content is in the neighborhood of 9000 Kilocalories (kcal.) but his tolerance for alterations in heat content is only about ± 150 kcal.

We shall look first at the systemic effects of heat, then its local effects. Cold, or insufficient heat, will be considered in the same way.

Heat. Acute Systemic Effects. Whenever man is exposed to heat stress, a number of systems respond in an effort to rid the body of the thermal load. Peripheral vasodilatation occurs; as peripheral resistance falls, heart rate and cardiac output increase. If temperature gradients between the skin and the surrounding air are adequate, convective heat dissipation increases enough to restore balance. If not, or if the thermal load is large, sweating occurs. Evaporation is an extremely effective method of heat dissipation because of the high latent heat of vaporization of water. For evaporation to occur, however, the air surrounding the body must have a vapor pressure below the saturation vapor pressure at skin temperature.

If these mechanisms for heat loss are not adequate to keep pace with the rate of heat input to the body, heat storage must occur; the core temperature will rise. A number of symptom complexes are seen when man encounters heat stress beyond his capacities.

Heat stroke is the most serious of these syndromes. Its presence is made known by anxiety, irritability, visual disturbances, delirium, collapse, coma, and death if treatment is inadequate. The skin is dry, hot, and flushed. The rectal temperature is very high (40 to 43° C.). Cessation of sweating in the presence of continued thermal stress, probably owing to failure of central thermoregulatory centers, allows a very rapid increase in the rate of heat storage.

Heat stroke constitutes a true medical emergency. Removal of the patient from the source of the heat stress followed by vigorous attempts to cool the body are the first measures to be instituted. Rapid cooling should be used, though it must be realized that skin cooling induces peripheral vasoconstriction, which inhibits conduction of core heat to the surface.

As the rectal and core temperature begin to fall, it becomes necessary to moderate treatment so that one does not induce hypothermia, for it must be realized that the thermoregulatory mechanisms which retain heat are also ineffective in protecting against cold. In essence, the therapist must take over the task of maintaining thermal homeostasis until the patient recovers that capacity. Persons who have had heat stroke may tolerate severe heat poorly thereafter, because of permanent damage in the thermoregulatory centers.

Heat exhaustion is characterized by weakness, hypotension and elevated temperature. The skin is not dry, however; the patient has often been sweating vigorously. The condition is probably caused by moderate dehydration and salt imbalance. Removal from heat and treatment with fluid and electrolytes (the intravenous route may be necessary if the patient is nauseated) usually produce prompt recovery. There are no sequelae.

Heat cramps are seen in unacclimatized subjects doing strenuous work in hot environments. These cramps are attributed to salt depletion. The oral administration of dilute salt solution, or intravenous administration of physiologic saline, produces dramatic relief. These symptoms can be prevented by acclimatization (see later).

Thermogenic anhidrosis has been observed in healthy, acclimatized subjects after a considerable period of heat exposure. Profuse sweating for a prolonged period suddenly terminates except on the face and neck. Patients complain of malaise, warmth, fatigue, shakiness, and lightheadedness. The rectal temperature is usually normal. The skin is dry. Severe prickly heat is invariably present. The cause of the disorder appears to be either physical obstruction or physiologic exhaustion of sweat glands. Treatment consists of rest and return to a cooler environment.

Chronic Systemic Effects. Even physically fit men cannot work long or strenuously when they are first exposed to a very hot environment. If, however, they are allowed to perform work of gradually increasing intensity during the first 1 to 2 weeks of exposure, their work tolerance increases markedly. A number of physiologic changes are observed in the course of this acclimatization process. The volume of sweat increases; its electrolyte concentration decreases. Heart rates at given work loads decrease sharply. Postural hypotension no longer occurs. Work tolerance approaches values previously obtained in cool environments. Water intake increases sharply, though thirst still is not an adequate guide for fluid replacement.

Acclimatization is impeded or reversed, once present, by fatigue, ingestion of alcohol, restriction of water, systemic illness, or temporary removal from exposure.

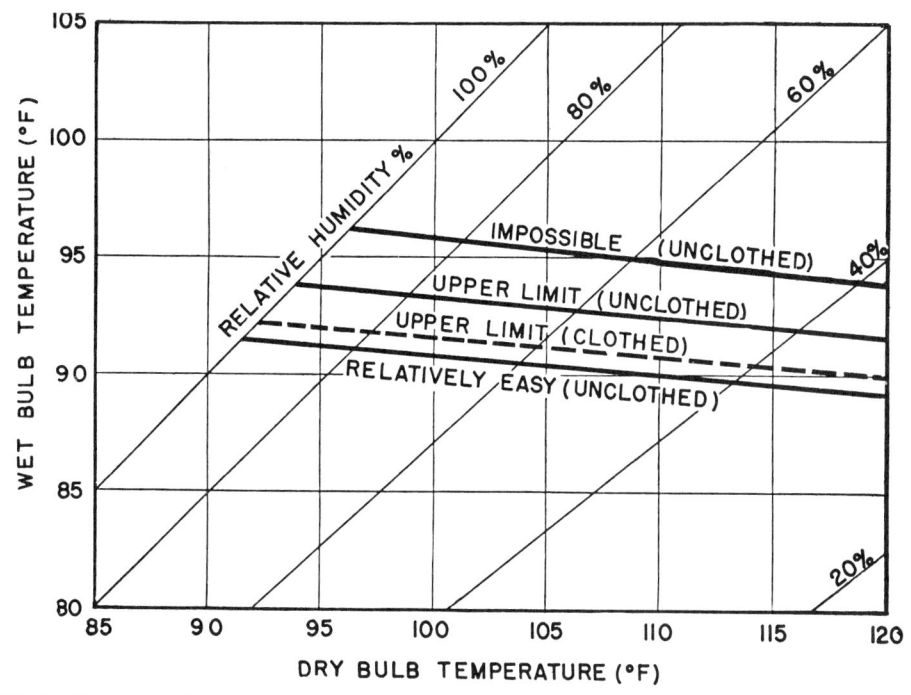

Figure 33-3 Diagram indicating equivalent zones of "impossible," difficult (upper limit), and relatively easy combinations of dry and wet bulb temperatures; the effect of relative humidity and of clothing on acclimatized men working for 4 hours at an energy expenditure of about 300 calories per hour. (From Largent and Ashe, 1958.)

Tolerance for work in hot environments has been studied by many authors. The data shown in Figure 33-3 are representative.

LOCAL EFFECTS. It has been noted repeatedly here that the radiant energy transferred to a volume of tissue, relative to the capacity of that tissue and its perfusing blood to remove heat, will determine whether heat storage and a temperature rise will occur. Most human proteins are easily denatured by heat; thus, the thermal capacity of living tissue is rather small.

If the rate of heat input to the skin is high, local heating occurs. Histamine and other vasodilator substances are released, producing erythema. If the temperature rises further, local vesication occurs. If the temperature continues to rise, coagulation necrosis of the germinal epithelium results and the skin will slough. At still higher temperatures, charring is observed. This, in brief, is the sequence seen when the skin is burned. The relationship between the rate of energy input and duration of input is logarithmic.

The secondary and tertiary adjustments in fluid and electrolyte balance which occur following burns of considerable extent are beyond the scope of this survey. References to recent reviews of the topic will be found at the end of this chapter.

There is evidence that increases in the temperature of the testes in man inhibit spermatogenesis. This is thought to be one of the reasons why spermatogenesis is inhibited in an undescended testicle. Increases in testicular temperature may also increase the rate of "spontaneous" mutations in the germinal cells, though the quantum energies in this portion of the electromagnetic spectrum are very low.

Infrared Radiation: Effects on the Eye. The cornea is virtually transparent to the highest portion of the IR spectrum (wavelengths shorter than 19,000 A.U.). The crystalline lens has a similar but not identical transmissibility characteristic; it becomes increasingly transparent at wavelengths shorter than 15,000 A.U.

There is, therefore, a range of wavelengths in the high infrared portion of the spectrum for which the cornea and aqueous are more transparent than the lens. As a result, heating of the lens occurs, both directly and secondarily as a result of absorption of the same wavelengths by the iris.

The industrial phenomenon now known as "glass-blower's cataract" was described in the 18th century. Since that time, many workers have studied these lesions and have established conclusively that they are caused by thermal radiation rather than by light, as was first thought. The cataracts typically begin to form at the posterior pole of the lens and develop slowly after months or years of exposure to intense thermal radiation from industrial furnaces or other similar sources. Similar lesions would likely be produced by lasers radiating at appropriate wavelengths.

Normal Thermal Environments for Man. Much research has been done on the limits of environmental comfort for man under various conditions of activity. Since comfort is a subjective phenomenon, most of this research has necessarily made use of subjective indices. A unit of thermal insulation has been developed, the clo, which is "the amount of insulation necessary to maintain comfort in a seated, resting subject in a normally ventilated room (air movement 20 ft. per min. or 10 cm. per sec.) at a temperature of 70° F. (21° C.) and a relative humidity of the air of less than 50 per cent." For American men and women wearing 1 clo of insulation, thermal comfort ranges are 70 to 85° F. (21 to 29° C.).

As environmental temperature falls, man's thermal environment begins to require him to cope with an inadequate thermal input. We call this *cold*.

Cold. SYSTEMIC EFFECTS. In general, where man faces, lives with, and can acclimatize to heat, he tends to avoid or circumvent the effects of cold. Man has only a limited number of ways of coping with the lack of environmental heat; in the course of evolution, he has lost many of the mechanisms available to other mammals.

Man can increase his insulation somewhat by peripheral vasoconstriction: skin temperature drops and skin-environment gradients decrease. If cold air is flowing by the skin, however, convective losses are still considerable. The thick blanket of hair and the piloerector mechanisms of our mammalian cousins have long since been lost to man, as has the ability to vasoconstrict the rich blanket of scalp vessels in response to cold.

We do retain the ability to increase our rate of heat production, either by moving muscles in doing work or by shivering. We can also increase our effective insulation blanket by wearing clothing. The disadvantage of clothing is that the amount of insulation necessary to maintain comfort at rest is entirely too much when strenuous work is performed. Also, the insulating value of clothing is considerably reduced as it becomes wetted by sweat. It is thus necessary to maintain air flow over the skin to aid in evaporation while such work is being performed.

When man is unable to maintain thermal balance, his core temperature begins to drop. Severe shivering and exhaustion induced by voluntary work give way to profound feelings of lassitude and an overwhelming desire to sleep. More prolonged exposure causes continued body cooling and usually death by ventricular fibrillation when the cardiac temperature reaches 27° C., though survival has been reported after rapid rewarming of humans whose core temperature was as low as 18° C.

Just as rapidly moving air removes heat from a warm object more rapidly than still air, so water, with its high specific heat, removes heat from the body very much more rapidly than air. Immersion in water at near-freezing temperature renders a man incapable of helping himself within a very few minutes and is usually fatal in less than an hour, whereas he will survive in still air at this temperature for many hours.

LOCAL EFFECTS. When an extremity or other body part with the exception of the scalp is exposed to cold, piloerection ("goose pimples") and vasoconstriction occur. As the skin temperature approaches 0° C., metabolic needs are maintained for a time; pain in the area gives way to numbness. Thereafter, edema and blistering may appear. Gangrene, with or without infection, will occur if the part is allowed to remain cold; if rapid rewarming is instituted, permanent injury is minimized, though the part may be painful for a considerable time. If cell disruption due to formation of ice crystals has occurred, permanent disability of some degree is likely. This is the picture of *frostbite*.

Exposure of extremities (most often the feet) to cold, wet environments gives rise to a related disorder known as *trench foot* or shelter foot. In this condition, actual tissue freezing is rare, but tissue maceration may be extreme, and permanen disability is not uncommon.

There is some evidence that local adaptation to cold may occur, especially in the hands. Massey's data suggest that such adaptation proceeds over a period of perhaps seven weeks. Other studies indicate that there may be seasonal fluctuations in hand blood flow in cold climates, larger flows being observed in the coldest seasons.

Visible Radiation: Light

The narrow band of electromagnetic waves lying between 7.7 and 3.8×10^8 MHz (wavelengths between about 3900 and 7700 A.U.) has an importance to man out of all proportion to its miniscule contribution to the total energy flux within the universe. It is important because our eyes can sense this band; visible radiation illuminates our world and thus gives us the mobility which has made us what we are. No less important, it is a portion of this band which provides the specific energy levels required for photosynthesis, the basic source of all our nutritive needs.

The physiology of the eye is adequately described in textbooks; it will be alluded to only briefly here. More important in terms of pathologic physiology are the tolerable range of light intensities and man's efforts to adapt to levels outside this range.

The human retina has two types of sensors: rods, or scotopic sensors, and cones, or photopic sensors. The rods are found in greatest numbers at distances of about 10 degrees from the center of the fovea; their numbers remain relatively constant for a considerable distance toward the periphery. There are no rods at the center of the fovea, however, where cone cells are found in greatest density.

The rod cells in the completely dark-adapted eye have a threshold on the order of 5×10^{-6} millilamberts (mL.). Cones reach their maximum acuity at illumination intensities above 10^5 mL. The retina's visual range is thus at least 10 orders of magnitude.

After prolonged exposure to bright light, the retinal sensors require a finite time to become maximally adapted to low levels of light. It is presumed that this adaptation time reflects the time necessary for complete regeneration of the photosensitive pigments within the sensors. Cone cells reach maximum sensitivity (0.001 to 0.01 mL.) within 6 to 8 minutes, whereas the more sensitive rods require about 30 minutes of darkness (or of dim red light, to which they are insensitive) to reach maximum sensitivity (less than 0.00001 mL.). Many environmental and endogenous factors influence these values; the effect of hypoxia has been mentioned, as an instance.

The eye and brain can perceive, though not in fine detail, objects illuminated by starlight. Given this incredible sensitivity, it is fair to ask whether this sensing mechanism is damaged by complete darkness: by the total absence of light.

If one eye of certain mammals is covered for even a few days or weeks during early postnatal development, there is an almost complete shift of ocular dominance to the contralateral eye. These effects appear to be permanent. Although comparable data are not available for man, Weisel suggests that a child whose eye is covered for a short period during the critical phase of postnatal central nervous system development may well end up with a permanent visual defect in that eye. The initial period in monkeys is the first 6 weeks of life; it may well be longer in man.

At the other end of the range of light intensities, we must consider the effects of exceedingly intense levels of illumination. The luminance of a nuclear fireball viewed from 4 miles away may exceed 10^8 mL.; the sun, viewed from earth, has a luminance of 4×10^8 mL. In evaluating the effects of those intensities, we must consider two factors peculiar to visible radiation and the eye. First, the cornea, aqueous, lens, and vitreous are all relatively transparent to electromagnetic waves in the visible band. Second, and perhaps more important, the eye is not merely a sensing system; it focuses a point source of light on the retina. For this reason, very intense light sources concentrate their energy on a very small area of the retina and choroid, where pigment absorbs nearly all visible radiation which reaches it. Thus, nearly all the energy incident upon this small area is converted to heat, in amounts which very rapidly produce irreversible changes in the affected cells.

Retinal burns from solar, nuclear, or laser radiation produce permanent visual field defects or blind spots. If these are in the periphery, they represent no great problem. Unfortunately, it is also "only human" to look directly toward the source of intense light, which focuses the radiation directly on the fovea. The central field defect thus produced severely limits the visual acuity of the eye—or of both eyes—thereafter, because acuity rapidly declines at angular distances of even a few degrees from the fovea. Eclipse blindness, caused by viewing solar eclipses through inadequate filters, is a form of this lesion. Even the image of the solar corona, still visible at the moment of total eclipse, is bright enough to cause such burns.

Lasers (*L*ight *a*mplification by *s*timulated *e*mission of *r*adiation) represent a special hazard. Because the energy emitted by these devices is coherent (all of one frequency), there is almost no beam divergence, and unbelievably energetic pulses of radiation can be generated. These can literally vaporize any matter not transparent to them. The increasing use of such devices in science, industry, and military applications multiplies the hazards to which workers, or troops, may be subjected.

Ultraviolet Radiation

Visible radiation is energetic enough to trigger photosynthesis, as well as a variety of oxidative reactions in inorganic chemicals. Since the energy content of radiation is directly proportional to its frequency, the ultraviolet band (wavelengths from roughly 3900 to 1000 A.U.) contains increasingly energetic radiation, whose energies are powerful enough to disrupt various types of intramolecular chemical bonds. Indeed, the considerable germicidal effectiveness of UV is due to its ability to disrupt the helical structure of DNA.

Fortunately, earth's atmosphere absorbs nearly all the very considerable flux of ultraviolet radiation which reaches it. Wavelengths shorter than 2400 A.U. are strongly absorbed by molecular oxygen, with the production of ozone in the upper atmosphere. Ozone itself absorbs all UV radiation shorter than 2900 A.U. and some of that between 2900 and 3200 A.U. Water vapor and dust in the troposphere absorb more, so that the flux of ultraviolet light at the earth's surface is very small. Nonetheless, enough reaches us to cause a variety of physiologic and pathologic effects. In the former category, we may place the conversion of provitamin D to vitamin D; in the latter, the production of sunburn and tanning.

Vitamin D is produced in the human epidermis from 7-dehydrocholesterol by ultraviolet radiation in the 2900 to 3200 A.U. band (see p. 856). Since little UV reaches the surface of the earth when the sun is less than 20 degrees above the horizon (owing to atmospheric scattering), it is clear that people living in the high north latitudes may be at risk of vitamin D deficiency for a substantial part of each year. This is especially true in industrial urban areas, where air pollution by dust is considerable and where people may have little exposure to sunlight. In these days of vitamin D-supplemented milk, one seldom recalls how serious a problem rickets was and for how long.

Sunburn is produced by ultraviolet light in the band of 2900 to 3200 A.U., though large doses of radiation longer than 3200 A.U. do produce erythema. After a latent period of up to several hours following exposure, cutaneous blood vessels dilate, with resultant erythema over the exposed area, and discomfort and pain. The erythema reaches a peak between 8 and 24 hours following exposure and then gradually fades. If the burn is severe, vesiculation may occur, followed after a variable time by desquamation. A suntan of variable degree replaces the burn. Adaptation of the skin to repeated UV exposure occurs, manifested by deposition of melanin in the skin, though other adaptive mechanisms may be involved as well.

It should be emphasized that these signs are manifestations of injury to the dermis. Increases in mitotic activity are seen as desquamation takes place, together with marked thickening of the Malpighian layer of the epidermis. The relationship between such changes and the eventual development of cancers is not known, though it is clear that repeated sunburn causes degenerative changes in both dermis and epidermis. It has also been shown, both experimentally in animals and by epidemiologic studies in man, that ultraviolet radiation in the 2800 to 3150 A.U. band does produce skin cancer.

Ionizing Radiation*

The Nature of Ionizing Radiation. Even while the primordial cosmic gases were condensing to form the earth, radioactive decay of atomic nuclei was taking place, as it does today. Thus even before man's "recent" appearance, these spontaneous changes occurring within atomic nuclei were emitting particulates (alpha, beta) or photons (gamma) of an energetic nature. A geometric increase in possible sources of ionizing radiation occurred with the technological applications that followed the discovery and isolation of radium by the Curies. A further quantum increase in this potential for human exposure ensued as a result of the harnessing of atomic energy stemming from nuclear weapon technology. With further application of this Promethean reproduction of solar energetics to meet the energy demands of man, the potential for ionizing radiation exposure can predictably be expected to develop apace.

Exposure of man can take place either through externally encountered ionizing radiation or through absorption of radioactive elements in the form of radionuclides which enter the body. The former event will produce consequences dependent solely upon the basis of the specific physical nature of such radiation. The latter occurrence, internal deposition, will produce specific biological effects which are dependent upon metabolic handling of the specific radionuclide, since the course of such elements through the body proceeds without regard by the organism for the unstable nature of the element. That is, although ^{24}Na will produce both beta and gamma radiation, the body "sees" such atoms only as sodium per se. Hence, this radioactive sodium will distribute itself through the body as any sodium molecule, i.e., to a greater extent in the extracellular rather than intracellular compartment. Accordingly, understanding of the effects of absorbed radiation (as radionuclides) will depend upon knowledge of the metabolic handling of the element in question. The duration of possible effects within the body can be seen to extend from short-lived effects stemming from ^{24}Na (half-life in the body = 15 hours) absorption which distributes itself widely, to the other extreme in the case of strontium 90, which is deposited in bone and but slowly turned over, i.e., half-life in the body = 5700 days.

Physical Aspects of Ionizing Radiation. Regardless of whether radiation impinges upon the body externally or internally, knowledge of the physical properties of the various forms of either particulate or photon produced ionizing radiation is necessary for understanding radiobiological effects. The major particulate types of radiation are:

Alpha Particles — Identical to a helium nucleus in atomic structure, these have relatively high masses which can produce severe cellular disruption because of their vigorous ionizing effects. However, such particulates have relatively short ranges, and even the most energetic fail to penetrate past the stratum corneum of the skin. Hence, the greatest danger results from internal deposition where metabolically active cells are intimately in association with elements producing this type of radiation.

Beta Particles — Identical to electrons, these may be associated with negative or positive charges. Although they have less ionizing poten-

---

*This section was written by Bertram D. Dinman.

past 25 years permits a high degree of predictability of clinical response.

The degree of injury being dependent upon the amount of radiation incurred, one can clinically describe a dose-derived spectrum of response. Although the acute radiation syndrome has been described as demonstrating the cerebral, gastrointestinal, or hematopoietic form, in actuality this syndrome consists of combinations of such "target-organ" effects. It has been suggested that on the basis of dose one can expect five injury groups, which are as follows:

Group I: Most patients are asymptomatic, while a few have minimal prodromal symptoms; dose = less than 150 rads.*

Group II: Mild form of the acute radiation syndrome, associated with transient prodromal nausea and vomiting, with mild clinical and laboratory evidence of hematopoietic alteration; dose = 200 to 400 rads.

Group III: Serious effects associated with complications of severe hematopoietic damage and some evidence of gastrointestinal alteration; dose = 400 to 600 rads.

Group IV: Accelerated version of the acute disorder dominated by complications of gastrointestinal injury. Length of survival is determined by the severity of gastrointestinal damage; dose = 600 to 1400 rads.

Group V: Fulminating course with severe central nervous system manifestations; dose = greater than 2000 rads.

Figures 33–5 to 33–8 summarize the various dose responses in terms of clinical manifestations, history, and duration of effects. All these groups pass through four clinical stages which will now be described.

CLINICAL STAGE 1 – INITIAL OR PRODROMAL STAGE. Regardless of dose, the psychological concomitants of a known exposure may tend to obscure the pathologic significance of events in this stage. With this in mind, it can be stated in general that the earlier the onset of signs and symptoms, the higher the likely dose. Thus, if no nausea and vomiting occur within the first few hours, the patient is more likely in Group I, whereas in Groups II and III these symptoms occur within one hour of exposure. By contrast, in Groups IV and V, there is rapid onset of diarrhea, ataxia, disorientation, coma, and shock. The earlier this occurs, i.e., within the first hour, the more likely it is that the patient has been exposed to an overwhelming dose, i.e., Group V.

By the first 6 to 8 hours postexposure, the prodromal symptoms reach their maximum. During this time, Group III, IV, and V patients show weakness and fatigue, conjunctivitis, sweating, and paresthesias; these symptoms can be severe among those in Groups IV and V.

Finally, within 24 to 48 hours, Groups I and II show a subsidence of symptoms; Group III shows tailing off; Groups IV and V will merge without a latent period into the manifest illness. Group V patients having suffered massive exposures, e.g., greater than 10,000 rads, may rapidly progress through stages 2 and 3 in as short a time as hours or as long as half a day.

CLINICAL STAGE 2 – LATENT PERIOD. In both Groups I and V there may be no latent period. In the former, there are no symptoms that follow the prodrome, while in Group V fever, profuse sweating, insomnia, disorientation, cardiovascular shock, watery diarrhea and vomiting, and coma may continue unabated.

In those groups exposed to intermediate doses of ionizing radiation, the latent asymptomatic period – except for weakness and fatigue – reflects the dose. Thus, for Group II, the latent period is 2 to 3 weeks, while for Groups III and IV there is a shorter asymptomatic interval of 5 to 14 days.

CLINICAL STAGES 3 AND 4 – MANIFEST ILLNESS AND RECOVERY. Group I patients continue to be asymptomatic. An early lymphocytic elevation may be seen, but otherwise little abnormality in any parameter appears in this group. By contrast, the hematopoietic manifestations in Group II occur in a mild to moderate degree. After a latent period, chills, fever, weight loss, fatigue, and epilation are seen. The latter has an apparent threshold of 350 rads, while the loss of hair is complete with single doses of 450 to 600 rads. However, beta radiation alone may produce this effect. Hematopoietic damage is manifest by pharyngitis, secondary infections of the upper respiratory tract, melena, hematuria, gingival bleeding, and mild purpura. Forty to 50 days after exposure, clinical manifestations begin to remit, with convalescence beginning between 2 and 3 months after the exposure. Although some weakness may persist, clinical recovery is apparent within 6 months.

Group III patients show similar manifestations of a hematopoietic nature as those in Group II. However, the onset of these changes as well as the other associated clinical alterations is more rapid, i.e., within 12 to 18 days postexposure. Furthermore, the degree of sign and symptom alteration is more severe. Accordingly, the patient demonstrates a marked depression of platelets and leukocytes.

In addition, within one month after exposure gastrointestinal damage becomes manifest. A severe, bloody diarrhea, progressively worse abdominal pain, hematemesis, and hematuria with oliguria supervene. Between 25 and 40 days, despite vigorous measures, death may occur preceded by profound shock and coma.

(Text continued on page 940.)

---

*Rad = unit of absorbed dose, expressed in terms of amount of energy absorbed per unit of tissue; 1 rad = 100 ergs per gram.

Figure 33–5 Group II exposure (200 to 400 rads).

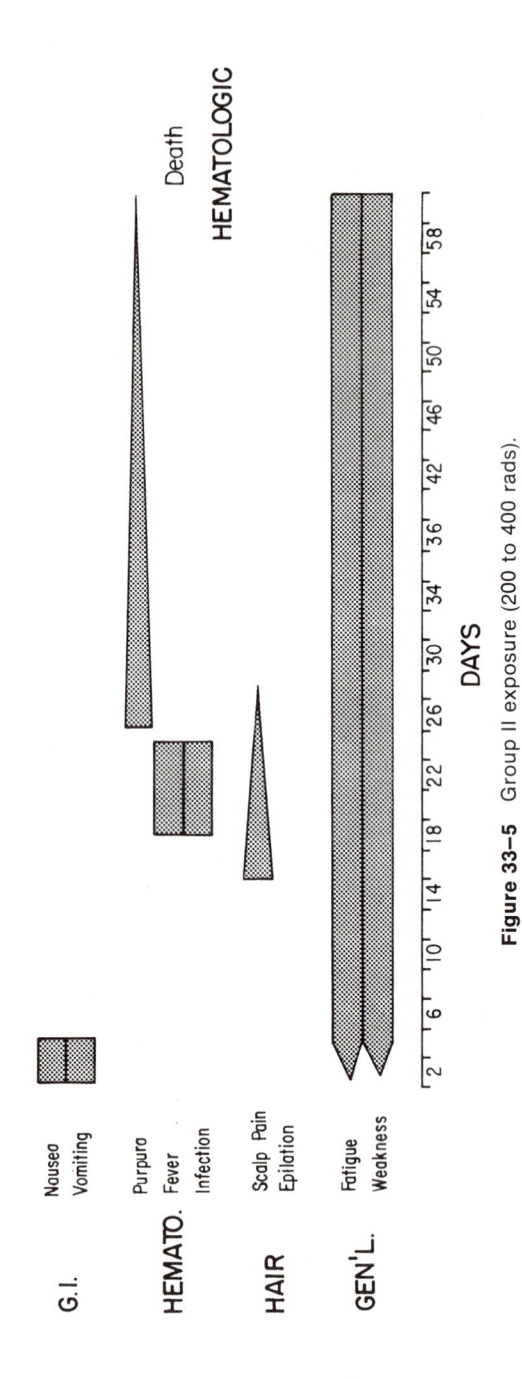

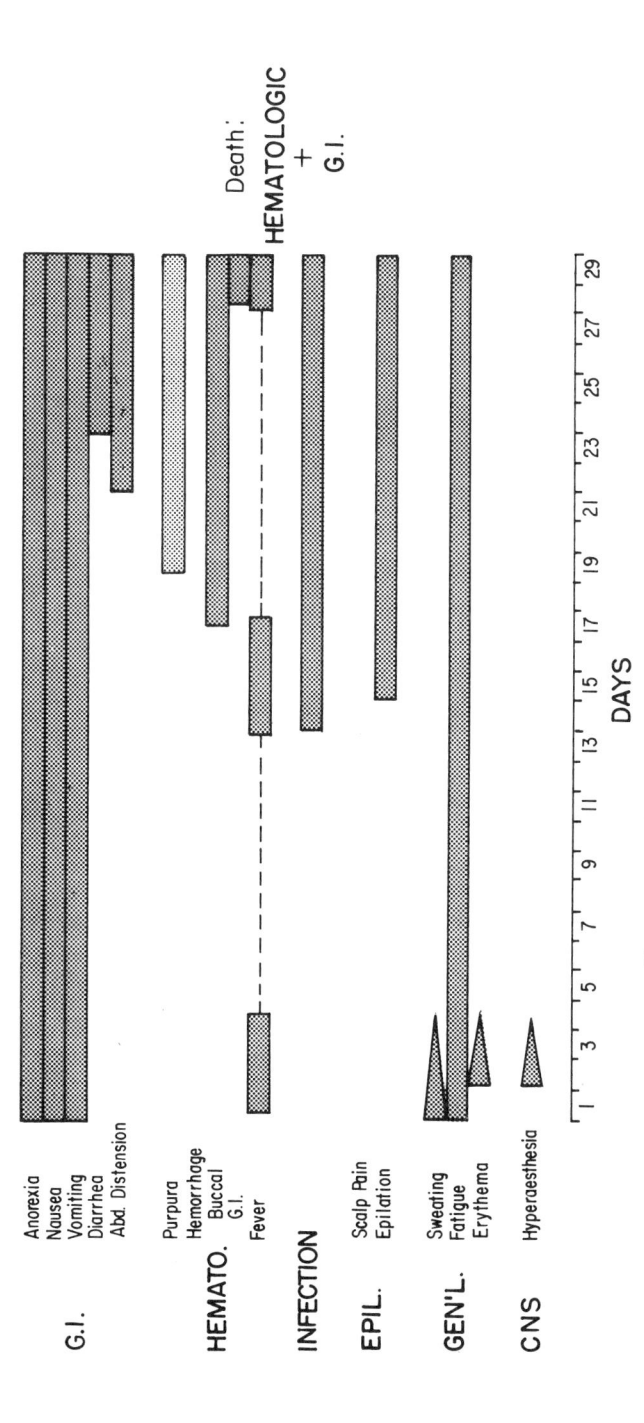

Figure 33-6 Group III exposure (400 to 600 rads).

Figure 33–7 Group IV exposure (600 to 1400 rads).

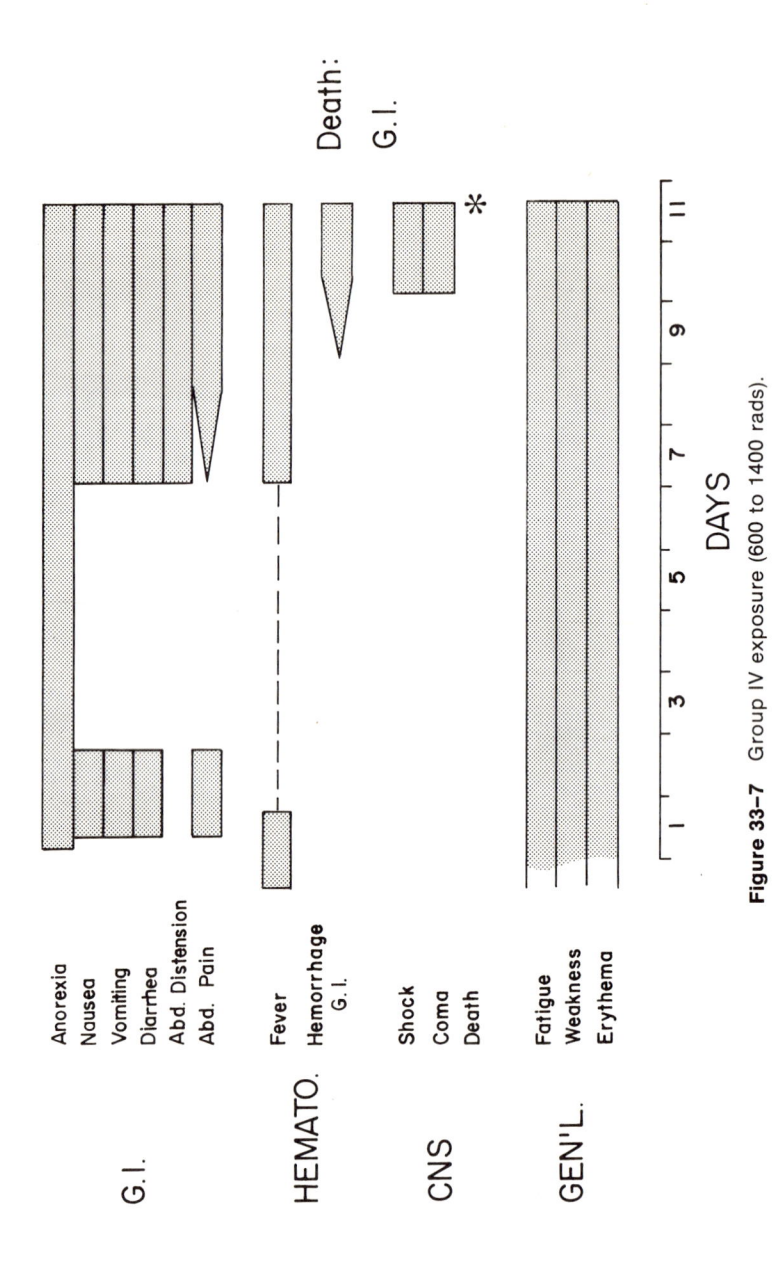

EFFECTS OF PHYSICAL AGENTS

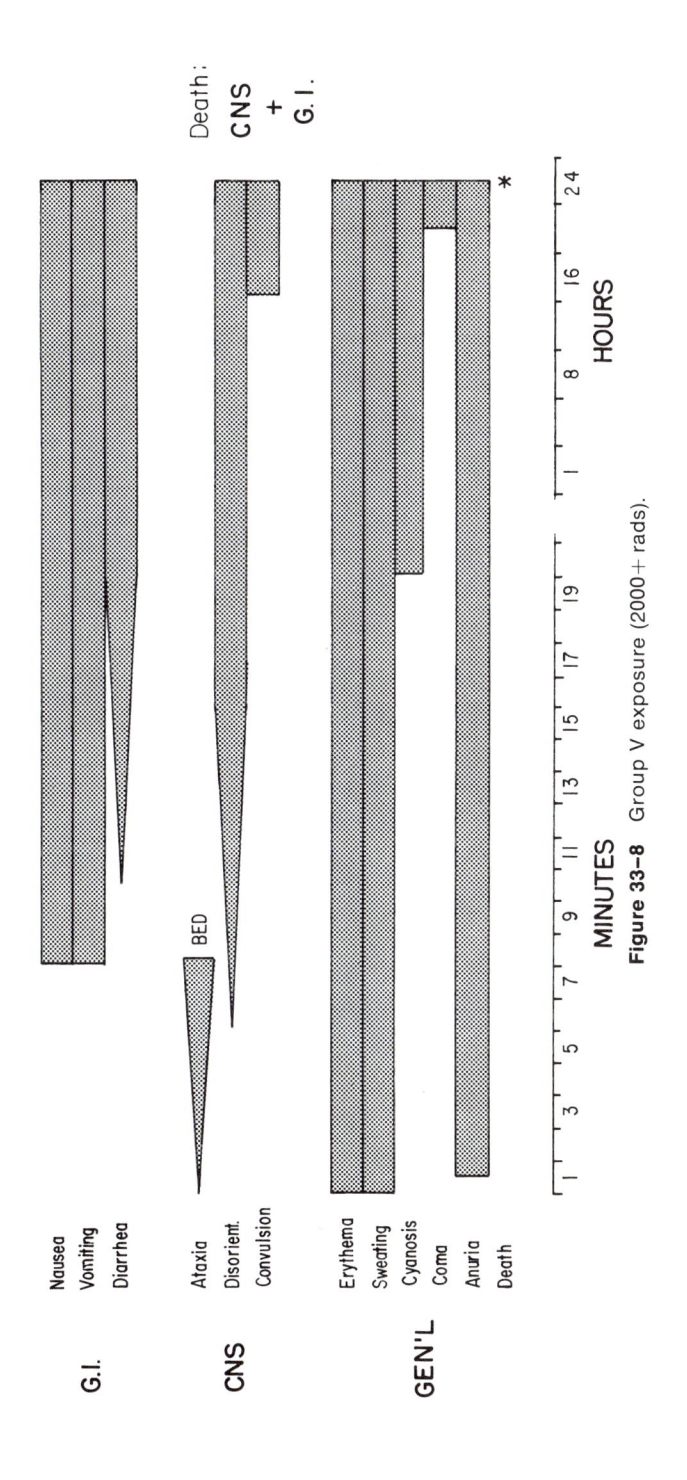

Figure 33-8 Group V exposure (2000+ rads).

Group IV patients usually run an abbreviated course of some 15 to 30 days. Since gastrointestinal symptoms occur early, the patient may not survive sufficiently long for the hematopoietic response to be seen. However, pancytopenia developing within the first week may combine with gastrointestinal damage to produce a hemorrhagic gastroenteritis, melena, and extreme prostration. Despite vigorous measures, these patients usually die 15 to 30 days after exposure with all the gastrointestinal signs and symptoms noted previously but in a more severe form.

Group V patients demonstrate the rapid downhill course previously mentioned. Since the late hematologic changes are not seen, the clinical manifestations revolve about gastrointestinal and central nervous system damage. Thus, mental incapacitation, shown by ataxia, incoherence, hyperventilation, and disorientation, and vomiting, diarrhea, and abdominal cramps occur within the first hour or two following exposure. While a brief interlude of mental coherence may intervene, the usual course is rapid and inexorably downhill, regardless of treatment.

Therapeutic Principles. From the foregoing it can be seen that doses in the range producing a gastrointestinal syndrome (Groups III and IV) pose severe if not insuperable problems. Whereas measures designed to replace blood elements are feasible, no therapeutic resources are available for the correction of the gastrointestinal defect. Thus, the ineffectiveness or unavailability of remedial measures reflects the 50 per cent mortality rate in this range of dosage, while lethality is probably inevitable at 800 to 1000 rad levels.

Group I patients, by contrast, can be followed as outpatients, with the extent of rest and clinical supervision dependent upon the individual's physical and psychological reactions.

Group II or higher patients require hospitalization. Measures directed toward protection against effects of leukopenia (e.g., infection) and thrombocytopenia (bleeding phenomenon) are indicated. For the former, antibiotics, strict antisepsis, and isolation are required; hemorrhages may require enriched plasma or platelet transfusions for temporary relief. Blood transfusions are useful. Homologous bone marrow transplants have been useful for as long as a month after exposure in tiding the patient over the period of blood cell element depletion.

Radiation by Beta and Electron Beams. Whereas external gamma and/or neutron radiation is capable of producing internal body change, radiation produced by beta or linear accelerators usually produces change restricted to skin depth. Furthermore, because the beams produced are usually narrow, damage is frequently localized.

The net effect is the production of a local burn, similar in appearance and clinical course to a thermal burn. As in the case of severe local burns from any cause, a systemic reaction may be seen. However, some of the features of the acute radiation syndrome may occur.

Internal Deposition of Radionuclides. In general, alpha emitters are found in the naturally occurring radioactive elements (U, Th, Ac) and in association with the artificially produced transuranic elements. Most other radionuclides emit beta radiations, while some others also produce gamma. Although not usually hazardous outside the body (except when daughter products may be gamma emitters), such radionuclides when ingested in the gastrointestinal tract in chemically soluble forms may be absorbed and distributed systemically. Even more serious consequences may ensue when such materials are inhaled, since even the insoluble forms may be trapped in the lungs; the inspired soluble compounds can be absorbed and widely distributed throughout the body. Thus, irradiation of pulmonary lymph nodes and lung tissue occurs following the former occurrence, or distribution to various organs will result from the uptake of the short-range but intensely ionizing alpha emissions.

In general, radiation hazards associated with internal deposition depend largely upon the physical properties (e.g., half-life, decay mode, radiation produced) and the metabolic pathway in the body (e.g., critical organs, biological half-life). The chemical characteristics, route of entry, and quantity entering the body also determine damage potentials.

The physical half-life will determine how long radioactive emission occurs; this may be as short as 37 minutes (^{38}Cl) or as long as 16.4 million years (^{129}I). Equally important in determining how long an absorbed nuclide may exert an effect in the body is the concept of "biological half-life." For example, 50 per cent of the molecules presented in a dose of iodine will within 20 to 50 days have been taken up, incorporated in various thyroid products which eventually will be degraded, and excreted from the body. All molecules that enter the body economy will have a metabolic turnover rate which may be referred to in terms of "biological half-life," i.e., the time necessary for 50 per cent of the molecules taken up to have been incorporated into various cellular components and be excreted following the usual degradation and replacement of such body components. Thus, by combining the "physical half-life" and the "biological half-life" one can mathematically calculate an "effective half-life" which is the product of these two functions. This expression thus considers both physical radiation half-life and rate of biological turnover in defining the duration of risk from absorbed radionuclides.

In addition to biological properties determining how long a radioactive element remains in the body, these biological characteristics also determine which organs will selectively absorb them. The concentration in these "selective" organs will vary with time. It can be clearly seen that a complete time dependent description of the passage of radionuclides through the body is complex. By sampling the various body products and fluids some estimations can be made of radionuclide burdens. While this is feasible (by whole-body counting) for gamma emitters, radioanalysis of breath, blood, urine, feces, or tissue may be necessary for determination of body burden in the case of alpha- or beta-emitting radionuclides.

The ability to take therapeutic action is limited by the ability to "selectively" remove specific elements from the body. Aside from permitting natural turnover to run its course, use of chelating agents (EDTA, DPTA) have been advocated to achieve this end. More recently, pulmonary lavage has been used immediately after inhalation of radionuclides to limit the absorbed dose.

Delayed Radiation Effects

Whereas the immediate effects of acute ionizing injury in man are dramatic and clearly defined, the consequences which may follow long after acute radiation or repeated small doses are less readily apparent. Indeed, attributing such effects to radiation becomes difficult, since most of such delayed effects are due to unknown causes, e.g., aging, cancer, cataracts.

Local Irradiation and Delayed Effects. There is evidence which appears to indict whole body radiation as being a more effective inducer of life-span shortening than local radiation. However, cataracts may result from local lenticular radiation, although fractionation of dose appears to both decrease their size and retard their onset. It has been estimated that clinically significant cataracts are produced by 600 to 1000 rads to the eye. The mechanism causing such change is not known.

Other delayed effects have some elements which suggest a common mechanistic denominator. For example, delayed but ultimate parenchymal cell destruction is usually associated with degenerative changes in the vascular bed. Thus, the skin changes which occur late after exposure are characterized by atrophy of the epithelial cells and the dermal appendages, although local hypertrophy of skin may also occur. As is the case with whole body irradiation, changes are seen in the vascular bed; this later may be manifest by either scarring and sclerosis or compensatory hypertrophy of local vascular tissues resulting in telangiectasia. In addition, as a consequence of local irradiation of the kidneys, arterionephrosclerosis and resultant hypertension may eventually occur; similarly in the lung progressive fibrosis and vascular sclerosis ensue.

Whole Body Radiation and Late Effects. One of the most difficult late effects to verify in man is that of shortening of life span. The evidence is quite strong in experimental animals exposed to fast neutrons; the life-shortening is essentially linear from the lowest measurable dose. Similarly, the longevity of radiologists in past years, when compared to life spans of other specialists at no special risk, strongly suggests a life-shortening effect resulting from prolonged exposure to relatively small doses of ionizing radiation.

As described in the section on radiobiology (see earlier) the critical target organelles are those in which one finds DNA. With the occurrence of interactions these centers of cellular control—both of ongoing metabolic function as well as of replication and organization—are affected. Such structural-chemical effects may be immediate, but if these changes are small they may not be immediately expressed. Rather, each minimal insult, being cumulative, may not be expressed in the cell until generations of accumulating defects are incurred. Although the germ cells are especially vulnerable targets, effects in somatic cells some generations later are also equally possible. Such resulting rearrangements of genetic material are probably permanent, although autorepair of DNA has recently been described. However, the great majority of reorganized mutations do not appear to reverse themselves and are generally believed to be deleterious.

The net results will be found among a whole range of effects under genetic control (e.g., life span, birth weight, fertility, intelligence). How much of an increase in radiation burden is needed to double the present rate of inheritable defects is not known. Certainly, given omnipresent natural radiation background, it is some figure greater than the 3 rads incurred over a generation (30 years) because of such background.

Radiation Carcinogenesis. Many years of uncontrolled radiation among the early roentgenologists have produced numerous end results. The skin cancers have been obvious; the demonstration that leukemia was a consequence of such exposure followed much later. Finally, similar results, i.e., leukemia, emerged among survivors of the atomic bombarding of Hiroshima and Nagasaki. The result of ^{223}Ra absorption and bone deposition with later development of osteosarcoma have been extensively documented. The thyroid adenocarcinoma appearing in later life following childhood irradiation of the neck; and the lung tumors among uranium miners in Colorado and Schneeburg (Joachimstal) exposed to radium daughter products also attest to the carcinogenic potential of ionizing radiation. In each of these instances the dose required to produce such results has been estimated; whether a threshold for carcinogenic effect exists and what it might be are open to question. Such questions are probably not susceptible to a ready answer, since if by chance a single ionizing event occurred at *the* appropriate locus in *one* cell in any individual, any consequent malignant change could not be statistically detected. Obviously, while a "single" hit could occur, the statistical probability for detecting such a consequence becomes attainable only as more events—in more people—occur. Accordingly, with the necessity for more "hits" to occur, estimates of thresholds for effect become inflated. Thus, in the final analysis, present approaches which depend upon statistical bases for resolution of the problem of thresholds for radiation effects are inadequate to answer these questions.

THE KINETIC ENVIRONMENT

In a previous section, we referred to man's mobility as one of the attributes which has made him what he is. In his constant attempts to master and control his environment, man has found mobility to be an absolute essential since earliest times. He cannot synthesize glucose from readily available simpler compounds; he must therefore search out plants which do so. He is puny, compared to some of the animal predators (including his fellow man), so he must be able to flee from them. He reproduces rapidly; crowding and his own desire to know the unknown have led him to explore his entire planet, and recently to go even beyond its confines.

Movement requires work—kinetic energy. To understand man with respect to his physical environment, we must understand how he is affected by force fields, either natural or of his own making. That is the purpose of this section. We shall first consider the effects of gravity and its absence, together with the effects of activity and inactivity. The effects of supragravitational force fields will be discussed. Thereafter, vibration and noise will be considered, for they are inevitable concomitants of an industrial society. Finally, we must discuss briefly man's responses to combinations of stresses, since he rarely encounters environmental stress in isolation.

Gravity

Man, and every other biological organism on earth, has evolved under the constant influence of the acceleration of gravity, a force field which pulls us toward the earth's center of mass at roughly 32 ft. per sec.[2] Each time man rises from the supine to the erect position, the column of blood within him is accelerated toward his feet; each time he raises his arms, the action is resisted. When he climbs a hill, he gains potential energy at the cost of an expenditure of roughly 5 times as much energy, for the human organism works at only about 20 per cent efficiency.

The constant pull of gravity has profound effects on a motile organism, and especially on one which normally extends itself to its full height. The column of blood in the venous reservoir is 5 to 6 feet high; there is, therefore, a gradient in pressure from the top to the bottom of that column of 5 to 6 feet of water, or about 120 mm. Hg. Were it not for the valves in our veins, this entire pressure would be exerted on the vessels in our lower legs whenever we are erect. The heart must supply the brain with blood at adequate perfusion pressures both when the body is supine and the hydrostatic column is horizontal, and when it is upright, with a hydrostatic column over a foot high.

Man has learned to cope with this situation, though not without cost to himself. One instance of this cost is varicose veins in the lower extremities, a serious and disfiguring problem for many. Stasis ulcers of the skin over the legs are another probably allied problem. More serious for some is postural hypotension, an inability to maintain adequate cardiac output and peripheral resistance in the upright position.

Even in those of us who can cope with sudden changes in position, fairly major physiologic responses are involved. When we assume the recumbent position for any period of time, venous return is improved. The volume receptors in the right atrium sense this, and a water diuresis results. Over a longer period of time, calcium mobilization and excretion lead to demineralization of bone. The muscles, especially the antigravity muscles, lose strength and mass. The smooth muscle in the walls of blood vessels may also lose tone and the capacity to respond to changes in posture.

All these changes make little difference—as long as we remain supine. If, however, we return to the erect posture, we find ourselves unable to cope with gravitational stress. Bed rest for prolonged periods robs man of many of his normal modes of coping with his environment.

Weightlessness. Bed rest is *not* weightlessness, though it is tempting to consider them together. As man began to explore the space above our atmosphere, medical support personnel began to worry about whether the deadaptive changes seen in prolonged recumbency would appear in astronauts, when the centrifugal accelerations involved in orbital flight exactly balanced the centripedal acceleration due to gravity. It has been found that many of the changes observed are indeed similar, though the data are far from conclusive. Man has thus far experienced weightlessness for over 7 weeks. Bone densitometry has suggested that a degree of demineralization occurs; physical deconditioning with diminished exercise tolerance has been observed. Intolerance to upright tilt has in some cases been profound, though short-lived. Decreases in circulating red cell mass and plasma volume have been noted.

The importance of these and other related findings is still disputed. Some believe that prolonged weightlessness will have profound and dangerous effects on man; others feel that by two weeks of exposure, man begins to readapt despite his altered environment. One of the principal purposes of NASA's Skylab program, involving 28- and 56-day exposures, was to explore this matter further.

Little research has been done on man in supragravity force fields, in part because of the very elaborate equipment required. Smith and others have exposed animals, notably fowl, to long periods in strong gravitational fields. They find evidence of adaptation, notably in bone structure, antigravity muscle mass, and postural reflexes.

One of the major factors inhibiting research in this area is that weightlessness cannot be simulated on earth for more than a few seconds. To date, the best tool for such research has been suspension under water at neutral buoyancy in a pressurized space suit. This technique, however well it simulates the difficulties of moving and working in a zero-G field, has severe drawbacks for physiologic experimentation.

Physical Activity. It was noted above that prolonged bed rest causes a variety of deadaptive changes in the human organism. The fullest development of heat acclimatization requires both heat and physical work. The importance of physical activity in maintaining the adaptability of the human organism has become a popular topic of discussion in recent years; many easily available scientific and popular texts consider this topic in detail. It is necessary, however, that it receive at least brief consideration here as well.

Just as musculoskeletal inactivity causes disuse atrophy and skeletal demineralization, so the performance of musculoskeletal work produces, over a period of time, hypertrophy and increased capillarity of skeletal muscles, optimal mineralization of long bones, and a number of adaptive alterations in the heart and cardiovascular system, including greater cardiac volume and output per stroke, lower resting heart rates, greater work capacity, higher oxygen uptake during work (with consequent sparing of the less efficient anaerobic energy sources), and often an increased sense of well-being.

The induction of these changes requires that the organism be stressed repeatedly by the performance of strenuous physical work. A number of carefully controlled studies indicate that optimal cardiorespiratory fitness can better be achieved and maintained by relatively brief spurts of fairly intense exercise than by much longer periods of less intense exercise. It seems certain, however, that the maintenance of man's reserve capacity to deal with physiologic stress requires that man be stressed on a continuing basis; this truism is nowhere more clear than with respect to man's capacity to perform muscular work.

Prolonged Acceleration. Aircraft have freedom of motion in all spatial axes. As a result of this freedom, they are capable of accelerations, especially angular, which significantly displace or alter the magnitude of the apparent normal G vector. Detailed consideration of this field, in which much research has been done, is beyond the scope of this review. It will simply be said here that, as an instance, in a 60-degree banked turn in level flight an acceleration of twice normal gravity (2 G) is imparted to the occupants of an aircraft. The acceleration in this case is parallel to the long axis of the body. Exactly the same acceleration may occur when an airplane pulls out of a dive into level flight or into a climb.

Since the net G vector is the same in both instances, the pilot or occupant may be unable to differentiate those two quite dissimilar situations unless he is provided with gyroscopic instruments to tell him what is occurring. The result is spatial disorientation, a common and dangerous problem in flight. If the natural horizon is not visible, the pilot must use instruments, which are not affected as are his semicircular canals and otoliths by angular and linear accelerations.

With respect to both orientation and cardiovascular physiology, prolonged linear and radial accelerations induce changes which may be adaptive or deadaptive. Several references are provided; standard texts cover these topics in detail.

Abrupt Accelerations; Impact

Whenever a body acquires momentum, it must dissipate that momentum to return to rest. Since momentum is the product of mass times velocity, the faster we go the more dangerous it becomes to stop abruptly.

Any consideration of the effects of impact upon man must take into account the rate of onset of the decelerative impulse, the peak magnitude of the deceleration, its duration, the orientation of the man with respect to the force field, and the nature of any protective equipment and of the environment around him.

The average magnitude of an impact may be simply estimated in terms of the initial velocity, the final velocity (usually zero), and the distance over which the vehicle or man came to rest. The deceleration thus derived is usually expressed as a ratio, the denominator of which is the acceleration due to gravity. Figure 33-9 shows a variety of deceleration and impact experiences in terms of initial velocity and stopping distance. Body orientation differs in these experiences; the approximate survival limits shown must be interpreted cautiously.

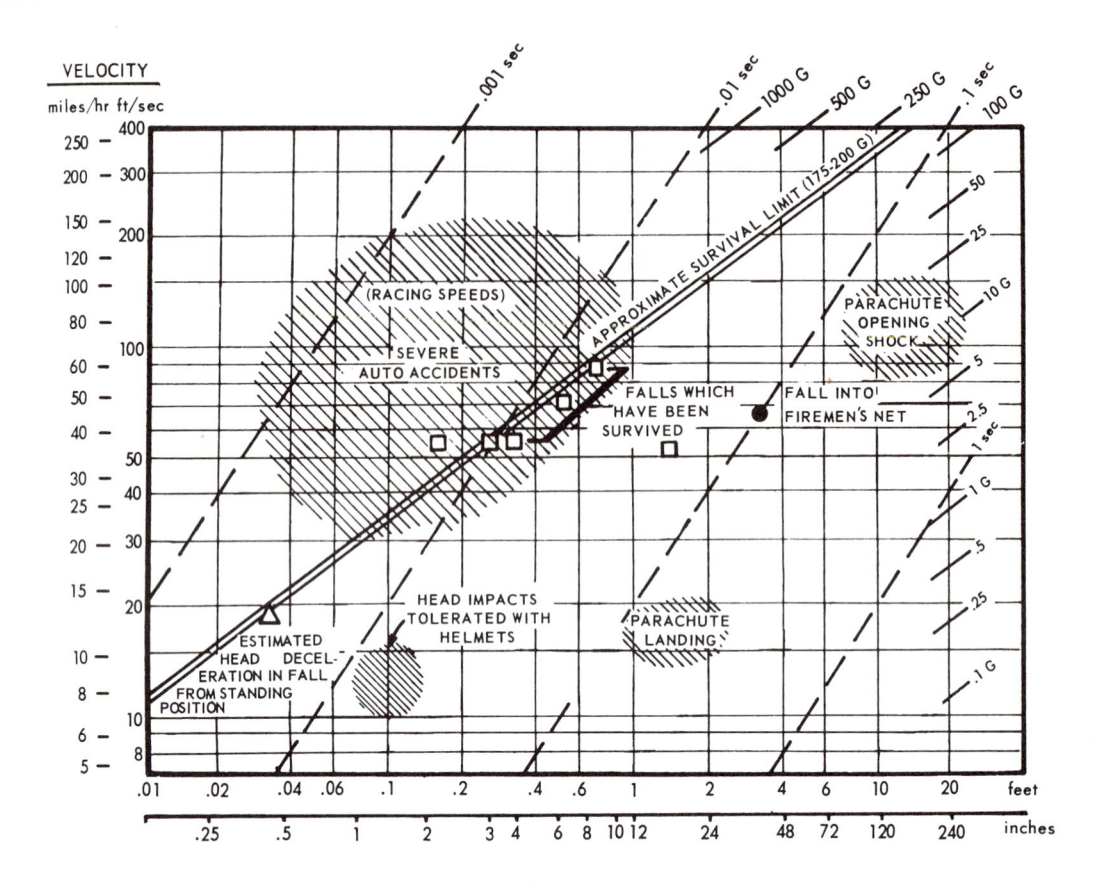

Figure 33-9 This figure brings together a variety of impact and deceleration experiences by plotting the data from a number of sources on the common axes of deceleration distance and velocity. Stopping time and impact force in G units are shown as secondary scales. The data points with hollow squares are for free falls of 50 to 150 ft. with survival. The line labeled "approximate survival limit" must be used with caution, since many biophysical factors influence the injury due to deceleration. (From Parker, J. F., and West, V. R. (Eds.): Bioastronautics Data Book. 2nd ed. Washington, D.C., U.S. Government Printing Office, 1973.)

Tolerance limits depend to a considerable extent on the peak acceleration during an impact. Peak transverse accelerations of 100 to 200 G for 0.01 seconds are tolerated without injury, whereas only 20 to 30 G can be tolerated for 1 second. The duration of an applied acceleration determines whether the body acts as a rigid, or a viscoelastic, object. During accelerations or decelerations longer than 0.05 to 0.10 sec., the internal organs and blood are significantly affected; physiologic adaptations begin to occur.

Tolerance for vertical or longitudinal impact is substantially less than for transverse (anteroposterior) forces. The outcome of such an impact depends to a considerable extent on whether one's knees are locked or are allowed to flex (thus increasing the distance over which the trunk is decelerated).

Following moderate transverse impacts (15 to 25 G with onset rates from 400 to 1000 G per sec.), a number of transient physiologic changes are seen in subjects who are free from structural damage. These include hypotension, bradycardia (a vagal effect which is blocked by atropine), transient neurologic changes, changes in blood platelets, psychological changes, and generalized stress reactions. These effects must be taken into account when evaluating the condition of persons involved in auto accidents.

It should be pointed out here that in auto crashes, the most serious injuries are usually caused by a secondary impact of occupants with steering wheel, interior structure, windshield, or objects in the vicinity, if the occupants are ejected from the vehicle. Adequate restraint systems are now available in new automobiles; the decline in fatalities and in the number and severity of injuries which would result from their universal use would be startling. While auto manufacturers, prodded by new federal standards, have made considerable strides in delethalizing interiors, the simplest way to avoid injury from impacting vehicle parts is not to contact them; there is no substitute for an adequate restraint system in this regard.

Vibration

Vibration may be thought of as repeated brief accelerations; these may be sinusoidal or random in character and may be applied to a part of the body (as when vibrating hand tools are used) or to the whole body.

Human responses to vibration depend to a considerable extent upon the frequency of the vibration with respect to the resonance frequencies of various body organs. All studies of whole-body vibration show a sharp decrease in voluntary tolerance at frequencies of 4 to 7 cycles per sec. owing to resonance of the abdominal organs, as an instance.

G forces during vibration are a function of frequency and amplitude of the applied acceleration. The amplitude of the seat or platform, however, is usually damped considerably by the body. Head movement, for instance, is usually very much less than seat movement.

Limits of voluntary tolerance for longitudinal vibration in the seated position are from 0.1 to 0.4 G at frequencies of 1 to 40 cycles per sec. Minor injury begins to occur at levels of 2 to 5 G, depending on exposure time. Such injuries are the result of mechanical deformation and shear forces upon adjacent tissues of differing densities and masses.

A different sort of injury pattern is seen in some workers whose jobs involve prolonged contact with vibrating hand tools. After a variable period of exposure, usually in cold environments, a proportion of these workers will begin to show vascular changes in the hands, with vascular spasm typical of Raynaud's phenomenon. It is not certain whether the changes seen in the arteries are primary or secondary to nerve injury, but considerable thickening of arterial walls has been demonstrated. The disorder is disabling, since once present, it is exacerbated by exposure of the individual or of his hand to cold, as well as to vibration.

Noise

The human ear, like the eye, has an enormous tolerance for cyclic pressure changes which reach the eardrum through the air. The auditory threshold in normal young persons is in the neighborhood of 10^{-4} dynes per cm.^{2}; the ear can tolerate sound pressure levels as high as 10^3 dynes per cm.^{2} In contemporary society, however, much louder sound pressure levels are produced by certain machines and by explosives; these sounds and others of lesser magnitude for longer periods of exposure can cause harm. Both acute dysfunction and chronic damage of the very sensitive auditory mechanism result from exposure to high sound pressure levels.

Because of the very wide range of pressures to which the ear can respond, it is conventional to express sound pressure levels in decibels (dB) relative to the threshold of hearing. Figure 33–10 shows the overall SPLs of a variety of common environmental sources of sound.

The frequency spectrum to which the normal ear responds is roughly 30 to 12,000 cycles per second (hertz). Since sounds containing substantial proportions of high-frequency energy are somewhat more injurious than predominantly low-frequency sounds, it is necessary to evaluate the sound environment in terms of its frequency components as well as its overall sound pressure levels.

Noise has been defined as "unwanted sound." It has become common practice, therefore, to talk of "noisy environments" and of "the effects of noise." It will be immediately obvious to those who have been exposed to rock-and-roll music in close quarters that one man's sound may be another's noise, however. The damage caused by sound, or noise, is a function of its energy content, not its information content.

Intense sound (SPL greater than 85 to 95 dB) causes, after a period of exposure, an upward shift in auditory thresholds for pure tones. If sound exposure is terminated or interrupted, this "temporary threshold shift" disappears over a period of hours or a few days and auditory acuity again becomes normal. The exact physiologic nature of this phenomenon is not known, though it appears to be an end-organ rather than a central response. Regardless of the frequency content of the sound which induces the temporary shift, the shift itself is seen earliest and to the greatest degrees in the range of frequencies between 1500 and 4000 Hz.

If exposures to sound pressure levels of this magnitude are continued over a long time period, a gradual permanent threshold shift occurs. The rate of onset and magnitude of this shift vary considerably, but they are roughly proportional to the intensity of the sound to which persons are exposed. Fairly good normative data are available for continuous noise exposure; the effects of exposure to impulse noise are less well understood.

The permanent threshold shift (which may have a further temporary shift superimposed upon it) represents true neural deafness and is irreversible. It results from degeneration of the

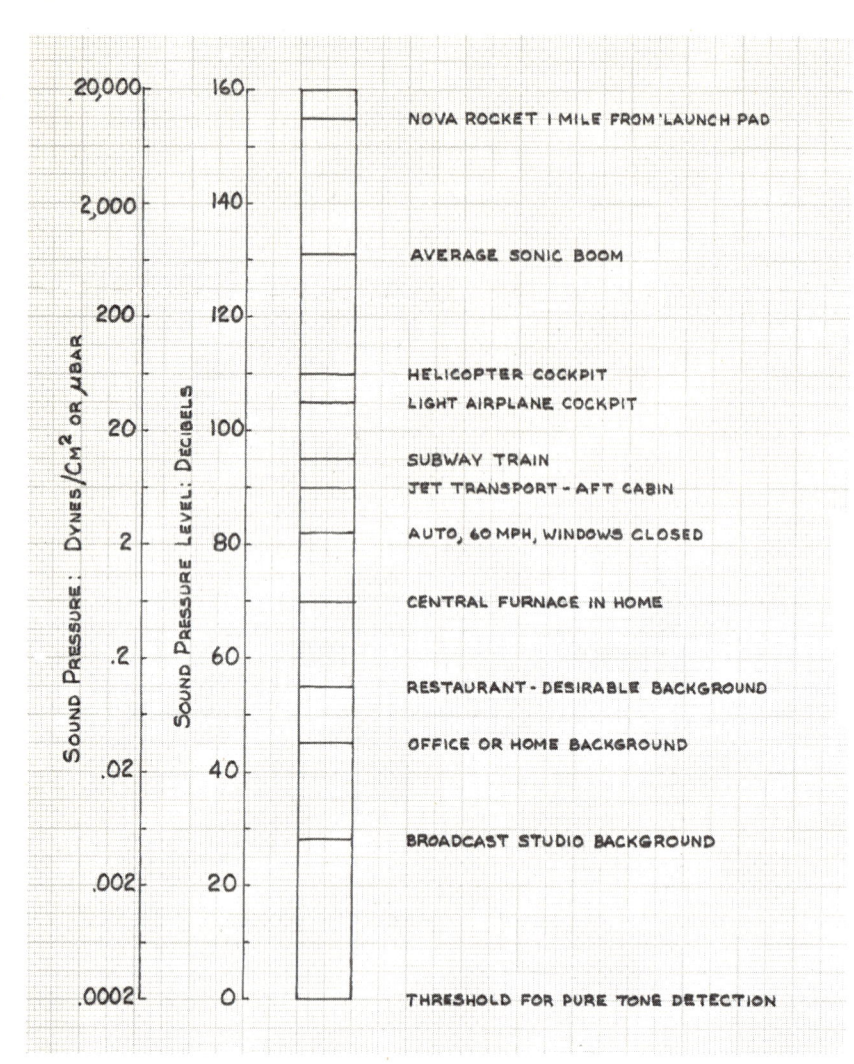

Figure 33-10 Range of auditory sensitivity showing sound pressure levels generated by various sources.

sensory cells in the organ of Corti. Deafness from noise exposure may be difficult to differentiate from presbycusis, the usual decrease in auditory acuity seen in older people, since both forms cause greater deficits in acuity for tones of high frequencies (4000 to 12,000 Hz). Indeed, some have argued that presbycusis itself is induced by exposure to high sound pressures over a lifetime. (This may be true in part, but it is probably not a full explanation; genetic factors are certainly involved.)

Temporary deafness of a different sort results from obstruction in the external ear canal (water or cerumen), from fluid in the middle ear due to barotitis, or from a ruptured tympanic membrane. Although the human tympanum is very resistant to rupture, an explosive blast or very high pressure differential across the drum may cause traumatic rupture. The lesion is self-limiting, and spontaneous healing ordinarily occurs within a few days. Repeated episodes of serous otitis media, however, may cause thickening of the eardrum, with damping of its motion and loss of elasticity. The threshold shift seen in such cases tends to be roughly uniform across low and high frequencies. A similar picture is seen in otosclerosis. Such hearing losses are characteristic of conductive, as opposed to neural, or perceptive, deafness and are sometimes amenable to medical or surgical treatment.

Ultrasound

Mechanical vibrations with frequencies above about 15,000 Hz are not detected by the human ear; such waves therefore are called ultrasonic.

As frequency increases, propagation through air decreases; extremely high ultrasonic vibrations are readily transmitted only by relatively incompressible (liquid or solid) materials. The energy contained in such waves can, however, be converted to thermal energy in the tissues; this is the basis of continuous output ultrasonic diathermy units. Alternatively, again by proper selection of frequencies and with use of a pulsed wave transmitter and receiver, ultrasound can be used to visualize tissue discontinuities within the body. It is used, for instance, to determine the location of the placenta prior to amniocentesis. The power outputs used in such studies are not hazardous. It has also been suggested that changes in cell membrane permeability can be induced by ultrasound without destruction or denaturation of cell proteins.

COMBINED STRESSES

In this brief review of man's responses to his physical environment, most of our discussion has dealt with the effects of single stressors. No such discussion can be complete, however, if it does not emphasize that man rarely encounters these stressors in isolation. We normally live and work and play in the presence of a great variety of physical, chemical, biological, and sociocultural stressors, some antagonistic, others additive or synergistic. Indeed, we know from sensory deprivation experiments that too little stress may be at least as damaging to man as too much stress, that man functions best in a fairly rich environment.

The aluminum foundry worker must perform strenuous work in the face of often severe thermal stress; the mountain climber must exert himself while affected by both hypoxia and cold. Operators of heavy equipment are exposed to high levels of noise and vibration under a wide range of climatic conditions. Each of these persons is working under the influence as well of biological and socioeconomic factors which may or may not impose additional stress upon him.

In dealing with disorders caused by environmental stresses, the physician must keep in mind the pathologic physiology of these disorders if his therapeutic efforts are to be effective. The person who performs muscular work in a hot environment must share his cardiac output between his working muscles, which depend on the blood for oxygen, and his skin, to which heat is carried from the core by blood. These two stresses therefore are additive with respect to their physiologic demands. Their combined effects are multiplied when fluid must be expended for evaporative cooling, reducing the plasma volume.

Many other examples could be cited; the important point is simply that such problems as these are amenable to rational treatment aimed at restoring the body to its normal homeostatic condition, or at supporting the patient until he can again adapt to stress. This is the essence of environmental medicine once injury has occurred. The same reasoning, however, based on knowledge of physiology, can as easily be applied to the prevention of such injuries. Herein lie our most stimulating challenges in the field of environmental health.

REFERENCES

Literature concerning this broad area of study is widely spread among journals devoted to medicine, physiology, psychology, and engineering. There are a few publications in which reports relating to a variety of environmental stressors are gathered together. Because of their particular value, they are listed here; individual reports follow in alphabetical order.

Bedwell, T. C., and Strughold, H. (Eds.): Bioastronautics and the Exploration of Space. Available from Clearinghouse for Federal Scientific and Technical Information, Springfield, Virginia, 1965.
Bennett, P. B., and Elliott, D. H.: The Physiology and Medicine of Diving and Compressed Air Work. Baltimore, Williams and Wilkins Co., 1969.
Dill, D. B. (Ed.): Handbook of Physiology. Section 4, Adaptation to the Environment. Washington, D.C., American Physiological Society, 1964.
Lambertsen, C. J. (Ed.): Proceedings of the Third Symposium on Underwater Physiology. Baltimore, Williams and Wilkins Co., 1967.
Lambertsen, C. J. (Ed.): Proceedings of the Fourth Symposium on Underwater Physiology. New York, Academic Press, 1971.

Leithead, C. S., and Lind, A. R.: Heat Stress and Heat Disorders. Philadelphia, F. A. Davis Co., 1964.
McFarland, A.: Human Factors in Air Transportation. New York, McGraw-Hill Book Co., 1953.
Randel, H. W. (Ed.): Aerospace Medicine. 2nd ed. Baltimore, Williams and Wilkins Co., 1971.
Parker, J. F., Jr., and West, V. R. (Eds.): Bioastronautics Data Book. 2nd ed. NASA SP-3006. Washington, D.C., U.S. Government Printing Office, 1973.

Allen, S. C.: A comparison of the effects of nitrogen lack and hyperoxia on the vascular development of the chick embryo. Aerospace Med. 34:897, 1963.
Anonymous: Radiation Induced Cancer. Proceedings Series. International Atomic Energy Agency, Vienna, Austria, 1969.
Bartleson, C. J.: Retinal burns from intense light sources. Amer. Industr. Hyg. Assoc. J., 29:415, 1968.
Bass, D. E., Kleeman, R., Quinn, M., Henschel, A., and Hegnauer, H.: Mechanisms of acclimatization to heat in man. Medicine, 34:323, 1955.
Billings, C. E., Brashear, R. E., Bason, R., and Mathews, D. K.: Medical observations during 20 days at 3800 meters. Arch. Environ. Health, 18:987, 1969.
Boerema, I., et al. (Eds.): Clinical Applications of Hyperbaric Oxygen. Amsterdam, Elsevier Publishing Co., 1964.

Burton, A. C. and Edholm, O. G.: Man in a Cold Environment. London, Edward Arnold, 1955.

Clark, J. M., and Lambertsen, C. J.: Pulmonary oxygen toxicity: A review. Pharmacol. Rev., *23*:37, 1971.

Cogan, D. G.: Lesions of the eye from radiant energy. J.A.M.A., *142*:145, 1950.

DiGiovanni, C., Jr., and Chambers, R. M.: Physiologic and psychologic aspects of the gravity spectrum. New Eng. J. Med., *270*:35, 88, 134; 1964.

Fenn, W. O.: Possible role of hydrostatic pressure in diving. *In* Lambertsen, C. J. (Ed.): Underwater Physiology. Baltimore, Williams and Wilkins Co., 1967.

Folk, G. E., Jr.: Introduction to Environmental Physiology: Environmental Extremes and Mammalian Survival. Philadelphia, Lea and Febiger, 1966.

Fox, R. H., Goldsmith, R., Hampton, I. F. G., and Hunt, J. J.: Heat acclimatization by controlled hyperthermia in hot-dry and hot-wet climates. J. Appl. Physiol., *22*:39, 1967.

Fox, R. H., Goldsmith, R., Kidd, D. J., and Lewis, H. E.: Acclimatization to heat in man by controlled elevation of body temperature. J. Physiol., *166*:530, 1963.

Fryer, D. I.: Subatmospheric Decompression Sickness in Man. Slough, England, Technivision Services, 1969.

Gauer, O. H. and Zuidema, G. D.: Gravitational Stress in Aerospace Medicine. Boston, Little, Brown and Co., 1961.

Glorig, A., Ward, W. D., and Nixon, J.: Damage risk criteria and noise-induced hearing loss. Arch. Otolaryngol., *74*:413, 1961.

Hopps, J. A.: The electric shock hazard in hospitals. Canad. Med. Assoc. J., *98*:1002, 1968.

Howath, S. M. (Ed.): Cold Injury. Transactions of the Sixth Conference, New York, Josiah Macy, Jr., Foundation, 1960.

Hultgren, H. N., Spickard, W., and Lopez, C.: Further studies of high-altitude pulmonary oedema. Brit. Heart J., *24*:95, 1962.

International Commission on Radiological Protection: The Evaluation of Risks from Radiation. ICRP Publication No. 8. Oxford, Pergamon Press, 1966.

Kryter, K. D.: The Effects of Noise on Man. New York, Academic Press, 1970.

Largent, E. J. and Ashe, W. F.: Upper limits of thermal stress for workmen. Amer. Industr. Hyg. Assoc. J., *19*:246, 1958.

Levi, L. (Ed.): Emotional Stress. New York, American Elsevier Publishing Co., 1967.

Lichter, I., Borrie, J., and Miller, W. M.: Radio-frequency hazards with cardiac pacemakers. Brit. Med. J., *1*:1513, 1965.

Linder, G. S.: Mechanical vibration effects on human beings. Aerospace Med., *33*:939, 1962.

Margaria, R.: Exercise at Altitude. New York, Excerpta Medica Foundation, 1967.

Mathews, D. K., Stacy, R. W., and Hoover, G. N.: Physiology of Muscular Activity and Exercise. New York, Ronald Press, 1964.

McCally, M., and Graveline, D. E.: Physiologic aspects of prolonged weightlessness. New Eng. J. Med., *269*:508, 1963.

Menon, N. D.: High-altitude edema. New Eng. J. Med., *273*:66, 1965.

Peyton, M. F. (Ed.): Biological Effects of Microwave Radiation. Vol. I. New York, Plenum Press, 1961.

Roy, S.: Acute mountain sickness in Himalayan terrain. *In* Hegnauer, A. H. (Ed.): Biomedicine of High Terrestrial Elevations. Washington, D.C., U.S. Army Medical Research and Development Command, January, 1969.

Sacq, Z. M., and Alexander, P. A.: Fundamentals of Radiobiology. Oxford, Pergamon Press, 1961.

Schaefer, K. E., et al.: Pulmonary and circulatory adjustments determining the limits of depth in breathhold diving. Science, *162*:1020, 1968.

Saenger, E. L. (Ed.): Medical Aspects of Radiation Accidents. A Handbook for Physicians, Health Physicists and Industrial Hygienists. U.S. Atomic Energy Commission, 1963.

Sugimoto, T., Schall, S. F., and Wallace, A. G.: Factors determining vulnerability to ventricular fibrillation induced by 60-CPS alternating current. Circ. Res., *21*:601, 1967.

Webb, P.: Body heat loss in undersea gaseous environment. Aerospace Med., *41*:1283, 1970.

Weisel, T. N.: Effects of monocular deprivation on the cat's visual cortex. Trans. Amer. Acad. Ophthal. Otolaryng., *75*:1186, 1971.

Wood, J. E. and Bass, D. E.: Thermoregulatory and circulatory adjustments during acclimatization to heat in man. J. Clin. Invest., *39*:825, 1960.

CHAPTER 34 CHEMICAL AGENTS AND DISEASE

B. D. DINMAN

INTRODUCTION

Early man, by trial and error, was able to classify botanical and biological materials as safe or harmful (food or poison). However, today we know that we cannot distinguish clearly between such substances. We recognize degrees of harm and degrees of safety. Some substances or chemicals considered innocuous may, in sufficient quantities, cause harmful effects, whereas some agents considered definitely harmful may be taken safely in minute quantities. Thus, we have the concept of dose; almost all beneficial agents in certain doses may cause untoward effects.

In his attempt to gain mastery over the environment, man and his technology have also brought into being new molecules which the world has never before known. In the latter half of the twentieth century, new chemical agents have been synthesized which have the ability to regulate the growth rates of plants and animals, or which can differentially cause weeds to wither while sparing crop growth. A host of such agents ubiquitously find their way into channels of commerce leading directly to the household, whether intended for domestic use, e.g., detergents, or as a residue associated with foodstuffs. Hence all physicians should have some understanding of the interaction of such exogenous chemical agents with biological systems.

Of great interest today is the field of *environmental toxicology*. This area includes incidental encounters with chemicals, for example, in the atmosphere or by contact at work or play, or by ingestion in the form of food additives. These chemicals may be considered basically as contaminants of the environment or of food and water. Some are chemicals added to animal feeds which are later consumed when such animals are used as a food source for man. Pesticides and insecticides used in agriculture may be left as residues on or in food. Some chemicals are deliberately added to foods as preservatives. Others may be absorbed from the environment, for example, the consumption of fish contaminated with mercury.

There is growing concern regarding the pollution of water by industrial wastes and inadequate sewage disposal and of air by automobile exhausts or industrial wastes, with concentrations of pollutants reaching levels that may affect health. Such pollutants include carbon monoxide and sulfur dioxide, chlorides, oxidants and organic acids, solids of smoke and dust, and other compounds.

Accidental or deliberate ingestion of chemicals used as drugs is another form of toxicity. Children may ingest drugs, cleaning agents used in the home, and lead paint, for example. In adults, use of barbiturates, alcohol, and addictive drugs can be lethal when abused. Automobile accidents are often an indirect result of such abuse. Chemicals with beneficial effects used as therapeutic agents may, in certain individuals, have undesirable or unwanted effects to possibly dangerous degrees as well as the primary effects of excessive dosage. The route of administration may have an important bearing on concentration reached in certain parts of the body and consequently on actions and reactions.

Before this era, relatively few chemicals were readily available to the public at large, while food additives were of simple nature and frequently of biological origin. Formerly the study of the effect of chemicals was directed toward post-mortem examination of end results of tissue response. This yielded a static visualization of both agent-specific and nonspecific tissue alteration. But with advent of the doctrine of "prevention of occurrence" or "prevention of progression" of disease, only a conceptualization of the dynamic functional changes induced by a chemical at *all* stages of tissue response will permit the development of effective clinical preventatives. It should be apparent that study of chemically induced lesions seen from the viewpoint of morphology alone can give little insight into the early clinical events associated with chemical intoxication. Thus if we are to intervene effectively to prevent these pathologic processes, an understanding of the earliest functional events is required.

Relation of Dose to Tissue Response

Basic to this chapter is the concept that dose as a function of time is the determinant of tissue response. While this is almost a priori recognized by the practitioner dealing with therapeutic chemicals, for some unknown reason dose as a determinant of response is ignored when he considers chemical "poisons." It will become apparent in this chapter that enzymatically controlled metabolic systems capable of handling exogenous chemicals have rate limits. These systems are to varying degrees self replicative, and may be supplemented by alternate metabolic pathways which also operate under similar limitations. If in general these limitations in the rate of metabolic transformation or regeneration of metabolic pathways are not exceeded by the dose or the time over which the dose is given, there are few if any chemical agents with which a biological system cannot cope. From another viewpoint, quantitative factors inevitably influence the interaction between chemicals and the cell. Such agents exert their effects by physicochemical interactions with "target sites," e.g., binding of sulfhydryl radicals in close proximity to the active site of an enzyme (see p. 961). However, if these chemicals combine with a sulfhydryl radical spatially removed from an active site, or with another nonessential material present in excess in the cell, e.g., substrate, such bindings have little or no effect upon cellular structure or function. Thus, it is apparent that stochastic considerations will determine the probability of interaction of chemical agents with "target sites," i.e., the more molecules of the foreign agent present in the cell, the greater the probability of interaction with "target sites."

Whether these determinants apply to the case of carcinogenic chemical agents is open to question. The Millers have suggested such a possibility on the basis of a carcinogen interacting with nonessential nucleophilic materials in the cell. The problem with carcinogens is further complicated by the apparently different mode of action of such agents as compared with the action of other chemicals. With the latter, the outcome of the toxic chemical-cellular molecule interaction is either fatal for the cell or followed by replacement or repair of the affected cellular component. Similar consequences of the carcinogen-cellular interaction do not, apparently, occur. It appears at present that nonfatal but permanent damage can ensue, especially involving those sites controlling cellular activities, e.g., metabolic, replicative. Thus, potentially vital functions may be damaged without expression of harm until such control systems are activated. Further, such potential control defects may persist long after the carcinogen is gone from the cell; this persistence of damage can be permanent, since the defective control molecule may be replicated with successive mitotic events. In this fashion, multiple, insidious intracellular functional "scars" may accumulate on repeated contacts with carcinogens, yet expression of such functional aberrations may not be apparent until years later.

Genetically Determined Enzyme Response

In addition to these determinants of the dose-response relationship, still another factor controls the course and outcome of an individual's reaction to chemical agents. This response is based upon the genetically determined availability of an enzyme(s) required for metabolic degradation or detoxification. Such a genetically determined phenomenon is exemplified by the case of those enzymes responsible for the splitting of the bond between choline and its ester, i.e., the cholinesterases. Whereas most individuals have the usual form of this enzyme that attacks the choline-ester bond readily, some small group (1:5100) within the population is endowed with a relatively large proportion of an atypical form of this enzyme exhibiting a *lower* affinity for cleavage of this bond. It must be pointed out that the normal process producing hydrolytic cleavage of the ester-choline bond is to some extent available to such persons, so that physiologic concentrations of acetylcholine normally present can be degraded and inactivated. Only upon administration of the muscle relaxant succinylcholine is there clinical manifestation of the presence of this atypical catalyst among these persons. As a result of the failure of enzymatic breakdown of this compound, such patients given the agent at surgery respond with a severe, persistent apnea.

Utilizing special techniques, Kalow has shown that acetylcholine esterase distributes itself within a population in three groupings, i.e., a rare number of individuals (1:5100) with little of the "normal" enzyme activity, a second (and major) group with the usual enzyme activity, and a third, infrequent group (1:30) whose enzyme activity is intermediate in "quantity". Most observations on the inheritance of these characteristics indicate the presence of two autosomal allelic genes without dominance, with each gene causing the formation of one of the two types of enzyme. The typical genotype leading to "usual" enzyme elaboration can be expressed as AA; the atypical, low enzyme activity is expressed by the genotype BB, while intermediate enzyme activity would possess one of each allele, i.e., AB (Fig. 34-1). Except under conditions of drug administration discussed earlier there probably would not be clinical expression of this defect in the heterozygous group AB. Nevertheless, by appropriate techniques an intermediate amount of enzyme activity can be demonstrated. Other inborn errors of metabolism, e.g., phenylketonuria, galactosemia, in general appear to distribute and express themselves similarly in large populations.

The foregoing bears directly upon the concept of the genetically determined variation of response to chemicals. The statistical origin of the concept of "normal" is clinically all too often forgotten. Thus, while the "normal" individual represents the population within the large middle portion of the bell-shaped curve or "gaussian" distribution, there still remain those persons at the upper and lower portions (or "tails") of this distribution of occurrences. Accordingly, if the physician gives a similar dose of therapeutic agent to enough patients over the years, eventually he will be faced with a patient who responds as if he were given gross overdosage. This person probably represents one of the few such individuals at the lower tail of the distribution of responses normally found in the population. Such a clinically susceptible individual may not possess the necessary enzymatic integrity of a chemical degradation pathway to the required extent, and thus the chemical agent may persist over a longer period of time in relatively high concentrations. It appears that the efficacy with which a metabolic pathway carries out its function is related in part to genetic endowment. Just as this atypical individual expresses a homozygosity (BB) of allelic endowment, the vast majority of individuals in the population on the rising slope of the normal curve are either heterozygous or more frequently homozygous in their genetic endowment. While the heterozygous may have somewhat less of the usual form of the enzyme, nevertheless such patients in the main have sufficient catalyst to escape clinical detection.

When one considers the foregoing, it can be seen that probabilistic and genetic factors largely

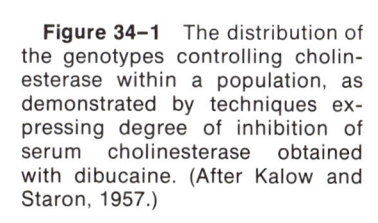

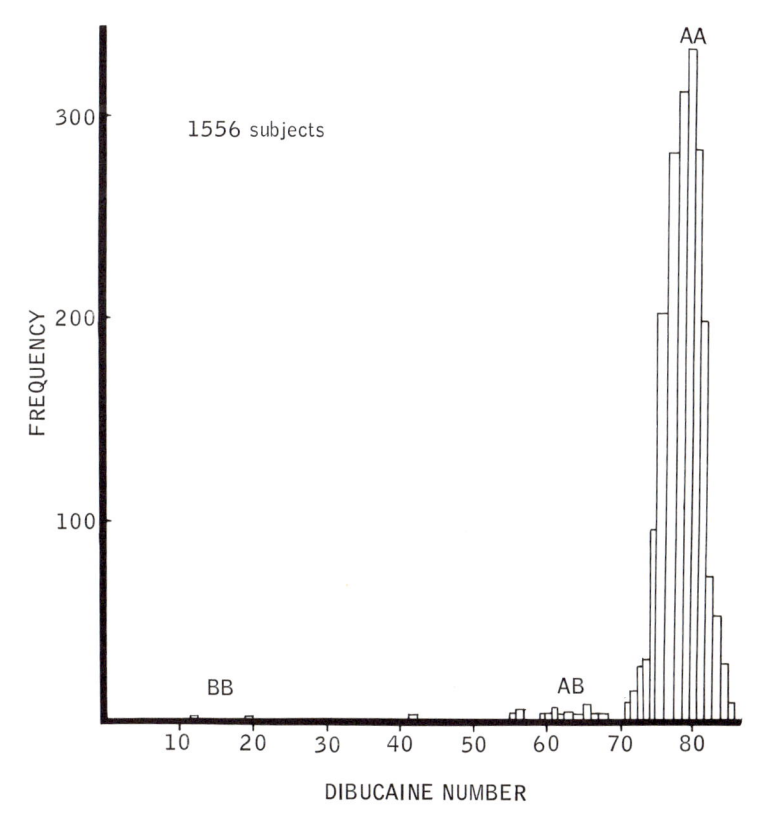

Figure 34-1 The distribution of the genotypes controlling cholinesterase within a population, as demonstrated by techniques expressing degree of inhibition of serum cholinesterase obtained with dibucaine. (After Kalow and Staron, 1957.)

determine the outcome of cellular-chemical interactions. The dose-dependent stochastic parameter is basic to the acceptance of the concept of environmental threshold limits, i.e., the borderline between safety and hazard with chemical contacts. Although it is essentially true that for every foreign molecule entering the cell there will be an interaction, it does not follow that deleterious effects will ensue, unless an excess intrudes. For example, since man throughout his existence absorbs definite quantities of lead, mercury, and so on, it is reasonable to assume that undesirable effects will not occur until too many of such molecules enter the cell. Admittedly, the picture may be somewhat different for compounds produced by technology which have had no prior existence in nature, e.g., polychlorinated biphenyls (PCB). Man has not had the opportunity to develop in the course of evolution metabolic mechanisms for dealing with such relatively new materials. But even here the picture is complicated by the observation that capabilities for enzyme induction exist, making possible metabolic handling potentials for such "new" materials.

THE INTERACTION OF BIOLOGICAL SYSTEMS AND CHEMICAL AGENTS

INTRODUCTION

For rational understanding of the clinical response resulting from the encounter of a biological system with a toxic chemical agent, insight into the characteristics of the two interacting components is necessary. The delicately balanced, energy-dependent biological host with its range of compensatory mechanisms can only return to a position of homeostasis from within certain limits; the chemical agent can effect a change upon such systems only as a function of certain physicochemical characteristics. Study of the effect of each of these variables can lead to discernment of the essentials producing the symptom complex or the diffuse clinical picture resulting from such an encounter.

CHARACTERISTICS OF CHEMICAL INTOXICANTS GOVERNING THEIR BIOLOGICAL ACTIVITY

The effect that a chemical agent may exert upon the body economy is dependent not only upon the host's biological characteristics, but also upon the physicochemical nature of that exogenous agent. A three-dimensional matrix might be constructed consisting of the physicochemical, quantitative, and temporal parameters responsible for the specific effects of these agents.

As for the first of these, the physicochemical, given a compound whose energy state is close to or at ground level, such material is less capable of transferring energy to another compound. The energy state of a chemical compound, in terms of everyday language, is usually referred to as its "reactivity." If a chemical is relatively insoluble or inert in reference to other adjacent molecules, it may act simply as a foreign body by virtue of its low reactivity. However, it must be understood that the inertness or minimal reactivity of any specific chemical compound in a relatively simple in-vitro system frequently bears no relevance to the complex and relatively reactive biological milieu. Thus, silica dioxide outside the body is extremely insoluble; its capability of inciting a severe pulmonary proliferative reaction is well established.

The potential for chemical reaction occurs if an exogenous chemical is less stable energetically or is more highly soluble and is made available to the normal constituents of a cell. However, both conditions of "availability" and solubility must be met before any interaction can occur. It is not surprising therefore, in view of the predominantly aqueous internal environment, that chemical agents which have relatively higher levels of biological activity usually ionize and are water soluble. By contrast, truly nonpolar compounds should less readily interact with cellular constituents unless these cellular components are themselves nonpolar. However, such lipid-soluble compounds react with aqueous cellular components because of the presence of naturally occurring emulsifying components such as phospholipids, or because of the presence of lipid components in subcellular structures.

The molecular configuration of an exogenous chemical agent can markedly alter tissue response. This is exemplified by the naphthylamines, wherein the position of the amine substituent on the naphthylic nucleus determines whether this chemical is carcinogenic. With the amine substituted at the alpha position this agent does not produce bladder tumors; amine substitution at the beta position produces a potent carcinogen (Fig. 34–2). Since the same applies with benzidine, the accessibility of the *para* position for further metabolic alteration (hydroxylation?) may aid in determining carcinogenic behavior.

The principle that pharmacodynamic response is dose dependent is clearly applicable to the area of toxicology. The observation of Hutchinson, that a biological system will interact only when 10^4 atoms of an element are present within a cell, might well set a lower limit of dosage. From this level and upward, the net result of the presence of a foreign compound to the host organism becomes dependent upon quantitative considerations, such as degree of energy change in a cell system, the numbers of cells involved and the primacy of

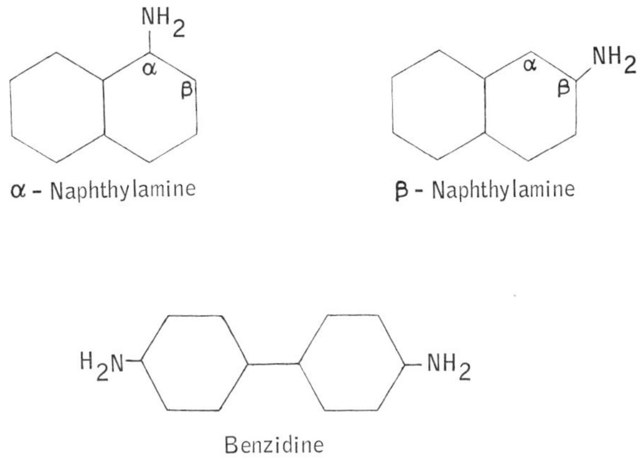

Figure 34-2 While the α-naphthylamine is not carcinogenic, the β isomer is clearly oncogenic, as is benzidine. Note that the *para* positions of both carcinogenic materials are inaccessible to metabolic alteration, in contrast to the noncarcinogenic α isomer.

α - Naphthylamine

β - Naphthylamine

Benzidine

the organ at risk. Thus, given the most toxic chemical known, there appears to be a dose level below which no detectable signs or symptoms appear. Though there may be functional biochemical or anatomic change at the cellular level, unless relatively large numbers of cells are altered clinical response will not be manifest. With the passage of time, the extraneous detritus resulting from such an interaction may be excreted or deactivated and the damaged cell ultimately replaced (except in the central nervous system). With these adjustments the total body economy returns to normal without any residual evidence of chemical damage. Accordingly it can be stated that for *any* chemical there is a lower limit below which toxicity cannot be demonstrated in the intact animal except by the most subtle and sophisticated methodologies. And even with these techniques, with small doses no meaningful functional alteration can be defined.

In addition to the chemical reactivity of the material in question, the wide variation in toxic potential among any large numbers of chemicals (e.g., hydrogen sulfide in contrast to sulfur dioxide) is also a reflection of the relative rates of operation of available detoxification pathways. Considered from a different viewpoint, chemical intoxication will result only when the rate at which the agent or its metabolite is presented to the body is in excess of rate limits placed on the pertinent degradative or excretory processes that inactivate the chemical.

This principle can be clearly demonstrated in the case of exposure to soluble lead acetate. If an individual ingests this compound at levels which exceed 2.0 mg. daily, he can be shown to be slowly and progressively increasing his body burden of lead. His blood lead level will slowly rise over a 4-week period from a level within the normal range of 0.02 to 0.05 mg. per 100 grams of blood to a new level of the order of 0.07 to 0.09 mg. per 100 grams of blood. While this laboratory indicator demonstrates absorption of lead, in many cases there will be no distinctive clinical alteration, even though there may be an elevation of coproporphyrin and disturbances in delta-amino levulinic acid metabolism. Under these conditions of dosage, it can be seen that the metabolic reaction rates controlling bone sequestration of lead have not been exceeded. Accordingly the amount of lead presented over the time period under consideration can be stored at this site where it is relatively inert. Rapid removal of this individual from exposure will be followed over several weeks by a gradual decrease in blood and bone lead levels, without his being aware that exposure to a toxic chemical has occurred. If the dose is doubled, over a shorter period of time lead absorption sufficient to elevate blood lead levels to 0.1 to 0.12 mg. per 100 grams of blood will occur, and the individual so exposed might well have symptoms. In this case the rate of absorption exceeds the gross rate of bony uptake. Consequently, the lead which remains outside the bony matrix has a greater opportunity to wreak clinical mischief.

Given a still larger dose in the same short time period, the rate at which lead can be stored in the bony matrix is rapidly exceeded. Whereas clinical lead intoxication makes its appearance after several weeks of low level exposure, under these conditions of acute dosing clinical alterations rapidly become manifest. Thus the third component of our chemical agent matrix, i.e., the time parameter, is interdependent in the main on the quantitative consideration of dose. That is, the occurrence of an acute biological response is dependent upon the algebraic sum* of (a) the

---

*In other than short-term, acute conditions of exposure, such algebraic summation of these two factors, i.e, dose vs. deactivation rate, requires that the dose response curve be linear. With chronic dosing this straight-line relationship between dose and response is usually not linear; accordingly under such chronic conditions these relationships cannot be expressed by simple algebraic summation.

amount of chemical presented to the body economy per unit time minus (b) the *rate* of metabolic deactivation or sequestration and excretion. Ultimately these rates are dependent upon the rate characteristics of each individual enzyme-mediated metabolic reaction occurring as one step in a multiple sequence of biochemical events.

Inherent, of course, in the concept of rate is the basic premise that time is its prime component, this variable being an integral member of the physicochemical and quantitative factors of our triad.

ENERGETICS OF CELLULAR ACTIVITY AND CONTROL OF ITS EQUILIBRIUM

The multiple, complex processes whereby a cell reproduces itself, constructs new or replacement components or communicates, are ultimately dependent upon the availability of usable energy. Further, in addition to the driving forces necessary to run these processes, their effectiveness depends upon the integration of intracellular control mechanisms which initiate, moderate the rate of, and terminate these activities in ordered sequences.

It should be apparent that if an exogenous chemical is introduced into this delicately balanced interdependent cellular system, potentials for interruption and disorder exist. The mechanisms that produce energy to sustain these processes are a particularly crucial point at which potential chemical interference may occur. The energy utilized to drive the engines of our civilization is derived from the chemical bonds of fossil fuels. The degradation of these bonds unlocks these bonds with the attendant release of heat. Living systems similarly obtain free energy by opening the chemical bonds of fuel stuffs, and utilize this energy or store it as its needs dictate. However, since the cell can only operate within a relatively narrow temperature range, it is unable to use heat energy to function, since thermal energy is usable only when it can be passed from one locus to a second when the latter is at lower temperature. The cell cannot burn its fuel at the 1400° F. combustion temperature of fossil fuels. Thus within a relatively low, constant temperature range, within a narrow range of hydrogen ion concentration and in a dilute aqueous medium, a more sophisticated means of energy extraction has evolved.

Free energy extracted from foodstuffs by oxidation is stored in the physiologically usable form as the bond of the terminal phosphate group of the adenosine triphosphate (ATP) molecule, rather than liberated as heat. The process of glycolysis, whereby glucose is broken down and energy potentials extracted, is not simply brought about by a drastic hydrolysis of this energy source, but rather occurs in a stepwise, ordered manner proceeding through at least 11 stages, each catalyzed by a specific enzyme, the process finally ending in pyruvate.

Following glycolysis, pyruvate is broken down, and the two carbon products are recombined with a four-carbon moiety, oxalacetate, in the Krebs or citric acid cycle. Energized electrons are extracted from the intermediates of this cycle by specific enzymes and are fed into a series of electron carrier molecules of the respiratory chain. These are once more available for storage as available energy in the form of the high energy phosphate bond of ATP. The Krebs cycle and this latter process, referred to as oxidative phosphorylation, both occur within specific structural components of the mitochondria.

It should be apparent that this orderly process is dependent upon the integrity of enzymes that initiate and control the rate of each intervening step. Clearly, each succeeding step in this multiphase process is dependent upon the successful completion of the immediately prior process. These crucial enzymes may be readily altered, since functioning of these proteins depends upon the integrity of a specific amino acid sequence, active site relationships, three-dimensional spatial configuration of their molecular arrangements, and so forth.

When a heavy metal ion is brought into contact with such an enzyme molecule, a binding site is usually available to the metal. This binding site may take the form of a ligand, e.g., –SH, –NH$_2$, –OH, and so on. The resulting complexing or ionic binding of such a heavy metal to the enzyme molecule may change this catalyst's functional characteristics. In the case of any one step of the energy-producing processes described above, if a single enzyme necessary for any one step is blocked, this imperatively requisite source of power will cease to operate and the dependent process will run down and cease.

These enzymatically controlled processes depend not only upon the stereochemical intactness of the protein molecule; in many cases enzymes require specific spatial relationships to subcellular structural entities. Thus, while the molecular integrity of the enzyme glucose-6-phosphatase may not be compromised, this enzyme also appears to require an intact endoplasmic reticulum or ergastoplasmic membrane system. If these membranes, or the plasma membrane, are considered a bimolecular layer of a lipoprotein nature, such exogenous chemicals as nonpolar lipid solvents (e.g., CCl_4) may readily be seen to possess considerable potentials for damaging effects. By changing this membrane's physical-chemical state, morphologic integrity is compromised; but in addition there is impairment of the activity of those enzyme systems dependent upon the intactness of this structure.

The electron-transport chain, the final step in

this energy-producing mechanism, has been shown to be located within an elementary particle on another lipoprotein membrane within the mitochondria. These particles too are apparently dependent upon an organized and ordered three-dimensional pattern. The specific spatial separation of these particles bearing the electron transport process allows enzymes of the citric acid cycle (contained in the nonparticulate matrix of the mitochondria) "access" to the elementary particles. If a lipid solvent disrupts these mitochondrial membranes, the structural relationships of the electron transfer particles to the membrane are destroyed. In the absence of the electron transport system, any precedent energy-yielding reactions (e.g., glycolysis or Krebs citrate cycle) that yield energized electrons are less effective, since transfer of this energy—as in the formation of ATP from ADP—is no longer as effectively accomplished. Under such conditions less usable energy is stored or accumulated. Thus, as previously accumulated high energy phosphate bonds are utilized, in the absence of their replacement the energy level of the cell runs down. Accordingly, such vital energy-dependent functions, such as control of permeability, synthesis, and so forth, are impaired and finally blocked, with cell breakdown following apace.

In the test tube, as the products of a chemical reaction accumulate, a gradual slowing of interaction occurs in keeping with physicochemical laws. Within the cell the products of one reaction sequentially enter into successive reactions, so that ultimately the products of this activity are either synthesized into a cell component, serve as a source of energy or are transferred from the cell. If a reaction product accumulates within a cell, one can conclude that the reaction yielding this material is operating at a rate in excess of the capability of the succeeding process. In vitro, physicochemical considerations would eventually halt the reaction producing this product, but not until considerable product accumulates. Within the cell, however, while it appears that metabolic processes are responsive to such reaction dynamics, more subtle means of cellular function control are also available. The key to these control devices lies in the fact that enzymes influence both the quantitative and qualitative functions of metabolic pathways. Thus any mechanism that can influence activity of enzymes in turn controls cellular metabolic processes.

The concept of "end-product inhibition" provides one such mechanism for influencing enzyme action (Fig. 34-3). This device is brought into play by the accumulation of a product which may be elaborated as a result of a sequence of enzymatically mediated chemical transformations. This accumulation of product appears to inhibit the synthesis of new enzyme and/or its activity per se. It should be noted that the enzyme so influenced is usually not directly involved with the elaboration of the triggering product, but rather is several reactions precedent to the "product." Thus the process of "end-product inhibition," by acting upon the enzyme mediating one step in a chain of metabolic activity, can bring to a halt or control the rate of this cellular sequence of chemical events.

Another mechanism whereby an enzyme's activity may be regulated has been demonstrated in the case of glutamic dehydrogenase. It appears that this enzyme under the proper conditions may have its catalytic activity abolished upon depolymerization into four smaller molecular fragments. Quite remarkably these four monomeric forms still are active enzymes, but now act in quite another reaction involving the oxidation of alanine. But given the proper conditions within the cell, these four fragments can again

Figure 34-3 End-product inhibition mechanisms. The product (P) of a series of enzymatically mediated reactions may inhibit or moderate the reaction A → B by means of two possible mechanisms. It can inhibit synthesis of E_1 from its precursors p_2 and p or it can join with the enzyme E_1 to form the inactive complex E_1P.

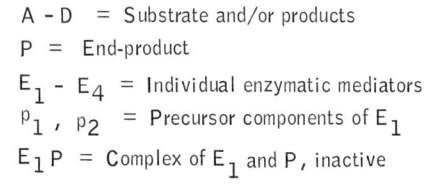

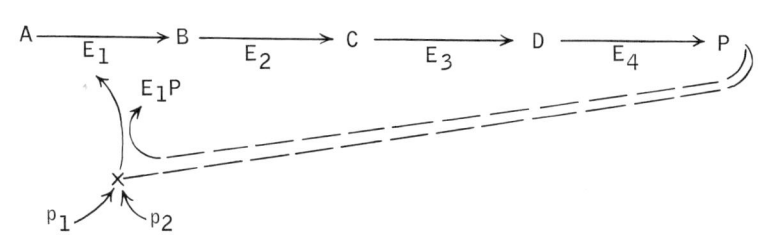

A - D = Substrate and/or products
P = End-product
E_1 - E_4 = Individual enzymatic mediators
p_1, p_2 = Precursor components of E_1
E_1P = Complex of E_1 and P, inactive

polymerize to express their presence as the enzyme glutamic dehydrogenase once more. This unique chain of events provides still another autoregulatory method whereby metabolic activity controlled by enzymes may be controlled within the cell. It should be pointed out that the quantitative aspects of many factors controlling this remarkable depolymerization and repolymerization are critically controlling parameters.

In summary, these brief discussions suggest various sites at which the cell's dynamic equilibrium may be disturbed by structural as well as biochemical alteration. Agents which affect the molecular arrangement of the structural components of the cell may ultimately alter specific enzymatically controlled function. The physicochemical arrangement of the protein molecules that constitute the enzymes may be altered directly by chemical agents, leading to loss of catalytic activity. We have seen but a few examples of how metabolic activity is controlled by exquisitely balanced autoregulatory systems which utilize enzymes as their operants.

These quantitative and time-dependent variables all may apparently affect the delicate interactions required to maintain a state of dynamic equilibrium in conformation with general laws of physics and chemistry. This equilibrium is not static as is a stone lying on a flat level surface; rather it is similar to the equilibrium of a tightrope walker who sways to one side and then another, but necessarily about a single balance point. These cellular systems are similarly in a dynamic equilibrium, with the degree of stability of this system similarly limited by an allowable degree of "sway" which will or will not permit restoration toward an equilibrium point when such displacements occur.

PORTALS OF ENTRY OF CHEMICALS

Dependent upon physiochemical considerations previously discussed, chemicals can enter the body through (1) the lungs, (2) the skin and mucous membranes and (3) the gastrointestinal tract. Aside from medicaments, the entry of a chemical agent through this last route was formerly either the result of criminal or suicidal intent. However, with modern advances in the development of chemical agents for multiple applications in agriculture (e.g., selective plant poisons, defoliants, pesticides, growth accelerators) or in the household (detergents, polishes, chemical bleaches and whiteners), there exist numerous opportunities for chemical compounds to enter the body through the gastrointestinal tract. By contrast, occupational exposure to chemicals usually leads to absorption in the order of frequency indicated by the three portals of entry mentioned above.

INHALATION OF CHEMICALS

While entry of chemicals into the body is commonly thought of as pursuing the oral pathway, entry through the respiratory tract affords a remarkably effective route of ingress. The surface area of the pulmonary capillary-gas exchange surface has been estimated to cover approximately 140 square meters. This compares favorably with the gastrointestinal absorptive surface, and is at least 50 times greater than the adult skin surface area. Thus, given the proper physicochemical circumstances, the pulmonary portal represents a considerable potential exchange surface for gas, vapors, fumes and even particulates.

Furthermore, following lung absorption, carriage of chemicals directly to the brain and other vital organs occurs without prior passage through the liver, in which organ detoxification mechanisms might inactivate the agent. Accordingly possibilities are enhanced for exposure to the undegraded chemical in these organs.

The degree of absorption through the pulmonary portal of entry is primarily dependent upon the physical state of the chemical under consideration. Fumes, vapors, mists and gases, being molecular or in the submicron size range, are absorbed into the capillary bed of the lungs in accordance with definite physiochemical laws. While in the main the locus of action of materials in these physical states is determined by their solubility, the dose of such materials presented to the respiratory tract may also play a role in determining the site of damage.

Given a highly soluble vapor, e.g., hydrochloric acid or ammonia, unless the respiratory tract is presented with large doses, there is "scrubbing out" of this irritant gas in the aqueous mucus cover of the turbinates and pharynx, with the consequence that little if any of the vapor reaches the lower respiratory tract. Under these conditions, the effects of small doses of such highly soluble irritant gases are mainly manifest by erythema and discomfort in the nose and throat and of the conjunctiva. If presented in large doses, however, the "scrubbing" capacity of the upper respiratory tract may be overwhelmed, with the result that sufficient of the irritant gases reach the lower respiratory tract to produce a chemical burn of the lungs. Under these conditions patchy or—in very large doses—massive pulmonary edema occurs. By contrast, gases of relatively low solubility in aqueous media will produce little upper respiratory tract irritation, though they quite readily reach the lower branches of the pulmonary tree—even in small doses—producing lung pathology here. This is exemplified by relatively insoluble phosgene gas, which even in small doses will largely reach the alveoli, gradually go into solution, slowly hydrolyze to HCl and some hours later produce pulmonary edema. Thus, mol for mol, such gases or vapors of lower water solubility are frequently more capable than the more water-soluble gases of producing serious pathologic alterations in the lower reaches of the respiratory tree, since the former readily by-pass the protective aqueous mucus layer serving as an absorptive medium in the upper respiratory tract.

Rates of diffusion of vapors or gases are dependent upon the partial pressure differentials between the alveolar air and vascular compartment. The instantaneous partial pressure of such gases or vapors in the blood is in the main a function of their solubilities in what is essentially an aqueous medium. Accordingly, though fresh blood rapidly replaces aerated blood in the pulmonary capillaries, if the vapor is nonpolar – and thus only slightly soluble in this aqueous system – saturation of the blood occurs at a rate directly proportional to pulmonary blood flow. Because of this marked limitation placed on uptake by low solubility in blood, nonpolar vapors or gases in the alveoli rapidly come into equilibrium with the vascular compartment, in contrast to the more water-soluble (polar) vapors or gases. As this equilibrium approaches, the pressure differential between blood and alveolar air decreases, and there is less of the driving force from ambient air to the body interior. In the case of the soluble gases or vapors, the rate of blood saturation is directly proportional to alveolar partial pressure, since the rate of uptake is not limited by solubility considerations.

This rate of pulmonary uptake may be altered by extrapulmonary considerations. The rate of movement of these dissolved vapors or gases from the vascular compartment to the internal milieu directly affects the blood partial pressure of these materials. Such movement from the liquid phase of the circulation may be due to renal excretion, specific tissue pick-up (e.g., CO by the erythrocyte) or a partition coefficient more favorable to extravascular localization. This last case is seen when DDT appears to move selectively from the blood to organs of relatively higher lipid concentration than the blood, e.g., the mesenteric fat depots.

While the rate of absorption is to a large degree a function of the specific physicochemical nature of the material under consideration, this rate can be altered by physiologic activity or pathologic alteration. If blood flow and ventilation rates are altered by physical activity, the rate of absorption is increased as larger volumes of relatively unsaturated blood are presented to more alveoli containing the gas in question. The rate of absorption accordingly is greatly increased with increased physical exertion. Among individuals with impairment in excretory (i.e., kidney) or detoxification (i.e., liver) function, a more rapid buildup of toxicants occurs on respiratory exposure than is the case among normals. Though equilibrium is reached more rapidly, nevertheless smaller doses produce toxicity in such persons more rapidly, as the net gain in retention of the chemical toxicant occurs more promptly.

The lungs should also be considered as a potential organ of passive excretion following exposure to gases or vapors. If a person so exposed is removed to a contaminant-free atmosphere, this effectively diminishes the alveolar partial pressure of the gas in question, assuming continued ventilation and lung perfusion. With a gradient now established in the direction *from* the capillary to the alveolus, the absorbed gas or vapor leaves the blood. While maintenance of ventilation and circulation permits body desaturation of such gaseous contaminants, measures intended to stimulate either respiration or circulation should be considered with reservation, as the toxic properties of the inhaled gas may have imposed an undue circulatory load. Under these circumstances, any attempt to drive these functions more vigorously may precipitate decompensation.

The ability of particulate matter entering the pulmonary tree to produce a local and systemic effect depends largely upon its physical nature. The chemical nature of such materials may be of secondary importance, since particles too large to reach the lower segments of the lungs have relatively less pathologic potential, regardless of chemical properties. Thus size, density and surface area of particulates determine biological activity to a large extent. Particles larger than 5 microns in size are usually not particularly active as far as inciting pulmonary disease or permitting absorption. As mass usually is related to size, large particles, once set in motion, have a higher inertia than smaller particles. In view of the numerous changes of direction of air flow in the pulmonary tree, it follows that particles having a high kinetic energy and inertia (i.e., having less physical ability to change direction of motion) also have a greater probability of impingement, and lesser probabilities of deeper penetration of the lungs. It should also be apparent that variations in particle density may determine impingement probabilities. Thus, given a particle of uranium oxide with a density of 11 and a diameter of 1 micron, it will behave in the respiratory tract as a particle of lower density several microns larger in diameter. From this stems the observation that, given a similarity in particle size, deep pulmonary penetration and deposition of uranium oxide (which particle is of high density) are less than those of a low density particle. Another factor making large particles more likely to impinge on a portion of the tracheobronchial tree is the fact that larger and/or denser particles tend to remain suspended in air for only a short period in contrast to smaller or lighter ones. Both these factors, size and density, combine to determine probability of deposition. Impaction in the air conduction passages leads ultimately to pulmonary cleansing effected by the upward-moving escalator of the cilia-propelled tracheobronchial mucus. This "moving stairway" acts from the alveolar duct level upward, continuously carrying out of the lung those particulates entrapped in this tenacious moving carpet.

Other physical properties of particulates appear to be determinants of biological activity. The crystalline lattice structure peculiar to silica, which exists chemically as free silicon dioxide, elicits a potent fibrogenic response in the lung. By contrast, noncrystalline amorphous silicates are essentially inert. It has been pointed out that the intra-atomic distance of the two oxygen atoms of this crystal is similar to the relationship of similar atoms on the surface of the endotoxin molecule of the pneumococcus bacillus. What relationship this may have to the immune nature of the response, which in some aspects is common to these dissimilar agents, is as yet obscure.

In addition, the elastic properties of the particulate may play a role in determining biological response, since particulate fibers of similar sizes, e.g., fiberglass and asbestos, produce quite different results in the lung. While fiberglass responds to elastic deformation quite readily and does not produce pulmonary damage, asbestos fibers are relatively inelastic and do produce pathologic alteration when they lodge in the constantly changing diameters of bronchioles. Undoubtedly, the specific chemical nature of the asbestos fiber plays a role in inciting pathologic alteration. Indeed, the chemical nature of the asbestos fiber in contrast to the glass fiber may be the major determinant of the pulmonary reaction. However, such response may well be also dependent upon its peculiar mechanical properties.

Finally, the chemical nature of the particle which impinges in the lungs may determine the nature of the biological response. Particulates of lead oxide impinging on alveolar surfaces allow for leaching and systemic absorption, while similar particles of lead sulfide are associated with little if any absorption.

The ultimate fate of particles that impinge on the pulmonary surfaces is variable, though such final disposal loci also determine the site of response. Particulates which are deposited in the alveoli may be phagocytized by macrophages. In the case of crystalline silica, these particles most frequently are conveyed by dust cells along the peribronchial and perivascular lymphatics, though some few of these cells may migrate upward through the air conduction pathways.

Phagocytes that have ingested such crystals eventually reach the hilar lymph nodes where they are filtered out. This accumulation leads to a fibrous response, which in turn produces enlargement of these nodes early in the disease. Subsequent distortion of the tracheobronchial tree may lead to inadequate drainage with accumulation of small amounts of mucus and a scanty cough. Many of the phagocytes—for reasons yet unclear—break down in the course of this passage through these lymphatic channels, with the development of a localized inflammatory response in association with this necrotic debris. With the inflammatory response there is an impairment of lymphatic movement and phagocytic activity, resulting in stasis, retention of silica locally and the formation of fibrotic nodules at these sites. Later, after years of exposure to free silica, increased lung markings and typical fibrotic nodules of silicosis are found along the course of the lymphatics. The typical silica nodule of the lung parenchyma, characterized by a circumferentially oriented, onion-skin-like hyalin deposition, is also seen in the hilar lymph node. In addition such individuals appear to be highly susceptible to tuberculous infection. When this complication supervenes, a more diffuse fibrosis and associated pulmonary obstructive disorder result. As these dense nodules begin to calcify, the roentgenogram will clearly demonstrate these radiopaque nodular structures, each of which might be considered the tombstone of a silica crystal.

ABSORPTION VIA THE CUTANEOUS ROUTE

The skin is usually considered as constituting an effective barrier to entry into the internal milieu. Inorganic electrolytes, high molecular weight substances, molecular aggregates and particulates quite clearly cannot penetrate the uninjured epidermal layer. To a very slight extent some gases may pass directly through the cutaneous barricade.

The barriers to transcutaneous movement are found at several points in and on the skin. Immediately on the epidermal surface is a water and oil emulsion, liberated by keratinizing cells and secretions of the sebaceous and sweat glands. While the pH (4.5 to 6.0) of this "acid mantle" is said to have antifungal and antibacterial properties, it poses little resistance to passage of most compounds. Since the keratin layer is fairly porous, it is at the area directly above the granular layer (between the stratum granulosum and stratum corneum) that one finds the first major mechanism appearing to block further passage of many compounds across the skin barrier.

The causes of the relatively high degree of impermeability found here are not fully understood.

These cells have been shown by electron microscopy to be extremely dense, consisting of a uniform keratin material, and to contain less than 10 per cent water. Furthermore, at this location there has been demonstrated an electronegatively charged, horizontally oriented field which is believed to repel anions and prevent cations from penetrating more deeply. Furthermore, passage around these cells becomes more difficult since at this level the cells are most densely packed.

However, for certain groups of chemicals the skin poses no significant hindrance to percutaneous passage. Nonpolar materials of an ether:water partition coefficient greater than 1 most readily traverse this percutaneous route. It is assumed that, since most such lipid-like materials pass directly through cells, the lipid content of these cutaneous cell membranes permits such passage. In the case of aniline or carbon tetrachloride, this apparently appears to be true, since these nonpolar compounds pass through the intact skin almost as readily as any other portal. Though this theory applies in many cases, there are, however, some exceptions to this concept. Indeed, phenol, which is soluble in both aqueous and lipid media, passes extremely readily through the skin barrier.

While the skin surface per se is the major entry route as a result of its larger surface area, the dermal appendages also permit entrance to the internal environment of the body. The termination of the granulosum barrier described above occurs at the level where the sebaceous gland enters the follicle. This barrier layer may thus be by-passed, for chemicals can diffuse through the continuum of the liquid phase or mantle on the skin surface and thence eventually to these glands. The cells of the pilosebaceous apparatus with their extensive blood supply appear to be quite permeable. By contrast, it is believed that the sweat glands do not provide a significant portal of entry.

In addition, the foregoing premises are based upon an intact skin surface. Therefore, breaks in the epidermal continuity may afford a significant portal of entry for highly toxic chemicals. Systemic distribution may occur following penetration of the skin by flying objects contaminated by such agents, or through lacerations or abrasions. However, here again systemic absorption usually is dependent upon solubility and particle size, since these determine the potential for leaching of the chemical constituents of such bodies.

GASTROINTESTINAL TRACT AND MUCOUS MEMBRANE ABSORPTION

As previously noted, absorption via this route is a result of specific and peculiar situations rather than occurrences that usually arise from occupational or the more common environmental exposures. The potential for gastrointestinal tract absorption must be considered, however, under such circumstances when toxic materials are inadvertently carried to the mouth by contamination of cigarettes, food or the hands themselves. Such contamination is commonly noted in work places characterized by inadequate environmental hygiene.

While the rate of absorption for numerous materials is variable, the small intestine is apparently the major site of gastrointestinal absorption. Except for ethyl alcohol, few if any chemical agents are absorbed directly through the gastric mucosa. Those agents absorbed at the remainder of the small intestine do so as a function of various physicochemical factors.

The rate of absorption is frequently decreased in the presence of food, since liquids dilute and solid particulates may react to form insoluble complexes or allow adsorption of toxic materials onto their surfaces. Thus the presence of the casein of milk on contacting caustics forms a curd-like mass due to protein coagulation, thus leading to adsorption and decreased gastrointestinal tract absorption.

Solubility also plays a role in the rate of gastrointestinal absorption. More carbon tetrachloride is absorbed in the presence of a fatty meal or alcohol, as the concentration of this solvent per unit volume of gastrointestinal contents is decreased. In the presence of a relatively high concentration at an absorbing surface, transmembrane movement is impeded by rate limits of absorption in contrast to low concentrations. Such rate limits appear to be operative in the gastrointestinal tract. The "selectivity" of absorption that prevents the uptake of "unnatural" substances appears to be an expression of such concentration-dependent rate limits.

Systemic effects are also modified by the fact that materials absorbed through the gastrointestinal tract must first pass through the liver via the portal system. This transit introduces the potential for metabolic transformations such as detoxification or degradation and/or excretion via the biliary duct. Thus, in the case of lead and arsenic, entry into the general circulation is prevented to a degree by excretion into the biliary system.

Absorption of various chemicals at the surfaces of the gastrointestinal tract, as with any body interface, may lead to local damage. With ingestion of corrosive agents, irreversible alteration of protein components may readily occur, leading to the potentials for discontinuity of such epithelial surfaces. The clinical expression of this change is seen in the denaturation of the protein of the mucosa by caustics, resulting in a typical white, friable appearance. Since coagulated protein is relatively less elastic, normal gastrointestinal movement may lead to disruption of the mucosa. If these destructive corrosive effects extend deeper than the superficial mucosa, rupture of the superficial blood vessels with associated hemorrhage may develop.

What is frequently considered a local effect in the gastrointestinal tract may actually be an expression of a systemic alteration in which the intestinal tract may also participate. Such is the case with the ulcerations of the upper bowel seen in arsenic ingestion. Apparently one of the basic lesions of arsenic intoxication is a marked alteration in capillary permeability. This primary lesion is expressed by leakage at the glomerular tuft with the resultant hematuria and proteinuria. However, because of the dramatic changes within the gastrointestinal tract, the renal lesion usually present is not sought and thus not detected. In the gut, leakage of the fluid phase from the superficial capillary bed leads to extravasation and collection of serum in the submucosa. With further accumulation, stretching of the mucosa continues until rupture occurs, which in turn leads to frank bleeding from what appears to be an ulcerated mucosa. Fluid and protein continue to be lost via this discontinuity, while hypermotility, cramping and severe abdominal pain appear due to the irritation produced by such luminal contents and rupture of the mucosa. In acute arsenic intoxication a fatal termination may supervene due to fluid losses from the vascular bed, shock and circulatory collapse. Yet that which is seen as a local effect is in fact a manifestation of a systemic alteration in capillary permeability at the molecular level. Since permeability maintenance is energy dependent, it has been suggested that the known interference by arsenic with pyruvate dehydrogenase activity in the Embden-Meyerhof pathway may reduce energy availability to endothelial cells. With ensuing entropy, loss of permeability control in such structures may be one of the earliest functional alterations.

The mucous membranes offer a varying degree of protection of the internal environment from hostile agents. Women with no known contact to mercury other than certain mercury-containing contraceptive preparations can be demonstrated to absorb considerable amounts of inorganic mercury salts; a degree of absorption via this route is possible even to the point of producing a fatal outcome. The absorption of nitroglycerin or even larger molecules, e.g., progesterone, via the buccal mucous membrane is well known. In former years the absorption of silver salts following nasal instillation was sufficient to cause the generalized body discoloration of argyria. While these portals of entry are well demonstrated, the elucidation of the mechanism of absorption and factors affecting this process are not clear at this time.

CELLULAR BIOLOGY AND ENZYMATIC ALTERATION AS DETERMINANT OF CLINICAL RESPONSE TO TOXIC CHEMICAL ABSORPTION

For the rational understanding of the clinical symptom complex which may result from absorption of a toxic chemical, the study of the interrelations between organ systems, i.e., physiologic response, is of itself inadequate. That this is true arises from knowledge that chemical-induced alteration of organ function may stem from causes other than direct modification of its constituent cells. Changes in any one of several organs demonstrating a pathologic alteration may result from changes far removed from that organ, e.g., changes in blood flow, or hormone-mediated and/or direct neurogenic activity. Such changes are seen following absorption of hexavalent uranium producing renal tubular damage and resultant accumulation of waste products of metabolism. Their buildup in the circulation appears to play a role in liver injury with resultant fatty metamorphosis. Yet study of hepatic physiology would provide an inadequate basis for building a rational, mechanistic understanding of the clinical complex stemming from uranium intoxication.

Similarly, pathologic alteration described in terms of structural change contributes only in part to comprehension of the mechanisms underlying clinical response. The structural entities contained within the cell are not the static, fixed entities suggested by morphologic study. The delimiting boundary of the cell, i.e., the plasma membrane, cytoplasm and associated organelles, the nucleus and its contents—all these cell components in health and disease are constantly in a state of flux or turnover. The replacement and renewal inherent in this state are clearly dependent upon energy sources. This driving force is necessary for the activity involved in synthesis of replacement components and the dynamic functions carried out by and among these structures. The integration of this system and its synthetic or energy-producing activity are ultimately dependent upon catalysts which determine the rate of these reactions. Accordingly, in the final analyses, these crucial activities are dependent upon enzymatic control. While it must be understood that enzymes do not contribute to the net energy required for such chemical reactions, it should be pointed out that such catalysis accelerates such reactions, permitting them to proceed within restricted temperature and concentration ranges.

Thus we have arrived at our premise, i.e., that much of the clinical picture of chemically induced morbidity will be more clearly explicable when we can describe the interactions of toxic agents on enzymes and the metabolic systems they control. Though the details of such interactions constitute an as yet ill-perceived horizon, undoubtedly the biochemical approach will in turn be succeeded by the viewpoint that considers such dynamics purely in a biophysical frame of reference. Since these intimate biophysical insights are not yet within our grasp, our discussion here centers mainly about the mechanisms whereby chemicals alter intracellular enzymatic processes.

MODE OF ACTION OF CHEMICALS UPON ENZYME SYSTEMS

Enzymatic Inactivation or Denaturation

As is the case with other proteins, the functional status of an enzyme is dependent upon its three-dimensional structural integrity. Exposure of any protein system to drastic chemical or thermal conditions may produce irreversible alteration of these requisite spatial relationships. On contact with strong acids or alkaline agents skin surfaces and mucous membranes demonstrate the formation of an irreversible protein coagulum. The changes induced by thermal coagulation of egg white are clearly analogous to alterations seen following tissue contact by chemical coagulants. Thus there are similar alterations of the structural characteristics (e.g., elasticity, flexibility) and the functional nature (e.g., permeability) of the target tissues. These become whitened, biologically insert and readily friable. Given undue mechanical stress, such surfaces can be ruptured readily. This clearly serves to explain the clinical basis for the contraindication of gastric tube passage through an alkali-burned esophagus; such a devitalized organ is structurally weakened and presents a high risk of perforation. With the passage of time, phagocytic removal of detritus occurs, and this protein coagulum is replaced by fibrous tissue, scarring and subsequent contracture. All these changes can occur at any body surface so contacted.

However, enzymatic activity can be irreversibly inactivated by means less drastic than protein denaturation. Such interactions are at the root of chemical toxicity, and their specific mechanisms are here considered individually.

Direct Enzyme-Chemical Combination

This type of interaction is one of the most obvious manners in which toxicity may be produced. A chemical agent may combine with an enzyme so as to alter the catalyst's structural relationships, and especially its active-site or active-group spatial associations. The significance of such alterations is readily apparent, since it is at such sites that the substrate (i.e., the material acted upon and changed by the enzyme) combines with the enzyme. The very brief association of these two components (enzyme and substrate) leads to the formation of a complex. This combination is succeeded by a change in the substrate, which becomes "activated," i.e., the substrate becomes particularly susceptible to chemical reaction or change.

The combination of the cyanide ion with an atom of iron produces a metal-cyanide complex; this combination inhibits the activity of cytochrome A_3 in the terminal segment of the electron transfer chain. With inhibition of this reaction, there is a cessation of the oxidative mechanism. This process plays a vital role in the metabolic reaction providing a major source of energy for cellular activity. Clinically, the first symptom of mild poisoning is manifest by that system with the highest level of oxidative metabolic needs and whose aberration is most rapidly reflected by clinical alteration. Given these requirements, one expects the central nervous system to be the first to demonstrate clearly symptomatic alterations analogous to a lack of oxygen, since the net effect of impairment of cellular oxidation (or the ability to utilize oxygen) is essentially the same as that produced by hypoxia. Thus headache, lassitude and nausea appear as manifestations of nerve cell hypoxia, but in more severe poisonings—as anoxia, in this peculiar sense, supervenes—these manifestations are replaced by signs of oxygen lack at motor centers. The convulsions resulting from this type of cellular "anoxia" at these sites are succeeded by collapse and respiratory paralysis. Death may occur quite rapidly as a consequence of anoxia of the vital brain stem nuclei controlling cardiovascular and respiratory functions.

The lethal propensities of cyanide are somewhat unusual, since the block of a critical step in the electron transfer chain cannot be readily by-passed by a shunt or alternate pathway. Arsenic by contrast is lethal only in relatively larger doses than cyanide, since enzymatic blocks produced by its salts or oxides may be by-passed. Arsenic, by combining with the sulfhydryl groups associated with numerous enzymes, e.g., pyruvate oxidase, forms an inactive complex. However, in those organs which can utilize fatty acids as a source of energy substrate, these lipid moieties may be utilized in energy production by their entry into the citric acid cycle independent of carbohydrate sources. Accordingly an arsenic-induced block in carbohydrate oxidative energy metabolism at the point of pyruvate oxidation can be by-passed and energy needs met. Thus in chronic arsenic poisoning the myocardium demonstrates only minor clinical manifestations of functional change because of the existence of such shunts in these cells. This alternate energy source may not be as readily available to peripheral nervous tissue. Such possibility of "by-pass" potential may account for the observation that in subacute and chronic arsenic intoxication, peripheral nerve degeneration produces clinical symptoms of motor and sensory dysfunction in contrast to relatively few changes in cardiac function.

An exceptionally clear picture of direct enzyme inhibition is afforded by examination of the effects of the organophosphate insecticides upon the enzyme acetylcholine esterase (AChE). It should be recalled that acetylcholine acts as the chemical mediator transmitting nervous impulses across the synapse. This enzyme AChE causes hydrolysis or breakdown of acetylcholine secreted at such neural synapses. By virtue of this usual action of AChE at these sites there is termination of the nerve impulse at the synaptic junction or motor end-plate.

The organophosphate pesticides are of such a molecular size and configuration that they attach at the two active sites of the AChE molecule whereat acetylcholine ordinarily would be bound, activated and then cleaved by this esterase. This phosphorylated enzyme complex (i.e., the AChE-organophosphate combination) is quite abnormally stable. Furthermore, access to the active site on AChE where acetylcholine normally is cleaved, is blocked, leading to failure of acetylcholine breakdown. Therefore this mediator acetylcholine persists and continues to stimulate at postganglionic parasympathetic synapses and striated muscle motor end-plates. Protracted stimulation of the motor nerves of the gastrointestinal tract produces vomiting, diarrhea and abdominal cramps, while continued ciliary body stimulation causes contraction and resultant blurring of vision and miosis. Persistent parasympathetic stimulation leads to increased secretions by glandular cells, as manifested by salivation, lacrimation and diaphoresis. In addition parasympathetically induced bronchoconstriction causes airway obstruction and increased secretions in the tracheobronchial tree, so that expiratory wheezing and moist rales are heard. Persons thus affected complain of a tightness in the chest (bronchoconstriction?) and dyspnea. With progression of this intoxication resulting from enzyme inhibition, the fine muscle tremors or fasciculation caused by continuous motor end-plate stimulation are succeeded by gross convulsions, stemming from both central motor stimulation and continued peripheral nerve activity. Ultimately, malcoordinated respiratory muscle activity and central nervous system hyperactivity lead to impaired respiratory exchange with cyanosis, exhaustion, coma and death. That all of these result mainly from continued acetylcholine-mediated activity at these various receptor sites of the involved synapses is clearly demonstrated by administration of large doses of atropine. This compound produces a striking reversal of the signs of toxicity described above by blocking responsiveness to acetylcholine at receptor portions of the synaptic junction.

Competitive Inhibition

This mechanism applies to that situation wherein a toxic material competes with other metabolites or cofactors for the active site of an enzyme. Such competitive inhibition reaches a maximum when the competing material structurally is highly similar to the chemical configuration of the constituent (i.e., metabolite or cofactor) normally acted upon by the enzyme (see above).

An unusual but probably not unique example of pharmacologic competitive inhibition is seen in the behavior of two organophosphate pesticides which compete for a single specific enzymatic detoxification system. One of these, malathion, is approximately 30 times less toxic than another such pesticide, EPN. Yet when given in combination, the toxicity of malathion is remarkably enhanced. It appears that EPN more successfully competes for the same enzyme that ordinarily would rapidly hydrolize malathion. It is believed that malathion cannot be acted upon by this enzyme that would ordinarily render it metabolically inactive, i.e., reduce its toxicity. Accordingly, this unsuccessful competition of malathion for the degrading enzyme leads to its persistence and accumulation as a toxicologically active agent. Though other similar combinations of organic thiophosphates are known to produce similar enhancements of toxicity, similar situations not involving organic thiophosphates undoubtedly exist.

INDUCTION OF TOXICITY BY METABOLIC ALTERATION OF CHEMICALS

Though the word "detoxification" implies a mechanism that reduces toxic potentials inherent in a compound, it should be understood that these processes whereby the animal economy produces such metabolic transformations phylogenetically stem mainly from an ability to utilize food substances. Thus "detoxification" pathways that exist do so largely insofar as nonfood substances exhibiting structural similarities to food components may be acted upon. Indeed, these relatively nondiscriminating biological enzyme systems may produce the apparent paradox of enhanced toxicity following this peculiar metabolic transformation, i.e., "detoxification."

Oxidation

This is one of the most common mechanisms whereby metabolic transformations may be achieved. For example, toluene is oxidized to benzoic acid, biologically a relatively innocuous compound. However, such metabolic oxidations may form products of greatly enhanced toxicity, a conspicuous example being the product of methanol oxidation, formaldehyde. This oxidative product is of relatively high cytotoxic potential, causing irreversible alteration of protein. The specific effect of wood alcohol on the retina is explained in part on the basis that retinal cells—as well as hepatocytes—are believed to be specific loci whereat the enzyme alcohol dehydrogenase catalyzes the biological oxidation of alcohols. Accordingly it has been suggested that intracellular oxidation by the enzyme produces within the retinal cells minute quantities of formaldehyde. However, despite the small quantities elaborated, such intracellular formation of formaldehyde is sufficient to produce cellular damage. The blindness that may follow methanol intoxication is an expression of the minimal capacity for regeneration of injured central nervous system tissue. Concurrently, hepatocytic death is readily succeeded by regenerative replacement of necrotized liver cells so that permanent liver damage does not ensue following such an insult. Other examples of enhanced toxicity following oxidative change are found following successive oxidation of the benzene molecule to di- and trihydroxybenzene. This successive transformation appears to lead to successively increasing acute toxicity. In yet another instance, the replacement of sulfur by oxygen leads to the oxidation of inert parathion to the highly toxic paraoxon with resultant severe physiologic embarrassment (see discussion of acetylcholine esterase inhibition).

Reduction

Though reduction represents a somewhat less frequent body metabolic activity than oxidation, several groups of foreign compounds are altered by this mechanism. Nitrobenzenes or certain organic compounds composed of an aromatic ring with an attached nitrogen (e.g., primaquine, sulfanilimide) ordinarily can be metabolized by reduction without serious consequences. The additional hydrogen atom to carry out this reduction is ordinarily supplied by reduced triphosphopyridine nucleotide (TPNH) which normally is in adequate supply in most tissues. The formation of TPNH is in certain cells, e.g., erythrocytes, probably dependent in the main upon the action of the enzyme glucose-6-phosphate dehydrogenase (G-6-PD).

An unusual example of failure of the reductive process stems from a genetically determined metabolic defect. This abnormality occurs in certain racial groups which genetically develop erythrocytes deficient in G-6-PD. As a consequence of deficiency there is a diminution of red cell TPNH. Because of the deficiency of TPNH, there is a concurrent diminution in the rate of glutathione reduction, the hydrogen ion donated by TPNH being required to carry out this reduction. Both of these compounds, TPNH and reduced glutathione, are in turn required to maintain hemoglobin and ferro-catalase in the reduced state. This defect and the attendant deficiencies are not expressed under normal conditions in individuals carrying this genetic abnormality.

However, with the absorption of oxidizing chemicals there is a conversion of hemoglobin to the oxidized form, i.e., methemoglobin. To reduce this oxidized hemoglobin to the physiologically functional (i.e., reduced) form requires an increased supply of hydrogen atoms. Among persons having decreased G-6-PD and resultant diminished TPNH to act as a hydrogen ion donor, this peculiar enzyme deficiency leads to serious consequences. With impairment of erythrocytic ability to re-establish a reducing environment, the rate of reduction of this oxidized hemoglobin (i.e., methemoglobin) formed by nitrogen-containing aromatic chemicals is markedly decreased. This ultimately leads to a temporal persistence of methemoglobin in persons with this genetic defect in contrast to individuals possessing normal G-6-PD activity in the erythrocyte. Furthermore, reduced glutathione appears to be required for cellular integrity. Among such susceptibles, with both of these loads upon cellular homeostasis, absorption of these oxidizing compounds frequently results in massive hemolysis and/or prolonged methemoglobinemia. Thus what had previously been empirically described as "hypersensitivity" can be explained by hereditary factors determining the integrity of this metabolic pathway.

As previously noted in the discussion of oxidation reactions, a reductive type alteration resulting in a more toxic product is seen in the reduction of nitrobenzene to aminobenzene and coincident oxidation to para-aminophenol. This metabolic product is approximately 50 to 80 times more toxic than the parent material, nitrobenzene.

Conjugation

Conjugative metabolic alterations resulting in synthesis of new compounds occur commonly in the course of normal body activity. Such additions of normal tissue constituents, e.g., glucuronate or sulfate, to the molecule of a foreign material usually result in solubilization of the original exogenous molecule. While in most cases this results in a compound of lesser toxicity, continued utilization of the endogenous constituent involved in conjugative processes may lead to depletion of these vital substances. A depletion of cysteine, utilized in the conjugation of p-bromobenzene, is seen when this chemical is fed to growing animals in excess of certain quantities. These feedings lead to a cessation of growth, since the animal is unable to provide sufficient cysteine for both growth and conjugation of the excessive amounts of p-bromobenzene.

The fact that cysteine is utilized for detoxification of p-bromobenzene has been utilized in the treatment of selenium intoxication. In areas where selenium is present in soils, body burdens of this element become relatively high. The selenium ingested in vegetation and water in such locations displaces the sulfur of cysteine and methionine of body tissues with a resultant deficiency of these amino acids. Selenized individuals have been given p-bromobenzene in the hope of removing from their bodies some of the selenium-containing cysteine. In these cases conjugation of the selenium-containing cysteine with the p-bromobenzene occurred. This was confirmed by the observation that selenium blood levels dropped considerably and that urinary excretion of selenium as a mercapturic acid rose with this therapy.

Lethal Synthesis

In contrast to detoxification effected by conjugative synthesis, the metabolic transformation by the body of one chemical into a new compound can have untoward results. In addition to the oxidative, reductive and conjugative processes previously considered, a somewhat different type of synthesis by the body has been demonstrated following absorption of sodium fluoroacetate (1080). The metabolic transfer to citric acid of the fluorine atoms in this toxic compound leads to the biological synthesis of fluorocitrate. This citrate is an inhibitor of the enzyme aconitase, with the result that the normal product of this enzyme's activity, cis-aconitate, is not formed. This deficiency of cis-aconitate blocks the completion of the Krebs or citric acid cycle necessary for oxidative energy metabolism and cell respiration. Those cells requiring the highest rates of oxidation, i.e., myocardial and central nervous system cells, are the first to demonstrate this energy source depletion. Absorption of 1080 leads to severe cardiac irregularities of rhythm, failure and collapse, accompanied by a rapid onset of convulsions and finally coma. The result of this block of the Krebs cycle apparently cannot be effectively reversed, since the fluorocitrate aconitase complex formed cannot be degraded by any known enzyme system. The possibility exists for entry into the Krebs cycle of other normally available metabolites, e.g., α-ketoglutarate, oxaloacetate, beyond the point of the fluorocitrate-induced block. However, the potential for such by-passes appears limited in view of the extreme toxicity of this compound 1080.

SOME BIOPHYSICAL DETERMINANTS OF CHEMICAL INTOXICATION

A mechanism of toxicity due to direct combination by an exogenous chemical with a body component is clearly illustrated by the remarkable affinity of carbon monoxide for hemoglobin. Carbon monoxide forms a moderately stable complex with the ferrous tetrapyrrole respiratory pigment hemoglobin. As a result of this association CO blocks the accessibility of reactive sites on the hemoglobin molecule ordinarily available for oxygen carriage. In such a competition between CO and O_2, the attraction of carbon monoxide for hemoglobin is approximately 240 times greater than that of oxygen.

From these considerations it follows that while this affinity of CO for hemoglobin is so much greater than that of oxygen, nevertheless this is a *relative* affinity for the hemoglobin molecule. Accordingly the partial pressures of these two gases act as determinants of the quantities of each gas taken up. Thus, given a fixed concentration of carbon monoxide in the ambient air (and concurrently in the alveolus), ultimately a point of equilibrium between CO in blood and alveolar air is reached. As this event approaches, the rate of hemoglobin conversion gradually decreases, since the "back pressure" of CO in the blood approaches the alveolar CO partial pressure. This increasing "back pressure" gradually decreases the pressure differential or gradient across the alveolar membrane, with the result that the rate of CO absorption slows, and the proportion of CO absorbed from the inspired mixture decreases steadily from its initial value of about 50 per cent. When equilibrium is reached, the net transfer of CO between blood and air and the rate of increase in carboxyhemoglobin become zero.

Achievement of this steady state can readily serve to illustrate the concept of dose dependency in a responsive biological system at the molecular and physiologic levels. If the concentrations of CO in air occur in the range of 50 parts per million (0.005 per cent), an equilibrium between blood and ambient air is eventually reached. This event occurs with conversion of approximately 8 per cent of the available hemoglobin. At such time, if the exposure concentration remains at 50 ppm, there is no longer an increase or decrease in the net amount of hemoglobin existing as the carboxyhemoglobin form.

Furthermore, this example of the conversion of hemoglobin by carbon monoxide can serve also to illustrate clearly the time parameter which is a major determinant of chemical intoxication. As previously stated, this conversion occurs at a rate dependent upon the alveolar partial pressure. At a concentration of approximately 50 ppm, approximately 9 hours must elapse for this concentration to come into equilibrium, i.e., the 8 per cent carboxyhemoglobin conversion level. By contrast, because of the CO arising from tobacco combustion, moderately heavy cigarette smokers are commonly found to have this concentration of carboxyhemoglobin. Yet Goldsmith and co-workers have shown that levels of 400 to 450 ppm (0.04 to 0.045 per cent) CO are attained in the inhaled cigarette smoke stream. In the face of such relatively higher CO exposure levels of cigarette smokers, one is led to inquire why smokers have a level of carboxyhemoglobin formation comparable to that of individuals exposed to 50 ppm. Plainly, what is occurring with cigarette-induced CO exposure is repeated *short-term* peak concentration exposures. The result is a high gradient of short duration across the alveolar membrane during the act of smoke inhalation. As smoking ceases this gradient is subsequently reversed because of a relatively high "back pressure" from the blood to the alveoli. Over several hours of intermittent smoking the net effect results in an equilibration at approximately 8 per cent hemoglobin conversion, despite the peak exposure levels. Thus the high peaks over a period of time average out to levels which only very indirectly reflect these high levels of CO found in the cigarette smoke stream.

However, these hemoglobin conversion rates are also dependent upon physiologic factors, a prime consideration being the pulmonary ventilation parameter. Thus, by increasing the volume of air moved per unit time, one readily sees that a greater quantity of CO can be presented to the gas exchange membrane per unit time. Consequently, rates of hemoglobin conversion can reflect a change in physical activity, since in going from the resting state to one of heavy work it has been found that the rate of conversion is increased by a factor of 366 per cent.

The fact that this alteration of an intrinsic property of hemoglobin, i.e., its ability to carry oxygen, does not produce a permanent structural change in the hemoglobin molecule points up another possible manner by which chemicals may interact with many biological molecules. This CO-hemoglobin molecular complex is an example of an interaction that produces only a functional modification of the hemoglobin molecule. Concurrently the underlying structural nature of the hemoglobin molecule remains relatively intact and can express its preintoxication functional characteristics given once more the proper conditions of oxygen tension.

There is yet another functional change in hemoglobin as a result of its combination with CO. Douglas and Haldane quite clearly stated that "oxygen is given off from oxyhemoglobin in a totally abnormal manner when the blood is highly saturated with carbon monoxide... the dissociation of oxygen being altered in such a way that the oxygen comes off less readily, or only at a lower pressure than in normal bloods." As a consequence of the reluctance to give up oxygen peculiar to this mixture of oxygenated and carbon monoxide-heme complexes on a single hemoglobin molecule, the release of oxygen from such erythrocytes to the tissue goes on much less *readily*. The rate of release of oxygen normally required by the tissues occurs in the presence of carboxyhemoglobin only when tissue oxygen pressure falls to very low tensions. That this shift in the oxyhemoglobin dissociation curve becomes significant only with relatively high carboxyhemoglobin levels (i.e., greater than 20 to 30 per cent conversion) is not clearly appreciated. Nevertheless this shift in the oxygen dissociation curve can pose problems if a sudden increased tissue demand—as with exercise—is imposed upon this already fragilely balanced system of oxygen supply and demand at the tissues. A clinical example of this impediment to oxygen release is seen in those individuals who have suffered CO intoxication. On attempting to rise and walk about from the semiconscious state, they may take only a few steps before they once more collapse. Thus, while their tissue needs are met at rest, the increased tissue demand associated with work of motion cannot be met due to this oxygen dissociation shift and lowered O_2 carrying capacity.

Depending on several circumstances, such combinations of chemicals and body constituents may have either a beneficial or deleterious effect. Most drugs form reversible complexes with plasma proteins and intracellular components. These nonspecific, loose chemical attachments may provide a reservoir from which the compound can be released in response to a decrease in the circulating, unbound form of the chemical in question. This dynamic equilibrium may ultimately serve to permit prolongation of drug action as a consequence of slow release from such binding stores. In the case of lead, the storage of this ion in the bony matrix may permit buildup in concentration of this potentially toxic agent in this depot without the manifestation of intoxication despite prolonged low level absorption. However, with stress situations, e.g., heat (?), mobilization of such stores leads to symptoms of acute intoxication, though the patient may no longer be in lead exposure. Such a dynamic equilibrium between the lead bound in the bony compartment and that in the vascular compartment has implications in regard to chelation therapy.

Chelation has been defined as the incorporation of a metal ion into a heterocyclic ring structure. The metal is bound by two or more ions of the complexing molecule, the latter being referred to as a ligand. Certain atoms in the ligand "donate" electrons to the metal atoms and thus "share" electron pairs with the metal ions. By reason of this electron "sharing," the metal ion is sequestered within the "ionic cage" of the donor molecule, inhibiting expression of the toxic nature of many metal ions.

At present, available chelating agents, e.g., Versene, or calcium disodium ethylenediaminetetracetic acid (EDTA), are capable of chelating only circulating lead and other ions. While the acute symptoms due to unsequestered lead are rapidly abated by chelation, therapy directed toward removal of body burdens of lead outside the vascular compartment is ineffectual. Thus, if the patient is given a rest period of about 1 week, an equilibrium between lead bound in bone and circulating lead will be re-established. At this time another 3 to 5 days of EDTA therapy leads to chelation of the circulating lead with diminution of this compartment's loading. By such an alternating, stepwise program the clinician may achieve diminution of the total body burden of lead.

METALS IN THE ENVIRONMENT

Principles of Bioconcentration and Biotransformation

The earth's crust is the source of all metallic elements which man encounters. Since man is a creature of that crust, it follows that the waters and plants of the earth's surface, which eventually take up these elements, will convey them to man. In addition, since the forces of weather continually wear away the crust, aerosols and dusts containing metallic elements are eventually taken up by the human respiratory tract. The nature of such ecologic flows for lead are depicted in Figure 34–4; consideration of this diagram will indicate the multiple possibilities for human uptake through air, water and plant, and animal life.

Such natural fluxes have continued over the millennia. Since this process was characterized by a slow turnover, the distribution media (e.g., air, water) permitted slow but ready dilution. High concentrations in any locale were uncommon until the intrusion of man's technology. By virtue of man's extractive capacity (e.g., mining, smelting, and redistribution) relatively more concentrated quantities of crustal elements were introduced into the environment. It is such activities which pose potential threats to human health, since evolutionarily determined metabolic capabilities for coping with these heavier loadings of metallic elements may be exceeded.

Another factor which may pose a threat to man derives from the phenomenon of biological concentration. This depends upon food chains through which elemental materials are passed.

With each successive step from lower organism to higher (i.e., as each predator feeds on lower forms) there may be successive concentration of certain elements. Thus, as bottom-dwelling bacteria bearing mercury are eaten by worms, which are fed upon by smaller fish, which are in turn fed upon by still larger fish, increasingly more mercury is borne to the higher predator. When ultimately man consumes the largest predacious fish, he may also be taking up a dangerous amount of mercury as a result of this bioconcentration process via the food chain.

These concentrating food chains with man at the apex are further complicated by the phenomenon of biotransformation. In this process, lower organisms may convert a relatively inert element to a more toxic form, which then may be passed up the food chain to man. Such was seen when relatively large concentrations of mercury deposited in bodies of water by industrial operations were converted from elemental forms to relatively more toxic organic compounds, i.e., from inorganic mercury to methyl mercury. Although such transformations were probably for microorganisms a form of detoxification, the net result for man was the introduction of a highly poisonous compound into his body following consumption of fish so contaminated. The consequences of such human uptake were seen in Minimata and Niigata, Japan, where serious neurotoxicity occurred following inorganic mercury pollution of coastal fishing grounds and biotransformation among marine biota.

At present it appears that metallic bioconcentration through food chains poses a limited threat to man. Since multiple successive steps are required, short food chains (e.g., soil to plant to grazing animals to man) do not appear to present a threat. By contrast, where man is at the apex of a multi-step food chain (with marine food sources) such potential threats to human health may apply. Fortunately, at this time it appears that bioconcentration by plant forms is a relatively uncommon phenomenon, e.g., translocation of lead and mercury from the soil to plant parenchyma is minimal.

Consequences of Metallic Contamination of the Environment

The threat posed by mercury contamination of the environment is relatively well understood at the present time. The phenomena of bioconcentration and biotransformation have caused severe local problems where mercury was allowed to escape into water courses. It was formerly believed that such elemental mercury effluents were not hazardous to man, since in this form they were not believed to be biologically accessible to the

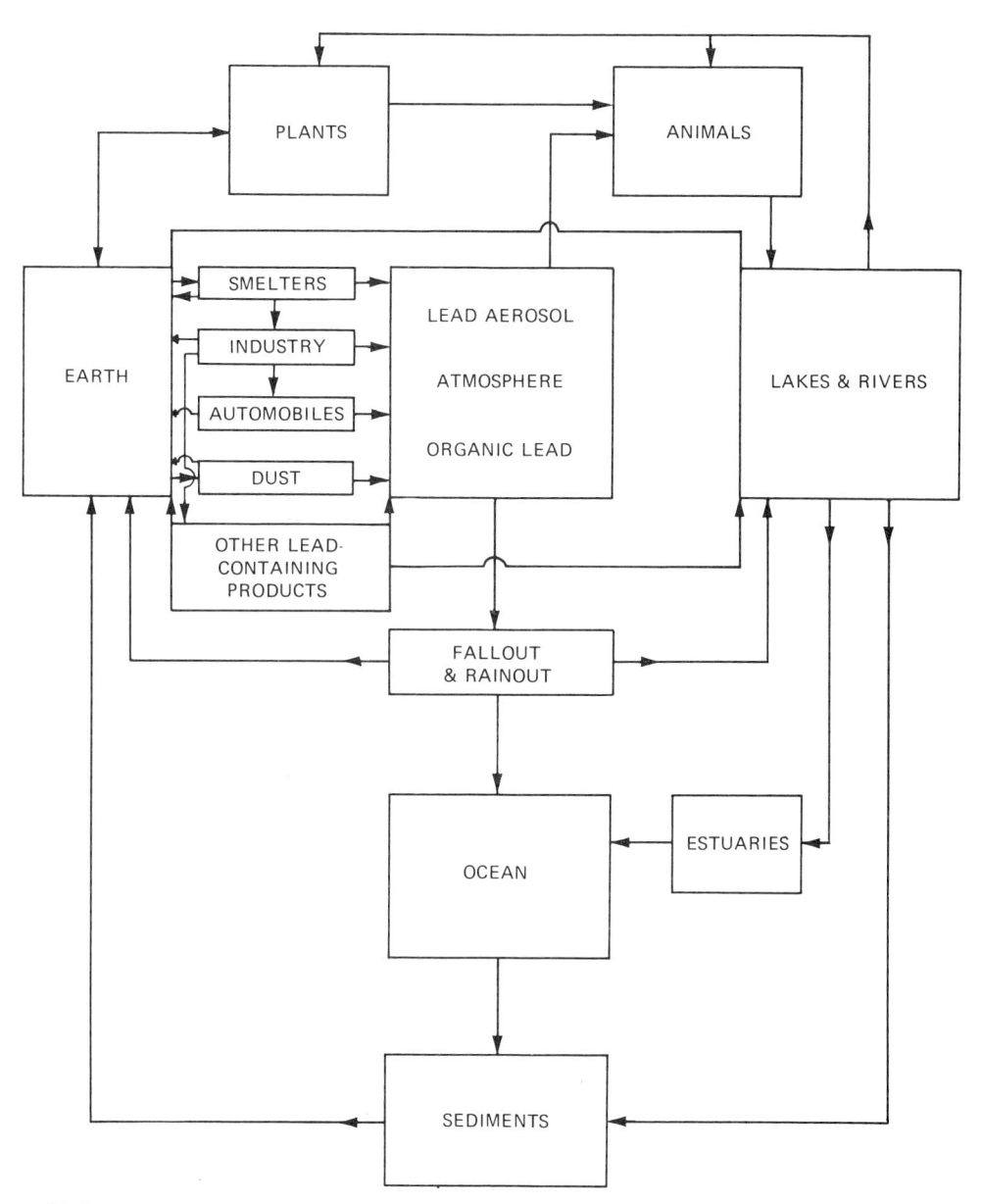

Figure 34-4 Ecologic flow chart for lead, showing possible cycling pathways and compartments. Man may be at risk of uptake via the atmospheric or various aqueous compartments in addition to the floral and faunal compartments. (Lead: Airborne Lead in Perspective, Publication ISBN 0-309-01941-9, Committee on Biologic Effects of Atmospheric Pollutants, National Academy of Sciences—National Research Council, Washington, D.C., 1972.)

food chain or to man. The severe consequences of our ignorance of such biotransformation processes for mercury led to over 100 cases of severe methyl mercury intoxication in Japan. Because the biotransformed methyl mercury is relatively poorly degraded by man, it persists for long periods of time in tissues having a high lipid partition coefficient. Thus, it finds its way to the brain, where it is diffusely distributed producing severe extensive brain damage. The clinical result of such central nervous system deposition was motor defects, blindness, and sensory aberrations. Particularly distressing was the observation that fetal brain development was at a particularly high risk. Whereas in a number of cases pregnant women did not manifest neurotoxicity, their subsequently delivered infants were found to suffer severe dysplastic and atrophic brain abnormalities of a permanent, disabling nature.

Although severe cases of methyl mercury intoxication can be readily detected, the consequences of less severe mercury loadings are unclear. For example, could less severe mercury uptake produce minimal but disabling deficiencies of cognition or motor function? At present the answer to such a question is unknown.

Further problems regarding mercury pollution revolve about the possible effects of this element upon germ tissues. Experiments with onion root-tip cells have demonstrated disturbances in c-mitoses and chromosome breakages at extremely low mercury concentrations, e.g., 0.25×10^{-6} molar phenyl and methyl mercury. What the significance of such findings is for man may be problematic. Nevertheless, some similar hazard to man because of environmental mercury contamination cannot be ignored at this time.

While the threat to man posed by mercury contamination is clearly related to biotransformation and bioconcentration, similar phenomena do not appear to play a role for other metals, e.g., lead or cadmium. At present, neither food-chain concentration nor biotransformation has been demonstrated for other metals. Translocation from soil or leaf surfaces to plant parenchyma does not appear to be appreciable despite heavy lead loadings from auto exhausts. Although the concentration of lead in air over urban areas is 20 times greater than that over sparsely populated regions, there is little evidence that the lead content in city air has increased over the past 15 years. Because of the high degree of exhaust pipe lead dispersion, we do not appear to be facing an increasingly higher burden of airborne lead.

In consideration of the potential for total lead loadings in man, two specific populations may be at some risk. A small number of men engaged in work with lead or exposed to auto exhausts continually (e.g., garage workers, traffic policemen) may bear some risk of increased lead absorption. City-dwelling children may experience more significant consequences associated with pica for lead painted chips and street dirt. Lead contents as high as 2000 micrograms per gram of street dirt have been demonstrated. Ingestion of such dirt, e.g., as little as 0.41 gram per day, could result in clinical lead intoxication. Even this amount of intake does not allow for normal dietary or leaded paint ingestion.

As with mercury, serious questions can be raised concerning the consequences of undetected or subclinical lead intoxication. Because of the proclivity for lead deposition in a child's brain, subclinical intoxication may readily go undiagnosed. Such affected children may be misjudged as having "behavior problems" or may be dismissed as merely "clumsy." Although the extent of such problems is poorly defined, mass screening studies have revealed that as high as 5 to 8 per cent of urban children have blood lead levels of 50 micrograms per 100 grams of blood or higher. Such studies barely indicate the scope of the problem but do suggest that a high index of suspicion of subclinical lead intoxication in children is warranted in urban areas.

The hazards that have been described with regard to lead and mercury may apply in the future to other environmental metallic contaminants, e.g., cadmium, arsenic, selenium, vanadium, and so on. Although specific human hazards due to such environmental pollutants have not been described (with the exception of cadmium), such situations offer little comfort. Preliminary evidence strongly suggests that the increase in the levels of environmental cadmium during the last 50 years has been more rapid than for other metals. The role of this element in chronic renal, cardiovascular, and mineral metabolic disturbances is just becoming discernible. That human damage has occurred is clear. However, the gross contamination by cadmium of water courses responsible for Itai-Itai disease in Japan appears unique. Nevertheless, while such dramatic events are rare but discernible, the question of the effects of long-term, low-level cadmium or other heavy metal pollution is imperfectly understood.

Although the ramifications of metal-biotransformation have been extensively studied since 1965, nothing thus far precludes the possibility of the occurrence of unknown modes of biotransformation. Certainly prior to that time this particular phenomenon, as it involved metals in the environment, was unknown; similarly, the possibility that other unpleasant surprises on the part of nature will be discovered should not be unexpected. In the light of our present ignorance, it behooves man to control totally unnecessary ecosystem pollution in order to hopefully obviate future disasters such as that at Minimata.

THE STRUCTURAL AND FUNCTIONAL CONSEQUENCES OF CHEMICAL TOXICITY

RELATIONSHIP OF ULTRASTRUCTURE TO CELL FUNCTION

The cell membrane may be considered as constituting the interface of the cell with the external environment. This applies even to innermost cells of the body, since the extracellular fluid medium serving as a transport medium produces relatively little change in chemicals of extracorporeal origin. Most frequently exogenous materials carried in the extracellular compartment are only moderately and/or reversibly altered, e.g., the loosely bound complexes of drugs and plasma protein.

The cell membrane takes the form of a double-layered structure. Each of the two layers is 35 to 40 angstroms thick and consists of a lipoprotein complex. Various modifications of these layers occur in specific cell types, e.g., microvilli in secretive and absorptive cells, or invaginations of various other plasma membranes. Transport across physically unaltered membranes is achieved as the result of active, energy-dependent and probably enzymatically controlled activity. The process of phagocytosis or pinocytosis, whereby materials are transported across the membrane, produces a physical modification of these membranes. Phagocytosis causes incorporation of particulate material, while the pinocytosis incorporates extracellular fluid. These processes are probably a common method whereby most cells take up water and solutes.

Though the enzymatic processes controlling and mediating these activities are as yet not clear, it appears that this complex activity can be readily disturbed by chemical agents. Additionally it is obvious that alteration of structural integrity may also produce changes in cell wall function. In the case of mercuric or cupric chloride, changes in potassium and phosphate concentrations within the cell probably stem from the alteration of the membrane's normal cross-linking of sulfhydryl groups. The effects of lipid solvent, e.g., CCl_4, may also stem from a disturbance of the physical stability of the cell membrane's lipid components.

The endoplasmic reticula or ergastoplasm, membranous channels which dip down into and course through the cell matrix, are considered by some to be an invagination of the cell membrane. Both morphologically and functionally these are differentiated into two specific types. One of these is associated with electron-dense particles that lie on what might be considered the intracellular side of these membranous channels. These particles, the polyribosomes, are one of the sites of intracellular protein synthesis. Here messenger RNA from the nucleus meets the activated amino acids carried by transfer RNA. Linkage of these amino acid moieties into the proper sequence, as directed by the sequence code carried by messenger RNA, leads to the synthesis of a specific protein. If this concept is real, that the interior of the endoplasmic reticular channel does represent an intruding continuum of the cell membrane, and this communicates with the external cell environment, synthesis of protein occurring at this locus on the endoplasmic reticulum would provide for ready egress of such newly formed protein from the interior milieu of the cell.

Another portion of these membranes has no associated granules. These smooth membranes appear to be the site of numerous processes. The enzyme glucose-6-phosphatase (G-6-Pase) is located on these smooth membranes. The spatial association of the enzyme with this membrane appears to be prerequisite for its catalytic function. For the transport of glucose out of liver cells for use in other organs of the body, dephosphorylation of glucose-6-phosphate by this enzyme is required before secretion from the cell can occur. Once more, the location of G-6-Pase at the endoplasmic reticulum may afford a convenient site for communication with the external environment. In addition several enzymatically controlled detoxification processes such as oxidation of hexobarbital, dealkylation of codeine and aminopyrine and hydroxylation of acetanilid are localized in these smooth membranes. Undoubtedly many more chemical agents will be found to be structurally altered or transformed in this portion of the cell. Also inherent in such structural association is the implication that any chemical agent affecting this locus may cause unexpected drug responses. Exposure to chlordane or DDT appears to stimulate the detoxifying enzyme activities associated with these structures. Accordingly, drugs given to animals pretreated with these pesticides have been shown to be metabolized at an accelerated rate for some months after this pretreatment.

Equally as important might be the inhibition of metabolic transformation activity in this structure. The result of such enzyme inhibition on the detoxification process has been previously considered.

Other functions have been ascribed to this reticulum. It has been suggested by Siekevitz that control of cell permeability also resides in part in this structure. If indeed the reticulum is an extension of the plasma membrane into the cell, control of movement to and from the cell at this interface would not be unreasonable.

The mitochondria are another of the cytoplasmic organelles affording a structural matrix upon which are placed vital biochemical functions. These structures within the cytoplasm are variegated in shape and size in life. They consist of a dual membrane, the inner membrane being involuted into "shelves" or cristae. On these shelves are seen "elementary particles," approximately 80 to 100 angstroms in diameter. These particles apparently are the site of the respiratory (or electron-transport chain) and phosphorylating enzymes. The semifluid matrix within the mitochondria carries the Krebs (citric acid) cycle enzymes. Thus within this organelle is found an important part of the process mediating oxidation of foodstuffs and yielding electrons, which are in turn transferred to the respiratory enzyme chain. It is at this elementary particle in the mitochondria that the cyanide ion complexes with the iron-containing cytochrome enzymes of the electron-transfer chain, leading in turn to cessation of cellular respiration.

There also occurs within the mitochondria the transfer of electrons that provide the energy to be stored in ATP. The process whereby energy is stored as high energy chemical bonds for later release is referred to as oxidative phosphorylation. This process is susceptible to an interference that may be exerted by several chemicals, such as dinitrophenol and dinitro-ortho-cresol. Absorption of these chemicals results in failure of ATP formation. Under these conditions oxidative processes continue to operate in the absence of ATP formation. As a result heat, rather than energy-rich phosphate bonds, is produced. The clinical picture of acute hyperthermia and a rapid increase of 20 to 30 per cent in metabolic rate reflects an ill-fated attempt to replace ATP stores. There is a marked tachycardia, perspiration and eventual collapse. Though this picture simulates hyperthyroid crisis, there is no elevation in cardiac output and no alleviation of the symptoms of myxedema, and in contrast to such crises there is depression of levels of circulating protein-bound iodine and decreased I^{131} uptake.

CELL TOXICITY—A CHEMICOPHYSIOLOGIC SYNTHESIS

The effects at the cell level of a typical hepatotoxin, carbon tetrachloride, and the physiologic consequences of its cellular effect serve as a possible prototype of integrated response to toxic agents occurring at multiple levels. It appears that a major change in permeability occurs, possibly due to this compound's lipid solvent effect at the cell membrane and at the endoplasmic reticulum. While the intimate mechanisms of this alteration in permeability are not clear, the consequences are rather well defined. One of the earliest changes consists of increases in intracellular calcium, water and sodium and a loss of potassium. Each of these shifts represents an impairment of the processes responsible for normal permeability maintenance. The increase in calcium and decrease in potassium potentially lead to diminution of oxidative phosphorylation. (However, this is not actually seen till later in the course of this process.) The increase in intracellular sodium and water in turn produces the microscopic picture of a swollen hydropic cell.

As another consequence of damage to the endoplasmic reticulum, there is a decrease in glucose-6-phosphatase (G-6-Pase) activity concurrent to or following apace with a rapid diminution in hepatic glycogen. It should be recalled that before glucose can be secreted from a hepatocyte, the enzyme G-6-Pase must dephosphorylate (remove phosphate) from glucose-6-phosphate. Accordingly, damage to the endoplasmic reticulum and its associated enzyme G-6-Pase probably leads to failure of glucose secretion by the liver, with a concurrent drop in blood glucose noted. At the same time there is evidence of a stress response characterized by increased adrenal cortical and medullary activity. The adrenal medullary release of such catecholamines as norepinephrine and epinephrine may represent a response of failure of hepatic glucose secretion and the resultant hypoglycemia. At the same time, the adrenal cortical response may represent another attempt to correct the diminished oxidizable circulating substrate, i.e., glucose. The glucosteroids, by activating and/or leading to synthesis of the transaminases (pyruvic, oxaloacetic) bring about conversion of the amino acids alanine and aspartic acid (aspartate) to pyruvate and oxaloacetate respectively. Thus products resulting from these transformations can be utilized in the Krebs cycle. The end result is conversion of protein (i.e., gluconeogenesis). Thus a noncarbohydrate source can provide an oxidizable substrate.

Unfortunately the secretion of epinephrine and related neurohumors secreted in response to CCl_4 absorption may cause other untoward effects. Brody has suggested that stimulation of the nerves to the hepatic blood vessels produces restriction of blood supply to the liver, hypoxia and central lobular necrosis. In addition the catecholamines appear to mobilize nonesterified fatty acids from depots. These lipid precursors presented in large quantities to a damaged liver play an important role in the etiology of "fatty" liver associated with this type of intoxication.

Hypoxia in turn leads to a shift toward utilization of anaerobic pathways. This in turn produces a decrease in pH, due to an accumulation of lactate and because the process of glycolysis produces phosphate by-products. The change in cell pH plays a role in the breakdown of lysosomes which release their proteolytic enzymes; in addition, lowering of pH activates these catalysts. These proteolytic enzymes cause a breakdown of cell structure protein, which leads in turn to accumulation of osmotically active molecules. Despite a leaky membrane this damaged cell continues the swelling which previously had been precipitated by calcium and sodium uptake noted above.

Concurrently, other energy-dependent processes begin to fail. Protein synthesis slows and then is practically halted. While many enzyme systems continue to operate — especially those in the mitochondria until relatively late in the course of cell damage — there begins a fragmentation of the coordinated multilinked activity characteristic of the normal organized, metabolic system. With a failure of this coordination, structure begins to fragment and nuclear breakdown is seen. This results in the spill of nucleoprotein into the extracellular spaces among other cellular debris. Before this stage, examination of the cell demonstrates persistence of nuclear outlines. Nevertheless this unit has become an inert, foreign object which then becomes the subject of phagocytosis or "heterolysis."

Though this sequence of morphologic breakdown may take 8 to 12 hours, in the course of the alterations herein described the cell actually has reached a point of no return at about the second or third hour. It is noteworthy that while structurally the hepatocyte might have appeared intact or at worst reversibly altered (e.g., hydropic and/or granular alteration), functionally this unit of life has advanced far down the road toward cell death.

The net result of these changes is an area of necrosis within the liver. If this area is small, detection of this damage may be demonstrable only by an increased serum enzyme activity, a change in alpha globulin synthesis or a qualitative change in albumin. These latter two changes, which reflect a defect in protein synthesis, are expressed by a positive cephalin-cholesterol flocculation test. This abnormality probably results from damage to the rough-surfaced endoplasmic reticulum where protein synthesis occurred (see above). Such structural alteration as seen by electron microscopy correlates quite clearly with early failure in protein synthesis by the liver resulting from CCl_4 poisoning.

If, however, the quantitative volume of cell damage is larger, breakdown of the parenchymal cells leads to decreased synthesis of osmotically active molecules with a resultant edema. In addition, defects in coagulation due to the failure of synthesis of prothrombin and other clotting factors may lead to intravascular thrombosis. With cell breakdown, physical obstruction to biliary egress via the bile radicles produces clinical jaundice.

It should be pointed out that the effect of CCl_4 in acute intoxication is not limited to hepatic alteration. Indeed, in acute cases in the absence of lethal central nervous system depression, the cause of death is usually renal failure. While the sequence of changes described here has been more clearly elaborated for the hepatocyte, future investigations will undoubtedly cast more light upon renal alteration that frequently leads to demise in acute CCl_4 poisoning.

REFERENCES

Belknap, E. L., and Belknap, E. L., Jr.: Clinical control of health in the storage battery industry. Indust. Med. Surg., 28:94, 1959.

Beutler, E.: The hemolytic effect of primaquine and related compounds: A review. Blood, 24:103, 1959.

Boyer, P. D.: Mechanisms of enzyme action. Ann. Rev. Biochem., 29:15, 1960.

Brodie, B. B., Cosmides, G. J., and Rael, D. P.: Toxicology and the biomedical sciences. Science, 148:1547, 1965.

Brody, T. M., Calvert, D. N., and Schneider, A. F.: Alterations of carbon tetrachloride-induced pathologic changes in the rat by spinal transection, adrenalectomy and adrenergic blocking agents. J. Pharmacol. Exper. Therap., 131:341, 1961.

Cell Regulatory Mechanisms. Cold Spring Harbor Symposia on Quantitative Biology, Volume XXVI. Cold Spring Harbor, N.Y., Long Island Biologic Association, 1961.

Chenoweth, M. B.: Monofluoroacetic acid and related compounds. Pharmacol. Rev., 1:383, 1949.

Coburn, R. F.: Biological effects of carbon monoxide. Ann. N.Y. Acad. Sci., 174:430, 1970.

Dinman, B. D., and Ashe, W. F.: Arsenic intoxication. In Harvey, J. C. (Ed.): Tice's Practice of Medicine. Hagerstown, Md., W. F. Prior Co., 1962.

Dinman, B. D.: "Non-concept" of "no-threshold": chemicals in the environment. Science, 175:495, 1972.

Douglas, C. G., and Haldane, J. B. S.: The laws of combination of hemaglobin with carbon monoxide and oxygen. J. Physiol., 44:275, 1912.

Durham, W. F., and Hayes, W. J., Jr.: Organic phosphorus poisoning and its therapy; with special reference to modes of action and compounds that reactivate inhibited cholinesterase. Arch. Environ. Health, 5:21, 1962.

Fernández-Morán, H.: Cell-membrane ultrastructure. Low-temperature microscopy and x-ray diffraction studies of lipoprotein components in lamellar systems. Circulation, 26:1039 (supplement, part II) 1962.

Fouts, J. R.: Interaction of drugs and hepatic microsomes. Fed. Proc., 21:1107, 1962.

Fox, C. F., Dinman, B. D., and Frajola, W. J.: CCl_4 poisoning: II. Serum enzymes, free fatty acids and liver pathology; effects of phenoxybenzamine and Phenergan. Proc. Soc. Exper. Biol. Med., 111:721, 1962.

Goldsmith, J. R., Terzaghi, J., and Hackney, J. D.: Evaluation of fluctuating carbon monoxide exposure. Arch. Environ. Health, 7:647, 1963.

Henderson, Y., and Haggard, H. W.: Noxious Gases and the Principles of Respiration Influencing Their Action. 2nd ed. New York, Reinhold Publishing Corp., 1943.

Hutchinson, G. E.: The influence of the environment. Proc. Nat. Acad. Sc., 51:930, 1964.

Kalow, W.: Pharmacogenetics: Heredity and the Response to Drugs. Philadelphia, W. B. Saunders Co., 1962.

Lanza, A. J. (Ed.): The Pneumoconioses. New York, Grune and Stratton, 1963.

Loomis, T. A.: Essentials of Toxicology. Philadelphia, Lea and Febiger, 1968.

Majno, G.: Death of liver tissue. In Rouiller, C. (Ed.): The Liver. Vol. II. New York, Academic Press, 1964.

Malkinson, F. D.: Permeability of the stratum corneum. *In* Montagna, W., and Lobitz, W. C. (Eds.): The Epidermis. New York, Academic Press, 1964, p. 435.

Miller, J. A., and Miller, E. C.: Guest Editorial. Chemical carcinogenesis: Mechanisms – approaches to control. J. Natl. Cancer Inst., 47:v, 1971.

Passow, H., and Rothstein, A.: The binding of mercury by the yeast cell in relation to changes in permeability. J. Gen. Physiol., 43:621, 1960.

Patty, F. A. (Ed.): Industrial Hygiene and Toxicology. Vol. II. 2nd ed. New York, Interscience Publishers, 1963.

Peters, R. A.: The study of enzymes in relation to selective toxicity in animal tissues. Sympos. Soc. Exper. Biol., 3:36, 1949.

Ponder, E.: The cell membrane and its properties. In Brachet, J., and Mirsky, A. E. (Eds.): The Cell. Vol. II. New York, Academic Press, 1961, pp. 1–84.

Report of the Committee on Biological Effects of Atmospheric Pollutants. Lead: Airborne lead in perspective. Washington, D.C., National Academy of Sciences, 1972.

Report on Methyl Mercury in Fish. A toxicologic-epidemiologic evaluation of risks. Nordisk Hygienisk Tidskrift (Stockholm), Suppl. 4, November, 1971.

Reynolds, E. S.: Liver parenchymal injury. J. Cell. Biol., 19:139, 1963.

Rouiller, C.: Experimental toxic injury of the liver. *In* Rouiller, C. (Ed.): The Liver. Vol. II. New York, Academic Press, 1964.

Rosen, F., Roberts, N. R., and Nichol, C. A.: Glucocorticosteroids and transaminase activity. J. Biol. Chem., 234:476, 1959.

Schotz, M. C., and Recknagel, R. O.: Rapid increase of rat liver triglycerides following CCl_4 poisoning. Biochim. Biophys. Acta, 41:151, 1960.

Siekevitz, P.: On the meaning of intracellular structure for metabolic regulation. *In* Wolstenholme, G. E. W., and O'Connor, C. M. (Eds.): Ciba Foundation Symposium on The Regulation of Cell Metabolism. Boston, Little, Brown and Co., 1959.

Stokinger, H. E.: Means of contact and entry of toxic agents. *In* Occupational Diseases, A Guide To Their Recognition. U.S. Public Health Service Publication 1097. Washington, D.C., U.S. Government Printing Office, 1964.

Thiers, R. E., Reynolds, E. S., and Vallee, B. L.: The effect of carbon tetrachloride poisoning on subcellular metal distribution in rat liver. J. Biol. Chem., 253:2130, 1960.

Umbarger, H. E.: Endproduct inhibition of the initial enzyme in a biosynthetic sequence as a mechanism of feedback control. *In* Bonner, D. M. (Ed.): Control Mechanisms in Cellular Processes. New York, Ronald Press, 1961, pp. 67–85.

Williams, R. J. P.: Nature and properties of metal ions of biological interest and their coordination compounds. Fed. Proc., 20:5 (supplement 10, part II), 1961.

Williams, T. R.: Detoxification Mechanisms. The Metabolism and Detoxification of Drugs, Toxic Substances and Other Organic Compounds. 2nd ed. London, Chapman and Hall, 1959.

Yielding, K. L., and Tomkins, G. M.: Structural alteration in crystalline glutamic dehydrogenase induced by steroid hormones. Proc. Nat. Acad. Sc., 46:1483, 1960.

INDEX

Note: Page numbers in *italics* refer to material in illustrations; page numbers followed by (t) refer to tables.

A-beta-lipoproteinemia, 752, 756
Abortion, septic, with septicemia, DIC in, 652
Abruptio placentae, DIC in, 652
Abscess(es), liver, 810
  lung, 406
    in pneumococcal pneumonia, 498
    tumor of lung, and, 404
  myocardial, 491
Absorption, 745
  abnormalities of, 751–759
  carbohydrate, *746*, 747–748, *749*
  folic acid, 750–751
  normal, 746
  of fat, 746–747, *746*, *748*
  of protein, *746*, 748–750
  of vitamin B_{12}, 750–751
Acanthocytes, distortion of erythrocytes into, 595, *595*
Acanthocytosis, hereditary, 595
Acceleration, abrupt, 943–945
  prolonged, 943
  vibration as, 945
Accessory spleen, 680
Acetyl-CoA, production of, 7–8, 12
Achalasia, 704
Achlorhydria, 716
  in gastric carcinoma, 731
Achylia gastrica, 716
Acid(s). See also specific acids; e.g., *Pantothenic acid.*
  amino, 750(t)
  ascorbic, 855
  cholic, 775
  ethacrynic, 353
  folic, 855
  hexuronic, 420
  hyaluronic, 420
  nicotinic, 854
  pantothenic, 854–855
  para-aminohippuric, 347
  tetrahydrofolic, 750
Acid-base disturbances, of lungs, 390
Acidification, 350–352
  sodium conservation by, 351(t)
Acidosis, 390
  in chronic renal failure, 369
  renal tubular, 367, 815

Acrocentric chromosomes, definition of, 51, 90
Acromegaly, 426, 874–875
ACTH, effect of on lipid metabolism, 18
Actin, myocardial, 207, *208*, 215, *216*
Actinomycin D, 856
Actinomycosis, 410
Action potential, configurations of, *333*
Active transport, 347
Actomyosin-ATPase, in cardiac failure, 283
Acute bronchitis, 453
Acute gouty arthritis, 431–434
Acute granulocytic leukemia, 609–613
  signs and symptoms of, 611
Acute leukemia, chemotherapeutic agents in treatment of, 613(t)
Acute liver cell failure, 811–812
Acute lymphocytic leukemia, 609
Acute nephritis, edema in, 363
Acute renal failure, 368
Addison's disease, 886
  clinical findings in, 887
Adenine, 71
Adenocarcinoma, of colon, 786
  of esophagus, 701
  radiation, of thyroid, 941
Adenohypophyseal hormones, hyperglycemic effects of, 10
Adenoma, in primary hyperparathyroidism, 893
  islet cell, of pancreas, 836
  of colon, 786
  toxic, 883
  villous, 786
Adenomatous polyps, 729
  of colon, 786
Adenomyomatosis, 824
Adenosine, and vasodilatation, 151
Adenovirus, and interstitial pneumonia, 499
Adenylate cyclase-cyclic AMP system, 867–868
Adipocyte(s), 843, *844*
  in anorexia nervosa, 849
Adjuvants, 98–99
Adrenal cortex, biological actions of, 884–885
  clinical entities in, 886–890
  physiology of, 884–885

INDEX

Adrenal cortical hormones, secretory rates and body fluid concentrations of, 885(t)
Adrenal glands, hyperplasia of, 887
Adrenal glucocorticoids, effect on connective tissue, 421
Adrenal hyperplasia, congenital, 82
Adrenal medulla, 896–898
  clinical entities in, 898
  physiology of, 896–898
Adrenal steroids, biosynthesis, transport, and metabolism of, 885
Adrenal steroidogenesis, defects in, 889
Adrenergic receptors, 896
Adrenocortical hormones. See *Glucocorticoids*.
Adrenocorticotropic hormone, 872
Adrenogenital syndrome, 83
Afibrinogenemia, congenital, 84
Afterload, 220
  in mechanical function of heart, 291
Agammaglobulinemia, B-cell system in, 129
  pneumocystis pneumonia in, 126, *127*
  Swiss type, 130
Age, advancing, and salmonella bacteremia, 494
  effect of on blood pressure, 182, *183*
Agglutination, antibody induced, 485
Aging, chromosomes in, 70
Airway resistance, 375, 378
Airways, collapse of, 376, *376*
  obstruction of, measurement of, 377–379
Albinism, 79, 82
Albumin, in cirrhosis, 797
Alcohol, toxic effects of, on pancreas, 830
Alcoholic pancreatitis, 830–831
Alcoholism, and pancreatitis, 828
  and vitamin deficiency, 858
Aldosterone, biological activities of, 884–885
  excessive secretion of, chronic, 889
  in colon, 774
  in regulation of arterial pressure, 159, *160*
  regulation of secretion of, 884
Aldosteronism, potassium deficit in, 351
  primary, 885, 889–890
    and hypertension, 195–196
Alkaline phosphatase, placental, 810
Alkalosis, 390
Alkaptonuria, 24, 79, *79*, 426
Allele(s), definition of, 90
  silent, definition of, 92
Allergic hepatitis, 813
Allergic purpura, 658
Allergin-reagin tissue reactions, 447–448
Allergy, alpha-adrenergic participation in, 452
  autonomic imbalance in, 451–452
  beta-adrenergic blockade theory in, 451–452
  cholinergic participation in, 452
  definition of term, 445
  nature of and relation to other immunologically induced diseases, 445–456
Allosteric regulation, of protein function, 37
Alpha particles, in ionizing radiation, 932
Alpha receptors, 739
Alpha-tocopherol, 857
Alpha toxin, of *Clostridium perfringens*, 458, 460, 461
  action of on lecithin, 461, *462*

Alveolar capillary block syndrome, 384
Alveolar hypoventilation, of high altitude, 549
Alveolar membrane leakage, in pulmonary edema, 173
Alveolar ventilation, 387–388
  abnormalities of, 388
  defined by arterial P_{CO_2}, 387–388
Alveolar volume, 387
Alveoli, 394–395
  as pulmonary protective mechanisms, 395
  hypoxic, and vasoconstriction, 172
Amenorrhea, primary, in Turner's syndrome, 910
Amino acids, in protein synthesis, 20–24, *25*, 34
  metabolism of, 23–24, *25*
  transport of, and malabsorption, 757
Ammonia, in amino acid metabolism, 23
  metabolism of in liver, 792
Amniotic fluid embolism, DIC in, 652
AMP, cyclic, in myocardial metabolism, 214
Amphenone, 353
Amylase, serum, in diagnosis of pancreatitis, 834
Amyloid disease, as host response, 485–486
Amyloidosis, 485, 752
  splenomegaly in, 679
Amylopectin, 747
Amylopectinosis, 7
Anacidity, 716
Anaphase lag, 56
Anaphylactic reaction, DIC in, 652
Anaphylactic shock, with cold urticaria, 453
Anaphylactic system, 113–115, *114*
Anaphylaxis, 452–453
Andersen's disease, 7
Androgens, in Fanconi's anemia, 537
  red cell production and, 543, *544*
Anemia(s). See also specific entities; e.g., *Aplastic anemia*.
  and congenital heart disease, in heart failure, 282
  and cyanosis, 390
  and hypersplenism, 682
  aplastic, 532–537
  cardiac output in, 531
  chronic hereditary nonspherocytic hemolytic, 590, *591*
  classification of, 529–530, 530(t)
  cold agglutinin hemolytic, 596
  Cooley's, 534, 576
  definition of, 529–530
  endocrine disorders and, 542–546
  Fanconi's, 537, 609
  general effects of, 530–531
  in acute granulocytic leukopenia, 611
  in carcinoma of stomach, 732
  in chronic infection, 480–481
  in chronic lymphatic leukemia, 625
  in cirrhosis, 594–595
  in gonadal dysfunction, 543
  in pregnancy, 543–544
  in red cell aplasia, 544, *545*
  in ulcerative colitis, 782
  mechanism of, in splenomegaly, 682
  Mediterranean, 590, *591*
  megaloblastic, 555–556
  microangiopathic hemolytic, 594

INDEX

Anemia(s) (*Continued*)
   of chronic disorders, 541–542
   oxygen perfusion of tissues in, 531
   pernicious, 427
   red cell production in, 531
   renal disease, 539, *539*
   severe, cardiac output in, 238
   sickle cell, 534, 574, 680
     and salmonella bacteremia, 494
   sideroblastic, 569
   warm antibody autoimmune hemolytic, 596
Anemic anoxia, 389
Aneuploidy, 55
   autosomal, 57
   definition of, 90
   in acute lymphatic leukemia, 626
   sex chromosomal, 59–65
Aneurysms, mycotic, in bacterial endocarditis, 493
   of left ventricle, 256
Angina, in aortic regurgitation, 262
   intestinal, 763
Angina pectoris, arteriography in, 253
   beta-adrenergic blockers in, 292
   contraction pattern after, 254
   in aortic stenosis, 260
   propranolol in, 292
Angiocardiogram, and left ventricular hypertrophy, 255
   with left ventricle and segment of left ventricular wall outlined, *243*
Angiocardiography, in determining left ventricular chamber volume, 243
   in segmental abnormalities of left ventricular contraction, 253
   left ventricular, techniques in, 254
Angiography, quantitative, in ischemic heart disease, 256
Angiotensin, 188–189, *188*
   effect of arterial pressure, 193, *194*
Angiotensin II, 357
Angiotensinogen, 357
Ångstrom units, 927
Anhidrosis, thermogenic, 928
Ankylosis, fibrous, 428
Anorexia, in carcinoma of pancreas, 836
   in carcinoma of stomach, 731
   in chronic renal failure, 369
Anorexia nervosa, 711, 847(t), 849
Anosmia, 877
   in hypogonadism, 908
Anoxia, 389–390, 922
Anterior pituitary, clinical entities in, 873–877
   control of secretion of, 872–873
   physiology of, 872
Anterior pituitary-testicular relationships, 907
Anthrax, 471
Antibiotics, effect of on protein synthesis, 30(t), 32
Antibody(ies), anti-intrinsic factor, 557, *557*
   antimitochondrial, 810
   anti-Rh, 597, 598
   cytophilic, 114
   cytotropic, 113
   IgE type, in allergy, 446

Antibody(ies) (*Continued*)
   natural, 98
   specific, 113
Antibody production, in cell clusters, 109, *110*
Antibody response, 102–104, *103*
Antibody synthesis, cellular aspects of, 104–109
Anticholinergics, in cramping abdominal pain, 778
Antidiuresis, 352
Antidiuretic hormone, 348, 349, 352
   secretion of, 877
     inappropriate, 878–879
Antigen(s), 98–99
   binding of, 100, 102, *103*
   carcinoembryonic, 810
   hepatitis associated, 810
   tumor-associated, 138–140
   virus-specific, 139
Antigen-antibody complex, and eosinophilia, 484
Antilymphocyte serum, 112
Antimetabolites, and vitamin deficiency, 858
Antimicrobial agents, and gastroenteritis, 494
   and salmonella bacteremia, 494
Antimitochondrial antibody, 810
Antiplatelet antibody, disorders producing, 677, 677(t)
Anuria, 362
Aorta, arteriosclerotic aneurysm of, and salmonella bacteremia, 495
   coarctation of, hypertension in, 194
   in blood pressure regulation, 184
Aortic compliance, 182
Aortic disease, combined with mitral valve disease, 263–264
Aortic regurgitation, 261–263
   combined with aortic stenosis, 263
   left ventricular and aortic pressures in, *263*
   left ventricular pressure-volume curves in, *249*
   severe, apex impulse tracing of, *309*
   treatment of, 263
   ventricular and regurgitation volumes in, *262*
Aortic stenosis, 257
   combined with aortic regurgitation, 263
   left ventricular pressure-volume curves in, *249*
   myocardial function in, 260–261
   pressure-volume diagram, *261*
   recording of left ventricular and aortic pressure in, 239, *240*
   treatment of, 260–261
Aortic stenosis and regurgitation, left ventricular pressure-volume curves in, *249*
Aortic valve, bacterial endocarditis of, 262
   incompetence of, volume overload and, 281
Aortic valve disease, 260–264
Aortic valve prosthesis, ventricular pressure in, *223*
   with isoproterenol, *224*
Apathy, in chronic renal failure, 369
Apex cardiogram, *307*

Apex cardiography, to record chest wall motion, 306
Apex kinetocardiogram, *308, 309*
Aplasia, gonadal, 910-912
  red cell, anemia in, 544, *545*
    thymomas in, 544
Aplastic anemia, 532-537
  bone marrow transplantation in, 537
  drugs associated with development of, 535-536, 535(t)
  etiologic classification of, 535(t)
  etiology and pathogenesis of, 535
  immunologic rejection in, 537
  plasma iron and erythropoietin in, 534
  radiation caused, 536
Apoferritin, in formation of ferritin, 565, *565*
Appetite, loss of, 711
  and hunger, 710-711
Argon, 924
Argyll Robertson pupil, in late syphilis, 496
Arm, of chromosome, definition of, 90
Arrhythmia(s). See also *Cardiac arrhythmias.*
  automaticity as mechanism of impulse formation in, 329
  mechanisms and pathogenesis of, 329-344
  primary, 282
Arterial pressure, and blood volume, 184-185
  control of, feedback gain in, 159-161, *160*
  long-term determinants of, 161, *162*
  decreased. See *Hypotension.*
  determination of, direct, 178, *179*, 181
    indirect, 178-181
  effect of angiotensin on, 193, *194*
  effect of total peripheral resistance on, 150
  elevated. See *Hypertension.*
  factors determining, 181-183
  hemodynamic factors in, 158-162
  physical and environmental effect on, 182-183
  pulmonary, 172
  regulation of, 183-190
    central reactions, 187
    hemodynamics of, 183-184
    intravascular volume, 184-185
    kidneys in, 187-190
    neural reflexes, 185-187
    vascular control, 185
  systemic, 177-205
Arterial pulsation, 174-175
Arteries, in blood pressure regulation, 184
Arteriograms, of liver, 791
Arteriosclerosis, in essential hypertension, 366
Arteriovenous fistula, effect on circulatory function, *153*
Arteriovenous shunt, cardiac output in, 238
Arthralgia, in serum sickness, 435
Arthritis, characteristics of synovial fluid in, 424(t)
  gouty, acute, 431-433
    chronic, 433
    in fasting, 848
  hypertrophic, 426
  infectious, specific, 430-431

Arthritis (*Continued*)
  in pneumococcal pneumonia, 499
  in rheumatic fever, 435
  rheumatoid, 435-439
  severe degenerative, in hemophilia, 427
Arthus reaction, 449
Articular cartilage, 422-423
  expansion and contraction of with pressure, 422, *423*
Articular nerves, 422
Artificial heart, 292
Artificial respiration, in poliomyelitis, 505
Asbestosis, 403
Ascites, in acute pancreatitis, 833
Ascorbic acid, 855
Ash, percentage of in human body weight, 840, *840*
Aspergillosis, 410
Aspiration, and lung abscess, 406
  in Zenker's diverticulum, 699
Aspiration pneumonia, 408
Asplenism, hematologic findings in, 672(t)
Asterixis, in hepatic encephalopathy, 812
Asthma, 397-398
  bronchial. See *Bronchial asthma.*
  chronic, long-term management of, 451
  reagin mediated, 453
Ataxia-telangiectasia, *130, 134, 135*
Ataxia-telangiectasia syndrome, 69
Atelectasis, 403-404
  effect of on local blood flow, 173
  pneumonia and, 404
Atherosclerosis, and ischemic heart disease, 253
Atopic sensitization, nature of, 446-447
ATPase, membrane bound, in alpha adrenergic activity, 452
ATP production, in myocardial metabolism, 212-214, *213*
Atransferrinemia, 84
Atresia, esophageal, 705
Atrial enlargement, electrocardiograph in, 324-325
Atrial fibrillation, in mitral stenosis, 257
  tachysystole in, 339
Atrial myxoma, 257
Atrial pressure, right, effect on blood volume, 172
Atrium, enlargement of, excitation in, 324, *324, 325*
  left, enlargement of in mitral regurgitation, 259
Atrophic gastritis, 719
  and carcinoma of stomach, 730
Atropine, in bronchial asthma, 452
Auditory sensitivity, range of, *946*
Auscultatory gap, 180
Australia antigen, 810
Autoantibodies, 440
Autoimmune disease, 440
Autoimmune hemolytic anemia, antiplatelet antibody in, 677, 677(t)
Autoimmune hemolytic disease of newborn, 596
Autoimmunity, 98
Automaticity, as mechanism of impulse formation in cardiac arrhythmias, 329

INDEX

Autonomic nervous system, influence of, on cardiac output, 237
Autoregulation, circulatory, 150, 184
Autosomal dominant inheritance, 42-43, *42, 43*
Autosomal recessive inheritance, 43-45, *44*
Autosome, definition of, 90
Auto-splenectomy, 680
A-V conduction, 332, 335, *336*
Azotemia, 356, 362, 815
Azulfidine, 783

Babinski sign, in spinal cord degeneration, 555
Bacillus anthracis, 471
  exotoxin of, 458(t)
Back, stiff, in bacterial meningitis, 500
Bacteremia, hypotension in, 478
  in pneumonia, 407
  pseudomonas, blood vessel involvement in, 479
  Pseudomonas aeruginosa, 469
  salmonella, 494-495
  shock in, 477
  Staphylococcus aureus, 468
Bacteria, basic mechanisms of pathogenicity of, 458
  invasion of tissues by, 468-469
    effects of widespread dissemination, 468-469
    local effects of, 468
  toxigenic, exotoxins of, 458(t)
Bacterial endocarditis, embolic phenomena in, 492
  immune complexes in, 485
  immunological aspects and hypersensitivity phenomena of, 493
  in pneumococcal pneumonia, 499
  metastatic infections in, 492
  of aortic valve, 262
Bacterial meningitis, 500-504
  abnormalities of cerebrospinal fluid in, 500
  manifestations of infection in, 500
Bacterial septicemia, DIC in, 652
Bacterial toxins, production of, 458-468
Balanced translocation, definition of, 90
Barodontalgia, 920
Barometric pressure, altitude, and depth in sea water, relationships of, *919*
  decompression sickness and, 921-922
  decreasing, effects of, 920-921
  fluctuations of, effects of on earth, 918-919
  high, effects of, 919-920
  increasing, effects of, 920
  low, tolerance limits for, 918
  man's tolerance to, 917-918
  normal range of, 918
  rapid changes in, effects of, 920
Baroreceptors, 186
Baroreceptor reflex, 158, *160*
Barosinusitis, 920
Barr body(ies), 59, *60*, 889
  definition of, 92
Base pairing, 71

B cells, 108, 109, 124-126
  evaluation of, 126, 128(t)
Belching, 711-712
Bence Jones protein, 358
  in amyloidosis, 486
  in M-component disorders, 631
Bence Jones proteinuria, 358, 631
Bends, 921
Benemid, 347
Benign monoclonal gammopathy, 633
Beta-adrenergic blockade theory, 451-452
Beta adrenergic blockers, in angina pectoris, 292
Beta-globin, subunit of, *572*
Beta particles, in ionizing radiation, 932
Beta radiation, 940
Beta receptors, 739
Biliary cirrhosis, 814
Biliary colic, 823
Biliary ducts, gallstones in, 823
Bile, approximate composition of, 819(t)
  cholesterol in, 821
  concentration of, 818-819
  flow of, 800
  formation of, mechanism of, 799-800
  human, composition of, 799(t)
Bile acids, chemical structure of, *822*
  formation of, *801*
Bile acid diarrhea, 778
Bile duct, common, anatomic course of, *803*
  obstructed, in wall of duodenum *803*
Bile salts, alteration of in disease, 800-801
  and bile salt metabolism, 800-801
  and fat absorption, 747
Bilirubin, metabolism of, in liver, production of, 579, *580*
  tests of metabolism of, 795-796, 795(t)
Binding, in regulation of protein function, 36
  of base pairs, 28
Biochemical processes, molecular regulation of, 36-38
Biochemistry, metabolic, 3-26
Bioconcentration, principle of, 966
Biology, molecular, 27-39
  in disease, 38
Biopsy, of liver, 809
  in cholestasis, 804
Biosynthesis, of catecholamines, 896
Biotin, 854-855
Biotransformation, principle of, 966
Black tongue, in niacin deficiency, 854
Blastomycosis, 410
Bleeding, in peptic ulcer, 727
Blind loop syndrome, 558, 559, 754
Block, local, with micro-entry, 337, *338*
Block-in-reaction sequence, 40, 75-76
Blood, capillary flow of, 386
  changes in, as host response to infection, 479-484
  disorders of, pathophysiology of, 511-644
  glucose levels of, in diagnosis of pancreatitis, 835
  loss of, and iron deficiency, 567
  major lipid components of, 850(t)
  oxygen dissociation curve of, *519*
  oxygen-hemoglobin equilibrium curves for, 380, *380*

Blood (*Continued*)
  sequestration of, in spleen, 669
  volume of, and hematocrit, 532, *533*
    in polycythemia, 532, *532*
Blood cells, formation of, 511, *512, 513*
  in urine, 361–362
Blood circulation, peripheral, control of, 284–285
Blood clotting systems, activation of, 481–484
Blood CO_2, 379–383
Blood factors, 481, *482, 483*
Blood O_2, 379–383
Blood flow, and arterial pressure, 181
  cardiac, in cardiac failure, 285
  cerebral, in cardiac failure, 285
  in intestines, 763
  in polycythemia, 532
  local, regulation of, 150–151
  through liver, 804–805
    methods to measure, 804(t)
Blood platelets, 633–646. See also *Thrombocytes*.
  aggregation of, *635*
  classification of disorders in, 639–640, 640(t)
  core of, *634*
  count of, in massive splenomegaly, *676*
  destruction of, in idiopathic thrombocytopenic purpura, 676
  disc-shaped and spiny, *635*
  feedback control system for, *639*
  function of, 634–636
  kinetics of, 636–639
  life span of, *637*
  pathophysiology of, 639–646
  qualitative abnormalities in, 645–646
  quantitative abnormalities in, 640–645
  relation of spleen to, 674–678
  sequestration of, with increased destruction, 676–678
    without premature destruction, 674–676
  transfused, recovery of in circulating blood, *645*
Blood pressure, effect of physical and environmental factors on, 182–183
  high. See *Hypertension*.
  low. See *Hypotension*.
Blood sugar concentration, 8, 10
Blood volume, and arterial pressure, 184–185
  in cardiac output regulation, 153
  in essential hypertension, 198–199
  regulation of, 170–172
Blood volume measurement, vs. circulatory filling pressure measurement, 171
Blood volume regulation, vs. interstitial fluid volume regulation, 170
Bloom's syndrome, 69
  leukemia in, 609
Blue diaper syndrome, 77(t)
Body, analysis of components of, *840*
  composition of, isotope dilution in measurement of, 840
  resistance of to cancer, 731
Bohr effect, *380*
Bone, abnormal formation of, as effect of trauma, 427

Bone (*Continued*)
  calcium in, 891
  comparison of major metabolic diseases of, 892(t)
  effect of renal failure on, *894*
  long, blood supply to, *508*
  metabolic disease of, 891–892
Bone, remodeling of, calcitonin in, 891
  parathyroid hormone and, 891
  vitamin D and, 856
Bone marrow, cells of, 512, 513, 514, *514*
  destruction of by radiation, 536
  fibrosis of, 608–609
  hematology of, 511–517
  transplantation of, 135
    in aplastic anemia, 537
Bornholm disease, 413
Botulinum toxin, 464
Botulism, 464
Bowel. See *Colon*, and *Small intestine*.
Bowel sounds, in pancreatitis, 832
Bradycardia, in infections, 478
Bradykinin, formation of, 745, *745*
Brain. See also *Cerebral*.
  effects of poliomyelitis on, 505
Branched-chain α-keto acidemia, 80–81, *81*
Break, in chromosome, definition of, 90
Breathing, mechanics of, 371–382
  work of, 378
Bronchi, 393–394
  as pulmonary protective mechanisms, 395
Bronchial asthma, 397, 453
  atropine in, 452
Bronchial obstruction, and bronchiectasis, 406
Bronchiectasis, 406–407
  amyloidosis in, 485
  dry, 407
Bronchioles, respiratory, 394
Bronchitis, acute, 453
  chronic, 405–406, 453
Bronchopneumonia, 408
Brucella, endotoxin of, 466
Bruton agammaglobulinemia, 622
BTPS, 371
Burns, immunodeficiency disease in, 138
  of retina, 931
Burr cells, in uremia, 539, *540*
Bursa equivalent lymphocytes, 615
Bursa of Fabricius, 106–108
Bursal system development, *125*
Bursitis, subacromial, 434
Busulfan, and interstitial pneumonia, 499

Cabot's rings, 555
Caerulein, amino acid sequence of, *713*
Calcareous tendinitis, with subacromial bursitis, 434
Calcinosis, pancreatic, 831
Calcitonin, in bone remodeling, 891
  in kidneys, 891
Calcium, 856
  and coagulation, 648
  conservation of, in kidneys, 891
  homeostasis, sites of parathyroid action in, 891(t)

Calcium (*Continued*)
  in bone, 891
  in cardiac contraction, 216–217
  in gastrointestinal tract, 890
  in parathyroids, 890
  mobilization of from bones, in poliomyelitis, 506
Calcium deficiency, in osteoporosis, 896
Calcium metabolism, effect of renal failure on, *894*
Calculography, 820
Calories, deficiency of, 846–849
  intake and expenditure of, *843*
    imbalance between, 841–842
  storage and utilization of, 843–845
Cancer, chromosomal abnormalities and, 69
  in immunodeficiency diseases, 142
  resistance of body to, 731
Candidiasis, 410
Capacity, vital, 372
Capillaries, in blood pressure regulation, 184
Capillary blood flow, 386
Capillary drainage, in edema, 169
Capillary exchange, 162–163, *163*
Capillary-fluid shift mechanism, 159, *160*
Capsule, of joint, 422
Carbohydrate(s), absorption of, *746*, 747–748, *749*
  attached to proteins, 35
  ingestion of, in kwashiorkor, 849
  metabolism of, 3–10, *4, 6, 9, 19, 20, 26*
    aerobic, 7–8
    anaerobic, 5–7, *6*
    hormonal effects in, 10
    in liver, 799
  storage of, 843
    insulin in, 845
Carbon dioxide, effect on local blood flow, 151
Carbon monoxide poisoning, cardiac output in, 238
Carbon skeleton, disposition of, 24
Carbon tetrachloride, effects of on cell, 970
Carcinoid tumors, 744
Carcinoma, gastric, 716, 758
  in primary hyperparathyroidism, 893
  islet cell, of pancreas, 836
  metastatic, DIC in, 652
  of colon, 758, 787
  of esophagus, 701
  of gallbladder, 825
  of pancreas, 836
  of stomach, 730–732
    symptoms of, 731–732
Carcinoembryonic antigen, 810
Cardia, disorders of, interfering with transport of ingested material, 704–705
  mechanisms for competency of, 705–708
Cardiac arrhythmias, automaticity as mechanism of impulse formation in, 329
  classification of, 329(t)
  mechanisms and pathogenesis of, 329–344
Cardiac catheterization, 239–243
  in cyanotic heart disease, 242–243
  in intracardiac shunts, 241
  in left-to-right shunts, 241–242

Cardiac catheterization (*Continued*)
  intracardiac pressure recordings in, 239–241
  in nonobstructive cardiomyopathies, 266
  Seldinger technique in, 239
Cardiac contraction, mechanisms of, 206–230
Cardiac enlargement, 268
  in heart failure, 252
Cardiac failure, alterations of preload, afterload and contractile state in, 290, 290(t)
  biochemical and mechanical alterations in, 282–284
  cardiac output and, 285
  clinical, underlying mechanisms in, 280–282
  exogenous factors in, 283–284
  factors in causation of, 280(t)
  hypertrophy in, 282
  increased metabolic demands in, 260–261
  mechanical factors in, 282
  multiple factors causing, 282
  primary arrhythmias in, 282
  right and left, symptoms and signs of, 289(t)
  physiologic principles in therapy of, 290–292
  symptoms and signs of, 289
Cardiac hypertrophy, effect on pumping capacity, 152
Cardiac insufficiency, 157
Cardiac output, 235–239
  and arterial pressure, 181
  and heart failure, 285
  and total peripheral resistance, 183, *184*
  autonomic control of, 237
  effect on total peripheral resistance, 150
  heart in, 152, 154–156, *155*
  hemodynamic factors in, 151–157
  in high-output states, 156
  in low-output states, 157
  in febrile state, 475
  measurement of, 235–239
  measurement of, Fick method of, 236
  measurement of, indicator dilution method in, 236–237
  normal, 237
  peripheral circulation in, 153–156, *155*
  peripheral oxygen requirement and, 237–238
  regional distribution of, 285(t)
  regulation of, 237
  therapeutic control of, 238
  vascular resistance and, 238
Cardiac performance, normal, 274–277
  normal values for, 274(t)
Cardiac replacement, total, 292
Cardiac reserve, 152
Cardiac sound, and human hearing spectrum, *296*
Cardiac valves, diseases of, 256–259
Cardiomyopathies, 264–266
  idiopathic, 265–266
  nonobstructive, 265
  obstructive, 265
  precordial movement abnormalities in, 310

Cardiomyopathies (*Continued*)
  secondary, 266
  table of, 264
Cardiopulmonary bypass, in mitral regurgitation, 259
Cardiovascular disease, high altitude, 548
Cardiovascular reflexes, in heart failure, 155-156
Cardiovascular system, in late syphilis, 496
Carditis, in rheumatic fever, 435
Cartilage, arrangement of collagen fibrils in, 422, *422*
  articular, 422-423
Casts, in urine, 360
  types of, 360-361
Cataracts, galactose accumulation and, 80, 81
  glass-blower's, 929
Catecholamines, biosynthesis of, 896
  calorigenic effects of, 842
  degradation of, 897-898
  in joint inflammation, 430
Cathepsins, 21
Catheterization, cardiac, 239-243
Celiac disease, 755
Cell(s). See also specific cells; e.g., *Kupffer cells, Paneth cells.*
  blood, formation of, 511, *512, 513*
  bone marrow, 512, 513, 514, *514*
  burr, 539, *540*
  chemistry of, 27
  connective tissue, 418
  Kupffer, 665, 689, 792
  liver, schematic model of, *791*
  Paneth, 736
  plasma, 666(t)
  proliferation of, DNA replication and, 30
  reticuloendothelial, 523, *523*, 666
  stem, 418
  structure of, 969
Cell function, relation of ultrastructure to, 969-970
Cell life cycle, definition of, 90
Cell organelles, 35-36
Cell toxicity, 970
Cellular activity, energetics of, and control of equilibrium, 954-956
Cellular damage, in liver, tests of, 809(t)
Cellular necrosis, in liver, tests of, 809-810
Central nervous system, chronic viral infections of, 486
  in late syphilis, 496
  niacin deficiency and, 854
  pyridoxine deficiency and, 854
  thiamin deficiency in, 853
Centromere, definition of, 51, 90
Cephalic tetanus, 463
Cephalins, 15
Cerebral circulation, 202
Cerebral edema, in bacterial meningitis, 500
Cerebrospinal fluid, abnormalities of, in bacterial meningitis, 501
Cerebrosides, 16
Cerebrovascular disease, hypotension in, 204-205
Charcot's joints, 427
Chediak-Higashi syndrome, 604, 605
Chemical agents, and disease, 949-971

Chemical agents (*Continued*)
  cell response to, 950
  cutaneous absorption of, 958-959
  energetics of cellular activity in, 954-956
  gastrointestinal tract and mucous membrane absorption of, 959-960
  genetically determined enzyme response to, 950-952
  induction of toxicity by metabolic alteration of, 962-964
  inhalation of, 956-958
  interaction of biological systems and, 952-956
  mode of action of, on enzyme system, 961-962
  portals of entry of, 956-960
  toxic, 949-972
    absorption of, cellular biology and enzymatic alteration as determinant of, 960-966
Chemical intoxicants, characteristics governing biological activity of, 952-954
  biological determinants of, 964-966
Chemical toxicity, structural and functional consequences of, 969-971
Chemoreceptors, 187
Chemoreceptor reflex, 158, *160*
Chemotherapy, effect of on DNA synthesis, 38
Chest wall, motion of, 306
  relation of to diaphragm and lungs, *372*
Chlamydia, and interstitial pneumonia, 499
Chlordane, 969
Chloride, transport of, in colon, 774
Chloridorrhea, 785-786
  congenital, 77(t), 79
Chlorothiazide, 353
Chokes, 921
Cholagogues, 819
Cholangiography, 820
  transhepatic, in cholestasis, 804
Cholecystectomy, 836
Cholecystitis, 820, 824
Cholecystography, oral, 820
Cholecystokinin-pancreozymin, 760
  amino acid sequence of, *713*
Cholecystoses, hyperplastic, 824
Cholelithiasis, 820
Cholera, 464-466
  diarrhea of, 759
  precolonic, 776-777
Cholera enterotoxin, 464-466
Cholestasis, 801-804
  findings sometimes present in, *802*
  levels of abnormality producing, *802*
Cholesterol, 849
  chemical structure of, *822*
  formation of bile acids from, *801*
  in bile, 821
  in steroid biosynthesis, 885
  metabolism of, 16-18, *17*
Cholesterolosis, 824
Cholesterol stones, 821
Cholestyramine, and malabsorption, 756
Cholic acid, 775
Cholinesterase, genotypes controlling, distribution of, *951*

INDEX

Chondroitin, 420
Chondroitin-4-sulfate, 420
Chondroitin-6-sulfate, 420
Chordae tendinae, ruptured, and mitral regurgitation, 258
Christmas disease, 84
Christmas factor, 481
Chromatid, definition of, 51, 90
Chromatin, definition of, 90
  sex, 59, *60*
Chromium, deficiencies of, 860–861
Chromophobe adenoma, nonsecretory, 873
Chromosomes, 51, *52*, 52(t), *53*, 905
  abnormalities of, 54–70
    cytogenetic shorthand for, 54
    in acute lymphatic leukemia, 626
    numerical, 55–66, 55(t)
    structural, 55(t), 66–69, 67(t), *68*
  and cancer, 69
  breakage of, 69
  human metaphase, *51*, 52(t)
  in aging, 70
  pattern of, in chronic granulocytic leukemia, *607*
Chromosome ring, definition of, 91
Chronic asthma, long term management of, 451
Chronic bronchitis, 405–406, 453
Chronic erythroleukemia, 609
Chronic granulocytic leukemia, 606–608
  chromosomal pattern in, *607*
Chronic granulomatous disease of childhood, 691
Chronic obstructive lung disease, 453
Chronic renal failure, 368–370
  uremia in, 369
Chylomicrons, 850, 851
Circulation, cerebral, 202
  changes in, in pneumonia, 498
  coronary, 280
  enterohepatic, 800
  hemodynamic factors in, 149, *150*
  peripheral, in cardiac output regulation, 153–156, *155*
  pulmonary, 172–174, 385–386
  systemic, pressure variations in, 177, *179*
Circulatory assist, mechanical, 292–293
Circulatory changes, as host response to infection, 478
Circulatory filling pressure, in cardiac output regulation, 153
  in shock and heart failure, 154
  measurement of, 171
Circulatory system, abnormal structure and function of, 650–657
  intrinsic and extrinsic disorders of, 654–657
  normal function and structure of, 646–650
Cirrhosis, 813–814
  albumin in, 797
  and secondary hypersplenism, 684
  anemia in, 594–595
  hepatic, and salmonella bacteremia, 494
Cis, definition of, 90
Cistron, definition of, 90
Citrate, as anticoagulant, 648
Citric acid cycle, 3, 5, 7–8, *9*
Clostridium botulinum, exotoxin of, 458(t)

Clostridium perfringens, 760
  alpha toxin of, 458, 460, 461
  exotoxin of, 458(t)
  toxins of, 460
Clostridium perfringens bacteremia, erythrocyte destruction in, 480
Clostridium tetani, 458
  exotoxin of, 458(t)
Clostridium welchii, septicemia of, 592
Clotting, blood. See *Coagulation*.
CO, diffusion of in lung, 383
CO_2, blood, 379–383
  diffusion of in lung, 384
  equilibration curve for, 381, *381*
  in arterial and mixed venous blood, 382(t)
Coagulation, abnormalities of in liver, 797
  in pancreatitis, 833
  cascade concept of, 646
  difficulties in, in hepatic disease, 815
  disseminated intravascular, 651
  electrical, 927
  intravascular, disseminated, 481
  irregularities in, endotoxin induced, 467
Coagulation defects, in bacterial uremia, 481–484
Coagulation factors, biologic half-lives of, 650(t)
  disorders of, classification of, 651(t)
  extrinsic and intrinsic, 654–657
  hereditary abnormalities of, 650
  measurement of, *655*
  sequence of reactions in, *649*
Cobamide, 855
Coccidioidomycosis, 410
Codon(s), definition of, 90
  triplet, 73, *74*
Coenzyme A, pantothenic acid in, 854
Coenzyme binding, reduced, and inborn errors, 85
Colchicine, and malabsorption, 756
COLD, 453
Cold, effects of, 930
Cold agglutinin hemolytic anemia, 596
Cold agglutinins, 485
Cold urticaria, allergen in, 452
Colic, biliary, 823
Colitis, granulomatous, 781
  transmural, 781
  ulcerative, 758, 781, 782–783
Collagen, 418
  fibrils of, arrangement in cartilage, 422, *422*
Collagenases, 419, 458
Collagen diseases, 440
Collagen vascular diseases, and interstitial pneumonia, 499
Colon, anatomy of, 767
  carcinoma of, 758
  Crohn's disease in, 783–785
  disorders of secretory function in, 785–786
  diverticular disease of, 779–781
  electrolyte and fluid balance in, 773, 774
  gas in, 775–776
  greedy, 774
  idiopathic chronic inflammatory disease of, 781–782
  inflammatory disease of wall of, 778
  innervation of, 769

Colon (*Continued*)
  microflora of, 788
  motility of, 770
    distribution of activity in, 772(t)
    types of contractions in, 771(t)
  normal-appearing, diarrhea with, 776-778
  normal function of, 769
  progressive contraction of, 770
  sigmoid, hypertrophy of circular muscle of, *781*
    in diverticulitis, *780*
  smooth muscle of, electrical properties of, 769
  tumors of, 786-788
  volume overload of, 776
  wall of, layers of, 767
Colonoscopy, 787
Colony-inhibition assay, 140, *141*
Coma, as host response to infection, 478
  hyperosmolar nonketotic, 902
  in hypoglycemia, 904
  ketoacidotic, vs. hypoglycemia, differential diagnosis of, 904(t)
  liver, 812
Compensatory emphysema, 399
Competitive inhibitors, 36, 37(t)
Complementation, definition of, 90
Complement system, 115-119, 116(t), *118*
  alternate pathways in, 117-119, *118*
  disorders of, 136
  homeostatic control of, 119
Compliance, aortic, 182
Concentration-dilution tests, of renal function, 356-357
Conduction, supernormal A-V, 335, *335*
Conduction, V-A, 335, *335*
Conduction block, escape beat and, 330, *331*
  simple, 332-336
Conduction disorders, intraventricular, and QRS waveform, 327-328
Confusion, as host response to infection, 478
Congenital cystic disease, 401
Congenital heart disease, left-to-right shunts in, 280
Congenital syphilis, 496-497
Congestion, pulmonary venous, 289-290
  venous, systemic, 290
Congestive heart failure, 273-294, 758
  in aortic regurgitation, 262
  renal physiology in, 284
Congestive splenomegaly, splenectomy in, 684
Conjugate gaze, disorders of, in bacterial meningitis, 500
Conjugation, process of, 963-964
Connective tissue, cells of, 418
  fibrillar components of, 418-419
  formation of, 420-421
  structure and function of, 417-421
Conn's disease, and hypertension, 195-196
Conn's syndrome, 889-890
Constipation, 785
Constriction, primary. See *Centromere*.
  secondary, definition of, 91
Constrictive pericarditis, 268-269, 758
Consumption coagulopathy, 651
Continence, fecal, 773

Continuous heart murmur, of patent ductus arteriosus, *306*
Contractile proteins, in contraction, 215, *216*
  of myocardium, 207-210, *210*
Contractile state, in mechanical function of heart, 291
Contractility, of myocardium, 219-220, *219*
  ejection indices in, 227
  evaluation of, 221-229
    force-velocity curve in, 221-222, *222, 223*
    isovolumic indices in, 222-227, *223, 224, 225, 226, 228*
Convulsions, in chronic renal failure, 369
  pyridoxine and, 854
Cooley's anemia, 534, 576
Copper, deficiencies in, 860
Coronary artery disease, 281
Coronary circulation, 280
Coronary heart disease, changes in myocardium in, *286*
  relation of ventricular performance to filling pressure in, *287*
Coronary insufficiency, in acute pancreatitis, 833
Cor pulmonale, in pneumoconiosis, 403
Corpus luteum, formation of, 908-909
Corticosteroids, 112
  and gastroenteritis, 494
  and salmonella bacteremia, 494
Corticotropin, 872
Cortisol, and Cushing's syndrome, 887
  biological activities of, 884-885
  metabolism of, 885
  regulation of secretion of, 884
Cough, as pulmonary protective mechanism, 395
Countercurrent exhange, in intestinal blood, 763, *763*
Counterpulsation, mechanical, 293
  mechanical consequences of, *293*
Corynebacterium diphtheriae, 470
  exotoxin of, 458(t)
Cough, in pulmonary disease, 378-379
Coxa vara, congenital, 427
Cramps, heat, 928
Cranial nerve, dysfunction of, in bacterial meningitis, 500
Craniopharyngiomas, 873
Creatine phosphate, in myocardial metabolism, *213*, 214
Creatinine, 24
Creatinine clearance test, 356
Crepitus, in osteoarthritis, 427
Cretinism, 882
Creutzfeld-Jacob disease, 486
Cricopharyngeal diverticulum, 699
Cricopharyngeal sphincter, disorders of, 699-700
Cri du chat syndrome, genetics of, 66
Crigler-Najjar syndrome, 794
Crohn's disease, 757, 758, 781, 783-785
  pathologic features of, 782(t)
  surgical management of, 783-785
Crossing-over, definition of, 90
Cross-reactivity, antigenic, 139, 140(t)
Cryoglobulin, 632

Cryptococcosis, 410
Crystal-induced synovitis, 431–434
Cubitus valgus, 910
Cushing's syndrome, 658, 871, 887–888
   and osteoporosis, 896
   potassium deficit in, 351
   typical laboratory findings in, 888(t)
Cyanide, 961
Cyanosis, 242, 390
   in pneumonia, 498
   low affinity hemoglobin with, 572
Cyanotic heart disease, cardiac catheterization in, 242–243
Cyclic AMP, 867
   as messenger, hormones using, 867(t)
   in myocardial metabolism, 214
Cystadenocarcinoma, of pancreas, 836
Cystathioninuria, 85
Cystic disease, congenital, 401
Cystic duct, obstruction of, 824
Cystic fibrosis, 836–837
   pancreatic insufficiency in, 837
   sweat test for, 837
Cystinuria, 757
   genetics of, 76–77, 77(t)
Cytogenetics, 50–54
Cytopenia, cure of by splenectomy, and hypersplenism, 682
Cytoplasm, erythrocyte, maturation disorders of, 560–577
Cytoplasmic inheritance, 36
Cytosine, 71
Cytotoxicity, in cellular immunity, 120, *121*
Cytotoxins, general, 459–462

Daughter cell, definition of, 90
DDT, 969
Dead space, anatomical respiratory, 387
Deamination, oxidative, 23
Deceleration, and impact, data on, *944*
Decompression sickness, 921–922
Defecation, 772–773
Defibrillation, electrical, 927
Deletion, of chromosomes, 66, 67(t)
   definition of, 90
Delirium, as host response to infection, 478
Demyelinization, 486
Denaturation, protein, 34
Dental caries, effect of fluoride on, 861(t)
Deoxyadenosyl cobalamine, structure of, *551*
Deoxycholic acid, secondary, chemical structure of, *822*
Deoxyribonucleic acid. See *DNA*.
Deoxysugar, 28
Dermatan-4-sulfate, 420
Dermatitis herpetiformis, 752
Detoxification, 962
Diabetes, 427
Diabetes insipidus, 878
   nephrogenic, 367
   pitressin-resistant, 350
Diabetes mellitus, 10, 878, 900–903
   hyperlipidemia in, 902–903
   hyperosmolar nonketotic coma in, 902

Diabetes mellitus (*Continued*)
   ketoacidosis in, 901–902
   natural history and sequelae of, *901*
Diabetic ketoacidosis, in pancreatitis, 832
Diaphragm, relationship of to chest wall and lungs, *372*
Diarrhea, bile acid, 778
   chronic, in immunodeficiency syndromes, 762
   in carcinoma of stomach, 732
   in chronic renal failure, 369
   in peptic ulcer, 724
   in ulcerative colitis, 782
   initiation of, 741
   of cholera, 759
   simple, 776–777
   with normal-appearing colon, 776–778
   with structural changes in colon, 778–785
Diarthrodial joint, 421, *421*
Diarthroses, 421
Diastolic heart murmur, 304
   decrescendo, of aortic regurgitation, *305*
Diastolic hypertension, 190
Diastolic work, of left ventricle, determining, 246–250
DIC, 651–654
Diet, lack in, and vitamin B_{12} deficiency, 556
DiGeorge syndrome, 622
Digestion, 745
   abnormalities of, 751–759
   normal, 746
Di Guglielmo syndrome, 560
Diodrast, in kidney excretion test, 354
Diphtheria, cardiac involvement in, 459
Diphtheria toxin, 459
Diplococcus pneumoniae, 458
   invasion of tissues by, 468
Diploid, definition of, 54, 90
Disaccharidases, deficiencies of, and malabsorption, 757
Discontinuous traits, definition of, 90
Disease. See also specific disease; e.g., *Crohn's disease, Hodgkin's disease*.
   Addison's, 886–887
   alteration of bile salts in, 800–801
   autoimmune, 440
   autoimmune hemolytic, of newborn, 596
   Bornholm, 413
   cardiovascular, of high altitude, 548
   celiac, 755
   chemical agents and, 949–971
   chronic granulomatous of childhood, 691
   collagen, 440
   Creutzfeld-Jacob, 486
   Crohn's, 757, 758, 781, 783–785
   cystic, congenital, 401
   gallbladder, pathophysiology of, 818–826
   Gaucher's, 679, 693
   Graves', 882–884
   heavy chain, 633
   Hodgkin's, 628–629, 685
   hyaline membrane, 401
   immune complex, 485
   immunologically induced, conceptual evolution for, 450–451, *450*

Disease (*Continued*)
  infectious, localized in specific organs, 489–510
  Kaschin-Beck, 426
  Legg-Perthes, 427
  lipids in, 849–852
  liver, 810–812
  Lyell's, 471
  mast cell, 752
  Menetrier's, 719
  metabolic, of bone, 891–892
  mitral valve, left atrial volume in, 259(t)
  Monge's, 548
  neuropathic joint, 427
  Niemann-Pick, 679
  nutritional factors in, 839–864
  pleural. See *Pleural disease.*
  pulmonary. See *Pulmonary disease.*
  reagin mediated, 452
  renal, 345–370, 540
  reversible obstructive airway, 453
  rheumatic, 417–444. See also *Rheumatic diseases.*
  trace elements in, 859–863
  viral, 486–487
  vitamins in, 852–959
  Von Willebrand's, 654
  Whipple's, 752
Disorders, pleural, 411–413
Disseminated intravascular coagulation, 481, 651
  classification of syndromes of, 652(t)
  pathogenesis of, *483*
Diuresis, 352–354
  in constrictive pericarditis, 269
Diuretics, 352–354
Diuretic agents, classification of, 353(t)
Diuretic drugs, 352
  functional classification of, 353(t)
Diuretic therapy, of hypertension, 353
Diverticulum(a), cricopharyngeal, 699
  of colon, 779
  of stomach, 709–710
  pulsion, 700
Diverticulitis, noninflammatory, 781
  sigmoid colon in, *780*
Diverticulosis, 779
  spastic, 780
Dizziness, in pleuritis, 412
DNA, 28–32, *29, 31*
  definition of, 90
  effect of drugs on, 30(t)
  in myocardium, 214
  in protein synthesis, 21, *22*
  mutation in, 71
  replication of, 30, *31*, 71, *71*
  structure of, *70*
  synthesis of, regulation of, 28, *31*
    repair *31*, 32
  transcription and translation of into proteins, 72, *72*
  vs. RNA, 28
DNA labeling, in lymphocyte kinetics, 620
Dominant, definition of, 90
Dose, relation of to tissue response, 950
Down's syndrome, 57–58, *57*
  karyotype in, *53*
  leukemia in, 609

Dp/dt, 222–227, *223, 224, 225, 226*
Drowning, DIC in, 652
Drugs, cytotoxic, 112
  diuretic, 352
  effect of on chromosomes, 69
  via colon, 775
Drug sensitivity, and interstitial pneumonia, 499
Drug tolerance, 38
Dry bronchiectasis, 407
Duct, cystic, obstruction of, *824*
Dumping syndrome, 729
Duodenal obstruction, in peptic ulcer, 727
Duodenal ulcer, hydrochloric acid output in, 726(t)
  perforation in, 728
Duodenum. See also *Small intestine.*
  bile duct obstructed in wall of, *803*
  distention in obstruction of, 741
Dwarfism, sexual ateliotic, 875, 876(t)
  zinc deficiency and, 860
Dysfibrinogenemia(s), 84, 653
Dysfunctions, tubular, 367
Dysphagia, 698
  and pulsion diverticulum, 700
Dyspnea, 390
  exertional, in mitral stenosis, 257
  in carcinoma of esophagus, 701
Dyssynergy, of contraction, 220, *221*

Ebullism, 918
ECG, in patient with mitral stenosis, *244*
Eclamptogenic toxemia, edema in, 363
E. coli, 760
Ectopic pacemaker, 339
Ectopic tachycardia, 339
Edema, 165–170
  cerebral, in bacterial meningitis, 500
  in acute nephritis, 363
  in constrictive pericarditis, 269
  in eclamptogenic toxemia, 363
  in kwashiorkor, 849
  in pancreatitis, 828
  in serum sickness, 435
  nephrotic syndrome and, 363–365
  of renal origin, 363
  physiological basis of, 167–170
  pitting, 168
  pulmonary, 173, 384
  in poliomyelitis, 506
  safety factors against, 170
  tissue compliance change in, 171
  tissue nutrition in, 169
Edematous pancreatitis, 829
Edwards' syndrome, 58, *59*
Effusion, pericardial, 267–268
Ehlers-Danlos syndrome, 658
Elastic fibers, 419
Electricity, 925–927
Electrocardiogram, 312–328
  and left ventricular hypertrophy, 255
  and vectorcardiogram, *313*
  atrial excitation and P wave in, 318–320
    diagrammatic representation of, 319
  cardiac basis of, 317–318
  electrical axis of, 316–317

INDEX

Electrocardiogram (*Continued*)
   in myocardial infarction, 325–327
   ventricular excitation and QRS complex in, 320
Electrocardiograph, in atrial enlargement, 324–325
Electrocardiographic leads, 314–317
   types of, 315, *315*
Electrocardiographic system, 314, *314, 317*
Electrocautery, 927
Electroconvulsive therapy, 927
Electrolytes, concentrations of, in colon, 774
   secretion of, in small intestine, 759–760
Electromagnetic energy, frequency, wavelength, and energy of, *926*
Electromagnetic environment, 925–942
Electromagnetic waves, 927
Electrophoresis, detection of defects in fat metabolism by, 850–852
Elliptocytosis, hereditary, 587
Embden-Meyerhof pathway, 3, 4, 5–7, 600, *601*
Embolism, in bacterial endocarditis, 492
   pulmonary, 401–402
Emphysema, 398–400
   and empyema, 413
   chronic bronchitis and, 405
   compensatory, 399
   interstitial, 399–400
Empyema, 412–413
Encephalitis, demyelinating, following viral disease, 486
Encephalomyelitides, postinfectious, 486
Encephalopathy, acute toxic, 478
   hepatic, 812
End-diastolic pressure, left ventricular, 222–229
Endocarditis, infectious process of infected heart valve in, 491
   pathogenesis of, 490
   pathophysiology of clinical features of, 490–493
   rheumatic, 256
Endocrine functions, renal, 357–358
Endocrine system, composition of, 865
   disorders of, 869
   elements of, 865
   functions of, 865
Endocrinology, 865–914
   laboratory procedures in, 870
Endocytosis, 689–691
   intracellular digestion in, 691
   mechanism of, *690*
   metabolic requirements of, 691
Endogenous pyrogen, 475
   site of action of, 476
   sources of, 476
Endoplasmic reticulum, 35
   electron transport in, *798*
   rough, in protein synthesis, 796
   smooth, function of, 797–798
Endotoxins, 458, 466–468
   biological effects of, 466–468
   tolerance to, 466
End-product inhibition, mechanisms of, *955*
Energy, average expenditure of, *842*
   electromagnetic, frequency, wavelength, and energy of, *926*
   storage of, in man, 843, 844(t)

Enteric fever, 494
Enterogastrone, 760
Enterohepatic circulation, 800
Enterokinase, 761
Enterotoxins, 464–468
   cholera, 464–466
Enthalpy, in biosystems, 27
Entropy, in biosystems, 27
Environment, electromagnetic, 925–942
   gaseous, 917–925
   kinetic, 942–947
   metals in, 966–968
   metallic contamination of, consequences of, 966–968
   physical, combined stresses in, 947
Environmental toxicology, 949
Enzymes, as mutant gene products, 75–76, 76(t)
   in protein regulation, 37
   in urine, 362
   pancreatic, function of, 828
   regulating drug metabolism, disorders caused by, 86–88, *87*
   secretion of, in small intestine, 760–761
   serum, in diagnosis of pancreatitis, 834
Enzyme induction and repression, 32, *33*, 38
Enzyme precursors, in complement system, 115
Enzyme system, mode of action of chemicals upon, 961–962
Eosinophilia, 400
   as host response, 484
Eosinophilic gastroenteritis, 752
Eosinophilic tumors, 873
Epidemic pleurodynia, 413
Epinephrine, 866
   and hyperglycemia, 897
   calorigenic effects of, 842
   effect of, on glucose metabolism, 10
      on lipid metabolism, 18
   in pheochromocytoma, 898
   mechanism of action of, 896–897
   pathways for biochemical disposal of, 897
Epstein-Barr virus, 623
Ergastoplasm, 969
Erythroblasts, function of, 517
   multinucleated, in bone marrow, *610*
Erythrocyte(s), 517–599. See also *Red cells.*
   as transporter of oxygen, 584
   circulation of through spleen, 669
   classification of hemolytic states in, 584
   destruction of, in splenic sequestration, 673–674
   energy source of, 584
   extrinsic disorders of, 592–599
   fragmentation of on fibrin strands, *594*
   function of, 517–520
   general signs of hemolysis in, 577–582
   hemolysis of, 485
   IgG coated, adherence of to macrophages, 597
   inclusion granules of, removal of by normal spleen, *672*
   injured, temporary sequestration of, *671*
   intrinsic disorders of, 585–592
   intrinsic enzyme deficiency of, 589
   intrinsically defective, survival of, *586*
   irregular distortion of, *594*
   kinetics of, 520–529

Erythrocyte(s) (*Continued*)
  maturation disorders of, 560–577
  mature, glycolytic pathways in, *585*
  membrane function and energy metabolism of, 582–584
  membrane of, 582, *582*
  mildly injured, selective splenic sequestration of, *673*
  mixing of, in normal and enlarged spleens, *669*
  pathophysiology of, 529–599
  pliability of, *588*
  production of, in anephric patient, 541, *541*
  relationship of to spleen, 669–674
  rigid, splenic effects on, *675*
  sickled, *573*
  structure of, 517
  survival disorders of, 577–599
Erythrocytosis, hepatocarcinoma and, 550
  high affinity hemoglobin with, 572
  of high altitude, 546–548
Erythroid hyperplasia, plasma clearance and red cell utilization in, 533, *533*
Erythroid pools, 524(t)
Erythroleukemia, chronic, 609
Erythropoietic feedback, 524, 525, *525*, 529
Erythropoietin, 358, 526–529, *526*, *528*
  blast formation and, 520
Erythrostasis, 673
Escape beat, conduction block and, 330, *331*
Escherichia coli, endotoxin of, 466
  exotoxin of, 458(t)
  in cholecystitis, 824
Esophageal atresia, 705
Esophageal muscles, disorders of, 700–701
Esophageal ring, 702
Esophageal spasm, 700–701
Esophageal stricture, 702–704
Esophageal web, 702
Esophagitis, in gastroesophageal reflux, 707
  reflux, 702
Esophagogastric junction, 698
Esophagoscopy, in gastroesophageal reflux, 707
Esophagus, 697–708
  diseases affecting, 705
  disorders of mucosa of, 701–704
  distal, as sphincter, 698
  functions of, 697
  neoplasms of, 701–702
  rupture of, 705
  structure of, 697–698
  transport of ingested material in, 698–705
Essential hypertension, 365–366, 890
  arteriosclerosis in, 366
  nephrosclerosis in, 366
  pyelonephritis in, 366
Essential thrombocythemia, 609
Estrogen, biosynthesis, transport, mechanisms of action, and disposal of, 910
Ethacrynic acid, 353
Euglobulin, in rheumatoid arthritis, 436
Eunuchism, 904
Eustachian tube, effects of barometric pressures on, 920
Excitation-contraction coupling, 215–217, *216*

Excretory function, renal, 345–354
  tests of, 354–357
Exfoliatin, 471
Exhaustion, heat, 928
Exophthalmos, in Graves' disease, 882
Exotoxins, 458
Expiratory flow rates, 377
Extrinsic clotting system, activation of, 481
Extrinsic factor, 648
Eye, infrared effects on, 929–930
  physiology of, 931

Factor(s), blood, 481, *482*, *483*
  leukocyte, and arthritis, 431
  plasma, in inflammation of joints, 430
  rheumatoid, 435
Factor VIII, method of measurement of, *655*
Factor IX, method of measurement of, *655*
Faintness, in pleuritis, 412
Fanconi's anemia, 537
  acute leukemia in, 609
Fanconi's syndrome, 69, 367
Fasting, 846–849
  effect of on substrate utilization, *848*
Fat, absorption of, 746–747, *746*, 748
  ingestion and metabolism of, 850
  metabolism of, 10–14, *12, 13, 14, 15*
    determination of defects in, 850–852
  percentage of in human body weight, 840, *840*
Fat cells, 843, 844, *844*
  effect of weight loss on size of, *844*
Fatness, techniques for measuring, 840(t)
Fats, storage of, insulin in, 845
Fat-soluble vitamins, 855–857
  toxicity from, 855
Fatty acids, breakdown of, 11–12, *14*
  oxidation of, *839*
  synthesis of, 10–11, *12, 13*
Febrile disease states, thermoregulation in, 474
Febrile headache, 477
Fecal continence, 773
Feedback gain, in arterial pressure control, 159–161, *160*
Feedback inhibition, 36
  loss of, and inherited disorders, 82
Fenn effect, 212
Felty's syndrome, and hypersplenism, 683
Ferritin, formation of, 565, *565*
Fertile eunuch syndrome, 908
Fetoglobin, 810
Fever, as defense mechanism, 474
  as host response to infection, 473
  cardiac output and, 238, 475
  cardiorespiratory changes in, 475
  endotoxin induced, 466
  enteric, 494
  epidemic hemorrhagic, DIC in, 652
  in acute granulocytic leukemia, effect of prednisone on, *612*
  in bacterial meningitis, 500
  in cholecystitis, 824
  in pneumonia, 497
  in serum sickness, 435
  in ulcerative colitis, 782

INDEX

Fever (*Continued*)
  mechanism of production in, overt infections, 476
  mediators of, 475–476
  Oroya, and salmonella bacteremia, 494
  paratyphoid, 494
  Q, 499
  relapsing, louse-borne, 494
  rheumatic, 256, 435
  Rocky Mountain spotted, 481
    DIC in, 652
  scarlet, 470
  typhoid, 494
F_1 generation, definition of, 90
Fibers, elastic, 419
Fibrillation, 339–343
  atrial, tachysystole in, 339
  of cartilage, 425
  ventricular, 925
    spontaneous termination of, *341*, 342
    type A, *341*, 342
Fibrin stabilizing factor, 481
Fibrinogen, 646
  action of thrombin on, 647
  degradation of, by plasmin, *649*
  disorders of, 651–654
  structure of, *647*
Fibrinolysin, 647
Fibroblasts, 418
Fibromas, of pleura, 411
Fibrosarcomas, of pleura, 411
Fibrosis, 403
  of bone marrow, 608–609
  retroperitoneal, 758
Fibrositis, primary, 442
Fibrous ankylosis, 428
Fick method, in measurement of cardiac output, 236
Fingers, clubbing of in pulmonary neoplasm, 411
First heart sound, (S-1), 295
Fistula, arteriovenous, effect of on circulatory function, *153*
  gastrojejunocolic, in peptic ulcer, 728
  tracheo-esophageal, 701, 705
Flaking, of cartilage, 425
Flavin mononucleotide, 854
Fluid, retention of, in liver disease, 812
  synovial, 423–425
Fluoride, effect of on dental caries, 861(t)
  metabolism of, 861
Folate deficiency, dietary lack in, 559
  drugs and, 560
  malabsorption and, 558–559
  serum folate and red cell folate in, 558, *559*
  serum vitamin B_{12} levels in, 557, *558*
Folic acid, 855
  absorption of, 750–751
  as anti-anemic principle, 550–555
  description of, 552
  structure of, *553*
Follicle, ovarian, development of, 908–909
Follicle-stimulating hormone, 872
Food, intake of, external environment and, 843
  metabolic factors in, 843
  regulation of, 842

Fragment, chromosome, definition of, 90
Frank-Starling mechanism, 252
Frank-Starling principle, 218
Frank-Starling relationship, *277*
FRC, 372, 373, *373*
Frostbite, 930
Fungus infections, of lung, 410–411
Furosemide, 353

Galactokinase deficiency, 80
Galactose-1-phosphate accumulation, 80
Galactosemia, 80, 81
Gallbladder, carcinoma of, 825
  function of, 818–820
  inflammation of, 824
  less common diseases of, 824–825
  structure of, 818
  tests of function of, 820
Gallbladder disease, pathophysiology of, 818–826
Gallop heart sound, *301*
Gallstone(s), and cholestasis, 802
  and pancreatitis, 828
  clinical significance of, 823–824
  formation of, 820–824
  types of, 821
Ganglia, spinal, in herpes zoster, 507
Gangrene, gas, 460
Gap, chromosome, definition of, 69, 90
Garrod, A. E., 40, 75–76
Gas(es), dissolved in liquid, partial pressure of, 379
  inert, role of, 924
  inhalation of, 956
Gas gangrene, 460
Gaseous environment, 917–925
Gastrectomy, subtotal, serum vitamin B_{12} levels after, 557, *558*
Gastric carcinoma, 716, 758
  pain in, 718
Gastric fluid, aspiration of, in aspiration pneumonia, 408
Gastric mucosa, giant hypertrophy of mucosal folds of, 719
Gastric neoplasm, loss of appetite in, 711
Gastric resection, nutritional and metabolic problems related to, 728
Gastric secretion, 712–717
  disturbances in, 716
  physiologic considerations, 712
  principal components of, 715
  sources of products of, *715*
Gastric tone, 712
Gastric torsion, 710
Gastric tumors, benign, 729–730
Gastric ulcer, 723–724
  hydrochloric acid output in, 726(t)
Gastrin, 712, 713
  amino acid sequence of, *713*
Gastritis, acute erosive, 721
  chronic, nonspecific, 719–722
    pathogenesis of, 720
  in gastric ulcer, 724
  Menetrier's giant hypertrophic, 758
Gastroenteritis, acute, 758
  eosinophilic, 752
  salmonella, 493–494

Gastroenterology, endocrinology and metabolism, 695–914
Gastroenteropathies, protein losing, 758–759
　classification of, 758(t)
Gastroesophageal reflux, 707–708
　prevention of, 705–708
Gastrointestinal tract, calcium in, 890
　chemical absorption in, 959–960
　gas in, 775–776
　vitamin D in, 890
Gastrojejunocolic fistula, in peptic ulcer, 728
Gastrones, 761
Gaucher's disease, 16, 693
　splenomegaly in, 679
Gel, in interstitial spaces, 169
Gene, definition of, 90
Gene insertion, in treatment of inborn errors, 89
Gene products, defective, and inborn errors of metabolism, 75–76, 76(t)
General cytotoxins, 459–462
General paresis, in late syphilis, 496
Genetics, medical, 40–96
　terminology in, 90–92
Genetic disorders, multifactorial, 47–50, 48, 49(t), 50
Genetic variability, and DNA mutations, 28
Genitalia, embryogenesis of, 905
Genome, definition of, 90
Genotype, definition of, 90
Geotrichosis, 410
Giant follicular lymphoma, 630–631
Giant hemangioma, DIC in, 652
Giardia lambiia, 762
Gland(s). See specific gland; e.g., *Thyroid, Parathyroid.*
Gigantism, 874–875
Glanzmann's thrombasthenia, 645
Glass blower's cataract, 929
Globin, 569–577
　normal structure and synthesis of, 569–571
Globin chains, changes in, during intrauterine development, *570*
Glomerular filtration, 346–347
Glomerular proteinuria, 359
Glomerulonephritis, 359
　acute, edema in, 363
　poststreptococcal, 485
Glomerulus, schematic view of, *346*
Glucagon, 10
Glucocorticoids, and osteoporosis, 896
　effects of, on carbohydrate metabolism, 10
　on lipid metabolism, 18
　on protein metabolism, 23
Gluconeogenesis, 8, 24, 847
　impaired, 812
Glucose, as energy source of erythrocyte, 584
　concentration in blood, 8, 10
　conversion of to other metabolites, 3–4
　oxidation of, 3, 4–8
　uses of, 3–4
Glucose-galactose malabsorption, 77, *78*
Glucose-6-phosphatase deficiency, 7

Glucose-6-phosphate dehydrogenase deficiency, 86, 590–592
　drug-induced hemolysis in, *592*
　genetic types of, *591*
Glutamine formation, 23
Gluten enteropathy, 755
Glycine conjugate, chemical structure of, *822*
Glycocalyx, 736, *737*
Glycogen, 843
Glycogenesis, 3
Glycogenolysis, 8
Glycogen storage diseases, 7
Glycolipids, metabolism of, 16
Glycolysis, 3, 4, 5–7, *6*
　anaerobic, in myocardial metabolism, 213
Glycosaminoglycan, 420
Glycosuria, 347, *348*
　renal, 77(t), 78, *78*
Goiter, iodine deficiency and, 861–862
　multinodular toxic, 883
　toxic diffused, 882–884
Gonads, embryogenesis of, 905
Gonadal aplasia, 910–912
Gonadal dysfunction, anemia in, 543
Gonadotropins, 908
Gonococcus, and arthritis, 431
Goose pimples, 930
Gout, urate crystals in, 431, 433
Gouty arthritis, acute, 431–434
　pathogenesis of, 432, *432*
　chronic, 433
G-6-PD deficiency, 590–592, *591, 592*
Granulocyte(s), 599–612
　after phagocytosis, *600*
　classification of disorders in, 604, 604(t)
　myeloproliferative disorders of, 605–613
　pathophysiology of, 604–613
　production of, 602, *603*
　qualitative abnormalities in, 605
　quantitative abnormalities of, 604–605
　relation of spleen to, 678
　structure of, 599
Granulocyte pools, size of, 602(t)
Granulocytic leukemia, acute, 609–613
Granulocytopenia, 604–605
　endotoxin induced, 467
　in chronic lymphatic leukemia, 625
Granulocytosis, 605
Granulomatous colitis, 781
Graves' disease, 882–884
Gravity, 942–943
　physical activity and, 943
　prolonged acceleration and, 943
Gray hepatization, in lobar pneumonia, 497
Greedy colon, 774
Ground substance, 417, 419–420
Growth, disturbances of, in high magnetic fields, 925
　zinc deficiency and, 860
Growth hormone, 866, 872
　and acromegaly and gigantism, 874
　dwarfism and, 875
　effect of on protein metabolism, 21
　mechanism of action of, 875
Guanine, 71
Guillain-Barré syndrome, in diphtheria, 459
Gumma, in late syphilis, 496
Gynecomastia, 906

Haemophilus influenzae, and interstitial pneumonia, 499
Haemophilus influenzae meningitis, 503
Hageman factor, 481
 in joint inflammation, 430
Hamman-Rich syndrome, 403
Haploid, definition of, 54, 90
Haptens, 98
Haptoglobin, 797
Hartnup disease, 77, 77(t)
Haustra, 767
 barium enema showing, *768*
Haustral movement, types of, 771(t)
Haustral systole, 770
Headache, as host response to infection, 477
 as symptom of systemic infection, 477
 in bacterial meningitis, 500
Hearing, human, frequency spectrum of, *296*
Heart. See also entries under *Cardiac* and under *Cardio-*.
 artificial, 292
 as muscle, performance of, 278–280
 biochemical and functional relations in, 206–230
 contraction of, mechanisms of, 206–230
 excitation-contraction coupling in, 215–217
 function of, afterload in, 291
  contractile state in, 291
  preload in, 290
 in cardiac output regulation, 152, 154–156, *155*
 output of. See *Cardiac output.*
 pumping capacity of, 152
 size of, relation to oxygen consumption, *278*
Heart disease, chronic, distensibility of left ventricle in, 246
 growth of myocardium in, 249
 hypertrophy of left ventricle in, 247
 cyanotic, cardiac catheterization in, 242–243
 ischemic, 253–256
  left ventricular pressure, volume and pressure-volume curves in, *250*
  left ventricular end-diastolic volume and mass in, *250*
  left ventricular pressure and volume in, *248, 249*
 valvular, 256–259
  left ventricular stroke work and mass in, *250*
Heart failure, cardiac enlargement in, 252
 circulatory changes following, 155–156, *155*
 circulatory filling pressure in, 154
 circulatory recovery following, 156
 congestive, 273–294
 definition of, 273–274
 factors in causation of, 280(t)
 hemodynamics of, 252–253
 in diphtheria, 459
 in ischemic heart disease and acute myocardial infarction, 286–289
 malignant hypertension and, 279
 myocardial activity in, 217
 symptoms of, arteriography in, 253

Heart-lung bypass machine, as temporary circulatory support, 293
Heart murmur, 301
 diastolic, 304
 ejection systole of aortic and pulmonary valve stenosis, *303*
 functional, 303
 holosystolic, *302*
 systolic, 302
Heart muscle. See *Myocardium.*
Heart pumps, 292
Heart rate, 220
Heart sound(s), and murmurs, 295–306
 as heard over different valve areas, *298*
 at apex, *297*
 first, (S1), 295
 murmurs, and precordial movements, 295–310
 opening snap, 301
 over pulmonary area, *299*
 over tricuspid region, *299*
 second (S2), 297
 sound tracings of, *297, 299*
 third (S3), 299
Heat, acute systemic effects of, 928
 chronic systemic effects of, 928–929
 local effects of, 929
Heat cramps, 928
Heat exhaustion, 928
Heat stroke, 928
 DIC in, 652
Heavy chains, designations of, 99–100
Heavy chain diseases, 137–138, 633
Heberden's nodes, 426
Heinz bodies, 591, *593*
 breaking from red cell, *675*
Heister, valves of, 818
Helium, effects of high pressures on, 924
Hemangioma, cerebellar, and polycythemia vera, 550
Hematemesis, in carcinoma of esophagus, 701
Hematochezia, in ulcerative colitis, 782
Hematocrit, blood volume and, 532, *533*
Hematogenous osteomyelitis, 507
Hematologic disorders, pathophysiology of, 511–644
Hematology, study of, 511
Hematopoiesis, 512–517
 dynamic model of, *516*
Hematopoietic tissue, composition of, 517(t)
 morphology of, *516*
Hematuria, 361
Heme, formation of, 522, *522*
 structure of, *561*
 synthesis of, 560, *561*
Hemiparesis, in bacterial meningitis, 500
Hemizygous, definition of, 90
Hemochromatosis, 568, 569, 814
Hemodialysis, in acute renal failure, 368
Hemodynamics, in circulatory function, integrative, 149–176
 in essential hypertension, 196
 of arterial pressure regulation, 183–184
Hemoglobin, disorders in synthesis of, 560
 exterior mutants and, 573–575
 high affinity, with erythrocytosis, 572

Hemoglobin (*Continued*)
  intravascular handling of, *578*
  Lepore, examples of, *576*
  low affinity, with cyanosis, 572
  molecule of, *571*
  mutations in, 73–75, 75(t)
  oxygen affinity of, and sickling, *575*
  polypeptide chain of, 518, *518*
  renal handling of, *579*
  structures and structural mutations of, 571(t)
  unstable, with congenital Heinz body hemolytic anemia, 572–573
  with abnormal oxygen affinity, *572*
Hemoglobin defects, genetic errors and, 34
Hemoglobin molecule, 518, *519*
  composition of, 518
Hemoglobin synthesis, 522, *522*, 523
  iron in, 562–569
Hemoglobinopathy(ies), and gastroenteritis, 494
  due to quantitative defects, 575–577
  due to structural defects, 571–575, 571(t)
  nomenclature in, 571
  population genetics, 577
Hemoglobinuria, march, 593
Hemolysis, general signs of in erythrocyte, 577–582
  jaundice as sign of, 579
  mechanisms of, 674(t)
  rate of, measurement of, with radioactive hematin, *580*
  traumatic, 593
Hemolytic anemias, genetic error and, 34
Hemolytic uremic syndrome, 539
  DIC in, 652
Hemophilia, intra-articular hemorrhage in, 650
  severe degenerative arthritis in, 427
Hemophilia A, 654
  classic, 84
Hemophilia B, 654
Hemorrhage, after heparin therapy, 657
  gastrointestinal, in cirrhosis, 814
  in acute granulocytic leukemia, 611
  in chronic renal disease, 540
  in disseminated intravascular coagulation, 483
  in liver disease, 797
  intercranial, in acute lymphatic leukemia, 626
  intra-articular, in hemophilia, 650
Hemostasis, 634, 646–658
  vascular factors in, 657–658
Henle, loop of, 348–350
Heparin, 420
Heparitin sulfate, 420
Hepatic artery, flow of through liver, 804
Hepatic blood flow and portal hypertension, 804–809
Hepatic cirrhosis, and salmonella bacteremia, 494
Hepatitis, 813
  antiplatelet antibody in, 677, 677(t)
  in diphtheria, 459
  in secondary syphilis, 495
  loss of appetite in, 711
  viral, 485

Hepatocarcinoma, and erythrocytosis, 550
Hepatoma, 814
Hepatomegaly, 811
Hereditary acanthocytosis, 595
Hereditary elliptocytosis, 587
Hereditary spherocytosis, 585–587
  splenectomy in, 684
Herellea, 457
Hernia, hiatal, 706–707
Herniation, and obstruction of small intestine, 742
Herpes hominis, and interstitial pneumonia, 499
  viremia from, 469
Herpes simplex, 479
Herpes zoster, 506–507
Herpes zoster ophthalmicus, 507
Herpes zoster sine eruptione, 507
Heterochromatin, definition of, 90
Heterogeneity, definition of, 91
Heterokaryon, definition of, 91
Heterozygote(s), definition of, 91
  detection of, 43, 45
Hexosamine, 420
Hexose, 420
  transport of, and malabsorption, 757
Hexose monophosphate shunt, 600, *601*
Hexuronic acid, 420
Hiatal hernia, 706–707
High altitude, alveolar hypoventilation of, 549
  and arterial P_{O_2}, 392
  chronic acclimatization to, clinical features of, 547–548
  defective oxygen transport of, 549
  polycythemia of, 546–548
Hippuran, in kidney excretion test, 354
His-Purkinje fibers, rapid impulse formation in, 330, *331*
  transmembrane potentials of, 329, *330*
Histalog, 714
Histamine, 114
  in joint inflammation, 430
Histiocytosis, and interstitial pneumonia, 499
Histoplasma capsulatum, and interstitial pneumonia, 499
Histoplasmosis, 410
Histotoxic anoxia, 390
Hodgkin's disease, splenectomy in, 685
  stages of, *630*
  survival in after radiation, *629*
Hodgkin's lymphoma, 628–629
  Lukes-Butler classification, 630(t)
Homeostasis, 97, 119
Homocystinuria, 85
Homogentisic acid, accumulation of, 79, *79*
Homozygote, definition of, 91
Hormone(s), adrenocorticotropic, 872
  analysis of, competitive protein-binding assay in, 870
    radioimmunoassay in, 870
  anterior pituitary, parameters of, 874(t)
  antidiuretic, 348, 349, 352, 877
  calorigenic effects of, 841–842
  categories of, 866
  chemical nature, elaboration, secretion, and transport of, 866–867

Hormone(s) (*Continued*)
  cyclic AMP-mediated, action of, *868*
  definition and basic characterization of, 866
  follicle-stimulating, 872
  growth, 866, 872, 875
  interaction of, with cytoplasmic receptor protein and nuclear acceptors, 868–869
  intestinal, physiologic effects of, 760(t)
  lactogenic, 872
  luteinizing, 872
  mechanisms of action of, 867–869
  melanocyte-stimulating, 872
  parathyroid, 866, 891
  secretion of, in small intestine, 760–761
  secretory activity of, feedback control in, 866
  thyroid, transport of, 880
  thyrotropin-releasing, 871, 872
  thyroid-stimulating, 872
Hormone deficiency, in osteoporosis, 896
Horner's syndrome, in carcinoma of esophagus, 701
Host response, to infection, 473–488
  circulatory changes as, 478
  eosinophilia as, 484
  fever as, 473
  general, 473–484
  headache as, 477
  hematologic changes as, 479–484
  hypotension and shock as, 477–478
  immune, alterations due to, 484–486
  lymphocytosis as, 484
  reversible alterations of sensorium as, 478
  special, 484–487
  unusual, to viral disease, 486–487
Host-tumor relationships, 141–144
Howard test, in renal artery occlusion, 366
Howell-Jolly bodies, 555, 670
Hunger and appetite, 710–711
Hyaline membrane disease, 401
Hyaluronic acid, 420
Hydatidiform mole, DIC in, 652
Hydrochloric acid, and pain of peptic ulcer, 717
  hypersecretion of, 717
  secretion of, 712
  stimulation of by histamine, *551*
Hydrophobic interactions, in protein structure, 34
Hydrostatic pressure, effect on pulmonary blood flow, 173
Hyperbilirubinemia, 796
Hypercalcemia, in primary hyperparathyroidism, 893
Hyperdiploidy, definition of, 91
Hyperferremia, and salmonella bacteremia, 494
Hypergammaglobulinemia, 623–624
Hyperglycemia, 10
Hyperinsulinemia, 845
Hyperkalemia, in acute renal failure, 368
  in chronic renal failure, 368
Hyperlipidemia, 902–903
Hyperlipoproteinemia, classification of, 852(t)
Hyperosmolar nonketotic coma, and ketoacidosis, hormonal and metabolic differences, 903(t)

Hyperoxaluria, 82
Hyperoxia, 923–924
Hyperparathyroidism, primary, 893–894
Hyperpericardium, 268
Hyperplasia, adrenal congenital, 888–889
  nodular lymphoid, 762
Hyperplastic cholecystoses, 824–825
Hypersensitivity pneumonitis, 400
Hypersensitivity reactions, delayed, 119
Hypersplenism, 681–685
  indications for splenectomy in, 684
  mechanism of hemolysis in, 682–683
  mechanism of leukopenia in, 683–684
  mechanism of thrombocytopenia in, 683–684
  principal features of, 682
Hypersthenic oliguria, 363
Hypertension, 190–199
  arterial, etiology of, 191
  definition of, 190
  diastolic, 190
  diuretic therapy of, 353
  essential, *195*, 196–199, 365–366, 890. See also *Essential hypertension*.
    extracellular fluid and blood volume in, 198
    hemodynamic factors in, 196
    neurogenic factors in, 198
    renal pressor system in, 199
  etiologic classification of, 191(t)
  in coarctation of the aorta, 194
  in mineralocorticoid excess, 196, *197*
  in pheochromocytoma, 195, 898
  in primary aldosteronism, 195–196
  in renal parenchymal disease, 193–194, *195*
  lymphatic, 758
  malignant, and heart failure, 279
  orthostatic, *200, 201, 202*
  pathophysiological aspects of, 191–192
  postcausal, 192
  potassium deficit in, 352
  reflex adaptation in, 187, 192
  renal, 192–194, *193*, 366–370. See also *Renal hypertension*.
  renal excretory function and, 357
  renal pressor system in, 189
  renoprival, 358
  renovascular, 192–193, *194*, 357
  secondary, 192–196
  systolic, 190, 191(t)
Hyperthyroidism, apathetic, 883
  diarrhea associated with, 776
  Graves' disease and, 882
  masked, 883
Hypertrophic arthritis, 426
Hypertrophic gastritis, 719
Hypertrophy, in cardiac failure, 282
  of left ventricle, and chronic left ventricular dilatation, 249
    electrocardiogram and, 255
    in chronic heart disease, 247
    in ischemic heart disease, 254
    in mitral stenosis, 257
  of pylorus, 709
  of right ventricle, in mitral stenosis, 258
  ventricular, 245, 279
    and chronic ventricular chamber volume and work load, 252

INDEX

Hyperviscosity syndrome, 632
Hypoalbuminemia, 758
Hypocalcemia, in acute pancreatitis, 833
  in hypoparathyroidism, 892
  in malabsorption syndromes, 752
Hypochloridemia, in infectious disease, 487
Hypochromic microcytic anemia, copper deficiency and, 860
Hypodiploidy, definition of, 91
Hypogammaglobulinemia, 622-623, 752, 758
Hypoglycemia, 812, 903-904
  principal causes of, 903(t)
Hypogonadism, 877
  hypogonadotropic, 908
  hyposmia in, 908
  in female. See *Turner's syndrome.*
  in male. See *Klinefelter's syndrome.*
  Klinefelter's syndrome and, 906
  zinc deficiency and, 860
Hypokalemia, in hypertension, and primary aldosteronism, 889
  severe, from villous adenoma, 786
Hyponatremia, in chronic infections, 487
  in infectious disease, 487
Hypoparathyroidism, 892
Hypophosphaturia, in pseudohypoparathyroidism, 893
Hypopituitarism, monotropic, 877
Hypoproteinemia, 363
Hyposmia, 877
  in hypogonadism, 908
Hyposthenic oliguria, 363
Hyposthenuria, 362
Hypotension, 199-205
  as host response to infection, 477-478
  chronic, 200
  endotoxin induced, 467
  in aortic stenosis, 260
  in cerebrovascular disease, 204-205
  in shock, 200
  orthostatic, idiopathic, 204, 204(t)
  postural, 200, *200, 201*
    in fasting, 848
  pathophysiology of, 201-204, 203(t)
Hypothalamic, pituitary, and adrenal cortical relations, *887*
Hypothalamus, 870-871
  injury to, and obesity, 842
  neuroendocrine disorders in, 871
  physiology of, 870-871
  pituitary, ovaries, interactions of, 909-910
Hypothyroidism, and hyperthyroidism, contrasting features of, 882(t)
  juvenile, 882
  primary adult, 881
Hypovolemic shock, in acute pancreatitis, 832
Hypoxanthine-guanine-phosphoribosyl-transferase deficiency, 83-84
Hypoxia, 922-923
  alveolar, and vasoconstriction, 172
  effect of on local blood flow, 151
  in lobar pneumonia, 498

Idiopathic cardiomyopathy, 265-266
Idiopathic hypoparathyroidism, 892

Idiopathic thrombocytopenic purpura, 642
  antiplatelet antibody in, 677, 677(t)
  chronic, platelet destruction in, 676
  clinical manifestations of, 643
  splenectomy in, 680, 684
Idiosyncratic hepatitis, 813
Idioventricular tachycardia, 342, *342*
IgA, 99, 101, *102*
IgA deficiency, 129, *130*
IgD, 102, *102*
IgE, 102, *102*
IgG, 99, 101, *102*
IgG antibody, 596, *597*
IgG immunoglobulin, 595
IgM, 99-101, *102*
Ileocolitis, 781
Ileum. See also *Small intestine.*
  removal of, malabsorption after, 756
Ileus, 741-744
  consequences of, 743
  in pneumonia, 498
  postoperative, 742
Immobilization, and osteoporosis, 896
Immune complex diseases, 485
Immune mechanisms, and joint inflammation, 430
Immune response, 615
  cell-mediated, *617*
  effector mechanisms of, 113-122
  humoral, *617*
  induction of, 102-104, *103*
Immune system, cells of, 104-106, *105, 106*
  functions of, 97
Immunity, 691-693
  cell-mediated, biological amplification of, 119-122, *121*
  types of, 97-98
Immunobiology, 97-123
  tumor, 138-145
    clinical applications of, 144
Immunocytes, 613-633
  classification of disorders of, 621(t)
  function of, 615-620
  immunoproliferative disorders of, 625-633
  in RES, 666(t)
  memory of, 615
  qualitative disorders of, 624-625
  structure of, 613-615
  subclassification of, 614
Immunodeficiency diseases, 124-138
  autosomal recessive combined, *130,* 134, *134*
  malignant conditions in, 142(t)
  primary, 129-135
    cellular defect in, 129(t), *130*
    lymph node histology in, 129, *131*
  secondary, 136-138
  treatment of, 135
Immunodeficiency syndromes, 108
Immunoenhancement, 143
Immunogens, 98-99
  tumor, 143
Immunogenicity, 98-99
Immunoglobulins, 99-102
  biological properties of, 100-102, 101(t)
  classes of, 618
    comparison of, 618(t)
  kinetics of, 620-621
  pathophysiology of, 621-633

INDEX

Immunoglobulins (*Continued*)
  7S, assembly of in higher molecular weight immunoglobulins, *619*
    structure of, *619*
  structure of, 99, *100, 102*
Immunoglobulin metabolism, disorders of, 135–136
Immunologic memory, 109–112
Immunoproliferative diseases, 137
Immunosuppression, 112–113
Immunosurveillance, 141–144
Immunotherapy, nature of, 451
Impact, 943–945
  and deceleration, data on, *944*
Impulse formation and conduction, combined disturbances of, 338–339
Indicator dilution method, for determining left ventricular chamber volume, 243
Indigestion, and gallstones, 823–824
  in carcinoma of stomach, 731
Indigo carmine dye, in kidney excretion test, 354
Indocyanine green test, 795
Inert gases, role of, 924
Infancy, physiologic agammaglobulinemia of, 623
Infants, hyaline membrane disease in, 401
Infantilism, pituitary, 875
Infarction, in small intestine, 763–764
    nonocclusive, 764
  mesenteric, 808
Infection(s), bradycardia in, 478
  chronic, anemia in, 480–481
  disseminated, skin reactions in, 478–479
  fungus, of lung, 410–411
  host responses to, 473–488
  in acute granulocytic leukemia, 611
  intracranial, 500
  localization in specific organs, 489–510
  metabolic alterations in, 487
  metastatic, secondary to meningococcemia, 502–503
  overt, mechanism of fever production in, 476
  pulmonary, 405
  Salmonella, 493–495
  systemic, headache as indicator of, 477
  viral, thrombocytopenia after, 642
Infectious disease, localized in specific organs, 489–510
Infectious mononucleosis, aad lymphocytosis, 623
  headache in, 477
  splenic rupture in, 680, 681, *681*
Infective endocarditis, consequences of in multiple organ systems, 490–493
Infertility, male, Klinefelter's syndrome and, 906
Inflammation, immunologically mediated, 434–440
  of gallbladder, 824
  of joints, 428
    pathogenesis of, 430
  of pancreas, 828–836
  of tendon sheaths, 441
Inflammatory bowel disease, 778–785
Influenza, and interstitial pneumonia, 499
  headache in, 477
Infrared radiation, effects of on eye, 929–930

Inheritance, autosomal dominant, 42–43, *42, 43*
  autosomal recessive, 43–45, *44*
  biochemical basis for, 70–75
  mendelian, 41–47
  X-linked, 45–47, *46, 47*
Inherited disorders, applications to management of, 88–89, 88(t)
  defective membrane transport and, 76
  deficiencies of end product and, 82
  deficient or abnormal circulating proteins and, 84
  enzymes regulating drug metabolism and, 86
  loss of feedback inhibition and, 82
  mutant gene products and, 75
  precursor accumulation and, 79
  products of minor pathways and, 81
  reduced coenzyme binding or production and, 85
Inhibitors, competitive, 36, 37(t)
Insulin, 866
  action of, 899–900
  and adipose tissue, 899
  and liver, 900
  and muscle, 899
  biosynthesis and release of, 898–899
  effect of, on glucose metabolism, 10
    on lipid metabolism, 18
    on protein metabolism, 23
  in carbohydrate and fat storage, 845
  in liver, 799
  overdosage of, and hypoglycemia, 903
  radioimmunoassay in measurement of, 870
  relation of to body weight, *845*
Insulin deficiency, and ketoacidosis, 901–902
  in diabetes mellitus, 900
Intercalated disc, 210
Interferon, action of, 32
Interstitial emphysema, 399–400
Interstitial fluid pressure, dynamics of, 165–170
  effect of on lymph flow, 164
  regulation of, 167
Interstitial fluid protein, regulation of, 166–167
Interstitial fluid spaces, in blood volume regulation, 171
Interstitial fluid volume, regulation of, 167
  regulation of, vs. blood volume regulation, 170
Interstitial pneumonia, 499–500
Interventricular septum, rupture of, in myocardial infarction, 256
Intestinal absorption, of glucose, 8
Intestinal angina, 763
Intestinal ischemia, 763
Intestinal motility, 740
Intestinal mucosa, absorption of iron at, *563*
Intestinal transport mechanisms of, amino acid, 750(t)
Intestinal villi, 735–737
Intestine, large. See *Bowel, Colon, Large intestine.*
  membrane transport defects in, 76–79, 77(t), *78*

Intestine (*Continued*)
  small. See *Duodenum, Ileum, Jejunum,* and *Small intestine.*
Intoxication, chemical, biological determinants of, 964–966
  lead, 968
  vitamin D, 856
Intra-atrial block, 333, *334*
Intracardiac pressures, normal values of, 238(t)
Intracardiac pressure recordings, in cardiac catheterization, 239–241
Intracardiac shunts, cardiac catheterization in, 241
Intracellular digestion, 691
Intracranial hemorrhage, in acute lymphatic leukemia, 626
Intrapleural pressure, 372
Intrathoracic pressure, 372
Intrinsic clotting system, activation of, 481, *482*
Intrinsic factor, 648
  antibodies to, 557, *557*
  in absorption of vitamin B_{12}, 550
  lack of, in vitamin B_{12} deficiency, 556
  stimulation of secretion of by histamine, *551*
Intussusception, and obstruction of small intestine, 742
Inversions, of chromosomes, 67
Iodine, 861–863
  deficiency of, 862
    mechanisms in uptake in, 863
  intake of in U.S., *862*
  metabolism of, 879–880
    pathways of, *873*
  oxidation and organification of, 879
  storage and release of, 879–880
  uptake of, 879
Ion exchange, 350–352
  potassium in, 351
Ion transport, 350
Ionizing radiation, 932–941
  alpha particles in, 932
  beta particles in, 932–933
  biological bases of, 933
  cell biology of, 933
  nature of, 932
  neutrons in, 933
  physical aspects of, 932–933
IPP, 372
Iritis, in secondary syphilis, 495
Iron, absorption of, changes in, 563, *564*
  dose augmentation in, 563, *563*
  importance of gastric juices in, 564, *564*
  regulation of at intestinal mucosa, 563
  binding capacity of, changes in, in various disorders, 567
  changes in requirement during pregnancy, 568
  excess of, 568–569
    general effects of, 568
    pathogenesis of, 568–569
  in hemoglobin synthesis, 562–569
  metabolic pathways of, *566*
  normal metabolism of, 562–565
  serum, changes in, in various disorders, 567
  transport of, transferrin in, 565

Iron deficiency, blood loss and, 567
  general effects of, 566–567
  in anemia of chronic disorders, 542, *542*
  pathogenesis of, 567–568
Irritable colon syndrome, 777–778
Ischemia, in small intestine, 763–764
  long-term vascular effects of, 151
  of extremities, 175
Ischemic heart disease, 253–256
  angiographic assessment in, 256
  atherosclerosis and, 253
  mitral regurgitation in, 255
  reduced contraction of left ventricle in, 253
  ventricular performance in, 254–255
Ischemic response, CNS, 159, *160*
Islet cell adenoma, of pancreas, 836
Islet cell carcinoma, of pancreas, 836
Islets of Langerhans, 827, 898
Isochromosome, definition of, 91
Isochromosome X, 61, *62*
Isometric contraction, 221
Isoniazid, and inherited disease, 87
Isoproterenol, 897
  effect of on cardiac contractility, *224, 225*
Isosthenuria, pitressin resistant, 351
Isotonic contraction, 222
Isotope dilution, in measurement of body composition, 840

Janeway's lesions, 493
Jaundice, 811
  and cholestasis, 801
  classification of, in first year of life, 796, 796(t)
    in older children and adults, 797
  in carcinoma of pancreas, 836
  in cholecystitis, 824
  in pancreatitis, 832
  in scarlet fever, 471
Jejunal ulcer, 722, 728
  pain in, 727
Jejunum. See also *Small intestine.*
  human, biopsy of, *735, 736*
  proximal, distention in obstruction of, 741
  removal of, malabsorption after, 756
  tumors of, 744
Joint(s), abnormalities of, progression of, *426*
  as functional units, 425
  capsule of, 422
  Charcot's, 427
  degenerative changes in, 425–427
  diarthrodial, *421*
  effects of trauma on, 427–428
  inflammation of, 428
    pathogenesis of, 430
  lubrication of, 425
  mycotic infections of, 431
  neuropathic disease of, 427
  normal, characteristics of synovial fluid in, 424(t)
  pain in, 422
  structure and function of, 421–425
Joint disease, alterations in joint fluid produced by, 428–429

Joint disease (*Continued*)
　in rheumatoid arthritis, 429, *429*
　pathologic changes in, 425–429
Joint fluid, alterations in, from disease, 428–429
Juvenile hypothyroidism, 882
Juxtaglomerular apparatus, 188–189, 346

Kallikrein, 481, 828
Kallman's syndrome, 877
Karyolysis, in pancreatitis, 828
Karyotype, definition of, 91
　in Down's syndrome, *53*
　normal male, *52, 53*
　shorthand for, 54
Kaschin-Beck disease, 426
Keratosulfate, 420
Kernicterus, 794
Ketoacidosis, 901–902
　and hyperosmolar nonketotic coma, hormonal and metabolic differences, 903(t)
　diabetic, in pancreatitis, 832
　pathogenesis of, *902*
Ketone body formation, 12–13, 24
Kidney(s). See also *Renal.*
　blood flow of, 345–346
　　regulation in, 151
　blood volume of, 345
　calcitonin in, 891
　conservation of calcium in, 891
　disease of, clinical manifestations of, 358–365
　effect of arterial pressure on, 159
　endocrine functions of, 357–358
　excretion rate tests in, 354–355
　excretory functions of, 345–354
　　hemolysis in, 539
　formation of erythropoietin in, 358
　ion exchange in, 350–352
　in hyperglycemia, 10
　membrane transport defects in, 76–79, 77(t), *78*
　proximal tubule of, 347–348
　tests of excretory functions of, 354–357
Kidney stones, in hyperparathyroidism, 893
Kinetics, cellular, in immune response, 108–109
　in biological processes, 27
　of disease development, 39
Kinetic environment, 942–947
Kinetocardiography, to record chest wall function, 306
Kinetochore. See *Centromere.*
Kinins, in acute gouty arthritis, 432
Kinin peptides, in joint inflammation, 430
Kininogen system, in joint inflammation, 430
Klebsiella pneumoniae, 497
Klinefelter's syndrome, 63–64, 906–908
Knees, synovitis of, in congenital syphilis, 497
Koch phenomenon, 410
Krebs cycle, 3, 5, 7–8, *9*
Krypton, 925
Kupffer cells, 665, 792
　increase of in liver, 689

Kuru, 486
Kwashiorkor, 847(t), 849
　and pancreatitis, 831

Lactase, deficiency of, and malabsorption, 757
Lactate, production of, 5, *6*
Lactogenic hormone, 872
Lamina fenestra, 346
Langerhans, islets of, 827, 898–899
Laparotomy, in cholestasis, 804
Laplace relation, 220
Large intestine, 767–789. See also *Colon.*
　Crohn's disease in, 783–785
　disorders of motor and absorptive functions of, 776–788
　disorders of secretory function in, 785–786
　drugs and, 775
　electrical activity in, 769
　gas in, 775–776
　microflora of, 788
　motility mechanisms in, 770–771
　normal absorption and secretion in, 773–776
　normal motor function of, 769–773
　nutrients and metabolic products in, 774–775
　transit in, 771–772
　tumors of, 786–788
Lasers, 931
Law of Marfan, 409
Lead, contamination of environment by, 968
　ecologic flow chart for, *967*
Lead intoxication, 968
Lecithins, 15
Lecithinase, 458
Left bundle branch block, QRS waveform in, 328, *328*
Left heart failure, symptoms and signs of, 289(t)
Left-to-right shunt(s), conditions occurring in, 241
　in congenital heart disease, 280
Left ventricle, aneurysms of, 256
　contraction abnormalities of, 254
　determining volume and mass of, 243–244
　diastolic pressure pulses in, *287*
　diastolic work of, determining, 246–250
　dilatation of, and mitral regurgitation, 255
　distensibility of, chronic disease and, 246
　ejection characteristics of, 274–275
　failure of, 289
　function of, in ischemic heart disease, 253
　hypertrophy of, and chronic left ventricular dilatation, 249
　in mitral stenosis, pressure in, *244*
　rate of filling and rejection in, *247*
　reduced contraction in, in ischemic heart disease, 253
　relation between performance and filling pressure, *277*
　systolic work of, determining, 246–250
　time plot of pressure and volume curves in, *248*

Left ventricle (*Continued*)
　values in, in mitral valve insufficiency, 245, 246, *246*
　　normal, 245(t)
　volume curve in, *245*
Left ventricular end-diastolic pressure, 222–229
Left ventricular pump, function of, 244–252
Legg-Perthes disease, 427
Leiomyoma, 701, 729
Leprosy, amyloidosis in, 485
Lesions, Janeway's, 493
　mechanical, and ventricular contraction, 281
　of herpes zoster, 507
　of skin and mucous membranes, in late syphilis, 496
　renal, 549–550
　　in bacterial endocarditis, 493
Lethal synthesis, 964
Leukemia(s), acute, granulocytic, 609–613
　　lymphatic, 626–628
　　lymphocytic, 609
　　promyelocytic, DIC in, 652
　chronic, drugs used in, 608(t)
　　granulocytic, 606–608
　　　genetics of, 67–69, *68*, *70*
　　lymphatic, 625–626
　in polycythemia, 538
　radiation, 941
　splenic rupture in, 680
　splenomegaly in, 679
Leukocidin, 430
Leukocytes, in gouty arthritis, 431
Leukocyte factors, and arthritis, 431
Leukocytosis, in bacterial endocarditis, 492
　in cholecystitis, 824
　in ulcerative colitis, 782
Leukoencephalopathy, progressive multifocal, 486
Leukopenia, and hypersplenism, 682
　in typhoid fever, 480
　role of spleen in, 678
Light chains, designations of, 99–100
Lignac-Debré-de Toni-Fanconi tubular defects, 367
Linkage, definition of, 91
Lipids, 849–852
　metabolism of, 10–18, *11*, *12*, *13*, *14*, *15*, *17*, *19*, *20*, *26*, 850
　　hormonal effects on, 18
Lipidoses, 693
Lipoid pneumonia, 408
Lipolysis, 747
Lipomas, of pleura, 411
Lipoproteins, electrophoretic pattern for, *851*
　transport of, 851
　　function of, 35
β-Lipoprotein deficiency, congenital, 84
Liver. See also entries under *Hepat-*.
　acute cell failure in, 811–812
　ammonia and purine metabolism in, 792
　anatomic considerations and information techniques, 790–792
　appraisal of status of, 790(t)
　arteriograms of, 791
　bile formation, bile flow, and cholestasis in, 799–804

Liver (*Continued*)
　bilirubin metabolism in, 793
　biochemistry of, 792–799
　biopsy of, 809
　blood flow through, 804–805, 804(t)
　carbohydrate metabolism in, 799
　cells of, tests of insufficient functioning of, 810
　cirrhosis of, 813–814
　coagulation abnormalities in, 797
　disease of, approach to problem of, 810–812
　　cardiovascular effects of, 814
　　coagulation difficulties in, 815
　　effect of on other organs, 815–816
　　endocrine changes in, 815
　　hemorrhage in, 797
　　renal changes in, 814–815
　enlarged, in carcinoma of pancreas, 836
　fluid retention in, 812
　focal disease of, and syndromes of, 810–811
　functions of, 793–794
　　conjugation, 793–794
　　secretion, 794
　　uptake, 793
　function tests of, 809–810
　generalized disease of, and typical syndromes, 811–812, 811(t)
　glycogen storage in, 3, 8
　histology of, 791–792
　impaired gluconeogenesis in, 812
　lymph flow in, 808
　normal and pathologic physiology of, 790–817
　peritoneoscopy of, 791
　portal pressure and blood flow, and liver collateral flow, 804(t)
　proteins made predominantly by, 797(t)
　regeneration of, 792
　representative diseases of, 813–814
　scans of, 791(t)
　size and shape of, 790
　synthesis of bile acids by, 775
　tests of cellular damage in, 809(t)
　tests of cellular necrosis in, 809–810
　tests of inflammation in, 810
　tests of special etiology in, 810
　vascular impairment of, 813
Liver biopsy, in cholestasis, 804
Liver cells, compounds actively excreted by, 800(t)
　schematic model of, *791*
Liver encephalopathy, 812
Lobar pneumonia, 497–499
Localized tetanus, 464
Locus, definition of, 91
Loeffler's syndrome, 400
Loop of Henle, 348–350
Lowe's syndrome, 757
LSD, and chromosome breakage, 69, 70
Lung(s), acid-base disturbances of, 390
　air flow in, dynamic mechanics of, 375–377
　circulation in, 172–174
　compliance of, 373, 374
　diffusion of gases in, 383–385
　eosinophilic infiltration, 400

Lung(s) (Continued)
  exposure of to gases, 957
  functional residual capacity of, 372
  protective mechanisms of, 393–414
  relation of to chest wall and diaphragm, 372
  residual volume of, 373
  tidal volumes of, 372, 373
  tissue-gas surface tension of, 375
  total capacity of, 373, 374
  tumor of, 404–405
Lung abscess, 406
  in pneumococcal pneumonia, 498
  tumor of lung and, 404
Lung surfactant, function of, 35
Lung volumes, 371–375
  spirometric tracing of, 373
Lupus erythematosus, systemic, 439–440
Luteinizing hormone, 872
Lyell's disease, 471
  flow of, determinants of, 164
  in liver, 808
  transport of, abnormalities of, 757–758
Lymph node, 616
Lymphadenopathy, of spleen, 678
Lymphangiectasia, 752
  intestinal, primary, 758
  lymphatic transport disorders and, 758
Lymphatic drainage, from tissues, 163–164
  in edema, 169
Lymphatic hypertension, 758
Lymphatic leukemia, acute, 626–628
    chemotherapy in, 626–628
      labeling of blast cells in, 627
      survival in, between 1956 and 1971, 628
    chronic, 625–626
Lymphoblastic lymphosarcoma, 631
Lymphocytes, 105, 106, 106
  B and T, 124–129
  bone marrow, 615
  bursa equivalent, 615
  classification and general considerations, 621
  disorders of, classification of, 621(t)
    quantitative, 622
  electron microscope picture of, 614
  immunoproliferative disorders of, 625–633
  in RES, 666(t)
  in target cell destruction, 120, 121
  kinetics of, 620–621
  pathophysiology of, 621–623
  qualitative disorders of, 624–625
  structure of, 613
  thymus-derived, 615
Lymphocytic anemia, acute, 609
Lymphocytic lymphosarcoma, 631
Lymphocytopenia, 622–623, 758
  in Hodgkin's lymphoma, 628
Lymphocytosis, 623–624
  as host response, 484
Lymphoid cells, 105, 106, 106
Lymphoid organs, primary, 106–108
  secondary, 108
Lymphoid system, 124–129, 125
  developmental defects in, and immuno-deficiency diseases, 124
Lymphoma, antiplatelet antibody in, 677, 677(t)

Lymphoma (Continued)
  gastrointestinal, 758
  giant follicular, 630–631
  histological classification of, 629
  malignant, Hodgkin's type, 628–629
    other than Hodgkin's, 629–631
  non-Hodgkin's, splenectomy in, 685
Lymphopoiesis, diagram of, 621
Lymphoreticular system, 104–109
Lymphosarcoma, 630
Lymphotoxin, 120
Lyon hypothesis, 59–60
Lyonization, 45
Lyon-Meltzer test of gallbladder function, 820
Lysosomes, 36
  in joint inflammation, 430

M component, disorders of, 631–633
Macroglobulinemia, of Waldenström, 632
Macromolecules, complex aggregates of, 35–36
  informational, 27
  structure of, 28, 29
Macrophage(s), 104, 104
  as attachment site for basophils and eosinophils, 600, 601
  cell division in, 686, 686
  origin and kinetics of, 685–691
  tissue, in RES, 666(t)
Macrospherocyte, 586
Magnesium, 856
  changes in, in fasting, 848
  deficiency of, 857
Magnetism, 925
Malabsorption, after gastric resection, 753
  after removal of jejunum, 756
  and folate deficiency, 558–559
  and vitamin deficiency, 858
  disorders associated with, 754(t)
  following intestinal resection, 756
  glucose-galactose, 77, 78
  normal pattern of, 753
Malabsorption syndromes, 745, 751–752
Malaise, in bacterial meningitis, 500
Malaria, and salmonella bacteremia, 494
  DIC in, 652
  quartan, immune complexes in, 485
  recurrent, splenic rupture in, 680
  splenic rupture in, 681
  widespread involvement of organs in, 469
Malathion, 962
Malignant hypertension, and heart failure, 279
Malignant lymphoma, Hodgkin's type, 628–629
  other than Hodgkin's, 629–631
Malnutrition, and pancreatitis, 831
  and vitamin deficiency, 857
  comparison of forms of, 847(t)
  obstruction of small intestine and, 742
Man, normal thermal environment for, 930
Manometer, catheter tip, in intracardiac pressure recording, 239
Manometry, esophageal, 704
Maple syrup disease, 24, 80–81, 81

Marasmus, 847(t), 849
  and pancreatitis, 831
  subcutaneous fat in, 849
March hemoglobinuria, 593
Marfan, Law of, 409
Marfan's syndrome, 261
Mast cell disease, 752
McArdle's disease, 7
Measles, skin lesions in, 479
  demyelinating encephalitis following, 486
Mechanical circulatory assist, 292–293
Mechanical counterpulsation, 293
Meckel's diverticulum, 726
Mediterranean anemia, 590, *591*
Mega-esophagus, 704
Megakaryoblast, 633
Megakaryocyte, 633
Megakaryocytic hyperplasia in, idiopathic thrombocytopenic purpura, *643*
Megaloblastic anemia(s), general effects of, 555–556
  miscellaneous, 560
  vitamin B_{12} deficiency in, 555
Meiosis, 53
  definition of, 91
  nondisjunction in, *63*, 64
Melanocyte-stimulating hormone, 872
Membranes, functions of, 35
  microvillous plasma, 736, *737*
Membrane transport, defective, and inherited disorders, 76–79, 77(t), *78*
Memory, immunologic, negative, 111–112
  positive, 109–111
Mendelian inheritance, 41–47
Menetrier's disease, 719
Meninges, irritation in, 500
Meningitis, bacterial, 500–504
  Haemophilus influenzae, 503
  in pneumococcal pneumonia, 499
  in secondary syphilis, 495
  meningococcal, 502–503
  pneumococcal, 503
  serous, 504
  of scarlet fever, 471
  tuberculous, 503–504
Meningococcal meningitis, 502–503
Meningococcemia, 502
  adrenal insufficiency of, 886
  disseminated intravascular coagulation in, 481
Meningococcus, and arthritis, 431
Meningovascular syphilis, 496
Menstrual cycle, 908–909
Menstruation, 908–909
Mercury, contamination of environment by, 966–967
Meromyosin, 207
Mesenteric artery, main stem occlusion of, 764
Mesenteric infarction, 808
Messenger RNA, 32
Messenger, secondary, 37
Metabolic bone disease, 891–892
Metabolism, alterations in, in infection, 487
  biochemistry of, 3–26
  hormone, in hepatic disease, 815
  inborn errors of, 40–89

Metabolism (*Continued*)
  iodine, 879–880
  myocardial, 212–215, *212, 213*
  of bile salts, 800–801
  of bilirubin, tests of, 795–796, 795(t)
  of carbohydrates, 3–10, *4, 6, 9, 19, 20, 26*
  of immunoglobulins, disorders of, 135–136
  of lipids, 10–18, *11, 12, 13, 14, 15, 17, 19, 20, 26*
  of proteins, 18–26, *22, 25, 26*
  tissue, increased, effect on local blood flow, 151
  tryptophan, outline of, 744
Metacentric chromosome, definition of, 51, 91
Metals, in environment, 966–968
Metastatic infections, in bacterial endocarditis, 492
Methemoglobinemia, 571–572
Methionine malabsorption, 77(t)
Methotrexate, and interstitial pneumonia, 499
Methylmalonic aciduria, 85
Micellular solution, relative concentrations of cholesterol, lecithin, and bile salts in, 822
Microangiopathic hemolytic anemia, 594
Microflora, of large intestine, 788
Microorganism, host response to, 473
  invading, pathogenic properties of, 457–472
Micropinocytosis, 689
Microspherocyte, 586, *587*
Middle-lobe syndrome, 404
Mid-systolic click, 301
Migration-inhibition factor, 121
Miliary tuberculosis, 810
  and aplastic anemia, 537
Mineralocorticoids, excess of, and hypertension, 196, *197*
  in colon, 774
Minute ventilation, 388
Mitochondria, 36
  biochemical functions of, 969
  in myocardium, 211
Mitogenic, definition of, 91
Mitosis, 53
  definition of, 91
  inhibition of, 30
Mitral annulus, dilatation of, and mitral regurgitation, 255, 258
Mitral insufficiency, left ventricular values in, 245, *246*
Mitral regurgitation, 258–259
  after myocardial infarction, 256
  angiographic studies in, 258
  combined with mitral stenosis, 259
  in ischemic heart disease, 255
  left ventricular pressure-volume curves in, *249*
  mechanism of, *255*
  severe, movement tracings of, *310*
Mitral stenosis, 257–258
  combined with mitral regurgitation, 259
  ECG and left ventricular pressure in, *244*
  left ventricular pressure-volume curves in, *249*

Mitral stenosis (*Continued*)
  pressure readings in left atrium and left ventricle in, 239, *240*
  surgical considerations in, 258
Mitral valve, infection involving, 491
  left atrial volume in disease of, 259(t)
Mitral valve disease, combined with aortic disease, 263–264
Mole, hydatidiform, DIC in, 652
Molecular biology, 27–39
  in disease, 38
Monge's disease, 548
Monoclonal components, in serum protein, *624*
Monocyte(s), 104
  in RES, 666(t)
  origin and kinetics of, 685–691
  transformation to macrophage, 686, *687, 688*
Monocyte-macrophages, 599–612
  function of, 599–612
  kinetics and regulation of, 603
  life span of, 603
  pathophysiology of, 604–613
  structure of, 599
Mononucleosis, headache in, 477
  infectious, and lymphocytosis, 623
Monosomy, 55
  definition of, 91
Monozygotic, definition of, 91
Mosaic, definition of, 91
Mosaic karyotype, 54
Motility, intestinal, 740
Mucin clot test, 424
Mucopolysaccharides, composition of carbohydrate component of, 420(t)
Mucormycosis, 410
Mucosa, of colon, 767
  normal, *768*
  of esophagus, 697
    disorders of, 701–704
  of small intestine, 734
Mucosal crypts, of small intestine, 735
Mucous membranes, chemical absorption in, 959–960
  lesions of, in late syphilis, 496
  of colon, 767
Multifactorial genetic disorders, 47–50, *48, 49*(t), *50*
Murmur, heart, 301
  changing, in subacute endocarditis, 491
Muscle, cardiac. See *Myocardium*.
  glycogen storage in, 3, 8
  intestinal smooth, conduction in, 738, *738*
Muscle tone, in tetanus, 463
Muscularis externa, of colon, 767
  of small intestine, 734, 735
Mutant, definition of, 91
Mutation, definition of, 91
  in DNA, 71
Myalgia, in bacterial meningitis, 500
Mycobacterium tuberculosis, 410, 503
  host response to, 473
Mycoplasmal pneumonia, headache in, 477
Mycoplasma pneumoniae, and interstitial pneumonia, 499
  cold agglutinins, in pneumonia of, 485

Mycotic aneurysms, in bacterial endocarditis, 493
Mycotic infections, of joints, 431
Myeloblasts, mitotic division of, 515, *516*
Myelofibrosis, 608–609
  splenectomy in, 685
Myeloma, multiple, 137
  plasma cell, 632
Myocardial abscess, 491
Myocardial cell, 207, *208*
Myocardial contractility, 251
Myocardial failure, in amyloidosis, 485
Myocardial function, in aortic stenosis, 260–261
Myocardial infarction, chest pain after, arteriography in, 253
  electrocardiogram in, 325–327
  in bacterial endocarditis, 492
  interventricular septal defect in, 256
  mitral regurgitation after, 256
  rupture of interventricular septum in, 256
  transmural, systolic bulge in, 310
  ventricular performance after, 254
Myocardial oxygen consumption, 277–278, *277*
  heart size and, *278*
  tension-time index in, 277
Myocardial performance, 251–252
Myocarditis, in diphtheria, 459
Myocardium, aerobic metabolism and, 282
  contractile state of, 251
  contractility of, 219–220, *219*
    evaluation of, 221–229
  failing, factors related to, 282(t)
  forces within, computing of, 251–252
  function of, 217–229
  growth of, in chronic heart disease, 249
  in coronary heart disease, changes in, *286*
  length-tension curve of, 218–219, *218, 219*
  metabolism of, 212–215, *212, 213*
    cyclic AMP in, 214
    energetics in, 212–214, *212, 213*
    norepinephrine in, 215
    protein synthesis in, 214
  ultrastructure of, 207–212, *208, 209, 210, 211*
Myofibrils, 207, *208*
Myofilaments, 207, *208*
Myosin, 739
  myocardial, 207, *208*, 215, *216*
Myxedema, 881
Myxoma, left atrial, 257

Naphthylamines, structure of, *953*
Narcosis, nitrogen, 924
Nasopharynx, 393
Nausea, 711
  in carcinoma of stomach, 732
Neck, stiff, in bacterial meningitis, 500
Necrolysis, toxic epidermal, 471
Necrosis, in pancreatitis, 828
Neisseria gonorrhoeae, endotoxin of, 466
Neisseria meningitides, endotoxin of, 466
Nelson's syndrome, tumors of, 873

Neo-iopax, in kidney excretion tests, 355
Neomycin, and malabsorption, 756
Neon, 924
Neoplasia, in immunodeficiency diseases, 142
Neoplastic disease, and salmonella bacteremia, 494
  and gastroenteritis, 494
Nephritis, acute, edema in, 363
  in diphtheria, 459
  interstitial, in secondary syphilis, 495
Nephrocalcinosis, in primary hyperparathyroidism, 893
Nephrosclerosis, in essential hypertension, 366
Nephrotic syndrome, 138, 363-365
  in amyloidosis, 485
  in secondary syphilis, 495
  sequential changes in, *365*
  treatment of, 365
Nerves, articular, 422
Nervous system, autonomic, controlling influence on cardiac output, 237
  complications of, in diphtheria, 459
  in blood volume regulation, 170
  in cardiac output regulation, 152
  response of to ischemia, 159, *160*
Neural circulatory reflexes, 185-187, *186, 187*
Neural reflexes, in hypertension, 187, 192
Neuropathic joint disease, 427
Neurotoxins, 462-464
Neutrons, in ionizing radiation, 933
Neutropenia, in pneumococcal pneumonia, 480
  splenic, splenectomy in, 684
Neutrophils, circulating, changes in, in infection, 479
Newborn, autoimmune hemolytic disease of, 596
Niacin, 854
Nicotinamide, 854
Nicotinic acid, 854
Niemann-Pick disease, 16
  splenomegaly in, 679
Nitrogen, disposition of, 23
  role of, 924
Nitrogen narcosis, 924
Nocardiosis, 410
Node(s), Heberden's, 426
  lymph, *616*
  Osler's, 493
Noise, 945-946
Nonarticular rheumatism, 441-442
Nondisjunction, 55-56
  meiotic, *63, 64*
Nongranulomatous ulcerative jejunitis, 752
Nonobstructive cardiomyopathies, 265-266
Nonsense mutation, definition of, 91
Nontropical sprue, 752, 755, 758
Nonuniform capillary ventilation/capillary blood flow, 386-388
Norepinephrine, calorigenic effects of, 842
  in myocardial metabolism, 215
  in pheochromocytoma, 898
  mechanism of action of, 896-897
  pathways for disposal of, 897

Nose, as pulmonary protective mechanism, 395
Nuclear pyknosis, in pancreatitis, 828
Nucleic acids, 28-32, *29, 31*
  drug interactions with, 28, 30(t), 31
Nucleotide bases, 28
Nutrition, of tissues, in edema, 169

O_2, blood, 379-383
  in arterial and mixed venous blood, 382(t)
Obesity, 839-846
  adrenocortical steroids and, 846
  and gallstones, 821
  criteria for, 839
  endocrine consequences of, 845-846
  growth hormone and, 846
  hypothalamic, 842
  metabolic factors in, 843
Obstruction, in peptic ulcer, 727
  in small intestine, 741-744
    consequences of, 743
Obstructive cardiomyopathy, 265
Obstructive pulmonary emphysema, 398-400
Ochronosis, 426
Occlusion, of renal arteries, in renal hypertension, 366
  of superior mesenteric vein, 764
Occlusive coronary artery disease, 286
Oddi, sphincter of, 819
  in pancreatitis, 830
Oligemia, 204(t)
Oliguria, 362, 815
  hypersthenic, 363
  hyposthenic, 363
Open-heart surgery, DIC in, 652
Operon, definition of, 91
Operon model for protein biosynthesis, 72, *73*
Opsonins, 689
Optic atrophy, in late syphilis, 496
Optic perineuritis, in secondary syphilis, 495
Oral cystography, 820
Organelles, cell, 35-36
Organized sediment, in urine, 360
Ornithine cycle, 23, *25*
Ornithosis, 499
Orotic aciduria, 83
Oroya fever, and salmonella bacteremia, 494
Orthostatic hypertension, *200, 201,* 202
Orthostatic hypotension, idiopathic, 204, 204(t)
Osler's nodes, 493
Osmolality, urine, measurement of, 357
  tests of, 357
Osmotic diuretics, 352
Osteitis fibrosa cystica, 891, 892(t)
Osteoarthritis, 426
  secondary, 427
Osteochondritis, in congenital syphilis, 496
Osteodystrophy, renal, 894-895
  biochemical findings in, 895(t)
Osteomalacia, 892, 892(t)
  in vitamin D deficiency, 858

INDEX

Osteomyelitis, 507–510
  associated with vascular insufficiency, 509
  chronic, amyloidosis in, 485
  hematogenous, 507
  in different age groups, 508
  secondary to contiguous focus of infection, 509
Osteoporosis, 891, 892(t), 895–896
Osteosarcoma, radiation, 941
Ovarian dysgenesis, 60–63, *61, 62, 63*
Ovarian follicle, development of, 908–909
Ovaries, 908–912
  clinical entities in, 910–912
  physiology of, 908–910
Ovulation, 908–909
Oxidation, of glucose, 3, 4–8
  process of, 962–963
Oxidative phosphorylation, in myocardial metabolism, 212–213, *213*
Oxygen, absence of, 922
  affinity of, in anemia, 530
  atmospheric, 922
    decreases in, 922–923
    increases in, 923–924
  blood, 518–520
  consumption of, myocardial, 277–278, *277*
  effect on local blood flow, 151
  erythrocyte as transporter of, 584
  peripheral tissue requirement, and cardiac output, 237–238
  pressures of, at various altitudes, *546, 547*
  tensions of, at sea level, 923
  tissue, erythrocyte production and, 525
  tissue perfusion of, in anemia, 531, *531*
Oxygen consumption, myocardial, 212, *212*
Oxygen toxicity, and arterial P_{O_2}, 392

P_{CO_2}, arterial, causes of abnormalities of, 391–392
  factors altering, 391(t)
  definition of alveolar ventilation by, 387–388
P_{O_2}, arterial, causes of abnormalities of, 391–392
Pacemaker, downward displacement of, 332, *332*
  ectopic, 339
Pacesetter potential, smooth muscle, 738, *738*
Pacing, right atrial, abnormal contraction pattern after, 254
PAH, 347, 348, 354, 355, 356
Pain, abdominal, transmission of, 718–719
  cramping lower abdominal, in ulcerative colitis, 782
  in acute pancreatitis, 832
  in biliary colic, 823
  in carcinoma of pancreas, 836
  in carcinoma of stomach, 732
  in cholecystitis, 824
  in gastric carcinoma, 718
  in gastroesophageal reflux, 707
  in hyperplastic cholecystosis, 825
  in joint, 422
  in liver syndromes, 811
  in obstruction of small intestine, 742

Pain (*Continued*)
  in osteoarthritis, 427
  in peptic ulcer, 726
  in pneumonia, 407
  in small intestine, 741
  in stomach, mechanism of, 717–719
  local, constipation and, 785
  low back, in osteoporosis, 896
  periumbilical, in intestinal ischemia, 763
    in main stem occlusion of mesenteric artery, 764
  pleuritic, in pneumonia, 498
  ulcer, location of, 718
Pancreas, 898–904
  biosynthesis and release of insulin in, 898–899
  carcinoma of, 836
  clinical entities in, 900–904
  cystadenocarcinoma of, 836
  cystic fibrosis of, 836–837
  endocrine insufficiency of, 834
  exocrine insufficiency of, 833
  functions of, 827, 898
  inflammation of, 828–836
  normal anatomy and physiology of, 827–828
  pathophysiology of, 827–838
  physiology of, 898–900
  toxic effects of alcohol on, 830
Pancreatic calcinosis, 831
Pancreatic enzymes, function of, 828
Pancreatic exocrine insufficiency, 753
Pancreatic insufficiency, in cystic fibrosis, 837
Pancreatic neoplasm, loss of appetite in, 711
Pancreaticojejunostomy, 836
Pancreatitis, 828–836
  alcoholic, 830–831
  causative factors in, 829(t)
  common channel theory of, 829
  diagnostic aspects in, 834–835
  duodenal reflux theory of, 830
  edematous, 828
  hereditary, 831
  mechanisms of clinical manifestations of, 832–834
  obstruction-hypersecretion theory of, 830
  pathogenesis of, 831–832
  postoperative, 831
  therapeutic considerations in, 835–836
Pancytopenia, 532
Panencephalitis, subacute sclerosing, 486
Paneth cells, 736
Panhypopituitarism, 876–877
Pannus formation, in synovitis, 428
Pantothenic acid, 854–855
Papillary muscle, dysfunction of, and mitral regurgitation, 255
  rupture of, and mitral regurgitation, 255
Para-aminohippuric acid, 347, 348, 354, 355, 356
Paralysis, from herpes zoster, 507
Paraplegia, in late syphilis, 496
Parasystole, ventricular, 339, *340*
Parathyroid adenoma, and pancreatitis, 831
Parathyroid hormone, 866
  in bone remodeling, 891
  sites of action of, 891(t)

Parathyroids, 890–896
  physiology of, 890–891
Paratyphoid fever, 494
Parinaud's syndrome, 507
Paroxysmal nocturnal hemoglobinuria, 587–589
Pasteurella pestis, exotoxin of, 458(t)
Pastia's lines, in scarlet fever, 470
Patent ductus arteriosus, continuous heart murmur of, *306*
Peak power, and myocardial performance in chronic heart disease, 253, *253*
Pedigree analysis, 40, 42, 45, 47
Pellagra, in niacin deficiency, 854
Pentose phosphate pathway, 3, 8
Peptic ulcer, 722–729
  endocrine relationships and, 724–726
  hunger in, 710
  in hyperparathyroidism, 894
  pain of, 717, 724
  pathogenesis of, 722–724
  surgical procedures for, 728
  symptoms of, 726–728
  tissue resistance in, 723
Perforation, in duodenal ulcer, 728
Periarteritis nodosa, 441
Pericardial disease, 266–269
Pericardial effusion, 267–268
Pericardial friction rub, 306, *307*
Pericardial tamponade, 267
  treatment of, 268
Pericarditis, 267
  constrictive, 268–269, 758
  in pneumococcal pneumonia, 499
Pericardium, disease of, 266
  pain in, 267
Perineuritis, optic, in secondary syphilis, 495
Periostitis, in congenital syphilis, 496
  in secondary syphilis, 495
Peripheral blood circulation, control of, 284–285
Peripheral resistance, total, and arterial pressure, 150, 181
  and cardiac output, 150, 183, *184*
Peristalsis, 698–699, 712
  in bowel, 771
Peritoneal dialysis, in acute renal failure, 368
Peritoneoscopy, of liver, 791
Peritonitis, 728
  in pneumococcal pneumonia, 499
Pernicious anemia, 427
Pesticides, enzyme inhibition in, 962
Peyer's patches, 761
Phagocytes, 599–613
  function of, 599–601
  kinetics of, 602
  pathophysiology of, 604–613
  structure of, 599
Phagocytosis, 685, 689
  granulocyte after, *600*
  metabolic requirements of, 691
Phenocopy, definition of, 91
Phenolsulfonphthalein, in kidney excretion test, 354
Phenotype, definition of, 91
Phentolamine, 897

Phenylalanine, 24
  normal metabolic pathway, *79*
Phenylketonuria, 24, 79, 82
Pheochromocytoma, 898
  and hypertension, 195
Philadelphia chromosome, 67–69, *68*
Phlebotomy, in primary polycythemia, 538
Phosphate metabolism, effect of renal failure on, *894*
Phosphenes, 925
Phospholipase A, in pancreatitis, 828
Phospholipids, 849
  metabolism of, 15–16
Physical agents, effects of, 917–948
  toxic, 915–948
Piloerection, 930
Pinocytosis, 689, 690
Pitressin-resistant isosthenuria, 351
Pituitary, posterior, physiology of, 877–879
  tumors of, 873–874
Pituitary hormones, anterior, effect of on lipid metabolism, 18
Pituitary infantilism, 875
  vs. Turner's syndrome, differential diagnosis, 911(t)
Pituitrin, 356
Plasma, effect of on selenomethionine-75, *639*
Plasmablasts, 614
Plasma cell(s), 106, *106*, 614
  electron microscope picture of, *615*
  in RES, 666(t)
Plasma cell myeloma, 632
Plasma coagulation factors, 646–658
Plasma colloid osmotic pressure, 167, 169
Plasmacytes, 614
  in joint inflammation, 430
Plasma kallikrein, 481
Plasma kallikrein system, activation of, 481–484
Plasma renin activity, 188–189
  in renovascular hypertension, 193
Plasma volume, in essential hypertension, 198–199
Plasmin, 647
  degradation of fibrinogen by, 649
Plasminogen, local activation of, *651*
Plasmodium falciparum, 469
Plasmodium malariae, 469
Plasmodium vivax, 469
Platelets. See *Blood platelets.*
Pleiotropy, definition of, 91
Pleura, description of, 411
  inflammation of, 412
  tumors of, 411–412
Pleural disease, 393–414
Pleural disorders, 411–413
Pleuritis, 412
Pleurodynia, epidemic, 413
Plummer-Vinson syndrome, 701, 702
Pneumococcal meningitis, 503
Pneumococcal pneumonia, 407
  complications of, 498–499
  neutropenia in, 480
Pneumococcus, and arthritis, 431
Pneumoconiosis(es), 402–403
  and interstitial pneumonia, 499

Pneumocystis carinii, and interstitial pneumonia, 499
Pneumocystis pneumonia, in immunodeficiency disease, 126, *127*
Pneumonia, 407–408
 and atelectasis, 404
 aspiration, 408
 clinical manifestations of, 497–498
 desquamative interstitial, 499
 interstitial, 499–500
 lipoid, 408
 lobar, 497–499
 lymphocytic interstitial, 499
 mycoplasmal, headache in, 477
 pneumococcal, 407
  complications of, 498–499
 varicella, 499
Pneumonia alba, in congenital syphilis, 496
Pneumonitis, hypersensitivity, 400
Pneumothorax, 413
Poietins, proposed actions of, 515, *515*
Point mutation, definition of, 91
Poliomyelitis, 504–506
Polyarteritis nodosa, 440, 441
 eosinophilia in, 484
Polychromasia, 585
Polycythemia(s), cerebellar hemangiomas and, 550
 classification of, 529–530, 530(t)
 definition of, 529–530
 differential diagnosis of, 538(t)
 disorders implicated in, 550
 general effects of, 531–532
 of high altitude, 546–548
 primary, 537–538
 secondary, inappropriate, 549–550, 549(t)
Polycythemia vera, 546–550
 red cell aplasia in, *545*
Polyendocrine adenomatosis, 725
Polymorphism, protein, 76
 definition of, 91
Polymyositis, 440, 441
Polyp(s), adenomatous, 729
 tumor of, 786
Polypeptide, definition of, 91
Polyploidy, 55, *56*
 definition of, 91
Polyposis, gastrointestinal, 758
Polyribosome, polypeptide synthesis on, *460*
Polyuria, differential diagnosis of, 878(t)
Pompe's disease, 7
Porphyria, acute intermittent, 83
Porphyrins, disorders in synthesis of, 560–562
 acquired and inherited, 562
 general effects of, 561–562
 normal synthesis of, 560–561
Portacaval shunts, 808–809
Portal hypertension, consequences of, 805–808
 obstructions of portal vein causing, *806*
 sequelae of, 807(t)
Portal systemic shunts, surgically constructed, *808*
Portal vein, flow of through liver, 804
 pressure elevation in, causes of, 806(t)
 pressure in, 805–809

Posterior pituitary, clinical entities in, 878–879
 physiology of, 877–879
Postoperative ileus, 742
Postprimary adult tuberculosis, 409, 410
Postural hypotension, in fasting, 848
Posture, upright, arterial pressure in, 201
Potassium, in colon, 774
 plasma, and aldosterone secretion, 884
Potassium deficit, in aldosteronism, 351
 in Cushing's syndrome, 351
 in hypertension, 352
 in ion exchange, 351
Potassium intoxication, in acute renal failure, 368
Potential difference, boundary of, 317, *317, 318*
Potentials, conduction, in smooth muscle, 738, *738*
Power, ventricular, 247
Precolonic cholera, 776–777
Precordial movements, 306–310
Precursor accumulation, and inherited disorders, 79–81, *79, 81*
Prednisone, in red cell aplasia, *545*
Preglomerular proteinuria, 358–359
Pregnancy, 908–909
 and osteoporosis, 896
 anemia in, 543–544
 changes in iron requirement during, *568*
Preload, 217–219, *218, 219*
 in mechanical function of heart, 290
Pressor-antipressor function, in renal endocrine functions, 357–358
 barometric. See *Barometric pressure.*
Pressure-velocity relation, in left ventricle systole, 226–227, *226*
Primary aldosteronism, 889–890
 scheme for evaluation of, 890
Primary arrhythmias, 282
Primary fibrositis, 442
Primary syphilis, 495
P-R interval, 296
Proaccelerin, 481
Proband, definition of, 91
Proerythroblasts, 517
 mitotic division of, 515, *516*
 multiplication and maturation of, 522–524
 renewal of, 520, *521*
Progesterone, biosynthesis, transport, mechanisms of action, and disposal of, 910
Proinsulin, 34
Prolactin, 872
Properdin, 118
Proplasmablasts, 614
Propositus, definition of, 91
Propranolol, 335
 in angina pectoris, 292
Prostaglandins, function of, 35
Prostatic surgery, DIC in, 652
Protein(s), absorption of, *746*, 748–750
 Bence Jones, 358
 concentration of, regulation of, 38
 contractile, 207, 215
  of myocardium, 207–210, *210*
 deficiency of, 846–849
  in kwashiorkor, 849

Protein(s) (Continued)
  deficient or abnormal circulating, and inherited diseases, 84–85
  function of, 32–35
  function of regulation of, 36–38, 37(t)
  interstitial fluid, regulation of, 166–167
  made predominantly by liver, 797(t)
  metabolism of, 18–26, *22, 25, 26*
    hormonal effects on, 21
    synthesis, 20, *22*
    nonprotein moieties in, 35
  percentage of in human body weight, 840, *840*
  polymorphism, definition of, 91
  serum, electrophoretic separation of, *624*
  turnover rate of, 21
Protein biosynthesis, mammalian vs. microbial, 73
  operon model for, 72, *73*
Protein depletion, and wounds, 421
Proteinosis, pulmonary alveolar, 400
Protein polymorphism, 76
Protein structure, effect of environment on, 34
  toxic effects on, 34
Protein synthesis, 32, *33*
  myocardial, 214
  rough endoplasmic reticulum in, 796
Proteinuria(s), 348, 358–360
  Bence Jones, 358
  cast formation in, 360
  clinical considerations in, 359–360
  glomerular, 359
  mechanisms of, *349*
  preglomerular, 358–359
  tubular, 359
Proteolysis, 34
Protoplasmic toxins, 458
Proximal tubule, ion-exchange in, 350–352
  secretory systems of, 348
Pruritus, bile salts and, 800
  in chronic renal failure, 369
Pseudogout, 433–434
Pseudohermaphroditism, female, 888
Pseudohyperparathyroidism, 893
Pseudohypoparathyroidism, 893
Pseudolymphoma, 729
Pseudomonas aeruginosa bacteremia, 469
Pseudopseudohypoparathyroidism, 893
Pseudotumors, inflammatory, 729
Psittacosis, 499
Psychosis, acute, in pancreatitis, 833
  in carcinoma of pancreas, 836
Pteroylpolyglutamates, 552
  absorption of, *553*
Pterygium colli, 910
Pulmonary alveolar proteinosis, 400
Pulmonary artery, total resistance of, calculation of, 238
Pulmonary circulation, 172–174, 385–386
  control of, 385–386
Pulmonary disease, 393–414
  cough in, 378–379
  high altitude, 548, *548*
Pulmonary edema, 384
  in poliomyelitis, 506
Pulmonary embolism, 401–402
Pulmonary fibrosis, 403
Pulmonary infections, 405
Pulmonary neoplasms, clubbing of fingers and toes in, 411
Pulmonary tuberculosis, primary, 408
Pulmonary valve insufficiency, 304
Pulmonary venous congestion, 289–290
Pulmonary ventilation and blood gas exchange, 371–392
Pulse, peripheral, diminished, 174
Pulse pressure, factors determining, 182
Pulse wave velocity, 178
Pulsion diverticula, 700
Pulsus alternans, 174, 180
Pulsus paradoxicus, 267
Purines, 28
  metabolism of in liver, 792
Purpura, allergic, 658
  Henoch-Schönlein, 658
  senile, 658
Purpura fulminans, DIC in, 652
P wave, 319, 320, *321*
Pyelonephritis, in essential hypertension, 366
  in renal hypertension, 366
Pyknosis, nuclear, in pancreatitis, 828
Pyloric obstruction, in peptic ulcer, 727
Pylorus, hypertrophic stenosis of, 709
Pyridoxine, 854
Pyrimidines, 28
Pyrogen, endogenous, 475–477
Pyruvate, production of, 5–7, *6*
Pyruvate kinase deficiency, 589–590
Pyruvic acid, levels of, thiamin and, 853

Q fever, 499
QRS complex, 320, 321
  alterations of, 325–327, *325*
  mechanism of alteration of, *325*
  waveform of, in left bundle branch block, 328, *328*
    in right bundle branch block, 327, *328*
    intraventricular conduction disorders and, 327–328
Quadriparesis, in bacterial meningitis, 500
Quaternary structure, of protein, 34
Quartan malaria, immune complexes in, 485
Quinacrine mustard, in chromosome differentiation, 51

Radiation, and aplastic anemia, 536
  average blood element values in people exposed to, *934*
  bone marrow destruction from, 536
  by beta and electron beams, 940
  delayed effects of, 941–942
  effect of, on cells, 28, 32
    on chromosomes, 69
    on immune response, 112
  infrared, 927–930
    effects of on eye, 929–930
  ionizing, 932–941
  local, delayed effects of, 941
  microwave, 927
  thermal, 927–930

INDEX

Radiation (Continued)
  ultraviolet, 931–932
  visible, 930–931
  whole body, late effects in, 941
Radiation carcinogenesis, 941–942
Radiation enteritis, 752
Radiation injury, clinical manifestations of, 934–940
  five injury groups in, 935
  Group II exposure in, *936*
  Group III exposure in, *937*
  Group IV exposure in, *938*
  Group V exposure in, *939*
  latent stage of, 935
  manifest illness and recovery in, 935
  physiological basis of, 933–934
  prodromal stage of, 935
  therapeutic principles of, 940
Radiation pneumonitis, and interstitial pneumonia, 499
Radio frequencies, 927
Radioimmunoassay, in endocrinology, 870
Radioisotope renogram, 355
Radionuclides, internal deposition of, 940–941
Raspberry tongue, in scarlet fever, 470
Raynaud's disease, 175
Reaction(s), anaphylactic, 452–453
  DIC in, 652
  Schwartzman, endotoxin induced, 467
  skin, in disseminated infection, 478–479
  tissue, antigen-IgB antibody, 449
    immunologically induced, 447–450
Reagin-mediated asthma, 453
Reagin-mediated diseases, 452
Recessive, definition of, 91
Reciprocal rhythm, 337
Recombination, definition of, 91
Rectal ampulla, 772
Rectosigmoid junction, 772
Rectum, 772
Red cell(s). See also *Erythrocyte(s)*.
  changes in membrane, 674
  defect in, genetic error and, 34
  destruction of, 683
    in splenic sequestration, 673–674
  differentiation of, 524
  general signs of hemolysis in, 577–582
  Heinz body breaking from, *675*
  in urine, 361
  maturation of, 524
  membrane function and energy metabolism in, 582–584
  membrane of, cholesterol exchange and, 582, *583*
    gas transport across, 583
  survival disorders of, 577–599
Red hepatization, in lobar pneumonia, 497
Red thrombus, 646
Reduction, process of, 963
Reflux, gastroesophageal, 707–708
  prevention of, 705–708
Reflux esophagitis, 702
Refractory period, relation to nonconducted premature systoles, 332, *334*
Regulation of protein concentration, 38
Regulation of protein function, 36–38
Regurgitation, aortic, 261–263

Regurgitation (Continued)
  in gastroesophageal reflux, 707
  mitral, 258–259
Renal. See also entries under *Kidney(s)*.
Renal arteries, occlusion of, in renal hypertension, 366
Renal blood flow, 345–346
Renal-body fluid pressure control (or regulating) mechanism, infinite gain in, 161
Renal-body fluid pressure regulating mechanism, 159, *160*
Renal clearance, tests of, 355–356
Renal disease, 345–370
  chronic, hemorrhage in, 540
  clinical manifestations of, 358–365
  functional patterns in, 365–370
  in stem cell disorders, 539, *539*
Renal disorders, and inappropriate secondary polycythemia, 549–550
Renal endocrine function, 357–358
Renal excretory functions, 345–354
  hypertension and, 357
Renal failure, 367–370
  acute, 368
  chronic, 368–370
    purpura in, 645
  effect of on calcium and phosphate metabolism and on bone, *894*
  in acute pancreatitis, 833
  red cell life span in, 539, *540*
  treatment of, 368–370
Renal function, approximate average values in, 354(t)
  concentration dilution tests of, 356–357
Renal glycosuria, 367
Renal hypertension, 192–194, *193*, 366–370
  pyelonephritis in, 366
  renal arterial occlusion in, 366
Renal lesions, and inappropriate secondary polycythemia, 549–550
  in bacterial endocarditis, 493
Renal osteodystrophy, 894–895
  biochemical findings in, 895(t)
Renal parenchymal disease, and hypertension, 193–194, *195*
Renal physiology, in congestive heart failure, 284
Renal pressor mechanisms, 187–190, *188*
Renal pressor system, in essential hypertension, 199
  in renovascular hypertension, 193
Renal scintiscan, 355
Renal tubular acidosis, 367, 815
Renaturation, protein, 34
Renin, 357
  source of, 188
Renin-angiotensin system, 187–190, *188*, 884
Renin-angiotensin-vasoconstrictor mechanism, *160*
Renogram, radioisotope, 355
Renoprival mechanism, in hypertension, 192, *193*
Repair synthesis, 32
Replication, DNA, 30
  definition of, 91
RES, 665–694

Residual volume of lungs, 373
  methods of measuring, 374
Respiration, abnormalities of, 389-391
  control of, 388-392
Respiratory bronchioles, 394
Respiratory distress syndrome, DIC in, 652
Retained dead fetus, DIC in, 652
Reticulin, 419
Reticulocyte count, feedback control systems in, 524, *525*
Reticuloendothelial cell(s), 523, *523*, 666(t)
Reticuloendothelial system, 665-694
  distribution and function of cells in, 666(t)
  function of, 665-666
  pathologic disorders of, 692-693
Reticulum cell sarcoma, 630, 631
Retina, burns of, 931
Reversible obstructive airway disease, 453, 454(t)-455(t)
Rheumatic diseases, 417-444
Rheumatic endocarditis, 256
Rheumatic fever, 256, 435
Rheumatism, nonarticular, 441-442
Rheumatoid arthritis, 435-439
  antiplatelet antibody in, 677, 677(t)
  complement activation in, 436-437, *437*
  extra-articular inflammatory lesions in, 438, *439*
  inflammation in, 428
  joint disease in, 429, *429*
Rheumatoid factor, 435
Rheumatoid nodule, in rheumatoid arthritis, 438, *439*
Rheumatoid synovitis, 437
Rheumatology, allergy, infectious disease, and hematology, 415-694
Rhythm, reciprocal, 337
Rhythmic segmentation, 740, *740*
Riboflavin, 853-854
Ribonuclease, effects of zinc on, 860
Ribonucleic acid. See *RNA*.
Ribosomes, 35
  polypeptide elongation on, *461*
Rickets, familial hypophosphatemic, 77(t), 79
  vitamin D in, 856
Rickettsia, and interstitial pneumonia, 499
Rickettsial diseases, headache in, 477
Right bundle branch block, QRS waveform in, 327, *328*
Right heart failure, in pneumoconiosis, 403
  symptoms and signs of, 289(t)
Right-to-left shunt, 242
Right ventricle, failure of, 289
Ring, chromosome, definition of, 91
RNA, 28-32, *29*, *31*
  effects of drugs on, 30(t)
  in myocardium, 214
  in protein synthesis, 20-21, *22*
  messenger, 72, *72*
    control of synthesis of, *73*
  ribosomal, 72
  synthesis of, 32
  transfer, 72
  vs. DNA, 28
ROAD, 453, 454(t)-455(t)
Rocky Mountain spotted fever, disseminated intravascular coagulation in, 481, 652

Rokitansky-Aschoff sinuses, 818, 824
Roth's spots, 493
Rubella, demyelinating encephalitis following, 486
  DIC in, 652

S-A block, 333, *334*
S-A nodal and His-Purkinje fibers, transmembrane potentials, 329, *330*
Saddle nose, in congenital syphilis, 497
Salmonella, and enteric fever, 494
  endotoxin of, 466
Salmonella bacteremia, 494-495
Salmonella gastroenteritis, 493-494
Salmonella infections, 493-495
Salmonella typhosa, in typhoid fever, continuing endotoxemia from, 476
Salmonellosis, 493-495
Saluresis, 353
Sarcoidosis, and interstitial pneumonia, 499
Sarcolemma membrane, *208*, 210, *211*
Sarcoma, reticulum cell, 630, 631
Sarcomere, 207, *208*, *209*
Sarcomere lengths, during preload, *218*
Sarcoplasmic reticulum, 211, *211*
  in contractile process, 215
Sarcotubule system, 210, *211*
Satellite, definition of, 91
Scans, liver, use of, 791(t)
Scarlet fever, 470
  serous meningitis of, 471
Schatzki ring, 702
Schilling test, of vitamin B_{12} absorption, 752
Schwartzman reaction, endotoxin induced, 467
Scintiscan, renal, 355
Scintiscanning, liver, 790
Scleroderma, 440, 752
  esophageal involvement, 700
Sclerosis, systemic, 700
  progressive, 440
Scoliosis, in empyema, 412
Second heart sound (S2), 297
  paradoxical splitting of, *300*
Secondary cardiomyopathies, 266
Secondary constriction, definition of, 91
Secondary messenger, 37
Secondary osteoarthritis, 427
Secondary structure of protein, 34
Secondary syphilis, 495
  immune complexes in, 485
Secretin, 760
Secretion, gastric, 712-717
  liver, 794
Segregation, definition of, 91
Seizures, in bacterial meningitis, 500
Self assembly, 27, 35
Sella turcica, 872
Seminiferous tubule, dysgenesis of, 906
Senile purpura, 658
Sensitization, atopic, nature of, 446-447
Sensorium, reversible alterations to, as host response to infection, 478
Sensory constipation, 785
Septicemia, bacterial, DIC in, 652
  Clostridium welchii, 592

INDEX

Serotonin, 657, 744
  in joint inflammation, 430
  metabolic pathway of, *744*
Serous meningitis, 504
  of scarlet fever, 471
Serratia, 457
Serum cholinesterase deficiency, 86, *87*
Serum sickness, 434–435
Sex, human, determination of, 905
Sex chromatin, 59, *60*
  definition of, 92
Sex chromosomal aneuploidy, 59–65
Sex chromosomes, definition of, 92
Sheehan's syndrome, 876–877
Shield chest, 910
Shigella, 760
  exotoxin of, 458(t)
Shivering, to maintain body heat balance, 474
Shock, as host response to infection, 477–478
  circulatory filling pressure in, 154
  endotoxin induced, 467
  hypotension in, 200
  hypovolemic, in acute pancreatitis, 832
  with high or normal cardiac output, 477
  with reduced cardiac output, 477–478
Shunt(s), intracardiac, cardiac catheterization in, 241
  left-to-right, in cardiac catheterization in, 241–242
    in congenital heart disease, 280
  portacaval, 808–809
  portal systemic, surgically constructed, *808*
  pentose, 3, 8
Sickle cell anemia, 534, 574
  and salmonella bacteremia, 494
  genetics of, 73–75
  splenomegaly in, 680
Sickle cell trait, 574
Sickle hemoglobin, 40, 73–75
  genetic error and, 34
Sickling, 573
Sideroblast, 569
Sideroblastic anemias, 569
Silicosis, 403
Single breath N_2 test, for distribution of inspired gas, 386
Single ventricle, cyanosis in, 242
Sinuses, Rokitansky-Aschoff, 818, 824
  of Valsalva, mycotic aneurysm of, 491
Skeletal system, trauma to, in late syphilis, 496
Skin, lesions of, in late syphilis, 496
  eruptions of, in serum sickness, 435
Skin reactions, in disseminated infection, 478–479
Small intestine, 734–766. See also *Duodenum, Ileum, Jejunum.*
  abnormal structure and function of, 762
  abnormalities of lymphatic transport in, 757–758
  abnormalities of mucosal transport in, 755–757
  basic electric rhythm of, 769
  digestive-absorptive function of, 745–759
  digestive-absorptive unit of, 736

Small intestine (*Continued*)
  immunologic function of, 761–762
  intraluminal abnormalities of, 752–755
  ischemia and infarction in, 763–764
  motor dysfunction due to humoral mechanisms in, 744–745
  motor function of, 738–745
    abnormal, 741
    normal, 738–741
  normal digestion and absorption in, 746
  normal structure of, 734–738
  normal structure and function of, 761–762
  normal vascular physiology of, 762–763
  obstruction and ileus in, 741–744
  pain in, 741
  protein-losing gastroenteropathies in, 758–759
  relative sterility of, 754
  secretion of hormones and enzymes in, 760–761
  secretory function of, 759–761
  vascular disorders of, 762–764
  water and electrolyte secretion in, 759–760
Smooth muscle, of colon, electrical properties of, 769
Snake bite, DIC in, 652
Sodium conservation, by acidofication, 351(t)
Somatic, definition of, 92
Somatotropin, 872
Spasm, esophageal, 700–701
  of cricopharyngeal sphincter, 699
  of entire stomach, 712
  painless, of pylorus, 712
Spastic constipation, 785
Specific gravity, urine, measurement of, 357
Spherocytosis, aplastic crisis following, *545*
  hereditary, 77(t), 79, 585, 681
  splenectomy in, 684
Sphincter(s), anal, 773
  cricopharyngeal, 697
  lower esophageal, hypertensive, 704–705
  of Oddi, 819
    in pancreatitis, 830
Sphingomyelins, 16
Sphygmomanometer, use of, 178, 180
Spike potential, smooth muscle, 738, *738, 739*
Spinal cord, degeneration of, 427, 555, *555*
Spinal ganglia, in herpes zoster, 507
Spirometer, in measurement of airway obstruction, 377, *377*
Splanchnic nerves, motor fibers in, 739
Spleen, accessory, 680
  as sequestrating organism, 674
  circulation of, *668*
  contractural ability of, 678
  enlargement of, 678
  historical perspectives, 666–667
  in primary immunodeficiency disease, 129, *132*
  in thrombocytopenia, 644
  lymphadenopathy of, 678
  normal, structure of, 667–669
  relation of to erythrocytes, 669–674
  relation of to granulocytes, 678
  relation of to platelets, 674–678

Spleen (*Continued*)
  role of in leukopenia, 678
  rupture of, 680–681
  sequestration of blood in, 669–674
    with destruction of erythrocytes, 673–674
    without destruction of erythrocytes, 669–672
  trauma to, splenic rupture in, 681
Spleen and reticuloendothelial system, 665–694
Splenectomy, effect of on peripheral platelet levels, *677*
  hematologic findings after, 672(t)
  in hereditary spherocytosis, 684
  in pyruvate kinase deficiency, 589
  in splenomegaly, 684
  indications for in hypersplenism, 684
Splenic neutropenia, splenectomy in, 684
Splenic sequestration, destruction of erythrocytes in, 673–674
  selective, *673*
Splenomegaly, 678–680
  and hypersplenism, 682
  common causes of, 679(t)
  congestive, splenectomy in, 684
    splenic rupture in, 680
  hemolytic anemia and red cell sequestration in, *682*
  in myelofibrosis, 608
  massive, platelet count in, *676*
  mixing of erythrocytes in, 670
  splenectomy in, 684
Splenosis, 680
Sprue, hypergammaglobulinemia, 762
  nontropical, 755, 758
  tropical, 752
Staphylococcus aureus, exotoxins of, 458(t)
  osteomyelitis and, 509
Staphylococcus aureus bacteremia, 468
Staphylococcus epidermidis, 457
Starvation, 846–849, 847(t)
S-T deflection, ventricular repolarization and, 322–324
Steatorrhea, 754, 758
  in hypogammaglobulinemic sprue, 762
Stem cell(s), 418
  disorders of, 532–550
  unipotential, disorders of, 539–550
Stenosis, aortic and pulmonary, heart murmurs of, 303
  hypertrophic, of pylorus, 709
  left ventricle end-diastolic pressure and volume in, *248*
  valvular, cardiac catheterization and, 239
Steroids, 866
  adrenocortical, and obesity, 846
  androgenic, calorigenic effects of, 842
Steroid biosynthesis, cholesterol in, 885
Sterol metabolism, 16–18, *17*
Stomach, 709–733. See also entries beginning *Gastr-*.
  anatomical variations of, 709
  carcinoma of, 730–732
  congenital anomalies of, 709–710
  diverticula of, 709–710
  mechanism of pain in, 717–719

Stomach (*Continued*)
  motor disturbances of, 712
  pain in, location of, 718
  sensory disturbances of, 710–712
Stomatitis, in chronic renal failure, 369
Strawberry tongue, in scarlet fever, 470
Streptococcus(i), Group A, 457
  exotoxin of, 458(t)
  hemolytic, in rheumatic fever, 435
Streptococcus pyogenes, 457, 458
  exotoxin of, 458(t)
Stress relaxation, 159, *160*
Stretch receptors, in arterial pressure regulation, 185–187
Stricture(s), esophageal, 702–704
  inflammatory, and obstruction of small intestine, 742
Stroke, heat, 928
Stroke work, and myocardial performance in chronic heart disease, 253
ST segment, 320, 321
ST-T abnormalities, transmembrane action potential alterations and, 326, 327, *327*
Stuart factor, 481
Stupor, as host response to infection, 478
Subacromial bursitis, 434
Subdural effusion, sterile, in bacterial meningitis, 501
Submucosa, of colon, 767
  of small intestine, 734, 735
Substrates, "fraudulent," 36
Subtotal gastrectomy, and salmonella gastroenteritis, 494
Sulfate formation, 24
Sulfobromophthalein test, 795
Sulfur, disposition of, 24
Sunburn, 932
Superficial gastritis, 719
Supernormal A-V conduction, 335, *335*
Surgery, open-heart, DIC in, 652
  prostatic, DIC in, 652
Surveillance, 97, 141–144
Swallowing, normal, 698–699
Sweat test, in cystic fibrosis, 837
Swiss type lymphocytic agammaglobulinemia, 622
Sympathectomy, abdominal, and paralytic ileus, 742
Syncope, 200, *201*
  in decompression sickness, 922
Syndrome, alveolar capillary block, 384
  blind loop, 558, 559, 754
  Bloom's, 609
  Chediak-Higashi, 604, 605
  Conn's, 889–890
  Crigler-Najjar, 794
  Cushing's, 658, 871, 887–888, 896
  DiGeorge's, 622
  Di Guglielmo's, 560
  Down's, 609
  dumping, 729
  Ehlers-Danlos, 658
  Fanconi's, 367
  Felty's, 683
  fertile eunuch, 908
  Guillain-Barré, in diphtheria, 459
  Hamman-Rich, 403

Syndrome (*Continued*)
  hemolytic uremic, 539
    DIC in, 652
  Horner's, 701
  irritable colon, 777–778
  Kallman's, 877
  Klinefelter's, 906–908
  Loeffler's, 400
  Lowe's, 757
  malabsorption, 745, 751–752
  Marfan's, 261
  middle-lobe, 404
  Nelson's, 873
  nephrotic, 353–365, 495
    in amyloidosis, 485
  Parinaud's, 507
  Plummer-Vinson, 701, 702
  respiratory distress, DIC in, 652
  Sheehan's, 876–877
  trisomy 13, 58
  trisomy 18, 58, 59
  Turner's, 910–912
  Waring blender, 594
  Waterhouse-Friderichsen, 502, 886
  Wermer's, 725
  Wiskott-Aldrich, 622
  Zollinger-Ellison, 714, 717, 724, 776
Synovial fluid, 423–425
  characteristics of in arthritis, 424(t)
Synovial tissue, 423
Synovitis, 428
  crystal induced, 431–434
  in serum sickness, 435
  in systemic lupus erythematosus, 439
  of knees, in congenital syphilis, 497
  rheumatoid, 437
  tuberculous, 431
Synovium, 423
  acute inflammation of, 428
Synthesis, lethal, 964
Syphilis, 495–497
  congenital, 496–497
  early, 495
  late, 496
  meningovascular, 496
  secondary, immune complexes in, 485
  secondary eruption of, 495
Syringomyelia, 427
Systemic lupus erythematosus, 439–440
  antiplatelet antibody in, 677, 677(t)
Systemic venous congestion, 290
Systole(s), haustral, 770
  myocardial chamber dimensions in, 251
  nonconducted premature, relation of refractory period to, 332, *334*
Systolic heart murmur, 302
Systolic hypertension, 190, 191(t)
Systolic pressure, mean, determination of, 178
Systolic work, of left ventricle, determining, 246–250

Ta wave, 320, *321*
T cells, 108, 109, 124–126
  evaluation of, 126, 128(t)

Tabes dorsalis, in late syphilis, 496
  neuropathic joints and, 427
Tachycardia, abnormal contraction pattern after, 254
  ectopic, 339
  ventricular, slow, 342, *342*
Taenia coli, 767
Tamponade, pericardial, 267
Target cell destruction, 120, *121*
Taurine conjugate, chemical structure of, *822*
Temporary circulatory assist, mechanical, 292–293
Tendinitis, calcareous, with subacromial bursitis, 434
Tendon sheaths, inflammation of, 441
Tenosynovitis, 441
Tension-time index, in myocardial oxygen consumption, 277–278
Tertiary structure of protein, 34
Test(s), liver function, 809–810
  sweat, in cystic fibrosis, 837
Testis(es), 904–908
  adult, biosynthesis, transport, and action of testosterone in, 906
  clinical entities in, 906
  feminizing, syndrome of, 908
  function of, 904
  physiology of, 904–906
  postnatal function of, 905–906
  regulation of function of, 906
Testosterone, biosynthesis, transport, and action of, 906
  effect of on protein metabolism, 21
Tetanus, 458
  cephalic, 463
  localized, 464
Tetanus toxin, 462–464
  site of action of, *463*
Tetrahydrofolic acid, 750
Tetralogy of Fallot, cyanosis in, 242
Tetraploid, definition of, 92
Tetraploidy, 55
Thalassemias, genetics of, 75
Thermodynamics, in biological processes, 27
Thermogenic anhidrosis, 928
Thermoregulation, in febrile disease states, 474
  normal, 474
Thiamin, 853
Third heart sound (S3), 299
Thirst, antidiuretic hormone and, 878
Thoracic empyema, 412–413
Thrill, in heart murmur, 302
Thrombasthenia, Glanzmann's, 645
Thrombin, action of on fibrinogen, 647
Thrombocyte(s), 633–646. See also *Platelets.*
  classification of disorders in, 639–640, 640(t)
  function of, 634–636
  kinetics of, 636–639
  pathophysiology of, 639–646
  qualitative abnormalities of, 645–646
  quantitative abnormalities in, 640–645
  structure of, 633–634
Thrombocythemia, essential, 609

Thrombocytopenia, 640–645
  and hypersplenism, 682
  in aplastic anemia, 534
  in chronic lymphatic leukemia, 625
  possible mechanisms for, *641*
  rebound, after platelet transfusion, *638*
Thrombocytosis, 645
  following splenectomy, in idiopathic thrombocytopenic purpura, *644*
  rebound, after platelet depletion, *638*
Thymic hypoplasia, 130, *130, 131, 134*
Thymidine, tritiated, in chromosome differentiation, 51
Thymine, 28, 71
Thymomas, in red cell aplasia, 544
Thymus, 106–108
  in ataxia-telangiectasia, 134, *135*
Thymus system development, 125
Thyroglobulin, organification in, *873*
Thyroid, clinical entities in, 881–884
  enlargement of, iodine deficiency and, 863
  medullary tumors of, diarrhea associated with, 776
  physiology of, 879–880
  radioactive scans of, 883
  tests of function of, 880–881
Thyroid hormone, deficiency of, 82
  calorigenic effect of, 841
  effect of, on glucose metabolism, 10
    on lipid metabolism, 18
    on protein metabolism, 23
  excess of, 883
  transport of, 880
Thyrotoxicosis, 882–883
  and osteoporosis, 896
  cardiac output and, 238
Thyrotropin, 872
Thyrotropin-releasing hormone, 871, 872
Thyroxine, 866
  cell entry, intracellular metabolism, and fate of, 880
Thyroxine-binding globulin, deficiency of, 84
Tibia, saber-shaped, in congenital syphilis, 497
Tidal volume, 372, *373*
Tissue, hematopoietic, composition of, 517(t)
  morphology of, *516*
  synovial, 423
Tissue colloid osmotic pressure, 169
Tissue fluids, mobility of, 167, *168*
Tissue hypoxia, at high altitude, 547
Tissue nutrition, in edema, 169
Tissue pressure, measurement of, 166
  types of, 165–166
Tissue, reaction, allergin-reagin, 447–448
  antigen-IgB antibody, 449
  Arthus, 449
  cell-mediated, 449
  immunologically induced, 447–450
  types of, 447(t)
Toes, clubbing of, in pulmonary neoplasm, 411
Tolerance, 111–112
  drug-induced, 113
Torsion, gastric, 710
  of spleen, splenic rupture in, 680
Total cardiac replacement, 292

Total lung capacity, 373
Toxemia, DIC in, 652
  eclamptogenic, edema in, 363
Toxic agents, chemical, 949–972
  physical, 915–948
Toxic epidermal necrolysis, 471
Toxicity, chemical, structural and functional consequences of, 969–971
  induction of, by metabolic alteration of chemicals, 962–964
  in fat-soluble vitamins, 855
Toxicology, environmental, 949
Toxin, anthrax, purified, 471
  bacterial, production of, 458–468
  botulinum, 464
  of *Clostridium perfringens*, 460
  production and invasiveness of, as basis of pathogenicity, 469–471
  tetanus, 462–464
Trace elements, 859–863, 859(t)
Trachea, 393–394
Tracheitis, acute, and bronchitis, 405
Tracheo-esophageal fistula, 705
Tract, gastrointestinal. See *Gastrointestinal tract.*
Trans, definition of, 92
Transamination, 23
Transcortin, 885
Transcription, definition of, 92
  genetic, *31, 32, 33*
Transduction, definition of, 92
Transfer factor, 120
Transferrin, in iron transport, 565
Transfusion, blood, antiplatelet antibody in, 677, 677(t)
Transfusion reaction, massive, DIC in, 652
Translation, definition of, 92
  genetic, *31,* 32
Translocation, balanced, definition of, 90
  definition of, 92
  of chromosomes, 66
Transmural colitis, 781
Transposition of great vessels, cyanosis in, 242
Trauma, effects of on joints, 427–428
  massive, DIC in, 652
Traumatic hemolysis, 593
Trench foot, 930
Treponema pallidum, 495
Treponemia, 495
Tricarboxylic acid cycle, 3, 5, 7–8, *9, 12, 14*
Trichinella spiralis, eosinophilia from infection by, 484
Tricuspid atresia, cyanosis in, 242
Triglycerides, 843–845
  breakdown of, 14
  synthesis of, 13–14, *15*
Triiodothyronine, 866
Triploidy, 55, *56*
  definition of, 92
Trisomy, 55
  definition of, 92
Trisomy 13 syndrome, 58
Trisomy 18 syndrome, 58, *59*
Trisomy 21, 57–58, *57*
Tropical sprue, 752
Tropocollagen, 418

INDEX

Tropomyosin, 210, *210*
Troponin, 210, *210*
Truncus arteriosus, cyanosis in, 242
Trypanosomiasis, cold agglutinins in, 485
Trypsin, 828
Trypsinogen, 828
Tryptophan metabolism, outline of, *744*
T system, of myocardium, 210, *211*
Tuberculin, 410
Tuberculosis, 408–410
   amyloidosis in, 485
   and meningitis, 504
   in pneumoconiosis, 403
   miliary, 537, 810
   protective mechanisms, 409
Tuberculous meningitis, 503–504
Tuberculous synovitis, 431
Tubular dysfunctions, 367
Tubular proteinuria, 359
Tubular, proximal of kidney, 347–348
Tubulorrhexis, 363
Tumors, and obstruction of small intestine, 742
   gastric, benign, 729–730
   of colon, 786–788
   of lung, 404
   of pleura, 411–412
   pedicle formation in, 786, *787*
   pituitary, 873–874
   retroperitoneal, 758
Tumor immunity, demonstration of, 140–141, *141*
Tumor immunobiology, 138–145
   clinical applications of, 144
Turner's syndrome, 60–63, *61, 62, 63,* 910–912
   principal clinical features in, 910
   vs. pituitary infantilism, differential diagnosis, 911(t)
Typhoid fever, 494
   headache in, 477
   leukopenia in, 480
Typhus, headache in, 477
Tyrosine, 24
Tyrosinosis, *79*

Ulcer, peptic, 722–729
   hunger in, 710
   perforation of, 718
   Zollinger-Ellison, 724–725
Ulcerative colitis, 758, 781, 782–783
   complications of, 783
   extracolonic manifestations of, 783(t)
   pathologic features of, 782(t)
Ultrasound, 946–947
Ultraviolet light, effect on DNA, 72
Ultraviolet radiation, 931–932
   effect on cells, 28, 32
Unidirectional block, and re-entry, 337–338 *337*, 338
Uracil, 72
Urate crystals, in gout, 431, 433
Urea clearance test, 356
Urea formation, 23, *25*

Uremia, 367–370
   bacterial, coagulation defects in, 481–484
   burr cells, in, 539, *540*
   erythropoietin response in, 540, *541*
   in systemic lupus erythematosus, 439
   vomiting, anorexia and apathy in, 369
Uric acid stones, in fasting, 848
Urine, casts in, 360
   enzymes in, 362
   organized sediment in, 360
   osmolality, measurement of, 357
   protein content of, 358
   red blood cells in, 361
   specific gravity of, 357
      measurement of, 357
      in diabetes insipidus, 878
   white blood cells in, 361–362
Urine concentration, countercurrent concept of, 349–350, *350*
   tests of, 356–357
Urine osmolality, relationship with specific gravity, *357*
Urine urobilinogen test, 796
Urobilinogen, excretion of, 794
Urticaria, cold, 452, 453

Vaccinia, demyelinating encephalitis following, 486
V-A conduction, 335, *335*
Valsalva maneuver, circulatory responses to, 186, *186*
Valvulae conniventes, 735
Valvular, ischemic heart, and pericardial disease, 235–272
Valvular heart disease, 256–259
Valvular incompetence, volume overload and, 281
Varicella, and interstitial pneumonia, 499
   and herpes zoster, 506
   demyelinating encephalitis following, 486
Varicella pneumonia, 499
Vascular bed, resistance of, calculation of, 238
Vascular capacity, effect on filling pressure, 154
Vascular control, principles of, 185
Vascular disease, peripheral, 175
Vascular insufficiency, and pancreatitis, 831
Vasodilatation, in local blood flow regulation, 151
Vasomotor activity, 185
Vasopressin, 356, 866
   secretion of, 877
Vectorcardiogram, and electrocardiogram, *313*
Veins, in blood pressure regulation, 184
Venous congestion, systemic, 290
Venous pressure, central vs. peripheral, 157
   measurement of, 158
   regulation and abnormalities of, 157–158
Venous return, 154, *155*
Ventilation, alveolar, 387–388
   maximal voluntary, 389
   minute, 388, 389

Ventricle(s), contraction patterns of, 275, *275*
  left, end-diastolic pressure in, 222-229
  normal and abnormal pressure-volume relationships for, *276*
  passive pressure-volume relationship of, *276*
Ventricular activation sequence, 321, *321*, 322, *322, 323*
Ventricular aneurysms, 256
Ventricular chamber, left, volume and mass of, 243-244
Ventricular contraction, abnormalities of, 254
  mechanical lesions and, 281
Ventricular ejection rate, 253
  and myocardial performance in chronic heart disease, 253
Ventricular excitation, and QRS complex, in electrocardiogram, 320
Ventricular fibrillation, 925
Ventricular filling, disorders of, 281
Ventricular function curve, 218-219, *219*
  normal and depressed, schematic representation of, 252
Ventricular hypertrophy, 245, 279
  pressure-velocity relation in, *226*
Ventricular parasystole, 339, *340*
Ventricular performance, after substituting noncontracting elements for contracting myocardium, *288*
Ventricular power, 247
Ventricular repolarization, and S-T deflection, 322-324
Ventricular systole, reduction of number of contractile elements activated during, *288*
Ventricular tachycardia, aneurysms in, 256
  slow, 342, *342*
Ventriculoatrial shunt, immune complexes in, 485
Vibration, 945
Vibrio cholerae, 759
  endotoxin of, 466
  enterotoxin of, 464-466
  exotoxin of, 458(t)
Villi, intestinal, 735-737
  leaf-shaped, in human jejunum, *735*
  various shapes of, in human jejunum, *736*
Villous adenoma, 786
Viral disease, unusual host responses to, 486-487
Viral hepatitis, 813
Viremia, from *Herpes hominis,* 469
Virilization, in congenital adrenal hyperplasia, 888
Virus(es), Epstein-Barr, 623
  effect of on chromosomes, 69
  hypersensitivity induced by, 486
  tumor, 138-140
Visible radiation, 930-931
Visual field defects, in bacterial meningitis, 500
Vital capacity, 372
  in emphysema, 399
  timed, 377
Vitamin A, 855-856
  toxicity from, 855

Vitamin B_1, 853
Vitamin B_2, 853-854
Vitamin B_6, 854
Vitamin B_{12}, 855
  absorption of, 550, 750-751
  as anti-anemia principle, 550-555
  malabsorption of, 77(t), 79
  mucosal absorption of in terminal ileum, 552
  role of in propionate metabolism, 554, *554*
Vitamin B_{12} deficiency, 556-558
  anatomic abnormalities and, 558
  and malabsorption, 757
  decreased ileal absorption in, 557-558
  dietary lack in, 556
  hematologic response to treatment of, *556*
  in megaloblastic anemia, 555
  intrinsic factor lack in, 556-557
Vitamin B_{12}-folate interrelationships, *554*
Vitamin C, 855
Vitamin D, 856-857
  in gastrointestinal tract, 890
  in kidneys, 891
  intoxication from, 856
  toxicity from, 855
Vitamin E, 857
Vitamin K, 857
  and blood coagulation factors, 657
  in synthesis of coagulation factors, 650
Vitamin dependent inborn errors, 85-86, *86*
Vitamins, 852-859
  deficiency of, 853-859
    in kwashiorkor, 849
    pathology in, 857-859
  definition of, 852
  fat-soluble, 855-857
  increased utilization of, and vitamin deficiency, 859
  recommended daily allowances for, 853(t)
  water-soluble, 853-855
Volume, tidal, 372, *373*
Volvulus, 710
  and obstruction of small intestine, 742
Vomiting, 711
  in carcinoma of stomach, 732
  in chronic renal failure, 369
Von Gierke's disease, 7
Von Willebrand's disease, 84, 654
  factor VIII level and bleeding time in, 656

Waldenström's macroglobulinemia, 137, 632
Warm antibody autoimmune hemolytic anemia, 596
Water, absorption of, by colon, 774
  percentage of in human body weight, 840, *840*
  retention of, in chronic infections, 487
  secretion of, in small intestine, 759-760
Water diuresis, 352
Water-soluble vitamins, 853-855
Water structure, effect of temperature on, 34
  in protein structure, 34
Waterhouse-Friderichsen syndrome, 502, 886

Weakness, in carcinoma of stomach, 732
Weight, desirable, in relation to height, 841(t)
  loss of, in anorexia nervosa, 849
Weightlessness, 942–943
Wenckebach phenomenon, 335, *336*
Wermer's syndrome, 725
Wharton's jelly, 417
Whipple's disease, 560, 752
  morphological changes in, 756
White cell(s). See *Leukocyte(s)*.
White thrombus, 646
Wilson's disease, 84
"Windkessel" function, 182, 184
Wiskott-Aldrich syndrome, 135, 662
Wounds, effect of protein depletion on, 421
  healing of, zinc deficiency and, 860

X chromosome, abnormal numbers of, 59–64
Xenon, 925
X-linked genes, definition of, 92
X-linked inheritance, 45–47, *46*, *47*

X-rays, effect on cells, 28, 32
  effect on immune response, 112
Xylose, 751

Y-body, 64, *66*
  definition of, 92
Y chromosome, 51, *52*
  abnormal number of, 64
Y protein, in liver uptake, 793
YY syndrome, 64, *65*

Zenker's diverticulum, 699
Zinc, 859–860
  deficiency of, 860
Zollinger-Ellison syndrome, 714, 717, 724, 776
  hydrochloric acid output in, 726(t)
Zoster sine herpete, 507
Zygote, definition of, 92